■ Richard S. Stack, MD
Associate Professor
Division of Cardiology
Department of Medicine
Duke University School of Medicine
Director
Interventional Cardiovascular Catheterization Program
Duke University Medical Center
Durham, North Carolina

■ Gary S. Roubin, MD, PhD
Director, Center for Endovascular Intervention
Department of Medicine
Lenox Hill Hospital
New York, New York

■ William W. O'Neill, MD
Director, Division of Cardiology
William Beaumont Hospital
Royal Oak, Michigan

# Interventional Cardiovascular Medicine

## Principles and Practice

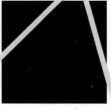

## 2nd Edition

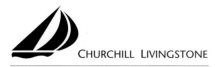 CHURCHILL LIVINGSTONE

*A Harcourt Health Sciences Company*
New York   Edinburgh   London   Philadelphia

**CHURCHILL LIVINGSTONE**
*A Harcourt Health Sciences Company*

The Curtis Center
Independence Square West
Philadelphia, Pennsylvania 19106

**Library of Congress Cataloging-in-Publication Data**

Interventional cardiovascular medicine: principles and practice / [edited by] Richard
S. Stack, Gary S. Roubin, William W. O'Neill.—2nd ed.

p.    cm.

Includes bibliographical references and index.

ISBN 0–443–07979–X

1. Blood vessels—Endoscopic surgery.    2. Angioplasty.    I. Stack, Richard
S.    II. Roubin, Gary S.    III. O'Neill, William W.    [DNLM: 1.
Cardiovascular diseases—therapy.    2. Catheterization.    WG 166 I617 2001]

RD598.5    .I623   2001      617.4′13—dc21

*Acquisitions Editor:*  Marc Strauss
*Developmental Editor:*  Faith Voit
*Manuscript Editor:*  Anne Ostroff
*Production Manager:*  Mary B. Stermel
*Illustration Specialist:*  Robert Quinn

INTERVENTIONAL CARDIOVASCULAR MEDICINE:
Principles and Practice                                            ISBN 0–443–07979–X

Printed in the United States of America.

Last digit is the print number:    9    8    7    6    5    4    3    2    1

# CONTRIBUTORS

FRANK V. AGUIRRE, MD
Clinical Associate Professor of Medicine, Southern Illinois University School of Medicine; Interventional Cardiologist, Prairie Cardiovascular Consultants, Springfield, Illinois
*Coronary Doppler Flow Measurements*

DARIUS ALIABADI, MD
Staff Cardiologist, Southeast Alabama Medical Center, Dothan, Alabama
*Stent Complications*

STEVEN L. ALMANY, MD, FACC
Medical Director, Department of Cardiology, William Beaumont Hospital, Royal Oak, Michigan
*Radial and Brachial Artery–Based Access for Diagnostic and Interventional Procedures*

HENNING RUD ANDERSEN, MD, PhD
Associate Professor, Aarhus University; Consultant Cardiologist, Aarhus University Hospital (Skejby), Aarhus, Denmark
*Pathology of Atherosclerotic Plaque: Stable, Unstable, and Infarctional*

PETER G. ANDERSON, DVM, PhD
Associate Professor of Pathology, University of Alabama at Birmingham, Birmingham, Alabama
*Pathology of Various Mechanical Interventional Procedures and Devices*

WAYNE B. BATCHELOR, MD, MHS
Assistant Professor of Medicine, Terrence Donnelly Heart Centre, St. Michael's Hospital, University of Toronto, Toronto, Ontario, Canada
*Perfusion Balloon Catheter*

ERIC R. BATES, MD
Professor, University of Michigan; Director, Cardiac Catheterization Laboratory, University of Michigan Hospital, Ann Arbor, Michigan
*Medical Versus Interventional Therapy for Stable Angina Pectoris*

WILLIAM A. BAXLEY, MD
Professor of Medicine, University of Alabama Medical Center, Birmingham, Alabama
*Support Systems for Percutaneous Cardiac Interventions*

GUIDO BELLI, MD
Rome, Italy
*Optimal Technique for Stent Deployment*

OLIVIER F. BERTRAND, MD, DPhil
Assistant Professor, Faculty of Medicine, University of Laval; Staff Cardiologist, Interventional Cardiology Laboratories, Quebec Heart-Lung Institute at University Hospital Laval, Ste. Foy, Québec, Canada
*Cutting Balloon Angioplasty*

MICHAEL A. BLAZING, MD
Assistant Professor of Medicine, Duke University Medical Center, Durham, North Carolina
*The Vascular Biology of Restenosis: An Overview*

RAOUL BONAN, MD
Associate Professor, Université de Montréal; Cardiologist (Interventional Cardiology), Institut de Cardiologie de Montréal, Montréal, Québec, Canada
*Cutting Balloon Angioplasty*

ROBERT M. CALIFF, MD
Professor of Medicine, Duke University Medical Center; Attending Physician and Chief Executive Officer, Clinical Research Institute, and Associate Vice Chancellor, Clinical Research, Duke University Medical Center, Durham, North Carolina
*Surgical Therapy Versus Interventional Therapy in Patients with Stable Coronary Ischemia*

M. LEE CHENEY, JD
Attorney, Womble Carlyle Sandridge & Rice, PLLC, Research Triangle Park, North Carolina
*Medicolegal Issues in Interventional Cardiology*

DAVID J. COHEN, MD
Assistant Professor of Medicine, Harvard Medical School; Associate Director of Interventional Cardiology, Beth Israel Deaconess Medical Center, Boston, Massachusetts
*The Economics of Percutaneous Coronary Intervention*

ANTONIO COLOMBO, MD
New York University, New York City; University of Milan, and University Vito-Solute, Milan, Italy; Director, Interventional Cardiology, San Raffaele Hospital and Columbus Hospital, Milan, Italy
*Selection of Coronary Stents for Particular Anatomy; The AVE Microstent: Evolutions in Design and Clinical Utility*

PETER J. CONLON, MB, MHS, FRCPI, FACP
Consulting Assistant Professor, Duke University Medical Center, Durham, North Carolina; Consultant Nephrologist/Renal Transplant Physician, Beaumont Hospital, Dublin, Ireland
*Management of Renal Artery Stenosis*

DAVID A. COX, MD
Mid-Carolina Cardiology, Charlotte, North Carolina
*Vascular Biology of Mechanical Intervention*

IAN R. CROCKER, MD
Department of Cardiology, Emory University School
of Medicine, Atlanta, Georgia
*Vascular Radiation Therapy to Reduce
Restenosis*

JAMES J. CROWLEY, MB, MD, MRCPI
Assistant Lecturer, Department of Medicine, University College; Consultant Cardiologist, University
College Hospital, Galway, Ireland
*The ACS MultiLink Stent; Management of Renal
Artery Stenosis*

LARRY S. DEAN, MD
Professor of Medicine and Surgery, University of
Washington School of Medicine; Director, University of Washington Regional Heart Center, University of Washington Academic Medical Center, Seattle, Washington
*Percutaneous Balloon Valvuloplasty*

JAMES M. DOUGLAS, Jr., MD, FACS
Director, Cardiothoracic Surgery, St. Joseph Hospital, Bellingham, Washington
*Emergency Coronary Artery Bypass Grafting*

STEPHEN G. ELLIS, MD
Professor of Medicine, The Ohio State University,
Columbus; Director, Jones Cardiac Catheterization
Laboratories, The Cleveland Clinic Foundation,
Cleveland, Ohio
*Left Main Coronary Interventions; Optimal
Technique for Stent Deployment*

ERLING FALK, MD, PhD
Professor of Cardiovascular Pathology, Aarhus University, Aarhus, Denmark
*Pathology of Atherosclerotic Plaque: Stable,
Unstable, and Infarctional*

DONALD D. GLOWER, MD
Professor of Surgery, Duke University Medical Center, Durham, North Carolina
*Emergency Coronary Artery Bypass Grafting*

CINDY L. GRINES, MD
Director, Cardiac Catheterization Laboratories, William Beaumont Hospital, Royal Oak, Michigan
*Primary Coronary Angioplasty in Acute
Myocardial Infarction: Comparative Analysis
with Thrombolytic Therapy; Beyond Primary
PTCA: New Approaches to Mechanical
Reperfusion Therapy in Acute Myocardial
Infarction; Left Main Coronary Interventions*

WILLIAM B. HILLEGASS, MD, MPH
Assistant Professor of Cardiovascular Medicine,
University of Alabama at Birmingham, Birmingham,
Alabama
*Endovascular Therapies for Diseases of the Aorta*

RAINER HOFFMANN, MD
University Hospital, Aachen, Germany
*In-Stent Restenosis: Mechanisms, Definitions,
and Treatment*

MUN K. HONG, MD
Director, Experimental Physiology and Pharmacology, Washington Cardiology Center/Washington
Hospital Center, Washington, D.C.
*In-Stent Restenosis: Mechanisms, Definitions,
and Treatment*

SRIRAM S. IYER, MD
Clinical Associate Professor of Medicine, New York
University School of Medicine; Associate Chief, Endovascular Section, Lenox Hill Heart and Vascular
Institute, Lenox Hill Hospital, New York, New York
*Carotid Artery Intervention*

JAMES G. JOLLIS, MD
Associate Professor, Department of Medicine, Division of Cardiology, Duke University Medical Center,
Durham, North Carolina
*Surgical Therapy Versus Interventional Therapy
in Patients with Stable Coronary Ischemia*

WILLIAM D. JORDAN, Jr., MD, FACS
Associate Professor and Chief, Section of Vascular
Surgery, University of Alabama at Birmingham, Birmingham, Alabama
*Endovascular Therapies for Diseases of the Aorta*

ELLEN C. KEELEY, MD
Assistant Professor of Medicine, University of Texas
Southwestern Medical School, Dallas, Texas
*Left Main Coronary Interventions*

KENNETH M. KENT, MD, PhD
Washington Cardiology Center, Washington, D.C.
*Intravascular Ultrasound Imaging in the
Evaluation and Interventional Treatment of
Coronary Artery Disease; In-Stent Restenosis:
Mechanisms, Definitions, and Treatment*

MORTON J. KERN, MD
Professor of Medicine, St. Louis University; Director, J.G. Mudd Cardiac Catheterization Laboratory,
St. Louis University, St. Louis, Missouri
*Coronary Doppler Flow Measurements*

SPENCER B. KING III, MD
Clinical Professor of Medicine, Emory University
School of Medicine; Fuqua Chair of Interventional
Cardiology, The Fuqua Heart Center at Piedmont
Hospital, Atlanta, Georgia
*Vascular Radiation Therapy to Reduce
Restenosis*

JOHNNIE KNOBLOCH, EMTP
Intervention Laboratory Technologist, University of
Alabama Medical Center, Birmingham, Alabama
*Support Systems for Percutaneous Cardiac
Interventions*

YOSHIO KOBAYASHI, MD
Assistant Director of Intravascular Ultrasound Laboratory, Cardiovascular Research Foundation, Lenox Hill Heart and Vascular Institute, New York, New York
*Selection of Coronary Stents for Particular Anatomy*

DAVID F. KONG, MD, AM
Fellow, Cardiovascular Diseases, and Summit Medical Outcomes Fellow, Duke University Medical Center, Durham, North Carolina
*Acute Closure, Dissection, and Perforation*

MARINO LABINAZ, MD, FRCP(C), FACC
Associate Professor of Medicine, University of Ottawa; Co-Director, Cardiac Catheterization Laboratory, and Program Director, Adult Cardiology, University of Ottawa Heart Institute, Ottawa, Ontario, Canada
*Coronary Transluminal Extraction Catheter Atherectomy*

ALEXANDRA J. LANSKY, MD
Director, Angiographic Core Laboratory and Women's Health Initiative, Cardiovascular Research Foundation, New York, New York
*The Gianturco-Roubin II Stent*

ROBERT J. LEDERMAN, MD
Assistant Professor, Division of Cardiology, Department of Internal Medicine, and Lecturer, Department of Radiology, University of Michigan Health System, Ann Arbor, Michigan; Director, Cardiovascular Interventions, National Heart, Lung and Blood Institute, National Institutes of Health, Bethesda, Maryland
*Medical Versus Interventional Therapy for Stable Angina Pectoris*

MARTIN B. LEON, MD
Staff Physician, Lenox Hill Hospital, New York, New York
*Intravascular Ultrasound Imaging in the Evaluation and Interventional Treatment of Coronary Artery Disease; The Gianturco-Roubin II Stent; In-Stent Restenosis: Mechanisms, Definitions, and Treatment*

MING W. LIU, MD
Associate Professor of Medicine, University of Alabama at Birmingham; Interventional Cardiologist, University of Alabama Hospital, Birmingham, Alabama
*Vascular Biology of Mechanical Intervention*

MINA MADAN, MD, MHS, FRCPC
Assistant Professor of Medicine, University of Toronto; Staff Interventional Cardiologist, Sunnybrook and Women's College Health Sciences Centre, Toronto, Ontario, Canada
*Interventional Strategy in Patients with Previous Coronary Bypass Surgery*

DANIEL B. MARK, MD, MPH
Professor of Medicine, Duke University Medical Center; Director, Outcomes Research and Assessment Group, Duke Clinical Research Institute, Durham, North Carolina
*Assessment of Prognosis in Patients with Coronary Artery Disease*

GIOVANNI MARTINI, CCP
Perfusionist, European Board of Cardiovascular Perfusionists, Milan, Italy
*Selection of Coronary Stents for Particular Anatomy*

PETER A. McCULLOUGH, MD, MPH
Associate Professor of Medicine, University of Missouri–Kansas City School of Medicine; Chief of Cardiology, Truman Medical Centers, Kansas City, Missouri
*Epidemiology of Coronary Heart Disease*

ROXANA MEHRAN, MD
Cardiology Research Foundation, Washington Hospital Center, Washington, D.C.
*In-Stent Restenosis: Mechanisms, Definitions, and Treatment*

GARY S. MINTZ, MD
Washington Hospital Center, Washington, D.C.
*Intravascular Ultrasound Imaging in the Evaluation and Interventional Treatment of Coronary Artery Disease; In-Stent Restenosis: Mechanisms, Definitions, and Treatment*

MEG B. MOLLOY, DrPH, MPH, RD
Executive Director, North Carolina Prevention Partners, Institute for Public Health, School of Public Health, University of North Carolina at Chapel Hill, Chapel Hill, North Carolina
*Coronary Artery Disease: The Basis for Secondary Prevention*

JEFFREY MOSES, MD
Clinical Professor of Medicine, New York University School of Medicine; Chief, Interventional Cardiology, Lenox Hill Heart and Vascular Institute, New York, New York
*The AVE Microstent: Evolutions in Design and Clinical Utility*

ISSAM MOUSSA, MD
Instructor in Medicine, New York University School of Medicine; Director, Clinical Outcome Research, Lenox Hill Heart and Vascular Institute, New York, New York
*Selection of Coronary Stents for Particular Anatomy; The AVE Microstent: Evolutions in Design and Clinical Utility*

JOSEPH B. MUHLESTEIN, MD
Associate Professor of Medicine, University of Utah
School of Medicine; Director of Cardiology Re-
search, LDS Hospital, Salt Lake City, Utah
*The Vascular Biology of Restenosis: An
Overview; Perfusion Balloon Catheter*

DAVID W. M. MULLER, MBBS, MD
Associate Professor of Medicine, University of New
South Wales; Director, Cardiac Catheterization Labo-
ratory, St. Vincent's Hospital, Sydney, New South
Wales, Australia
*Medical Versus Interventional Therapy for Stable
Angina Pectoris*

GISHEL NEW, MB, PhD
Director of Clinical Research, Lenox Hill Heart and
Vascular Institute of New York, New York, New York
*Carotid Artery Intervention*

STEVEN E. NISSEN, MD, FACC
Professor of Medicine, Ohio State University–CCF/
DIV; Vice Chairman, Department of Cardiology,
Cleveland Clinic Foundation, Cleveland, Ohio
*Physical Principles of Radiographic and Digital
Imaging in the Cardiac Catheterization
Laboratory*

JAMI M. NORRIS, MS, RCEP
Fitness Director, Duke Center for Living, Duke Uni-
versity, Durham, North Carolina
*Coronary Artery Disease: The Basis for
Secondary Prevention*

E. MAGNUS OHMAN, MD
Professor of Medicine, Chief of Cardiology, and Di-
rector, University of North Carolina Heart Center,
Chapel Hill, North Carolina
*Surgical Therapy Versus Interventional Therapy
in Patients with Stable Coronary Ischemia*

WILLIAM W. O'NEILL, MD, FACC
Director, Division of Cardiology, and Co-director,
Beaumont Heart Center, William Beaumont Hospi-
tal, Royal Oak, Michigan
*Interventional Therapy of Cardiogenic Shock;
Radial Artery Access for Diagnostic and
Interventional Procedures; Mechanical
Rotational Atherectomy*

JAMES M. PARKS, MD
Birmingham, Alabama
*Vascular Biology of Mechanical Intervention*

GREGORY S. PAVLIDES, MD
Vice Chief, Cardiology, and Director, Cardiac Cathe-
terization Laboratories, Onassis Cardiac Surgery
Center, Athens, Greece
*Local Drug Delivery*

GAIL E. PETERSON, MD
Fellow, Duke University Medical Center; Director of
Cardiology, Durham VA Medical Center, Durham,
North Carolina
*Surgical Therapy Versus Interventional Therapy
in Patients with Stable Coronary Ischemia*

HARRY R. PHILLIPS III, MD
Professor of Medicine, Duke University; Co-director
of Interventional Cardiovascular Program, Duke
University Medical Center, Durham, North Carolina
*Surgical Therapy Versus Interventional Therapy
in Patients with Stable Coronary Ischemia;
Coronary Angioplasty: Femoral Approach*

AUGUSTO D. PICHARD, MD
Washington Cardiology Center, Washington, D.C.
*Intravascular Ultrasound Imaging in the
Evaluation and Interventional Treatment of
Coronary Artery Disease; In-Stent Restenosis:
Mechanisms, Definitions, and Treatment*

JEFFREY J. POPMA, MD
Associate Professor of Medicine, Harvard Medical
School; Director, Interventional Cardiology, Brigham
and Women's Hospital, Boston, Massachusetts
*Intravascular Ultrasound Imaging in the
Evaluation and Interventional Treatment of
Coronary Artery Disease*

JOSEPH A. PUMA, DO, FACC
Associate Consulting Professor of Medicine, Duke
University Medical Center, Durham, North Carolina
*Chronic Total Occlusions; Coronary
Transluminal Extraction Catheter Atherectomy*

RUTH QUILLIAN, PhD
Duke University Medical Center, Durham, North
Carolina
*Coronary Artery Disease: The Basis for
Secondary Prevention*

J. G. REVES, MD
Professor and Chairman, Department of Anesthesi-
ology, Duke University Medical Center, Durham,
North Carolina
*Emergency Coronary Artery Bypass Grafting*

KEITH A. ROBINSON, PhD
Associate Professor of Medicine (Cardiology), Medical College of Georgia, Augusta; Director of Preclinical Research, Atlanta Cardiovascular Research Institute, Norcross, Georgia
*Vascular Radiation Therapy to Reduce
Restenosis*

GARY S. ROUBIN, MBBS, MD, PhD
Clinical Professor of Medicine, New York Univer-
sity; Chief, Endovascular Section, Lenox Hill Heart
and Vascular Institute of New York, New York,
New York
*Angiographic Views and Techniques for
Coronary Intervention; Support Systems for
Percutaneous Cardiac Interventions; Carotid
Artery Intervention*

ROBERT D. SAFIAN, MD
Director, Interventional Cardiology, William Beau-
mont Hospital, Royal Oak, Michigan
*Stent Complications*

RENATO M. SANTOS, MD
Cardiologist, Cardiovascular Associates, Kingsport, Tennessee
*Management of Renal Artery Stenosis*

LOWELL F. SATLER, MD
Georgetown University School of Medicine; Georgetown University Hospital, Washington, D.C.
*Intravascular Ultrasound Imaging in the Evaluation and Interventional Treatment of Coronary Artery Disease; In-Stent Restenosis: Mechanisms, Definitions, and Treatment*

RICHARD A. SCHATZ, MD
Research Director, Cardiovascular Interventions, Scripps Clinic, La Jolla, California
*The Palmaz-Schatz Stent*

U. SIGWART, MD, FRCP
Professor of Medicine, University of Düsseldorf, Düsseldorf, Germany; Director, Department of Invasive Cardiology, Royal Brompton Hospital, London, United Kingdom
*The Wallstent*

MICHAEL H. SKETCH, Jr., MD
Associate Professor of Medicine, Duke University Medical Center; Director, Diagnostic and Interventional Cardiac Catheterization Laboratories, Duke University Medical Center, Durham, North Carolina
*Interventional Strategy in Patients with Previous Coronary Bypass Surgery; Design of the Interventional Cardiac Catheterization Laboratory; Coronary Transluminal Extraction Catheter Atherectomy; Perfusion Balloon Catheter*

THOMAS F. SLAUGHTER, MD
Assistant Professor, Duke University Medical Center; Division of Veterans Affairs Anesthesia, Department of Veterans Affairs Medical Center, Durham, North Carolina
*Emergency Coronary Artery Bypass Grafting*

RICHARD S. STACK, MD
Professor of Medicine, Duke University; Duke University Hospital, Durham, North Carolina
*Comprehensive Interventional Therapy*

GREGG W. STONE, MD
Director of Cardiovascular Research and Education, Cardiovascular Research Foundation, Lenox Hill Heart and Vascular Institute, New York, New York
*Primary Coronary Angioplasty in Acute Myocardial Infarction: Comparative Analysis with Thrombolytic Therapy; Beyond Primary PTCA: New Approaches to Mechanical Reperfusion Therapy in Acute Myocardial Infarction*

CRAIG A. SUKIN, MD
Cardiology Associates of Cincinnati, Cincinnati, Ohio
*The Economics of Percutaneous Coronary Intervention*

MARTIN J. SULLIVAN, MD
Associate Professor of Medicine, Duke University Medical Center; Director, Science and Healing, Duke Center for Integrative Medicine, Duke University Health System, Durham, North Carolina
*Coronary Artery Disease: The Basis for Secondary Prevention*

JOHN P. SWEENEY, MD
Interventional Cardiology Fellow, Scripps Clinic, La Jolla, California
*The Palmaz-Schatz Stent*

JAMES E. TCHENG, MD
Associate Professor of Medicine, Duke University Medical Center; Duke Clinical Research Institute, Durham, North Carolina
*Design of the Interventional Cardiac Catheterization Laboratory; Coronary Angioplasty: Femoral Approach; Chronic Total Occlusions; Adjunctive Pharmacologic Support During Percutaneous Coronary Intervention; Direct Laser Ablation*

ALAN N. TENAGLIA, MD
Associate Professor of Medicine, Tulane University; Director, Cardiac Catheterization Laboratories and Interventional Cardiology Program, Tulane Hospital, New Orleans, Louisiana
*Coronary Angioplasty: Femoral Approach*

MARK C. THEL, MD
Chattanooga Heart Institute, Chattanooga, Tennessee
*Adjunctive Pharmacologic Support During Percutaneous Coronary Intervention*

FRANK V. TILLI, MD
Interventional Cardiologist, Allegheny General Hospital, Pittsburgh, Pennsylvania
*Coronary Angioscopy*

JIRI J. VITEK, MD, PhD
Neuroradiologist, Endovascular Section, Lenox Hill Heart and Vascular Institute of New York, New York, New York
*Carotid Artery Intervention*

RON WAKSMAN, MD
Washington Cardiology Center, Washington, D.C.
*In-Stent Restenosis: Mechanisms, Definitions, and Treatment*

BRUCE F. WALLER, MD
Clinical Professor of Medicine and Pathology, Indiana School of Medicine; Cardiologist and Medical Director, Clinical Laboratory, The Care Group, and Director, Cardiovascular Pathology Registry, Indianapolis, Indiana
*Pathology of Various Mechanical Interventional Procedures and Devices*

RICHARD P. WAWRZYNSKI, MBA
Administrator, Cardiac Catheterization Laboratories, Duke University Medical Center, Durham, North Carolina
*Design of the Interventional Cardiac Catheterization Laboratory*

DAVID J. WHELLAN, MD
Cardiology Fellow, Duke University Medical Center, Durham, North Carolina
*Coronary Artery Disease: The Basis for Secondary Prevention*

JAMES P. ZIDAR, MD, FACC
Associate Professor of Medicine, Cardiovascular Division, Department of Medicine, Duke University Medical Center, Durham, North Carolina
*The Vascular Biology of Restenosis: An Overview; Acute Closure, Dissection, and Perforation; The ACS MultiLink Stent*

# PREFACE

Since our first edition of *Interventional Cardiovascular Medicine: Principles and Practice,* major strides have been made to overcome the two main limitations of angioplasty: thrombosis and restenosis. Acute and subacute thrombosis have been largely overcome by the nearly routine use of advanced design stents in the great majority of patients, coupled with potent antiplatelet therapies. Restenosis rates have also been favorably modified by the frequent use of stents (overcoming recoil and geometric remodeling) and the more recent application of radiation and drug-eluting stents (inhibiting intimal proliferation). These breakthroughs have caused a steady and continuous growth of interventional procedures as an effective minimally invasive solution to obstructive coronary artery disease and as a choice increasingly favored over bypass surgery.

During the same time period, there has been a rapid growth in the number of cardiologists who have moved from a focus on the heart alone to a more global interventional treatment strategy for their patients with atherosclerotic disease. Coronary interventionalists are growing into *comprehensive* interventionalists. Although local politics involving radiologists and surgeons still sometimes inhibits practice in these areas, many institutions have evolved an acceptance of a multidisciplinary approach that allows all qualified practitioners to participate in the interventional treatment of their patients. Major advances in peripheral device development that have led to a more coronary-like feel and performance have helped fuel this advance.

Cardiologists have led the drive to find a safe, minimally invasive alternative to carotid endarterectomy. With the entry of cardiologists as leaders in this emerging field, and with their experience in the use of randomized trials to determine the best treatment strategies for subsets of patients with carotid artery disease, cardiologists are now well on the way to advancing carotid interventional techniques to the same state of the art as coronary interventional techniques. One has only to witness the rapid development of very low-profile self-expanding nitinol carotid stents with the use of coronary-based guide wire systems or the invention of sophisticated embolic protection devices to confirm the validity of this observation. The carotid interventional population could eventually approach the size of the coronary interventional population if carotid stents are shown to reduce stroke rates in comparison to medical therapy in asymptomatic patients as well as symptomatic patients. The routine use of effective embolic protection devices could potentially make this a much safer alternative than medical therapy alone.

As in the first edition, our aim has been to provide a state-of-the-art review of the major clinical subject areas of interventional cardiovascular medicine, relying both on the collective experience of the editors and on the expertise of the numerous internationally recognized leaders who have contributed chapters to this text. This 2nd edition again focuses on merging practical and pragmatic interventional techniques with sound scientific evidence to provide the reader with the most comprehensive review of this exciting and rapidly advancing field.

The editors wish to express their deep and sincere gratitude to Marc Strauss and Faith Voit at the W.B. Saunders Company, who have tirelessly supported the monumental task of publishing this text, as well as to the secretarial staff in the offices of each of the editors.

Richard S. Stack, MD
Gary S. Roubin, MD, PhD
William W. O'Neill, MD

# CONTENTS

**1**

# History and Development

# Comprehensive Interventional Therapy

*Richard S. Stack*

Andreas Gruentzig was the first comprehensive interventionist. As a pioneer in the field of interventional radiology, he recognized that the techniques that he originally developed for peripheral arteries would be equally applicable to the coronary arteries. By crossing traditional professional boundaries to enter into the field of cardiology he transformed the management of patients with coronary artery disease. Ironically, more than two decades after the original publication of his coronary work, his vision has come full circle.[1] Now, cardiologists from around the world are recrossing professional boundaries of radiology and surgery and are treating patients with peripheral vascular disease.

In this, the second edition of *Interventional Cardiovascular Medicine,* the authors recognize this major shift in the field of interventional revascularization. We have included numerous chapters on pragmatic approaches for the performance of peripheral vascular procedures, including the most up-to-date and comprehensive treatise available on carotid artery stenting by Dr. Gary Roubin. In the remainder of this introductory chapter, the factors motivating interventional cardiologists to enter the field of peripheral vascular intervention are identified. The traditional barriers that are currently being overcome to allow all qualified interventional cardiologists to perform these procedures are reviewed.

## FACTORS MOTIVATING CARDIOLOGISTS TO PERFORM VASCULAR INTERVENTIONS

Several major forces combine to motivate cardiologists to perform peripheral vascular interventional procedures (Table 1–1). Although each factor is important in its own right, the increasing awareness among cardiologists that the interaction between sites of atherosclerosis in different areas of the body (e.g., renal arteries or carotid arteries) can have profound implications for their ability to effectively manage coronary artery disease (CAD) in their pa-

tients may be the most important factor. Once this "disease management" approach to atherosclerosis is appreciated by cardiologists, the ability to optimally care for their patients is significantly enhanced. The American Board of Internal Medicine awards board certification to cardiologists in the subspecialty of cardiovascular disease, *not* in cardiology per se. In the past, the emphasis has been almost entirely on the cardiac aspect. This "cardiocentric" approach is now being abandoned in favor of a global, comprehensive approach to the treatment of cardiovascular disease.

## Patient Care: Comprehensive Atherosclerotic Disease Management

Many cardiologists do not recognize the fact that they are already experts in vascular medicine. The average interventional cardiologist spends virtually all of his or her time treating the *vessels* of the heart and not the myocardium per se. In fact, the myocardium is often just an innocent bystander, as

**TABLE 1–1. FACTORS DRIVING INTERVENTIONAL CARDIOLOGISTS TO PERFORM PERIPHERAL INTERVENTION**

*Patient Care: Global Disease Management*

Cardiologists recognize the need to treat all manifestations of atherosclerosis as systemic disease.

*Success of Coronary Stents*

Cardiologists can leverage the skill sets that they have mastered in placing stents in the coronary arteries.

*Political Influence*

Cardiologists have major political influence on their hospital administrations, allowing them to achieve compromises with the surgery and radiology departments.

*Economics*

There is a flattening of the growth curve in coronary interventional procedures, coupled with a major decrease in reimbursement. The ability to perform peripheral vascular procedures is an important way for cardiologists to expand their interventional practice.

in myocardial infarction, in the vascular disease. Thus, armed with the extensive knowledge that they have gained in treating the risk factors of coronary vascular disease, cardiologists represent the subspecialty that is in the best position to provide optimal medical management for all patients with atherosclerosis.

Numerous interactions of atherosclerosis in various areas of the body are seen constantly in the practice of the interventional cardiologist. Once these relationships and interactions are recognized, the potential for the interventional cardiologist to treat all important manifestations of atherosclerotic disease in patients becomes abundantly clear. Table 1–2 shows several examples of these interactions. Of importance is that the occurrence of other manifestations of atherosclerosis is much more common among the interventional cardiologist's patients than in the general population. These patients are already preselected to have significant systemic atherosclerotic disease by the time they first present with symptoms of angina or the occurrence of a myocardial infarction. As an illustration, Harding and associates performed a study in which they reviewed 1302 sequential aortograms performed at Duke University Medical Center during cardiac catheterization.[2] They found that there was some renal artery disease in 30% of the population and significant stenosis (>50% narrowing of the luminal diameter) in 15% (unilateral in 11%, bilateral in 4%). There was also a progressive and highly linear relationship between coronary artery disease and renal artery disease: Renal artery stenosis was present in 10.7% of patients with single-vessel CAD, in 17.6% of patients with two-vessel CAD, and in 29.9% of patients with three-vessel disease. Thirty-nine percent of patients with left main artery disease were found to have renal artery narrowing.

The clinical interactions of coronary artery disease with other manifestations of atherosclerotic disease are also very common. For example, in order to rehabilitate patients after myocardial infarction, it may be necessary to place stents into the iliac or femoral arteries in order to allow them to exercise. It may even be necessary to treat the iliac obstruction in order to gain access to the heart for coronary intervention. In patients with renal artery stenosis, it may be necessary to place stents into the renal arteries in order to manage blood pressure, improve renal function, allow the use of angiotensin-converting enzyme (ACE) inhibitors (for congestive heart failure or after myocardial infarction), or treat flash pulmonary edema.[3] In a study by Khosla and colleagues,[3] 120 patients with hypertension refractory to medical therapy underwent coronary artery stent placement. Forty-eight patients (40%) presented with either unstable angina (N = 20) or congestive heart failure (N = 28) as the predominant symptom. At a mean follow-up of 253 ± 192 days, there was sustained improvement in 72.5% of all patients, including 72% of the 20 patients with unstable angina and 73% of the 28 patients with congestive heart failure. In a similar study by Rajachandran and associates, 28% (20) of 72 patients who received stents for renal artery stenosis originally presented with flash pulmonary edema.[4] Of these patients, 60% (12 of 20) had global renal ischemia (bilateral lesions or lesions in a single kidney). Thirteen patients had normal ejection fractions, which suggested diastolic dysfunction, and 12 patients had left ventricular hypertrophy. At a follow-up period of 6 months, 90% (18 of 20) had no further episodes of congestive heart failure. Thus, it seems clear that the ability to treat patients with renal artery stenosis within cardiac interventionalists' practice is of significant benefit to their patients.

## Success of Coronary Stents

In addition to the recognition by interventional cardiologists of the benefit to their patients derived from managing all aspects of their atherosclerotic disease, several other factors motivate interventional cardiologists to perform peripheral intervention. One important reason is the success of coronary stent placement itself. In most institutions, stent placement is performed in the great majority of coronary interventional procedures. Improvements in guide catheters, guide wires, balloons, and stent technology have made the approach to even the most difficult lesions relatively easy. In recognition of the major movement of cardiologists into the field of peripheral vascular intervention, interventional device companies have provided major improvements in peripheral interventional equipment as well. It is now fairly easy for cardiologists to

**TABLE 1–2. INTERACTIONS OF VARIOUS MANIFESTATIONS OF ATHEROSCLEROSIS IN THE PATIENT WITH CORONARY DISEASE**

Iliac stenosis preventing catheterization, coronary intervention, or intra-aortic balloon pump placement
Claudication preventing effective exercise rehabilitation program after myocardial infarction
Subclavian stenosis preventing effective use of a LIMA graft
Renal artery stenosis causing hypertension or flash pulmonary edema; untreated renal artery stenosis may also prevent the use of ACE inhibitors for hypertension or for survival benefit after myocardial infarction

ACE, angiotensin-converting enzyme; LIMA, left internal mammary artery.

transfer the skills learned in the interventional coronary laboratory to the interventional treatment of patients with femoral, iliac, renal, and supra-aortic disease.

## Political Influence

Another factor motivating cardiologists to perform peripheral intervention is the fact that they exert significant political influence within the institutions in which they work. As opposed to the radiologists, they have a distinct advantage by virtue of the fact that they have final authority on the management of their own patients. Cardiologists are able to see patients in clinics and recognize manifestations of atherosclerosis in areas of the body other than the heart. They can order the appropriate noninvasive tests and perform appropriate invasive diagnostic testing as they deem necessary for their patients. Finally, as opposed to the radiologists, cardiologists have privileges to admit their own patients to the hospital. Although turf battles still rage over privileges for cardiologists to perform interventional peripheral procedures, there has been a steady increase in the number of cardiologists who are able to become credentialed.

## Economics

A final factor that is probably contributing to the movement of cardiologists into peripheral vascular intervention is economics. The decreasing reimbursement for coronary procedures and the increasing competition among the growing number of coronary interventionalists are motivating individual practitioners to seek new skills in order to treat a larger variety of lesions than those of CAD alone. Reimbursement for peripheral interventional procedures has traditionally not been as high as for coronary procedures; however, peripheral procedures have not been targeted for the dramatic cuts in the levels of reimbursement seen with Medicare reimbursement reductions for coronary interventions.

## TRADITIONAL BARRIERS TO CARDIOLOGISTS THAT ARE CURRENTLY BREAKING DOWN

### Turf Wars

Management of peripheral vascular disease has traditionally been the domain of the vascular surgeon. Vascular surgeons have maintained a strong relationship with vascular radiologists. If and when a vascular surgeon believed that a particular patient could benefit from a percutaneous intervention, it was the vascular radiologist who received the referral. In fact, vascular radiologists have been performing percutaneous vascular interventional procedures since before cardiologists ever considered coronary intervention a treatment. Thus, when all of the factors outlined in the previous section combined to create the current movement of cardiologists into the field of peripheral vascular disease, a major altercation among surgeons, radiologists, and cardiologists began. In most institutions, the cardiologists found themselves fighting a battle on two flanks: surgeons on one side and radiologists, who allied with the surgeons, on the other. Fortunately, after a few years of fruitless argument, many institutions have recognized that a multidisciplinary approach results in the best outcome for all concerned, particularly the patient. In order to achieve this result, however, cardiologists should be careful not to give the appearance of moving into the management of patients with peripheral vascular disease with the notion of putting their colleagues out of business. The truth is that there are more than enough patients who are in need of peripheral vascular treatment to keep all three specialties satisfied. In fact, peripheral vascular disease is one of the most underdiagnosed and undertreated of all disorders. Much of this underrecognition and undertreatment results from the fact that there were few minimally invasive and effective interventional treatment options available until as recently as the 1990s.

It is critical that cardiologists take the time and effort to learn how to manage all aspects of peripheral vascular disease in their patients. They must also spend the time to learn the numerous methodologic and procedural differences between coronary and peripheral vascular interventional procedures. One of the best ways to learn all aspects of peripheral vascular disease is to work together with members of the surgery and radiology departments. Once the members of the various disciplines learn to work together, it quickly becomes apparent that each specialty has an enormous amount to offer because of their different backgrounds and experience. Finally, by teaming up within an institution, the multidisciplinary approach will give all the physicians in that institution a significant strategic advantage over their competitors, who may be bogged down in turf wars instead of actively recruiting and treating patients.

### Equipment

Major changes have occurred in the availability of "coronary-like" peripheral vascular products for the interventionalist. In fact, the newest peripheral interventional equipment offers .014-inch–based technology similar to that used by cardiologists on a daily basis. Stents are now highly flexible, provide excellent coverage, and can be delivered easily to virtually any peripheral site within the body. One of the barriers to cardiologists' performing femoral procedures was the fact that the femoral artery was traditionally approached only via anterograde access. The cardiologist is much more familiar with the retrograde approach, which is generally easier (particularly in obese patients) and does not involve close proximity of the operator to the x-ray tube. Interventional device companies have developed flexible sheaths that allow the operator access to the contralateral femoral artery across the iliac bifurcation through a standard retrograde approach. This is preferable to the anterograde approach in many instances, particularly when the sheath is removed and compression occurs in the opposite leg from where the femoral intervention was performed. The retrograde approach avoids the need to occlude blood flow to the freshly treated site. Cardiologists should, however, become familiar with anterograde access techniques because they are sometimes the procedure of choice.

## Education

It is critical that cardiologists planning to perform peripheral vascular interventional procedures obtain proper instruction in the specific techniques. Peripheral intervention sometimes requires entirely different technical skills and judgment than those used in coronary intervention. Cardiologists performing peripheral vascular interventional procedures must develop expertise in how to avoid complications associated with each specific vascular region, in order to exercise proper judgment during interventional procedures.

Fortunately, virtually all major live demonstration courses now include extensive oral presentations as well as live case demonstrations for peripheral vascular intervention. In addition, all of the major coronary interventional textbooks now feature extensive sections on peripheral vascular intervention.

## CREDENTIALING

One of the greatest barriers to cardiologists' performing peripheral interventional procedures has been the inability to be credentialed at their individual hospitals. Radiologists and surgeons who often serve on the credentialing boards have created criteria designed to exclude cardiologists from performance of these procedures. An advance in credentialing guidelines put forward by the Society of Cardiac Angiography and Intervention has resulted in a highly achievable method for cardiologists to enter the field of peripheral intervention. In an article published in the Journal of Cardiac Catheteriza-

tion and Intervention, guidelines were developed both for limited competency and unrestricted clinical competency for peripheral intervention.[5] These criteria account for the need of cardiologists to perform limited peripheral interventional procedures for the legitimate management of their patients. Specifically, management of iliac and renal lesions is handled differently from the more complex peripheral vascular interventional procedures. These relatively straightforward procedures allow the cardiologist to begin accumulating experience in the peripheral vasculature. It is actually very important for cardiac interventionalists to at least learn iliac and renal procedures. For example, cardiologists may be called upon to treat patients for emergency interventional procedures during acute myocardial infarction. It can be argued that if the patient has a tight stenosis of one or both iliac arteries, the cardiologist should have the right to treat these lesions in order to adequately manage the patient. A clear example of this would be in the setting of acute myocardial infarction with cardiogenic shock when the cardiologist may need both iliac arteries to perform intra-aortic balloon pump insertion as well as coronary intervention. As for renal disease, as described earlier, there is a high incidence of clinically significant renal lesions among the coronary interventionalist's patients. The ability to treat these obstructions is in the very best interest of the patients. In the guidelines outlined by the Society for Cardiac Angiography and Interventions (SCA& I), cardiologists can achieve limited credentials for procedures involving iliac and renal arteries by having active credentials for coronary intervention, attending a live iliac or renal artery training course, and successfully performing three proctored cases as the primary operator. After gaining experience with these types of cases, the cardiologist can eventually finish the 50 peripheral vascular interventional procedures required for unrestricted clinical competency.

## CONCLUSION

There has been a major shift among interventional cardiologists into the field of peripheral vascular intervention. This movement should benefit patients by increasing the recognition of this highly underdiagnosed disease, thus allowing patients to receive treatment through minimally invasive interventional techniques. In addition, cardiologists can apply their skills in the medical management of the risk factors of atherosclerosis to help reduce the systemic manifestations of atherosclerosis wherever they occur.

## REFERENCES

1. Gruentzig AR: Transluminal dilation of coronary artery stenosis. Lancet 1:263, 1978.
2. Harding MB, Smith LR, Himmelstein SI, et al: Renal artery stenosis: Prevalence and associated risk factors in patients undergoing routine cardiac catheterization. J Am Soc Nephrol 2:1608–1616, 1992.
3. Khosla S, White CJ, Collins TJ, et al: Effects of renal artery stent implantation in patients with renovascular hypertension presenting with unstable angina or congestive heart failure. Am J Cardiol 80:363–366, 1997.
4. Rajachandran, Rosenfeld, et al: J Am Coll Cardiol 29:486A, 1997.
5. Babb JD, Collins TJ, Cowley MJ, et al: Revised guidelines for the performance of peripheral vascular intervention. Catheter Cardiovasc Interv 46:21–23, 1999.

# II

# Intervention and the Atherosclerotic Vessel

# 2

# Vascular Biology of Mechanical Intervention

*Ming W. Liu    James M. Parks    David A. Cox    François M. Booyse*

Interventional cardiologists become intimately involved in the biology of vascular endothelial and smooth muscle cells and activate platelets and coagulation mechanisms each time they perform an angioplasty. Mechanical interventions create immediate and prolonged demands on a segment of diseased vessel wall that has already altered its normal biologic function. Increasingly, it is recognized that vascular endothelial and smooth muscle cells undergo complex and intertwined responses to vascular injury that function in a reparative fashion. Understanding how these reparative responses relate to vascular injury from mechanical interventions offers the best opportunity to devise clinically effective strategies to prevent restenosis or alter the incidence of acute closure. Two caveats should be appreciated: First, much of the experimental biology involved after vascular injury has been described in animal models; second, its relevance to the human atherosclerotic plaque is unclear.

The formation of thrombus at the site of vascular injury in patients with unstable coronary syndromes and those undergoing mechanical vascular intervention often results in myocardial ischemia or infarction. Developments over the past decade have established the important role of platelets in the pathogenesis of thrombus formation in these patients. Advances in the understanding of the mechanism of platelet adhesion, activation, and aggregation have led to exciting avenues for the prevention of platelet-related complications. Normal hemostasis is a delicate balance between reactions favoring thrombin generation and clot formation (coagulation) and those favoring plasmin generation and clot lysis (fibrinolysis). The understanding of the mechanisms of platelet and hemostasis in forming thrombus is essential to interventional cardiologists.

This chapter reviews the following: (1) the role of endothelial cell in vascular injury; (2) the role of smooth muscle cell in reparative process after balloon injury; (3) the role of platelets in maintaining vascular integrity, as well as their response to injury; and (4) hemostasis and alterations that occur after various mechanical and pharmacologic interventions.

## ENDOTHELIAL CELLS

Endothelial cells (ECs) that line the luminal surface exist as a monolayer throughout the vascular tree. These cells can be readily identified by morphologic characteristics, by staining for factor VIII-related antigen (von Willebrand factor), or by the uptake of fluoresceinated acetylated low density lipoproteins, all of which provide specific evidence of endothelial origin.[1, 2] ECs sense flow and grow with their long axis oriented in the direction of flow, except in areas of turbulence.[3] Although ECs are firmly attached to each other and to their basement membrane, balloon injury denudes these cells from the vessel wall.

Rather than simply serving as a conduit for circulating blood, vascular ECs maintain several important metabolic functions that can be altered by atherosclerosis or mechanical injury[2] (Table 2–1). ECs actively modulate local hemostasis and thrombolysis and regulate vessel diameter through acute vasomotor mechanisms and long-term control of arterial wall thickness. Besides producing vasoactive compounds, ECs synthesize at least three growth factors (fibroblast growth factor [FGF], platelet-derived growth factor [PDGF], transforming growth factor-$\beta$ [TGF-$\beta$]), and maintain underlying smooth muscle cells [SMCs] in a quiescent state by releasing heparin. Finally, a significant number of components of EC basement membrane (types IV and V collagen, laminin, proteoglycans) and extracellular matrix (fibronectin) are produced by ECs.

## Vasoactive Compounds

Vascular ECs release numerous vasodilators, including endothelium-derived relaxing factor (EDRF) and prostacyclin, and also synthesize a class of vasoconstrictor agents known as endothelins (ETs) (Table

**TABLE 2–1. FUNCTIONAL PROPERTIES OF ENDOTHELIAL CELLS**

| FUNCTION | EXAMPLES |
|---|---|
| Permeability barrier | Surface charge and presence of glycocalyx<br>Tight junctions<br>Pore size of transcytotic vesicles<br>Basement membrane |
| Thromboresistance | Thrombomodulin content of plasma membrane<br>Rapid metabolism of platelet aggregating agents<br>Synthesis and secretion of prostacyclin and plasminogen activator |
| Mediation of vascular tone | Synthesis and secretion of prostacylin, endothelium-derived relaxing factor, and endothelin |
| Inflammatory and immune response | Expression of leukocyte adhesion molecules, leukocyte chemotactic proteins, growth factors, hematopoietic factors, growth inhibitory agents, scavenger receptors |

Modified from Stary HC, Blankenhorn DH, Chandler AB, et al: A definition of the intima of human arteries and of its atherosclerosis-prone regions. Circulation 85:391, 1992. By permission of the American Heart Association, Inc.

2–2). A local renin-angiotensin II system has also been identified in the vascular endothelium. Such agents are likely to be important in regulating local vascular tone after injury. Clinically, nitrate therapy results in vasodilation by increasing nitric oxide levels; nitric oxide relaxes vascular smooth muscle cells by increasing cyclic guanosine monophosphate. EDRF, a potent vasodilator produced from ECs, results in local (paracrine) vasodilation by the same mechanism. In fact, EDRF has been identified as nitric oxide or a closely related compound. The vascular tree likely maintains some level of continuous dilatation by local EDRF released by ECs; EDRF released into the bloodstream is immediately inactivated by hemoglobin, which also degrades nitric oxide.[4]

Some evidence exists that cyclic guanosine monophosphate and nitrovasodilators inhibit in vitro SMC proliferation, suggesting that EDRF could play

**TABLE 2–2. VASOACTIVE SUBSTANCES PRODUCED BY ENDOTHELIAL CELLS**

| SUBSTANCE | EFFECT |
|---|---|
| Endothelium-derived relaxing factor (EDRF) | Vasodilation; impedes platelet aggregation synergistically with prostacyclin |
| Prostacyclin | Vasodilation; impedes platelet aggregation |
| Endothelin | Vasoconstriction, production linked to EDRF |
| Angiotensin II | Vasoconstriction, modulates smooth muscle cell growth |

a role in SMC growth modulation.[5] After experimental balloon injury, regenerated endothelium produced less vasodilation in response to acetylcholine, with persistent dysfunction noted up to 4 weeks after injury. Increased intimal thickening occurred in arterial segments with less responsiveness to acetylcholine; these effects may result from reduced release of EDRF.[6] Whether EDRF exerts similar effects on atherosclerotic vessels is unclear. EDRF has been shown to result in attenuated vasodilation in human atherosclerotic arteries removed from transplanted hearts or even to produce paradoxical vasoconstriction in diseased vessels.[7, 8]

Prostacyclin is a prostaglandin hormone produced by EC that also has local rather than systemic effects.[4] Synergistically with EDRF, prostacyclin impedes platelet aggregation. Some evidence suggests that prostacyclin may also relax underlying vascular SMC. Although thromboxane $A_2$ released by platelets induces platelet aggregation and vasoconstriction, prostacyclin made by ECs has potent local antiplatelet and vasodilatory effects. Aspirin, used clinically to inhibit thromboxane production by platelets, unfortunately also inhibits EC production of prostacyclin, even in lower doses.

ETs are a newly recognized class of compounds with impressive vasoconstrictive properties. ET-I is a subtype made by ECs with pressor potency 10 times that of angiotensin II.[4] Diverse agents, including thrombin, TGF-β, and angiotensin II, elicit ET production.[9] However, ET production seems to be linked to EDRF; thrombin-induced production of ET is inhibited by EDRF.[10] ET can stimulate in vitro SMC proliferation.[11]

Evidence also suggests the existence of a localized renin angiotensin system in the vessel wall. Both angiotensin II and angiotensin-converting enzyme can be localized to the vascular endothelium, although their effects in maintaining local vascular tone are undefined.[12] Some reports have suggested that angiotensin II may function as a growth factor for vascular SMCs.[13] Angiotensin II and angiotensin-converting enzyme found in overlying ECs may modulate vascular SMC growth.

The relevance of EC synthesis of local vasoactive agents to vascular injury from mechanical intervention is speculative, although intriguing. Local vasoactive agents made by ECs may interact with other growth factors and modulated SMC proliferation. Vascular tone is an important determinant of shear stress, which can influence both EC regrowth and SMC proliferation. Vasoconstriction may occur when endothelial denudation results from mechanical intervention and local EDRF levels are diminished. Prostacyclin may serve as a reserve vasodilator when local endothelial damage has perturbed EDRF production.[4] The role of ET has not been defined, although a link to EDRF seems clear. ET may participate in vessel repair because other factors associated with vessel injury, such as thrombin and TGF-β, stimulate messenger RNA synthesis of ET precursors.[9]

## Endothelial Regeneration

ECs grow as a monolayer and, when confluent, cease replication. Disruption of cell contact inhibition results in rapid cell replication. Ingrowth occurs by replication of ECs from the proximal and distal untraumatized vessel segments.[14] Growth occurs at an approximate rate of 0.2 mm/day for 8 to 12 weeks, but in rat carotid arteries, growth stops at 10 to 12 mm, leaving a segment of vessel wall uncovered by ECs.[15] The same phenomenon of incomplete EC regeneration in humans is noted in vascular grafts when regenerating ECs fail to cover the prosthesis fully.

However, it is not clear to what extent incomplete EC regeneration after mechanical intervention occurs in humans. After placement of balloon-expandable stents, EC regeneration and coverage of strut wires appear complete at 4 weeks both in animals and in humans.[16, 17] Complete EC regrowth is noted in the middle of the stented segment. Autopsy evidence suggests that complete EC regrowth may occur in humans after angioplasty as well, with full EC regeneration noted as early as 1 month after the procedure.[18] Although some animal data support the notion that EC regeneration may not be complete, other experimental data do suggest that EC can cover the injured vessel wall by day 10 after balloon injury.[15] Because longer (3.0- and 4.0-cm) angioplasty balloons are becoming more available and likely create larger areas of EC denudement, a greater period for complete EC regeneration may be required, or incomplete regeneration may occur. Both results may have some influence on the degree of neointimal thickening seen with the use of these devices.

Numerous studies have shown that if ECs are gently denuded or removed with a nylon filament loop in a manner that does not damage the underlying media, an early platelet response occurs, followed by rapid EC regeneration and little neointimal proliferation.[19, 20] Presumably, placement of intracoronary guide wires results in the same minimal vessel wall damage as does the aforementioned experimental design. Experimental models involving more extensive EC denudation result in maximal neointimal proliferation where EC regeneration last occurred. Thus, a critical time may exist when EC regrowth could precede maximal SMC proliferation and arrest the development of neointimal formation.[21, 22] Overlying ECs likely play an important role in controlling SMC proliferation via secretion of heparin and other growth-inhibitory factors, with some evidence that neointimal proliferation ceases when ECs regenerate.[22] However, when deep medial injury accompanies EC denudation with balloon injury (as happens almost uniformly during clinical angioplasty), significant neointimal proliferation occurs in these experimental models.[23]

## Dysfunctional Regenerating Endothelium

Some experimental evidence exists that regenerating endothelium may be dysfunctional. In a rabbit iliac artery model, regenerating cells 2 and 4 weeks after balloon injury did stain for factor VIII antigen, suggesting an endothelial origin. However, this regenerating endothelium was shown to be less responsive to acetylcholine. Arterial segments with more severe endothelial dysfunction had greater intimal thickening; reduced release of EDRF may play a role in both reduced endothelium-dependent vasodilation and increased intimal thickening.[6] Regenerating dysfunctional endothelium may make less growth inhibitors (heparin, EDRF) or more growth promoters (PDGF, FGF, angiotensin II). Thus, even though regenerating endothelium may cover denuded vessel wall, such ECs may be dysfunctional. SMC proliferation and production of extracellular matrix could persist in the face of such a dysfunctional endothelium.

Incomplete EC regeneration may occur after balloon injury, leaving SMCs abutting the luminal surface. In areas of experimental chronic denudation in rat carotid arteries where EC regrowth does not occur, luminal SMCs resemble ECs morphologically but do not stain with antibody to factor VIII, nor do they stimulate thrombosis.[24] Whether such luminal SMCs are capable of generating growth inhibitors to the same extent as regenerating ECs is unclear. Luminal SMCs do differ from neointimal SMC in their expression of PDGF A-chain and PDGF receptors, suggesting that functional differences may exist.[25] Functional differences in these luminal SMCs may ultimately affect the degree of neointimal proliferation. The concept of dysfunctional endothelium is an important focus of current research, with efforts aimed at exploring differences in vascular tone.[26]

## Endothelial Cell Influence on Smooth Muscle Cells

The importance of EC regeneration relates to the observations that (1) heparin and heparin-like substances made by ECs inhibit SMC growth in vitro[27]; (2) heparin derived from ECs and SMCs likely is the major growth-inhibiting factor that maintains SMCs in a quiescent state[27, 28]; (3) as EC regeneration occurs, these cells synthesize heparin proteoglycans as they cease to proliferate[29]; (4) vascular SMCs begin to cease to proliferate when endothelium is fully regenerated, although extracellular matrix production continues[22]; and (5) experimental data suggest that EC regeneration and SMC proliferation may be closely linked because in vitro SMC proliferation appears to be greatly affected by the rate of EC proliferation.[30]

Heparin is a glycosaminoglycan with specific inhibitory effects on SMC growth. Heparin and related agents (heparan sulfate, heparan) inhibit SMC proliferation and migration in vitro and in vivo.[31, 32] Both ECs and SMCs can synthesize heparin, suggesting that SMCs may be able to modulate their own proliferation. The mechanisms involved have not been fully clarified; the exact block in the cell cycle is controversial.

## VASCULAR SMOOTH MUSCLE CELLS

The internal elastic lamina defines the border between intima and media. In normal vessels, the intima (from the internal elastic lamina to EC layer) is usually quite thin but thickens in atherosclerotic or restenotic vessels.[2] Many experimental results relating to restenosis have been extrapolated from atherosclerosis models; restenosis is viewed as an acceleration of the neointimal proliferation that occurs in atherosclerosis. Much attention is focused on vascular SMC proliferation, migration, and production of extracellular matrix, all of which can result in neointimal proliferation and luminal compromise. The biology of vascular SMCs is clearly involved in the pathogenesis of atherosclerotic plaques and in the maintenance of vascular tone. Our focus in this section, however, is on SMC involvement in vascular repair and restenosis after balloon injury.

### Regulation of SMC Growth: SMC Phenotypes

Vascular SMCs primarily function to maintain wall tension (Table 2–3). In this capacity, these cells exist in a contractile phenotype characterized by a markedly decreased ability to divide, little rough endoplasmic reticulum and synthetic organelles, and diminished production of extracellular matrix.[2, 21, 33] Quiescent SMCs (contractile phenotype) stain strongly for SM-actin because of an increased amount of contractile proteins. Contractile SMCs are less responsive to growth factors and exist primarily in the media of the vessel wall.

Should vascular injury occur, SMCs can revert to

**TABLE 2–3.   FUNCTIONAL PROPERTIES OF VASCULAR SMOOTH MUSCLE CELLS**

| FUNCTION | EXAMPLES |
| --- | --- |
| Contractility | Modulation of content of contractile proteins |
| | Responsiveness to mediators of vascular tone |
| Maintenance of structural integrity | Synthesis and secretion of connective tissues (collagen, elastin, and proteoglycan) |
| | Capacity to proliferate via expression of growth factor receptors and synthesis and secretion of growth factors |
| | Capacity to migrate |
| Lipid metabolism | Removal of deposited lipoproteins via expression of low-density lipoprotein receptors and/or phagocytosis |

Modified from Stary HC, Blankenhorn DH, Chandler AB, et al: A definition of the intima of human arteries and of its atherosclerosis-prone regions. Circulation 85:391, 1992. By permission of the American Heart Association, Inc.

a synthetic phenotype characterized by an increased ability to replicate, little contractile function, and a marked increase in synthetic function with increased amounts of rough endoplasmic reticulum (Fig. 2–1).[34] Extracellular matrix production is five times greater in synthetic SMCs.[33] Synthetic SMCs stain weaker for SM-actin because fewer contractile proteins are present (Table 2–4). These SMCs are found primarily in the intima. Data from immunohistochemical staining of atherectomy specimens suggest that proliferating SMCs can be identified by monoclonal antibody stains, which reflect a change in SMC-actin isoform expression.[35] Proliferating

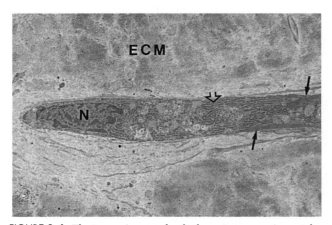

FIGURE 2–1. Electron micrograph of atherectomy specimen taken from the left anterior descending coronary artery of a patient who developed restenosis 4 weeks after angioplasty. The single smooth muscle cell is of the synthetic phenotype and contains abundant endoplasmic reticulum (*open arrow*) with very few myofilament bundles along the periphery of the cell (*arrows*). This smooth muscle cell is surrounded by amorphous extracellular matrix material (ECM). N, smooth muscle cell nucleus. (×12,000.) (Courtesy of Dr. Peter G. Anderson, Department of Pathology, University of Alabama at Birmingham.)

**TABLE 2–4.   SMOOTH MUSCLE CELL PHENOTYPES**

| CONTRACTILE PHENOTYPE | SYNTHETIC PHENOTYPE |
|---|---|
| Myofilament rich | Myofilament poor |
| Decreased capacity to divide | Increased ability to replicate |
| Less rough endoplasmic reticulum and synthetic organelles | Increased rough endoplasmic reticulum and synthetic organelles |
| Less extracellular matrix production | Increased matrix production |
| Stain strongly for SM-actin | Weaker stain for SM-actin |
| | Proliferating cells stain for cyclin and tenascin |

SMCs also stain for cyclin (proliferating cell nuclear antigen) and tenascin (an extracellular matrix protein).[36, 37]

Reversion of SMCs to a synthetic phenotype allows these cells to participate in tissue repair, or pathologically, atherosclerotic lesions. The ability to synthesize large amounts of collagen, elastin, or proteoglycans can be viewed as a normal reparative response to vessel injury. Heterogeneous populations of SMCs exist; that is, not all vascular SMCs respond to injury at the extreme spectrums of contractile or synthetic phenotypes.[38] The factors that elicit a change to the synthetic phenotype are undefined but may involve (1) removal of growth inhibitors as ECs are denuded; (2) release of growth factors from platelets, inflammatory cells, and injured or dying ECs and SMCs; or (3) production of autocrine/paracrine growth factors by proliferating SMCs themselves.

## Regulation of SMC Growth: SMC Proliferation

Quiescent SMCs proliferate at extremely low rates (0.06%/day), most likely because of growth inhibition from heparin made by ECs and SMCs.[39] In the animal model, the following events occur as a result of balloon injury in normal arteries. Significant EC loss and balloon injury result in SMC proliferation first in the media and then, after migration, in the intima. SMC proliferation after balloon injury in normal artery occurs in up to 30% to 50% of medial SMCs, which revert to a synthetic phenotype.[33] Entrance into the cell cycle occurs as soon as 2 to 3 days after injury, and maximal proliferation is completed between 7 to 14 days. SMCs undergo approximately three rounds of replication. Migration occurs at about day 4, most likely because of the chemotactic effects of PDGF. Approximately 50% of the cells that migrate into the intima never divide and make up about 10% of the final intimal population.[19, 39] After 2 weeks, the number of SMCs

in the neointima remains constant.[40] Further increases in neointimal proliferation result from increased cell volume from hypertrophy and accumulation of extracellular matrix rather than from further cell division and appear to peak at 2 to 3 months.[22] Morphologically, proliferating SMCs are scattered loosely in the extracellular matrix (Fig. 2–2). By 6 months, most SMCs have returned to the contractile phenotype and synthesize much less extracellular matrix.[21, 33]

Proliferating SMCs are found at both primary and restenotic percutaneous transluminal coronary angioplasty sites. The ability to retrieve tissue for sophisticated studies and in vitro culture has been greatly aided by atherectomy devices that obtain small fragments of tissue. When proliferating SMCs obtained with atherectomy from primary lesions are compared with those obtained from restenotic lesions, restenotic SMCs show a higher and more persistent rate of proliferation.[41] Further data suggest that proliferating SMCs alter actin isoform expression compared with quiescent SMCs.[42, 43] These results imply that SMC proliferation may involve activation of specific genes that result in phenotypic and functional changes.

## Determinant of SMC Growth: Stretch Injury

Experimental models have shown when EC denudation occurs without damage to underlying SMCs, platelets adhere to the subendothelium and degranulate, releasing multiple growth factors,[20] yet much less neointimal proliferation is noted, as compared with other models using balloon catheter injury involving SMC damage.[23] In a rabbit model,

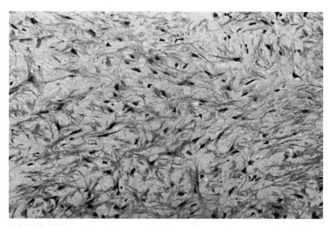

FIGURE 2–2. Photomicrograph of an atherectomy specimen from patient in Figure 2–1. This neointimal tissue consists of irregularly shaped smooth muscle cells with abundant eosinophilic extracellular matrix material. This pattern is consistent with the synthetic phenotype of smooth muscle cells seen in restenotic tissues. (H&E, ×300.) (Courtesy of Dr. Peter G. Anderson, Department of Pathology, University of Alabama at Birmingham.)

higher balloon pressures together with oversized balloon injury resulted in increased neointimal proliferation.[44] Oversized intracoronary stenting in a porcine model produces marked sustained tensile stress, which results in significant neointimal proliferation.[16] The extent of neointimal proliferation in this model appears to be proportional to the extent of injury when rupture of the internal elastic lamina is used as a marker.[45] Severe medial injury may trigger neointimal proliferation by direct effects on SMCs, increased infiltration of inflammatory cells and mediators, and increased deposition of platelets on a dissected vessel wall. Because percutaneous transluminal coronary angioplasty is performed on vessels that may have eccentric atherosclerotic plaques, marked stretching of medial SMCs in undiseased segments of vessel wall can occur during balloon inflation. An exuberant neointimal response beyond that expected in normal reparative function may result from severe stretch injury.[33]

## Determinant of SMC Growth: Shear Stress

Low or oscillatory shear stress results in greater intimal thickening.[19, 33] Experimentally, increased blood flow (higher shear stress) in endothelialized vascular grafts results in decreased neointimal thickening. Decreased neointimal thickness appeared to be caused by a reduction in SMC number, with resultant decreased matrix production.[46] In a similar study, SMC proliferative rates were decreased when shear stress was high but physiologic.[47] In another study in a canine femoral model, decreased blood flow resulted in significant neointimal thickening, regardless of laser or balloon injury.[48] Poor vascular flow was an important determinant of neointimal thickening when method and severity of injury were controlled.

Hemodynamic factors influence EC regrowth, SMC proliferation, and, ultimately, neointimal proliferation.[19, 33, 49] Low wall shear stress may inhibit EC regrowth and may result in a regenerated endothelium that produces less heparin and EDRF.[6, 50] Less growth inhibition of underlying SMCs would be expected from such an endothelium. Intact ECs likely sense changes in shear stress and modulate SMC proliferation because SMCs do not directly sense alterations in shear stress.[45, 46]

The levels of shear stress and disturbed flow may be important determinants of the likelihood of restenosis occurring after angioplasty. Even if appropriately functional endothelial regrowth has occurred and SMCs have undergone minimal stretch injury, a suboptimal angioplasty result that involves large areas of low shear stress or disturbed flow may enhance neointimal proliferation. A self-perpetuating cycle could ensue in which neointimal proliferation results in vascular remodeling, which produces even larger areas of low shear stress and increased luminal narrowing.[33]

## Growth Factors

The interactions between peptide growth factors in the control of vascular SMC proliferation and migration are complex and are not fully understood. Table 2–5 summarizes the growth factors likely to play a role in restenosis. Growth factors interact and often act synergistically. Many sources contribute growth factors, including platelets, neutrophils, macrophages, and SMCs (Table 2–6). Some growth factors have multiple targets; FGF affects both EC regeneration and SMC proliferation. Other growth factors, such as PDGF, come from multiple sources but seem

**TABLE 2–5.** **POTENTIAL ROLE OF GROWTH FACTORS IN CORONARY RESTENOSIS**

| GROWTH FACTOR | POTENTIAL ACTION IN RESTENOSIS |
|---|---|
| PDGF | Stimulates smooth muscle cell migration and proliferation |
| FGF | Stimulates endothelial cell and fibroblast proliferation |
| EGF | Replaces heparin on cell surface; promotes smooth muscle cell proliferation |
| IGF | Promotes smooth muscle cell proliferation and extracellular matrix production |
| TGF | Regulates matrix remodeling; likely to regulate other growth factors |

EGF, epidermal growth factor; FGF, fibroblast growth factor; IGF, insulin-like growth factor; PDGF, platelet-derived growth factor; TGF, transforming growth factor.

Adapted from Forrester JS, Fishbein M, Helfant R, et al: A paradigm for restenosis based on cell biology clues for the development of new preventive therapies. J Am Coll Cardiol 17:758, 1991. Reprinted with permission from the American College of Cardiology.

**TABLE 2–6.** **PRODUCTION OF GROWTH FACTORS BY CELLS ASSOCIATED WITH VASCULAR INJURY**

| CELLS | GROWTH FACTORS | | | |
|---|---|---|---|---|
| | PDGF | FGF | TGF-β | EGF |
| Platelets | + | − | + | + |
| Monocyte/macrophages | + | + | + | − |
| Endothelial cells | + | + | + | − |
| Smooth muscle cells | + | + | − | − |

EGF, epidermal growth factor; FGF, fibroblast growth factor; PDGF, platelet-derived growth factor; TGF-β, transforming growth factor-β.

+, growth factor production; −, no known growth factor production.

Adapted from Klagsbrun M, Edelman M: Biological and biochemical properties of fibroblast growth factors: Implications for the pathogenesis of atherosclerosis. Arteriosclerosis 9:269, 1989.

**TABLE 2–7.   TARGET CELLS FOR GROWTH FACTORS**

| GROWTH FACTOR | ENDOTHELIAL CELLS | SMOOTH MUSCLE CELLS |
|---|---|---|
| PDGF | − | + |
| FGF | + | + |
| TGF-β | Inhibitory | ? |
| EGF | ? | + |

EGF, epidermal growth factor; FGF, fibroblast growth factor; PDGF, platelet-derived growth factor; TGF-β, transforming growth factor-β.

+, mitogenic effect; −, nonmitogenic effect; ?, conflicting data.

Adapted from Klagsbrun M, Edelman M: Biological and biochemical properties of fibroblast growth factors: Implications for the pathogenesis of atherosclerosis. Arteriosclerosis 9:269, 1989.

to alter primarily SMC function; ECs do not have receptors for PDGF (Table 2–7).

### Platelet-Derived Growth Factor

PDGF is a disulfide-bonded dimer. This potent mitogen (promotes cell division) for SMCs is also chemotactic (directs cell migration) for SMCs, macrophages, and neutrophils. PDGF functions as competence factor and renders cells capable of moving from the arrested state to active cell cycling. Other growth factors, such as insulin-like growth factor-1 (IGF-1) and epidermal growth factor (EGF), function as progression factors and allow cells made competent by PDGF to enter the S phase and begin DNA synthesis. Balloon injury results in marked rises in the production of PDGF, with little PDGF production occurring in the uninjured vessel wall.[51] Also, PDGF production has been demonstrated in atherosclerotic plaques.[52, 53] Platelet-released growth factors stimulate in vitro SMC proliferation.[54] Intimal thickening after balloon injury in thrombocytopenic animals was reduced.[22] Experimentally, trapidil, a PDGF antagonist, has been shown to inhibit SMC proliferation.[55]

Intimal thickening was substantially reduced in these thrombocytopenic animals with antiplatelet antibodies. Interestingly, thymidine labeling of SMCs after balloon injury was unchanged between control and thrombocytopenic animals, showing no differences in SMC proliferation rates.[56] However, these data imply that growth factors released by platelets may affect SMC migration rather than proliferation. Furthermore, a study showed that anti-PDGF antibody resulted in marked reduction in neointima formation in a rat model without significant differences in mean thymidine labeling index (a measure of proliferation). This suggests a role for PDGF as a promoter of SMC migration rather than of proliferation.[57]

### Fibroblast Growth Factor

Two subtypes, acidic and basic FGF (aFGF, bFGF), exist and compete for receptor binding. aFGF appears to have biologic effects similar to those of bFGF, except for diminished potency. bFGF is synthesized by both ECs and vascular SMCs and is a potent EC and SMC mitogen. Both subtypes of FGF lack a signal peptide and therefore cannot normally cross cell membranes.[58] Evidence suggests that FGF is also a key factor in the control of SMC proliferation. FGF is released by dying or damaged ECs and SMCs but is not released by platelets. Both vascular SMCs and ECs synthesize and respond to FGF. Because this growth factor lacks a signal peptide and cannot be transported into the endoplasmic reticulum, it cannot be secreted from healthy cells. This is an important distinction; other peptide growth factors are secreted. Injury or cell death results in the rapid release of FGF. Experimentally, it has been shown that mechanical injury alone, rather than cell death, results in the release of bFGF.[59]

aFGF has little effect on quiescent uninjured vascular SMCs but acts as a potent mitogen for injured SMCs. aFGF exerts its effects by up-regulation of receptors for both aFGF and PDGF and by synergistic stimulation of SMC growth with PDGF.[57] Although bFGF has been shown to stimulate EC regrowth, it also stimulates growth of vascular SMC and of the vaso vasorum.[60] bFGF is localized in the vessel wall and is also a potent mitogen for injured SMCs. Data show that prolonged infusion of bFGF after balloon injury results in significant intimal thickening, with little effect of bFGF occurring on arteries with intact ECs.[61] Another study showed that infusion of an antibody to bFGF after balloon injury results in decreased SMC proliferation and neointimal thickening in a rat carotid artery model, although neointimal thickening was still produced.[62] These findings suggest that FGF may be a significant growth factor in the setting of vascular injury because increased levels are present when cell injury or death occurs.

### Insulin-like Growth Factors, Epidermal Growth Factor, and Transforming Growth Factor-β

Current data suggest that IGF-1 and EGF function as progression factors that allow DNA synthesis to occur in cells stimulated by PDGF and probably by FGF. IGF-1 (also known as somatomedin-C) may be an important rate-limiting step in SMC proliferation after exposure to PDGF. Experimentally, balloon injury results in increased IGF-1 levels.[63] Local tissue levels of IGF-1 are also stimulated by growth hormone, a process that can be blocked by angiopeptin. EGF is another known SMC mitogen, found primarily in platelets. Quiescent SMCs in vitro express approximately 4200 EGF receptors per cell, whereas proliferating SMCs demonstrate about 44,000 EGF receptors per cell.[64] This marked increase in receptor expression in proliferating cells has been taken advantage of; rapid proliferating SMCs can be targeted and selectively killed by conjugating a *Pseudomonas* exotoxin with TGF-β, which binds to the EGF receptor.[65] Little cytotoxicity was seen against quiescent SMCs compared with proliferating cells. A similar approach has been used with FGF by conjugating cell toxins, such as saporin and targeting proliferating SMCs, which also have significantly increased FGF receptors.[66]

TGF-β modulates EC regrowth by inhibiting bFGF and likely plays a significant role in SMC proliferation.[57] TGF-β can either stimulate or inhibit cell growth, modulates synthesis of growth factor receptors, and acts either cooperatively or antagonistically with other growth factors. Its effects can be contradictory; with a low density of SMCs, it inhibits growth, whereas confluent SMCs are stimulated by TGF-β.[57] Low concentrations of TGF-β stimulate SMC growth, and high concentrations of this growth factor inhibit proliferation.[67] Also, TGF-β is probably the major regulator of extracellular matrix production and stimulates synthesis of matrix proteins by ECs and SMCs.[21]

### Angiotensin II

Angiotensin II is a vasoconstrictor that is locally expressed in the vessel wall; it also functions in the control of SMC growth.[13] When angiotensin II was infused in a rat carotid model, SMC proliferative rates were increased in balloon-injured arterial segments. Surprisingly, increases in SMC proliferation were also noted in uninjured arterial segments, although not to the same extent as in injured segments.[68] In an in vivo model, it was shown that supraphysiologic doses of angiotensin-converting enzyme inhibitors markedly inhibited myointimal proliferation.[69]

## Migration of Smooth Muscle Cells

Not all SMCs present in the neointima have undergone replication.[39] PDGF likely regulates SMC migration in vivo. Intimal thickening seems to involve migration of SMCs from the media across the internal elastic lamina into the intima, even by cells that do not undergo mitosis. Data from atherectomy specimens show that restenotic SMCs increase their production of nonmuscle myosin as compared with quiescent SMCs.[70] Because nonmuscle myosin appears to be required for cell movement, such a change in isoform expression appears to be relevant to SMC proliferation and migration. Why some

SMCs migrate without undergoing mitotic division is unclear; the great majority of intimal SMCs do revert to a synthetic phenotype and produce increased amounts of extracellular matrix.

To move through the extracellular matrix, SMCs must degrade matrix proteins surrounding the cell and initiate directed motion. Many of the same mechanisms may also explain how tumor cells migrate, as well as how cell movement occurs during follicular rupture. The evidence suggests that migration may be mediated by the local generation of plasmin from plasminogen, with resultant degradation of matrix proteins.[71] Plasminogen is readily available, given the activation of intrinsic fibrinolytic components on the cell surface. Plasmin activates procollagenases and can degrade many matrix molecules itself. The generation of plasmin for cell migration involves the synthesis of functional plasminogen activators (urokinase [uPA] and tissue-type plasminogen activator [tPA]) at a local cell surface–associated level rather than in the bloodstream.

Data in the rat balloon injury model suggest that plasminogen activator (uPA and tPA) expression by SMCs is associated with SMC proliferation and migration.[72] In this model, uPA expression by SMCs was markedly increased early after balloon injury and remained high throughout both SMC proliferation and migration. Increased expression of tPA was not associated with cell proliferation, but expression rose in association with cell migration.

## Inflammatory Mediators

Cytokines and lymphokines are regulatory proteins that mediate inflammatory responses.[73] Balloon injury stimulates an inflammatory reaction involving migration of neutrophils, macrophages, and lymphocytes. Platelet release of growth factors and autocrine production of endogenous growth factors by SMCs probably interact with growth factors released by macrophages and neutrophils, but these mechanisms have not been defined. Macrophages do release specific growth factors, most notably macrophage-derived PDGF. There is evidence to suggest that leukocyte migration may modulate the proliferative response of SMCs.[74] Cytokines probably mediate these interactions, but their diverse biologic effects are only beginning to be understood.

Interleukin-1 (IL-1) is a cytokine synthesized by monocytes that stimulates prostanoids responsible for inhibiting SMC proliferation.[75] Like FGF, IL-1 lacks a signal peptide and cannot be secreted. Conversely, IL-1 functions as a potent mitogen for SMCs, primarily because IL-1 synergistically interacts with PDGF and FGF.[76, 77] Its effects extend beyond SMC proliferation; IL-1 stimulates platelet-activating factor and increases neutrophil adhesiveness. Interferon γ is a lymphokine secreted by T lymphocytes that inhibits SMC proliferation in culture. In a rat model, interferon γ given parenterally for 1 week after balloon injury resulted in inhibition of SMC replication at 7 days, as well as a reduction in neointimal proliferation at 2 weeks.[78]

## Extracellular Matrix

Once SMCs migrate into the intima, neointimal thickening ensues as a result of cellular proliferation, hypertrophy, and production of extracellular matrix. As noted earlier, 2 weeks after balloon injury, the rate of SMC proliferation markedly slows, and the number of neointimal SMCs remains constant. Synthesis of extracellular matrix components by these SMCs continues for months, however, and clearly contributes to the formation of restenotic lesions.[21, 34, 39] Ultimately, inhibiting neointimal proliferation and preventing restenosis may require strategies that affect both SMC proliferation and extracellular matrix production by synthetic phenotype SMCs (Fig. 2–3).

The extracellular matrix is composed of collagens,

proteoglycans, elastin, fibronectin, and laminin.[2] Production of these extracellular matrix components by SMCs occurs when they are stimulated by growth factors. Synthesis of extracellular matrix proteoglycans by SMCs is regulated primarily by TGF-β. The extracellular matrix is not an inert ground substance; it regulates the phenotypic expression of ECs and SMCs and undergoes structural changes over time. Fibronectin appears to modulate SMCs, so that they change from a contractile to a synthetic phenotype, whereas laminin maintains a contractile phenotype.[79] As proliferating SMCs cease to replicate, they produce significant amounts of proteoglycans (chondroitin sulfate and dermatan sulfate). Fibronectin becomes replaced by proteoglycans as extracellular matrix production continues.[21]

Heparin appears to modulate extracellular matrix composition in vivo by increasing proteoglycan content and diminishing relative amounts of elastin and collagen.[80] This modeling of matrix seems important in the healing of vascular injury. After several months, the extracellular matrix again undergoes a change in composition as SMCs shift back to a contractile phenotype. Collagen again replaces pro-

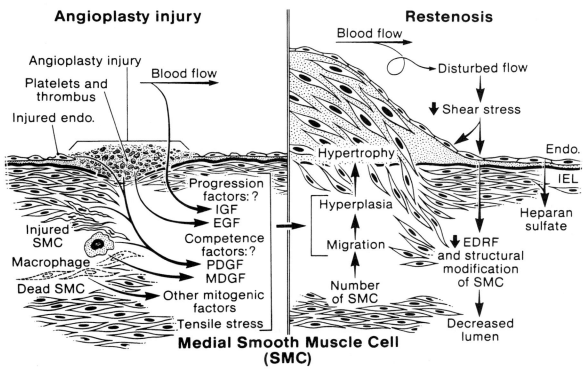

FIGURE 2–3. Postulated mechanisms for restenosis. After balloon injury, in addition to the immediate release of platelet-derived growth factor (PDGF) from platelets, injured endothelium, smooth muscle cells (SMC), and macrophages also produce PDGF or PDGF-like molecules. PDGF is a competence factor committing the cell to enter the replication cycle. Platelets and serum also provide progression factors that enable the cells to progress through the cell cycle. Multiple other mitogenic factors exist and, with PDGF, stimulate smooth muscle cell proliferation. If a sufficient number of activated smooth muscle cells undergo migration and proliferation with a later increase in their size and with production of extracellular matrix, a restenotic lesion can form. In addition, if there is disturbed flow and decreased shear stress, this would not only enhance intimal proliferation but also initiate structural change of the vascular wall to decrease the lumen. Endo, endothelial cells; IEL, internal elastic lamina; IGF, insulin-like growth factor; EDRF, endothelium-derived relaxing factor; EGF, epidermal growth factor; MDGF, macrophage-derived growth factor. (Adapted from Liu MW, Roubin GS, King SB: Restenosis after coronary angioplasty: Potential biologic determinants and role of intimal hyperplasia. Circulation 79:1374, 1989.)

**TABLE 2–8.    IN VIVO STUDIES OF PLATELET ACCUMULATION**

| TYPE INJURY | LIPID AND MONOCYTE ACCUMULATION | PLATELET DEPOSITION |
|---|---|---|
| I | + + | − |
| II | − | + |
| III | − | + + |

From Fuster V, Badimon L, Cohen M, et al: Insights into the pathogenesis of acute ischemic syndrome. Circulation 75:636, 1987.

teoglycans as the major component of extracellular matrix, although the factors controlling this process are unclear.

## PLATELETS

In vivo studies, primarily in rabbits and pigs, have suggested that the accumulation of platelets at the site of injury occurs rapidly.[81, 82] The peak of accumulation occurs within 2 hours of injury and is dependent on two factors: depth of injury and flow. Fuster and associates[83] have defined three levels of injury (Table 2–8): level I is limited to the EC and layer, level II injury is through the EC layer and into the intima, and level III injury is into the media. Level I injury does not induce platelet accumulation and results primarily in the local accumulation of lipids and monocytes. However, level II and III injuries similar to those induced during percutaneous transluminal coronary angioplasty do result in rapid platelet accumulation caused by the exposure of thrombogenic proteins present in the intima and media. In addition to the depth of injury, rheologic factors play a major role in the kinetics of platelet accumulation. Clinically, it has long been known that important thrombus formation occurs primarily at sites of luminal narrowing.[84] In the pig model with experimentally induced type II and III injury, platelet accumulation measured at sites of luminal narrowing increases as the percentage of stenosis increases.[83, 85] In similar experiments in which the degree of luminal narrowing is controlled, the amount of platelet accumulation at sites of type II and III injury has been found to be dependent on local shear rates. At shear rates of less than $850^{s-1}$, the deposition of platelets is not significant. However, at shear rates of greater than $1250^{s-1}$, marked increase in platelet deposition was noted.[86, 87] Therefore, the accumulation of platelets at the site of injury is dependent on the level of injury, as well as local rheologic factors. The mechanism of shear rate–dependent platelet adhesion has been partially clarified by the identification of several families of platelet receptors.

## Platelet Adhesion

Fundamental to the maintenance of normal vessel patency and hemostasis is the preservation of an intact layer of ECs. After injury, this protective layer of cells is removed, exposing the subendothelial proteins to circulating factors and ultimately leading to thrombus formation. A variety of platelet interactions are required for this phenomenon to occur. These include the adhesion of platelets to subendothelial proteins, the binding of platelets to other platelets (aggregation), and the adhesion of platelets to other cells. These adhesive functions are mediated by glycoproteins located on the platelet surface.[86, 87] These glycoproteins have been classified within three known gene families: integrin, leucine rich, and selectin (Table 2–9).

### Integrin Family

The most plentiful is the integrin family, which includes glycoproteins GP IIb/IIIa, GP Ia/IIa, and GP Ic/IIa. GP IIb/IIIa is the most abundant, with each platelet containing 50,000 receptors and accounting for 1% to 2% of the total platelet protein.[88] On activated platelets, the GP IIb/IIIa receptor binds to fibrinogen, fibronectin, immobilized von Willebrand factor, and thrombospondin in a calcium-dependent fashion.[89–91] However, the primary function appears to mediate platelet-platelet interaction (aggregation) by binding to fibrinogen. Each fibrinogen molecule contains multiple Arg-Gly-Asp sequences that serve as a recognition site for the IIb/IIIa receptor.[90, 92–94] This allows for the binding of platelets by way of a fibrinogen "bridge." Glanzmann's thrombasthenia, an autosomal recessive bleeding disorder, is characterized by a deficit in the ability of platelets to bind to adhesive proteins and been shown to be due to a lack of the IIb/IIIa receptor.[95] The second most abundant member of the integrin family is the GP Ia/IIa receptor. Approximately 2000 copies are found on the platelet surface[96, 97] but unlike the IIb/IIIa receptor, expression of the GP Ia/IIa receptor does not require activation of the platelet.[98] This

**TABLE 2–9.    GENE FAMILIES THAT MEDIATE ADHESIVE FUNCTIONS**

| GENE FAMILY | RECEPTOR | LIGAND |
|---|---|---|
| Integrin | IIb/IIIa | Fibronectin, vitronectin, fibrinogen, von Willebrand factor, thrombospondin |
| | Ia/IIa | Types I and III collagen |
| | Ic/IIa | Laminin |
| Leucine-rich | Ib/IX | Immobilized von Willebrand factor |
| Selectin | GMP-140 | Leukocytes and monocytes |

receptor has been isolated and shown to bind to type I and III collagen in a magnesium-dependent fashion.[99] This binding is not dependent on the amino acid sequence Arg-Gly-Asp (RGD) but does result in platelet activation, which may be its primary function.[99, 100] A mild bleeding disorder has been described in a patient whose platelets were refractory to collagen-induced aggregation and were deficient in GP Ia/IIa.[101]

Finally, the least abundant integrin receptor is the GP Ic/IIa receptor. Like the GP Ia/IIa receptor, the GP Ic/IIa receptor does not require platelet activation and binds to its ligand in a magnesium-dependent manner.[102, 103] GP Ic/IIa binds to laminin in low shear stress conditions and by an RGD-independent mechanism.[102]

### Leucine-Rich Family

The most abundant glycoprotein in this family is the GP Ib/IX complex, which has approximately 25,000 copies per platelet.[104] The major role of the GP Ib/IX complex is to bind to immobilized von Willebrand factor.[105–107] von Willebrand factor is a multimetric glycoprotein synthesized by the EC and secreted into the circulation and deposited in the subendothelium. The interaction between von Willebrand factor and the GP Ib/IX complex is mediated by a binding domain located near the amino-terminus of the von Willebrand molecule and is responsible for platelet binding in conditions of high shear stress.[108] However, the GP Ib/IX does not recognize circulating von Willebrand factor.[109] The reason for this observation is unknown but may have to do with high shear stress stimulating the binding of von Willebrand factor to the GP Ib/IX complex.[110] Unlike integrin receptors, the binding of the GP Ib/IX complex is not divalent cation dependent and also is a transmembrane complex, allowing for a coupling of adhesion to functions within the platelet.[109, 111] A rare autosomal bleeding disorder associated with prolonged bleeding time, known as Bernard-Soulier syndrome, has been shown to be due to a congenital lack of the GP Ib/IX complex.[105, 112] Platelets from these patients fail to aggregate in the presence of ristocetin and demonstrate defective adhesion in vitro.[113] The stimulation of binding at high shear rates of the Ib/IX receptor and von Willebrand factor explains the clinically observed "shear rate dependence" of platelets.

### Selectin Family

The most prevalent platelet receptor from this gene family is the granule membrane protein 140.[113, 114] Granule membrane protein has been shown to function as a receptor that binds to neutrophils and monocytes.[114, 115] This interaction between platelets and neutrophils/monocytes is calcium dependent and, like the IIb/IIIa receptor, requires platelet activation to be expressed on the platelet surface.[37] The role of the granule membrane protein 140 receptor is unknown. It has been suggested that its function is to localize leukocytes to the site of vascular injury, or is a means by which activated platelets may be recognized in the circulation by macrophages and removed, or both.

## Platelet Activation

The formation of a platelet monolayer at the site of vascular injury is a "passive" process and is only the first step in a complex series of reactions that lead to platelet-rich thrombus formation. The release of tissue factor (and subsequent thrombin formation by way of the extrinsic pathway) that occurs with deep vessel injury is potentiated by the formation of a platelet monolayer, because it serves as an excellent surface for the formation of the prothrombinase complex. Locally produced thrombin binds to the surface of the platelet, resulting in increased intracellular calcium and platelet to activate its neighbors, and results in the release of dense granules (Table 2–10). These dense granules contain adenosine diphosphate, serotonin, and calcium. In the presence of calcium, adenosine diphosphate and other agonists (serotonin, collagen, and platelet-activating factor) bind to the platelet surface and activate intracellular phospholipase C in a G protein–dependent manner. This in turn activates protein kinase C, which is responsible for the increase in calcium levels.[86] The increase in calcium allows for the IIb/IIIa receptor to undergo a conformational change, thereby allowing for platelet-fibrinogen-platelet binding (platelet aggregation).[98] The increase in intracellular calcium also activates phospholipase $A_2$, which catalyzes the release of arachidonic acid from membrane phospholipids and results in the synthesis of the potent platelet-aggregating substance thromboxane $A_2$ (Fig. 2–4). The secretion of such potent platelet aggregating agents by stimulated platelets allows for a single platelet to activate its neighbors and results in rapid thrombus growth.

## TABLE 2–10.  PLATELET GRANULES

| PLATELET GRANULES | CONTENTS |
| --- | --- |
| Dense | Adenosine diphosphate, serotonin, calcium, phosphate |
| Alpha | Fibrinogen, von Willebrand factor, platelet factor 4, beta-thromboglobulin, platelet-derived growth factor, fibronectin, thrombospondin, platelet factor 5 |

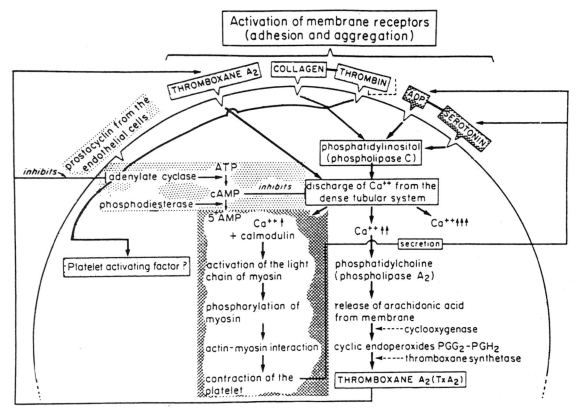

FIGURE 2–4. Schematic representing a summary of the mechanisms involved in platelet activation. Agonists (ADP, thrombin, collagen, serotonin, thromboxane $A_2$) bind to the platelet surface and lead to the mobilization of intracellular calcium. Cyclic adenosine monophosphate (cAMP) inhibits the mobilization from the dense tubular system. ADP, adenosine diphosphate; ATP, adenosine triphosphate; $PGE_1$, prostaglandin $E_1$; $PGG_2$, prostaglandin $G_2$; $PGH_2$, prostaglandin $H_2$. (From Stein B, Fuster V, Israel DH, et al: Platelet inhibitor agents in cardiovascular disease: An update. J Am Coll Cardiol 14:813, 1989.)

### Prostacyclin

Prostacyclin is a potent inhibitor of platelet aggregation and is synthesized by way of the arachidonic pathway primarily by ECs.[115] It acts to counterbalance the effects of thromboxane $A_2$ by stimulating adenyl cyclase, which results in the decrease in intracellular calcium.[108] The decrease in intracellular calcium inhibits both platelet secretion and aggregation.

### Leukotrienes

The other arm of the arachidonic pathway is controlled by the enzyme lipoxygenase, which is responsible for the production of leukotrienes. Our understanding of these compounds is limited, but they have been demonstrated to be potent mediators in chemotaxis and immune-mediated reactions. Leukotrienes have also been noted to have vasoconstrictor actions on coronary smooth muscles.[86] Because of the chemotaxic function, as well as their effects on smooth muscles, the role of leukotrienes in the process of SMC migration and proliferation after vascular injury has become an area of great interest.

### Alpha Granules

Like dense granules, alpha granules are present in platelet and are secreted on platelet activation. Alpha granules contain fibrinogen, fibronectin, and von Willebrand factor, which contribute to the process of platelet aggregation (see Table 2–10). However, these granules also contain PDGF and thrombospondin. PDGF is a potent chemotaxic agent for vascular SMCs and is involved in the migration and proliferation of smooth muscle cells after vascular injury. Thrombospondin is shown to participate in the regulation of smooth muscle growth.[116, 117] The presence of these agents in the platelet and their temporal release at the site of vascular injury is the cornerstone of the hypothesis that the platelet is a critical player in the migration and proliferation of medial SMCs after vascular injury.

## THROMBOSIS

Normal hemostasis (Fig. 2–5) is a delicate balance between reactions favoring thrombin generation and clot formation (coagulation) and those favoring plasmin generation and clot lysis (fibrinolysis).

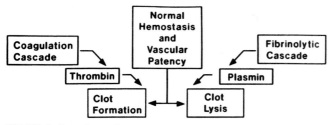

FIGURE 2–5. Balance between coagulation and fibrinolysis required to maintain normal hemostasis.

## Coagulation (Table 2–11)

After denudation of the endothelium and disruption of the atherosclerotic plaque and medial tissues, exposure of proteins, such as type II and IV collagen, immobilized von Willebrand factor, fibronectin, vitronectin and laminin, lead to the adhesion of a monolayer of platelets at the injury site.[118] Adhesion is mediated by a family of transmembrane receptors, known as integrin receptors, located on the surface of platelets. After integrin receptor–mediated adhesion, platelet activation occurs, exposing the glycoprotein IIb/IIIa receptor on the platelet surface responsible for platelet-fibrinogen interaction (platelet aggregation). Along with platelets, macrophages and monocytes converge at the injury site, leading to the assembly of enzyme complexes and surfaces necessary for the generation of insoluble fibrin. One of the earliest observations by investigators interested in coagulation was that blood would clot when exposed to damaged tissue. It was therefore believed that the factor or factors responsible were "extrinsic" to the blood. Similarly, it was noted that blood placed in a container would clot in the absence of damaged tissue, leading investigators to postulate that the factor or factors responsible were "intrinsic" to the blood itself. Since these early observations,

**TABLE 2–11.   PROPERTIES OF COAGULATION PROTEINS**

| FACTOR | MW (kd) | SERUM | TRADITIONAL NAMES |
|---|---|---|---|
| I | 340 | 7.5 | Fibrinogen |
| II* | 72 | 1.4 | Prothrombin |
| V | 330 | 0.02 | Proaccelerin |
| VII* | 47 | 0.01 | Proconvertin |
| VIII | 265 | 0.004 | Antihemophilic factor |
| IX* | 68 | 0.09 | Christmas factor |
| X* | 56 | 0.17 | Stuart-Prower factor |
| XI | 160 | 0.25 | PTA |
| XII | 80 | 0.4 | Hageman factor |
| XIII | 320 | 0.05 | |

PTA, plasma thromboplastin antecedent.
*Vitamin K–dependent factors.
From Harker LA, Mann KG: Thrombosis and fibrinolysis. *In* Fuster V, Verstraete M (eds): Thrombosis in Cardiovascular Disorders. Philadelphia: WB Saunders, 1992.

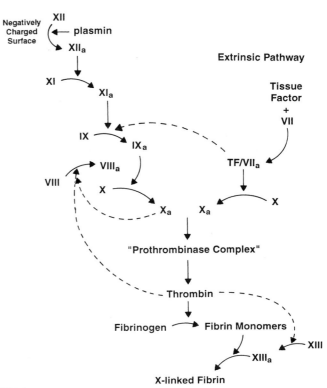

FIGURE 2–6. Extrinsic and intrinsic pathways of coagulation. (Activated forms of the factors are denoted with a subscripted *a*.)

the two pathways, historically termed the *intrinsic* and *extrinsic* pathways of coagulation, have been well studied and defined, as have their respective roles in normal hemostasis (Fig. 2–6).[119, 120]

### *Extrinsic Pathway*

Because coronary angioplasty involves the exposure of vessel wall tissues to the blood, the extrinsic pathway is of key interest to the interventional cardiologist. After vessel wall injury, a unique, approximately 50-kD protein, termed *tissue factor*, is exposed to the blood. Tissue factor is synthesized in various cell types that are not usually in contact with the blood and initiates the extrinsic pathway by forming a calcium-dependent complex with circulating factor VII.[121–123] After the binding of tissue factor to factor VII, factor VII undergoes a conformational change, exposing its active site and generating the active tissue factor/VII complex.[124] In the presence of tissue factor, the enzymatic activity factor VII for its substrate factor X is markedly increased.[121, 124, 125] It is factor Xa (activated X) that, along with its cofactor, factor Va, associates with various phospholipid surfaces (e.g., platelets, monocytes, lymphocytes), forming the prothrombinase complex[126–128] (Fig. 2–7). Surface localized factor Xa,

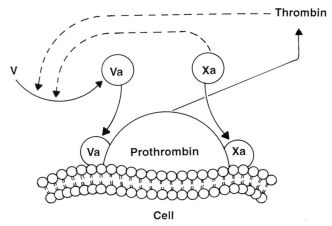

FIGURE 2–7. Prothrombinase complex.

factor Va, and prothrombin are then responsible for the generation of the fundamental enzyme thrombin.[129, 130] However, the key regulatory function of tissue factor and factor VII in coagulation is not exclusive to the extrinsic pathway. The tissue factor/factor VIIa complex is also capable of "crossing over" to the intrinsic pathway and activating factor IX directly,[131, 132] thereby bypassing the need for "contact" factors to stimulate the intrinsic pathway. This observation, in conjunction with studies on patients with various congenital factor deficiencies,[133, 134] has established the extrinsic pathway as being primarily responsible for the initiation of coagulation and the maintenance of normal hemostasis in vivo, as well as the mediation of the acute syndromes in patients with coronary artery disease with and without interventions.

### Intrinsic Pathway

Although previous studies have suggested that the extrinsic pathway may be primarily responsible for maintaining normal hemostasis, the intrinsic pathway may play a major role in situations where foreign surfaces are brought into contact with the blood (i.e., catheters, guide wires, balloons, and intracoronary stents) and therefore deserves special attention. The ongoing exposure of a foreign surface and the activation of the intrinsic pathway may explain, in part, the thrombogenicity of various intracoronary devices as well as the failure of aggressive antithrombotic therapies to inhibit acute or subacute closure of the "injured" vessel.

In contrast to the extrinsic pathway, the intrinsic pathway is more complex, consisting of a series of enzymatic reactions beginning with the activation of factor XII. In the presence of negatively charged surfaces, factor XII undergoes a conformational change, rendering it more sensitive to activation by plasma proteases, such as kallikrein and plasmin, to generate the activated factor XII (XIIa).[135, 136] Once formed, factor XIIa cleaves factor XI to its activated form (factor XIa). Factor XIa then activates IX by cleaving a small peptide (factor IX peptide) from factor IX, resulting in the active enzyme IXa. Factor IXa binds to various surfaces and, in the presence of its cofactor, factor VIIIa, and calcium, cleaves a small peptide (factor X peptide) from factor X, yielding factor Xa.[137] As described previously, factor Xa is then capable of generating thrombin by way of the prothrombinase complex. This cascade of reactions results in marked amplification at each successive step, allowing for an explosion of thrombin generation once the intrinsic pathway is activated. The amplification is further augmented by the presence of several positive feedback loops (see Fig. 2–6). Early in the cascade, factor XI feeds back and activates factor XII directly.[135, 136] In addition, both factor Xa and thrombin are capable of activating the cofactors VIII and V, which, when activated, increase the rate of their respective reactions more than 1000-fold.[130, 138] Factor VIIIa functions by selectively augmenting the binding of factor IXa, rather than factor IX, to the EC surface, allowing for the surface localization of subsequent factor X activation.[139, 140] Factor Va, as described previously, increases the efficiency of factor Xa conversion of prothrombin to thrombin and serves as the rate-limiting step in the formation of the prothrombinase complex.[127] The net effect of these positive feedback loops explains in part the difficulty of systemic pharmacologic therapy for complete control of the generation of thrombin.

### Thrombin

Regardless of the mode of initiation, the final result of the coagulation cascade is the production of thrombin. Because of the multiple functions of thrombin, understanding the role of thrombin after vascular injury is mandatory for anyone who treats patients after vascular intervention. Thrombin is a serine protease that is pivotal in normal hemostasis, having both procoagulant and anticoagulant functions. Thrombin can promote coagulation by several mechanisms. Thrombin cleaves the amino-terminal end of the alpha chain of fibrinogen to generate fibrinopeptide A. The remaining portion of the fibrinogen molecule polymerizes to form loosely associated monomers.[141] These intertwined monomers are then further cleaved by thrombin to yield fibrinopeptide B and insoluble fibrin monomers. Fibrin monomers, in the presence of thrombin-activated factor XIIIA, then polymerize and form a stable meshwork of crosslinked fibrin at the site of injury.[142] Morphologic and angioscopic studies have demonstrated that this fibrin meshwork visually correlates with the "red clot" seen angioscopically in acute coronary syndromes and after interventions.[118, 143] At the same time, thrombin can bind to a thrombin-specific transmembrane receptor on the platelet surface, which results in platelet activation and exposure on the surface of the IIb/IIIa receptor, which mediates subsequent platelet aggregation.[144] Finally, thrombin is capable of activating factors VIII and V directly that will allow for the marked amplification of thrombin generation and the coagulation process. In addition, thrombin plays a pivotal role in regulating its own generation by negative feedback inhibition. After the binding of factor Xa to the platelet surface, membrane-bound prothrombin is cleaved, yielding an intermediate meizothrombin.[145] Meizothrombin remains membrane bound and is unable to activate platelets or cleave fibrinogen. It does, however, have the ability to recognize and activate protein C bound to thrombomodulin, which in turn inactivates surface-localized factor Va and factor VIIIa (Fig. 2–8) and effectively inhibits thrombin generation. In addition to the generation of activated protein C, thrombin also is a potent stimulus for the release of tPA and uPA from vascular ECs.[145, 146] This activation of fibrinolysis leads to the local production of fibrin-associated plasmin, which is responsible for fibrin degradation and clot organization.

## Natural Anticoagulation Pathways

(Table 2–12)

For normal hemostasis, it is imperative that in addition to generating thrombin, multiple feedback actions not only allow for an exuberant and rapid

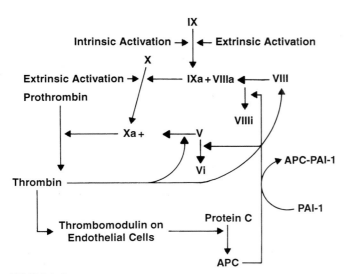

FIGURE 2–8. Role of protein C in the regulation of the coagulation cascade. APC, activated protein C; PAI-1, plasminogen activator inhibitor-1. (From Esmon CT: Protein-C: Biochemistry, physiology, and clinical implications. Blood 62:1155, 1983.)

### TABLE 2–12.    PROPERTIES OF NATURAL ANTICOAGULATION PROTEINS

| INHIBITOR | MW (kd) | SERUM CONCENTRATION (μmol) |
|---|---|---|
| Protein C | 56 | 0.08 |
| Protein S | 67 | 0.14 |
| Antithrombin III | 58 | 2–3 |
| Heparin cofactor II | 65 | 1–1.3 |
| Protease nexin I | 43 | —* |
| TFPI (LACI) | 34 | .003 |
| Thrombomodulin | 35 | —* |

LACI, lipid-associated coagulation inhibitor; TFPI, tissue factor pathway inhibitor.
*Surface localized only.
From Harker LA, Mann KG: Thrombosis and fibrinolysis. In Fuster V, Verstraete M (eds): Thrombosis in Cardiovascular Disorders. Philadelphia: WB Saunders, 1992.

response to vascular injury, but also simultaneously provide mechanisms to protect the vasculature from the consequences of excessive clotting. These natural anticoagulation pathways are responsible for this tight regulation, thrombin inhibition versus generation at several levels. Insights into these pathways have led to the development of new pharmacologic approaches that have shown promise in controlling the adverse consequences of thrombin after vascular intervention and thrombolysis.

### Antithrombin III

Antithrombin III is an approximately 58-kD glycoprotein synthesized by the liver and present in the circulation at a concentration of 0.15 to 0.18 mg/mL (2 to 3 μmol).[147, 148] Antithrombin III not only is an inhibitor of thrombin but also has activity against kallikrein; plasmin; factors XIIa, XIa, Xa, and IXa; and trypsin.[149, 150] Antithrombin III complexes with thrombin by binding to its serine active site and then forming a covalent bond between enzyme and inhibitor.[151] Once complexes are formed, the antithrombin III/thrombin complex is cleared from the circulation by the reticuloendothelial system. In the presence of heparin, the binding of antithrombin to thrombin is increased more than 1000-fold.[151] Kinetic studies have demonstrated that the unique 3-0 sulfate glucosamine group on the heparin molecule is responsible for the avid binding of heparin to antithrombin III.[152, 153] Antithrombin III then undergoes a conformational change that increases its efficiency for binding thrombin.[154] Once the antithrombin III/thrombin complex is formed, the heparin molecule is released and is available to bind antithrombin III again (Fig. 2–9).

### Heparin Cofactor II

Heparin cofactor II is an approximately 65-kD protein synthesized in the liver and present in the

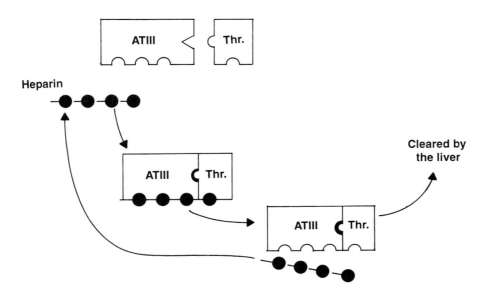

FIGURE 2–9. Mechanism by which heparin molecules of 18–20 residues enhance the interaction between antithrombin III (ATIII) and thrombin (Thr.).

circulation at a concentration of 0.06 to 0.08 mg/mL (1 to 1.3 μmol).[155, 156] Like antithrombin III, its inhibitory effect on thrombin is accelerated by heparin and, in fact, shares approximately 50% homology with antithrombin III in sequences flanking the active site.[157] Unlike antithrombin III, however, heparin cofactor II is specific for thrombin, having no activity against any other coagulation enzyme.[158]

### Protease Nexin I

Finally, protease nexin I is an approximately 43-kD protein identified in fibroblast cultures[159] as well as in SMCs and cells of epithelial origins.[160] In addition to inhibiting thrombin, protease nexin I also is capable of inhibiting both plasminogen activators uPA and tPA.[154] It, too, shares approximately 30% sequence homology with antithrombin III[161] but does not circulate in any appreciable amounts, suggesting that its primary role may be associated with inhibiting the protease-mediated degradation of extracellular matrix in the extravascular compartment.[162] Like heparin cofactor II and antithrombin, the affinity of protease nexin I for thrombin is increased approximately 200-fold in the presence of heparin.

### Protein C

Protein C is a two-chain, approximately 62-kD protein synthesized by the liver and present in the circulation at a concentration of approximately 0.08 μm.[163] To become activated, protein C requires the binding of calcium to a non–vitamin K dependent binding site located on the light chain of protein C.[163] This binding results in a conformational change of protein C,[163, 164] making it resistant to circulating thrombin but highly susceptible to thrombin bound to the membrane cofactor thrombomodulin. This allows thrombomodulin-bound thrombin to cleave a small peptide from the heavy chain of protein C, rendering it biologically active.[165] Activated protein C exerts its anticoagulation function by inactivating both factor Va and factor VIIIa, thereby markedly inhibiting subsequent thrombin generation. However, for optimal inhibition of factors Va and VIIIa, the cofactor protein S must be present along with protein C.[166] In addition to its anticoagulant properties, protein C also irreversibly binds and inhibits plasminogen activator inhibitor 1 (PAI-1).[167, 168] PAI-1 inhibits both plasminogen activators (uPA and tPA) and appears to be a major regulator of fibrinolytic activity (see later discussion). By inhibiting PAI-1, protein C serves to increase fibrinolytic activity (plasmin generation) and therefore clot lysis. Activated protein C is unique in that it expresses anticoagulant properties only when thrombin is present and has been an intense area of research as a potential therapeutic agent.

### Tissue Factor Pathway Inhibitor

At a different level, a newly described 34-kD protein, tissue factor pathway inhibitor (TFPI), or lipid-associated coagulation inhibitor, inhibits thrombin generation by binding and inhibiting factor Xa.[169] TFPI is found in platelets and subendothelial matrix and is associated with lipoproteins.[169] In addition to inhibiting factor Xa, the TFPI/Xa complex appears to associate with the tissue factor/VIIa complex, blocking further interaction between tissue factor/VIIa complex and substrates factor X and IX.[170, 171] TFPI appears to bind to its primary reservoir, subendothelial matrix, by way of its heparin binding sites and can be displaced by intravenous doses of heparin as low as 3000 units (total dose), resulting in up to a fivefold increase in the serum concentration of TFPI.[172] This displacement of TFPI by heparin explains in part the ability of heparin to effectively inhibit factor Xa activity.

## TABLE 2–13. PROPERTIES OF FIBRINOLYTIC PROTEINS

| PROTEIN | MW (kd) | SERUM CONCENTRATION (μg/μl) |
| --- | --- | --- |
| Plasminogen | 92 | 200 |
| scuPA | 54 | 0.008 |
| tPA | 67 | 0.005 |
| PAI-1 | 50 | 0.05 |
| Alpha-2 antiplasmin | 70 | 70 |

PAI-1, plasminogen activator inhibitor-1; scuPA, single-chain urokinase plasminogen activator; tPA, tissue plasminogen activator.

From Harker LA, Mann KG: Thrombosis and fibrinolysis. *In* Fuster V, Verstraete M (eds): Thrombosis in Cardiovascular Disorders. Philadelphia: WB Saunders, 1992.

## Fibrinolysis (Table 2–13)

Normal hemostasis is a delicate balance between the coagulation system (resulting in clot formation) and the fibrinolytic system (resulting in clot lysis). A clear understanding of natural and pharmacologically induced thrombolysis is as important to the cardiovascular interventionist as the understanding of thrombosis. In addition to the inhibitors of coagulation, the fibrinolytic system serves to counterbalance those factors that promote coagulation ultimately by producing plasmin, which is capable of dissolving insoluble fibrin. Thus, plasmin becomes pivotal in the maintenance of normal hemostasis and vessel patency. The components of the fibrinolytic system, like the coagulation system, consist of a series of surface-localized enzymatic reactions, ultimately resulting in the production of the serine protease plasmin (Fig. 2–10). Also, like the coagulation cascade, the fibrinolytic system has several natural inhibitors.

### Plasminogen

Plasminogen is a ubiquitous 92-kD protein present in the normal circulation at a concentration of approximately 2 μmol.[173] Plasminogen exists in the circulation with an amino terminal glutamic acid (Glu-plasminogen) but is easily converted by limited proteolysis to a modified form with a terminal ly-sine, valine, or methionine (Lys-plasminogen).[174] Even though Lys-plasminogen may bind more avidly to EC surfaces, Glu-plasminogen appears to be the predominant form in vivo.[175] Plasminogen binds specifically to several cell types, including monocytes, platelets, and ECs, and to fibrinogen via its lysine binding sites.

On exposure to catalytic amounts of plasminogen activators (uPA, tPA), the single-chain plasminogen is rapidly cleaved, resulting in the formation of the two-chain serine protease plasmin.[173] In addition to dissolving "insoluble fibrin," plasmin has multiple roles as the mediator of fibrinolysis. Associated with the EC surface, plasmin appears to play an important part in maintaining the antithrombotic nature of the vessel wall. In addition, plasmin is required for day-to-day cellular function, such as migration and proliferation.[176] The natural inhibitor of plasmin, a₂-antiplasmin, binds plasmin in serum but is unable to bind to plasmin associated with clot or cell surfaces.[177] This results in two unique functions of plasmin. First, it is capable of digesting insoluble crosslinked fibrin to soluble fibrin degradation products. Second, it is able to convert various cell-associated precursors to their active enzyme forms. For example, plasmin is responsible for the conversion of procollagenase to active collagenase.[178] This allows for the digestion of pericellular matrix, which is critical for cell functions such as migration and proliferation. uPA and tPA levels in the vessel wall have been shown in experimental models to increase significantly after balloon injury, and this rise precedes the onset of SMC migration.[179] In addition, plasmin is capable of inactivating factors Va[180] and VIIa,[181] resulting in the inhibition of further thrombin generation. Because plasmin is not consumed in these reactions, the generation of a small catalytic amount of plasmin is capable of profound biologic consequences.

### Tissue-type Plasminogen Activator

tPA is a 67-kD protein produced by many cell types and is present in the circulation at a concentration

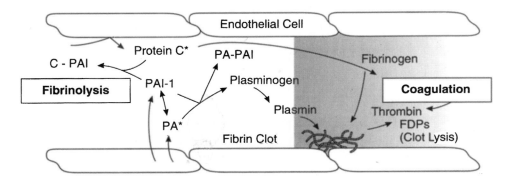

FIGURE 2–10. Fibrinolysis. PA, plasminogen activator; PAI-1, plasminogen activator inhibitor-1; FDP, fibrin degradation product.

of 0.005 $\mu g/\mu L$.[141] tPA functions as a serine protease with the ability to bind specifically to various cell types, including ECs, monocytes, and SMCs.[182–186] In the absence of fibrin, tPA is a relatively poor plasminogen activator; however, in the presence of fibrin, the rate of plasminogen activation is markedly increased. This enhanced ability of tPA to activate plasminogen comes from kinetic studies that suggest that the binding of tPA to fibrin lowers the $K_m$ (increases its affinity for its substrate) but not catalytic rate constant (a measure of the efficiency with which the enzyme acts on the substrate).[173, 187] In a sense, the fibrin meshwork at the site of thrombus formation increases the local concentration of plasminogen and its activators, thereby facilitating the optimal interaction between enzymes and substrate. This localization allows for efficient production of plasmin in a milieu protected from the plasmin inhibitor $a_2$-antiplasmin, thus enhancing rapid clot lysis. Mass production of tPA by recombinant technology has led to the use of this natural protein clinically as a fibrin-specific thrombolytic agent.

### Urokinase

uPA is a single-chain 54-kD protein (single-chain urokinase plasminogen activator) produced by many cell types, including ECs, monocytes, and SMCs.[182] Single-chain urokinase can be converted by catalytic levels of various proteases, including plasmin and kallikrein, to a highly active two-chain form (a 35-kD heavy chain and a 20-kD light chain) that lacks the fibrin specificity of tPA but has a catalytic rate constant that is approximately 1000 times more efficient than its single-chain precursor in activating plasminogen.[188, 189] All urokinase forms (single-chain urokinase and uPA) bind specifically to cell surfaces (monocytes, ECs, and SMCs) via a well characterized 55-kD receptor protein (UPAR) attached to the cell surface membrane by a phosphatidylinositol anchor.[190–192] Like clot-associated plasmin, receptors for both plasminogen activators allow for the regulated generation of cell surface-localized plasmin in a milieu protected from circulating $a_2$-antiplasmin. This contributes to the antithrombotic nature of the EC surface and provides protease activity necessary for other biologic functions, such as migration and proliferation.[176] Urokinase, like tPA, has been produced in large quantities and has been used clinically as a thrombolytic agent.

### Inhibitors of Fibrinolysis

Like the coagulation cascade, fibrinolysis is a highly regulated pathway with multiple inhibitors. Primary among these is $a_2$-antiplasmin. In the circulation, it exists at a concentration of approximately 1 $\mu m$[193]

and efficiently inhibits plasmin by binding to its active site via specific lysine binding sites.[194] Apparently, these sites are not available when plasmin is bound to, and associated with, the cell surface or fibrin clots; thus, $a_2$-antiplasmin is unable to neutralize plasmin on cell surfaces and is associated with clots. Perhaps the best way to understand the normal function of $a_2$-antiplasmin is to view the clinical situation (for acute myocardial infarction), in which sufficiently large doses of plasminogen activator have been given to completely overwhelm circulating levels of $a_2$-antiplasmin. This results in the net formation of active circulating plasmin and the existence of a systemic "lytic state," in which plasmin can degrade various plasma proteins, for example, factors Va and VIIa.[180, 181] It is this degradation of plasma proteins that is responsible for the bleeding complications associated with thrombolytic therapy. In addition to $a_2$-antiplasmin, antithrombin III is an inhibitor of plasmin, and this inhibition is accelerated by heparin.[195, 196] However, in vivo, this appears not to be a significant mechanism for plasmin clearance.[197] A similar nonspecific protease inhibitor, $a_2$-macroglobulin, is capable of binding and inhibiting plasmin in vitro. Its role in vivo remains less well defined. Several inhibitors of the plasminogen activators have also been described, including protease nexin I (see section on natural anticoagulant pathways), but chief among these is PAI-1. PAI-1 is a 50-kD protein synthesized by various cells types, including ECs and hepatic cells.[198, 199] PAI-1 is present in platelets and is bound to extracellular matrix–associated vitronectin.[200] It is an acute-phase reactant and is therefore released from ECs in response to various agents and cytokines, including endotoxin,[201] thrombin,[146] TGF-$\beta$,[202] IL-1,[203] and tumor necrosis factor-a.[204] The acute-phase response of PAI-1 has made it difficult to interpret clinical studies that have attempted to correlate PAI-1 activity with acute coronary syndromes. Unlike other inhibitors with which it shares some structural homology (antithrombin III and $a_2$-antiplasmin), PAI-1 is unique in that it exists in two forms, latent and active.[198] The mechanism for the conversion of latent to active form remains unknown, and the largest reservoir of PAI-1 that is bound to matrix-associated vitronectin appears to be active.[205] PAI-1 functions by binding to tPA and two-chain uPA (but not to single-chain uPA), forming a covalent PA/PAI-1 complex that is ultimately removed by the reticuloendothelial system.[206] Two other plasminogen activator inhibitors have been described: PAI-2 (isolated from placental tissue) and PAI-3 (initially discovered in urine and apparently similar to protein C inhibitor).[207, 208] However, PAI-1 appears to be primarily responsible for the regulation of plasminogen activator activity in the blood.

## CONCLUSION

The biology of endothelial and smooth muscle cells clearly becomes an integral part of every angioplasty procedure. Acute closure and restenosis remain important limitations, even with new interventional devices. These clinical events represent a complex biologic attempt by the vessel wall to heal a profound injury. Molecular biology and invasive cardiology are likely to become more intimately involved as progress in understanding these biologic responses translates into new clinical approaches.

Platelets are an active participant in the maintenance of normal hemostasis as well as the key mediator of complications after vascular intervention. Over the past decade, several platelet membrane receptors have been isolated and characterized. These receptors and their function explain at least in part the clinically observed dependence of the platelet aggregation on the degree of injury, and rheologic factors. The mechanical improvement in rheologic factors achieved with various interventional techniques is therefore tainted by the degree of injury required to obtain such an improved luminal diameter. Novel approaches stimulated by a better understanding of normal platelet function will undoubtedly contribute significantly to the care of interventional patients in the near future.

Acute thrombosis of the treated artery, as a primary or a secondary event, remains a major cause of the morbidity and mortality associated with intravascular intervention. Attempts to reduce this complication have centered on high-dose anticoagulation and antiplatelet therapy. A better understanding is needed in the molecular events involved in the maintenance of normal hemostasis as well as the series of reactions initiated when vessel injury is induced. Advances in this field have led to a better therapy for thrombotic complications in vascular intervention.

## REFERENCES

1. Jaffe EA: Endothelial cells and the biology of factor VIII. N Engl J Med 296:377, 1977.
2. Stary HC, Blankenhorn DH, Chandler AB, et al: A definition of the intima of human arteries and of its atherosclerosis-prone regions. Circulation 85:391, 1992.
3. Levesque MJ, Nerum RM: The elongation and organization of cultured endothelial cells in response to shear. J Biomech Eng 107:341, 1985.
4. Vane JR, Anggard EE, Botting RM: Regulatory functions of the vascular endothelium. N Engl J Med 323:27, 1990.
5. Garg UC, Hassid A: Nitric oxide-generating vasodilators and 8-bromo-cyclic guanosine monophosphate inhibit mitogenesis and proliferation of cultured rat vascular smooth muscle cells. J Clin Invest 83:1774, 1989.
6. Weidinger FF, McLenachan JM, Cybulsky MI, et al: Persistent dysfunction of regenerating endothelium after balloon angioplasty of rabbit iliac artery. Circulation 81:1667, 1990.
7. Furstermann V, Mugge A, Alheid U, et al: Selective attenuation of endothelial-mediated vasodilation in atherosclerotic human coronary arteries. Circ Res 62:185, 1988.
8. Ludmer PL, Selwyn AP, Shook TL, et al: Paradoxical vasoconstriction induced by acetylcholine in atherosclerotic coronary arteries. N Engl J Med 315:1046, 1986.
9. Makasi T, Kimura S, Yanagisawa M, et al: Molecular and cellular mechanism of endothelin regulation. Circulation 84:1457, 1991.
10. Boulanger C, Lushcer TF: Release of endothelin from the porcine aorta. J Clin Invest 85:587, 1990.
11. Komuro I, Kurihara H, Sugiyama T, et al: Endothelin stimulates c-fos and c-myc expression and proliferation of vascular smooth muscle cells. FEBS Lett 238:249, 1988.
12. Webb DJ, Cockroft JR: Circulating and tissue renin-angiotensin systems: the role of the endothelium. In Warren JB (ed): The Endothelium: An Introduction to Current Research, 1st ed, p 65. New York: Wiley-Liss, 1990.
13. Dzau VJ, Gibbons GH, Pratt RE: Molecular mechanisms of vascular renin-angiotensin system in myointimal hyperplasia. Hypertension 18(suppl II):11–100, 1991.
14. Haudenschild CC, Schwartz SM: Endothelial regeneration: II. Restitution of endothelial continuity. Lab Invest 41:407, 1979.
15. Reidy MA, Clowes AW, Schwartz SM: Endothelial regeneration: V. Inhibition of endothelial regeneration in arteries of rat and rabbit. Lab Invest 49:569, 1983.
16. Schwartz RS, Murphy JG, Edwards WD, et al: Restenosis after balloon angioplasty: A practical proliferative model in porcine coronary arteries. Circulation 82:2190, 1990.
17. Anderson PG, Bajaj RK, Baxley WA, et al: Vascular pathology of balloon-expandable flexible coil stents in humans. J Am Coll Cardiol 19:372, 1992.
18. Gravanis MB, Roubin GS: Histopathologic phenomena at the site of percutaneous transluminal coronary angioplasty: The problem of restenosis. Hum Pathol 20:477, 1989.
19. Ip JH, Fuster V, Badimon L, et al: Syndromes of accelerated atherosclerosis: Role of vascular injury and smooth muscle cell proliferation. J Am Coll Cardiol 15:1667, 1990.
20. Lindner V, Reidy MA, Fingerle J: Regrowth of arterial endothelium: Denudation with minimal trauma leads to complete endothelial cell regrowth. Lab Invest 61:556, 1989.
21. Forrester JS, Fishbein M, Helfant R, et al: A paradigm for restenosis based on cell biology clues for the development of new preventive therapies. J Am Coll Cardiol 17:758, 1991.
22. Clowes AW, Reidy MA: Prevention of stenosis after vascular reconstruction: Pharmacologic control of intimal hyperplasia. A review. J Vasc Surg 13:885, 1991.
23. Clowes AW, Reidy MA, Clowes MM: Mechanisms of stenosis after arterial injury. Lab Invest 49:208, 1983.
24. Clowes AW, Clowes MW, Reidy MA: Kinetics of cellular proliferation after arterial injury: III. Endothelial and smooth muscle growth in chronically denuded vessels. Lab Invest 54:295, 1986.
25. Majesky MW, Reidy MA, Bowen-Pope DF, et al: PDGF ligand and receptor gene expression during repair of arterial injury. J Cell Biol 111:2149, 1990.
26. Healy B: Endothelial cell dysfunction: An emerging endocrinopathy linked to coronary disease. J Am Coll Cardiol 16:357, 1990.
27. Castellot JJ, Addonizio MC, Rosenberg RD, et al: Cultured endothelial cells produce a heparin-like inhibitor of smooth muscle cell growth. J Cell Biol 90:372, 1981.
28. Fritze LMS, Reilly CR, Rosenberg RD: An antiproliferative heparan sulfate species produced by postconfluent smooth muscle cells. J Cell Biol 100:1041, 1985.
29. Kinsella MG, Wight TN: Modulation of sulfated proteoglycan synthesis by bovine aortic endothelial cells during migration. J Cell Biol 102:679, 1986.
30. Koo EWY, Gottlieb AI: Neointimal formation in the porcine aortic organ culture. Lab Invest 64:743, 1991.
31. Castellot JJ, Wright TC, Karnovsky MJ: Regulation of vascular smooth muscle cell growth by heparin and heparan sulfates. Semin Thromb Hemost 13:489, 1987.
32. Clowes AW, Clowes MM: Kinetics of cellular proliferation

after arterial injury: IV. Heparin inhibits rat smooth muscle mitogenesis and migration. Cir Res 58:839, 1986.

33. Liu MW, Roubin GS, King SB: Restenosis after coronary angioplasty: Potential biologic determinants and role of intimal hyperplasia. Circulation 79:1374, 1989.

34. Schwartz SM, Campbell GR, Campbell JH: Replication of smooth muscle cells in vascular disease. Circ Res 58:427, 1986.

35. Ueda M, Becker AE, Tsukada T, et al: Fibrocellular tissue responses after percutaneous transluminal coronary angioplasty. Circulation 83:1327, 1991.

36. Gordon D, Reidy MA, Bendiff EP, et al: Cell proliferation in human coronary arteries. Proc Natl Acad Sci USA 87:4600, 1990.

37. Hedin U, Holm J, Hanson GK: Induction of tenascin in rat arterial injury. Am J Pathol 139:649, 1991.

38. Haudenschild CC, Grunwald J: Proliferative heterogeneity of vascular smooth muscle cells and its alteration by injury. Exp Cell Res 157:364, 1985.

39. Clowes AW, Schwartz SM: Significance of quiescent smooth muscle migration in the injured rat carotid artery. Circ Res 56:139, 1985.

40. Hanke H, Strohschneider T, Oberhoff M, et al: Time course of smooth muscle cell proliferation in the intima and media of arteries following experimental angioplasty. Circ Res 67:651, 1990.

41. Dartsch PC, Voisard R, Bauriedel G: Growth characteristics and cytoskeletal organization of cultured smooth muscle cells from human primary and restenosing lesions. Arteriosclerosis 10:62, 1990.

42. Guyton J, Rosenberg R, Clowes AW, et al: Inhibition of rat arterial smooth muscle cell proliferation by heparin: In vivo studies with anticoagulant and nonanticoagulant heparin. Circ Res 46:625, 1980.

43. Clowes AW, Clowes MM, Kocker O, et al: Arterial smooth muscle cells in vivo: Relationship between actin isoform expression and mitogenesis and their modulation by heparin. J Cell Biol 107:1939, 1988.

44. Sarembock IJ, Laveau PJ, Sigal SL, et al: Influence of inflation pressure and balloon size on the development of intimal hyperplasia after balloon angioplasty. Circulation 80:1029, 1989.

45. Schwartz RS, Huber KC, Murphy JG, et al: Restenosis and the proportional neointimal response to coronary artery injury: Results in a porcine model. J Am Coll Cardiol 19:267, 1992.

46. Kohler TR, Kirman TR, Kraiss LW, et al: Increased blood flow inhibits neointimal hyperplasia in endothelialized vascular grafts. Circ Res 69:1557, 1991.

47. Kraiss LW, Kirkman TR, Kohler TR, et al: Shear stress regulates smooth muscle proliferation and neointimal thickness in porous polytetrafluorethylene grafts. Arterioscler Thromb 11:1844, 1991.

48. Hehrlein C, Chuang CH, Tuntelder JR, et al: Effects of vascular runoff on myointimal hyperplasia after mechanical balloon or thermal laser arterial injury in dogs. Circulation 84:884, 1991.

49. Davies PF, Remuzzi A, Gordon EJ, et al: Turbulent fluid shear stress induces vascular endothelial cell turnover in vitro. Proc Natl Acad Sci USA 83:2114, 1986.

50. Ando J, Nomura H, Kamiya S: The effect of fluid shear stress on the migration and proliferation after arterial injury: V. Role of acute distension in the induction of smooth muscle cell of cultured endothelial cells. Microvasc Res 33:62, 1987.

51. Walker LN, Bowen-Pope DF, Ross R, et al: Production of platelet-derived growth factor-like molecules by cultured arterial smooth muscle cells accompanies proliferation after arterial injury. Proc Natl Acad Sci USA 83:7311, 1986.

52. Libby P, Warner SJC, Salomon RN, et al: Production of platelet-derived growth factor-like mitogen by smooth muscle cells from human atheroma. N Engl J Med 318:1493, 1988.

53. Wilcox JN, Smith KM, Williams LT, et al: Platelet-derived growth factor MRNA detection in human atherosclerotic plaques by in situ hybridization. J Clin Invest 82:1134, 1988.

54. Bell L, Madri JA: Effect of platelet factors on migration of cultured bovine aortic endothelial and smooth muscle cells. Circ Res 65:1057, 1989.

55. Liu MW, Roubin GS, Robinson KA, et al: Trapidil in preventing restenosis after balloon angioplasty in the atherosclerotic rabbit. Circulation 81:1089, 1990.

56. Fingerle J, Johnson R, Clowes AW, et al: Role of platelets in smooth muscle cell proliferation and migration after vascular injury in rat carotid artery. Proc Natl Acad Sci USA 86:8412, 1989.

57. Fems GA, Raines EW, Sprugel KH, et al: Inhibition of neointimal smooth muscle accumulation after angioplasty by an antibody to PDGF. Science 253:1129, 1991.

58. Schneider MD, Parker TG: Cardiac myocytes as targets for the action of peptide growth factors. Circulation 81:1443, 1990.

59. McNeil PL, Muthukrishan L, Warder E, et al: Growth factors are released by mechanically wounded endothelial cells. J Cell Biol 109:811, 1989.

60. Cuevas P, Gonzalez AM, Carceller F, et al: Vascular response to basic fibroblast growth factor when infused onto the normal adventitia or into the injured media of the rat carotid artery. Circ Res 69:360, 1991.

61. Lindner V, Lappi DA, Baird A, et al: Role of basic fibroblast growth factor in vascular lesion formation. Circ Res 68:196, 1991.

62. Lindner V, Reidy MA: Proliferation of smooth muscle cells after vascular injury is inhibited by an antibody against basic fibroblast growth factor. Proc Natl Acad Sci USA 88:3739, 1991.

63. Cercek B, Fishbein MC, Forrester JS, et al: Induction of insulinlike growth factor I messenger RNA in rat aortas after balloon denudation. Circ Res 66:1755, 1990.

64. Nanney LB, Stoscheck CM, King LE: Characterization of binding and receptor for epidermal growth factor in smooth muscle. Cell Tissue Res 254:125, 1988.

65. Epstein SE, Siegall CB, Biro S, et al: Cytotoxic effects of a recombinant chimeric toxin on rapid proliferation vascular smooth muscle cells. Circulation 84:778, 1991.

66. Casscelis W, Wai C, Shrivastav S, et al: Smooth muscle proliferation in vessel injury is characterized by expression of fibroblast growth factor receptor and is inhibited by a toxin-fibroblast growth factor conjugate. Circulation 82:208A, 1990.

67. Battegay EJ, Raines EW, Seifert RA, et al: TGF-β induces bimodal proliferation of connective tissue cells via complex control of an autocrine PDGF loop. Cell 63:515, 1990.

68. Daemen MJAP, Lombardi DM, Bosman FT, et al: Angiotensin II induces smooth muscle cell proliferation in the normal and injured rat arterial wall. Circ Res 68:450, 1991.

69. Powell JS, Clozel JP, Muller RKM, et al: Inhibition of angiotensin converting enzyme prevents myointimal proliferation after vascular injury. Science 245:186, 1989.

70. Leclerc G, Isner JM, Keamery M, et al: Evidence implicating nonmuscle myosin in restenosis. Circulation 85:543, 1992.

71. Saksela O, Rifkin DB: Cell-associated plasminogen activators: Regulation and physiological functions. Annu Rev Cell Biol 4:93, 1988.

72. Clowes AW, Clowes MM, Au YPT, et al: Smooth muscle cells express urokinase during mitogenesis and tissue-type plasminogen activator during migration in injured rat carotid arteries. Circ Res 67:61, 1990.

73. Libby P, Friedman GB, Salomon RN: Cytokines as modulators of cell proliferation in fibrotic diseases. Am Rev Respir Dis 140:1114, 1989.

74. Prescott MF, Mcbride CK, Court M: Development of intimal lesions after leukocyte migration into the vessel wall. Am J Pathol 135:835, 1989.

75. Libby P, Warner SJC, Friedman GB: Interleukin 1: A mitogen for human vascular smooth muscle cell that induces the release of growth-inhibiting prostanoids. J Clin Invest 81:487, 1988.

76. Sawada H, Kan M, McKeehan WL: Opposite effects of monokines (interleukin-I and tissue necrosis factor) on

platelet and heparin-binding (fibroblast) growth factor binding to human aortic endothelial and smooth muscle cell. In Vitro Cell Dev Biol 26:213, 1990.

77. Raines EW, Dower SK, Ross R: Interleukin-I mitogenic activity for fibroblasts and smooth muscle cells is due to PDGFAA. Science 243:393, 1989.

78. Hansson GK, Holm J: Gamma-interferon inhibits arterial stenosis after injury. Circulation 84:1266, 1991.

79. Hedin U, Bottger BA, Forsberg E, et al: Diverse effects of fibronectin and laminin on phenotypic properties of cultured arterial smooth muscle cells. J Cell Biol 107:307, 1988.

80. Snow AD, Bolender RP, Wight TN, et al: Heparin modulates the composition of the extracellular matrix domain surrounding arterial smooth muscle cells. Am J Pathol 137:313, 1990.

81. Stockmans F, Deckmyn H, Gruwez J, et al: Continuous quantitative monitoring of mural platelet-dependent thrombus kinetics in the crushed rat femoral vein. Thromb Haemost 65:425, 1991.

82. Wilentz JR, Sanborn TA, Haudenschild CC, et al: Platelet accumulation in experimental angioplasty: Time course and relation to vascular injury. Circulation 75:636, 1987.

83. Fuster V, Badimon L, Cohen M, et al: Insights into the pathogenesis of acute ischemic syndrome. Circulation 77:1213, 1988.

84. Badimon L, Badimon JJ: Mechanisms of arterial thrombosis in non-parallel streamlines: Platelet thrombi grow on the apex of stenotic severely injured vessel wall. J Clin Invest 84:1134, 1989.

85. Lassila R, Badimon JJ, Vallabhajosula S, et al: Dynamic monitoring of platelet deposition on severely damaged vessel wall in flowing blood. Arteriosclerosis 10:306, 1990.

86. Stein B, Fuster V, Israel DH, et al: Platelet inhibitor agents in cardiovascular disease: An update. J Am Coll Cardiol 14:813, 1989.

87. Badimon L, Badimon JJ, Turitto VT, et al: Platelet thrombus formation on collagen type 1: A model of deep vessel injury. Circulation 78:1431, 1988.

88. Isenberg WM, McEver RP, Phillips DR, et al: The platelet fibrinogen receptor: An immunogold-surface replica study of agonist-induced ligand binding and receptor clustering. J Cell Biol 99:2140, 1987.

89. Fitzgerald LA, Phillips DR: Calcium regulation of the platelet membrane, glycoprotein IIb-IIIa complex. J Biol Chem 260:11366, 1985.

90. Plow EF, Pierschbacher MD, Ruoslahti E, et al: The effect of Arg-Gly-Asp-containing peptides on fibrinogen and von Willebrand factor binding to platelets. Proc Natl Acad Sci USA 82:8057, 1985.

91. Rybak ME: Glycoprotein IIb and IIIa and platelet thrombosis in a liposome model of platelet aggregation. Thromb Haemost 55:240, 1986.

92. Pierschbacher MD, Ruoslahti E: Influence of stereochemistry of the sequence Arg-Gly-Asp-Xaa on binding specificity in cell adhesion. J Biol Chem 262:17294, 1987.

93. Pierschbacher MD, Ruoslahti E: Cell attachment activity of fibronectin can be duplicated by small synthetic fragments of the molecule. Nature 309:30, 1984.

94. Gartner TK, Taylor DB: The amino acid sequence Gly-Ala-Pro-Leu appears to be a fibrinogen binding site in the platelet integrin, glycoprotein IIb. Thromb Res 60:291, 1990.

95. Ginsberg MH, Lightsey A, Kunicki TJ, et al: Divalent cation regulation of the surface orientation of platelet membrane glycoprotein IIb: Correlation with fibrinogen binding function and definition of a novel variant of Glanzmann's thrombasthenia. J Clin Invest 78:1103, 1986.

96. Pischel KD, Bluestein HG, Woods VL: Platelet glycoprotein Ia, Ic, and IIa are physiochemically indistinguishable from the very late activation antigens adhesion-related proteins of lymphocytes and other cell types. J Clin Invest 81:505, 1988.

97. Hemler ME, Crouse C, Takada Y, et al: Multiple very late antigen (VLA) heterodimers on platelets: Evidence for distinct VLA2, VLA-5 (fibronectin receptor) and VLA-6 structures. J Biol Chem 263:7660, 1988.

98. Hawiger J: Formation and regulation of platelet and fibrin hemostatic plug. Hum Pathol 18:111, 1987.

99. Staatz W, Rajpara SM, Wayner EA, et al: The membrane glycoprotein Ia-IIa (VLA-2) complex mediates the Mg + + - dependent adhesion of platelets to collagen. J Cell Biol 108:1917, 1989.

100. Staatz WD, Walsh JJ, Pexton T, et al: The alpha2 beta, integrin cell surface collagen receptor binds to the alpha, (I)-CB3 peptide of collagen. J Biol Chem 265:4778, 1990.

101. Nieuwenhuis HK, Akkerman JWN, Houdijk WPM, et al: Human blood platelets showing no response to collagen fail to express surface glycoprotein Ia. Nature 318:470, 1985.

102. Sonnenberg A, Modderman PW, Hogervorst F: Laminin receptor on platelets is the integrin VLA-6. Nature 360:487, 1988.

103. Sonnenberg A, Janssen H, Hogervorst F, et al: A complex of platelet glycoproteins Ic and IIa identified by a rat monoclonal antibody. J Biol Chem 262:10376, 1987.

104. Clemetson KJ: Glycoproteins of the platelet plasma membrane. In George JN, Nurden AT, Phillips DR (eds): Platelet Membrane Glycoproteins, p 51. New York: Plenum, 1990.

105. George JN, Nurden AT, Phillips DR: Molecular defects in interactions of platelets with the vessel wall. N Engl J Med 311:1084, 1984.

106. Weiss HJ, Turitto VT, Baumgartner HR: Platelet adhesion and thrombus formation on subendothelium in platelets deficient in glycoproteins IIb-IIIa, Ib and storage granules. Blood 67:322, 1986.

107. Hantgan RR, Hindriks G, Taylor RG, et al: Glycoprotein Ib, von Willebrand factor, and glycoprotein IIb:IIIa are all involved in platelet adhesion to fibrin in flowing whole blood. Blood 76:345, 1990.

108. Weiss HJ, Turitto VT, Baumgartner HR: Effect of shear rate on platelet interaction with subendothelium in citrated and native blood. J Lab Clin Med 92:750, 1978.

109. Roth GJ: Developing relationships: Arterial platelet adhesion, glycoprotein Ib, and leucine-rich glycoproteins. Blood 77:5, 1991.

110. Nievelstein PFEM, de Groot PG, D'Slessio P, et al: Platelet adhesion to vascular cells: The role of exogenous von Willebrand factor in platelet adhesion. Arteriosclerosis 10:462, 1990.

111. Lopez JA, Chung DW, Fujikawa K, et al: The alpha and beta chains of human platelet glycoprotein Ib are both transmembrane proteins containing a leucine-rich amino acid sequence. Proc Natl Acad Sci USA 85:2135, 1988.

112. Yamamoto N, Greco NJ, Barnard MR, et al: Glycoprotein Ib (GPIb)-dependent and GPIb-independent pathways of thrombin-induced platelet activation. Blood 77:1740, 1991.

113. McEver RJP, Beckstead JH, Moore KL, et al: GMP-140, a platelet alpha-granule membrane protein, is also synthesized by vascular endothelial cells and is localized in Veibel-Palade bodies. J Clin Invest 84:92, 1989.

114. Larson RS, Corbi AL, Berman L, et al: Primary structure of the LFA-I alpha subunit: An integrin with an embedded domain defining a protein superfamily. J Cell Biol 108:703, 1989.

115. Hamburger SA, McEver RP: GMP-140 mediated adhesion of stimulated platelets to neutrophils. Blood 75:550, 1990.

116. Asch AS, Barnwell J, Silverstein RL: Isolation of the thrombospondin membrane receptor. J Clin Invest 79:1054, 1987.

117. Majack RA, Cook SC, Bornstein P: Control of smooth muscle cell growth by components of the extracellular matrix: Autocrine role for thrombospondin. Proc Natl Acad Sci USA 83:9050, 1986.

118. Steele PM, Chesebro JH, Stanson AW, et al: Balloon angioplasty: Natural history of the pathophysiologic response to injury in a pig model. Circ Res 57:105, 1985.

119. Macfarlane RG: An enzyme cascade in the blood clotting mechanism and its function as a biochemical amplifier. Nature 202:498, 1964.

120. Dayer EW, Ratnoff OD: Waterfall sequence for intrinsic blood clotting. Science 145:1310, 1964.

121. Prydz H, Petterson KS: Synthesis of thromboplastin (tissue factor) by endothelial cells. Haemostasis 18:215, 1988.

122. Bjorklid E, Storm E: Purification and some properties of the

protein component of tissue thromboplastin from human brain. Biochem J 165:89, 1977.

123. Bjorklid E, Storm E, Prydz H: The protein component of human brain thromboplastin. Biochem Biophys Res Commun 55:969, 1973.

124. Broze GJ, Majerus PW: Purification and properties of human coagulation factor VII. J Biol Chem 255:1242, 1980.

125. Bach R, Nemerson Y, Kiningsberg W: Purification and characterization of bovine tissue factor. J Biol Chem 256:8324, 1981.

126. Tracy PB, Rohrbach MS, Mann KG: Functional prothrombinase complex assembly on isolated monocytes and lymphocytes. J Biol Chem 258:7264, 1983.

127. Tracy PB, Nesheim ME, Mann KG: Coordinate binding of factor Va and factor Xa to the unstimulated platelet. J Biol Chem 256:743, 1981.

128. Nesheim ME, Eid S, Mann KG: Assembly of the prothrombinase complex in the absence of prothrombin. J Biol Chem 256:9874, 1981.

129. Esmon CT, Owen WG, Jackson CM: A plausible mechanism for prothrombin activation by factor Xa, factor Va, phospholipid and calcium ions. J Biol Chem 249:8045, 1974.

130. Nesheim ME, Kettner C, Shaw E, et al: Cofactor dependence of factor Xa incorporation into the prothrombinase complex. J Biol Chem 256:6537, 1981.

131. Nemerson Y: Regulation of the initiation of coagulation by factor VIII. Haemostasis 13:150, 1983.

132. Osterud B, Rapaport SI: Activation of factor IX by the reaction product of tissue factor and factor VII. Proc Natl Acad Sci USA 74:5260, 1977.

133. Bauer KA, Kass BL, ten Cate H, et al: Detection of factor activation in humans. Blood 74:2007, 1989.

134. Bauer KA, Kass BL, ten Cate H, et al: Factor IX is activated in vivo by the tissue factor mechanism. Blood 76:731, 1990.

135. Griffin JH: The role of surface in the surface-dependent activation of Hageman factor (factor XII). Proc Natl Acad Sci USA 75:1998, 1978.

136. Griffin JH, Cochran CG: Recent advances in the understanding of contact activation reactions. Semin Thromb Hemost 5:254, 1979.

137. Meade TW, Miller GJ, Rosenberg RD: Characteristics associated with the risk of arterial thrombosis and the prethrombotic state. In Fuster V, Verstraete M (eds): Thrombosis in Cardiovascular Disorders, p 79. Philadelphia: WB Saunders, 1992.

138. Nesheim ME, Taswell JB, Mann KG: The contribution of bovine factor V and factor Va to the activity of prothrombinase. J Biol Chem 254:10952, 1979.

139. Heimeck R, Schwartz S: Binding of coagulation factors IX and X to the endothelial surface. Biochem Biophys Res Commun 111:723, 1983.

140. Stern D, Nawroth P, Kisiel W, et al: The binding of factor IXa to cultured bovine aortic endothelial cells. J Biol Chem 260:6717, 1985.

141. Harker LA, Mann KG: Thrombosis and fibrinolysis. In Fuster V, Verstraete M (eds): Thrombosis in Cardiovascular Disorders, p 1. Philadelphia: WB Saunders, 1992.

142. Olexa SA, Budzynski AZ: Evidence for four different polymerization sites involved in human fibrin formation. Proc Natl Acad Sci USA 77:1374, 1980.

143. Sherman CT, Litvack F, Grundsest U, et al: Coronary angioscopy in patients with unstable angina pectoris. N Engl J Med 315:913, 1986.

144. Thien-Khai HV, Hung DT, Wheaton VI, et al: Molecular cloning of a functional thrombin receptor reveals a novel proteolytic mechanism of receptor activation. Cell 64:1057, 1991.

145. Booyse FM, Bruce R, Dolenak D, et al: Rapid release and deactivation of plasminogen activators in human endothelial cell cultures in the presence of thrombin and ionophore A23187. Semin Thromb Hemost 12:228, 1986.

146. van Hinsbergh VWM, Sprengers BD, Kooistrat T: Effects of thrombin on the production of plasminogen activators and plasminogen activator inhibitor-I by human foreskin microvascular endothelial cells. Thromb Haemost 57:148, 1987.

147. Barrowcliffe TW, Johnson EA, Thomas D: Antithrombin III and heparin. Br Med Bull 34:143, 1978.

148. Murano G, William L, Miller-Anderson M, et al: Some properties of antithrombin-III and its concentration in human plasma. Thromb Res 18:259, 1980.

149. Olsen ST, Bjork I, Halvorson HR, et al: The role of heparin-protease interactions in heparin acceleration of thrombin inhibition by antithrombin III. Fed Proc 45:1637, 1986.

150. Marcum JA, Rosenberg RD: The biochemistry, cell biology, and pathophysiology of anticoagulantly active heparin-like molecules of the vessel wall. In Lane DA, Lindahl U (eds): Heparin, p 275. Boca Raton, FL: CRC Press, 1989.

151. Rosenberg RD, Damus PS: The purification and mechanism of action of human antithrombin-heparin cofactor. J Biol Chem 248:6490, 1973.

152. Lindahl U, Backstrom G, Thunberg L, et al: Evidence for a 3-0-sulfated D-glucosamine residue in the antithrombin binding sequence of heparin. Proc Natl Acad Sci USA 77:6651, 1980.

153. Lindahl U, Thunberg L, Backstrom G, et al: Extension and structural variability of the antithrombin-binding sequence in heparin. J Biol Chem 259:12368, 1984.

154. Preissner KT: Anticoagulant potential of endothelial cells membrane components. Haemostasis 18:271, 1988.

155. Bringshaw GF, Shanberge JN: Identification of two distinct heparin cofactors in human plasma: Separation and partial purification. Thromb Res 4:683, 1974.

156. Griffin MJ, Carraway T, White GC, et al: Heparin cofactor activities in a family with hereditary antithrombin III deficiency: Evidence for a second heparin cofactor in human plasma. Blood 61:111, 1983.

157. Griffin MJ, Noyes CM, Church FC: Reactive site peptide structural similarity between heparin cofactor II and antithrombin III. J Biol Chem 260:2218, 1985.

158. Parker KA, Toliefsen DM: The protease specificity of heparin cofactor II: Inhibition of thrombin generated during coagulation. J Biol Chem 260:3501, 1985.

159. Baker JB, Low DA, Simmer RL, et al: Protease nexin: A cellular component that links thrombin and plasminogen activator and mediates their binding to cells. Cell 21:37, 1980.

160. Eaton DL, Baker JB: Evidence that a variety of cultured cells secrete protease nexin and produce a distinct cytoplasmic serine protease-binding factor. J Cell Physiol 117:175, 1983.

161. Baker JB, Gronke RS: Protease nexins and cell regulation. Semin Thromb Hemost 12:216, 1987.

162. Bergman BL, Scott S, Watts S, et al: Inhibition of tumor cell-mediated extracellular matrix destruction by a fibroblast proteinase inhibitor, protease nexin 1. Proc Natl Acad Sci USA 83:996, 1986.

163. Esmon CT: Protein-C: Biochemistry, physiology, and clinical implications. Blood 62:1155, 1983.

164. Collen D: Fibrin-specific thrombolytic therapy. Thromb Res 53(suppl VIII):3, 1988.

165. Bauer KA, Rosenburg RD: The pathophysiology of the prethrombotic state in humans: Insights gained from studies using markers of hemostatic system activation. Blood 70:343, 1987.

166. Walker F: Regulation of activated protein C by a new protein: A possible function for bovine factor S. J Biol Chem 255:5521, 1980.

167. Fay WP, Owen WG: Platelet plasminogen activator inhibitor: Purification and characterization of interaction with plasminogen activators and activated protein C. Biochemistry 28:5773, 1989.

168. van Hinsbergh VWM, Bertina RM, van Wijngaarden A, et al: Activated protein C decreases plasminogen activator-inhibitor activity in endothelial cell-conditioned medium. Blood 65:444, 1985.

169. Novotny WF, Palmier M, Wun T, et al: Purification and properties of heparin-releasable lipoprotein-associated coagulation inhibitor. Blood 78:394, 1991.

170. Broze GJ, Miletich JP: Characterization of the inhibition of tissue factor in serum. Blood 69:150, 1987.

171. Rao LVM, Rapaport SI: Studies of a mechanism inhibiting

the initiation of the extrinsic pathway of coagulation. Blood 69:645, 1987.

172. Novotny WF, Brown SG, Miletich JP, et al: Plasma antigen levels of the lipoprotein-associated coagulation inhibitor in patient samples. Blood 78:387, 1991.

173. Collen D, Lijnen HR: Basic and clinical aspects of fibrinolysis and thrombolysis. Blood 78:3114, 1991.

174. Wallen D, Wiman B: Characterization of human plasminogen II: Separation and partial characterization of different molecular forms of human plasminogen. Biochim Biophys Acta 257:122, 1972.

175. Holvoet P, Lijnen HR, Colien D: A monoclonal antibody specific for Lys-plasminogen: Application to the study of the activation pathways of plasminogen in vivo. J Biol Chem 260:12106, 1985.

176. Schleef RR, Loskutoff DJ: Fibrinolytic system of vascular endothelial cells. Haemostasis 18:328, 1988.

177. Wiman R, Collen D: On the kinetics of the reaction between human antiplasmin and plasmin. Eur J Biochem 84:573, 1978.

178. Werb Z, Mainardi CL, Vater CA, et al: Endogenous activation of latent collagenase by rheumatoid synovial cells. N Engl J Med 296:1017, 1977.

179. Clowes AW, Clowes MM, Au YPT, et al: Smooth muscle cells express urokinase during mitogenesis and tissue-type plasminogen activator during migration in injured rat carotid artery. Circ Res 67:61, 1990.

180. Lee CD, Mann KG: Activation/inactivation of human factor V by plasmin. Blood 73:185, 1989.

181. Verstraete M, Vermylen J: Interaction between coagulation, fibrinolysis, complement and kinin systems. *In* Verstraete M, Vermylen J (eds): Thrombosis, p 48. Oxford: Pergamon Press, 1984.

182. Levin EG, Loskutoff DJ: Cultured bovine endothelial cells produce both urokinase and tissue-type plasminogen activators. J Cell Biol 94:631, 1982.

183. Barnathan ES, Koo A, van der Keyl H, et al: Tissue-type plasminogen activator binding to human endothelial cells. J Biol Chem 263:7792, 1988.

184. Russel ME, Quertermous T, Declerck PJ, et al: Binding of tissue-type plasminogen activator with human endothelial cell monolayers. J Biol Chem 265:2569, 1990.

185. Hajjar KA, Hamel NM, Harpel PC, et al: Binding of tissue plasminogen activator to cultured human endothelial cells. J Clin Invest 80:1712, 1987.

186. Hajjar KA: The endothelial cell tissue plasminogen activator receptor. J Biol Chem 266:21962, 1991.

187. Hoylaerts M, Rijken DC, Lijnen HR, et al: Kinetics of the activation of plasminogen by human tissue plasminogen activators: Role of fibrin. J Biol Chem 257:2912, 1982.

188. Manchanda N, Schwartz BS: Single chain urokinase. J Biol Chem 266:14580, 1991.

189. Booyse FM, Lin PH, Traylor M, et al: Purification and properties of a single-chain urokinase-type plasminogen activator form produced by subcultured human umbilical vein endothelial cells. J Biol Chem 263:15139, 1988.

190. Blasi F, Stoppelli P, Cubellis MV: The receptor for urokinaseplasminogen activator. J Cell Biochem 32:179, 1986.

191. Appella E, Robinson EA, Ulrich SJ, et al: The receptor-binding sequence of urokinase. J Biol Chem 262:4437, 1987.

192. Haddock RC, Spell ML, Baker CD, et al: Urokinase binding and receptor identification in cultured endothelial cells. J Biol Chem 266:21466, 1991.

193. Teger-Nilsson AC, Friberg P, Gyzander E: Determination of a new rapid plasmin inhibitor in human blood by means of a plasmin specific tripeptide substrate. Scand J Clin Lab Invest 3:403, 1977.

194. Moroi M, Aoki N: Isolation and characterization of alpha2-plasmin inhibitor from human plasma: A novel protease inhibitor which inhibits activator-induced clot lysis. J Biol Chem 251:5956, 1976.

195. Highsmith R, Rosenberg RD: The inhibition of human plasmin by human-antithrombin-heparin cofactor. J Biol Chem 249:4335, 1974.

196. Machovich R, Bauer RI, Aranyi P, et al: Kinetic analysis of the heparin-enhanced plasmin/antithrombin III reaction: Apparent catalytic role of heparin. Biochem J 199:521, 1981.

197. Collen D, Semerano N, Telesforo P, et al: The inhibition of plasmin by antithrombin III. Br J Haematol 39:101, 1978.

198. Katagiri K, Okada K, Hattori H, et al: Bovine endothelial cell plasminogen activator inhibitor. Eur J Biochem 176:81, 1988.

199. Loskutoff DJ, van Mourik JA, Erickson LA, et al: Detection of an unusually stable fibrinolytic inhibitor produced by bovine endothelial cells. Proc Natl Acad Sci USA 80:2956, 1983.

200. Preissner KT, Jenne D: Structure of vitronectin and its biological role in haemostasis. Thromb Haemost 66:123, 1991.

201. Colucci M, Daramow JA, Collen D: Generation in plasma of a fast-acting inhibitor of plasminogen activators in response to endotoxin stimulation. J Clin Invest 175:824, 1985.

202. Mimuro J, Loskutoff DJ: Effect of transforming growth factor beta (TGF beta) on the fibrinolytic system of cultured bovine aortic endothelial cells [Abstract]. Thromb Haemost 58:447, 1987.

203. Nachman RL, Hajjar KA, Silverstein RL, et al: Interleukin I induces endothelial cell synthesis of plasminogen activator inhibitor. J Exp Med 163:1595, 1986.

204. Schleef RR, Bevilacqua MP, Sawdeg M, et al: Cytokine activation of vascular endothelium: Effects on tissue-type plasminogen activator and type I plasminogen activator inhibitor. J Biol Chem 263:5797, 1988.

205. Burck PJ, Berg DH, Warrick MW, et al: Characterization of a modified human tissue plasminogen activator comprising a kringle-2 and a protease domain. J Biol Chem 265:5170, 1990.

206. Knudsen BS, Nachman RL: Matrix plasminogen activator inhibitor. J Biol Chem 263:9476, 1988.

207. Stump DC, Thienport M, Collen D: Purification and characterization of a novel inhibitor or urokinase from human urine. J Biol Chem 261:12759, 1986.

208. Suzuki K, Nishioka J, Hasimoto S: Protein C inhibitor: Purification from human plasma and characterization. J Biol Chem 258:163, 1983.

# 3

# Pathology of Atherosclerotic Plaque: Stable, Unstable, and Infarctional

*Erling Falk    Henning Rud Andersen*

The result of coronary balloon angioplasty (success versus failure, acute closure and restenosis) and probably also of other interventional coronary procedures depends on operator skills and experience, patient-related factors (e.g., age, gender, S-lipids, diabetes, smoking), the clinical syndrome (e.g., chronic angina, unstable angina, acute infarction), and lesion-related characteristics (location, degree of obstruction, length, eccentricity, calcification, composition, consistency, vulnerability, and irregularity of the target lesion[s]).[1–4] In experienced hands, lesion-related characteristics (i.e., plaque morphology) have emerged as the most important determinants of the outcome.[5, 6]

## LESION-RELATED CHARACTERISTICS

Atherosclerosis is primarily an intimal disease that, by definition, is characterized by atherosis and sclerosis. The former component (atherosis) is lipid-rich and "soft" like gruel, whereas the latter component (sclerosis) is collagen rich and "hard." There is considerable interplaque as well as intraplaque variability in plaque composition, but the hard sclerotic component is usually much more voluminous than the soft atheromatous. Some patients have only hard plaques, others only soft ones, but most patients have plaques containing variable amounts of both hard and soft components[7, 8] (Fig. 3–1). The reason is unknown, as is the relationship, if any, between the atheromatous and the sclerotic component. Secondarily, both components may become calcified, increasing the rigidity of the atherosclerotic plaque.

## Topography

Significant stenoses are found most frequently within the first few centimeters of the two left-sided branches (in particular, proximal in the left anterior descending artery), and the proximal and distal halves of the right coronary artery are nearly similarly affected.[9, 10] Circumferentially, atherosclerotic plaques tend to occur and progress at the outer (lateral) walls of bifurcations and on inner curvatures, regions characterized by reduced flow velocity and low/oscillating wall shear stress.[11–14] Thus, the flow-divider region between the two branches of the left main stem is usually free of disease, whereas atherosclerotic plaques preferentially involve the outer walls of the bifurcation and extend downstream on the myocardial (the inner curvature) rather than on the epicardial side of the arteries.[12, 13] In the right coronary artery, plaques tend to concentrate on the inner wall of the curvature adjacent to the myocardium as the artery runs around the heart within the atrioventricular groove.[12] Interestingly, atherosclerotic lesions are seldom found beneath myocardial bridges.[15]

## Left Main Stenosis

The left main stem is usually free of severe atherosclerotic involvement.[10] Left main stenosis may be particularly frequent in patients with hyperlipoproteinemia type II and is nearly always accompanied by severe disease of the other three major coronary arteries.[16] Isolated stenosis of the left main stem is very rare[16] and is usually confined to the ostium.[17]

## Ostial Lesion

Most often, coronary ostial narrowing is the result of primary disease of the aorta,[10] the classic example being syphilitic aortitis. Today it is most frequently caused by atherosclerosis, usually accompanied by severe involvement of the coronary arteries. Very rarely, and particularly in young women, isolated ostial stenosis may be present.[18] In the homozygous form of hyperlipoproteinemia type II, there is an unusual but highly characteristic plaque distribution, with striking involvement of the ascending

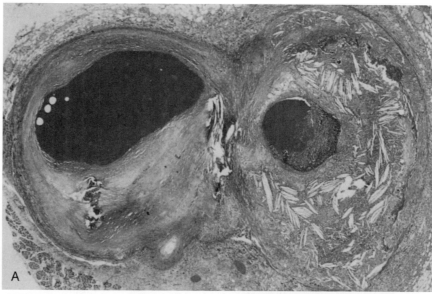

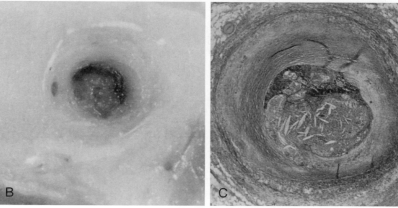

FIGURE 3–1. *A,* Plaque variability. Histologic cross section just distal to vessel bifurcation showing a hard collagenous plaque in the branch to the left and a soft atheromatous one with ruptured surface and mural thrombus (unstable plaque) to the right. (There is radiographic contrast medium in the lumen.) *B* and *C,* Atheroembolization. Downstream to the ruptured plaque, the right-sided branch is occluded by atheromatous plaque material with cholesterol crystal (*B* is a macroscopic view, *C* is microscopic).

aorta (including the aortic valve cusps), often causing severe ostial narrowing.[19]

## Length of Stenosis

Angiographically, the great majority of coronary lesions appear to be rather short, usually less than 10 mm in length.[6] By contrast, histologic examination reveals that most stenotic lesions are considerably longer because the adjacent angiographically normal vascular segments are also often severely diseased. Baroldi[10] examined 565 severe stenoses histologically and found a length less than 5 mm in 13%, of 5 to 20 mm in 38%, and of greater than 20 mm in 49%. Thus, nearly half of these severely stenotic segments were narrowed for a considerable length. There was no relationship to the clinical situation, that is, whether the death was of coronary (acute infarction or sudden death) or noncoronary (accident) origin.[10]

## Diffuseness of Disease

Evaluated angiographically, coronary atherosclerosis appears to be a focal disease, and it is so in the sense that it gives rise to intimal plaques that involve the coronary tree unevenly, longitudinally as well as circumferentially. However, in patients with atherosclerotic heart disease, the extent of "plaquing" is usually so widespread ("diffuse") that virtually no vascular segment is left entirely unaffected.[20] Coronary arteries undergo compensatory enlargement during early plaque growth and may thus preserve a normal lumen despite rather severe vessel wall disease.[11, 21–23] Therefore, angiography usually underestimates the extent of vessel wall involvement, and vascular segments judged normal (because the lumen appears normal) are frequently severely diseased[24, 25] (Fig. 3–2). In the legs, the atherosclerotic process seems to be more diffuse (and more distally located) in diabetic patients than in those without diabetes,[26] but whether the same is true for the coronary arteries remains controversial.[27, 28]

## Aneurysm/Ectasia

The two terms commonly used to describe focal or diffuse dilation of coronary arteries are *aneurysm*

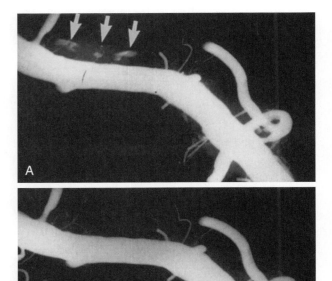

FIGURE 3–2. Angiography underestimates vessel wall disease. Postmortem angiogram of coronary segment before *(A)* and after *(B)* decalcification. Plaque calcifications *(arrows)* disclose severe vessel wall disease despite nearly normal vascular lumen.

and *ectasia*. In adults, atherosclerotic vessel wall destruction is the most frequent underlying cause, and aneurysms and stenotic lesions usually coexist.[29–31] The aneurysms nearly always contain thrombus that may occlude the lumen and/or embolize, but atherosclerotic coronary aneurysms do not rupture.[29, 31] Aneurysmal coronary artery disease is probably a subset or variant of coronary atherosclerosis and not a distinct clinical entity.[30]

## Luminal Shape and Position ("Eccentricity")

The extent of circumferential vessel wall involvement differs from plaque to plaque and along the course of a stenotic lesion, giving rise to quite variable shapes and position of the residual lumen. On cross section, the shape of the narrowed lumen may be round, oval or D-shaped, but it is virtually never crescentic or slit-like in pressure-fixed specimens,[11, 32] unless the underlying plaque is rapidly progressing because of ruptured surface, plaque hemorrhage, and/or luminal thrombosis.[33] It is stated that most hard fibrous plaques result in round rather than "ovoid" lumens, whereas the opposite applies to soft lipid-rich plaques.[33] Irrespective of luminal shape, the residual lumen may be positioned centrally encircled entirely by plaque or peripherally (with or without an adjacent plaque-free

arc of normal vessel wall). Baroldi[10] examined 1069 severe stenoses (greater than 70% diameter reduction) and found that 46% had a central lumen encircled by plaque (called "concentric"), whereas 54% had a more or less peripherally positioned lumen either with (called "semilunar") or without (called "eccentric") an adjacent plaque-free wall segment (30% and 24%, respectively). As plaques enlarge, more of the circumference is involved, so the proportion of plaques with a normal wall segment becomes lower with increasing severity of stenosis.[32–34] The muscular media is normal in plaque-free wall segments but is thinner and often totally destroyed beneath advanced atherosclerotic plaques.[34, 35]

Unfortunately, the term *eccentric* has been used to characterize quite different features of atherosclerotic lesions, making comparisons between studies difficult. It has, for example, been used for (1) all asymmetric plaques with the residual lumen off-center, evaluated on histologic cross sections[9, 11]; (2) only those asymmetric plaques that have a plaque-free wall segment with preserved media[8] (these constitute only a fraction of all asymmetric plaques,[10, 36] partly explaining why pathologists using this definition find more concentric than eccentric plaques[8]); (3) asymmetric stenoses, evaluated angiographically (probably representing asymmetric plaques with the residual lumen off-center)[1, 37]; and (4) noncircular luminal shapes, evaluated by biplane angiography[38] or by intravascular ultrasound.[39] Importantly, the latter (luminal shape "eccentricity") should not be equated with plaque eccentricity because, on cross section, the lumen may be circular, oval, or D-shaped, irrespective of its position, centrally or off-center.

## Calcification

In adults, coronary calcification is nearly always of atherosclerotic origin and indicates the presence of advanced intimal disease, but plaque calcification probably has little functional significance. The degree of plaque calcification increases with luminal narrowing,[40] but there is no strong correlation between the degree of calcification and (1) the severity of stenosis[41, 42]; (2) other plaque characteristics[10]; or (3) the length of symptoms or presenting symptoms (angina or acute myocardial infarction).[43] Plaque calcification appears to increase with patient age,[44] with lesion age,[9] and perhaps with diastolic blood-pressure.[43] In Roberts'[45] experience, heavily calcified coronary arteries are common in patients with diabetes mellitus. Although diabetes predisposes to medial calcification (Mönckeberg's calcinosis), especially of the muscular arteries of the legs, medial calcification is practically never seen in the coronary arteries of adults.[41, 46, 47]

# Vulnerability, Rupture, and Thrombogenesis

## Vulnerability

The composition, consistency, and vulnerability of atherosclerotic plaques differ. The main component of coronary plaques is usually hard collagenous tissue (sclerosis), which is stable and rather innocuous. By contrast, lipid accumulation (atherosis) is dangerous because it softens plaques, making them vulnerable, that is, prone to rupture, and ruptured plaques underlie the great majority of thrombus-related acute heart attacks.[48] Typically, a vulnerable plaque consists of a pool of soft extracellular lipid (the atheromatous gruel) separated from the vascular lumen by a cap of fibrous tissue (Fig. 3–3). The cap varies greatly in thickness, cellularity, strength, and stiffness but is often thinnest and most heavily infiltrated by foam cells at its junction with the adjacent more normal intima. Macrophage foam cells are frequently found at the plaque rupture site,[49] indicating ongoing disease activity, at least locally, which may have weakened the cap and predisposed it to rupture (see Fig. 3–3F). The soft atheromatous gruel is avascular, but a dense plexus of microvessels (neovascularization) frequently extends from the adventitia through the media and into the base of the plaque.[50] These small thin-walled vessels may give rise to minor hemorrhages at the base of the plaque, irrespective of the integrity of the plaque surface.[51]

On the basis of clinical experience it has been suggested that small (early) plaques are more susceptible to rupture than are larger, more advanced stenotic plaques. Another explanation could be that small nonstenotic plaques are not more susceptible to rupture than are larger plaques, but if a small plaque ruptures, the clinical consequences are more grave because it is "unprotected" by collateral vessels. Importantly, vulnerability is not a simple function of stenosis severity; that is, it is not the size (plaque volume) but the composition (plaque type) that matters.[52]

## Ruptured Surface

Rupture of the plaque surface (with or without thrombosis superimposed) occurs frequently during the evolution and growth of coronary lesions and is probably the most important mechanism underlying sudden and rapid plaque progression. Generally, the risk of plaque rupture increases with increasing severity of atherosclerotic changes: the more plaques, the higher risk of rupture. Davies and Thomas[51] found at least 103 ruptured coronary plaques (and 115 thrombi) in 74 patients who died suddenly of ischemic heart disease. They later found one or more ruptured plaques incidentally (unrelated to the cause of death) in 9% of persons dying suddenly of noncardiac causes without an atheroma-related disease, increasing to 22% in those with a disease such as hypertension or diabetes.[53] Clearly, the more meticulous the search for ruptured plaques, the more are found. As many as 103 ruptured plaques have been identified in 47 patients dying of coronary atherosclerosis.[54] Thus, although plaque rupture underlies most acute coronary syndromes, it is clearly clinically silent in the great majority of cases.

Ruptured plaques, stenotic lesions, and luminal thrombi are all found with the highest frequency in the same vascular segments.[55] Ruptures vary greatly in size, but most are microscopic and occur at the periphery of the fibrous cap. Progressive lipid accumulation (gruel formation) and cap weakening, possibly related to ongoing macrophage activity, predispose the plaque to rupture. The dynamic interplay between plaque vulnerability (which changes with time) and external "triggers" probably determines the particular moment and point of rupture. Of these, vulnerability is probably most important because only vulnerable plaques rupture; when they do, rupture usually occurs during normal daily activities, without any obvious precipitating causes.[56]

## Luminal Thrombus

Most (more than 75%) major coronary thrombi are precipitated by a sudden rupture of the plaque surface, exposing thrombogenic material to the flowing blood[48, 57] (see Fig. 3–3). Minor and superficial intimal irregularities (but no frank rupture, i.e., no deep injury) are found beneath the rest of the thrombi (20% to 25%), usually in combination with a severe atherosclerotic stenosis.[54]

Microscopic examination of the culprit lesion from patients dying soon after the onset of an acute heart attack reveals that the most recent part of the thrombus responsible for the final symptoms consists predominantly of aggregated platelets, often admixed with displaced atheromatous plaque material. The latter and/or intimal flaps may sometimes project into the narrowed lumen and thus give rise to a primarily nonthrombotic vascular occlusion.[44, 48, 58, 59] Fibrin subsequently infiltrates the early platelet-rich thrombus and eventually enmeshes the platelets, stabilizing the thrombus. Such a temporal interplay between platelets and fibrin agrees with experimental studies and also explains why fresh thrombi are more easily lysed than are older consolidated thrombi. Microscopic examination also shows that more than 80% of coronary thrombi have a layered structure, with thrombus material of dif-

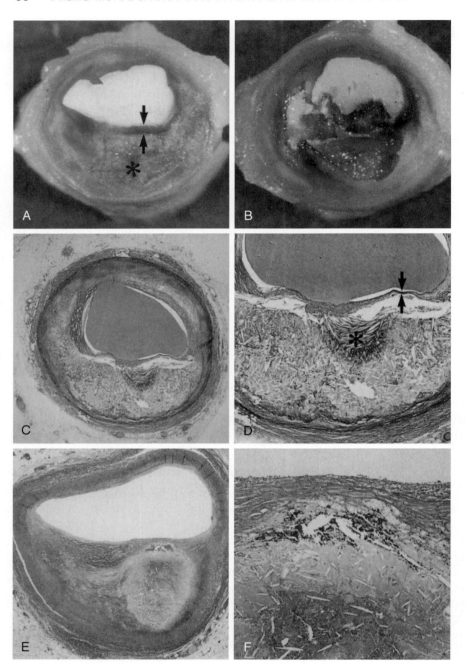

FIGURE 3–3. Vulnerable plaques. *A* and *B*, Adjacent cross sections (3 mm apart) showing a soft atheromatous plaque consisting of a lipid pool *(asterisk in A)* separated from the vascular lumen by a thin cap of fibrous tissue *(between arrows)*. The cap is intact in *A* (vulnerable) but ruptured in *B* (unstable). A small mural thrombus has evolved at the rupture site where thrombogenic material has been exposed. (Macroscopic view, white radiographic contrast medium in the lumen.) *C* and *D*, Extremely vulnerable plaque with a very thin fibrous cap *(between arrows)*. The small hemorrhage just beneath the cap *(asterisk)* indicates that it is probably ruptured nearby. *E* and *F*, One half of this plaque is soft and vulnerable. Macrophage foam cells are seen at the border between the gruel and the fibrous cap, indicating ongoing disease activity and maybe eroding the cap from beneath.

fering age, indicating an episodic growth by repeated mural deposits over time.[60] Furthermore, small fragments of thromboembolic material are frequently found impacted in intramyocardial arteries downstream to evolving coronary thrombi, often associated with microinfarcts.[60, 61] Consequently, coronary thrombosis is usually a dynamic process in which the thrombus size varies over time, causing intermittent coronary obstruction—thrombosis and thrombolysis are dynamic processes occurring simultaneously.[62] Endogenous thrombolysis gradually (usually over the course of weeks) reopens most thrombosed arteries, but it works slowly unaided,

and a severe stenosis often persists. Pharmacologic thrombolysis works faster, but the ultimate result is probably not much better than that achieved by endogenous thrombolysis, if the latter is aided by effective inhibition of the ongoing thrombotic component of this dynamic process (i.e., effective antithrombotic therapy).[62] Thus, the goal (reperfusion) may be reached by two different approaches: enhancing thrombolysis and/or inhibiting thrombosis.

Many atherosclerotic stenoses underlying coronary thrombi are only mild or moderate; that is, they are hemodynamically insignificant, indicating that reduced flow plays no major role for the initial evolution of a coronary thrombus. On the contrary, rapid blood velocity due to preexisting atherosclerotic stenosis seems to promote arterial thrombosis, probably via shear-induced platelet activation.[48] Furthermore, platelet aggregation and thrombus formation may take place not only within the stenosis but also poststenotically where flow separation, recirculation, and turbulence probably offer ideal fluid dynamic conditions for progressive growth of a thrombus (Fig. 3–4). Because the mural thrombus formed within the stenosis is often much smaller than the free-floating tail of thrombus extending

downstream, angiographic filling defects thought to represent nonoccluding thrombi are typically identified poststenotically.[63] Such free-floating tails of thrombi extending downstream poststenotically seem to have a high potential to embolize.[64] Secondary to the reduced flow caused by the platelet-rich thrombus at the rupture site, the blood proximal and distal to the occlusion may stagnate and coagulate (clot), giving rise to a stagnation thrombosis consisting predominantly of erythrocytes held together by fibrin membranes similar to a venous thrombus formed in stagnant blood[48] (Fig. 3–5). The

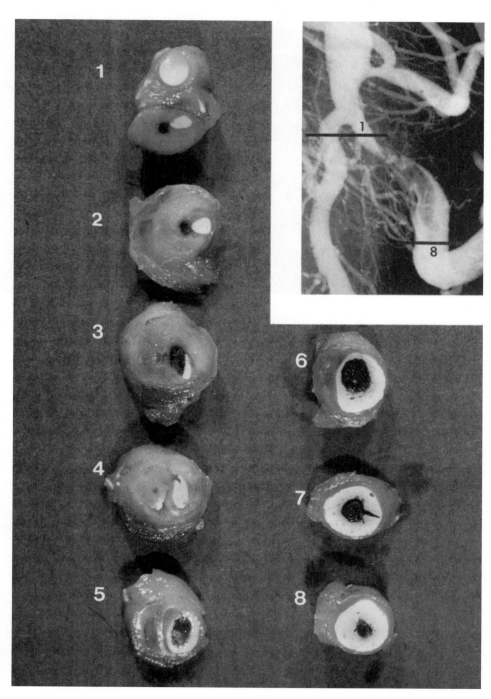

FIGURE 3–4. Thrombosis within and distal to stenosis. Postmortem angiogram *(inset)* from a patient who died after an acute heart attack, and the corresponding consecutive cross sections cut through the lesion at 2-mm intervals (from *1* to *8*). *2,* Ruptured plaque surface with hemorrhage into the plaque. *3,* Nonoccluding luminal thrombus within the stenosis. *4* to *8,* Freely floating tail of thrombus extending downstream to the stenosis into a normal vascular segment. The thrombus is surrounded by the white radiographic contrast medium injected post mortem.

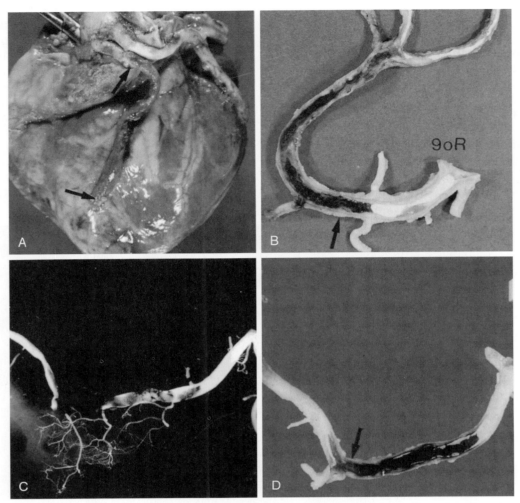

FIGURE 3–5. Secondary stagnation thrombosis. *A,* Saphenous vein graft to left anterior descending artery thrombosed in nearly its entire length *(between arrows).* The patient died soon after the operation, and autopsy revealed primary occlusion at the distal anastomotic site. *B,* Right coronary artery cut open longitudinally. A huge stagnation thrombosis blocks the artery between the rupture site *(arrow)* and the origin of the posterior descending branch. *C* and *D,* Postmortem angiogram and corresponding right coronary artery cut open longitudinally. An impressive stagnation thrombosis has propagated upstream from the primary platelet-rich thrombus at the *arrow.*

white platelet-rich thrombus at the rupture site is usually rather small, whereas the red erythrocyte-rich stagnation thrombus may be extensive, particularly in coronary vein grafts (Fig. 3–6*A, B*; see Fig. 3–5*A*) and in right coronary arteries, where there are no or only few side branches, respectively. Although the secondarily formed "clot" is probably more easily lysed than is the primary platelet-rich thrombus at the rupture site, a several-centimeter-long clot may contribute significantly to the "thrombotic burden" in these vessels.

Vasospasm may contribute to the dynamic flow obstruction, and often does so, before, during, and after an acute heart attack.[65] For initial reperfusion of occluded arteries, thrombolysis rather than spasmolysis is required, but spasmolytic agents may subsequently improve the result, indicating that thrombosis and vasospasm often coexist. The former may give rise to the latter.[56]

## Chronic Total Occlusion

Like severe stenoses, most complete occlusions are located within the first few centimeters of the coronary arteries and their branches (although the proximal excess is not so marked in the right coronary artery), and the proximal segment of the left anterior descending artery is the most frequently involved segment.[44, 66, 67] Most complete coronary occlusions, fresh as well as old, are short, generally less than 5 mm long.[58, 66, 67]

An occluding (nonrecanalized) thrombus within a diseased coronary artery may persist without significant light microscopic changes for weeks; ultimately, it is invaded by capillaries, smooth muscle cells, and macrophages and becomes organized. With age, the stroma becomes more fibrous (harder) and less cellular,[68] perhaps with one or more newly formed endothelialized channels passing through it. The appearances of healed (chronic) occlusions are,

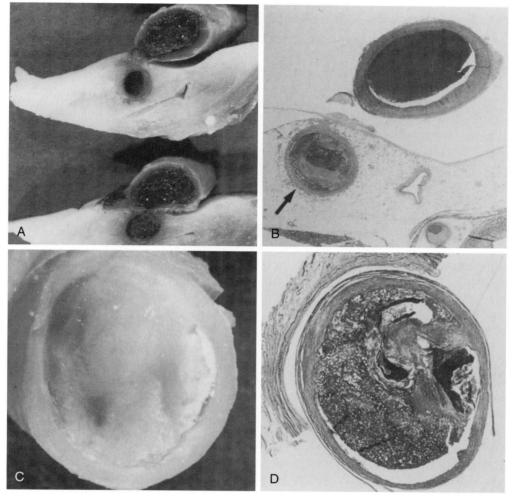

FIGURE 3–6. Vein graft thrombosis. *A* and *B,* Cross sections just proximal to the graft-coronary artery anastomosis (see Fig. 3–5*A*) showing huge thrombotic burden in the graft due to its caliber and its lack of side branches, causing extensive blood stagnation (and coagulation) in case of occlusion. Localized coronary dissection is seen in the grafted artery *(arrow)* just proximal to the anastomotic site. *C* and *D,* Soft atheromatous vein graft plaque developed in less than 4 years in a hyperlipidemic patient. The cause of death was plaque rupture with luminal thrombus superimposed *(D),* giving rise to cardiogenic shock.

however, extremely variable[68] (Fig. 3–7). At this stage, the atherosclerotic plaque may be softer than the organized thrombus blocking the original lumen, explaining why autopsy scissors often pass through the soft atheromatous gruel of such lesions, instead of opening the original lumen.

### *Tortuosity and Caliber*

The tortuosity and caliber of the artery harboring the target lesion may be of importance. Coronary arteries become more tortuous with age and with cardiac shrinkage.[69] They dilate, particularly non-sclerotic arteries, with increasing heart weight.[69–71] Generally, women have smaller hearts and coronary arteries than men[70] but, even with the same heart weight, the coronary arteries in women appear to be slightly smaller than those in men.[71] Coronary arteries lose their elasticity with age; if they are examined in undistended state postmortem, they appear

to become wider.[70] If, however, they are examined after pressure-fixation, a simple age-related dilatation is far less apparent, if it occurs at all.[69, 71] One clinical study suggests that the opposite may occur; that is, they may decrease in luminal size with age.[72]

## Graft Lesions

### *Lesions in Saphenous Vein Grafts*

A typically self-limited fibromuscular intimal thickening develops during the first year in all vein grafts patent at 1 month after surgery.[73] A preexisting atherosclerotic plaque in the grafted artery may, of course, be responsible for early atherosclerotic stenosis at the anastomotic site, but the graft itself is free of atherosclerosis during the first postoperative year. Thereafter, early atherosclerotic changes may be identified in the thickened intima, and within a few years, advanced plaques are responsible for

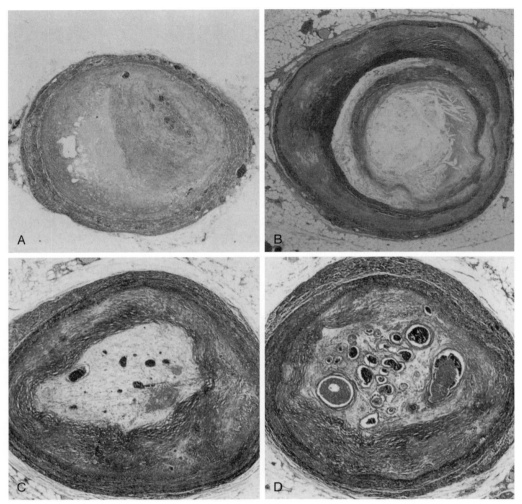

FIGURE 3–7. Chronic occlusions vary greatly. *A,* Atheromatous plaque (soft) and organized collagen-rich (firm) luminal thrombus. *B,* Predominantly collagenous plaque and soft atheromatous gruel displaced into the lumen, occluding it. *C,* Hard collagenous plaque and organized collagen-poor luminal thrombus. *D,* Organized and partly recanalized thrombus (i.e., the lesion is no longer totally occlusive).

most vein graft failures.[73–75] Morphologically, advanced plaques in vein grafts closely resemble those in native coronary arteries, but they are generally more voluminous, less calcified, and more rich in foam cells and extracellular lipid; that is, they are larger, softer, and more friable.[73, 74] Consequently, vein graft plaques are particularly vulnerable. Furthermore, atherosclerotic vein grafts appear to be particularly susceptible to aneurysm formation.[76]

Similar to sudden occlusion of native coronary arteries, spontaneous rupture of a soft atheromatous plaque with thrombosis superimposed is the most common mechanism of late acute graft occlusion[75, 77] (see Fig. 3–6C, D). The thrombotic component is, however, often much greater in vein grafts than in native arteries because of the greater caliber of vein grafts and the lack of sidebranches, conditions that promote blood stagnation and coagulation (i.e., secondary stagnation thrombus formation) (see Figs. 3–5A and 3–6A, B). Of interest for chronic graft

occlusions, poorly organized thrombus is often present in vein grafts known to have been occluded for a long period, indicating that vein graft thrombi organize slowly, if at all.[78]

### Lesions in Internal Mammary Arteries

In their natural position, the internal mammary arteries are nearly free of both the age-related diffuse intimal thickening (known from coronary arteries) and atherosclerosis.[79, 80] After grafting, some (usually minimal) fibrocellular intimal thickening may occur, but atherosclerosis is still extremely rare,[78, 81] in sharp contrast to saphenous vein grafts. The reason for the relative sparing of the internal mammary arteries from these processes is unclear.

## PATIENT-RELATED FACTORS AND LESION-RELATED CHARACTERISTICS

There is a well-known association between patient-related factors, such as age, sex, S-cholesterol, blood pressure, and diabetes (but not smoking), and the extent of coronary atherosclerosis (plaque volume),[82] but little is known about these same factors and specific lesion-related characteristics (plaque type). Two autopsy studies suggest that S-lipids correlate most strongly with fatty streaks (foam cell lesions), whereas blood pressure seems to correlate particularly with fibrous plaques.[83, 84] Surprisingly, hyperlipoproteinemia does not seem to give rise to particularly lipid-rich (soft), hence vulnerable, plaques.[19, 85] Consequently, patient-related factors are not very helpful in predicting the character of the target lesion or lesions.

## CLINICAL SYNDROMES AND LESION-RELATED CHARACTERISTICS

Unlike patient-related factors, the actual symptomatic status correlates strongly with the morphologic features (i.e., lesion-related characteristics) of the culprit lesion. In particular, the progression from stable to unstable coronary artery disease is clearly related to plaque vulnerability, plaque rupture and/or luminal thrombosis (plaque type) rather than to extent of disease (plaque volume).[60, 86, 87] These features are illustrated in Figure 3–8.

## Stable Angina Pectoris

In patients with stable angina, the composition and the eccentricity of atherosclerotic plaques vary greatly from individual to individual. Most patients have a mixture of plaque types in varying proportions, and the characteristics of one plaque often differ from those of another nearby plaque[8] (see Fig. 3–1). However, of importance, most high-grade stenoses (perhaps 60%) appear to be fibrous, and therefore stable, and rather innocuous; vulnerable rupture-prone plaques with a large pool of soft lipid may not be present at all in a great minority of patients, in perhaps as many as one third.[8] These patients are probably at low risk of experiencing a thrombus-related acute heart attack. Regarding plaque morphology and vasomotion, eccentric (asymmetric) coronary stenoses seem to have a higher dynamic potential than that of concentric (symmetric) coronary stenoses.[37]

## Unstable Coronary Syndromes

Rupture of hemodynamic insignificant lesions is probably silent clinically in the great majority of cases. Otherwise, unstable angina seems to be a good clinical marker of ruptured coronary plaques. The natural history of unstable angina probably mirrors that of the underlying ruptured plaque, that is, stabilization (resealing of the rupture), accentuation

of symptoms (mural thrombosis), or infarction (occlusive thrombosis). Typically, coronary angiography[88, 89] and angioscopy[87, 90] performed during acute heart attacks have demonstrated the presence of transient nonocclusive thrombi in unstable angina with pain at rest, severe stenoses (probably representing mural thrombosis or early spontaneous recanalized thrombi) that may progress to total occlusion in non–Q-wave infarction, and occlusive thrombi that may persist or lyse spontaneously (but too late for significant myocardial salvage) in Q-wave infarction. The culprit lesion responsible for out-of-hospital cardiac arrest or sudden death is apparently often similar to that of unstable angina: plaque rupture with mural thrombosis.[48] Thus, a ruptured plaque with a dynamic thrombosis superimposed (with or without concomitant vasospasm) seems to underlie the great majority of acute coronary syndromes, with the clinical presentation and the outcome, depending on the severity and duration of ischemia—whether the obstruction is occlusive or nonocclusive, transient or persistent—modified by the magnitude of collateral flow.

## Acute Myocardial Infarction
### Successful Thrombolysis

Spontaneous recanalization of thrombosed coronary arteries may occur early by retraction, fragmentation, and lysis of the thrombus and/or by "spasmolysis" or later by organization and remodeling. Endogenous thrombolysis aided by effective anticoagulation will probably open most thrombosed arteries before hospital discharge, but pharmacologic thrombolysis may accelerate this process significantly.[62] A severe stenosis is usually present immediately after otherwise successful thrombolysis, probably caused by preexisting atherosclerosis and residual thrombus. Particularly if severe, the residual stenosis may reocclude rapidly,[91] and marked irregularity of the infarct-related lesion seems to predispose to early clinical instability.[92] The unstable features may resolve, at least partially, over 5 to 10 days,[92] probably because of continuing endogenous thrombolysis; subsequent remodeling may further improve the result.

### Persistent Occlusion

Reopening of the occluded artery is important for survival after infarction.[62] Unfortunately, a substantial proportion of infarct-related vessels remains occluded despite thrombolytic treatment, probably 20% to 25%. An occluding thrombus is nearly always found at autopsy[62]; also, clinical studies indicate that a thrombus usually is present, despite the failure of standard thrombolytic treatment to reper-

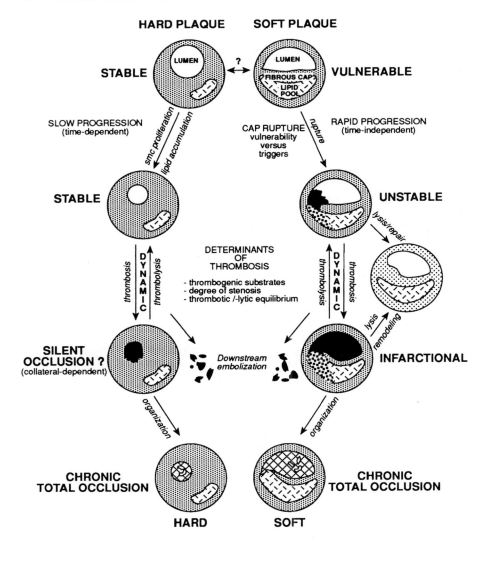

FIGURE 3–8. Plaque types and modes of progression.

fuse.[62] The reason for the partly age-dependent and apparently intrinsic thrombolytic resistance of some thrombi is unknown, but experimental data indicate that not all thrombi are equally susceptible to thrombolysis. Thus, thrombi formed within arterial stenoses and other platelet-rich thrombi appear to be particularly resistant to lysis, contrary to erythrocyte-rich clots formed in stagnant blood.[62] Accordingly, clinical data indicate that the relatively small but platelet-rich thrombus within the atherosclerotic stenosis disappears only slowly during thrombolysis and that it may resist even prolonged intracoronary streptokinase infusion, whereas the "tail" of thrombus extending downstream usually dissolves rapidly and completely.[64] That thrombi formed within severe stenoses are particularly difficult to lyse is consistent with the lower patency rate after infarction in patients with preceding chronic angina (indicating an underlying severe atherosclerotic stenosis), compared with that in patients without preceding angina.[62] Thus, the presence of a strong thrombogenic stimulus in the form of a tight atherosclerotic stenosis and/or extensive plaque disruption seems to be associated with lytic failure, probably because thrombi formed under such conditions are particularly rich in platelets. Other causes of unsuccessful thrombolysis could be extensive stagnation thrombosis or nonthrombotic obstructions in the form of major plaque hemorrhages (called "hemorrhagic dissection"[68]), intimal flaps, or displaced atheromatous plaque material[44, 48, 58, 59] (see Figs. 3–1B, C and 3–7B). Vasospasm probably plays no role in the persistency of the occlusion.

Thus, the character of the infarct-related lesions usually treated by "rescue" angioplasty (persistent occlusions despite thrombolysis), by "adjunctive" angioplasty (residual stenoses after thrombolytic reperfusion), and by "primary" angioplasty (all infarct-related lesions without antecedent thrombolytic therapy) probably differs significantly, as do the complication rates.

### Reocclusion

As for the initial thrombotic occlusion, thrombin and platelets seem to play key roles for early reocclusion, and rethrombosis depends probably on the same factors (although dissimilar qualitatively and/or quantitatively) as those responsible for the initial event, that is, the residual thrombogenic substrate, local flow disturbances (residual stenosis/flow), and the actual thrombotic-thrombolytic equilibrium.[62]

## IMPLICATIONS FOR MECHANICAL INTERVENTION

The results of interventional procedures depend primarily on the character of the target lesion or lesions, that is, lesion-related characteristics.[5] Therefore, knowledge of the specific pathoanatomy of the lesion or lesions in question is required for the proper application of this technology to patient management.

## Location

Size of vessel and the associated perfusion area correlate.[72] Therefore, the larger the caliber of the coronary segment harboring the target lesion, the greater amount of myocardium is at risk (if viable) during the procedure.[93] In addition, "distant" perfusion areas may also be at risk, if supplied by collaterals. Plaques preferentially occur on the inner wall of curvatures, that is, adjacent to the myocardium (opposite the epicardial surface), which may be of importance in reducing the risk of hemopericardium in case of vessel perforation during procedures aimed at removing/ablating plaques.

## Diffuse Disease

Patients with atherosclerotic heart disease usually have widespread "plaquing." Angiography often underestimates the extent of disease, as well as the degree and the length of stenoses (see Fig. 3–2).

## Degree of Stenosis

Severe and fibrous (hard) stenoses may be impossible to dilate,[5] particularly if the residual lumen is surrounded entirely by plaque tissue (concentric lesions).[94] By contrast, it may not be so risky to attack a high-grade stenosis, because the myocardium at risk is often "protected" by collateral perfusion in case of acute closure.

## Calcification

Calcification may hinder optimal dissection of the coronary arteries by surgeons and pathologists and may, of course, also constitute an obstacle to interventional procedures.[5]

## Eccentricity

The term eccentric should be used only to characterize plaque configuration (asymmetric plaques/stenoses) and should not be used for noncircular luminal shapes. Concentric stenoses are usually considered more fixed and rigid than eccentric ones. The latter may be more compliant according to the extent of the plaque-free (or at least less diseased) wall segment. It has been suggested that stretching of the plaque-free wall segment may be a more frequent mechanism underlying successful coronary angioplasty than previously thought,[34] but immediate or gradual return of the overstretched segment to its original state (recoil) could also explain some instances of failure or early restenosis.[34, 95] With current technique, eccentricity itself may, however, prove to have no major role in the outcome.[4, 5]

## Vulnerability, Rupture, and Thrombogenicity

The lesion responsible for stable angina is probably most often collagenous and lipid poor (i.e., hard and stable), whereas lipid-rich atheromatous (i.e., soft and vulnerable) plaques with or without superimposed thrombosis underlie the great majority of acute coronary syndromes. Because fibrous tissue, soft gruel, and thrombus have different mechanical as well as thrombogenic properties, and therefore different risk profiles, these features should be taken into account when interventional procedures are considered. Ruptured plaques with or without superimposed thrombus may be identified angiographically by their irregular luminal borders and/or intraluminal lucencies[96] (Figs. 3–9 and 3–10).

Importantly, spontaneous plaque rupture and iatrogenic vessel wall disruption differ significantly. For example, balloon dilatation of concentric lesions usually splits the plaque where it is thinnest (and less resistant), whereas eccentric lesions usu-

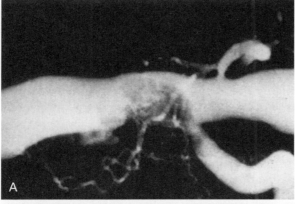

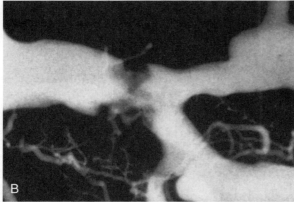

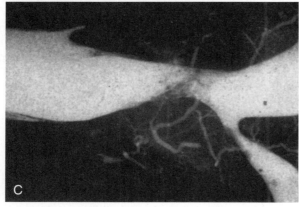

FIGURE 3–9. Unstable lesions. *A–C*, Postmortem angiograms from three patients who died after acute heart attacks. All three lesions have irregular borders, and intraluminal lucencies are seen within the stenoses. (Flow direction: from left to right.) The underlying pathoanatomy is revealed in Figure 3–10, in which the corresponding cross sections are shown.

ally split at their periphery, separating the entire rigid plaque from the adjacent much more pliable (expansible) plaque-free wall segment and media, often accompanied by localized medial disruption and dissection.[97–99] Thus, the plaque itself, including the fibrous cap of soft plaques, generally remains intact, unless the cap already was ruptured spontaneously before angioplasty, as in the case of unstable/infarctional culprit lesions.[100, 101] The integ-

rity of the fibrous cap of soft plaques and the mode of plaque splitting during mechanical intervention may be of vital importance for the acute (thrombus and dissection) as well as the long-term (restenosis) result.[99, 102]

## Thrombus

Atherothrombotic plaques, often present in patients with acute coronary syndromes, appear to be associated with a particularly high complication rate during intervention.[51, 103] The often huge "thrombotic burden" of thrombosed coronary vein grafts and, to some extent, right coronary arteries, may explain not only the lower reperfusion rates and higher reocclusion rate of these vessels with thrombolysis but also why mechanical intervention often fails as well. Although thrombolysis is usually effective in reopening occluded vessels, residual thrombus may persist for days, increasing the risk of complications during intervention. Angioplasty during or immediately after thrombolysis could also be dangerous because it may increase the risk of occluding vessel wall hemorrhage secondary to angioplasty-induced intimal/medial dissection.[104] If possible, mechanical intervention should be delayed because extensive remodeling may render the procedure unnecessary.

As mentioned, the character of the infarct-related lesions usually treated by rescue angioplasty (persistent occlusions despite thrombolysis), by adjunctive angioplasty (residual stenoses after thrombolytic reperfusion), and by primary angioplasty (all infarct-related lesions without antecedent thrombolytic therapy) probably differs significantly, which may explain the different complication rates.[105]

## Chronic Total Occlusion

The nature, particularly the age, of the thrombotic component of the occlusion is probably a very important factor in determining the outcome of recanalization procedures.[106, 107] An occluding thrombus within a diseased vessel may remain unorganized and susceptible to intracoronary thrombolysis for weeks,[108, 109] sometimes even months,[110] while the fully organized thrombus may be so hard that a guide wire may pass through the soft gruel of the underlying plaque (creating a new channel in the vessel wall), rather than through the organized thrombus blocking the lumen.[97, 106] Even if the occlusion is short, fully organized, and firm, thrombus surrounded by hard plaque tissue may be impossible to recanalize, or impossible to dilate, if perforated.[106]

## Vein Graft Lesions

Generally, plaques in vein grafts are larger, softer, and much more friable than are plaques in native

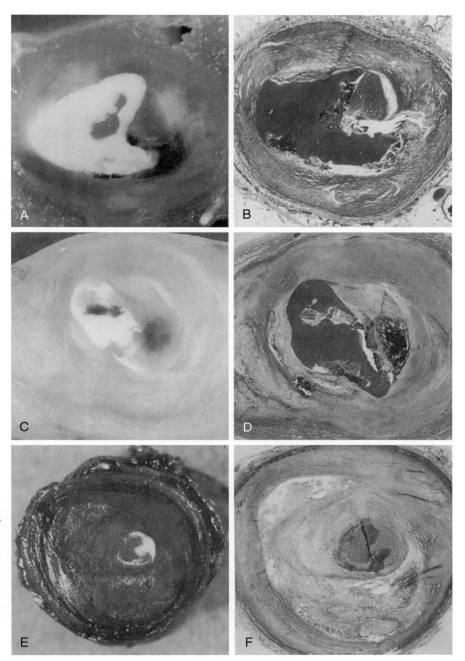

FIGURE 3–10. Unstable lesions. *A* and *B,* Ruptured plaque with missing atheromatous plaque material, plaque hemorrhage, and nonoccluding luminal thrombus (see Fig. 3–9*A*). The thrombus is white macroscopically *(A)* and platelet-rich microscopically *(B)*. *C* and *D,* Predominantly hard plaque with a rather small pool of soft lipid superficially in the plaque. The covering fibrous cap is ruptured, giving rise to hemorrhage into the lipid pool and nonoccluding luminal thrombosis (see Fig. 3–9*B*). *E* and *F,* Atherosclerotic stenosis with a small plaque rupture (not represented in these sections) and nonoccluding thrombus within the severely stenotic lumen (see Fig. 3–9*C*). The macroscopic section *(E)* has been stained with Oil Red O.

coronary arteries.[73, 74, 111] Consequently, vein graft plaques are particularly vulnerable and may easily disrupt either spontaneously or during intervention/manipulation, with high risk of life-threatening atheroembolization[111]—a fact realized for years by pathologists, as well as by cardiac surgeons.[73, 112] Lesion-associated thrombus seems to increase the complication and recurrence rate.[113]

## CONCLUSION

The natural progression of coronary atherosclerosis, particularly the risk of experiencing a rupture/

thrombus-related heart attack, and the result of interventional procedures depend primarily on lesion-related characteristics (i.e., plaque composition). Plaque size is not a good indicator of plaque vulnerability and rupture risk, illustrated by the fact that most acute heart attacks represent rapid progression of mild or moderate stenoses, which frequently are not the most severe stenoses present in these patients. Therefore, catheter-based interventions targeting the most severe stenoses only cannot stand alone. To prevent rupture/thrombus-related acute heart attacks, therapy needs to address the entire coronary tree ("systemic" intervention) to retard disease progression. High-resolution vascular imaging techniques may in the future be useful in assessing coronary lesion morphology, particularly to help identify the soft rupture-prone (high-risk) lesions and the complicated rapidly evolving plaques, thereby guiding catheter-based vascular interventions and choice of the most appropriate systemic therapy for the individual patient.

## ACKNOWLEDGMENTS

For assistance in preparing this article, we want to thank secretary Lis Schmidt, histotechnician Marianne Brosbøl, the photographers Doris Petersen and Inge Ravn, and illustrator Margrethe Krog Hansen.

## REFERENCES

1. Ellis SG, Roubin GS, King SB, et al: Angiographic and clinical predictors of acute closure after native vessel coronary angioplasty. Circulation 77:372, 1988.
2. Fisch C, DeSanctis RW, Dodge HT, et al: Guidelines for percutaneous transluminal coronary angioplasty: A report of the American College of Cardiology/American Heart Association Task Force on Assessment of Diagnostic and Therapeutic Cardiovascular Procedures (Subcommittee on Percutaneous Transluminal Coronary Angioplasty). Circulation 78:486, 1988.
3. Ryan TJ, Klocke FJ, Reynolds WA: Clinical competence in percutaneous transluminal coronary angioplasty: A statement for physicians from the ACP/ACC/AHA Task Force on Clinical Privileges in Cardiology. Circulation 81:2041, 1990.
4. Ellis SG, Vandormael MG, Cowley MJ, et al: Coronary morphologic and clinical determinants of procedural outcome with angioplasty for multivessel coronary disease: Implications for patient selection. Circulation 82:1193, 1990.
5. Savage MP, Goldberg S, Hirshfeld JW, et al: Clinical and angiographic determinants of primary coronary angioplasty success. J Am Coll Cardiol 17:22, 1991.
6. Hirshfeld JW, Schwartz S, Jugo R, et al: Restenosis after coronary angioplasty: A multivariate statistical model to relate lesion and procedure variables to restenosis. J Am Coll Cardiol 18:647, 1991.
7. Becker AE: Coronary morphology in unstable angina. In Bleifeld W, Hamm CW, Braunwald E (eds): Unstable Angina, p 52. New York: Springer-Verlag, 1990.
8. Hangartner JRW, Charleston AJ, Davies MJ, et al: Morphological characteristics of clinically significant coronary artery stenosis in stable angina. Br Heart J 56:501, 1986.
9. Vlodaver Z, Edwards JE: Pathology of coronary atherosclerosis. Prog Cardiovasc Dis 14:256, 1971.
10. Baroldi G: Diseases of the coronary arteries. In Silver MD (ed): Cardiovascular Pathology, vol 1, p VII:317. New York: Churchill Livingstone, 1983.
11. Glagov S, Zarins C, Giddens DP, et al: Hemodynamics and atherosclerosis: Insights and perspectives gained from studies of human arteries. Arch Pathol Lab Med 112:1018, 1988.
12. Fox B, James K, Morgan B, et al: Distribution of fatty and fibrous plaques in young human coronary arteries. Atherosclerosis 41:337, 1982.
13. Grøttum P, Svindland A, Walløe L: Localization of atherosclerotic lesions in the bifurcation of the main left coronary artery. Atherosclerosis 47:55, 1983.
14. Sabbah HN, Khaja F, Hawkins ET, et al: Relation of atherosclerosis to arterial wall shear in the left anterior descending coronary artery of man. Am Heart J 112:453, 1986.
15. Ishii T, Hosoda Y: The significance of myocardial bridge upon atherosclerosis in the left anterior descending coronary artery. J Pathol 148:279, 1986.
16. Bulkley BH, Roberts WC: Atherosclerotic narrowing of the left main coronary artery: A necropsy analysis of 152 patients with fatal coronary heart disease and varying degrees of left main narrowing. Circulation 53:823, 1976.
17. Topaz O, Warner M, Lanter P, et al: Isolated significant left main coronary artery stenosis: Angiographic, hemodynamic, and clinical findings in 16 patients. Am Heart J 122:1308, 1991.
18. Stewart JT, Ward DE, Davies MJ, et al: Isolated coronary ostial stenosis: Observations on the pathology. Eur Heart J 8:917, 1987.
19. Roberts WC, Ferrans VJ, Levy RI, et al: Cardiovascular pathology in hyperlipoproteinemia: Anatomic observations in 42 necropsy patients with normal or abnormal serum lipoprotein patterns. Am J Cardiol 31:557, 1973.
20. Roberts WC: Diffuse extent of coronary atherosclerosis in fatal coronary artery disease. Am J Cardiol 65:2F, 1990.
21. Glagov S, Weisenberg E, Christopher BA, et al: Compensatory enlargement of human atherosclerotic coronary arteries. N Engl J Med 316:1371, 1987.
22. Zarins CK, Weisenberg E, Kolettis G, et al: Differential enlargement of artery segments in response to enlarging atherosclerotic plaques. J Vasc Surg 7:386, 1988.
23. Stiel GM, Stiel LSG, Schofer J, et al: Impact of compensatory enlargement of atherosclerotic coronary arteries on angiographic assessment of coronary artery disease. Circulation 80:1603, 1989.
24. McPherson DD, Hiratzka LF, Lamberth WC, et al: Delineation of the extent of coronary atherosclerosis by high-frequency epicardial echocardiography. N Engl J Med 316:304, 1987.
25. Tobis JM, Mallery J, Mahon D, et al: Intravascular ultrasound imaging of human coronary arteries in vivo: Analysis of tissue characterizations with comparison to in vitro histological specimens. Circulation 83:913, 1991.
26. Haimovici H: Patterns of arteriosclerotic lesions of the lower extremity. Arch Surg 95:918, 1967.
27. Waller BF, Palumbo PJ, Lie JT, et al: Status of the coronary arteries at necropsy in diabetes mellitus with onset after age 30 years: Analysis of 229 diabetic patients with and without clinical evidence of coronary heart disease and comparison to 183 control subjects. Am J Med 69:498, 1980.
28. Vigorita VJ, Moore GW, Hutchins GM: Absence of correlation between coronary arterial atherosclerosis and severity or duration of diabetes mellitus of adult onset. Am J Cardiol 46:535, 1980.
29. Virmani R, Robinowitz M, Atkinson JB, et al: Acquired coronary arterial aneurysms: An autopsy study of 52 patients. Hum Pathol 17:575, 1986.
30. Robinson FC: Aneurysms of the coronary arteries. Am Heart J 109:129, 1985.
31. Tunick PA, Slater J, Kronzon I, et al: Discrete atherosclerotic coronary artery aneurysms: A study of 20 patients. J Am Coll Cardiol 15:279, 1990.
32. Freudenberg H, Lichtlen PR: Das normale Wandsegment bei Koronarstenosen—eine postmortale Studie. Z Kardiol 70:863, 1981.
33. Thomas AC, Davies MJ, Dilly S, et al: Potential errors in the estimation of coronary arterial stenosis from clinical arteriography with reference to the shape of the coronary arterial lumen. Br Heart J 55:129, 1986.
34. Waller BF: The eccentric coronary atherosclerotic plaque: Morphologic observations and clinical relevance. Clin Cardiol 12:14, 1989.
35. Isner JM, Donaldson RF, Fortin AH, et al: Attenuation of the media of coronary arteries in advanced atherosclerosis. Am J Cardiol 58:937, 1986.
36. Quyyumi AA, Al-rufaie HK, Olsen EGJ, et al: Coronary anatomy in patients with various manifestations of three vessel coronary artery disease. Br Heart J 54:362, 1985.
37. Kaski JC, Tousoulis D, Haider AW, et al: Reactivity of eccentric and concentric coronary stenoses in patients with chronic stable angina. J Am Coll Cardiol 17:627, 1991.
38. Lichtlen PR, Rafflenbeul W, Freudenberg H: Patho-anatomy and function of coronary obstructions leading to unstable angina pectoris, anatomical and angiographic studies. In Hugenholtz PG, Goldman BS (eds): Unstable Angina. Cur-

rent Concepts and Management, p 81. New York: Schattauer, 1985.

39. Nissen SE, Gurley JC, Grines CL, et al: Intravascular ultrasound assessment of lumen size and wall morphology in normal subjects and patients with coronary artery disease. Circulation 84:1087, 1991.

40. Gertz SD, Malekzadeh S, Dollar AL, et al: Composition of atherosclerotic plaques in the four major epicardial coronary arteries in patients ≥90 years of age. Am J Cardiol 67:1228, 1991.

41. Blankenhorn DH: Coronary arterial calcification: A review. Am J Med Sci 242:41, 1961.

42. Editorial: Ultrafest CT for coronary calcification. Lancet 1:1449, 1991.

43. Oliver MF, Samuel E, Morley P, et al: Detection of coronary-artery calcification during life. Lancet 1:891, 1964.

44. Crawford T, Dexter D, Teare RD: Coronary-artery pathology in sudden death from myocardial ischaemia. Lancet 1:181, 1961.

45. Roberts WC: The coronary arteries in fatal coronary events. *In* Chung EK (ed): Controversy in Cardiology. The Practical Clinical Approach, p 1. New York: Springer-Verlag, 1976.

46. Lachman AS, Spray TL, Kerwin DM, et al: Medial calcinosis of Mönckeberg: A review of the problem and a description of a patient with involvement of peripheral, visceral and coronary arteries. Am J Med 63:615, 1977.

47. Roberts WC, Waller BF: Effect of chronic hypercalcemia on the heart: An analysis of 18 necropsy patients. Am J Med 71:371, 1981.

48. Falk E: Coronary thrombosis: Pathogenesis and clinical manifestations. Am J Cardiol 68:28B, 1991.

49. Richardson PD, Davies MJ, Born GVR: Influence of plaque configuration and stress distribution on fissuring of coronary atherosclerotic plaques. Lancet 2:941, 1989.

50. Barger AC, Beeuwkes R, Lainey LL, et al: Hypothesis: Vasa vasorum and neovascularization of human coronary arteries: A possible role in the pathophysiology of atherosclerosis. N Engl J Med 310:175, 1984.

51. Davies MJ, Thomas A: Thrombosis and acute coronary-artery lesions in sudden cardiac ischemic death. N Engl J Med 30:1137, 1984.

52. Little WC: Angiographic assessment of the culprit coronary artery lesion before acute myocardial infarction. Am J Cardiol 66:44G, 1990.

53. Davies MJ, Bland JM, Hangartner JRW, et al: Factors influencing the presence or absence of acute coronary artery thrombi in sudden ischaemic death. Eur Heart J 10:203, 1989.

54. Falk E: Plaque rupture with severe pre-existing stenosis precipitating coronary thrombosis: Characteristics of coronary atherosclerotic plaques underlying fatal occlusive thrombi. Br Heart J 50:127, 1983.

55. el Fawal MA, Berg GA, Wheatley DJ, et al: Sudden coronary death in Glasgow: Nature and frequency of acute coronary lesions. Br Heart J 57:329, 1987.

56. Falk E: Why do plaques rupture? Circulation 86:III-30, 1992.

57. Davies MJ, Thomas AC: Plaque fissuring—The cause of acute myocardial infarction, sudden ischaemic death, and crescendo angina. Br Heart J 53:363, 1985.

58. Fulton WFM: The morphology of coronary thrombotic occlusions relevant to thrombolytic intervention. *In* Kaltenbach M et al (eds): Transluminal Coronary Angioplasty and Intracoronary Thrombolysis, p 244. New York: Springer-Verlag, 1982.

59. Davies MJ: A macro and micro view of coronary vascular insult in ischemic heart disease. Circulation 82(suppl II):S38, 1990.

60. Falk E: Unstable angina with fatal outcome: Dynamic coronary thrombosis leading to infarction and/or sudden death. Autopsy evidence of recurrent mural thrombosis with peripheral embolization culminating in total vascular occlusion. Circulation 71:699, 1985.

61. Davies MJ, Thomas AC, Knapman PA, et al: Intramyocardial platelet aggregation in patients with unstable angina suffering sudden ischemic cardiac death. Circulation 73:418, 1986.

62. Falk E: Dynamics in thrombus formation. Ann NY Acad Sci 667:204, 1992.

63. Ambrose JA, Hjemdahl-Monsen CE: Arteriographic anatomy and mechanisms of myocardial ischemia in unstable angina. J Am Coll Cardiol 9:1397, 1987.

64. Brown BG, Gallery CA, Badger RS, et al: Incomplete lysis of thrombus in the moderate underlying atherosclerotic lesion during intracoronary infusion of streptokinase for acute myocardial infarction: Quantitative angiographic observations. Circulation 73:653, 1986.

65. Hackett D, Davies G, Chierchia S, et al: Intermittent coronary occlusion in acute myocardial infarction: Value of combined thrombolytic and vasodilator therapy. N Engl J Med 317:1055, 1987.

66. Schlesinger MJ, Zoll PM: Incidence and localization of coronary artery occlusions. Arch Pathol 32:178, 1941.

67. Rodriguez FL, Robbins SL, Banasiewicz M: Postmortem antiographic studies on the coronary arterial circulation. Incidence and topography of occlusive coronary lesions: Relation to anatomic pattern of large coronary arteries. Am Heart J 68:490, 1964.

68. Friedman M: The coronary canalized thrombus: Provenance, structure, function, and relationship to death due to coronary artery disease. Br J Exp Pathol 48:556, 1967.

69. Hutchins GM, Bulkley BH, Miner MM, et al: Correlation of age and heart weight with tortuosity and caliber of normal human coronary arteries. Am Heart J 94:196, 1977.

70. Roberts CS, Roberts C: Cross-sectional area of the proximal portions of the three major epicardial coronary arteries in 98 necropsy patients with different coronary events. Relationship to heart weight, age, and sex. Circulation 62:953, 1980.

71. Hort W, Lichti H, Kalbfleisch H, et al: The size of human coronary arteries depending on the physiological and pathological growth of the heart, the age, the size of the supplying areas, and the degree of coronary sclerosis: A postmortem study. Virchows Arch [A] 397:37, 1982.

72. Leung WH, Stadius ML, Alderman EL: Determinants of normal coronary artery dimensions in humans. Circulation 84:2294, 1991.

73. Smith SH, Geer JC: Morphology of saphenous vein-coronary artery bypass grafts. Arch Pathol Lab Med 107:13, 1983.

74. Kern WH, Wells WJ, Meyer BW: The pathology of surgically excised aortocoronary saphenous vein bypass grafts. Am J Surg Pathol 5:491, 1981.

75. Walts AE, Fishbein MC, Matloff JM: Thrombosed, ruptured atheromatous plaques in saphenous vein coronary artery bypass grafts: Ten years' experience. Am Heart J 114:718, 1987.

76. Neitzel GF, Barboriak JJ, Pintar K, et al: Atherosclerosis in aortocoronary bypass grafts: Morphologic study and risk factor analysis 6 to 12 years after surgery. Atherosclerosis 6:594, 1986.

77. Falk E: Fatal atherosclerosis developed in less than 4 years in aortocoronary vein graft in a hyperlipidemic patient. Acta Pathol Microbiol Immunol Scand [A] 92:73, 1984.

78. Schoen FJ: Interventional and Surgical Cardiovascular Pathology. Clinical Correlations and Basic Principles. Philadelphia: WB Saunders, 1989.

79. Sims FH, Gavin JB, Vanderwee MA: The intima of human coronary arteries. Am Heart J 118:32, 1989.

80. Sisto T, Isola J: Incidence of atherosclerosis in the internal mammary artery. Ann Thorac Surg 47:884, 1989.

81. Shelton ME, Forman MB, Virmani R, et al: A comparison of morphologic and arteriographic findings in long-term internal mammary artery and saphenous vein bypass grafts. J Am Coll Cardiol 11:297, 1988.

82. Reed DM, Maclean CJ, Hayashi T: Predictors of atherosclerosis in the Honolulu heart program. I. Biologic, dietary, and lifestyle characteristics. Am J Epidemiol 126:214, 1987.

83. Newman WP, Freedman DS, Voors AW, et al: Relation of serum lipoprotein levels and systolic blood pressure to early atherosclerosis. N Engl J Med 314:138, 1986.

84. Tanaka K, Masuda J, Imamura T, et al: A nation-wide study of atherosclerosis in infants, children and young adults in Japan. Atherosclerosis 72:143, 1988.

85. Kragel AH, Roberts WC: Composition of atherosclerotic plaques in the coronary arteries in homozygous familial hypercholesterolemia. Am Heart J 121:210, 1991.

86. Ambrose JA, Israel DH: Angiography in unstable angina. Am J Cardiol 68:78B, 1991.

87. Forrester J: Intimal disruption and coronary thrombosis: Its role in the pathogenesis of human coronary disease. Am J Cardiol 68:69B, 1991.

88. DeWood MA, Spores J, Notske R, et al: Prevalence of total coronary occlusion during the early hours of transmural myocardial infarction. N Engl J Med 303:897, 1980.

89. DeWood MA, Stifter WF, Simpson CS, et al: Coronary arteriographic findings soon after non-Q-wave myocardial infarction. N Engl J Med 315:417, 1986.

90. Mizuno K, Miyamoto A, Satomura K, et al: Angioscopic coronary macromorphology in patients with acute coronary disorders. Lancet 1:809, 1991.

91. Harrison DG, Ferguson DW, Collins SM, et al: Rethrombosis after reperfusion with streptokinase: Importance of geometry of residual lesions. Circulation 69:991, 1984.

92. Davies SW, Marchant B, Lyons JP, et al: Irregular coronary lesion morphology after thrombolysis predicts early clinical instability. J Am Coll Cardiol 18:669, 1991.

93. Ellis SG, Myler RK, King SB, et al: Causes and correlates of death after unsupported coronary angioplasty: Implications for use of angioplasty and advanced support techniques in high-risk settings. Am J Cardiol 68:1447, 1991.

94. Farb A, Virmani R, Atkinson JB, et al: Plaque morphology and pathologic changes in arteries from patients dying after coronary balloon angioplasty. J Am Coll Cardiol 16:1421, 1990.

95. Hanet C, Wijns W, Michel X, et al: Influence of balloon size and stenosis morphology on immediate and delayed elastic recoil after percutaneous transluminal coronary angioplasty. J Am Coll Cardiol 18:506, 1991.

96. Levin D, Fallon JT: Significance of the angiographic morphology of localized coronary stenoses: Histopathologic correlations. Circulation 66:316, 1982.

97. Lyon RT, Zarins CK, Lu CT, et al: Vessel, plaque, and lumen morphology after transluminal balloon angioplasty: Quantitative study in distended human arteries. Atherosclerosis 7:306, 1987.

98. Gravanis MB, Roubin GS: Histopathologic phenomena at the site of percutaneous transluminal coronary angioplasty: The problem of restenosis. Hum Pathol 20:477, 1989.

99. Ueda M, Becker AE, Fujimoto T, et al: The early phenomena of restenosis following percutaneous transluminal coronary angioplasty. Eur Heart J 12:937, 1991.

100. Colavita PG, Ideker RE, Reimer KA, et al: The spectrum of pathology associated with percutaneous transluminal coronary angioplasty during acute myocardial infarction. J Am Coll Cardiol 8:855, 1986.

101. Kohchi K, Takebayashi S, Block PC, et al: Arterial changes after percutaneous transluminal coronary angioplasty: Results at autopsy. J Am Coll Cardiol 10:592, 1987.

102. Nobuyoshi M, Kimura T, Ohishi H, et al: Restenosis after percutaneous transluminal coronary angioplasty: Pathologic observations in 20 patients. J Am Coll Cardiol 17:433, 1991.

103. de Feyter PJ, van den Brand M, Jaarman GJ, et al: Acute coronary artery occlusion during and after percutaneous transluminal coronary angioplasty: Frequency, prediction, clinical course, management, and follow-up. Circulation 83:927, 1991.

104. Waller BF, Rothbaum DA, Pinkerton CA, et al: Status of the myocardium and infarct-related coronary artery in 19 necropsy patients with acute recanalization using pharmacologic (streptokinase, r-tissue plasminogen activator), mechanical (percutaneous transluminal coronary angioplasty) or combined types of reperfusion therapy. J Am Coll Cardiol 9:785, 1987.

105. Topol EJ, Gacioch GM: Discordance in results of right coronary intervention [Letter]. Circulation 84:955, 1991.

106. Sanborn TA: Recanalization of arterial occlusions: Pathologic basis and contributing factors [Editorial]. J Am Coll Cardiol 13:1558, 1989.

107. Kaltenbach M, Vallbracht C, Hartmann A: Chronic coronary occlusions—Reopening with low speed rotational angioplasty, abstracted. Circulation 84(suppl II):S250, 1991.

108. Ruocco NA, Currier JW, Jacobs AK, et al: Experience with low-dose intracoronary recombinant tissue-type plasminogen activator for nonacute total occlusions before percutaneous transluminal coronary angioplasty. Am J Cardiol 68:1609, 1991.

109. Hartmann J, McKeever L, Teran I, et al: Prolonged infusion of urokinase for chronically occluded aortocoronary bypass grafts. Am J Cardiol 61:189, 1988.

110. Vaska KJ, Whitlow PL: Selective tissue plasminogen activator infusion for chronic total occlusions of native coronary arteries failing angioplasty, abstracted. Circulation 84(suppl II):S250, 1991.

111. Saber RS, Edwards WD, Holmes DR, et al: Balloon angioplasty of aortocoronary saphenous vein bypass grafts: A histopathologic study of six grafts from five patients, with emphasis on restenosis and embolic complications. J Am Coll Cardiol 12:1501, 1988.

112. Keon WJ, Heggtveit HA, Leduc J: Perioperative myocardial infarction caused by atheroembolism. J Thorac Cardiovasc Surg 84:849, 1982.

113. Douglas JS: Angioplasty of saphenous vein and internal mammary artery bypass grafts. In Topol EJ (ed): Textbook of Interventional Cardiology, p 327. Philadelphia: WB Saunders, 1990.

# 4

# Pathology of Various Mechanical Interventional Procedures and Devices

*Bruce F. Waller    Peter G. Anderson*

Since 1980, there has been an explosive increase in the number of techniques and devices used to treat obstructed coronary arteries. Since its introduction in 1977,[1] catheter balloon angioplasty has gained wide acceptance as a nonsurgical form of therapy for acutely and chronically obstructed coronary arteries, and this technique is the cornerstone from which newer tools and techniques have been developed. Many interventional devices are currently used or under study; their morphologic effects on ("remodeling") vessel luminal shape or obstruction can be classified into two underlying processes[2]: (1) *remodeling* ("displacing," "expanding," "attaching") and (2) *removal* ("heating," "drilling," "excising") (Tables 4–1 and 4–2). This chapter reviews acute and chronic changes of remodeling after

**TABLE 4–1.** **MORPHOLOGIC EFFECTS OF INTERVENTIONAL DEVICES USED IN TREATING OBSTRUCTED CORONARY ARTERIES: REMODELING**

Alter the coronary luminal shape or amount of coronary luminal obstruction by
- Displacing atherosclerotic plaque, thrombus, or both
  Angioplasty
    Cracking
    Breaking
    Tearing
    Splitting
  Stent placement
- Expanding the arc of disease-free wall in eccentric atherosclerotic plaques or the entire circumference in concentric plaques
  Stretching
  Angioplasty
- Attaching portions of intimal flaps or other obstructing material against adjacent walls
  Thermal balloon, pyroplasty, thermal probes
    Welding
    Gluing
    Molding

**TABLE 4–2.** **MORPHOLOGIC EFFECTS OF INTERVENTIONAL DEVICES USED IN TREATING OBSTRUCTED CORONARY ARTERIES: REMOVAL**

Alter the amount of luminal obstruction by removal of obstructing atherosclerotic plaque, thrombus, or both by:
- Healing the obstructing material
  Thermal balloons, thermal probes, lasers
    Burning
    Melting
    Baking
- Drilling through totally obstructed vessels
  Grinding
  Drilling
- Excising a portion of the obstructing material
  Atherectomy
    Shaving
    Scraping
    Cutting

balloon angioplasty and other interventional techniques.

## REMODELING

Interventional devices that remodel the coronary lumen do so by (1) displacing atherosclerotic plaque, thrombus, or both by means of "cracking," "breaking," and "splitting" (through balloon angioplasty) or (2) stent implantation (intravascular stents). The coronary lumen also can be remodeled by expanding the vessel walls by means of stretching the arc of disease-free wall in eccentric plaques[3] or stretching the entire vessel circumference in concentric plaques. Coronary luminal obstruction can be remodeled by attaching portions of intimal flaps, thrombi, or other obstruction material to adjacent vessel walls by means of welding, gluing, or molding (through balloon pyroplasty, thermal balloons, hot-tip probes) (see Table 4–1). The newest technique in remodeling involves the use of cold temperatures to alter the tissue shape and response to balloon dilation.

## REMOVING

Interventional devices that alter the degree of luminal obstruction by removal of obstructing plaque, thrombus, or both do so by (1) heating, by means of burning, vaporizing, melting, or baking the obstructing material (thermal balloons, thermal probes); (2) drilling through total luminal occlusions; or (3) excising a portion of the occluding material, by means of cutting, shaving, or scraping (atherectomy) (see Table 4–2).

## BALLOON ANGIOPLASTY

### Historical Review of Morphologic Reports

Increased experience and advances in balloon angioplasty technology have resulted in an improved primary success rate (90% to 95%) and a lowered complication rate (4% to 5%).[4] Despite the therapeutic success of coronary balloon angioplasty, the exact mechanisms by which this technique improves vessel patency remain uncertain. Acute morphologic and histologic observations in coronary arteries of patients undergoing balloon angioplasty are limited[2] but provide clues regarding the mechanisms of action.

Block and colleagues[5] initially reported "splitting" of atherosclerotic plaque in two patients undergoing balloon angioplasty. In one patient, an extension of the plaque "splitting" into the coronary media resulted in a dissecting hematoma. Waller and associates[6, 7] described morphologic and histologic observations in several patients undergoing angioplasty procedures 4 hours to 30 days before tissue examination. In each patient, an intimal crack, tear, fracture, or break was recognized, and each had variable degrees of medial penetration. The medial involvement was localized (barely penetrating the internal elastic membrane) in some patients and extensive (antegrade, retrograde, or both forms of dissection) in others (Fig. 4–1). Adventitial disruption was not observed. Waller and associates[8] reported autopsy findings in nine additional patients who had undergone balloon angioplasty procedures alone or in conjunction with thrombolytic therapy for acute myocardial infarction (AMI). Each of these patients had intimal-medial tears; the four who had undergone both thrombolytic reperfusion and balloon angioplasty had associated coronary wall and luminal hemorrhage. Mizuno and cowork-

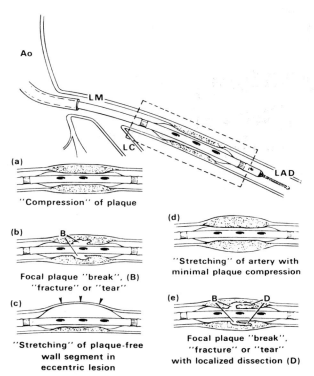

FIGURE 4–1. Diagram of five possible mechanisms of the success of coronary artery balloon angioplasty. Ao, aorta; LAD, left anterior descending artery; LC, left circumflex artery; LM, left main artery. (From Waller BF: Coronary luminal shape and the arc of disease-free wall: Morphologic observations and clinical relevance. J Am Coll Cardiol 6:1100–1101, 1985.)

ers[9] serially sectioned the balloon angioplasty site in one patient at necropsy and observed intimal and medial splitting, which led to coronary artery dissection. Soward and colleagues[10] reported plaque splitting, medial dissection, and "lifting" of the atherosclerotic plaque from the medial layer at the site of previous balloon angioplasty. La Delia and coauthors[11] described histologic findings in the left anterior descending coronary artery of a patient who had undergone angioplasty and streptokinase therapy for AMI. Atherosclerotic plaque cleavage, subintimal leukocytic infiltrations, and medial and adventitial fractures with hemorrhage were observed.

## Mechanisms

From these observations, several mechanisms of balloon angioplasty were identified (Fig. 4–2; see Fig. 4–1).

### Plaque Compression

Dotter and Judkins[12] as well as Gruentzig[13] initially attributed the success of balloon angioplasty to redistribution and compression of intimal atherosclerotic plaque. Inflation of the angioplasty balloon within an arterial stenosis was thought to compress

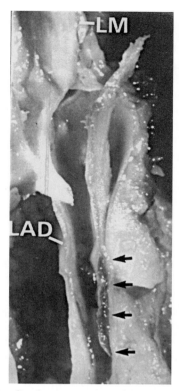

FIGURE 4–2. Localized coronary artery dissection *(arrows)* is present at the site of transluminal balloon angioplasty in the left anterior descending (LAD) coronary artery. LM, left main artery. (From Waller BF, McManus BM, Gorfinkel HJ, et al: Status of the major epicardial coronary arteries 80 to 150 days after percutaneous transluminal coronary angioplasty: Analysis of 3 necropsy patients. Am J Cardiol 51:81–84, 1983.)

atherosclerotic plaque components against the arterial wall, increasing the size of the vessel lumen. Most atherosclerotic plaque in human coronary arteries, however, is composed of dense fibrocollagenous tissue with varying amounts of calcific deposits (i.e., hard plaque) and far smaller amounts of intracellular and extracellular lipid (i.e., soft plaque). Thus, it seems unlikely that plaque compression plays a major role in dilation of human coronary arteries by balloon angioplasty. If compression were a mechanism of dilation, it would most likely occur in dilation of newly formed atherosclerotic plaque (primarily in young patients) or of recently deposited thrombus (as in saphenous vein bypass grafts).

### Plaque Fracture

Results of angioplasty in experimental models and in human vessels[2] suggest that an important mechanism of coronary angioplasty in humans is breaking, cracking, splitting, or fracturing of atherosclerotic plaque (see Figs. 4–1 and 4–2). Plaque fractures, breaks, dissection clefts, and cracks extending from the lumen for variable lengths into the plaque (inti-

mal only) improve vessel patency by creating additional channels for coronary blood flow.

### Plaque Fracture, Intimal Flaps, and Localized Medial Dissection

Waller and associates[6] described plaque fracture, intimal atherosclerotic flaps, and localized medial dissection as the major mechanisms of balloon angioplasty in human coronary arteries (see Figs. 4–1 and 4–2). Initial and persistent expansion of luminal cross-sectional area appears to require deep intimal fractures (occasionally creating intimal "flaps") with localized tears or dissection of the underlying vessel media.

### Stretching of Plaque-Free Wall Segment

An additional major mechanism of coronary artery dilation appears to be stretching of plaque-free wall segments of eccentric atherosclerotic lesions.[3, 14] Inflation of angioplasty balloons in eccentric lesions distends or stretches the normal wall segment but causes little or no damage to the plaque on the remaining portions of the arterial wall. This may result initially in an increase in coronary luminal diameter and cross-sectional area, but several days or weeks later, the gradual relaxation of this overstretched segment ("restitution of tone") reduces the coronary lumen to the predilation state. The high frequency (up to 73%) of eccentric-type coronary lesions in severely diseased vessels[3, 14] suggests that stretching of the plaque-free wall segment may be a more frequent mechanism of clinically successful coronary angioplasty than previously appreciated.

### Stretching and Compression

A fifth mechanism of balloon coronary angioplasty is the combination of vessel stretching with minimal plaque compression (see Fig. 4–1). In this situation, an oversized angioplasty balloon may stretch the entire coronary segment that is concentrically narrowed by fibrocollagenous plaque.

## Acute (Abrupt) Closure of the Angioplasty Site

Abrupt closure at the angioplasty site occurs in 2% to 6% of patients who undergo balloon angioplasty.[15–20] Clinical explanations for abrupt closure include coronary artery spasm (2%), localized thrombus (8%), and coronary dissection (34%).[19] Morphologic explanations for abrupt closure are depicted.[20] Acute vessel occlusion by a folded, curled-up, large intimal flap accounts for most of these cases. This morphologic finding may correspond to the clinical category of dissection in that a large intimal flap is created by an extensive intimal-medial dissection plane (Fig. 4–3; see Fig. 4–2). Abrupt relaxation of an overstretched disease-free wall of an eccentric plaque may also cause acute closure. Another possible mechanism for abrupt closure is coronary artery recoil or artery spasm. The coronary artery media of the disease-free wall in an eccentric plaque is functionally normal: capable of reacting to various humoral, neurogenic, or traumatic (e.g., balloon dilation) stimuli.[20–22] Balloon dilation of this eccentric lesion (Figure 9) stretches the arc of normal wall, which is conducive to acute recoil or spasm. Nonocclusive fibrin-platelet thrombus often layers the angioplasty site, but occlusive thrombus unassociated with intimal flaps at the angioplasty site is uncommon in patients who die within hours of coronary dilation.[20–22] Although thrombus may be associated with large, curled-up intimal flaps or intimal-medial flaps, the primary mechanism for abrupt closure is the tissue. Thrombus is a secondary factor. Subintimal hemorrhage as a result of traumatic balloon injury of atherosclerotic plaque is another possible cause of abrupt closure. Subintimal plaque bleeding may acutely expand the plaque and severely narrow or occlude the angioplasty site. Intraplaque and intraluminal bleeding can acutely occlude an angioplasty site, but this has been reported to occur only in patients who have undergone combined balloon angioplasty and thrombolytic therapy.[22]

Walter and associates reviewed autopsy findings in 130 patients who had undergone balloon angioplasty procedures and had abrupt or acute closure of the angioplasty site (Table 4–3; Figs. 4–4, 4–5, and 4–6; see Fig. 4–3). The patients' ages ranged from 41 to 78 years (mean, 54), and 88% were men. The vessel most commonly involved with angioplasty was the left anterior descending (LAD) artery (85%). By definition, early closure can occur up to 30 days after angioplasty. Abrupt closure occurred in 55 patients (42%) within the first day after angioplasty (see Table 4–3) and more than half of these closures occurred within the first 12 hours after angioplasty. In another 45 patients (35%), closure occurred within the first week after angioplasty. In summary, 77% of acute closures at the angioplasty site occurred within 1 week after balloon dilation. In the remaining 30 patients (23%), closure occurred 8 to 30 days after the procedure.

Morphologic bases for angioplasty site closure are depicted in Figure 4–3. The most common cause of abrupt or acute angioplasty closure was a large intimal or intimal-medial flap of tissue occluding the coronary artery lumen (see Table 4–3): 80 sites (62%). The second most common cause was recoil of a stretched eccentric lesion: 41 sites (32%). In only 7 patients (5%) were the sites occluded by thrombus (without associated intimal or intimal-medial flaps). Two patients had plaque hemorrhage and luminal thrombus, causing acute closure of the angioplasty site. Both of these patients had undergone emergency angioplasty and received thrombolytic agents in the treatment of AMI.[20]

Thrombus was also present at the sites of intimal and intimal-medial flaps, but the flap of tissue curled up within the coronary lumen was the pri-

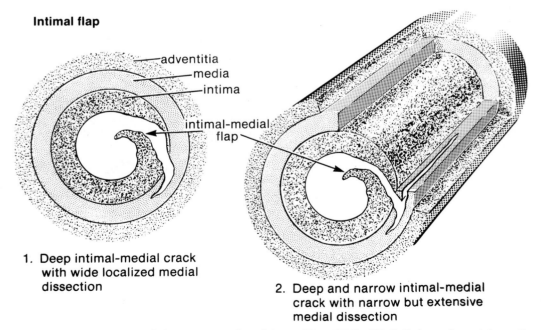

**Intimal flap**

adventitia
media
intima
intimal-medial flap

1. **Deep intimal-medial crack with wide localized medial dissection**

2. **Deep and narrow intimal-medial crack with narrow but extensive medial dissection**

FIGURE 4–3. Diagram showing intimal-medial tear creating flap of tissue. (From Waller BF: Pathology of new interventional procedures used in coronary disease. *In* Waller BF [ed]: Contemporary Issues in Cardiovascular Pathology. Philadelphia: FA Davis, 1988.)

**TABLE 4–3.    CERTAIN CLINICAL-MORPHOLOGIC OBSERVATIONS IN NECROPSY SPECIMENS FROM 130 PATIENTS WITH ACUTE CLOSURE AT THE SITE OF CORONARY BALLOON ANGIOPLASTY (PTCA) (BEFORE AVAILABILITY AND USE OF CORONARY STENTS)**

Number of patients: 130
Ages: 41–78 (M = 54)
Men-women ratio: 114 (88%): 16 (12%)
Artery of PTCA
    LAD: N = 110 (85%)
    RCA: N = 18 (14%)
    LC: N = 2 (1%)
Interval from PTCA to occlusion
  Abrupt
    0–12 hours: N = 31 (24%)
    13–23 hours: N = 24 (18%)
  Acute
    1–3 days: N = 28 (22%)
    4–7 days: N = 17 (13%)
  Early
    8–15 days: N = 12 (9%)
    16–23 days: N = 10 (8%)
    24–30 days: N = 8 (6%)
Interval from occlusion to death: 1–24 hours
Morphologic basis for closure
  Intimal flap ± thrombus: N = 4 (3%)
  Intimal-medial flap ± thrombus: N = 76 (59%)*
  Elastic recoil ("spasm") (no thrombus): N = 41 (32%)†
  Thrombus only, no flap (primary thrombus): N = 7 (5%)
  Plaque hemorrhage + luminal thrombus: N = 2 (1%)‡
Type of underlying atherosclerotic lesion
  Concentric: N = 85 (65%)
  Eccentric: N = 45 (35%)§

| Calcific deposits in plaque at site of acute PTCA closure | 0 | 1± | 2± | 3± |
|---|---|---|---|---|
| Intimal, intimal-medial flap (N = 80) | 0 | 22 | 42 | 16 |
| Elastic recoil (N = 41) | 12 | 8 | 17 | 4 |
| Thrombus only (N = 7) | 3 | 2 | 2 | 0 |
| Plaque hemorrhage and luminal thrombus (N = 2) | 1 | 0 | 1 | 0 |

LAD, left anterior descending artery; LC, left circumflex artery; MI, myocardial infarction; PTCA, percutaneous transluminal coronary angioplasty; RCA, right coronary artery.

*Includes 4 with extensive longitudinal dissection antegrade, retrograde, or both from the angioplasty site. †No intimal, internal-medial flaps, or cracks. ‡Both underwent emergency PTCA and received thrombolytic agents for acute MI. §Includes all 41 sites of elastic recoil and 4 sites of thrombus only (7c, 7d).

Data from Waller et al.[20]

mary reason for occlusion. Secondary thrombus resulted from reduced flow across the dilation site. In the 7 sites with thrombus only, no associated plaque flaps could be identified. Four of the seven sites were eccentric lesions. Acute elastic recoil (spasm) may have further precipitated acute primary thrombus formation.[20]

The type of underlying plaque at the site of acute closure was predominately concentric (65%). All of the 85 sites with concentric plaque had identifiable injuries from angioplasty. Of these lesions, 68 (85%) had 2 + or 3 + calcific deposits. In contrast, all of

the sites of abrupt closure without evidence of cracks, breaks, tears, or flaps were eccentric in nature. Of 7 primary thrombotic occlusions, 4 had underlying eccentric plaques. Of the 41 sites with elastic recoil or acute spasm, 30 (69%) had minimal (1 +) or no (0) calcific deposits (see Table 4–3).

In summary, the most common cause of acute, abrupt, or early closure at angioplasty sites is occluding intimal-medial flaps.[20]

## Treatment of Abrupt Closure

Abrupt closure has been treated with repeated balloon angioplasty and prolonged (30- to 60-minute) balloon inflation with perfusion catheters.[20, 23] Perfusion catheters are placed across the occluded angioplasty site so that arterial blood enters the catheter proximally and exits distally (see Fig. 4–6).

Newer interventional devices may also be useful in the treatment of abrupt closure (see Fig. 4–6). Thermal angioplasty balloons may be used to "seal" or "weld" large intimal flaps against the adjacent vessel wall. Pyroplasty techniques ("thermal weld-

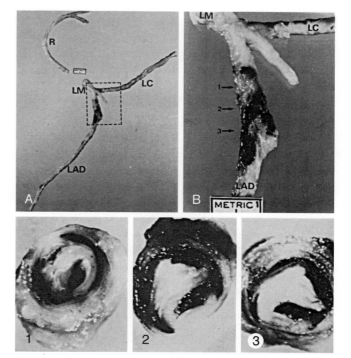

FIGURE 4–4. Composite views of artery of angioplasty *(A, B)* and cross sections through angioplasty site of acute occlusion *(1, 2, and 3)*. The patient had undergone acute angioplasty shortly after receiving a "systemic" thrombolytic agent. Acute occlusion develops as a result of plaque hemorrhage and luminal thrombus in the angioplasty "cracks." *1 to 3* are cross sections through the site of acute occlusion at zones marked 1, 2, and 3 in *B*, LAD, left anterior descending artery; LC, left circumflex artery; LM, left main artery; R, right. (From Waller BF, Rothbaum DA, Pinkerton CA, et al: Status of the myocardium and infarct-related coronary artery in 19 necropsy patients with acute recanalization using pharmacologic, mechanical or combined types of reperfusion therapy. J Am Coll Cardiol 9:785–801, 1987.)

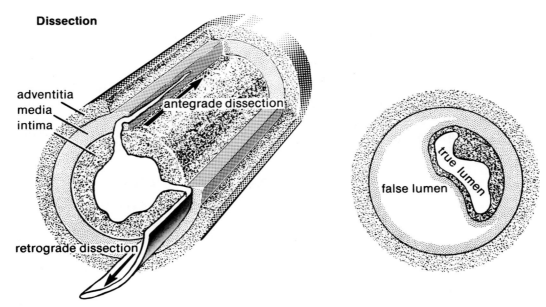

FIGURE 4–5. Diagram showing complications of intimal medial tears from angioplasty extending in an antegrade or retrograde direction within the media. A dissection channel is created in the media, closing off the true lumen. (From Waller BF: Pathology of new interventional procedures used in coronary disease. *In* Waller BF [ed]: Contemporary Issues in Cardiovascular Pathology. Philadelphia: FA Davis, 1988.)

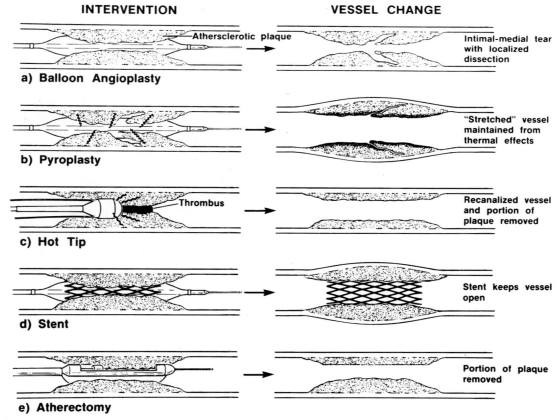

FIGURE 4–6. Diagram summarizing interventional techniques or devices or both used to treat abrupt, acute, or early closure at the balloon angioplasty site. (From Waller BF: "Crackers, breakers, stretchers, drillers, welders, melters"—The future treatment of atherosclerotic coronary artery disease? A clinical morphologic assessment. J Am Coll Cardiol 13:969–987, 1989.)

ing'') may involve the use of laser, radiofrequency, ultrasound, or chemically derived energy sources. Balloon-expandable intravascular stents have also been used to treat abrupt closure of an angioplasty site[22] (see Fig. 4–6). Intracoronary stents also offer a rapid percutaneous technique for holding the intimal-medial flap against the vessel wall permanently without the use of surgery or the extra equipment necessary for thermal angioplasty.[20]

Thermal angioplasty and stents may be used at the site of abrupt closure caused by spasm. Thermal injury to the segment of disease-free wall involved in spasm may permit long-term luminal distention. Thermal probes can be used to reopen an angioplasty site occluded by thrombus, with or without intimal flaps. Atherectomy devices can also be used to remove large intimal-medial flaps, thrombus, or both (see Fig. 4–6).

## BALLOON ANGIOPLASTY RESTENOSIS: INTIMAL PROLIFERATION AND CHRONIC ELASTIC RECOIL

Despite the widespread use of coronary balloon angioplasty, advances in angioplasty technology, improvements in operator techniques, and primary success rates of more than 90% in dilation, restenosis at the angioplasty site is the major problem limiting the long-term efficacy of this procedure. The frequency of restenosis ranges from 17% to 47%, depending on variations in definitions of restenosis: clinical, angiographic, physiologic, anatomic, and statistical.[22–31] Several studies were conducted to determine various factors that might predispose to or be associated with restenosis: (1) angiographic-hemodynamic factors (e.g., number of angioplasty sites, pre- and postdilation diameters, changes in trans-stenotic pressure gradients); (2) lesion characteristics (diffuse, long, eccentric, calcified); (3) the presence or absence of intimal flaps or dissection; (4) clinical factors (e.g., gender, presence or absence of unstable angina pectoris or of diabetes mellitus, whether patient smokes); and (5) technical factors (e.g., number, duration, and pressure of balloon inflations; ratio of balloon size to vessel size). This portion of the review describes previously reported[32] autopsy findings of clinical, morphologic, and histologic changes late (>30 days) after clinically successful coronary balloon angioplasty in 30 patients and classifies the restenosis lesions into two categories. This section also reviews autopsy results in 41 previously reported patients with coronary angioplasty restenosis lesions.[33–37]

Thirty patients had undergone previous coronary balloon angioplasty (Table 4–4). The dilation procedures were clinically successful in that symptoms

of myocardial ischemia were relieved and final angiographic diameter reduction at the angioplasty site was 30% or less (ranging from "luminal irregularities" to 30% narrowing). The interval from balloon angioplasty to morphologic examination at autopsy ranged from 1.6 months to 24.1 months (average 11.7 months). Restenosis occurred in 17 patients within 12 months of angioplasty and in 12 patients between 12 and 24 months after angioplasty; 1 patient was studied at 24.1 months. Clinical symptoms of restenosis occurred in 23 (77%); 5 patients (17%) had no clinical evidence of restenosis. Patients with clinical evidence of restenosis died sooner (8.2 months) after angioplasty than did those without clinical symptoms (14.5 months; $p < 0.05$).

### Medications after Angioplasty

Each of the 20 patients had had some type of pharmacologic therapy after angioplasty: nitrates, β blockers, calcium channel blockers, aspirin, dipyridamole, warfarin, or steroids. Five patients had used aspirin alone; the remaining 23 patients had used two or more drugs. No specific correlation existed between the interval before restenosis and the type of pharmacologic therapy employed. Two patients were treated with warfarin, and one patient received a course of prednisone (10 mg/day) tapering over 1 month.

### Mode of Death

Of the 30 patients, 22 (73%) had a cardiac mode of death: 2 (6%) had recurrent angina and subsequent fatal AMI; 9 (30%) had sudden coronary death (4 with preceding angina); and 11 (37%) had recurrent angina, underwent coronary artery bypass surgery, and died shortly thereafter. The remaining 8 (27%) patients had noncardiac causes of death: 3 died of neoplastic disease, 4 died in automobile accidents, and 1 had a fatal stroke. Of the 8 patients with noncardiac causes of death, 5 had no clinical evidence of myocardial ischemia, and 3 had recurrent angina pectoris.

### Autopsy Data

Of the 30 angioplasty-subjected coronary arteries examined, 18 (60%) showed gross evidence of the angioplasty sites, all of which had "whitish" material on the luminal surface corresponding to intimal proliferation. In the remaining 12 (40%) arteries, no gross evidence of previous angioplasty was identified. These angioplasty sites appeared as typical atherosclerotic plaques. Of the 30 balloon angioplasty sites, 15 (50%) were concentric and 15 (50%) were eccentric. Correlation of the interval before restenosis with the type of lumen disclosed no significant

**TABLE 4–4.** **SUMMARY OF CLINICAL AND MORPHOLOGIC FEATURES OF 10 ADDITIONAL AUTOPSY SPECIMENS FROM PATIENTS DYING LATE (>30 DAYS) AFTER CLINICALLY SUCCESSFUL BALLOON ANGIOPLASTY (PTCA)**

| | PATIENT | | | | | | | | | |
|---|---|---|---|---|---|---|---|---|---|---|
| FEATURE | 1 | 2 | 3 | 4 | 5 | 6 | 7 | 8 | 9 | 10 |
| Age (y), gender | 48, M | 53, M | 42, M | 55, M | 42, M | 48, F | 40, M | 56, M | 39, M | 51, M |
| Interval from PTCA to death (months) | 3.8 | 5.8 | 7.5 | 15.3 | 18.2 | 21.5 | 16.5 | 19.2 | 22.5 | 20.5 |
| Artery of PTCA | LAD | LAD | LAD | RCA | LAD | LAD | LAD | RCA | LAD | LAD |
| Clinical restenosis: Symptoms | | | | | | | | | | |
| Angina | Present | Present | Present | Present | Present | Present | 0 | Present | Present | Present |
| AMI | 0 | 0 | Present | 0 | 0 | 0 | 0 | 0 | 0 | 0 |
| SCD | 0 | 0 | 0 | 0 | 0 | Present | 0 | Present | Present | 0 |
| Mode of Death Cardiac | | | | | | | | | | |
| AMI | 0 | 0 | 0 | 0 | 0 | 0 | 0 | 0 | 0 | 0 |
| SCD | 0 | 0 | 0 | 0 | 0 | Present | 0 | Present | Present | 0 |
| AP+CABG | Present | Present | Present | Present | 0 | 0 | 0 | 0 | 0 | Present |
| Noncardiac | 0 | 0 | 0 | 0 | Present | 0 | Present | 0 | 0 | 0 |
| Auto Accident | | | | | Present | 0 | Present | 0 | | 0 |
| Type of coronary artery in women | C | E | E | C | E | C | C | E | E | C |
| Type of lesion | | | | | | | | | | |
| IP | Present | 0 | Present | Present | 0 | Present | Present | 0 | 0 | Present |
| AP | 0 | Present | 0 | 0 | Present | 0 | 0 | Present | Present | 0 |
| Evidence PTCA | Present | 0 | 0 | Present | 0 | Present | Present | 0 | 0 | Present |
| Restenosis mechanism | | | | | | | | | | |
| a) SMP | Present | 0 | Present | Present | 0 | Present | Present | 0 | 0 | Present |
| b) ER | 0 | Present | 0 | 0 | Present | 0 | 0 | Present | Present | 0 |

AMI, acute myocardial infarction; AP+CABG, angina pectoris plus coronary artery bypass grafting; C, concentric; E, eccentric; ER, elastic (chronic) recoil; F, female; LAD, left anterior descending artery; M, male; PTCA, percutaneous transluminal coronary angioplasty; RCA, right coronary artery; SCD, sudden coronary death; SMP, smooth muscle proliferation.

difference in the timing of restenosis: for concentric lesions, the interval was 8 to 20 months (average, 8.4); for eccentric lesions, 2.2 to 24 months (average, 8.5). Comparison of various intervals before restenosis also failed to disclose significant differences between concentric and eccentric plaques: less than 6 months: 1.6 to 5.0 months (average, 3.7) and 2.0 to 5.5 months (average, 3.9); 6 to 12 months: 6.8 months and 7.4 months; and more than 12 months: 17.2 to 20 months (average, 18.2) and 12.1 to 24.1 months (average 16.9), respectively. Thus, the intervals before restenosis were similar for eccentric and concentric lesions. Restenosis in eccentric lesions was similar in frequency regardless of whether the interval before restenosis was shorter than 6 months or longer than 1 year after balloon angioplasty.

## Type of Lesion at the Restenosis Site

Histologic analysis of the angioplasty sites disclosed that intimal proliferation was responsible for the restenosis in 18 patients (60%) (Figs. 4–7 and 4–8). Of the 18 sites with intimal proliferation, 14 (78%) had some evidence of previous intimal or intimal-medial tears, cracks, or breaks. Histologic analysis of the remaining 12 (40%) angioplasty sites disclosed typical atherosclerotic plaques (Fig. 4–9). Of these

12 sites, 10 had eccentric atherosclerotic lesions with a variable arc of disease-free or nearly disease-free wall (see Fig. 4–9). None of these 12 sites had evidence of previous angioplasty injury (crack, break, tear) or healed modification of previous injury. The atherosclerotic plaque was uniformly consistent without histologic evidence of a new, immature luminal layer. The plaque was uniformly densely fibrotic with occasional calcific deposits. Thus, no evidence of new or accelerated atherosclerotic plaque was observed in these 12 angioplasty sites. The arc of disease-free wall contained medial layers of normal thickness without evidence of scarring or atrophy.

## Clinical Pathologic Correlations

Morphologic and histologic observations at the angioplasty restenosis sites enable classification of the lesions into two distinct subgroups: (1) intimal proliferation with or without evidence of healed angioplasty injury (see Figs. 4–7 to 4–9) and (2) atherosclerotic plaques without evidence of previous balloon injury.

### Intimal Proliferation

In the study reported by Waller and associates,[32] 60% of restenosis angioplasty lesions had intimal

FIGURE 4–7. Sites of coronary angioplasty restenosis in four patients. *A,* No morphologic evidence of previous balloon angioplasty and no intimal fibrous proliferation (IFP) 150 days after successful balloon angioplasty. Note the eccentric lumen (L). AP, atherosclerotic plaque. Movat stain, ×10. *B,* IFP at 6.8 months. Minimal IFP coats a previously minimally dilated vessel with superficial intimal injury only. Elastic trichrome stain, ×10. *C,* IFP at 17.2 months in a patient with sudden coronary death as the first manifestation of angioplasty restenosis. Elastic trichrome stain, ×10. *D,* IFP with focal calcific deposits and lipid accumulation 24.1 months after successful balloon angioplasty. The patient died of gastrointestinal cancer. Elastic trichrome stain, ×10. (From Waller BF, Pinkerton CA, Orr CM, et al: Morphologic observations late [>30 days] after clinically successful coronary balloon angioplasty: An analysis of 20 necropsy patients and literature review of 41 necropsy patients with coronary angioplasty restenosis. Circulation [suppl I]:28–41, 1991.)

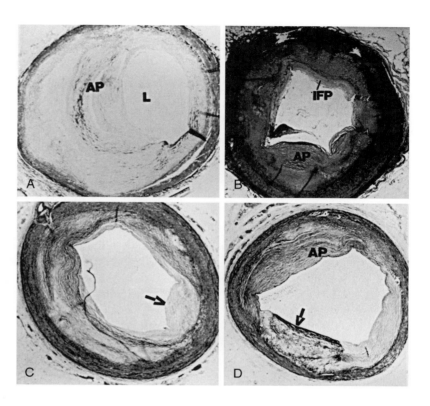

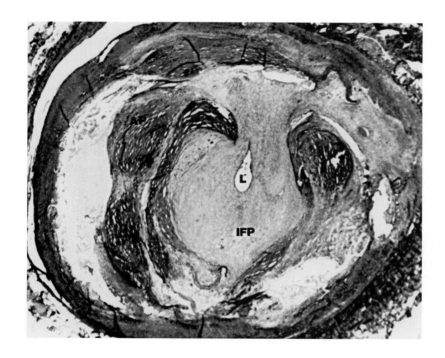

FIGURE 4–8. Intimal fibrous proliferation (IFP) of the left anterior descending artery "coating" underlying atherosclerotic plaque (AP) 4.5 months after balloon angioplasty. L, lumen. (From Waller BF, Pinkerton CA, Foster LN: Morphologic evidence of accelerated left main coronary artery disease: A late complication of percutaneous transluminal angioplasty of the proximal left anterior descending coronary artery. J Am Coll Cardiol 9:1019–1023, 1987.)

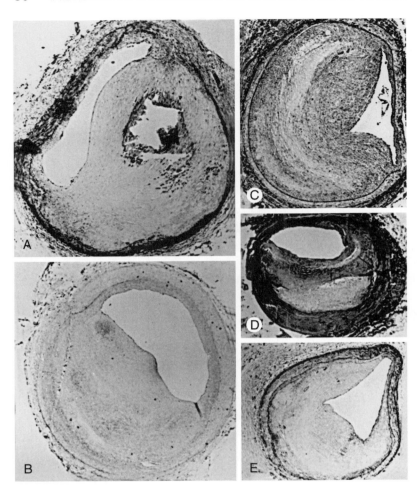

FIGURE 4–9. Sites of previous balloon angioplasty show no intimal fibrous proliferation and no evidence of previous balloon injury (cracks, breaks, or tears) or healed version. Instead, each is an eccentric atherosclerotic plaque (AP) with a variable arc of disease-free or nearly disease-free wall *(small arrows)*. Elastic recoil of the overstretched eccentric wall is the likely mechanism of restenosis in these patients. Note that the medial thickness *(arrows)* is normal in the eccentric wall. The patients whose sites are shown in *B, C,* and *E* had clinical symptoms of restenosis. *A* to *E:* elastic trichrome stains, ×10. (From Waller BF, Pinkerton CA, Orr CM, et al: Morphologic observations late [>30 days] after clinically successful coronary balloon angioplasty: An analysis of 20 necropsy patients and literature review of 41 necropsy patients with coronary angioplasty restenosis. Circulation [suppl I]:28–41, 1991.)

proliferation. Histologic features of the proliferation were similar despite differences in the interval before restenosis (short vs. long), the type of postangioplasty medical therapy (nitrates vs. blockers vs. aspirin), the artery subjected to angioplasty, the presence or absence of recurrent myocardial ischemia, and the mode of death (cardiac vs. noncardiac). The amount of proliferation tissue appeared greater in lesions with evidence of previous intimal-medial angioplasty injury than in lesions with only intimal injury. The most widely accepted theory about the development of intimal proliferation involves responses from damaged vessel endothelium and media (Figs. 4–10 to 4–12; see Figs. 4–7 to 4–9).[11, 26–28, 31] Components with a major role in this response appear to be smooth muscle cells in the media, diseased intima, and platelets. With plaque disruption, localized deposition of platelets occurs with subsequent release of thromboxane $A_2$, further platelet deposition, and subsequent release of growth factors such as platelet-derived growth factor. Vessel endothelium also releases various growth factors such as endothelial and fibroblast growth factors. This process appears to result in migration, proliferation, and alteration of the vessel wall smooth muscle

cells with fibrocellular tissue accumulation (see Figs. 4–10 to 4–12).

A review of previously published reports describing late findings after coronary balloon angioplasty[33–37, 40–49] (Table 4–5) described 41 patients with 44 lesions examined at autopsy. In 29 lesions (69%), the angioplasty site contained various amounts of intimal proliferation. The interval from angioplasty to death ranged from 2 to 9 months (see Table 4–5).

## Atherosclerotic Plaques Without Intimal Proliferation

In the study by Waller and associates,[32] eight (40%) restenosis angioplasty sites had only atherosclerotic plaques, without superimposed intimal fibrocellular proliferation, without evidence of previous angioplasty injury, and without evidence of newly developing atherosclerotic plaque. Of the 12 patients in this subgroup, 7 had clinical evidence of myocardial ischemia. Of the 12 late angioplasty lesions, 10 were eccentric and 2 were concentric. The arc of disease-free wall in 6 eccentric lesions had histologically normal-appearing media without atrophy and with-

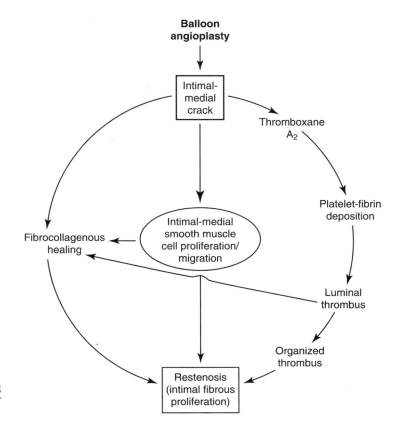

FIGURE 4–10. Diagram depicting current understanding of development of intimal-medial cell proliferation after balloon angioplasty.

out scarring. In contrast, the media of the diseased wall segments were atrophied and focally scarred. This observation suggests that disease-free wall segments may be dynamic segments reacting to various mechanical, neurogenic, or vasoactive stimuli (i.e., capable of stretch and elastic recoil) (Figs. 4–13 and 4–14).

**TABLE 4–5. SUMMARY OF CLINICAL AND AUTOPSY FEATURES OF PREVIOUSLY REPORTED PATIENTS (1979–1989) WITH RESTENOSIS LATE (>30 DAYS) AFTER CORONARY BALLOON ANGIOPLASTY**

| | |
|---|---|
| Number of studies (references 30–44) | 15 |
| Number of patients | 41 |
| Number of coronary sites | 44 |
| Ages (years) [mean] | 33–72 |
| Artery of restenosis | |
|    Left anterior descending | 68% |
|    Right coronary | 1% |
|    Left circumflex | 1% |
| Diagonal | 3% |
|    Left main | 3% |
| Lumen type (11/44 sites) | |
|    Concentric | 2/11 |
|    Eccentric | 9/11 |
| Changes at angioplasty site | |
|    Intimal proliferation | 69% |
|    Atherosclerotic plaques only | 31% |

The absence of morphologic signs of previous dilation injury or intimal proliferation tissue in this subgroup of patients who had previously undergone dilation can be explained in at least two ways: (1) stretching of diseased wall (concentric lesions) or disease-free wall (eccentric lesions) during the initial procedure with subsequent chronic elastic recoil (restenosis) (see Figs. 4–13 and 4–14) and (2) progression of atherosclerotic disease ("accelerated atherosclerosis"). Waller and associates[32] were among the first investigators to suggest that gradual (chronic) elastic recoil of overstretched vessel walls may represent an important subgroup of restenosis lesions after balloon angioplasty (see Figs. 4–13 and 4–14).

In reviews of results of autopsies on previously reported patients with late coronary balloon angioplasty sites, about one third of the sites were described as showing only atherosclerotic plaque (see Table 4–5). The specific type of coronary lumen was not described in most of these studies.[33–37, 40–49]

Although acute elastic recoil shortly after balloon angioplasty is a generally well-recognized mechanism of abrupt narrowing, chronic elastic recoil as a mechanism of late luminal narrowing is not well appreciated. Possible explanations for chronic recoil of overstretched eccentric segments involve recovery from temporary or permanent injury to medial smooth muscle cells (see Figs. 4–13 and 4–14).

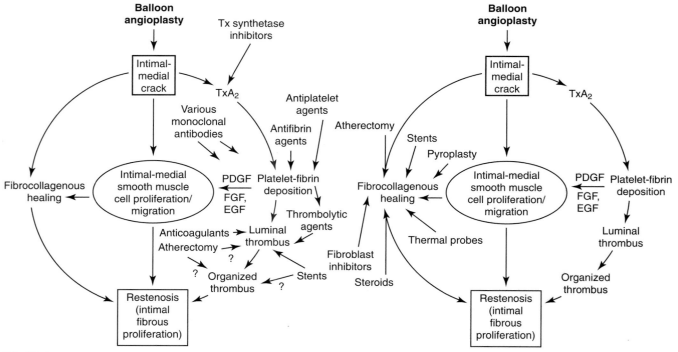

FIGURE 4–11. Development of intimal-medial cell proliferation with various interventional agents or devices focusing on the area of platelet-fibrin deposition *(left)* and fibrocellular healing phase *(right)*. EGF, endothelial cell–derived growth factor; FGF, fibroblast growth factor; PDGF, platelet-derived growth factor; Tx, thromboxane; TxA$_2$, thromboxane A$_2$.

Smooth muscle cells that are temporarily dysfunctional ("stunned") over a period of weeks to months may eventually regain their function, thereby setting the stage for late recoil. However, acute injury of the smooth muscle cells during dilation may result eventually in replacement rather than repair of these cells. Replacement with normally functioning smooth muscle cells over a period of weeks to months may allow recoil at a late basis.

The absence at autopsy of morphologic signs of previous balloon angioplasty in patients with restenosis also may be interpreted as indicating acceleration or progression of underlying atherosclerotic plaque.[50, 51] Two histologic features in the present study indicated that this is an unlikely explanation: (1) the atherosclerotic plaque is densely fibrotic with focal calcific deposits, indicating mature atherosclerotic lesions, and (2) the inner (luminal) layers of the atherosclerotic plaque are histologically similar to the outer layers of the plaque (i.e., no evidence of new vs. old plaque). It is conceivable that many months or years after balloon angioplasty, intimal proliferation tissue changes, converts, or degenerates to typical atherosclerotic plaque by incorporation of lipid. In the two oldest restenosis lesions, calcific deposits were noted in the intimal proliferation tissue. In one case, lipid accumulation had occurred. It is possible that mural thrombus becomes incorporated into the underlying plaque and later changes to atherosclerosis.

## Confirmation of Autopsy Restenosis Findings in the Living Patient with Angioplasty Restenosis

An interventional device used in the treatment of obstructed coronary arteries is the Simpson atherectomy device (DVI). This device alters luminal obstruction by removing obstructing material.[2] The atherectomy device has frequently been used to treat balloon angioplasty restenosis lesions. Tissue removed from angioplasty restenosis sites belongs to three categories[52]: (1) intimal proliferation (with or without thrombus), (2) atherosclerotic plaque with or without thrombus, and (3) thrombus only. The intimal proliferation tissue removed in the living patient is grossly and histologically identical to autopsy specimens of angioplasty restenosis tissue. Excised tissue from restenosis lesions consisting of only atherosclerotic plaque may correlate with the second groups of restenosis lesions described at autopsy: eccentric or concentric atherosclerotic lesions without intimal proliferation. The initial angioplasty mechanism in this instance would be inadequate or superficial dilation of the lesion, eccentric or concentric vessel wall stretching, or both. Thus, atherectomy samples obtained from living patients with angioplasty restenosis are identical to restenosis tissue obtained at autopsy (Fig. 4–15). The frequency of intimal proliferation samples obtained from atherectomy coronary restenosis sites is

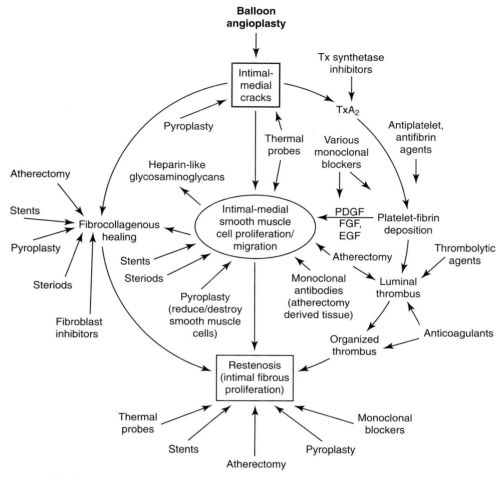

FIGURE 4–12. Diagram of development of intimal-medial cell proliferation with multiple areas of mechanical, pharmacologic, and immunologic (or combinations) intervention in the areas of smooth muscle migration, fibrin-platelet deposition, and fibrocollagenous healing. EGF, endothelial cell–derived growth factor; FGF, fibroblast growth factor; PDGF, platelet-derived growth factor; Tx, thromboxane; TxA₂, thromboxane A₂.

slightly less than that reported in the autopsy study by Waller and associates.[32, 53]

## Repeat Balloon Angioplasty

Patients undergoing repeat balloon angioplasty for one or more instances of restenosis generally have a higher success rate of dilation than do patients undergoing initial dilation (91% vs. 68%,[54] 97% vs. 85%,[55] 85% vs. 61%[56]). Major angioplasty complications are generally fewer.[56–63] However, restenosis rates after repeated balloon angioplasty tend to be slightly higher than with the primary angioplasty procedure (36%,[64] 51%,[56] 26%,[57] 37%,[62]). In one study, the mean interval between repeat angioplasty and a second recurrence of stenosis was longer than the interval between initial angioplasty and first recurrence.[55] In a study by Rapold and colleagues,[54] the interval from repeat dilation to restenosis was similar to the interval between initial angioplasty and first restenosis (96% and 85% of restenoses,

respectively, occurred within 8 months after dilation). As many as five angioplasty procedures have been performed with repeated episodes of restenosis.[54–63]

Figure 4–16 and Table 4–6 indicate the mechanisms of dilation in repeated balloon angioplasty with recurring restenosis.[65] Four basic mechanisms of dilation occur with a primary dilation: intimal-medial crack (intimal-medial injury), eccentric disease-free wall stretching, superficial intimal splitting (intimal injury only), and concentric stretching without cracks. Depending on the specific cause of subsequent restenosis (intimal proliferation, elastic recoil of eccentric lesions, progression of atherosclerotic plaque, or elastic recoil of concentric vessel stretching), subsequent balloon angioplasty procedures involve mechanisms similar to those in the primary dilation. Cracking or splitting of intimal hyperplasia may occur, but concentric stretching of this concentric fibrocollagenous tissue is also a possibility. Deeper splitting of underlying or adjacent athero-

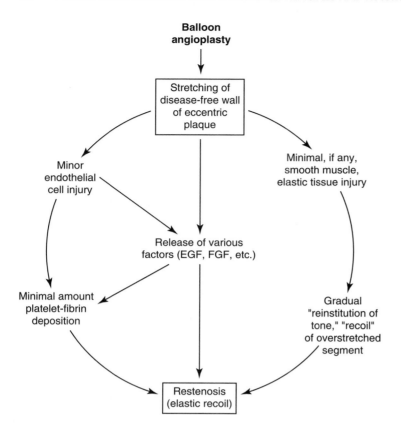

FIGURE 4–13. Diagram depicting the development of chronic elastic recoil of overstretched eccentric plaques during angioplasty. EGF, endothelial cell–derived growth factor; FGF, fibroblast growth factor.

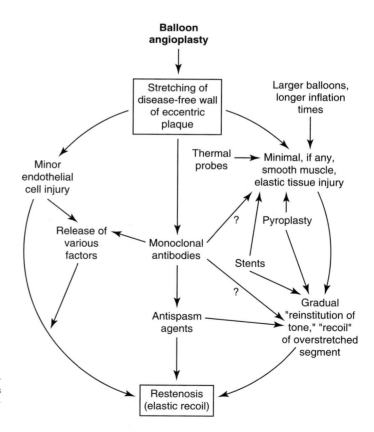

FIGURE 4–14. Diagram showing development of chronic elastic recoil (restenosis) at the site of angioplasty and various types of mechanical, pharmacologic, or immunologic intervention.

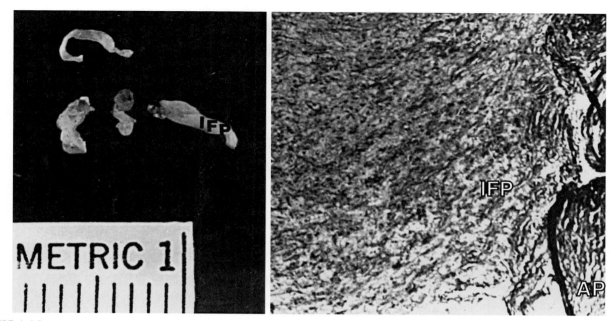

FIGURE 4–15. Coronary atherectomy specimen from a restenosis lesion in the left anterior descending artery. *Left,* The whitish material is intimal fibrous proliferation (IFP) tissue. The darker material is atherosclerotic plaque (AP). *Right,* Histologically, the IFP material is identical to that seen in autopsy specimens from patients with IFP restenosis and to that regard reported from peripheral atherectomy restenosis lesions. (From Waller BF: "Crackers, breakers, stretchers, drillers, welders, melters"—The future treatment of atherosclerotic coronary artery disease? A clinical morphologic assessment. J Am Coll Cardiol 13:969–987, 1989.)

sclerotic plaque also seems a likely mechanism of repeat dilations for restenosis. Repeated restretching of an eccentric lesion is possible (Fig. 4–16; see Table 4–6), but the formation of concentric intimal

### TABLE 4–6. POSSIBLE MECHANISMS OF DILATION IN SUBSEQUENT BALLOON ANGIOPLASTY AFTER ONE OR MORE INSTANCES OF RESTENOSIS

| CAUSE OF RESTENOSIS | MECHANISM OF ACTION |
| --- | --- |
| Intimal fibrinous proliferation (IFP) | Splitting or cracking of new IFP* |
| | Concentric stretching of restenosis lesion |
| | New or additional splitting or cracking of underlying plaque* |
| Elastic recoil of eccentric lesions | Restretching disease-free segment |
| | New splitting or cracking of underlying plaque* |
| | Splitting or cracking of new, minimal IFP* |
| Atherosclerotic plaque (superficial intimal splitting or inadequate dilation during initial angioplasty) | Deeper splitting or cracking of underlying plaque* |
| | Splitting or cracking of new IFP* |
| Elastic recoil of concentric vessel stretching | New cracking or splitting of underlying plaque* |
| | Cracking or splitting of new IFP* |
| | Restretching: concentric |

*New calcific deposits may enhance the effectiveness of redilation.

hyperplasia in this area may result in concentric stretching with or without minor cracking. New calcific deposits in underlying or adjacent atherosclerotic plaque or present in chronic intimal hyperplasia may enhance the effectiveness of redilation by promoting intimal-medial cracking.[65]

## MORPHOLOGIC CORRELATES OF CORONARY ANGIOGRAPHIC PATTERNS AT THE SITE OF PERCUTANEOUS TRANSLUMINAL CORONARY ANGIOPLASTY: ANGIOGRAPHIC-HISTOLOGIC CORRELATES OF REMODELING[66, 67]

Vessel injury at the site of balloon dilation produces a range of anatomic changes, including intimal splitting, intimal-medial splitting with localized dissection, extensive dissection, and, in rare cases, coronary artery rupture. These morphologic changes produce a range of angiographic appearances variously described as "haziness," "ground-glass," "splits," "flaps," "dissections," and "ruptures."[66, 67] To facilitate communication and evaluation of angiographic results of balloon angioplasty, Holmes and colleagues[68] provided a classification of the angiographic findings and their potential mechanisms in 100 consecutive patients. Waller[67] provided anatomic-angiographic correlations at the site of balloon angioplasty in 66 patients who had died within 30 days of coronary artery angioplasty.

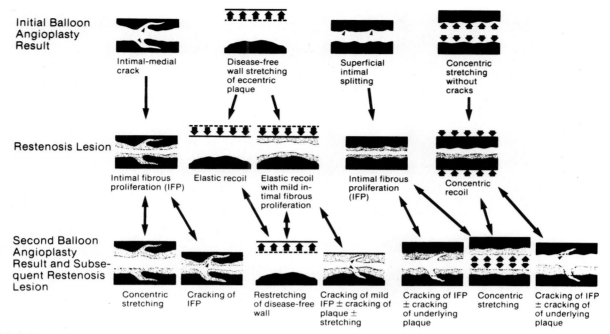

FIGURE 4–16. Possible explanations of balloon angioplasty restenosis and mechanism of subsequent successful repeat balloon angioplasty. (From Waller BF, Orr CM, Pinkerton CA, et al: Morphologic observations late after coronary balloon angioplasty; mechanisms of acute injury and relationship to restenosis. Radiology SCVIR Special Series 1991, in press.)

## Morphologic Patterns

Of the 76 coronary angioplasty sites in the 66 patients, evidence of angioplasty injury was found in 67 sites (88%) (Table 4–7): shallow, superficial intimal cracks or splits (intimal injury; 11 sites [16%]), deeper intimal cracks or splits with localized medial dissection (intimal-medial; 49 sites [73%]), intimal cracks with extensive medial dissection (5 sites [7%]), and adventitial perforation or rupture (intimal-medial-adventitial injury; 2 sites [3%]). Deep intimal-medial injury produced intimal flaps in 29 sites (43%). The remaining 9 angioplasty sites (12%) had no morphologic evidence of dilation injury. Of these 9 sites, 8 had eccentric lesions with an arc of disease-free wall,[66, 69] and 1 was a concentric atherosclerotic plaque lesion.

## Angiographic Patterns

In the 76 balloon dilation sites from the 66 patients, the angiographic patterns were classified as floods (see Table 4–7): smooth-walled dilation (10 sites [14%]), intraluminal haziness (29 sites [38%]), intimal flaps (33 sites [43%]), coronary dissection (1 site [1%]), extravasated contrast material (2 sites [3%]), and spasm (1 site [1%]). In the two cases of extravasated contrast material, the contrast material was confined to the coronary wall in one patient (vessel "staining") and leaked outside the vessel in the other (rupture into pericardial space).

## Morphologic-Angiographic Correlations

The corresponding morphologic-angiographic patterns are summarized in Table 4–7. Of the 10 angioplasty sites with a smooth-wall appearance on angiograms, 2 had shallow, superficial intimal cracks (intimal injury only) and 7 had eccentric lesions without morphologic evidence of injury (Fig. 4–17).[67] Of the 29 sites with angiographic intraluminal haziness or "ground-glass" appearance, 9 had intimal injuries only, 19 had intimal-medial injuries with localized medial dissection, and 1 had a similar intimal-medial tear, but the luminal surface was irregularly covered by fibrin-platelet thrombus. Of the dilation sites with an intimal flap or localized dissection, 29 had deep intimal-medial tears with extensive medial dissection (Fig. 4–18). In the single patient with a coronary dissection, the angioplasty site disclosed a deep intimal-medial tear with an extensive longitudinal medial dissection (see Fig. 4–18). Of the 2 patients with angiographic evidence of extravasated contrast material, both had intimal-medial-adventitial involvement of the coronary artery (see Fig. 4–18). One site had localized adventitial involvement, referred to as a "coronary perforation" or "confined rupture." The other site had adventitial separation (i.e., "frank rupture"). Only 1 coronary angioplasty site had angiographic evidence of coronary spasm, which correlated morphologically with an eccentric atherosclerotic plaque lesion

**TABLE 4–7. MORPHOLOGIC EXPLANATIONS FOR VARIOUS ANGIOGRAPHIC PATTERNS OBSERVED AT THE SITE OF CLINICAL PERCUTANEOUS TRANSLUMINAL CORONARY ANGIOPLASTY**

| ANGIOGRAPHIC OBSERVATION | MORPHOLOGIC-HISTOLOGIC CHANGES |
| --- | --- |
| Smooth-walled dilation | Superficial, shallow intimal cracks or splits |
| | Dilation of arc of diseased free wall in eccentric lesion |
| | Insensitivity of angiography to detect superficial intimal and/or shallow intimal/medial cracks |
| | Circumferential and concentric stretching of artery wall with or without minimal plaque compression |
| Intraluminal haziness | Intimal-medial cracks, splits with localized medial dissection channels |
| | Deep, intimal cracks without medial involvement |
| | Fibrin-platelet thrombi creating irregular or ragged luminal surfaces |
| "Intimal" flap ("intimal split"; localized dissection) | Deep intimal-medial crack with deep and wide but localized medial dissection creating an intimal-medial luminal flap |
| | Deep and narrow intimal-medial crack with narrow but extensive medial dissection creating a long intimal-medial luminal flap |
| Dissection "dissecting hematoma"; "coronary dissection"; "extensive dissection"; "antegrade dissection" | Deep and extensive intimal-medial cracks with antegrade and/or retrograde medial dissection |
| Extravasated contrast material localized to artery or escaping into pericardial space | Deep intimal-medial split with dissection involving adventitial layer (continued rupture; perforation) |
| | Deep intimal-medial split with dissection into adventitial layer with rupture (rupture) |

with an arc of disease-free wall and no evidence of atherosclerotic plaque injury.

In the study by Holmes and colleagues,[68] smooth-walled dilation was the most common angiographic pattern (41%), followed by intimal flaps (split) and dissection (22%) and intraluminal haziness (17%). Speculation for the anatomic basis of these various patterns included alterations in endothelium and disruption of intimal and medial layers of the coronary vessel with or without associated intraluminal thrombus. Angiographic results of Waller's study[67] indicated that intimal flaps and intraluminal hazi-

ness were the two most frequent angiographic coronary angioplasty patterns, accounting for 43% and 38% of the sites, respectively. The most common anatomic correlate for both of these angiographic patterns was an intimal-medial split or crack with localized medial dissection. Of the balloon dilation sites with angiographic "intimal flaps," all 33 had varying degrees of intimal-medial tears that produced the appearance of intraluminal flaps. The deep cracks or breaks created by the balloon dilation produced luminal channels associated with a flap of intimal (plaque) medial tissue. These flaps may be large at times and can result in sudden or abrupt closure of the dilation site.[2, 67]

Of the 29 angioplasty sites with angiographic patterns of "haziness," 19 (66%) had anatomic correlates of intimal-medial splits. However, the haziness pattern was also associated with purely intimal injuries (31%) and with laminated fibrin-platelet thrombus coating an underlying intimal-medial injury (3%). In the past,[68, 70, 71] angiographic "haziness" at the dilation site was attributed to the dispersion of contrast media down multiple fissures or channels. The present study indicates that intimal irregularities (shallow, superficial splits) and/or irregular surfaces produced by adherent thrombus also are explanations for this angiographic pattern.

Intimal flaps created by deep intimal-medial cracks may be interpreted angiographically as coronary dissections and/or intimal splits. The angiographic term *coronary dissection* generally has been reserved for the situation in which clinical symptoms of ischemia are associated with this pattern or in which an extensive coronary intramural channel of contrast material is angiographically visible. The terms *intimal dissection* and *intimal split,* however, are used for the situations in which the split is localized to the angioplasty site and is unassociated with clinical evidence of ischemia. From an anatomic point of view, these localized intimal flaps are the result of a desirable intimal-medial split with localized medial dissection.[67] Angiographic evidence of intimal flaps resulting from balloon angioplasty was initially considered an unfavorable outcome, but more recent clinical studies suggest that their presence may indicate a substantial increase in coronary luminal cross-sectional area[72] and are associated with a decrease in the frequency of restenosis.[73, 74]

Angiographic coronary artery dissection is associated with an extensive intramural channel that anatomically is located in the vessel media (see Fig. 4–18). The intramural channel (false lumen) may extend in an antegrade or retrograde direction from the angioplasty site. An extensive preexisting coronary artery dissection may be a relative contraindication to balloon angioplasty. Waller examined the

**Smooth-walled dilation**

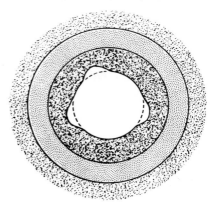 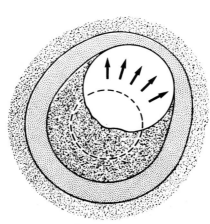 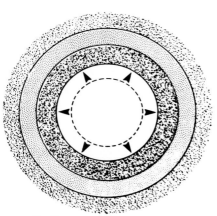

1. Superficial, shallow intimal splits

2. Dilation of arc of disease free wall (eccentric plaque)

3. Concentric stretching of entire vessel

FIGURE 4–17. Diagram showing three morphologic correlates for an angiographic smooth-walled appearance of the site of balloon angioplasty. Shallow, superficial intimal injuries and no injury at all are the most common explanations for the smooth-walled appearance. (From Waller BF: Pathology of new interventional procedures used in coronary disease. *In* Waller BF [ed]: Contemporary Issues in Cardiovascular Pathology. Philadelphia: FA Davis, 1988.)

right coronary artery of a 37-year-old woman who underwent balloon dilation for a focal, proximal, severe right coronary artery stenosis. Before the balloon angioplasty procedure, an extensive coronary artery dissection was created by the guiding catheter. The intimal layer essentially remained anchored to the vessel wall at the site of proximal stenosis. Subsequent successful dilation of the proximal ste-

nosis created the usual intimal-medial crack, but the intimal layer became free within the coronary lumen and collapsed upon itself, occluding the entire distal right coronary artery (intimal intussusception).[67]

Coronary artery aneurysm formation after balloon angioplasty, reported by Hill and colleagues,[75] is an uncommon angiographic pattern. Aneurysmal dila-

**Extravasated contrast material**

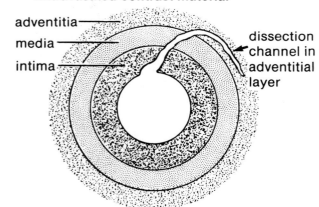

adventitia
media
intima

dissection channel in adventitial layer

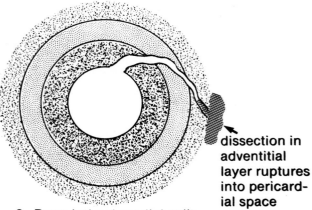

dissection in adventitial layer ruptures into pericardial space

1. Deep intimal-medial crack with dissection involving adventitial layer (confined rupture)(perforation)

2. Deep intimal-medial split with dissection into adventitial layer with rupture (rupture)

FIGURE 4–18. Diagram showing two morphologic correlates for extravasated contrast media at the site of percutaneous transluminal coronary angioplasty (PTCA): A dissection channel extends into the adventitial layer and remains confined to this zone *(left)*, or the dissection channel perforates the adventitial layer and enters the pericardial space *(right)*. (From Waller BF: Pathology of new interventional procedures used in coronary disease. *In* Waller BF [ed]: Contemporary Issues in Cardiovascular Pathology. Philadelphia: FA Davis, 1988.)

tion was not observed in the patients studied by Holmes and associates,[68] nor was it observed in the angiographic-morphologic study by Waller.[67] An anatomic explanation for the angiographic appearance of an aneurysm at the angioplasty site is probably related to overdilation of an arc of disease-free wall in an eccentric plaque[67, 76] (see Fig. 4–17) and less likely to be the result of perforation into the coronary adventitial layer (confined rupture, pseudoaneurysm). Thus, various angiographic patterns after balloon angioplasty are associated with a spectrum of anatomic findings, but the most frequent morphologic finding is an intimal-medial split with localized medial dissection.

## Effects of Balloon Angioplasty on Adjacent Nondilated Vessels

Angiographic reports[77–82] have noted accelerated development of coronary artery stenoses proximal to the site of previous dilation. In these reports, five patients underwent angioplasty in the proximal LAD coronary artery and returned 6 to 14 months later with a severe lesion in the left main coronary artery. Morphologic evaluation of these lesions was not available. Waller and associates[51] reported histologic observations in an accelerated stenosis occurring proximal to a previously dilated lesion. The patient had undergone balloon angioplasty of the proximal LAD artery 4 months before returning with severe stenosis of the left main coronary artery. At autopsy, two 5-mm-long segments of the left main coronary artery disclosed initial (old) atherosclerotic plaque that had narrowed the lumen 51% to 75% in cross-sectional area, with superimposed (new) fibrocellular material that had further narrowed the cross-sectional luminal area 77% to 100%. The fibrocellular tissue in the left main coronary artery was histologically identical to that observed in the proximal LAD artery at the site of previous balloon angioplasty.

Acceleration of left main coronary artery narrowing by fibrocellular tissue proliferation may have resulted from several possible mechanisms: intimal injury (caused by the guiding catheter, the guide wire, or the dilating balloon) and retrograde extension of the fibrocellular tissue from an adjacent site without left main arterial wall injury. The incidence of progressive left main coronary artery narrowing after angioplasty of the LAD or left circumflex artery or both is unknown but is probably low. Of more than 344 patients restudied angiographically within 1 year of previous coronary dilation in whom specific attention was given to the left main coronary artery, only 4 patients (1%) were recognized to have accelerated left main coronary artery narrowing.[77, 78]

Zamorano and associates[82] reported vessel wall changes in the proximal nontreated segment after balloon angioplasty with the use of intracoronary ultrasound study. Of 18 patients undergoing intravascular ultrasound study immediately after angioplasty and 6 months later, 7 (38%) had stenosis at the follow-up ultrasound study. Luminal narrowing proximal to the angioplasty site was angiographically documented in 2 patients, and new intimal thickening in the proximal nondilated segment was shown by ultrasound study in all 7. This study demonstrated a correlation between restenosis at the angioplasty site and increased new proximal intimal thickening.

Desai and colleagues[83] reported aneurysm formation in the left main artery after angioplasty for a mid–left circumflex lesion 6 months earlier. This represents another effect of balloon angioplasty on adjacent nondilated vessels.

## Infarcted Artery Undergoing Acute Balloon Angioplasty With or Without Preceding Thrombolysis

Waller and associates[22] reviewed the morphologic status of infarcted coronary arteries at autopsy from 19 patients with evolving AMI in whom the infarcted artery was acutely dilated with or without preceding thrombolytic therapy. The infarcted vessel was the LAD artery in 13 patients, the right anterior descending artery in 4, the left main coronary artery in 1, and the left circumflex artery in 1. In 16 arteries, residual thrombus was present at the site of previous occlusion; thrombus was occlusive in 9. The degree of underlying atherosclerotic plaque present after thrombolysis therapy varied slightly, depending on the form of therapy. All reperfused arteries had more than 50% cross-sectional area narrowing at the site of previous occlusion, and 10 had 76% to 100% cross-sectional area narrowing. Of the 9 patients who had undergone balloon angioplasty with or without lytic agents, 8 had 51% to 75% narrowing in the cross-sectional area by plaque, and 1 had more than 75% narrowing. In contrast, of the 9 patients who received streptokinase infusion without balloon angioplasty, 8 had more than 75% narrowing in cross-sectional areas by atherosclerotic plaque, and one had 51% to 75% narrowing. The presence of intraplaque hemorrhage and plaque fracture also varied, depending on the use of balloon angioplasty with or without lytic agents. Each of the 9 patients who had undergone percutaneous transluminal coronary angioplasty (PTCA) had histologic evidence of intimal-medial plaque fractures, tears, or cracks. In one patient, the fracture extended into the adventitia and caused coronary artery rupture. Of the nine arteries with evidence of angioplasty procedures, four had intraplaque hemorrhage in the area of angioplasty, and all had been subjected to the additional use of a lytic agent (streptokinase in three, tissue-type plasminogen activator [tPA] in one). Intraplaque hemorrhage was absent in patients who had received streptokinase infusion alone. These observations suggest that the use of combined angioplasty and a lytic agent may produce localized bleeding at a site of angioplasty injury, which may cause additional coronary luminal narrowing.[22]

## Intraplaque Hemorrhage in the Infarct-Related Artery

The 9 patients receiving acute angioplasty reperfusion therapy also can be categorized in two distinct subgroups: those treated with angioplasty alone and those treated with angioplasty plus thrombolytic agents. In the 5 patients treated with angioplasty alone, there were plaque fractures and cracks at the site of angioplasty without intimal or medial hemorrhage. In contrast, in the 4 patients treated with angioplasty plus thrombolytic therapy, there were plaque fractures and cracks at the site of angioplasty with hemorrhage involving the intimal, medial, and adventitial layers of the coronary artery. In one patient, the hemorrhage was so extensive that it narrowed the coronary lumen at the angioplasty site. In the 10 patients who had received streptokinase therapy alone, intraplaque hemorrhage was absent. Thus, the use of combined angioplasty and thrombolytic agents in acute reperfusion therapy may produce localized bleeding at the angioplasty site, and the bleeding may cause additional luminal narrowing.[22]

## DISTAL EMBOLIZATION OF ATHEROSCLEROTIC PLAQUE, THROMBUS, OR BOTH

## Balloon Angioplasty of Coronary Arteries

Embolic complications during or immediately after balloon angioplasty of stenotic coronary arteries have been reported in experimental animals[84] and in 0.06% to 1.0% of patients.[85–90] Pathologic documentation of the embolic complication after balloon angioplasty, thrombolytic therapy, or both has been reported in at least 39 patients.[91–94]

## Acute Reperfusion Therapy

Coronary embolization is a rare angiographically documented complication of angioplasty, thrombolytic therapy, or both.[93–97] Menke and colleagues[93] were among the first to document at autopsy the final location or end point of fragments of thrombus that were angiographically observed to stream distally after thrombolytic therapy. Menke and colleagues[93] studied a 44-year-old patient at autopsy who had histologic evidence of distal embolization after thrombolytic therapy for the proximal left main artery. Histologic sections of the anterolateral papillary muscle disclosed that several intramyocardial coronary arteries were occluded by thrombotic material identical in composition to that remaining in the left main artery.

More recently, Saber and associates[94] reported autopsy findings in 32 patients with coronary embolization after balloon angioplasty, thrombolytic therapy, or both. Of these 32 patients, 26 (81%) had evidence of one or 4 more emboli within the intramural coronary arteries (number of emboli ranged from 1 to 6, mean 3). Emboli consisted of thrombus (41 [5%]).[94] The number of emboli was greater in the artery of intervention. Infarction extension or new infarction was related to the presence of postinterventional coronary microemboli. New electrocardiographic changes were strongly associated with the presence of emboli.

Consequences of distal migration of occluding coronary thrombus fragmented during pharmacologic or mechanical thrombolysis therapy for evolving myocardial infarction remain unclear. The observation of multiple occluded intramyocardial vessels suggests that the consequences of distal embolization may be similar to those of primary coronary embolism.[98, 99] In primary coronary embolism, the smaller the embolus, the greater the chance that it will travel distally and lodge in a small coronary artery. Conversely, the larger the embolus, the greater the likelihood that it will lodge proximally in a large coronary artery. An embolus so small that it affects a single intramural coronary artery and is observed at autopsy only on histologic examination probably has little clinical or morphologic significance, whereas a larger embolus may occlude multiple intramural vessels and produce new or added clinical myocardial dysfunction. In the setting of an evolving myocardial infarction, migration of a single small fragment of occluding thrombus into the distal portion of the infarcted artery is likely to be clinically silent or clinically inseparable from the ongoing infarction and to produce little additional myocardial damage. Migration of a single larger fragment of thrombus may lodge more proximally in the infarcted artery and result in continuation of myocardial necrosis already in progress. Alternatively, larger thrombi may fragment and occlude multiple intramyocardial arteries, producing secondary thrombus of the epicardial coronary vessel that feeds the obstructed arterioles, compromising collateral flow from other major coronary arteries, or both.

In either situation, myocardial necrosis may extend.[98, 99]

## Balloon Angioplasty of Aortocoronary Saphenous Vein Bypass Grafts

Several investigators have noted coronary embolization to be a complication of balloon angioplasty of saphenous vein grafts.[100–103] Its frequency, which is higher than that in balloon angioplasty of native coronary arteries, accounts for 2 (1.9%) of 103 cases reported by Saber and associates,[102] who also reported pathologic documentation of coronary embolization after balloon angioplasty of aortocoronary saphenous vein bypass grafts. In one of their two cases, a large thromboatheromatous embolus obstructed the proximal left anterior descending artery and was removed at the time of operation. In the second case, embolization of atheromatous and thrombotic debris resulted in obstruction of many intramural coronary artery branches and was considered contributory to the death of the patient.

Embolization of thrombotic or atheromatous material probably occurs more frequently after balloon angioplasty than has been recognized, inasmuch as it is clinically asymptomatic in most cases because of the small size and number of emboli. Balloon dilation of saphenous vein grafts, however, is probably more likely to produce symptomatic embolization because vein grafts and their atheromatous plaques are generally larger than the coronary arteries to which they are anastomosed. In addition, atherosclerosis in vein grafts tends to be more friable and less fibrocalcific than its counterpart in the native coronary arteries.[100] Saber and associates[102] recommended that balloon angioplasty be performed for aortocoronary saphenous vein bypass grafts that are more than 1 year of age, with the realization that involvement by friable atherosclerosis is likely and that atheroembolization represents a risk.[102]

## MORPHOLOGIC CHANGES OF BALLOON ANGIOPLASTY OF AORTOCORONARY SAPHENOUS VEIN BYPASS GRAFTS

Morphologic changes in aortocoronary saphenous vein bypass grafts after balloon angioplasty have been reported.[102, 104] This section summarizes clinical and morphologic observations in two patients previously reported[104] and 12 additional patients (Tables 4–8 and 4–9) undergoing saphenous vein bypass graft angioplasty early and late after graft insertion.[104] Operatively excised segments of saphenous vein bypass grafts from 14 patients undergoing balloon angioplasty of the bypass graft either early ("young" grafts; i.e., ≤1 year [8 patients]) and late (old grafts; i.e., ≥1 year [6 patients]) after aortocoronary bypass surgery was the basis of this study (see Tables 4–8 and 4–9).

## Angioplasty of Saphenous Vein Graft Early After Bypass Surgery: Morphologic Features

An operatively excised portion of saphenous vein graft (see Tables 4–8 and 4–9) measured 40 mm in length and was free of calcific deposits. The excised segment included the site of maximal balloon inflation and a short distal portion through which the

**TABLE 4–8.  CLINICAL OBSERVATIONS IN 12 PATIENTS WHO UNDERWENT PERCUTANEOUS BALLOON ANGIOPLASTY OF STENOTIC SAPHENOUS VEIN BYPASS GRAFTS EARLY (≤1 YEAR) AND LATE (>1 YEAR) AFTER AORTOCORONARY BYPASS OPERATION**

| OBSERVATION | EARLY GRAFTS | LATE GRAFTS |
|---|---|---|
| Number of grafts | 7 | 5 |
| Interval (months) from bypass (CABG) to balloon angioplasty (PTA) | 1–8 | 28–120 |
|  | (mean = 4) | (mean = 71) |
| Interval (months) from PTA to SV graft excision | 0.5–1 | 2–8 |
|  | (mean = .7) | (mean = 5) |
| Angiography-angioplasty data |  |  |
|   Maximum SV graft narrowing (% DR) before PTA | 90–99 | 95–99 |
|  | (mean = 95) | (mean = 97) |
|   Maximum SV graft narrowing (% DR after PTA; % decrease) | 10–20 | 10–20 |
|  | (mean = 15) | (mean = 12) |
|   Angiographic evidence of "dissection" or "split" | 1*/7 | 5/5 |
|   Maximum SV graft narrowing (% DR) before SV excision | 95%–100% | 95%–100% |
| Site of PTCA |  |  |
|   Aortic-SV anastomotic site | 3 | 0 |
|   Body of SV | 2 | 5 |
|   Coronary-SV anastomotic site | 2 | 0 |

CABG, coronary artery bypass grafting; DR, diameter reduction; PTA, percutaneous transluminal angioplasty; PTCA, percutaneous transluminal coronary angioplasty; SV, saphenous vein.
*One of two patients had angiographic evidence of "split" in coronary artery lesion.

**TABLE 4–9.** **MORPHOLOGIC OBSERVATIONS IN 12 PATIENTS UNDERGOING PERCUTANEOUS BALLOON ANGIOPLASTY OF STENOTIC SAPHENOUS VEIN BYPASS GRAFTS EARLY (≤1 YEAR) AND LATE (>1 YEAR) AFTER AORTOCORONARY BYPASS OPERATION**

| OBSERVATION | EARLY GRAFTS | LATE GRAFTS |
|---|---|---|
| Number | 7 | 5 |
| Maximal SV graft narrowing (% cross-sectional area [xsa]) at site of PTA | 76–100 | 76–100 |
| Cause of graft narrowing | | |
|    Thrombus only (T) | 1 | 0 |
|    Intimal proliferation ± T only | 2 | 0 |
|    Atherosclerotic plaques ± T only | 2 | 0 |
|    Both intimal proliferation and atherosclerotic plaques ± T | 0 | 5 |
|    Mechanical (technical) problem at graft insertion site | 2 | 0 |
|    Calcific deposits in graft | 0/7* | 5/5 |
| Mechanism of initial PTA success | | |
|    Stretching | 6† | 0 |
|    Cracking, splitting | 1‡ | 5/5 |
|    Morphologic evidence of crack | 1/1‡ | |
| Mechanism of restenosis after PTA success | | |
|    Thrombosis (primary) | 1‡ | 0 |
|    Spasm (recoil) | 6† | 0 |
|    New atherosclerotic plaque | 0 | 0 |
|    Smooth muscle proliferation | 0 | 5/5 |

*No calcific deposits were identified in saphenous vein graft but mild (+1/4+)

catheter and guide wire had passed but in which balloon inflation did not occur. The external diameter (about 7 mm) of the proximal 30 mm of graft (the portion subjected to angioplasty) was slightly wider than the external diameter (about 5 mm) of the distal nondilated segment. The entire specimen was cut transversely into eight 5-mm segments and numbered 1 to 8. Segments 1 to 6 were from areas of previous balloon angioplasty, and segments 7 and 8 were from nondilated areas.

## Angioplasty of Saphenous Vein Graft Late After Bypass Surgery: Morphologic Features

An operatively excised portion of saphenous graft measured 42 mm in length and had foci of calcific deposits in the area of dilation. The entire specimen was cut transversely into eight 5-mm long segments and numbered 1 to 8. Segments 4 to 6 were from the site of maximal balloon inflation. The area of the angioplasty dissection noted angiographically was localized specifically on the excised saphenous vein specimen.

## Morphologic Observations in the Early (Young) Saphenous Vein Graft

The lumen of each of the eight 5-mm saphenous vein segments was narrowed more than 75% in cross-sectional area by intimal thickening (Fig. 4–19; see Tables 4–8 and 4–9). Histologically, the diffuse intimal thickening of both dilated and nondilated segments consisted of cellular fibrocollagenous tissue without foam cells or cholesterol clefts (intimal fibrous hyperplasia, fibrous proliferation). Segments 1 to 6 were serially sectioned at 10 μm intervals to search for sites of splits, tears, cracks, or other morphologic evidence of previous balloon angioplasty. Control segments 7 and 8 were also sectioned in a similar manner. Histologic assessment by light microscopy did not disclose any distinctive morphologic lesions in the intimal, medial, or adventitial layers of dilated or nondilated segments of the saphenous vein graft.

Ultrastructural evaluation of segments 2 (dilated) and 6 (nondilated) disclosed the absence of endothelial luminal cells in the dilated segment; in contrast, they were present in the nondilated segment. Cells lining the graft lumen in the dilated segment had features of myofibroblasts (cytoplasmic filaments with focal condensations and abundant rough endoplasmic reticulum). Fibrin-like extracellular material (possibly representing residual basement membrane) condensed along the luminal border of these myofibroblasts. The endothelial cells lining the lumen of the distal nondilated segment had luminal and abluminal micropinocytotic vesicles and well-formed intercellular junctions. No distinctive differences in myofibroblasts or collagen fibrils were noted between segments 2 and 8.

## Morphologic Observations in the Late (Old) Saphenous Vein Graft

The lumen of each of the eight 5-mm saphenous vein segments had diffuse but variable degrees of intimal thickening (Figs. 4–20 and 4–21). The maximal cross-sectional area luminal reduction by inti-

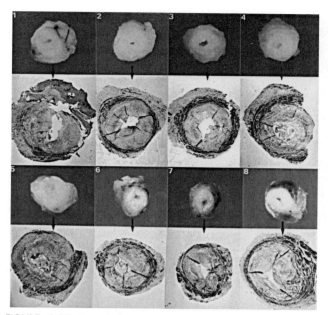

FIGURE 4–19. Morphologic and histologic photographs of the eight segments of saphenous vein graft. Segments 1 to 6 are from the area of balloon inflation and dilation, and segments 7 and 8 are from nondilated portions of the graft ("controls"). Each of the eight segments had diffuse and severe cross-sectional area luminal narrowing by intimal thickening consisting of fibrocollagenous tissue. No segments contained atherosclerotic plaque or calcium deposits. No distinctive histologic changes were observed in the segments subjected to transluminal balloon angioplasty in comparison with control segments. Elastic stains, ×6. (From Waller BF, Rothbaum DA, Gorfinkel HJ, et al: Morphologic observations after percutaneous transluminal balloon angioplasty of early and late aortocoronary saphenous vein bypass grafts. J Am Coll Cardiol 4:784–792, 1984.)

mal thickening occurred in segments 3, 4, and 6. Histologically, the intimal thickening in segments 4 to 6 consisted of foam cells, cholesterol clefts, fibrocollagenous tissue, foci of myofibroblasts, and calcific deposits characteristic of atherosclerotic plaque (see Figs. 4–20 and 4–21). Intimal thickening of segments 1 to 3 and 7 and 8 was predominantly fibrocollagenous in nature except for occasional foci of foam cells, cholesterol clefts, and calcium. In the site of angioplasty dissection (segments 4 to 6) (see Figs. 4–20 and 4–21), the intima was partially separated from the media. This "intimal flap" had begun to reattach to the wall of the graft, representing healing of a localized plaque tear or fracture[5] (see Tables 4–8 and 4–9).

## Clinical Morphologic Correlations

Each of the patients just described had undergone one or more clinically successful percutaneous transluminal angioplasty dilations of a stenotic saphenous vein bypass graft early (1 to 8 months) or late (28 to 120 months) after graft insertion (see

Tables 4–8 and 4–9). Angiographic similarities between the early and late saphenous vein grafts included an increase in luminal diameter associated with a decrease in mean trans-stenotic pressure gradient after angioplasty and with restenosis of the graft at the site of previous dilation 1 or 2 months later. Angiographic differences between the grafts included the absence of cracks, breaks, or splits after dilation in the early grafts (except in one in which a native coronary lesion was dilated) but the presence of an intimal split after the angioplasty procedures in the late grafts. An additional angiographic difference between the grafts was the location of stenosis. The site of stenosis in the early grafts was at the proximal end of the graft (aortic anastomosis) in 4 patients, coronary anastomosis in 2, and within the body of the grafts in 2, whereas the site of stenosis in the late grafts was in the graft body

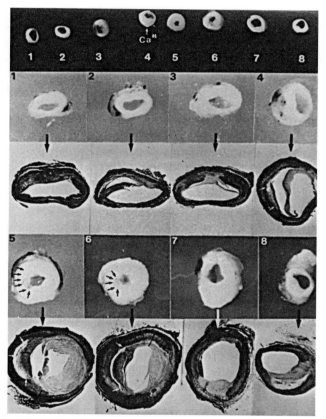

FIGURE 4–20. Photographs of morphologic and histologic segments of saphenous vein graft. Each of the segments shows diffuse but variable degrees of intimal thickening composed of atherosclerotic plaque. The segment with the most severe luminal narrowing (5) corresponds to the area of previous transluminal balloon angioplasty procedures *(small arrows)*. The top panel represents radiographs of the individual cross sections (1 to 8) showing calcific deposits Ca#). (From Waller BF, Rothbaum DA, Gorfinkel HJ, et al: Morphologic observations after percutaneous transluminal balloon angioplasty of early and late aortocoronary saphenous vein bypass grafts. J Am Coll Cardiol 4:784–792, 1984.)

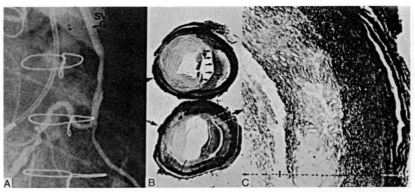

FIGURE 4–21. Angiographic morphologic-histologic correlation at the site of angioplasty dissection 2 months before graft excision. *A*, Angiographic frame of saphenous vein bypass graft (SVG) after transluminal balloon angioplasty, showing a line of dissection. *B*, Corresponding morphologic segments *(large arrows)* of SVG in area of angiographic dissection, showing severe luminal cross-sectional area narrowing with an intimal flap *(small arrows)* and a partially healed intimal fracture. *C*, Higher magnification (×80) of boxed area in *B* showing the intimal (I) fracture site. The intimal thickening is composed of fibrocollagenous tissue, foam cells, and cholesterol clefts. A, adventitia; M, media. *A* to *C:* elastic stains. (From Waller BF, Rothbaum DA, Gorfinkel HJ, et al: Morphologic observations after percutaneous transluminal balloon angioplasty of early and late aortocoronary saphenous vein bypass grafts. J Am Coll Cardiol 4:784–792, 1984.)

(midportion) in all 6. Morphologic similarities between the grafts included diffuse intimal thickening by fibrocollagenous tissue with fibrotic medial and adventitial layers. Morphologic differences between the grafts were distinctive: The early grafts had thickened intima without atherosclerotic plaque changes or calcific deposits and no morphologic evidence of previous dilation, whereas the late grafts had thickened intima typical of atherosclerotic plaque with focal calcific deposits and morphologic evidence of angioplasty injury.[104]

## Therapeutic Implications for Saphenous Vein Angioplasty Derived from Morphologic Observations

The fate of an aortocoronary saphenous vein bypass graft appears to be dependent on several factors relevant to the time interval from bypass grafting to graft obstruction. Graft occlusion developing within 1 month of bypass graft insertion is almost invariably secondary to graft thrombosis that is related to technical factors such as stenosis at the aortic or coronary anastomotic site, intraoperative vein trauma, or poor distal runoff secondary to severe atherosclerosis or reduced caliber of the distal native vessel.[104] These technical factors and the nature of the obstructing material (thrombus) appear to limit the role of balloon angioplasty in successfully relieving saphenous vein graft obstruction that occurs within 1 month of bypass operation.[104]

Functionally significant graft stenoses developing between 1 month and 1 year after graft insertion are nearly always characterized by intimal thickening histologically composed of cellular or acellular fibrocollagenous tissue. The venous medial and ad-

ventitial layers become fibrotic, and the graft resembles a thick, fibrous tube. Focally stenotic lesions produced by this intimal thickening appear amenable to dilation by balloon angioplasty, as illustrated in the first patient described earlier. However, in view of the histologic composition of the intima, the dilating mechanism is probably not intimal compression[104] but rather graft "stretching" (Fig. 4–22). Depending on the degree of graft stretching, the dilating procedure may have limited therapeutic success (weeks to months) with graft "restenosis" representing gradual "restitution of tone" of an overstretched graft segment.[104]

Saphenous vein graft stenoses occurring after 1 year and generally after 3 years after graft insertion usually consist of atherosclerotic plaque in addition to intimal fibrous thickening.[105–110] The atherosclerotic plaque in saphenous vein grafts appears morphologically similar to that observed in native coronary arteries: foam cells, cholesterol clefts, blood product debris, fibrocollagenous tissue, and calcific deposits.[108, 110] Focal stenoses produced by this type of lesion also appear amenable to dilation by balloon angioplasty, as illustrated in the second patient described earlier. The mechanism of conduit dilation in this setting appears similar to that proposed for coronary artery angioplasty: plaque splitting, cracking, or breaking with or without localized intimal-medial dissection (Fig. 4–23).[104] Therapeutic limitations in dilating saphenous vein grafts narrowed by atherosclerotic plaque are probably similar to those observed in atherosclerotic coronary arteries subjected to balloon angioplasty.

In addition to the age of the bypass graft, at least two other anatomic factors appear to influence the therapeutic success of balloon angioplasty of saphe-

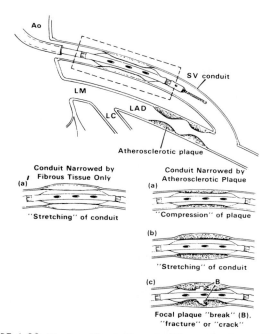

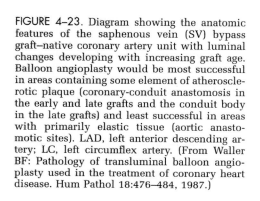

FIGURE 4–22. Diagram illustrating possible mechanisms of luminal balloon angioplasty in stenotic aortocoronary saphenous vein (SV) bypass grafts. Two types of lesions characterized the SV stenoses, depending on the interval from graft insertion to early obstruction. Early (<1 year) (a, left) contain intimal thickening composed primarily of fibrocollagenous tissue without calcium, and dilatation is accomplished by conduit "stretching." Late (>1 year) grafts (a, b, and c, right) contain intimal thickening composed of atherosclerotic plaque and calcium, and dilatation is accomplished by plaque compression (unlikely), graft stretching, or plaque fracture or break (most likely). Ao, aorta; LAD, left anterior descending artery; LC, left circumflex artery; LM, left main artery. (From Waller BF, Rothbaum DA, Gorfinkel HJ, et al: Morphologic observations after percutaneous transluminal balloon angioplasty of early and late aortocoronary saphenous vein bypass grafts. J Am Coll Cardiol 4:784–792, 1984.)

nous vein grafts: the length and location of stenosis.[104] Long stenotic segments of saphenous vein (>15 to 20 mm) are often technically more difficult to dilate and are associated with a lower rate of primary therapeutic success than are short stenotic segments (<5 mm). Graft stenoses may be located at the anastomotic sites (aorta-graft or coronary artery–graft) or within the body of the graft (see Fig. 4–23). Angiographic studies[111–114] have suggested that saphenous vein graft stenoses at the coronary artery–graft anastomotic site have the best therapeutic results, followed by lesions in the graft body and at the aorta-graft anastomotic site, respectively. An anatomic factor supporting the relatively high rate of success in dilating stenotic coronary artery–graft anastomotic sites is the presence of atherosclerotic plaque in the coronary portion of the anastomosis.[115–117] Stenoses in the graft body or at the aortic-graft anastomotic site are less likely to have the potential angioplasty advantage of associated atherosclerotic plaque unless the graft is more than 3 years old.[101–104, 107–109, 116, 117]

## Clinical Results of Percutaneous Transluminal Angioplasty of Saphenous Vein Grafts

Gruentzig and associates[118] reported as early as 1979 that vein graft angioplasty was successful in five of seven attempts. However, three of the five successful grafts demonstrated "restenosis" during follow-up, prompting Gruentzig to suggest that there was a different kind of disease[103, 116] in the bypass graft. Ford and associates[113, 114] dilated nine saphenous vein grafts 4 to 84 months (mean, 46 months) after graft insertion. Primary angiographic success occurred in six of the nine grafts with only late success (>9 months) in two of the six initial successes. Of the two late successes, one graft was 18 months old at initial angioplasty and the second was 5 months old. Famularo and colleagues[119] reported morphologic observations in an unsuccessful dilation of a saphenous vein conduit with atherosclerotic plaque.

FIGURE 4–23. Diagram showing the anatomic features of the saphenous vein (SV) bypass graft–native coronary artery unit with luminal changes developing with increasing graft age. Balloon angioplasty would be most successful in areas containing some element of atherosclerotic plaque (coronary-conduit anastomosis in the early and late grafts and the conduit body in the late grafts) and least successful in areas with primarily elastic tissue (aortic anastomotic sites). LAD, left anterior descending artery; LC, left circumflex artery. (From Waller BF: Pathology of transluminal balloon angioplasty used in the treatment of coronary heart disease. Hum Pathol 18:476–484, 1987.)

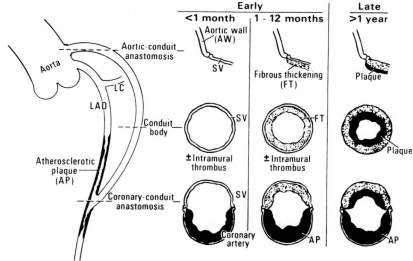

The age of the graft was not provided; morphologic study of the angioplasty site revealed intimal tears of atherosclerotic plaque. Douglas and associates[112] reported their angioplasty results in 62 bypass grafts. Of the 62 grafts, 40 (65%) were dilated early after insertion (>1 year) and 22 (35%) were dilated late after insertion (>1 year). Primary success occurred in 37 early grafts (93%), with restenosis 6 months or later in 9 (24%), and in 21 late grafts (95%), with the same restenosis rate as with the early grafts (24%).

Famularo and colleagues[103] reported a clinical review of saphenous vein angioplasty studies of 1571 patients undergoing saphenous vein angioplasty (various graft ages); the initial success rate ranged from 75% to 94% (average, 88%).[103] Embolization rates ranged from 0% to 7% (average, >3%).

As suggested first by Waller and associates,[104] the site of balloon angioplasty in the aortocoronary bypass graft unit—aorta–saphenous vein anastomotic site (proximal), body of graft, or coronary artery–saphenous vein anastomotic site (distal)—influences the initial success of angioplasty and subsequent type and frequency of restenosis (see Fig. 4–23).[104]

Breakdown of the early and late grafts according to stenosis location revealed that the distal graft stenoses (early and late) had a high initial dilation success rate and a lower restenosis rate. Graft stenoses located in the body or proximal end had a slightly lower initial dilation success rate but three times the restenosis frequency in the distal sites (39% vs. 13%).

A review[103] of 15 studies[112, 120–133] reporting initial success rate of dilation and subsequent restenosis rate according to site dilated disclosed average initial success rates of 93% (body), 90% (distal site), and 86% (proximal site). Restenosis rates according to site of dilation were lowest in the body (28%) and much higher in the distal (42%) and proximal (58%) sites. Variability in definitions of "proximal," "body," and "distal" and the considerable variability in ages of saphenous vein grafts account for the differences between morphologic studies[102, 104] and clinical studies.[103, 112, 120, 143]

## Acute Closure at the Site of Balloon Angioplasty in Saphenous Vein Bypass Grafts

In comparison to acute closure at the angioplasty site in coronary arteries undergoing balloon angioplasty procedures (see earlier discussion), relatively little morphologic information is available concerning acute closure at angioplasty sites in saphenous vein bypass grafts.[144] We reviewed autopsy findings in nine patients who had abrupt or acute closure of angioplasty sites in either young (≤1 year) and old

(>1 year) saphenous vein bypass grafts (see Table 4–9).

In the young graft group (graft age, >1 month to 1 year), six patients died within 24 hours (mean, 11 hours) of balloon angioplasty. Morphologic causes of the closure included intimal-medial flap (with or without thrombus) in zero, elastic recoil in three and primary thrombus alone in three. The underlying pathologic process was intimal proliferation in all six patients. Acute or abrupt closure occurred at the aortic anastomotic site in two, in the body of the graft in three, and at the coronary artery anastomotic site in one (Table 4–10). Morphologic study of closure and the site of angioplasty revealed that elastic recoil occurred at both aortic anastomotic sites dilated, acute thrombosis occurred in the body of the graft, and a large intimal-medial flap was part of the underlying atherosclerotic plaque in the native coronary artery at the saphenous vein anastomotic site. Thus, acute or abrupt closure in saphenous vein bypass graft angioplasty sites was the result of spasm or thrombosis in five of the six patients with grafts aged 1 year or less.

**TABLE 4–10.  CERTAIN CLINICAL-MORPHOLOGIC OBSERVATIONS IN AUTOPSY SPECIMENS FROM 9 PATIENTS WITH ACUTE CLOSURE AT THE SITE OF BALLOON ANGIOPLASTY (PTA)**

| OBSERVATION | EARLY (≤1 YEAR) | LATE (>1 YEAR) |
|---|---|---|
| No. of patients | 6 | 3 |
| Age range | 52–77 | 54–75 |
| Gender | | |
| No. of men | 6 | 3 |
| No. of women | 0 | 0 |
| Type of CABG | Saphenous vein | Saphenous vein |
| Age of graft | | |
| <1 month | N = 3 | N = 2 |
| 1–6 months | N = 2 | N = 1 |
| 7–12 months | N = 1 | N = 0 |
| Interval from PTA to death | 0–24 h | 0–2 days |
| Mean | 11 h | 18 h |
| Morphologic basis for closure | | |
| Intimal flap ± thrombus | 0 | 0 |
| Intimal-medial flap ± thrombus | 10* | 2 |
| Elastic recoil | 20† | 0 |
| Thrombosis only | 3‡ | 1 |
| Plaque hemorrhage | 0 | 0 |
| Underlying vessel lesion | | |
| Intimal proliferation | 6 | 0 |
| Atherosclerotic plaque | 0 | 3 |
| Site of obstruction | | |
| Aortic anastomotic site | 2† | 0 |
| Body of graft | 3‡ | 3 |
| Coronary anastomosis site | 1* | 0 |

CABG, coronary artery bypass grafting; PTA, percutaneous transluminal angioplasty.

In the old graft group (graft age, >1 to 10 years; see Table 4–10), three patients died within 2 days (mean, 18 hours) of balloon angioplasty. Morphologic bases for the closure included intimal-medial flaps (with or without thrombus) in two, elastic recoil in 0, and primary thrombus alone in one. The underlying pathologic process was atherosclerotic plaque in all three patients. All sites of acute or abrupt closure were in the body of the saphenous vein graft (see Table 4–9). Examination of the cause and site of acute or abrupt angioplasty closure revealed that large atherosclerotic flaps (with or without thrombus) curled up within the body of the graft in two patients, and acute primary thrombosis occurred in the third patient. Thus, acute or abrupt closure in saphenous vein bypass graft angioplasty sites had causes similar to those seen in acute or abrupt closure of coronary artery angioplasty sites: large intimal-medial flaps or primary thrombosis (grafts aged >1 year).

## NEW INTERVENTIONAL TECHNIQUES FOR TREATMENT OF OBSTRUCTED SAPHENOUS VEIN BYPASS GRAFTS

Several new interventional devices (stents, atherectomy, laser) have been used in the treatment of obstructed saphenous vein bypass grafts.

### Stents

Intracoronary stents were applied to saphenous vein bypass graft treatment strategies as early as 1989.[134] Several studies[134–139] indicated that the success rate was high (>95%) but that there was a high incidence of subacute thrombosis and bleeding complications from anticoagulation.[103] In addition, the incidence of restenosis remained high, ranging from 21% to 47%, depending on the type of stent employed (Wallstent, Palmaz-Schatz stent, Cook stent). Restenosis was more frequent in the Wallstent studies (36%[134] and 47%[136]), less so the Cook (flexible coil) stent studies (35%[137]), and least frequent in the Palmaz-Schatz stent studies (21%[138] and 26%[139]). In studies by Eeckhout and colleagues[140] and Vaishnav and coworkers,[141] the Wiktor (tantalum wire) stent has been employed in treatment of obstructed saphenous vein bypass grafts. Initial results indicate a high initial success rate and a lower restenosis rate in comparison with other stents. One advantage of the Wiktor stent is its radiopaque nature. "Biliary" stents have also been used in large saphenous vein bypass grafts.[142, 143] Initial results are encouraging.

Van Beusekom and colleagues[144] conducted histologic studies after Wallstent placement in human saphenous vein bypass grafts that were excised surgically 3 to 320 days after stent implantation.

Twenty-one stents from 10 patients were examined. It was observed that large amounts of platelets and leukocytes adhered to the stent wires during the first few days. At 3 months, the wires were embedded in a layered new intimal thickening, consisting of smooth muscle cells in a collagenous matrix. In addition, foam cells were abundant near the wires. Extracellular lipids and cholesterol crystals were found after 6 months. Smooth muscle cells and extracellular matrix were the predominant components of restenosis. This new intimal thickening was lined with endothelium, in some cases showing defect intercellular junctions and abnormal adherence of leukocytes and platelets as late as 10 months after implantation. Van Beusekom and colleagues concluded that this type of stent was potentially thrombogenic and seemed to be associated with extracellular lipid accumulation in venous aortocoronary bypass grafts.

### Atherectomy: Directional and Extractional

Atherectomy devices have also been used in treatment of obstructed saphenous vein bypass grafts.[138, 145–147] With directional atherectomy, the initial success rates were high (91% to 93%), but so were the restenosis rates (31% to 63%).[138, 145, 146] Embolization rates were also high, ranging from 7%[138, 145] to 11.5%.[146] Extractional atherectomy was successful in 89% of patients,[147] but the restenosis rate was still high, at 53%.[147] The embolization rate (3.5%[147]) was about half that with the directional atherectomy device, probably because of its mechanism of use: suction, extraction, and removal of material through the device.[147]

### Excimer Laser

Initial results with the use of excimer laser angioplasty in obstructed (old) saphenous vein grafts was favorable (97%),[148] but the restenosis rate was still very high (61%).[148] In a report of the Percutaneous Excimer Laser Coronary Angioplasty Registry,[149] 545 saphenous vein graft stenoses were treated with excimer laser angioplasty. Ostial lesions (i.e., proximal aortic anastomotic sites) had a higher degree of success (95%) than did lesions in the body of the graft. Lesions larger than 10 mm had a lower success rate (84%) and higher complication rate (12%) than did discrete lesions. Lesions in smaller vein grafts had higher success and lower complication rates than did those in larger grafts.[149]

### Stent Placement for Internal Mammary Graft Stenosis

The major problem associated with long-term patency of internal mammary arteries used as bypass grafts is the early occurrence of stenosis at the distal coronary anastomotic site.[150] Balloon angioplasty has (as expected in view of the anatomy at the site discussed earlier) been highly successful. Stent placement at this site for internal mammary graft stenosis has been reported.[150]

## ATHERECTOMY

Atherectomy is a new mechanical technique capable of removing luminal obstructions (atherosclerotic plaque, smooth muscle proliferation, thrombus, combinations). Various cutting, scraping, shaving, and pulverizing devices have been developed: the Simpson atherotome (DVI), the Rotablade, and the transluminal extraction catheter (TEC). Atherectomy devices also have been used to excise intimal-medial flaps that cause acute occlusion after balloon angioplasty procedures. Tissue samples can be obtained with the Simpson AtheroCath (directional atherectomy[151, 152]) or the TEC. Specimens obtained with the AtheroCath average 12 mm long, 2 mm wide, and 0.25 mm deep; samples obtained with the TEC are much smaller and fragmented. Findings of histologic analysis of excised tissue include atherosclerotic plaque with and without calcific deposits, thrombus, and smooth muscle "restenosis" tissue. Actual removal of plaque by atherectomy rather than simply cracking atheroma by angioplasty increases the luminal cross-sectional area.

Garratt and colleagues[153] reported clinical and autopsy features of three patients who died after undergoing coronary atherectomy. At autopsy, treated vessel wall segments (LAD artery in two patients, vein graft in one) showed discrete defects extending into atheroma, media, or adventitia, corresponding with the presence of these tissue types in the atherectomy specimens. Late findings including proliferating tissue extending from the resected areas into the vessel lumen. In one patient, the intimal hyperplasia was sufficient to narrow the vessel lumen by more than 75% and was complicated in subsequent myocardial ischemia and infarction. Plaque fracturing and medial dissection were not observed in the treated vessels, which indicates that any associated use of a dilating balloon (as part of the atherectomy device or after atherectomy) did not create additional injury typical of balloon angioplasty. Garratt and colleagues suggested, however, that balloon stretching of vessel wall structures could contribute to the mechanism of successful atherectomy with the DVI device.[152] Acute mural thrombus deposition was present in the resection zone of one patient who died 12 hours after atherectomy. This finding suggests that mural thrombus may develop acutely over the area of resection.

## Restenosis After Directional Atherectomy: Tissue Analysis

Garratt and colleagues[154] reported rates of restenosis after successful directional coronary atherectomy and examined the correlation between the coronary and vein bypass graft restenosis rate and the extent of vascular injury. After 6 months, the overall restenosis rate was 50% (37 of 74 lesions). The restenosis rate was 42% when intima alone was resected, 50% when media was resected, and 63% when adventitia was resected—the rate increasing with increasing depth of vessel injury. Tissues from patients undergoing a second atherectomy for restenosis after initial atherectomy (i.e., atherectomy restenosis) demonstrated neointimal hyperplasia that appeared histologically identical to restenosis tissue after balloon angioplasty.

Waller and associates[155] reported results of histologic analysis from more than 400 patients who received directional coronary atherectomy at three separate institutions—St. Vincent Hospital (Indianapolis, Indiana),[156] Sequoia Hospital (Redwood, California),[157] and Beth Israel Hospital (Boston, Massachusetts)[158, 159]—between 1986 and 1990 (Table 4–11).

Coronary atherectomy samples were obtained from approximately 500 stenotic coronary artery lesions involving the left anterior descending (54% to 75%), right (12% to 32%) or branch (0 to 2%) coronary arteries (see Table 4–11). Of the coronary atherectomy tissue, 28%[156] to 66%[158, 159] was obtained from native coronary arteries without a prior intervention and was classified as "primary" or "de novo" lesions, and 34%[158, 159] to 65%[156] of samples were obtained from coronary artery sites that had undergone a prior intervention (most commonly, balloon angioplasty; less frequently, primary atherectomy) and were categorized as "restenosis" lesions (see Table 4–11).[155]

Information concerning number of atherectomy samples obtained per patient was available from two[156, 157] of the three studies. Of 1264 atherectomy samples from two studies of nearly 400 patients,[156, 157] between 1 and 26 atherectomy samples (average, 8 and 10 samples) per patient were obtained per procedure (see Table 4–11). The average number of samples obtained during atherectomy in the third study[158, 159] was 11.6 (standard deviation, 6.5).

### Histologic Definitions[155]

Stenotic lesions were histologically classified into two major types: atherosclerotic plaque and intimal proliferation. Lesions classified as atherosclerotic plaque included samples consisting of fibrous connective tissue with or without associated foam cells,

**TABLE 4–11.    SELECTED CLINICAL OBSERVATIONS OF PATIENTS UNDERGOING PERCUTANEOUS DIRECTION CORONARY ATHERECTOMY**

| CHARACTERISTIC | ATHERECTOMY STUDY | | | TOTAL |
| --- | --- | --- | --- | --- |
| | WALLER ET AL[6] | JOHNSON ET AL[7] | SCHNITT ET AL[8, 9] | |
| No. of patients | 119 | 260* | 151† | 530 |
| Age (years) | | | | |
| Range | 35–87 | 18–85 | 34–87 | 18–85 |
| Mean | 58 | 59 | 58 | |
| Men | 104 (87%) | 23 (8.9%) | 73% | |
| Women | 15 (13%) | 29 (11%) | 27% | |
| Total no. of atherectomy samples | | | | |
| Range per patient | 2–25 | 1–26 | — | 1–26 |
| Average per patient | 8 | 10 | 11.6 ± 6 | |
| Subgroups of patients undergoing atherectomy | | | | |
| Primary (de novo) lesions | 33 (28%) | 109 (40%) | 105 (69%) | 247 (47%) |
| Restenosis lesions (PTCA, atherectomy, or both) | 77 (65%) | 161 (60%) | 56 (31%) | 294 (53%) |
| Coronary artery of atherectomy‡ | | | | |
| Left main | 0 | 9 (3%) | 4 (2%) | 13 |
| LAD | 64 (54%) | 103 (61%) | 143 (75%) | 310 |
| Left circumflex | 17 (14%) | 12 (4%) | 21 (11%) | 50 |
| Right | 38 (32%) | 80 (30%) | 22 (12%) | 140 |
| Branch | 0 | 6 (2%) | 0 | 6 |

LAD, left anterior descending artery; PTCA, percutaneous transluminal coronary angioplasty.

*Includes an unspecified number of patients with aortocoronary saphenous vein bypass graft atherectomy procedures. †Excludes 27 saphenous vein graft lesions. ‡Coronary atherectomy performed on 190 lesions in 151 patients in Schnitt et al's study.

From Waller BF, Pinkerton CA, Kereiakes D, et al: Morphologic analysis of 506 coronary atherectomy specimens from 107 patient: Histologically similar findings of restenosis following primary balloon angioplasty versus primary atherectomy. J Am Coll Cardiol 15:197A, 1990.

cholesterol clefts, lipid cores of pale granular material, or lymphocytes. Lesions classified as intimal proliferation (hyperplasia) were characterized by a proliferation of stellate to spindle-shaped smooth muscle cells within a loose to mildly fibrotic myxoid stroma rich in acid proteoglycan material. Intimal proliferation lesions were more cellular and generally less fibrotic than atherosclerotic plaques and often appeared as a discrete layer coating or covering the surface of markedly collagenous atherosclerotic plaques. Another histologic feature assessed was the presence or absence of calcific deposits and thrombus. Variations in classification of the major tissue types with or without calcium and thrombus make specific category comparisons difficult (Table 4–12).[155]

Vessel wall layers (media and adventitia) were also identified. Media was defined as fragments of atherectomy tissue with randomly oriented fragments of smooth muscle, demarcated in some instances from overlying plaque or proliferation tissue by an internal elastic layer (membrane lamina). Adventitia was defined as a vessel layer consisting of fibrous connective tissue with occasional small blood vessels or nerves. In some samples, fragments of an external elastic membrane were identified. The presence or absence of media and adventitia was documented by means of specialized elastic stained sections. Two studies[156, 157] provided specific quantification of amount and/or length and/or thickness (i.e., depth) of media obtained per sample.[155]

## Primary Versus Restenotic Lesions

The predominant tissue type in atherectomy tissue from native or primary coronary artery lesions was atherosclerotic plaque with or without thrombus (78%[156] to 98%[158, 159]; mean, 93%) (see Table 4–12). A major difference among the three studies concerned the presence or absence and frequency of proliferation tissue in the native or primary atherectomy subgroup. In the study by Waller and associates,[156] none of the native stenotic lesions excised by atherectomy catheters contained intimal proliferation tissue. In contrast, Johnson and associates[157] and Schnitt and colleagues[158, 159] found that 22% to 42%, respectively, of primary atherectomy samples contained variable amount of intimal proliferation. Both of the latter studies[157–159] indicated that the intimal proliferative tissue obtained from native (de novo) stenotic lesions was histologically[157–159] and immunologically[158] identical to that seen in the intimal proliferation lesions of restenosis after angioplasty or after atherectomy.

The overwhelming tissue type seen in the atherectomy samples from restenosed coronary artery sites was intimal proliferation (hyperplasia), with or without associated atherosclerotic plaque or thrombus (83%[156] to 95%[158, 159]; mean, 88%) (Table 4–13). All three studies found that most lesions with intimal proliferation lesions also contained some atherosclerotic plaque (66%[156] to 95%[158, 159]). One study[156] indicated 17% of atherectomy samples con-

**TABLE 4–12. HISTOLOGIC OBSERVATIONS OF CORONARY ATHERECTOMY TISSUE OBTAINED BY PERCUTANEOUS DIRECTIONAL ATHERECTOMY: NATIVE (DE NOVO) LESIONS**

| TISSUE FEATURES | PRIMARY (DE NOVO) STENOTIC LESIONS | | | TOTALS |
| --- | --- | --- | --- | --- |
| | WALLER ET AL[6] (N = 33) | JOHNSON ET AL[7] (N = 109) | SCHNITT ET AL[8, 9] (N = 105) | |
| Atherosclerotic plaque (AP) ± thrombus | 33 patients (268 [97%] samples) | 85 (78%) | 103 (98%) | 247 |
| Intimal proliferation (IP) ± thrombus | 0 | 24 (22%) | 44 (42%) | 68 |
| AP + IP ± thrombus | 0 | —‡ | —‡ | — |
| Thrombus only | 2 patients (6%) | 67 (61%) | 0† | 69 |
| Calcific deposits | | | | |
| Present | 25 (76%) | 50 (47%) | —‡ | 75 |
| Absent | 8 (24%) | 59 (54%) | —‡ | 67 |
| Vessel media | | | | |
| Present | 13 patients (39%) | 51 (47%) | 72 (69%) | 136 |
| Absent | 20 patients (61%) | 58 (53%) | 33 (31%) | 111 |
| Vessel adventitia | | | | |
| Present | 1 patient (3%), 1/276 samples (0.4%) | 21 (20%) | 36 (34%) | 58 |
| Absent | 32 patients (97%) | 88 (81%) | 69 (66%) | 189 |

*Data exclude saphenous vein graft specimens.

†Personal communication with SJS and DB. Breakdown into subgroups of intimal proliferation (hyperplasia) only, with or without thrombus, is not available. No patient had thrombus only.

‡Data not available or specific subgroups not identified. Number represents total lesions with varying amounts of thrombus with or without atherosclerotic plaques or intimal proliferation.

From Waller BF, Pinkerton CA, Kereiakes D, et al: Morphologic analysis of 506 coronary atherectomy specimens from 107 patients: Histologically similar findings of restenosis following primary balloon angioplasty versus primary atherectomy. J Am Coll Cardiol 15:197A, 1990.

tained only proliferative tissue, whereas two studies[156, 157] identified a specific subgroup of restenotic lesions that contained only atherosclerotic plaque, with or without thrombus (14%[157] and 17%[156]) (see Table 4–13). The atherosclerotic plaques in this subgroup were histologically identical to other fragments of plaque in restenosis lesions and to de novo or primary stenotic lesions.[155]

Calcific deposits were identified in patients with primary and restenotic lesion subgroups[156, 157] but

**TABLE 4–13. HISTOLOGIC OBSERVATIONS OF CORONARY ATHERECTOMY TISSUE OBTAINED BY PERCUTANEOUS DIRECTIONAL ATHERECTOMY: RESTENOSIS LESIONS**

| TISSUE FEATURES | RESTENOSIS OF STENOTIC LESIONS | | | TOTALS |
| --- | --- | --- | --- | --- |
| | WALLER ET AL[6] (N = 77) | JOHNSON ET AL[7] (N = 161) | SCHNITT ET AL[8, 9] (N = 56) | |
| Atherosclerotic plaque (AP) ± thrombus | 13 (17%) | 23 (14%) | 53 (95%) | 89 |
| Intimal proliferation (IP) ± thrombus | 13 (17%) | 138 (86%) | 51 (91%) | 202 |
| AP + IP ± thrombus | 51 (66%) | 0 | 0 | 51 |
| Thrombus only | 0 | 63 (39%)† | 0* | 63 |
| Calcific deposits | | | | |
| Present | 49 (64%) | 72 (45%) | —‡ | 121 |
| Absent | 28 (36%) | 89 (55%) | —‡ | 117 |
| Vessel media | | | | |
| Present | 30 (39%) | 64 (40%) | 35 (63%) | 129 |
| Absent | 47 (61%) | 97 (60%) | 21 (38%) | 165 |
| Vessel adventitia | | | | |
| Present | — 0 | 27 (17%) | 11 (20%) | 38 |
| Absent | 77 (100%) | 134 (83%) | 45 (80%) | 256 |

*Personal communication with SJS and DB. Breakdown of subgroup with atherosclerotic plaque only in restenosis lesions is not available. No patient had thrombus only.

†Number represents total lesions with varying amounts of thrombus ± atherosclerotic plaque, with or without intimal proliferation.

‡Data not available or specific subgroups not identified.

From Waller BF, Pinkerton CA, Kereiakes D, et al: Morphologic analysis of 506 coronary atherectomy specimens from 107 patients: Histologically similar findings of restenosis following primary balloon angioplasty versus primary atherectomy. J Am Coll Cardiol 15:197A, 1990.

were more frequent in the patients with native lesion atherectomy: 47%[157] to 76%[156] and 45%[157] to 64%,[156] respectively (Tables 4–11 and 4–13). The calcific deposits were found primarily in atherosclerotic plaque components in restenosis lesions but were occasionally found within intimal proliferation zones.[156]

Fragments of thrombus were found in variable frequencies among the three studies (see Tables 4–11 and 4–12). In most instances, the thrombotic material showed at least focal evidence of organization (ingrowth of fibroblasts and/or capillaries). Aggregates of fibrin, admixed with erythrocytes and leukocytes but without evidence of organization 3, were not recorded as thrombus because such aggregates may have been related to the atherectomy procedure.[155]

## Vessel Wall Layers[155]

Variable degrees of media were identified in both tissue subgroups of atherectomy samples (see Tables 4–11 and 4–13). In the primary, native, or de novo lesion subgroup, vessel media was identified in viable amounts: 39%[156] to 69%[157, 158] (mean 52%). In the restenosis lesion subgroup, vessel media was identified histologically in 39%[156] to 63%[158, 159] (mean, 48%) of patients. In the study by Johnson and associates,[157] the aggregate length of media was slightly greater in the primary lesions (4.8 mm) than in the restenosis lesions (4.1 mm). Despite identical frequencies (39%) of media identified in native and restenosis lesions in the study by Waller and associates[156] maximal thickness ("depth") of media was greater in the primary lesions (199.7 $\mu$m) than in restenosis lesions (144.8 $\mu$m).

Vessel adventitia was also identified with variable frequency among the three studies (see Tables 4–11 and 4–13). Two major categories of tissue were found: (1) atherosclerotic plaque with or without thrombus, and (2) intimal proliferation (intimal hyperplasia) with or without atherosclerotic plaque and/or thrombus.[157] Of native (primary, de novo) stenotic coronary lesions treated with directional atherectomy, more than 90% of the tissue samples contained typical atherosclerotic plaque. In contrast, of the tissue obtained from stenotic coronary lesions after intervention (restenosis after primary balloon angioplasty, primary atherectomy or both), more than 88% consisted of intimal proliferation. The remaining atherectomy samples from de novo coronary stenoses consisted of thrombi[156] or intimal proliferation,[157–159] whereas remaining atherectomy samples from restenosis lesions consisted of atherosclerotic plaque without associated intimal proliferation.[156, 157]

## Clinically Relevant Conclusions Derived From Histologic Observations

Several observations are clinically relevant to the morphologic histologic findings reviewed in the present study.[155]

1. Intimal proliferation (hyperplasia; "restenosis") lesions in living patients with previous balloon angioplasty procedures are histologically identical to those reported in autopsy specimens.[160] Johnson and associates[161] were the first researchers to document the identical nature of angioplasty restenotic tissue from both living and dead patients with peripheral vascular disease. Waller and associates confirmed the identical nature of angioplasty restenosis tissue in both living and dead patients in the coronary arterial system.[155]

2. Restenosis tissue after coronary atherectomy is histologically identical to intimal proliferation tissue after conventional balloon angioplasty.[160] As a potential alternative or adjunctive therapy with balloon angioplasty, directional atherectomy still carries the risk of restenosis. Findings of clinical and angiographic follow-up of patients with primary atherectomy procedures suggest that the frequency of restenosis is similar to that after standard balloon angioplasty.[158, 159] Moreover, restenosis tissue at sites of primary atherectomy is histologically identical to that after primary balloon angioplasty. Intimal proliferative tissue from both procedures was similar in cellularity, vascularity, degree of fibrosis, content of inflammatory cells, and presence of thrombus. This finding confirms suggestions that smooth muscle migration and proliferation are nonspecific reactions to vascular injury.[162] A preliminary report of atherectomy restenosis tissue from patients treated with laser-assisted balloon angioplasty or "stand-alone" laser therapy or obtained from stenotic Gianturco-Roubin stents indicates histologic similarity to primary atherectomy or primary balloon angioplasty restenosis tissue.[155, 163]

3. Restenosis lesions occurring after balloon angioplasty do not consist exclusively of intimal proliferation tissue.[160, 161] Some studies of angioplasty restenosis at autopsy have shown only atherosclerotic plaques (with or without thrombus), with no morphologic evidence of lesion disruption (or healed version of injury) or intimal hyperplasia.[160, 164, 165] Waller and associates'[155] histologic study of atherectomy tissue from restenosis sites of previous balloon angioplasty, however, showed that atherosclerotic plaque alone (i.e., without associated intimal proliferative tissue) is observed in 14% to 17% of patients.[156, 157] Possible explanations for restenosis in this sub-

group of patients include (1) elastic recoil of overstretched normal vessel wall of eccentric atherosclerotic lesions,[164, 166] (2) technically inadequate balloon dilation, (3) tissue sampling error, and (4) progression of intimal proliferation lesions to atherosclerotic plaques. Tissue sampling error seems unlikely in that the procedure of atherectomy entails circumferential rotation of the cutting edge. Progressive fibrosis accompanied by loss of smooth muscle cells could conceivably transform areas of intimal proliferation into typical atherosclerotic plaque, but this explanation seems unlikely for sites dilated less than 4 months earlier. A more likely explanation for restenosis in this group of patients is chronic recoil of eccentric atherosclerotic lesions.[155]

4. Deep vessel wall components (media, adventitia) are observed frequently in atherectomized tissue. In three large series of patients with coronary atherectomy-derived tissue, summarized in Waller and associates'[155] report, vessel media was identified in 39%[6] to 69%.[156–159] Localized fragments of media were seen either juxtaposed to abnormal intima (demarcated from it by an internal elastic membrane) or as part of a full-thickness vessel wall excision. The frequency of excised media in de novo (primary, de novo) coronary stenoses was similar to that of excised media in restenosis sites in one study (39%[156]) but tended to be slightly higher in the other two studies (47% vs. 69% and 40% vs. 63%,[156–158] respectively). Two[156, 157] of the three studies also indicate quantization of media thickness (depth)[156] or length[157] is greater in de novo than in restenosis lesions. One explanation for this difference is that the diseased intima is thicker in restenosis lesions and thus provides less opportunity for penetration of the underlying vessel media. Alternatively, primary lesions may be more eccentric in nature, containing areas of media without much overlying plaque.[155] It is uncertain whether resection of media and adventitia components influence the degree of subsequent restenosis and/or atherectomy procedural complications. The relationship between presence and amount of media on atherectomy samples and subsequent frequency of restenosis is being discussed.[156, 159, 167, 168] At present, three studies[158, 159, 166] have indicated no significant relationship between the presence of atherectomy media and the frequency of subsequent restenosis.[155]

5. Native coronary stenotic lesions do not consist exclusively of atherosclerotic plaque (with or without thrombus).[155] Although intimal proliferation (hyperplasia) had been observed previously in atherectomy tissue from restenosis after a prior intervention, the finding of intimal proliferation with plaque in atherectomy specimens from primary (de novo) lesions has more recently been reported. Although more than 75% of atherectomy samples from primary or de novo lesions consist of atherosclerotic plaque (with or without thrombus), 22%[157] to 42%[158] of primary atherectomy lesions also contain intimal proliferative tissue (see Table 4–10). Selected specialized immunologic testing of intimal proliferative tissue from both de novo and restenosis lesions confirms their identity.[159] In contrast to the studies by Johnson and associates[157] and Schnitt and colleagues[158, 159] Waller and associates[166] found no instance of intimal proliferation in 268 atherectomy samples from 33 patients with de novo coronary stenosis. In further analysis of their 24 (22%) cases of native atherectomy stenoses with intimal hyperplasia, Johnson and associates[157] found that angioplasty or atherectomy had been previously performed proximal or distal to the hyperplastic lesion in 11 patients (46%), simulation of intimal hyperplasia by focal in-growth of myofibroblasts at the periphery of organizing thrombi occurred in 5 (21%), and possible simulation of the hyperplasia by relatively young atherosclerotic lesions still in an active growth phase were found in the remaining 8 de novo lesions (33%). Schnitt and colleagues[159] provided no further details regarding their 29 (45%) sites of primary stenoses with intimal proliferation, but many such lesions were from patients with unstable angina, unstable angina which suggests that spontaneous plaque injury (fissure) may stimulate a spontaneous and progressive hyperplastic response like that seen in restenosis lesions. Miller and colleagues[169] provided further information about these de novo lesions. Intimal hyperplasia was found in 42 (40%) of 105 of de novo coronary artery stenoses excised during directional atherectomy. Of these 42 lesions (45 patients), the frequencies of younger age of the lesion and location of the lesion in the left anterior descending artery were greater than in 57 lesions with de novo atherectomy tissue consisting of atherosclerotic plaque without associated intimal proliferation. No other differences in baseline characteristics (including unstable angina), angiographic findings, or clinical outcome were identified between the two subgroups of de novo lesions.[169]

# STENTS

## Morphology[171]

Intravascular implants have been designed to reverse the untoward effects of balloon angioplasty by acting as a scaffold to "tack up" the intimal dissections, mechanically prevent elastic recoil and vascular spasm, and possibly limit thrombus formation by increasing vessel blood flow.[170–175] Clinical studies have demonstrated that intravascular stents do indeed improve stenosis geometry after angioplasty.[176–182] These studies also suggest that intracoronary stents may be effective in maintaining long-term vessel patency. Because it has been well documented that restenosis rates are higher in patients with greater residual stenoses immediately after the vascular intervention (i.e., a post-PTCA stenosis rate of >30%),[181–185] use of intravascular stents to improve postprocedural vessel lumen diameter may lead to a reduced restenosis rate.

Numerous experimental animal studies have examined the short- and long-term morphologic effects of intravascular stents in coronary arteries[178, 187–191]; however, few studies have evaluated the morphologic characteristics of intravascular stents in human atherosclerotic vessels or saphenous vein grafts.[171, 192–194] Because of the relatively low number of patients who have undergone stent implantation and the success rate of this procedure, few pathologic specimens from humans are available for evaluation. This section reviews morphologic findings in human vessels after stent placement as well as reports from other investigators.

## Morphology of Intravascular Stents in Humans

Studies of the vascular response to intravascular stents in humans has been limited by the paucity of material for evaluation. The combined cases from both authors include five specimens of stent-implanted coronary arteries ranging from 1 day to 10 months after implantation. In one earlier report, Schatz and coworkers[192] described the morphologic features of a stent-implanted coronary artery 8 weeks after implantation. Surgical retrieval of stent-implanted saphenous vein grafts has also provided pathologic specimens for evaluation. The authors examined four specimens from stented saphenous vein bypass grafts, and von Beusekom and coauthors[194] described the morphology of 10 specimens from stent-implanted vein grafts.

### Coronary Artery Specimens with Stents

#### Stent Age: Less than 24 Hours

One stent-implanted coronary artery specimen was obtained within the first 24 hours after stent implantation.[170] The patient was an 80-year-old woman with a long history of coronary artery disease and 95% stenosis of the ostium of the left main coronary artery. Angioplasty of the ostial lesion was unsuc-

cessful, so a 20-mm-long, 3.5-mm-diameter balloon-expandable flexible coil stent (Gianturco-Roubin Flex-Stent) was placed in the left main coronary artery. Despite deployment of the stent, there was a residual ostial stenosis. The patient died 12 hours after stent placement. At autopsy the aortic root was found to contain extensive atherosclerosis with ulcerated plaques. These atherosclerotic plaques produced the ostial stenosis of the left main coronary artery. The proximal portion of the stent extended into the aortic lumen, but the atherosclerotic plaque tissue interdigitated between two coils of the stent and continued to compromise the ostium of the artery. Just distal to the ostium, the stent-implanted segment of the left main coronary artery was patent with no evidence of thrombotic material associated with the stent wires or the vessel wall. There was histologic evidence of angioplasty-induced injury with dissection of the atheroma and the vessel wall. There were also focal indentations in the vessel wall produced by the stent wires.

#### Stent Age: 7 Days

The second patient was a 73-year-old female physician with a long history of atherosclerotic coronary artery disease, including past myocardial infarction and coronary bypass grafting.[195] About 1 week before death, she had recurrent angina and underwent coronary angiography. A lesion occluding 90% of the proximal LAD artery was identified. Angioplasty was attempted with multiple inflations and balloons. The lesion was "hard" and heavily calcified, and a large plaque fracture resulted. With a threat of abrupt closure, a 20-mm-long, 3.0-mm-diameter intracoronary Gianturco-Roubin Flex-Stent was implanted. Seven days after placement of the stent and nearing hospital discharge, the patient experienced sudden recurrent chest pain and ventricular fibrillation and died. Her prothrombin time on the day of death was 17 seconds (control value, 11 seconds).

At autopsy, the heart was radiographed to identify the site of stent placement. A "hook-like" proximal extension of the stent was visible, the proximalmost tip located in the distal left main coronary artery and ostium of the left circumflex artery. The epicardial coronary arteries were removed intact and again radiographed. Subsequent transverse sectioning of the coronary arteries revealed occlusion of the stent by thrombus. Fragments of thrombus were also present on the hooklike proximal tip of the stent. The underlying atherosclerotic plaque showed evidence of balloon angioplasty–related dissection. The anterior wall of the left ventricle showed evidence of acute infarction.

#### Stent Age: 21 Days

The third patient was a 71-year-old man with stenosis involving 80% of the LAD lumen.[170] Angioplasty of the LAD lesion was performed with moderate success, but because of sluggish flow and threatened closure, a 20-mm-long, 3.0-mm-diameter Gianturco-Roubin Flex-Stent was deployed. The patient died 3 weeks later from complications of aspiration pneumonia, renal failure, and a lateral wall myocardial infarction. The LAD artery was isolated, and the region containing the intracoronary stent was identified. The vessel was patent and contained no thrombotic material. Sections of the LAD artery proximal to the stent-implanted region, which had undergone balloon angioplasty, demonstrated an intimal tear and a dissection flap. The proximal portion of the stent-implanted artery was sectioned transversely, and the region containing the diagonal artery was sectioned longitudinally. The stent wires could be visualized through a thin neointimal covering (Fig. 4–24). Scanning electron microscopy of this region demonstrated a thin neointima covering the stent wires (Fig. 4–25). The disruption of the neointima in these scanning electron micrographs was caused by postmortem autolysis and processing artifact. The stent wires were embedded into the wall of the artery, and the neointima was covered by endothelial cells (see Fig. 4–25C,D). The endothelial cells were slightly rounded and raised, but the endothelial covering was complete in all sections examined. Photomicrographs of histologic cross sections of the stent-implanted LAD artery just distal to the diagonal artery are shown in Figure 4–26. In these sections, the hole left by the stent wire is marked by an asterisk. A neointima that was only 30 to 50 μm thick was overlying and adjacent to the stent wires. The stent wire acted as a scaffold, holding the intimal flap against the wall of the vessel. There was a small amount of thrombotic material and smooth muscle cells within the dissection plane between the intimal flap and the wall of the vessel (see Fig. 4–26B). Longitudinal sections of the stent-implanted LAD segment (see Fig. 4–26C,D) again demonstrated the dissection plane as well as the indentations in the media (asterisks) where the stent wires held the dissection flap against the vessel wall. The neointimal tissue overlying the stent wire consists of spindle-shaped cells with eosinophilic interstitial tissue. These formalin-fixed, paraffin-embedded slides were immunostained with smooth muscle α-actin, desmin, vimentin, and factor VIII. The spindle-shaped cells in the neointima reacted positively with smooth muscle α-actin, vimentin, and desmin antibody. This morphologic picture and the immunohistochemical staining characteristics are consistent with smooth muscle cells of the secretory phenotype. The cells lining the vessel lumen, including the neointimal area overlying the stent wires, reacted with factor VIII, which is characteristic of endothelial cells. Serial sections throughout the stent-implanted region of the LAD artery demonstrated evidence of the PTCA dissection and disruption of the media. There was only mild residual stenosis, which did not affect more than 20% to 30% of the luminal diameter.

### Stent Age: 6 Months

The fourth patient was a 75-year-old man who underwent coronary arteriography for chest pain.[196] A totally occluded right coronary artery was successfully reopened and dilated. Four months later the patient returned with recurrent chest pain. A repeat angiogram disclosed restenosis of the right coronary artery angioplasty site. A second attempt at angio-

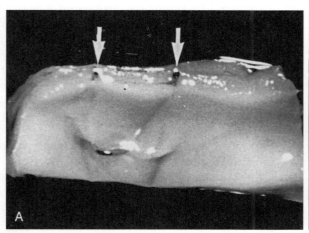
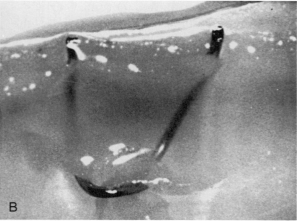

FIGURE 4–24. Photographs of the luminal surface of the stent-implanted region of the left anterior descending artery from the third patient (71-year-old man with stenosis of the left anterior descending artery), 3 weeks after placement of a Gianturco-Roubin Flex-Stent. *A,* The stent wires were cut with fine wire cutters, and the cut ends of the wires can be seen embedded into the vessel wall *(arrows). B,* Higher power photograph demonstrating the smooth neointima covering the stent wire. The curved end of the stent wire has artifactually torn through the neointima during dissection. (From Anderson PG, Bajaj RK, Baxley WA, et al: Vascular pathology of balloon-expandable flexible coil stents in humans. J Am Coll Cardiol 19:372–381, 1992.)

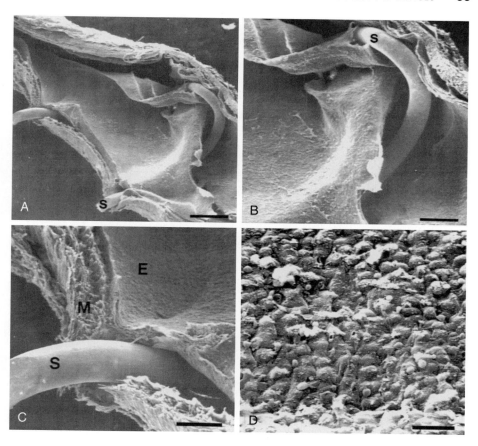

FIGURE 4–25. Scanning electron micrographs of the luminal surface of the left anterior descending artery from the third patient (71-year-old man with stenosis of the left anterior descending artery), 3 weeks after placement of a Gianturco-Roubin Flex-Stent. *A,* Low-power view of the opened vessel showing the stent wires (S) covered by neointima. The neointima covering the stent wires has pulled away from the vessel wall during processing. *B,* A higher power micrograph showing the neointima covering the stent wire. *C,* The stent is embedded into the media of the vessel (M). The neointima covers the stent wire and is re-endothelialized (E). *D,* Endothelial cells on the surface of the neointima are slightly rounded and raised, but they do form a contiguous endothelial covering within the vessel lumen of the stented region. (From Anderson PG, Bajaj RK, Baxley WA, et al: Vascular pathology of balloon expandable flexible coil stents in humans. J Am Coll Cardiol 19:372–381, 1992.)

plasty was associated with lesion recoil. Therefore, a 20-mm-long, 3.5-mm-diameter stent was placed. Six months later the patient again experienced chest discomfort. Angiography revealed stenosis occluding 75% of the midportion of the stent. The patient underwent atherectomy of the stenotic site with a Simpson Coronary AtheroCath (Devices for Vascular Intervention, Inc.; Redwood City CA). Three cuts were made. During the last cut, the distal portion of the stent was entrapped in the cutter and snapped. That portion of the stent uncoiled and was removed. Fluoroscopy showed that the remainder of the stent was intact. An angioplasty balloon was then used to dilate within the stent to "recompress" any dislodged portion of the stent.

Six pieces of restenotic tissue from within the stented vessel were recovered. Histologic examination disclosed smooth muscle cell intimal proliferation characteristic of restenosis tissue. Fragments of thrombus were also present. No calcific deposits or atherosclerotic plaque was present.

### Stent Age: 10 Months

The fifth patient was a 71-year-old woman with type II diabetes mellitus, hypertension, and a history of two previous myocardial infarctions, who presented with unstable angina. The patient underwent angio-

plasty of a lesion in the left circumflex artery and a lesion in the mid-LAD artery at the branch point of the first diagonal, with subsequent placement of a 20-mm-long, 3.0-mm-diameter Gianturco-Roubin Flex-Stent at the LAD site. There was evidence of thrombotic material within the stent, so a perfusion catheter was deployed to deliver urokinase at 160,000 U/hour for 2 hours, followed by 80,000 U/hour overnight. The next day a hazy lesion occluding 30% to 40% of the middle of the stent was present and angioplasty was performed inside the stent, alleviating the stenosis. Six months later the patient again experienced unstable angina, and a repeat angiogram demonstrated 100% occlusion of the LAD artery at the stent site. Angioplasty was successfully performed inside the stent; residual stenosis produced 40% occlusion. Four months later, the patient again developed unstable angina, and an angiogram revealed stenosis of the LAD artery involving 80% of the stent site. The patient opted for saphenous vein bypass grafting but died shortly after the operation.

At autopsy, the LAD artery was found to be patent with no evidence of thrombus. The stent wires were covered by re-endothelialized neointima, and the wires were incorporated into the vessel wall (Figs. 4–27 and 4–28). The LAD artery contained areas of atherosclerotic disease (Fig. 4–29; see Fig. 4–27), in

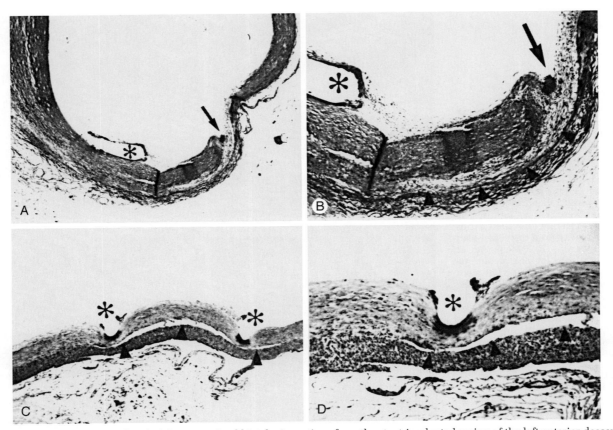

FIGURE 4–26. Photomicrographs of trichrome-stained histologic sections from the stent-implanted region of the left anterior descending artery from the third patient (71-year-old man with stenosis of the left anterior descending artery), 3 weeks after placement of a Gianturco-Roubin Flex-Stent. The stent wire had been carefully removed before processing for histology. *A,* The thin neointimal covering can be seen overlying the area where the stent wire has been removed *(asterisk).* The intimal flap *(arrow)* has been held against the vessel wall by the stent. *B,* The dissection plane of the intimal flap *(arrowheads)* is clearly visible; however, the stent *(asterisk)* has held the flap against the vessel wall, and neointimal tissue has reattached the flap to the vessel wall *(arrow). C,* Longitudinal sections of the vessel demonstrate the indentations left by the stent wires *(asterisks)* and the dissection plane *(arrowheads).* The neointima was accidentally removed with the stent wires during preparation of the specimen for microscopy. *D,* The stent wire *(asterisk)* compressed the media and held this tissue against the vessel wall. (From Anderson PG, Bajaj RK, Baxley WA, et al: Vascular pathology of balloon expandable flexible coil stents in humans. J Am Coll Cardiol 19:372–381, 1992.)

addition to the neointimal proliferative reaction. The neointima comprised primarily smooth muscle cells, as demonstrated by immunohistochemical staining with smooth muscle α-actin, with fewer numbers of macrophages and lymphocytes (see Fig. 4–29E,F). This inflammatory reaction was present within or adjacent to areas of atherosclerosis. There was a mild inflammatory reaction immediately surrounding the stent wires (see Fig. 4–29), and in some cases this consisted of macrophages, occasional multinucleated giant cells ("foreign body giant cells"), and lymphocytes (see Fig. 4–29D). Also, within the neointima there were areas of thrombotic material that appeared to be incorporated into the neointima.

## Summary of Stented Coronary Artery Morphology

Morphologic evaluation of five cases of intravascular stents in human coronary arteries[171] suggests that the flexible coil stents are re-endothelialized by 3 weeks in situ and are completely covered by neointima. This neointima consists of primarily smooth muscle cells with few inflammatory cells. There was evidence of thrombotic material incorporated into the neointima. These findings are similar to those seen by Schatz and coworkers[192] 8 weeks after placement of two Palmaz-Schatz stents in the left circumflex coronary artery of a patient who had undergone two previous angioplasty procedures. Even the aforementioned patient examined 10 months after stent placement, the inflammatory response to the stent wire was minimal, and there was no evidence of unusual degeneration of the vessel wall in association with stent placement. In the case in which the stent wires were not properly deployed and the wires were not embedded into the wall of the vessel, there was thrombosis of the stented vessel despite adequate anticoagulation. The presence of the stent wires within the vessel lumen undoubtedly predisposed the vessel to thrombosis. This demonstrates the need to ensure proper stent delivery with close apposition of the stent wires to the vessel wall.

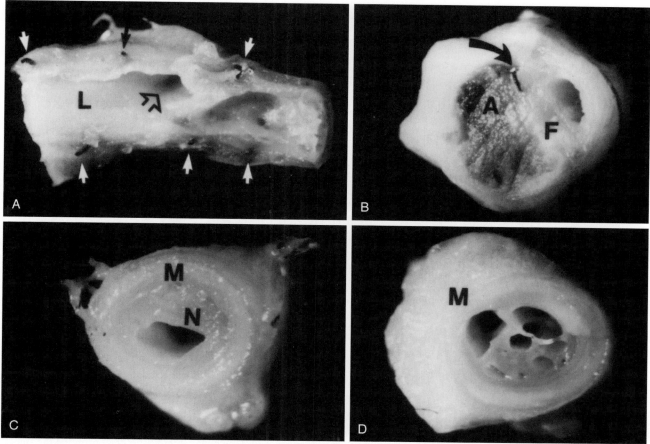

FIGURE 4–27. Gross photographs of left anterior descending artery (LAD) from the fifth patient (71-year-old woman with diabetes mellitus), 10 months after placement of a Gianturco-Roubin Flex-Stent. *A,* The stent-implanted vessel segment was opened longitudinally with the proximal portion of the vessel on the left side of the picture. The vessel lumen (L) is patent, and the stent wires are visible *(arrows)* in the vessel wall. The diagonal artery *(open arrowhead)* is patent at its origin in the LAD segment with the stent; however, atherosclerotic and restenotic tissue significantly compromised the lumen of the diagonal artery distally. *B,* A cross section of the artery segment with the stent, just proximal to the artery segment pictured in *A,* demonstrates an eccentric atheroma (A), covered by fibrous cap (F) and a patent lumen (L) that is severely compromised. The stent wire *(curved arrow),* which is embedded in the fibrous cap, is covered by neointima. *C,* Cross section of artery with the stent, without significant atheroma, demonstrating the vessel media (M) and the neointimal tissue (N) that is partially occluding the vessel lumen (L). *D,* Distal to the artery segment with the stent, the LAD contained numerous vascular channels (center of vessel segment) that are indicative of a recanalized thrombus. M, vessel media.

## Saphenous Vein Bypass Graft Biopsy Specimens

Saphenous vein grafts develop diffuse stenosis with age and have a propensity for developing stenotic lesions at the anastomotic sites.[197, 198] Angioplasty has been used to alleviate the clinical symptoms associated with these stenoses, and, as might be expected, acute closure and restenosis can occur after intervention. Various types of stents, including balloon expandable and self-expanding wire stents, have been implanted in saphenous vein grafts. The pathologic findings have been described both in stent-implanted vein grafts from autopsy specimens and in vein grafts removed from patients who underwent a second bypass grafting operation.[170, 194] The specimens described herein represent one stent-implanted vein graft obtained at autopsy 20 days

after implantation and three specimens from patients who underwent a second bypass operation 3, 5, and 6 months after stent implantation because of restenosis within the stented vein graft segment.[171]

### Stent Age: 20 Days

In the first patient, a Gianturco-Roubin Flex-Stent had been in place for 20 days, but the stent coils were not completely embedded in the wall of the vessel. Despite the presence of stent coils in the vessel lumen, there was no evidence of thrombotic material. Histologically, the vessel wall contained areas of injury caused by angioplasty and stent placement. There was a mild accumulation of thrombotic material adjacent to the indentations left by the stent wire, but there was little or no neointima. Throughout the stent-implanted region, there

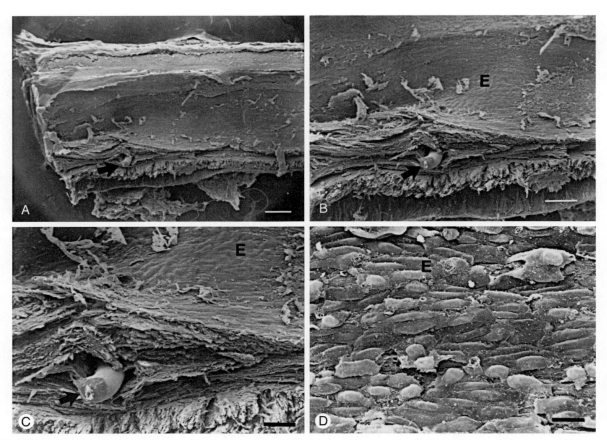

FIGURE 4–28. Scanning electron micrographs of the left anterior descending artery from the fifth patient (71-year-old woman with diabetes mellitus), 10 months after placement of a Gianturco-Roubin Flex-Stent. *A,* Low-power micrograph demonstrating the smooth, clean luminal surface with a piece of the stent wire protruding from the vessel wall *(arrow).* The bar in the lower right corner represents 500 μm. *B* and *C,* Closer views of stent wire *(arrow)* that has compressed the media and is covered by neointima. The continuous endothelial layer (E) is evident on the surface of the neointima. In *B,* the bar indicates 300 μm; in *C,* 150 μm. *D,* High-power view of endothelial cells covering the neointima. The bar indicates 20 μm.

was very minimal neointimal growth and no inflammation associated with the injury.

### Stent Age: 3 Months

The second patient had undergone angioplasty of a stenosed saphenous vein graft to the mid-LAD artery with placement of PS-20 Palmaz-Schatz biliary stents (Johnson & Johnson Interventional Systems) at the proximal and distal ends of the graft. Three months later the patient again developed unstable angina, caused by thrombosis of the stent-implanted vein graft, and underwent a second bypass grafting operation with removal of the original stent-implanted saphenous vein graft at the time of reoperation. The vessels were opened longitudinally by the surgeon. There was thrombotic material within the lumen of the vessel closely associated with the distal portion of the saphenous vein graft. The distal stent was not embedded in the wall of the vein graft, and there was no gross or microscopic evidence of re-endothelialization or neointimal formation in association with the stent. The segment of vein graft containing the proximal stent also contained thrombotic material, but this thrombus did not occlude the vessel (Fig. 4–30). In this specimen, the stent wires were embedded in the wall of the vessel, and neointimal tissue had grown over the stent wires to a thickness ranging from 400 to 1150 μm. This neointimal tissue contained organizing thrombotic material with smooth muscle cells, fibroblasts, and inflammatory cells (Fig. 4–31). In some areas the neointima was entirely cellular, consisting primarily of smooth muscle cells, with little evidence of thrombotic material (see Fig. 4–31). There was little if any inflammatory response to the stent wires.

### Stent Age: 5 Months

The third patient was a 65-year-old man with a history of saphenous vein bypass grafting to the LAD artery who had undergone angioplasty of the proximal and distal anastomotic sites of the graft. Ten days later he had undergone a second angioplasty procedure with placement of 20-mm-long,

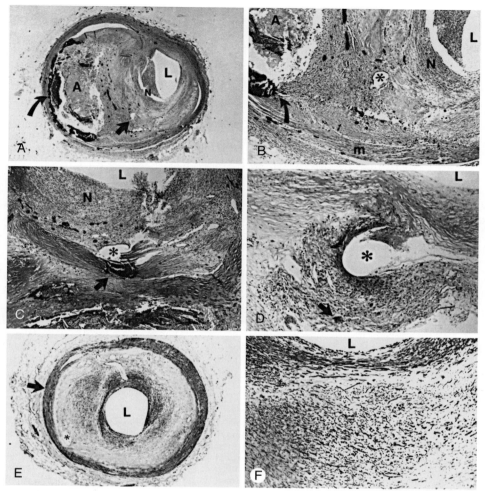

FIGURE 4–29. Photographs of the left anterior descending artery (LAD) from the fifth patient (71-year-old woman with diabetes mellitus), 10 months after placement of a Gianturco-Roubin Flex-Stent. *A,* This cross section from the stent-implanted LAD (same as in Fig. 4–28*B*) contains a large eccentric atheroma (A) with areas of calcification (darker material, *curved arrow*). In addition to the atheroma, the vessel lumen (L) is also partially occluded by neointimal tissue (N). The hole left after removal of the stent wire is stent marked by the *arrow. B,* Higher power view of the specimen in *A* demonstrating the location of the stent wire *(asterisk)* and the neointimal proliferative tissue (N). The atheroma (A) and the calcification *(curved arrow)* are also visible. L, vessel lumen; M, media. *C,* Section of LAD where the stent wire *(asterisk)* had compressed the fibrous cap overlying the atheroma (A). This is associated with a focal area of calcification immediately under the stent wire *(arrow).* The neointima (N) is seen above the stent wire. Note the lack of inflammatory reaction adjacent to the stent wire. L, lumen. *D,* High-power photomicrograph of an adjacent histologic section demonstrating a mild inflammatory reaction, consisting of lymphocytes, macrophages, and foreign body giant cells *(arrow),* around the stent wire *(asterisk).* L, lumen. *E,* Photomicrograph of a stent-implanted artery section that was reacted with an antibody to smooth muscle α-actin. The dark color is a positive reaction for smooth muscle α-actin. The media *(arrow)* stained intensely, whereas the neointima stained less intensely except immediately around the vessel lumen (L). The hole left after stent removal is marked with an *asterisk. F,* Higher magnification of the neointima from *E* shows that within the pale staining area of the neointima, there are numerous cells that stain positively for smooth muscle α-actin. The loose arrangement of these cells and the abundant extracellular matrix, which does not stain, results in the pale staining of the neointima seen in the low-power photomicrograph in panel *E.*

2.5-mm-diameter Gianturco-Roubin Flex-Stents, at both the proximal and distal anastomotic sites.[170] After 5 months, the patient again developed chest pain, caused by stenoses at the anastomotic sites. The patient then underwent a repeat saphenous vein bypass grafting operation with removal of the stent-implanted vein graft. The sections of saphenous vein graft submitted for pathologic examination were patent; however, the vessel walls were markedly thickened by fibrous connective tissue. Light microscopic evaluation of these specimens

demonstrated the thickened intima and a large eccentric atherosclerotic plaque in the proximal segment of the vein graft (Fig. 4–32*A*). Longitudinal sections of the graft (see Fig. 4–32*B*) demonstrated the marked thickening of the vessel wall, the indentations produced by the stent wires, and the stent wire compressing the fibrous cap overlying the atheromatous lesions. In some areas the neointima overlying the stent wire was intact, and its thickness ranged from 100 to 150 μm. It was composed of fusiform-shaped cells that stained positively with

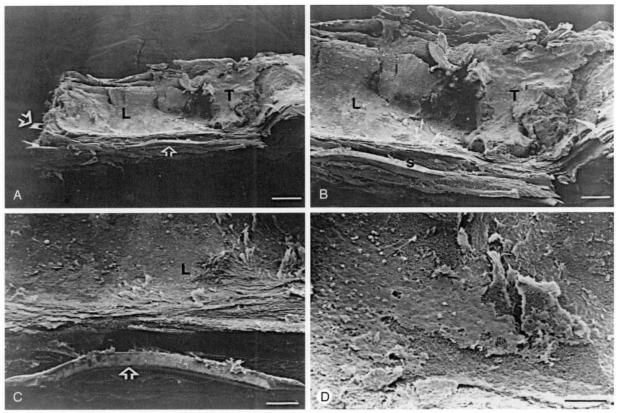

FIGURE 4–30. Scanning electron micrography of saphenous vein graft 2 months after placement of PS-20 Palmaz-Schatz biliary stents (Johnson & Johnson Interventional Systems). *A,* Low-power photomicrograph demonstrating the thrombotic material (T) partially occluding the vessel lumen (L). The stent wires *(open arrows)* are visible under the neointima. The bar in the lower right corner represents 1 mm. *B,* Higher power micrograph demonstrating the thrombotic material (T) partially occluding the vessel lumen (L). The stent wire (S) is visible under the neointima. The bar represents 500 μm. *C,* Close-up view of stent wires *(open arrow)* covered by neointima. L, vessel lumen. The bar represents 300 μm. *D,* The surface of the vessel lumen contains sheets of endothelial cells and thrombotic material. The bar represents 200 μm.

smooth muscle α-actin. These smooth muscle cells had very little extracellular matrix, and they have a more mature (contractile type) morphologic profile, in comparison with the secretory phenotype cells seen in the previous case, in which the stent had been implanted for only 3 weeks. There were also occasional lymphocytes and macrophages within the neointima covering the stent wire. The cells were diffusely distributed within the neointima and were not associated with or concentrated around the stent wire. This suggests that this inflammatory reaction is a general reaction within the vessel wall and is not associated with a rejection reaction to the wire. There was no evidence of inflammatory reaction associated with the stent wires in these specimens.

### Stent Age: 6 Months

The fourth patient was a man who, 10 years after saphenous vein bypass grafting, developed a non–Q-wave myocardial infarction; catheterization study revealed severe stenoses of the grafts to the left circumflex and LAD arteries.[170] Angioplasty of the circumflex and LAD lesions was successfully performed with adjunctive use of an eximer laser. Two months later the patient developed angina, and stenosis involving 90% of the diameter of the circumflex artery was relieved by angioplasty and placement of a 20-mm-long, 3.0-mm-diameter Gianturco-Roubin Flex-Stent. Five months later the patient again developed angina, and angioplasty was performed inside the stent. One month later (6 months after stent placement), the patient again developed angina, and at this time internal mammary artery bypass grafting was performed. During surgery the saphenous vein bypass graft containing the stent was retrieved and was subjected to morphologic examination. The saphenous vein bypass graft was markedly thickened and contained extensive neointimal proliferation (Fig. 4–33*A,B*). The thickness of the neointima ranged from 250 to 500 μm. This neointimal tissue obstructed the lumen of the saphenous vein graft. The neointima contained spindle-shaped smooth muscle cells and a mild lymphocytic infiltration. There was minimal in-

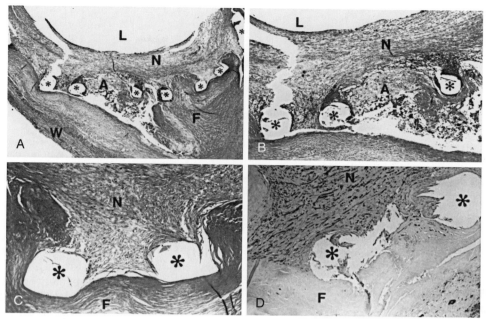

FIGURE 4–31. Photomicrograph of saphenous vein graft 2 months after placement of a PS-20 Palmaz-Schatz biliary stent (Johnson & Johnson Interventional Systems). *A,* In this low-power micrograph of a hematoxylin and eosin–stained section, the holes left after removal of the stent wires are labeled with *asterisks.* There is a layer of neointima (N) overlying the stent, and the lumen (L) is patent. An area of atheroma (A) is present in the intima of the vein graft along with areas of fibrous connective tissue (F). Smooth muscle cells make up the wall (W) of the vein graft. *B,* Higher power photomicrograph of tissue section in *A,* demonstrating the holes left by the stent wires *(asterisks),* the atheroma (A), the neointima (N), and the patent lumen (L). *C,* The stent wires *(asterisks)* compress the fibrous tissue (F) in the wall of the vein graft. The neointima (N) is composed of a loose arrangement of smooth muscle cells and abundant extracellular matrix material. Note the absence of inflammation around the holes left by the stent wires. *D,* Same section as in *C* reacted with an antibody to smooth muscle α-actin. The fusiform cells in the neointima react strongly with the antibody for smooth muscle α-actin and are surrounded by abundant extracellular matrix material. F, fibrous tissue; *asterisks* represent holes left after stent wires were removed.

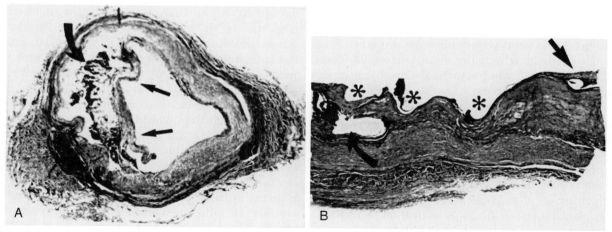

FIGURE 4–32. *A,* Photomicrograph of a hematoxylin and eosin–stained cross section of saphenous vein graft 5 months after placement of a Gianturco-Roubin Flex-Stent. The vessel wall is thickened, and there is an eccentric atheromatous lesion *(curved arrow)* with a fibrous cap *(straight arrows).* This lesion contained fresh hemorrhage. *B,* Longitudinal section of stented portion of vein graft just proximal to the segment shown in *A.* The atheromatous lesion *(curved arrow)* with the fibrous cap can be seen. The indentations left by the stent wires *(asterisks)* are visible on the luminal surface of the vessel. One of these stent wires (left side of figure) compresses the fibrous cap overlying the atheromatous lesion. The neointima was artifactually removed over most of this specimen during processing of the tissue samples, except in the far right side of this photograph *(arrow).* In this region, the hole left by the stent wire is visible, and the neointima has grown over this stent wire *(arrow).* (From Anderson PG, Bajaj RK, Baxley WA, et al: Vascular pathology of balloon expandable flexible coil stents in humans. J Am Coll Cardiol 19:372–381, 1992.)

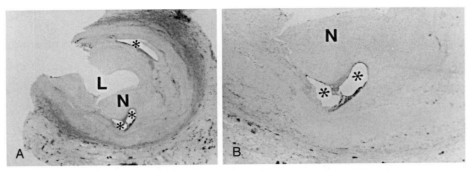

FIGURE 4–33. *A*, Photomicrograph of a hematoxylin and eosin–stained cross section of the saphenous vein graft 6 months after placement of a Gianturco-Roubin Flex-Stent. The holes left after stent wire removal *(asterisks)* are seen, and the neointimal tissue (N) can be seen overlying the stent. L, lumen. *B*, High-power photomicrograph of the saphenous vein graft wall with the holes left by the stent wires *(asterisks)* and the neointimal covering (N). (From Anderson PG, Bajaj RK, Baxley WA, et al: Vascular pathology of balloon expandable flexible coil stents in humans. J Am Coll Cardiol 19:372–381, 1992.)

flammation in association with the stent wires in the vessel wall.

### *Summary of Stented Saphenous Vein Graft Morphology*

The morphologic features in the preceding cases of stented saphenous vein grafts, evaluated from 20 days to 6 months after placement, demonstrate (1) some thrombus formation associated with the stent wires and (2) neointimal proliferation comprising smooth muscle cells and few inflammatory cells. In the two cases in which the stent wires were not clearly embedded into the wall of the vessel, there was little if any neointimal tissue and no evidence of re-endothelialization of the stent. This lack of neointimal response in the stents that were not embedded into the vessel wall may have resulted from movement of the stent wire inside the lumen of the vessel. In cases in which the stent was embedded into the vessel wall, the neointimal tissue was able to surround and grow over the stent wires. This later observation of neointimal response to stents is consistent with findings by van Beusekom and coauthors,[194] who evaluated saphenous vein grafts after implantation of self-expanding Wallstents. They observed thrombotic material adjacent to the stent wires and neointima consisting of primarily smooth muscle cells. Their findings with the Wallstent are similar to our findings with the Gianturco-Roubin Flex-Stent and the Palmaz-Schatz stent.

## Summary of Current Stent Pathology

Intravascular stent implantation has proved to be an important addition to the armamentarium of the interventional cardiologist. The clinical utility of stents in preventing acute closure after PTCA is promising, and the role of stents in preventing or decreasing the clinical impact of restenosis remains to be determined. It is clear from the available hu-

man pathologic material that intravascular stents do act as a scaffold to hold open the vessel after the injury produced during angioplasty. Current data also demonstrate that the stent wires are initially covered with a thin platelet fibrin coating, if the patient has received adequate anticoagulation to prevent acute thrombotic occlusion, and within 2 to 3 weeks, the stent wires are covered by re-endothelialized neointima. The only exceptions to this time scale of re-endothelialization were the two cases in which the stent wires were not firmly embedded into the vessel wall. In these cases there was an increased risk of thrombosis, and re-endothelialization did not take place, possibly because of the movement of the stent wires in the vessel lumen. From our series of patients, and according to observations by others, there was very little inflammatory response to the stent wire. Even in our case in which the stent had been in place for 10 months, the inflammatory response was minimal, and there was no deterioration of the vessel media. Because stents are placed in diseased arteries, the stent wires are often embedded into fibrous tissue and atheroma, in which they would not be expected to cause medial injury. In the few instances in which stent wires were in contact with the media, there was compression and focal thinning of the media but no evidence of severe degeneration. These results in humans are similar to those of experimental animal studies. Despite the variety of animal species and model systems used, the basic vascular response to stent implantation is fairly uniform and is similar to observations in humans. Thus, the available data from animals and humans suggest that intravascular stents are well tolerated by the blood vessel, and no untoward degenerative or inflammatory response has been observed. It is apparent that the process of restenosis is not completely prevented by stenting. However, the increased lumen diameter produced after stent implantation may lead to a decrease in the incidence of clinical symptoms caused by restenosis. Well-designed prospective, randomized, clinical trials are necessary to answer specific questions about the clinical efficacy of intravascular stents.

## BALLOON PYROPLASTY

## Thermal Balloon Angioplasty, "Biologic Stent" Implantation

Thermal balloon angioplasty, originally developed as laser balloon angioplasty,[199, 200] is a method of remolding or remodeling a stenotic atherosclerotic vessel in order to increase luminal area. Various energy sources can be used to produce a thermal injury on vessel walls or adjacent plaque. Results of animal and cadaver[201, 202] studies indicate that thermal balloon angioplasty decreases vessel elasticity at the dilation site, and heat molds the arterial segment to the size and shape of the inflated angioplasty balloon. This process creates, in effect, a "biologic stent." In addition to the acute remolding effects, thermal effects on the underlying media may destroy smooth muscle cells involved in the late restenosis process.[202]

Lee and colleagues[202] evaluated radiofrequency as an energy source for balloon pyroplasty. Delivery of radiofrequency in combination with balloon inflation pressure effectively molded atherosclerotic plaque and vessels. Experimental studies on layers of human cadaver aorta showed tissue fusion ("welding") of previously separated layers, thus indicating the usefulness of this technique in treatment of intraluminal intimal flaps. In the experimental model, balloon pyroplasty has not been associated with subsequent vessel aneurysm or ruptures.

Becker and colleagues[203] established several principles of interaction between radiofrequency current and vascular tissues: feasibility of fusion of tissue layers (intima-media, media-adventitia), vascular molding, and destruction of cellular elements of the media. Each of these interactions through a radiofrequency heated balloon may provide solutions toward angioplasty dissection and acute closure, dilation and elastic recoil of eccentric plaques, and medial smooth muscle proliferation after angioplasty (restenosis).

## Thermal Probes

### Glazing

Thermal probes may be used after coronary balloon angioplasty in an attempt to seal off superficial intimal disruptions. The low-powered probe skims through the treated vessel, "glazing" the new lumen. No tissue is removed, but a "finishing-touch" type of remodeling occurs.[204]

## REFERENCES

1. Gruentzig AR, Myler RK, Hanna EH, et al: Coronary transluminal angioplasty [Abstract]. Circulation 84(suppl II):55–56, 1977.
2. Waller BF: "Crackers, breakers, stretchers, drillers, scrapers, shavers, burners, welders, melters"—The future treatment of atherosclerotic coronary artery disease? A clinical morphologic assessment. J Am Coll Cardiol 13:969–987, 1989.
3. Waller BF: The eccentric coronary atherosclerotic plaque: Morphologic observations and clinical relevance. Clin Cardiol 12:14–20, 1989.
4. Baim DS (ed): A symposium: Interventional cardiology 1987. Am J Cardiol 61:1G–117G, 1988.
5. Block PC, Myler RK, Stertzer S, et al: Morphology after transluminal angioplasty in human beings. N Engl J Med 305:382–385, 1981.
6. Waller BF, Dillon JC, Cowley MH: Plaque hematoma and coronary dissection with percutaneous transluminal angioplasty (PTCA) of severely stenotic lesions: Morphologic coronary observations in 5 men within 30 days of PTCA [Abstract]. Circulation 68:III-144, 1983.
7. Waller BF: Pathology of transluminal balloon angioplasty used in the treatment of coronary heart disease. Hum Pathol 18:476–484, 1987.
8. Waller BF, Rothbaum DA, Pinkerton CA, et al: Status of the myocardium and infarct-related coronary artery in 19 necropsy patients with acute recanalization using pharmacologic, mechanical or combined types of reperfusion therapy. J Am Coll Cardiol 9:785–801, 1987.
9. Mizuno K, Jurita A, Imazeki N: Pathologic findings after percutaneous transluminal coronary angioplasty. Br Heart J 52:588–590, 1984.
10. Soward AL, Essed CE, Serruys PW: Coronary arterial findings after accidental death immediately after successful percutaneous transluminal coronary angioplasty. Am J Cardiol 56:794–795, 1985.
11. La Delia V, Rossi PA, Sommers S, et al: Coronary histology after percutaneous transluminal coronary angioplasty. Texas Heart Inst J 15:113–116, 1988.
12. Dotter CT, Judkins MP: Transluminal treatment of atherosclerotic obstructions: Description of new technic and a preliminary report of its application. Circulation 30:654–670, 1964.
13. Gruentzig AR: Transluminal dilatation of coronary artery stenosis. Lancet 1:263–266, 1978.
14. Waller BF: Coronary luminal shape and the arc of disease-free wall: Morphologic observations and clinical relevance. J Am Coll Cardiol 6:1100–1101, 1985.
15. Cowley MJ, Dovros G, Kelsey SF, et al: Emergency coronary bypass surgery after coronary angioplasty: The National Heart, Lung and Blood Institute's Percutaneous Transluminal Coronary Angioplasty Registry experience. Am J Cardiol 53:22C–26C, 1984.
16. Bredlau CE, Roubin GS, Leimgruber PP, et al: In-hospital morbidity and mortality in patients undergoing elective coronary angioplasty. Circulation 72:1044–1052, 1985.
17. Simpfendorfer C, Belardi J, Bellamy G, et al: Frequency, management and follow-up of patients with acute coronary occlusions after percutaneous coronary angioplasty. Am J Cardiol 59:267–269, 1987.
18. Sinclair IN, McCabe CH, Sipperly ME, et al: Predictors, therapeutic options and long-term outcome of abrupt reclosure. Am J Cardiol 61:615–665, 1988.
19. Baim DS, Ignatius EJ: Use of percutaneous transluminal coronary angioplasty: Results of a current survey. Am J Cardiol 61:3G–8G, 1988.
20. Waller BF, Fry E, Peters T, et al: Abrupt (<1 day), acute (<1 week) and early (<1 month) vessel closure at the angioplasty site. Morphologic observations and causes of closure in 130 necropsy patients undergoing coronary angioplasty. Clin Cardiol, in press.
21. Waller BF: Coronary luminal shape and the arc of disease-free wall: Morphologic observations and clinical relevance. J Am Coll Cardiol 6:1100–1101, 1985.
22. Waller BF, Rothbaum DA, Pinkerton CA, et al: Status of

the myocardium and infarct-related coronary artery in 19 necropsy patients with acute recanalization using pharmacologic, mechanical or combined types of reperfusion therapy. J Am Coll Cardiol 9:785–801, 1987.

23. Erbel R, Clas W, Busch U, et al: New balloon catheter for prolonged percutaneous transluminal coronary angioplasty and bypass flow in occluded vessels. Catheter Cardiovasc Diagn 12:116–123, 1986.

24. Myler RM, Shaw RE, Stertzler SH, et al: Recurrence after coronary angioplasty. Catheter Cardiovasc Diagn 13:77–86, 1987.

25. Haudenschild CC: Restenosis: Basic considerations. In Topol EJ (ed): Textbook of Interventional Cardiology, pp 344–362. Philadelphia: WB Saunders, 1990.

26. Califf RM, Ohman EM, Frid DJ, et al: Restenosis: The clinical issues. In Topol EJ (ed): Textbook of Interventional Cardiology, pp 363–394. Philadelphia: WB Saunders, 1990.

27. Blackshear JL, O'Callaghan WG, Califf RM: Medical approaches to prevention of restenosis after coronary angioplasty. J Am Coll Cardiol 9:834–848, 1987.

28. Waller BF, Orr CM, Pinkerton CA, et al: Morphologic observations late after coronary balloon angioplasty; mechanisms of acute injury and relationship to restenosis. Radiology SCVIR Special Series 1991, in press.

29. Waller BF, Pinkerton CA: Coronary balloon angioplasty restenosis: Definitions, pathogenesis, and treatment strategies. J Interv Cardiol, in press.

30. Waller BF: PTCA: Mechanisms of dilation and causes of acute and late closures. Cardiovasc Rev Report 10:35–47, 1989.

31. Liu MW, Roubin GS, King SB: Restenosis after coronary angioplasty. Potential biologic determinants and role of intima hyperplasia. Point of view. Circulation 79:1374–1387, 1989.

32. Waller BF, Pinkerton CA, Orr CM, et al: Morphologic observations late (>30 days) after clinically successful coronary balloon angioplasty: An analysis of 20 necropsy patients and literature review of 41 necropsy patients with coronary angioplasty restenosis. Circulation (suppl I):28–41, 1991.

33. Gruentzig AR, Senning A, Siegenthaler WE: Nonoperative dilatation of coronary-artery stenosis. N Engl J Med 301:61–68, 1979.

34. Essed CE, Van Den Brand M, Becker AE: Transluminal coronary angioplasty and early restenosis. Fibrocellular occlusion after wall laceration. Br Heart J 49:393–396, 1983.

35. Hollman J, Austin GE, Gruentzig AR, et al: Coronary artery spasm at the site of angioplasty in the first 12 months after successful percutaneous transluminal coronary angioplasty. J Am Coll Cardiol 6:1039–1045, 1983.

36. Giraldo A, Esposo OM, Meis JM: Intimal hyperplasia as a cause of restenosis after percutaneous transluminal coronary angioplasty. Arch Pathol Lab Med 109:173–175, 1985.

37. Schneider J, Gruentzig A: Percutaneous transluminal angioplasty: Morphologic findings in 3 patients. Pathol Res Pract 180:348–352, 1985.

38. Waller BF, Pinkerton CA, Foster LN: Morphologic evidence of accelerated left main coronary artery disease: A late complication of percutaneous transluminal angioplasty of the proximal left anterior descending coronary artery. J Am Coll Cardiol 9:1019–1023, 1987.

39. Lee BI, Becker GJ, Waller BF, et al: Thermal compression and molding of atherosclerotic vascular tissue with use of radiofrequency energy: Implications for radiofrequency balloon angioplasty. J Am Coll Cardiol 13:1167–1175, 1989.

40. de Morais CF, Lopes EA, Checchi H, et al: Percutaneous transluminal coronary angioplasty—Histopathological analysis of 9 necropsy cases. Virchows Arch 410:195–202, 1989.

41. Duber C, Jungbluth A, Rumpelt HJ, et al: Morphology of the coronary arteries after combined thrombolysis and percutaneous transluminal coronary angioplasty for acute myocardial infarction. Am J Cardiol 58:698–703, 1986.

42. Bruneval P, Guermonpres JL, Perrier P, et al: Coronary artery restenosis following transluminal coronary angioplasty. Arch Pathol Lab Med 110:1186–1187, 1986.

43. Ueda M, Becker AE, Fujimoto T: Pathological changes in-

duced by repeated percutaneous transluminal coronary angioplasty. Br Heart J 58:635–643, 1987.

44. Morimoto SI, Sekiguchi M, Endo M, et al: Mechanism of luminal enlargement in PTCA and restenosis: A histopathological study of necropsied coronary arteries collected from various centers in Japan. Jpn Circ J 51:1101–1115, 1987.

45. Kohchi K, Takebayashi S, Block PC, et al: Arterial changes after percutaneous transluminal coronary angioplasty: Results at autopsy. J Am Coll Cardiol 10:592–599, 1987.

46. Walley VA, Higginson LAJ, Marguis JF, et al: Local morphologic effects of coronary balloon angioplasty. Can J Cardiol 4:17–24, 1988.

47. Potkin BN, Roberts WC: Effects of percutaneous transluminal coronary angioplasty on atherosclerotic plaques and relation of plaque composition and arterial size to outcome. Am J Cardiol 62:41–50, 1988.

48. Gravanis MB, Roubin GS: Histopathologic phenomena at the site of percutaneous transluminal coronary angioplasty: The problem of restenosis. Human Pathol 20:477–485, 1989.

49. Morimoto SI, Kajita A, Sekiguchi M, et al: Histologic observations of restenosis following angioplasty where PTCA percutaneous transluminal coronary angioplasty was successful but where the patient died seven months later of a non-associated cause. Respir Circulation 41C8:708–718, 1993.

50. Waller BF, McManus BM, Gorfinkel HJ, et al: Status of the major epicardial coronary arteries 80 to 150 days after percutaneous transluminal coronary angioplasty: Analysis of 3 necropsy patients. Am J Cardiol 51:81–84, 1983.

51. Waller BF, Pinkerton CA, Foster LN: Morphologic evidence of accelerated left main coronary artery disease: A late complication of percutaneous transluminal angioplasty of the proximal left anterior descending coronary artery. J Am Coll Cardiol 9:1019–1023, 1987.

52. Waller BF, Pinkerton CA: "Cutters, scoopers, shavers, and scrapers"—The importance of atherectomy devices and clinical relevance of tissue removed. J Am Coll Cardiol 15:426–428, 1990.

53. Waller BF, Johnson DE, Schnitt SJ, et al: Histologic analysis of directional coronary atherectomy samples. A review of findings and their clinical relevance. Am J Cardiol 72:80E–87E, 1993.

54. Rapold HJ, David PR, Vai PG, et al: Restenosis and its determinants in first and repeat coronary angioplasty. Eur Heart J 8:575–586, 1987.

55. Meier B, King SB, Gruentzig AR, et al: Repeat coronary angioplasty. J Am Coll Cardiol 4:463, 1984.

56. Williams DO, Gruentzig AR, Kent KM, et al: Efficacy of repeat PTCA for coronary restenosis. Am J Cardiol 53:32C–35C, 1984.

57. Giorgi LV, Hartzler GO, Rutherford BD, et al: Should repeat PTCA be performed on patients with multiple recurring restenoses? [Abstract]. Circulation 70(suppl):II-177, 1984.

58. Teirstein PS, Hoover CA, Ligon RW, et al: Repeat coronary angioplasty efficacy of a third angioplasty for a second restenosis. J Am Coll Cardiol 13:291–296, 1989.

59. Black AJ, Anderson HV, Roubin GS, et al: Repeat coronary angioplasty: Correlates of a second restenosis. J Am Coll Cardiol 11:714–718, 1988.

60. Valibracht C, Kober G, Klepzig H, et al: Recurrent restenosis after transluminal coronary angioplasty: Dilation or surgery? Eur Heart J 9(suppl C):7–10, 1988.

61. Finci L, Meier B, Steffenino G, et al: Restenosis and repeat coronary angioplasty in Genevea. Eur Heart J 9(suppl C):11–13, 1988.

62. Quigley PJ, Hlatky MA, Hinohara T, et al: Repeat percutaneous transluminal coronary angioplasty and predictors of recurrent restenosis. Am J Cardiol 63:409–413, 1989.

63. Sugrue DD, Vlietstra RE, Hammes LN, et al: Repeat balloon coronary angioplasty for symptomatic restenosis: a not of caution. Eur Heart J 8:697–701, 1987.

64. Majack RA: Toward a molecular understanding of vascular smooth muscle growth control. Cardiovasc Rev Rep 7:731–737, 1986.

65. Waller BF, Orr CM, Pinkerton CA, et al: Part 12: Balloon angioplasty restenosis: Proliferation and chronic elastic re-

coil. *In* Castaneda-Zuniga WR, Tadarvarthy SM (eds): Interventional Radiology, pp 451–460. Baltimore: Williams & Wilkins, 1992.

66. Waller BF: Pathology of new interventional procedures used in coronary disease. *In* Waller BF (ed): Contemporary Issues in Cardiovascular Pathology. Philadelphia: FA Davis, 1988.

67. Waller BF: Morphologic correlates of coronary angiographic patterns at the site of percutaneous transluminal coronary angioplasty. Clin Cardiol 11:817–822, 1988.

68. Holmes DR Jr, Vlietstra RE, Mock MB, et al: Angiographic changes produced by percutaneous transluminal coronary angioplasty. Am J Cardiol 51:676–683, 1983.

69. Saner HE, Gobel FL, Salomonowitz E, et al: The disease-free wall in coronary atherosclerosis: Its relation to degree of obstruction. J Am Coll Cardiol 6:1096–1099, 1985.

70. Castenada-Zunida WR, Formanek A, Tadavarthy M, et al: The mechanism of balloon angioplasty. Radiology 135:565, 1980.

71. Block PC, Fallon JT, Elmer D: Experimental angioplasty: Lesions from the laboratory. Am J Radiol 135:907, 1980.

72. Zarkins CK, Lu CT, Gewertz BL, et al: Arterial disruption and remodeling following balloon dilation. Surgery 92:1086, 1982.

73. Mathews BJ, Ewels CJ, Kent KM: Coronary dissection: A predictor of restenosis? Am Heart J 115:547, 1988.

74. Leimgruber PP, Roubin GS, Anderson HV, et al: Influence of intimal dissection on restenosis after successful coronary angioplasty. Circulation 72:530, 1985.

75. Hill JA, Margolis JR, Feldman RL, et al: Coronary arterial aneurysm formation after balloon angioplasty. Am J Cardiol 52:261, 1983.

76. Waller BF: Coronary luminal shape and the arc of disease-free wall: Morphologic observations and clinical relevance. J Am Coll Cardiol 6:1100–1101, 1985.

77. Graf RH, Verani MS: Left main coronary artery stenosis: A possible complication of transluminal coronary angioplasty. Catheter Cardiovasc Diagn 10:163–166, 1984.

78. Slack JD, Pinkerton CA: Subacute left main coronary stenosis: An unusual but serious complication of percutaneous transluminal angioplasty. Angiology 36:130–136, 1985.

79. Hamad N, Pichard A, Oboler A, et al: Left main coronary artery stenosis as a late complication of percutaneous transluminal coronary angioplasty. Am J Cardiol 60:1183–1184, 1987.

80. Haraphongse M, Rossall RE: Subacute left main coronary stenosis following percutaneous transluminal coronary angioplasty. Catheter Cardiovasc Diagn 13:401–404, 1987.

81. Harper JM, Shah Y, Kern MJ, et al: Progression of left main coronary artery stenosis following left anterior descending coronary artery angioplasty. Catheter Cardiovasc Diagn 13:398–400, 1987.

82. Zamorano J, Erbel R, Ge J, et al: Vessel wall changes in the proximal non-treated segment after PTCA. An in vivo intracoronary ultrasound study. European Heart J 15:105–1511, 1994.

83. Desai PK, Ro JH, Pucillo A, et al: Left main coronary artery aneurysm following percutaneous transluminal angioplasty: A report of a case and review of the literature. Catheter Cardiovasc Diagn 27:113–116, 1992.

84. Block PC, Elmer D, Fallon JT: Release of atherosclerotic debris after transluminal angioplasty. Circulation 65:950–952, 1982.

85. Hall DP, Gruentzig AR: Percutaneous transluminal coronary angioplasty: An update on indications, techniques, and results. Cardiol Clin 3:37–48, 1985.

86. Holmes DR Jr, Vlietstra RE, Mock MB, et al: Angiographic changes produced by percutaneous transluminal coronary angioplasty. Am J Cardiol 51:676–683, 1983.

87. Dorros G, Cowley MJ, Simpson J, et al: Percutaneous transluminal coronary angioplasty: Report of complications from the National Heart, Lung and Blood Institute PTCA Registry. Circulation 67:723–730, 1983.

88. Holmes DR, Holubkov R, Vlietstra RE, et al: Comparison of complications during percutaneous transluminal coronary angioplasty from 1977 to 1981 and from 1985 to 1986. The National Heart Lung, and Blood Institute PTCA Registry. J Am Coll Cardiol 12:1149–1155, 1988.

89. MacDonald RG, Feldman RL, Conti CR, et al: Thromboembolic complications of coronary angioplasty. Am J Cardiol 54:916–917, 1984.

90. Keon WJ, Heggtveit HA, Leduc J: Perioperative myocardial infarction caused by atheroembolism. J Thorac Cardiovasc Surg 84:849–855, 1982.

91. Colavita PG, Ideker RE, Reimer KA, et al: The spectrum of pathology associated with percutaneous transluminal coronary angioplasty during acute myocardial infarction. J Am Coll Cardiol 8:855–860, 1986.

92. de Morais CF, Lopez EA, Checchi H, et al: Percutaneous transluminal coronary angioplasty: Histolopathological analysis of nine necropsy cases. Virchows Arch 410:195–202, 1986.

93. Menke DM, Jordan MD, Aust CH, et al: Histologic evidence of distal coronary thromboembolism: A complication of acute proximal coronary artery thrombolysis therapy. Chest 9:614–616, 1986.

94. Saber RS, Edwards WD, Bailey KR, et al: Coronary embolization after balloon angioplasty or thrombolytic therapy: An autopsy study of 32 cases. J Am Coll Cardiol 22:1283–1288, 1993.

95. Saenz CB, Harrell RR, Sawyer JA, et al: Acute percutaneous transluminal coronary angioplasty complicated by embolism to a coronary artery remote from the site of infarction. Catheter Cardiovasc Diagn 13:266–268, 1987.

96. Cameron J, Buchbinder M, Wexler L, et al: Thromboembolic complications of percutaneous transluminal coronary angioplasty for myocardial infarction. Catheter Cardiovasc Diagn 13:100–106, 1987.

97. Richardson SG, Callen D, Morton P, et al: Pathological changes after intravenous streptokinase treatment in eight patients with acute myocardial infarction. Br Heart J 61:390–395, 1989.

98. Roberts WC: Coronary embolism: A review of causes, consequences and diagnostic considerations. Cardiovasc Med 3:699–710, 1978.

99. Waller BF, Dixon DS, Kim RW, et al: Embolus to the left main coronary artery. Am J Cardiol 50:658–660, 1982.

100. Aueron F, Gruentzig A: Distal embolization of a coronary artery bypass graft atheroma during percutaneous transluminal coronary angioplasty. Am J Cardiol 53:953–954, 1984.

101. Reeder GS, Bresnahan JF, Holmes DR Jr, et al: Angioplasty for aortocoronary bypass graft stenosis. Mayo Clin Proc 61:14–19, 1986.

102. Saber RS, Edwards WD, Holmes DR, et al: Balloon angioplasty of aortocoronary saphenous vein bypass grafts: A histopathologic study of six grafts from five patients with emphasis on restenosis and embolic complications. J Am Coll Cardiol 12:1501–1509, 1988.

103. De Feyter PJ, Van Suylen RJ, De Jaegere PPT, et al: Balloon angioplasty for the treatment of lesions in saphenous vein bypass grafts. J Am Coll Cardiol 21:1539–1549, 1993.

104. Waller BF, Rothbaum DA, Gorfinkel HJ, et al: Morphologic observations after percutaneous transluminal balloon angioplasty of early and late aortocoronary saphenous vein bypass grafts. J Am Coll Cardiol 4:784–792, 1984.

105. Batayias GE, Barboriak JJ, Korns ME, et al: The spectrum of pathologic changes in aortocoronary saphenous vein grafts. Circulation 56(suppl II):18–22, 1977.

106. Bulkey BH, Hutchins GM: Accelerated "atherosclerosis." A morphologic study of 97 saphenous vein coronary artery bypass grafts. Circulation 55:163–169, 1977.

107. Campeau L, Lesperance J, Corbara F, et al: Aortocoronary saphenous vein bypass graft changes 5 to 7 years after surgery. Circulation 58(suppl I):170–175, 1978.

108. Lie JT, Lawrie GM, Morris GC: Aortocoronary bypass saphenous vein graft atherosclerosis. Anatomic study of 99 vein grafts from normal and hyperlipoproteinemic patients up to 75 months postoperatively. Am J Cardiol 40:906–913, 1977.

109. Smith SH, Greer JC: Morphology of saphenous vein–coronary artery bypass grafts. Seven to 116 months after surgery. Arch Pathol Lab Med 107:13–18, 1983.

110. World Health Organization: Classification of atherosclerotic

lesions—Report of a study group. Technical Report Series 143, pp 3–20. Geneva: World Health Organization, 1958.

111. Baughman KL, Pasternak RC, Fallon JT, et al: Transluminal coronary angioplasty of postmortem human hearts. Am J Cardiol 48:1044–1047, 1981.

112. Douglas JS, Gruentzig AR, King SB III, et al: Percutaneous transluminal coronary angioplasty in patients with prior coronary surgery. J Am Coll Cardiol 2:745–754, 1983.

113. Ford WB, Wholey MH, Zikria EA, et al: Percutaneous transluminal angioplasty in the management of occlusive disease involving the coronary arteries and saphenous vein bypass grafts. J Thorac Cardiovasc Surg 79:1–11, 1980.

114. Ford WB, Wholey MH, Zikria EA, et al: Percutaneous transluminal dilation of aortocoronary saphenous vein bypass grafts. Chest 79:529–535, 1981.

115. Waller BF, Roberts WC: Amount of luminal narrowing in bypassed and nonbypassed native coronary arteries in necropsy patients early and late after aorto-coronary bypass operations. *In* Mason DT, Collins JT (eds): Myocardial Revascularization. Medical and Surgical Advances in Coronary Disease, pp 503–513. New York: Yorke Medical Books, 1981.

116. Marti MC, Bouchardy B, Cox JN: Aorto-coronary bypass with autogenous saphenous vein grafts: Histological aspects. Virchows Arch 352:255–266, 1971.

117. Vlodaver Z, Edwards JE: Pathologic analysis in fatal cases following saphenous vein coronary arterial bypass. Chest 64:555–563, 1973.

118. Gruentzig AR, Senning A, Siengenthaler WE: Nonoperative dilatation of coronary artery stenosis: Percutaneous transluminal coronary angioplasty. N Engl J Med 301:61–68, 1979.

119. Famularo M, Vasilomanolakis EC, Schrager B, et al: Percutaneous transluminal angioplasty of aortocoronary saphenous vein graft: morphologic observations. JAMA 249:3347–3350, 1983.

120. Dorros G, Johnson WD, Tector AJ, et al: Percutaneous transluminal coronary angioplasty in patients with prior coronary artery bypass grafting. J Thorac Cardiovasc Surg 87:17–26, 1984.

121. Corbelli J, Franco I, Hollman J, et al: Percutaneous transluminal coronary angioplasty after previous coronary artery bypass surgery. Am J Cardiol 56:398–403, 1985.

122. Pinkerton CA, Slack JD, Orr CM, et al: Percutaneous transluminal angioplasty in patients with prior myocardial revascularization surgery. Am J Cardiol 61:15G–22G, 1988.

123. Cooper I, Ineson N, Demirtas E, et al: Role of angioplasty in patients with previous coronary artery bypass surgery. Catheter Cardiovasc Diagn 16:81–86, 1989.

124. Platko WP, Hollman J, Whitlow PL, et al: Percutaneous transluminal coronary angioplasty of saphenous vein graft stenosis: Long term follow-up. J Am Coll Cardiol 14:1645–1650, 1989.

125. Webb JG, Myler RK, Shaw RE, et al: Coronary angioplasty after coronary bypass surgery: Initial results and late outcome in 422 patients. J Am Coll Cardiol 16:812–820, 1990.

126. Meester BH, Samson M, Suryapranata H, et al: Long term follow-up after attempted angioplasty of saphenous vein grafts: The Thoraxcenter experience 1981–1988. Eur Heart J 12:648–653, 1991.

127. El Gamal M, Bonnier H, Michels R, et al: Percutaneous transluminal angioplasty of stenosed aortocoronary bypass grafts. Br Heart J 52:617–620, 1984.

128. Block PC, Cowley MJ, Kaltenbach M, et al: Percutaneous angioplasty of stenoses of bypass grafts or of bypass graft anastomotic sites. Am J Cardiol 53:666–668, 1984.

129. Reeder GS, Bresnahan JF, Holmes DR, et al: Angioplasty for aortocoronary bypass graft stenosis. Mayo Clin Proc 61:14–19, 1986.

130. Douglas JS: Angioplasty of saphenous vein and internal mammary artery bypass grafts. *In* Topol EJ (ed): Textbook of Interventional Cardiology. Philadelphia: WB Saunders, 1990.

131. Cote G, Myler RK, Stertzer SH, et al: Percutaneous transluminal angioplasty of stenotic coronary artery bypass grafts: 5 years experience. J Am Coll Cardiol 9:8–17, 1987.

132. Dorros G, Lewin RF, Mathiak LM, et al: Percutaneous trans-

luminal coronary angioplasty in patients with two or more previous coronary artery bypass grafting operations. Am J Cardiol 61:1243–1247, 1988.

133. Reeves F, Bonan R, Cote H, et al: Long term angiographic follow-up after angioplasty or venous coronary bypass grafts. Am Heart J 122:620–627, 1991.

134. Urban P, Sigwart U, Golf S, et al: Intravascular stenting for stenosis of aortocoronary venous bypass grafts. J Am Coll Cardiol 13:1085–1091, 1989.

135. Serruys PW, Strauss BH, Beatt KJ, et al: Angiographic follow-up after placement of a self-expanding coronary artery stent. N Engl J Med 324:13–17, 1991.

136. de Scheerder IK, Strauss BH, de Feyter PJ, et al: Stenting of venous bypass grafts: A new treatment modality for patients who are poor candidates for reintervention. Am Heart J 123:1046–1054, 1992.

137. Bilodeau L, Iyer S, Cannon AD, et al: Flexible coil stent (Cook, Inc.) in saphenous vein grafts: Clinical and angiographic follow-up [Abstract]. J Am Coll Cardiol 19:264A, 1992.

138. Pomerantz R, Kuntz R, Carrozza J, et al: Treatment of vein graft stenoses by stents or directional atherectomy [Abstract]. Circulation 84:II-249, 1991.

139. Leon MB, Ellis SG, Pickard AD, et al: Stents may be the preferred treatment for focal aortocoronary vein graft disease [Abstract]. Circulation 84:II-249, 1991.

140. Eeckhout E, Goy JJ, Stauffer JC, et al: Endoluminal stenting of narrowed saphenous vein grafts: Long-term clinical and angiographic follow-up. Catheter Cardiovasc Diagn 32:139–146, 1994.

141. Vaishnav S, Aziz S, Layton C: Clinical experience with the Wiktor stent in native coronary arteries and coronary bypass grafts. Br Heart J 72:288–293, 1994.

142. White CJ, Ramee SR, Collins TJ, et al: Placement of "biliary" stents in saphenous vein coronary bypass grafts. Catheter Cardiovasc Diagn 30:91–95, 1993.

143. Nunez BD, Simari RD, Keelan ET, et al: A novel approach to the placement of Palmaz-Schatz biliary stents in saphenous vein grafts. Catheter Cardiovasc Diagn 35:350–353, 1995.

144. van Beusekom HM, van der Giessen WJ, van Suylen R, et al: Histology after stenting of human saphenous vein bypass grafts: Observations from surgically excised grafts 3 to 320 days after stent implantation. J Am Coll Cardiol 21:45–54, 1993.

145. Kaufmann UP, Garratt KN, Vlietstra RE, et al: Transluminal atherectomy of saphenous vein aortocoronary bypass grafts. Am J Cardiol 65:1430–1433, 1990.

146. Selmon MR, Hinohara T, Robertson GC, et al: Directional coronary atherectomy for saphenous vein graft stenoses [Abstract]. J Am Coll Cardiol 17:23A, 1991.

147. Meany T, Kramer B, Knopf W, et al: Multicenter experience of atherectomy of saphenous vein grafts: Immediate results and follow-up [Abstract]. J Am Coll Cardiol 19:262A, 1992.

148. Untereker WJ, Litvack F, Margolis JR, et al: Excimer laser coronary angioplasty of saphenous vein grafts [Abstract]. Circulation 84:II-249, 1991.

149. Bittl JA, Sanborn TA, Yardley DE, et al: Predictors of outcome of percutaneous excimer laser coronary angioplasty of saphenous vein bypass graft lesions. The Percutaneous Excimer Laser Coronary Angioplasty Registry. Am J Cardiol 74:144–148, 1994.

150. Hadjimiltiades S, Gourassas J, Louridas G, et al: Stenting the distal anastomotic site of the left internal mammary artery graft: A case report. Catheter Cardiovasc Diagn 32:157–161, 1994.

151. Simpson JB, Selmon MR, Robertson GC: Transluminal atherectomy for occlusive peripheral vascular disease. Am J Cardiol 61:965–1015, 1988.

152. Graor RA, Whitlow PL: Transluminal atherectomy for occlusive peripheral vascular disease. J Am Coll Cardiol 15:1551–1558, 1990.

153. Garratt KN, Edwards WD, Vlietstra RE, et al: Coronary morphology after percutaneous directional atherectomy in humans: Autopsy analysis of three patients. J Am Coll Cardiol 16:1432–1436, 1990.

154. Garratt KN, Holmes DR, Bell MR, et al: Restenosis after directional coronary atherectomy: Differences between primary atheromatous and restenosis lesions and influence of subintimal tissue resection. J Am Coll Cardiol 16:1665–1671, 1990.
155. Waller BF, Johnson DE, Schnitt SJ, et al: Histologic analysis of directional coronary atherectomy samples. A review of findings and their clinical relevance. Am J Cardiol 72:80E–87E, 1993.
156. Waller BF, Pinkerton CA, Kereiakes D, et al: Morphologic analysis of 506 coronary atherectomy specimens from 107 patients: Histologically similar findings of restenosis following primary balloon angioplasty versus primary atherectomy. J Am Coll Cardiol 15:197A, 1990.
157. Johnson DE, Hinohara T, Robertson GC, et al: Coronary vascular lesions resected by directional coronary atherectomy. The histopathology of 328 successfully excised primary and recurrent stenoses. Circulation, in press.
158. Fishman RF, Kuntz RE, Carrozza JP, et al: Long-term results of directional coronary atherectomy: Predictors of restenosis. J Am Coll Cardiol 20:1101–1110, 1992.
159. Schnitt SJ, Safian RD, Kuntz RE, et al: Histologic findings in specimens obtained by percutaneous directional coronary atherectomy. Hum Pathol 23:415–420, 1992.
160. Waller BF, Pinkerton CA: "Cutters, scoopers, shavers, and scrapers": the importance of atherectomy devices and clinical relevance of tissue removed. J Am Coll Cardiol 15:426–428, 1990.
161. Johnson DE, Hinohara T, Selmon MR, et al: Primary peripheral arterial stenoses and restenoses excised by transluminal atherectomy: A histopathologic study. J Am Coll Cardiol 15:419–425, 1990.
162. Ip JH, Fuster V, Badimon L, et al: Syndromes of accelerated atherosclerosis: Role of vascular injury and smooth muscle cell proliferation. J Am Coll Cardiol 15:1667–1687, 1990.
163. Waller BF, Pinkerton CA, Rothbaum DA, et al: Restenosis tissue following hot tip laser, excimer laser, primary atherectomy and balloon angioplasty procedures: Histologically similar intimal proliferation in 33 atherectomy patients. Circulation 82(suppl III):312A.
164. Waller BF, Pinkerton CA, Orr CM, et al: Morphological observations late (>30 days) after clinically successful coronary balloon angioplasty. Circulation 83(suppl I):28–41, 1991.
165. Safian RA, Gelbfish JS, Erny RE, et al: Coronary atherectomy. Clinical, angiographic and histological findings and observations regarding potential mechanisms. Circulation 82:69–79, 1990.
166. Waller BF: The eccentric coronary atherosclerotic plaque: Morphologic observations and clinical relevance. Clin Cardiol 12:14–20, 1989.
167. Kuntz RE, Hinohara T, Safian RD, et al: Restenosis after directional coronary atherectomy. Effects of luminal diameter and deep wall excision. Circulation 86:1394–1399, 1992.
168. Garratt KN, Kaufmann WP, Edwards WD, et al: Safety of percutaneous coronary atherectomy with deep arterial resection. Am J Cardiol 64:538–540, 1989.
169. Miller MJ, Kuntz RE, Friedrich SP, et al: Frequency and consequences of intimal hyperplasia in specimens retrieved by directional atherectomy of native primary coronary artery stenoses and subsequent restenoses. Am J Cardiol 71:652–658, 1993.
170. Anderson PG, Bajaj RK, Baxley WA, et al: Vascular pathology of balloon-expandable flexible coil stents in humans. J Am Coll Cardiol 19:372–381, 1992.
171. Ellis SG, Topol EJ: Intracoronary stents: Will they fulfill their promise as an adjunct to angioplasty? J Am Coll Cardiol 13:1425–1430, 1989.
172. Murphy JG, Garratt KN, Schwartz RS, et al: Intracoronary stenting: Bailout or bypass? Catheter Cardiovasc Diagn 21:260–262, 1990.
173. Lembo NJ, Roubin GS: Intravascular stents. Cardiol Clin 7:877–894, 1989.
174. Schatz RA: A view of vascular stents. Circulation 79:445–457, 1989.
175. Sigwart U, Urban P, Golf S, et al: Emergency coronary artery stenting for acute occlusion after coronary balloon angioplasty. Circulation 78:1121–1127, 1988.
176. Serruys PW, Juilliere Y, Bertrand ME, et al: Additional improvement of stenosis geometry in human coronary arteries by stenting after balloon dilation. Am J Cardiol 61:71G–76G, 1988.
177. Levine MD, Leonard BM, Burke JA, et al: Clinical and angiographic results of balloon-expandable intracoronary stents in right coronary artery stenoses. J Am Coll Cardiol 16:332–339, 1990.
178. Roubin GS, Robinson KS: The Gianturco-Roubin stent. In Topol EJ (ed): Textbook of Interventional Cardiology, pp 663–646. Philadelphia: WB Saunders, 1990.
179. Haude M, Erbel R, Straub U, et al: Results of intracoronary stents for management of coronary dissection after balloon angioplasty. Am J Cardiol 67:691–696, 1991.
180. Kuntz RE, Safian RD, Carrozza JP, et al: The importance of acute luminal diameter in determining restenosis after coronary atherectomy or stenting. Circulation 86:1827–1835, 1992.
181. Kuntz RE, Gibson M, Nobuyoshi M, et al: Generalized model of restenosis after conventional balloon angioplasty, stenting, and directional atherectomy. J Am Coll Cardiol 21:15–25, 1993.
182. Roubin GS, Cannon AD, Agrawal SK, et al: Intracoronary stenting for acute and threatened closure complicating percutaneous transluminal coronary angioplasty. Circulation 85:916–927, 1992.
183. Ellis SG, Shaw RE, Gershony G, et al: Risk factors, time course and treatment effect for restenosis after successful percutaneous transluminal coronary angioplasty of chronic total occlusion. Am J Cardiol 63:897–901, 1989.
184. Ellis SG, Roubin GS, King SB III, et al: Importance of stenosis morphology in the estimation of restenosis risk after elective percutaneous transluminal coronary angioplasty. Am J Cardiol 63:30–34, 1989.
185. Fishman RF, Kuntz RE, Carrozza JP Jr, et al: Long-term results of directional coronary atherectomy: Predictors of restenosis. J Am Coll Cardiol 20:1101–1110, 1992.
186. Cox DA, Anderson PG, Roubin GS, et al: Effect of local delivery of heparin and methotrexate on neointimal proliferation in stented porcine coronary arteries. Coron Artery Dis 3:237–248, 1992.
187. Anderson PG: Restenosis: Animal models and morphometric techniques in studies of the vascular response to injury. Cardiovasc Pathol 1:263–278, 1992.
188. Agrawal SK, Anderson PG, Roubin GS, et al: Effect of repeat angioplasty of stented coronary arteries in a swine model. 1993 Submitted.
189. Roubin GS, Robinson KA, King SB III, et al: Early and late results of intracoronary arterial stenting after coronary angioplasty in dogs. Circulation 76:891–897, 1987.
190. Schwartz RS, Murphy JG, Edwards WD, et al: Restenosis after balloon angioplasty. A practical proliferative model in porcine coronary arteries. Circulation 82:2190–2200, 1990.
191. Rodgers GP, Minor ST, Robinson K, et al: Adjuvant therapy for intracoronary stents. Investigations in atherosclerotic swine. Circulation 82:560–569, 1990.
192. Schatz RA, Baim DS, Leon M, et al: Clinical experience with the Palmaz-Schatz coronary stent. Initial results of a multicenter study. Circulation 83:148–161, 1991.
193. Serruys PW, Strauss BH, Beatt KJ, et al: Angiographic follow-up after placement of a self-expanding coronary artery stent. N Engl J Med 324:13–17, 1991.
194. van Beusekom HMM, van der Giessen WJ, van Suylen RJ, et al: Histology after stenting of human saphenous vein bypass grafts: Observations from surgically excised grafts 3 to 320 days after stent implantation. J Am Coll Cardiol 21:45–54, 1993.
195. Waller BF, Pinkerton C, Van Tassel J, et al: Early and late morphologic changes following intracoronary stenting with the Gianturco-Roubin flexible stent. Clin Cardiol 1993; (in press).
196. Bowerman RE, Pinkerton CA, Kirk B, et al: Disruption of a coronary stent during atherectomy for restenosis. Catheter Cardiovasc Diagn 24:248–251, 1991.

197. Smith SH, Geer JC: Morphology of saphenous vein–coronary bypass grafts. Seven to 116 months after surgery. Arch Pathol Lab Med 107:13–18, 1983.
198. Garratt KN, Edwards WD, Kaufmann UP, et al: Differential histopathology of primary atherosclerotic and restenotic lesions in coronary arteries and saphenous vein bypass grafts: Analysis of tissue obtained from 73 patients by directional atherectomy. J Am Coll Cardiol 17(2):442–448, 1991.
199. Spears JR: Percutaneous transluminal coronary angioplasty restenosis: Potential prevention with laser balloon angioplasty. Am J Cardiol 60:61b–64b, 1987.
200. Litvack F, Grundfest W, Mohr F, et al: "Hot-tip" angioplasty by a novel radiofrequency catheter [Abstract]. Circulation 76(suppl IV):47, 1987.
201. Jenkins RD, Sinclair IN, Leonard BM, et al: Laser balloon angioplasty vs balloon angioplasty in normal iliac arteries [Abstract]. Circulation 76(suppl IV):47, 1987.
202. Lee BI, Becker GJ, Waller BF, et al: Thermal compression and molding of atherosclerotic vascular tissue with use of radiofrequency energy: Implications for radiofrequency balloon angioplasty. J Am Coll Cardiol 13:1167–1175, 1989.
203. Becker GJ, Lee BI, Waller BF, et al: Potential of radio-frequency balloon angioplasty: Weld strengths, dose-response relationship, and correlative histology. Radiology 174:1003–1008, 1990.
204. Myler RK, Cumberland DA, Clark DA, et al: High and low power thermal laser angioplasty for total occlusions and restenosis in man [Abstract]. Circulation 76(suppl IV):230, 1987.
205. Waller BF, Pinkerton CA, Orr CM, et al: Morphologic analysis of 2053 coronary atherectomy samples from 274 patients. Clin Cardiol, in preparation.

# 5

# Coronary Artery Disease: The Basis for Secondary Prevention

*David J. Whellan*     *Meg B. Molloy*     *Ruth Quillian*     *Jami M. Norris*
*Martin J. Sullivan*

Until the late 1980s, most investigators thought atherosclerosis was a relentlessly progressive process that could not be altered by modifying risk factors. As stated in the *British Medical Journal* in 1977, "Only the optimists among us believe that obstructive atheroma in the coronary arteries of our patients with angina might regress if we could persuade them to reduce the load of adverse factors in their lifestyle."[1] The first indication of coronary lesion regression came from case studies in the 1970s and the early 1980s.[2–6] Nevertheless, patients who underwent serial angiography had less than 6% regression of lesions with standard medical therapy.[7–19] In contrast to these earlier findings, later studies showed that lowering cholesterol levels through intensive risk factor management and lipid-lowering therapy significantly deters progression of atherosclerosis and promotes its regression. Even though the changes in coronary lesions are small, they translate into significant improvement in outcome.[20, 21]

From the 1960s to the early 1980s, the primary role of cardiac rehabilitation was the exercise training of patients who had experienced myocardial infarction (MI). However, the emphasis has shifted over the last 15 years to include a multidisciplinary approach to reduce risk factors and improve diet, psychosocial functioning, and exercise performance. At least 16 clinical trials using serial angiography have demonstrated that intensive risk factor intervention programs can increase coronary artery luminal diameter, improve myocardial blood flow, reduce myocardial ischemia and infarction, and decrease the rate of coronary death in patients with coronary artery disease (CAD).[22–46] Although meta-analysis in this area is subject to difficulties in interpretation, one such analysis found that treatment reduced the odds for progression of coronary lesions by 49%, increased the odds for no change by 33%, and raised the odds for coronary artery regression by 219%. Cardiovascular events declined by 47%.[47]

These studies have heightened interest in medically modifying the progression of atherosclerosis. Lifestyle changes, exercise, and antihyperlipidemic therapy improve both coronary anatomy and outcome when compared with usual care. Whereas 10 years ago, the role of secondary prevention in CAD was unclear, intensive risk factor reduction has now emerged as important and standard therapy in this disorder. The evidence for secondary prevention as a means of limiting coronary artery atherosclerosis, decreasing recurrent MI, and improving survival has grown to the point that standard of care dictates that cardiologists incorporate these interventions into their practice. In 1994, the American Heart Association (AHA) recommended that patients with known CAD undergo a comprehensive risk factor reduction program centered on lipid-lowering therapy, blood pressure control, smoking cessation, diet, exercise, weight loss, and stress reduction.[48]

## RISK FACTORS FOR CAD

Nearly three fourths of what influences the health status of the population is rooted in the lifestyle of individuals and in the environments in which they live. From this population perspective, only 10% of health determinants are linked to health care delivery.[49] These data suggest that altering lifestyle and environmental factors may have the largest impact on health outcomes in the long term. When one considers a prevalent and costly condition such as CAD, this perspective makes even more compelling the need to offer a multiple-intervention program to the individual with CAD and CAD risk factors.

During the 1970s and 1980s, many epidemiologic studies identified the risk factors associated with

CAD. A pioneering study, the Seven Countries Study,[50, 51] found that in populations in which CAD is a major cause of death, eating diets with lower content of saturated fat tended to reduce blood cholesterol levels and decrease the risk of death. The population effort utilized in a Finnish study consisted of environmental supports for healthy behaviors and educational efforts to help individuals adopt more healthful lifestyles.[52] This model is nearly twice as effective in reducing acute MI rates as the strategy used in the United States, Great Britain, and Canada, which targets high-risk patients only.

By the 1980s, strong evidence from epidemiologic studies, including the Framingham study, showed a significant association between elevated serum cholesterol levels and atherosclerosis.[53–59] With the discovery of the low density lipoprotein (LDL) receptor by Brown and Goldstein[60] and the association among defects in LDL receptor activity, familial hypercholesterolemia, and early atherosclerosis, population studies began to examine cholesterol as a risk factor for CAD. Three primary prevention trials published in the early to middle 1980s, the Helsinki Heart Study,[61] the Oslo intervention trial,[62] and the Lipid Research Clinics Coronary Primary Prevention Trial,[63] were able to demonstrate that atherosclerosis-related mortality could be lowered by a reduction of plasma cholesterol. Total mortality was generally unchanged in these studies. The West of Scotland Coronary Prevention Study confirmed these earlier findings.[64, 65] Use of pravastatin in middle-aged men with hypercholesterolemia and no history of myocardial infarction significantly reduced coronary events, including nonfatal MIs, death from coronary heart disease, and death from all cardiovascular causes. In addition, death from any cause declined by 22% ($p = 0.051$).

Lifestyle factors, such as smoking, obesity, and physical inactivity, and psychosocial factors, including social isolation and lower socioeconomic status, play a role in the development of CAD.[66–82] Another compelling view of how lifestyles and behaviors contribute to health is McGinnis and Foege's[83] estimates of the actual causes of death in the United States. Although we typically view heart disease, cancer, stroke, pulmonary disease, accidents, and diabetes as causes of death, the "real causes" are rooted in lifestyle and behaviors.

Once a patient has CAD, the relative risk of an MI is five to seven times higher than in persons without overt coronary disease.[84–90] In the Framingham study, infarction rates for men and women who previously had an infarction were 22% and 24%, respectively, over a 6-year period versus 7% and 3% in men and women, respectively, who started the study free of CAD.[87] This higher risk for patients with CAD compared with patients without CAD holds true for any level of plasma cholesterol.[91] In addition, once a patient suffers a myocardial infarct, an increase in plasma cholesterol level predicts an increase in likelihood of death.[87, 91–93] The 10-year risk of death from cardiovascular disease for a man with preexisting CAD increased from 3.8% to almost 19.6% with a rise in levels of total cholesterol from "desirable" to "high," whereas the corresponding risk for a man without CAD at the beginning of the 10-year study increased from 1.7% to 4.9%.[87] Reduced high density lipoprotein (HDL) cholesterol (HDL-C) is strongly predictive of cardiovascular events in patients with CAD independent of total cholesterol.[94] The Montreal Heart Study found levels of HDL-C and plasma LDL apolipoprotein-B to be powerful predictors of progression of CAD in saphenous grafts and native vessels.[95]

## EXERCISE AND CORONARY HEART DISEASE (CHD)

Sedentary lifestyle is an independent risk factor for coronary artery disease.[96–100] The relative risk of a CHD death during 8.5 years of follow-up was 4.3, least-fit quartile compared with most-fit quartile, adjusted for other risk factors.[98] This risk is similar to the relative risks for current smoking, high blood pressure, and 1 mmol/L higher LDL cholesterol (LDL-C) (4.3, 1.5, and 2.4, respectively). The Multiple Risk Factor Intervention Trial, a randomized trial of 12,138 middle-aged men, found that moderate leisure-time physical activity was associated with 63% as many fatal CHD events and sudden deaths, and 70% as many total deaths as low leisure-time physical activity.[96] An 8-year follow-up study examined physical fitness and the risk of all-cause and cause-specific mortality in a group of 13,344 men and women.[96] The results showed a decline in age-adjusted all-cause mortality rates across fitness quintiles, low fit to high fit, for both men and women. These trends remained after adjustment for other potentially confounding variables. Whaley and Blair[101] reviewed 18 studies published since 1990, finding that 17 showed an inverse association between physical activity or fitness and risk of CHD or fatal cardiovascular disease.

Haskell[102, 103] has extensively analyzed the data from epidemiologic studies to determine the characteristics and dose of physical activity related to health consequences, including risk of CHD. He observed that in most of these studies, reduced risk of CHD mortality has been associated with predominantly light to moderate physical activity. The estimated difference in energy expenditure between the least active participants at increased risk of CHD mortality and the moderately active participants with a lower CHD mortality rate was 150 to 400 kcal/day or 1050 to 2800 kcal/week for an average-sized person.[104, 105] The largest reduction in all-cause mortality was seen between the first and second quintiles in the follow-up study to the Multiple Risk Factor Intervention Trial.[96]

Exercise leads to an increase in HDL-C[106, 107] and an improvement in glucose tolerance,[108] and facilitates weight loss, which may lower LDL-C. In studies reporting beneficial changes in HDL triglyceride or levels, the training period is usually at least 12 weeks in length and is often accompanied by significant fat weight loss. Cross-sectional studies have shown that middle-aged and older men and women who reported engaging in regular physical activity on a wide variety of questionnaires and surveys have HDL-C levels that are typically 20% to 30% higher than those who are sedentary. These studies also report lower triglyceride and very low density lipoprotein cholesterol (VLDL-C) levels in active than in inactive adults.[109–111]

Exercise may also provide psychological benefits. In patients with CAD, several studies have shown a decrease in depression and anxiety, which is associated with an improved quality of life,[112, 113] after exercise in a cardiac rehabilitation program.

## PSYCHOSOCIAL FUNCTION AND CAD

In the late 1950s, cardiologists Meyer Friedman and Ray Rosenman, working together with biochemist Sanford O. Byers, began to focus attention on a series of behaviors in their cardiac patients that they eventually demonstrated to be an independent predictor of later development of heart disease.[114, 115] This cluster of behaviors, termed the *type A behavior profile,* centered on an individual's struggle to achieve or accomplish more and more in less and less time, often in the face of perceived opposition from other people. The men in the Western Collaborative Group Study who demonstrated the type A profile were 1.7 to 4.5 times as likely to have some manifestation of heart disease than subjects who did not show the same behavioral profile *(type B profile); the increased risk ratios for type A men held true for every CHD category—overt MI, silent MI, angina, CHD death, and second MI for those who had experienced MI during the study.*[114] In addition to this work, other researchers noted that the type A profile was strongly associated with the degree of coronary artery blockage in patients undergoing angiography.[116] These studies led a 1981 National Institutes of Health (NIH) panel to conclude that the type A profile was a separate risk factor for CHD.[117]

Researchers began to study the components of the profile separately after the publication of equivocal findings on the predictive validity of the type A profile in CAD.[118, 119] Although some of the controversy stemmed from differences in the difficult measurement of type A characteristics, it also became clear that the type A profile was not the seminal psychosocial risk factor. The three components that are manifested by this type A struggle are (1) a sense of time urgency *(hurry sickness),* (2) free-floating hostility, and (3) intense competitiveness. Williams and colleagues[120, 121] surmised that hostility and bottled-up anger may have more damaging effects on the heart, whereas hurry sickness and competitiveness may have beneficial social or psychological value. The first two features may thus increase circulating stress hormones that can have a long-term effect on the cardiovascular system. Hostility had even greater predictive validity for CAD than did the type A profile for both men and women.[120, 121] Indeed, Dembroski and associates[122] found that hostility measures were valid predictors of CHD outcomes, such as MI and CHD mortality, even in epidemiologic data sets that failed to show the type A–CAD relationship.[122] Their study also clarified that it is the overt expression of hostility, in terms of antagonism and interpersonal disagreeableness, that drives the hostility-CHD relationship, rather than the tendency to experience distressing emotions such as anger, resentment, and suspicion.

The importance of social and emotional connection has long been known clinically, yet its systematic study is relatively new. One early epidemiologic study of 4775 middle-aged adults assessed social networks (presence and extent of connection through marriage, extended family, friends, churches, and group affiliations) upon entry into the study and assessed mortality 9 years later.[123] These researchers found that subjects with lower social network scores were twice as likely to die from CHD and all causes as subjects with higher scores. Although the mechanisms of the social support–heart disease relationship are unclear, later researchers have more directly studied this phenomenon, theorizing that if poor social support is linked to heart disease incidence in primary populations, strong social and emotional support might buffer disease progression in other populations.

Orth-Gomer and colleagues[124] took this issue up in a prospective study of 736 randomly selected, middle-aged men who were monitored for 6 years. Low social support scores reliably predicted CHD incidence, even after control for traditional risk factors. The relationship between heart disease incidence and social support was as strong as the relationship between heart disease and smoking in this sample.[124] These researchers had earlier investigated the social support–heart disease relationship in a secondary population.[125] They noted that social isolation independently predicted mortality in men with the type A profile but not in men with the type B profile. Moreover, 69% of the socially isolated type A men had died at 10 years, compared with only 17% of the socially integrated type A men, after control for traditional risk factors.[125] Although it is not yet clear whether strengthening interpersonal connections will prove beneficial in survival studies, an NIH multicenter trial is currently under way to see whether such intervention for cardiac patients indeed improves prognosis.

Depression was identified as a psychosocial risk factor in CHD as early as 1987 and has received growing attention since the mid-1990s. Booth-Kewley and Friedman,[126] in a meta-analytic review of 13 studies, noted that depression (as defined by multiple different instruments) was a reliable predictor of heart disease incidence, as strongly related to heart disease (combined effect size = 0.225; $p <$ 0.0000001) as type A characteristics and traditional risk factors. When the meta-analysis was repeated, however, with stricter decision rules and with weighting of the included studies according to sample size, depression no longer held as a significant predictor.[127] Later studies that directly tested the hypothesis that depression predicts heart disease incidence nevertheless confirmed the importance of depression in primary and secondary prevention. In a study monitoring physical health from 1964 until 1991, 730 Danish men and women reported numerous symptoms of depression and were shown to have a higher risk of developing heart disease.[128] The long-lasting nature of the depressive symptoms was more important in prediction than the severity of the symptoms.

Using a prospective design and more stringent diagnostic criteria for clinical depression, Frasure-Smith and colleagues[129, 130] conducted a study of 222 male and female patients who had been hospitalized for MI and discharged; they found that depression after MI predicted survival at 6 months and at 18 months. Similarly, patients with established CAD who rated themselves as having moderate to severe depression had 72% and 84% greater risks of cardiac death 5 to 10 years after assessment and more than 10 years after assessment, respectively.[131] Although it has yet to be empirically determined that treatment of depression will enhance prognosis for patients, results of these studies would suggest the usefulness of such therapy. As mentioned previously, an NIH multicenter trial is currently under way to determine whether psychosocial intervention for cardiac patients indeed improves not only quality of life but also survival.

One construct that may link these psychosocial risk factors has to do with the presence of psychological or interpersonal stress. It is hypothesized that the links from type A behavior and hostility to cardiovascular disease are mediated through the autonomic and neuroendocrine systems and are manifested as extreme cardiovascular reactivity to stress.[132, 133] Thus, one way that social support[134–137] and depression[138–140] may enter the equation is through their ability to affect an individual's response to stress. There is also evidence that the relationship between psychological stress and cardiac events may be mediated by the occurrence of myocardial ischemia in patients with documented CAD. Mental stress–induced ischemia has been found to be associated with significantly higher rates of subsequent fatal and nonfatal cardiac events (odds ratio 2.8).[141]

Although the exact mechanisms of the link between psychosocial risk factors and cardiac disease are unclear at this time, it is evident that these factors contribute to heart disease incidence in both primary and secondary populations and to prognosis in tertiary samples. However, the potential impact of psychosocial intervention in these populations is currently under study.

## CLINICAL NUTRITION MANAGEMENT OF CAD

In the clinical setting, nutrition intervention programs are a cornerstone of therapy in the prevention and treatment of CAD.[142–147] CAD risk factors that respond to nutrition intervention include lipoproteins, body weight, hypertension, and diabetes[148] as well as progression of coronary atherosclerotic disease.[149] The AHA and the National Heart, Lung, and Blood Institute's National Cholesterol Education Program (NCEP) promote medical nutrition therapy as the first line of treatment for hypercholesterolemia.[150, 151] According to NCEP criteria, 29% of all the U.S. populations are candidates for nutrition intervention; among people 55 years or older, this figure is greater than 50%.[152] Although many individuals who have just experienced a heart attack or heart surgery are ready to change their eating patterns, they do not have the knowledge or behavioral skills to do so in a therapeutically appropriate manner.

Three leading nutritional factors have been identified as atherogenic in humans[142, 146, 153]:

1. Dietary saturated fatty acids (found in coconut and palm oil, animal fat and hydrogenated fat, shortening, and cocoa butter), which are the principal nutritional culprits in hyperlipidemia.
2. Excess caloric intake leading to obesity.
3. Dietary cholesterol (found in meats, poultry, egg yolks, and dairy foods), which has an effect on

lipids that is half that of the effect of saturated fat intake.

Decreasing these three factors has been shown to significantly reduce plasma total cholesterol levels and LDL-C and so is the main thrust of nutritional counseling in these patients. The NCEP suggests that for patients with hypercholesterolemia, step I and step II diets are the first level of intervention. For persons with genetic hyperlipidemia or established CAD, a more restrictive diet is recommended at the outset.[151, 154] For persons who show excessively high triglyceride levels in response to either a step I or step II diet, a diet high in monounsaturated fat and low in saturated fat and cholesterol is recommended. If the response to these diets is insufficient, more intensive efforts to lower dietary fat should be tried in motivated patients before the initiation of pharmacologic therapy. A step 1 diet calls for an intake of saturated fat to be less than 10% of calories, of total fat, less than 30% of calories, and of dietary cholesterol, less than 300 mg/day. A step II diet calls for further reduction of saturated fat intake to less than 7% of calories and of dietary cholesterol to less than 200 mg/day.[145]

Very low fat, high-carbohydrate diets are generally defined as obtaining less than 20% of calories from fat, like the AHA phase III diet. More restrictive diets obtaining less than 10% of calories from fat include the Pritikin Diet and Dean Ornish's Reversal Diet. The angiographic trials described here have noted that the lower the dietary fat, the greater the amount of disease regression. This effect is hypothesized to result from a host of factors, including coagulation factors, postprandial lipemia, chylomicron remnants, and elevated serum LDL-C. Very low fat diets should not be considered appropriate for persons with impaired glucose tolerance, non–insulin-dependent diabetes mellitus (NIDDM), or hypertriglyceridemia, because of growing evidence that a very high carbohydrate intake worsens glucose tolerance.[154, 155]

In addition to the amount of dietary saturated fats and cholesterol, several other nutritional factors may alter serum lipids and possibly promote disease regression. The omega-6 class of polyunsaturated fats (corn oil, safflower oil, cottonseed oil) have been shown to reduce total and LDL-C. However, these oils may also lower HDL-C and are linked with free radical injury, a process that may be atherogenic because it is linked to oxidative modification of LDL-C.[156] When substituted for saturated fatty acids, monounsaturated fatty acids (MUFAs), found in canola oil, olive oil, sesame oil, and peanut oil and the foods from which these oils are extracted, are known to lower total cholesterol and LDL-C, yet do not lower HDL-C.[142, 145, 153] Also, there is interest in

the use of high-MUFA diets in patients with NIDDM and hypertriglyceridemia to favorably influence lipids without creating glucose intolerance.[155, 157] A high-MUFA diet, which has become popularly known as the "Mediterranean diet" and is rich in olive oil, is a natural diet found in Greece, Italy, southern France, and Northern Africa. The eating pattern in this region is correlated with low rates of CAD and other chronic diseases related to diet.[158] Omega-3 fatty acids (found in cold-water fish such as mackerel, tuna, salmon, and bluefish) (1) reduce the synthesis of triglycerides and VLDL in the liver, (2) shorten the turnover of VLDL in the plasma, an effect that may be hypocholesterolemic,[143] and (3) decrease platelet aggregation.[159] Soluble fiber (found in barley, oats, legumes, pectin, gums, oranges, and apples), when added to a low-fat diet, can reduce plasma total cholesterol by 6% to 19%.[144]

When individuals are guided to lower the fat in their diet, a reciprocal relationship with dietary carbohydrate is invoked that has been shown to improve lipid levels and other cardiovascular risk factors. Most Americans consume approximately 45% of calories from carbohydrate and would benefit from increasing their carbohydrate intake to at least 55% of calories. However, a dramatic and rapid increase in carbohydrate intake can raise plasma triglycerides and lower the plasma HDL in some individuals[146]; therefore, gradual dietary changes and blood glucose monitoring for diabetics should be encouraged. A vegetarian pattern of eating, which usually incorporates the dietary guidelines for preventing and treating hyperlipidemia described previously, has been shown to be lipid lowering.[142, 144] Some studies also suggest that vegetarianism may favorably affect the lipid profile independent of the factors already listed.[160] Careful planning of a vegetarian diet is required to ensure an adequate intake of vitamins and nutrients, and to avoid a high-fat, high saturated fat intake, which may occur when an individual omits meat but unknowingly selects snacks, desserts, and condiments high in saturated fat.

Proceedings from a 1991 National Heart, Lung and Blood Institute (NHLBI) Consensus Workshop on the role of antioxidants in the prevention of human atherosclerosis suggested that antioxidants may favorably affect the progression of atherosclerosis.[161] Several lines of evidence have continued to support the concept that antioxidants are beneficial in humans. Vitamin E intake has been demonstrated to be associated with reduced rates of ischemic heart disease and cardiovascular mortality, and in the Cambridge Heart Antioxidant Study (CHAOS),[162] a 77% reduction in nonfatal heart attacks was seen among persons with CAD taking vitamin E versus those receiving placebo. The incidence of CAD and all-cause deaths was higher, although nonsignificantly, in the vitamin E group, however. Current studies are exploring the benefits of using vitamin E supplements in earlier stages of the disease, when atheroma formation could be prevented. Therapeutic levels of vitamin E in clinical trials range from 100 to 1000 IU/day and are known to be nontoxic.

Some, but not all, studies suggest an association between high plasma vitamin C and elevated HDL. An intake of vitamin C exceeding 1 g has little or no additional effect on plasma levels of vitamin C.[161] In light of data indicating that high levels of plasma ferritin are linked to oxidation of LDL, large doses of vitamin C must be viewed with caution, because ascorbic acid increases iron absorption. For persons with genetic predisposition for iron overload diseases such as hemochromatosis, megadoses of vitamin C can lead to high ferritin levels and actually promote LDL oxidation and atherosclerosis.[163]

β-Carotene supplementation may reduce the incidence of recurrent myocardial infarct in men.[161] Controversy surrounding β-carotene, however, arose from the cancer prevention β-Carotene and Retinol Efficacy Trial (CARET),[164, 165] which was terminated in January 1996 after preliminary data showed that supplements had no beneficial effect and may actually be more harmful (although the data were found among smokers, a feature that may confound the findings). Because of this finding, Harvard's Women's Health Study, involving 20,000 female health professionals, has removed β-carotene as an intervention.[166] Although selenium, zinc, and copper have been implicated as having a role in oxidation and antioxidation,[161] more research is needed to make possible recommendations about these trace minerals other than the recommended dietary allowances. Angiographic studies are currently under way to examine the role of antioxidants in altering atherosclerosis progression in man.

It has become increasingly evident that acute thrombosis plays a major role in the development of an MI. Accordingly, the roles of thrombosis and hemostatic factors and their interaction with nutrients have become the subject of intense research. Limited data suggest that excessive intakes of saturated fatty acids are associated with an increased tendency for thrombosis. In contrast, high intakes of omega-3 fatty acids have been shown to be antithrombogenic.[146] Although these doses of omega-3 fatty acids cannot be obtained from the diet, it is reasonable to suggest frequent consumption of seafood, which is rich in omega-3 fatty acids. Studies have indicated that a component of red wine also has an effect on platelet activity and, therefore, that moderate intake of red wine may have an antithrombogenic effect.[167–169]

The effects of obesity in coronary heart disease

are disputed.[146] Although it has been demonstrated that being overweight is linked with the development of type II diabetes and hypertension, its effect on lipoproteins is mixed.[146] The effects of excessive caloric intake on raising plasma triglyceride levels and lowering HDL-C levels have been demonstrated. Current research is examining the effect on abdominal fat lipoprotein metabolism and other cardiovascular risk factors. Dietary fat has been linked with the deposition of body fat[170] and, as the most calorically dense nutrient, is targeted for reduction in the effort to reduce weight. A moderate weight loss rate (0.5 to 2 lb per week) is optimal for maintaining muscle, bone mass, and metabolic rate and for promoting long-term behavioral changes.

The optimal dietary fat intake for patients with CAD has yet to be determined. There are mixed angiographic data showing that both progression and regression of atherosclerosis have been found with diets obtaining 25% to 30% of calories from fat.[171–174] It should be noted that very low fat diets can result in an increase in plasma triglyercide levels and a reduction in HDL levels.[142] However, the consequences of these changes for atherosclerosis are not defined. For persons with advanced CAD, it is prudent to advise a fat intake in the range of 15% to 25% fat, with the inclusion of MUFAs and omega-3 fatty acids. Regardless of the dietary fat level, there is an enormous amount of data supporting the benefits of adding nutrient-rich, phytoestrogen-containing foods to the diet, particularly fruits, vegetables, grains, and low-fat dairy foods. Data are emerging to support the addition of these foods, which have antioxidant, antithrombotic, and phytoestrogen-containing properties and so may directly mediate cellular and metabolic changes to promote optimal lipid and glucose levels, blood pressure, body weight, and cardiovascular anatomy and to reduce CAD morbidity and mortality.

## EXERCISE TRAINING AND PATIENTS WITH CAD

The almost 1 million survivors and 7 million patients with stable angina pectoris are candidates for cardiac rehabilitation, as are the nearly 700,000 patients who undergo coronary revascularization procedures annually. An estimated 4.7 million patients with heart failure may also be eligible. However, Only 15% to 20% of all patients with heart disease who are candidates for cardiac rehabilitation actually participate in formal programs.[175]

Cardiac rehabilitation and exercise training in patients after MI may decrease mortality and fatal reinfarction by approximately 20%.[176–179] Although most single-center studies have not shown a statistically significant treatment effect of cardiac rehabilitation because of their small sample sizes, studies that pooled the results from several samples found a 20% to 29% reduction in mortality in patients who exercised when compared with controls who did not.[176, 179] A meta-analysis of 22 randomized trials of rehabilitation of 4544 post-MI patients provided further evidence of the benefit of cardiac rehabilitation.[178] Most studies showed an overall beneficial effect on survival, although the confidence interval (CI) for individual studies was wide. During a 3-year follow-up period, the overall odds ratio was 0.80 for total mortality, 0.78 for cardiovascular mortality, and 0.75 for fatal reinfarction. In a second meta-analysis, similar reduction in mortality in pooled data from 10 studies confirmed this finding.[177] A later study of 182 post-MI patients younger than 65 years who were not included in the two meta-analyses showed that training significantly improved mortality in comparison with usual care and risk factor counseling ($p < 0.03$). The reduction in mortality achieved by cardiac rehabilitation with a focus on exercise training is similar to the reduction seen with β-blocker therapy.

The benefit of exercise training appears to come predominantly from peripheral adaptations. Although exercise stroke volume in certain patients may improve after 12 months of intense exercise training,[181] stroke volume, left ventricular (LV) ejection fraction, and intracardiac filling pressures do not improve after long-term exercise in most studies.[83, 84, 182–187] After long-term exercise, thallium perfusion defects during stress testing tend to improve in patients.[188, 189] There is no improvement, however, in exercise-induced wall motion abnormalities with exercise training.[187] The exact mechanism for improved myocardial perfusion during exercise remains undetermined. The findings may be due to improved collateral flow, increased coronary artery diameter, or better coronary vasomotor tone.[190] Nonetheless, the majority of the benefit derived from exercise training is secondary not to improved myocardial oxygen delivery but to peripheral changes.

Exercise training causes an increase in peak oxygen consumption, a training bradycardia, and a rise in peak arteriovenous oxygen difference.[182–185] These changes are believed to be derived from peripheral adaptations, including an increase in peak muscle blood flow[185] and higher aerobic enzyme content in skeletal muscle,[191] which lead to more efficient oxygen extraction play. In addition, patients with CAD can raise the work rate at which myocardial ischemia or angina occurs through exercise training.[95, 188–190, 192–197] The mechanism by which this benefit takes place is not completely understood. There is an increase in the rate-pressure product at which

ischemia occurs after intensive training.[190, 192, 196, 197] However, the onset of ischemia occurs at the same rate-pressure product but a higher work rate after training, as a result of the improved heart rate response caused by training.[193–195] The benefits of exercise training extend to elderly cardiac patients. After a 12-week exercise program initiated within 6 weeks of an acute MI or coronary artery bypass surgery, patients 65 years or older were found to have improved their physical work capacity by 53%, compared with 48% for patients 40 to 64 years old.[198]

## THE ROLE OF LIPID-LOWERING DRUG THERAPY

A number of secondary prevention trials using diet, drugs, or both to lower cholesterol levels provide ample evidence for the importance of such therapies. However, initial studies had difficulty relating lipid-lowering therapies to reductions in total mortality. The Coronary Drug Project[199, 200] was one of these initial studies that investigated drug therapy and outcome. At 6 years, use of clofibrate and niacin achieved no change in mortality; and only niacin had no significant benefit in decreasing nonfatal recurrent myocardial infarct. However, at 15 years, which was 9 years after discontinuation of the drug, the use of niacin had achieved an 11% reduction in mortality versus placebo.[199]

The first double-blind randomized controlled trial to demonstrate an improved outcome from lowering of cholesterol levels was the National Heart, Lung, and Blood Institute Type II Coronary Intervention Study,[22, 23] published in 1984. The intervention, consisting of diet and cholestyramine, altered coronary lesions as documented by serial angiography. Although the study did not show a lowering of LDL-C to levels currently achieved by intensive lifestyle changes and drug therapy, it was the first study to suggest that lowering LDL-C could retard the rate of progression of CHD in patients with type II hyperlipoproteinemia.

Further analysis of the subjects in this study revealed that the progression of CAD was inversely related to the combination of an increase in HDL-C and a decrease in LDL-C.[201] Changes in the rations of HDL-C to total cholesterol and HDL-C to LDL-C were the best predictors of CAD change. Using a vegetarian diet to significantly decrease total cholesterol in patients with CAD ($\geq$ 50% stenosis on angiogram) in one or more major coronary arteries, the Leiden Intervention Trial[46] confirmed the relationship of serum cholesterol changes with progression of atherosclerosis. In this study, growth of coronary lesions correlated only with total/HDL cholesterol ratio ($r = 0.05$, $p = 0.001$) but not with blood pressure, smoking status, alcohol intake, weight, or drug treatment.

The Cholesterol Lowering Atherosclerosis Study (CLAS),[24, 25] which randomly assigned 188 nonsmoking, white males who had undergone coronary artery bypass surgery for treatment with diet plus colestipol and niacin or diet alone, provided further evidence that lowering cholesterol could affect CAD. CLAS was the first study to show a higher rate of CAD regression with a lowering of cholesterol. After 2 years, visually estimated regression of coronary atherosclerosis, as assessed from lumen diameter, was seen in 16% of the treatment group (diet plus colestipol and niacin) versus 2% in the placebo group (diet alone). Although subjects in both groups showed progression of atherosclerosis, fewer patients showed progression in the treatment group (39%) than in the placebo group (61%) ($p < 0.001$). Further analysis of the 82 subjects in the placebo group revealed that 64 of the patients did not have new lesions during the 2-year period.[202] The analysis compared the placebo group subjects who did not have new lesions to those who did to evaluate dietary differences between them. Each quartile increase in consumption of total fat and polyunsaturated fat was associated with a significant increase in risk of new lesion development (odds ratio of 1.11 and 1.28, with 95% CI 1.02–1.20 and 1.07–1.53, respectively), confirming the importance of diet in progression of lesions.

The double-blind, randomized, controlled Familial Atherosclerosis Treatment Study (FATS)[27] examined changes over 2.5 years in coronary anatomy in patients treated with lipid-lowering drugs. Subjects were randomly assigned to three treatments: (1) lovastatin and colestipol (N = 38), (2) niacin and colestipol (N = 36), and (3) conventional therapy with placebo and colestipol if the LDL level exceeded the 90th percentile for age (N = 46). With regression or progression of disease defined as a change of 10% or more in lumen diameter, quantitative arteriography demonstrated disease regression in 32% of the lovastatin-colestipol group, 39% of the niacin-colestipol group, and 11% of the control group; disease progression occurred in 21%, 25%, and 46%, respectively. Regression of coronary lesions correlated independently with reductions in apolipoprotein B (LDL) and systolic blood pressure and with increases in HDL-C. In addition, the study revealed a direct relationship between the severity of stenosis and the number of clinical events.

Evaluating a combination of colestipol, niacin, and lovastatin, the UCSF Arteriosclerosis Specialized Center of Research Intervention Trial (SCOR)[28] demonstrated similar beneficial changes in lesion progression (20% in the treated group vs. 41% in controls) in patients with documented coronary atherosclerosis and heterozygous familial hypercholesterolemia (average total cholesterol ≥ 373 mg/dL).

As evidence for the beneficial effect of hydroxymethylglutaryl coenzyme A (HMG CoA) reductase inhibitors became apparent, a large number of studies examined the effect of this class of drugs on atherosclerosis progression.[35–37, 42–45] Trials such as Pravastatin Limitation of Atherosclerosis in the Coronary Arteries (PLAC I) Trial,[44, 45] the Monitored Atherosclerosis Regression Study (MARS),[37] The Canadian Coronary Atherosclerosis Intervention Trial,[35, 36] and the Multicentre Anti-Atheroma Study (MAAS)[42, 43] used HMG CoA reductase inhibitors to lower total cholesterol and HDL-C levels by an average of 24.5% and 30%, respectively, and to raise HDL cholesterol levels 8%. Each study showed a significant decrease in lesion progression and coronary events, including fatal and nonfatal MI.

A number of studies have attempted to apply the concept of lowering cholesterol with statins to patients with coronary atherosclerosis and normal to moderately elevated serum cholesterol levels. The Harvard Atherosclerosis Reversibility Project (HARP)[203] studied 79 patients who had CHD and a mean cholesterol concentration of 5.5 mmol/L over 2.5 years. Active treatment, consisting of pravastatin, nicotinic acid, cholestyramine, and gemfibrozil used in stepwise maner in addition to dietary therapy, significantly decreased plasma lipid levels but had little effect on coronary artery lesions. Contradicting the outcomes of the HARP study was the conclusion of the Regression Growth Evaluation Statin Study (REGRESS).[46] Patients taking pravastatin in addition to dietary therapy had less decrease in the mean segment diameter than controls (0.06 vs. 0.10; $p = 0.019$). In addition, treatment caused a significant decrease in cardiovascular events (p = 0.002). It remains unclear, however, whether treating patients with normal cholesterol levels changes the anatomy of coronary lesions.

In a meta-analysis of early secondary prevention trials using diet, drugs, or both to lower cholesterol levels, Rousouw and associates[204] found that a significant reduction in the nonfatal, fatal, and total MIs (odds ratios of 0.75, 0.84, and 0.78, respectively) was obtained with a reduction in serum cholesterol. When mortality was taken into consideration, the researchers found a significant decrease in cardiovascular deaths (odds ratio 0.88; $p < 0.05$) but a small, nonsignificant increase in noncardiovascular deaths (odds ratio 1.30). Overall mortality did decrease because cardiovascular deaths made a higher percentage of deaths (82%), but this change was not significant.

Later studies not used in the preceding meta-analysis confirmed the argument that lowering cholesterol in post-MI patients reduces the number of cardiac events, but once again, reductions of total mortality were not obtained. For 3 years, the Pravastatin, Lipids, and Atherosclerosis in the Carotid Arteries (PLAC II) Trial[205–207] monitored 151 patients with previous CAD, LDL values between the 60th and 90th percentiles for age and gender, and carotid artery atherosclerotic plaques with an intimal medial thickness 1.3 mm or greater. In the pravastatin-treated patients, total cholesterol and LDL-C levels were lower then those in the control patients (22% and 29%, respectively; $p < 0.001$ for both). HDL-C levels increased 7% ($p < 0.001$). Lowering serum cholesterol and LDL and increasing HDL resulted in (1) a 60% reduction in the rate of nonfatal MIs plus deaths caused by CAD ($p = 0.09$), (2) a 61% reduction in the rate of any fatal event plus any nonfatal MI ($p = 0.04$), and (3) an 80% reduction in the rate of fatal plus any nonfatal MI ($p = 0.03$). When the databases of the PLAC I and PLAC II trials were pooled (559 coronary patients), a 55% reduction in coronary incidence ($p = 0.014$) and a 67% reduction in the rate of nonfatal MI ($p = 0.006$), with an even more significant decrease in patients 65 years or older, were noted.[208] Although a 40% reduction in deaths was noted, this finding was not significant. The Pravastatin Multinational Study Group for Cardiac Risk Patients[209] was a larger study of 1062 patients with hypercholesterolemia and two or more additional risk factors for atherosclerotic CAD. Although this was not strictly a secondary prevention study, the number of serious cardiovascular adverse events was significantly lower in the subjects taking pravastatin.

The Scandinavian Simvastatin Survival Study (4S)[210–212] is a landmark study that conclusively showed that decreasing total cholesterol and LDL-C and increasing HDL-C through the use of simvastatin improved total mortality. In 4S, 4444 patients with angina pectoris or previous MI and moderate hypercholesterolemia were randomly assigned to double-blind treatment with simvastatin or placebo. The baseline serum lipid levels were total cholesterol, 261 mg/dL; LDL-C, 188 mg/dL; HDL-C, 46 mg/dL; and triglycerides, 132 mg/dL. The patients also followed a lipid-lowering diet during the study. The changes in total cholesterol, LDL-C, and HDL-C with simvastatin were $-25\%$, $-35\%$, and $+8\%$, respectively. Over a 5.4-year median follow-up period, simvastatin significantly reduced coronary deaths and all cardiac events (42% and 34%, respectively). Most importantly, simvastatin improved 6-year probabilities of survival from 87.6% to 91.3%, with a relative risk of 0.70 (95% CI 0.58–0.85; $p = 0.0003$).

The 4S had several significant results.[212, 213] First is the significant reduction in total mortality, which was obtained because the trial was continued be-yond the time at which significant differences in coronary events were observed. Second, no excess in noncardiovascular deaths occurred. Third, for the first time in a clinical trial of lipid-lowering therapy, there was a significant reduction in cerebrovascular events. Fourth, a wide range of subjects (men and women both younger and older than 60 years) benefited from the therapy. The analysis by quartile of baseline LDL-C levels found that the percentage of patients with major coronary events tended to be higher with increasing quartile of total and LDL cholesterol levels as well as LDL-C/HDL-C ratio, and with decreasing quartile of HDL-C.[212–214] The effect of simvastatin in reducing major coronary events was similar in all quartiles of baseline total cholesterol, HDL-C, and LDL-C levels.

The Cholesterol and Recurrent Events Trial[215, 216] studied the effect of 40 mg of pravastatin over 5 years in 4159 patients with MI who had plasma total cholesterol levels less than 240 mg/dL and LDL-C levels between 115 and 174 mg/dL. All patients in the study received the NCEP step I diet. Pravastatin decreased LDL-C levels from a mean of 139 mg/dL to 98 mg/dL (32% decline), which was 28% lower than the mean in the placebo group. The total cholesterol level was 20% lower, and the HDL-C level was 5% higher in treated patients than in control patients. Over 5 years, the patients who received pravastatin experienced a 24% lower rate of fatal CHD or confirmed MI, the primary end points, than the control group ($p = 0.003$). Reductions also occurred in rates of nonfatal MIs, (23%; $p = 0.02$), coronary bypass surgery (26%; $p = 0.005$) and angioplasty (23%; $p = 0.01$) as well as the incidence of stroke (31%; $p = 0.03$). Neither patient's age, the presence of hypertension or diabetes, smoking status, nor the patient's LV ejection fraction altered the beneficial effect of pravastatin. However, patient's baseline LDL-C level did influence the amount of reduction in the rate of coronary events. Patients with baseline LDL-C levels in excess of 150 mg/dL showed a 35% reduction in rate of coronary events versus a 3% reduction in patients with baseline LDL-C levels lower than 125 mg/dL ($p = 0.03$ for the interaction of baseline LDL-C level and risk reduction). No significant difference in the overall death rate between treated and control subjects was observed.

The Long-Term Intervention with Pravastatin in Ischaemic Disease (LIPID) Study[217, 218] was begun in 1990. Between June 1990 and December 1992, 9014 patients who had experienced either an acute MI or unstable angina within the preceding 3 months to 3 years and had a total cholesterol level of 155 to 271 mg/dL were enrolled. Patients were randomly assigned to receive either pravastatin 40 mg once daily or placebo. The researchers observed a 24%

relative risk reduction in total mortality with pravastatin versus placebo (95% CI 12% to 35%; $p <$ 0.001) over 6 years. The overall mortality rates of the intervention and control groups were 11.0% and 14.1%, respectively. This figure translates into 31 deaths avoided per 1000 patients treated. There was a 24% relative risk reduction in CHD mortality over 6 years (6.4% vs. 8.3%, pravastatin vs. placebo; $p$, 0.001). The benefit of taking pravastatin was independent of any subgroupings, including gender, age, cardiac event, level of total cholesterol, and level of LDL-C. Important differences exist between the LIPID study and 4S cohorts. More than 80% of the LIPID subjects could not have been enrolled in the 4S on the basis of their cholesterol level, age, or history of CAD.

## MULTIPLE-INTERVENTION APPROACHES AND CORONARY LESIONS

The blinded, randomized, controlled Lifestyle Heart Trial[31] examined coronary anatomy before and after a comprehensive set of diet, exercise, and behavioral interventions. All participants in this 1-year study had significant coronary atherosclerosis, had an LV ejection fraction greater than 25%, and were not taking lipid-lowering medications. The treatment group (N = 22) was assigned to a low-fat (10% of calories from fat) vegetarian diet, 1 hour a day of stress management, and 3 hours or more of aerobic exercise per week. Control subjects (N = 19) were given usual care and were counseled to follow a 30% fat diet and to exercise.

The benefit of the nonpharmacologic therapies was evident in the significant differences between experimental and control groups in levels of total cholesterol (24% vs. 5%; $p = 0.02$) and LDL-C (37% vs. 6%; $p = 0.007$). Treatment subjects also lost an average of 10 kg, whereas control subjects gained 1 kg ($p < 0.0001$). The incidence of angina was lower in the treatment group compared with controls (91% vs. 165%, respectively; $p = 0.06$) with additional reductions in angina severity ($p < 0.001$) and duration ($p = 0.14$) in comparison with controls. The improvement in CAD lesion mirrored the clinical improvements. The average percentage diameter stenosis decreased from 40% to 37.8% in the treatment group, but an increase in this parameter was seen in the control group (42.7% and 46.1%, respectively; $p = 0.001$). The Lifestyle Heart Trial was the first study to demonstrate that progression of CAD lesions could be slowed through the use of dietary and lifestyle changes alone. In addition, the level of compliance with the treatment program correlated with lesion changes in a dose-response fashion.

The Stanford Coronary Risk Intervention Project (SCRIP)[41] confirmed the beneficial impact that a multidisciplinary approach could have on CAD. This study randomly assigned 300 men and women to receive either the usual care of their own physician or multifactor risk reduction, which consisted of diet education, exercise, weight loss, smoking cessation, and lipid-lowering medical therapy. A significant difference in the use of lipid-lowering therapy was seen between the two groups. In the risk reduction group, significant differences from the usual care group were observed in levels of LDL-C and apolipoprotein-B ($-22\%$), HDL-C cholesterol ($+12\%$), and plasma triglycerides ($-20\%$), body weight ($-4\%$), and exercise capacity ($+20\%$). The rate of coronary artery narrowing was 47% less in the risk reduction group ($p < 0.02$). Further analysis of the coronary lesions found that new lesions tended to occur in the usual care patients rather than the risk reduction patients (new lesions per patient, 0.47 vs. 0.30; $p = 0.06$).[134] Although there was no significant difference between the two groups in the rates of overall mortality or cardiac death, there was a significant difference in the combined end point of cardiac deaths and hospitalizations for nonfatal MI, percutaneous transluminal, coronary angioplasty (PTCA), and coronary artery bypass graft (25 vs. 44; $p = .05$).

The St. Thomas' Atherosclerosis Regression Study (STARS)[33] examined the effects of dietary changes with or without cholestyramine versus usual care in men with angina or previous MI. By decreasing total cholesterol and LDL levels in treatment groups more than in control subjects, the study achieved a decline in the progression of coronary atherosclerosis from almost half (46%) in those receiving usual care to only 12% in those receiving diet and cholestyramine and to 15% in those receiving diet alone. Regression of atherosclerosis was seen in 4% of the usual care group and in 33% and 38% of the diet plus cholestyramine and diet alone groups, respectively. As in previous studies, lesions with greater than 50% stenosis demonstrated the most improvement. In addition to demonstrating the anatomic effects of these diet-based therapies, the study showed that the two treatment groups had fewer clinical cardiac events than the usual care group ($p < 0.05$); also, the treatment group had less angina compared with baseline ($p < 0.05$), whereas angina in control subjects did not change.

Schuler and associates[32, 39] examined the effects of exercise and a 20% fat diet in patients with CAD. The study design gave control subjects a 1-week hospitalization for instructions about the need for regular exercise and a low-fat diet (AHA phase 1 diet) 0 and then discharged them to the care of their private physician. The intervention group received 3 weeks of in-hospital instruction about a diet with less than 20% of calories from fat and less than 200 mg cholesterol per day. In addition, they were asked to exercise at home on a bicycle ergometer for a minimum of 30 minutes a day and to attend two 60-minute group exercise sessions per week. Patients were seen at the clinic at least four times a year.

The first study in which Schuler and associates used this design was a case-controlled study of 36 patients.[32] Quantitative angiographic analysis found increased regression of coronary atherosclerosis (39% vs. 6%) and decreased progression (28% vs. 33%) in the treated versus the control groups, respectively. A direct relationship was found between the extent of progression in the lesions and the total cholesterol level in the control group, but the same relationship was not seen in the treatment group. There was no difference in lipid levels between treatment patients who had lesion progression and treatment patients who experienced lesion regression. In addition, other risk factors could not account for this difference.

In a larger randomized study involving 111 men, known as the Heidelberg Study, these researchers again found overall delayed lesion progression in the exercise and diet group versus controls.[39] Decreasing levels of total cholesterol by 11% and of LDL-C by 9%, with no change in HDL-C, achieved an increase in regression (32% vs. 17%; $p < 0.05$) and a decrease in progression (23% vs. 48%; $p < 0.05$) of coronary lesions in the treatment group versus the control group, who showed no change in lipid profiles. In addition, myocardial ischemia improved after the intervention but there was no change in control subjects (no $p$ value given).

## LESION PROGRESSION AND OUTCOMES

Several possible mechanisms may contribute to the reported clinical improvements. As the described studies show, lipid-lowering therapy allows plaque stabilization, leading to a reduction in the incidence of plaque rupture and increases in coronary luminal diameter. In addition, coronary artery endothelium becomes dysfunctional in terms of vasomotor response in the presence of hypercholesterolemia with or without atherosclerosis.[219–223] When the hypercholesterolemia is treated with either cholestyramine[224] or an HMG CoA reductase inhibitor,[222, 223, 225] endothelial dysfunction reverses in response to intracoronary injection of acetylcholine within 6 months[222, 224, 225] or 1 year.[223]

An additional benefit of decreasing coronary lesion progression and increasing regression is the improved flow reserve that is obtained from small changes in luminal diameter. Gould and colleagues[173] reanalyzed the angiograms of patients in the Lifestyle Heart Trial to assess coronary reserve flow. Coronary flow reserve was derived from lesion geometry, including entrance and exit angles, in both groups before and after the study. Patients in the treatment group showed progression in the distal segment only, whereas control patients had progression in both the proximal and distal portions of the lesion. The differences in lesion changes caused a larger decrease in flow reserve in mild lesions in control patients. The remodeling brought on by the interventions in the Lifestyle Heart Trial improved minimal luminal diameter, diminished entrance and exit angles, and reduced percentage stenosis from 66.5% to 57.5%, leading to a significant improvement in calculated coronary flow reserve.

In a small study using exercise and diet, Czernin and associates[226] provided further evidence that lowering resting blood flow and increasing coronary vasodilatory capacity improves myocardial flow reserve. This analysis suggests that small to moderate changes in significant coronary stenosis due to intensive risk factor modification may be accompanied by physiologically significant improvements in coronary flow reserve.

Further evidence supporting the concept of improved coronary flow reserve is the finding of a reduction in induced ischemia, measured by exercise testing and thallium scintigraphy, in patients treated with exercise and diet in the Heidelberg Study.[39] In addition, this study demonstrated a significant improvement in myocardial oxygen consumption, estimated from the rate-pressure product, in treated subjects versus controls ($p < 0.05$). In the small study by Czernin and associates,[226] the better flow reserve caused by the intervention correlated with improved ischemia, as measured by positron emission tomography after pharmacologic stress testing. Although the overall changes in minimal luminal areas were small in most treated patients in the trial, these minor changes appeared to be translated into a significant improvement in clinical outcome. Interestingly, the amount of collateral vessel formation increased with progression of the disease and decreased with its regressions.[227] This observation is supported by the findings that cardiovascular morbidity,[27, 34] angina frequency,[27, 31] and stress-induced myocardial ischemia[31, 32, 39] are reduced after intensive risk factor management.

In CLAS-II,[26] the follow-up study to CLAS, 103 men underwent a third angiogram, which demonstrated continuing favorable results for the drug-treated group. In addition to less angiographic progression (48% for treated group vs. 87% for controls), patients in the treatment group also demonstrated a reduction in the formation of new lesions in both grafted and nongrafted native coronary arteries. However, the number of new arterial occlusions was not different. This supports the concept that progression to occlusion may be "thrombosis driven" whereas progression of luminal stenosis may be "lipid driven."

An important finding of FATS[27] was association of the extent of lesion progression and the number of clinical events. As previously stated, there was a reduction in adverse clinical events in treated patients compared with controls ($p < 0.05$). With each increase in stenosis, which was divided into the three categories small, moderate, and large, an increase in clinical events was seen—1, 5, and 9, respectively. Once again, minor angiographic changes corresponded to changes in clinical events. The use of coronary progression as an end point was further established by Waters and colleagues,[21] who showed that coronary progression is a strong independent predictor of future coronary events (relative risk 1.7; $p < 0.001$), particularly cardiac death (relative risk 7.3; $p < 0.001$).

## IMPLICATIONS FOR TREATMENT

The nutrition and health research described in this chapter can be translated into specific cardiac rehabilitation dietary guidelines. For example, within the cardiac rehabilitation program at the Duke University Center for Living, the Sarah W. Stedman Nutrition Center has developed a nonjudgmental, positive approach to help each client develop the nutritional knowledge, skills, and behaviors to promote optimal health. Clients can choose to participate in an intensive 2-week retreat, Healing the Heart, or in an ongoing cardiac rehabilitation program. The program provides individuals with the tools they need to begin assessing their eating patterns and developing their individual nutrition prescriptions. Because dietary fat is a major focus of this approach, patients are made aware of their fat gram "budget" for each day. At the Duke University Center for Living, clients are guided to lower their fat intake to at least 20% of total calories while making changes at their own pace in the Healing the Heart program and to 25% in the cardiac rehabilitation program. At the end of this initial program, each client design a personal nutrition plan that includes his or her goals for changing specific food patterns and identifies additional nutrition skills and behaviors the client is required to implement to fulfill the nutrition prescription.

Perhaps the most difficult task a health professional must deal with is that of patient compliance with a health care prescription, whether it be medication, smoking cessation, nutrition, exercise, stress management, or other therapy. Several factors have been shown to dramatically enhance patient compliance in the area of nutrition. These factors include, but are certainly not limited to the following:

- The individual's readiness to change[228]
- A participatory, problem-solving mode of nutrition education with frequent follow-up[229]
- A focus on skill-building, activities[230]
- Social support and reinforcement[231]
- Individualization
- An emphasis on a positive approach (instead of promoting negative words, such as "no," "stop," and "don't," therapy concentrates on guiding the person to focus on what to eat, e.g., "I will eat fruit and popcorn for snacks") that allows the individual to move at his or her own pace and make personal decisions about nutritional patterns

The process of dietary change is not an overnight one. Continuous support, reinforcement, and goal setting are necessary for long-term dietary changes. The health professional should suggest skill-building and learning opportunities, such as restaurant or supermarket programs and cooking schools that offer a new style of food purchasing, cooking, and dining out. A participatory style of assessment using a few simple questions to determine what changes the individual has already made may better facilitate nutrition behavior changes. Finally, family members should be involved in the treatment program, because social support for nutrition changes enhances and sustains nutrition behavior change.

## PSYCHOSOCIAL COUNSELING

Relational intimacy is at risk in many aspects of the psychosocial risk factors for coronary artery disease—hostility, social isolation, depression, and interpersonal stress. Hostile patients tend to be emotionally isolated, as are many depressed patients. Socially isolated patients are often physically as well as emotionally isolated. Furthermore, interpersonally stressed patients may have difficulties expressing their own needs in respectful ways in order to increase intimacy rather than isolate themselves. Because this theme of interpersonal connection links the psychosocial risk factors, we have developed a program at Duke University Center for Living that addresses the importance of developing and enhancing interpersonal relationships in coping with heart disease.

The more intense and short-term version of this program, Healing the Heart, is designed as a 2-week retreat in which cardiovascular patients and their partners immerse themselves in an intensive lifestyle management program as an adjunct to their usual care. Patients work through the program in a group setting within an emotionally safe, nurturing environment where bonding is encouraged through the use of communication skills. The psychosocial components of the program center on the importance of intrapersonal and interpersonal stress management, learning to recognize stress signals, exploring coping strategies, and practicing them in the group.

The longer-term version of this program, which does not require a 2-week immersion at the Center for Living, is offered as an integral part of our outpatient cardiac rehabilitation program. Upon entry into the program, each patient receives an individualized psychosocial assessment by a health psychologist. At this assessment, type A characteristics, hostility, depression, social isolation, and stress level are evaluated. Immediate feedback is provided verbally to the patient, and an individualized treatment plan is developed. The psychosocial recommendations are then discussed with the cardiac rehabilitation team, and written feedback is given to the team and referring physician as well. Most patients then participate in a 4-hour introduction to stress management course, which is taught in an experimental group format. This class focuses on helping patients understand the rationale for developing multiple stress management strategies and the skills to put these strategies in place. The interpersonal nature of the class combines with the interpersonal connection that is encouraged among patients during weekly meetings, where risk factor interventions, medical advances, and coping strategies are presented by various members of the cardiac rehabilitation staff (health psychologists, exercise physiologists, physician assistants, nurses, and cardiologists). In addition, participants are encouraged to attend the weekly lunch and open-discussion support group. Family members are invited to attend the stress management class and open-discussion groups. Finally, patients are tracked by the health psychologist during weekly "walk-throughs," wherein the psychologist briefly touches base with higher-risk patients during their exercise sessions to ensure that they are following through on their individual treatment plans. It is also useful to have the psychologist available during these weekly walk-throughs, so that he or she may demonstrate the importance of psychosocial intervention and help normalize the psychosocial reactions many people experience while coping with cardiac illness.

## SMOKING AND CAD

There is growing evidence that a brief physician-delivered intervention can have a positive effect on smoking cessation.[232–235] Reviews support the use of brief physician counseling in combination with nicotine replacement when indicated.[234, 236] For example, a well-designed randomized trial monitoring 1261 smokers has suggested that the most effective approach is brief physician counseling combined with the availability of nicotine-containing gum.[233] The gum was provided only for those patients who set a quit date and were receptive to use of the gum.[233] Nicotine replacement in other studies was found to be effective in 13% of quitters and noted to be most effective with patients who are nicotine dependent.[234] Although not all patients in these studies had cardiovascular disease, reviews of the cardiovascular toxicity of nicotine indicate that the benefits of smoking cessation outweigh the negligible risks of nicotine replacement therapy, even for patients with coronary disease.[235, 237]

Confidence in ability to quit is consistently predictive of new quitting and of maintained abstinence.[233, 238] More specifically, confidence in ability to quit (self-efficacy) is likely to be predictive once the patient is contemplating quitting, but not at earlier stages.

This issue is best understood through the Prochaska and DiClemente[239] stage-of-change model, which proposes that smoking cessation involves movement through various stages, not necessarily in linear order. This model suggests that smokers go through five stages as follows:

1. *Precontemplation*: The smoker is not even considering quitting.
2. *Contemplation*: The smoker has some thought about and interest in quitting but has taken no behavioral steps.
3. *Preparation*: The smoker actually gets ready to stop smoking.
4. *Action*: The smoker begins cutting back gradually or sets a quit date.
5. *Maintenance*: The smoker has stopped smoking and is in the maintenance stage, working on continuing abstinence.

Patients' honest answers to two questions can help distinguish their stage and provide cues to the best approach to further helping the patient move along the change continuum[240]; "Do you seriously intend to quit smoking in the next 6 months?" and "Do you plan to quit in the next 30 days?" The patient who gives two negative responses is at the precontemplation stage. A positive response to the first question and a negative response to the second indicate the contemplation stage. Two positive responses suggest that the patient is at the preparation stage. If the patient has stopped smoking in the past 6 months, he or she is in the action stage. If the patient has quit smoking more than 6 months ago but is still tempted to smoke, even occasionally, he or she is in the maintenance phase. Thus, asking these few questions to determine the patient's current stage appears to identify who is likely to profit from which interventions.[240, 241]

Physicians can best help patients in the precontemplation stage by increasing their awareness, pointing out the "cold, hard facts" about the dangers of smoking in spite of patients' denial and rationalization skills. Patients in the contemplation stage are helped more by hearing specific information on the pros of quitting as well as the cons of smoking. In the preparation stage, physicians can help the patient formulate an individualized plan and select a quit date. Finally, in the action and maintenance stages, physicians can reinforce change by recognizing the patient's success despite continued struggle and encouraging him or her to persevere. In terms of helping patients formulate specific cessation plans, the physician should consider a patient's preference about nicotine replacement therapy and the choice between gradual and sudden cessation. Research suggests that the success rates for gradual cessation and sudden cessation are similar.[234]

Although the magnitude of the effect of physician involvement in well-designed smoking cessation programs may appear small (e.g., 12.9% to 16.7% 1-week point prevalence cessation rate for three distinct physician-delivered treatments; and 6.0% to 10.0% 1-year maintained cessation rates[233]), it is greater than the average found among self-quitters in the general population (4.3%).[242] Quit rates for heart patients involved in cardiac rehabilitation are somewhat higher, estimated at 17% to 26%.[243] Among post-MI patients, self-quitting rates are significantly better (45% to 55%), and cessation interventions involving health professionals (physician or nurse) augment these rates to as high as 69% to 71% at 1-year follow-up.[244, 245]

It is noteworthy that even simple personalized advice provided by a physician helps smokers quit smoking and maintain abstinence.[234] The success rate, though low (2%), is no different from that seen with more intense behavior modification programs and is considerably more cost effective.[234] Thus, even if a physician is unable to make time to counsel patients, it is worthwhile for the physician to simply advise patients to quit and then ask, at each visit, whether they have questions about smoking risks. Helping a patient move to the next stage of change, and closer to quitting, is success itself, because the literature shows that patients move through cognitive readiness stages of some sort before quitting.[240, 246, 247]

## EXERCISE PRESCRIPTION FOR PATIENTS WITH CAD

The primary goals of an exercise program are (1) to reduce cardiovascular morbidity,[176–178] (2) to increase the angina threshold,[188–190, 192–197] and (3) to improve aerobic fitness, muscle strength, muscle endurance, and flexibility.[248] Most exercise programs are based on supervised outpatient activities, with the patient coming to the rehabilitation center three times per week for 1 to 1.5 hours.

Some hospitals use home-based exercise programs for low-risk patients.[249, 250] The patient exercises at home on a stationary bike or by walking while using a portable heart rate monitor. To enhance compliance and review progress, a staff person telephones twice a week, and the patient transmits his or her EKG by telephone during 1 minute of exercise and during 1 minute immediately after exercise. In two studies comparing home exercise with supervised facility-based training for post-MI patients without clinical complications, no difference was seen in the increase in functional capacity.[249, 250] Although this approach has the advantage of being cost effective and may reach patients from a wider geographic area, it may not meet the needs of high-risk patients.

Facility-based programs, such as the Duke University Center for Living and the Toronto Rehabilitation Center, represent the opposite end of the spectrum from home-based exercise programs. The exercise prescription for cardiovascular fitness consists of the following four components: intensity, duration, frequency, and mode of activity. Usually, exercise intensity is prescribed as a percentage of individual functional capacity with the use of heart rate to calculate the appropriate level. The general recommendation for exercise intensity is 60% to 85% of maximal oxygen uptake,[248] although several studies suggest potential health benefits of regular exercise at lower intensity levels if they are performed for longer duration and at higher frequency than discussed here.[96, 251] For totally sedentary individuals, even a moderate level of activity, like walking, may be beneficial in reducing cardiovascular events.[96] The most accurate way to calculate the prescribed intensity level, or training range (TR), is to obtain data from an exercise stress test and use the heart rate (HR) reserve method (Karvonen formula), as follows:

$$\text{Maximal HR (from exercise test)} - \text{Resting HR} = \text{HR Reserve}$$

$$\text{HR Reserve} \times (0.6\text{–}0.85) + \text{Resting HR} = \text{TR}$$

This calculation will give a training intensity of approximately 60% to 85% of maximal oxygen uptake.[248] Higher-intensity exercise is often associated with greater risk of orthopedic injuries and lower rate of compliance.[172, 252]

To optimize aerobic capacity, patients should exercise 20 to 45 minutes a day, 3 to 5 days per week. Any activity that uses large muscle groups in rhythmic, dynamic movements, such as walking, jogging, cycling, swimming, calisthenics, or cross-country skiing, leads to aerobic conditioning. Aerobic exercise as well as strength and flexibility training should begin with an initial 5- to 10-minute warm-up period, to adapt the cardiovascular system to the workout. It is equally important to allow 5 to 10 minutes at the end of the session for cooling down. Proper footwear should be emphasized when a weight-bearing activity, such as walking, jogging, or running, is the aerobic exercise of choice. A properly fitted running shoe together with a gradually increased exercise prescription is the best way to prevent foot, leg, and knee injuries. Exercise clothes should be made of breathable, sweat-absorbent material and worn in layers according to the air temperature, humidity, and wind-chill factor.

Many vocational tasks and activities of daily life include various types of lifting, carrying, or pushing. Therefore, it is important that the exercise program also improves muscle strength and endurance. Resistance exercise has been shown to be safe for patients with cardiovascular disease, even at a relatively high percentage of maximum voluntary contraction.[253, 254] To avoid an excessive blood pressure response, the patient should use rhythmic, dynamic movements during calisthenics or weightlifting. Patients should emphasize the number of repetitions completed rather than the amount of weight lifted and should perform full range of motion in each exercise. Strengthening exercises should be performed two to three times per week with a rest day in between. The stiffness and lack of normal range of motion in joints seen among the elderly are not entirely a function of age but, rather, may result from a sedentary lifestyle. This condition may predispose the individual to exercise-related injuries. Therefore, flexibility exercises designed to increase the extensibility of the muscles and ligaments through active or passive movements should be performed three times per week.

## CONCLUSION

The evidence for treating patients with CHD in a multidisciplinary approach is overwhelming. But now that we know lowering cholesterol and improving psychosocial function and exercise capacity can improve survival and quality of life, the next step is implementing interventions that incorporate proven strategies. As already mentioned, only a minority of patients eligible for cardiac rehabilitation participate in formal programs.[175] The reason may be that patients do not have access to formal programs and instead perform exercise therapy in a local setting. In addition, patients may be noncompliant with therapies recommended by their physicians. Patients' medication nonadherence is a common problem that may affect their survival.[255]

Part of the blame for the failure of patients to receive adequate therapy, however, rests with physicians. In one study conducted in a teaching hospital, only 17% of patients with CAD, and high levels of total cholesterol, LDL-C, or both were being actively treated with diet, drug therapy, or both.[256] In the past, cardiologists have been resistant to treating hypercholesterolemia for a number of reasons.[257–259] However, many of their questions and concerns have been laid to rest. Although there are still a few controversies regarding the appropriate population to screen and treat,[260–262] no one doubts the need to screen and treat patients who have CAD or are at high risk for CAD, as stated in the American College of Physicians Guidelines for Cholesterol Screening[263] and the NCEP Guidelines.[264]

This chapter gives the physician the background necessary to feel comfortable about initiating long-term interventions for a patient suffering from CAD. Although there are a multitude of new devices and medicines on the horizon, a huge impact on survival can be achieved by implementing therapies already proven to save lives and improve patients' quality of life.

## REFERENCES

1. Anonymous: Regression of atheroma. BMJ 2:1–2, 1977.
2. Basta LL, Williams C, Kioschos JM, Spector AA: Regression of atherosclerotic stenosing lesions of the renal arteries and spontaneous cure of systemic hypertension through control of hyperlipidemia. Am J Med 61:420–423, 1976.
3. Conti CR: Myocardial revascularization without surgery: Angiographic evidence of regression of coronary artery occlusive disease associated with clinical and objective improvement. Adv Cardiol 26:110–117, 1979.
4. Crawford DW, Sanmarco ME, Blankenhorn DH: Spatial reconstruction of human femoral atheromas showing regression. Am J Med 66:784–789, 1979.
5. Bassler TJ: "Regression" of atheroma. West J Med 132:474–475, 1980.
6. Roth D, Kostuk WK: Noninvasive and invasive demonstration of spontaneous regression of coronary artery disease. Circulation 62:888–896, 1980.
7. Gensini GG, Esente P, Kelly A: Natural history of coronary disease in patients with and without bypass graft surgery. Circulation 49(suppl II): II-98–II-102, 1974.
8. Landmann J, Kolsters W, Bruschke AVG: Regression of coronary artery obstructions demonstrated by coronary arteriography. Eur J Cardiol 4:475–479, 1976.
9. Tillgren C, Sténson S, Lund F: Obliterative arterial disease of the lower limbs studied by means of repeated femoral arteriography: An attempt to evaluate the effect of long-term anticoagulant therapy. Acta Radiol 1:1161–1178, 1963.
10. Bemis CE, Gorlin R, Kemp HG, Herman MV: Progression of coronary artery disease: A clinical arteriographic study. Circulation 47:455–464, 1973.
11. Nash DT, Caldwell N, Ancona D: Accelerated coronary artery disease arteriographically proved. N Y State J Med 74:947–950, 1974.

12. Nash DT, Gensini G, Simon H, et al: Progression of coronary atherosclerosis and dietary hyperlipidemia. Circulation 56:363–365, 1977.
13. Bruschke AV, Wijers TS, Kolsters W, et al: The anatomic evolution of coronary artery disease demonstrated by coronary arteriography in 256 nonoperated patients. Circulation 63:527–536, 1981.
14. Palac RT, Hwang MH, Meadows WR, et al: Progression of coronary artery disease in medically and surgically treated patients. Circulation 64(suppl II):II-17–II-21, 1981.
15. Kramer JR, Kitazume H, Proudfit WL, et al: Progression and regression of coronary atherosclerosis: Relation to risk factors. Am Heart J 105:134–144, 1983.
16. Singh RN: Progression of coronary atherosclerosis: Clues to pathogenesis from serial coronary arteriography. Br Heart J 52:451–461, 1984.
17. Moise A, Goulet C, Théroux P, et al: Spontaneous regression of coronary artery obstructions. Catheter Cardiovasc Diagn 11:235–245, 1985.
18. Bruschke AVG, Kramer JR Jr, Bal ET, et al: The dynamics of progression of coronary atherosclerosis studies in 168 medically treated patients who underwent coronary arteriography three times. Am Heart J 117:296–305, 1989.
19. Kuthan F, Burkhalter A, Baitsch R, et al: Development of occlusive arterial disease in lower limbs: Angiographic follow-up of 705 medical patients. Arch Surg 103:545–547, 1971.
20. Brown BG, Zhao XQ, Sacco DE, et al: Lipid lowering and plaque regression: New insights into prevention of plaque disruption and clinical events in coronary artery disease. Clinical Progress Series 1781–1785.
21. Waters D, Craven TE, Lesperance J: Prognostic significance of progression of coronary atherosclerosis. Circulation 87:1067–1075, 1993.
22. Brensike JF, Levy RI, Kelsey SF: Effects of therapy with cholestyramine on progression of coronary arteriosclerosis: Results of the NHLBI Type II Coronary Intervention Study. Circulation 69:313–324, 1984.
23. Brensike JF, Kelsey SF, Passamani ER: National Heart, Lung, and Blood Institute Type II Coronary Intervention Study: Design, methods, and baseline characteristics. Control Clin Trials 3:91–111, 1982.
24. Blankenhorn DH, Nessim SA, Johnson RL: Beneficial effects of combined colestipol-niacin therapy on coronary atherosclerosis and coronary venous bypass grafts. JAMA 257:3233–3240, 1987.
25. Blankenhorn DH, Johnson RL, Nessim SA: The Cholesterol Lowering Atherosclerosis Study (CLAS): Design, methods, and baseline results. Control Clin Trials 8:354–387, 1987.
26. Cashin-Hemphill L, Mack WJ, Pogoda JM: Beneficial effects of colestipol-niacin on coronary atherosclerosis: A 4-year follow-up. JAMA 264:3013–3017, 1990.
27. Brown G, Albers JJ, Fisher LD: Regression of coronary artery disease as a result of intensive lipid-lowering therapy in men with high levels of apolipoprotein B. N Engl J Med 323:1289–1298, 1990.
28. Kane JP, Malloy MJ, Ports TA: Regression of coronary atherosclerosis during treatment of familial hypercholesterolemia with combined drug regimens. JAMA 264:3007–3012, 1990.
29. Buchwald H, Varco RL, Matts JP: Effect of partial ileal bypass surgery on mortality and morbidity from coronary heart disease in patients with hypercholesterolemia: Report of the Program on the Surgical Control of the Hyperlipidemias (POSCH). N Engl J Med 323:946–955, 1990.
30. Buchwald H, Matts JP, Fitch LL: Program on the surgical control of the hyperlipidemias (POSCH): Design and methodology. J Clin Epidemiol 42(12):1111–1127, 1989.
31. Ornish D, Brown SE, Scherwitz LW: Can lifestyle changes reverse coronary heart disease? The Lifestyle Heart Trial. Lancet 336:129–133, 1990.
32. Schuler G, Hambrecht R, Schlierf G: Myocardial perfusion and regression of coronary artery disease in patients on a regimen of intensive physical exercise and low fat diet. J Am Coll Cardiol 19:34–42, 1992.
33. Watts GF, Lewis B, Brunt JNH: Effects on coronary artery disease of lipid-lowering diet, or diet plus cholestyramine, in the St. Thomas' Atherosclerosis Regression Study (STARS). Lancet 339:563–569, 1992.
34. Arntzenius AC, Kromhout D, Barth JD: Diet, lipoproteins, and the progression of coronary atherosclerosis: The Leiden Intervention Trial. N Engl J Med 312:805–811, 1985.
35. Waters D, Higginson L, Gladstone P, et al: Effects of monotherapy with an HMG-CoA reductase inhibitor on the progression of coronary atherosclerosis as assessed by serial quantitative arteriography: The Canadian Coronary Atherosclerosis Intervention Trial. Circulation 89:959–968, 1994.
36. Waters D, Higginson L, Gladstone P, et al: Design features of a controlled clinical trial to assess the effect of an HMG CoA reductase inhibitor on the progression of coronary artery disease. Control Clin Trials 14:45–74, 1993.
37. Blankenhorn DH, Azen SP, Kramsch DM, et al: Coronary angiographic changes with lovastatin therapy: The Monitored Atherosclerosis Regression Study (MARS). Ann Intern Med 119:969–976, 1993.
38. Arntzenius AC, Kromhout D, Barth JD, et al: Diet, lipoproteins and the progression of coronary atherosclerosis: The Leiden Intervention Trial. N Engl J Med 312:805–811, 1985.
39. Schuler G, Hambrecht R, Schlierf G, et al: Regular physical exercise and low-fat diet: Effects on progression of coronary artery disease. Circulation 86:1–11, 1992.
40. Gould KL, Ornish D, Kirkeeide R, et al: Improved stenosis geometry by quantitative coronary arteriography after vigorous risk factor modification. Am J Cardiol 69:845–853, 1992.
41. Haskell WL, Alderman EL, Fair JM, et al: Effects of intensive multiple risk factor reduction on coronary atherosclerosis and clinical cardiac events in men and women with coronary artery disease: The Stanford Coronary Risk Intervention Project (SCRIP). Circulation 89:975–990, 1994.
42. Oliver MF, MAAS Investigators: Effect of simvastatin on coronary atheroma: The Multicentre Anti-Atheroma Study (MAAS). Lancet 344:633–638, 1994.
43. Dumont JM, and the MAAS Research Group: Effect of cholesterol reduction by simvastatin on progression of coronary atherosclerosis. Control Clin Trials 14:209–228, 1993.
44. Pitt B, Mancini GBJ, Ellis SG, et al, for the PLAC-I Investigators: Pravastatin limitation of atherosclerosis in the coronary arteries (PLAC-I): Reduction in atherosclerosis progression and clinical events. J Am Coll Cardiol 26:1133–1139, 1995.
45. Pitt B, Ellis SG, Mancini GBJ, et al, for the PLAC I Investigators: Design and recruitment in the United States of a multicenter quantitative angiographic trial of pravastatin to limit atherosclerosis in the coronary arteries (PLAC I). Am J Cardiol 72:31–35, 1993.
46. Jukema JW, Bruschke AVG, van Boven AJ, et al: Coronary artery disease/myocardial infarction: Effects of lipid lowering by pravastatin on progression and regression of coronary artery disease in symptomatic men with normal to moderately elevated serum cholesterol levels: The Regression Growth Evaluation Statin Study (REGRESS). Circulation 91:2528–2540, 1995.
47. Rossouw JE: Lipid-lowering interventions in angiographic trials. Am J Cardiol 76:86C–92C, 1995.
48. Pearson T, Rapaport E, Criqui M, et al: Optimal risk factor management in the patients after coronary revascularization: A statement for healthcare professionals from an American Heart Association writing group. Circulation 90:3125–3133, 1994.
49. Wenger NC, Froelicher ES, Smith LK, et al: Cardiac Rehabilitation as Secondary Prevention. Clinical Practice Guideline: Quick Reference Guide for Clinicians, No. 17. Rockville, MD: U.S. Dept. of Health and Human Services, Public Health Service, Agency for Health Care Policy and Research and National Heart, Lung, and Blood Institute, 1995. Publication AHCPR 96-0673.
50. Keys A (ed): Coronary Heart Disease in Seven Countries. Circulation 41(suppl I):I-1–I-198, 1970.
51. Keys A, Aravanis C, Van Buchem FSP, et al: The diet and all-causes death rate in the Seven Countries Study. Lancet 2:58–61, 1981.

52. Puska P, Nissinen A, Tuomilehto J, et al: The community-based strategy to prevent coronary artery disease: Conclusions from the 10 years of the North Karelia Project. *In* Health Promotion: An Anthology, pp 89–125. Washington, DC: Pan American Health Organization, Pan American Sanitary Bureau, Regional Office of the World Health Organization, 1996. Scientific Publication No. 557.

53. Carlson LA, Bottiger LE: Ischaemic heart-disease in relation to fasting values of plasma triglycerides and cholesterol: Stockholm Prospective Study. Lancet 1:865–868, 1972.

54. Castelli WP, Doyle JT, Gordon T, et al: HDL cholesterol and other lipids in coronary heart disease: The Cooperative Lipoprotein Phenotyping Study. Circulation 55:767–772, 1977.

55. Dawber TR: The Framingham Study: The Epidemiology of Atherosclerotic Disease. Cambridge, MA: Harvard University Press, 1980.

56. Shekelle RB, Shryock AM, Paul O, et al: Diet, serum cholesterol, and death from coronary heart disease: The Western Electric Study. N Engl J Med 304:65–70, 1981.

57. Castelli WP, Garrison RJ, Wilson PWF, et al: Incidence of coronary heart disease and lipoprotein cholesterol levels: The Framingham Study. JAMA 256:2835–2838, 1986.

58. Martin MJ, Browner WS, Hulley SB, et al: Serum cholesterol, blood pressure and mortality: Implications from a cohort of 361 662 men. Lancet 1:933–936, 1986.

59. Shipley MJ, Pocock SJ, Marmot MG: Does plasma cholesterol concentration predict mortality from coronary heart disease in elderly people? 18 year follow up in Whitehall study. BMJ 303:89–92, 1991.

60. Brown MS, Goldstein JL: A receptor-mediated pathway for cholesterol homeostasis. Science 232:34–47, 1986.

61. Frick MH, Elo O, Haapa K, et al: Helsinki Heart Study: Primary-prevention trial with gemfibrozil in middle-aged men with dyslipidemia: Safety of treatment, changes in risk factors, and incidence of coronary heart disease. N Engl J Med 317:1237–1245, 1987.

62. Hjermann I, Holme I, Velve Byre K, et al: Effect of diet and smoking intervention on the incidence of coronary heart disease: Report from the Oslo Study Group of a randomized trial in healthy men. Lancet 2:1303–1310, 1981.

63. Lipid Research Clinics Program: The Lipid Research Clinics Coronary Primary Prevention Trial results: I. Reduction in incidence of coronary heart disease. JAMA 251:351–364, 1984.

64. Shepherd J, Cobbe SM, Ford I, et al, for the West of Scotland Coronary Prevention Study Group: Prevention of coronary heart disease with pravastatin in men with hypercholesterolemia. N Engl J Med 333:1301–1307, 1995.

65. West of Scotland Coronary Prevention Study Group: A coronary primary prevention study of Scottish men age 45–64 years: Trial design. J Clin Epidemiol 45:849–860, 1992.

66. Rosenman RH, Brand RJ, Jenkins D, et al: Coronary heart disease in the Western Collaborative Group Study. JAMA 233(8):872–877, 1975.

67. Friedman GD, Petitti DB, Bawol RD, et al: Mortality in cigarette smokers and quitters: Effect of base-line differences. N Engl J Med 304:1407–1410, 1981.

68. Neaton JD, Kuller LH, Wentworth D, et al: Total and cardiovascular mortality in relation to cigarette smoking, serum cholesterol concentration, and diastolic blood pressure among black and white males followed up for five years. Am Heart J 108(3, pt 2):759–769, 1984.

69. Selzer CC: Framingham Study data and "established wisdom" about cigarette smoking and coronary heart disease. J Clin Epidemiol 42:743–750, 1989.

70. Hubert HB, Feinleib M, McNamara PM, et al: Obesity as an independent risk factor for cardiovascular disease: A 26-year follow-up of participants in the Framingham Heart Study. Circulation 67:968–977, 1983.

71. Bray AB: Complications of obesity. Ann Intern Med 103:1052–1062, 1985.

72. Reed D, Yano K: Predictors of arteriographically defined coronary stenosis in the Honolulu Heart Program: Comparisons of cohort and arteriography series analyses. Am J Epidemiol 134:111–122, 1991.

73. Fletcher GF, Blair SN, Blumenthal J, et al: Benefits and recommendations for physical activity programs for all Americans: A statement for health professionals by the Committee on Exercise and Cardiac Rehabilitation of the Council on Clinical Cardiology, American Heart Association. Circulation 86:340–344, 1992.

74. Paffenbarger RS, Hyde RT, Wing AL, et al: A natural history of athleticism and cardiovascular health. JAMA 252:491–495, 1984.

75. Leon AS, Connett J, Jacobs DR Jr, et al: Leisure-time physical activity levels and risk of coronary heart disease and death: The Multiple Risk Factor Intervention Trial. JAMA 258:2388–2395, 1987.

76. Blair SN, Kohl HW III, Paffenbarger RS, et al: Physical fitness and all-cause mortality: A prospective study of healthy men and women. JAMA 262:2395–2401, 1989.

77. Marmot MG, Syme SL, Kagan A, et al: Epidemiologic studies of coronary heart disease and stroke in Japanese men living in Japan, Hawaii and California: Prevalence of coronary and hypertensive heart disease and associated risk factors. Am J Epidemiol 102:514–525, 1975.

78. Ruberman W, Weinblatt E, Goldberg JD, et al: Psychosocial influences on mortality after myocardial infarction. N Engl J Med 311:552–559, 1984.

79. Reed D, McGee D, Yano K, Feinleib M: Social networks and coronary heart disease among Japanese men in Hawaii. Am J Epidemiol 117:384–396, 1983.

80. Kaplan GA: Social contacts and ischaemic heart disease. Ann Clin Res 20:131–136, 1988.

81. Cassel J, Heyden S, Bartel AG, et al: Incidence of coronary heart disease by ethnic group, social class, and sex. Arch Intern Med 128:901–906, 1971.

82. Williams RB, Barefoot JC, Califf RM, et al: Prognostic importance of social and economic resources among medically treated patients with angiography documented coronary artery disease. JAMA 267:520–524, 1992.

83. McGinnis M, Foege WH: Actual causes of death in the United States. JAMA 270:2207–2212, 1993.

84. Heliovaara M, Karvonen MJ, Punsar S, et al: Importance of coronary risk factors in the presence or absence of myocardial ischemia. Am J Cardiol 50:1248–1252, 1982.

85. Shaper AG, Pocock SJ, Walker M, et al: Risk factors for ischaemic heart disease: The prospective phase of the British Regional Heart Study. J Epidemiol Community Health 39:197–209, 1985.

86. Gordon DJ, Ekelund LG, Karon JM, et al: Predictive value of exercise tolerance test for mortality in North American men: The Lipid Research Clinics Mortality Follow-up Study. Circulation 74:252–261, 1986.

87. Pekkanen J, Linn S, Geiss G, et al: Ten-year mortality from cardiovascular disease in relation to cholesterol level among men with and without preexisting cardiovascular disease. N Engl J Med 322:1700–1707, 1990.

88. Williams OD, Stinnett S, Chambless LE, et al: Populations and methods for assessing dyslipoproteinemia and its correlates: The Lipid Research Clinics Program Prevalence Study. Circulation 73(Suppl I): I-4–I-11, 1986.

89. Central Patient Registry and Coordinating Center for the Lipid Research Clinics: Reference Manual for Lipid Research Clinics Program Prevalence Study, vol I. Chapel Hill, University of North Carolina, 1974.

90. The Lipid Research Clinics Program Epidemiology Committee: Plasma lipid distributions in selected North American populations: The Lipid Research Clinics Prevalence Study. Circulation 60:427–439, 1979.

91. Coronary Drug Project Research Group: Natural history of myocardial infarction in the Coronary Drug Project: Long-term prognostic importance of serum lipid levels. Am J Cardiol 42:489–498, 1978.

92. Schlant RC, Forman S, Stamler J, et al, for the Coronary Drug Project Research Group: The natural history of coronary heart disease: Prognostic factors after recovery from myocardial infarction in 2789 men: The 5-year findings of the Coronary Drug Project. Circulation 66:401–414, 1982.

93. Stamler J, Wentworth D, Neaton JD, for the MRFIT Research Group: Is relationship between serum cholesterol and risk

of premature death from coronary heart disease continuous or graded? Findings in 356,222 primary screenees of the Multiple Risk Factor Intervention Trial (MRFIT). JAMA 256:2823–2828, 1986.

94. Miller M, Seidler A, Kwiterovich PO, et al: Long-term predictors of subsequent cardiovascular events with coronary artery disease and "desirable" levels of plasma total cholesterol. Circulation 86:1165–1170, 1992.

95. Campeau L, Enjalbert M, Lesperance J, et al: The relation of risk factors to the development of atherosclerosis in saphenous-vein bypass grafts and the progression of disease in the native circulation: A study of 10 years after aortocoronary bypass surgery. N Engl J Med 311:1329–1332, 1984.

96. Blair SN, Kohl HW, Paffenbarger RS, et al: Physical fitness and all-cause mortality. JAMA 262:2395–2401, 1989.

97. Berlin HA, Colditz GA: A meta-analysis of physical activity in the prevention of coronary heart attacks. Am J Epidemiol 132:612–628, 1987.

98. Ekelund L-G, Haskell WL, Johnson SL, et al: Physical fitness as a predictor of cardiovascular mortality in asymptomatic North American men. N Engl J Med 319:1379–1384, 1988.

99. Ekelund L-G, Haskell WL, Troung YL, et al: Physical fitness as predictor of cardiovascular mortality in asymptomatic females [Abstract]. Circulation 78(suppl II):110, 1988.

100. Leon AS, Connett J, Jacobs DR, et al: Leisure-time physical activity levels and risk of coronary heart disease and death: The Multiple Risk Factor Intervention Trial. JAMA 258:2388–2395, 1987.

101. Whaley MH, Blair SN: Epidemiology of physical activity, physical fitness, and coronary heart disease. Am Coll Sports Med Certified News 5:1, 1995.

102. Haskell WL: Dose response of physical activity and disease risk factors. In Pekka O, Telma R (eds): Sport for All, pp 125–134. Amsterdam: Elsevier Science, 1991.

103. Haskell WL: Health consequences of physical activity: Understanding and challenges regarding dose response. Med Sci Sports Exerc 26:649–660, 1994.

104. Oldridge N, Furlong W, Feeny D, et al: Economic evaluation of cardiac rehabilitation soon after acute myocardial infarction. Am J Cardiol 72:154–161, 1993.

105. Bonestam E, Breikks A, Hartford M: Effects of early rehabilitation on consumption of medical care during the first year after acute myocardial infarction in patients > 65 years of age. Am J Cardiol 75:767–771, 1995.

106. Haskell WL: The influence of exercise training on plasma lipids and lipoproteins in health and disease. Acta Med Scand 711(suppl):25–37, 1986.

107. Thompson PD, Cullinane EM, Sady SP, et al: High density lipoprotein metabolism in endurance athletes and sedentary men. Circulation 84:140–152, 1991.

108. Holloszy JO, Shult J, Kusnierkiewicz A, et al: Effects of exercise on glucose tolerance and insulin resistance. Acta Med Scand 711(suppl):55–65, 1986.

109. Durstine JL, WL Haskell: Effect of exercise training on plasma lipids and lipoproteins. Exer Sport Sci Rev: 44:477–521, 1994.

110. Stefanick ML: Exercise, lipoproteins, and cardiovascular disease. In Fletcher GF (ed): Cardiovascular Response to Exercise, pp 325–345. Mount Kisco, NY: Futura, 1994.

111. Etherton TD, Peterson S, Kris-Etherton PM: Effects of exercise on plasma lipids and lipoproteins of women. Proc Soc Exp Biol Med 240:123–137, 1993.

112. Cardiac rehabilitation services. Health and Public Policy Committee, American College of Physicians. Ann Intern Med 109:671–673, 1988.

113. Taylor CB, Houston-Miller N, Ahn DK, et al: The effects of exercise training programs on psychosocial improvement in uncomplicated postmyocardial infarction patients. J Psychosom Res 30:581–587, 1986.

114. Rosenman RH, Brand RJ, Jenkins CD, et al: Coronary heart disease in the Western Collaborative Group Study: Final follow-up experience of 8.5 years. JAMA 233:872–877, 1975.

115. Friedman M, Ulmer D: Treating Type A Behavior and Your Heart. New York: Fawcett Crest, 1984.

116. Blumenthal JA, Williams RB, Kong Y, et al: Type A behavior pattern and atherosclerosis. Circulation 58:634–649, 1978.

117. Review Panel on Coronary-Prone Behavior and Coronary Heart Disease: A critical review. Circulation 63:1199–1215, 1981.

118. Shekelle RB, Hulley S, Neaton J, et al: The MRFIT behavior pattern study: II. Type A behavior pattern and incidence of coronary heart disease. Am J Epidemiol 122:559–570, 1985.

119. Ragland DR, Brand RJ: Coronary heart disease mortality in the Western Collaborative Group Study. Am J Epidemiol 127:462–475, 1988.

120. Williams RB, Haney TL, Lee KL, et al: Type A behavior, hostility and coronary atherosclerosis. Psychosom Med 42:539–549, 1980.

121. Barefoot JC, Dahlstrom WG, Williams RB: Hostility, CHD incidence, and total mortality: A 25-year follow-up study of 255 physicians. Psychosom Med 45:59–63, 1983.

122. Dembroski TM, MacDougall JM, Costa PT, Grandits GA: Components of hostility as predictors of sudden death and myocardial infarction in the Multiple Risk Factors Intervention Trial. Psychosom Med 51:514–522, 1989.

123. Berkman LF, Syme SL: Social networks, host resistance, and mortality: A nine-year follow-up of Alameda County residents. Am J Epidemiol 109:186–204, 1979.

124. Orth-Gomer K, Rosengren A, Wilhelmsen L: Lack of social support and incidence of coronary heart disease in middle-aged Swedish men. Psychosom Med 55:37–43, 1993.

125. Orth-Gomer K, Unden AL: Type A behavior, social support, and coronary risk: Interaction and significance for mortality in cardiac patients. Psychosom Med 52:59–72, 1990.

126. Booth-Kewley S, Friedman H: Psychological predictors of heart disease: A quantitative review. Psychol Bull 101(3):343–362, 1987.

127. Matthew KA: Coronary hear disease and type A behaviors: Update on and alternative to the Booth-Kewley and Friedman (1987) quantitative review. Psychol Bull 104(3):373–380, 1988.

128. Barefoot JC, Schroll M: Symptoms of depression, acute myocardial infarction, and total mortality in a community sample. Circulation 93:1976–1980, 1996.

129. Frasure-Smith N, Lesperance F, Talajic M: Depression following myocardial infarction: Impact on 6-month survival. JAMA 270:1819–1825, 1993.

130. Frasure-Smith N, Lesperance F, Talajic M: Depression and 18 month prognosis after myocardial infarction. Circulation 91:999–1005, 1995.

131. Barefoot JC, Helms MJ, Mark DB, et al: Depression and long-term mortality risk in patients with coronary artery disease. Am J Cardiol 78:613–617, 1996.

132. Turner JR, Sherwood A, Light KC: Individual differences in cardiovascular response to stress. New York: Plenum, 1992.

133. Turner JR: Cardiovascular Reactivity and Stress: Patterns of Physiological Response. New York: Plenum, 1994.

134. Cohen S, Wills TA: Stress, social support, and the buffering hypothesis. Psychol Bull 98:310–357, 1985.

135. Blumenthal JA, Burg MM, Barefoot I, et al: Social support, type A behavior, and coronary artery disease. Psychosom Med 49:331–340, 1987.

136. Suarez EC, Williams RB: Situational determinants of cardiovascular and emotional reactivity in high and low hostile men. Psychosom Med 51:404–418, 1989.

137. Williams R, Barefoot J, Califf R, et al: Prognostic importance of social and economic resources among patients with angiographically documented coronary artery disease. JAMA 267:520–524, 1992.

138. Gold P, Goodwin F, Chrousos G: Clinical and biochemical manifestations of depression: Relation to the neurobiology of stress. N Engl J Med 319:348–353, 1988.

139. Holahan CJ, Moos RH, Holahan CK, et al: Social support, coping, and depressive symptoms in a late-middle-aged sample of patients reporting cardiac illness. Health Psychol 14(2):152–163, 1995.

140. Carney RM, Freedland KE, Rich MW, et al: Depression as a risk factor for cardiac events in established coronary heart disease: A review of possible mechanisms. Ann Behav Med 17:142–129, 1995.

141. Jiang W, Babyak M, Krantz DS, et al: Mental stress-induced myocardial ischemia and cardiac events. JAMA 275:1651–1656, 1996.

142. Grundy SM, Denke MA: Dietary influences on serum lipids and lipoproteins. J Lipid Res 31:1149–1172, 1990.

143. Connor WE, Connor SL: The dietary prevention and treatment of coronary heart disease. In Connor WE, Bristow JD (eds): Coronary Heart Disease. Philadelphia: JB Lippincott, 1984.

144. Kris-Etherton PM, Krummel D, Russel M, et al: The effect of diet on plasma lipids, lipoprotein, and coronary heart disease. J Am Diet Assoc: 1373–1400, 1988.

145. Report of the National Cholesterol Education Program Expert Panel on Detection, Evaluation and Treatment of High Blood Cholesterol in Adults. Arch Intern Med 148:36–69, 1988.

146. Grundy SM, Brown WV, Dietschy JM, et al: Workshop III: Basis for dietary treatment. Circulation 80:729–734, 1989.

147. The Nutrition Committee, American Heart Association: Dietary guidelines for healthy American adults. Circulation 77:721A–724A, 1988.

148. Kris-Etherton PM, Krummel DA: Role of nutrition in the prevention and treatment of coronary artery disease in women. J Am Diet Assoc 93:987–993, 1993.

149. Watts GF, Jackson P, Burke V, et al: Dietary fatty acids and progression of coronary artery disease in men. Am J Clin Nutr 64:202–209, 1996.

150. Chait A, Brunzell JD, Denke MA, et al: Rationale of the Diet-Heart Statement of the American Heart Association: Report of the Nutrition Committee. Circulation 88:3008–3029, 1993.

151. Second Report of the Expert Panel on Detection, Evaluation, and Treatment of High Blood Cholesterol in Adults (Adult Treatment Panel II). Bethesda, MD: National Institutes of Health, National Heart, Lung and Blood Institute, 1993. Publication NIH 93-3095.

152. Sempos CT, Cleeman JI, Caroll MD, et al: Prevalence of high blood cholesterol among US adults. JAMA 269:3009–3014, 1993.

153. Grundy SM, Barrett-Connor E, Rudel LL, et al: Workshop on the impact of dietary cholesterol on plasma lipoproteins and atherogenesis. Arteriosclerosis 8(1):95–101, 1988.

154. Connor WE, Connor SL: Importance of diet in the treatment of familial hypercholesterolemia. Am J Cardiol 72:42D–53D, 1993.

155. Coulston AM, Hollenbeck CB, Swislocki AL, et al: Persistence of hypertriglyceridemic effects of low-fat, high carbohydrate diets in NIDDM patients. JAMA 12:94–101, 1989.

156. Steinberg D, Parthasarathy S, Carew TE, et al: Beyond cholesterol: Modifications of low-density lipoprotein that increase its atherogenicity. N Engl J Med 320:915–924, 1989.

157. Rasumssen OW, Thomsen C, Hansen KW, et al: Effects on blood pressure, glucose, and lipid levels of a high-monounsatured fat diet compared with a high-carbohydrate diet in NIDDM subjects. Diabetes Care 16:1565–1571, 1993.

158. Kushi LH, Lenart EB, Willett WC: Health implications of Mediterranean diets in light of contemporary knowledge: 1. Plant foods and dairy products. Am J Clin Nutr 61:1402S–1406S, 1995.

159. Davidson MH, Liebson PR: Marine lipids and atherosclerosis: A review. Cardiol Rev Rep 7(5):461–472, 1986.

160. Sirtori CR, Gatti E, Mantero O, et al: Clinical experience with the soybean protein diet in the treatment of hypercholesterolemia. Am J Clin Nutr 32:1645–1658, 1979.

161. Steinberg D: Antioxidants in the prevention of human atherosclerosis: Summary of the proceedings of a National Heart, Lung and Blood Institute Workshop: Sept. 5–6, 1991, Bethesda, MD. Circulation 85:2338–2344, 1992.

162. Stephens NG, Parsons A, Schofield PM, et al: Randomised controlled trial of vitamin E in patients with coronary disease: Cambridge Heart Antioxidant Study (CHAOS). Lancet 347:781–786, 1996.

163. Herbert V: Iron disorders can mimic anything, so always test for them. Blood Rev 3:125–132, 1992.

164. Omenn GS, Goodman GE, Thornquist MD, et al: Effects of a combination of beta carotene and vitamin A on lung cancer and cardiovascular disease. N Engl J Med 334:1150–1155, 1996.

165. Thornquist MD, Omenn GS, Goodman GE, et al: Statistical design and monitoring of the Carotene and Retinol Efficacy Trial (CARET). Control Clin Trials 14:308–324, 1993.

166. Clinical Investigator News 1996; 4(2):1.

167. Renaud S, De Lorgeril M: Wine, alcohol, platelets, and the French paradox for coronary heart disease. Lancet 339:1523–1526, 1992.

168. Frankel EN, Waterhouse AL, Kinsella JE: Inhibition of human LDL oxidation by resveratrol. Lancet 341:1103–1104, 1993.

169. Frankel EN, Kanner J, Gliman JB, et al: Inhibition of human low-density lipoprotein by phenol substances in red wine. Lancet 341:454–457, 1993.

170. Flatt JP: Importance of nutrient balance in bodyweight regulation. Diabetes Metab Rev 4:571–581, 1985.

171. Lopez JAG, Armstrong ML, Piegors DJ, et al: Effect of early and advanced atherosclerosis on vascular responses to serotonin, thromboxane A2, and adenosine diphosphate (ADP). Circulation 79:698–705, 1989.

172. Dishman RK, Sallis J, Orenstein D: The determinants of physical activity and exercise. Public Health Rep 100:158–180, 1985.

173. Gould KL, Ornish D, Kirkeeide R, et al: Improved stenosis geometry by quantitative coronary arteriography after vigorous risk factor modification. Am J Cardiol 69:845–853, 1992.

174. Zeiher AM, Drexler H, Wollschlaeger H, et al: Coronary vasomotion in response to sympathetic stimulation in humans: Importance of the functional integrity of the endothelium. J Am Coll Cardiol 14:1181–1190, 1989.

175. Wenger NK, Froelicher ES, Smith LK, et al: Cardiac Rehabilitation. Clinical Practice Guideline No. 17. Rockville, MD: U.S. Dept of Health and Human Services, Public Health Service, Agency for Health Care Policy and Research and National Heart, lung and Blood Institute, 1995 Publication AHCPR 96-0672.

176. Collins R, Yusuf S, Peto R: Exercise after myocardial infarction reduces mortality: Evidence from randomized controlled trails [Abstract]. J Am Coll Cardiol 3:622, 1984.

177. Oldridge NB, Guyatt GH, Fischer ME, et al: Cardiac rehabilitation after myocardial infarction: Combined experience of randomized clinical trials. JAMA 260:945–950, 1988.

178. O'Connor GT: An overview of randomized trials of rehabilitation with exercise after myocardial infarction. Circulation 80:235–244, 1989.

179. Shephard RJ: The value of exercise in ischemic heart disease: A cumulative analysis. J Cardiac Rehabil 3:294–298, 1983.

180. P.R.E.COR Group: Comparison of a rehabilitation programme, a counseling programme and usual care after an acute myocardial infarction: Results of a long-term randomized trial. Eur Heart J 12:612–616, 1991.

181. Hagberg JM, Ehsani AA, Holloszy JO: Effect of 12 months of intense exercise training on stroke volume in patients with coronary artery disease. Circulation 67:1194–1199, 1983.

182. Clausen JP: Circulatory adjustments to dynamic exercise and effect of physical training in normal subjects and patients with coronary artery disease. Prog Cardiovasc Dis 18:459–495, 1976.

183. Varnauskas E, Bergman H, Houk P, Bjorntorp P: Hemodynamic effects of physical training in coronary patients. Lancet 2:8–12, 1986.

184. Detry JM, Rousseau M, Vandenbroucke G, et al: Increased arteriovenous oxygen difference after physical training in coronary heart disease. Circulation 44:109–118, 1971.

185. Clausen JP, Trap-Jensen J: Effects of training on the distribution of cardiac output in patients with coronary artery disease. Circulation 42:611–624, 1970.

186. Letac B, Cribier A, Desplanches JF: A study of left ventricular function in coronary patients before and after physical training. Circulation 56:375–378, 1977.

187. Cobb FR, Williams RS, McEwan P, et al: Effects of exercise

training on ventricular function in patients with recent myocardial infarction. Circulation 66:100–108, 1982.

188. Froelicher V, Jensen D, Genter F, et al: A randomized trial of exercise training in patients with coronary artery disease. JAMA 252:1291–1297, 1984.

189. Sebrechts CP, Klein JL, Ahnve S, et al: Myocardial perfusion changes following 1 year of exercise training assessed by thallium-201 circumferential count profiles. Am Heart J 112:1217–1225, 1986.

190. Hagberg JM: Physiologic adaptations to prolonged high-intensity exercise training in patients with coronary artery disease. Med Sci Sports Exerc 23:661–667, 1991.

191. Ferguson RJ, Taylor AW, Cote P, et al: Skeletal muscle and cardiac changes with training in patients with angina pectoris. Am J Physiol 243:H830–H836, 1982.

192. Sim DN, Neill WA: Investigation of the physiological basis for increased exercise threshold for angina pectoris and physical conditioning. J Clin Invest 54:763–770, 1974.

193. Myers J, Ahnve S, Froelicher V, et al: A randomized trial of the effects of 1 year of exercise training on computer-measured ST segment displacement in patients with coronary artery disease. J Am Coll Cardiol 4:1094–1102, 1984.

194. Detry JMR, Bruce RA: Effects of physical training on exertional ST-segment depression in coronary artery disease. Circulation 44:390–398, 1971.

195. Nolewajka AJ, Kostuk WL, Rechnitzer PA, et al: Exercise and human collateralization: An angiographic and scintigraphic assessment. Circulation 60:114–121, 1979.

196. Amsterdam EA, Laslett LJ, Dressendorfer RH, et al: Exercise training in coronary artery disease: Is there a cardiac effect? Am Heart J 101:870–873, 1981.

197. Ehsani AA, Heath GW, Hagberg JM, et al: Effects of 12 months of intense exercise training on ischemic ST-segment depression in patients with coronary artery disease. Circulation 64:1116–1124, 1981.

198. Williams MA, Maresh CM, Esterbrooks DJ, et al: Early exercise training in patients older than age 65 years compared with that in younger patients after acute myocardial infarction or coronary bypass grafting. Am J Cardiol 55:263–266, 1985.

199. Canner PL, Berge KG, Wenger NK, et al: Fifteen year mortality in Coronary Drug Project patients: Long-term benefit with niacin. J Am Coll Cardiol 8:1245–1255, 1986.

200. The Coronary Drug Project Research Group: Clofibrate and niacin in coronary heart disease. JAMA 231:360–381, 1975.

201. Levy RI, Brensike JF, Eptstein SE, et al: The influence of changes in lipid values induced by cholestyramine and diet on progression of coronary artery disease: Results of the NHLBI Type II Coronary Intervention Study. Circulation 69:325–337, 1984.

202. Blankenhorn DH, Johnson RL, Mack WJ, et al: The influence of diet on the appearance of new lesions in human coronary arteries. JAMA 263:1646–1652, 1990.

203. Sacks FM, Paternak RC, Gibson CM, et al, for the Harvard Atherosclerosis Reversibility Project: Effect on coronary atherosclerosis of decrease in plasma cholesterol concentrations in normocholesterolaemic patients. Lancet 344:1182–1186, 1994.

204. Rousouw JE, Lewis B, Rifkind BM: The values of lowering cholesterol after myocardial infarction. N Engl J Med 323:1112–1119, 1990.

205. Furberg CD, Byington RP, Crouse JR, et al: Pravastatin, lipids, and major coronary events. Am J Cardiol 73:1133–1134, 1994.

206. Crouse JR, Byington RP, Bond MG, et al: Pravastatin, lipids, and atherosclerosis outcome. Control Clin Trials 13:495–506, 1992.

207. Byington RP, Furberg CD, Crouse JR, et al: Pravastatin, lipids, and atherosclerosis in the carotid arteries (PLAC-II). Am J Cardiol 76:54C–59C, 1995.

208. Furberg CD, Pitt B, Byington RP, et al, for the PLAC I and PLAC II Investigators: Reduction in coronary events during treatment with pravastatin. Am J Cardiol 76:60C–63C, 1995.

209. The Pravastatin Multinational Study Group for Cardiac Risk Patients: Effects of pravastatin in patients with serum total cholesterol levels from 5.2 to 7.8 mmol/liter (200 to 300 mg/dl) plus two additional atherosclerotic risk factors. Am J Cardiol 72:1031–1037, 1993.

210. Scandinavian Simvastatin Survival Study Group: Randomised trial of cholesterol lowering in 4444 patients with coronary heart disease: The Scandinavian Simvastatin Survival Study (4S). Lancet 344:1383–1389, 1994.

211. The Scandinavian Simvastatin Survival Study Group: Design and baseline results of the Scandinavian Simvastatin Survival Study of patients with stable angina and/or previous myocardial infarction. Am J Cardiol 71:393–400, 1993.

212. Kjekshus J, Pedersen TR, for the Scandinavian Simvastatin Survival Study Group: Reducing the risk of coronary events: Evidence from the Scandinavian Simvastatin Survival Study (4S). Am J Cardiol 76:64C–68C, 1995.

213. Pearson TA, Swan HJC: Lipid lowering: The case for identifying and treating the high-risk patients. Cardiol Clin 14:117–130, 1996.

214. Scandinavian Simvastatin Survival Study Group: Baseline serum cholesterol and treatment effect in the Scandinavian Simvastatin Survival Study (4S). Lancet 345:1274–1275, 1995.

215. Sacks FM, Pfeffer MA, Moye LA, et al, for the Cholesterol and Recurrent Events Trial Investigators: The effect of pravastatin on coronary events after myocardial infarction in patients with average cholesterol levels. N Engl J Med 335:1001–1009, 1996.

216. Sacks FM, Pfeffer MA, Moye L, et al: Rationale and design of a secondary prevention trial of lowering normal plasma cholesterol levels after acute myocardial infarction: The Cholesterol and Recurrent Events trial (CARE). Am J Cardiol 68:1436–1446, 1991.

217. The Long-Term Intervention with Pravastatin in Ischaemic Disease (LIPID) Study Group: Prevention of cardiovascular events and death with pravastatin in patients with coronary heart disease and a broad range of initial cholesterol levels. N Engl J Med 339:1349–1357, 1998.

218. The LIPID Study Investigators: Design features and baseline characteristics of the LIPID (Long-Term Intervention with Pravastatin in Ischaemic Disease) study: A randomised trial in patients from Australia and New Zealand with previous myocardial infarction and/or unstable angina. Am J Cardiol 76:474–479, 1995.

219. Golino P, Piscione F, Willerson JT, et al: Divergent effects of serotonin on coronary-artery dimensions and blood flow in patients with coronary atherosclerosis and control patients. N Engl J Med 324:641–648, 1991.

220. Ludmer PL, Selwyn AP, Shook TL, et al: Paradoxical vasoconstriction induced by acetylcholine in atherosclerotic coronary arteries. N Engl J Med 315:1046–1051, 1986.

221. Zeiher AM, Drexler H, Saurbier B, et al: Endothelium-mediated coronary blood flow modulation in humans: Effects of age, atherosclerosis, hypercholesterolemia, and hypertension. J Clin Invest 92:652–662, 1993.

222. Treasure CB, Klein JL, Wientraub WS, et al: Beneficial effects of cholesterol-lowering therapy on the coronary endothelium in patients with coronary artery disease. N Engl J Med 332:481–487, 1995.

223. Anderson, TJ, Meredith IT, Yeung AC, et al: The effect of cholesterol-lowering and antioxidant therapy on endothelium-dependent coronary vasomotion. N Engl J Med 332:488–493, 1995.

224. Leung WH, Lau CP, Wong CK: Beneficial effect of cholesterol-lowering therapy on coronary endothelium-dependent relaxation in hypercholesterolaemic patients. Lancet 341:1496–1500, 1993.

225. Egashira K, Hirooka Y, Kai H, et al: Reduction in serum cholesterol with pravastatin improves endothelium-dependent coronary vasomotion in patients with hypercholesterolemia. Circulation 89:2519–2524, 1994.

226. Czernin J, Barnard RJ, Sun KT, et al: Effect of short-term cardiovascular conditioning and low-fat diet on myocardial blood flow and flow reserve. Circulation 92:197–204, 1995.

227. Niebauer J, Hambrecht R, Marburger C, et al: Impact of intensive physical exercise and low-fat diet on collateral vessel formation in stable angina pectoris and angiographi-

cally confirmed coronary artery disease. Am J Cardiol 76:771–775, 1995.

228. Kristal AR, White E, Shattuck AL, et al: Long-term maintenance of a low-fat diet: Durability of fat-related dietary habits in the Women's Health Trial. J Am Diet Assoc 92:553–559, 1992.

229. Kelman HC: Compliance, identification, and internalization: Three processes of attitude change. In Hinto BL, Reitz HJ (eds): Groups and Organizations: Integrated Readings in the Analysis of Social Behavior. California: Wadsworth, 1971.

230. Barnes MS, Terry RD: Adherence to the cardiac diet: Attitudes of patients after myocardial infarction. J Am Diet Assoc 91:1435–1439, 1991.

231. Shannon B, Bagby R, Want MQ, et al: Self-efficacy: A contributor to the explanation of eating behavior. Health Educ Res 5:395–407, 1990.

232. Wilson D, Taylor W, Gilbert R, et al: A randomized trial of a family physician intervention for smoking cessation. JAMA 160:1570–1574, 1988.

233. Ockene JK, Kristeller J, Pbert L, et al: The physician-delivered smoking intervention project: Can short-term interventions produce long-term effects for a general outpatients population? Health Psychol 13(3):278–281, 1994.

234. Law M, Tang JL: An analysis of the effectiveness of interventions intended to help people stop smoking. Arch Intern Med 155:1933–1941, 1995.

235. Rigotti NA, Pasternak RC: Cigarette smoking and coronary heart disease: Risks and management. Cardiol Clin 14:51–68, 1996.

236. Timmreck TC, Randolph JF: Smoking cessation: Clinical steps to improve compliance. Geriatrics 48(4):63–70, 1993.

237. Benowitz NL, Gourlay SG: Cardiovascular toxicity of nicotine: Implications for nicotine replacement therapy. J Am Col Cardiol 29:1422–1431, 1997.

238. U.S. Surgeon General: Reducing the Health Consequences of Smoking: 25 Years of Progress: A Report of the Surgeon General. 1989, Rockville, MD: Centers for Disease Control, Center for Chronic Disease Prevention and Health Promotion, Office on Smoking and Health, 1989. DHHS Publication No. CDC 87-8398.

239. Prochaska JO, DiClemente CC: Stages and processes of self-change in smoking: Toward an integrative model of change. J Consult Clin Psychol 5:390–395, 1983.

240. Prochaska JO, Norcross JC, DiClemente CC: Changing for Good: The Revolutionary Program that Explains the Six Stages of Change and Teaches You How to Free Yourself from Bad Habits. New York: William Morrow, 1994.

241. Perz CA, DiClemente CC, Carbonari JP: Doing the right thing? The interaction of stages and processes of change in successful smoking cessation. Health Psychol 15(6):462–468, 1996.

242. Cohen S, Lichtenstein E, Prochaska JO, et al: Debunking myths about self-quitting. Am Psychol 44:1355–1366, 1989.

243. Wenger NK, Froelicher ES, Kent Smith L, et al: Cardiac Rehabilitation. Clinical Practice Guideline, No. 17. Rockville, MD: U.S. Dept of Health and Human Services, Public Health Service, Agency for Health Care Policy and Research and National Heart, Lung, and Blood Institute, 1995. Publication AHCPR 96-0672.

244. Taylor CB, Houston-Miller N, Killen JD, et al: Smoking cessation after acute myocardial infarction: Effects of a nurse-managed intervention. Ann Intern Med 113:118–123, 1990.

245. DeBusk RF, Houston-Miller N, Superko HR, et al: A case-management system for coronary risk factor modification after acute myocardial infarction. Ann Intern Med 120:721–729, 1994.

246. Lichtenstein E, Lando HA, Nothwehr F: Readiness to quit as a predictor of smoking changes in the Minnesota Heart Health Program. Health Psychol 13(5):393–396, 1994.

247. Hughes JR: An algorithm for smoking cessation. Arch Fam Med 3(3):280–285, 1994.

248. American College of Sports Medicine position stand. The recommended quantity of exercise for developing and maintaining cardiorespiratory and muscular fitness in healthy adults. Med Sci Sports Exerc 22:265–274, 1990.

249. Kugler J, Dimsdale JE, Hartley H, et al: Hospital supervised vs home exercise in cardiac rehabilitation effects on aerobic fitness, anxiety, and depression. Arch Phys Med Rehabil 71:322–325, 1990.

250. Miller NH, Haskell WL, Berra K, et al: Home versus group exercise for increasing functional capacity after myocardial infarction. Circulation 70:645–649, 1984.

251. Haskell WL: Physical activity and health: Need to define the required stimulus. Am J Cardiol 55:4D–9D, 1985.

252. Pollock ML, Wilmore JH: Exercise in Health and Disease: Evaluation and Prescription for Prevention and Rehabilitation, 2nd ed. Philadelphia: WB Saunders, 1990.

253. Sparling PB, Cantwell JD, Dolan CM, et al: Strength training in a cardiac rehabilitation program: A six-month follow-up. Arch Phys Med Rehab 71:148–152, 1990.

254. Ghilarducci LE, Holly RG, Amsterdam EA: Effects of high resistance training in coronary artery disease. Am J Cardiol 64:866–870, 1989.

255. McDermott MM, Schmitt B, Wallner E: Impact of medication nonadherence on coronary heart disease outcomes: A critical review. Arch Intern Med 157:1921–1929, 1997.

256. Cohen MV, Byrne M, Levine B, et al: Low rate of treatment of hypercholesterolemia by cardiologists in patients with suspected and proven coronary artery disease. Circulation 83:1294–1304, 1991.

257. Roberts WC: Getting cardiologists interested in lipids. Am J Cardiol 72:744–745, 1993.

258. Stevenson JC, Godsland IF, Wynn V: Cardiologists rebuked. Lancet 344:1557, 1994.

259. Swann HJC: Why cardiologists must be interested in lipids. Am J Cardiol 75:1067–1068, 1995.

260. Garber AM, Browner WS: Cholesterol screening guidelines: Consensus, evidence, and common sense. Circulation 95:1642–1645, 1997.

261. Cleeman JI, Grundy SM: National Cholesterol Education Program recommendations for cholesterol testing in young adults: A science-based approach. Circulation 95:1646–1650, 1997.

262. LaRosa JC, Pearson TA: Cholesterol screening guidelines: Consensus, evidence, and the departure from common sense. Circulation 95:1651–1653, 1997.

263. Garber AM, Browner WS: American College of Physicians guidelines for using serum cholesterol, high-density lipoprotein cholesterol, and triglyceride levels as screening tests for preventing coronary heart disease in adults. Ann Intern Med 124:515–517, 1996.

264. Expert Panel on Detection, Evaluation, and Treatment of High Blood Cholesterol in Adults: National Cholesterol Education Program: Second report of the Expert Panel on Detection, Evaluation, and Treatment of High Blood Cholesterol in Adults (Adult Treatment Panel II). Circulation 89:1329–1445, 1994.

# The Vascular Biology of Restenosis: An Overview

*Joseph B. Muhlestein*     *James P. Zidar*     *Michael A. Blazing*

Dr. Andreas Gruentzig reported the first successful percutaneous transluminal coronary angioplasty (PTCA) in 1977.[1] In the 20 years since his report, the application of percutaneous intravascular revascularization has evolved greatly. More than 300,000 percutaneous intravascular interventions are performed each year, and this procedure is now a standard part of therapy.[2] Current methods of mechanically altering or removing the obstructive atherosclerotic plaque within coronary arteries include standard balloon angioplasty, atherectomy, laser angioplasty, and intravascular stent implantation.[3]

Although advances in technology and technique have increased the number and the kinds of lesions that can be percutaneously approached, science has failed to solve the "Achilles heel" of all intravascular mechanical interventions—restenosis. Initial restenosis rates for angioplasty were estimated to be about 33%,[4] but large follow-up studies have documented restenosis rates as high as 43%[5]. With this large percentage of patients often requiring repeat angioplasty or coronary artery bypass surgery,[6] restenosis remains a significant problem. Some trials have shown that intravascular stenting and adjunctive treatment with a monoclonal antibody to a platelet integrin receptor reduce the rate of restenosis, but the residual rates of restenosis with these treatments remain significant.[7, 8] Consequently, much effort has been exerted to discover risk factors that predispose patients to restenosis as well as basic mechanisms driving that process.

Multiple large retrospective studies have been performed to evaluate possible technical and clinical features that may increase the risk of restenosis after intravascular intervention.[9–18] In general, the epidemiology of restenosis after PTCA is complex and multifactorial, and multivariate analysis has revealed some predisposing factors. To date, only three clinical factors have been found to be independent predictors of restenosis. These and other technical factors that have independent predictive value are shown in Table 6–1, This information has not proved to be highly sensitive or specific in prospectively predicting restenosis, nor does this information assist significantly in elucidating the underlying mechanisms involved with restenosis. Understanding these mechanisms is essential to the goal of developing strategies for the reduction and prevention of post-PTCA restenosis. Much effort has been expended in the search of the basic mechanisms at work within the diseased vessel during restenosis. The purpose of this chapter is to describe the information known to date concerning these potential mechanisms.

## OVERVIEW

Arteries have three basic layers: the intima, the media, and the adventitia. The intima is the innermost layer of the artery, which includes endothelial cells and the potential or real space between these cells and the internal elastic lamina. The second layer is the muscular media, which is composed primarily of smooth muscle cells (SMCs). This layer may not be as uniform as once suspected because evidence suggests that multiple phenotypes of SMCs exist within this layer.[19] The third layer is the adventitia, which is composed of fibroblasts and matrix proteins. This last layer is not just a passive capsule but instead appears to play an important role in the vessel's response to flow, injury, or disease by in-

**TABLE 6–1.     PREDICTORS OF RESTENOSIS**

| CLINICAL PREDICTORS | TECHNICAL PREDICTORS |
|---|---|
| Diabetes mellitus | Less than optimal initial result |
| Unstable angina | Low final transluminal pressure gradient |
| Male sex | Prolonged single inflation time |
| | High-grade preprocedural stenosis |
| | Absence of dissection |
| | Long lesions |
| | Total occlusions |

fluencing the process of geometric remodeling.[20, 21] It is likely that both the intima and the adventitia have important roles in restenosis, whereas the media does not.[21–23] The time course and the extent of the change in the shape and size of an artery therefore depend on the relative involvement of these two arterial layers and on other ongoing factors. These can be segregated into two major categories by whether they act mainly as mechanical or biologic factors.

## MECHANICAL FACTORS INVOLVED IN RESTENOSIS

Local mechanical factors associated with restenosis are summarized in Table 6–2. These include elastic recoil, pathologic late remodeling (healing)/contraction, residual plaque, and thrombus. These factors are discussed in more detail in the following sections.

### Elastic Recoil

The mechanisms of lesion dilation in balloon angioplasty are multiple, complex, variable, and still controversial. Initially, it was believed that the dilating pressure of the balloon caused vessel remodeling by compression of the atheroma.[24] Later, in vitro studies suggested that fluid expression from atherosclerotic tissue, especially that consisting mainly of soft plaque, could also play a role.[25] However, pathologic studies after PTCA have found that most plaques in human coronary arteries are composed of dense fibrous and occasionally calcified tissue that is typically incompressible, and the most consistent finding after angioplasty is disruption and splitting of the neointima, localized intimal dissection, and some degree of stretching of the media and adventitia.[3, 26] In addition, especially in cases in which the atherosclerotic plaque is eccentrically located within the vessel, passive stretching of the uninvolved portion of the vessel wall may also play a role.

Thus, elastic recoil of a stretched vessel is one mechanism that plays a role in the development of restenosis. To evaluate the degree to which elastic recoil occurs immediately after angioplasty, Rensing and associates[27] evaluated the minimal luminal cross-sectional areas of 151 successfully dilated lesions in 136 patients during balloon inflation and directly after withdrawal of the balloon. A videodensitometric analysis technique was used for the assessment of vascular cross-sectional areas. Elastic recoil was defined as the difference between balloon cross-sectional area of the largest balloon used at the highest pressure and minimal luminal cross-sectional area after PTCA. Mean balloon cross-sectional area was $5.2 \pm 1.6$ mm$^2$ during inflation, compared with $2.6 \pm 1.4$ mm$^2$ minimal luminal cross-sectional area immediately after inflation. Oversizing of the balloon (balloon artery ratio > 1) led to more recoil ($0.8 \pm 0.3$ versus $0.6 \pm 0.3$ mm, $p < 0.001$), suggesting an elastic phenomenon. Thus, nearly 50% of the theoretically achievable cross-sectional area (i.e., balloon cross-sectional area) is lost shortly after balloon deflation, and this is even greater if oversized balloons are used. A larger study was then performed on 607 lesions in 526 patients.[28] This larger study confirmed their initial results. In addition, univariate analysis revealed that asymmetric lesions (lesions located in less angulated parts of the artery and lesions with a low plaque content) showed more elastic recoil. The investigators believed that eccentric lesions showed significantly more elastic recoil because of preferential stretching of the nondiseased portion of the vessel with subsequently more elastic recoil. Lesions located in distal parts of the coronary tree were also associated with more elastic recoil, probably related to relative balloon oversizing in these distal lesions.

More angulated lesions and those with larger plaque mass showed less elastic recoil because intervention in these lesions released a constricting effect of plaque (cicatrization) that prevents normal compensatory vessel enlargement.[20] The postulated mechanism for the release is that angiographically visible dissection (which is more common in these types of lesions[29]), causes gross disruption of both the vessel wall and the associated plaque, which allows the media to return to its normal outer diameter. This outward recoil thus reduced the amount of inward recoil usually associated with vessel stretching.

To determine the effect of elastic recoil on post angioplasty luminal diameter over time, Hanet and colleagues[30] performed arteriography on 28 patients immediately after angioplasty and again 24 hours

## TABLE 6–2. LOCAL MECHANICAL FACTORS INVOLVED IN RESTENOSIS AFTER CORONARY BALLOON ANGIOPLASTY

| FACTOR | COMMENTS |
| --- | --- |
| Elastic recoil | Leads to immediate loss of nearly 50% of theoretically achieved cross-sectional area |
| Pathologic remodeling | May lead to chronic significant loss of luminal area |
| Residual plaque | Is found to be a major component of restenotic tissue in many cases |
| Thrombus | May contribute to both early and late restenosis |

later. Immediately after the procedure, the difference between inflated balloon diameter and minimal luminal diameter averaged 0.93 ± 0.43 mm for the entire group and was greater both in eccentric stenoses (1.13 ± 0.39 vs. 0.7 ± 0.36 mm; $p < 0.01$) and after angioplasty with an oversized balloon (1.20 ± 0.37 vs. 0.71 ± 0.33 mm; $p < 0.005$). At 24 hours, the balloon minus minimal luminal diameter difference was unchanged at the group level (0.86 ± 0.38 mm), but the absolute minimal luminal diameter increased significantly in the subgroup of coronary segments dilated with an oversized balloon (1.97 ± 0.37 vs. 1.81 ± 0.28 mm; $p < 0.05$). From these data, the investigators confirmed the importance of lesion eccentricity and balloon-artery ratios in the degree of immediate elastic recoil. Importantly, they also concluded that nearly universally, elastic recoil is an immediate phenomenon whose effects on atrial segment diameter are maximal at the end of the angioplasty procedure, and in some cases, arterial segment diameter may actually improve over the first 24 hours.

The extent of elastic recoil has important prognostic implications. Kuntz and coworkers[31] used a continuous regression model to analyze the results of pre-, post-, and 3- to 6-month quantitative coronary angiograms in 524 consecutive patients after they underwent PTCA, directional atherectomy, or stenting. This analysis found that restenosis was dependent only on the residual stenosis (result after recoil) immediately after the procedure. The extent of restenosis was not dependent on the device used, and all three devices were found to produce similar degrees of restenosis.[31]

In summary, elastic recoil has a significantly negative effect on the immediate results of PTCA, with a loss of nearly 50% of the theoretically achieved cross-sectional area. This is more pronounced when eccentric lesions are approached or when oversized balloons are used. There is no significant further effect of elastic recoil on restenosis over the next 24 hours, but the extent of residual stenosis that remains after elastic recoil is an important prognostic determinant of restenosis.

## Pathologic Late Remodeling: Healing/Contraction

It is postulated that part of the phenomenon of restenosis may well be viewed simply as an overshoot of the natural healing process after vascular injury. In this light, it is useful to evaluate data gained concerning the healing process in general. Studies in this regard have often noted the initial development of disorganized exuberant granulation connective tissue that, over time, organizes more fully into fibrocytic tissue, commonly referred to as scar tissue. During this process, the tissue is found to shrink and also contract down on itself, pulling the margins of normal tissue into more close approximation. This process is often referred to as healing contracture, or cicatrization.[32]

This process has a role in the adventitia and perhaps in the intima during the development of restenosis after interventional coronary procedures.[21] In the pig model, coronary angioplasty causes a rapid development of a hypercellular response in the adventitia.[21] This response is more marked than that seen in the media or the intima. Cell proliferation peaks at 14 days and comes back to baseline by 28 days. Coincident with the cell proliferation is phenotypic modulation of normal fibroblasts to myofibroblasts. In this modulated state, these cells produce abnormal and abundant amounts of type I and type III collagen, which is deposited in the adventitia. This collagen deposition leads to significant focal thickening of the adventitia. The authors of this study postulated that this thickened fibrotic adventitia adversely affects the usual ability of vessels to preserve lumen size by limiting compensatory enlargement.[20] The cicatrization effect may also produce a circumferential shortening of the adventitia, thus reducing the intraluminal diameter (increasing stenosis) by constriction. This last assumption is supported by a rabbit model of restenosis studied by Lafont and associates,[33] in which the degree of restenosis found after angioplasty (of a "diseased" arterial segment) correlated with an index of constriction. It is further supported by an intravascular ultrasound study in humans with clinical signs of restenosis.[34] In this study, total cross-sectional area (CSA), or area within the external elastic lamina, was measured in the affected portion of the vessel and in reference portions above and below the affected area. Persons who had undergone angioplasty but had no symptoms were also examined in a similar manner as a second set of controls. In patients with symptoms, the total CSA at the angioplasty site was significantly smaller than the CSA at the reference areas. This difference in CSA accounted for 83% of the loss in lumenal area, whereas only 17% was due to increases in vessel wall area (neointima). In the control patients who underwent angioplasty but had no symptoms, there was no significant difference between total CSA at the angioplasty and the reference sites. This loss of CSA resulting in luminal restenosis has been termed pathologic arterial remodeling.[35] In an individual patient, it is often difficult to ascertain angiographically whether intimal hyperplasia or pathologic arterial remodeling is the major factor causing restenosis. This often becomes more clear after the vessel is viewed with intravascular ultrasound. This may have significant impact on the effectiveness of certain forms of revascularization, especially atherectomy.

In summary, angioplasty results in an injury to the vessel wall that elicits a response to injury that is similar to wound healing. Fibroblasts are activated, replicate, and deposit collagen to heal the wound. A consequence of this healing process is a thickened adventitia. This change in the adventitia impairs the normal process, which is responsible for maintaining lumen size—compensatory enlargement. It may also lead to vessel contraction, which would be additive to any intimal hyperplastic process with regard to lumen narrowing.

STENTS AND REMODELING. In theory, one way to overcome elastic recoil would be to use a stent to support the initial gain associated with angioplasty. Results from the BENESTENT I trial, in which 520 patients were randomly assigned to either a stent or standard balloon angioplasty, support this assumption.[36] In this study, stenting was associated with a 40% better gain in diameter and a 21% improvement in absolute minimum lumen diameter. Although there was more loss in lumen diameter after stenting than after angioplasty, patients who received stents were more likely ($p < 0.003$) not to have restenosis (vessel stenosis > 50%). Of more importance, patients who received stents were less likely to need revascularization at 6 months and at 1 year.[37] This trial validated a belief that stenting would lead to greater initial gain, which in turn would lead to less restenosis and need for repeat revascularization. The 1-year follow-up also validates the assumption that the process of restenosis is largely complete by 6 months.

The finding that stenting may have stimulated a more vigorous restenotic response was not unexpected, given earlier findings regarding the stimulation of neointimal proliferation by stents in animal models.[38, 39] Hoffmann and colleagues[40] used intravascular ultrasound to investigate the patterns and mechanisms of stent restenosis in 142 stents. They found that late lumen loss in the stented segment was due primarily to neointimal tissue growth (follow-up plaque size minus postprocedure plaque size), whereas late lumen loss outside the stented area (on either end of the stent) was due to remodeling (loss in CSA of the external lamina). They concluded that stenting effectively prevented constrictive remodeling but was associated with significant neointimal proliferation, which was the major cause of late lumen loss. However, because greater initial gain can be obtained with a stent, the degree of lumen loss was not pathologic. They also commented that stenting had a negative effect on remodeling in that it prevented the process of compensatory enlargement.

In summary, stenting improves initial gain in lumen diameter by at least partially overcoming immediate elastic recoil. This improved immediate gain has been associated with a decreased need for future angioplasty procedures. Stenting also limits pathologic remodeling (chronic recoil), which is a consequence of arterial injury and a significant contributory factor to late lumen loss in angioplasty. Stenting is not without problems, however, because this procedure appears to more vigorously stimulate neointimal hyperplasia and prevents the beneficial remodeling process of compensatory enlargement.

## Residual Plaque

Particularly in relation to balloon coronary angioplasty, the continued presence of residual atherosclerotic plaque whose bulk is not changed by the procedure may contribute to the development of restenosis. Haudenschild[41] has reported the presence, in tissue removed from restenosis sites, of large amounts of old plaque components, indicating that loose parts of the old vessel wall can contribute substantially to the restenosis by displacement. Excessive catheter trauma favors this reocclusion process by creating large dissections; however, insufficient dilatation does not leave enough space for the necessary fibrocellular healing. An obvious approach to eliminating this problem has been the development of various atherectomy devices that actually excise and remove the bulk of the atherosclerotic plaque either in mass, such as with directional coronary atherectomy,[42] or piecemeal, as with transluminal extraction catheter atherectomy.[43] Unfortunately, although these approaches have shown promise in producing better immediate results in select circumstances, they have shown little effect on the overall restenosis rate.[44] Ablation of residual plaque mass has also been attempted through the use of laser energy, but again with little effect on restenosis.[45, 46]

In summary, the presence of residual atherosclerotic plaque or an interventional coronary procedure can contribute to the development of restenosis. However, attempts to address this problem have not resulted in a significant reduction in the ultimate restenosis rate.

## Thrombus

Thrombus formation is an inevitable consequence of the current methods of percutaneous intervention. All of these procedures disrupt normal vessel architecture, exposing the inner layers of the vessel wall, including the media and the adventitia, to blood products. Components of these layers, especially type II collagen[47] and tissue factor,[48] are highly thrombogenic. Atherectomy, PTCA, and laser procedures create clefts or dissections in the plaque mass; these are initially covered by platelets, then filled in by thrombus.[49] Stent placement adds the additional thrombogenic component of a foreign object (the stent) to this already hypercoagulable environment. Given the fact that some thrombus is inevitable, the important question (which is not yet resolved) is how does the extent and duration of its presence influence restenosis?

A porcine coronary angioplasty and stent model provides important insight into a potential three-stage hypothesis that examines the effect of thrombus on restenosis.[50] In the first stage of this model, PTCA or stent placement is associated with an immediate response of "thrombus" formation, which is composed of aggregated platelets at sites of deep injury covered by a combination of fibrin and trapped erythrocytes. In the next stage, which is over the next 3 to 4 days, the thrombus is covered by endothelium and invaded by white cells. These mononuclear leukocytes invade the thrombus in a lumenal to adventitial direction and are often surrounded by clear zones, which may represent clot lysis and resorption. Both the leukocytes and the degenerating thrombus release potent stimuli for the last phase of this model, which is SMC recruitment and proliferation. During SMC proliferation, the remaining thrombus initially provides a matrix for migration, then is resorbed and replaced by neointima.

The relative importance of thrombus in this model can be ascertained by measuring the effect on restenosis of interventions that effect thrombus formation. Direct and indirect thrombin inhibitors, such as hirudin and heparin, have proved not to be efficacious in human trials.[51, 52] Molecular size limitations (heparin) and dose and bleeding complications (hirudin) have been advanced as reasons why these treatments were ineffective. Animal studies suggest that blockade of the coagulation pathway further upstream to prevent the generation of thrombin will have better safety profile and will be more efficacious.[53, 54] Specific targets include factor VIIa inhibitors and tissue factor inhibitors.[54] The most promising agent is the monoclonal antibody abciximab, which binds to and blocks the key protein receptor (integrin $\alpha_2\beta_3$, also called GPIIbIIIa) responsible for activation and attachment of platelets.[55] Two separate studies in humans have shown that use of this antibody during angioplasty reduces the need for future revascularization and hence is clinically preventing restenosis.[56–58] Besides decreasing platelet adherence, mechanisms invoked for the effect of this antibody include the dose-dependent inhibition of thrombin generation by tissue factor, thrombin incorporation into clot, and cross-reactiv-

ity with the $\alpha_5\beta_3$ integrin, which is important for SMC migration as well as thrombin generation.[59]

In summary, thrombus formation, occurring as a result of the trauma sustained to the vessel during coronary angioplasty, contributes to the development of restenosis. Mechanisms for this contribution include stimulating leukocyte migration and providing growth factors, matrix, and support for SMC migration. Inhibition of thrombus formation with c7E3 monoclonal antibodies, which affect both the platelet and the fibrin components of a clot, has been shown to clinically reduce restenosis. Further human studies using intravascular ultrasound and pathologic specimens are needed to provide histologic confirmation of these clinical findings. Future targets to prevent thrombus formation are currently focused on inhibiting the formation of early factors in the clotting cascade.

## PATHOGENESIS OF RESTENOSIS

The process of restenosis appears to be fundamentally different from that of primary atherosclerosis. Whereas primary atherosclerotic plaque consists of varying amounts of cholesterol clefts, calcification, and a modest cellular component (Fig. 6–1A), restenotic plaque generally shows dense intimal hyperplasia with marked cellular and fibrous components, but without cholesterol clefts or calcification (Fig. 6–1B).

Vessel injury sets in motion an orderly progression of events, which can be divided into three general stages: (1) acute injury, (2) early healing, and (3) late healing. These stages occur after all interventional procedures in all cases; however, the magnitude of the response can be different in each case. In this context, restenosis can be defined as the overexuberant healing response of an artery to injury. Given the variability of this response between patients and even within different vessels of the same patient, it is unlikely that any one factor or simple combination of factors completely controls this process.

Various cell types, growth factors, circulating proteins, and cytokines have important roles in controlling the process of restenosis. Important cell types include SMCs, mononuclear and polynuclear white cells, platelets, and fibroblasts. Important growth factors include platelet-derived growth factor (PDGF), fibroblast growth factor (FGF), and transforming growth factor (TGF). Significant circulating proteins include thrombin and angiotensin II. Key cytokines include interferon $\gamma$ and the interleukins. Determining the significance of the role of each of these elements is further complicated by the fact that the importance of each element varies from

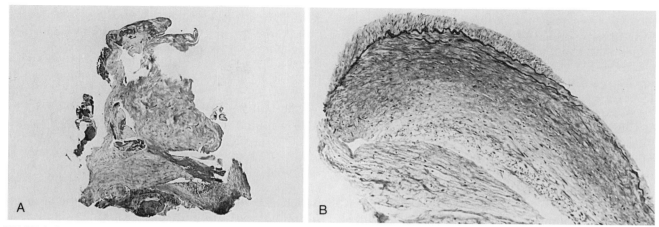

FIGURE 6–1. *(A)* Primary atherosclerotic plaque atherectomy specimen containing cholesterol clefts, calcification, and modest cellularity. *(B)* Coronary restenotic lesion atherectomy specimen. The internal elastic lamina *(dark wavy line)* separates a thin rim of media *(above)* from a thick dense layer of intimal hyperplasia with marked cellular and fibrous components.

species to species. Therefore, findings from the current animal models of restenosis have limitations with regard to their relevance to human restenosis. The failure of heparin,[52] angiotensin-converting enzyme inhibitors[60] and fluvastatin[61] to impair restenosis in human trials highlight these limitations. The remainder of this chapter focuses on describing the animal models and human pathologic correlates of restenosis. Special emphasis is placed on the potential significance of each key element as it pertains to restenosis.

## Animal Models

The rat carotid artery model has been the most extensively studied animal model of restenosis. This model has yielded important information about molecular and pharmacologic mechanisms purportedly involved in neointimal formation.[22, 62–64] However, these findings need to be interpreted with some caution, given the context of the injury in this model. First, injury in this model takes place in a normal artery, where, unlike in human coronaries (especially atherosclerotic ones), the intima is a potential space that is essentially free of cells.[65] Second, injury results in lamellar platelet formation with little fibrin deposition and little or no leukocyte infiltration.[66, 67] Thus, the potential impact of these elements (thrombus and leukocytes) on the restenotic process is not addressed by this model. What this simple model addresses well (and possibly overemphasizes) is the role of SMCs in the restenotic process.

The SMC response to injury in this model can be broken down into four partially overlapping stages: (1) injury-elicited proliferation of SMCs, (2) SMC migration into the intima, (3) intimal proliferation of SMCs, and (4) extracellular matrix synthesis and deposition.[68] Injury resulting in removal of the en-

dothelium and disrupting the internal elastic lamina causes the death of 15% to 25% of medial SMCs.[69] Cell death is essential because it results in the release of basic FGF (bFGF) from dying SMCs; bFGF has been shown to be a key stimulant for the first wave of medial SMC proliferation.[70] This wave of proliferation begins at 6 to 24 hours and peaks at 48 hours after injury. Thymidine labeling to detect DNA synthesis indicates that 20% to 40% of medial SMCs enter S phase after balloon dilatation. If gentle injury is sustained that removes only the endothelium, then this first wave of SMC response is largely abolished.[71] SMC migration into the intima is the second stage. This stage begins at 4 days after injury, but the duration of this phase is unknown. In the rat, PDGF plays an important role in this stage as infusion of this growth factor enhances migration and antibodies against it reduce the size of the intimal lesion.[72]

The third stage, intimal proliferation of SMCs, peaks at 4 to 7 days and continues up to 12 weeks after injury. This proliferation occurs primarily at the luminal surface of the neointima and may involve a special type of SMC.[73, 74] These SMCs overexpress numerous growth factors and other growth control receptors, like the angiotensin II receptor.[64, 75] The fourth stage is one of extracellular matrix synthesis and deposition, which is responsible for a further modest increase in intimal thickness from 2 weeks to 3 months after injury. After 3 months, the intimal thickness remains fairly constant.

As alluded to earlier, the response of the rat carotid to balloon injury may be significantly modified by several manipulations. Thrombocytopenia or PDGF depletion induced by specific monoclonal antibodies does not alter the initial proliferative event but does reduce SMC migration and matrix formation.[76] Platelet-derived products thus appear to mediate the later stages of the vascular response but not the initial proliferative response in the rat. Endothelial removal by nylon loop abrasion in contrast to balloon dilatation results in denudation with substantial platelet accumulation but without medial barotrauma injury. In this case, the initial proliferative response is diminished, endothelium regenerates within 4 days, and there is no migration of SMCs and hence no intimal thickening.[77] Hydrostatic stretching of the carotid causes vessel distention and only minimal patchy endothelial loss. Endothelial regeneration occurs over the course of 3 days before the onset of SMC migration. The initial proliferative response in this injury model, which is at least partially mediated by stretch, is not much different from that seen with balloon dilatation. However, the regeneration of endothelium before SMC migration substantially reduces both SMC migration and neointimal formation.[78] Additional evidence. that re-endothelialization is important in this system comes from investigations of heparin infusion. Heparin administered at 50 U/kg/hour or 100 U/kg/hour led to complete re-endothelialization and significantly less myointimal thickening in rat carotids subjected to balloon injury or air drying compared with controls.[79] Use of an angiotensin-converting enzyme inhibitor, cilazapril (10 mg/kg/day), to block the proliferation of SMCs in stage three has also been shown to decrease the amount and the extent of neointimal proliferation.[80] In addition, angiotensin-converting enzyme inhibitors were shown to reduce smooth muscle cell content and matrix formation, as well as to preserve luminal patency compared with placebo in this study.[80]

In summary, in the rat model, medial arterial vascular injury results in an initial proliferative event that centers around SMCs in the media. The absence of endothelium and the presence of platelets mediate migration and degree of intimal thickening. Intimal thickening is further effected by the proliferation of SMCs in the intima. Finally, in the intima, these SMCs produce significant matrix, which further contributes to intimal thickening.

In contrast to the rat model, the porcine model of restenosis has been divided into three stages: (1) thrombotic, (2) cellular recruitment, and (3) proliferative.[49, 81] The pathology associated with the thrombotic and early cellular recruitment stages of the pig model differs substantially from that of the rat model, whereas the proliferative stage is similar to the last two (proliferative and matrix) stages of the rat model. These differences are undoubtedly important because the histopathology of the neointima that develops in the pig is nearly identical to that which develops after angioplasty in a human artery.[49]

Significant differences in the pathology of these two models (pig vs. rat) include early SMC activation (none versus substantial), platelet deposition (aggregates versus lamellar), fibrin deposition (marked versus minimal), leukocyte infiltration (present vs. absent), rate and extent of re-endothelialization (fast and complete vs. slower and often incomplete), and timing and route of SMC migration/proliferation (day 7, intimal to medial, vs. day 4 to 7, medial to intimal).[22, 49, 81] The fibrin- and platelet-rich thrombus of this model may affect the restenosis process in multiple ways. It may serve as a reservoir for growth factors and chemoattractants, which may originate from trapped platelets or serum.[82] It traps thrombin, which stimulates leukocyte migration and leukocyte proliferation[83] and acts as a mitogen for SMCs.[84] The thrombus also appears to serve as a biodegradable scaffold that directs SMC migration from the lumen toward the media.[81] The potential importance of thrombus has been further enhanced by the effects of recombinant hirudin in the pig angioplasty model. In these studies, hirudin treatment significantly decreased platelet and fibrinogen deposition and prevented mural thrombus formation as well as decreased restenosis.[85, 86]

Despite the nearly identical histopathology of pig and human neointima, these lesions must differ because the findings with hirudin have not been reproducible in humans.[51] One key difference is that the restenotic lesion in humans arises from injury to a previously diseased vessel, whereas the process of restenosis that has been studied in most pig models arises from injury to healthy or minimally diseased vessel. A double-injury model has been developed to try to circumvent this problem. In this model, normal vessel is injured, and then the animal is fed cholesterol before the second experimental injury is caused.[87] Wilensky and cowokers[88] used a double-injury model in rabbit femoral arteries to characterize the repair response of an abnormal vessel to angioplasty injury. They found that angioplasty in this setting resulted in significant dissection into the intima and media rather than simple crush of the intima and media. As in the normal pig model, thrombus filled the dissection planes, cellular infiltration of the thrombus repaired the dissection, and peak SMC and macrophage proliferation occurred at 3 to 5 days. They also noted that angioplasty resulted in adventitial injury with concomitant adventitial cellular proliferation (primarily fibroblasts) and matrix deposition. Lumen loss early after the procedure was due to a combination of immediate recoil and or thrombus filling the dissection planes. Only a minority (<33%) of late lumen loss was accounted for by increases in intimal area or neointimal formation.

Atherectomy and autopsy studies have yielded some important information regarding human neointima.[89] An autopsy study of six patients who died between 2 days and 4 months after single-vessel angioplasty has given support to the pig model of restenosis. This study found the presence of fibrin-platelet thrombus at 2 days after PTCA, influx of leukocytes (macrophages) at 5 days, and dedifferentiation of SMCs at the border of the PTCA site by 12 days. A significant difference between the pig model and this autopsy study was that endothelium was not identified on the luminal surface except in patients who had undergone angioplasty more than 4 months previously. Multiple atherectomy studies of restenotic lesions have shown that cellular replication in restenotic lesions, as measured by staining for proliferating cell nuclear antigen (a cellular marker for entry into the cell cycle), occurs infrequently and at low levels.[90,91] Of 100 consecutive restenotic leions, 74 had no evidence of proliferation, and most of the rest had only sparse evidence of proliferation.[91] In this study, there was no proliferative peak, and positive staining specimens were found over the period of 1 to 390 days. This finding is in marked contrast to the rat models, in which 15% to 30% of cells can be found to be proliferating cell nuclear antigen positive at early times.[62–64] One possible explanation for the low levels of proliferating cell nuclear antigen staining in human samples is that the proliferation of human SMCs is rapidly modulated by the process of apoptosis (programmed cell death).[92]

One final and interesting postulation for human susceptibility to restenosis is that prior infection with cytomegalovirus (CMV) virus leaves arteries susceptible to the process of proliferation. CMV, like other herpes viruses, can persist indefinitely in some host cells. CMV DNA has been found in smooth muscle cells from restenotic lesions.[93] Furthermore, the CMV immediate early gene products are known to interfere with the tumor suppresser gene *p53*; therefore, local reactivation of CMV by trauma could impair the usual block that *p53* imposes on the cell cycle and/or its ability to induce apoptosis, which in turn would lead to clonal proliferation and accumulation of SMCs.[93] In support of this hypothesis is a small prospective study of 75 consecutive patients who underwent directional atherectomy. These patients had CMV titers checked before the procedure, then underwent atherectomy, then were recatheterized 6 months later. The initial mean minimal lumen diameter of the target vessel was greater in the CMV seropositive group; however, at 6 months, this group had a much greater reduction in luminal diameter, resulting in a significantly higher rate of restenosis (43% vs. 8%).[94] Logistic regression analysis found CMV seropositivity and CMV titer to be predictive of restenosis. The authors did not comment on a possible effect of an increase in initial minimal lumen diameter on the rate and the extent of restenosis.

## Cells Involved in Restenosis

At one time, the pathogenesis of restenosis was believed to be primarily a result of the proliferation and migration of medial SMCs. This reasoning grew out of investigations that examined the process of restenosis in the rat model. Investigations in other animal models and in human atherectomy specimens have implicated important roles for other cell types, including endothelial cells, platelets, leukocytes, and fibroblasts.

### Smooth Muscle Cells

SMCs have multiple potential roles in the process of restenosis. This cell type is the most common type found in neointima.[92] They produce growth factors that support the process of restenosis.[67] They also serve as the primary source of neointimal matrix proteins, which form the bulk of the volume of the mature neointima.[95]

Evidence suggests that the media of normal arteries is populated by multiple phenotypes of SMCs.[63] Whether these phenotypes represent a spectrum of dedifferentiation (from contractile to synthetic) or distinct lineages is controversial.[63, 70, 96] In the uninjured vessel wall, contractile phenotype cells predominate, but cells that lack the characteristic proteins of the contractile phenotype can be identified.[97] In the intima, both contractile and synthetic types of SMCs are common, depending on the age of the lesion.[67, 78] Vessel injury increases the proportion of synthetic type cells, either by initiating dedifferentiation or by providing a favorable growth environment for the synthetic lineage.[98] These synthetic cells fail to express SMC-specific actins and express other unique genes, such as growth factors, which may play important roles in determining the proliferative extent of the neointima.[67] In human arteries, this dedifferentiation is seen as early as 2 days after angioplasty.[97]

Injury also induces other important responses in medial SMCs. These responses occur in a series of overlapping phases. The first phase is medial SMC proliferation.[69] In rat and rabbit models, early proliferation (1 to 3 days) occurs in 20% to 40% of medial SMCs.[88] Atherectomy data suggest that this initial stage of proliferation may be much less prominent in humans.[91] The second phase is SMC migration. The exact origin of SMCs that have migrated into the intima is still controversial, but the porcine model suggests that most SMCs migrate from the adjacent uninjured media rather than from the media directly beneath the injury.[51] Analysis of human vessels at autopsy appears to confirm this site as the likely origin of intimal SMCs.[97] The third phase of SMC response is intimal proliferation and matrix formation. In all animal models, proliferation of intimal SMCs is most pronounced near the luminal surface.[73, 88] However, the time course of this proliferation varies dramatically between species. For example, in the rat, significant levels of proliferation can be seen at 12 weeks, whereas in the rabbit, less than 1% of intimal SMCs were seen to be actively dividing at 4 weeks.[73, 88] Matrix formation increases in all species between 14 and 28 days after the initial injury.[88, 97, 99] Increased formation of matrix in the neointima has been attributed to a both a decrease in matrix protein degradation and a change in the primary type of matrix proteins expressed.[88, 100–102]

### Endothelial Cells

Evidence that the endothelium effects the process of restenosis stems from observations in the rat model, where intimal hyperplasia is limited when the endothelium is minimally disrupted or if re-endothelialization occurs quickly.[77, 78] To what extent this limited hyperplasia is a function of minimized SMC damage, accelerated reconstitution of the barrier function of endothelium, or accelerated reconstitution of the SMC growth inhibitory function of the endothelium in this model is unknown. Furthermore, re-endothelialization is not the only determinant of the degree of final intimal thickening, because intimal thickening appears to cease after 3 months, even in the absence of endothelium.[99]

Two important growth inhibitory molecules, nitric oxide (NO) and heparin sulfate, are lost when the endothelium is disrupted. Heparin sulfate, which is secreted by endothelial cells into the intimal space, inhibits SMC proliferation by blocking the transition of cells from the $G_1$ to the S phase.[62] This compound has proved to be an effective antiproliferative agent in various animal models.[99] Paradoxically, in humans, it has not.[49] Evidence suggests that this may be because human SMCs are preferentially activated by factors (e.g., PDGF) that bypass the growth-inhibitory effects of heparin.[103]

NO is a very small very reactive molecule produced by endothelial cells from the amino acid arginine. It has been shown to inhibit SMC proliferation, platelet adhesion, and leukocyte margination.[104] In a rabbit model of restenosis, large doses of arginine given after endothelial denudation have resulted in a significant reduction in neointimal thickening.[105] In the rat carotid model, vessel injury has been shown to trigger nitric oxide production from SMCs through the induction of a protein that generates NO. This protein is the inducible form of NO synthase (iNOS).[106] Inhibition of NO production from this protein was associated with a threefold

increase in platelet deposition on the artery surface and a 24% reduction in flow across the artery bed. The authors speculated that the expression of iNOS in SMCs represented a protective mechanism that may compensate for endothelial loss.

### Platelets

Platelet adhesion, secretion, and aggregation are key initial steps in the process of restenosis. Resting platelets circulate freely in the blood until they are exposed to specific substrates, such as collagen, von Willebrand factor, fibronectin, and other subendothelial substrates. Exposure results in adhesion, which activates the platelet. Activation results in secretion of vasoactive, mitogenic, and thrombogenic substances, which are the true initiators of the restenotic process. These substances, along with fibrinogen, contribute to the activation of additional surrounding platelets and clotting proteins. The end result is the formation at the site of injury of a mixed thrombus, which contains multiple growth factors, chemokines, and other mitogenic substances that may affect restenosis.

Severe thrombocytopenia inhibits the formation of neointimal lesions in rabbit and rat models of restenosis.[107] Agents that effect platelet secretion, such as aspirin and dipyridamole, have been ineffective inhibitors of neointimal proliferation in humans.[108] At least one agent that affects platelet aggregation, abciximab, has been shown to effectively inhibit restenosis.[8] This agent is the chimeric monoclonal antibody fragment abciximab, which binds to and blocks the function of the GPIIb/IIIa protein complex, which is the major platelet aggregation receptor.[54] It also cross-reacts with a minor adhesion receptor $\alpha_v\beta_3$, the vitronectin receptor, on the platelet.[54] The vitronectin receptor is also found on SMCs and monocytes, where it is believed to be important for adhesion and migration of these cells.[109] Because other agents that selectively block the GPIIb/IIIa receptor have not been found to significantly inhibit restenosis,[8] it is unclear whether the inhibitory growth action of abciximab is due to inhibition of platelet aggregation, inhibition of SMC (or white blood cell) migration, or some combination of both functions.

### Leukocytes

Our understanding of the role of leukocytes in restenosis remains rudimentary. Some studies have indicated that coronary angioplasty triggers both neutrophil and monocyte adhesion and activation.[110, 111] Neutrophil activation has been inversely associated with late lumen loss.[112] The speculated mechanisms for this association are that neutrophil adherence may decrease platelet adherence through release of platelet-inhibitory molecules and that release of proteases by neutrophils may alter late vascular remodeling and thus prevent contraction.[113]

The monocytes that have been best characterized are macrophages. Macrophages have been known to play an important role in atherosclerosis for years.[114] These mononuclear immune cells express tissue factor and release cytokines, metalloproteinases, and growth factors, all of which can affect the processes of restenosis. In the atherosclerotic rabbit model of restenosis, a significant percentage of the early replicating cells in the neointima are monocytes.[88] One human study has found the content of macrophages in primary plaque material to be a predictor for restenosis after directional atherectomy.[115] This study examined specimens from 50 patients who had unstable angina, no previous intervention at the suspected culprit site, at least 1.5 mm$^2$ of specimen area for pathologic examination, and relook angiography within 12 months of the directional atherectomy procedure. At relook angiography, 30 of these 50 patients had restenosis (>50% stenosis diameter). Retrospective analysis of the plaque material from the restenosis ($n = 30$) and no restenosis ($n = 20$) groups revealed that the cohort that developed restenosis had a twofold greater content of macrophages in their plaques before directional atherectomy. The percentage of SMC area in the two groups was equivalent at about 55%. Logistic regression analysis of the data identified macrophages as an independent predictor for restenosis.[115] This linkage of monocytes to restenosis is further supported by the rabbit carotid model, in which inhibition of monocytes reduced intimal SMC accumulation by 70%.[116]

### Fibroblasts

Adventitial fibroblasts have been implicated as important contributors to restenosis.[21] Vessel injury induces replication of adventitial fibroblasts and phenotypic modulation to a myofibroblastic cell type. These changes have been postulated to be key events in the vascular remodeling processes that lead to late lumen loss.[32, 33] These modulated cells express abundant amounts of collagen, which leaves the "repaired" adventia fibrotic. This fibrosis can impair the normal response of compensatory enlargement.[20] And it may contribute further to late lumen loss by contracting and thus constricting the vessel.[21, 33]

In summary, the typical restenotic lesion differs from the usual atherosclerotic plaque both in architecture and in lipid content, although both contain SMCs and fibrous tissue.[117, 118] Arterial injury stimulates the migration and the growth of SMCs in all patients, but the extent of neointimal proliferation varies dramatically between individuals. Mechanical stretch and/or vessel fracturing directly damages cells and the normal matrix, resulting in growth factor release.[119] Injury causes platelet adhesion, secretion, and aggregation. These platelets release PDGF, epidermal growth factor, serotonin, and thromboxane, all stimulants of SMC chemotaxis and migration. Injury causes inflammatory macrophages and other leukocytes to accumulate along the injured vessel wall. These cells secrete macrophage-derived growth factor, interleukin-1, and cyclo-oxygenase. Finally, injury activates and phenotypically transforms fibroblasts, which contribute to the process of restenosis by affecting vessel remodeling.

## Growth Factors

Growth factors play an important regulatory role in the process of restenosis. These factors affect the migration, proliferation, and phenotypic modulation of the cells that populate the neointima and the regenerating adventitia. Which factors are most important in human restenosis has been difficult to establish because of the interspecies variability of the types and the proportions of cells in the neointima. The search for and the study of important growth factors in human restenosis is still ongoing. The factors that have the most potential importance include PDGF, TGF, interferon γ, and FGF. These are discussed separately in greater detail.

### Platelet-Derived Growth Factor

PDGF affects both SMC migration and proliferation.[120] It was first described by Ross and Glomset[121] while they were studying wound healing and atherogenesis. The association between platelet adhesion to the damaged arterial wall and the marked increase in SMC and fibroblast proliferation led investigators to postulate that platelets were the source of this growth-promoting activity. At that time, it was also known that serum from clotted blood contained elements required for the successful growth of fibroblasts in culture. Because cell-free, plasma-derived serum lacked growth-promoting activity, this suggested that some cell-derived factor was elaborated on clotting. Furthermore, because this activity could be restored only by platelets, the name *platelet-derived growth factor* was coined.[122]

There are two PDGF genes; *PDGF-A* and *PDGF-B*.[123, 124] These genes code for protein chains that bear 60% homology to each other, are highly cationic, and contain eight highly conserved cysteine residues. The cysteine residues are critical for biologic activity.[125] They are involved in intrachain and interchain disulfide bond formation, which is necessary for the production of the active form of PDGF, which is a dimer. The affinity of the PDGF-A and PDGF-B chains for one another results in the potential formation of three different covalent dimers: PDGF-AA, a covalently linked homodimer of two A chains; PDGF-BB, a covalently linked homodimer of two B chains; and PDGF-AB, a covalently linked heterodimer of one A and one B chain.[126] All three isoforms of PDGF are present in equal amounts in human platelets, whereas the PDGF-BB isoform predominates in rat, pig, and baboon platelets.[127]

PDGF exhibits biologic activity through binding and bringing together of specific transmembrane receptor polypeptides—the PDGF receptors (PDGFRs). There are two receptor polypeptides, called PDGFR-$\alpha$ and PDGFR-$\beta$.[128] The receptor polypeptides are inactive until they are brought together into a dimer by the binding action of PDGF. These polypeptides can form one of three noncovalently associated complexes: $\alpha/\alpha$, $\beta/\beta$, or $\alpha/\beta$. The $\alpha$ receptor can bind PDGF A or B chains, whereas the $\beta$ receptor can bind only PDGF-B chains. These receptors are present on the cell surfaces of all vascular wall cells.[129] Cell response is therefore determined by receptor type as follows: cells with $\alpha/\alpha$ receptors can respond to any PDGF signal, cells with $\alpha/\beta$ receptors can respond to PDGF-AB or PDGF-BB signals, and cells with $\beta/\beta$ receptors can respond only to a PDGF-BB signal.[130] Dimerization of these polypeptides results in autophosphorylation of the receptor at specific tyrosine residues. This autophosphorylation sets off a series of kinase reactions, which then lead to gene activation.[131]

Biologic activities reported for PDGF include induction of early biochemical events required for the growth and proliferation of various cell types. In particular, PDGF induces the turnover of phosphatidyl inositol, increases intracellular calcium levels, induces the expression of c-*myc* and c-*fos* messenger RNA in quiescent fibroblasts in culture,[132] modulates prostaglandin synthesis,[133] up-regulates the expression of low-density lipoprotein receptors,[134] stimulates vasoconstriction,[135] increases endocytosis, and induces chemotaxis in smooth muscle cells, macrophages, and neutrophils.[136] Evidence suggests that chemotaxis is associated with activation of the $\beta\beta$-receptor.[72, 137]

PDGF ligand and receptor expression changes in response to injury.[138] These changes occur at specific times and locations in the injured and healing vessel and appear to vary from species to species.[139] In the rat, injury led to two phases of PDGF ligand and receptor gene expression.[138] In the first 48 hours, there was a rapid increase in PDGF-A transcript and a large decrease in PDGF-$\beta$ receptor messenger RNA levels. At two weeks, PDGF-$\beta$ receptor levels rebounded to three to five times control levels, whereas PDGFR-$\alpha$ receptor levels fell to three times

below control. Luminal SMCs produced PDGF-A ligand and PDGFR-$\beta$ transcripts but little or no PDGF-B or PDGFR-$\alpha$ transcript. Medial SMC ligand and receptor expression returned to control levels.[138] These data suggest that autocrine PDGF loops do not drive intimal proliferation in the rat, because the A ligand cannot activate the $\beta\beta$ receptor. In the rabbit, injury resulted in progressive increases in PDGF-B transcript and protein, which peaked at day 7.[139] Transcripts of PDGFR-$\beta$ were also found to increase. Cell proliferation in neointimal SMCs coincided with the peak in PDGF-B levels. In this system, PDGF-B expression and PDGFR-$\beta$ immunoreactivity colocalized, which implied that an autocrine loop possibly was driving cellular proliferation.

The lack of an autocrine loop in the rat model is perplexing because both PDGF-B and PDGFR-$\beta\beta$ have been shown to be important for migration and hence intimal proliferation. Infusion of PDGF-BB increases neointimal cellularity,[72] antibodies against its PDGF-BB reduce neointimal size,[140] and antisense oligonucleotides, which prevent the expression of the $\beta\beta$ receptor, reduce neointimal size.[137] Paracrine loops appear to be more important in this model because the time course and expression of PDGF-BB ligands from regenerating endothelial cells have been shown to mirror the increased expression of $\beta\beta$ receptor in intimal SMCs.[141] The role of PDGF-A in this model is unclear but may involve differentiation or proliferation.

The time course and expression levels of PDGF ligand and receptor are not known in human neointimas. In human atheroma, PDGF-B expression has been localized to macrophage.[142] Ross[126] postulated in his rat carotid model that macrophages may actually be the most important early source of PDGF. Regardless of its source, PDGF stimulates specific target cells by binding to cell surface receptors and initiating a cascade of events that lead to DNA synthesis and cellular proliferation. However, PDGF may be a ubiquitous growth factor that promotes atherosclerotic plaque expansion by a second group of progressive factors that initiate DNA synthesis and cell division.[143] Stiles and colleagues[143] described PDGF as "competence factor" that allows cells to move from a quiescent state to active cell cycling.

A more complete understanding of this factor may lead to the development of therapeutic agents for retarding restenosis. Triazolopyrimidine, a PDGF antagonist, has been demonstrated in an in vitro rabbit model to inhibit SMC proliferation. Experimentally induced atherosclerotic iliac artery lesions in New Zealand white rabbits were treated with triazolopyrimidine at 60 mg/kg/day from 2 days before until 4 weeks after percutaneous transluminal angioplasty. When compared with a control group, triazolopyrimidine significantly increased the luminal area and reduced the intimal thickness in the atherosclerotic rabbit iliac artery after balloon angioplasty.[144] This finding has been confirmed in humans in the Studio Tropidil versus Aspirin nella Restenosis Coronarica (STARC) study, in which this agent reduced restenosis rates from 40% to 24%.[145] A 17.9% absolute reduction (41% relative reduction) in recurrent angina was associated with active treatment. Whether the GPIIb/IIIa-inhibiting agents affect PDGF secretion as a part of their mechanism of restenosis inhibition is unknown.

### Transforming Growth Factor

TGF belongs to a growing family of polypeptide factors that share certain structural and function characteristics.[146] Types $\alpha$ and $\beta$ have been described and so named for their ability to transform fibroblasts, despite their remote structural relationship. These two factors may have synergistic, antagonistic, or completely dissociated actions in various cell systems.

TGF-$\beta$ was discovered as a product of murine sarcoma virus–transformed cells and named for its ability to stimulate anchorage-independent growth of normal fibroblasts.[147] This 112-amino-acid peptide is found abundantly at cell surfaces and in the extracellular matrix in an inactive propeptide form. Proteolytic cleavage activates the growth factor.[148] Like PDGF, TGF-$\beta$ has three forms in humans and are composed of combinations of the $\beta_1$ and $\beta_2$ subunits. TGF-$\beta_1$ is the most active form of this growth factor in vascular repair. Its sequences are highly conserved and exhibit a 99% sequence homology between human and mouse.[149] Infusions of this growth factor or transfection of the TGF-$\beta_1$ complementary DNA into injured arteries accelerates intimal formation.[150] Antibodies to TGF-$\beta_1$ retard this process.[151]

The active TGF-$\beta_1$ peptide interacts with a group of three receptors, called the type I, II, or III TGF-$\beta$ receptors.[148] Effects elicited by ligand-receptor interactions include mediation of fibrosis, angiogenesis, stimulation of plasminogen activator inhibitor levels, stimulation of SMC proliferation, excessive SMC matrix production, and paradoxically, growth inhibition of SMCs.[148] The combination of intracellular signals generated by the relative stimulation of these three receptors appears to determine the affect that this growth factor has on a cell.[148] For example, human SMCs from normal arteries express all three types of TGF-$\beta$ receptor, but human SMCs grown from vascular lesions are deficient in type II receptors. Normal SMCs are growth inhibited by TGF-$\beta_1$, but cells grown from human vascular lesions are

growth stimulated and are induced to produce vast amounts of collagen by this growth factor.[148] Reconstitution of normal levels of TGF-$\beta$ type II receptor levels in lesion cells makes TGF-$\beta_1$ growth inhibitory for this cell type. This lack of type II receptors does not affect all of the potential effects of TGF-$\beta_1$, because TGF-$\beta_1$ induces plasminogen activator inhibitor production in both cell types.[148]

An additional function of TGF-$\beta$ appears to be as a potent chemotactic factor for fibroblasts and monocytes.[152] It also has been shown to inhibit T and B cell proliferation without affecting interleukin-2 or interleukin-2 receptor expression.[153] TGF-$\beta_1$ mediates some of these effects at levels in the femtomolar range, making it one of the most potent immunomodulators.

## Interferon-$\gamma$

As reviewed earlier, several studies using cell-specific monoclonal antibodies have shown that monocyte-derived macrophages and T lymphocytes are present in significant numbers in the atherosclerotic and restenotic plaque.[149] Jonasson and colleagues[54] described T lymphocytes constituting 20% of the cell population in the fibrous cap of the human atherosclerotic plaque. Immunocytochemical data suggest that T cells can modulate the growth properties and other functions of SMCs. Many smooth muscle cells within atherosclerotic plaque express class II major histocompatibility complex antigens, although they lack these antigens in nonatherosclerotic arteries.[155] Although these Ia antigens play a basic role in the presentation of foreign antigens to T cells, their expression by macrophages and endothelial cells is induced by interferon-$\gamma$.[156]

The interferons were originally identified and characterized according to their ability to induce the production of RNA and protein in target cells. Interferon-$\alpha$ (leukocyte derived) and interferon-$\beta$ (fibroblast derived) are produced during viral or bacterial infections. Immune or interferon-$\gamma$ is produced primarily by T lymphocytes on mitogen or antigen stimulation. Human interferon-$\gamma$ is a 166-amino-acid polypeptide, whereas murine interferon $\gamma$ is a 136-amino-acid polypeptide that exhibits a 40% homology with the human form. This low degree of homology is believed to contribute to the apparent lack of species cross-reactivity.

Interferon-$\gamma$ is a lymphokine secreted by activated T cells that inhibits cellular proliferation in cultured rat aortic smooth muscle cells and induces Ia antigen expression. Hansson and coworkers[157] described an in vivo rat model in which they denuded carotid arteries via balloon injury and replicating cells were radiolabeled by $^3$H-thymidine that was continuously infused via intraperitoneal osmotic pumps over 2 weeks. They noted that Ia-positive, [3]H-thymidine–positive cells had undergone fewer rounds of replication than Ia-negative ones, which suggests that Ia antigen might be selectively expressed by nonproliferating SMCs. In addition, they noted recombinant interferon-γ inhibited SMC proliferation in a dose-dependent fashion. These results suggest that interferon-γ acts as a natural regulator of SMC growth and Ia expression in injury-induced intimal thickening of atherosclerotic plaque in a rat carotid injury model.

Wilson and colleagues[158] have completed a study to evaluate the antiatherogenic effectiveness of the administration of purified rabbit interferon in a cholesterol-fed rabbit model. New Zealand White rabbits were fed a 1% cholesterol diet, and a subgroup of animals received intramuscular injections of 1 million units of interferon twice a week. Both the interferon-treated and the control groups had average serum cholesterol levels above 2000 mg/dL during the 8-week study. Although no significant change in serum lipids occurred between the two groups, interferon treatment did result in a significant reduction (25% to 8%) in lesion size, as measured by aortic cross-section. These data suggest that the mechanism of atherosclerosis suppression in these cholesterol-fed rabbits is not related to the lowering of serum cholesterol levels, but it may be associated with inhibition of lesion initiation. However, the rabbit interferon was purified from RK13 rabbit kidney cultures stimulated with parainfluenza virus–1. The possibility exists that this preparation contained other biologic response modifiers, which could account for the observed effects, and thus may be unrelated to interferon. A subsequent study in rats supports the inhibitory effect of interferon-γ on lesion initiation.[159]

## Fibroblast Growth Factor

Acidic and basic fibroblast growth factors (aFGF and bFGF) are members of a family of heparin-binding growth factors. Although initially described as factors capable of inducing fibroblast proliferation in neural tissue, these angiogenic peptides are potent mitogens for endothelial cells and SMCs.[160] Both aFGF and bFGF exert their mitogenic influence via saturable high-affinity receptors on various cells. Published in vivo data for aFGF are scarce. However, in a canine model, Banai and associates[161] demonstrated that aFGF can cause vascular SMC hyperplasia in areas subjected to ischemic injury. In this study, aFGF was delivered to the myocardium via an epicardial sponge in dogs whose coronary flow was compromised.

bFGF is an 118,00-D peptide that shares 55% sequence homology with aFGF and remains highly conserved among species. This growth factor has been localized to the nuclei of both endothelial and SMCs.[70] It is also present complexed to heparin in basement membranes and extracellular matrices in vivo.[162] Injury during angioplasty leads to the release of this potent SMC and endothelial cell mitogen from these stores.[163]

bFGF binds to specific cell receptors that, like PDGF receptors, are tyrosine kinase receptors.[164–166] Binding of bFGF to this specific receptor requires that bFGF be complexed to heparin sulfate.[167] Evidence suggests that heparin use during angioplasty may lead to the displacement of bFGF from luminal surfaces. This displaced bFGF has been shown to be preferentially sequestered by injured vessels, where it may potentiate proliferation.[166]

Lindner and Reidy[168] demonstrated that bFGF is angiogenic in vivo. Their model involved rat carotid arteries that underwent balloon catheter denudation, with subsequent cessation of re-endothelialization. This cessation could be overcome by the systemic administration of bFGF.[167] The systemic administration of bFGF also has been shown to stimulate SMC proliferation.[71] Administration of a neutralizing bFGF antibody decreased injury-induced (first-wave) SMC proliferation by 80% in the rat carotid injury model when it was given before angioplasty.[70] This 80% reduction in proliferation with antibodies did not affect the development or extent of neointimal formation. In contrast, treatment of injured rat artery segments with an adenovirus carrying an antisense bFGF transcript has led to a significant reduction in neointimal formation.[168] The authors suggested that this inhibition was effective because of prolonged inhibition of bFGF synthesis.

Casscells and colleagues[169] explored a unique approach for antiproliferative therapy that utilized FGF receptor expression. They found increased expression of FGF in proliferating SMCs in vivo and in vitro. The ribosome inhibitor saporin, when conjugated to bFGF, killed proliferating, FGF receptor–expressing SMCs, but not quiescent receptor–negative SMCs. These investigators demonstrated via radioligand binding and immunocytochemistry that no high-affinity FGF receptors were present in normal adult rat tissues, except brain. However, FGF receptors were detected 1 to 7 days after aortic crush injury. A single dose of the bFGF-saporin construct delivered 1 to 2 days after injury inhibited DNA synthesis and intimal thickening but had no effect on uninjured vessels or evident toxicity. These data suggest that expression of FGF receptors in vascular injury may provide a selective approach for the ablation of proliferating smooth muscle cells. Further investigation is needed.

## CONCLUSION

Despite the continually improving acute results associated with percutaneous interventional revascularization procedures, restenosis of the coronary artery at the procedure site remains a significant problem. The vascular biology associated with restenosis is complicated and still not well understood. Early and late elastic recoil, pathologic remodeling/healing contraction, and residual plaque and thrombus formation all appear to play a mechanical role in the development of restenosis. Cells that appear to play an important role in the vascular biology of restenosis include SMC, endothelial cells, platelets, leukocytes, and fibroblasts. When stimulated, each has the capacity to elaborate any number of protein factors that may play important roles in the initiation and perpetuation of the hyperplastic or remodeling responses that result in restenosis. As a greater understanding of the basic mechanisms behind restenosis is gained, strategies to prevent, inhibit, or limit the process are being developed and tested.

## REFERENCES

1. Gruentzig AR, Myler RK, Hanna EH, et al: Coronary transluminal angioplasty [Abstract]. Circulation 55–56(suppl III):III-84, 1977.
2. ACC/AHA Task Force Report. Guidelines for percutaneous transluminal coronary angioplasty. J Am Coll Cardiol 22(7):2033–2054, 1993.
3. Waller BF: "Crackers, breakers, stretcher, drillers, scrapers, shavers, burners, welders, and melters"—the future treatment of atherosclerotic coronary disease? A clinical-morphologic assessment. J Am Coll Cardiol 13:969, 1989.
4. Gruentzig AR, King SB, Schlumpf M, et al: Long-term follow-up after percutaneous transluminal coronary angioplasty. N Engl J Med 316:1127, 1987.
5. Tcheng JE, Fortin DF, Frid DJ, et al: Conditional probabilities of restenosis following coronary angioplasty [Abstract]. Circulation 82(suppl III):III-1, 1990.
6. Hlatky MA, Lipscomb J, Nelson C, et al: Resource use and cost of initial coronary revascularization: Coronary angioplasty vs coronary bypass surgery. Circulation 82(suppl 5):IV-208, 1990.
7. Serruys PW, Jaegere P, Kiemenji F, et al: A comparison of balloon-expandable stent implantation with balloon angioplasty in patients with coronary artery disease. N Engl J Med 331:489–495, 1994.
8. Tcheng JE: Glycoprotein IIb/IIIa receptor inhibitors: Putting the EPIC, IMPACT II, RESTORE, and EPILOG Trials into perspective. Am J Cardiol 78(suppl 3A):35–40, 1996.
9. Roubin GS, King SB 3d, Douglas JS Jr: Restenosis after percutaneous transluminal coronary angioplasty: The Emory University Hospital experience. Am J Cardiol 60(3):39B–43B, 1987.
10. Douglas JS Jr, King SB 3d, Roubin GS: Influence of the methodology of percutaneous transluminal coronary angioplasty on restenosis. Am J Cardiol 60(3):29B–33B, 1987.
11. Arora RR, Konrad K, Badhwar K, et al: Restenosis after transluminal coronary angioplasty: A risk factor analysis. Cathet Cardiovasc Diagn 19(1):17–22, 1990.
12. Rupprecht HJ, Brennecke R, Bernhard G et al: Analysis of risk factors for restenosis after PTCA. Cathet Cardiovasc Diagn 19(3):151–159, 1990.
13. Fleck E, Regitz V, Lehnert A, et al: Restenosis after balloon dilatation of coronary stenosis, multivariate analysis of potential risk factors. Eur Heart J 9(suppl C):15–18, 1988.
14. Meier B: Restenosis after coronary angioplasty: Review of the literature. Eur Heart J 9(suppl C):1–6, 1988.
15. Blackshear JL, O'Callaghan WG, Califf RM: Medical approaches to prevention of restenosis after coronary angioplasty. J Am Coll Cardiol 9(4):834–848, 1987.
16. Ellis SG, Shaw RE, Gershony G, et al: Risk factors, time course and treatment effect for restenosis after successful percutaneous transluminal coronary angioplasty of chronic total occlusion. Am J Cardiol 63(13):897–901, 1989.
17. Pepine CJ, Hirshfeld JW, Macdonald RG, et al: A controlled trial of corticosteroids to prevent restenosis after coronary angioplasty. Circulation 81(6):1753–1761, 1990.
18. Ellis SG, Shaw RE, Gershony G, et al: Risk factors, time course and treatment effect for restenosis after successful percutaneous transluminal coronary angioplasty of chronic total occlusion. Am J Cardiol 63(13):897–901, 1989.
19. Scwartz SM, Majesky MW, Murry CE: The intima: Development and monoclonal responses to injury. Atherosclerosis 118(suppl):S125–S140, 1995.
20. Glagov S, Weisenberg E, Zarnes CK, et al: Compensatory enlargement of human atherosclerotic coronary arteries. N Engl Med 316:1371–1375, 1987.
21. Shi Y, Pieniek M, Fard A, et al: Adventitial remodeling after coronary arterial injury. Circulation 93:340–348, 1996.
22. Schwartz SM, Reidy MA, O'Brien ER: Assessment of factors important in atherosclerotic occlusion and restenosis. Thromb Haemost 74:541–551, 1995.
23. Forester JS, Fishbien M, Helfant R et al: A paradigm for restenosis based on cell biology clues for the development of new preventive therapies. J Am Cardiol 17:758–769, 1991.
24. Dotter CT, Judkins MP: Transluminal treatment of atherosclerotic obstructions: Description of new technique and a preliminary report of its application. Circulation 30:654–670, 1964.
25. Kaltenbach M, Beyer J, Walter S, et al: Prolonged application of pressure in transluminal coronary angioplasty. Cathet Cardiovasc Diagn 10:213–219, 1984.
26. Block PC, Myler RK, Stertzer S, et al: Morphology after transluminal angioplasty in human beings. N Engl J Med 305:382–385, 1981.
27. Rensing BJ, Hermans WR, Beatt KJ, et al: Quantitative angiographic assessment of elastic recoil after percutaneous transluminal coronary angioplasty. Am J Cardiol 66(15):1039–1044, 1990.
28. Rensing BJ, Hermans WR, Strauss BH, et al: Regional differences in elastic recoil after percutaneous transluminal coronary angioplasty: A quantitative angiographic study. J Am Coll Cardiol 17(6 suppl B):34B–38B, 1991.
29. Ellis SG, Roubin GS, King SB III, et al: Angiographic and clinical predictors of acute closure after native vessel coronary angioplasty. Circulation 77:372–379, 1988.
30. Hanet C, Wijns W, Michel X, et al: Influence of balloon size and stenosis morphology on immediate and delayed elastic recoil after percutaneous transluminal coronary angioplasty. J Am Coll Cardiol 18(2):506–511, 1991.
31. Kuntz RE, Gibson M, Nobuyoshi M, et al: Generalized model of restenosis after conventional balloon angioplasty, stenting and directional atherectomy. J Am Coll Cardiol 21:15, 1993.
32. Montessano R, Orci L: Transforming growth factor beta stimulates collagen-matrix contraction by fibroblasts: Implications for wound healing. Proc Nat Acad Sci USA 85(13):4894–4897, 1988.
33. Lafont A, Gusman LA, Whitlow PL, et al: Restenosis after experimental angioplasty: Intimal, medial and adventitial changes associated with constrictive remodeling. Circ Res 76:996–1002, 1995.
34. Luo H, Nishioka T, Eigler NL, et al: Coronary artery restenosis after balloon angioplasty in humans is associated with circumferential coronary constriction. Arterioscler Thromb Vasc Biol 16:1393–1398, 1996.
35. Mintz GS, Kent KM, Pichard AD, et al: Intravascular ultrasound insights into mechanism of stenosis formation and restenosis. Cardiol Clin 15(1):17–29, 1997.
36. Serruys PW, Jaegere P, Kiemenji F, et al: A comparison of

balloon expandable stent implantation with balloon angioplasty in patients with coronary artery disease. N Engl J Med 331:489–495, 1994.

37. Macaya C, Serruys PW, Ruygrok P, et al, for the Benestent Study Group: Continued benefit of coronary stenting vs balloon angioplasty: One-year clinical follow-up of Benestent Trial. J Am Coll Cardiol 27:255–261, 1996.

38. Edelman ER, Rogers C: Hoop dreams, stents without restenosis. Circulation 94:1199–1202, 1996.

39. Grinstead WC, Rodgers GP, Mazur W, et al: Comparison of three porcine restenosis models: The relative importance of hypercholesterolemia, endothelial abrasion, and stenting. Coron Artery Dis 5:425–434, 1994.

40. Hoffman R, Mintz GS, Dussaillant GR, et al: Patterns and mechanisms of in-stent restenosis, a serial intravascular ultrasound study. Circulation 94:1247–1254, 1996.

41. Haudenschild CC: Pathogenesis of restenosis: A correlation of clinical observations with cellular responses. Kardiol 79(suppl 3):17–22, 1990.

42. Hinohara T, Robertson GC, Selmon MR, et al: Directional coronary atherectomy. J Intervent Cardiol 2(5):217–226, 1990.

43. Sketch MH Jr, Phillips HP, Lee M, et al: Coronary transluminal extraction-endarterectomy. J Invasive Cardiol 3:13–18, 1991.

44. Safian RD, Gelbfish JS, Erny RE, et al: Coronary atherectomy: Clinical, angiographic, and histological finding and observations regarding potential mechanisms. Circulation 82:69–79, 1990.

45. Buchwald AB, Werner GS, Unterberg C, et al: Restenosis after excimer laser angioplasty of coronary stenoses and chronic total occlusions. Am Heart J 123:878, 1992.

46. Werner G, Buchwald A, Unterberg C, et al: Excimer laser angioplasty in coronary artery disease. Eur Heart J 12:24, 1991.

47. Badimon L, Turitto VT, Rosemark JA, et al: Characterization of tubular flow chamber for studying platelet interaction with biologic and prosthetic materials: Deposition of indium-111-labeled platelets oncology subendothelium and expanded polytetrafluoroethylene. J Lab Clin Med 110:706, 1987.

48. Speidel CM, Eisenberg PR, Ruf W, et al: Tissue factor mediates prolonged procoagulant activity on the luminal surface of balloon injured aortas in rabbits. Circulation 92:3323–3330, 1995.

49. Wilensky RL, Pizlo IG, Sandusky G, et al: Vascular repair mechanisms after directional atherectomy of percutaneous transluminal coronary angioplasty in atherosclerotic rabbit iliac arteries. Am Heart J 132:13–22, 1996.

50. Scwartz, RS, Edwards WD, Antoniades LC, et al: Coronary restenosis: Prospects for solution and new perspectives from a porcine model. Mayo Clin Proc 68:54–62, 1993.

51. Ellis SG, Reubin GS, Willentz J, et al: Effect of 18- to 24-hour heparin administration for prevention of restenosis after uncomplicated coronary angioplasty. Am Heart J 117:777, 1989.

52. van den Bos AA, Deckers J, Heyndricks G, et al: Safety and efficacy of recombinant hirudin vs heparin in patient with stable angina undergoing coronary angioplasty. Circulation 88:2058, 1993.

53. Harker LA, Hanson SR, Wilcox JN, et al: Antithrombotic and antilesion benefits without hemorrhagic risks by inhibiting tissue factor pathway. Haemostasis 26(suppl 1):76–82, 1996.

54. Jang Y, Guzman LA, Lincoff M, et al: Influence of blockade at specific levels of the coagulation cascade on restenosis in a rabbit atherosclerotic femoral artery injury model. Circulation 92:3041–3050, 1995.

55. Coller, Scudder LE, Beer J, et al: Monoclonal antibodies to platelet glycoprotein IIb/IIIa as antithrombotic agents. Ann NY Acad Sci 614:193–213, 1991.

56. Topol EJ, Califf RM, Weisman HF, et al: On behalf of the EPIC investigators. Lancet 343:881–886, 1994.

57. van de Werf F: More evidence for beneficial effect of platelet glycoprotein IIb/IIIa-blockage during coronary intervention: Latest results from the EPILOG and CAPTURE trials [Hotline Editorial]. Eur Heart J 325–326, 1996.

58. Tcheng JE: Glycoprotein IIb/IIIa receptor inhibitors: Putting the EPIC, IMPACT II, RESTORE, and EPILOG Trials into perspective. Am J Cardiol 78(suppl 3A):35–40, 1996.

59. Reverter JC, Beguin S, Kessels H, et al: Inhibition of platelet-mediated tissue factor-induced thrombin generation by the mouse/human chimeric 7E3 antibody. J Clin Invest 98:868–874, 1996.

60. MERCATORS Study Group: Does the new angiotensin-converting enzyme inhibitor cilazapril prevent restenosis after percutaneous transluminal coronary angioplasty? Circulation 86:100, 1992.

61. FLARE Trial. Presented at the American College of Cardiology, 1997.

62. Majesky MW, Schwartz SM, Clowes MM, et al: Heparin regulates smooth muscle S phase entry in the injured rat carotid artery. Circ Res 61:296–300, 1987.

63. Schwartz SM, Majesky MW, Murry CE: The intima: Development and monoclonal responses to injury. Atherosclerosis 118(suppl):S125–S140, 1995.

64. Daemen MJAP, Lombardi DM, Bosman FT et al: Angiotensin II induces smooth muscle cell proliferation in the normal and injured rat arterial wall. Circ Res 68:450–456, 1991.

65. Vesselinovitch D: Animal models and the study of atherosclerosis. Arch Pathol Lab Med 112:1011, 1988.

66. Clowes AW, Reidy MA: Prevention of stenosis after vascular reconstruction: Pharmacologic control of intimal hyperplasia—A review. J Vas Surg 13:885, 1991.

67. Schwartz SM, deBlois D, O'Brien RM: The intima: Soil for atherosclerosis and restenosis. Circ Res 77:445–465, 1995.

68. Clowes AW, Clowes MM, Fingerle J, et al: Regulation of smooth muscle growth in injured artery. J Cardiovasc Pharmacol 14(suppl):S12, 1989.

69. Clowes AW, Clowes MM, Reidy MA: Kinetics of cellular proliferation after arterial injury. I: Smooth muscle growth in the absence of endothelium. Lab Invest 49:327, 1983.

70. Lindner V, Reidy MA: Proliferation of smooth muscle cells after vascular injury is inhibited by an antibody against basic fibroblast growth factor. Proc Natl Acad Sci USA 88:3739–3743, 1991.

71. Fingerle J, Au YP, Clowes AW, et al: Intimal lesion formation in rat carotid arteries after endothelial denudation in absence of medial injury. Arteriosclerosis 10:1082, 1990.

72. Fingerle J, Johnson R, Clowes AW, et al: Role of platelets in smooth muscle cell proliferation and migration after vascular injury in rat carotid artery. Proc Natl Acad Sci USA 86:8412–8416, 1989.

73. Clowes AW, Clowes MM, Reidy MA: Kinetics of cellular proliferation after arterial injury. III: Endothelial and smooth muscle growth in chronically denuded vessels. Lab Invest 54:295, 1986.

74. Schwartz SM, Foy L, Bowen-Pope DF, et al: Derivation and properties of platelet-derived growth factor-independent rat smooth muscle cells. Am J Pathol 136:1417, 1990.

75. Prescott MF, Webb RL, Reidy MA: Angiotensin-converting enzyme inhibitor vs angiotensin II, $AT_1$ receptor antagonist: Effects on smooth muscle cell migration and proliferation after balloon catheter injury. Am J Pathol 139:1291–1296, 1991.

76. Fingerle J, Johnson R, Couser W, et al: Effects of thrombocytopenia on smooth muscle proliferation and intima formation in injured rat carotid. FASEB J 2:1077, 1988.

77. Tada T, Reidy MA: Endothelial regeneration. IX: Arterial injury followed by rapid endothelial repair induces smooth-muscle-cell proliferation but not intimal thickening. Am J Pathol 129:429, 1987.

78. Clowes AW, Clowes MM, Reidy MA: Role of acute distention in the induction of smooth muscle proliferation after arterial denudation. Fed Proc 46:720, 1987.

79. Clowes AW: Suppression by heparin of smooth muscle cell proliferation in injured arteries. Nature 265:625, 1977.

80. Powell JS, Clozel JP, Muller RK, et al: Inhibitors of angiotensin-converting enzyme prevent myointimal proliferation after vascular injury. Science 245:186, 1989.

81. Schwartz RS, Holmes DR, Topol EJ. The restenosis para-

digm revisited: An alternative proposal for cellular mechanisms. J Am Coll Cardiol 20:1284–1293, 1992.

82. Ip JH, Fouster V, Israel D, et al: The role of platelet thrombin and hyperplasia in restenosis after coronary angioplasty. J Am Coll Cardiol 17(suppl B):77B, 1991.

83. Bar-Shavit R, Benezra M, Eldor A, et al: Thrombin immobilized to extra cellular matrix is potent mitogen for vascular SMC: Nonenzymatic model of action. Cell Reg 1:453, 1990.

84. McNamara Ca, Sarembock IJ, Bachhuber BG, et al: Thrombin and vascular smooth muscle cell proliferation: Implications for atherosclerosis and restenosis. Semin Thromb Hemost 22(2):139–144, 1996.

85. Heras M, Chesebro JH, Penny WJ, et al: Effects of thrombin inhibition on the development of acute platelet-thrombus deposition during angioplasty in pigs. Heparin vs. recombinant hirudin, a specific thrombin inhibitor. Circulation 79:657, 1989.

86. Heras M, Chesebro JH, Webster MW, et al: Hirudin, heparin and placebo during deep arterial injury in the pig: The in vivo role of thrombin in platelet-mediated thrombus. Circulation 82:1476, 1990.

87. Faxon DP, Weber VJ, Handenschild C, et al: Acute effects of transluminal angioplasty in three experimental models of atherosclerosis. Arteriosclerosis 2:125, 1982.

88. Wilensky RL, March KL, Gradus-Pizlo I, et al: Vascular injury, repair, and restenosis after percutaneous transluminal angioplasty in the atherosclerotic rabbit. Circulation 92:2995–3005, 1995.

89. Ueda M, Becker AE, Naruko T, et al: Smooth muscle cell dedifferentiation is a fundamental change preceding wound healing after percutaneous transluminal coronary angioplasty in humans. Coron Artery Dis 6:71–81, 1995.

90. Taylor AJ, Farb AA, Angello DA, et al: Proliferative activity in coronary atherectomy tissue: Clinical histopathologic and immunohistochemical correlates. Chest 108:815–820, 1995.

91. O'Brien ER, Alpers CE, Stewart DL, et al: Proliferation in primary and restenotic coronary atherectomy tissue: Implications for antiproliferative therapy. Circ Res 73:223–231, 1993.

92. Isner JM, Kearney M, Bortman S, et al: Apoptosis in human atherosclerosis and restenosis. Circulation 9191:2703–2711, 1995.

93. Speir E, Modali R, Haung ES, et al: Potential role of human cytomegalovirus and p53 interaction in coronary restenosis. Science 265:391–394, 1994.

94. Zhou YF, Leon MB, Waclawiw MA, et al: Association between prior cytomegalovirus infection and the risk of restenosis after coronary atherectomy. N Engl J Med 335:624–630, 1996.

95. Meyers P: Vascular wound healing and restenosis following revascularization. *In* Weber (ed): Wound Healing Responses in Cardiovascular Disease, p. 137, Mt Kisco, NY: Futura Publishing, 1995.

96. Ueda M, Becker AE, Naruko T, et al: Smooth muscle cell de differentiation is a fundamental change preceding wound healing after percutaneous transluminal coronary angioplasty in humans. Coron Artery Dis 6:71–81, 1995.

97. Frid MG, Moiseeva EP, Stenmark KR: Multiple phenotypically distinct smooth muscle cell populations exist in the adult and developing pulmonary arterial media in vivo. Circ Res 75:669, 1994.

98. Chen YH, Chen YL, Lin SJ, et al: Electron microscopic studies of phenotypic modulation of smooth muscle cells in coronary arteries of patients with unstable angina pectoris and postangioplasty restenosis. Circulation 95:1169–1175, 1997.

99. Hamon M, Bauters C, McFadden EP, et al: Restenosis after coronary angioplasty. Eur Heart J 16(suppl I): 33–48, 1995.

100. Guarda E, Katwa LC, Campbell SE et al: Extracellular matrix collagen synthesis and degradation following coronary balloon angioplasty. J Mol Cell Cardiol 28:699–706, 1996.

101. Tyagi SC, Meyers L, Schmaltz RA, et al: Proteinases and restenosis in the human coronary artery. Extracellular matrix production exceeds the expression of proteolytic activity. Atherosclerosis 116:43–57, 1997.

102. Coats WD, Whittaker P, Cheung DT, et al: Collagen content is significantly lower in restenotic vs nonrestenotic vessel after balloon angioplasty in the atherosclerotic rabbit model. Circulation 95:1293–1300, 1997.

103. Geary RL, Koyama N, Wang TW, et al: Failure of heparin to inhibit intimal hyperplasia in injured baboon arteries: The role of heparin-sensitive and insensitive pathways in the stimulation of smooth muscle cell migration and proliferation. Circulation 91:2972–2981, 1995.

104. Ignarro L, Murad F (eds): Nitric oxide: Biochemistry, molecular biology, land therapeutic implications. Adv Pharmacol 34:1–516, 1995.

105. McNamara DB, Dedi B, Bauters C, et al: L-Arginine inhibits balloon catheter-induced intimal hyperplasia. Biochem Biophys Res Commun 193:291, 1993.

106. Yan ZQ, Yokota T, Zhang W, et al: Expression of inducible nitric oxide synthase inhibits platelet adhesion and restores blood flow in the injured artery. Circ Res 79:38, 1996.

107. Clowes AW, Clowes MM, Fingerle J, et al: Restenosis of smooth muscle cell growth in injured artery. J Cardiovasc Pharmacol 14(suppl 6): S12, 1989.

108. Chan P, Patel M, Betteridge L, et al: Abnormal growth regulation of vascular smooth muscle cells by heparin in patients with restenosis. Lancet 341:341, 1993.

109. Brown SL, Lundgren CH, Nordt T, et al: Stimulation of migration of human aortic smooth muscle cells by vitronectin: Implications for atherosclerosis. Cardiovasc Res 28:1815, 1994.

110. Serrano C, Ramires SAF, Venturinelli M, et al: Coronary angioplasty results in leukocyte and platelet activation with adhesion molecule expression. J Am Coll Cardiol 29:1276–1283, 1997.

111. Neuman FJ, Ott I, Gawaz M, et al: Neutrophil and platelet activation at balloon-injured coronary artery plaque in patients undergoing angioplasty. J Am Coll Cardiol 27819–27824, 1996.

112. Pieterma A, Kofflard M, De Wit LEA, et al: Late lumen loss after coronary angioplasty is associated with the activation status of circulating phagocytes before treatment. Circulation 91:1320–1325, 1995.

113. Sluiter W, de Vree WJ, Pietersma A, et al: Prevention of late lumen loss after coronary angioplasty by photodynamic therapy: Role of activated neutrophils. Mol Cell Biochem 157:233–238, 1996.

114. Stary HC, Chandler AB, Dinsmore RE, et al: A definition of advanced types of atherosclerotic lesions and a histological classification of atherosclerosis. A report from the Committee on Vascular Lesions of the Council on Arteriosclerosis, American Heart Association. Circulation 92:1355–1374, 1995.

115. Moreno PR, Bernardi VH, Lopez-Cuellar J, et al: Macrophage infiltration predicts restenosis after coronary intervention in patients with unstable angina. Circulation 94:3098–3102, 1996.

116. Kling D, Fingerle J, Harlan JM, et al: Mononuclear leukocytes invade rabbit arterial intima thickening formation via CD 18- and VLA-4-dependent mechanisms and stimulate smooth muscle migration. Circ Res 77:1121–1228, 1995.

117. Essed CE, Van der Brand M, Becker AE: Transluminal coronary angioplasty and early restenosis: Fibrocellular occlusion after wall laceration. Br Heart J 49:393–396, 1983.

118. Austin GE, Ratliff NB, Hooman J, et al: Intimal proliferation of smooth muscle cells as an explanation for recurrent coronary artery restenosis after percutaneous transluminal angioplasty. J Am Coll Cardiol 6(2):369–375, 1985.

119. Berk BC, Alexander RW, Brock TA, et al: Vasoconstriction: A new activity for platelet-derived growth factor. Science 232:87–90, 1986.

120. Fingerle J, Johnson R, Clowes AW, et al: Role of platelets in smooth muscle cell proliferation and migration after vascular injury in rat carotid artery. Proc Natl Acad Sci USA 86:8412–8416, 1989.

121. Ross R, Glomset JA: Atherosclerosis and the arterial smooth muscle cell. Science 180:1332–1339, 1973.

122. Ross R, Glomset J, Karaya B, et al: A platelet-dependent serum factor that stimulates the proliferation of arterial

smooth muscle cells in vitro. Proc Natl Acad Sci USA 71:1207–1210, 1974.

123. Betsholtz C, Johnsson A, Heldin CH, et al: cDNA sequence and chromosomal localization of human platelet-derived growth factor A-chain and its expression in tumor cell lines. Nature 320:695–699, 1986.

124. Collins T, Ginsburg D, Boss JM, et al: Cultured human endothelial cells express platelet-derived growth factor B chain: cDNA cloning and structural analysis. Nature 316:748–750, 1985.

125. Robbins KC, Antoniades HN, Devare SG, et al: Structural and immunological similarities between simian sarcoma virus gene products and human platelet-derived growth factor. Nature 305:605–608, 1983.

126. Ross R: Platelet-derived growth factor. Lancet 1(8648):1179–1182, 1989.

127. Hart CE, Clowes AW: Platelet-derived growth factor and arterial response to injury. Circulation 95:555–556, 1997.

128. Glenn K, Bowen-Pope DF, Ross R: Platelet-derived growth factor. J Biol Chem 257:5172–5176, 1982.

129. Boynton AL, Leffert HL (eds): Control of Animal Cell Proliferation. New York: Academic Press, 1985, pp 281–316.

130. Hart CE, Forstrom JW, Kelly JD, et al: Two classes of PDGF receptor recognize different isoforms of PDGF. Science 240:1529–1531, 1988.

131. Claesson-Welch L: Mechanism of action platelet-derived growth factor. Int J Biochem Cell Biol 28(4):373–385, 1996.

132. Kelly K, Cochran BH, Stiles CD, et al: Cell-specific regulation of c-*myc* gene by lymphocyte mitogens and platelet-derived growth factor. Cell 35:603–610, 1983.

133. Habenicht AJ, Georig M, Grulich J, et al: Human platelet-derived growth factor stimulates prostaglandin synthesis by activation and by rapid de novo synthesis of cyclooxygenase. J Clin Invest 75:1381–1387, 1985.

134. Habenicht AJ, Dresel HA, Goerig M, et al: Low-density lipoprotein receptor-dependent prostaglandin synthesis in Swiss 3T3 cells stimulated by platelet-derived growth factor. Proc Natl Acad Sci USA 83:1344–1348, 1986.

135. Berk BC, Alexander RW, Brock TA, et al: Vasoconstriction: A new activity for platelet-derived growth factor. Science 232:87–90, 1986.

136. Seppa H, Grotendorst G, Seppa S, et al: Platelet-derived growth factor is chemotactic for fibroblasts. J Cell Biol 92:584–588, 1982.

137. Sirois MG, Simons M, Edelman ER: Antisense oligonucleotide inhibition of PDGR-β receptor subunit expression directs suppression of intimal thickening. Circulation 95:669–676, 1997.

138. Majesky MW, Reidy MA, Bowen-Pope DF, et al: PDGF ligand and receptor gene expression during repair of arterial injury. J Cell Biol 111:2149–2158, 1990.

139. Uchida K, Sasahara M, Morigami N, et al: Expression of platelet-derived growth factor β-chain in neointimal smooth muscle cells of balloon injured rabbit femoral arteries. Atherosclerosis 124:9–23, 1996.

140. Ferns GA, Raines EW, Sprugel KH, et al: Inhibition of neointimal smooth muscle accumulation after angioplasty by an antibody to PDGF. Science 253(5024):1129–1132, 1991.

141. Lindner V, Reidy MA: Platelet-derived growth factor ligand and receptor expression by large vessel endothelium in vivo. Am J Pathol 1946:1488–1497, 1995.

142. Ross R, Masuda J, Raines EW, et al: Localization of PDGF-β protein in macrophages in all phases of atherogenesis. Science 248:1009, 1990.

143. Stiles CD, Pledger WJ, Tucker RW, et al: Regulation of the Balb/C-3T3 cell cycle effects of growth factors. J Supramol Struct 13:489–499, 1980.

144. Liu MW, Roubin GS, Robinson KA, et al: Trapidil in preventing restenosis after balloon angioplasty in the atherosclerotic rabbit. Circulation 81:1089–1093, 1990.

145. Maresta A, Balducelli M, Cantini L, et al, for the STARC Investigators. Trapidil (triazolopyrimidine), a platelet-derived growth factor antagonist, reduces restenosis after percutaneous transluminal coronary angioplasty: Results of the randomized double-blind STARC Study. Circulation 90:2710–2715, 1994.

146. Massague J: The TGF-β family of growth and differentiation factors. Cell 49:437–438, 1987.

147. De Larco JE, Todoro GJ: Growth factors from murine sarcoma virus-transformed cells. Proc Natl Acad Sci 75(8):4001–4005, 1978.

148. McCaffrey TA, Consigli S, Baoheng D, et al: Decreased type II/type I TGF-β receptor ratio in cells derived from human atherosclerosis lesion. J Clin Invest 96:2667–2675, 1995.

149. Gown AM, Tsukada T, Ross R: Human atherosclerosis II: Immunocytochemical analysis of the cellular composition of human atherosclerotic lesions. Am J Pathol 125:191–207, 1986.

150. Majesky MW, Lindner V, Twardzik DR, et al: Production of transforming growth factor beta 1 during repair of arterial injury. J Clin Invest 88:904–910, 1991.

151. Wolf YG, Ramussen LM, Ruoslahit E: Antibodies against transforming growth factor β1 suppress intima hyperplasia in a rat model. J Clin Invest 93:1172–1178, 1994.

152. Wahl SM, Hunt DE, Wakefield LM, et al: Transforming growth factor type β induces monocyte chemotaxis and growth factor production. Proc Natl Acad Sci USA 84:5788–5792, 1987.

153. Wahl SM, Hunt DA, Wong HL, et al: Transforming growth factor-β is a potent immunosuppressive agent that inhibits IL-1 dependent lymphocyte proliferation. J Immunol 140:3026–3032, 1988.

154. Jonasson L, Holm J, Skalli O, et al: Regional accumulations of T cells, macrophages, and smooth muscle cells in the human atherosclerotic plaque. Arteriosclerosis 6:131–140, 1986.

155. Jonasson L, Holm J, Skalli O, et al: Expression of class II transplantation antigen on vascular smooth muscle cells in human atherosclerosis. J Clin Invest 76:125–131, 1985.

156. Pober JS, Gimbrone MA, Cotran RS, et al: Ia expression by vascular endothelium is inducible by activated T cells and by human gamma-interferon. J Exp Med 157:1339–1353, 1983.

157. Hansson GK, Jonasson L, Holm J, et al: Gamma-interferon regulates vascular smooth muscle proliferation and Ia antigen expression in vivo and in vitro. Circ Res 63:712–719, 1988.

158. Wilson AC, Schaub RG, Goldstein RC, et al: Suppression of aortic atherosclerosis in cholesterol-fed rabbits by purified rabbit interferon. Arteriosclerosis 10:208–214, 1990.

159. Castronuovo JJ, Guss SB, Mysh D, et al: Cytokine therapy for arterial restenosis: Inhibition of neointimal hyperplasia by gamma-interferon. Cardiovasc Surg 3(5):463–468, 1995.

160. Folkman J, Klagsburn M: Angiogenic factors. Science 235:442–447, 1987.

161. Banai S, Jaklitsch MT, Casscells W, et al: Effects of acidic fibroblast growth factor on normal and ischemic myocardium. Circ Res 69:76–85, 1991.

162. Folkman J, Klagsbrun M, Sasse J, et al: A heparin-binding angiogenic protein-basic fibroblast growth factor is stored within basement membrane. Am J Pathol 130:393–400, 1988.

163. Burgess WH, Maciag T: The heparin binding (fibroblast) growth factor family of proteins. Annu Rev Biochem 58:575–606, 1989.

164. Yayon A, Klagsbrun M, Esko JD, et al: Cell surface, heparin like molecules are required for binding of basic fibroblast growth factor to its high affinity receptor. Cell 64:841–848, 1991.

165. Ornitz DM, Yayon A, Flanagan JG, et al: Heparin is required for cell-free binding of basic fibroblast growth factor to soluble receptor and for myogenesis in whole cells. Mol Cell Biol 12:240–247, 1992.

166. Medalion B, Merin G, Aingorn H, et al: Endogenous basic fibroblast growth factor displaced by heparin from the lumenal surface of human blood vessels is preferentially seques-

tered by injured regions of the vessel wall. Circulation 95:1853–1862, 1997.

167. Lindner V, Reidy MA: Expression of basic fibroblast growth factor and its receptor by smooth muscle cells and endothelium in injured rat arteries. An en face study. Circ Res 73(3):589–595, 1993.

168. Hanna AK, Fox JC, Neshis D, et al: Antisense basic fibroblast growth factor gene transfer reduces neointimal thickening after arterial injury. J Vasc Surg 25(2):320–325, 1997.

169. Casscells W, Wai C, Shrivaastav S, et al: Smooth muscle proliferation in vessel injury is characterized by expression of fibroblast growth factor receptors and is inhibited by a toxin-fibroblast growth factor conjugate. Circulation 82:4(suppl3) III-208, 1990.

**III**

# Intervention and the Patient with Cardiovascular Disease

# 7

# Epidemiology of Coronary Heart Disease

*Peter A. McCullough*

Coronary heart disease (CHD) is the leading killer and the largest public health problem in the United States today. Historical advances since 1950, including the development of pharmacologic therapy, coronary care units, and revascularization procedures, have contributed to the decline in overall cardiovascular disease–related mortality observed since the 1960s. Since 1980, the rate of this mortality has declined approximately 30% (Fig. 7–1).[1] Increasing recognition of hypertension and its treatment, resulting in a reduction in stroke deaths, and the decline in new cases of rheumatic valvular disease since the advent of penicillin have contributed to this overall reduction in cardiovascular disease–related mortality. This reduction, with little change in the incidence rates, has led to an increase in the number of patients with CHD. In addition, the high numbers of middle-aged people ("baby boomers"), in combination with their expected increase in longevity, will result in a sharp increase in the population over the age of 65 by the year 2040 (Fig. 7–2A,B). Therefore, both future incidence and prevalence rates for CHD are expected to increase well into the 21st century.

It is known that the atherosclerotic process begins in early adulthood and that symptomatic disease appears much later.[2, 3] The average American male has a 20% chance of developing overt CHD before the age of 60, whereas this chance is approximately 6% for the average American female.[4] On the basis of the Framingham Heart Study, it is known that CHD rates increase linearly for both sexes, with the peak in incidence for males in the fifth and sixth decades and the peak for females 10 years after that of males.[5] The current estimated prevalence of cardiovascular disease in the United States is 57,490,000, approximately 25% of the entire population. This prevalence can be divided into four categories: hypertension, 50,000,000; CHD, 13,670,000; stroke, 3,820,000; and rheumatic heart disease, 1,380,000.[6, 7] These statistics take into account overlap between the categories. The number of deaths attributable to cardiovascular disease in 1994 was 954,720, representing 42% of all deaths

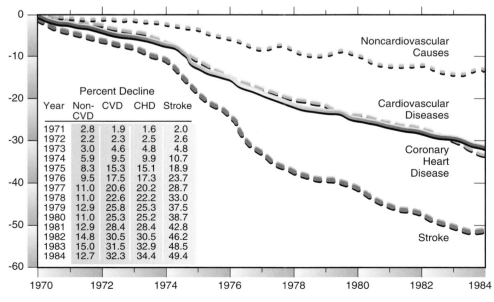

| | Percent Decline | | | |
|---|---|---|---|---|
| Year | Non-CVD | CVD | CHD | Stroke |
| 1971 | 2.8 | 1.9 | 1.6 | 2.0 |
| 1972 | 2.2 | 2.3 | 2.5 | 2.6 |
| 1973 | 3.0 | 4.6 | 4.8 | 4.8 |
| 1974 | 5.9 | 9.5 | 9.9 | 10.7 |
| 1975 | 8.3 | 15.3 | 15.1 | 18.9 |
| 1976 | 9.5 | 17.5 | 17.3 | 23.7 |
| 1977 | 11.0 | 20.6 | 20.2 | 28.7 |
| 1978 | 11.0 | 22.6 | 22.2 | 33.0 |
| 1979 | 12.9 | 25.8 | 25.3 | 37.5 |
| 1980 | 11.0 | 25.3 | 25.2 | 38.7 |
| 1981 | 12.9 | 28.4 | 28.4 | 42.8 |
| 1982 | 14.8 | 30.5 | 30.5 | 46.2 |
| 1983 | 15.0 | 31.5 | 32.9 | 48.5 |
| 1984 | 12.7 | 32.3 | 34.4 | 49.4 |

FIGURE 7–1. Declining mortality from cardiovascular disease from 1970 to 1984. (Adapted from the National Heart, Lung, and Blood Institute Center for National Health Statistics.)

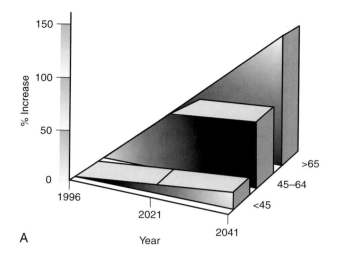

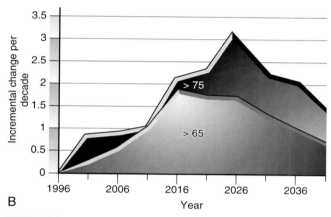

FIGURE 7–2. Projected population growth from 1996 to 2041 (*A*) and 1996 to 2036 (*B*) by age group. (Adapted from Kelly DT: Paul Dudley White International Lecture. Our future society. A global challenge. Circulation 95[11]:2459–2464, 1997.)

that year. The cause of death is depicted in Figure 7–3. In 1993, 37% of all cardiovascular disease–related deaths occurred in patients younger than 75 years, which was the average life expectancy for that year.[1]

It is clear that cardiovascular disease remains a primary public health problem in the United States. The magnitude of the problem appears to be increasing as a result of changes in population age structure and an increasing number of patients with CHD who are living longer.

## THE EPIDEMIOLOGIC EVIDENCE

History has shown the importance of cardiovascular disease in industrialized society for more than a century. In fact, since 1900, cardiovascular disease has been the leading killer of adults in every year except in 1918 (exceeded by trauma deaths in World

War I).[1] Factors associated with an industrialized lifestyle were first clearly shown, in migration and international cross-sectional studies, to have an impact over and above genetic background.

The Ni-Hon-San and the Honolulu Heart Studies demonstrated that Japanese people who migrated from Japan to Hawaii and then from Hawaii to the U.S. mainland had an increasing incidence of CHD. This natural experiment showed that with genetic background held relatively constant, increasing risk could be attributable to dietary and lifestyle factors associated with industrialized living, including increasing fat consumption, increased serum cholesterol, development of hypertension, and the initiation of tobacco abuse.[8–14] The Puerto Rico Heart Health Study revealed that CHD was linked to urban living situations, which were associated with increased levels of cholesterol, increased smoking, and decreased activity levels.[15, 16] The Seven Countries Study, a cohort study of 9780 men aged 40 to 59 in Yugoslavia, Finland, Italy, The Netherlands, Greece, the United States, and Japan, showed that risk factors such as age, high serum cholesterol, high systolic blood pressure, smoking, obesity, and reduced physical activity all have an impact on cardiovascular risk, including incident cases of acute myocardial infarction and cardiac death. However, in a multivariate analysis, only the risk factors of age, high cholesterol, and hypertension were shown to extend across cultures and geographic regions.[17] In addition, this study revealed that incidence rates had variability between northern and southern latitudes, particularly in Europe.[18]

The World Health Organization Monitoring Trends and Determinants in Cardiovascular Disease (MONICA) Project is a 26-country observational study of risk factor differences among countries and is designed to measure trends in population characteristics, in detection of clinical disease, and in differences in CHD mortality over time. This study has described decreasing rates of mortality from myocardial infarction and stroke; the decreases are attributed to improved treatment in Europe.[19–25] Unfortunately, the incidence of CHD appears to be increasing in Far Eastern countries such as Japan, Taiwan, and Korea as a result of increases in total dietary fat and a rise in the population mean cholesterol level.[26] These epidemiologic observations from international studies, along with those of prospective cohort studies, have provided the basis for risk factor analysis and description of the natural history and treatment of CHD.

The best known and most extensive cardiovascular cohort investigation is the Framingham Heart Study. Beginning in 1947 in Framingham, Massachusetts, an effort to enlist all patients within the city limits into a lifelong cohort study was under-

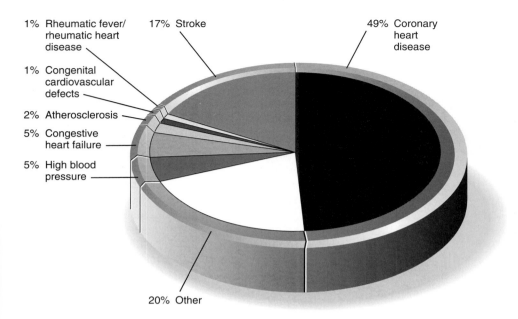

1% Rheumatic fever/rheumatic heart disease

1% Congenital cardiovascular defects

2% Atherosclerosis

5% Congestive heart failure

5% High blood pressure

17% Stroke

49% Coronary heart disease

20% Other

FIGURE 7–3. Percentage breakdown of deaths from cardiovascular disease in the United States, 1993. (Adapted from the American Heart Association: 1997 Heart and Stroke Statistical Update. Dallas: American Heart Association, 1997.)

taken. Men and women aged 30 to 59 were screened, and 5127 were found to be disease-free and were monitored over time with a variety of serial examinations and interviews.[4, 5, 27, 28] From this study, hundreds of scientific publications have come forth elucidating the relationship between risk factors, incidence rates, biologic responses (such as left ventricular hypertrophy and dysfunction), and mortality rates.[29–31] In addition, the Framingham cohort has given investigators the opportunity to identify trends in risk factor profiles over time.[32–34]

The Multiple Risk Factor Intervention Trial (MRFIT) is another inception cohort study in which 361,662 men aged 35 to 57 were screened and randomly assigned either to a multifactorial risk factor reduction program or to usual care; the entire group underwent long-term follow-up. Analyses of the study cohort and the screened participants provided the basis for a variety of risk factor observations, particularly the quantitative relationship between serum cholesterol and mortality (see Fig. 7–3).[35–42] A partial list of cohort studies that have contributed to the body of knowledge regarding risk factors and the epidemiology of CHD is given in Table 7–1.[39, 43–52]

Patterns of disease observed over time in cohort studies provided evidence that factors including hyperlipidemia, smoking, hypertension, diabetes, family history of cardiovascular disease, obesity, male gender, physical inactivity, low fiber intake, estrogen use in women, vitamin consumption, and aspirin use were related in various ways to CHD. These studies, combined with intervention trials, have helped to define and test risk factor hypotheses, confirm the causal relationships, and provide the basis for treatment and prevention.

## RISK FACTOR ANALYSIS AND MODIFICATION

Risk factors for CHD are defined as attributes or personal traits that are directly related to the probability of developing the disease. Widely recognized risk factors and their public health importance are listed in Table 7–2. In general, the interaction of multiple risk factors or their effect indicates substantial risk for a given individual. This is relevant to most people in industrialized countries, in as much as any person is likely to compile multiple risk factors over a life span. The following text is a brief summary of the known independent effects of risk factors from the epidemiologic literature discussed earlier.

## Primary Risk Factors

### Age

The individual risk and population prevalence of CHD increase with age. The incidence of multivessel disease and left ventricular impairment increases with age as well.[53, 54] Accordingly, the prognosis is worse with advancing age after treatment for virtually any cardiac event.[55, 56] Current guidelines consider age over 45 for men and age over 55 for women singular risk factors for the development of CHD.[57] Age is one of the most important covariates for the interventional cardiologist to consider, in view of its strong relationship to outcomes after procedures.

### Gender

At all ages, the risk of developing CHD is greater in men than in women, although this difference in risk

**TABLE 7–1.   SELECTED LARGE-SCALE EPIDEMIOLOGIC AND EXPERIMENTAL STUDIES OF CORONARY HEART DISEASE**

| STUDY | DESIGN | MEN | WOMEN | DIETARY DATA | MORTALITY | PRINCIPAL ACTIVITY |
|---|---|---|---|---|---|---|
| Seven Countries | 10-yr cohort | 9780 | — | + | + | Risk factors |
| Framingham | 50-yr cohort | 2282 | 2845 | + | + | Risk factors |
| Harvard Alumni | Cross-sectional | 16,936 | — | + | + | Physical activity |
| Western Collaborative | 5-yr cohort | 3524 | — | − | + | Psychosocial factors |
| U.S. Railroad | 20-yr cohort | 3049 | — | + | + | Risk factors |
| Puerto Rico | 17-yr cohort | 8783 | — | + | + | Risk factors, urban/rural |
| Western Electric | 25-yr cohort | 2107 | — | + | + | Risk factors |
| Honolulu | 10-yr cohort | 7705 | — | + | + | Risk factors, migration |
| Evans County | 9-yr cohort | 1157 | 1343 | + | + | Risk factors, ethnicity |
| Charleston | Cross-sectional | 986 | 1195 | + | + | Risk factors, ethnicity |
| Ireland-Boston Diet | 20-yr cohort | 1001 | — | + | + | Risk factors, diet |
| LRC Prevalence | Cross-sectional | ~3700 | ~3700 | + | + | Risk factors, lipids |
| Tecumseh | 9-yr cohort | ~4000 | ~4000 | + | + | Risk factors, general health |
| Ni-Ho-San | Cross-sectional | 11,991 | — | + | + | Diet, migration |
| Framingham Offspring | Longitudinal | 1341 | 1530 | + | − | Genetic risk |
| Kuopio | Cross-sectional | 2682 | — | + | − | Risk factors, carotid disease |
| Minnesota | Cross-sectional | 3828 | 4260 | + | − | Psychosocial factors |
| Manitoba | 26-yr cohort | 3983 | — | − | + | Body weight |
| Rancho Bernardo | 7-yr cohort | 2322 | 2730 | + | + | Risk factors, estrogen |
| Alameda County | Cross-sectional | 3158 | 3770 | + | + | General health |
| Pawtucket | Longitudinal | ~42% | ~58% | + | − | CHD education |
| Tokelau Island | 14-yr cohort | 370 | 440 | + | − | Lifestyle, migration |
| San Antonio | 13-yr cohort | 1176 | 1041 | + | − | Risk factors, ethnicity |
| Stanford Three | Longitudinal | 1018 | 1133 | + | − | CHD education |
| MRFIT | RCT/25-yr cohort | 12,866 | — | + | + | Risk factor reduction |
| Muscatine | Longitudinal | 2500 | 2500 | + | − | Lipids in children |
| Bogalusa | Longitudinal cross-sectional | 2433 | 2245 | + | + | Children, ethnicity |
| Intersalt | Cross-sectional | 5045 | 5034 | + | − | HTN, dietary sodium |
| Nurses Health Study | 10-yr cohort | 39,910 | 87,245 | + | − | Dietary vitamin A, C, E |
| MONICA | 10-yr initial cohort | yes | yes | + | + | Risk factor trends |
| Gothenburg | Longitudinal | — | 1622 | + | + | Risk factors, women |
| Tromsco | Cross-sectional | 8867 | — | + | − | Risk factors |
| EWPHE | RCT | 400 | 440 | + | + | HTN primary prevention diuretic |
| IPPPSH | RCT | 3194 | 3163 | − | − | HTN primary prevention beta-blocker |
| HTN Detection & Follow-up | RCT | 5901 | 5039 | − | − | HTN primary prevention stepped care |
| VA Cooperative HTN | RCT | 523 | — | − | − | HTN blood pressure control |
| SHEP | RCT | 2242 | 2494 | − | − | HTN cardiovascular events stepped care |
| LRC Primary Prevention | RCT | 3806 | — | + | + | Primary prevention cholestyramine |
| WHO clofibrate | RCT | 15,745 | — | − | + | Primary prevention |
| Helsinki Heart | RCT | 4081 | — | + | − | Primary prevention gemfibrozol |
| West of Scotland | RCT | 6595 | — | − | + | Primary prevention pravastatin |
| AMIS | RCT | 4021 | 503 | − | − | Primary prevention ASA |
| Physicians Health | RCT | 22,701 | — | − | + | Primary prevention ASA/Vit A |
| 4S | RCT | 3599 | 845 | − | + | Secondary prevention simvastatin |
| CARE | RCT | 3583 | 576 | − | + | Secondary prevention pravastatin |

AMIS, Aspirin in Myocardial Infarction Study; CARE, Cholesterol and Recurrent Events; CHD, coronary heart disease; EWPHE, European Working Party on Hypertension in the Elderly; HTN, hypertension; IPPPSH, Interventional Prospective Primary Prevention Study in Hypertension; LRC, Lipid Research Clinics; MONICA, Monitoring Trends and Determinants in Cardiovascular Disease; MRFIT, Multiple Risk Factor Intervention Trial; RCT, Randomized Controlled Trial; 4S, Scandinavian Simvastatin Survival Study; SHEP, Systolic Hypertension in the Elderly Program; VA, Veterans Affairs; WHO, World Health Organization.

**TABLE 7–2. COMMON CARDIAC RISK FACTORS AND THEIR MEASURES OF ASSOCIATION WITH CORONARY HEART DISEASE AND ESTIMATES OF PUBLIC HEALTH IMPORTANCE IN TERMS OF PREVENTABLE DEATHS**

| RISK FACTOR | PREVALENCE (%) | CRUDE RELATIVE RISK | POPULATION ATTRIBUTABLE RISK (%) | ESTIMATED PREVENTABLE DEATHS |
|---|---|---|---|---|
| Cigarette smoking | | | | |
| Males | 31.2 | 1.9 | 20.8 | 64,302 |
| Females | 26.5 | 1.8 | 16.4 | 46,570 |
| Hypertension (>159/>94 mm Hg) | 17.7 | 2.8 | 23.0 | 136,416 |
| Diabetes mellitus | | | | |
| Males | 5.7 | 2.1 | 5.6 | 17,312 |
| Females | 7.4 | 4.7 | 21.6 | 61,336 |
| Cholesterol | | | | |
| Total ≥240 mg/dL | 26.7 | 3.0 | 29.8 | 176,747 |
| HDL <35 mg/dL | 11.2 | 2.4 | 13.5 | 80,070 |
| Inactivity | 58.8 | 1.9 | 34.6 | 205,216 |
| Overweight | | | | |
| RW ≥ 59 kg (130 lb) | 26.6 | 2.0 | 18.1 | 107,353 |

HDL, high-density lipoprotein cholesterol; RW, relative weight.
Adapted from Bittner V, Oberman A: Epidemiology of coronary heart disease. *In* Roubin GS, Califf RM, O'Neill WW, et al (eds): Interventional Cardiovascular Medicine: Principles and Practice, pp 147–164. New York: Churchill Livingstone, 1994.

is narrowed approximately 10 years after menopause (age 60).[58, 59] Population studies have shown that a consistent gender difference can be observed in countries with quite different overall rates of CHD (Fig. 7–4). Most models of CHD consider male gender a singular risk factor, the relative risk of male gender being approximately 2.5 to 4.5.[49] It is estimated that 30% of the gender difference can be explained by estrogen status.[60, 61] Estrogen replace-

ment has been related to lessened CHD risk, and several ongoing randomized trials are evaluating the potential protective role of these hormones.

The first of these trials to be reported was the Heart and Estrogen/progestin Replacement Study (HERS). In contrast to prior nonrandomized studies, HERS found no benefit from estrogen replacement as secondary prevention in 2763 women at five years follow-up.[61a] The most notable current study

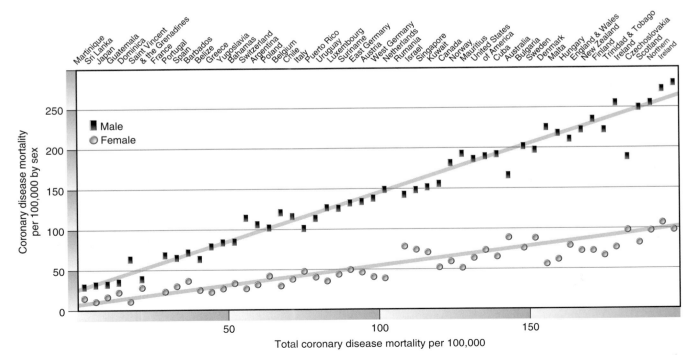

FIGURE 7–4. Consistent male-to-female ratio of 2.5 to 4.5 for fatal coronary heart disease (CHD) in countries with different rates of CHD. (Adapted from Barrett-Connor E: Sex differences in coronary heart disease. Why are women so superior? The 1995 Ancel Keys Lecture. Circulation 95[1]:252–264, 1997.)

is the Women's Health Initiative, a 15-year National Institutes of Health project, which focuses on the relationship of estrogen and CHD death in 164,500 postmenopausal women (aged 50 to 79). Female gender as a clinical variable poses an unusual proposition in that it is protective against developing CHD; however, it has been reported that once the disease is overt, women have higher complication rates after virtually all cardiac events and procedures.[62–66] This observation has led to many investigations into gender bias in referral for procedures.[67] Most well-controlled analyses agree that when all confounders are accounted for, women are not currently underreferred for cardiac procedures.[68–71]

### Family History

The relative risk of CHD is 2 to 5 for a person with a first-degree relative who has premature CHD and is younger than the age of 55.[30, 72–75] Furthermore, a family history of premature myocardial infarction is an independent predictor of overall mortality.[76]

### Hypertension

Diastolic and systolic hypertension, defined as pressures consistently over 80 and 140, respectively, are accepted risk factors for CHD development, congestive heart failure (CHF), and stroke.[77] Intervention trials have confirmed that hypertension control reduces the risks of stoke and cardiac events in all ages.[78, 79] Although the incidence of stroke and CHF are more closely related to hypertension, an estimated 15% of the excess incidence of CHD is attributable to the presence of hypertension.[80] One potential linked variable to consider in the relationship between hypertension and CHD events is left ventricular hypertrophy (LVH), which is discussed later.

### Diabetes

Diabetes mellitus, defined as a fasting plasma glucose level higher than 126 mg/dL or documented glucose intolerance, is, like age, a well-recognized risk factor for CHD development and increased morbidity and mortality with virtually any cardiac event or procedure.[81, 82] The relative risk for cardiac death in diabetic patients is between 2 and 5.[83] Hyperinsulinemia, a preclinical marker of diabetes, has been clearly associated with increased cardiac risk.[84, 85] The clustering of insulin resistance, dyslipidemia, hypertension, and truncal obesity has been termed *familial dyslipidemic hypertension*, or the *deadly quartet*, and is related to high rates of CHD development.[86] Interventional studies of enhanced diabetic control have shown only modest improvements in cardiac outcome. Diabetes is a common comorbidity; approximately 25% of interventional cardiolo-

gists' patients who undergo procedures have diabetes.[87–89] Finally, diabetes has been shown to be directly and independently linked to the development of contrast nephropathy and mortality after cardiac procedures.[89]

### Dyslipidemia

The causative role of elevations in serum lipid levels is probably the best proven of all cardiac risk factor hypotheses. The diagnosis and treatment of lipid disorders is beyond the scope of this text. Figure 7–5 contains a summary of current guidelines regarding lipid management and cardiovascular risk for patients without CHD (primary prevention). Guidelines for comprehensive medical management of the patient with overt CHD is given in Figure 7–6 (secondary prevention). The following text is a brief discussion of individual parameters and cardiac risk.

TOTAL CHOLESTEROL. A high total cholesterol level is a powerful predictor of the development of CHD and its morbidity and mortality. A continuous and nonlinear relationship between cholesterol and cardiac events has been shown in hundreds of thousands of patients (Fig. 7–7).[42, 90–96] Furthermore, there is conclusive evidence that reduction in serum cholesterol levels reduces cardiac morbidity and mortality, regardless of whether CHD is clinically overt. This was demonstrated in the West of Scotland trial, in which 6595 men aged 45 to 64 with hypercholesterolemia (mean serum cholesterol level, 272 mg/dL) were randomly assigned to receive either pravastatin, 40 mg/day, or placebo.[97] Those receiving pravastatin were observed to have significant risk reductions in nonfatal myocardial infarction and cardiac death over 5 years (Fig. 7–8). The mechanism of the lipid-lowering benefit appears to involve more than the modest plaque regression or stabilization in progression rates observed in many trials (Fig. 7–9).[98–108] These trials have consistently shown that despite a modest effect on the angiographic appearance of the coronaries, lipid-lowering therapy significantly reduces the long-term incidence of cardiac events (Table 7–3). Newer data indicate a relationship between reduced lipoprotein levels and improved endothelial function, reduced plaque vulnerability to rupture, and more favorable blood clotting profiles.[109–113]

LDL CHOLESTEROL. Low-density lipoprotein (LDL) particles appear to be the most atherogenic factor. The numbers of these particles in the serum is related to the quantity of apolipoprotein B (apo-B). Smaller LDL particles appear to be more atherogenic than larger ones, and for this reason, the apo-B level may be a better indicator of atherosclerosis risk than

| Risk Intervention | Recommendations | | | |
|---|---|---|---|---|
| **Smoking:**<br>__Goal__<br>**complete cessation** | Ask about smoking status as part of routine evaluation. Reinforce nonsmoking status.<br>Strongly encourage patient and family to stop smoking.<br>Provide counseling, nicotine replacement, and formal cessation programs as appropriate. | | | |
| **Blood pressure control:**<br>__Goal__<br>≤140/90 mm Hg | Measure blood pressure in all adults at least every 2½ years<br>Promote lifestyle modification: weight control, physical activity, moderation in alcohol intake, moderate sodium restriction.<br>If blood pressure ≥140/90 mm Hg after 3 months of life habit modification or if initial blood pressure >160/100 mm Hg: add blood pressure medication, individualize therapy to patient's other requirements and characteristics. | | | |
| **Cholesterol management:**<br>__Primary goal__<br>**LDL < 160 mg/dL if 0–1 risk factors**<br>**or**<br>**LDL < 130 mg/dL if ≥2 risk factors**<br>__Secondary goals__<br>**HDL > 35 mg/dL**<br>**TG < 200 mg/dL** | Ask about dietary habits as part of routine evaluation.<br>Measure total and HDL cholesterol in all adults ≥20 y and assess positive and negative risk factors at least every 5 years.<br>For all persons: promote AHA Step I Diet (≤30% fat, <10% saturated fat, <300 mg/d cholesterol), weight control, and physical activity.<br>Measure LDL if total cholesterol ≥ 240 mg/dL or ≥ 200 mg/dL with ≥2 risk factors or if HDL < 35 mg/dL | | | |

| | | | | |
|---|---|---|---|---|
| | If LDL:<br>≥160 mg/dL with 0–1 risk factors or<br>≥130 mg/dL on two occasions with ≥2 risk factors; then<br><br>Start Step II Diet (≤30% fat, <7% saturated fat, <200 mg/dL cholesterol) and weight control.<br><br>Rule out secondary causes of high LDL (LFTs, TFTs, UA).<br><br>If LDL:<br>≥160 mg/dL plus 2 risk factors; or<br>≥190 mg/dL; or<br>≥220 mg/dL in men <35 y or in premenopausal women; then<br><br>Consider adding drug therapy to diet therapy for LDL levels > those listed above that persist despite Step II Diet. | | | Risk factors: age (men ≥45 y, women ≥55 y or post-menopausal), hypertension, diabetes, smoking, HDL <35 mg/dL, family history of CHD in first-degree relatives (in male relatives <55 y, female relatives <65 y)<br>HDL ≥60 mg/dL: Subtract 1 risk factor from the number of positive risk factors. |
| | **Suggested drug therapy for high LDL levels (≥160 mg/dL)**<br>**(drug selection priority modified according to TG level)** | | | |
| | TG < 200 mg/dL | TG 200–400 mg/dL | TG > 400 mg/dL | HDL < 35 mg/dL: |
| | Statin<br>Resin<br>Niacin | Statin<br>Niacin | Consider combined drug therapy (niacin, fibrates, statin) | Emphasize weight management and physical activity, avoidance of cigarette smoking. Niacin raises HDL. Consider niacin if patient has ≥2 risk factors and high LDL (except patients with diabetes). |
| | If LDL goal not achieved, consider combination drug therapy. | | | |

| Risk Intervention | Recommendations | | | |
|---|---|---|---|---|
| **Physical activity:**<br>__Goal__<br>**Increase amount**<br>**Exercise regularly**<br>**3–4 times per**<br>**week for 30 minutes** | Ask about physical activity status and exercise habits as part of routine evaluation.<br>Encourage 30 minutes of moderate-intensity dynamic exercise 3–4 times per week as well as increased physical activity in daily life habits for persons who are inactive.<br>Encourage regular exercise to improve conditioning and optimize fitness level.<br>Advise medically supervised programs for those with low functional capacity and/or comorbidities.<br>Promote environmental factors conducive to health (i.e., golf courses that permit walking). | | | |
| **Weight management:**<br>__Goal__<br>**Achieve and maintain desirable weight**<br>**(BMI 21–25 kg/m²)** | Measure patient's weight and height, BMI, and waist-to-hip ratio at each visit as part of routine evaluation.<br>Start weight management and physical activity as appropriate. Desirable BMI range: 21–25 kg/m².<br>BMI of 25 kg/m² corresponds to percentage desirable body weight of 110%; desirable waist-to-hip ratio for men, <0.9; for middle-aged and elderly woman, <0.8. | | | |
| **Estrogens:** | Consider estrogen replacement therapy in postmenopausal women, especially those with multiple CHD risk factors, such as elevated LDL.<br>Individualize recommendation consistent with other health risks. | | | |

TG, triglycerides; LFTs, liver function tests; TFTs, thyroid function tests;
UA, uric acid; CHD, coronary heart disease; BMI, body mass index.

FIGURE 7–5. Clinical guidelines for primary prevention of coronary heart disease (CHD), based on risk factors and lipid profiles. (Adapted from Grundy SM, Balady GJ, Criqui MH, et al: When to start cholesterol-lowering therapy in patients with coronary heart disease. A statement for healthcare professionals from the American Heart Association Task Force on Risk Reduction. Circulation 95(1):1683–1685, 1997.)

**Guide to Comprehensive Risk Reduction
for Patients With Coronary and Other Vascular Disease**

| Risk Intervention | Recommendations |
|---|---|
| **Smoking:**<br>Goal<br>complete cessation | Strongly encourage patient and family to stop smoking.<br>Provide counseling, nicotine replacement, and formal cessation programs as appropriate. |
| **Lipid management:**<br>Primary goal<br>LDL < 100 mg/dL<br><br>Secondary goals<br>HDL > 35 mg/dL<br>TG < 200 mg/dL | Start AHA Step II Diet in all patients: ≤30% fat, <7% saturated fat, <200mg/d cholesterol.<br>Assess fasting lipid profile. In post-MI patients, lipid profile may take 4–6 weeks to stabilize. Add drug therapy according to the following guide:<br><br>LDL < 100 mg/dL — No drug therapy<br>LDL 100–130 mg/dL — Consider adding drug therapy to diet as follows:<br>LDL > 130 mg/dL — Add drug therapy to diet, as follows:<br>HDL < 35 mg/dL — Emphasize weight management and physical activity. Advise smoking cessation. If needed to achieve LDL goals, consider niacin, statin, fibrate.<br><br>Suggested drug therapy<br><br>TG < 200 mg/dL — Statin, Resin, Niacin<br>TG 200–400 mg/dL — Statin, Niacin<br>TG > 400 mg/dL — Consider combined drug therapy (niacin, fibrate, statin)<br><br>If LDL goal not achieved, consider combination therapy. |
| **Physical activity:**<br>Minimum goal<br>30 minutes 3–4<br>times per week | Assess risk, preferably with exercise test, to guide prescription.<br>Encourage minimum of 30–60 minutes of moderate-intensity activity 3 or 4 times weekly (walking, jogging, cycling, or other aerobic activity) supplemented by an increase in daily lifestyle activites (e.g., walking breaks at work, using stairs, gardening, household work). Maximum benefit 5–6 hours a week.<br>Advise medically supervised programs for moderate- to high-risk patients. |
| **Weight management** | Start intensive diet and appropriate physical activity intervention, as outlined above, in patients >120% of ideal weight for height.<br>Particularly emphasize need for weight loss in patients with hypertension, elevated triglycerides, or elevated glucose levels. |
| **Antiplatelet agents/ anticoagulants** | Start aspirin 80–325 mg/d if not contraindicated.<br>Manage warfarin to international normalized ratio = 2 to 3.5 for post-MI patients not able to take aspirin. |
| **ACE inhibitors post-MI:** | Start early post-MI in stable high-risk patients (anterior MI, previous MI, Killip class II [$S_3$ gallop, rales, radiographic CHF]).<br>Continue indefinitely for all with LV dysfunction (ejection fraction ≤ 40%) or failure.<br>Use as needed to manage blood pressure or symptoms in all other patients. |
| **Beta-blockers:** | Start in high-risk post-MI patients (arrhythmia, LV dysfunction, inducible ischemia) at 5–28 days. Continue 6 months minimum. Observe usual contraindications.<br>Use as needed to manage angina, rhythm, or blood pressure in all other patients. |
| **Estrogens:** | Consider estrogen replacement in all postmenopausal women.<br>Individualize recommendation consistent with other health risks. |
| **Blood pressure control:**<br>Goal<br>≤140/90 mm Hg | Initiate lifestyle modification—weight control, physical activity, alcohol moderation, and moderate sodium restriction—in all patients with blood pressure >140 mm Hg systolic or 90 mm Hg diastolic.<br>Add blood pressure medication, individualized to other patient requirements and characteristics (i.e., age, race, need for drugs with specific benefits) if blood pressure is not less than 140 mm Hg systolic or 90 mm Hg diastolic in 3 months or if *initial* blood pressure is > 160 mm Hg systolic or 100 mm Hg diastolic. |

ACE, angiotensin-converting enzyme; MI, myocardial infarction; TG, triglycerides; LV, left ventricular.

FIGURE 7–6. Comprehensive guidelines for medical management and risk reduction in patients with overt coronary heart disease. (Adapted from Smith SC Jr: Risk-reduction therapy: The challenge to change. Presented at the 68th scientific sessions of the American Heart Association, November 13, 1995, Anaheim, California. Circulation 93[12]:2205–2211, 1996.)

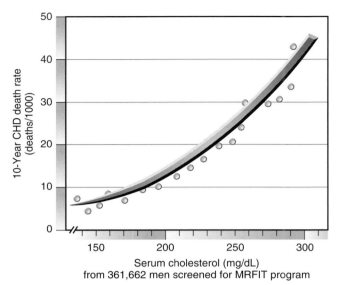

FIGURE 7–7. The relationship between serum cholesterol and subsequent death from coronary heart disease over 10 years. (Adapted from National Institutes of Health: Publication No. 90–3047, 1990.)

is the LDL level itself. The incidence of new and recurrent cardiac events is strongly related to the LDL and apo-B levels, as demonstrated in the regression and prevention trials cited above. The current National Cholesterol Education Program (NCEP) guidelines focus on management of the LDL levels according to individual risk.[57] The part of those guidelines that is relevant to interventional cardiology is that concerning patients with demonstrated coronary disease. Current recommendations include diet and usually drug therapy to achieve an LDL level less than 100 mg/dL.

**HDL CHOLESTEROL.** High-density lipoprotein (HDL), which contains apolipoprotein-A1, is inversely related to cardiovascular risk. A low HDL level (<35 mg/dL in men and <45 mg/dL in women) and an elevated triglyceride level constitute the most common lipid profile among interventional cardiology patients.[114, 115] To date, several randomized trials have been completed that support the concept of raising HDL as a cardiovascular intervention. The Veterans Affairs High-Density Lipoprotein Cholesterol Intervention Trial (VA-HIT) demonstrated that a 6% rise in HDL and a 31% decrease in triglycerides with gemfibrozil led to a 22% reduction in nonfatal myocardial infarction and cardiac deaths.[115a] However, patients with a high HDL (>65 mg/dL) have a reduced CHD risk, and this is considered a negative risk factor. Because of the complementary information, the LDL/HDL ratio is considered the strongest index of CHD risk (e.g., a ratio >5 predicts risk in an asymptomatic person).[115]

**TRIGLYCERIDES.** The relationship between triglycerides and CHD has probably been underestimated because of the linkage between depressed HDL levels and elevated triglyceride levels. Several studies have shown fewer cardiac events with therapy aimed at lowering elevated triglyceride levels.[115, 116] The relevant consideration for the interventional cardiologist is that the patient with low HDL and elevated triglyceride levels (>200 mg/dL) is most likely to have an LDL level above the target, and therapy can still be guided by the NCEP guidelines.

**LIPOPROTEIN A (LP[a]).** Lp(a) particles contain apolipoprotein-A (apo-A), which has structural similarities to plasminogen. Lp(a) levels appear to be governed primarily by genetic determinants and are clearly related to risk of cardiac events (at levels >30 mg/dL) in white persons.[117] Lp(a) does not have strong predictive value in African-Americans.[117] Niacin, estrogens, and alcohol all lower Lp(a) modestly; however, there have been no intervention trials targeting Lp(a). There has been great research interest in measuring other newly discovered lipoproteins and their relationship to CHD. Currently, the value of measuring other lipoproteins in clinical practice is controversial.

**SMOKING.** Smoking remains the most preventable cause of premature death in the North American population. There is a dose-response relationship between the number of cigarettes smoked per day

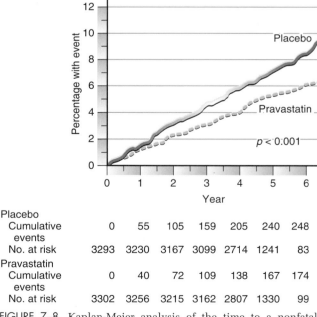

| | | | | | | | |
|---|---|---|---|---|---|---|---|
| **Placebo** | | | | | | | |
| Cumulative events | 0 | 55 | 105 | 159 | 205 | 240 | 248 |
| No. at risk | 3293 | 3230 | 3167 | 3099 | 2714 | 1241 | 83 |
| **Pravastatin** | | | | | | | |
| Cumulative events | 0 | 40 | 72 | 109 | 138 | 167 | 174 |
| No. at risk | 3302 | 3256 | 3215 | 3162 | 2807 | 1330 | 99 |

FIGURE 7–8. Kaplan-Meier analysis of the time to a nonfatal myocardial infarction or cardiac death in the West of Scotland trial. (Adapted from Shepherd J, Cobbe SM, Ford I, et al: Prevention of coronary heart disease with pravastatin in men with hypercholesterolemia. West of Scotland Coronary Prevention Study Group. N Engl J Med 333:1301–1307, 1995.)

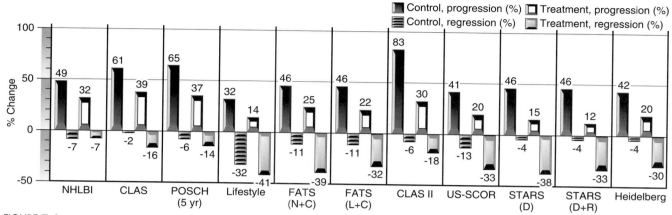

FIGURE 7–9. Summary of the regression and progression of atherosclerosis measured by angiography in controlled trials. C, cholestyramine; CLAS II, Cholesterol Lowering Atherosclerosis Study; D, diet; FATS, Familial Atherosclerosis Treatment Study; L, lovastatin; N, niacin; NHLBI, National Heart, Lung, and Blood Institute; POSCH, Program on the Surgical Control of the Hyperlipidemias; R, resin; STARS, St Thomas' Atherosclerosis Regression Study; US-SCOR, Specialized Center of Research Intervention Trial.

and CHD risk.[118] Smoking also increases mortality rates among patients with coronary disease that is documented angiographically and after revascularization.[119] Passive smoking also appears to increase the risk of CHD development and is relevant to angioplasty patients whose households include smokers.[120] Obviously, all patients are strongly advised during routine health visits, and especially after a cardiac event such as revascularization, to stop smoking.

## Secondary Risk Factors

### Ethnic Background

Life expectancy is shorter and mortality rates are higher for black than for white Americans.[121, 122] Be-

cause cardiovascular disease is the leading cause of death overall, it is not surprising that CHD epidemiologic studies have revealed higher death rates for black people.[123] Similarly, persons of Hispanic descent have exhibited high rates of glucose intolerance, dyslipidemia, and CHD.[124–126] Although race and ethnic background have not been considered traditional risk factors because of primarily study design issues, they are clearly linked to CHD in part through genetic background and in part by socioeconomic status. Further work in this area is needed to quantitate the independent effects of these variables.

### Obesity

The body mass index (BMI)—weight in kilograms divided by the height in meters squared—is an ex-

**TABLE 7–3.    SUMMARY OF THE CARDIAC EVENT REDUCTIONS OBSERVED IN CORONARY REGRESSION TRIALS: CLINICAL CORONARY EVENT OUTCOMES IN LIPID INTERVENTION TRIALS***

| STUDY | TREATMENTS | YEARS | % EVENT REDUCTION |
|---|---|---|---|
| NHLBI Type II | Diet + resin | 5 | 33 |
| CLAS | Diet + resin + niacin | 2 | 25 |
| POSCH | Diet + surgery ± resin | 9.7 | 35† |
| FATS | Diet + resin + niacin | 2.5 | 80† |
| FATS | Diet + niacin + lovastatin | 2.5 | 70 |
| CLAS II | Diet + resin + niacin | 4 | 43 |
| STARS | Diet | 3 | 69† |
| STARS | Diet + resin | 3 | 89† |
| SCRIP | Diet + drugs + exercise | 4 | 39† |
| MARS | Diet + lovastatin | 2 | 24 |
| PLAC-I | Diet + pravastatin | 3 | 61† |
| PLAC-II | Diet + pravastatin | 3 | 60 |
| CCAIT | Diet + lovastatin | 2 | 25 |

CCAIT, Canadian Coronary Atherosclerosis Intervention Trial; CLAS, Cholesterol Lowering Atherosclerosis Trial; FATS, Familial Atherosclerosis Treatment Study; MARS, Monitored Atherosclerosis Regression Study; NHLBI, National Heart, Lung, and Blood Institute; PLAC, Pravastatin Limitation of Atherosclerosis in the Coronary Arteries; POSCH, Program of the Surgical Control of the Hyperlipidemias; SCRIP, Stanford Coronary Risk Intervention Project; STARS, St Thomas' Atherosclerosis Regression Study.

*In which angiographic criteria for entry were used.

†Statistically significant.

Adapted from Waters D, Lesperance J: Regression of coronary atherosclerosis: An achievable goal? Review of results from recent clinical trials. Am J Med 91:10S–17S, 1991.

cellent measure of obesity. An easy-to-use nomogram for calculation of BMI is given in Figure 7–10. In general, a person is considered obese when the BMI exceeds 27, which is true of about 25% of the North American population. Obesity contributes to CHD by affecting other factors (hypertension, diabetes, dyslipidemia) and has a weak independent relationship to CHD itself.[127] Central obesity, the typical pattern in men, carries a higher risk of CHD events in both genders than does peripheral obesity. A waist-to-hip ratio greater than 0.8 in women and greater than 1.0 in men indicates elevated CHD risk. A nomogram for calculating the waist-to-hip ratio is given in Figure 7–11. Weight reduction is advised in both primary and secondary prevention populations to achieve a BMI of less than 27.

### Physical Inactivity

More than half of the North American population does not exercise regularly. Although physical inactivity, like obesity, contributes to CHD risk through other risk factors, there is a measurable independent effect of a sedentary lifestyle on cardiovascular mortality reproduced in multiple studies.[128–131] Pooled results from multiple studies show improved fitness and reduced mortality with exercise training programs in patients with established CHD.[132] On the basis of these data, an exercise program for all patients after revascularization is recommended.

### Type A Personality

A hard-driving, ambitious, aggressive, and hostile personality type appears to have an independent effect on the development of CHD.[133] There have been no definitive studies regarding behavior modification and reduction of risk.

### Elevated C-Reactive Protein

Multiple studies have confirmed a relationship between elevated levels of high-sensitivity C-reactive protein (hs-CRP) and nonfatal myocardial infarction and cardiac death. These data have been confounded by the observation that those with elevated hs-CRP have markedly attenuated risk when taking aspirin. Because aspirin is currently recommended as primary prevention for those older than age 45 and for all secondary prevention patients, the role of hs-CRP in patient management remains unclear.[133a]

### Hyperhomocysteinemia

There has been a large effort in the research community to evaluate the relationship between serum homocysteine levels and atherosclerotic disease.[134–137] A large number of studies consistently indicate that elevated levels of homocysteine (>14 nmol/mL) are strongly related to CHD, cerebrovascular disease, and peripheral vascular disease (Fig. 7–12). It is estimated that for every 5 nmol/mL increase in serum homocysteine, the odds ratio for CHD is 1.6 to 1.8, equivalent to an elevation of 20 mg/dL of total cholesterol.[138] There are multiple randomized trials under way of vitamin supplementation (folate, vitamin $B_6$, vitamin $B_{12}$) to reduce homocysteine levels and hence reduce risk.[138a] General recommendations regarding vitamin use are given later.

### Alcohol Consumption

The relationship between alcohol consumption and CHD has received great interest in the medical community. Moderate intake of alcohol (2 ounces, or two drinks, per day) is associated with a reduced risk of CHD. This benefit may be mediated through mild elevations in HDL levels.[139–145] There is a clear U-shaped curve for alcohol and mortality. Moderate consumption appears to reduce CHD risk; higher consumption is clearly related to an increase in mortality from noncardiac causes.

### Diet and Vitamins

There is a clear association between a high-fat diet and CHD risk. Diet is correlated with other risk factors such as serum lipid levels, obesity, physical inactivity, and hypertension. High-fiber diets appear to be associated with lower CHD risk.[146–148] Also, intake of nuts has been related to reduced risk.[149] Diets high in fish consumption, at least in some studies, have been related to lower CHD risk.[150, 151] Epidemiologic and angiographic data further suggest that diets supplemented with vitamin A, C, and E, may be cardioprotective.[152–155] Two definitive trials have weighed in on the benefit of vitamins. The Heart Outcomes Protection Evaluation (HOPE) randomized 2545 women and 6996 men to 400 IU of vitamin E versus placebo and found no benefit. The Physicians' Health Study, in a similar fashion, tested the benefits of β-carotene (50 mg qod) in 22,071 male physicians and found no benefit.[156, 157] On the basis of the data available, most experts recommend an American Heart Association Step II diet (less than 7% of calories derived from saturated fat, and less than 200 mg of cholesterol) and a multivitamin with B complex and folate (400 μg) for all patients after revascularization. There appear to be no disadvantages to this approach besides cost at this time.

### Other Potential Factors

Although deficiency of selenium, a natural antioxidant, has been suggested as a potential risk factor, multiple studies have shown no clear relation-

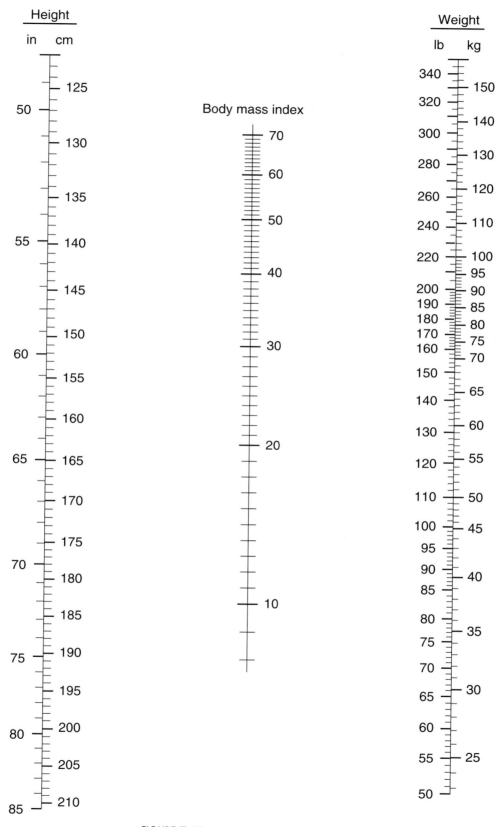

FIGURE 7–10. Body mass index nomogram.

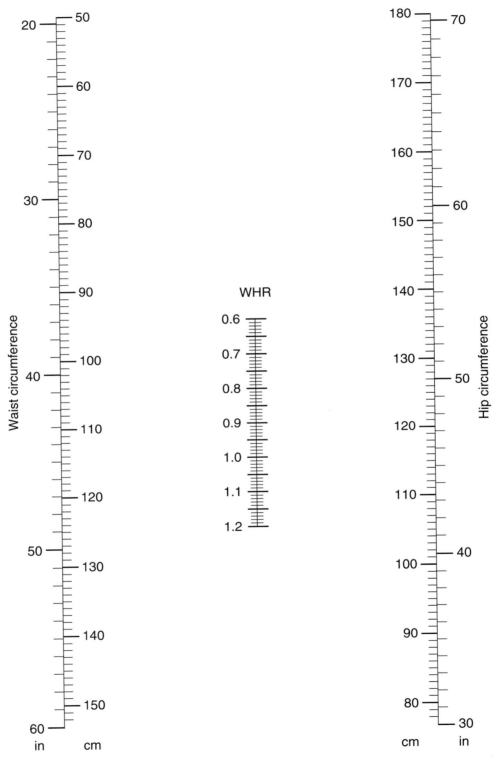

FIGURE 7–11. Waist-to-hip ratio (WHR) nomogram. A ratio exceeding 0.8 in women and exceeding 1.0 in men is predictive of increased risk of coronary heart disease.

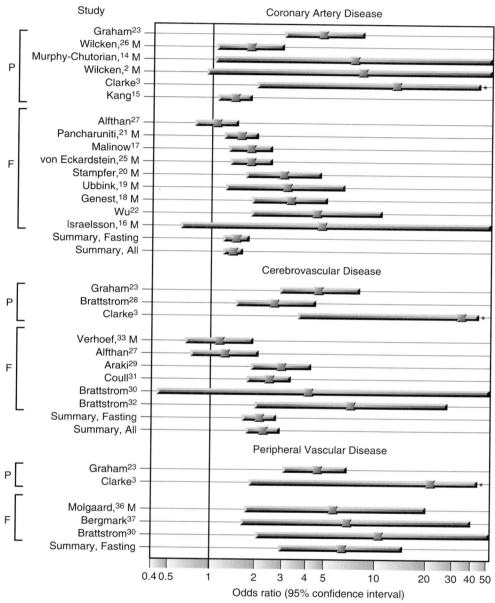

FIGURE 7–12. Odds ratio display for the relationship between fasting plasma (F) and post–methionine load test (P) measurements of homocysteine and vascular disease. (Adapted from Boushey CJ, Beresford SA, Omenn GS, et al: A quantitative assessment of plasma homocysteine as a risk factor for vascular disease. Probable benefits of increasing folic acid intake. JAMA 274:1049–1057, 1995.)

ship.[160-164] One small randomized trial suggested a benefit of selenium supplementation after myocardial infarction.[165] Epidemiologic and angiographic data do suggest that elevated fibrinogen levels and serum viscosity are related to cardiac events.[166, 168-170] There are a variety of other dietary and rheologic parameters under investigation, but they are beyond the scope of this text. For the interested reader, Hopkins and Williams have summarized more than 200 suggested coronary risk factors.[171]

## Risk Factors Assessed by Noninvasive Imaging

### Left Ventricular Hypertrophy

The prevalence of LVH as documented by echocardiography is approximately 15% of the U.S. population. Prevalence rates are higher in patients with obesity and hypertension. Left ventricular mass, whether inferred from LVH through electrocardiography or measured by echocardiography, has been shown to be an independent predictor of CHD (Fig. 7–13).[29, 172, 173] This relationship appears to be valid across age groups.[174] This finding has clinical importance in that LVH can be reduced by antihypertensive therapy, and this form of ventricular remodeling may be a mechanism for the reduced cardiac event rates observed in some hypertension trials. The mechanisms by which LVH and cardiac events may be related including modulation of angiotensin-converting enzyme, nitric oxide, and endothelin, with their corresponding influences on endothelial function, shear stress, and plaque stability, are the focus of several National Institutes of Health protocols.

### Coronary Calcification

In addition to LVH, coronary calcification represents a biologic variable measured with new technology that can be considered a risk factor in—or, more precisely, a marker of—early coronary disease.[175-177] Electron beam computed tomography of the chest has been shown to be a sensitive tool in identifying the presence of calcium in the coronary tree.[178-180] Studies are in progress to determine the population-based significance of screening and how it fits into traditional risk factor modification.

In summary, a large body of observational and experimental data supports risk factor analysis and coronary prevention measures. Preventive cardiology starts with primary care screening of blood pressure, lipid profiles, and glucose intolerance and counseling with regard to smoking cessation. Risk factor analysis aids in prediction of future CHD and cardiac events. Many risk factors (age, gender, diabetes, smoking, hypertension, LVH) contribute not only to atherosclerosis risk but also to revascularization morbidity and mortality. Unfortunately, patients have overt CHD by the time they reach the interventional cardiologist, and secondary prevention along with revascularization is the central issue. Reduction in cardiac risk factors and secondary prevention are now considered integral parts of care for the interventional cardiology patient.

## EPIDEMIOLOGY AND CORONARY INTERVENTION

Since the 1960s, the focus of cardiovascular epidemiologists has been on describing risk of CHD development in individuals and populations. More recent efforts in cardiovascular epidemiology have been aimed at describing relationships between various treatments administered and population outcomes. The aspect of epidemiology that has been of great interest to interventional cardiologists involves the observations of expanding interventional practice since 1980 both in the United States and abroad (Fig. 7–14). These observations have described large variations in procedure use between regions within the United States and between countries. As costs and efficiency in care move to the forefront of policy discussions, outcomes studies will play a critical role in shaping the future of interventional practice. This section highlights a few areas of investigation regarding epidemiology as it relates to interventional treatment.

## Use of Angiography After Myocardial Infarction

As of 1997, patients with acute transmural infarction who present early and without contraindications are usually considered for reperfusion therapy. Other areas in this book deal with the issues of

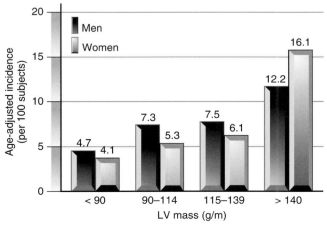

FIGURE 7–13. Relationship between left ventricular (LV) mass and 4-year age-adjusted incidence of coronary heart disease.

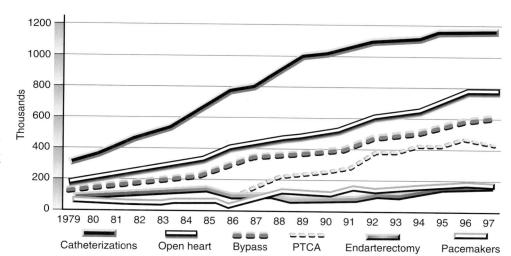

FIGURE 7–14. Trends in cardio-vascular procedure utilization in the United States over a 15-year period. PTCA, percutaneous transluminal coronary angio-plasty. (Adapted from the American Heart Association: 2000 Heart and Stroke Statistical Update. Dallas: American Heart Association, 1997.)

primary angioplasty. However, the most commonly used strategy worldwide is still thrombolytic therapy. Studies have shown wide national and global discrepancies with regard to the routine use of angiography after thrombolysis.[181, 182] When all clinical variables have been accounted for, these differences have been attributed to factors such as availability of angiography, specialty of treating physician, regional practice patterns, and patient's socioeconomic status.[182–187] Comparative studies between the United States and Canada, where the rates of angiography use are high and low, respectively, have shown no differences in population mortality (Fig. 7–15A–C).[188] However, several studies indicate that CHD patients in the United States have better functional status with less angina, improved quality of life measures, and higher return-to-work rates.[189] Examination of the elderly subgroup has revealed lower in-hospital mortality rates in the United States, but this benefit does not persist beyond 1 year; this outcome reflects the confounding effect of competing mortality from other illnesses.[190] Because multiple factors are involved, it has been difficult to isolate the independent effect of more aggressive practice patterns on positive patient outcomes over time, despite increasing use of angiography.[191]

## Use of Angioplasty in Stable and Unstable Coronary Syndromes

Multiple studies have shown that the number of angioplasty procedures performed each year in the United States continues to rise. In 1994, an estimated 428,000 angioplasty procedures were performed.[1] Use of interventional management in the treatment of stable angina and silent ischemia has been rising, according to several relatively small studies showing positive benefit in terms of morbidity and mortality.[192, 193] The rate of primary angioplasty for treatment of acute myocardial infarction

has been steadily growing despite a lack of growth of new catheterization laboratories or bypass surgery programs.[194] The use of primary angioplasty has been linked to urban centers with bypass surgery programs; however, determinants of its use on a patient basis have shown that in general, younger, lower risk patients have been receiving this form of treatment rather than thrombolytics.[195, 196] Studies from the mid-1990s indicate that early angiography and intervention for patients with acute coronary syndromes who are ineligible for thrombolysis are beneficial in terms of reducing morbidity and may constitute a future acceptable protocol, especially for the elderly, who are commonly excluded from thrombolysis.[197, 198] The American College of Cardiology National Cardiovascular Data Registry reported the procedural outcomes from 67 institutions involving 137,598 patients from 1991 to 1996 and provides an excellent source of future outcomes data with regard to the expanding use of coronary intervention.[199]

## Use of Bypass Surgery

The number of total bypass procedures still exceeds the number of angioplasties; an estimated 501,000 operations were carried out in 1994. The growth in bypass surgery appears to be much slower than that of percutaneous intervention, although with the advent of "mini-bypass" procedures, this rate can be expected to increase. As with angioplasty, there are differences in usage by various regions and countries. One comparative study between New York State and Ontario showed that adjusted rates of bypass surgery were higher in New York State, despite patients' having higher risk profiles.[200] There are clear trends for more bypass surgery in the elderly and in diabetic patients, according to the results of multiple clinical trials.[81, 88, 201–204] Public reporting of patient outcomes after surgery listed by individual

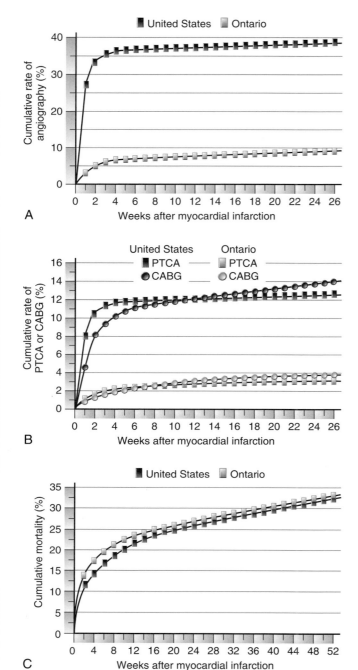

FIGURE 7-15. Procedure utilization rates (angiography, percutaneous transluminal coronary angioplasty [PTCA], or coronary artery bypass grafting [CABG]) and cumulative mortality plotted over the 2 to 4 years after myocardial infarction in the United States and Canada. These graphs represent 224,258 Medicare recipients in the United States and 9444 patients in Ontario, Canada, adjusted for age and sex. (Adapted from Tu JV, Pashos CL, Naylor CD, et al: Use of cardiac procedures and outcomes in elderly patients with myocardial infarction in the United States and Canada. N Engl J Med 336:1500–1505, 1997.)

surgeon in several states has raised concerns regarding future selection criteria for bypass candidates. Outcomes studies regarding the impact of this process from a public health perspective are not available at the time of this writing.

## SUMMARY

Knowledge regarding the epidemiology of CHD has become extensive and has provided the basis for risk factor analysis and ultimately successful coronary intervention from a medical and revascularization standpoint. All coronary risk models imply that prevention measures should be applied to patients under the care of the interventional cardiologist if they are not already in place. The epidemiology of CHD and the changing characteristics of the U.S. population have driven up rates of all cardiovascular procedures. Individual and population inequities exist with regard to the use of these procedures in the United States and elsewhere. Future outcomes studies and clinical trials are expected to provide a basis for refined local and national policy regarding procedure use integrated with secondary prevention in the treatment of stable and unstable coronary syndromes.

## REFERENCES

1. American Heart Association 1997 Heart and Stroke Statistical Update. Dallas: American Heart Association, 1997.
2. Fuster V, Badimon L, Badimon JJ, et al: The pathogenesis of coronary artery disease and the acute coronary syndromes (2). N Engl J Med 326:310–318, 1992.
3. Fuster V, Badimon L, Badimon JJ, et al: The pathogenesis of coronary artery disease and the acute coronary syndromes (1). N Engl J Med 326:242–250, 1992.
4. Castelli WP: Epidemiology of coronary heart disease: The Framingham study. Am J Med 76:4, 1984.
5. National Heart, Lung, and Blood Institute: The Framingham study: An epidemiological investigation of cardiovascular disease (Publication No. 87–2703). Washington DC: U.S. Government Printing Office, 1987.
8. Yano K, Reed DM, Kagan A: Coronary heart disease, hypertension and stroke among Japanese-American men in Hawaii: The Honolulu Heart Program. Hawaii Med J 44:297–300, 312, 1985.
9. Carter C, McGee D, Yano K: Morbidity and mortality rates in Okinawan Japanese vs. mainland Japanese: The Honolulu Heart Program. Hum Biol 56:339–353, 1984.
10. McGee DL, Reed DM, Yano K, et al: Ten-year incidence of coronary heart disease in the Honolulu Heart Program. Relationship to nutrient intake. Am J Epidemiol 119:667–676, 1984.
11. Benfante RJ, Reed DM, MacLean CJ, et al: Risk factors in middle age that predict early and late onset of coronary heart disease. J Clin Epidemiol 42:95–104, 1989.
12. Donahue RP, Abbott RD, Reed DM, et al: Physical activity and coronary heart disease in middle-aged and elderly men: The Honolulu Heart Program. Am J Public Health 78:683–685, 1988.
13. Benfante R, Yano K, Hwang LJ, et al: Elevated serum cholesterol is a risk factor for both coronary heart disease and thromboembolic stroke in Hawaiian Japanese men. Implications of shared risk. Stroke 25:814–820, 1994.
14. Reed D, Yano K: Predictors of arteriographically defined coronary stenosis in the Honolulu Heart Program. Comparisons of cohort and arteriography series analyses. Am J Epidemiol 134:111–122, 1991.
15. Garcia-Palmieri MR, Costas R Jr, Cruz-Vidal M, et al: Urban-rural differences in coronary heart disease in a low incidence area. The Puerto Rico heart study. Am J Epidemiol 107:206–215, 1978.
16. Garcia-Palmieri MR, Sorlie PD, Havlik RJ, et al: Urban-rural differences in 12 year coronary heart disease mortality: The

Puerto Rico Heart Health Program. J Clin Epidemiol 41:285–292, 1988.

17. Conti S, Farchi G, Menotti A: Coronary risk factors and excess mortality from all causes and specific causes. Int J Epidemiol 12:301–307, 1983.

18. Yano K, Rhoads G, Kagan A: Epidemiology of serum uric acid among 8000 Japanese-American men in Hawaii. J Chronic Dis 30:171–184, 1977.

19. Bothing S: WHO MONICA Project: Objectives and design. Int J Epidemiol 18:S29–S37, 1989.

20. The World Health Organization MONICA Project (Monitoring Trends and Determinants in Cardiovascular Disease): A major international collaboration. WHO MONICA Project Principal Investigators. J Clin Epidemiol 41:105–114, 1988.

21. Keil U, Kuulasmaa K: WHO MONICA Project: Risk factors. Int J Epidemiol 18:S46–S55, 1989 [published erratum, Int J Epidemiol 19:775, 1990].

22. Tunstall-Pedoe H, Kuulasmaa K, Amouyel P, et al: Myocardial infarction and coronary deaths in the World Health Organization MONICA Project. Registration procedures, event rates, and case-fatality rates in 38 populations from 21 countries in four continents. Circulation 90:583–612, 1994.

23. Heller RF, Dobson AJ, Alexander HM, et al: Changes in drug treatment and case fatality of patients with acute myocardial infarction. Observations from the Newcastle MONICA Project, 1984/1985 to 1988/1990. Med J Aust 157:83–86, 1992.

24. Thorvaldsen P, Asplund K, Kuulasmaa K, et al: Stroke incidence, case fatality, and mortality in the WHO MONICA project. World Health Organization Monitoring Trends and Determinants in Cardiovascular Disease. Stroke 26:361–367, 1995 [published errata, Stroke 26:1504, 2376, 1995].

25. Stegmayr B, Asplund K: Exploring the declining case fatality in acute stroke. Population-based observation in the northern Sweden MONICA Project. J Intern Med 240:143–149, 1996.

26. Janus ED, Postiglione A, Singh RB, et al: The modernization of Asia: Implications for coronary heart disease. Circulation 94:2671–2673, 1996.

27. Feinleib M: The Framingham study: Sample selection, follow-up, and methods of analyses. Natl Cancer Inst Monogr 67:59–64, 1985.

28. Higgins MW: The Framingham Heart Study: Review of epidemiological design and data, limitations and prospects. Prog Clin Biol Res 147:51–64, 1984.

29. Kannel WB: Left ventricular hypertrophy as a risk factor: The Framingham experience. J Hypertens Suppl 9:S3–S8, 1991 [discussion, J Hypertens Suppl S8–S9, 1991].

30. Myers RH, Kiely DK, Cupples LA, et al: Parental history is an independent risk factor for coronary artery disease: The Framingham study. Am Heart J 120:963–969, 1990.

31. Galderisi M, Lauer MS, Levy D: Echocardiographic determinants of clinical outcome in subjects with coronary artery disease (the Framingham Heart Study). Am J Cardiol 70:971–976, 1992.

32. Castelli WP, Garrison RJ, Wilson PW, et al: Incidence of coronary heart disease and lipoprotein cholesterol levels. The Framingham study. JAMA 256:2835–2838, 1986.

33. D'Agostino RB, Kannel WB, Belanger AJ, et al: Trends in CHD and risk factors at age 55–64 in the Framingham study. Int J Epidemiol 18:S67–S72, 1989.

34. Wilson PW, Anderson KM, Castelli WP: Twelve-year incidence of coronary heart disease in middle-aged adults during the era of hypertensive therapy: The Framingham offspring study. Am J Med 90:11–16, 1991 [published erratum, Am J Med 90:537, 1991].

35. The Multiple Risk Factor Intervention Trial (MRFIT). A national study of primary prevention of coronary heart disease. JAMA 235:825–827, 1976.

36. Zukel WJ, Paul O, Schnaper HW: The Multiple Risk Factor Intervention Trial (MRFIT): I. Historical perspective. Prev Med 10:387–401, 1981.

37. Sherwin R, Kaelber CT, Kezdi P, et al: The Multiple Risk Factor Intervention Trial (MRFIT): II. The development of the protocol. Prev Med 10:402–425, 1981.

38. Benfari RC: The Multiple Risk Factor Intervention Trial (MRFIT): III. The model for intervention. Prev Med 10:426–442, 1981.

39. Caggiula AW, Christakis G, Farrand M, et al: The Multiple Risk Factor Intervention Trial (MRFIT): IV. Intervention on blood lipids. Prev Med 10:443–475, 1981.

40. Hughes GH, Hymowitz N, Ockene JK, et al: The Multiple Risk Factor Intervention Trial (MRFIT): V. Intervention on smoking. Prev Med 10:476–500, 1981.

41. Neaton JD, Broste S, Cohen L, et al: The Multiple Risk Factor Intervention Trial (MRFIT): VII. A comparison of risk factor changes between the two study groups. Prev Med 10:519–543, 1981.

42. Stamler J, Wentworth D, Neaton JD: Is relationship between serum cholesterol and risk of premature death from coronary heart disease continuous and graded? Findings in 356,222 primary screenees of the Multiple Risk Factor Intervention Trial (MRFIT). JAMA 256:2823–2828, 1986.

43. Rosenman RH, Brand RJ, Jenkins D, et al: Coronary heart disease in Western Collaborative Group Study. Final follow-up experience of 8 1/2 years. JAMA 233:872–877, 1975.

44. Stamler J, Dyer AR, Shekelle RB, et al: Relationship of baseline major risk factors to coronary and all-cause mortality, and to longevity: Findings from long-term follow-up of Chicago cohorts. Cardiology 82:191–222, 1993.

45. Keil JE, Sutherland SE, Knapp RG, et al: Mortality rates and risk factors for coronary disease in black as compared with white men and women. N Engl J Med 329:73–78, 1993.

46. Ostrander LD Jr, Lamphiear DE: Coronary risk factors in a community. Findings in Tecumseh, Michigan. Circulation 53:152–156, 1976.

47. McGovern PG, Pankow JS, Shahar E, et al: Recent trends in acute coronary heart disease—Mortality, morbidity, medical care, and risk factors. The Minnesota Heart Survey Investigators. N Engl J Med 334:884–890, 1996.

48. Rabkin SW, Mathewson FA, Hsu PH: Relation of body weight to development of ischemic heart disease in a cohort of young North American men after a 26 year observation period: The Manitoba study. Am J Cardiol 39:452–458, 1977.

49. Wingard DL, Suarez L, Barrett-Connor E: The sex differential in mortality from all causes and ischemic heart disease. Am J Epidemiol 117:165–172, 1983.

50. Kaplan GA, Cohn BA, Cohen RD, et al: The decline in ischemic heart disease mortality: Prospective evidence from the Alameda County Study. Am J Epidemiol 127:1131–1142, 1988.

51. Wilhelmsen L, Johansson S, Ulvenstam G, et al: CHD in Sweden: Mortality, incidence and risk factors over 20 years in Gothenburg. Int J Epidemiol 18:S101–S108, 1989.

52. Hazuda HP, Stern MP, Gaskill SP, et al: Ethnic differences in health knowledge and behaviors related to the prevention and treatment of coronary heart disease. The San Antonio Heart Study. Am J Epidemiol 117:717–728, 1983.

53. Loaldi A, Annoni L, Apostolo A, et al: Coronary angiographic features in 2,234 patients with clinical suspicion of coronary heart disease without modifiable risk factors. Jpn Heart J 34:11–21, 1993.

54. Lesnefsky EJ, Lundergan CF, Hodgson JM, et al: Increased left ventricular dysfunction in elderly patients despite successful thrombolysis: The GUSTO-I angiographic experience. J Am Coll Cardiol 28:331–337, 1996.

55. Smith SC, Gilpin E, Ahnve S, et al: Outlook after acute myocardial infarction in the very elderly compared with that in patients aged 65 to 75 years. J Am Coll Cardiol 16:784–792, 1990.

56. Aguirre FV, McMahon RP, Mueller H, et al: Impact of age on clinical outcome and postlytic management strategies in patients treated with intravenous thrombolytic therapy. Results from the TIMI II Study. TIMI II Investigators. Circulation 90:78–86, 1994.

57. Summary of the second report of the National Cholesterol Education Program (NCEP) Expert Panel on Detection, Evaluation, and Treatment of High Blood Cholesterol in Adults (Adult Treatment Panel II) [Comment]. JAMA 269:3015–3023, 1993.

58. Lerner DJ, Kannel WB: Patterns of coronary heart disease

morbidity and mortality in the sexes: A 26-year follow-up of the Framingham population. Am Heart J 111:383–390, 1986.

59. Lapidus L, Bengtsson C, Lindquist O: Menopausal age and risk of cardiovascular disease and death. A 12-year follow-up of participants in the population study of women in Gothenburg, Sweden. Acta Obstet Gynecol Scand Suppl 130:37–41, 1985.

60. Criqui MH, Suarez L, Barrett-Connor E, et al: Postmenopausal estrogen use and mortality. Results from a prospective study in a defined, homogeneous community. Am J Epidemiol 128:606–614, 1988.

61. Gorodeski GI: Impact of the menopause on the epidemiology and risk factors of coronary artery heart disease in women. Exp Gerontol 29:357–375, 1994.

61a. Hulley S, Grady D, Bush T, et al: Randomized trial of estrogen plus progestin for secondary prevention of coronary heart disease in postmenopausal women. Heart and Estrogen/progestin Replacement Study (HERS) Research Group. JAMA 280:605–613, 1998.

62. Greenland P, Reicher-Reiss H, Goldbourt U, et al: In-hospital and 1-year mortality in 1,524 women after myocardial infarction. Comparison with 4,315 men. Circulation 83:484–491, 1991.

63. Cameron AA, Davis KB, Rogers WJ: Recurrence of angina after coronary artery bypass surgery: Predictors and prognosis (CASS Registry). Coronary Artery Surgery Study. J Am Coll Cardiol 26:895–899, 1995.

64. Craddock D, Iyer VS, Russell WJ: Factors influencing mortality and myocardial infarction after coronary artery bypass grafting. Curr Opin Cardiol 9:664–669, 1994.

65. Oweida SW, Roubin GS, Smith RB, et al: Postcatheterization vascular complications associated with percutaneous transluminal coronary angioplasty. J Vasc Surg 12:310–315, 1990.

66. Jenkins JS, Flaker GC, Nolte B, et al: Causes of higher in-hospital mortality in women than in men after acute myocardial infarction. Am J Cardiol 73:319–322, 1994.

67. Eysmann SB, Douglas PS: Reperfusion and revascularization strategies for coronary artery disease in women. JAMA 268:1903–1907, 1992.

68. Lincoff AM, Califf RM, Ellis SG, et al: Thrombolytic therapy for women with myocardial infarction: Is there a gender gap? Thrombolysis and Angioplasty in Myocardial Infarction Study Group. J Am Coll Cardiol 22:1780–1787, 1993.

69. Bell MR, Berger PB, Holmes DR, et al: Referral for coronary artery revascularization procedures after diagnostic coronary angiography: Evidence for gender bias? J Am Coll Cardiol 25:1650–1655, 1995.

70. Hutchinson LA, Pasternack PF, Baumann FG, et al: Is there detrimental gender bias in preoperative cardiac management of patients undergoing vascular surgery? Circulation 90:II-220–II-223, 1994.

71. Krumholz HM, Douglas PS, Lauer MS, et al: Selection of patients for coronary angiography and coronary revascularization early after myocardial infarction: Is there evidence for a gender bias? Ann Intern Med 116:785–790, 1992.

72. Schildkraut JM, Myers RH, Cupples LA, et al: Coronary risk associated with age and sex of parental heart disease in the Framingham Study. Am J Cardiol 64:555–559, 1989.

73. Hopkins PN, Williams RR, Kuida H, et al: Family history as an independent risk factor for incident coronary artery disease in a high-risk cohort in Utah. Am J Cardiol 62:703–707, 1988.

74. Grech ED, Ramsdale DR, Bray CL, et al: Family history as an independent risk factor of coronary artery disease. Eur Heart J 13:1311–1315, 1992.

75. Reed T, Fabsitz RR, Quiroga J: Family history of ischemic heart disease with respect to mean twin-pair cholesterol and subsequent ischemic heart disease in the NHLBI twin study. Genet Epidemiol 7:335–347, 1990.

76. Barrett-Connor E, Khaw K: Family history of heart attack as an independent predictor of death due to cardiovascular disease. Circulation 69:1065–1069, 1984.

77. Stamler J, Neaton JD, Wentworth DN: Blood pressure (systolic and diastolic) and risk of fatal coronary heart disease. Hypertension 13:I-2–I-12, 1989.

78. Collins R, Peto R, MacMahon S, et al: Blood pressure, stroke, and coronary heart disease: Part 2. Short-term reductions in blood pressure: Overview of randomised drug trials in their epidemiological context. Lancet 335:827–838, 1990.

79. Perry HM Jr, McDonald RH, Hulley SB, et al: Systolic Hypertension in the Elderly Program, Pilot Study (SHEP-PS): Morbidity and mortality experience. J Hypertens Suppl 4:S21–S23, 1986.

80. Carman WJ, Barrett-Connor E, Sowers M, et al: Higher risk of cardiovascular mortality among lean hypertensive individuals in Tecumseh, Michigan. Circulation 89:703–711, 1994.

81. Stein B, Weintraub WS, Gebhart SP, et al: Influence of diabetes mellitus on early and late outcome after percutaneous transluminal coronary angioplasty. Circulation 91:979–989, 1995.

82. Barrett-Connor E, Orchard TJ: Insulin-dependent diabetes mellitus and ischemic heart disease. Diabetes Care 8(suppl 1):65–70, 1985.

83. Barrett-Connor EL, Cohn BA, Wingard DL, et al: Why is diabetes mellitus a stronger risk factor for fatal ischemic heart disease in women than in men? The Rancho Bernardo Study. JAMA 265:627–631, 1991 [published erratum, JAMA 265:3249, 1991].

84. Perry IJ, Wannamethee SG, Whincup PH, et al: Serum insulin and incident coronary heart disease in middle-aged British men. Am J Epidemiol 144:224–234, 1996.

85. Despres JP, Marette A: Relation of components of insulin resistance syndrome to coronary disease risk. Curr Opin Lipidol 5:274–289, 1994.

86. Sharp SD, Williams RR, Hunt SC, et al: Coronary risk factors and the severity of angiographic coronary artery disease in members of high-risk pedigrees. Am Heart J 123:279–285, 1992.

87. Frye RL, Sopko G, Detre KM: The BARI trial: Baseline observations. The BARI Investigators. Trans Am Clin Climatol Assoc 104:26–30, 1992.

88. Comparison of coronary bypass surgery with angioplasty in patients with multivessel disease. The Bypass Angioplasty Revascularization Investigation (BARI) Investigators. N Engl J Med 335:217–225, 1996.

89. McCullough PA, Wolyn R, Rocher LL, et al: Acute contrast nephropathy after coronary intervention: Incidence, risk factors, and relationship to mortality [Abstract]. J Am Coll Cardiol 27:304A–305A, 1996.

90. Stemmermann GN, Chyou PH, Kagan A, et al: Serum cholesterol and mortality among Japanese-American men. The Honolulu (Hawaii) Heart Program. Arch Intern Med 151:969–972, 1991.

91. Reed D, Yano K, Kagan A: Lipids and lipoproteins as predictors of coronary heart disease, stroke, and cancer in the Honolulu Heart Program. Am J Med 80:871–878, 1986.

92. Carmelli D, Halpern J, Swan GE, et al: 27-Year mortality in the Western Collaborative Group Study: Construction of risk groups by recursive partitioning. J Clin Epidemiol 44:1341–1351, 1991.

93. Dyer AR, Stamler J, Shekelle RB: Serum cholesterol and mortality from coronary heart disease in young, middle-aged, and older men and women from three Chicago epidemiologic studies. Ann Epidemiol 2:51–57, 1992.

94. Keil JE, Sutherland SE, Knapp RG, et al: Serum cholesterol—Risk factor for coronary disease mortality in younger and older blacks and whites. The Charleston Heart Study, 1960–1988. Ann Epidemiol 2:93–99, 1992.

95. Higgins M, Keller JB: Cholesterol, coronary heart disease, and total mortality in middle-aged and elderly men and women in Tecumseh. Ann Epidemiol 2:69–76, 1992.

96. Waters D, Pedersen TR: Review of cholesterol-lowering therapy: Coronary angiographic and events trials. Am J Med 101:4A34S–38S, 1996.

97. Shepherd J, Cobbe SM, Ford I, et al: Prevention of coronary heart disease with pravastin in men with hypercholesterolemia. West of Scotland Coronary Prevention Study Group. N Engl J Med 333:1301–1307, 1995.

98. Sacks FM, Pfeffer MA, Moye LA, et al: The effect of pravastatin on coronary events after myocardial infarction in

patients with average cholesterol levels. Cholesterol and Recurrent Events Trial investigators. N Engl J Med 335:1001–1009, 1996.

99. Buchwald H, Varco RL, Matts JP, et al: Effect of partial ileal bypass surgery on mortality and morbidity from coronary heart disease in patients with hypercholesterolemia. Report of the Program on the Surgical Control of the Hyperlipidemias (POSCH). N Engl J Med 323:946–955, 1990.

100. Buchwald H, Matts JP, Fitch LL, et al: Changes in sequential coronary arteriograms and subsequent coronary events. Surgical Control of the Hyperlipidemias (POSCH) Group. JAMA 268:1429–1433, 1992.

101. Brown G, Albers JJ, Fisher LD, et al: Regression of coronary artery disease as a result of intensive lipid-lowering therapy in men with high levels of apolipoprotein B. N Engl J Med 323:1289–1298, 1990.

102. Maher VM, Brown BG, Marcovina SM, et al: Effects of lowering elevated LDL cholesterol on the cardiovascular risk of lipoprotein(a). JAMA 274:1771–1774, 1995.

103. Kroon AA, Aengevaeren WR, van-der-Werf T, et al: LDL-Apheresis Atherosclerosis Regression Study (LAARS). Effect of aggressive versus conventional lipid lowering treatment on coronary atherosclerosis. Circulation 93:1826–1835, 1996.

104. Jukema JW, Bruschke AV, van-Boven AJ, et al: Effects of lipid lowering by pravastatin on progression and regression of coronary artery disease in symptomatic men with normal to moderately elevated serum cholesterol levels. The Regression Growth Evaluation Statin Study (REGRESS). Circulation 91:2528–2540, 1995.

105. Blankenhorn DH, Azen SP, Kramsch DM, et al: Coronary angiographic changes with lovastatin therapy. The Monitored Atherosclerosis Regression Study (MARS). The MARS Research Group. Ann Intern Med 119:969–976, 1993.

106. Watts GF, Lewis B, Brunt JN, et al: Effects on coronary artery disease of lipid-lowering diet, or diet plus cholestyramine, in the St Thomas' Atherosclerosis Regression Study (STARS). Lancet 339:563–569, 1992.

107. Waters D, Lesperance J: Regression of coronary atherosclerosis: An achievable goal? Review of results from recent clinical trials. Am J Med 91:10S–17S, 1991.

108. Thompson GR, Maher VM, Matthews S, et al: Familial Hypercholesterolaemia Regression Study: A randomised trial of low-density-lipoprotein apheresis. Lancet 345:811–816, 1995.

109. Anderson TJ, Meredith IT, Yeung AC, et al: The effect of cholesterol-lowering and antioxidant therapy on endothelium-dependent coronary vasomotion. N Engl J Med 332:488–493, 1995.

110. Treasure CB, Klein JL, Weintraub WS, et al: Beneficial effects of cholesterol-lowering therapy on the coronary endothelium in patients with coronary artery disease. N Engl J Med 332:481–487, 1995.

111. Sacks FM, Gerhard M, Walsh BW: Sex hormones, lipoproteins, and vascular reactivity. Curr Opin Lipidol 6:161–166, 1995.

112. Ridker PM, Vaughan DE, Stampfer MJ, et al: A cross-sectional study of endogenous tissue plasminogen activator, total cholesterol, HDL cholesterol, and apolipoproteins A-I, A-II, and B-100. Arterioscler Thromb 13:1587–1592, 1993.

113. Koenig W, Sund M, Ernst E, et al: Association between rheology and components of lipoproteins in human blood. Results from the MONICA project. Circulation 85:2197–2204, 1992.

114. Murie J, Tuohy AP, Carroll D: Impact of a health promotion programme on multiple risk factors for CHD: A preliminary evaluation. Scott Med J 39:12–16, 1994.

115. Manninen V, Tenkanen L, Koskinen P, et al: Joint effects of serum triglyceride and LDL cholesterol and HDL cholesterol concentrations on coronary heart disease risk in the Helsinki Heart Study. Implications for treatment. Circulation 85:37–45, 1992.

115a. Rubins HB, Robins SJ, Collins D, et al: Gemfibrozil for the secondary prevention of coronary heart disease in men with low levels of high-density lipoprotein cholesterol. Veterans

Affairs High-Density Lipoprotein Cholesterol Intervention Trial Study Group. N Engl J Med 341:410–418, 1999.

116. Carlson LA, Rosenhamer G: Reduction of mortality in the Stockholm Ischaemic Heart Disease Secondary Prevention Study by combined treatment with clofibrate and nicotinic acid. Acta Med Scand 223:405–418, 1988.

117. Sorrentino MJ, Vielhauer C, Eisenbart JD, et al: Plasma lipoprotein (a) protein concentration and coronary artery disease in black patients compared with white patients. Am J Med 93:658–662, 1992.

118. Kannel WB, Neaton JD, Wentworth D, et al: Overall and coronary heart disease mortality rates in relation to major risk factors in 325,348 men screened for the MRFIT. Multiple Risk Factor Intervention Trial. Am Heart J 112:825–836, 1986.

119. Vlietstra RE, Kronmal RA, Oberman A, et al: Effect of cigarette smoking on survival of patients with angiographically documented coronary artery disease. Report from the CASS registry. JAMA 255:1023–1027, 1986.

120. Steenland K, Thun M, Lally C, et al: Environmental tobacco smoke and coronary heart disease in the American Cancer Society CPS-II cohort. Circulation 94:622–628, 1996.

121. Cooper RS, Ford E: Comparability of risk factors for coronary heart disease among blacks and whites in the NHANES-I Epidemiologic Follow-up Study. Ann Epidemiol 2:637–645, 1992.

122. Cooper RS, Ghali JK: Coronary heart disease: Black-white differences. Cardiovasc Clin 21:205–225, 1991.

123. Fang J, Madhavan S, Alderman MH: The association between birthplace and mortality from cardiovascular causes among black and white residents of New York City. N Engl J Med 335:1545–1551, 1996.

124. Mitchell BD, Haffner SM, Hazuda HP, et al: Diabetes and coronary heart disease risk in Mexican Americans. Ann Epidemiol 2:101–106, 1996 [published erratum, Ann Epidemiol 3:117, 1993].

125. Kurita A, Takase B, Uehata A, et al: Differences in plasma beta-endorphin and bradykinin levels between patients with painless or with painful myocardial ischemia. Am Heart J 123:304–309, 1992.

126. Posadas-Romero C, Tapia-Conyer R, Lerman-Garber I, et al: Cholesterol levels and prevalence of hypercholesterolemia in a Mexican adult population. Atherosclerosis 118:275–284, 1995.

127. Hubert HB, Feinleib M, McNamara PM, et al: Obesity as an independent risk factor for cardiovascular disease: A 26-year follow-up of participants in the Framingham Heart Study. Circulation 67:968–977, 1983.

128. Costas P Jr, Garcia-Palmieri MR, Nazario E, et al: Relation of lipids, weight and physical activity to incidence of coronary heart disease: The Puerto Rico heart study. Am J Cardiol 42:653–658, 1978.

129. Paffenbarger RS Jr, Hyde RT, Wing AL, et al: The association of changes in physical-activity level and other lifestyle characteristics with mortality among men. N Engl J Med 328:538–545, 1993.

130. Paffenbarger RS Jr, Hyde RT, Wing AL, et al: A natural history of athleticism and cardiovascular health. JAMA 252:491–495, 1984.

131. Garcia-Palmieri MR, Costas R Jr, Cruz-Vidal M, et al: Increased physical activity: A protective factor against heart attacks in Puerto Rico. Am J Cardiol 50:749–755, 1982.

132. O'Connor GT, Buring JE, Yusuf S, et al: An overview of randomized trials of rehabilitation with exercise after myocardial infarction. Circulation 80:234–244, 1989.

133. Siegler IC, Peterson BL, Barefoot JC, et al: Hostility during late adolescence predicts coronary risk factors at mid-life. Am J Epidemiol 136:146–154, 1992.

133a. Ridker PM, Cushman M, Stampfer MJ, et al: Inflammation, aspirin, and the risk of cardiovascular disease in apparently healthy men. N Engl J Med 336:973–979, 1997.

134. Genest JJ, McNamara JR, Salem DN, et al: Plasma homocyst(e)ine levels in men with premature coronary artery disease. J Am Coll Cardiol 16:1114–1119, 1990.

135. Gallagher PM, Meleady R, Shields DC, et al: Homocysteine

and risk of premature coronary heart disease. Evidence for a common gene mutation. Circulation 94:2154–2158, 1996.

136. Arnesen E, Refsum H, Bonaa KH, et al: Serum total homocysteine and coronary heart disease. Int J Epidemiol 24:704–709, 1995.

137. Gunby P: Lipoprotein patterns, plaque, homocysteine, and hormones among ongoing cardiology studies [News]. JAMA 276:1122–1127, 1996.

138. Boushey CJ, Beresford SA, Omenn GS, et al: A quantitative assessment of plasma homocysteine as a risk factor for vascular disease. Probable benefits of increasing folic acid intake. JAMA 274:1049–1057, 1995.

138a. Eikelboom JW, Lonn E, Genest J Jr, et al: Homocyst(e)ine and cardiovascular disease: A critical review of the epidemiologic evidence. Ann Intern Med 131:363–375, 1999.

139. Renaud S, De-Lorgeril M: Wine, alcohol, platelets, and the French paradox for coronary heart disease. Lancet 339:1523–1526, 1992.

140. Langer RD, Criqui MH, Reed DM: Lipoproteins and blood pressure as biological pathways for effect of moderate alcohol consumption on coronary heart disease. Circulation 85:910–915, 1992.

141. Boffetta P, Garfinkel L: Alcohol drinking and mortality among men enrolled in an American Cancer Society prospective study. Epidemiology 1:342–348, 1990.

142. Stampfer MJ, Colditz GA, Willett WC, et al: A prospective study of moderate alcohol consumption and the risk of coronary disease and stroke in women. N Engl J Med 319:267–273, 1988.

143. Woodward M, Tunstall-Pedoe H: Alcohol consumption, diet, coronary risk factors, and prevalent coronary heart disease in men and women in the Scottish heart health study. J Epidemiol Community Health 49:354–362, 1995.

144. Ducimetiere P, Guize L, Marciniak A, et al: Arteriographically documented coronary artery disease and alcohol consumption in French men. The CORALI Study. Eur Heart J 14:727–733, 1993.

145. Friedman LA, Kimball AW. Coronary heart disease mortality and alcohol consumption in Framingham. Am J Epidemiol 124:481–489, 1986.

146. Rimm EB, Ascherio A, Giovannucci E, et al: Vegetable, fruit, and cereal fiber intake and risk of coronary heart disease among men. JAMA 275:447–451, 1996.

147. Khaw KT, Barrett-Connor E: Dietary fiber and reduced ischemic heart disease mortality rates in men and women: A 12-year prospective study. Am J Epidemiol 126:1093–1102, 1987.

148. Marckmann P, Sandstrom B, Jespersen J: Low-fat, high-fiber diet favorably affects several independent risk markers of ischemic heart disease: Observations on blood lipids, coagulation, and fibrinolysis from a trial of middle-aged Danes. Am J Clin Nutr 59:935–939, 1994.

149. Fraser GE, Sabate J, Beeson WL, et al: A possible protective effect of nut consumption on risk of coronary heart disease. The Adventist Health Study. Arch Intern Med 152:1416–1424, 1992.

150. Morris MC, Manson JE, Rosner B, et al: Fish consumption and cardiovascular disease in the Physicians' Health Study: A prospective study. Am J Epidemiol 142:166–175, 1995.

151. Daviglus ML, Stamler J, Orencia AJ, et al: Fish consumption and the 30-year risk of fatal myocardial infarction. N Engl J Med 336:1046–1053, 1997.

152. Todd S, Woodward M, Bolton-Smith C: An investigation of the relationship between antioxidant vitamin intake and coronary heart disease in men and women using logistic regression analysis. J Clin Epidemiol 48:307–316, 1995.

153. Gaziano JM: Antioxidant vitamins and coronary artery disease risk. Am J Med 97:18S–21S, 1994.

154. Pandey DK, Shekelle R, Selwyn BJ, et al: Dietary vitamin C and beta-carotene and risk of death in middle-aged men. The Western Electric Study. Am J Epidemiol 142:1269–1278, 1995.

155. Hodis HN, Mack WJ, LaBree L, et al: Serial coronary angiographic evidence that antioxidant vitamin intake reduces progression of coronary artery atherosclerosis. JAMA 273:1849–1854, 1995.

156. Yusuf S, Dagenais G, Pogue J, et al: Vitamin E supplementation and cardiovascular events in high-risk patients. The Heart Outcomes Prevention Evaluation Study Investigators. N Engl J Med 342:154–160, 2000.

157. Hennekens CH, Buring JE, Manson JE, et al: Lack of effect of long-term supplementation with beta carotene on the incidence of malignant neoplasms and cardiovascular disease. N Engl J Med 334:1145–1149, 1996.

160. Luoma PV, Nayha S, Sikkila K, et al: High serum alpha-tocopherol, albumin, selenium and cholesterol, and low mortality from coronary heart disease in northern Finland. J Intern Med 237:49–54, 1995.

161. Bukkens SG, de Vos N, Kok FJ, et al: Selenium status and cardiovascular risk factors in healthy Dutch subjects. J Am Coll Nutr 9:128–135, 1990.

162. Jossa F, Trevisan M, Krogh V, et al: Serum selenium and coronary heart disease risk factors in southern Italian men. Atherosclerosis 87:129–134, 1991.

163. Salonen JT: Selenium in ischaemic heart disease. Int J Epidemiol 16:323–328, 1987.

164. Virtamo J, Valkeila E, Alfthan G, et al: Serum selenium and the risk of coronary heart disease and stroke. Am J Epidemiol 122:276–282, 1985.

165. Korpela H, Kumpulainen J, Jussila E, et al: Effect of selenium supplementation after acute myocardial infarction. Res Commun Chem Pathol Pharmacol 65:249–252, 1989.

166. Yarnell JW, Baker IA, Sweetnam PM, et al: Fibrinogen, viscosity, and white blood cell count are major risk factors for ischemic heart disease. The Caerphilly and Speedwell collaborative heart disease studies. Circulation 83:836–844, 1991.

168. Eichner JE, Moore WE, McKee PA, et al: Fibrinogen levels in women having coronary angiography. Am J Cardiol 78:15–18, 1996.

169. Becker RC, Cannon CP, Bovill EG, et al: Prognostic value of plasma fibrinogen concentration in patients with unstable angina and non-Q-wave myocardial infarction (TIMI IIIB Trial). Am J Cardiol 78:142–147, 1996.

170. Barasch E, Benderly M, Graff E, et al: Plasma fibrinogen levels and their correlates in 6457 coronary heart disease patients. The Bezafibrate Infarction Prevention (BIP) Study. J Clin Epidemiol 48:757–765, 1995.

171. Hopkins PN, Williams RR: A survey of 246 suggested coronary risk factors. Atherosclerosis 40:1–52, 1981.

172. Levy D, Garrison RJ, Savage DD, et al: Left ventricular mass and incidence of coronary heart disease in an elderly cohort. The Framingham Heart Study. Ann Intern Med 110:101–107, 1989.

173. Galderisi M, Lauer MS, Levy D: Echocardiographic determinants of clinical outcome in subjects with coronary artery disease (the Framingham Heart Study). Am J Cardiol 70:971–976, 1992.

174. Gardin JM, Siscovick D, Anton-Culver H, et al: Sex, age, and disease affect echocardiographic left ventricular mass and systolic function in the free-living elderly. The Cardiovascular Health Study. Circulation 91:1739–1748, 1995.

175. Detrano R, Hsiai T, Wang S, et al: Prognostic value of coronary calcification and angiographic stenoses in patients undergoing coronary angiography. J Am Coll Cardiol 27:285–290, 1996.

176. Fallavollita JA, Brody AS, Bunnell IL, et al: Fast computed tomography detection of coronary calcification in the diagnosis of coronary artery disease. Comparison with angiography in patients <50 years old. Circulation 89:285–290, 1994.

177. Loecker TH, Schwartz RS, Cotta CW, et al: Fluoroscopic coronary artery calcification and associated coronary disease in asymptomatic young men. J Am Coll Cardiol 19:1167–1172, 1992.

178. Wexler L, Brundage B, Crouse J, et al: Coronary artery calcification: Pathophysiology, epidemiology, imaging methods, and clinical implications. A statement for health professionals from the American Heart Association Writing Group. Circulation 94:1175–1192, 1996.

179. Mahoney LT, Burns TL, Stanford W, et al: Coronary risk factors measured in childhood and young adult life are

associated with coronary artery calcification in young adults: The Muscatine Study. J Am Coll Cardiol 27:277–284, 1996.

180. Kajinami K, Seki H, Takekoshi N, et al: Noninvasive prediction of coronary atherosclerosis by quantification of coronary artery calcification using electron beam computed tomography: Comparison with electrocardiographic and thallium exercise stress test results. J Am Coll Cardiol 26:1209–1221, 1995.

181. Pilote L, Califf RM, Sapp S, et al: Regional variation across the United States in the management of acute myocardial infarction. GUSTO-1 Investigators. Global Utilization of Streptokinase and Tissue Plasminogen Activator for Occluded Coronary Arteries. N Engl J Med 333:565–572, 1995.

182. McCullough PA, O'Neill WW: Influence of regional cardiovascular mortality on the use of angiography after acute myocardial infarction. Am J Cardiol 79:575–580, 1997.

183. Rogers WJ, Bowlby LJ, Chandra NC, et al: Treatment of myocardial infarction in the United States (1990 to 1993). Observations from the National Registry of Myocardial Infarction. Circulation 90:2103–2114, 1994.

184. Henderson RA, Raskino CL, Hampton JR: Variations in the use of coronary arteriography in the UK: The RITA trial coronary arteriogram register. Q J Med 88:167–173, 1995.

185. Spertus JA, Weiss NS, Every NR, et al: The influence of clinical risk factors on the use of angiography and revascularization after acute myocardial infarction. Myocardial Infarction Triage and Intervention Project Investigators. Arch Intern Med 155:2309–2316, 1995.

186. Every NR, Fihn SD, Maynard C, et al: Resource utilization in treatment of acute myocardial infarction: Staff-model health maintenance organization versus fee-for-service hospitals. The MITI Investigators. Myocardial Infarction Triage and Intervention. J Am Coll Cardiol 26:401–406, 1995.

187. Pilote L, Granger C, Armstrong PW, et al: Differences in the treatment of myocardial infarction between the United States and Canada. A survey of physicians in the GUSTO trial. Med Care 33:598–610, 1995.

188. Pilote L, Racine N, Hlatky MA: Differences in the treatment of myocardial infarction in the United States and Canada. A comparison of two university hospitals. Arch Intern Med 154:1090–1096, 1994.

189. Pilote L, Bourassa MG, Bacon C, et al: Better functional status in American than Canadian patients with heart disease: An effect of medical care? J Am Coll Cardiol 26:1115–1120, 1995.

190. Tu JV, Pashos CL, Naylor CD, et al: Use of cardiac procedures and outcomes in elderly patients with myocardial infarction in the United States and Canada. N Engl J Med 336:1500–1505, 1997.

191. Nicod P, Gilpin EA, Dittrich H, et al: Trends in use of coronary angiography in subacute phase of myocardial infarction. Circulation 84:1004–1015, 1991.

192. Bourassa MG, Knatterud GL, Pepine CJ, et al: Asymptomatic Cardiac Ischemia Pilot (ACIP) Study. Improvement of cardiac ischemia at 1 year after PTCA and CABG. Circulation 92:II-1–II-7, 1995.

193. Rogers WJ, Bourassa MG, Andrews TC, et al: Asymptomatic Cardiac Ischemia Pilot (ACIP) study: Outcome at 1 year for patients with asymptomatic cardiac ischemia randomized to medical therapy or revascularization. The ACIP Investigators. J Am Coll Cardiol 26:594–605, 1995.

194. Rogers WJ, Chandra NC, French WJ, et al: Trends in the use of reperfusion therapy: Experience from the Second National Registry of Myocardial Infarction (NRMI-2) [Abstract]. Circulation 94:I-196, 1996.

195. Sada MJ, French WJ, Gore JM, et al: Primary PTCA in the United States: Determinants of use [Abstract]. Circulation 94:I-532, 1996.

196. Paul SD, Lambrew CT, Rogers WJ, et al: A study of 118,276 patients with acute myocardial infarction in the United States in 1995: Less aggressive care, worse prognosis, and longer hospital stay in diabetics [Abstract]. Circulation 94:I-610–I-611, 1996.

197. McCullough PA, O'Neill WW, Graham M, et al: A prospective randomized trial of triage angiography in suspected acute myocardial infarction patients who are considered ineligible for reperfusion therapy [Abstract]. Circulation 94:I-570, 1996.

198. Ellerbeck EF, Jencks SF, Radford MJ, et al: Quality of care for Medicare patients with acute myocardial infarction. A four-state pilot study from the Cooperative Cardiovascular Project. JAMA 273:1509–1514, 1995.

199. Weintraub WS: Data management, outcomes assessment and information in cardiovascular practice. J Invasive Cardiol 8:127–131, 1996.

200. Tu JV, Naylor CD, Kumar D, et al: Coronary artery bypass graft surgery in Ontario and New York State: Which rate is right? Steering Committee of the Cardiac Care Network of Ontario. Ann Intern Med 126:13–19, 1997.

201. Weintraub WS, Wenger NK, Jones EL, et al: Changing clinical characteristics of coronary surgery patients. Differences between men and women. Circulation 88:II-79–II-86, 1993.

202. Weintraub WS, Jones EL, King SB, et al: Changing use of coronary angioplasty and coronary bypass surgery in the treatment of chronic coronary artery disease. Am J Cardiol 65:183–188, 1990.

203. King SB 3rd, Lembo NJ, Weintraub WS, et al: A randomized trial comparing coronary angioplasty with coronary bypass surgery. Emory Angioplasty versus Surgery Trial (EAST). N Engl J Med 331:1044–1050, 1994.

204. Coronary angioplasty versus coronary artery bypass surgery: The Randomised Intervention Treatment of Angina (RITA) trial. Lancet 341:573–580, 1993.

# 8

# Assessment of Prognosis in Patients with Coronary Artery Disease

*Daniel B. Mark*

Coronary artery disease (CAD) is a chronic illness with which many patients must live for decades. During the life span of a given patient, the disease typically cycles in and out of a number of clinically defined phases, such as unstable angina and acute myocardial infarction (MI).[1, 2] Each phase provides new hazards for the patient and new challenges for the physician. Understanding the risks present at each point in the patient's illness and the likely effects of available treatments on these risks is a crucial part of medical practice. Furthermore, because all clinical decision-making is ultimately driven by the clinician's and patient's assessments of risk[3] (Fig. 8–1), either explicit or implicit, a careful study of prognostic assessment is essential to understanding the proper role of interventional cardiology in the care of patients with CAD.

Since the previous edition of this book was published in 1994, the tools and techniques of interventional cardiology have continued to demonstrate dramatic evolution. Although such innovations have undoubtedly improved the procedures and broadened the population for whom such therapy is an option, they have also created a moving target for those wishing to link individual technologic advances to clinical outcomes. Often, techniques or approaches are rendered obsolete by "new technology" before we have accumulated a full picture of

the outcomes associated with the "old technology." Thus, prognostic assessment, of necessity, blends empirical observations with models specifying structural or functional links among patient characteristics, treatment effects, and clinical outcomes.

This chapter reviews the prognostic assessment of the patient with CAD. Five main topics are considered. First, aspects of the history of prognostic assessment in cardiology are highlighted to provide a contextual framework for the remaining discussion. Second, general methodologic issues relating to risk assessment in CAD are discussed. Third, the main clinical syndromes of CAD are reviewed, with primary concentration on the medically treated patient and emphasis on the continuum of risk that exists in this disease. Fourth, the effects of medical therapy itself on the natural history of CAD are examined. Finally, a general introduction to the ways in which coronary revascularization may affect patient outcomes is provided. The benefits of revascularization therapy are discussed further in subsequent chapters.

## HISTORICAL BACKGROUND

At its inception, cardiology was largely a diagnostic or observational discipline. Physicians monitored

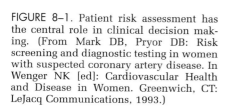

FIGURE 8–1. Patient risk assessment has the central role in clinical decision making. (From Mark DB, Pryor DB: Risk screening and diagnostic testing in women with suspected coronary artery disease. In Wenger NK [ed]: Cardiovascular Health and Disease in Women. Greenwich, CT: LeJacq Communications, 1993.)

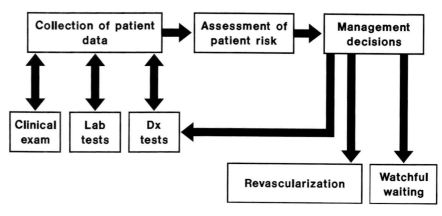

patients for many years and watched as the natural history of the disease unfolded. After their patients died, doctors used the autopsy examination to validate suppositions developed during those years of follow-up. The careful and insightful natural history observations of the most gifted clinical investigators, Paul Dudley White, Samuel Levine, and Paul Woods, among others, were published in classic papers and textbooks, establishing the foundation for the modern discipline of cardiology. Many of their ideas can still be found in current textbooks.

The development of selective coronary angiography by Sones in 1958 provided clinicians with a more accessible method than autopsy for confirming diagnostic suppositions.[4] Angiography also allowed them to study the natural history of the disease as a function of different levels of anatomic disease severity.[5, 6] With the introduction of coronary bypass surgery by Favoloro, Sabiston, and others during the mid-1960s, clinicians obtained a powerful tool for altering that natural history.

Around this time, Eugene Stead became one of the first modern physicians to recognize the limitations of the clinician's memory as the primary source of data about patient outcomes with alternative treatments. During the mid-1960s, he pioneered the clinical use of computers to supplement physicians in developing a complete picture of outcomes after different treatments. The result was the Duke Databank for Cardiovascular Disease, now the oldest and largest ongoing registry of cardiovascular patients in the world.[7] Stead's original idea was that having all clinicians at Duke record the details of their patients directly in the Databank and then monitoring these patients systematically over time would enable the rapid development of a depth and breadth of information that would exceed that of the most experienced clinician.[8–11] Furthermore, the computerized Databank was not unduly influenced by the experience of a recent "miraculous save" or a terrible complication and did not suffer from selective recall problems, as most clinicians do.

At the same time that Stead and colleagues were initiating the use of computers in clinical medicine, the disciplines of biostatistics and clinical epidemiology were developing more structured, scientific methods for using clinical experience to make accurate prognostic predictions.[12–16] The next section reviews some basic methodologic issues related to the epidemiologic and statistical aspects of risk assessment.

## METHODOLOGIC PRINCIPLES

### General Issues

All prognostic assessment is, in essence, an attempt to predict the future from a knowledge of the past.

Traditionally, physicians have approached this area quite informally, relying heavily on their own remembered clinical experiences, their understanding of relevant pathophysiology (i.e., their conceptual model of what is going on), and their interpretation of selected portions of the medical literature.[17–19] Informal methods of prognostic prediction often involve forming a gestalt impression of risk (e.g., "high" or "low" risk) through the use of simple heuristics or rules of thumb and past experience, both personal and literature based. For example, in patients with suspected CAD presenting for initial evaluation, a clinician might decide that any patient with an "early positive" exercise treadmill test value (or some such equivalent result) is at "high risk" and deserves prompt invasive evaluation but that other patients can be managed less aggressively. Or a clinician might maintain that a patient with an ulcerated plaque in the proximal right coronary artery and good left ventricular (LV) function is at "high risk" and requires immediate revascularization, because the clinician can remember two previous patients with a "similar" picture who died suddenly while being treated medically.

Informal risk assessments pose several potential problems that can ultimately affect the quality of clinical care. For example, in the preceding situations, the clinician is rarely required to specify what is meant by *high risk*, and the term clearly has different meanings for different physicians. The management decisions that flow from such informal risk assessments, therefore, may vary substantially from one clinician to the next and even over time for an individual clinician. In addition, clinicians virtually never formally evaluate the accuracy of the risk stratification algorithms they use in their own practices. Finally, in assessing risk or any other probabilistic event, clinicians can consider only a small number of characteristics at one time and are unable to account for overlapping prognostic information coming from highly correlated measures.

Unrecognized or unaccounted-for correlations among variables can lead a clinician using informal risk assessment to overestimate the importance of characteristics, resulting in biased projections. For example, the LV ejection fraction and the number of diseased vessels are two of the most important prognostic variables in a CAD population. They are also at least moderately correlated, meaning that to some extent they provide the same rather than independent prognostic information. In CAD, the ejection fraction is depressed because of prior MIs or "hibernating" myocardium[20] due to severe coronary lesions in the vessels supplying the areas in question. Thus, the higher the number of segments of the left ventricle that are damaged (with consequent depression of the ejection fraction), the greater the likelihood of multivessel disease.

Similar types of overlap exist for a host of other prognostic variables. There is, for example, a great deal of overlap between catheterization and exercise test variables. We conceptualize the former as "anatomic data" and the latter as "functional data," but in reality the divisions are not so clear-cut. Exercise ejection fraction and the change in ejection fractions from rest to peak exercise (measures of function) are substantially correlated with resting ejection fraction and number of diseased vessels (measures of anatomy). Each provides unique information as well, but again, the situation is not entirely straightforward. Whether prognostic information is unique or not largely depends on what is already known about a patient. An exercise test may provide a great deal of new information about a patient if the only evaluations performed thus far are a history and physical examination or relatively little if the results of cardiac catheterization are already known.

Any discipline or activity that depends on the ability to make predictions of future outcomes from past experience requires a formal methodology for developing predictions that are accurate and reproducible.[15, 16, 21] This is true for such seemingly disparate activities as weather forecasting and prognostic assessment of patients with CAD. The use of more formal risk stratification tools provides the clinician with additional accuracy and standardization over unguided gestalt impressions. Examples of such tools are diagnostic and therapeutic algorithms and prognostic nomograms (Fig. 8–2). Statistical models go even further in providing the clinician with state-of-the-art tools for assessing prognosis (see later discussion). The advantages of such models are that they can take into account many important pieces of clinical data that have been collected on the patient, attribute to each its proper weight or importance, and account for the overlap of information resulting from the correlations present among variables.

There are three major limitations of statistical models for prognostic assessment. First, they are computationally complex, making them unappealing and inconvenient for busy clinicians to use. Implementation of the model calculations on a computer can overcome at least some of this problem. Second, prognostic statistical models may provide detailed, accurate predictions of outcome, but they offer no accompanying advice to the clinician about what management decision to make. Perhaps it is not so important to be able to distinguish a patient

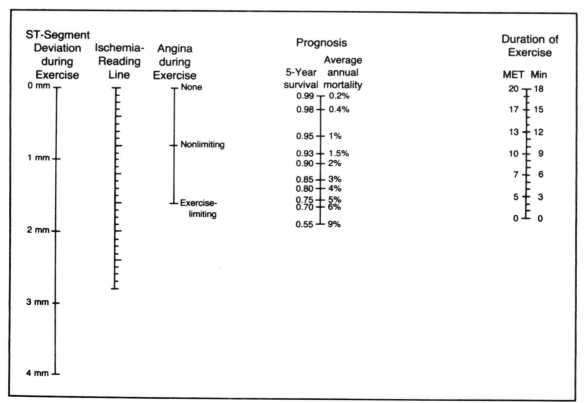

FIGURE 8–2. Duke prognostic treadmill score nomogram provides an example of a method for structuring risk stratification when only a limited number of variables need to be considered. Using the exercise ST response, the occurrence of exercise-induced angina, and the duration of exercise, it is possible to estimate 5-year survival or average annual mortality. MET, maximal exercise tolerance. (From Mark DB, Shaw L, Harrell FE, et al: Prognostic value of a treadmill exercise score in outpatients with suspected coronary artery disease. N Engl J Med 325:849, 1991.)

with a 75% 5-year survival estimate from one with a 65% 5-year survival estimate if they are both to be regarded as "high risk" and managed according to a clinician's "high-risk" algorithm. Although this observation may certainly be true at present, current pressures on the health care system to contain costs may soon persuade doctors of the value of going beyond simple algorithms and predicting how much benefit or value will be associated with a given management decision. Finally, there is no agreement on a uniform set of standards for evaluating the quality of predictions generated by a prognostic model, as would be required for any new laboratory test to be used in medical practice.[15, 22] In the absence of such standards and associated quality control, it is not clear that the use by an individual practitioner of a prognostic model derived from the medical literature would automatically ensure better risk stratification and subsequent decision-making than the less quantitative methods discussed previously.

Two main types of problems can interfere with valid generalization (with the use of either formal models or informal or gestalt assessments) from one patient group to another.

1. The biology of the disease process differs between groups in ways that affect outcome importantly.
2. In one or both of the groups, selection and other biases may alter the apparent relationship between prognostic factors and outcome in ways that are difficult to recognize and quantify.

Differences in biology can be accounted for in prognostic studies if the differences are properly recognized and understood. Failure to understand the underlying biology adequately is one of the main sources of inaccuracy in prognostic assessment. Selection bias and other sources of bias are equally problematic, because there is no easy test for their presence and no clear way to estimate the magnitude of their effect.

In the absence of definitive tests of the quality of prognostic studies, one must rely rather heavily on an evaluation of research methodology. The following three areas are of particular importance:

1. Was the population chosen for the study appropriate to the questions being posed?
2. Were the proper statistical methods used in analyzing the results?
3. Have the observations been validated in an appropriate independent sample?

These issues are briefly reviewed in the next three sections.

## Patient Samples for Prognostic Stratification

Several main types of patient samples have been used to study the prognosis of CAD (Table 8–1). Population-based outcome data are theoretically the most valid, because they are free of any type of selection or referral bias and the group of patients to whom such data pertains is usually clear. The Framingham Study is a leading example of this type of prognostic study,[23] although there are many others. The primary drawback of population-based studies is that confirmation of disease status is usually based solely on clinical criteria. Such a study cannot, therefore, address the proper role of interventional cardiology in patients with three-vessel disease, for example, because there is no way to identify all the individuals in the population who fit into this angiographic subgroup. Another problem with population studies is that substantial numbers of individuals selected to participate (often before disease has become clinically evident) may refuse. One third of the subjects invited to participate in the Framingham Study declined and had to be replaced with volunteers, who typically have better than average outcomes.

In recent years, administrative or insurance claims data have been applied with growing frequency to study clinical outcomes.[24, 25] Advantages of these data sources include massive numbers of patients, a clear reference population, and often freedom from referral or selection bias. There are some notable disadvantages as well, particularly the poor quality of many of the individual variables collected in such databases and the restricted types of information available. For example, administrative databases of patients undergoing percutaneous transluminal coronary angioplasty (PTCA) or coronary artery bypass grafting (CABG) contain no information about number of diseased vessels or ejection fraction, because there are no International Classification of Diseases, Revision (ICD-9) codes for these variables. Despite this deficiency, such data are currently being used to compare alternative treatment

**TABLE 8–1. PATIENT SAMPLES USED FOR PROGNOSTIC ASSESSMENT**

Population-based (e.g., Framingham)
Multicenter clinical trial (e.g., CASS, MRFIT)
Multicenter registry (e.g., CASS, BARI, RITA)
Single-center registry (e.g., Duke, Mayo, Emory, University of Alabama, Cleveland Clinic)
Single investigator or group
Undefined

*Abbreviations:* BARI, Bypass Angioplasty Revascularization Investigation; CASS, Coronary Artery Surgery Study; MRFIT, Multiple Risk Factor Intervention Trial; RITA, Randomised Intervention Treatment of Angina study.

strategies in patients with CAD.[26, 27] In view of current limitations, perhaps the best use of administrative data is to generate hypotheses and to point out geographic differences in practice patterns or outcomes that can then be evaluated with more detailed, focused data collection and analysis.[24, 25]

Multicenter randomized clinical trials often provide detailed outcome and therapeutic efficacy information about a very narrow, highly selected segment of the potential patient population and are usually drawn from academic and other tertiary care hospitals. The main exceptions to this generalization are the megatrials that have been performed to evaluate various therapeutic strategies for acute coronary disease. Megatrials can provide a much broader picture of the benefits of therapy, often combining results from hundreds of hospitals in many countries. However, not all megatrials are equally informative. The amount of data collected, the extent to which the data have been subjected to quality control, and the amount and type of follow-up available can all substantially influence the degree to which the results of a given megatrial will influence clinical practice.

A number of multicenter randomized trials have included registries of nonrandomized patients to evaluate outcomes in "randomizable versus randomized" patients and to perform observational analyses in other subgroups of interest.[28–30] The importance of such registries is highlighted by the fact that fewer than 15% of patients with CAD referred to Duke University for coronary angiography during the 1970s would have been eligible for any of the three major randomized trials of CABG versus medical therapy conducted during that period. Furthermore, the largest treatment differences between CABG and medical therapy found by the Coronary Artery Surgery Study (CASS) Investigators in their observational registry occurred in patients specifically excluded from the randomized trial portion of their study.[31–33]

Single-center registries have much in common with clinical trials and multicenter registries but reflect only the experience of a single institution.[34] Nevertheless, the leading registries employ most of the rigorous data collection techniques and operating standards of clinical trials without incorporating their restrictive entry and exclusion criteria. For example, long-term follow-up of patients receiving interventional procedures at Duke University is performed by a group in the Duke Databank who are totally separate from the interventional cardiologists performing the procedures. The goal is always 100% follow-up (i.e., no detection bias for cardiac events); in practice, it has been possible to achieve approximately 98% follow-up for mortality status. Any follow-up hospitalizations of a cardiac nature prompt requests for additional information to determine whether criteria for an acute MI have been met. In general, both single-center and multicenter registries tend to reflect the best care and best outcomes available to patients with CAD and not the average or "typical" care provided in a given area or to a particular segment of the population. Thus, such data alone may not be entirely suitable for health policy analyses, because the reported results are not representative of the health care in the country as a whole.[27] In addition, both types of registries are subject to referral or selection biases, the effects of which are hard to quantify.

One of the oldest types of patient samples used to study outcomes is that drawn from the practice of an individual or group of physicians. These case series do not usually include all patients referred to a given institution. The reference group is presumed to be composed of patients from similar practices in similar geographic areas. One concern about these studies is that the same individuals who are providing the care are also usually judging the quality of the outcomes. It is noteworthy that many of the advances in interventional cardiology have been reported first as case series by groups of physicians practicing outside traditional academic settings. However, the value of such advances is not established until larger multicenter studies can evaluate and replicate the benefits seen in these initial reports.

Besides considering the patient sample involved in a particular study of CAD outcomes, it is important to note the time period in which the study was conducted. Observations from the Duke Databank have documented a significant improvement between 1969 and 1984 in the outcomes of patients treated with bypass surgery, presumably relating to technologic advances in the procedure, such as internal mammary artery grafting and cold potassium cardioplegia.[35] Substantial improvements have been recorded in success rates of percutaneous coronary revascularization over the past 10 years, although it is still unclear whether there are associated trends in long-term outcome. At a minimum, therefore, these sorts of secular improvements in outcome over time underscore the need for great caution when one is comparing patients in current practice with any sort of historical control population.

## Statistical Analysis

Two main statistical approaches are used to examine prognostic issues in CAD: subgrouping and modeling.[16] Each has important advantages and disadvantages. *Subgrouping* is the traditional approach that clinicians have employed from the earliest years of medical practice. A few key characteristics of a current patient are identified to allow that patient to be linked with "similar" previous patients from either the physician's past experience or the literature. The number of characteristics that can be used to specify a subgroup is limited by the complexity that each additional factor introduces and by the diminishing numbers of past patients who can be classified into that more precisely defined subgroup. The underlying assumption is that subgrouping creates subsets of patients with a homogeneous prognosis. This assumption is clearly incorrect—almost any subgroup of patients with CAD defined by three to five clinical characteristics (e.g., age, sex, symptom course, number of diseased vessels, ejection fraction) can be shown to be prognostically heterogeneous through examination of other important variables (e.g., diabetes, symptoms of congestive heart failure, comorbidity). Conceptually, subgrouping carries the strong assumption that different subgroups (e.g., men vs. women, older vs. younger patients) are so different that the findings from one cannot be safely extrapolated to the other.

*Statistical modeling,* by contrast, starts from the position that coronary artery disease patients are more similar than not and allows the importance of specific characteristics to vary from one type of patient to another only when there is strong evidence that such is the case.[16] Modeling is a much more powerful technique for analyzing prognosis, in part because it can consider the effects of dozens of characteristics simultaneously compared with the handful of factors considered by subgrouping.

Clinicians are often uncomfortable with modeling, however, because the underlying mathematics is obscure and because the results seem remote from the "real" (i.e., subgroup) data. In fact, all prognostic assessment involves some underlying "model." The subgrouping model, as noted previously, assumes that patients in different subgroups are biologically dissimilar with regard to prognosis and that, within a given subgroup, patients are homogeneous. Furthermore, relationships "observed" in subgroup data are actually just an estimate of the true biologic and epidemiologic relationships existing in the underlying population. Statistical models simply provide alternative conceptual specifications about the relationships present in the underlying data. Some models make fairly restrictive assumptions about the behavior of the variables being modeled (so-called parametric statistical techniques), whereas others have relatively few such assumptions (nonparametric techniques). In the latter category are the Cox proportional hazards model used to study prognosis with varying lengths of follow-up[12, 14, 16] and the logistic model often used to study short-term (e.g., 30-day) survival.[36]

A potential disadvantage of statistical modeling is the greater sophistication required of the analyst constructing the model and of the audience attempting to apply the results in clinical practice. The ready availability of statistical analysis computer software that can be easily used by researchers who have only a minimal grasp of underlying assumptions and technical limitations may represent an additional liability, because the medical audience for this work is usually in no position to distinguish a well-done from a poorly done analysis.

## Validation of Prognostic Assessments

The process of predicting outcomes in patients with CAD has many features in common with the performance of a laboratory or diagnostic test. Although a given risk stratification algorithm or prognostic model may work exceedingly well at the tertiary care hospital that derived it and published an enthusiastic report about it, there is no guarantee that the algorithm or model will perform even approximately as well in a new site or even at the same site in a new group of patients. The reasons for this situation include the following[16]:

1. The researchers who derived the algorithm or model inadvertently incorporated a nonbiologic effect or "noise" (often referred to as *overfitting*), making it appear to work better than it actually does in that group and ensuring that it will work substantially less well in any other group.
2. The types of patients seen in a new site differ in some important way(s) from the patients seen at the site of the original study.
3. The data collected at new sites as part of the algorithm or model differ systematically in either meaning or measurement quality from those collected at the original site. For example, if a study describing the use of exercise thallium testing for prognostic stratification identified a particular variable, say, the quantitative heart-to-lung thallium ratio, as being most important for identifying high-risk patients, it may be difficult for other sites to identify a similar high-risk group if they do not have the technology or the expertise to perform the necessary calculations.

*Validation* is a process of demonstrating that a prognostic stratification rule (or a diagnostic test) works sufficiently well in settings and patient samples independent of those in which it was derived to provide confidence that it can be used in clinical management.[16, 22] Of the many prognostic models, algorithms, and rules of thumb published each year, only a very small percentage are ever subjected to any kind of validation. Validation can be performed for both the prognostic stratification rule itself (i.e., its components and their specified relationships) and its predictive abilities, but usually we are most concerned about the latter. The following three components can be assessed in evaluating the quality of prognostic predictions[15]:

- Precision, or test-retest repeatability (usually evaluated by calculating confidence limits around predictions)
- Calibration, or how close a given prediction lies to the actual value for a given patient
- Discrimination, or the ability to separate patients with and without the outcome of interest (e.g., cardiac death)

Prognostic rules or models that do not perform well according to these criteria are akin to unreliable laboratory tests. Neverthless, although clinical laboratories are regulated and required to perform up to prespecified standards, relatively little attention has been paid to the quality of clinical decision-making that is based on inadequately validated models or algorithms.

## PROGNOSIS IN THE MEDICALLY TREATED PATIENT

The prognosis of the medically treated patient with CAD is a function of a set of variables or characteristics that collectively describe the current state and progressive nature of the patient's disease.[1] Most of the research on prognosis in CAD has focused on survival, the primary focus of this discussion. It should be remembered, however, that other outcomes, such as MI, angina, and quality of life, are often equally important to clinical decision-making.

Although most prognostic studies of CAD tend to treat the different clinical phases of the disease as distinct problems, each with its own unique set of risk factors, there is growing evidence that CAD can best be understood by viewing the disease as a continuum.[1, 37] This discussion therefore starts by reviewing the basic components of this risk continuum and then attempts to place observations on specific phases of CAD (e.g., unstable angina, acute MI) into this perspective.

## CAD Risk Continuum

Conceptually, the probability of cardiac death in coronary disease can be viewed as the sum of the risks attributable to the patient's current state and the risks that the patient's disease will progress to a different state (of higher or lower risk). Although this classification necessarily oversimplifies a complex problem, it is helpful in pointing out the types of questions clinicians must address to assess the prognosis of their patients.

**TABLE 8–2.    MAJOR PROGNOSTIC FACTORS IN CORONARY DISEASE RELATING TO CURRENT RISK STATE**

Left ventricular function/damage
    History of prior MI
    CHF symptoms
    Cardiomegaly on chest radiography
    Ejection fraction
    Regional LV wall-motion abnormalities
    LV diastolic function
    LV end-systolic and end-diastolic volumes
    Mitral regurgitation
    Atrial fibrillation
    Conduction disturbances on ECG
Coronary disease severity
    Anatomic extent of CAD
    Transient ischemia
    Collateral vessels
Coronary plaque event
    Symptom course (unstable, progressive, stable)
    Transient ischemia
    Hematologic milieu
Electrical event
    Ventricular arrhythmias
    Late potentials
    Decreased heart rate variability

*Abbreviations:* CAD, coronary artery disease; CHF, congestive heart failure; ECG, electrocardiography; LV, left ventricular; MI, myocardial infarction.

### Current Risk State

The patient's current risk state is primarily a function of four types of prognostic measures, which are listed in Table 8–2.[1, 37]

#### LV Function

Most important are variables describing the amount of LV damage present (Fig. 8–3) and the success of

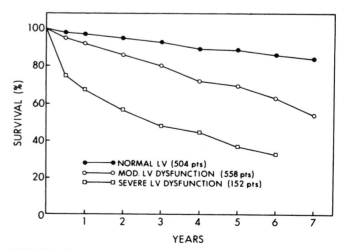

FIGURE 8–3. Survival curves (unadjusted) for 1214 CAD patients in the Duke Databank stratified according to the degree of left ventricular (LV) dysfunction present. (From Harris PJ, Harrell FE Jr, Lee KL, et al: Survival in medically treated coronary artery disease. Circulation 60:1259–1269, 1979.)

mechanisms activated to compensate for that damage. Although the ejection fraction is the summary measure most often employed in prognostic assessment, it is clearly not a comprehensive description of ventricular function.[37] Part of the reason is that a damaged heart can maintain an approximately normal ejection fraction by dilation through the use of the Frank-Starling mechanism.[38] Thus, a number of studies have suggested that ventricular volumes, particularly the end-systolic volume, are stronger prognostic factors than the ejection fraction.[39, 40] Ventricular volumes are more difficult to measure accurately, however, and their value in routine clinical practice has not yet been established.

In addition, the presence and severity of symptoms of congestive heart failure (CHF) have been repeatedly shown to add independent prognostic information to the ejection fraction. Thus, a patient with a given ejection fraction value and symptomatic heart failure is clearly at a substantially greater risk than a similar patient without CHF symptoms.[41, 42] Presumably, the presence of CHF symptoms provides information that is not available from the ejection fraction about the inability of the left ventricle to compensate fully for cumulative damage experienced. The hemodynamic correlate of CHF symptoms is found in measures of LV diastolic function, and there is now evidence that such measures also provide prognostic information independent of the ejection fraction.[43]

Similarly, the presence and extent of regional LV wall-motion abnormalities provides prognostic information beyond that available in the ejection fraction, especially in acute MI, in which hyperdynamic activity in the uninvolved segments can compensate for impaired function in the infarct zone.[44] As discussed later in this section, there is an ongoing debate about whether ventricular arrhythmias are an independent prognostic marker of myocardial electrical instability or are simply a manifestation of LV dysfunction. Several electrical manifestations of coronary heart disease in addition to ventricular arrhythmias are commonly associated with LV damage, including atrial fibrillation and conduction disturbances. Atrial fibrillation is an uncommon arrhythmia in CAD, with a prevalence of 0.6% estimated from 18,343 patients in the CASS registry.[45] The presence of atrial fibrillation in this population correlated particularly with ischemic mitral regurgitation and with symptomatic CHF. Even after these factors were accounted for, however, atrial fibrillation was an independent prognostic factor, approximately doubling a patient's risk of dying compared with the risk effect of sinus rhythm.[44] Similar considerations apply to interventricular conduction disturbances, particularly left bundle branch blocks and interventricular conduction defects that do not meet full criteria for left bundle branch block.[46]

Ischemic mitral regurgitation emerged during the 1990s as an important and frequently underdiagnosed problem in coronary disease.[47, 48] Overall, about 20% of patients with CAD presenting for diagnostic cardiac catheterization have some degree of mitral regurgitation, and 3% have severe (i.e., 3 + to 4 +) regurgitation.[47, 48] Pathophysiologically, there are three main forms of the disease.[48] The most common is *papillary muscle dysfunction*, which is typically initiated by an inferior or posterior wall MI involving the posterior descending artery[49] and the posteromedial papillary muscle.[49] The anterolateral papillary muscle is much less commonly involved, probably because of its dual blood supply from diagonal branches of the left anterior descending (LAD) artery and marginal branches from the left circumflex (LCX) artery. The second and least common type of ischemic mitral regurgitation is *papillary muscle rupture*. The prevalence of this condition, which can be viewed as an extreme form of papillary muscle dysfunction, is less than 1% in most acute MI populations. The third type of mitral regurgitation is that due to LV *dilatation and regional wall-motion abnormalities* with secondary disruption of proper mitral valve function.

Prognostically, mitral regurgitation of any degree is a significant adverse factor, and severe regurgitation is a major independent determinant of survival (Fig. 8–4). For the acute forms of the disease, short-term risk may be substantially increased, but if proper mitral valve function can be promptly restored with reperfusion therapy and revascularization, long-term prognosis may not be affected. This is particularly true for patients with otherwise small infarctions and limited atherosclerotic involvement of the noninfarct coronary arteries. On the other hand, many patients with severe mitral regurgitation in the setting of acute MI have three-vessel disease and a substantially depressed ejection fraction.[49–51] For these patients, long-term prognosis is also poor, especially in the absence of revascularization therapy and mitral repair or replacement.[47]

In patients with chronic ischemic mitral regurgitation, the valve dysfunction is often secondary to the cumulative effects of multiple infarctions on LV function, and the prognosis is usually quite poor. Part of the reason is that once mitral regurgitation develops in a damaged heart, it tends to promote further LV dilatation as compensation for the diminished forward stroke volume, worsening the amount of regurgitation (hence the saying "mitral regurgitation begets more mitral regurgitation") and accelerating the clinical deterioration of the patient.

*Severity of Coronary Disease*

After LV function, the most important prognostic characteristics of the CAD patient relate to the

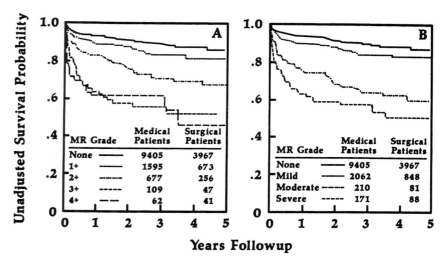

FIGURE 8–4. Survival curves (unadjusted) for 11,848 CAD patients in the Duke Databank demonstrating the relationship between degree of ischemic mitral regurgitation (MR) and prognosis in medically treated patients. Mitral regurgitation is graded as 0 to 4 + *(A)* or none to severe *(B)*. (From Hickey MS, Smith LR, Muhlbaier LH, et al: Current prognosis of ischemic mitral regurgitation: Implications for future management. Circulation 78(suppl I):I-51–I-59, 1988.)

anatomic extent and severity of atherosclerotic involvement of the coronary tree.[1, 37] Typically, this is measured as *the number of diseased vessels*, a classification system popularized during the early 1970s at the Cleveland Clinic.[52] In this classification, the coronary tree is divided into three major segments[4]: the LAD system, including the large diagonal branches; the LCX system, including large optional diagonal and obtuse marginal branches; and the right coronary system, including the posterior descending artery and any large posterolateral LV branches. Conceptually, the number of diseased vessels classification is intended to convey the magnitude of jeopardy faced by the corresponding three major segments of the left ventricle. Left main coronary disease, which jeopardizes the territory of the LAD and LCX, counts as two-vessel disease; in patients with a left dominant circulation, all three territories are jeopardized, and significant left main coronary disease counts as three-vessel disease.

Although the number of diseased vessels classification is widely used in prognostic studies (Fig. 8–5) and in clinical decision-making, it is insufficiently informative for both purposes. For example, a patient with a 99% proximal LAD lesion and a patient with a 75% lesion of a medium-sized third obtuse marginal coronary artery both have "one-vessel disease" but clearly have different prognoses and may require different therapeutic strategies. Later advances in quantitative angiography have challenged the primacy of the long-accepted "significant" coronary stenosis as judged arteriographically,[52] but the advantages of quantitative angiography for prognostic assessment have yet to be established.

Since the 1970s, many investigators have tried to create a more informative and prognostically useful classification of coronary disease severity, but no such effort has met with general clinical acceptance.

A system that has achieved some use in research studies is the coronary artery jeopardy score derived by investigators at the Massachusetts General Hospital and validated independently by Califf and co-workers[53] at Duke University. This score divides the coronary tree into six major segments and assigns two points to each segment with a 75% or greater stenosis (Fig. 8–6). Thus, the score values range from 0 (no significant CAD) to 12 (left main and right coronary artery [RCA] disease) and stratify prognosis significantly better than the classification using the number of diseased vessels (Fig. 8–7).[53] However, this score has several important limitations that are generally characteristic of all attempts in this area, as follows:

1. All lesions of 75% or greater are treated as prognostically equivalent without consideration

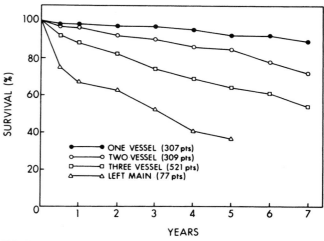

FIGURE 8–5. Survival curves (unadjusted) for 1214 CAD patients in the Duke Databank stratified according to the number of diseased vessels. (From Harris PJ, Harrell FE Jr, Lee KL, et al: Survival in medically treated coronary artery disease. Circulation 60:1259–1269, 1979.)

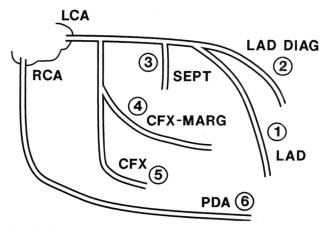

FIGURE 8–6. Coronary artery jeopardy score derived by R. Johnson and colleagues at the Massachusetts General Hospital and validated in the Duke Databank population. Each of the six major segments indicated is assigned two points if it contains a ≥75% stenosis. CFX, circumflex; DIAG, diagonal; LAD, left anterior descending; LCA, left coronary artery; MARG, margin; PDA, posterior descending artery; RCA, right coronary artery; SEPT, septum. (From Califf RM, Phillips HR, Hindman MC, et al: Prognostic value of a coronary artery jeopardy score. J Am Coll Cardiol 5:1055–1063, 1985.)

given to the actual amount of myocardium at risk.[54]

2. The presence of serial lesions and collateral vessels is not taken into account.
3. The variable branching pattern of the coronary tree in different patients is not accounted for.
4. The viability of myocardium downstream from each lesion is not considered.

Any system that did meet all these objectives, however, would likely be much too complex for routine clinical use. Current attempts in this area involve taking advantage of new flexible computerized coronary tree programs that are growing in use.

Smith and colleagues[55] from Duke University have proposed a new prognostic CAD index designed to overcome some of the deficiencies of the number of diseased vessels classification (Table 8–3). This index, which is hierarchical and assigns the patient to the worst category applicable, takes into account prognostically important data about lesion severity (a 95% lesion is higher risk than a 75% stenosis) and location (a proximal lesion is higher risk than a nonproximal lesion, especially in the LAD). Categories with similar prognoses have been collapsed together to reduce the complexity of the final index, and prognostic weights have been assigned ranging from 0 (no CAD) to 100 (at least 95% left main coronary disease). Experience with this new index suggests that it may identify anatomic subsets of patients who could derive particular benefit from revascularization strategies with PTCA or CABG that were not evident with classification of the number of diseased vessels.[56]

Another prognostic measure related to the coronary anatomy is the occurrence of transient ischemia, often called *silent ischemia.* Although it is now well established that in many patients with CAD, the majority of ischemic electrocardiographic (ECG) events recorded by ambulatory monitoring are not accompanied by symptoms,[57] the use of the term *silent ischemia* emphasizes an artificial dichotomy between silent and symptomatic episodes. The original hypothesis of Cohn, that silent ischemia might reflect a defective anginal warning system that would place patients at increased risk relative to their symptomatic counterparts,[58] has generally not been supported by the data. Growing evidence now suggests that ischemia occurs on a continuum and that the frequency and magnitude of transient ischemic episodes (both symptomatic and silent) correlate strongly with the severity of underlying CAD.[59, 60] Frequent or profound transient ischemia appears to

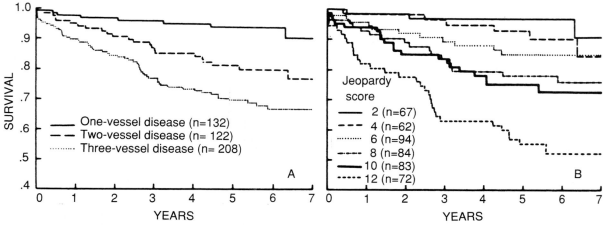

FIGURE 8–7. Survival stratified by the jeopardy score *(B)* compared with the number of diseased vessels *(A)* in 462 CAD patients from the Duke Databank. Note that the jeopardy score provides more prognostic distinctions. (From Califf RM, Phillips HR, Hindman MC, et al: Prognostic value of a coronary artery jeopardy score. J Am Coll Cardiol 5:1055–1063, 1985.)

## TABLE 8–3.    DUKE PROGNOSTIC CAD INDEX

| EXTENT OF CAD | PROGNOSTIC WEIGHT (0–100) |
|---|---|
| No CAD, ≥50% | 0 |
| 1 VD, 50–74% | 19 |
| >1 VD, 50–74% | 23 |
| 1 VD, 75% | 23 |
| 1 VD, ≥95% | 32 |
| 2 VD | 37 |
| 2 VD, both ≥95% | 42 |
| 1 VD, ≥95% proximal LAD | 48 |
| 2 VD, 95% LAD | 48 |
| 2 VD, ≥95% proximal LAD | 56 |
| 3 VD | 56 |
| 3 VD, ≥95% in at least one | 63 |
| 3 VD, proximal LAD | 67 |
| 3 VD, ≥95% proximal LAD | 74 |
| Left main, 75% | 82 |
| Left main, ≥95% | 100 |

*Abbreviations:* 1 VD, one-vessel disease; 2 VD, two-vessel disease; 3 VD, three-vessel disease; CAD, coronary artery disease; LAD, left anterior descending.

From Smith LR, Harrell FE Jr, Rankin JS, et al: Determinants of early versus late cardiac death in patients undergoing coronary artery bypass graft surgery. Circulation 84(suppl III):245–253, 1991.

have prognostic implications similar to those of an early positive treadmill test result.[60, 61] Much of the prognostic content of transient ischemia therefore relates to CAD severity.[62, 63] This is true both for ischemia detected during ambulatory monitoring and for that occurring during an exercise or pharmacologic stress test. Several studies have proposed that there is an independent prognostic component

as well.[64–67] It is possible that transient ischemia, during ambulatory monitoring or exercise testing, may differentiate similar-appearing coronary lesions with differing "functional" importance.[68]

One aspect of coronary anatomy that appears to be important in understanding CAD prognosis is the physical characteristics of the coronary tree. Specifically, the size of the coronary vessels (which is at least partly a function of body size), the number of branches present and the pattern of branching, the presence of collateral vessels,[69–74] and the development of compensatory enlargement[75] have all been considered potential determinants of outcome. Of these, collateral coronary vessels have received the most study, albeit much of it in animal models. Interestingly, Epstein and colleagues[2] from the National Institutes of Health (NIH) and Greenfield (personal communication) from Duke University have suggested that transient (silent) ischemia may actually provide prognostic benefits in CAD by stimulating formation of collateral vessels, thereby possibly reducing the likelihood of a fatal cardiac event (Fig. 8–8)[2] and decreasing the size of nonfatal myocardial infarctions.[76]

### Coronary Plaque Event

A third major domain of prognostic variables in CAD is the coronary plaque event. A growing body of pathologic, angioscopic, and ultrasound data supports the notion that plaque rupture is the initiating

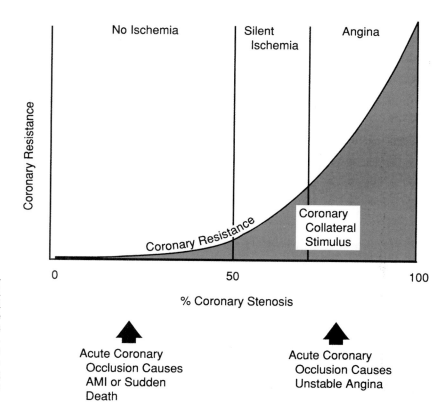

FIGURE 8–8. Relationship between coronary stenosis severity, the development of collateral circulation, and the occurrence of silent and symptomatic ischemia. The more severe the ischemia, the more collateral circulation is formed. AMI, acute myocardial infarction. (From Epstein SE, Quyyumi AA, Bonow A: Sudden cardiac death without warning: Possible mechanisms and implications for screening symptomatic populations. N Engl J Med 321: 320–324, 1989.)

event for most of the adverse consequences of CAD.[77–83] Coronary plaque rupture may be microscopic, with the only sequela being an asymptomatic enlargement of the involved plaque, or it may be substantial, initiating formation of an obstructive coronary thrombus. Some plaques, particularly those with a cholesterol-rich core and a thin fibrous cap, are more likely to rupture than others. Importantly, these plaques are often judged to be "insignificant" on coronary angiography,[3] whereas the "significant" plaques (i.e., at least 75% stenosis) appear much less likely to rupture.[83–85] The specific triggers of plaque rupture and the subsequent thrombotic and fibrinolytic responses all remain incompletely understood.[86, 87]

Clinicians have long recognized that some patients appear to form plaques with a low likelihood of rupture, so that over time, these patients progress to having extensive atherosclerotic involvement of the coronary tree that may cause severe angina, but they continue to have well-preserved LV function. Others progress early to major plaque rupture with MI and subsequent LV dysfunction. Whether there are actually such distinct subtypes of patients and whether these differences in disease course are specifically due to variations in plaque biology remain unsettled. We currently have no way of prospectively identifying patients with differing prognoses according to specific plaque characteristics. Coronary angiography is a notoriously insensitive method of studying individual plaques. Advances in coronary angioscopy and coronary ultrasound techniques may eventually change our understanding of coronary plaque events and prognosis.[82, 88–90]

Since about 1985, an intriguing body of epidemiologic and pathophysiologic data has been accumulating that suggests that the outcome of a given plaque event may be determined to a significant extent by the hematologic milieu. The outcome of a plaque event depends, at least partially, on how severely the cap of the plaque is disrupted and on how much underlying material is thereby exposed to or extruded into the blood stream.[78] However, what happens after plaque rupture seems to be modulated by several hematologic factors, including levels of fibrinogen and factor VII, plasma viscosity, white blood cell count, platelet count and activity, and the state of the fibrinolytic system.[78, 91–97]

Many of these hematologic factors are correlated with one another and with more traditional cardiovascular risk factors, particularly smoking and cholesterol levels, so that the details of these relationships in causal terms have not yet been clearly established. For example, it is possible that smoking exerts its deleterious effects in CAD[96] by creating a hypercoagulable state with raised levels of fibrinogen, plasma viscosity, and platelet activation. In this way, smoking may convert a plaque event that is self-limited into one that has major clinical sequelae. An alternative proposal is that the atherogenic effects of smoking are mediated, at least in part, through the production of oxygen free radicals that create oxidized low density lipoprotein (LDL) cholesterol.[98] Observations suggest that the hematologic response to plaque events may be different in patients presenting with unstable angina and those presenting with an acute MI, with more platelet-rich thrombi in the former and more fibrin-rich thrombi in the latter.[81, 82] Other lines of evidence point to the inflammatory response as a major mechanism of acute coronary disease.[99]

Clinically, the major markers of an unstable coronary plaque are a change in the patient's symptom pattern and, possibly, a change in the pattern of transient ischemia experienced by the patient. Our research group has evaluated the prognostic information available from the patient's routine angina history in detail.[100, 101] The course of the patient's symptoms over the preceding 6 weeks (i.e., stable, progressive without nocturnal symptoms, progressive with nocturnal symptoms, or unstable) and the average frequency of anginal episodes per day were both strong predictors of prognosis even when information on LV function and CAD severity from catheterization was taken into account. A distinct change in the patient's symptom pattern strongly suggests a recent plaque event with an increase in the size of a coronary plaque that has caused a reduction in myocardial blood flow and ischemia thresholds.[102, 103] Conversely, a stable symptom pattern suggests the absence of recent plaque events of consequence.

Falk[83] and Davies and Thomas[104] have hypothesized, on the basis of pathologic data, that plaque events occur relatively frequently in atherosclerotic plaques and that only a small fraction of such events result in clinically detectable changes in patient status. Changes in symptoms reported by the patient are clearly insensitive markers of consequential plaque events at a stage early enough to abort their consequences with appropriate therapy. Approximately one half of all patients in whom an acute MI develops do not have a preceding history of any CAD symptoms.[23, 105] Despite this substantial limitation of symptom status as a measure of disease activity, there is currently no more efficient objective method of identifying patients with CAD in whom impending or fresh plaque events require aggressive therapy to minimize the consequences of an enlarging coronary thrombus. Neither exercise testing nor ambulatory monitoring is practical for screening, as they cannot be repeated frequently enough to provide adequate surveillance. Given the rapidity with which a plaque event can develop and progress, it is quite possible for a patient who has a negative adequate exercise test result to experience a massive anterior MI 2 weeks later.[106] Future technologic advances may eventually provide a means for very early identification of high-risk plaque events; for now, however, the most efficient method available to clinicians is still a careful cardiac history, with the protean manifestations of early unstable ischemic disease kept in mind.

Initial work on the relationship of anginal symptoms and transient ischemia recorded by ambulatory monitoring showed a poor correspondence between the occurrence of symptoms and objective measures of ischemia.[107, 108] In addition, a number of studies found no relationship between the presence of symptoms and measures of ischemic severity.[109] However, no study has yet rigorously tested the comparative prognostic value of detailed symptom information (as contained, for example, in the Duke Angina score[101]) against an objective measure of ischemia, such as ambulatory monitoring, in a sufficiently large population of patients with CAD undergoing medical treatment with adequate follow-up. Studies on transient ischemia in acute ischemic heart disease have shown a correlation between the frequency and duration of ischemic episodes and the presence of an angiographically visible thrombus.[110, 111] Transient ischemia in this setting does stratify the risk of cardiac events,[112–115] probably by identifying the patients with more unstable plaques whose disease is not responding adequately to therapy. However, the added value of ambulatory monitoring as a routine practice in patients with acute ischemic heart disease has not yet been established.[116, 117] Furthermore, the value of monitoring transient ischemia to stratify the risk of a patient with a plaque known to be unstable on clinical grounds does not extend to surveillance for the presence of unstable plaques among patients with stable or asymptomatic disease.

### Electrical Stability of Myocardium

The last major domain of CAD current risk state relates to the electrical stability (or lack thereof) of the myocardium.[118] A large number of studies has examined the relationships between various forms of ventricular arrhythmia and survival in CAD.[117, 118] In general, malignant ventricular arrhythmias (e.g., sustained ventricular tachycardia [VT], ventricular fibrillation) are significant adverse prognostic markers except when they occur in the earliest hours of acute MI.[119, 120] The importance of lesser degrees of ventricular arrhythmia, such as frequent premature ventricular contractions (PVCs) or nonsustained VT, remains more controversial, especially regarding their therapeutic implications.

There has been a long-standing debate in the literature on CAD prognosis about the relationship between ventricular arrhythmias and the severity of LV dysfunction. The presence of electrical instability in patients with CAD correlates strongly with the extent of LV damage. Malignant ventricular arrhythmias are uncommon in patients with normal left ventricles, even in the presence of extensive CAD, but are a routine finding in patients with ejection fractions of less than 20%. This strong linkage has fueled a debate about whether ventricular arrhythmias are an independent risk factor or are merely another marker of the presence and extent of ischemic LV dysfunction.[118, 121] This debate has been complicated by reports from the Cardiac Arrhythmia Suppression Trial (CAST) showing that antiarrhythmic drugs that are quite effective in suppressing ventricular arrhythmias actually increase mortality in post-MI patients.[122, 123] By contrast, β-blockers and coronary bypass surgery, two therapies whose primary impact is believed to be on ischemia, have both been reported to diminish the risk of sudden cardiac death.[124–127]

In addition, a randomized trial comparing empirical metoprolol therapy with an electrophysiologic study–guided selection of antiarrhythmics for patients with sustained symptomatic VT found no difference in outcome between the two approaches.[128] Certainly, the demonstration that interventions directed specifically at ventricular arrhythmias improve survival would strongly support the thesis that such arrhythmias are independent prognostic factors. Studies with implantable defibrillators have shown that potentially fatal ventricular arrhythmias can be successfully aborted, but the issue of whether suppressing "warning arrhythmias" with pharmacotherapy can prevent the more serious arrhythmic episode remains unsettled.[129]

Two types of measures have been proposed to evaluate the risk of malignant ventricular arrhythmias and sudden cardiac death in patients with CAD, late potentials on the signal-averaged ECG and diminished heart rate variability. Late potentials are believed to indicate the electrophysiologic substrate for reentrant VT[130]; numerous studies have now shown this finding to be independent of ambulatory monitoring and LV function in assessing prognosis.[131] Heart rate variability reflects the combined activity of the parasympathetic and sympathetic nervous systems, both of which can affect the threshold for ventricular fibrillation. Multiple studies have now confirmed the independent prognostic importance of heart rate variability in patients who have experienced MI and sudden cardiac death.[132–135]

### Progression of Coronary Disease

Along with measures of current risk state, prognosis in CAD depends on the likelihood that the disease will progress to a higher or a lower risk state.[136] Coronary disease progression is believed to occur through two basic mechanisms.[79] First, plaque events create abrupt stepwise shifts in disease activity and risk. Through a series of plaque events, a patient can evolve, over a period of years, from having insignificant CAD to having severe multivessel disease. As noted previously, plaque events are still largely unpredictable, and their pathogenesis is incompletely defined.

The second major mechanism of CAD progression involves a more gradual "silting up" of atherosclerotic plaques from lipid accumulation and smooth muscle cell proliferation over a long period. Predictors of this form of disease progression are believed to include most of the standard cardiovascular risk factors, such as smoking, diabetes, hypertension, and hypercholesterolemia.[137] Reversal of this process by risk factor modification and pharmacotherapy is one of the primary pathways for regression of atherosclerosis.[79, 138] Although a conceptual distinction between plaque events and lipid accumulation–smooth muscle proliferation as alternative mechanisms for disease progression appears useful at present, one should keep in mind that both may actually be aspects of a common process and may be driven by the same risk factors.

## CAD Syndromes

Clinically, the manifestations of CAD are usually segregated into a number of broad categories according to the major symptomatic manifestations of the disease: *Asymptomatic* or *presymptomatic* describes the latent or quiescent phase of the disease, wheareas *stable angina, progressive angina* (often included by many as part of unstable angina), *unstable angina, acute MI,* and *postinfarction angina* describe the symptomatic phases and carry important prognostic implications, as discussed in the previous section. *Sudden cardiac death* and *malignant ventricular arrhythmias* refer to two aspects of the disease with prominent manifestations of electrical myocardial instability. *Ischemic cardiomyopathy* refers to the disease state in which major damage to the left ventricle has taken place. All these syndromes are defined with approximate or informal clinical criteria, and the boundaries distinguishing them are often not sharply delineated.

Viewing these CAD syndromes as a set of unrelated or only minimally related conditions sets the stage for generating a great deal of confusing and contradictory information about prognosis. Among other things, this approach necessitates identifying separate (and often different) prognostic factors for each syndrome and subsyndrome. Thus, one may conclude, for example, that LV function is not a prognostic factor in low-risk patients, identified on the basis of clinical or exercise data or both, but is a prognostic factor for high-risk patients.[139] Although such distinctions may actually have a biologic basis, the vast majority of those reported in the literature are almost certainly products of the vagaries of statistical analysis of subgroups and of the variations seen in individual data sets.[140]

By contrast, in terms of the continuum of CAD presented in the last section of this chapter, LV function is always an important prognostic factor, but for an individual patient or a group of patients with normal LV function, one can conclude that (1) the prognosis will generally be quite good, and (2) other domains (see Table 8–2) must be examined to understand where the risks lie. Furthermore, such a unifying approach to CAD prognosis gives us a much more secure framework on which to base treatment decisions, because we can extrapolate the available comparative treatment data but are not limited by the small amount of subset data available in the literature. This topic is considered further in the later section discussing the effects of revascularization therapy.

## Effects of Medical Therapy on CAD Outcomes

Much of the literature on the prognosis of CAD avoids dealing with the issue of whether medical therapy itself alters the natural history of the disease. In fact, researchers have often tacitly assumed that medical therapy does not affect outcome (particularly survival) and that all forms of medical therapy are equivalent in this regard. However, these are largely pragmatic rather than scientific decisions. With hundreds of individual therapeutic agents constituting at least six main classes of drugs now available for treatment of the patient with CAD and a lack of clear consensus on the optimal sequence of use or combinations of agents, analysis of the effects of medical therapy becomes a formidable task. Yet there is strong evidence that many agents do affect survival in CAD.[141–143] A comprehensive review of the evidence is beyond the scope of this chapter, but some of the most important data in this area are highlighted here.

Some of the strongest evidence available about the prognostic effects of medical therapy pertain to aspirin.[144–146] Aspirin inhibits the formation of thromboxane $A_2$, thereby diminishing platelet aggregation promoted by some but not all physiologic stimuli. Because platelets are some of the main participants in the thrombotic consequences of a coronary plaque event, platelet inhibition is a plausible mechanism for clinical benefit. Evidence about the survival benefits of aspirin in subjects with preclinical CAD (i.e., primary prevention) is inconclusive, but aspirin has been shown in two large trials to reduce the risk of a first nonfatal MI by 33%.[147] In patients with chronic stable angina, the Physician's Health Study reported an 87% reduction in the risk of a first nonfatal MI that was statistically significant and a 49% reduction in mortality that was not.[146] In unstable angina, aspirin has been shown to have significant benefit for stabilizing an acutely unstable coronary plaque, producing reductions of 50% or more in mortality and MI rates.[143, 148–152] In acute MI, the Second International Study of Infarct Survival (ISIS-2)[153] showed conclusively that low-dose aspirin given immediately reduced 30-day mortality and had an additive effect to that of thrombolytic therapy. At least eight trials have evaluated the role of aspirin after acute MI.[142, 144] Although individually they have arrived at conflicting conclusions, their pooled data suggest a 10% to 14% reduction in long-term mortality and a 20% to 30% reduction in rate of reinfarction.

There has been much debate about the relationship of aspirin dose with potential prognostic benefits. Although some theoretical arguments have been made in favor of low-dose aspirin, little empirical evidence supports the dominance of any individual dosing strategy. Doses in the range of 160 to 325 mg/day, however, provide the same risk reduction as higher doses with fewer side effects.[154]

Later work demonstrated that the prognostic benefits of aspirin in CAD may well extend to a newer class of antiplatelet agents, the glycoprotein IIb/IIIa (GP IIb/IIIa) receptor blockers. A meta-analysis of all randomized trials of GP IIb/IIIa receptor blockers has shown a significant reduction in rates of death and nonfatal MI for this class of antiplatelet agents in patients undergoing coronary intervention and in acute coronary syndrome patients.[154a]

β-Adrenergic blockers are another class of agents for which there is good evidence of prognostic benefit in CAD.[142] However, the available data are largely confined to the acute MI and post-MI phases of the disease. There are no data either supporting the prophylactic use of β blockers in completely asymptomatic subjects or from adequately controlled studies about the survival effects in stable angina. In patients with acute MI not receiving thrombolytic therapy, β blockers lower mortality by approximately 15% when given immediately.[142] They also lower mortality by about 20% and reduce the risk of reinfarction by around 25% when started before hospital discharge and continued for at least the first 2 years after MI.[127, 142, 155] The long-term survival benefits of β blockers given to patients treated with reperfusion therapy have been less well studied.[156] The mechanism of benefit of β blockers in survival is uncertain, may be multifactorial, and is believed

to be a class effect, rather than a property, of individual agents in this class.

Nitrates are the oldest class of agents used for the treatment of ischemic heart disease. There are no controlled trial data evaluating their prognostic effects on asymptomatic subjects or patients with stable angina. Seven randomized trials involving approximately 900 patients were conducted to evaluate intravenous nitroglycerin in acute MI during the prethrombolytic era.[157] In aggregate, these data suggest a 49% reduction in mortality associated with early nitrate therapy. The long-term prognostic effects of such agents after MI remain undefined, although one retrospective study suggested continued benefit.[158] Nitrates have several effects on the heart that may lead to clinical benefit, including decreasing preload and afterload and dilating epicardial coronary vessels and collaterals. In addition, an antiplatelet effect has been suggested.[158]

Calcium channel blocking drugs represent the newest class of antianginal agents developed for ischemic heart disease. An overview of the available randomized trial data on these drugs has raised concerns about an adverse effect on survival.[159] Five trials of nifedipine in acute MI have all shown better survival in the placebo-treated patients. One large trial of diltiazem in acute MI showed no difference in overall mortality but higher mortality in the subgroup with well-preserved LV function.[160, 161] Two trials of verapamil in acute MI have reported beneficial trends for the treatment group. Diltiazem has been shown to reduce early (i.e., same ECG region) nonfatal reinfarction in patients with non–Q wave MIs.[162, 163] However, in three randomized trials involving about 900 patients, nifedipine did not affect the risk of death or nonfatal infarction. Amlodipine had no effect on survival in patients with ischemic cardiomyopathy.[164]

Calcium channel blocking agents are theoretically quite attractive drugs for the treatment of CAD. Their vasodilatory properties make them potent antianginal agents. In addition, preliminary work suggested that these drugs may inhibit the progression of atherosclerosis.[165] However, there is the strong suggestion in the available literature of long-term harm from both diltiazem and nifedipine, particularly in the setting of significant LV damage.[159] Additional studies are clearly required in this area.

Angiotensin-converting enzyme (ACE) inhibitors are not antianginal agents but are now commonly used in patients with CAD and hypertension or CHF. Controlled trials using these agents demonstrated a significant reduction in mortality in patients with significant LV dysfunction (both symptomatic and asymptomatic).[166–170] Furthermore, two trials showed a reduction in the rate of nonfatal MI with these drugs.[166, 168] Statin therapy in patients with varying degrees of hyperlipidemia has also been shown to reduce the rates of MI and to prolong survival in patients with CAD.[171]

In summary, there is good evidence that medical therapy alters the prognosis of CAD but not always in a beneficial way. Also, it is highly likely that medical therapy has improved since the 1970s in its capacity to alter prognosis, although few direct empirical data have been published to support this contention.

## Effects of Revascularization Therapy on CAD Outcomes

Having considered the general methodology of prognostic stratification and the factors most important to that process, one is now faced with the challenge of relating the predicted prognoses of individual patients to appropriate therapeutic decisions. Although the specifics of this area are discussed in detail in subsequent chapters, some general comments are warranted here. The basic issue is understanding how therapy affects risk so as to be able to predict, for an individual or a group, expected outcomes with alternative treatment strategies. To achieve this understanding, one must make a distinction between relative risk and absolute risk.

*Absolute risk* is the risk for a patient of having some outcomes (often death) at a defined point in time (e.g., 5-year mortality rate or 5-year survival). The absolute survival benefits of CABG relative to medicine can be measured as the difference in the proportions of patients alive at 5 years (or some other arbitrary point) with CABG and with medical therapy. *Relative risk,* by contrast, is the risk that patients with a certain characteristic (e.g., diabetes) or with a certain therapy (e.g., CABG) have for a given outcome (e.g., cardiac death) divided by the

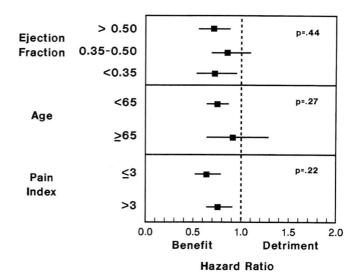

FIGURE 8–10. CABG-medicine hazard (mortality) ratios with 95% confidence limits for 5809 CAD patients in the Duke Databank (1969–1984) according to levels of major noncoronary prognostic factors. Note that the patient's age, ejection fraction, and tempo of angina do not influence the effectiveness of CABG in improving survival on a relative scale. (From Califf RM, Harrell FE Jr, Lee KL, et al: The evolution of medical and surgical therapy for coronary artery disease: A 15-year perspective. JAMA 261: 2077–2086, 1989.)

risk of an appropriate comparison group (e.g., no diabetes, medical therapy). In some types of survival analysis, the term *hazard ratio* is often used instead of *relative risk.* For example, the hazard ratio for CABG versus medical therapy in patients with three-vessel disease in the Duke Databank is approximately 0.50; this means that the risk of dying from cardiac causes was 50% less with CABG than with medical therapy over the follow-up period.

In clinical decision-making, both relative risk and absolute risk are important. In patients with CAD, revascularization therapy acts to reduce mortality risk attributable to the CAD present by an amount proportional to the extent of the CAD (Fig. 8–9). In other words, an effective CABG procedure neutralizes or substantially mitigates the risk of dying attributable to the amount of significant CAD present. This risk reduction is summarized in the relative risk or hazard ratio measure, which expresses (along with appropriate confidence limits) how well the therapy works, as judged from the available data.

After having their CAD "fixed," patients are still at risk from their noncoronary prognostic factors, which are not generally altered by revascularization. Thus, on an absolute survival scale, noncoronary prognostic factors, such as older age or a low ejection fraction, act to magnify the differences between therapies,[31–33] but on a relative scale, their effect on prognosis does not differ according to different levels of the factors (Fig. 8–10).[34] For example, CABG

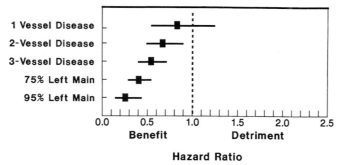

FIGURE 8–9. CABG-medicine hazard (mortality) ratios with 95% confidence limits for 5809 CAD patients in the Duke Databank (1969–1984) according to the number of diseased vessels present. The effectiveness of CABG in improving survival is clearly a function of CAD severity. (From Califf RM, Harrell FE Jr, Lee KL, et al: The evolution of medical and surgical therapy for coronary artery disease: A 15-year perspective. JAMA 261:2077–2086, 1989.)

reduces the risk of three-vessel disease by about 50%, on average, relative to medical therapy, regardless of the patient's age or ejection fraction. However, older patients with three-vessel disease who have poor LV function experience a larger absolute improvement in survival with CABG than young patients with three-vessel disease who have well-preserved LV function. This is not because CABG works better in patients with low ejection fractions but because the benefits of CABG in coronary disease are magnified in nonspecific ways by factors that increase the medical patient's risk of cardiovascular death (Fig. 8–11). The biggest therapeutic benefits of revascularization are typically observed in the patients with the most severe CAD (lowest CABG–medical therapy relative risk or hazard ratio) and the highest absolute medical therapy risk.[34, 172]

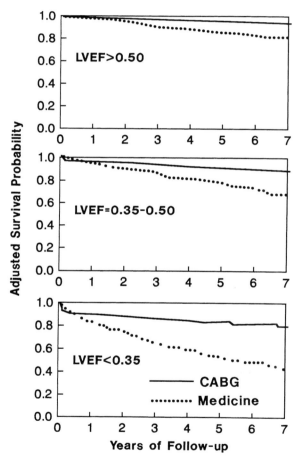

FIGURE 8–11. CABG-medicine hazard (mortality) ratios with 95% confidence limits for patients with coronary artery disease in the Duke Databank (1969–1984) according to level of ejection fraction. Note that while CABG does not differentially affect survival on a relative scale according to the degree of left ventricular dysfunction present (see Fig. 8–7), it does have a magnifying effect on the absolute survival differences observed. CABG, coronary artery bypass grafting; LVEF, left ventricular ejection fraction. (From Califf RM, Harrell FE Jr, Lee KL, et al: The evolution of medical and surgical therapy for coronary artery disease: A 15-year perspective. JAMA 261:2077–2086, 1989.)

Statistical tests of survival differences in different treatment groups using the Cox proportional hazards model specifically evaluate whether the treatment pair (e.g., CABG–medical therapy) hazard ratio is different from a ratio of 1.0 (i.e., no difference), given the actual survival outcomes observed. If the associated $p$ value is less than 0.05, the new therapy is declared to be effective; otherwise, it is often concluded that no therapeutic benefit was observed. Although such testing is given prominence in evaluation of therapeutic efficacy, much of the emphasis on the $p$ value is misplaced. Much more important is the magnitude of benefit provided by the therapy (with associated confidence limits).[173] A 25% reduction in the risk of death may appear enormously significant when observed in a megatrial of 20,000 patients (i.e., $p < 0.0001$) but may fail to reach statistical significance in a study of only a few hundred patients (i.e., $p > 0.05$). The higher the mortality rate of the population, the smaller the requisite sample size, because it is actually the number of events (deaths) observed that defines the statistical power of the analysis rather than the total population size. Thus, although statistical testing of survival differences is helpful, it should never be viewed as a substitute for evaluating the relative and absolute magnitudes of benefit provided and judging the clinical value of this benefit.

It is reasonable to presume that any percutaneous therapeutic strategy that provides revascularization with a success rate approximating that of CABG and with a procedural mortality at or below that of CABG should provide survival benefits similar to those seen with CABG. However, none of the randomized trials of PTCA conducted to date was large enough to detect any underlying survival differences with confidence.[30] In the case of CABG, it is now clear that the largest survival benefits in comparison with medical therapy are seen in patients with the most extensive CAD (left main coronary or three-vessel disease), along with the highest noncoronary medical risk (i.e., poor LV function).[34] This is true even though these are also the patients with the highest procedural risks[173] (Fig. 8–12). Extrapolating these results to interventional cardiology is complicated by the fact that the sorts of patients showing the greatest benefits with CABG are infrequently selected for PTCA or stenting. The patients typically selected for percutaneous intervention are relatively low risk, making it difficult for clinical trials of the usual size (i.e., 1000 patients or fewer per treatment group) to demonstrate a survival benefit. Careful analysis of more than 9000 patients with CAD in the Duke Databank treated with CABG, PTCA, or medical therapy has shown modest survival benefits for PTCA compared with medical

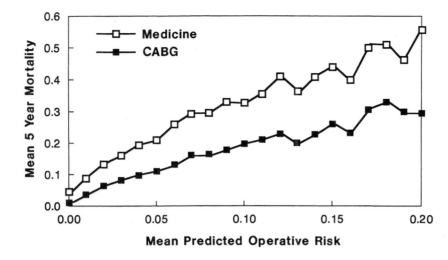

FIGURE 8–12. Coronary artery bypass grafting (CABG) risk versus benefit in 5809 patients with coronary artery disease in the Duke Databank (1969–1984). The y-axis shows the average 5-year mortality rate for the CABG and medical patients, whereas the x-axis shows the average predicted operative risk (Cox regression model) for these patients (both medical and CABG). Note that the separation between the medical and CABG curves increases (i.e., greater CABG benefit) as the predicted operative mortality rises (higher-risk patients). (From Califf RM, Harrell FE Jr, Lee KL, et al: Changing efficacy of coronary revascularization: Implications for patient selection. Circulation 78[suppl I]:I-185, 1988.)

therapy.[56] However, the major challenge that all revascularization strategies pose for cardiologists in the new millennium is not only to show that their survival benefits are real (i.e., statistically significant) but also to understand when they are worthwhile for the patient.

## ACKNOWLEDGMENTS

I appreciate the careful review and the excellent technical support of Tracey Dryden in the preparation of this chapter.

## REFERENCES

1. Working Group on Rehabilitation of the European Society of Cardiology: Risk of cardiac events (in patients with established ischaemic heart disease). Eur Heart J 13(suppl C):14–19, 1992.
2. Epstein SE, Quyyumi AA, Bonow RO: Sudden cardiac death without warning: Possible mechanisms and implications for screening asymptomatic populations. N Engl J Med 321:320–324, 1989.
3. Giroud D, Li JM, Urban P, et al: Relation of the site of acute myocardial infarction to the most severe coronary arterial stenosis at prior angiography. Am J Cardiol 69:729–732, 1992.
4. Mark DB, Califf RM, Stack RS, et al: Cardiac catheterization. In Sabiston DC (ed): The Davis-Christopher Textbook of Surgery, 13th ed, pp 2135–2165. Philadelphia: WB Saunders, 1986.
5. Favaloro RG: The developmental phase of modern coronary artery surgery. Am J Cardiol 66:1496–1503, 1990.
6. Schiff A: The development of coronary artery bypass surgery. Coron Artery Dis 1(1):121–132, 1990.
7. Rosati RA, McNeer JF, Starmer CF, et al: A new information system for medical practice. Arch Intern Med 135:1017–1024, 1975.
8. Rosati RA, Wallace AG, Stead EA: The way of the future. Arch Intern Med 131:285–287, 1973.
9. Harris PJ, Harrell FE Jr, Lee KL, et al: Survival in medically treated coronary artery disease. Circulation 60:1259–1269, 1979.
10. Harris PJ, Harrell FE Jr, Lee KL, et al: Nonfatal myocardial infarction in medically treated patients with coronary artery disease. Am J Cardiol 46:937–942, 1980.
11. Harris PJ, Lee KL, Harrell FE Jr, et al: Outcome in medically treated coronary artery disease. Ischemic events: Nonfatal infarction and death. Circulation 62:718–726, 1980.

12. Cox DR: Regression models and life-tables (with discussion). J Roy Stat Soc 34:187–220, 1972.
13. Kaplan EL, Meier P: Nonparametric estimation from incomplete observations. J Am Stat Assoc 53:457–481, 1958.
14. Harrell FE Jr, Lee KL, Califf RM, et al: Regression modeling strategies for improved prognostic prediction. Stat Med 3:143–152, 1984.
15. Pryor DB, Lee KL: Methods for the analysis and assessment of clinical databases: The clinician's perspective. Stat Med 10:617–628, 1991.
16. Harrell FE Jr, Lee KL, Mark DB: Multivariate prognostic models: Measuring and reducing errors. Stat Med 15:361–387, 1996.
17. Mark DB: Ischemic heart disease. In Conn RB (ed): Current Diagnosis 8, pp 416–427. Philadelphia: WB Saunders, 1991.
18. Lee KL, Pryor DB, Harrell FE Jr, et al: Predicting outcome in coronary disease: Statistical models versus expert clinicians. Am J Med 80:553–560, 1986.
19. Kong DF, Lee KL, Harrell FE Jr, et al: Clinical experience and predicting survival in coronary disease. Arch Intern Med 149:1177–1181, 1989.
20. Rahimtoola SH: The hibernating myocardium. Am Heart J 117:211–221, 1989.
21. Harrell FE Jr, Califf RM, Pryor DB, et al: Evaluating the yield of medical tests. JAMA 247:2543–2546, 1982.
22. Wasson JH, Sox HC, Neff RK, et al: Clinical prediction rules. N Engl J Med 313:793–799, 1985.
23. Kannel WB, Manning F: Natural history of angina pectoris in the Framingham study. Am J Cardiol 29:154–163, 1972.
24. Jollis JG, Ancukiewicz M, DeLong E, et al: Discordance of databases designed for claims payment versus clinical information systems: Implications for outcomes research. Ann Intern Med 119:844–850, 1993.
25. Fisher ES, Whaley FS, Krushat M, et al: The accuracy of Medicare's hospital claims data: Progress has been made, but problems remain. Am J Public Health 82:243–248, 1992.
26. Roper WL, Winkenwerder W, Hackbarth GM, et al: Effectiveness in health care: An initiative to evaluate and improve medical practice. N Engl J Med 319:1197–1202, 1988.
27. Hartz AJ, Kuhn EM, Pryor DB, et al: Mortality after coronary angioplasty and coronary artery bypass surgery (the national Medicare experience). Am J Cardiol 70:179–185, 1992.
28. Chaitman BR, Ryan TJ, Kronmal RA, et al: Coronary artery surgery study (CASS): Comparability of 10 year survival in randomized and randomizable patients. J Am Coll Cardiol 16:1071–1078, 1990.
29. Henderson RA: The Randomised Intervention Treatment of Angina (RITA) trial protocol: A long term study of coronary angioplasty and coronary artery bypass surgery in patients with angina. Br Heart J 62:411–414, 1989.
30. The BARI Investigators: Protocol for the Bypass Angioplasty

Revascularization Investigation. Circulation 84(suppl V): V-1–V-27, 1991.

31. Alderman EL, Fisher LD, Litwin P, et al: Results of coronary artery surgery in patients with poor left ventricular function (CASS). Circulation 68:785–795, 1983.
32. Kaiser GC, Davis KB, Fisher LD, et al: Survival following coronary artery bypass grafting in patients with severe angina pectoris (CASS). J Thorac Cardiovasc Surg 89:513–524, 1985.
33. Gersh BJ, Phil D, Kronmal RA, et al: Comparison of coronary artery bypass surgery and medical therapy in patients 65 years of age or older: A nonrandomized study from the Coronary Artery Surgery Study (CASS) registry. N Engl J Med 313:217–224, 1985.
34. Califf RM, Harrell FE Jr, Lee KL, et al: The evolution of medical and surgical therapy for coronary artery disease: A 15-year perspective. JAMA 261:2077–2086, 1989.
35. Pryor DB, Harrell FE Jr, Rankin JS, et al: The changing survival benefits of coronary revascularization over time. Circulation 76(suppl V):V-13–V-21, 1987.
36. Walker SH: Estimation of the probability of an event as a function of several independent variables. Biometrika 54:167–179, 1967.
37. Pryor DB, Bruce RA, Chaitman BR, et al: Task force I: Determination of prognosis in patients with ischemic heart disease. J Am Coll Cardiol 14:1016–1025, 1989.
38. Eng C: Enlargement of the heart. Heart Failure 15–24, 1991.
39. White HD: Relation of thrombolysis during acute myocardial infarction to left ventricular function and mortality. Am J Cardiol 66:92–95, 1990.
40. Konstam MA, Kronenberg MW, Udelson JE, et al: Effectiveness of preload reserve as a determinant of clinical status in patients with left ventricular systolic dysfunction. Am J Cardiol 69:1591–1595, 1992.
41. Bounous EP Jr, Mark DB, Pollock BG, et al: Surgical survival benefits for coronary disease patients with left ventricular dysfunction. Circulation 78(suppl I):I-151–I-157, 1988.
42. Gradman A, Deedwania P, Cody R, et al: Predictors of total mortality and sudden death in mild to moderate heart failure. J Am Coll Cardiol 14:564–570, 1989.
43. Clements IP, Brown ML, Zinsmeister AR, et al: Influence of left ventricular diastolic filling on symptoms and survival in patients with decreased left ventricular systolic function. Am J Cardiol 67:1245–1250, 1991.
44. Grines CL, Topol EJ, Califf RM, et al: Prognostic implications and predictors of enhanced regional wall motion of the noninfarct zone after thrombolysis and angioplasty therapy of acute myocardial infarction. Circulation 80:245–253, 1989.
45. Cameron A, Schwartz MJ, Kronmal RA, et al: Prevalence and significance of atrial fibrillation in coronary artery disease (CASS Registry). Am J Cardiol 61:714–717, 1988.
46. Bateman TM, Weiss MH, Czer LSC, et al: Fascicular conduction disturbances and ischemic heart disease: Adverse prognosis despite coronary revascularization. J Am Coll Cardiol 5:632–639, 1985.
47. Hickey MS, Smith LR, Muhlbaier LH, et al: Current prognosis of ischemic mitral regurgitation: Implications for future management. Circulation 78(suppl I):I-51–I-59, 1988.
48. Rankin JS, Livesey SA, Smith LR, et al: Trends in the surgical treatment of ischemic mitral regurgitation: Effects of mitral valve repair on hospital mortality. Semin Thorac Cardiovasc Surg 1:149–163, 1989.
49. Sharma SK, Seckler J, Israel DH, et al: Clinical, angiographic and anatomic findings in acute severe ischemic mitral regurgitation. Am J Cardiol 70:277–280, 1992.
50. Tcheng JE, Jackman JD, Nelson CL, et al: Outcome of patients sustaining acute ischemic mitral regurgitation during myocardial infarction. Ann Intern Med 117:18–24, 1992.
51. Lehmann KG, Francis CK, Dodge HT, et al: Mitral regurgitation in early myocardial infarction: Incidence, clinical detection, and prognostic implications. Ann Intern Med 117:10–17, 1992.
52. Bruschke AVG, Proudfit WL, Sones FM Jr: Progress study of 590 consecutive nonsurgical cases of coronary disease followed 5-9 years: II. Ventriculographic and other correlations. Circulation 158:1154–1163, 1973.
53. Califf RM, Phillips HR, Hindman MC, et al: Prognostic value of a coronary artery jeopardy score. J Am Coll Cardiol 5:1055–1063, 1985.
54. Huber KC, Bresnahan JF, Bresnahan DR, et al: Measurement of myocardium at risk by technetium-99m sestamibi: Correlation with coronary angiography. J Am Coll Cardiol 19:67–73, 1992.
55. Smith LR, Harrell FE Jr, Rankin JS, et al: Determinants of early versus late cardiac death in patients undergoing coronary artery bypass graft surgery. Circulation 84(suppl III):245–253, 1991.
56. Mark DB, Nelson CL, Califf RM, et al: The continuing evolution of therapy for coronary artery disease: Initial results from the era of coronary angioplasty. Circulation 89:2015–2025, 1994.
57. Nabel EG, Rocco MB, Barry J, et al: Asymptomatic ischemia in patients with coronary artery disease. JAMA 257:1923–1928, 1987.
58. Cohn PF: Silent myocardial ischemia in patients with a defective anginal warning system. Am J Cardiol 45:697–702, 1980.
59. Mark DB, Hlatky MA, Califf RM, et al: Painless exercise ST deviation on the treadmill: Long-term prognosis. J Am Coll Cardiol 14:885–892, 1989.
60. Mulcahy D, Keegan J, Crean P, et al: Silent myocardial ischaemia in chronic stable angina: A study of its frequency and characteristics in 150 patients. Br Heart J 60:417–423, 1988.
61. Mulcahy D, Keegan J, Sparrow J, et al: Ischemia in the ambulatory setting—The total ischemic burden: Relation to exercise testing and investigative and therapeutic implications. J Am Coll Cardiol 14:1166–1172, 1989.
62. Weiner DA, Ryan TJ, McCabe CH, et al: Significance of silent myocardial ischemia during exercise testing in patients with coronary artery disease. Am J Cardiol 59:725–729, 1987.
63. Weiner DA, Ryan TJ, McCabe CH, et al: Risk of developing an acute myocardial infarction or sudden coronary death in patients with exercise-induced silent myocardial ischemia: A report from the Coronary Artery Surgery Study (CASS) registry. Am J Cardiol 62:1155–1158, 1988.
64. Deedwania PC, Carbajal EV: Silent ischemia during daily life is an independent predictor of mortality in stable angina. Circulation 81:748–756, 1990.
65. Rocco MB, Nabel EG, Campbell S, et al: Prognostic importance of myocardial ischemia detected by ambulatory monitoring in patients with stable coronary artery disease. Circulation 78:877–884, 1988.
66. Yeung AC, Barry J, Orav J, et al: Effects of asymptomatic ischemia on long-term prognosis in chronic stable coronary disease. Circulation 83:1598–1604, 1991.
67. Raby KE, Goldman L, Cook EF, et al: Long-term prognosis of myocardial ischemia detected by Holter monitoring in peripheral vascular disease. Am J Cardiol 66:1309–1313, 1990.
68. Deedwania PC, Carbajal EV: Usefulness of ambulatory silent myocardial ischemia added to the prognostic value of exercise test parameters in predicting risk of cardiac death in patients with stable angina pectoris and exercise-induced myocardial ischemia. Am J Cardiol 68:1279–1286, 1991.
69. Rentrop KP, Thornton JC, Feit F, et al: Determinants and protective potential of coronary arterial collaterals as assessed by an angioplasty model. Am J Cardiol 61:677–684, 1988.
70. Dilsizian V, Cannon RO III, Tracy CM, et al: Enhanced regional left ventricular function after distant coronary bypass by means of improved collateral blood flow. J Am Coll Cardiol 14:312–318, 1989.
71. Gregg DE, Patterson RE: Functional importance of the coronary collaterals. N Engl J Med 303:1404–1406, 1980.
72. Topol EJ, Ellis SG: Coronary collaterals revisited: Accessory pathway to myocardial preservation during infarction. Circulation 83:1084–1086, 1991.
73. Cohen M, Rentrop KP: Limitation of myocardial ischemia

by collateral circulation during sudden controlled coronary artery occlusion in human subjects: A prospective study. Circulation 74:469–476, 1986.

74. Norell MS, Lyons JP, Gardener JE, et al: Protective effect of collateral vessels during coronary angioplasty. Br Heart J 62:241–245, 1989.

75. Glagov S, Weisenberg E, Zarins CK, et al: Compensatory enlargement of human atherosclerotic coronary arteries. N Engl J Med 316:1371–1375, 1987.

76. Habib GB, Heibig J, Forman SA, et al: Influence of coronary collateral vessels on myocardial infarct size in humans: Results of Phase I Thrombolysis in Myocardial Infarction (TIMI) trial. Circulation 83:739–746, 1991.

77. Davies MJ, Thomas A: Thrombosis and acute coronary-artery lesions in sudden cardiac ischemic death. N Engl J Med 310:1137–1140, 1984.

78. Fuster V, Badimon L, Badimon JJ, et al: The pathogenesis of coronary artery disease and the acute coronary syndromes (Second of two parts). N Engl J Med 326:310–318, 1992.

79. Davies MJ, Krikler DM, Katz D: Atherosclerosis: Inhibition or regression as therapeutic possibilities. Br Heart J 65:302–310, 1991.

80. Richardson PD, Davies MJ, Born GVR: Influence of plaque configuration and stress distribution on fissuring of coronary atherosclerotic plaques. Lancet 2:941–944, 1989.

81. Ambrose JA: Plaque disruption and the acute coronary syndromes of unstable angina and myocardial infarction: If the substrate is similar, why is the clinical presentation different? J Am Coll Cardiol 19:1653–1658, 1992.

82. Mizuno K, Satomura K, Miyamoto A, et al: Angioscopic evaluation of coronary-artery thrombi in acute coronary syndromes. N Engl J Med 326:287–291, 1992.

83. Falk E: Morphologic features of unstable atherothrombotic plaques underlying acute coronary syndromes. Am J Cardiol 63:114E–120E, 1989.

84. Hackett D, Davies G, Maseri A: Pre-existing coronary stenoses in patients with first myocardial infarction are not necessarily severe. Eur Heart J 9:1317–1323, 1988.

85. Little WC, Constantinescu M, Applegate RJ, et al: Can coronary angiography predict the site of a subsequent myocardial infarction in patients with mild-to-moderate coronary artery disease? Circulation 78:1157–1166, 1988.

86. Gertz SD, Roberts WC: Hemodynamic shear force in rupture of coronary arterial atherosclerotic plaques. Am J Cardiol 66:1368–1372, 1990.

87. Lee RT, Grodzinsky AJ, Frank EH, et al: Structure-dependent dynamic mechanical behavior of fibrous caps from human atherosclerotic plaques. Circulation 83:1764–1770, 1991.

88. Peduzzi P, Detre K, Wittes J, et al: Intent-to-treat analysis and the problem of crossovers. J Thorac Cardiovasc Surg 101:481–487, 1991.

89. McPherson DD, Johnson MR, Alvarez NM, et al: Variable morphology of coronary atherosclerosis: Characterization of atherosclerotic plaque and residual arterial lumen size and shape by epicardial echocardiography. J Am Coll Cardiol 19:593–599, 1992.

90. Mizuno K, Miyamoto A, Satomura K, et al: Angioscopic coronary macromorphology in patients with acute coronary disorders. Lancet 337:809–812, 1991.

91. Ridker PM, Hennekens CH: Hemostatic risk factors for coronary heart disease. Circulation 83:1098–1100, 1991.

92. Meade TW, Brozovic M, Chakrabarti RR, et al: Haemostatic function and ischaemic heart disease: Principal results of the Northwick Park Heart Study. Lancet 2:533–537, 1986.

93. Wilhelmsen L, Svardsudd K, Korsan-Bengtsen K, et al: Fibrinogen as a risk factor for stroke and myocardial infarction. N Engl J Med 311:501–505, 1984.

94. Elwood PC, Renaud S, Sharp DS, et al: Ischemic heart disease and platelet aggregation: The Caerphilly Collaborative Heart Disease Study. Circulation 83:38–44, 1991.

95. Yarnell JWG, Baker IA, Sweetnam PM, et al: Fibrinogen, viscosity, and white blood cell count are major risk factors for ischemic heart disease: The Caerphilly and Speedwell Collaborative Heart Disease Studies. Circulation 83:836–844, 1991.

96. Fitzgerald DJ, Roy L, Catella F, et al: Platelet activation in unstable coronary disease. N Engl J Med 315:983–999, 1986.

97. Held C, Hjemdahl P, Rehnquist N, et al: Fibrinolytic variables and cardiovascular prognosis in patients with stable angina pectoris treated with verapamil or metoprolol: Results from the Angina Prognosis Study in Stockholm. Circulation 95:2380–2386, 1997.

98. Miller ER, Appel LJ, Jiang L, et al: Association between cigarette smoking and lipid peroxidation in a controlled feeding study. Circulation 96:1097–1101, 1997.

99. Serneri GGN, Prisco D, Martini F, et al: Acute T-cell activation is detectable in unstable angina. Circulation 95:1806–1812, 1997.

100. Cohn PF, Harris P, Barry WH, et al: Prognostic importance of anginal symptoms in angiographically defined coronary artery disease. Am J Cardiol 47:233–237, 1981.

101. Califf RM, Mark DB, Harrell FE Jr, et al: Importance of clinical measures of ischemia in the prognosis of patients with documented coronary artery disease. J Am Coll Cardiol 11:20–26, 1988.

102. Ambrose JA, Winters SL, Arora RR, et al: Angiographic evolution of coronary artery morphology in unstable angina. J Am Coll Cardiol 7:472–478, 1986.

103. Depre C, Wijns W, Robert AM, et al: Pathology of unstable plaque: Correlation with the clinical severity of acute coronary syndromes. J Am Coll Cardiol 30:694–702, 1997.

104. Davies MJ, Thomas AC: Plaque fissuring: The cause of acute myocardial infarction, sudden ischemic death, and crescendo angina. Br Heart J 53:363–373, 1985.

105. Gordon T, Kannel WB: Premature mortality from coronary heart disease. JAMA 215:1617–1625, 1971.

106. Coplan NL, Fuster V: Limitations of the exercise test as a screen for acute cardiac events in asymptomatic patients. Am Heart J 119:987–990, 1990.

107. Epstein SE, Quyyumi AA, Bonow RO: Myocardial ischemia—Silent or symptomatic. N Engl J Med 318:1038–1043, 1988.

108. Nabel EG, Barry J, Rocco MB, et al: Variability of transient myocardial ischemia in ambulatory patients with coronary artery disease. Circulation 78:60–67, 1988.

109. Gasperetti CM, Burwell LR, Beller GA: Prevalence of and variables associated with silent myocardial ischemia on exercise thallium-201 stress testing. J Am Coll Cardiol 16:115–123, 1990.

110. Langer A, Freeman MR, Armstrong PW: Relation of angiographic detected intracoronary thrombus and silent myocardial ischemia in unstable angina pectoris. Am J Cardiol 66:1381–1382, 1990.

111. Freeman MR, Williams AE, Chisholm RJ, et al: Intracoronary thrombus and complex plaque morphology in unstable angina: Relation to timing of angiography and in-hospital cardiac events. Circulation 80:17–23, 1989.

112. Larsson H, Jonasson T, Ringqvist I, et al: Diagnostic and prognostic importance of ST recording after an episode of unstable angina or non–Q-wave myocardial infarction. Eur Heart J 13:207–212, 1992.

113. Betriu A, Heras M, Cohen M, et al: Unstable angina: Outcome according to clinical presentation. J Am Coll Cardiol 19:1659–1663, 1992.

114. Gottlieb SO, Weisfeldt ML, Ouyang P, et al: Silent ischemia predicts infarction and death during 2 year follow-up of unstable angina. J Am Coll Cardiol 10:756–760, 1987.

115. Romeo F, Rosano GMC, Martuscelli E, et al: Unstable angina: Role of silent ischemia and total ischemic time (silent plus painful ischemia), a 6-year follow-up. J Am Coll Cardiol 19:1173–1179, 1992.

116. Wilcox I, Ben Freedman S, Kelly DT, et al: Clinical significance of silent ischemia in unstable angina pectoris. Am J Cardiol 65:1313–1316, 1990.

117. Wilcox I, Freedman SB, Li J, et al: Comparison of exercise stress testing with ambulatory electrocardiographic monitoring in the detection of myocardial ischemia after unstable angina pectoris. Am J Cardiol 67:89–91, 1991.

118. Califf RM, McKinnis RA, Burks J, et al: Prognostic implications of ventricular arrhythmias during 24 hour ambulatory

monitoring in patients undergoing cardiac catheterization for coronary artery disease. Am J Cardiol 50:23–31, 1982.

119. Eldar M, Sievner Z, Goldbourt U, et al: Primary ventricular tachycardia in acute myocardial infarction: Clinical characteristics and mortality. Ann Intern Med 117:31–36, 1992.

120. Volpi A, Cavalli A, Santoro E, et al: Incidence and prognosis of secondary ventricular fibrillation in acute myocardial infarction. Circulation 82:1279–1288, 1990.

121. Andresen D, Steinbeck G, Bruggemann T, et al: Prognosis of patients with sustained ventricular tachycardia and of survivors of cardiac arrest not inducible by programmed stimulation. Am J Cardiol 70:1250–1254, 1992.

122. The Cardiac Arrhythmia Pilot Study (CAPS) Investigators: Effects of encainide, flecainide, imipramine and moricizine on ventricular arrhythmias during the year after acute myocardial infarction: The CAPS. Am J Cardiol 61:501–509, 1988.

123. Echt DS, Liebson PR, Mitchell LB, et al, and the CAST Investigators: Mortality and morbidity in patients receiving encainide, flecainide, or placebo: The Cardiac Arrhythmia Suppression Trial. N Engl J Med 324:781–788, 1991.

124. Holmes DR, Davis KB, Mock MB, et al: The effect of medical and surgical treatment on subsequent sudden cardiac death in patients with coronary artery disease: A report from the coronary artery surgery study. Circulation 73:1254–1263, 1986.

125. Kelly P, Ruskin JN, Vlahakes GJ, et al: Surgical coronary revascularization in survivors of prehospital cardiac arrest: Its effect on inducible ventricular arrhythmias and long-term survival. J Am Coll Cardiol 15:267–273, 1990.

126. Every NR, Fahrenbruch CE, Hallstrom AP, et al: Influence of coronary bypass surgery on subsequent outcome of patients resuscitated from out of hospital cardiac arrest. J Am Coll Cardiol 19:1435–1439, 1992.

127. Furberg CD, Hawkins CM, Lichstein E: Effect of propranolol in postinfarction patients with mechanical or electrical complications. Circulation 69:761–765, 1984.

128. Steinbeck G, Andresen D, Bach P, et al: A comparison of electrophysiologically guided antiarrhythmic drug therapy with beta-blocker therapy in patients with symptomatic, sustained ventricular tachyarrhythmias. N Engl J Med 327:987–992, 1992.

129. Moss AJ, Hall WJ, Cannom DS, et al: Improved survival with an implanted defibrillator in patients with coronary disease at high risk for ventricular arrhythmia. N Engl J Med 335:1933–1940, 1996.

130. Worley SJ, Mark DB, Smith WM, et al: Comparison of time domain and frequency domain variables from the signal-averaged electrocardiogram: A multivariable analysis. J Am Coll Cardiol 11:1041–1051, 1988.

131. Steinberg JS, Regan A, Sciacca RR, et al: Predicting arrhythmic events after acute myocardial infarction using the signal-averaged electrocardiogram. Am J Cardiol 69:13–21, 1992.

132. Dougherty CM, Burr RL: Comparison of heart rate variability in survivors and nonsurvivors of sudden cardiac arrest. Am J Cardiol 70:441–448, 1992.

133. Odemuyiwa O, Malik M, Farrell T, et al: Comparison of the predictive characteristics of heart rate variability index and left ventricular ejection fraction for all-cause mortality, arrhythmic events and sudden death after acute myocardial infarction. Am J Cardiol 68:434–439, 1991.

134. Farrell TG, Bashir Y, Cripps T, et al: Risk stratification for arrhythmic events in postinfarction patients based on heart rate variability, ambulatory electrocardiographic variables and the signal-averaged electrocardiogram. J Am Coll Cardiol 18:687–697, 1991.

135. Bigger JT Jr, Fleiss JL, Steinman RC, et al: Correlations among time and frequency domain measures of heart period variability two weeks after acute myocardial infarction. Am J Cardiol 69:891–898, 1992.

136. Working Group on Rehabilitation of the European Society of Cardiology: Ischaemic heart disease: Risk stratification and intervention. Risk of progression of coronary artery disease. Eur Heart J 13(suppl C):3–13, 1992.

137. Mack WJ, Blankenhorn DH: Factors influencing the forma-

tion of new human coronary lesions: Age, blood pressure, and blood cholesterol. Am J Public Health 81:1180–1184, 1991.

138. Collins P, Fox K: The pathogenesis of atheroma and the rationale for its treatment. Eur Heart J 13:560–565, 1992.

139. Brunelli C, Cristofani R, L'Abbate A: Long-term survival in medically treated patients with ischaemic heart disease and prognostic importance of clinical and electrocardiographic data (the Italian CNR multicentre prospective study 0D1). Eur Heart J 10:292–303, 1989.

140. Oxman AD, Guyatt GH: A consumer's guide to subgroup analyses. Ann Intern Med 116:78–84, 1992.

141. Goldman GJ, Pichard AD: The natural history of coronary artery disease: Does medical therapy improve the prognosis? Prog Cardiovasc Dis 25:513–552, 1983.

142. Yusuf S, Wittes J, Friedman L: Overview of results of randomized clinical trials in heart disease: I. Treatments following myocardial infarction. JAMA 260:2088–2093, 1988.

143. Yusuf S, Wittes J, Friedman L: Overview of results of randomized clinical trials in heart disease: II. Unstable angina, heart failure, primary prevention with aspirin, and risk factor modification. JAMA 260:2259–2263, 1988.

144. Willard JE, Lange RA, Hillis LD: The use of aspirin in ischemic heart disease. N Engl J Med 327:175–181, 1992.

145. Steering Committee of the Physicians' Health Study Research Group: Final report on the aspirin component of the ongoing physicians' health study. N Engl J Med 321:129–135, 1989.

146. Ridker PM, Manson JE, Gaziano M, et al: Low-dose aspirin therapy for chronic stable angina: A randomized, placebo-controlled clinical trial. Ann Intern Med 114:835–839, 1991.

147. Manson JE, Tosteson H, Ridker PM, et al: The primary prevention of myocardial infarction. N Engl J Med 326:1406–1416, 1992.

148. Lewis HD, Davis JW, Archibald DG, et al: Protective effects of aspirin against acute myocardial infarction and death in men with unstable angina. N Engl J Med 309:396–403, 1983.

149. Nyman I, Larsson H, Wallentin L, et al: Prevention of serious cardiac events by low-dose aspirin in patients with silent myocardial ischaemia. Lancet 340:497–501, 1992.

150. Wallentin LC, The Research Group on Instability in Coronary Artery Disease in Southeast Sweden: Aspirin (75 mg/day) after an episode of unstable coronary artery disease: Long-term effects on the risk for myocardial infarction, occurrence of severe angina and the need for revascularization. J Am Coll Cardiol 18:1587–1593, 1991.

151. Cairns JA, Gent M, Singer J, et al: Aspirin, sulfinpyrazone, or both in unstable angina. N Engl J Med 313:1369–1375, 1985.

152. Theroux P, Ouimet H, McCans J, et al: Aspirin, heparin, or both to treat acute unstable angina. N Engl J Med 319:1105–1111, 1988.

153. ISIS-2 (Second International Study of Infarct Survival): Investigators: Randomised trial of intravenous streptokinase, oral aspirin, both, or neither among 17,187 cases of suspected acute myocardial infarction: ISIS-2. Lancet 2:349–360, 1988.

154. Braunwald E, Mark DB, Jones RH, et al: Unstable Angina: Diagnosis and Management, 1994. Publication AHCPR, 94-0682. Bethesda, MD: Agency for Health Care Policy & Research, 1994.

154a. Kong DF, Califf RM, Miller DP, et al: Clinical outcomes of therapeutic agents that block the platelet glycoprotein IIb/IIa integrin in ischemic heart disease. Circulation 98:2829–2835, 1998.

155. Yusuf S, Wittes J, Probstfield J: Evaluating effects of treatment in subgroups of patients within a clinical trial: The case of non–Q-wave myocardial infarction and beta blockers. Am J Cardiol 66:220–222, 1990.

156. TIMI Study Group: Comparison of invasive and conservative strategies after treatment with intravenous tissue plasminogen activator in acute myocardial infarction: Results of the Thrombolysis in Myocardial Infarction (TIMI) Phase II Trial. N Engl J Med 320:618–627, 1989.

157. Yusuf S, MacMahon S, Collins R, et al: Effect of intravenous

nitrates on mortality in acute myocardial infarction: An overview of the randomised trials. Lancet 1:1088–1092, 1988.

158. Rapaport E: Influence of long-acting nitrate therapy on the risk of reinfarction, sudden death, and total mortality in survivors of acute myocardial infarction. Am Heart J 110:276–280, 1983.

159. Held PH, Yusuf S, Furberg CD: Calcium channel blockers in acute myocardial infarction and unstable angina: An overview. Br Med J 299:1187–1192, 1989.

160. The Multicenter Diltiazem Postinfarction Trial Research Group: The effect of diltiazem on mortality and reinfarction after myocardial infarction. N Engl J Med 319:385–392, 1988.

161. Boden WE, Krone RJ, Kleiger RE, et al: Electrocardiographic subset analysis of diltiazem administration on long-term outcome after acute myocardial infarction. Am J Cardiol 67:335–342, 1991.

162. Wong SC, Greenberg H, Hager WD, et al: Effects of diltiazem on recurrent myocardial infarction in patients with non–Q wave myocardial infarction. J Am Coll Cardiol 19:1421–1425, 1992.

163. Gibson RS, Boden WE, Theroux P, et al: Diltiazem and reinfarction in patients with non–Q-wave myocardial infarction. N Engl J Med 315:423–429, 1986.

164. Packer M, O'Connor CM, Ghali JK, et al: Effect of amlodipine on morbidity and mortality in severe chronic heart failure. N Engl J Med 335:1107–1114, 1996.

165. Henry PD: Calcium channel blockers and progression of coronary artery disease. Circulation 82:2251–2253, 1990.

166. Pfeffer MA, Braunwald E, Moye LA, et al: Effect of captopril on mortality and morbidity in patients with left ventricular dysfunction after myocardial infarction: Results of the survival and ventricular enlargement trial. N Engl J Med 327:669–677, 1992.

167. SOLVD Investigators: Effect of enalapril on mortality and the development of heart failure in asymptomatic patients with reduced left ventricular ejection fractions. N Engl J Med 327:685–691, 1992.

168. Yusuf S, Pepine CJ, Garces C, et al: Effect of enalapril on myocardial infarction and unstable angina in patients with low ejection fractions. Lancet 340:1173–1178, 1992.

169. SOLVD Investigators: Effect of enalapril on survival in patients with reduced left ventricular ejection fractions and congestive heart failure. N Engl J Med 325:293–302, 1991.

170. Kjekshus J, Swedberg K, Snapinn S: Effects of enalapril on long-term mortality in severe congestive heart failure. Am J Cardiol 69:103–117, 1992.

171. Pedersen TR, Kjekshus J, Berg K, et al, for the Scandinavian Simvastatin Survival Group: Cholesterol lowering and the use of healthcare resources: Results of the Scandinavian Simvastatin Survival Study. Circulation 93:1796–1802, 1996.

172. Gersh BJ, Califf RM, Loop FD, et al: Coronary bypass surgery in chronic stable angina. Circulation 79(suppl I):I-46–I-59, 1989.

173. Braitman LE: Confidence intervals assess both clinical significance and statistical significance. Ann Intern Med 114:515–517, 1991.

# Medical Versus Interventional Therapy for Stable Angina Pectoris

*Robert J. Lederman*     *Eric R. Bates*     *David W. M. Muller*

Since the first aortocoronary bypass surgery in 1967[1] and the first percutaneous transluminal coronary angioplasty (PTCA) in 1977,[2] revascularization options for patients with coronary artery disease (CAD) have proliferated to include atherectomy and endoluminal stenting. Concurrent advances in medical therapy include wider application of antiplatelet therapy, β-adrenergic blockade, calcium channel blockade, angiotensin-converting enzyme (ACE) inhibition, and aggressive risk factor modification. Unfortunately, few contemporary data are available comparing PTCA with medical therapy for the treatment of stable angina pectoris.

This review considers the relative merits of the two treatment strategies. It describes, first, the pathogenesis of coronary atherosclerosis and disease progression; second, the natural history of CAD through the use of historical clinical data; third, the evolution of medical therapies since 1990 and the potential impact of contemporary therapies on clinical outcome; and finally, the effects of percutaneous coronary interventions on symptom status and patient survival.

## CORONARY ARTERY DISEASE

### Pathology of Disease Progression

Any therapy of coronary disease not only should relieve symptoms but also, ideally, should alter the underlying disease process and avert progressive coronary obstruction, myocardial infarction (MI), and premature death. Pathologic studies have improved our understanding of CAD progression. Atherosclerotic plaques consist principally of extracellular lipid and fibrous connective tissue. The plaque itself tends to have a crescent shape with a central lipid pool interposed between the arterial media and a fibrous cap. The lipid component consists of cholesterol and cholesterol esters in an extracellular

pool or within the vacuolated cytoplasm of foam cells.[3] The connective tissue matrix consists of collagen types I and III, with a variable amount of elastin, proteoglycans including tissue factor, and degradative matrix metalloproteinases including stromelysin and gelatinases. Plaques also contain numerous inflammatory cells, such as macrophages, lymphocytes, and mast cells. Disease progression appears to be related not only to the slow accumulation of lipid in the central pool but also to sudden fissuring or rupture of a fragile fibrous cap overlying the lipid pool. Such plaque disruption exposes the highly thrombogenic lipid core and connective tissue matrix to blood, leading to platelet accumulation and thrombus formation both within the plaque and adherent to the plaque surface, encroaching further on the arterial lumen and potentially restricting coronary blood flow.

Triggers for plaque fissuring or rupture are poorly understood.[4] Plaques usually rupture along the "shoulder" between the fibrous cap of an eccentric plaque and the adjacent, relatively normal arterial wall, where circumferential stress is maximal.[5] Infiltrating inflammatory cells, particularly macrophages, elaborate degradative enzymes, which may compromise the integrity of the fibrous cap. Lipid-rich plaques appear to be particularly susceptible to rupture, perhaps because of abrupt regional changes in arterial wall compliance.[6]

Pathologic studies suggest that plaque fissuring is a relatively common event, even in patients dying from noncardiac causes, and is not necessarily associated with thrombotic coronary occlusion and acceleration of symptoms.[7] In some patients, the adherent mural thrombus may incorporate within the plaque and organize through the formation of new connective tissue matrix. Disease progression tends, therefore, to be episodic and unpredictable. The clinical correlate of these events is the sudden appearance of new high-grade obstructive stenoses at sites previously shown to have only minimal disease.[8] These new lesions may or may not be associated with the development of unstable angina or acute MI. Even without causing symptoms, such disrupted plaques are thought more likely to progress than "smooth" or angiographically nondisrupted plaques.[9]

Furthermore, although coronary occlusion occurs frequently in patients with critically narrowed coronary arteries,[10] the severity of stenosis as determined by angiography poorly predicts the site of future coronary occlusion and acute MI. Coronary occlusion occurs as frequently at sites of previously minor, nonobstructive stenoses as at sites with moderately severe flow-limiting disease.[11, 12] Similarly, after successful thrombolytic therapy for acute MI, the mean diameter of stenosis of the underlying plaque tends to be relatively mild.[13]

## Natural History

In the absence of appropriate therapy, symptomatic CAD is associated with a poor clinical outcome. Although no true control group of patients has been studied, epidemiologic studies from the early 1970s, performed before the widespread use of antiplatelet and contemporary antianginal therapy, provide some insight into the natural history of CAD. Data from the Framingham Study,[14] for example, indicate a 25% 5-year MI rate in symptomatic patients, and a 30% 8-year mortality rate in patients older than 55 years; 44% of all cardiac deaths were sudden. Coronary arteriography was shown to predict survival in a series of 590 patients studied at the Cleveland Clinic[15] (Fig. 9–1). The overall 5-year cardiac mortality was 34.4% for the total population, but this parameter ranged from 14.6% in patients with one-vessel disease to 37.8% in patients with two-vessel disease, to 53.8% in patients with three-vessel disease, and to 56.8% in patients with significant left main CAD; 15-year overall mortality rates were

52%, 72%, 82%, and 91%, respectively.[16] Left ventricular (LV) function was also shown to be predictive, with a 25% 5-year mortality in patients with normal LV systolic function and a 69% mortality in patients with severe global LV dysfunction.[17]

From 1977 to 1984, the clinical outcomes of patients treated in three randomized medicine versus surgery trials were reported.[18–20] The medical therapy for the nonsurgical patients was not dictated by protocol but consisted predominantly of oral nitrates and β-adrenergic blocking agents (β blockers). Calcium channel antagonists were not yet available in the United States, and the value of antiplatelet therapy, lipid-lowering therapy, angiotensin-converting enzyme (ACE) inhibitor therapy, and aggressive risk factor modification had not yet been fully appreciated. In the Veterans Administration Cooperative Study,[18, 21] 686 patients with stable angina and documented CAD (at least one-vessel disease and LV ejection fraction greater than 25% to 30%) were assigned to medical therapy or surgical revascularization between 1972 and 1974. In the medically treated patients, the overall 6-year survival was 75%, but this parameter ranged from 87% in patients with one-vessel disease to 60% in patients with left main disease.

Similar results were reported in the European Coronary Surgery Study.[19] Among 768 patients with at least two-vessel disease and preserved LV function (ejection fraction of 50% or greater), the overall 6-year survival for medically treated patients was 81% and was inversely proportional to the extent of coronary disease. Subgroup analysis highlighted the importance of proximal left anterior descending (LAD) coronary disease. Patients with two-vessel disease that did not include disease in the proximal third of the LAD had a 6-year survival of 95%, compared with 80.2% in patients with proximal LAD disease, the latter being comparable to the survival of patients with three-vessel disease (80.4%).

In the Coronary Artery Surgery Study (CASS), 780 patients were assigned to medical or surgical therapy between 1975 and 1979.[20] The patients enrolled in the study had mild stable angina (Canadian Cardiovascular Society [CCS] class I or II), and relatively well-preserved LV function (80% had an ejection fraction of 50% or greater); patients with 70% or greater left main coronary stenosis or a LV ejection fraction less than 35% were excluded. The annual risk of nonfatal infarction in the 390 patients assigned to medical therapy was 2.2% per year, a somewhat lower incidence than the 2.8% reported from the Duke Database[22] and the 5% in the Framingham Study.[14] The overall annual mortality rate in medically treated patients was 1.6%, with rates of 1.4%, 1.2%, and 2.1% in patients with one-, two-, and three-vessel disease, respectively.[23] These rates were considerably lower than the 3.3% annual

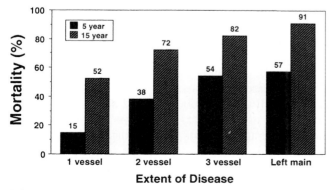

FIGURE 9–1. Relationship between angiographic extent of coronary artery disease and long-term survival for 590 patients treated at the Cleveland Clinic, 1963–1965. (Data from Bruschke et al[15] and Proudfit et al[16].)

medical mortality in the European Coronary Surgery Study[19] and the 4.3% annual mortality in the Veterans Administration Cooperative Study,[18] a difference that reflects the clinical stability of patients in CASS and the exclusion of high-risk patients from that study. After 10 years, 40% of patients initially given medical treatment in the CASS had undergone bypass surgery. The overall mortality was 21%, 69% of patients were free of death or nonfatal reinfarction, and 42% were free of angina.[24, 25]

The higher-risk patients excluded from the CASS randomized study were included in the CASS Registry.[26] Of the 24,959 patients who underwent evaluation during the study period, 20,088 had no prior history of bypass surgery and were initially treated medically. In this large population of patients, 4-year survival was again shown to be closely associated with the extent of disease and of LV dysfunction. The overall annual mortality rate was 3.7%, considerably higher than in the selected, low-risk population in the randomized study. Patients with no significant CAD had a 4-year survival of 97%, compared with survival rates of 92%, 84%, and 68% for patients with one-, two-, and three-vessel disease, respectively. The survival was 92% for patients with LV ejection fractions of 50% or greater, 83% for those with LV ejection fractions of 35% to 49%, and 58% for those with LV ejection fractions less than 35%.

## MEDICAL THERAPY FOR STABLE ANGINA PECTORIS

### Epidemiologic Trends in Chronic Coronary Artery Disease

Since the time of the studies just described, which were conducted in the early and middle 1970s, there

has been a progressive decline in the annual mortality rate from acute MI in the United States. The death rate for acute MI has fallen from 226 per 100,000 men in 1950 to 166 per 100,000 in 1979, to 93 per 100,000 in 1994. The decline for women has been less dramatic, from 125 per 100,000 in 1950 to 103 per 100,000 in 1979, to 78 100,000 in 1994[27, 28] (Fig. 9–2). This reduction in mortality is attributed to both better prevention and better treatment of CAD.[29] It is important to note that the mortality decline antedates the widespread application of both surgical and percutaneous revascularization procedures and thus appears to be related to changes in lifestyle, modification of coronary risk factors, and perhaps other, unrecognized epidemiologic influences.

The impact of preventive measures on cardiac mortality has been reviewed and is outlined in Table 9–1.[30] Clearly, these measures are equally as important as management strategies for patients with established CAD, whether the disease is treated with antianginal therapy, percutaneous intervention, or surgical revascularization. Meticulous attention to the factors discussed in the following sections constitutes the minimum standard of care for patients with CAD.

## Smoking Cessation

Convincing observational case-control and cohort data show that smoking tobacco doubles the incidence and mortality of cardiovascular disease.[31] The likelihood of cardiovascular events increases in proportion to the "dose" of tobacco,[32] which magnifies other coronary risk factors.[33]

Smoking accelerates coronary atherosclerosis[34] through mechanisms that may involve enhanced

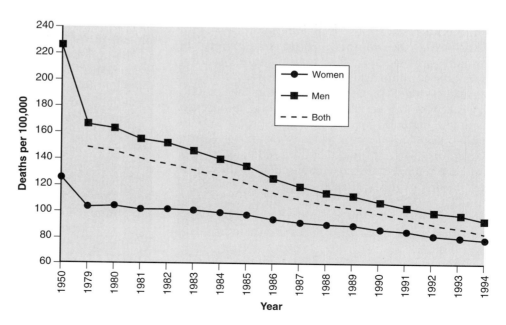

FIGURE 9–2. Mortality of acute myocardial infarction, 1950 to 1994. (From National Center for Health Statistics.[28])

**TABLE 9–1.  RISK REDUCTION AND ESTIMATED IMPROVEMENT IN LIFE EXPECTANCY AFTER RISK FACTOR REDUCTION MODIFICATION IN A TYPICAL 35-YEAR-OLD PATIENT**

| MEDICAL INTERVENTION | RISK REDUCTION | CHANGE IN LIFE EXPECTANCY (YEARS) |
|---|---|---|
| Smoking cessation | 50%–70% within 5 y | +2.3 |
| Reduction in LDL cholesterol (to <125 mg/dL) | 29% over 5 y | +0.5–4.2 |
| Treatment of hypertension (to diastolic BP < 88 mm Hg) | 2%–3% per 1-mm decrease in diastolic BP | +1.1–5.3 |
| Weight reduction to ideal | 33%–55% | +0.7–1.7 |
| Regular exercise | 45% | NA |
| Mild to moderate alcohol consumption | 25%–45% | NA |

BP, blood pressure; LDL, low-density lipoprotein; NA, not applicable.
Data from Manson et al.,[35] Tsevat et al,[42] and 4S Investigators.[43]

platelet aggregability,[35] increased plasma fibrinogen and decreased fibrinolytic activity,[36] increased sympathomimetic activity and catecholamine release,[37] reduced high density lipoprotein (HDL),[38] and endothelial injury.[39] In addition, tobacco smoke may trigger acute coronary events by (1) altering adrenergic and endothelial tone, plasma free fatty acids, and myocardial oxygen consumption and (2) decreasing the ventricular fibrillation threshold.

Fortunately, cardiovascular risk rapidly returns toward baseline within 3 to 5 years of smoking cessation.[40, 41] Thus, smoking cessation not only is inexpensive but also probably is the intervention with the greatest potential effect on cardiac mortality. A 35-year-old man who stops smoking can be expected to live 2.3 years longer.[42]

## Treatment of Hyperlipidemia

Numerous quantitative arteriographic studies have demonstrated that moderate lowering of serum cholesterol alters the natural history of atherosclerosis by slowing its progression and, in some patients, reducing the volume of atherosclerotic plaque.[43] Compared with angioplasty, the luminal alteration is quite modest.

In the Regression Growth Evaluation Statin Study (REGRESS),[44] for example, 778 patients undergoing coronary arteriography had paired arteriograms 2 years after random assignment to receive either pravastatin 40 mg or placebo. Baseline total serum cholesterol was 155 to 310 mg/dL. Total cholesterol level fell by 20% in the treatment group and remained unchanged in the placebo group. Mean arteriographic segment diameter (an index of overall coronary plaque burden) decreased by 0.10 mm in the placebo group and 0.06 mm in the pravastatin group ($p = 0.019$). Median maximum stenosis diameter decreased by 0.09 mm in the placebo group compared with 0.03 mm in the pravastatin group ($p = 0.001$).

Nonpharmacologic approaches to lipid lowering have also been shown to effectively reduce disease progression. In the Lifestyle Heart Trial (LHT),[45] 28 patients with angiographically documented CAD were treated with a stringent low-fat vegetarian diet, moderate exercise, and stress management; 20 patients were treated by conventional means. In the experimental group, the average percent diameter stenosis, as determined on quantitative coronary angiography, diminished over the 12-month study period from 40.0% to 37.8%, whereas the stenosis severity increased from 42.7% to 46.1% in the group receiving conventional care. The magnitude of the change was similar when analysis of only the single tightest stenosis was performed. The experimental group showed other changes in plaque morphology, including improvements in stenosis length and inflow and exit angles.[46]

It is important to note that in the majority of patients, coronary atherosclerosis progresses inexorably. In most angiographic regression trials, more patients showed quantitatively defined "progression" of coronary stenoses than "regression," whether they were randomly assigned to receive lipid-lowering therapy or placebo. Moreover, MI remains a risk even in treated patients (Table 9–2).

The most important effects of lipid-lowering therapy probably are not hemodynamically significant alterations in luminal caliber but, rather, alterations in the biology of atherosclerotic plaques. After 6 to 12 months, pharmacologic lipid lowering improves acetylcholine-induced vasoconstriction (a marker of endothelial dysfunction) in patients with hypercholesterolemia and normal[47] or diseased[48, 49] coronary arteries (Fig. 9–3). Moreover, forearm endothelium-dependent vasomotion is improved within only 2 to 12 weeks by medications[50] and within minutes after low density lipoprotein (LDL) apheresis.[51]

Furthermore, and in striking contrast to the modest influence on coronary lumen diameter, lipid-lowering therapy substantially reduces the rate of clinical events. In the Scandinavian Simvastatin Survival Study (4S),[52] 4444 patients with angina or a previous infarction and a mean LDL-cholesterol

**TABLE 9–2.    LIPID-LOWERING THERAPY AND INCIDENCE OF NONFATAL MI IN PATIENTS WITH HYPERCHOLESTEROLEMIA**

| STUDY | YEARS | N | INCIDENCE OF NONFATAL MI (%) | |
|-------|-------|---|------------------------------|---|
| | | | CONTROL GROUP | TREATMENT GROUP |
| CDP-NA[154] | 5 | 3908 | 12% | 9% |
| LRC-CPPT[155] | 7.4 | 3806 | 8% | 7% |
| Helsinki[156] | 5 | 4081 | 4% | 2% |
| Oslo[157] | 5 | 1232 | 4% | 2% |
| 4S[52] | 5 | 4444 | 19% | 13% |
| WOSCOPS[53] | 5 | 6595 | 6% | 4% |
| CARE[53] | 5 | 4159 | 8% | 6% |
| *Total* | | 28,194 | 9.9% | 6.9% |

CARE, Cholesterol and Recurrent Events trial; CDP-NA, Coronary Drug Project Nicotinic Acid group; LRC-CPPT, Lipid Research Clinics Coronary Primary Prevention Trial; Helsinki, Helsinki Heart Study; MI, myocardial infarction; Oslo, Oslo Study Group; 4S, Scandinavian Simvastatin Survival Study; WOSCOPS, West of Scotland Coronary Prevention Study.

Adapted from Superko H: Lipid disorders contributing to coronary heart disease: An update. Curr Probl Cardiol 21:736–780, 1996.

level of 188 mg/dL were treated with simvastatin, 10 to 40 mg/day, or placebo. After 5 years, simvastatin reduced LDL cholesterol by 35%, mortality by 30% ($p = 0.0003$; Fig. 9–4), and the rate of major coronary events by 31% ($p < 0.00001$). In the West of Scotland Coronary Prevention Study,[53] 6595 patients without known coronary disease and with a mean LDL-cholesterol level of 192 mg/dL were randomly assigned to receive pravastatin, 40 mg/day, or placebo. After an average of 5 years, pravastatin had lowered LDL-cholesterol level by 26% and the rates of cardiac death by 33% ($p = 0.042$) and of major coronary events by 31% ($p < 0.001$).

Even patients with "average" North American cholesterol levels derive benefit from lipid lowering. In the Cholesterol and Recurrent Events (CARE) trial,[54] 4159 patients, averaging 10 months after MI and having LDL-cholesterol levels of 115 to 174

mg/dL (average, 139 mg/dL) were randomly assigned to receive 40 mg/day of pravastatin or placebo. LDL-cholesterol level was reduced 32% during the 5-year follow-up. The primary end point of combined cardiac mortality and nonfatal infarction was reduced by 24% ($p = 0.003$), cardiac mortality was reduced by 20% ($p = 0.10$), and the rates of nonfatal infarction and mechanical revascularization were reduced by 23% ($p = 0.02$) and 27% ($p < 0.001$), respectively. Benefit seemed confined to patients with a baseline LDL-cholesterol level exceeding 125 mg/dL. All three studies showed benefit in women as well as men and in younger as well as older patients. However, patients older than 75 years were not studied. Previous reports, of excess rates of neoplastic and violent deaths in patients treated with lipid-lowering drugs,[55] were not substantiated.[52, 53] Thus, unlike conventional anti-ische-

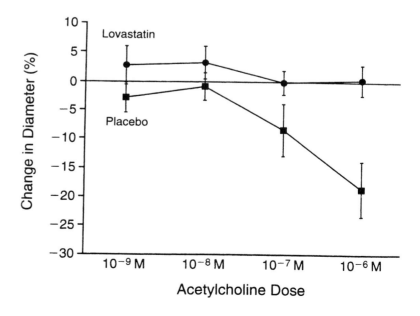

FIGURE 9–3. Responses of the most constricting segment of the epicardial coronary artery to serial infusions of acetylcholine in hypercholesterolemic patients treated with lovastatin or placebo. The pathologic vasoconstrictor response to acetylcholine (expressed as percentage change from baseline diameter in the most constricting segment) was significantly attenuated in the lovastatin group ($p = 0.004$). Negative numbers indicate vasoconstriction. (From Treasure CB, Klein JL, Weintraub WS, et al: Beneficial effects of cholesterol-lowering therapy on the coronary endothelium in patients with coronary artery disease. N Engl J Med 332:481–487, 1995.)

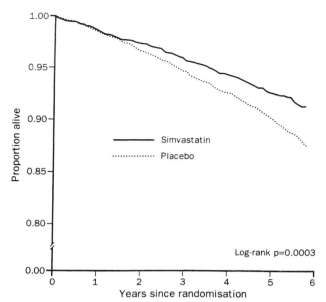

FIGURE 9–4. Mortality after lipid-lowering therapy in patients with coronary artery disease. (From 4S Investigators: Randomised trial of cholesterol lowering in 4444 patients with coronary heart disease: The Scandinavian Simvastatin Survival Study [4S]. Lancet 344:1383–1389, 1994.)

mic therapy, lipid-lowering therapy may alter the propensity for atherosclerotic plaques to progress and, possibly, to rupture.

Lowering serum cholesterol level from more than 200 mg/dL to less than 200 mg/dL in a 35-year-old man could be expected to achieve an increase in survival of 0.5 to 4.2 years.[42]

## Treatment of Hypertension

Although individual randomized trials have often failed to show a reduction in cardiac mortality for patients receiving medical therapy for mild hypertension, a meta-analysis of 14 published randomized trials showed a 21% reduction in overall vascular mortality ($p < 0.0002$), a 42% reduction in the incidence of stroke ($p < 0.0001$), and a 14% reduction in the incidence of MI ($p < 0.01$) in a total population of 37,000 patients.[56] The mean fall in diastolic blood pressure in the treated patients during the 5-year study period was 5 to 6 mm Hg. This benefit also appears to be evident in elderly patients with systolic hypertension. In one study of elderly patients, antihypertensive therapy reduced the incidence of nonfatal infarction and coronary death by 27% ($p = 0.02$).[57]

## Treatment of Diabetes Mellitus

Microvascular complications of diabetes (nephropathy, retinopathy, neuropathy) are clearly related to the level of hyperglycemia and are reduced by me-

ticulous glycemic control in patients with type I diabetes.[58] Macrovascular complications, including incidence and fatality from acute and chronic MI, stroke, and peripheral vascular disease, also are increased in patients with both type I and type II diabetes.[59–62] Endothelial dysfunction is readily demonstrable[63] and appears related to duration of diabetes and to concurrent dyslipidemia.[64] Reversal of experimental diabetes in rats normalizes endothelial function.[65] However, it remains to be established whether intensified hypoglycemic therapy will attenuate macrovascular complications in humans.

The Diabetes Control and Complications Trial,[58] which evaluated intensive insulin therapy in type I diabetes, showed a reduction in the rate of cardiovascular events by 41% during a 6-year period compared with standard insulin therapy. However, the events were too few to reach statistical significance. Two prospective observational Finnish studies of glycemia control in more than 350 patients with type II diabetes showed a progressive decline in cardiovascular mortality among tertiles with lower fasting blood glucose and glycohemoglobin, both among patients treated with diet alone and among those treated with hypoglycemic medications, including insulin.[66–68]

Insulin therapy can conceivably induce weight gain and exacerbate hypertension and dyslipidemia, and itself may be atherogenic.[69, 70] Therefore, patients with CAD and type II diabetes may benefit from "insulin-sparing" strategies. Metformin combined with sulfonylureas may confer adequate glycemic control.[71] The intestinal disaccharidase inhibitor acarbose may be synergistic.[72] In patients requiring insulin, combination therapy with sulfonylureas[73] or troglitazone[74] is effective and may reduce insulin "toxicity."

## Antiplatelet Therapy

Low-dose aspirin therapy is used both to prevent coronary disease in healthy patients and to treat established disease. In the U.S. Physicians' Health Study,[75] prophylactic aspirin therapy was associated with a 44% reduction in the incidence of first infarction ($p < 0.00001$) in 22,071 men aged 40 to 84 years. Meta-analysis of antiplatelet therapy (primarily aspirin) in more than 140,000 patients with angina, prior MI, or prior aortocoronary bypass surgery showed that rates of death, nonfatal MI, and stroke were each reduced by one third (each $2p < 0.00001$).[76] Benefits were significant in middle and old age, in men and women, in hypertensive and normotensive patients, and in diabetic and nondiabetic patients. Patients intolerant of aspirin can be treated with ticlopidine,[77] which is potentially myelotoxic, or dipyridamole, which is less potent. Other antiplatelet agents are promising. In the Clopidogrel versus Aspirin in Patients at Risk of Ischaemic Events (CAPRIE) trial,[78] patients with known vascular disease who were randomly assigned to receive clopidogrel, 75 mg/day, had a 8.7% ($p = 0.043$) reduction in rate of stroke, MI, or vascular death over 3 years compared with those who received aspirin, 325 mg/day, with no recognizable difference in safety of the two agents.

## β-Adrenergic Antagonists

β Blockers are offered to patients with stable CAD to control symptoms and possibly to improve prognosis. They may reduce ischemia by lowering heart rate, diminishing inotropy, and favorably altering cardiac loading conditions. They also may alter prognosis by suppressing tachyarrhythmia and reducing triggers of atheromatous plaque rupture. β blockers unequivocally reduce mortality after MI[79] and are probably a treatment of first choice in patients who tolerate them in stable angina. The intriguing observation that β blockade reduces the rate of late but not early coronary events after noncardiac surgery[80] invites the hypothesis that this class of drug blocks triggers of atherosclerotic plaque instability and may have long-term benefit in stable coronary disease.

## ACE Inhibitors

ACE inhibitors clearly reduce mortality in patients with depressed LV function after MI,[81–83] and they also lower the rate of recurrent ischemic events, including MI.[82] The reduction in renin-angiotensin activation may lower circumferential plaque stress and may even improve coronary vasomotor tone.[84] The utility of ACE inhibitors in the patient without LV dysfunction who has evidence of vascular disease or diabetes plus one other cardiovascular risk factor has been demonstrated.[85]

## Postmenopausal Hormone Replacement Therapy

Manifest CAD is uncommon in women before menopause. Conversely, premature surgical menopause without estrogen replacement doubles the risk of significant CAD.[86] A meta-analysis of 31 observational studies estimated that a 44% reduction in CAD could be achieved with postmenopausal estrogen replacement therapy.[87]

The exact mechanism of potential benefit is uncertain. Estrogen modestly reduces serum LDL-cholesterol and lipoprotein Lp(a) levels, increases high density lipoprotein (HDL) cholesterol, may protect against lipoprotein oxidation, and may lower levels of serum fibrinogen and other hemostatic factors.[88] Estrogens may improve endothelial dysfunction. Intracoronary administration of 17-beta-estradiol at physiologic concentrations attenuates acetylcholine-induced vasoconstriction in normal[89] and diseased[89, 90] coronary arteries in postmenopausal women but not in men. The improved vasomotor function may explain an anti-ischemic effect. Sublingual 17-beta-estradiol improved duration of treadmill exercise and time to ischemia compared with placebo in a randomized, double-blind study of postmenopausal women with coronary disease.[91]

Unfortunately, the promise of hormone replacement therapy has not been realized in randomized trials. The Heart and Estrogen/Progestin Replacement Study (HERS)[92] found that 4 years of treatment with conjugated estrogen plus medroxyprogesterone acetate had no effect on nonfatal myocardial infarction or death in women with established coronary artery disease. Closer evaluation of the data revealed increased risk for thromboembolic events in the first year of active treatment and fewer coronary events in years 4 and 5. The Women's Health Initiative Hormone Replacement Trial[93] is ongoing. Women who have had hysterectomies receive unopposed estrogen or placebo, whereas women with intact uteruses receive either the same estrogen plus progestin as used in HERS or placebo. A preliminary safety report noted a slight increase in cardiovascular events in the first 2 years with active treatment, as was seen in HERS.

More recently, the Estrogen Replacement and Atherosclerosis (ERA) trial[94] found no effect of estrogen alone or in combination with progesterone on angiographic lesion development or progression. The Raloxifene Use for The Heart (RUTH) trial is testing whether a selective estrogen receptor modulator will have a role in secondary prevention of coronary disease.

## Antioxidant and Other Vitamin Therapy

Dietary or pharmacologic antioxidants (vitamin E, β-carotene, ascorbic acid, flavanoids) may inhibit oxidative modification of LDL and may reduce atherogenesis. Epidemiologic studies show a 30% to 40% reduction in death or infarction risk in people whose dietary diaries suggest higher intake of vitamin E.[95, 96] In the Alpha Tocopherol Beta Carotene (ATBC) study,[97] vitamin E was associated with a very modest reduction in the incidence of angina (relative risk, 0.91; 95% CI 0.83 to 0.99). β-Carotene had no effect, nor was benefit found for it in other studies.[98, 99] In the Cambridge Heart Antioxidant Study (CHAOS),[100] 2002 men with angiographically proven coronary disease were randomly assigned to receive either placebo or a significantly higher dose of vitamin E (400 to 800 IU/day, reduced in midstudy for lack of funds). Over 1 year, vitamin E reduced the combined end point of mortality and nonfatal infarction from 7% to 4% ($p = 0.005$) and nonfatal infarction by two thirds, from 4.2% to 1.4% ($p = 0.005$). However, the rate of cardiovascular deaths was nonsignificantly higher in the vitamin E group than in the placebo group (2.6% versus 2.4%; $p = 0.61$).

Two more studies demonstrated no benefit on cardiovascular outcomes with vitamin E treatment.[101, 102]

Elevated plasma homocysteine is an independent risk factor for coronary, cerebral, and peripheral vascular disease,[103] although the mechanism is unclear. In the U.S. Physicians' Health Study, men with fasting homocysteine levels above the 95th percentile were 3.4 times more likely to experience coronary disease than those with levels below the 90th percentile ($p = 0.03$).[104] Plasma homocysteine levels after methionine loading increases diagnostic sensitivity. Deficiency of folic acid, pyridoxine, and cobalamin induce elevations in plasma homocysteine values; supplementation with any of these substances reduces plasma homocysteine levels. Whether such supplementation lowers the risk for cardiovascular disease awaits further study.[105]

## Calcium Channel Blockers

Calcium channel antagonists, in theory, may prevent progression of atherosclerosis through a number of mechanisms, including inhibition of lipid accumulation, reduction of endothelial injury, and lessening of vasoconstriction.[106] Two clinical studies have suggested that the calcium channel antagonists nifedipine[107] and nicardipine[108] have no effect on progression of established atherosclerotic disease but may inhibit the development of new lesions. In the Prospective Randomized Evaluation of the Vascular Effects of Norvasc Trial (PREVENT),[108] amlodipine had no effect on angiographic progression of coronary disease or rates of myocardial infarction or death, but it did reduce hospitalizations for unstable angina and revascularization. The routine clinical use of calcium channel antagonists as a secondary preventive measure has been tempered by the findings of the Multicenter Diltiazem Postinfarction Trial Research Group.[110] In this study, treatment with diltiazem was associated with no improvement in overall survival after MI.

## Other, Nonpharmacologic Therapies

Several other approaches to treatment and prevention of CAD also appear to have favorable effects on clinical outcome. They are regular physical activity, treatment of obesity, and the consumption of small to moderate amounts of alcohol.[30]

## PERCUTANEOUS REVASCULARIZATION FOR STABLE ANGINA PECTORIS

## ACIP Study

Evidence on electrogram (ECG) of provocable or spontaneous ischemia confers an adverse prognosis in patients with stable CAD,[111–113] and suppression of ischemia identifies patients with stable angina at reduced risk for adverse outcomes.[114] However, it has not been clearly established whether the goal of anti-ischemic therapy should be solely palliative (to control angina) or whether more aggressive suppression even of asymptomatic myocardial ischemia (evident on ambulatory ECG, for example) will improve outcome.

To this end, the Asymptomatic Cardiac Ischemia Pilot (ACIP) study sponsored by the National Institutes of Health[115] compared three antianginal strategies in 558 patients with stable angina. Most were white and male and had good functional status, preserved LV function, multivessel CAD, and evidence of ischemia after approximately 4 metabolic equivalents (METS) of exercise. They were randomly assigned to be treated by (1) nonblind use of medications titrated over 4 weeks to suppress angina (angina-guided treatment), (2) additional blind use of medications titrated to suppress ischemia on serial ambulatory ECGs over 8 weeks (ischemia-guided treatment), or (3) nonblind use of medications and mechanical revascularization, either PTCA or coronary artery bypass grafting (CABG), as determined from suitable anatomy and likelihood of complete revascularization. Anti-ischemic regimens consisted of escalating doses of atenolol plus nifedipine or of diltiazem plus nitroglycerin. Second medications were added according to a predetermined protocol. Lipid-lowering therapy was not specified.

At 12 weeks, all groups had fewer episodes of daily-life ischemia, reduced cumulative ischemic time during ambulatory ECG, and improved performance on treadmill testing.[116, 117] The ischemia-guided strategy was no more successful than the angina-guided strategy in eliminating daily-life ischemia, which persisted in the majority of patients (61% and 59%, respectively). However, only 45% of the patients treated with mechanical revascularization continued to have ischemia triggered by activities of daily living. Patients who had undergone revascularization also had significantly better times to ischemia and times to angina on treadmill testing than either of the patient groups receiving medical treatment. After 1 year, 61% of patients in the revascularization group did not require antianginal medications, compared with 28% of patients in the two medical treatment groups. Mortality was 4.4% in the angina-guided treatment group, 1.6% in the ischemia-guided treatment group, and 0 in the revascularization group.[118] Similarly, the cumulative end point of death, infarction, nonprotocol revascularization, and hospital admission was 32% in the angina-guided treatment group, 31% in the ischemia-guided treatment group, and 18% in the revascularization group.[119, 120]

## ACME Study

The Angioplasty Compared to Medicine (ACME) trial[121] was a Veterans Affairs Cooperative Studies multicenter, randomized study. Its premise was that although PTCA was unlikely to reduce the already very low mortality of patients with one-vessel disease, the procedure would achieve a lower frequency of angina and better exercise tolerance than antianginal therapy over a 6-month study period. Patients were eligible for participation in the ACME study if they had stable angina, recent MI, or silent ischemia with 3-mm or greater ST segment depression on exercise stress testing. Angiograms in eligible patients showed a 70% to 99% stenosis in the proximal two thirds of one major epicardial coronary artery. Eligible patients also had at least a 1-mm ST segment depression on treadmill testing or a reversible perfusion defect on thallium scintigraphy.

During the study period, between 1986 and 1990, almost 10,000 patients were screened, 371 eligible patients were identified, and 212 patients agreed to be assigned randomly either to PTCA or to medical therapy. Medical therapy consisted of aspirin, oral nitrates, β blockers, and calcium channel blockers. No other specific attempts were made to control baseline risk factors, including hyperlipidemia. Patients who underwent PTCA also received calcium channel blockers for 1 month after the procedure. All patients were reevaluated with exercise stress testing and coronary angiography after 6 months. To isolate the effect of PTCA on exercise performance, the researchers temporarily discontinued all antianginal drugs in the PTCA group before stress testing, even though these agents were continued in the medical therapy group. The primary end points for the study were the change in exercise tolerance, frequency of angina, and use of sublingual nitroglycerin from baseline to the final month of the study.

Of the 100 patients in whom PTCA was attempted, success (defined as a greater than 20% reduction in diameter stenosis of the index lesion

**TABLE 9–3.  IMMEDIATE PTCA OUTCOME AND 6-MONTH EVENT RATE IN PATIENTS ASSIGNED TO MEDICAL THERAPY OR TO PTCA IN THE ACME STUDY**

|  | PTCA (N = 105) | MEDICINE (N = 107) |
|---|---|---|
| PTCA attempted | 100 | — |
| PTCA successful | 80 | — |
| Emergency CABG | 2 | 0 |
| Acute MI | 4 | 0 |
| Death | 0 | 1 |
| Repeat or late PTCA | 16 | 11 |
| Elective CABG | 5 | 0 |
| Late MI | 1 | 3 |

ACME, Angioplasty compared to medicine; CABG, coronary artery bypass graft surgery; MI, myocardial infarction; PTCA, percutaneous transluminal coronary angioplasty.

without MI or the need for emergency CABG surgery) was achieved in 80. Emergency surgery was required in two patients, and four had Q-wave or non–Q-wave MIs (Table 9–3). During the follow-up period, PTCA for restenosis was performed in 16 patients, 5 underwent elective coronary artery surgery, and 1 patient had an acute MI; there were no procedural or late deaths in this group (see Table 9–3). Of the 107 patients assigned to medical therapy, 11 underwent PTCA during the follow-up period, but none underwent bypass graft surgery. MI occurred in 3 patients, and 1 patient died during an elective coronary angioplasty procedure (see Table 9–3).

At 6 months, 64% of patients in the PTCA group were angina free compared with 46% in the medical treatment group ($p = 0.01$) (Fig. 9–5). This difference was associated with a greater reduction in the number of angina episodes per month and a statistically nonsignificant decrease in the use of nitroglycerin. Functional capacity, as assessed by the total duration of exercise, the maximal heart rate–blood

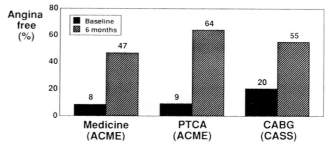

FIGURE 9–5. Improvement in symptom status from baseline to 6-month follow-up in the medicine and PTCA treatment arms of the ACME study. For comparison, baseline and 12-month follow-up data are included for patients with one-vessel disease treated by bypass graft surgery in the Coronary Artery Surgery Study (CASS). (Data from Parisi et al[121] and Coronary Artery Surgery Study investigators.[23])

pressure product, and the time to onset of chest pain, improved in both groups, but the improvement was significantly greater in the PTCA group (Fig. 9–6). As expected, index lesion severity at follow-up angiography was significantly less in the PTCA group (54% vs. 75%; $p < 0.001$). During this short follow-up period, the incidence of disease progression to 70% or greater diameter stenosis in other vessels was relatively high in both groups (10% vs. 7%; $p = 0.50$). PTCA was associated with a smaller need for antianginal medications and with a better overall psychologic well-being score and index of general health and vitality[122] but also with a greater need for rehospitalization during the follow-up period and no better rate of return to employment.

Thus, mechanical treatment of stable coronary stenoses in patients with one-vessel disease was shown in this study to improve overall quality of life and symptom status, at the expense of a higher rate of initial procedural complications. Several inherent limitations of the study warrant further comment. The clinical success rate for PTCA in this study was only 80%, which is comparable to the success rate in the National Heart, Lung, and Blood Institute PTCA Registry from the same period[123] but low by contemporary standards. The availability of bail-out stenting would probably have reduced the need for emergency bypass graft surgery, and a higher primary success rate would have reduced the need for elective surgery and would perhaps have further increased the difference in functional capacity between the two groups. Similarly, in clinical practice,

PTCA and medical therapy are not mutually exclusive. Had patients in the PTCA group been exercising while receiving medical therapy, the difference in exercise capacity might have been even greater. Finally, the difference in hospitalization may have been somewhat exaggerated by the study design, which sought to minimize mechanical revascularization in the medically treated patients. In fact, patients in this treatment arm frequently underwent revascularization procedures immediately after completion of the study, for symptomatic relief.

## MASS

The Medicine Angioplasty Surgery Study (MASS)[124] also found medications to be substantially less effective than revascularization in controlling angina but that angioplasty did not reduce composite end points. In the study, 214 patients with stable angina, severe proximal LAD stenosis, and preserved LV systolic function were randomly assigned to receive (1) internal mammary coronary bypass surgery, all procedures of which were conducted by the same surgeon, (2) balloon angioplasty, all procedures of which were conducted by the same interventionist, or (3) medical therapy. Angioplasty did not involve endoluminal stenting. Medical therapy consisted of aspirin and anti-ischemics, but not necessarily β blockers. Two patients died, each late after angioplasty or bypass surgery. Of the 72 patients assigned to receive medical therapy, 4 had nonfatal infarctions and 7 had refractory angina requiring surgery or angioplasty. Of the 72 patients assigned to un-

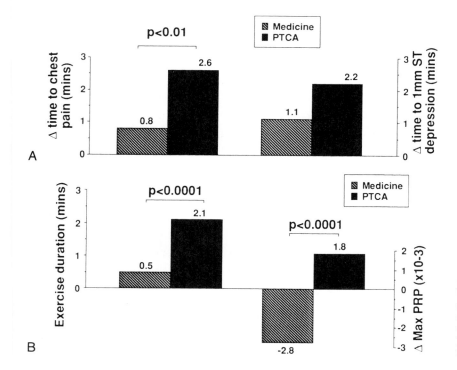

FIGURE 9–6. Change in exercise tolerance from baseline to 6-month follow-up in the two treatment arms of the ACME Study. PTCA was associated with a significantly greater increase in exercise duration, maximum pressure-rate product (PRP), and time to chest pain. (Data from Parisi et al.[121])

dergo angioplasty, 2 had periprocedural infarctions and required emergency surgery, and 1 had unsuccessful angioplasty. Angiography was performed in 27 patients (37.5%) with recurrent angina after PTCA, of whom 21 had second PTCA procedures and 8 underwent elective coronary bypass surgery.

PTCA was more effective than medical therapy in controlling angina. After 3 years, 18% of the patients assigned to undergo angioplasty and 68% of the patients assigned to receive medical therapy had angina ($p < 0.01$). Cumulative likelihood of death, infarction, or second revascularization procedure (not including second angioplasty in the PTCA arm of the study) was 24% among PTCA patients and 17% among medical patients ($p = $ NS).

## RITA-2

In the second Randomised Intervention Treatment of Angina study (RITA-2),[125] 70,000 patients were screened for eligibility during angiography in Ireland or the United Kingdom. Of 2750 patients considered eligible, 1018 were randomly assigned either to conventional medical therapy or to PTCA. Aggressive cholesterol-lowering treatment was not instituted, but aspirin and β blockers were used widely. Most patients had stable angina, although 21% had CCS class III angina or worse, and 20% had no angina upon entry into the study; 66% had one-vessel disease and 33% two-vessel disease; most had nearly normal LV systolic function. Angioplasty strategy was left to the operators' discretion, and although stents were apparently available for bail-out at some centers, they were employed in only 9% of protocol interventions.

During a median 2.7-year follow-up period, death or nonfatal MI occurred in 32 patients (6.3%) undergoing PTCA compared with 17 patients (3.3%) receiving medical therapy ($p = 0.02$). Most of the difference is attributed to periprocedural complications, which led to death in 1 patient and to nonfatal infarction in 7 patients undergoing PTCA. Ninety-six patients in the PTCA group (19%) underwent subsequent PTCA or CABG, in comparison with 118 (23%) in the medical therapy arm.

After 6 months, 80% of patients in the PTCA group were angina free, in comparison with 67% of patients in the medical therapy group ($p < 0.001$). After 2 years, 82% were angina free in the PTCA group, in comparison with 74% in the medical therapy group ($p = 0.02$). This progressively narrowing difference between groups is attributed to the performance of nonprotocol mechanical revascularization in all patients whose symptoms worsened during the follow-up period. Post hoc analysis revealed greater symptomatic benefit of PTCA than of medical therapy for patients with CCS class II or greater angina at baseline and for patients who were unable to exercise more than 9 minutes at baseline.

In summary, this larger randomized trial of selected patients with comparatively low mortality risk showed a modest symptomatic advantage of PTCA over medical therapy, again at the expense of periprocedural morbidity and mortality. Not surprisingly, benefit was confined to patients who had significant symptoms.

## AVERT Study

The Atorvastatin Versus Revascularization Treatment (AVERT) study[126] enrolled 341 low-risk patients with one- or two-vessel disease, ejection fractions exceeding 40%, class 0 to 2 angina, and an LDL cholesterol level (LDL-C) exceeding 115 mg/dL. Subjects were assigned either to atorvastatin, 80 mg, plus usual care, including β blockers or nitrates, or to PTCA (which could include lipid-lowering medications). The primary end point included the composite of cardiac death, cardiac arrest, nonfatal myocardial infarction, stroke, PTCA, CABG, or hospitalization for angina. Atorvastatin reduced LDL-C by 40% to 77 mg/dL, in comparison with an LDL-C level of 119 mg/dL in the PTCA group. Twenty-two patients (13%) treated with atorvastatin had ischemic events during the 18-month follow-up, in comparison with 37 patients (21%) in the PTCA group. No difference in cardiac death or nonfatal myocardial infarction was found between the two groups. More CABG procedures and more hospitalization for angina occurred in the PTCA group. However, the study was limited by small sample size, selective recruitment, short duration of follow-up, lack of ischemia-guided revascularization, open-label design, lack of information on antianginal medication dosing, and the subjective end point of "worsening angina."

## Percutaneous Interventions for Multivessel CAD

As noted previously, the number of major epicardial coronary arteries with obstructive stenoses is a powerful predictor of long-term survival[14–16]; surgical revascularization has been shown to provide very satisfactory symptom relief in patients with two- or three-vessel disease.[18, 19, 127] The use of percutaneous coronary interventions for patients with multivessel disease has grown considerably, on the assumption that this approach may provide adequate symptom relief and may defer eventual coronary bypass surgery, at a lower cost and lower morbidity than the surgical alternative.

Several studies have reported very high initial success rates for multivessel PTCA and have suggested that the immediate outcome for this procedure is similar to that observed after one-vessel PTCA.[128–130] Patients with multivessel disease now constitute approximately 40% of all patients undergoing PTCA, but in contrast to patients undergoing bypass surgery, the majority (60% to 80%) undergoing PTCA have two-vessel rather than three-vessel disease.[131–133]

An important factor in determining the suitability of percutaneous intervention in patients with multivessel disease is the likelihood of functionally complete myocardial revascularization. Complete revascularization is attempted in relatively few patients with multivessel disease and is achieved in only 20% to 60% of these patients.[123, 128, 131–138] Nonrandomized studies have suggested, however, that incomplete revascularization can provide satisfactory symptom relief with a good functional outcome when all vessels supplying viable myocardium can be satisfactorily treated.[132, 139–141] Of patients in whom complete revascularization is not achieved, only about a third have had inducible myocardial ischemia after the procedure.[132, 139–141]

In a small pilot companion to the ACME trial, 101 patients who had been ineligible for inclusion in the study because of two-vessel CAD were randomly assigned to receive PTCA or medical therapy.[142] After 6 months, there was a statistically nonsignificant difference between the PTCA and medical groups in freedom from angina (53% and 36%, respectively; $p = 0.09$), but no important difference in exercise duration ($+1.2$ minutes and $+1.3$ minutes, respectively; $p = 0.89$), myocardial perfusion image score, or improvement of quality of life score in comparison with baseline. There also was no significant difference in rates of cumulative death, MI, or unstable angina after 6 months (30% and 30%, respectively) or after a median 60 months (74% and 80%, respectively). No patients required emergency CABG, but 28% of patients undergoing PTCA required second revascularization procedures, in comparison with 16% of medically treated patients who underwent mechanical revascularization in the first 6 months. In more than a third of the angioplasty group, one vessel was considered untreatable by PTCA (usually an old occlusion). Complete revascularization was achieved in only the minority of patients: PTCA was considered successful in only 45% of patients with two treated vessels and in 80% of those in whom an occluded vessel was not treated.

Prospective nonrandomized data from Duke University collected between 1984 and 1990[143] suggest that the extent of CAD determines the impact of revascularization on survival. For single-vessel disease, PTCA had no 5-year survival advantage over medical therapy (95% and 94%, respectively) but a modest benefit in comparison with CABG (95% and 93%, respectively). For two-vessel disease, revascularization was associated with higher adjusted survival than medical therapy (PTCA 91%, CABG 91%, medicine 86%). For three-vessel disease, CABG had superior 5-year adjusted survival (PTCA 81%, CABG 89%, medicine 72%).

## Limitations of Clinical Trials of Percutaneous Coronary Interventions

An important finding in the ACME study was the failure of both medical therapy and angioplasty to prevent progression of nonindex coronary stenoses in the other coronary arteries even during the short follow-up period.[121] Previous studies have suggested that neither coronary angioplasty nor CABG reduces the net incidence of MI in comparison with medical therapy.[19–21, 24, 123] However, these studies were performed before the recognition that aggressive risk factor modification can slow disease progression and may indeed reduce the propensity for acute ischemic events.[52, 54, 144]

Randomized studies are plagued by evolutionary changes in therapeutics that often make a trial obsolete even before it is completed. Certainly, both angioplasty and coronary pharmacotherapy have changed since the early 1990s. At present, the applicability of percutaneous revascularization is limited by (1) chronic total coronary occlusions, for which percutaneous revascularization is often or usually unsuccessful, (2) the propensity for abrupt coronary occlusion, which results in serious early complications, and (3) recurrent stenosis, which negates the benefits of a successful procedure and affects approximately one third of patients undergoing percutaneous revascularization.

Newer approaches to the latter two problems markedly increase the safety and net benefit of percutaneous revascularization. Abciximab (ReoPro), a platelet glycoprotein IIb/IIIa (GPIIb/IIIa) receptor antagonist, reduces the rate of major ischemic events after angioplasty[145, 146] and may reduce the incidence of clinical restenosis at 6 months.[147] Endoluminal coronary stenting dramatically reduces angiographic and clinical restenosis in comparison with balloon angioplasty.[148, 149] The rate of adverse coronary events, including second revascularization procedure, is lowered further by technical improvements, including high-pressure balloon inflation,[150] postprocedural administration of aspirin and ticlopidine or clopidogrel without warfarin,[151] and, possibly, heparin-coated stents.[152] Bail-out stenting for obstructive dissection during angioplasty reduces the need for emergency aortocoronary bypass and now is employed widely.[153] Having stents available for emergency bail-out—even when not used—may permit more aggressive device sizing, improved postprocedural lumen diameter, and, possibly, less restenosis. This practice may account in part for the 50% difference in clinical restenosis rates between the control groups of the sequentially conducted antiplatelet trials EPIC (Evaluation of 7E3 for the Prevention of Ischemic Complications)[147] and EPI-LOG (Evaluation of PTCA to Improve Long-term Outcome by c7E3 GP IIB/IIIA Receptor Blockade).[146]

## CONCLUSIONS

Although relatively few randomized comparative data are available, it seems likely that a percutaneous interventional approach is appropriate for certain subgroups of patients with symptomatic CAD. In patients with one-vessel disease, PTCA has been shown to improve functional capacity and to reduce the frequency of angina pectoris. Randomized trials comparing angioplasty with aortocoronary bypass suggest that this improvement is also possible for patients with two-vessel, and possibly three-vessel, disease. There are no data to suggest that PTCA reduces the likelihood of subsequent MI, probably because acute thrombotic closure commonly occurs in arteries with nonobstructive disease detected on baseline angiography. Whether percutaneous interventional procedures actually improve survival remains unclear and awaits more definitive clinical trials. The Clinical Outcomes Utilizing Revascularization and Aggressive Drug Evaluation (COURAGE) trial is randomly assigning moderate-risk and low-risk patients with clear indications for PTCA to receive intensive medical therapy (including aspirin, anti-ischemic medications, and, when appropriate, a hydroxymethyl coenzyme A reductase inhibitor, and an ACE inhibitor), with or without "modern" percutaneous revascularization.

Although mechanical therapies, such as PTCA, may successfully treat symptoms of established and stable CAD, elective revascularization alone does not prevent disease progression or the morbidity and mortality associated with acute ischemic syndromes. Conversely, whereas intensive medical therapies may improve plaque stability, reduce the propensity for disease progression, and lower the rate of acute ischemic complications in the remainder of the coronary arterial tree, they do not offer the extent of symptom relief from established coronary stenoses attainable with mechanical revascularization.

## REFERENCES

1. Favaloro RG: Saphenous vein autograft replacement of severe segmental coronary artery occlusion: Operative technique. Ann Thorac Surg 5:334–339, 1968.
2. Gruntzig A: Transluminal dilatation of coronary-artery stenosis [Letter]. Lancet 1:263, 1978.
3. Davies MJ: A macro and micro view of coronary vascular insult in ischemic heart disease. Circulation 82:II-38–II-46, 1990.
4. Falk E, Shah PK, Fuster V: Coronary plaque disruption. Circulation 92:657–671, 1995.
5. Cheng GC, Loree HM, Kamm RD, et al: Distribution of circumferential stress in ruptured and stable atherosclerotic lesions. A structural analysis with histopathological correlation. Circulation 87:1179–1187, 1993.
6. Falk E: Plaque rupture with severe pre-existing stenosis precipitating coronary thrombosis. Characteristics of coronary atherosclerotic plaques underlying fatal occlusive thrombi. Br Heart J 50:127–134, 1983.
7. Davies MJ, Bland JM, Hangartner JR, et al: Factors influencing the presence or absence of acute coronary artery thrombi in sudden ischaemic death. Eur Heart J 10:203–208, 1989.
8. Haft JI, Haik BJ, Goldstein JE, et al: Development of significant coronary artery lesions in areas of minimal disease. A common mechanism for coronary disease progression. Chest 94:731–736, 1988.
9. Chester MR, Chen L, Kaski JC: The natural history of unheralded complex coronary plaques. J Am Coll Cardiol 28:604–608, 1996.
10. Ellis S, Alderman E, Cain K, et al: Prediction of risk of anterior myocardial infarction by lesion severity and measurement method of stenoses in the left anterior descending coronary distribution: A CASS Registry Study. J Am Coll Cardiol 11:908–916, 1988.
11. Ambrose JA, Tannenbaum MA, Alexopoulos D, et al: Angiographic progression of coronary artery disease and the development of myocardial infarction. J Am Coll Cardiol 12:56–62, 1988.
12. Little WC, Constantinescu M, Applegate RJ, et al: Can coronary angiography predict the site of a subsequent myocardial infarction in patients with mild-to-moderate coronary artery disease? Circulation 78:1157–1166, 1988.
13. Serruys PW, Arnold AE, Brower RW, et al: Effect of continued rt-PA administration on the residual stenosis after initially successful recanalization in acute myocardial infarction—A quantitative coronary angiography study of a randomized trial. Eur Heart J 8:1172–1181, 1987.
14. Kannel WB, Feinleib M: Natural history of angina pectoris in the Framingham Study. Prognosis and survival. Am J Cardiol 29:154–163, 1972.
15. Bruschke AV, Proudfit WL, Sones FM, Jr: Progress study of 590 consecutive nonsurgical cases of coronary disease followed 5–9 years: I. Arteriographic correlations. Circulation 47:1147–1153, 1973.
16. Proudfit WJ, Bruschke AV, MacMillan JP, et al: Fifteen year survival study of patients with obstructive coronary artery disease. Circulation 68:986–997, 1983.
17. Bruschke AV, Proudfit WL, Sones FM Jr: Progress study of 590 consecutive nonsurgical cases of coronary disease followed 5–9 years: II. Ventriculographic and other correlations. Circulation 47:1154–1163, 1973.
18. Veterans Administration Cooperative Group for the Study of Surgery for Coronary Arterial Occlusive Disease: Veterans Administration Cooperative Study of Surgery for Coronary Arterial Occlusive Disease: III. Methods and baseline characteristics, including experience with medical treatment. Am J Cardiol 40:212–225, 1977.
19. European Coronary Surgery Study Group: Prospective randomized study of coronary artery bypass surgery in stable angina pectoris: A progress report on survival. Circulation 65:67–71, 1982.
20. Coronary Artery Surgery Study investigators: Myocardial infarction and mortality in the Coronary Artery Surgery Study (CASS) randomized trial. N Engl J Med 310:750–758, 1984.
21. Takaro T, Hultgren HN, Detre KM, et al: The Veterans Administration Cooperative Study of stable angina: Current status. Circulation 65:60–67, 1982.
22. Harris PJ, Lee KL, Harrell FE Jr, et al: Outcome in medically treated coronary artery disease: Ischemic events: Nonfatal infarction and death. Circulation 62:718–726, 1980.
23. Coronary Artery Surgery Study Investigators: A randomized trial of coronary artery bypass surgery. Survival data. Circulation 68:939–950, 1983.
24. Alderman EL, Bourassa MG, Cohen LS, et al: Ten-year fol-

low-up of survival and myocardial infarction in the randomized Coronary Artery Surgery Study. Circulation 82:1629–1646, 1990.

25. Rogers WJ, Coggin CJ, Gersh BJ, et al: Ten-year follow-up of quality of life in patients randomized to receive medical therapy or coronary artery bypass graft surgery. The Coronary Artery Surgery Study (CASS). Circulation 82:1647–1658, 1990.

26. Mock MB, Ringqvist I, Fisher LD, et al: Survival of medically treated patients in the coronary artery surgery study (CASS) registry. Circulation 66:562–568, 1982.

27. U.S. Centers for Disease Control and Prevention: CDC WONDER Mortality Query [program], 1997. www.wonder.cdc.gov

28. National Center for Health Statistics: Vital Statistics of the United States, 1995 Life Tables, Vol II, Section 6. PHS 98-1104, Washington, DC: U.S. Government Printing Office, 1995.

29. Hunink M, Goldman L, Tosteson A, et al: The recent decline in mortality from coronary heart disease, 1980–1990. The effect of secular trends in risk factors and treatment. JAMA 277:535–542, 1997.

30. Manson JE, Tosteson H, Ridker PM, et al: The primary prevention of myocardial infarction. N Engl J Med 326:1406–1416, 1992.

31. United States Surgeon General: Reducing the Health Consequences of Smoking: 25 Years of Progress [Publication No. 017-001-00469-3]. Washington, DC: U.S. Department of Health and Human Services, 1989.

32. Doll R, Peto R: Mortality in relation to smoking: 20 years' observations on male British doctors. Br Med J 2:1525–1536, 1976.

33. Neaton JD, Wentworth D: Serum cholesterol, blood pressure, cigarette smoking, and death from coronary heart disease. Overall findings and differences by age for 316,099 white men. Multiple Risk Factor Intervention Trial Research Group. Arch Intern Med 152:56–64, 1992.

34. Waters D, Lesperance J, Gladstone P, et al: Effects of cigarette smoking on the angiographic evolution of coronary atherosclerosis. A Canadian Coronary Atherosclerosis Intervention Trial (CCAIT) Substudy. Circulation 94:614–621, 1996.

35. Hung J, Lam JY, Lacoste L, et al: Cigarette smoking acutely increases platelet thrombus formation in patients with coronary artery disease taking aspirin. Circulation 92:2432–2436, 1995.

36. Meade TW, Imeson J, Stirling Y: Effects of changes in smoking and other characteristics on clotting factors and the risk of ischaemic heart disease. Lancet 2:986–988, 1987.

37. Cryer PE, Haymond MW, Santiago JV, et al: Norepinephrine and epinephrine release and adrenergic mediation of smoking-associated hemodynamic and metabolic events. N Engl J Med 295:573–577, 1976.

38. Sigurdsson G Jr, Gudnason V, Sigurdsson G, et al: Interaction between a polymorphism of the apo A-I promoter region and smoking determines plasma levels of HDL and apo A-I. Arterioscler Thromb 12:1017–1022, 1992.

39. Celermajer DS, Sorensen KE, Georgakopoulos D, et al: Cigarette smoking is associated with dose-related and potentially reversible impairment of endothelium-dependent dilation in healthy young adults. Circulation 88:2149–2155, 1993.

40. Rosenberg L, Kaufman DW, Helmrich SP, et al: The risk of myocardial infarction after quitting smoking in men under 55 years of age. N Engl J Med 313:1511–1514, 1985.

41. Rosenberg L, Palmer JR, Shapiro S: Decline in the risk of myocardial infarction among women who stop smoking. N Engl J Med 322:213–217, 1990.

42. Tsevat J, Weinstein MC, Williams LW, et al: Expected gains in life expectancy from various coronary heart disease risk factor modifications. Circulation 83:1194–1201, 1991.

43. Superko H: Lipid disorders contributing to coronary heart disease: An update. Curr Probl Cardiol 21:736–780, 1996.

44. Jukema JW, Bruschke AV, van Boven AJ, et al: Effects of lipid lowering by pravastatin on progression and regression of coronary artery disease in symptomatic men with normal

to moderately elevated serum cholesterol levels. The Regression Growth Evaluation Statin Study (REGRESS). Circulation 91:2528–2540, 1995.

45. Ornish D, Brown SE, Scherwitz LW, et al: Can lifestyle changes reverse coronary heart disease? The Lifestyle Heart Trial. Lancet 336:129–133, 1990.

46. Gould KL, Ornish D, Kirkeeide R, et al: Improved stenosis geometry by quantitative coronary arteriography after vigorous risk factor modification. Am J Cardiol 69:845–853, 1992.

47. Leung WH, Lau CP, Wong CK: Beneficial effect of cholesterol-lowering therapy on coronary endothelium-dependent relaxation in hypercholesterolaemic patients. Lancet 341:1496–1500, 1993.

48. Anderson TJ, Meredith IT, Yeung AC, et al: The effect of cholesterol-lowering and antioxidant therapy on endothelium-dependent coronary vasomotion. N Engl J Med 332:488–493, 1995.

49. Treasure CB, Klein JL, Weintraub WS, et al: Beneficial effects of cholesterol-lowering therapy on the coronary endothelium in patients with coronary artery disease. N Engl J Med 332:481–487, 1995.

50. Stroes ES, Koomans HA, de Bruin TW, et al: Vascular function in the forearm of hypercholesterolaemic patients off and on lipid-lowering medication. Lancet 346:467–471, 1995.

51. Tamai O, Matsuoka H, Itabe H, et al: Single LDL apheresis improves endothelium-dependent vasodilatation in hypercholesterolemic humans. Circulation 95:76–82, 1997.

52. 4S Investigators: Randomised trial of cholesterol lowering in 4444 patients with coronary heart disease: The Scandinavian Simvastatin Survival Study (4S). Lancet 344:1383–1389, 1994.

53. Shepherd J, Cobbe SM, Ford I, et al: Prevention of coronary heart disease with pravastatin in men with hypercholesterolemia. West of Scotland Coronary Prevention Study Group. N Engl J Med 333:1301–1307, 1995.

54. Sacks FM, Pfeffer MA, Moye LA, et al: The effect of pravastatin on coronary events after myocardial infarction in patients with average cholesterol levels. Cholesterol and Recurrent Events Trial investigators. N Engl J Med 335:1001–1009, 1996.

55. Muldoon MF, Manuck SB, Matthews KA: Lowering cholesterol concentrations and mortality: A quantitative review of primary prevention trials. BMJ 301:309–314, 1990.

56. Collins R, Peto R, MacMahon S, et al: Blood pressure, stroke, and coronary heart disease: Part 2. Short-term reductions in blood pressure: Overview of randomised drug trials in their epidemiological context. Lancet 335:827–838, 1990.

57. SHEP Cooperative Research Group: Prevention of stroke by antihypertensive drug treatment in older persons with isolated systolic hypertension. Final results of the Systolic Hypertension in the Elderly Program (SHEP). JAMA 265:3255–3264, 1991.

58. The Diabetes Control and Complications Trial Research Group: The effect of intensive treatment of diabetes on the development and progression of long-term complications in insulin-dependent diabetes mellitus. N Engl J Med 329:977–986, 1993.

59. Kannel WB, McGee DL: Diabetes and cardiovascular risk factors: The Framingham study. Circulation 59:8–13, 1979.

60. Stamler J, Vaccaro O, Neaton JD, et al: Diabetes, other risk factors, and 12-yr cardiovascular mortality for men screened in the Multiple Risk Factor Intervention Trial. Diabetes Care 16:434–444, 1993.

61. Stein B, Weintraub WS, Gebhart SP, et al: Influence of diabetes mellitus on early and late outcome after percutaneous transluminal coronary angioplasty. Circulation 91:979–989, 1995.

62. The Bypass Angioplasty Revascularization Investigation (BARI) Investigators: Comparison of coronary bypass surgery with angioplasty in patients with multivessel disease. N Engl J Med 335:217–225, 1996.

63. Johnstone MT, Creager SJ, Scales KM, et al: Impaired endothelium-dependent vasodilation in patients with insulin-

dependent diabetes mellitus. Circulation 88:2510–2516, 1993.

64. Clarkson P, Celermajer DS, Donald AE, et al: Impaired vascular reactivity in insulin-dependent diabetes mellitus is related to disease duration and low density lipoprotein cholesterol levels. J Am Coll Cardiol 28:573–579, 1996.

65. Pieper GM, Jordan M, Adams MB, Roza AM: Syngeneic pancreatic islet transplantation reverses endothelial dysfunction in experimental diabetes. Diabetes 44:1106–1113, 1995.

66. Uusitupa MI, Niskanen LK, Siitonen O, et al: Ten-year cardiovascular mortality in relation to risk factors and abnormalities in lipoprotein composition in type 2 (non-insulin-dependent) diabetic and non-diabetic subjects. Diabetologia 36:1175–1184, 1993.

67. Kuusisto J, Mykkanen L, Pyorala K, et al: NIDDM and its metabolic control predict coronary heart disease in elderly subjects. Diabetes 43:960–967, 1994.

68. Laakso M: Glycemic control and the risk for coronary heart disease in patients with non-insulin-dependent diabetes mellitus. The Finnish studies. Ann Intern Med 124:127–130, 1996.

69. Genuth S: Exogenous insulin administration and cardiovascular risk in non-insulin-dependent and insulin-dependent diabetes mellitus. Ann Intern Med 124:104–109, 1996.

70. Sobel BE: Potentiation of vasculopathy by insulin: Implications from an NHLBI clinical alert. Circulation 93:1613–1615, 1996.

71. DeFronzo RA, Goodman AM: Efficacy of metformin in patients with non-insulin-dependent diabetes mellitus. The Multicenter Metformin Study Group. N Engl J Med 333:541–549, 1995.

72. Chiasson JL, Josse RG, Hunt JA, et al: The efficacy of acarbose in the treatment of patients with non-insulin-dependent diabetes mellitus. A multicenter controlled clinical trial. Ann Intern Med 121:928–935, 1994.

73. Johnson JL, Wolf SL, Kabadi UM: Efficacy of insulin and sulfonylurea combination therapy in type II diabetes. A meta-analysis of the randomized placebo-controlled trials. Arch Intern Med 156:259–264, 1996.

74. Nolan JJ, Ludvik B, Beerdsen P, et al: Improvement in glucose tolerance and insulin resistance in obese subjects treated with troglitazone. N Engl J Med 331:1188–1193, 1994.

75. Steering Committee of the Physicians' Health Study Research Group: Final report on the aspirin component of the ongoing Physicians' Health Study. N Engl J Med 321:129–135, 1989.

76. Antiplatelet Trialists' Collaboration: Collaborative overview of randomised trials of antiplatelet therapy—I: Prevention of death, myocardial infarction, and stroke by prolonged antiplatelet therapy in various categories of patients. BMJ 308:81–106, 1994.

77. Balsano F, Rizzon P, Violi F, et al: Antiplatelet treatment with ticlopidine in unstable angina: A controlled multicenter clinical trial. The Studio della Ticlopidina nell'Angina Instabile Group. Circulation 82:17–26, 1990.

78. CAPRIE Steering Committee: A randomised, blinded, trial of clopidogrel versus aspirin in patients at risk of ischaemic events (CAPRIE). Lancet 348:1329–1339, 1996.

79. Yusuf S, Peto R, Lewis J, et al: Beta blockade during and after myocardial infarction: An overview of the randomized trials. Prog Cardiovasc Dis 27:335–371, 1985.

80. Mangano DT, Layug EL, Wallace A, et al: Effect of atenolol on mortality and cardiovascular morbidity after noncardiac surgery. Multicenter Study of Perioperative Ischemia Research Group. N Engl J Med 335:1713–1720, 1996.

81. The SOLVD Investigators: Effect of enalapril on mortality and the development of heart failure in asymptomatic patients with reduced left ventricular ejection fractions. N Engl J Med 327:685–691, 1992.

82. Pfeffer MA, Braunwald E, Moye LA, et al: Effect of captopril on mortality and morbidity in patients with left ventricular dysfunction after myocardial infarction. Results of the survival and ventricular enlargement trial. The SAVE Investigators. N Engl J Med 327:669–677, 1992.

83. Kober L, Torp-Pedersen C, Carlsen JE, et al: A clinical trial of the angiotensin-converting-enzyme inhibitor trandolapril in patients with left ventricular dysfunction after myocardial infarction. Trandolapril Cardiac Evaluation (TRACE) Study Group. N Engl J Med 333:1670–1676, 1995.

84. Mancini GB, Henry GC, Macaya C, et al: Angiotensin-converting enzyme inhibition with quinapril improves endothelial vasomotor dysfunction in patients with coronary artery disease. The TREND (Trial on Reversing ENdothelial Dysfunction) Study. Circulation 94:258–265, 1996.

85. The Heart Outcomes Prevention Evaluation Study Investigators: Effects of an angiotensin-converting-enzyme inhibitor, ramipril, on cardiovascular events in high-risk patients. N Engl J Med 342:145–153, 2000.

86. Colditz GA, Willett WC, Stampfer MJ, et al: Menopause and the risk of coronary heart disease in women. N Engl J Med 316:1105–1110, 1987.

87. Stampfer MJ, Colditz GA: Estrogen replacement therapy and coronary heart disease: A quantitative assessment of the epidemiologic evidence. Prev Med 20:47–63, 1991.

88. Guetta V, Cannon RO 3rd: Cardiovascular effects of estrogen and lipid-lowering therapies in postmenopausal women. Circulation 93:1928–1937, 1996.

89. Gilligan DM, Quyyumi AA, Cannon RO 3rd: Effects of physiological levels of estrogen on coronary vasomotor function in postmenopausal women. Circulation 89:2545–2551, 1994.

90. Collins P, Rosano GM, Sarrel PM, et al: 17 beta-Estradiol attenuates acetylcholine-induced coronary arterial constriction in women but not men with coronary heart disease. Circulation 92:24–30, 1995.

91. Rosano GM, Sarrel PM, Poole-Wilson PA, et al: Beneficial effect of oestrogen on exercise-induced myocardial ischaemia in women with coronary artery disease. Lancet 342:133–136, 1993.

92. Hulley S, Grady D, Bush T: Randomized trial of estrogen plus progestin for secondary prevention of coronary disease in postmenopausal women. JAMA 280:605–613, 1998.

93. Rossouw JE: National Heart, Lung, and Blood Institute press statement, April 3, 2000.

94. Herrington DM, Reboussin DM, Brosnihan KB, et al: Effects of estrogen replacement on the progression of coronary artery atherosclerosis. N Engl J Med 343:522–529, 2000.

95. Stampfer MJ, Hennekens CH, Manson JE, et al: Vitamin E consumption and the risk of coronary disease in women. N Engl J Med 328:1444–1449, 1993.

96. Rimm EB, Stampfer MJ, Ascherio A, et al: Vitamin E consumption and the risk of coronary heart disease in men. N Engl J Med 328:1450–1456, 1993.

97. Rapola JM, Virtamo J, Haukka JK, et al: Effect of vitamin E and beta carotene on the incidence of angina pectoris. A randomized, double-blind, controlled trial. JAMA 275:693–698, 1996.

98. Hennekens CH, Buring JE, Manson JE, et al: Lack of effect of long-term supplementation with beta carotene on the incidence of malignant neoplasms and cardiovascular disease. N Engl J Med 334:1145–1149, 1996.

99. Omenn GS, Goodman GE, Thornquist MD, et al: Effects of a combination of beta carotene and vitamin A on lung cancer and cardiovascular disease. N Engl J Med 334:1150–1155, 1996.

100. Stephens NG, Parsons A, Schofield PM, et al: Randomised controlled trial of vitamin E in patients with coronary disease: Cambridge Heart Antioxidant Study (CHAOS). Lancet 347:781–786, 1996.

101. GISSI-Prevenzione Investigators: Dietary supplementation with n-3 polyunsaturated fatty acids and vitamin E after myocardial infarction: Results of the GISSI-Prevenzione trial. Lancet 354:447–455, 1999.

102. The Heart Outcomes Prevention Evaluation Study Investigators: Vitamin E supplementation and cardiovascular events in high-risk patients. N Engl J Med 342:154–160, 2000.

103. Boushey CJ, Beresford SA, Omenn GS, et al: A quantitative assessment of plasma homocysteine as a risk factor for

vascular disease. Probable benefits of increasing folic acid intakes. JAMA 274:1049–1057, 1995.

104. Stampfer MJ, Malinow MR, Willett WC, et al: A prospective study of plasma homocyst(e)ine and risk of myocardial infarction in US physicians. JAMA 268:877–881, 1992.

105. Mayer EL, Jacobsen DW, Robinson K: Homocysteine and coronary atherosclerosis. J Am Coll Cardiol 27:517–527, 1996.

106. Armstrong ML, Heistad DD, Lopez JA: Regression of atherosclerosis. A role for calcium antagonists. Am J Hypertens 4:503S–511S, 1991.

107. Lichtlen PR, Hugenholtz PG, Rafflenbeul W, et al: Retardation of angiographic progression of coronary artery disease by nifedipine. Results of the International Nifedipine Trial on Antiatherosclerotic Therapy (INTACT). Lancet 335:1109–1113, 1990.

108. Waters D, Lesperance J, Francetich M, et al: A controlled clinical trial to assess the effect of a calcium channel blocker on the progression of coronary atherosclerosis. Circulation 82:1940–1953, 1990.

109. Pitt B, Byington RP, Furberg CD, et al: Effect of amlodipine on the progression of atherosclerosis and the occurrence of clinical events. Circulation 102:1503–1510, 2000.

110. The Multicenter Diltiazem Postinfarction Trial Research Group: The effect of diltiazem on mortality and reinfarction after myocardial infarction. N Engl J Med 319:385–392, 1988.

111. Rocco MB, Nabel EG, Campbell S, et al: Prognostic importance of myocardial ischemia detected by ambulatory monitoring in patients with stable coronary artery disease. Circulation 78:877–884, 1988.

112. Deedwania PC, Carbajal EV: Silent ischemia during daily life is an independent predictor of mortality in stable angina. Circulation 81:748–756, 1990.

113. Yeung AC, Barry J, Orav J, et al: Effects of asymptomatic ischemia on long-term prognosis in chronic stable coronary disease. Circulation 83:1598–1604, 1991.

114. Pepine CJ, Cohn PF, Deedwania PC, et al: Effects of treatment on outcome in mildly symptomatic patients with ischemia during daily life. The Atenolol Silent Ischemia Study (ASIST). Circulation 90:762–768, 1994.

115. Pepine CJ, Geller NL, Knatterud GL, et al: The Asymptomatic Cardiac Ischemia Pilot (ACIP) study: Design of a randomized clinical trial, baseline data and implications for a long-term outcome trial. J Am Coll Cardiol 24:1–10, 1994.

116. Knatterud GL, Bourassa MG, Pepine CJ, et al: Effects of treatment strategies to suppress ischemia in patients with coronary artery disease: 12-week results of the Asymptomatic Cardiac Ischemia Pilot (ACIP) study. J Am Coll Cardiol 24:11–20, 1994.

117. Chaitman BR, Stone PH, Knatterud GL, et al: Asymptomatic Cardiac Ischemia Pilot (ACIP) study: Impact of anti-ischemia therapy on 12-week rest electrocardiogram and exercise test outcomes. The ACIP Investigators. J Am Coll Cardiol 26:585–593, 1995.

118. Rogers WJ, Bourassa MG, Andrews TC, et al: Asymptomatic Cardiac Ischemia Pilot (ACIP) study: Outcome at 1 year for patients with asymptomatic cardiac ischemia randomized to medical therapy or revascularization. The ACIP Investigators. J Am Coll Cardiol 26:594–605, 1995.

119. Bourassa MG, Pepine CJ, Forman SA, et al: Asymptomatic Cardiac Ischemia Pilot (ACIP) study: Effects of coronary angioplasty and coronary artery bypass graft surgery on recurrent angina and ischemia. The ACIP Investigators. J Am Coll Cardiol 26:606–614, 1995.

120. Bourassa MG, Knatterud GL, Pepine CJ, et al: Asymptomatic Cardiac Ischemia Pilot (ACIP) Study. Improvement of cardiac ischemia at 1 year after PTCA and CABG. Circulation 92:II-1–II-7, 1995.

121. Parisi AF, Folland ED, Hartigan P: A comparison of angioplasty with medical therapy in the treatment of single-vessel coronary artery disease. Veterans Affairs ACME Investigators. N Engl J Med 326:10–16, 1992.

122. Strauss WE, Fortin T, Hartigan P, et al: A comparison of quality of life scores in patients with angina pectoris after angioplasty compared with after medical therapy. Outcomes

of a randomized clinical trial. Veterans Affairs Study of Angioplasty Compared to Medical Therapy Investigators. Circulation 92:1710–1719, 1995.

123. Holmes DR Jr, Holubkov R, Vlietstra RE, et al: Comparison of complications during percutaneous transluminal coronary angioplasty from 1977 to 1981 and from 1985 to 1986: The National Heart, Lung, and Blood Institute Percutaneous Transluminal Coronary Angioplasty Registry. J Am Coll Cardiol 12:1149–1155, 1988.

124. Hueb WA, Bellotti G, de Oliveira SA, et al: The Medicine, Angioplasty or Surgery Study (MASS): A prospective, randomized trial of medical therapy, balloon angioplasty or bypass surgery for single proximal left anterior descending artery stenoses. J Am Coll Cardiol 26:1600–1605, 1995.

125. RITA-2 trial participants: Coronary angioplasty versus medical therapy for angina: The Second Randomised Intervention Treatment of Angina (RITA-2) trial. Lancet 350:461–468, 1997.

126. Pitt B, Waters D, Brown WV, et al: Aggressive lipid-lowering therapy compared with angioplasty in stable coronary artery disease. N Engl J Med 34:70–76, 1999.

127. Coronary Artery Surgery Study investigators: A randomized trial of coronary artery bypass surgery. Quality of life in patients randomly assigned to treatment groups. Circulation 68:951–960, 1983.

128. O'Keefe JH Jr, Rutherford BD, McConahay DR, et al: Multivessel coronary angioplasty from 1980 to 1989: Procedural results and long-term outcome. J Am Coll Cardiol 16:1097–1102, 1990.

129. Hollman J, Simpfendorfer C, Franco I, et al: Multivessel and single-vessel coronary angioplasty: A comparative study. Am Heart J 124:9–12, 1992.

130. Detre K, Holubkov R, Kelsey S, et al: Percutaneous transluminal coronary angioplasty in 1985–1986 and 1977–1981. The National Heart, Lung, and Blood Institute Registry. N Engl J Med 318:265–270, 1988.

131. Detre K, Holubkov R, Kelsey S, et al: One-year follow-up results of the 1985–1986 National Heart, Lung, and Blood Institute's Percutaneous Transluminal Coronary Angioplasty Registry. Circulation 80:421–428, 1989.

132. Deligonul U, Vandormael MG, Shah Y, et al: Prognostic value of early exercise stress testing after successful coronary angioplasty: Importance of the degree of revascularization. Am Heart J 117:509–514, 1989.

133. Weintraub WS, Jones EL, King SB, et al: Changing use of coronary angioplasty and coronary bypass surgery in the treatment of chronic coronary artery disease. Am J Cardiol 65:183–188, 1990.

134. Reeder GS, Holmes DR Jr, Detre K, et al: Degree of revascularization in patients with multivessel coronary disease: A report from the National Heart, Lung, and Blood Institute Percutaneous Transluminal Coronary Angioplasty Registry. Circulation 77:638–644, 1988.

135. Bourassa MG, Holubkov R, Yeh W, et al: Strategy of complete revascularization in patients with multivessel coronary artery disease (a report from the 1985–1986 NHLBI PTCA Registry). Am J Cardiol 70:174–178, 1992.

136. Bell MR, Bailey KR, Reeder GS, et al: Percutaneous transluminal angioplasty in patients with multivessel coronary disease: How important is complete revascularization for cardiac event-free survival? J Am Coll Cardiol 16:553–562, 1990.

137. Faxon DP, Ghalilli K, Jacobs AK, et al: The degree of revascularization and outcome after multivessel coronary angioplasty. Am Heart J 123:854–859, 1992.

138. Samson M, Meester HJ, De Feyter PJ, et al: Successful multiple segment coronary angioplasty: Effect of completeness of revascularization in single-vessel multilesions and multivessels. Am Heart J 120:1–12, 1990.

139. de Feyter PJ, Serruys PW, Arnold A, et al: Coronary angioplasty of the unstable angina related vessel in patients with multivessel disease. Eur Heart J 7:460–467, 1986.

140. de Feyter PJ: PTCA in patients with stable angina pectoris and multivessel disease: Is incomplete revascularization acceptable? Clin Cardiol 15:317–322, 1992.

141. Thomas ES, Most AS, Williams DO: Objective assessment

of coronary angioplasty for multivessel disease: Results of exercise stress testing. J Am Coll Cardiol 11:217–222, 1988.

142. Folland ED, Hartigan PM, Parisi AF: Percutaneous transluminal coronary angioplasty versus medical therapy for stable angina pectoris: Outcomes for patients with double-vessel versus single-vessel coronary artery disease in a Veterans Affairs Cooperative randomized trial. Veterans Affairs ACME Investigators [see comments]. J Am Coll Cardiol 29:1505–1511, 1997.

143. Mark DB, Nelson CL, Califf RM, et al: Continuing evolution of therapy for coronary artery disease. Initial results from the era of coronary angioplasty. Circulation 89:2015–2025, 1994.

144. Brown G, Albers JJ, Fisher LD, et al: Regression of coronary artery disease as a result of intensive lipid-lowering therapy in men with high levels of apolipoprotein B. N Engl J Med 323:1289–1298, 1990.

145. EPIC Investigators: Use of a monoclonal antibody directed against the platelet glycoprotein IIb/IIIa receptor in high-risk coronary angioplasty. N Engl J Med 330:956–961, 1994.

146. EPILOG Investigators: Platelet glycoprotein IIb/IIIa receptor blockade and low-dose heparin during percutaneous coronary revascularization. N Engl J Med 336:1689–1696, 1997.

147. Topol EJ, Califf RM, Weisman HF, et al: Randomised trial of coronary intervention with antibody against platelet IIb/IIIa integrin for reduction of clinical restenosis: Results at six months: The EPIC Investigators. Lancet 343:881–886, 1994.

148. Serruys PW, de Jaegere P, Kiemeneij F, et al: A comparison of balloon-expandable-stent implantation with balloon angioplasty in patients with coronary artery disease. Benestent Study Group. N Engl J Med 331:489–495, 1994.

149. Fischman DL, Leon MB, Baim DS, et al: A randomized comparison of coronary-stent placement and balloon angioplasty in the treatment of coronary artery disease. Stent Restenosis Study Investigators. N Engl J Med 331:496–501, 1994.

150. Colombo A, Hall P, Nakamura S, et al: Intracoronary stenting without anticoagulation accomplished with intravascular ultrasound guidance. Circulation 91:1676–1688, 1995.

151. Schomig A, Neumann FJ, Kastrati A, et al: A randomized comparison of antiplatelet and anticoagulant therapy after the placement of coronary-artery stents. N Engl J Med 334:1084–1089, 1996.

152. Serruys PW, Emanuelsson H, van der Giessen W, et al: Heparin-coated Palmaz-Schatz stents in human coronary arteries. Early outcome of the Benestent-II Pilot Study. Circulation 93:412–422, 1996.

153. George BS, Voorhees WD 3d, Roubin GS, et al: Multicenter investigation of coronary stenting to treat acute or threatened closure after percutaneous transluminal coronary angioplasty: Clinical and angiographic outcomes. J Am Coll Cardiol 22:135–143, 1993.

154. Berge KG, Canner PL: Coronary drug project: Experience with niacin. Coronary Drug Project Research Group. Eur J Clin Pharmacol 40(suppl 1):S49–S51, 1991.

155. Lipid Research Clinics Investigators: The Lipid Research Clinics Coronary Primary Prevention Trial results: I. Reduction in incidence of coronary heart disease. JAMA 251:351–364, 1984.

156. Frick MH, Elo O, Haapa K, et al: Helsinki Heart Study: Primary-prevention trial with gemfibrozil in middle-aged men with dyslipidemia. Safety of treatment, changes in risk factors, and incidence of coronary heart disease. N Engl J Med 317:1237–1245, 1987.

157. Hjermann I, Velve Byre K, Holme I, et al: Effect of diet and smoking intervention on the incidence of coronary heart disease. Report from the Oslo Study Group of a randomised trial in healthy men. Lancet 2:1303–1310, 1981.

# Surgical Therapy Versus Interventional Therapy in Patients with Stable Coronary Ischemia

Gail E. Peterson     Harry R. Phillips III     James Jollis     Robert M. Califf
E. Magnus Ohman

Medical management was the only therapy available to patients with coronary artery disease before 1964. In 1964, coronary artery bypass grafting (CABG) was first performed, and it quickly became a widely accepted alternative to medical management.[1] During the 1970s, multiple studies were done to elucidate which patients would benefit from CABG and which patients would be better served by medical management. A less invasive option for revascularization was introduced in 1977, when Andreas Gruentzig performed the first percutaneous transluminal coronary angioplasty (PTCA).[2] Since then, PTCA has come into widespread use. However, there have only been a few randomized trials comparing it with medical therapy.

Physicians now have many therapeutic options for their patients with stable coronary artery disease, ranging from medical management to percutaneous interventions to surgical revascularization. Multiple factors may influence this decision; in many patients, any of the three therapeutic options may be effective. Choosing the best mode of therapy is often not straightforward because the relative merits of these various modes remain controversial. In addition, the steady improvement in length of survival with the different treatment modalities makes comparing clinical trials difficult. Consequently, the treatment of coronary artery disease varies considerably among practitioners. This chapter reviews therapeutic options for patients with stable angina, concentrating on comparative studies of coronary bypass surgery, angioplasty, and medical management; we also evaluate the effects of completeness of revascularization, left ventricular function, age, diabetes mellitus, relative treatment costs, and new therapeutic developments on treatment choice.

## CABG VERSUS MEDICAL MANAGEMENT

Seven randomized trials involving more than 2600 patients explored the indications for CABG. The three largest randomized trials comparing CABG with medical therapy are the Veterans Administration Cooperative Study, the European Coronary Surgery Study, and the Coronary Artery Surgery Study (CASS). Although these studies identified certain groups of patients who would benefit from one form of therapy or another, for other patient groups the optimal form of therapy remained unclear. Three major randomized trials helped define the indications for surgical therapy for coronary disease. Between 1972 and 1974, the Veterans Administration Cooperative Study randomly assigned 686 men with stable angina and coronary disease in at least one vessel to receive either medical or CABG therapy. There were improved outcomes in the CABG recipients. After 7 years, patients treated surgically had improved survival rates (77%) in comparison with patients treated medically (70%; $p = 0.043$), but this survival benefit diminished with time. Annual mortality rates in the surgery recipients increased from 3.3% to 4.8% over the 7 years, whereas mortality rates for medical therapy decreased from 4.3% to 3% per year. By the 11-year[3] and 18-year[4] follow-ups, survival rates were essentially the same for both groups (58% and 30% among those who underwent CABG, and 57% and 33% among those who received medical therapy).

There was a statistically significant survival benefit with surgery in the 91 patients with left main coronary artery disease.[5] The analysis was based on intent to treat, and close to 80% of patients with left main coronary artery disease initially treated medically crossed over to surgical therapy. Despite this high crossover rate, better outcomes with surgical therapy indicate that patients with left main coronary disease should undergo early surgical therapy.

In addition, a high-risk group of patients was found to have decreased rates of mortality with CABG.[3] High risk was defined angiographically as having left ventricular dysfunction and three-vessel disease, or it was defined clinically as having two or more of the following: New York Heart Association classification III or IV disease, a history of hypertension, previous myocardial infarction, or ST depression documented on resting electrocardiography (ECG). Again, a significant survival benefit was seen among the high-risk patients at the 7-year follow-up, but this benefit was no longer evident at 11 years.[3] For the majority of patients without left main coronary artery disease or who did not belong to one of these high-risk subgroups, surgery offered no survival advantage over medical treatment (81% cumulative surgical survival rate vs. 90% medical survival rate at 7 years; $p = 0.079$). The numbers in the subgroups were small, insufficiently powered to detect a difference.

Between 1973 and 1976, the European Coronary Surgery Study enrolled 767 men younger than 65 years with stable angina, at least two-vessel disease, and normal left ventricular function.[6] At 8 years, survival rates were higher with CABG than with medical therapy (89% vs. 80%). At 12 years, the difference in survival rates had narrowed but was still evident (71% vs. 67%).[7] Subgroup analysis at 8 years revealed a survival benefit in surgically treated patients with three-vessel disease (92% with surgery vs. 77% with medical therapy) and in patients with two-vessel disease when the proximal left anterior descending (LAD) coronary artery was involved (90% with surgery vs. 79% with medicine). No benefit was evident in patients with two-vessel disease in the absence of proximal LAD disease (95% rate of 5-year survival with medicine vs. 91.1% with surgery) or in patients with single-vessel disease.

Between 1975 and 1979, the CASS enrolled 780 patients who were 65 years of age or younger and who had mild angina or had had a prior myocardial infarction. There was no difference in survival at 10 years between the two treatment groups (79% with medical therapy vs. 82% with surgery).[8] However, a significant survival advantage with surgery was seen in patients with left ventricular dysfunction (79% vs. 61% among those who took medications; $p = 0.01$). When patients with left ventricular dysfunction were evaluated in terms of coronary artery disease severity, a significant benefit was seen only among patients with three-vessel disease.

On the basis of these trials, certain patients were thought to have improved rates of survival with CABG over medical therapy: specifically, those with three-vessel disease, those with significant disease and decreased left ventricular function, and those with significant left main coronary artery disease. However, the effect of CABG on prognosis for patients with less significant coronary disease is more difficult to establish, because the individual trials included a relatively small number of these patients. Although it was possible to assess the effect of CABG on large reductions in mortality (for example, 50% reduction in 5 years), smaller and yet clinically important reductions in mortality could have been missed.[9]

A large number of patients was evaluated in Yusuf and colleagues' meta-analysis of trials randomly assigning patients with stable coronary disease to receive either medical or surgical therapy.[9] A total of 2649 patients constituted the overall population; three quarters of them were enrolled in the three large trials. There were 1324 patients randomly assigned to undergo CABG and 1325 patients randomly assigned to receive medical therapy. Table 10–1 shows baseline data of the patients enrolled.

Of the patients assigned to CABG, 93.7% actually underwent the surgery, and only 10% of surgically treated patients received an internal mammary graft.

## TABLE 10–1.   META-ANALYSIS OF THE CABG VERSUS MEDICINE TRIALS

| PATIENT CHARACTERISTICS | % OF PATIENTS |
| --- | --- |
| **Age Distribution** | |
| <40 | 8.5 |
| 41–50 | 38.2 |
| 51–60 | 46 |
| >60 | 7.3 |
| **Ejection Fraction (N = 2474)** | |
| <40 | 7.2 |
| 40–49 | 12.5 |
| 50–59 | 28 |
| >60 | 52.3 |
| **Male** | 96.8 |
| **Severity of Angina** | |
| None | 11.2 |
| Class I or II | 53.8 |
| Class III or IV | 35 |
| **No. of Vessels Diseased** | |
| Left main artery | 6.6 |
| One | 10.2 |
| Two | 32.4 |
| Three | 50.6 |
| **Location of Disease** | |
| Proximal LAD | 59.4 |
| LAD diagonal | 60.4 |
| Left circumflex | 73.8 |
| RCA | 81.6 |

CABG, coronary artery bypass grafting; LAD, left anterior descending artery; RCA, right coronary artery.

Adapted from Yusuf S, Zucker D, Peduzzi P, et al: Effect of coronary artery bypass graft surgery on survival: Overview of 10-year results from randomized trials by the Coronary Artery Bypass Graft Surgery Trialists Collaboration. Lancet 344:563–570, 1994.

The rate of early mortality was higher among the surgically treated patients: Within the first 30 days, 3.2% of patients randomly assigned to undergo CABG died, and at 1 year after surgery, the Kaplan-Meier rate of myocardial infarction or death was significantly higher among the CABG recipients (11.6%) than among the medication recipients (8.0%; $p < 0.001$). This outcome is attributable in part to the up-front perioperative risks with CABG. Early occlusion occurs in 8% to 12% of vein grafts, often as a result of technical factors.[10, 11] In addition, early thrombosis and fibrointimal proliferation may occur in grafts during the first 12 to 18 months, causing some attrition of graft patency.[12] However, with time, the survival curves cross between the first and second year after treatment, and a survival benefit with CABG is apparent. Between 18 months and 5 years after treatment, graft attrition is minimal, and the benefit of surgery appears to be greatest at 5 years. Overall, the CABG recipients had a significantly lower rate of mortality at 5 years (10.2% vs. 15.8%; $p = 0.0001$), as shown in Figure 10–1. With the longer duration of follow-up, the differences in mortality between the treatments narrow; at 10 years, the mortality rates were 26.4% with surgery and 30.5% with medicine ($p = 0.03$). After 5 years, the rates of graft occlusion increase to 4% to 5% per year,[11] and at 10 years, 50% of vein grafts

may be occluded.[13] In addition, disease progresses in vessels not subjected to CABG.

The survival benefit of CABG was greatest in patients with more extensive coronary artery disease.[9] Among patients with three-vessel disease, mortality reduction with CABG was 42% at 5 years ($p = 0.001$) and 24% at 10 years ($p = 0.02$). For patients with left main coronary artery disease, bypass surgery reduced mortality by 68% at 5 years ($p = 0.004$) and by 33% at 10 years ($p = 0.24$). Patients with proximal LAD disease also tended to benefit from surgery. In the absence of proximal LAD involvement, significant reductions in mortality with surgery were seen only in patients with three-vessel or left main coronary artery disease. There was a nonsignificant trend toward lower mortality rates with CABG among patients with one- and two-vessel disease at 5 years, and there was no difference at 10 years. Of the 1130 patients with one- or two-vessel disease, only 606 did not have proximal LAD involvement. Because of this small number and the low rate of adverse events in these patients, important differences in mortality may have been missed.

Although these studies provided some useful information, there are several confounding factors that make the conclusions less clear. The analysis was based on intention to treat, but approximately 41%

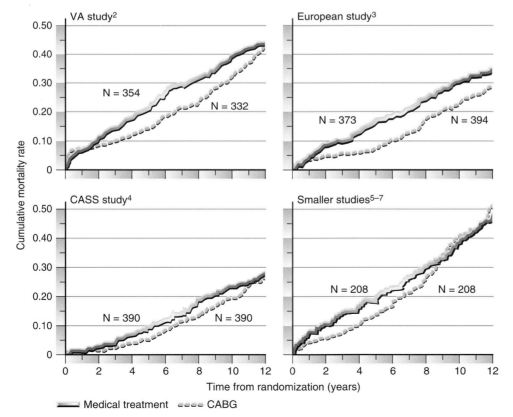

FIGURE 10–1. Survival curve for overall population evaluated in the studies comparing medical and surgical therapy. CABG, coronary artery bypass graftings; CASS, Coronary Artery Surgery Study; VA, Veterans Administration. (From Yusuf S, Zucker D, Peduzzi P, et al: Effect of coronary artery bypass graft surgery on survival: Overview of 10-year results from randomized trials by the Coronary Artery Bypass Graft Surgery Trialists Collaboration. Lancet 344:563–570, 1994.)

of patients randomly assigned to receive medical management crossed over to surgery by 10 years. The crossover rate was highest for patients with left main coronary artery disease and lowest for patients with one- or two-vessel disease. Because of the high crossover rate, the surgical benefit in patients overall, and particularly in those with more severe coronary disease, may have been underestimated.

Although surgery improves survival in certain groups of patients, it does not reduce the incidence of nonfatal myocardial infarctions. Myocardial infarctions are usually caused by plaque rupture, which can occur in insignificant lesions not likely to have been subjected to bypass surgery. However, surgical revascularization does increase the likelihood of surviving a myocardial infarction, inasmuch as it provides conduits for perfusing the viable myocardium, which must compensate for the acutely damaged myocardium during an infarction. Although surgery has not been shown to improve left ventricular function or result in greater employment rates, it is superior to medical therapy in relieving angina, regardless of the extent of coronary disease.[9] Surgery also reduces the incidence of sudden death in patients with coronary disease.[14, 15] Of importance is that the mechanism of preventing sudden death does not appear to be related to improvements in left ventricular function.

The benefits of CABG have increased over time,[16] despite the fact that surgery is increasingly being performed on patients with higher operative risks such as advanced age, abnormal left ventricular function, and more extensive coronary disease.[17] The use of internal thoracic artery grafts has improved rates of both early and late mortality.[18, 19] The 10-year survival rate after CABG is 89% when an internal mammary artery is used, in comparison with 71% when vein grafts are used alone.[18] Antiplatelet therapy and better intraoperative protection of the heart have contributed to improved survival and decreased morbidity. In addition, aggressive lowering of low-density lipoprotein cholesterol levels (to below 100 mg/dL) reduces progression of atherosclerosis in saphenous vein grafts.[20] Medical therapy has also improved, with widespread use of β blockers, angiotensin-converting enzyme (ACE) inhibitors, and cholesterol-lowering medications improving survival in patients with coronary disease. With the major improvements in both surgical and medical management of coronary artery disease since 1980, it is debatable whether the results of the early trials comparing surgical and medical management remain clinically applicable. Despite the improvements in therapy, as well as the introduction of alternative interventional therapies for coronary artery disease, clinical decision making today continues to be based largely on the results of these early trials.[8]

## PTCA

During the 1980s, angioplasty came into widespread use as an alternative form of therapy for coronary artery disease. Initially used only for a single proximal coronary lesion, it has been increasingly used for more complex lesions, for distal lesions, and in patients with multivessel disease. In spite of its use in more complex coronary lesions and in a higher risk patient population, the procedural success of PTCA has continued to increase.[21] The reason for this increasing success is multifactorial, but the primary factors are improved technology and better operator experience.

The predictors of periprocedural mortality with PTCA are the same as predictors of mortality with medical treatment[17, 22] and in the perioperative period of bypass surgery.[17, 23–25] The risk of procedure-related mortality with PTCA is a function of age, sex, baseline severity of illness, the likelihood of acute vessel closure, and the likelihood of hemodynamic collapse in the event of acute closure (Table 10–2). An excessive rate of procedure-related mortality independent of other patient characteristics is seen in women[26–30] and in older patients.[27, 30–32] Other baseline prognostic factors are left ventricular dysfunction,[27, 29] multivessel disease, and unstable anginal symptoms.[33, 34] Severe comorbidity is also important prognostically because of the impairment of compensatory physiologic responses in patients with other life-threatening illnesses. Predictors of major periprocedural complications include shock, unstable angina, dilatation of AHA/ACC type C lesions, and the presence of multivessel disease.[31]

Large numbers of patients have been studied to examine the outcomes of angioplasty. The Consensus Project is an American College of Cardiology–sponsored cooperative effort analyzing data from more than 200,000 patients from eight of the nations' largest databases, to establish standardized predictors of interventional outcomes (Table 10–3).[35] The reported occurrence of major adverse events is low (Table 10–4). If the New Approaches to Coronary Intervention (NACI) Registry—which reports outcomes of the use of newer devices and procedures (directional atherectomy, transluminal extraction atherectomy, rotational atherectomy, Palmaz-Schatz stents, the Gianturco-Roubin stent, and Advanced Interventional Systems or Spectranetics excimer lasers)—is excluded from the analysis, in-hospital myocardial infarction rates are found to be 1.1%, emergency CABG for failed PTCA occurs at a rate of 2.7%, and the in-hospital mortality rate is

**TABLE 10–2.    PREDICTORS OF IN-HOSPITAL MORTALITY**

| STUDY | NUMBER | MORTALITY (%) | CLINICAL CHARACTERISTICS | ANATOMIC CHARACTERISTICS |
|---|---|---|---|---|
| NHLBI[27] | 1801 | 1.0 | History of CHF, age ≥65, female gender | Three-vessel or left main artery disease |
| Kahn et al[33] | 9175 | 0.9 | Age ≥70, unstable angina, absence of prior CABG | LVEF ≤30%, multivessel disease |
| Ellis et al[28] | 8052 | 0.4 | Female gender | Jeopardy score, PTCA of proximal RCA |
| New York State[29] | 5827 | 0.6 | Cardiogenic shock, hemodynamic instability, female gender | LVEF <50% |
| NNE[26, 30] | 12,232 | 1.0 | Female gender | Multivessel disease |
| Weintraub et al[34] | 10,783 | 0.3 | Unstable angina, short stature | Multivessel disease, LVEF <50% |
| Rozenman[132] | 2067 | 0.8 | Female gender | |
| Combined | 49,937 | 0.7 | Female gender, advanced age, heart failure | Multivessel disease, left ventricular dysfunction |

CABG, coronary artery bypass grafting; CHF, congestive heart failure; LVEF, left ventricular ejection fraction; NHLBI, National Heart, Lung, and Blood Institute; NNE = Northern New England Cardiovascular Disease Study Group; PTCA, percutaneous transluminal coronary angioplasty; RCA, right coronary artery.

**TABLE 10–3.    DATABASES IN THE CONSENSUS PROJECT**

| DATABASE | YEARS | N | DESCRIPTION |
|---|---|---|---|
| National Cardiovascular Network (NCN) | 1994–1996 | 66,358 | Multicenter Registry |
| National Heart, Lung and Blood Institute (NHLBI) Coronary Angioplasty Registry | 1985–1986 | 2431 | Multicenter Registry |
| New Approaches to Coronary Intervention (NACI) Registry | 1990–1994 | 3561 | Multicenter Registry (new devices only) |
| New York State Cardiac Database | 1991–1994 | 62,670 | Multicenter Registry |
| Society for Coronary Angioplasty and Intervention (SCAI) Registry | 1993–1995 | 31,455 | Multicenter Registry |
| Duke Cardiovascular Database | 1991–1995 | 9462 | Single-Center Registry |
| Northern New England Cardiac Database | 1987–1996 | 23,252 | Multicenter Registry |
| Cooperative Cardiac Project Database (CCP) | 1994–1995 | 3196 | Multicenter Registry (patient age 65 or older) |

**TABLE 10–4.    CONSENSUS PROJECT: IN-HOSPITAL OUTCOMES**

| DATABASE | N | MORTALITY (%) | EMERGENCY CABG (%) | Q-WAVE MI (%) |
|---|---|---|---|---|
| NCN | 66,358 | 1.3 | 2.1 | 1.0 |
| NHLBI | 2431 | 1.4 | 6.0 | N/A |
| NACI | 3561 | 1.3 | 2.4 | 1.1 |
| NY | 62,670 | 0.9 | 3.4 | N/A |
| SCAI | 31,455 | 0.4 | 2.2 | 1.0 |
| Duke | 9462 | 1.1 | 2.4 | N/A |
| NNE | 12,232 | 1.1 | 2.8 | 1.7 |
| CCP | 3196 | 3.5 | 3.3 | 1.4 |

CABG, coronary artery bypass grafting; CCP, Cooperative Cardiac Project Database; Duke, Duke Cardiovascular Database; MI, myocardial infarction; N/A, not available; NACI, New Approaches to Coronary Intervention; NCN, National Cardiovascular Network; NHLBI, National Heart, Lung, and Blood Institute Coronary Angioplasty Registry; NNE, Northern New England Cardiac Database; NY, New York State Cardiac Database; SCAI, Society for Coronary Angioplasty and Intervention Registry.

1.0%. These low event rates may be partially biased, as the data are obtained from reports from individual hospitals and physicians and have not been independently reviewed. The Angioplasty Trials Pool,[35] involving almost 11,000 patients, is based on prospectively collected information from seven interventional randomized trials and one observational database. Unlike the data from the registries, the outcomes from the Angioplasty Trials Pool have been independently reviewed for accuracy as part of routine clinical trial data management. According to this database, the 6-month death rate is 1.3%, the myocardial infarction rate is 6.8%, and repeat revascularization rate is 17.4% (for CABG, the rate is 5.3%; for repeat PTCA, 13.4%).

Factors important in predicting intermediate to long-term mortality with PTCA are also similar to those predicting mortality with medical and surgical therapy (Table 10–5). Risk factors for survival in patients with coronary artery disease can be divided into five basic categories: *left ventricular function*, which is the most important factor in the short term; the *extent of coronary artery disease*; the presence of *risk factors for disease progression*, which is important for longer term survival; *age*, which exerts an independent effect on the risk of death even after the greater extent of coronary disease and the higher prevalence of left ventricular dysfunction in the elderly are accounted for; and the presence of *comorbid illness*, which is an important determinant of survival.

In most studies, left ventricular function at rest or during exercise is the most important predictor of survival in patients treated medically or surgically. Reports by Ellis and colleagues,[36] Vandormael and coworkers,[37] and Anderson and associates[38] have confirmed the prognostic importance of left ventricular function at rest in terms of intermediate (1- to 3-year) survival in patients treated with PTCA. Restenosis in multiple lesions supplying territories

necessary for marginal compensation of a ventricle may possibly lead to hemodynamic collapse if a new coronary event occurs as a result of plaque rupture.

The extent of coronary artery disease and the degree of ischemia present are important determinants of survival after PTCA as well as with medical therapy and after CABG.[17, 22] Ellis and colleagues[36] found significant stenosis of the LAD to be an important predictor of mortality in patients undergoing multivessel PTCA. In addition, patients undergoing angioplasty of more than one vessel have higher restenosis rates. Multilesion restenosis is significantly more common in patients with three-vessel disease.[39] Over a mean follow-up of 27 months, restenosis of at least one lesion occurred in 54% of patients with two-vessel disease and in 58% of patients with three-vessel disease. Restenosis of single lesions occurred in 40% of patients with two-vessel disease and in 29% of patients with three-vessel disease. Restenosis of more than one lesion occurred in 9% of patients with two-vessel disease and in 26% of patients with three-vessel disease (Fig. 10–2).

It is difficult to evaluate the significance of risk factors for progression of coronary disease in patients undergoing PTCA, because PTCA series record few deaths and have limited duration of follow-up. However, the presence of diabetes mellitus has emerged as an important factor associated with adverse outcomes after percutaneous interventions. Diabetes mellitus is an independent predictor of restenosis after PTCA[40] and of loss of initial gain in luminal diameter after coronary stent placement.[41] In addition, diabetes mellitus is an independent predictor of mortality and total coronary events (death, infarction, or need for CABG) after angioplasty.[36, 42]

Although age does not appear to be independently related to periprocedural mortality,[29] age is a risk factor for intermediate to long-term mortality in an-

## TABLE 10–5.    FACTORS PREDICTING INTERMEDIATE TO LONG-TERM MORTALITY WITH PTCA

| STUDY | FOLLOW-UP | MORTALITY | | CHARACTERISTICS |
|---|---|---|---|---|
| Ellis et al[36] | 22 months | | N/A | Left ventricular dysfunction |
| | | 8.5% vs. 2.5% | | Proximal LAD disease |
| | | | N/A | Diabetes |
| Weintraub et al[42] | 5 years | 17% vs. 3% | | Diabetes |
| | | 17% (≥70 yrs) vs. <5% (<70 yrs) | | Age |
| Kelsey et al[32] | 2 years | 8.8% (≥65 yrs) vs. 2.9% (<65 yrs) | | Age |
| Vandormael et al[37] | 5 years | 41% vs. 11% in multivessel disease | | Left ventricular dysfunction |
| Anderson et al[38] | 9 months | | N/A | Decreased LVEF |
| | | 9% vs. 2%† | | CHF |
| Holmes et al[99] | 4 years | 13% vs. 7% | | Decreased LVEF |
| Detre et al[45] | 1 year | 4.5% vs. 1.8% | | Multivessel disease |
| Barsness et al[104] | 5 years | 14% vs. 8% | | Diabetes |

CHF, congestive heart failure; LAD, left anterior descending artery; LVEF, left ventricular ejection fraction; PTCA, percutaneous transluminal coronary angioplasty.

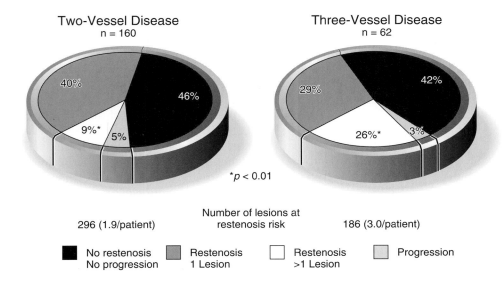

Two-Vessel Disease
n = 160

Three-Vessel Disease
n = 62

40%

46%

9%*

5%

29%

42%

26%*

3%

*p < 0.01

296 (1.9/patient)

Number of lesions at
restenosis risk

186 (3.0/patient)

■ No restenosis
No progression

▨ Restenosis
1 Lesion

☐ Restenosis
>1 Lesion

▨ Progression

FIGURE 10–2. Angiographic results after a mean follow-up of 27 months after multivessel angioplasty. (From Deligonul U, Vandormael MG, Kern MJ, et al: Coronary angioplasty: A therapeutic option for symptomatic patients with two and three vessel coronary disease. J Am Coll Cardiol 11:1173–1179, 1988.)

gioplasty even after adjustment for extent of coronary disease. One study found a 2.4-fold increase in risk of 2-year mortality with each decade of life at the time of PTCA, after adjustment for other factors.[32]

Comorbid illnesses also contribute to mortality in the population with coronary disease. The Charlson score, a simple index counting comorbid illnesses (diabetes mellitus, peptic ulcer disease, chronic obstructive pulmonary disease, malignancy, cerebrovascular disease, connective tissue disease, and renal disease), was found to be highly correlated with mortality.[43] In an analysis of long-term survival for patients in the Duke Cardiovascular Disease Database, comorbidity was the second most important prognostic factor (after left ventricular ejection fraction).[44] Patients with no comorbid diseases had improved cardiovascular survival at 4 years (93%) in comparison with patients who had two (78%) or three or more of these diagnoses (68%). Diabetes with end-organ damage was the most important comorbid illness in the index.

Despite the increasing risk of death, emergency CABG, or myocardial infarction with increasing number of diseased vessels, PTCA outcomes in patients with multivessel disease are similar to those of CABG, according to historical data.[30] Interpreting studies of multivessel angioplasty is complicated by difficulties with nomenclature. Most studies have reported outcomes in patients with multivessel disease, many of whom had undergone revascularization of only one part of the coronary tree. Clinical success rates, defined as successful dilatation of at least two vessels without major complications, have been 80% to 90%, and mortality rates are generally less than 2%.[30, 37, 39, 45–56] Most of these series selected low-risk patients for multivessel angioplasty, which accounts for the high success rates and low event rates reported.

Over time, long-term prognosis after PTCA has continued to improve. In a comparison of 5-year outcomes in the 1977–1981 National Heart, Lung, and Blood Institute (NHLBI) registry and the 1985–1986 registry,[21] patients in the later registry were, on average, older and had more diseased vessels, a higher incidence of abnormal left ventricular function, more prior myocardial infarctions, and higher incidences of heart failure, diabetes, and hypertension. Despite these greater risk factors, angiographic and clinical success rates were higher in the later cohort. No difference in in-hospital myocardial infarctions or mortality was evident, but more patients in the earlier cohort underwent same-stay CABG. After adjustment for baseline variables, the 5-year mortality rates were similar in the two registry cohorts (Table 10–6). Rates of myocardial infarction and CABG at 5-year follow-up were significantly lower in the later cohort.

## PTCA VERSUS MEDICAL MANAGEMENT

The use of PTCA evolved without guidance from randomized trials. Few studies have directly compared angioplasty with medical therapy. The first major randomized trial involving PTCA, the Angioplasty Compared to Medicine (ACME) trial,[57] was published in 1992. Men with one- or two-vessel disease, stable angina, and a positive functional study were randomly assigned to receive either PTCA or a stepped-care approach to medical therapy with the goal of eliminating angina. There was no significant difference in the incidence of myocardial infarctions or death between the two groups, although the size of the trial (212 patients) was not large enough to address these issues. The PTCA-treated patients were more likely to be free of angina, to require fewer antianginal medications, and

**TABLE 10–6.    FIVE-YEAR CUMULATIVE EVENT RATES OF NHLBI REGISTRY 2 COMPARED WITH REGISTRY 1**

| | 5-YEAR RATE, % UNADJUSTED RISK | | | | ADJUSTED RISK | |
| --- | --- | --- | --- | --- | --- | --- |
| EVENT | REG. 2 | REG. 1 | REG. 2 VS. REG. 1 | 95% CI | REG. 2 VS. REG. 1 | 95% CI |
| Death | 9.8 | 6.4 | 1.72 | 1.32–2.23 | 1.01 | 0.72–1.41 |
| MI | 13.6 | 14.5 | 0.95 | 0.79–1.14 | 0.67 | 0.53–0.85 |
| Death or MI | 20.5 | 18.7 | 1.13 | 0.97–1.33 | 0.77 | 0.63–0.94 |
| CABG | 19.2 | 39.4 | 0.42 | 0.37–0.48 | 0.33 | 0.27–0.39 |
| Death, MI, or CABG | 32.9 | 47.4 | 0.58 | 0.51–0.66 | 0.45 | 0.38–0.52 |
| Repeated PTCA | 27.8 | 17.2 | 1.80 | 1.54–2.10 | 1.41 | 1.16–1.71 |
| Any revascularization | 41.4 | 51.2 | 0.69 | 0.63–0.77 | 0.55 | 0.48–0.63 |

CABG, coronary artery bypass grafting; CI, confidence interval; MI, myocardial infarction; NHLBI, National Heart, Blood, and Lung Institute; PTCA, percutaneous transluminal coronary angioplasty.

Adapted from Detre K, Yeh W, Kelsey S, et al, for the Investigators of the NHLBI Percutaneous Transluminal Coronary Angioplasty Registry: Has improvement in PTCA intervention affected long-term prognosis? The NHLBI PTCA Registry experience. Circulation 91:2868–2875, 1995.

to have longer exercise times and significantly better physiologic well-being scores than were the medically treated patients. However, this came at the price of a greater need for procedures during follow-up and a greater initial expense.

A pilot study comparing angioplasty with medicine in patients with two-vessel disease revealed that both treatment groups had improved exercise duration, improved quality of life, and reduced angina.[58] This trial failed to find an advantage of angioplasty over medicine, as was seen in the patients with single-vessel disease. The small number of patients enrolled in the trial, less complete revascularization, and higher rates of restenosis in patients with two-vessel disease may have contributed to this outcome.

The second Randomised Intervention Treatment of Angina (RITA-2) trial evaluated patients with multivessel disease who were deemed appropriate for treatment with either medicine or PTCA.[59] The PTCA-treated patients had a significantly greater risk of death or nonfatal myocardial infarction than did the medically treated patients, although the risk of events in both groups was relatively low (6.3% and 3.3%, respectively). Although both treatment modalities ameliorated symptoms and improved exercise tolerance, angioplasty resulted in greater amelioration of symptoms, greater improvement in exercise tolerance, and a decrease in the amount of antianginal use in comparison with medical therapy in the group as a whole. However, these differences were not seen in patients with good exercise tolerance and mild angina at baseline. These results indicate that patients without severe angina at baseline may benefit from a trial of medical therapy, revascularization being reserved for patients without amelioration of symptoms.

With its expanded use, PTCA has become another therapeutic option for certain patients who pre-

viously would have had only the options of surgery or medication alone. There are patients for whom CABG is clearly the therapy of choice; for other patients, PTCA may be more suitable. However, until the 1990s, no prospective, randomized trial had investigated the best therapeutic choice for those patients in whom either revascularization approach may be chosen.

## RANDOMIZED TRIALS OF PTCA VERSUS CABG

Coronary artery bypass surgery has been clearly shown to be effective at treating symptoms and prolonging survival in certain patient subgroups.[3, 5, 6, 8] Although multivessel angioplasty is relatively low in risk and appears to have a remarkable success rate, its efficacy in the longer term treatment of multivessel disease, particularly in comparison with bypass grafting, was unclear. A task force was therefore organized by the NHLBI in 1985 to determine the need for a randomized trial investigating whether coronary angioplasty is a viable alternative to bypass surgery in patients who are suitable candidates for either procedure. Recommendations from the task force led to funding of two such trials: the Bypass Angioplasty Revascularization Investigation (BARI) and the Emory Angioplasty versus Surgery Trial (EAST). To date, nine randomized trials have compared angioplasty with bypass surgery in patients with coronary disease, as summarized in Table 10–7.

The initial RITA trial was the first published trial comparing angioplasty with CABG.[60] RITA was the only trial to include both single- and multivessel disease. In fact, more than one third of the 1011 patients enrolled had single-vessel disease. The two treatment groups had similar rates of the primary

**TABLE 10–7.    CHARACTERISTICS OF RANDOMIZED TRIALS COMPARING PTCA AND CABG**

| STUDY | ENROLLMENT PERIOD | NO. OF PATIENTS | FOLLOW-UP (YEARS) | PRIMARY END POINT | SECONDARY END POINTS |
|---|---|---|---|---|---|
| CABRI | 1988–1991 | 1054 | 1 | Angina, death | MI, antianginal requirement, revascularization |
| BARI | 1988–1991 | 1829 | 5 | Death | |
| RITA | 1988–1991 | 1011 | 2.5 | Death, MI | USA, arrhythmia, CHF, CVA |
| EAST | 1987–1990 | 392 | 3 | Death, MI, ischemia (thallium) (composite) | Degree of revascularization, Lvfxn, ETT, revascularization, quality of life, cost |
| GABI | 1988–1990 | 359 | 1 | Angina | Death, MI, procedure complications, revascularization |
| ERACI | 1988–1990 | 127 | 5 | Death, MI, angina, revascularization (combined) | In-hospital events (death, MI, revascularization), complete revascularization, costs |
| MASS | 1988–1991 | 214 | 3 | Cardiac death, MI, revascularization (combined) | Angina, employment status, ETT, atherosclerosis at 2-yr catheterization |
| Lausanne study | 1989–1993 | 134 | 5 | Death, MI, revascularization (combined) | Angina, ETT, medications, repeat catheterization |

BARI, Bypass Angioplasty Revascularization Investigation; CABG, coronary artery bypass grafting; CABRI, Coronary Angioplasty versus Bypass Revascularization Investigation; CHF, congestive heart failure; CVA, cerebrovascular accident; EAST, Emory Angioplasty versus Surgery Trial; ERACI, Argentine Randomized Trial of Percutaneous Transluminal Coronary Angioplasty versus Coronary Artery Bypass Surgery in Multivessel Disease; ETT, exercise tolerance test; GABI, German Angioplasty Bypass Surgery Investigation; MASS, Medicine, Angioplasty or Surgery Study; MI, myocardial infarction; PTCA, percutaneous transluminal coronary angioplasty; RITA, Randomised Intervention Treatment of Angina; USA, unstable angina.

trial end point, mortality and recurrent myocardial infarction combined, after 2.5 years of follow-up.

The Coronary Angioplasty versus Bypass Revascularization Investigation (CABRI) recruited 1054 patients from 26 high-volume European hospitals and reported results from the first year of a planned 10-year follow-up.[61] The primary outcomes evaluated were mortality and anginal class; no significant difference in mortality between the groups was evident at 1 year, but patients who underwent CABG had better relief of angina.

The BARI study was the largest of the randomized trials, enrolling 1829 patients from 18 clinical centers throughout the United States and Canada.[62] It was the only one of the randomized trials in which mortality alone was the predefined primary end point. Over a mean follow-up period of 5.4 years, there was no significant difference in mortality between the two treatment groups; cumulative survival rates were 89.3% for those assigned to bypass surgery and 86.3% for those assigned to angioplasty ($p = 0.19$).

The EAST study was performed at a single center, where 392 patients were randomly assigned to undergo CABG or angioplasty.[63] Outcomes were monitored over a 5-year period. The primary end point in this trial was a composite of death, myocardial infarction, and ischemia as seen on stress thallium images. At 3 years, there was no difference in the occurrence of a composite end point, which occurred in 27.3% of patients who underwent CABG and in 28.8% of those who underwent PTCA.

The German Angioplasty Bypass Surgery Investi-gation (GABI), a multicenter trial enrolling 359 patients at eight clinical sites in Germany,[64] recruited more patients with severe angina than did the other trials. Rates of occurrence of the primary end point, freedom from angina 1 year after treatment, were not significantly different between the two groups. Freedom from angina occurred in 74% of patients who underwent CABG and in 71% of patients who underwent PTCA.

The Argentine Randomized Trial of Percutaneous Transluminal Coronary Angioplasty versus Coronary Artery Bypass Surgery in Multivessel Disease (ERACI) was conducted at the Anchorena Hospital in Buenos Aires to compare rates of freedom from combined coronary events in patients undergoing PTCA or CABG.[65] The investigators enrolled 127 patients with either severe angina refractory to medications or a large area of ischemia identified by imaging studies. At 1 year, freedom from the combined end point of death, myocardial infarction, angina, and revascularization was more common among patients undergoing bypass grafting (83.5%) than among those treated with angioplasty (63.7%; $p < 0.005$). At 5 years, freedom from combined events continued to be significantly more common among those who had undergone CABG (68% vs. 40%; $p < 0.001$).[66]

A trial conducted in Toulouse, France, randomly assigned patients with multivessel disease to undergo PTCA (N = 57) or CABG (N = 52).[67] In-hospital complications occurred significantly more often in patients who underwent bypass (12 of 52, or 23%) than in those who underwent angioplasty

(5 of 57, or 8.8%; $p < 0.05$). However, only minimal additional in-hospital and follow-up information is available.[68]

Two studies examined treatment outcomes in the subgroup of patients with single-vessel coronary disease involving the proximal LAD. In a study conducted in Lausanne, Switzerland, 134 patients with proximal LAD disease and stable angina were randomly assigned to undergo internal mammary bypass grafting or PTCA. After a median follow-up period of 2.5 years, 86% of patients who underwent CABG and 43% of those who underwent PTCA were free of adverse effects ($p < 0.01$).[69] These results were similar to those in the Medicine Angioplasty or Surgery Study (MASS), in which patients with LAD disease and stable angina were randomly assigned to undergo mammary bypass surgery, undergo PTCA, or receive medical therapy.[70] At an average follow-up period of 3 years, 97% of patients undergoing CABG were free of events, in comparison with 76% of patients undergoing PTCA ($p < 0.01$). Neither study demonstrated a difference in mortality or cardiac death between the treatment groups, and both studies showed a similar reduction in angina.

Baseline demographics from the different trials are shown in Table 10–8. The average age of patients enrolled in the trials was 60 years. Three quarters of the patients were men. The proportion of patients with unstable angina varied widely, from as low as 14% in GABI to 83% in ERACI; unstable angina patients were excluded from enrollment in the Lausanne and MASS trials. The proportion of patients with three-vessel disease also varied among the trials; RITA and GABI had low percentages of patients with three-vessel disease in comparison with the other multivessel trials. Most patients enrolled had normal left ventricular function, the average ejection fraction being 60%.

The majority of results in the trials were analyzed according to intent to treat. Most of the patients enrolled underwent their assigned treatment; 96% of patients randomly assigned to undergo CABG actually underwent the surgery, and 97.5% of patients randomly assigned to undergo angioplasty underwent the procedure (Table 10–9). The angiographic PTCA success rate in the multivessel trials ranged from 78% in BARI to 92% in GABI, ERACI, and CABRI. As would be expected, higher angiographic success rates were seen in the single-vessel trials. The proportion of patients in whom internal mammary conduits were used varied from 37% in GABI to 82% in BARI.

Data on in-hospital events are available for all the trials with the exception of CABRI, which reported limited periprocedural data. In no trial was the periprocedural mortality rate significantly different between CABG and PTCA (Table 10–10). In the multivessel trials, mortality rates averaged 1.1% of PTCA-treated patients and 1.4% of CABG-treated patients. In GABI and ERACI, the mortality rates among CABG-treated patients were slightly but not significantly higher. There were no reported deaths in the single-vessel trials; however, the number of patients enrolled was relatively small.

Although there was no difference in early mortality, the number of periprocedural myocardial infarctions was significantly higher with surgery than with angioplasty in three trials (BARI, EAST, and GABI). The true incidence of periprocedural myocardial infarctions was probably underestimated, inasmuch as many of the trials[62–65] defined myocardial infarctions as new Q-waves on the electrocardiogram and periprocedural cardiac enzymes were not routinely measured. Therefore, non–Q-wave myocardial infarctions were either not diagnosed or not reported in these trials. In addition, perioperative myocardial infarctions are difficult to determine electrocardiographically in many bypass patients because of the effects of cardioplegia on the conduc-

## TABLE 10–8.   BASELINE DEMOGRAPHICS OF ENROLLED PATIENTS

| STUDY | MEAN AGE | % MEN | % WITH TWO-VESSEL DISEASE | % WITH THREE-VESSEL DISEASE | EJECTION FRACTION | UNSTABLE ANGINA |
|---|---|---|---|---|---|---|
| CABRI (N = 1054) | 60 | 78 | 57 | 41.5 | 63 | 14.5 |
| BARI (N = 1829) | 61 | 74 | 59 | 41 | 57 | 64 |
| RITA (N = 1011) | 57 | 81 | 43 | 12 | N/A | 55 |
| EAST (N = 392) | 62 | 74 | 60 | 40 | 61 | N/A |
| GABI (N = 359) | 59 | 79 | 82 | 18 | 56 | 14 |
| ERACI (N = 127) | 58 | 85 | 55 | 45 | 61 | 83 |
| MASS (N = 142) | 55 | 57 | 0 | 0 | 76 | 0 |
| Lausanne (N = 134) | 56 | 80 | 0 | 0 | N/A | 0 |
| Total (N = 5048) | 60 | 76.6 | 56.9 | 33.3 | 59.8 | 43.7 |

BARI, Bypass Angioplasty Revascularization Investigation; CABRI, Coronary Angioplasty versus Bypass Revascularization Investigation; EAST, Emory Angioplasty versus Surgery Trial; ERACI, Argentine Randomized Trial of Percutaneous Transluminal Coronary Angioplasty versus Coronary Artery Bypass Surgery in Multivessel Disease; GABI, German Angioplasty Bypass Surgery Investigation; MASS, Medicine, Angioplasty or Surgery Study; N/A, not available; RITA, Randomised Intervention Treatment of Angina.

**TABLE 10–9.  PROCEDURAL OUTCOMES**

| TRIAL | % UNDERGOING ASSIGNED PROCEDURE | | PTCA SUCCESS RATE (%) | USE OF IMA GRAFTS (%) |
|---|---|---|---|---|
| | PTCA | CABG | | |
| CABRI | 96.5 | 93.2 | 92 | 81 |
| BARI | 98.8 | 97.6 | 78 | 82 |
| RITA | 96.7 | 97.8 | 87 | 74 |
| EAST | 99 | 99.5 | 88 | N/A |
| GABI | 96.7 | 90.1 | 92 | 37 |
| ERACI | N/A | N/A | 92 | 76.5 |
| MASS | 100 | 100 | 92 | 100 |
| Lausanne | 100 | 89.4 | 97* | 100 |

BARI, Bypass Angioplasty Revascularization Investigation; CABG, coronary artery bypass grafting; CABRI, Coronary Angioplasty versus Bypass Revascularization; EAST, Emory Angioplasty versus Surgery Trial; ERACI, Argentine Randomized Trial of Percutaneous Transluminal Coronary Angioplasty versus Coronary Artery Bypass Surgery in Multivessel Disease; GABI, German Angioplasty Bypass Surgery Investigation; IMA, internal mammary artery; MASS, Medicine, Angioplasty or Surgery Study; N/A, not available; PTCA, percutaneous transluminal coronary angioplasty; RITA, Randomised Intervention Treatment of Angina.
*97% if stents are included, 94% if stents are excluded.

tion system. Overall, the rate of periprocedural myocardial infarctions in the PTCA recipients was 1.4%, in comparison with 2.4% of the CABG recipients.

The most significant difference between the two treatment modalities was the rate of repeat revascularization procedures. Of the multivessel trials, only ERACI found similar in-hospital revascularization rates between the two treatment groups. As a group, the multivessel trials had revascularization rates of 5.4% after PTCA, in comparison with 0.1% after CABG. The single-vessel trials observed higher in-hospital reintervention rates in the PTCA-treated

patients as well. The majority of reinterventions in the PTCA-treated patients were subsequent bypass operations. Often, these were emergency procedures necessitated by acute closure. Few patients who underwent CABG also underwent repeat revascularization during the initial hospitalization; the majority of those who did underwent PTCA.

Not surprisingly, hospital stays were longer after bypass surgery than after angioplasty.[60, 62, 64] In addition to the postoperative recovery period's being longer, complications associated with bypass surgery contributed to extended hospital stays. Periop-

**TABLE 10–10.  ANGIOPLASTY VERSUS CABG RANDOMIZED TRIALS: IN-HOSPITAL EVENTS**

| TRIAL | DEATH (%) | | MI (%) | | REVASCULARIZATION (%) | | CABG (%) | | PTCA (%) | |
|---|---|---|---|---|---|---|---|---|---|---|
| | PTCA | CABG | PTCA | CABG | PTCA | CABG | PTCA | CABG | PTCA | CABG |
| CABRI (N = 1054) | 1.3 | 1.3 | N/A | N/A | N/A | N/A | N/A | N/A | N/A | N/A |
| BARI (N = 1829) | 1.1 | 1.3 | 2.1 | 4.6* | 12.8 | 0.1† | 10.2 | 0.1 | 3.4 | 0 |
| RITA (N = 1011) | 0.8 | 1.2 | 3.5 | 2.4 | 6.9 | 0 | 5.9 | 0 | 1 | 0 |
| EAST (N = 392) | 1 | 1 | 3 | 10.3* | 10.1 | 0 | 10.1 | 0 | 0 | 0 |
| GABI (N = 359) | 1.1 | 2.5 | 2.3 | 8.1‡ | 11.4 | 1.9 | 8.2 | 1.1 | 2.8 | 0.6 |
| ERACI (N = 127) | 1.5 | 4.6 | 6.3 | 6.2 | 1.5 | 1.5 | 1.5 | 0 | 0 | 1.5 |
| MASS (N = 142) | 0 | 0 | 2.8 | 1.4 | 2.8 | 0 | 2.8 | 0 | 0 | 0 |
| Lausanne (N = 134) | 0 | 0 | 2.9 | 1.5 | 5.9 | 0 | 5.9 | 0 | 0 | 0 |
| Total (N = 5048) | 1 | 1.4 | 1.4 | 2.4 | 5 | 0.1 | 4.1 | 0.07 | 1 | 0.05 |
| Multivessel total (N = 4772) | 1.1 | 1.4 | 1.5 | 2.5 | 5.4 | 0.1 | 4.4 | 0.08 | 1.1 | 0.05 |

BARI, Bypass Angioplasty Revascularization Investigation; CABG, coronary artery bypass grafting; CABRI, Coronary Angioplasty versus Bypass Revascularization; EAST, Emory Angioplasty versus Surgery Trial; ERACI, Argentine Randomized Trial of Percutaneous Transluminal Coronary Angioplasty versus Coronary Artery Bypass Surgery in Multivessel Disease; GABI, German Angioplasty Bypass Surgery Investigation; MASS, Medicine, Angioplasty or Surgery Study; MI, myocardial infarction; N/A, not available; PTCA, percutaneous transluminal coronary angioplasty; RITA, Randomised Intervention Treatment of Angina.
*$p = 0.004$. †$p < 0.001$. ‡$p = 0.022$.

erative complications such as stroke, hemorrhage, arrhythmias, pulmonary embolism, and infections are not uncommon after bypass surgery, but they were not uniformly reported in the trials. In trials that did report complications, there was no detectable difference in the rate of procedure-related strokes.[60, 62–65, 70] In BARI, respiratory failure, wound dehiscence or infection, and reoperation for hemorrhage were statistically more common in the CABG-treated patients.[62] In GABI, significantly more patients who underwent CABG developed postoperative pneumonia.[64] RITA documented significantly more arrhythmias in the CABG-treated patients but noted more predischarge unstable angina in the angioplasty-treated patients.[60]

Follow-up duration varied; the longest reported follow-up was 5 years, in the BARI, EAST, and ERACI trials. A treatment-related difference in mortality or late myocardial infarctions was not evident in any of the trials (Table 10–11). Freedom from death and myocardial infarction combined was also similar in the two treatment groups. RITA reported that 1 year after treatment, infarction-free survival rates were 90.2% of patients randomly assigned to undergo PTCA and 91.4% of patients randomly assigned to undergo CABG.[60] BARI found that 5 years after treatment, 78.7% of patients randomly assigned to undergo PTCA were alive and free of infarction, in comparison with 80.4% of patients assigned to undergo CABG.[62]

Some of the trials included events such as revascularization or angina in the combined outcomes. The predefined combined end point in EAST was death, Q-wave myocardial infarction, or a large ischemic defect identified by thallium. At 3-year follow-up, 71.2% of patients randomly assigned to undergo PTCA were free from this end point, in comparison with 72.7% of patients randomly assigned to undergo CABG.[63] ERACI reported that 40% of patients assigned to undergo PTCA were alive and free from myocardial infarction, repeat revascularization, and angina after 5 years, in comparison with 68% of those assigned to undergo CABG ($p < 0.001$).[66] The Lausanne and MASS trials found freedom from death, myocardial infarction, or revascularization in more patients who underwent PTCA than patients treated surgically. At an average follow-up period of 2 years, 97% of patients randomly assigned to undergo CABG in the MASS trial were free of death, myocardial infarction, or revascularization, in comparison with 76% of patients assigned to undergo PTCA ($p = 0.0002$)[70]; in the Lausanne study, 86% of patients were free from such events, in comparison with 43% of patients treated with PTCA.[69] Although most trials showed a higher rate of posttreatment events among the patients treated with PTCA, this difference was driven by the higher revascularization rate. In the trials that did not include repeat revascularization in the combined outcome, no treatment-related difference was evident.

There was a major difference between the two procedures in the need for additional revascularization during the follow-up period. Subsequent revascularizations occurred much more frequently among the patients who underwent PTCA in every trial (Table 10–12). Most of the subsequent revascularization procedures were angioplasty. However, the rate of subsequent bypass surgery in the PTCA-treated patients was significant, ranging from 15% to 22% at 1 year[68] and from 25% to 31% at 5 years in the multivessel trials. Most revascularizations occurred within the first year. Despite this higher reintervention rate among the patients who had undergone

## TABLE 10–11.   FOLLOW-UP EVENTS

| STUDY | FOLLOW-UP (YEARS) | DEATH (%) | | LATE MI (%) | |
|---|---|---|---|---|---|
| | | PTCA | CABG | PTCA | CABG |
| CABRI | 1 | 3.9 | 2.7 | 4.9 | 3.5 |
| BARI | 5 | 13.7* | 10.7* | 10.9* | 11.7* |
| RITA | 2.5 | 3.1 | 3.6 | 6.7† | 5.2† |
| EAST | 3 | 6.2 | 7.1 | 14.6 | 19.6 |
| EAST | 5 | 12.1 | 8.8 | N/A | N/A |
| GABI | 1 | 2.2 | 5.1 | 3.8 | 7.3 |
| ERACI, 3-year | 3 | 9.5 | 4.7 | 7.8 | 7.8 |
| ERACI, 5-year | 5 | 12.7 | 9.4 | 11.1 | 9.4 |
| MASS | 3.5 | 1.4 | 1.4 | 2.8† | 1.4† |
| Lausanne | 2 | 4.4 | 1.4 | 11.8† | 3† |

BARI, Bypass Angioplasty Revascularization Investigation; CABG, coronary artery bypass grafting; CABRI, Coronary Angioplasty versus Bypass Revascularization; EAST, Emory Angioplasty versus Surgery Trial; ERACI, Argentine Randomized Trial of Percutaneous Transluminal Coronary Angioplasty versus Coronary Artery Bypass Surgery in Multivessel Disease; GABI, German Angioplasty Bypass Surgery Investigation; MASS, Medicine, Angioplasty or Surgery Study; MI, myocardial infarction; N/A, not available; PTCA, percutaneous transluminal coronary angioplasty; RITA, Randomised Intervention Treatment of Angina.

*Cumulative rates.
†Non–Q-wave MI included.

**TABLE 10–12.    FOLLOW-UP REVASCULARIZATION RATES**

| STUDY | FOLLOW-UP (YEARS) | REVASCULARIZATION (%) | | FOLLOW-UP PTCA (%) | | FOLLOW-UP CABG (%) | |
|---|---|---|---|---|---|---|---|
| | | PTCA | CABG | PTCA | CABG | PTCA | CABG |
| CABRI | 1 | 33.7 | 6.5 | 20.8 | 2.7 | 15.7 | 0.8 |
| BARI | 5 | 54 | 8 | 34 | 7 | 31 | 1 |
| RITA | 2 | 31 | 5 | 18 | 4.2 | 19 | 0.8 |
| EAST | 3 | 54 | 13 | 41 | 13 | 22 | 0.5 |
| EAST | 5 | N/A | N/A | 48.6 | 15.5 | 25.1 | 0.5 |
| GABI | 1 | 44 | 6 | 27 | 5.0 | 22 | 1 |
| ERACI | 3 | 37 | 6.3 | 14.3 | 6.3 | 22 | 0 |
| ERACI | 5 | 38 | 6.3 | N/A | N/A | N/A | N/A |
| MASS | 3.5 | N/A | 0 | 29 | 0 | 13.8 | 0 |
| Lausanne | 2 | 34 | 4.5 | 25 | 4.5 | 16 | 0 |

BARI, Bypass Angioplasty Revascularization Investigation; CABG, coronary artery bypass grafting; CABRI, Coronary Angioplasty versus Bypass Revascularization; EAST, Emory Angioplasty versus Surgery Trial; ERACI, Argentine Randomized Trial of Percutaneous Transluminal Coronary Angioplasty versus Coronary Artery Bypass Surgery in Multivessel Disease; GABI, German Angioplasty Bypass Surgery Investigation; MASS, Medicine, Angioplasty on Surgery Study; MI, myocardial infarction; N/A, not available; PTCA, percutaneous transluminal coronary angioplasty; RITA, Randomised Intervention Treatment of Angina.

PTCA, there was no increased risk of major cardiac events.

Patients in both treatment groups achieved substantial reductions in angina. Early on, surgery tended to be more effective at relieving angina. Despite more angina in the PTCA-treated patients at 3 years, the percentage of patients with ischemia as measured by stress thallium images was not statistically different between the two treatments in EAST.[63] Over time, the treatment-related difference in angina diminished. Five years into the EAST[71] and ERACI[66] trials, the prevalence of angina was low and not significantly different between treatment groups (Table 10–13). The progressive reduction in angina in the PTCA group was accompanied by a higher rate of reinterventions. However, much of the angina was treated effectively without surgery. In fact, 70% of the PTCA patients in BARI who were free of angina 5 years after treatment required no bypass surgery.[72]

## META-ANALYSIS OF CABG VERSUS PTCA

In 1995, Pocock and coworkers published a meta-analysis of eight of the nine randomized trials.[68] This meta-analysis included results obtained from the Toulouse investigators, but the results of the BARI trial were not available at the time of analysis. At a mean follow-up of 2.7 years, no difference in prognosis between the two therapies was detected. The total number of deaths was 79 (4.6%) of the 1710 PTCA-treated patients and 73 (4.4%) of the 1661 CABG-treated patients. Most deaths occurred in the first year of follow-up; myocardial infarction or cardiac death occurred in a total of 135 (7.9%)

**TABLE 10–13.    SYMPTOMS AT FOLLOW-UP**

| STUDY | FOLLOW-UP (YEARS) | ANGINA AT ENROLLMENT (%) | | PREVALENCE OF ANGINA (%) | | | ANTIANGINAL USE (%) | | |
|---|---|---|---|---|---|---|---|---|---|
| | | PTCA | CABG | PTCA | CABG | p | PTCA | CABG | p |
| CABRI | 1 | 84 | 88* | 13.9 | 10.1* | 0.012 | 70 | 53 | <0.001 |
| BARI | 5 | 100 | 100 | 22 | 14 | 0.003 | 76 | 57 | <0.001 |
| RITA | 2 | 92.9 | 93.4 | 31.3 | 21.5 | 0.007 | 61 | 34 | — |
| EAST | 3 | 89.9 | 91.1* | 20 | 12* | 0.039 | 66 | 51 | 0.005 |
| EAST | 5 | 89.9 | 91.1* | 4.7 | 8* | NS | N/A | N/A | — |
| GABI | 1 | N/A | N/A† | 29 | 26* | NS | 88 | 78 | 0.041 |
| ERACI | 3 | N/A | N/A | 4.8 | 3.2 | NS | N/A | N/A | — |
| ERACI | 5 | N/A | N/A | 6.3 | 9.4 | NS | N/A | N/A | — |
| MASS | 3 | 100 | 100 | 18 | 2 | <0.01 | N/A | N/A | — |
| Lausanne | 2 | 100 | 100 | 23 | 11 | 0.07 | 85 | 43 | <0.01 |

BARI, Bypass Angioplasty Revascularization Investigation; CABG, coronary artery bypass grafting; CABRI, Coronary Angioplasty versus Bypass Revascularization; EAST, Emory Angioplasty versus Surgery Trial; ERACI, Argentine Randomized Trial of Percutaneous Transluminal Coronary Angioplasty versus Coronary Artery Bypass Surgery in Multivessel Disease; GABI, German Angioplasty Bypass Surgery Investigation; MASS, Medicine, Angioplasty or Surgery Study; MI, myocardial infarction; N/A, not available; PTCA, percutaneous transluminal coronary angioplasty; RITA, Randomised Intervention Treatment of Angina.

*Angina class > I. †Patients enrolled were required to be "symptomatic."

patients who had undergone PTCA and 127 (7.6%) patients who had undergone CABG. After the first year, the risk of death or myocardial infarction was much lower for both groups.

There were marked differences between the two groups in the need for additional revascularization and in the relief of angina. In all trials combined, 33.7% of the patients randomly assigned to undergo PTCA required at least one additonal revascularization procedure during the first year of follow-up, in comparison with 3.3% of patients randomly assigned to undergo CABG. After the first year of follow-up, this difference diminished; revascularization occurred at a rate of 1.8 per 100 patient-years in the CABG-treated patients, in comparison with 4.5 per 100 patient-years in the PTCA-treated patients. The prevalence of NYHA anginal class 2 or greater was higher 1 year after PTCA, with a relative risk of 1.56 (10.8% of the CABG-treated patients vs. 17.6% of the PTCA-treated patients). After the first year, this relative risk decreased to 1.23 (12.7% vs. 15.8%).

The risk of cardiac death and myocardial infarction in single-vessel disease was lower with CABG than with PTCA. Patients with single-vessel disease had lower 1-year mortality rates than did those with multivessel disease, and they demonstrated a nonsignificant trend toward a lesser need for additional reinterventions (30.5% vs. 34.5%; $p = 0.2$). The prevalence of angina at 1- and 3-year follow-up was also lower in patients with single-vessel disease in both treatment groups ($p < 0.01$ and $p = 0.11$, respectively).

A second meta-analysis of five of the randomized trials involving only multivessel disease (ERACI,

RITA, CABRI, GABI, and EAST) indicated similar results.[73] There was a nonsignificant trend for lower rates of death or nonfatal myocardial infarctions ($p = 0.09$) and significantly lower rates of angina and revascularization in the CABG recipients over the 1- to 3-year follow-up period.

## LIMITATIONS OF THE TRIALS

There are several problems inherent in the trials comparing coronary bypass grafting with angioplasty. A bias occurs before randomization, inasmuch as many patients and their physicians are hesitant to participate in a trial involving a major surgical procedure. As a result, these trials have randomly assigned fewer than half of eligible patients (Table 10–14).[16] Therefore, the patients randomly assigned may not be a representative mix of the general population. For example, eligible patients not randomly assigned in BARI had higher educational levels than those randomly assigned and therefore may have been more compliant with diet, exercise, and medications during follow-up.[16] The trials also have strict eligibility criteria (Table 10–15), leading to final results that apply to a small fraction of the patients with coronary artery disease.

Another limitation is that the follow-up in these trials is not long-term. In general, vein graft occlusion rates increase after 5 years, and progression of coronary disease in ungrafted vessels may lead to an increase in symptoms and need for repeat revascularization in CABG recipients. Rates of morbidity and mortality are higher with second bypass operations than with the first, and there is no evidence

## TABLE 10–14. LIMITATIONS OF TRIALS: NUMBERS OF PATIENTS SCREENED VERSUS NUMBERS OF PATIENTS ENROLLED

| STUDY | UNDERWENT CATHETERIZATION | CAD | REQUIRED REVASCULARIZATION | MET CRITERIA | | ENROLLED |
|---|---|---|---|---|---|---|
| | | | | N | % | |
| CABRI | N/A | N/A | 42,580 | 23,047 | 54.1* | 1054 |
| BARI | N/A | 25,200† | N/A | 4110 | 16.3 | 1829 |
| RITA | N/A | 27,975 | 17,239 | N/A | N/A | 1011 |
| EAST | N/A | 5118† | N/A | 842 | 16.5 | 392 |
| GABI | N/A | 8981‡ | N/A | 359 | 4.0 | 359 |
| ERACI | 1409 | N/A | 748 | 301 | 21.4 | 127 |
| MASS | N/A | N/A | N/A | N/A | N/A | 213§ |
| Lausanne | 5119 | 1786‖ | N/A | 142 | 8.0 | 134 |

Results are presented as number of patients except where indicated.

BARI, Bypass Angioplasty Revascularization Investigation; CABRI, Coronary Angioplasty versus Bypass Revascularization; CAD, coronary artery disease; EAST, Emory Angioplasty versus Surgery Trial; ERACI, Argentine Randomized Trial of Percutaneous Transluminal Coronary Angioplasty versus Coronary Artery Bypass Surgery in Multivessel Disease; GABI, German Angioplasty Bypass Surgery Investigation; MASS, Medicine, Angioplasty or Surgery Study; N/A, not available; RITA, Randomised Intervention Treatment of Angina.

*Percentage of patients requiring revascularization. †Patients with multivessel disease and no prior revascularization. ‡Patients with multivessel disease only. §Of the patients screened, 20% refused participation, 5% participated in other trials, 5% had unstable angina, 6% had previous percutaneous transluminal coronary angioplasty, 2% had congestive heart failure, 28% had unsuitable lesions, 19% had lesions <70% vessel diameter, 8% had multivessel disease, 10% involved the first diagonal, and some patients had multiple reasons for not enrolling. ‖Patients with single-vessel disease only.

**TABLE 10–15. EXCLUSION CRITERIA OF THE RANDOMIZED TRIALS**

| STUDY | EXCLUSION CRITERIA |
|---|---|
| CABRI | One-VD, three-VD with two occluded vessels, left main coronary artery disease, ejection fraction < 35%, >76 years old, acute MI within 10 days, previous revascularization, recent cardiovascular accident, congestive heart failure |
| BARI | Insufficient angina or ischemia, unstable angina, acute MI, left main coronary artery disease, limited life expectancy, ascending aortic calcification, one-VD, prior revascularization |
| RITA | Left main coronary artery disease, previous revascularization, valvular disease |
| EAST | Chronic total occlusion, left main coronary artery disease, ejection fraction < 25%, insufficient symptoms or myocardium at risk, acute MI within the past 5 days, previous revascularization |
| GABI | Left main coronary artery disease, age > 74, occluded lesions, >50% of myocardium at risk, previous revascularization, MI within the past 4 weeks, unsuitable coronary features |
| ERACI | Left main coronary artery disease, ejection fraction < 35%, severe valvular disease, hypertrophic heart disease, acute MI, limited life expectancy |
| MASS | Unstable angina, prior MI, left ventricular dysfunction, prior revascularization, occluded lesions |
| Lausanne | Unstable angina, previous anterior MI, acute MI, ejection fraction < 50% |

BARI, Bypass Angioplasty Revascularization Investigation; CABRI, Coronary Angioplasty versus Bypass Revascularization; EAST, Emory Angioplasty versus Surgery Trial; ERACI, Argentine Randomized Trial of Percutaneous Transluminal Coronary Angioplasty versus Coronary Artery Bypass Surgery in Multivessel Disease; GABI, German Angioplasty Bypass Surgery Investigation; MASS, Medicine, Angioplasty or Surgery Study; MI, myocardial infarction; RITA, Randomised Intervention Treatment of Angina; VD, vessel disease.

that a second bypass operation increases the patient's chances of survival. In contrast, restenosis of vessels that have undergone angioplasty occurs within the first year. Follow-up studies of PTCA have suggested that after the first 6 months, dilated arteries are likely to remain patent for years.[74] If late symptoms develop in these patients, they often result from new coronary lesions rather than restenosis of the previous site of intervention.[74] There-

fore, the relatively short follow-up period of these trials may bias decisions in favor of CABG. The follow-up period in BARI is continuing for a total of 10 years to help address the issue of late attrition of saphenous vein grafts.

None of these trials had sufficient statistical power to evaluate differences in mortality. Even the meta-analyses had limited statistical power to detect clinically important differences in mortality between the two treatment strategies. Despite their lack of statistical power, the trial results are strikingly similar. This similarity exists even though there is considerable clinical heterogeneity among the trials, bringing added strength to their conclusions.

A final limitation common to all randomized trials comparing long-term outcomes concerns advances in technology. By the time the long-term results are available, advances in surgical and angioplasty technique limit application of the findings to current practice. In the case of CABG, surgical mortality rates have decreased since the initiation of the trials. In the case of PTCA, stents and platelet inhibitors are likely to have improved outcomes. These advances in technology need to be considered when revascularization strategies are compared.

## DUKE DATABASE

Observational studies support the conclusions of the randomized trials. Since 1971, the Duke Databank for Cardiovascular Diseases has maintained a registry containing detailed patient information and outcomes collected prospectively on patients undergoing cardiac catheterization at Duke.[75, 76] This information was used to develop a more extensive coronary artery classification system. Combinations of coronary lesions were ranked and weighted by means of a Cox regression analysis of medical prognosis in patients treated at Duke between 1969 and 1984.[77] In addition to the number of diseased vessels, this system takes into account the severity of lesions and whether the proximal LAD is involved (Table 10–16). This scoring system may define treatment differences more accurately than the tradi-

**TABLE 10–16. CORONARY ARTERY ANATOMY SCORE**

| CORONARY ANATOMY | PROGNOSTIC GROUP | | | | | | | | | | |
|---|---|---|---|---|---|---|---|---|---|---|---|
| | 1 | 2 | 3 | 4 | 5 | 5a | 6 | 6a | 7 | 8 | 9 |
| Number of stenoses ≥ 75% | 1 | 1 | 2 | 2 | 1 | 2 | 2 | 3 | 3 | 3 | 3 |
| Number of stenoses ≥ 95% | 0 | 1 | 0–1 | 2 | 1 | 1 | 1 | 0 | 1 | 0–2 | 0–3 |
| Any LAD location | ± | N | ± | N | Y | Y | Y | Y | Y | Y | Y |
| ≥75% stenosis of the proximal LAD | N | N | ± | N | Y | N | Y | N | N | Y | Y |
| ≥95% stenosis of the proximal LAD | N | N | N | N | Y | N | Y | N | N | N | Y |

LAD, left anterior descending artery; N, no; Y, yes.

tional one-, two-, and three-vessel classification system.

At Duke University, an observational study was performed on prospectively collected data from 9263 patients with coronary disease treated with medicine, PTCA, or CABG between 1984 and 1990.[78] These data reveal a modest but significant reduction in the risk of death with CABG in comparison with medical therapy.[78] As seen in the randomized trials, this reduction first becomes evident after 18 months; after 5 years, the survival curves again converge (Fig. 10–3). The medical and surgical survival curves in patients in the database who meet CASS eligibility criteria is strikingly similar to those of patients actually enrolled in CASS (Fig. 10–4). The anatomic extent of coronary disease is the dominant variable predicting treatment-related differences in survival, which are greatest in left main coronary artery disease, followed by three-, two-, and one-vessel disease. Figure 10–5 displays the trend favoring medical management over CABG in patients with the least severe coronary artery disease. In the most severe forms of single-vessel disease and the less severe forms of two-vessel disease, the effects of the two treatment strategies appear equivalent. In two-vessel disease with stenosis affecting 95% of the proximal LAD and in three-vessel disease, CABG improves survival.

A comparison of medical therapy with PTCA reveals a trend for PTCA to improve survival in relation to medicine for less severe forms of coronary artery disease (Fig. 10–6).[78] In contrast, in severe two-vessel disease (with stenosis affecting 95% of the proximal LAD) and all forms of three-vessel

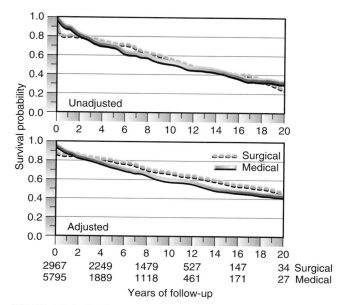

FIGURE 10–4. Kaplan-Meier unadjusted event-free survival of Duke patients meeting Coronary Artery Surgery Study (CASS) eligibility criteria: Comparison to 5- and 10-year event-free survival rates in patients reported by CASS. (From Muhlbaier LH, Pryor DB, Rankin JS, et al: Observational comparison of event-free survival with medical and surgical therapy in patients with coronary artery disease. 20 years of follow-up. Circulation 86:II-198–II-204, 1992.)

disease, the two therapeutic modalities appear to have equivalent effects on survival.

Over a follow-up period as long as 10 years (mean 5.3 years), there was no difference in cardiovascular mortality for patients with multivessel disease treated with PTCA or CABG.[78] When patients were

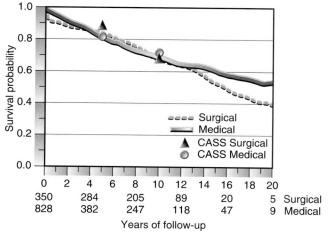

FIGURE 10–3. Kaplan-Meier event-free survival of patients treated medically and surgically from 1969 through 1984. Survival curves unadjusted and adjusted for important baseline characteristics are shown. CASS, Coronary Artery Surgery Study. (From Muhlbaier LH, Pryor DB, Rankin JS, et al: Observational comparison of event-free survival with medical and surgical therapy in patients with coronary artery disease. 20 years of follow-up. Circulation 86:II-198–II-204, 1992.)

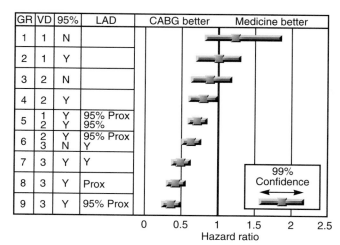

FIGURE 10–5. Medicine versus coronary artery bypass graft (CABG): hazard ratios and 99% confidence intervals. GR, prognostic group; LAD, left anterior descending artery; Prox, proximal; VD, vessel disease. (From Jones RH, Kesler K, Phillips HR III, et al: Long-term survival benefits of coronary artery bypass grafting and percutaneous transluminal angioplasty in patients with coronary artery disease. J Thorac Cardiovasc Surg 111:1013–1025, 1996.)

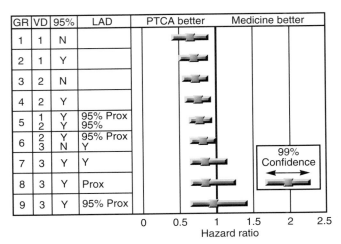

FIGURE 10–6. Medicine versus percutaneous transluminal coronary angioplasty (PTCA): hazard ratios and 99% confidence intervals.[78] GR, prognostic group; LAD, left anterior descending artery; Prox, proximal; VD, vessel disease. (From Jones RH, Kesler K, Phillips HR III, et al: Long-term survival benefits of coronary artery bypass grafting and percutaneous transluminal angioplasty in patients with coronary artery disease. J Thorac Cardiovasc Surg 111:1013–1025, 1996.)

categorized according to a coronary anatomy score, however, differences between the two treatment strategies in terms of cardiovascular mortality were appreciated (Fig. 10–7). All patients with single-vessel disease not involving the proximal LAD benefited from PTCA more than from CABG. Patients with three-vessel disease and those with two-vessel disease that included stenosis affecting at least 95% of proximal LAD benefited from CABG more than from PTCA. Similar survival rates with either treat-

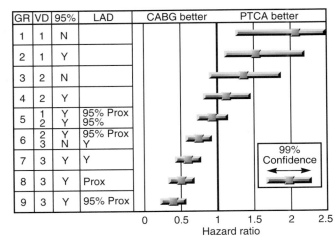

FIGURE 10–7. Percutaneous transluminal coronary angioplasty (PTCA) versus coronary artery bypass graft (CABG): hazard ratios and 99% confidence intervals.[78] GR, prognostic group; LAD, left anterior descending artery; Prox, proximal; VD, vessel disease. (From Jones RH, Kesler K, Phillips HR III, et al: Long-term survival benefits of coronary artery bypass grafting and percutaneous transluminal angioplasty in patients with coronary artery disease. J Thorac Cardiovasc Surg 111:1013–1025, 1996.)

ment modality were seen in other patients with two-vessel disease and in patients with stenosis affecting at least 95% of the proximal LAD. Absolute survival benefits increased with increasing severity of coronary disease in both treatment groups. Had patients been categorized according to the coronary anatomy score in randomized trials, a survival benefit with CABG may have been seen for patients with three-vessel disease and for some patients with two-vessel disease.

## COST COMPARISONS

If the clinical outcomes of PTCA and CABG are indeed similar, their relative cost becomes an important issue. Hospital costs in ERACI were, not surprisingly, significantly higher for patients undergoing CABG. At 1-year follow-up, costs remained almost twice as high for bypass surgery ($p < 0.01$).[65] In GABI, costs were also found to be lower for PTCA.[64] In RITA, the initial cost of PTCA—including that of the initial procedure, subsequent revascularization, needed stay in the intensive care unit, number of angiograms, and the use of drugs—was 52% of the cost of bypass grafting.[79] An accurate assessment of costs was difficult because the information was collected in the British National Health System, in which bills are not collected and resources must be estimated. Furthermore, the information collected did not include costs of therapy by primary physicians or costs related to patients' loss of work time. Because of the additional revascularization procedures required after PTCA, the relative cost rose to 80% of that of CABG at 2 years.

The relative costs were evaluated prospectively in a substudy of BARI.[80] The initial cost of angioplasty was significantly lower than that of CABG. This difference in cost narrowed with time as a result of the need for subsequent hospitalizations and cardiac medications in the patients who underwent angioplasty. However, after 5 years of follow-up, the total cost of angioplasty remained significantly (5%) lower than the total cost of bypass grafting ($p = 0.047$). Long-term costs varied with differing baseline characteristics. Four-year cumulative costs were significantly higher for patients with heart failure, diabetes, and other coexisting illnesses after adjustment for the clinical site and the length of hospitalization before random assignment. The cost benefit with angioplasty was significant only among patients with two-vessel disease; 5-year costs of the two procedures in patients with three-vessel disease were similar.

In the Duke database, the costs of PTCA were 66% of the costs of CABG at 1 year after the procedures.[81] The cost of angioplasty increased with increasing extent of disease. Therefore, in patients treated with angioplasty in the randomized trials, the cost of PTCA would likely approach that of CABG with increasing numbers of diseased vessels.

## QUALITY OF LIFE

Important quality-of-life issues were evaluated in the BARI substudy.[80] The functional status as measured by the Duke Activity Status Index[82, 83] improved in all patients during follow-up. The improvement in functional status in patients undergoing bypass surgery was significantly more than the improvement in those undergoing angioplasty during the first 3 years after treatment, but there was no difference in improvement after 4 or 5 years. Emotional health (as measured by the RAND Mental Health Inventory[84]) improved significantly in both groups after revascularization, with no significant difference between the two treatment groups. Baseline characteristics of patients influenced the amount of physical and emotional improvement after revascularization. Men were more likely to experience improvements in both physical and emotional function than were women. Patients with heart failure at baseline experienced less improvement in physical function, and patients with diabetes experienced less improvement in physical function at 4-year follow-up. Older patients experienced less improvement than did younger patients in terms of physical function but significantly more improvement in emotional function.

Patients who underwent angioplasty returned to work earlier than did those who underwent bypass grafting (medians, 6 vs. 11 weeks). At 6 months, 83% of patients initially employed returned to work at least part time. With time, fewer patients remained employed: 73% after 1 year and 45% after 5 years. There was no significant difference in employment between the two groups during follow-up and no difference in the number of hours spent at work.

Similar outcomes were found in other trials with employment information available. Employment rates at the 3-year follow-up in the EAST trial were low in both groups (36.5% of patients who had undergone PTCA vs. 38.5% of those who had undergone CABG) but may be explained in part by the average patient age of 62 at enrollment.[63] MASS enrolled patients with an average age of 55 years, and rates of employment at the 3-year follow-up were higher for both the PTCA-treated patients (64%) and CABG-treated patients (80%; $p$ = NS).[70] In RITA, employment rates were higher for the PTCA-treated patients at 1 month (46%, vs. 21% of

the CABG-treated patients) and increased to 75% (PTCA) and 77% (CABG) at 2 years.[60]

## STROKE

Pertinent to quality-of-life issues is the incidence of stroke after revascularization. The CASS registry reported 3.4% stroke rate at 1 year after bypass surgery.[85] In a large multicenter prospective trial, adverse cerebral perioperative outcomes occurred in 6.1% of patients undergoing CABG.[86] A total of 3.1% died from cerebral injury, suffered nonfatal strokes, or suffered transient ischemic attacks. The other 3% demonstrated deterioration of intellectual function or had seizures. Risk of adverse cerebral outcomes increased with age; approximately 8% of patients over the age of 80 experienced strokes or transient ischemic attacks. Stroke rates after angioplasty are much lower. In the Angioplasty Trials Pool database, three trials—Integrilin to Minimize Platelet Aggregation and Prevent Coronary Thrombosis (IMPACT) II and Coronary Angioplasty versus Excisional Atherectomy Trial (CAVEAT) 1 and 2—reported early stroke rates after PTCA. Within the first 24 hours of the procedure, 0.1% of 6058 patients experienced strokes, and 0.5% of 5327 patients had strokes within the first 30 days. Six-month follow-up data from CAVEAT 1 and CAVEAT 2 revealed a 0.5% stroke rate in 1291 patients. In the few randomized trials that compared PTCA and CABG and reported strokes, no difference in in-hospital stroke rates were found.[86a–86c]

## EFFECT OF COMPLETENESS OF REVASCULARIZATION ON TREATMENT OUTCOME

One important difference between surgical and percutaneous therapy is the ability to achieve complete revascularization. Complete revascularization is often defined as restoration of blood flow to areas of myocardium supplied by stenotic vessels or previously supplied by vessels that are occluded. Complete revascularization has been advocated as the goal of CABG but is not always possible in patients with multivessel disease that results from small coronary vessels or the presence of diffuse disease. Several studies have shown that patients who are completely revascularized by CABG have improved survival in comparison with those not completely revascularized.[87–89] According to the CASS registry, patients with only mild angina derived no added benefit from complete over partial revascularization. Patients with three-vessel disease and severe angina, however, showed significant improvement in late survival when three or more vessels were bypassed, in comparison with when only two vessels were bypassed; this effect was magnified when left ventricular dysfunction was present.[89] Although complete revascularization achieved by CABG has been shown to be superior to partial revascularization in patients with more severe disease, the advantage of complete over partial revascularization with PTCA is more difficult to discern.

Whether complete revascularization after angioplasty confers a survival benefit has been of particular interest, because complete revascularization with PTCA is achieved in fewer than 50% of patients with two-vessel disease and in only 20% of patients with three-vessel disease.[37, 39, 52, 90–92] Chronic total occlusions, unfavorable lesion morphology, and diffuse disease contribute to this low rate of complete revascularization with multivessel PTCA. In addition, in view of the risk of restenosis after PTCA, physicians may choose not to dilate noncritical lesions.

Mabin and associates[93] and Vandormael and colleagues[49] found higher rates of angina[93] and subsequent bypass surgery[49, 93] in patients who were incompletely revascularized. Differences in baseline characteristics between patients who are completely revascularized percutaneously and those who are incompletely revascularized may account for the differences in outcomes. Reeder and associates[94] noted important differences in baseline characteristics between patients completely revascularized and those incompletely revascularized. After adjustment for these baseline variables, there was no difference in rates of death, myocardial infarction, or angina between the groups, although the group with incomplete revascularization had higher rates of subsequent bypass surgery. Reports from the Mayo Clinic indicate that after adjustment for age, prior infarction, history of heart failure, severity of coronary artery disease, previous CABG, and baseline left ventricular function, an independent effect of completeness of revascularization on outcome was not evident.[52]

The functional significance of a lesion may help determine whether angioplasty will be attempted. In a study by Faxon and associates, patients with incomplete but functionally adequate multivessel revascularization (in which all viable myocardium was revascularized) with PTCA had 1-year outcomes similar to those in patients who had complete anatomic revascularization (in which all stenotic vessels opened regardless of whether the myocardium they supplied was viable).[95] In fact, fewer adverse events (death, myocardial infarction, or the need for CABG) occurred in patients who had incomplete revascularization but successful dilatation of bypassable vessels supporting viable myocardium (6%) than in patients who did not have revascularization of functionally significant areas (27%; $p <$ 0.04).[95] This was true even if the vessel dilated was completely occluded before the procedure.

In evaluating the studies that directly compare CABG with PTCA, the differing revascularization strategies in the trials must be carefully considered. For example, RITA required equivalent revascularization between the two treatments, and partial revascularization was allowed in EAST and CABRI, whereas the goal in GABI and ERACI was complete revascularization. The definition of complete revascularization is also important. GABI required the revascularization to be complete anatomically. However, ERACI allowed for functional revascularization, meaning that if the myocardium was not viable, revascularization to that area was not necessary. In ERACI, anatomic revascularization was complete in 88% of bypass-treated patients, in comparison with 51% of angioplasty-treated patients, but the rate of complete functional revascularization with PTCA (89%) was similar to that with CABG. In the PTCA-treated patients, there was no significant difference in freedom from combined ischemic events between those with complete functional revascularization and those with complete anatomic revascularization. In BARI, patients assigned to PTCA were not required to have all significant lesions dilated. Despite incomplete revascularization in the PTCA group, the rates of survival and freedom from myocardial infarctions were similar to those in patients more completely revascularized by CABG.[72]

## EFFECTS OF LEFT VENTRICULAR DYSFUNCTION

In most studies of survival with medical or surgical therapy, left ventricular function at rest (baseline) or during exercise is the most important predictor of survival. Likewise, several series suggest that at-rest left ventricular function is important to both periprocedural[27, 29] and late survival after angioplasty.[36, 37, 96–98] Surgical revascularization is known to improve outcome in patients with poor left ventricular function and multivessel disease, in comparison with medical therapy.[3] In contrast, Ellis and associates reported a 2-year mortality rate of 25% to 30% among patients with multivessel PTCA and ejection fractions less than 40%, higher than that expected with surgery.[36]

Outcomes of the 244 (of 1802) patients in the NHLBI 1985–1986 PTCA registry with left ventricular dysfunction (ejection fraction $\leq$ 45%) have been described.[99] There were important baseline differences: Patients with left ventricular dysfunction were more likely to have had a prior myocardial infarction and to have more extensive coronary artery disease, total coronary occlusions, a history of congestive heart disease, a history of CABG, and lower rates of complete revascularization than were patients with ejection fractions above 45%. Although there was no difference in in-hospital events, including death (0.8% vs. 0.7%), nonfatal myocardial infarctions (4.9% vs. 4.5%), acute closure (2.5% vs. 2.1%), and emergency CABG rates (4.5% vs. 3.2%), there was a difference in survival with time. At a mean follow-up of 4 years, 87% of patients with left ventricular dysfunction were alive, in comparison with 93% of patients with preserved left ventricular function ($p < 0.001$). This difference remained significant after adjustment for differences in baseline variables (age, diabetes, history of congestive heart failure, clinical success, and multivessel disease). However, event-free survival was no longer significantly different after adjustment for prior CABG (along with the aforementioned baseline variables).

A history of congestive heart failure, independent of left ventricular ejection fraction, also has important prognostic value in patients undergoing percutaneous interventions.[38] Patients with a history of congestive heart failure who undergo an intervention had increased intermediate (9-month) mortality in comparison with patients with no clinical history of congestive heart failure, even after ejection fraction was taken into account.

There is little information available on the comparison of surgical versus interventional therapy for patients with coronary disease and left ventricular dysfunction. Munger compared 166 patients with a mean ejection fraction of 31% who were treated with PTCA with 166 patients with similar ejection fractions who were treated surgically.[100] The 1-, 3-, and 5-year survival rates of patients treated with PTCA (85%, 77%, and 64%) were significantly lower than those of patients treated surgically (88%, 83%, and 69%).

Unfortunately, patients with left ventricular dysfunction were not well represented in the randomized trials comparing PTCA with CABG outcomes. In RITA, ejection fraction data were not presented. In the other trials, the mean ejection fraction was normal. The MASS and Lausanne trials excluded patients with left ventricular dysfunction. Therefore, the effect of left ventricular dysfunction on outcomes in the two treatment groups could not be evaluated in the randomized trials.

## EFFECTS OF AGE

The Mid-America Heart Institute has reported a 96% success rate among 1373 elderly patients undergoing PTCA.[56] Of these patients, 1.4% had a myocardial infarction, 0.8% required emergency CABG, and 1.6% died. In New York State, the 30-day mortality rate was 1.23% among patients 65 years of age or older, in comparison with 0.37% among those younger than 65[29]; this difference was not statistically different after gender, left ventricular function, and hemodynamic status were taken into account. With coronary bypass surgery, however, patients older than 65 years have higher rates of complications and mortality than do younger patients.[101] According to Medicare data, mortality rates at 30 days and 1 year were higher after CABG (6.5% and 12%) than after PTCA (4.4% and 8%).[102] Therefore, among the elderly, PTCA may be a preferable form of initial treatment when technically feasible.

## EFFECTS OF DIABETES

Diabetes is a predictor of poor outcome after angioplasty and coronary bypass grafting. A subgroup analysis from BARI indicated that there may be a survival advantage for diabetic patients undergoing surgical revascularization in comparison with diabetic patients undergoing percutaneous revascularization.[62] Although in-hospital survival rates in the two treatment groups were similar, the 5-year survival rate for diabetic patients was significantly lower among those who underwent PTCA (65.5%) than among those who underwent CABG (80.6%). In other studies, a survival difference between treatment groups was not evident. Weintraub and associates compared 2641 diabetic patients who had multivessel disease and no prior revascularization, treated with PTCA (836 patients) or CABG (1805 patients).[103] Because the study was not randomized, there were important differences in the treatment groups. The CABG-treated patients included fewer women and had less severe angina, lower ejection fractions, more heart failure, more prior myocardial infarctions, more three-vessel disease, and more urgent or emergency procedures than did the PTCA-treated patients. In-hospital mortality rates were higher after CABG (5% vs. 0.4%), but 5- and 10-year survival rates were similar (77% and 44% after PTCA, in comparison with 73% and 46% after CABG; $p = 0.05$). In a retrospective study, Barsness and associates obtained similar findings.[104] The study group consisted of 3220 patients with symptomatic multivessel disease undergoing PTCA (N = 704, 144 of whom had diabetes) or CABG (N = 2516, 625 of whom had diabetes). After adjustment for baseline characteristics, diabetic patients had lower rates of 5-year survival than did nondiabetic patients, regardless of therapy. Of patients undergoing angioplasty, those with diabetes had an adjusted 5-year survival rate of 86%, in comparison with 92% in patients without diabetes. Diabetic patients undergoing surgical revascularization had an adjusted 5-year survival rate of 89%, in comparison with 93% of nondiabetics. The type of revascularization selected (surgical vs. percutaneous) did not have a bearing on survival. Diabetes therefore appears to be a marker for poor outcome, regardless of revascularization mode, even after adjustment for differences in important prognostic characteristics. Thus, with the use of current available information, the mode of revascularization for diabetic patients with multivessel disease should be based on other clinical and technical considerations rather than simply on the presence or absence of diabetes.

## EFFECT OF HOSPITAL AND OPERATOR VOLUMES

Hospital and operator volumes have an important effect on procedural outcomes. Luft found higher surgical-related mortality rates in hospitals performing fewer than 200 coronary bypass procedures per year (5.7%) than in hospitals performing more than 200 procedures (3.4%).[105] Data from the California Health Facilities Commission revealed a strong association of hospital volume with death rate, adjusted for patient characteristics. Patients undergoing CABG in hospitals that performed fewer than 100 operations per year had an adjusted death rate of 0.052, with rates of 0.039, 0.041, and 0.031 among patients undergoing surgery in hospitals performing 101 to 200, 201 to 350, and 351 or more operations respectively, per year.[106] New York State's database demonstrated that both higher hospital volumes and higher surgical volumes are associated with lower procedural mortality rates but that the number of procedures performed by a given surgeon (surgeon volume) is the more important of the two measures.[107] More recent information from this database indicates that mortality rates have improved for both low- and high-volume surgeons, and the gap in risk-adjusted mortality between the two groups has remained but narrowed.[108] This narrowing has been postulated to result from good performance of physicians new to the system (and therefore performing fewer procedures their first year) and from the performance of surgeons who did not consistently have low numbers of procedures. However, the patients of the subgroup of low-volume surgeons who consistently perform few bypass procedures (50 or fewer annually) continue to experience high risk-adjusted mortality rates (8.96%).

Likewise, both cardiologist volume and hospital PTCA volume are significantly and inversely proportionate to in-hospital mortality rates and need for surgical revascularization during the same hospital stay.[109-111] Ritchie and associates evaluated outcomes from nearly 25,000 angioplasty procedures in the state of California in 1989.[110] Significantly more patients were referred for CABG during the same hospitalization in which angioplasty was performed in hospitals with lower volumes (≥200 procedures per year) than in higher-volume hospitals. Jollis and associates, using Medicare patient information, evaluated outcomes and found differences between hospitals with lower volume (50 angioplasty procedures in Medicare patients, corresponding to a total of approximately 100 to 200 angioplasty procedures annually) and those with higher volume (100 procedures in Medicare patients, or an estimated total of 200 to 400 angioplasty procedures per year).[111] Unadjusted in-hospital mortality rates were 3.9% in hospitals with lower annual volumes and 2.5% in hospitals with higher volumes. In addition, there was a higher rate of same-stay CABG surgery in patients in the lower volume hospitals (5.3% vs. 3.5%). The New York State Registry, involving more than 62,000 patients, evaluated the effects of physician volumes, in addition to hospital volumes, on outcomes. There were higher mortality and same-stay surgical rates when annual hospital procedural volumes were less than 600 and physician volumes were less than 75 per year.[109] These results may be explained in part by the effect of skills and experience (including the experience of support staff) on mortality and by referral of a larger volume of patients to hospitals or operators who produced better outcomes.

In the debate regarding angioplasty procedural volume, there are two opposing points of view. Those who oppose volume standards point out that the findings regarding volume and outcome are averaged, and among these low-volume operators, there are some physicians and hospitals with above-average performance. They also point to new technologies, such as stents and platelet inhibitors, that have reduced the rate of abrupt closure and emergency surgery. The studies cited previously were conducted before these technologies were available, and the volume-outcome relationship may no longer be apparent in more recent experience. Those who favor volume standards point to the difficulty in identifying low-volume operators with above-average performance as a result of the statistical limitations of small sample size. They also believe that until the new technologies have been shown to reduce complications by less experienced operators, the current weight of evidence supports volume limits.

## NEW ADVANCES

Multiple new devices are currently being evaluated as alternatives or adjuncts to angioplasty. The New

**TABLE 10–17.    IN-HOSPITAL EVENTS IN NACI REGISTRY**

| VARIABLE | TOTAL | DCA | TEC USED | ROTA | PSS USED | GRS USED | ELCAa | ELCAs |
|---|---|---|---|---|---|---|---|---|
| Number of patients | 2835 | 987 | 211 | 266 | 615 | 196 | 401 | 159 |
| Number of lesions | 3201 | 1084 | 240 | 349 | 674 | 213 | 474 | 167 |
| Device success (%) | 66.5 | 73.9 | 47.5 | 71.9 | 76.0 | 73.2 | 46.4 | 45.4 |
| Adjunctive PTCA (%) | 75.5 | 46.4 | 88.8 | 81.9 | 93.2 | 95.8 | 92.2 | 86.8 |
| Lesion success (%) | 92.2 | 94.3 | 80.4 | 97.1 | 97.3 | 88.3 | 85.2 | 88.6 |
| Death (%) | 1.6 | 0.6 | 5.7 | 0.8 | 2.3 | 1.5 | 1.2 | 1.3 |
| Q-wave MI (%) | 1.3 | 1.0 | 1.4 | 1.5 | 1.6 | 3.1 | 0.7 | 0.6 |
| Emergency CABG (%) | 1.7 | 1.6 | 0.9 | 0.4 | 0.7 | 4.1 | 2.0 | 5.0 |

CABG, coronary artery bypass grafting; DCA, directional coronary atherectomy; ELCA, excimer laser coronary angioplasty; GRS, Gianturco-Rubin stent; MI, myocardial infarction; NACI, New Approaches to Coronary Intervention; PSS, Palmaz-Schatz stent; PTCA, percutaneous transluminal coronary angioplasty; ROTA, Rotablator; TEC, transluminal extraction catheter.

Modified from Baim DS, Kent KM, King SB III, et al: Evaluating new devices. Acute (in-hospital) results from the New Approaches to Coronary Intervention Registry. Circulation 89:471–481, 1994.

Approaches to Coronary Intervention (NACI) registry is funded by the NHLBI to evaluate new devices.[112] Since 1990, participating centers have voluntarily reported results of the use of the various devices. In-hospital events reported to the NACI registry are shown in Table 10–17. Because patients are not randomly assigned, there are considerable differences between the devices with regard to baseline patient characteristics and types of lesions subjected to attempted repair. For example, the transluminal extraction catheter (TEC) was used mostly in thrombotic vein grafts; Rotablator and excimer laser coronary angioplasty (ELCAa) were used more commonly in calcified native vessel lesions; and the use of β-glucoronidase was more likely to be unplanned (after an angioplasty or new device attempt that was unsuccessful, suboptimal, or complicated by acute closure) than planned. Because of the different patient baseline characteristics, it is impossible to directly compare outcomes among the devices.

The use of stents has led to an improvement in outcomes in percutaneous interventions, as discussed in Chapter 36, Selection of Coronary Stents for Particular Anatomy. For example, the rate of urgent bypass surgery has been reduced from 3% to 1% with stent use.[113] More complete revascularization may result from stent use, because physicians are more likely to dilate long or complex lesions. In addition, restenosis rates have decreased from 32% to 22%.[113] The rates of restenosis may have decreased even more as a result of the use of high-pressure intrastent balloon inflation. Multivessel stent implantation is associated with high success rates and appears to be associated with decreased need for repeat revascularization at follow-up.[114] The use of intracoronary stents was not routine in the trials discussed earlier. This fact has important implications because the use of stents in the randomized trials may have led to reduced event rates and more complete revascularization in the PTCA group and may have even changed outcomes in

relation to surgery. Randomized trials are under way in South America, Europe, Canada, New Zealand, Israel, and England to compare multivessel stent implantation with coronary bypass grafting. The Arterial Revascularization Therapies Study (ARTS), a multicenter trial designed to compare the use of the Crown stent and the Cordis Crossflex stent with surgery in 1200 patients with multivessel disease, began enrolling patients in May 1997 and was published in May 2001.[114a] ERACI II, in which multivessel stent implantation with the Gianturco-Roubin II stent is compared with surgery, has been published.[114b]

Patients with diabetes mellitus are at increased risk for restenosis after coronary stent placement in comparison with those without diabetes.[115] Procedural factors predicting restenosis after stent placement are placement of multiple stents and a minimal lumen diameter of less than 3 mm immediately after stent placement. The incidence of restenosis after stent placement may be as low as 16% in the absence of these risk factors but as high as 54% with all three factors. Until randomized trial data concerning multivessel stenting and surgery become available, criteria such as these should be considered in predicting procedural outcomes for patients.

Coronary stent implantation has allowed successful percutaneous revascularization of patients previously considered to be candidates for surgical revascularization only. Although two of the five patients in Andreas Gruentzig's original report of angioplasty underwent dilatation of left main artery stenoses, the poor immediate and long-term outcomes in patients undergoing percutaneous revascularization of the unprotected left main artery led the American College of Cardiology/American Heart Association Task Force to regard angioplasty for unprotected left main artery stenosis an absolute contraindication.[116] The risks of left main artery angioplasty include the devastating consequences of dissection and abrupt closure and the common occurrence of elastic recoil, which is related to the high content of elastic fibers at the left main ostium. Since the advent of new technologies such as coronary stent implantation, scattered reports of percutaneous revascularization of left main artery stenosis began to appear increasingly in the literature.[117–120] A study of 42 consecutive patients with unprotected left main artery stenoses who declined surgical therapy reported a procedural success rate of 100%, with a 22% rate of restenosis occurring 6 months after stent placement.[121] A multicenter registry of 107 patients undergoing unprotected percutaneous revascularization of the left main artery has indicated excellent technical success rates (96.2%) and a 60.7% rate of 9-month survival free of events (death, infarction, bypass surgery).[122] Patients treated for acute infarction had a high in-hospital mortality rate (69%) and a low 9-month event-free survival rate (12.5%). Patients not initially presenting with infarction had an in-hospital mortality rate of 12% and both 6- and 12-month event-free survival rates of 68.1%. Higher 9-month event-free survival rates were seen in patients with stable angina (87.9%) and with preserved left ventricular function (86%). Therefore, unprotected percutaneous revascularization of the left main artery may be a reasonable option for certain subsets of patients in highly experienced centers.

Pharmacologic approaches that may reduce restenosis rates and improve outcomes are now being developed. Agents that target the integrin glycoprotein (GP) IIb/IIIa, a receptor for fibrinogen on the platelet cell membrane, appear to improve clinical outcomes after percutaneous interventions. Three agents have undergone phase III testing in humans: abciximab (ReoPro), eptifibatide (Integrilin), and tirofiban (Aggrastat).[123] The Evaluation of c7E3 in Preventing Ischemic Complications (EPIC) trial[124] determined that patients at high risk for complications after PTCA or directional coronary atherectomy (DCA) had significant reductions in events (including death, nonfatal myocardial infarctions, repeat revascularization, and procedural failure) at 30 days and 6 months when given abciximab via bolus and 12-hour infusion. However, an increase in hemorrhage and transfusion requirement was evident in the treated group. The Evaluation of PTCA to Improve Long-term Outcome by c7E3 GP IIB/IIIA Receptor Blockade (EPILOG) trial evaluated abciximab in patients of all levels of risk; lower doses of adjunctive heparin were used. The treatment group experienced a significant reduction in the incidences of death and myocardial infarction, along with a reduction in the rates of major hemorrhage, in comparison with the placebo recipients.[125, 126] Integrilin was evaluated in the Integrilin to Minimize Platelet Aggregation and Prevent Coronary Throm-

bosis II (IMPACT II) trial, which found a significant reduction in events at 24 hours in the treatment group with no increase in transfusions or major hemorrhage.[127] Tirofiban, evaluated in the Randomized Efficacy Study of Tirofiban for Outcomes and Restenosis (RESTORE) trial, resulted in a significant reduction in clinical events at two days.[128] Orally active agents have been evaluated in the role of long-term GP IIb/IIIa inhibition and found to be harmful at 6 month follow-up.[128a]

Other pharmacologic agents are being tested in an attempt to improve outcomes after angioplasty. Estrogen therapy appears to improve long-term outcomes with regard to restenosis, myocardial infarction, stroke, and death in postmenopausal women undergoing coronary angioplasty.[129] Probucol, which has both antioxidant and cholesterol-lowering properties, has been shown to reduce restenosis after angioplasty, although the drug was administered to the patients for 30 days before revascularization.[130] Surgical advances also continue. Analysis from the Duke Cardiovascular Disease Database has shown that survival rates after CABG have improved over time. The use of internal mammary artery (IMA) grafts specifically has improved both early and late survival.[18, 19] The 10-year survival rate when IMA grafts are used is 89%, in comparison with 71% with vein grafts alone.[18]

## CONCLUSION

In patients for whom medical therapy is deemed no longer an effective treatment, and when the coronary disease is amenable to equivalent revascularization by either angioplasty or surgery, outcomes within the first 5 years in terms of death and myocardial infarction are similar regardless of the intervention chosen. During the first 5 years after a procedure, patients undergoing PTCA have a greater number of subsequent interventions. However, after 10 years, the efficacy of CABG may decline as vein grafts occlude and disease elsewhere progresses; surgically treated patients are likely to undergo further interventions at that time. Both types of therapy are effective at relieving angina. Although angina is, early in the follow-up period, more prevalent in patients treated with angioplasty, the treatment-related differences in angina decrease with time.[131] Despite higher rates of angina early, there are no differences in employment rates or quality-of-life measures.[72]

CABG is still the procedure of choice for many patients with severe multivessel disease or left main artery disease. In many trials, patients were excluded from random assignment because of the presence of factors such as occluded vessels, complex coronary lesions, or left main artery stenosis, making angioplasty less safe or less likely to be successful. In these patients, as well as those with severely impaired left ventricular function, and perhaps in those with severe three-vessel disease or proximal LAD disease, bypass surgery would be preferable. Angioplasty may be a better option particularly for patients with single-vessel or less severe two-vessel disease, because of lower cost and less time for rehabilitation. New devices and pharmacotherapy may expand the settings in which percutaneous interventions may be useful. However, the potential for overuse of both forms of treatment for coronary disease exists. Whether the chosen therapy will provide symptom relief, correct a large ischemic burden, or result in a survival benefit in a given patient should be strongly considered. Therapeutic decisions should also take into account the patient's age, comorbid status, personal preferences, and the tradeoff between short-term procedural risk and long-term benefit.[132] Finally, the indications for revascularization and the benefits of medical therapy should not be forgotten.

## REFERENCES

1. Favaloro RG: Saphenous vein graft in the surgical treatment of coronary artery disease. J Thorac Cardiovasc Surg 58:178–185, 1969.
2. Gruentzig AR: Transluminal dilatation of coronary-artery stenosis [Abstract]. Lancet 1:263, 1978.
3. Veterans Administration Coronary Artery Bypass Surgery Cooperative Study Group: Eleven-year survival in the Veterans Administration randomized trial of coronary bypass surgery for stable angina. N Engl J Med 311:1333–1339, 1984.
4. Veterans Administration Coronary Artery Bypass Surgery Cooperative Study Group: Eighteen-year follow-up in the Veterans Affairs Cooperative Study of Coronary Artery Bypass Surgery for stable angina. Circulation 86.1:121–130, 1992.
5. Takaro T, Hultgren HN, Lipton MJ, et al: The VA cooperative randomized study of surgery for coronary arterial occlusive disease: II. Subgroup with significant left main lesions. Circulation 54(suppl 6):III-107–III-117, 1976.
6. European Coronary Surgery Study Group: Long-term results of prospective randomised study of coronary artery bypass surgery in stable angina pectoris. Lancet 2:1173–1180, 1982.
7. Varnauskas E: Twelve-year follow-up of survival in the randomized European Coronary Surgery Study. N Engl J Med 319:332–337, 1988.
8. Alderman EL, Bourassa MG, Cohen LS, et al: Ten-year follow-up of survival and myocardial infarction in the randomized Coronary Artery Surgery Study. Circulation 82:1629–1646, 1990.
9. Yusuf S, Zucker D, Peduzzi P, et al: Effect of coronary artery bypass graft surgery on survival: Overview of 10-year results from randomized trials by the Coronary Artery Bypass Graft Surgery Trialists Collaboration. Lancet 344:563–570, 1994.
10. Grondin CM, Campeau L, Thornton JC, et al: Coronary artery bypass grafting with saphenous vein. Circulation 79:I-24–I-29, 1989.
11. Campeau L, Enjalbert M, Lesperance J, et al: Atherosclerosis and late closure of aortocoronary saphenous vein grafts: Sequential angiographic studies at 2 weeks, 1 year, 5 to 7 years, and 10 to 12 years after surgery. Circulation 68:II-1–II-7, 1983.
12. Vlodaver Z, Edwards JE: Pathologic changes in aortic-coronary arterial saphenous vein grafts. Circulation 44:719–728, 1971.
13. FitzGibbon GM, Leach AJ, Kafka HP, et al: Coronary bypass graft fate: Long-term angiographic study. J Am Coll Cardiol 17:1075–1080, 1991.
14. Holmes DR Jr, Davis KB, Mock MB, et al: The effect of medical and surgical treatment on subsequent sudden cardiac death in patients with coronary artery disease: A report from the Coronary Artery Surgery Study. Circulation 73:1254–1263, 1986.
15. Hammermeister KE: Effect of aortocoronary saphenous vein bypass grafting on death and sudden death. Comparison of nonrandomized medically and surgically treated cohorts with comparable coronary disease and left ventricular function. Am J Cardiol 39:925, 1977.
16. Califf RM, Mark DB: Percutaneous intervention, surgery, and medical therapy: A perspective from the Duke Databank for Cardiovascular Diseases. Semin Thorac Cardiovasc Surg 6:120–128, 1994.
17. Califf RM, Harrell FE Jr, Lee KL, et al: The evolution of medical and surgical therapy for coronary artery disease. A 15-year perspective. JAMA 261:2077–2086, 1989.
18. Kirklin JW, Naftel CD, Blackstone EH, et al: Summary of a consensus concerning death and ischemic events after coronary artery bypass grafting. Circulation 79:I-81–I-91, 1989.
19. Cameron A, Davis KB, Green GE, et al: Clinical implications of internal mammary artery bypass grafts: The Coronary Artery Surgery Study experience. Circulation 77:815–819, 1988.
20. The Post Coronary Artery Bypass Graft Trial Investigators: The effect of aggressive lowering of low-density lipoprotein cholesterol levels and low-dose anticoagulation on obstructive changes in saphenous-vein coronary-artery bypass grafts. N Engl J Med 336:153–162, 1997.
21. Detre K, Yeh W, Kelsey S, et al, for the Investigators of the NHLBI Percutaneous Transluminal Coronary Angioplasty Registry: Has improvement in PTCA intervention affected long-term prognosis? The NHLBI PTCA Registry experience. Circulation 91:2868–2875, 1995.
22. Califf RM, Mark DB, Harrell FE Jr, et al: Importance of clinical measures of ischemia in the prognosis of patients with documented coronary artery disease. J Am Coll Cardiol 11:20–26, 1988.
23. Higgins TL, Estafanous FG, Loop FD, et al: Stratification of morbidity and mortality outcome by preoperative risk factors in coronary artery bypass patients: A clinical severity score. JAMA 267:2344–2348, 1992.
24. O'Connor GT, Plume SK, Olmstead EM, et al: Multivariate prediction of in-hospital mortality associated with coronary artery bypass graft surgery. Northern New England Cardiovascular Disease Study Group. Circulation 85:2110–2118, 1992.
25. ACC/AHA guidelines and indications for coronary artery bypass graft surgery. A report of the American College of Cardiology/American Heart Association Task Force on Assessment of Diagnostic and Therapeutic Cardiovascular Procedures (Subcommittee on Coronary Artery Bypass Graft Surgery). Circulation 83:1125–1173, 1991.
26. Malenka DJ, O'Connor GT, Quinton H, et al, for the Northern New England Cardiovascular Disease Study Group: Differences in outcomes between women and men associated with percutaneous transluminal coronary angioplasty. A regional prospective study of 13,061 procedures. Circulation 94(suppl II):II-99–II-104, 1996.
27. Holmes DR Jr, Holubkov R, Vlietstra RE, et al: Comparison of complications during percutaneous transluminal coronary angioplasty from 1977 to 1981 and from 1985 to 1986: The National Heart, Lung, and Blood Institute Percutaneous Transluminal Coronary Angioplasty Registry. J Am Coll Cardiol 12:1149–1155, 1988.
28. Ellis SG, Myler RK, King SB III, et al: Causes and correlates of death after unsupported coronary angioplasty: Implications for use of angioplasty and advanced support tech-

niques in high-risk settings. Am J Cardiol 68:1447–1451, 1991.

29. Hannan EL, Arani DT, Johnson LW, et al: Percutaneous transluminal coronary angioplasty in New York State. Risk factors and outcomes. JAMA 268:3092–3097, 1992.

30. Malenka DJ: Indications, practice and procedural outcomes of percutaneous transluminal coronary angioplasty in northern New England in the early 1990s. The Northern New England Cardiovascular Disease Study Group. Am J Cardiol 78:260–265, 1996.

31. Kimmel SE, Berlin JA, Strom BL, et al: Development and validation of simplified predictive index for major complications in contemporary percutaneous transluminal coronary angioplasty practice. The Registry Committee of the Society for Cardiac Angiography and Interventions. J Am Coll Cardiol 26:931–938, 1995.

32. Kelsey SF, Miller DP, Holubkov R, et al: Results of percutaneous transluminal coronary angioplasty in patients greater than or equal to 65 years of age (from the 1985 to 1986 National Heart, Lung, and Blood Institute's Coronary Angioplasty Registry). Am J Cardiol 66:1033–1038, 1990.

33. Kahn JK, Rutherford BD, McConahay DR, et al: Comparison of procedural results and risks of coronary angioplasty in men and women for conditions other than acute myocardial infarction. Am J Cardiol 69:1241–1242, 1992.

34. Weintraub WS, King SB III, Douglas JS Jr, et al: Percutaneous transluminal coronary angioplasty as a first revascularization procedure in single-, double- and triple-vessel coronary artery disease. J Am Coll Cardiol 26:142–151, 1995.

35. Block PC, Peterson ED, Krone RJ, et al: Developing a standard dataset for interventional cardiology [Abstract]. J Am Coll Cardiol 29(suppl A):316A, 1997.

36. Ellis SG, Cowley MJ, DiSciascio G, et al: Determinants of 2-year outcome after coronary angioplasty in patients with multivessel disease on the basis of comprehensive preprocedural evaluation. Implications for patient selection. The Multivessel Angioplasty Prognosis Study Group. Circulation 83:1905–1914, 1991.

37. Vandormael M, Deligonul U, Taussig S, et al: Predictors of long-term cardiac survival in patients with multivessel coronary artery disease undergoing percutaneous transluminal coronary angioplasty. Am J Cardiol 67:1–6, 1991.

38. Anderson RD, Ohman EM, Holmes DR Jr, et al: The prognostic value of congestive heart failure history in patients undergoing percutaneous coronary interventions. J Am Coll Cardiol 32:936–941, 1998.

39. Deligonul U, Vandormael MG, Kern MJ, et al: Coronary angioplasty: A therapeutic option for symptomatic patients with two and three vessel coronary disease. J Am Coll Cardiol 11:1173–1179, 1988.

40. Frid DJ, Fortin DF, Gardner LH, et al: The effect of diabetes on restenosis [Abstract]. J Am Coll Cardiol 17:268A, 1991.

41. Carrozza JP Jr, Kuntz RE, Fishman RF, et al: Restenosis after arterial injury caused by coronary stenting in patients with diabetes mellitus. Ann Intern Med 118:344–349, 1993.

42. Weintraub WS, Ghazzal ZMB, Douglas JS, et al: Initial management and long-term clinical outcome of restenosis after initially successful percutaneous transluminal coronary angioplasty. Am J Cardiol 70:47–55, 1992.

43. Charlson ME, Pompei P, Ales KL, et al: A new method of classifying prognostic comorbidity in longitudinal studies: Development and validation. J Chronic Dis 40:373–383, 1987.

44. Jollis JG, Lam LC, Lee KL, et al: Comorbidity has major prognostic importance in patients with coronary disease [Abstract]. Circulation 84:II-679, 1991.

45. Detre K, Holubkov R, Kelsey S, et al: Percutaneous transluminal coronary angioplasty in 1985–1986 and 1977–1981. The National Heart, Lung, and Blood Institute Registry. N Engl J Med 318:265–270, 1988.

46. Finci L, Meier B, de Bruyne B, et al: Angiographic follow-up after multivessel percutaneous transluminal coronary angioplasty. Am J Cardiol 60:467–470, 1987.

47. Myler RK, Topol EJ, Shaw RE, et al: Multiple vessel coronary angioplasty: Classification, results, and patterns of re-

stenosis in 494 consecutive patients. Catheter Cardiovasc Diagn 13:1–15, 1987.

48. Cowley MJ, Vetrovec GW, DiSciascio G, et al: Coronary angioplasty of multiple vessels: Short-term outcome and long-term results. Circulation 72:1314–1320, 1985.

49. Vandormael MG, Chaitman BR, Ischinger T, et al: Immediate and short-term benefit of multilesion coronary angioplasty: Influence of degree of revascularization. J Am Coll Cardiol 6:983–991, 1985.

50. Mata LA, Bosch X, David PR, et al: Clinical and angiographic assessment 6 months after double vessel percutaneous coronary angioplasty. J Am Coll Cardiol 6:1239–1244, 1985.

51. O'Keefe JH Jr, Rutherford BD, McConahay DR, et al: Multivessel coronary angioplasty from 1980 to 1989: Procedural results and long-term outcome. J Am Coll Cardiol 16:1097–1102, 1990.

52. Bell MR, Bailey KR, Reeder GS, et al: Percutaneous transluminal angioplasty in patients with multivessel coronary disease: How important is complete revascularization for cardiac event-free survival? J Am Coll Cardiol 16:553–562, 1990.

53. DiSciascio G, Cowley MJ, Vetrovec GW, et al: Triple vessel coronary angioplasty: Acute outcome and long-term results. J Am Coll Cardiol 12:42–48, 1988.

54. Ellis SG, Vandormael MG, Cowley MJ: Coronary morphologic and clinical determinants of procedural outcome with angioplasty for multivessel coronary disease: Implications for patient selection. Circulation 82:1193–1202, 1990.

55. Hubner PJ: Cardiac interventional procedures in the United Kingdom in 1989. Br Heart J 66:469–471, 1991.

56. Bedotto JB, Rutherford BD, McConahay DR, et al: Results of multivessel percutaneous transluminal coronary angioplasty in persons aged 65 years and older. Am J Cardiol 67:1051–1055, 1991.

57. Parisi AF, Folland ED, Hartigan P: A comparison of angioplasty with medical therapy in the treatment of single-vessel coronary artery disease. Veterans Affairs ACME Investigators. N Engl J Med 326:10–16, 1992.

58. Folland ED, Hartigan PM, Parisi AF, for the Veterans Affairs ACME Investigators: Percutaneous transluminal coronary angioplasty versus medical therapy for stable angina pectoris. Outcomes for patients with double-vessel single-vessel coronary artery disease in a Veterans Affairs cooperative randomized trial. J Am Coll Cardiol 29:1505–1511, 1997.

59. RITA-2 Trial Participants: Coronary angioplasty versus medical therapy for angina: The second Randomised Intervention Treatment of Angina (RITA-2) trial. Lancet 350:461–468, 1997.

60. RITA Trial Participants: Coronary angioplasty versus coronary artery bypass surgery: The Randomised Intervention Treatment of Angina (RITA) trial. Lancet 341:573–580, 1993.

61. CABRI Trial Participants: First-year results of CABRI (Coronary Angioplasty versus Bypass Revascularization Investigation). Lancet 346:1179–1184, 1995.

62. The Bypass Angioplasty Revascularization Investigation (BARI) Investigators: Comparison of coronary bypass surgery with angioplasty in patients with multivessel disease. N Engl J Med 335:217–225, 1996.

63. King SB III, Lembo NJ, Weintraub WS, et al: A randomized trial comparing coronary angioplasty with coronary bypass surgery. Emory Angioplasty versus Surgery Trial (EAST). N Engl J Med 331:1044–1050, 1994.

64. Hamm CW, Reimers J, Ischinger T, et al, for the German Angioplasty Bypass Surgery Investigation: A randomized study of coronary angioplasty compared with bypass surgery in patients with symptomatic multivessel coronary disease. German Angioplasty Bypass Surgery Investigation (GABI). N Engl J Med 331:1037–1043, 1994.

65. Rodriguez A, Boullon F, Perez-Balino N, et al: Argentine Randomized Trial of Percutaneous Transluminal Coronary Angioplasty versus Coronary Artery Bypass Surgery in Multivessel Disease (ERACI): In-hospital results and 1-year follow-up. J Am Coll Cardiol 22:1060–1067, 1993.

66. Mele E, Rodriguez AE, Peyregne E, et al: Final follow up of Argentine Randomized Trial of Percutaneous Transluminal

Coronary Angioplasty versus Coronary Artery Bypass Surgery in Multivessel Disease (ERACI): Clinical outcome and cost analysis [Abstract]. Circulation 94:I-435, 1996.

67. Puel J, Karouny E, Marco F, et al: Angioplasty versus surgery in multi-vessel disease: Immediate results and in-hospital outcome in a randomized prospective study [Abstract]. Circulation 86(suppl I):I-372, 1992.

68. Pocock SJ, Henderson RA, Rickards AF, et al: Meta-analysis of randomised trials comparing coronary angioplasty with bypass surgery. Lancet 346:1184–1189, 1995.

69. Goy JJ, Eeckhout E, Burnand B, et al: Coronary angioplasty versus left internal mammary artery grafting for isolated proximal left anterior descending artery stenosis. Lancet 343:1449–1453, 1994.

70. Hueb WA, Bellotti G, de Oliveira SA, et al: The Medicine, Angioplasty or Surgery Study (MASS): A prospective, randomized trial of medical therapy, balloon angioplasty or bypass surgery for single proximal left anterior descending artery stenoses. J Am Coll Cardiol 26:1600–1605, 1995.

71. Kosinski AS, Barnhart HX, Weintraub WS, et al, for EAST Investigators: Five year outcome after coronary surgery or coronary angioplasty: Results from the Emory Angioplasty vs. Surgery Trial (EAST) [Abstract]. Circulation 92:I-543, 1995.

72. The Writing Group for the Bypass Angioplasty Revascularization Investigation (BARI): Five-year clinical and functional outcome comparing bypass surgery and angioplasty in patients with multivessel coronary disease: A multicenter randomized trial. JAMA 277:715–721, 1997.

73. Sim I, Gupta M, McDonald K, et al: A meta-analysis of randomized trials comparing coronary artery bypass grafting with percutaneous transluminal coronary angioplasty in multivessel coronary artery disease. Am J Cardiol 76:1025–1029, 1995.

74. King SB III, Schlumpf M: Ten-year completed follow-up of percutaneous transluminal coronary angioplasty: The early Zurich experience. J Am Coll Cardiol 22:353–360, 1993.

75. Rosati RA, Wallace AG, Stead EA: The way of the future. Arch Intern Med 131:285, 1973.

76. Pryor DB, Califf RM, Harrell FE Jr, et al: Clinical data bases. Accomplishments and unrealized potential. Med Care 23:623–647, 1985.

77. Smith LR, Harrell FE Jr, Rankin JS, et al: Determinants of early versus late cardiac death in patients undergoing coronary artery bypass graft surgery. Circulation 84(suppl 5):III-245–III-253, 1991.

78. Jones RH, Kesler K, Phillips HR III, et al: Long-term survival benefits of coronary artery bypass grafting and percutaneous transluminal angioplasty in patients with coronary artery disease. J Thorac Cardiovasc Surg 111:1013–1025, 1996.

79. Sculpher MJ, Seed P, Henderson RA, et al: Health service costs of coronary angioplasty and coronary artery bypass surgery: The Randomised Intervention Treatment of Angina (RITA) trial. Lancet 344:927–930, 1994.

80. Hlatky MA, Rogers WJ, Johnstone I, et al, for the Bypass Angioplasty Revascularization Investigation (BARI): Medical care costs and quality of life after randomization to coronary angioplasty or coronary bypass surgery. N Engl J Med 336:92–99, 1997.

81. Mark DB: Implications of cost in treatment selection for patients with coronary heart disease. Ann Thorac Surg 61:S12–S15, 1996.

82. Hlatky MA, Boineau RE, Higginbotham MB, et al: A brief self-administered questionnaire to determine functional capacity (the Duke Activity Status Index). Am J Cardiol 64:651–654, 1989.

83. Nelson CL, Herndon JE, Mark DB, et al: Relation of clinical and angiographic factors to functional capacity as measured by the Duke Activity Status Index. Am J Cardiol 68:973–975, 1991.

84. Stewart AL: The MOS short-form general health survey: Reliability and validity in a patient population. Med Care 26:724, 1988.

85. Frye RL: Stroke in coronary artery bypass graft surgery: An analysis of the CASS experience. The participants in the Coronary Artery Surgery Study. Int J Cardiol 36:213–221, 1992.

86. Roach GW: Adverse cerebral outcomes after coronary bypass surgery. N Engl J Med 335:1857–1863, 1996.

86a. Kleiman NS: Primary and secondary safety endpoints from IMPACT II. Integrilin to Minimize Platelet Aggregation and Coronary Thrombosis. Am J Cardiol 80(4A):29B–33B, 1997.

86b. Holmes DR Jr, Topol EJ, Califf RM, et al: A multicenter, randomized trial of coronary angioplasty versus directional atherectomy for patients with saphenous vein bypass graft lesions. CAVEAT-II Investigators. Circulation 91:1966–1974, 1995.

86c. Elliott JM, Berdan LG, Holmes DR, et al: One-year follow-up in the Coronary Angioplasty Versus Excisional Atherectomy Trial (CAVEAT I). Circulation 91:2158–2166, 1995.

87. Cukingman RA, Carey JS, Wittig JH, et al: Influence of complete coronary revascularization on relief of angina. J Thorac Cardiovasc Surg 79:188–193, 1980.

88. Lavee J, Rath S, Quang-Hoa T, et al: Does complete revascularization by the conventional method truly provide the best possible results? Analysis of results and comparison with revascularization of infarct-prone segments (systematic segmental myocardial revascularization): The Sheba Study. J Thorac Cardiovasc Surg 92:279–290, 1986.

89. Bell MR, Gersh BJ, Schaff HV, et al, and the Investigators of the Coronary Artery Surgery Study: Effect of completeness of revascularization on long-term outcome of patients with three-vessel disease undergoing coronary artery bypass surgery: A report from the Coronary Artery Surgery Study (CASS) Registry. Circ Res 86:446–457, 1992.

90. Whitlow PL: Percutaneous transluminal coronary angioplasty in two and three vessel coronary disease: Information and speculation. J Am Coll Cardiol 11:1180–1182, 1988.

91. Bourassa MG, Holubkov R, Yeh W, et al, Co-investigators of the National Heart, Lung, and Blood Institute Percutaneous Transluminal Coronary Angioplasty Registry: Strategy of complete revascularization in patients with multivessel coronary artery disease (a report from the 1985–1986 NHLBI PTCA Registry). Am J Cardiol 70:174–178, 1992.

92. Bell MR, Berger PB, Bresnahan JF, et al: Initial and long-term outcome of 354 patients after coronary balloon angioplasty of total coronary artery occlusions. Circulation 85:1003–1011, 1992.

93. Mabin TA, Holmes DR, Smith HC, et al: Follow-up clinical results in patients undergoing percutaneous transluminal coronary angioplasty. Circulation 71:754–760, 1985.

94. Reeder GS, Holmes DR Jr, Detre K, et al: Degree of revascularization in patients with multivessel coronary disease: A report from the National Heart, Lung, and Blood Institute Percutaneous Transluminal Coronary Angioplasty Registry. Circulation 77:638–644, 1988.

95. Faxon DP, Ghalilli K, Jacobs AK, et al: The degree of revascularization and outcome after multivessel coronary angioplasty. Am Heart J 123:854–859, 1992.

96. Faxon DP, Ruocco N, Jacobs AK: Long-term outcome of patients after percutaneous transluminal coronary angioplasty. Circulation 81:IV-9–IV-13, 1990.

97. Stevens T, Kahn JK, McCallister BD, et al: Safety and efficacy of percutaneous transluminal coronary angioplasty in patients with left ventricular dysfunction. Am J Cardiol 68:313–319, 1991.

98. Serota H, Deligonul U, Lee WH, et al: Predictors of cardiac survival after percutaneous transluminal coronary angioplasty in patients with severe left ventricular dysfunction. Am J Cardiol 67:367–372, 1991.

99. Holmes DR Jr, Detre KM, Williams DO, et al: Long-term outcome of patients with depressed left ventricular function undergoing percutaneous transluminal coronary angioplasty. The NHLBI PTCA Registry. Circulation 87:21–29, 1993.

100. Munger TM: Long-term retrospective follow-up for outcome of percutaneous transluminal coronary angioplasty versus coronary artery bypass surgery in patients with severely depressed left ventricular function. J Am Coll Cardiol 17:63A, 1991.

101. Weintraub WS, Craver JM, Cohen CL, et al: Influence of age

on results of coronary artery surgery. Circulation 84:III-226–III-235, 1991.

102. Hartz AJ, Kuhn EM, Pryor DB, et al: Mortality after coronary angioplasty and coronary artery bypass surgery. Am J Cardiol 70:179–185, 1992.

103. Weintraub WS, King SB III, Guyton RA, et al: Coronary surgery and PTCA in diabetics with multivessel disease: Can the BARI results be generalized? [Abstract]. Circulation 94:I-435, 1996.

104. Barsness GW, Peterson ED, Ohman EM, et al: Relationship between diabetes mellitus and long-term survival after coronary bypass and angioplasty. Circulation 96:2551–2556, 1997.

105. Luft HS: Should operations be regionalized? The empirical relation between surgical volume and mortality. N Engl J Med 301:1364, 1979.

106. Showstack EL: Association of volume with outcome of coronary artery bypass graft surgery: Scheduled vs. nonscheduled operations. JAMA 257:785, 1987.

107. Hannan EL, O'Donnell JF, Kilburn H, et al: Investigation of the relationship between volume and mortality for surgical procedures performed in New York state hospitals. JAMA 262:503–510, 1989.

108. Hannan EL, Siu AL, Kumar D, et al: The decline in coronary artery bypass graft surgery mortality in New York state: The role of surgeon volume. JAMA 273:209–213, 1995.

109. Hannan EL, Racz M, Ryan TJ: Coronary angioplasty volume-outcome relationships for hospitals and cardiologists [Abstract]. JAMA 279:802, 1997.

110. Ritchie JL, Phillips KA, Luft HS: Coronary angioplasty: Statewide experience in California. Circulation 88:2735–2743, 1993.

111. Jollis JG, Peterson ED, DeLong ER, et al: The relation between the volume of coronary angioplasty procedures at hospitals treating Medicare beneficiaries and short-term mortality. N Engl J Med 331:1625–1629, 1994.

112. Baim DS, Kent KM, King SB III, et al: Evaluating new devices. Acute (in-hospital) results from the New Approaches to Coronary Intervention Registry. Circulation 89:471–481, 1994.

113. Serruys PW, de Jaegere P, Kiemeneij F, et al, for the Benestent Study Group: A comparison of balloon-expandable stent implantation with balloon angioplasty in patients with coronary artery disease. N Engl J Med 331:489–495, 1994.

114. Moussa I, Reimers B, Moses J, et al: Long-term angiographic and clinical outcome of patients undergoing multivessel coronary stenting. Circulation 96:3873–3879, 1997.

114a. Serruys PW, Unger F, Sousa JE, et al: Comparison of coronary artery bypass surgery and stenting for the treatment of multivessel disease. N Engl J Med 344:1117–1124, 2001.

114b. Rodriguez A, Bernardi V, Navia J, et al: Argentine Randomized Study: Coronary Bypass Surgery in patients with Multiple-Vessel Disease (ERACI II): 30-day and one-year follow-up results. J Am Coll Cardiol 37:51–58, 2001.

115. Kastrati A, Schomig A, Elezi S, et al: Predictive factors of restenosis after coronary stent placement. J Am Coll Cardiol 30:1428–1436, 1997.

116. Ryan TJ, Faxon DP, Gunnar RM, et al: Guidelines for percutaneous transluminal coronary angioplasty: A report of the American College of Cardiology/American Heart Association task force on assessment of diagnostic and therapeutic cardiovascular procedures (Subcommittee on Percutaneous

Transluminal Coronary Angioplasty). J Am Coll Cardiol 12:529–545, 1988.

117. Wong P, Wong C-W, Ko P, et al: Elective stenting of unprotected left main coronary disease. Catheter Cardiovasc Diagn 39:347–354, 1996.

118. Laham RJ, Carrozza JP, Baim DS: Treatment of unprotected left main stenoses with Palmaz-Schatz stenting. Catheter Cardiovasc Diagn 37:77–80, 1996.

119. Macaya C, Alfonso F, Iniqueq A, et al: Stenting for elastic recoil during coronary angioplasty of the left main coronary artery. Am J Cardiol 70:105–107, 1992.

120. Tommaso CL, Vogel JH, Vogel RA: Coronary angioplasty in high-risk patients with left main coronary stenosis: Results from the National Registry of Elective Supported Angioplasty. Catheter Cardiovasc Diagn 25:169–173, 1992.

121. Park S-J: Stenting of unprotected left main coronary artery stenoses: Immediate and late outcomes. J Am Coll Cardiol 31:37–42, 1998.

122. Ellis SG, Tamai H, Nobuyoshi M, et al: Contemporary percutaneous treatment of unprotected left main coronary stenoses: Initial results from a multicenter registry analysis 1994–1996. Circulation 96:3867–3872, 1997.

123. Tcheng JE: Glycoprotein IIb/IIIa receptor inhibitors: Putting the EPIC, IMPACT II, RESTORE, and EPILOG trials into perspective. Am J Cardiol 78:35–40, 1996.

124. The EPIC Investigators: Use of a monoclonal antibody directed against the platelet glycoprotein IIb/IIIa receptor in high-risk coronary angioplasty. N Engl J Med 330:956–961, 1994.

125. Lincoff AM, Tcheng JE, Califf RM, et al: Abciximab (c7E3 Fab, ReoPro) with reduced heparin dosing during coronary intervention: Final results of the EPILOG trial [Abstract]. J Am Coll Cardiol 29(suppl A):187A, 1997.

126. The EPILOG Investigators: Platelet glycoprotein IIb/IIIa receptor blockade and low-dose heparin during percutaneous coronary revascularization. N Engl J Med 336:1689–1696, 1997.

127. Tcheng JE, Lincoff AM, Sigmon KN, et al, for the IMPACT II Investigators: Platelet glycoprotein IIb/IIIa inhibition with Integrelin™ during percutaneous coronary intervention: The IMPACT II trial [Abstract]. Circulation 92(suppl I): I-543, 1995.

128. King SBI III: Administration of Tirofiban (MK-0383) will reduce the incidence of adverse cardiac outcome following PTCA/DCA (RESTORE) [Abstract]. J Am Coll Cardiol 27(suppl A):21, 1996.

128a. O'Neill WW, Serruys P, Knudtson M, et al: Long-term treatment with a platelet glycoprotein-receptor antagonist after percutaneous coronary revascularization. EXCITE trial investigators. N Engl J Med 342:1316–1324, 2000.

129. O'Keefe JH: Estrogen replacement therapy after coronary angioplasty in women. J Am Coll Cardiol 29:1, 1997.

130. Tardif J-C, Cote G, Lesperance J, et al, for the Multivitamins and Probucol Study Group: Probucol and multivitamins in the prevention of restenosis after coronary angioplasty. N Engl J Med 331:365–372, 1997.

131. Muhlbaier LH, Pryor DB, Rankin JS, et al: Observational comparison of event-free survival with medical and surgical therapy in patients with coronary artery disease. 20 years of follow-up. Circulation 86:II-198–II-204, 1992.

132. Rozenman Y: Age- and gender-related differences in success, major and minor complication rates and the duration of hospitalization after percutaneous transluminal coronary angioplasty. Cardiology 87:396, 1996.

# 11

# Primary Coronary Angioplasty in Acute Myocardial Infarction: Comparative Analysis with Thrombolytic Therapy

*Gregg W. Stone    Cindy L. Grines*

Acute myocardial infarction (AMI) is initiated by ulceration or fissuring of a previously stable atherosclerotic plaque, upon which superimposed thrombus formation results in coronary occlusion.[1, 2] Restoring antegrade blood flow during the first few hours after AMI results in improved survival rates and myocardial salvage.[3–7] Consequently, reperfusion therapy has become widely accepted as the cornerstone of treatment after AMI.

The major decision facing the physician when presented with a patient with evolving AMI is therefore the choice of a reperfusion strategy that will maximize the likelihood of restoring vessel patency and improving clinical outcomes with minimal adverse side effects. The ideal reperfusion modality would be widely available and simple to administer; would effectively restore antegrade flow in the occluded coronary artery in all patients, thereby resulting in maximal myocardial recovery and survival; would passivate the inherently unstable atherosclerotic plaque to minimize the incidence of recurrent ischemia and reinfarction, thereby facilitating early discharge; would have a favorable side effect profile, including minimal risk of reperfusion injury to the myocardium; would result in long-term patency of the infarcted vessel with improved infarct-free late survival; and would be cost effective. Two reperfusion strategies have become widely available for the treatment of AMI: thrombolytic therapy and primary percutaneous transluminal angioplasty (PTCA). In this chapter, the development, method, and outcomes of primary PTCA in patients with AMI are reviewed thoroughly, and the relative advantages and disadvantages of reperfusion with primary PTCA and with thrombolytic therapy are discussed in depth.

## EVOLUTION OF PRIMARY PTCA

## Limitations of Thrombolytic Therapy

Indisputable advantages of thrombolytic therapy are its universal availability and the fact that thrombolytic administration requires no particular expertise and may be initiated relatively rapidly after the patient arrives at the hospital. Several drawbacks of thrombolytic therapy, however, must be acknowledged; their existence spurred the development of primary PTCA (Table 11–1). The limitations of thrombolytic therapy must be understood in detail if the relative benefits of primary PTCA in comparison with thrombolysis are to be fully appreciated.

### Patency After Thrombolytic Therapy

The mechanism by which reperfusion therapy reduces infarct size and mortality is through the early restoration of rapid and effective antegrade perfusion in the infarcted vessel. In this regard, thrombolytic therapy is effective in, at most, one third to half of patients in whom it is administered. The concept of flow as graded by the Thrombolysis In Myocardial Infarction (TIMI) trial is central in understanding this issue. In the early thrombolytic trials, angiographically determined flow in the infarcted artery was graded according to the TIMI scale (Table 11–2).[8] Historically, patency was considered to be present if an angiogram demonstrated either TIMI grade 2 or 3 flow in the infarcted vessel,[8] which is true for 50% to 80% of patients after thrombolytic therapy. Multiple thrombolytic trials since have convincingly demonstrated, however, that restoration of normal, brisk antegrade flow in the infarcted vessel (TIMI grade 3 flow) within 90 minutes of therapy is required for maximal myocar-

**TABLE 11-1. LIMITATIONS OF THROMBOLYTIC THERAPY IN ACUTE MYOCARDIAL INFARCTION**

Low rates of early and sustained patency of the infarcted vessel after thrombolysis:
- 90-minute patency is restored in only 40%–85% of patients
- 90-minute TIMI grade 3 flow rates are restored in only 20%–60% of patients
- Myocardial blood flow and tissue metabolism remain abnormal in 20%–40% of patients despite TIMI-3 flow
- Predischarge reocclusion of the infarcted artery occurs in 10%–20% of patients
- Late reocclusion of the infarcted artery occurs in 25%–41% of previously patent infarct vessels

No reliable bedside markers of thrombolytic success are currently available:
- It is difficult to selectively apply a rescue PTCA strategy to further improve acute patency rates

Increased rate of reinfarction after thrombolytic therapy in comparison with placebo results in blunted myocardial recovery and increased early and late mortality

Increased rate of recurrent ischemia after thrombolytic therapy in comparison with placebo prolongs the duration of hospitalization, necessitates predischarge revascularization procedures, and increases costs

Hemorrhagic complications of thrombolytic therapy:
- Life-threatening or disabling bleeding in 0.5%–1.5% of patients
- Minor hemorrhagic complications in 5%–30% of patients

Limited efficacy in the patients at highest risk (e.g., those in cardiogenic shock)

Frequent contraindications to use

PTCA, percutaneous transluminal coronary angioplasty; TIMI, Thrombolysis in Myocardial Infarction (flow).

dial salvage and improved survival.[9–20] TIMI-2 flow results in outcomes only slightly better than if the infarcted artery remains occluded (TIMI grade 0 or 1 flow). In the 41,021-patient Global Utilization of Streptokinase and Tissue Plasminogen Activator for Occluded Coronary Arteries (GUSTO) study,[7] 2431 patients were enrolled in a substudy in which angiography was routinely performed 90 minutes, 180 minutes, 24 hours, or 5 to 7 days after initiation of thrombolytic therapy.[10, 15] Only the presence of brisk antegrade TIMI grade 3 flow on the 90-minute angiogram was correlated with improved survival. The

**TABLE 11-2. THE THROMBOLYSIS IN MYOCARDIAL INFARCTION (TIMI) FLOW SCALE**

TIMI grade 0: absence of antegrade flow beyond the point of occlusion

TIMI grade 1: partial penetration of contrast beyond the obstruction with absence of filling of the distal vessel

TIMI grade 2: patency of the vessel but with delayed filling or washout

TIMI grade 3: normal brisk antegrade flow and washout

Modified from the TIMI Study Group: The Thrombolysis in Myocardial Infarction (TIMI) trial: Phase 1 findings. N Engl J Med 312:932–936, 1985.

30-day mortality rate was 4.0% if TIMI grade 3 flow was restored, 7.9% if TIMI grade 2 flow was restored, and 8.6% if TIMI grade 0 or 1 flow was present. Furthermore, patients in whom TIMI grade 3 as opposed to grades 0 to 2 flow was restored had greater myocardial salvage, less frequent reocclusion of the infarcted artery, and a reduced need for subsequent revascularization procedures after admission.[9–20] The effect of TIMI flow on mortality and on other adverse outcomes according to a pooled analysis of thrombolytic trials is shown in Figure 11–1.[20]

Studies in which angiography has been performed 90 to 120 minutes after thrombolytic administration have documented TIMI grade 3 flow rates in only 20% to 40% of patients treated with non–fibrin-selective agents such as streptokinase, urokinase, and/or anisoylated plasminogen streptokinase activator complex (APSAC) and in 40% to 60% of patients treated with fibrin-specific agents such as tissue plasminogen activator (tPA) or reteplase (rPA).[9–25] Thus, with regard only to the ability to restore TIMI grade 3 flow, at most half of patients treated with intravenous thrombolytic agents may be considered to have achieved successful reperfusion.

Furthermore, myocardial tissue perfusion at a subcellular level may remain impaired despite the restoration of TIMI grade 3 antegrade flow. Maes and associates found that 11 (37%) of 30 patients had diminished myocardial blood flow, as assessed by positron emission tomography (PET), despite the presence of TIMI grade 3 flow 90 minutes after thrombolysis.[26] Regional left ventricular function was not recovered in any of these patients, as assessed by evaluation of paired radionuclide ventriculograms from 5 days to 3 months after treatment. In contrast, patients with normal myocardial blood flow, as assessed by PET imaging, 90 minutes after thrombolytic administration, had preserved or improved regional ventricular function 3 months later. Similar findings have been demonstrated by Ito and coworkers,[27, 28] who observed a dissociation between brisk antegrade angiographic flow and diminished myocardial perfusion in 23% of patients, as assessed by contrast echocardiography. Finally, Kern and colleagues showed that Doppler coronary flow velocity is reduced in a substantial percentage of patients with TIMI-3 flow after reperfusion in AMI.[29] In this series of 41 patients, reduced coronary flow velocity was a better predictor of recurrent angina and the need for revascularization than was the TIMI flow grade. The mechanism of inadequate microcirculating perfusion in the presence of brisk epicardial coronary blood flow may relate to myocellular damage or edema, microvascular spasm or disease, or distal thromboemboli.

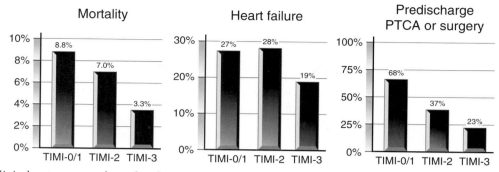

FIGURE 11–1. Clinical outcomes 30 days after thrombolytic therapy, stratified by TIMI flow present in the infarcted vessel on a 90-minute angiogram. PTCA, percutaneous transluminal coronary angioplasty; TIMI, Thrombolysis In Myocardial Infarction. (Data from Anderson et al.[20])

Thus, fewer than half of patients receiving thrombolytic therapy immediately achieve adequate tissue perfusion. In addition, these initial reperfusion rates are further degraded by reocclusion of the infarcted vessel.[30, 31] Because the majority of infarcted artery reocclusions after thrombolysis are clinically silent (as a result of significant collateral development, earlier completed infarction, or true "silent" ischemia or reinfarction),[32–34] routine follow-up angiography is necessary to assess the true incidence of late closure of infarcted vessels. Studies have shown that after successful thrombolysis, 10% to 20% of previously patent infarcted vessels have reoccluded at the time of predischarge angiography 7 to 14 days later.[22, 30–43] The incidence of reocclusion of infarcted arteries is higher after thrombolysis with fibrin-specific agents, such as tPA, than with non–fibrin-selective agents.[22, 30, 31, 37, 41–43] The consequences of reocclusion are significant. Ohman and associates found that early reocclusion of the infarcted vessel was the second most common cause of mortality after thrombolysis in AMI.[33] In this analysis of 810 patients from the Thrombolysis and Angioplasty in Myocardial Infarction (TAMI) trials,[33] early reocclu-

sion of the infarcted vessel occurred in 12.4% of patients and was associated with significantly higher rates of mortality, pulmonary edema, respiratory failure, and second- or third-degree atrioventricular block than in patients with sustained patency of the infarcted artery (Fig. 11–2). Similarly, in the GUSTO-I trial, the 30-day mortality rate among patients with documented reocclusion of the infarcted artery was 12.0%, in contrast to 1.1% of patients with sustained patency ($p < 0.001$). Indeed, this high rate of mortality in patients with reocclusion was similar to the 8.9% mortality rate among patients in whom thrombolysis was initially unsuccessful.[44]

In addition to the adverse consequences of early reocclusion of the infarcted vessel, late reocclusion within 3 to 12 months after hospital discharge has been documented in an additional 25% to 41% of patients after initial restoration of patency by thrombolytic therapy.[45–49] Late reocclusion of the infarcted vessel frequently results in reinfarction, blunted myocardial recovery, and late mortality. In the Antithrombotics in the Prevention of Reocclusion in Coronary Thrombolysis (APRICOT) trial,[32, 47] reoc-

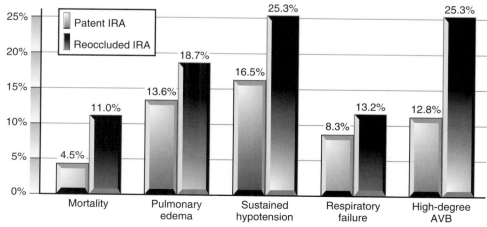

FIGURE 11–2. Consequences of infarcted artery reocclusion after successful reperfusion. AVB, atrioventricular block; IRA, infarct-related artery. (Data from the TAMI trials.[33])

clusion occurred in 71 (29%) of 248 lytic-treated patients who had undergone angiographic follow-up at a mean time of 77 ± 23 days after treatment. By actuarial analysis, the 1-year rate of survival free from reinfarction or the need for repeat revascularization procedures was 63% among patients with infarcted artery reocclusion, in contrast to 83% among those without reocclusion ($p < 0.001$). In comparison with patients without reocclusion, patients with infarcted artery reocclusion had higher 3-year rates of death (9% vs. 3%), reinfarction (27% vs. 9%), and the need for PTCA (30% vs. 14%). Only patients with sustained late patency of the infarcted vessel had an improvement in late left ventricular ejection fraction (LVEF) and preservation of end-systolic volume index (ESVI),[50] both of which are major predictors of late survival after AMI.[51, 52]

Prior studies have disagreed on whether reliable predictors of infarcted artery reocclusion after thrombolytic therapy can be identified.[31] Some reports found a greater likelihood of infarcted artery reocclusion in patients with intermittent coronary patency,[53] TIMI grade 2 flow (as opposed to grade 3 flow),[53–55] complex angiographic lesion morphology,[54–56] or high-grade residual stenosis after reperfusion[55–59]; other trials[60, 61] have been unable to identify clinical or angiographic correlates of infarcted artery reocclusion. It is therefore difficult to identify which patients may benefit from adjunctive pharmacologic or mechanical strategies to prevent reocclusion after successful thrombolysis in AMI.

Considering the relatively low rates of early TIMI grade 3 flow, the even lower rates of restoration of normal myocardial tissue perfusion, and the high rates of early and late reocclusion of the infarct vessel, Lincoff and Topol concluded that fewer than 25% of all patients receiving thrombolytic therapy achieve optimal reperfusion.[31]

### Difficulty in Assessing Thrombolytic Success

Patients with a persistently occluded infarcted artery 90 minutes after thrombolytic therapy have worse left ventricular function; are at increased risk of developing mechanical complications of AMI such as ventricular septal defect, papillary muscle, and free wall rupture; and have an increased incidence of early mortality.[10, 62] Studies in the early 1990s suggested that "rescue" PTCA to open coronary arteries that remain occluded shortly after thrombolytic therapy may be effective in improving myocardial function and clinical outcomes.[63, 64] In the TAMI-5 study,[63] 575 patients treated with thrombolytic therapy were randomly assigned to undergo immediate catheterization, with rescue PTCA if persistent coronary occlusion was demonstrated, or to undergo deferred catheterization. Rescue PTCA was performed in 18% of the patients who underwent immediate catheterization, with an 83% success rate. As a result, 96% of the patients who underwent immediate catheterization left the catheterization laboratory with a patent infarcted vessel. Patients who underwent immediate catheterization and rescue PTCA had greater predischarge patency (94% vs. 90%; $p = 0.065$), improved regional wall motion in the infarcted zone, and a reduced rate of recurrent ischemia in comparison to the delayed group. In the Randomized Evaluation of Salvage Angioplasty with Combined Utilization of Endpoints (RESCUE) study, 151 patients with a first anterior myocardial infarction and angiographically documented TIMI grade 0 or 1 flow after thrombolytic therapy were randomly assigned to receive rescue PTCA or conservative care.[64] PTCA was successful (TIMI grade 2 or 3 flow was restored) in 92% of patients, and TIMI grade 3 flow with residual stenosis of less than 50% of the luminal diameter was achieved in 68% of patients. At 30 days, the patients who underwent rescue PTCA had a higher exercise LVEF (45% vs. 40%; $p = 0.04$) and a reduction in the combined end point of death or New York Heart Association (NYHA) class III or IV heart failure (6.4% vs. 16.6%; $p = 0.05$). Because the investigators in this study excluded many high-risk patients who had the most to gain from a rescue strategy, including those with ongoing ischemia, occlusion of the proximal left anterior descending artery, or hemodynamic compromise, the benefits of rescue PTCA were probably underestimated in this trial.

If rescue PTCA is to be considered, routine angiography must be performed shortly after thrombolytic administration. The use of a femoral approach shortly after thrombolytic therapy, however, exposes the patient to significant risks of blood loss at the access site and should therefore be performed only in patients with a persistently occluded infarcted vessel. Unfortunately, there currently are no reliable bedside markers of reperfusion after intravenous thrombolysis, which would allow catheterization to be selectively performed only in patients in whom reperfusion has not occurred.[65] In this regard, continuous digital ST segment monitoring[66] and early measurement of serum creatine kinase MM-III isoforms, myoglobin, troponin-T, and troponin-I are promising[67–72] but still entail an unacceptable period of delay and do not yet possess sufficient sensitivity and specificity to be clinically dependable in the individual patient.

### Reinfarction After Thrombolytic Therapy

After successful thrombolysis, a high-grade, potentially unstable atherosclerotic plaque remains in the majority of patients[73-76]; this plaque results in blunted myocardial recovery and a twofold increased incidence of recurrent ischemia, postinfarction angina, and reinfarction in comparison to placebo.[3, 4, 77-79] Although infarcted artery reocclusion is often asymptomatic,[30, 31, 50, 79] clinically evident reinfarction after thrombolysis occurs twice as frequently as in placebo-treated controls[3, 4, 79] and has particularly ominous implications. In the TIMI-II trial,[80] reinfarction occurred in 10.4% of 3339 patients during 3-year follow-up. The 3-year mortality rate was 14.1% in patients with reinfarction, in contrast to 7.9% in a matched control group ($p < 0.01$). Kornowski and coworkers found reinfarction to be the most powerful determinant of late mortality after thrombolysis for a first myocardial infarction, with a relative risk of 4.7.[81]

### Recurrent Ischemia After Thrombolytic Therapy

In addition to the heightened risk of reinfarction after thrombolytic therapy, recurrent ischemia is also extremely common, occurring in 18% to 32% of patients after successful thrombolysis before hospital discharge.[60] The development of recurrent ischemia (with or without reinfarction) after reperfusion prolongs the hospital stay; necessitates cardiac catheterization and revascularization procedures before discharge; is associated with increased morbidity, mortality, and loss of ventricular function; and increases costs.[82-88] Califf and colleagues, reporting on the outcomes involving 1221 patients in the TAMI trials,[82] found that recurrent ischemia developed in 21% of thrombolytic-treated patients, including 2.5% of patients in whom reinfarction occurred. The prognosis of patients in whom recurrent ischemia develops without reinfarction was intermediate between the prognosis of stable patients and that of patients in whom reinfarction developed (Table 11–3). Similarly, Ellis and associates[87] re-

ported that of 405 patients undergoing angiography (with or without adjunctive PTCA) 120 minutes after thrombolysis, 303 patients (75%) had successful reperfusion without recurrent ischemia (group 1), 74 patients (18%) had successful reperfusion but later developed recurrent ischemia (group 2), and 28 patients (7%) had unsuccessful reperfusion (group 3). In-hospital mortality rates were 2% of group 1 patients, 15% of group 2 patients, and 32% of group 3 patients ($p < 0.001$). Furthermore, serial LVEF from admission to discharge improved by 1.2% in patients with successful reperfusion without recurrent ischemia, did not change in patients in whom recurrent ischemia developed, and worsened by 4.3% in patients in whom reperfusion was unsuccessful.

Unfortunately, as with infarct artery reocclusion, it has also proved difficult to predict which patients will develop recurrent ischemia after successful thrombolytic therapy. Some studies have noted that the likelihood of recurrent ischemia is increased in the presence of high-grade residual stenosis, TIMI grade 2 flow, use of tPA,[54, 88] or post-PTCA dissection in patients undergoing salvage angioplasty[86]; other studies have found no reliable clinical or angiographic predictors of this adverse event.[61, 62] In addition, the timing of recurrent ischemia after thrombolytic therapy is unpredictable; many events occur as late as 1 week or more after thrombolytic administration.[60, 84, 89] The high rate of recurrent ischemia after thrombolysis, in concert with its unpredictable nature and variable time course, precludes the safe implementation of an early discharge strategy in the large majority of thrombolytic-treated patients.[90, 91]

### Hemorrhagic Complications of Thrombolytic Therapy

The potential benefits of any reperfusion modality must be weighed against its side effects. Hemorrhagic complications are, of course, the major drawback of thrombolytic therapy. The most feared hemorrhagic complication of fibrinolysis is intracranial bleeding, which has occurred in approximately 0.5% to 1.0% of patients in most studies, despite the fact that most thrombolytic trials have had restrictive entry criteria specifically tailored to minimize this adverse event.[92-99] Mortality after intracranial hemorrhage in the setting of thrombolytic administration occurs in 40% to 75% of patients; the majority of survivors are severely disabled.[92-103] The incidence of intracranial bleeding after thrombolysis rises with advancing age, female gender, the use of tPA, greater tPA doses, concurrent warfarin use, higher heparin levels, lower body weight, prior cerebrovascular disease, and accelerated hypertension.[92-105]

**TABLE 11–3. OUTCOMES FOLLOWING RECURRENT ISCHEMIA AND REINFARCTION IN THE TAMI TRIALS**

| OUTCOME | RI AND REPEAT MI (N = 31 [2.5%]) | RI ONLY (N = 226 [18.5%]) | NEITHER (N = 964 [79%]) |
|---|---|---|---|
| Death | 23% | 11% | 4% |
| Heart failure | 48% | 31% | 17% |
| ICU days (median) | 6 | 4 | 3 |
| Hospital days (median) | 14 | 10 | 9 |
| Charges (mean) | $24,690 | $23,609 | $19,721 |

ICU, intensive care unit; MI, myocardial infarction; RI, recurrent ischemia; TAMI, Thrombolysis and Angioplasty in Myocardial Infarction.

Furthermore, the inherent risk of intracranial hemorrhage with thrombolytic drugs increases as more potent dosing regimens and adjunctive antithrombin agents are used in an effort to improve patency. Rates of intracerebral hemorrhage as high as 3.4% have occurred in studies in which higher doses of tPA, heparin, or hirudin were used, which necessitated the early termination or modification of the TIMI-I, GUSTO-IIa, TIMI-IXA, and r-Hirudin for Improvement of Thrombolysis (HIT-III) trials[106–111] (Fig. 11–3). Even with modified dosing regimens and carefully regulated inclusion criteria, intracranial bleeding nonetheless occurred in 0.9% of 15,060 patients enrolled in the GUSTO-III study, in which tPA was compared with reteplase (no treatment-related differences in hemorrhagic complications were evident between the two agents).[112]

Additional hazards of thrombolytic therapy include reperfusion injury[113] and the conversion of an otherwise bland infarction into a hemorrhagic infarction, which increases myocardial necrosis and the rates of cardiac rupture and mortality in the first 24 hours after treatment, in comparison with non–lytic-treated controls.[3, 4, 114–116] Other hemorrhagic complications of thrombolysis include gastrointestinal and genitourinary bleeding, hemoptysis, hemorrhagic tamponade, and major access site–related bleeding in as many as 25% of patients undergoing cardiac catheterization soon after drug administration.[117–122] Thus, in view of the narrow difference between toxic and therapeutic levels of these agents, safety considerations may prevent any thrombolytic drug from producing higher patency rates than are currently achieved. Indeed, considering the devastating consequences of intracerebral bleeding alone, physicians can question whether any rate of intracranial hemorrhage should be tolerated at all if there exist safer reperfusion alternatives that offer at least similar clinical outcomes without this iatrogenic complication.

## Limited Efficacy of Thrombolytic Therapy in Patients at High Risk

The short-term prognosis in AMI may be predicted by simple clinical variables present at the time of admission; features predictive of adverse outcomes include advanced age, female gender, the presence of diabetes mellitus, prior myocardial infarction, anterior infarction location, late presentation, and either congestive heart failure or tachycardia on admission.[123] Early mortality rates remain high after thrombolytic therapy in these patient subsets. In the GUSTO-I trial, 30-day mortality rates after thrombolytic therapy were 20% of patients 75 years or more of age, 32% of patients presenting in Killip class III, 10% of patients with anterior myocardial infarction, and 20% of patients with tachycardia on admission.[124]

Cardiogenic shock, which develops in 8% to 15% of patients with AMI, carries the worst prognosis of all subgroups thus far examined: an expected mortality rate of 70% to 90% with conservative medical therapy.[125, 126] The effective restoration of antegrade coronary flow and myocardial salvage in patients with shock is therefore especially crucial if this dismal prognosis is to be reversed. Unfortunately, thrombolytic therapy is largely ineffective in patients with cardiogenic shock (Fig. 11–4). Of 1029 patients treated with intracoronary streptokinase in the Society for Cardiac Angiography Registry,[127] the in-hospital mortality rate was 67% of patients in shock. The poor survival rate may be explained by the markedly lower rate of reperfusion achieved in patients in shock in comparison with the entire registry (44% vs. 71%), which may be a consequence of low perfusion pressure.[128] However, the in-hospital survival rate was 58% of patients in shock in whom patency was restored, in contrast to 16% of patients in whom the infarcted vessel remained occluded; this finding demonstrates the potential of successful reperfusion for improving

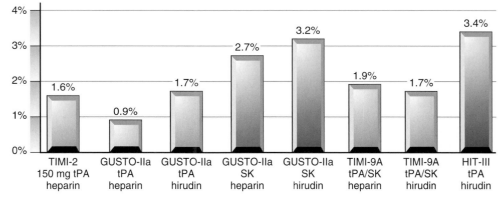

FIGURE 11–3. High rates of intracranial hemorrhage in several studies after thrombolysis with more aggressive thrombolytic regimens. See text for details. GUSTO, Global Utilization of Streptokinase and Tissue Plasminogen Activator for Occluded Coronary Arteries; HIT, r-Hirudin for Improvement of Thrombolysis; SK, streptokinase; TIMI, Thrombolysis In Myocardial Infarction; tPA, tissue-type plasminogen activator.

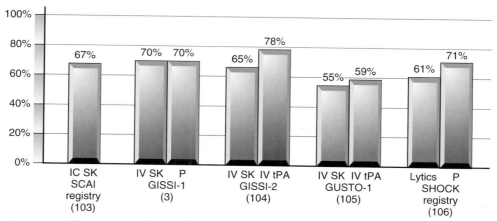

FIGURE 11–4. Short-term mortality rates after thrombolytic therapy in cardiogenic shock; GISSI, Gruppo Italiano per lo Studio della Streptochinasi nell'Infarto Miocardico; GUSTO, Global Utilization of Streptokinase and Tissue Plasminogen Activator for Occluded Coronary Arteries; IC, intracoronary; IV, intravenous; P, placebo; SCA&I, Society for Cardiac Angiography and Interventions; SHOCK, SHould we emergently revascularize Occluded Coronaries for cardiogenic Shock?; SK, streptokinase; tPA, tissue-type plasminogen activator.

the prognosis of cardiogenic shock. In the first Gruppo Italiano per lo Studio della Streptochinasi nell'Infarto Miocardico (GISSI-1) trial, the only placebo-controlled thrombolytic trial to enroll patients in cardiogenic shock, the mortality rate among patients in shock who received either intravenous streptokinase or placebo was 70%.[3] In the GISSI-2 study,[129] mortality was high among patients in shock after administration of tPA or streptokinase (78% vs. 65%, respectively; $p$ = NS). In the GUSTO-I trial, 315 patients presenting in shock were enrolled and treated with thrombolytic therapy, and shock developed in an additional 2657 lytic-treated patients after hospital admission.[130] In-hospital mortality rates were 57% and 56% in these patient groups, respectively. In a 19-center international prospective registry of 251 patients with cardiogenic shock, the short-term mortality rate among patients receiving thrombolytic therapy was similar to that among patients treated conservatively without lytic therapy (61% vs. 71%; $p$ = NS).[131] Thus, patients presenting with cardiogenic shock and other high-risk comorbid features have high mortality rates despite thrombolytic administration, partly as a result of decreased success of reperfusion.

## Frequent Contraindications to Thrombolytic Administration

Finally, because of concerns about lack of efficacy or hemorrhagic complications, many high-risk patients have been excluded from most prior trials of thrombolytic therapy.[3–9, 132, 133] Prior exclusion criteria in different studies have included advanced age, late presentation, prior coronary artery bypass graft surgery, either the absence of electrocardiographic ST segment elevation or the presence of bundle branch block, either hemorrhagic diathesis or prior cerebro-

vascular disease, and cardiogenic shock. Of 1471 consecutive patients with AMI treated at William Beaumont Hospital, Royal Oak, Michigan, over a 2-year period during which the TIMI trials were being performed, only 16% of patients were considered eligible for and received thrombolytic therapy.[133] Among the 84% of patients excluded from lytic administration, the mortality rate was nearly five-fold higher than that among thrombolytic-eligible patients (19% vs. 4%, $p$ < 0.001). Specifically, the mortality rates were 27% of patients more than 70 years of age, 14% of patients with prior stroke or hemorrhagic contraindications to thrombolysis, 21% of patients presenting more than 4 hours after symptom onset, 46% of patients with electrocardiographic results that rendered them ineligible for lytic treatment and 17% of patients with other miscellaneous exclusion criteria.[133]

Studies have shown that even when the inclusion criteria for thrombolytic therapy are broadened to include higher risk subsets, such as patients of any age (e.g., as in the GUSTO[7] trial) and patients presenting within 24 hours after symptom onset (e.g., as in the Late Assessment of Thrombolytic Efficacy [LATE] trial[134]), a minority of patients with AMI are treated with thrombolytic therapy, and these are, again, primarily patients at low risk. Analysis from the 30 centers in Ontario, Canada, participating in the GUSTO trial and the 10 centers participating in the LATE trial revealed that only 1304 (9%) of 13,961 patients presenting with AMI at the GUSTO hospitals during the study period were enrolled, and only 249 (4%) of 6246 patients with AMI at the LATE hospitals were enrolled.[135] Patients not treated in each study were more likely to be older, to be female, and to have more comorbid conditions. In comparison with enrolled patients, nonenrolled patients had markedly higher in-hospital mortality rates (16.8% vs. 6.9% in GUSTO, $p < 0.001$, and 19.7% vs. 6.6% in LATE, $p < 0.001$); these differences persisted after adjustment for age, gender, revascularization status, and comorbidity status.

Thus, restrictive inclusion criteria and concerns about hemorrhagic complications have ensured enrollment of a relatively low-risk cohort into most prior thrombolytic studies. Patients at high risk, those most likely to benefit from effective reperfusion, are often denied thrombolytic therapy and suffer high morbidity and mortality rates. Despite recommendations to broaden thrombolytic eligibility to include patients of any age presenting within 12 hours of symptom onset, large U.S. registries have revealed that currently only 22% to 35% of patients with AMI receive thrombolytic therapy.[136–139]

## PRIMARY PTCA APPROACH

To overcome the limitations of thrombolytic therapy, selected centers shifted to a mechanical approach to reperfusion in AMI, using balloon angioplasty. In the "primary," or "direct," PTCA strategy, thrombolytic therapy is expressly withheld, and the patient is transferred on an emergency basis to the cardiac catheterization laboratory for left ventriculography and selective coronary arteriography. The infarcted artery is identified, and PTCA is performed if appropriate. The term *primary PTCA* is actually somewhat of a misnomer, because the strategy is, in fact, emergency cardiac catheterization followed by the most appropriate means of obtaining reperfusion, tailored to the specific clinical and anatomic findings of each individual patient. Although prior studies have demonstrated that PTCA is performed in approximately 90% of patients, approximately 5% of patients have severe left main coronary artery disease or other features highly unfavorable for PTCA; these patients are best served by urgent or emergency bypass surgery. An additional 5% of patients exhibit spontaneous reperfusion, with residual stenosis affecting less than 70% of the vessel diameter and TIMI grade 3 flow; these patients are treated conservatively, and potential complications from either PTCA or thrombolysis are avoided. A rare patient is identified with minimal atherosclerosis and primary coronary thrombosis, most effectively treated by local intracoronary thrombolysis. Finally, coronary arteriography occasionally reveals normal left ventricular function without obstructive coronary artery disease, prompting the search for other conditions that may clinically and electrocardiographically mimic AMI, such as dissecting aortic aneurysm, myocarditis, pericarditis, or cholecystitis, thereby avoiding the potentially hazardous application of thrombolytic

therapy in these patients.[140] This situation is not trivial; in the Anglo-Scandinavian Study of Early Thrombosis (ASSET) trial,[5] 4.1% of patients enrolled with suspected AMI had noncoronary conditions, and an additional 6.4% had coronary artery disease without AMI. The 30-day mortality rates were 1.2% of patients randomly assigned to receive placebo and 9.5% of those receiving tPA. Thus, unlike the thrombolytic approach, wherein all patients are blindly treated with a pharmacologic agent, the primary PTCA approach is similar to the elective management of the nonemergency patient with a chest pain syndrome; the most appropriate treatment modality—whether it be percutaneous intervention, medication, or surgery—is chosen dictated by the baseline clinical, functional, and angiographic findings.

After the performance of the first primary PTCA by the group at the Mid America Heart Institute in November 1980,[141] the technique was rapidly adopted by other centers and is now the sole method used for reperfusion at selected institutions around the world. From the outset, it became evident that primary PTCA offered several notable advantages compared to thrombolysis. First and foremost, by withholding thrombolytic therapy, the occurrence of major hemorrhagic complications are markedly reduced, and the risk of intracerebral bleeding is essentially eliminated. Left ventriculography affords assessment of hemodynamic parameters and the determination of ventricular and valvular function, which are of powerful prognostic importance and clinically useful in patient management.[9, 142–152] In addition to identifying the infarcted vessel and the amount of myocardium at risk, coronary arteriography also reveals the extent of coronary artery disease and the status of collateral blood flow, the presence of which may prolong myocardial viability. PTCA, unlike thrombolysis, treats the underlying ruptured atherosclerotic plaque as well as the occlusive clot, thereby enhancing myocardial recovery and decreasing recurrent ischemia.[58, 153] In addition, the outcome of the attempted reperfusion is immediately known, as is the post-PTCA residual stenosis, presence or absence of residual thrombus or dissection, and the TIMI flow grade. A final difference from thrombolytic therapy is that most patients with AMI may benefit from primary PTCA; the only absolute contraindications are total absence of vascular access (e.g., as in Takayasu's arteritis), previous anaphylactoid contrast allergy, and absolute contraindications to heparin. Marked renal insufficiency in a patient not yet on dialysis constitutes a relative contraindication.

## Results of Primary PTCA in AMI

The publication of large, single-center observational series, prospective multicenter registry data, and multiple randomized comparisons of primary PTCA with thrombolytic therapy has contributed to the knowledge about the use of primary PTCA in AMI.

### Single-Center, Observational Series of Primary PTCA in AMI

The results of primary PTCA in a total of 2768 patients with AMI have been reported from 15 single-center experiences[141, 154–167] (Table 11–4). It must be recognized that the patients treated in these studies were quite different from those enrolled in thrombolytic trials. In general, patients undergoing primary PTCA represent an unselected population without exclusion criteria applied. Thus, analysis of the overall results must take into account the absence of age or symptom duration limitation, the relatively high percentage of enrolled patients who have undergone bypass surgery and those in cardiogenic shock, and the large percentage of patients included who otherwise would have been ineligible for thrombolytic therapy. Nonetheless, the short-term outcomes are quite favorable; patency has been achieved in 93% of patients, a greater percentage than that achieved by thrombolytic therapy alone[9, 10, 42, 168–170] (see Table 11–4). The short-term mortality rate of only 7.2% is also significantly less than that of historical controls, in view of the high-risk baseline features of the treated cohort. In patients undergoing immediate and predischarge left ventriculography, the paired LVEF rose from a mean of 49% on admission to 57% at discharge, which is consistent with marked myocardial recovery. In contrast, serial in-hospital measures of left ventricular function have not been shown to improve after thrombolytic therapy without adjunctive angioplasty.[171] The mean incidence of infarcted artery reocclusion after primary PTCA has been reported to be 10%; as dis-

cussed later, this relatively high rate in the early studies may reflect the lack of use of aspirin[172, 173] or of ionic contrast agents[144–177] or inadequate heparinization in many patients.[178–182]

### Lessons from Kansas City

Significant lessons can be learned from the Mid America Heart Institute practice, the single center with the most extensive experience (>2200 primary PTCA procedures have been performed).[141, 183–191] At this institution, 96% of patients with AMI who were eligible for reperfusion have been treated by primary PTCA.[141, 183] High-risk adverse features present at baseline in the patient population included cardiogenic shock (in 8% of patients), LVEF of less than 40% (in 29%), age of more than 70 years (in 22%), multivessel disease (in 57%), history of bypass surgery (in 13%), and one or more conditions contraindicating thrombolytic therapy (in 43%). The rate of successful recanalization in the infarcted artery was high (94%), whether the artery was initially occluded (TIMI grade 0 flow, 93% patency restored) or patent (TIMI grade 1 or higher flow, 96% patency achieved). In contrast, infarcted artery recanalization rates after thrombolytic therapy are significantly lower if the infarcted artery is initially totally occluded.[8] Primary PTCA was particularly efficacious in patients with single-vessel disease, in whom a 99% success rate was reported.[182] The success rate of primary PTCA did not vary among the three native epicardial coronary arteries, although immediate patency was lower in saphenous vein grafts and in patients with cardiogenic shock or multivessel disease (Table 11–5).[141, 184, 186, 189] According to logistic regression analysis, independent predictors of in-hospital mortality after primary PTCA were cardiogenic shock, failure to recanalize

### TABLE 11–4. SINGLE CENTER SERIES OF PRIMARY PTCA

| SERIES | N | VESSEL PATENCY | IN-HOSPITAL MORTALITY RATE | REOCCLUSION RATE | ACUTE LVEF | PREDISCHARGE LVEF |
|---|---|---|---|---|---|---|
| O'Keefe et al[141] | 1000 | 94% | 7.7% | 13% | 50% | 57% |
| Brodie et al[154] | 383 | 91% | 9.0% | NR | NR | NR |
| Beauchamp et al[155] | 214 | 92% | 7.9% | NR | NR | NR |
| Hanlon et al[156] | 204 | 94% | 3.4% | NR | NR | NR |
| Nakagawa et al[157] | 190 | 90% | 4.0% | NR | NR | NR |
| Rothbaum et al[158] | 151 | 87% | 9.0% | 9% | 39% | 50% |
| Zimarino et al[159] | 132 | 86% | 3.0% | NR | NR | NR |
| Miller et al[160] | 127 | 92% | 8.6% | 8% | NR | NR |
| Dageford et al[161] | 65 | 97% | 1.5% | 9% | NR | NR |
| O'Neill et al[162] | 63 | 92% | 6.3% | NR | NR | NR |
| Brush et al[163] | 62 | 96% | 3.2% | 0% | NR | NR |
| Kimura et al[164] | 58 | 88% | NR | 2% | NR | NR |
| Topol[165] | 47 | 86% | 6.3% | 13% | NR | NR |
| Marco et al[166] | 43 | 95% | 9.3% | NR | 54% | 58% |
| O'Neill et al[167] | 29 | 83% | 6.8% | 8% | 50% | 58% |
| Pooled | 2768 | 93% | 7.2% | 10% | 49% | 57% |

LVEF, left ventricular or ejection fraction; NR = not reported; PTCA, percutaneous transluminal coronary angioplasty.

**TABLE 11–5. PTCA SUCCESS AND IN-HOSPITAL MORTALITY RATES AMONG 1000 CONSECUTIVE PATIENTS UNDERGOING PRIMARY PTCA AT THE MID AMERICA HEART INSTITUTE[141]**

| MEASUREMENT | N | PTCA | | IN-HOSPITAL | |
| --- | --- | --- | --- | --- | --- |
| | | SUCCESS RATE | p | MORTALITY RATE | p |
| **Demographic** | | | | | |
| All | 1000 | 94% | — | 8% | — |
| Men | 723 | 94% | — | 7% | |
| Women | 277 | 94% | NS | 11% | 0.04 |
| Age < 70 | 778 | 94% | | 6% | |
| Age ≥ 70 | 222 | 93% | NS | 13% | <0.001 |
| **Event** | | | | | |
| Anterior MI | 424 | 92% | | 11% | |
| Nonanterior MI | 576 | 95% | 0.04 | 6% | 0.003 |
| Initial TIMI-0 | 629 | 93% | | 8% | |
| Initial TIMI-1 to -3 | 371 | 96% | 0.07 | 8% | NS |
| Reperfusion in <6 h | 729 | 94% | | 8% | |
| Reperfusion in ≥6 h | 211 | 95% | NS | 8% | NS |
| LVEF ≥ 40% | 709 | 95% | | 4% | |
| LVEF < 40% | 291 | 92% | 0.06 | 17% | 0.0001 |
| Cardiogenic shock | 79 | 82% | | 44% | |
| No cardiogenic shock | 921 | 95% | 0.001 | 5% | <0.0001 |
| Thrombolytic exclusions | 432 | 92% | | 14% | |
| Thrombolytic eligible | 568 | 96% | 0.01 | 3% | <0.0001 |
| No prior bypass surgery | 870 | 95% | | 8% | |
| Prior bypass surgery | 130 | 90% | 0.05 | 10% | NS |

LVEF, left ventricular ejection fraction; MI, myocardial infarction; NS, nonsignificant; PTCA, percutaneous transluminal coronary angioplasty; TIMI, Thrombolysis In Myocardial Infarction (flow).

the infarcted vessel, baseline LVEF of 40% or less, triple-vessel disease, anterior infarction, and age of more than 70 years (see Table 11–5). Other investigators have reached similar conclusions.[154, 158, 160] Paired admission and predischarge left ventriculograms were present for analysis in 88% of patients at the Mid America Heart Institute. The global LVEF rose from 49.7% at baseline to 57.4% at discharge. Independent correlates of improved global left ventricular function after primary PTCA included baseline LVEF of less than 40%, anterior myocardial infarction, sustained patency of the infarcted vessel (at predischarge angiography), and baseline TIMI flow of higher than grade 1. The improvement in LVEF was particularly gratifying in patients with cardiogenic shock; the mean LVEF was 30% on admission and rose to 42% at the time of discharge ($p < 0.0001$). The mean 7-year survival rate according to actuarial analysis was 80%; LVEF of less than 40%, presence of triple-vessel disease, age of more than 70 years, and presence of cardiogenic shock were identified as multivariate predictors of late mortality. During a mean follow-up period of 3.6 years, 53% of patients required repeat PTCA, 16% underwent late bypass surgery, and 13% experienced a Q-wave myocardial infarction.

The rate of mortality after failed primary PTCA is high, ranging from 34% to 39% in large series.[141, 154, 155] It has therefore been suggested that the stress of cardiac catheterization, the adverse effects of radiocontrast agents, and reperfusion arrhythmias may be inherent dangers to the patient with AMI. To address this issue, Bedotto and associates examined the presenting characteristics and hospital course of patients in whom primary PTCA was unsuccessful.[186] In this series, the in-hospital mortality rate was 5% among the 94% of patients in whom PTCA was successful, in contrast to 31% among patients in whom PTCA failed ($p < 0.0001$). Patients with failed PTCA were more likely than patients with successful PTCA to have triple-vessel disease (44% vs. 23%; $p < 0.003$), to have had a prior myocardial infarction (44% vs. 28%; $p < 0.03$), to have cardiogenic shock on admission (22% vs. 7%; $p < 0.003$), and to require emergency coronary artery bypass grafting (CABG) (27% vs. 0.5%; $p < 0.0001$). The only independent predictors of PTCA failure were the presence of cardiogenic shock and the presence of multivessel disease. Multiple high-risk features were present in patients dying after PTCA, including cardiogenic shock (50%), a history of prior myocardial infarction (43%), and multivessel disease (93%). Similarly, Zimarino and colleagues found that cardiogenic shock and left ventricular dysfunction were the strongest independent predictors of both angioplasty failure and untoward events (death or need for emergency CABG) after primary PTCA.[159] Thus, it is likely that the high mortality rate in this setting results from high-risk factors that are present in patients in whom PTCA fails, rather than from adverse effects of the procedure itself.

### The Primary Angioplasty Revascularization (PAR) Registry

The PAR registry was organized to further investigate the relative advantages of primary PTCA as an alternative to thrombolytic therapy at experienced centers. Emergency cardiac catheterization was prospectively performed at six clinical sites in 271 consecutive patients of any age who had suffered AMI within the previous 12 hours and who otherwise would have been eligible to receive thrombolytic therapy.[192] PTCA was performed in 245 patients (90%). The mean time from symptom onset to emergency room presentation was 108 minutes; from presentation to catheterization, 84 minutes; and from catheterization to reperfusion, 34 minutes. According to independent core laboratory analysis at the Duke University Medical Center, patency was restored in 99% of all patients; 97% achieved TIMI grade 3 flow, and 88% achieved residual stenosis affecting less than 50% of the vessel diameter. In-hospital mortality occurred in 3.7% of patients, reinfarction in 2.6%, stroke in 1.1%, and recurrent ischemia in 9.6%.

At the end of the 6-month follow-up period,[193] the mortality rate was 1.9%, the rate of nonfatal reinfarction was 3.1%, and repeat PTCA was performed in 16.3% of the group. Follow-up angiography was performed in 76% of surviving patients and demonstrated restenosis in 45% of infarcted vessels, including reocclusion in 13%. The majority of infarcted artery reocclusions were asymptomatic; only 35% resulted in reinfarction. In addition, however, late sustained patency of the infarcted vessel was an important determinant of ultimate myocardial salvage. The serial improvement in LVEF from the initial to the follow-up study was 8% for infarcted arteries that remained patent but 0% for those that reoccluded.[193] Thus, the results of the PAR Registry, in concert with earlier single-center observational series, supported the position that in comparison with thrombolytic therapy, primary PTCA at experienced centers results in greater patency and higher TIMI grade 3 flow rates; in low subsequent rates of mortality, reinfarction, and recurrent ischemia; and in improved late patency of the infarcted vessel, a major determinant of sustained myocardial recovery.

### Roadblocks to the Acceptance of Primary PTCA

Despite these favorable results, the widespread acceptance of primary PTCA for use in AMI was hindered by relatively disappointing outcomes of adjunctive PTCA after thrombolysis. Three trials of immediate PTCA after thrombolysis found increased rates of acute closure, need for emergency bypass surgery, hemorrhagic and vascular complications, and a disturbing trend toward increased mortality among the invasively managed patients.[194–196] Five trials examining the routine performance of delayed PTCA before hospital discharge in thrombolytic-treated patients were unable to demonstrate convincing evidence of benefit of the PTCA strategy.[197–201] Even the approach of rescue PTCA after failed thrombolysis, evaluated in a meta-analysis of 12 observational series and two moderate-sized randomized trials, demonstrated at most marginal advantages in terms of improved regional wall motion and LVEF, reduced rate of recurrent ischemia, and reduced rate of congestive heart failure, the benefits of which were offset by high rates of mortality and infarcted artery reocclusion.[63, 64, 202]

### The SAMI Trial

The equivocal results of intervention in AMI after thrombolytic therapy were initially difficult to place in perspective, in view of the otherwise excellent results of primary PTCA. Ultimately, O'Neill and colleagues hypothesized that the addition of thrombolytic therapy to PTCA in AMI not only was *not* beneficial but was actually harmful, serving to erode the otherwise salutary outcomes of primary PTCA when performed without antecedent thrombolysis. This theory was tested in the Streptokinase Angioplasty in Myocardial Infarction (SAMI) trial.[203] In this prospective, randomized study, 121 thrombolytic-eligible patients presenting within 4 hours of AMI onset were treated with aspirin and heparin and then, in a blinded manner, were randomly assigned to receive either intravenous streptokinase or placebo, after which they were immediately transferred to the cardiac catheterization laboratory for angiography and, if appropriate, PTCA. There were no baseline clinical or angiographic differences between the two groups. In comparison with patients treated with placebo and PTCA (i.e., primary PTCA), patients treated with streptokinase followed by immediate PTCA had higher rates of infarct artery reocclusion (necessitating emergency bypass surgery), more numerous hemorrhagic and vascular complications, and a more prolonged and expensive hospital course (Table 11–6). No differences in immediate or late infarcted artery patency, left ventricular function, rates of restenosis, or mortality were apparent.

### The TAUSA and TIMI-IIIB Trials

Two other well-designed, randomized studies also found worse outcomes when PTCA was combined

**TABLE 11–6.    RESULTS OF THE STREPTOKINASE ANGIOPLASTY MYOCARDIAL INFARCTON (SAMI) TRIAL**

| OUTCOME | STREPTOKINASE + PTCA (N = 58) | PTCA ALONE (N = 63) | p |
|---|---|---|---|
| **In-Hospital Outcomes** | | | |
| Eligible for PTCA | 81% | 92% | 0.08 |
| Successful PTCA | 98% | 92% | NS |
| Mortality | 5.1% | 6.5% | NS |
| Bypass surgery within 24 h | 10.3% | 1.6% | 0.03 |
| Recurerent ischemia | 12% | 16% | NS |
| Nadir hemoglobin level | 10.5 ± 1.8 | 11.9 ± 1.7 | 0.03 |
| Blood transfusion | 39% | 8% | 0.0001 |
| Vascular complications | 29% | 5% | 0.004 |
| Systemic bleeding complications | 10% | 0% | 0.01 |
| Radionuclide LVEF at 24 hours | 50% ± 12% | 52% ± 12% | NS |
| Length of hospital stay (days) | 9.3 ± 5.0 | 7.7 ± 4.0 | 0.046 |
| Hospital charges | $25,191 ± $15,368 | $19,643 ± $7,250 | 0.02 |
| **6-Month Outcomes** | | | |
| Radionuclide LVEF at 6 months | 51% ± 13% | 51% ± 12% | NS |
| Arterial patency | 86% | 89% | NS |
| Restenosis | 31% | 37% | NS |

LVEF, left ventricular ejection fraction; NS, nonsignificant; PTCA, percutaneous transluminal coronary angioplasty.

with thrombolytic therapy than when PTCA was used alone in acute ischemic syndromes. In the Thrombolysis and Angioplasty in UnStable Angina (TAUSA) trial, 469 patients with unstable angina, non–Q-wave myocardial infarction, or post-myocardial infarction angina were randomly assigned to receive 250,000 to 500,000 units of intracoronary urokinase or placebo before PTCA.[204] In comparison with placebo recipients, patients treated with urokinase experienced *increased* incidences of acute closure (10.2% vs. 4.3%; p = 0.02) and major cardiac events (12.9% vs. 6.3%; p = 0.02). The increased rate of abrupt closure with urokinase was especially marked in lesions with angiographic characteristics most likely to benefit from thrombolysis,[205] including complex lesions (15.0% abrupt closure with urokinase vs. 5.9% without urokinase), and filling defects (18.8% vs. 8.3%, respectively). Spielberg and associates also reported that acute closure rates were increased by the adjunctive use of intracoronary urokinase during PTCA.[206] Similarly, in the TIMI-IIIB trial,[207, 208] among 471 patients with at-rest angina or non–Q-wave myocardial infarction treated with PTCA, those randomly assigned to receive intravenous tPA 1 to 2 days before PTCA had higher rates of major adverse cardiac events (death, myocardial infarction, need for bypass surgery, or abrupt closure) than did those treated with PTCA alone (11% vs. 4%; p = 0.06).

### Explanation for the Worsened Outcomes of PTCA with Adjunctive Thrombolysis

Thus, it has been demonstrated clearly that the addition of thrombolytic therapy worsens the otherwise favorable results expected with PTCA alone in acute ischemic syndromes. Both pathologic and hematologic mechanisms may underlie this phenomenon. Waller and coworkers performed autopsies on 19 patients who had died shortly after initially successful thrombolysis, PTCA, or the combination.[209] Hemorrhagic infarction was present in all patients who had received thrombolytic therapy (with or without adjunctive PTCA) but was not seen in any patient treated with primary PTCA alone. In addition, hemorrhage into the plaque and arterial media was present only in coronary arteries treated with the combination of thrombolysis and PTCA. These findings have been confirmed by Colavita and colleagues.[210] In addition, in the TAUSA trial, post-PTCA dissections became increasingly severe over a 15-minute period if intracoronary thrombolytics had previously been given.[211] Furthermore, the administration of thrombolytic therapy results in platelet activation and a procoagulant effect, which may be particularly deleterious, in view of the increased platelet aggregation induced by PTCA.[212–215] Together, the combination of intraplaque and intramural hemorrhage, propagating dissection and enhancing platelet activation, is the likely explanation for the increased rate of abrupt closure after PTCA when thrombolytics are given. Finally, in an open-chest canine model, reperfusion injury after PTCA-mediated recanalization of an occluded infarcted vessel, negligible after primary PTCA alone, was markedly increased in severity if a systemic lytic state was also present.[216] Reperfusion injury, in combination with myocardial hemorrhage,[210, 211] may result in blunted myocardial recovery or increased myocardial necrosis with infarction extension when

PTCA is performed in concert with thrombolytic therapy.

## Randomized Trials of Primary PTCA and Thrombolytic Therapy

The widespread recognition of primary PTCA as a superior reperfusion modality awaited the results of prospective, randomized trials in which primary PTCA was compared directly with thrombolytic therapy. The first such trial was performed in 1984 and reported in 1986.[167, 217] In this pilot study, 56 patients presenting within 12 hours of onset of AMI were randomly assigned to receive intracoronary streptokinase or undergo primary PTCA.[167, 217] The time to reperfusion (4.8 vs. 4.1 hours, respectively) and the degree of patency achieved (85% vs. 83%) were similar with the two strategies. The residual stenosis, however, was significantly lower in the PTCA group (43% vs. 83%; $p < 0.001$), which was associated with significantly greater serial improvement in mean regional wall motion as assessed by the Sheehan-Dodge (SD) method (+1.32 vs. +0.59 SD/chord; $p < 0.05$) and global LVEF (+8% vs. +1%; $p < 0.001$). PTCA also resulted in less peri-infarction ischemia on predischarge exercise thallium 201 testing than after thrombolysis (14% vs. 45%; $p < 0.05$). Despite these encouraging results, however, additional randomized trials were not begun for 7 years, partly because of the reluctance of many physicians regularly performing primary PTCA to randomly assign patients to treatment, in view of ethical concerns.

Since 1994, however, a total of 10 randomized trials involving 2606 patients have prospectively compared primary PTCA with several different intravenous regimens of thrombolytic therapy. The thrombolytic agent used was streptokinase in four trials (608 patients randomly selected),[218-222] tPA dosed over 3 to 4 hours in three trials (588 patients randomly selected),[223-225] and front-loaded "accelerated" tPA in three trials (1410 patients randomly selected).[226-228] A comparison of the entry criteria for these studies appears in Table 11-7. Aspirin was given in all trials, as was intravenous heparin, except in the GUSTO-IIb angioplasty substudy, in which half of the patients in each group received hirudin rather than heparin.[226] The three accelerated tPA trials are notable in that approximately half of all the patients enrolled in the entire meta-analysis were from one of these studies,[226] whereas in the other two trials the entry criteria were tailored to randomly assign patients at predominantly high risk, either all with anterior myocardial infarctions[227] or all with inferior myocardial infarctions with reciprocal anterior ST segment depression.[228]

### Meta-analysis of the 10 PTCA-Thrombolysis Trials

A meta-analysis of the short-term outcomes from these trials was completed by Douglas Weaver, working in concert with the principal investigators from each study. On average, thrombolysis was initiated 26 minutes earlier than PTCA. The overall mortality rate at the end of the study period, however, was reduced from 6.6% after thrombolytic therapy

## TABLE 11-7. RANDOMIZED TRIALS OF PRIMARY PTCA VERSUS THROMBOLYTIC THERAPY

| | | | | | NO. PATIENTS | | TIME TO TREATMENT | |
|---|---|---|---|---|---|---|---|---|
| TRIAL | PATIENT POPULATION | LYTIC AGENT | SYMPTOM DURATION | STUDY PERIOD | PTCA | THROM-BOLYSIS | PTCA | THROM-BOLYSIS |
| Zjilstra et al[218] and De Boer et al[219] | ≤75 y, ST ↑ | 1.5 MU SK over 1 h | <6 h | Hospital discharge | 152 | 149 | 62 min* | 30 min* |
| Ribeiro et al[220] | <75 y, ST ↑ | 1.2 MU SK over 1 h | <12 h | Hospital discharge | 50 | 50 | 238 min† | 179 min† |
| Grinfeld et al[221] | Any age, ST ↑ | 1.5 MU SK over 1 h | <12 h | 30 days | 54 | 58 | 63 min‡ | 18 min‡ |
| Zjilstra et al[222] | Low risk, ST ↑ | 1.5 MU SK over 1 h | <12 h | 30 days | 45 | 50 | 68 min* | 29 min* |
| Grines[223]: The PAMI Trial | Any age, ST ↑ | Alteplase, 100 mg, over 3 h | <12 h | Hospital discharge | 195 | 200 | 60 min* | 32 min* |
| Gibbons et al[224] | <80 y, ST ↑ | Duteplase over 4 h | <12 h | Hospital discharge | 47 | 56 | 45 min* | 20 min* |
| DeWood[225] | <77 y, ST ↑ | Duteplase over 4 h | <12 h | 30 days | 46 | 44 | 126 min* | 84 min* |
| GUSTO-IIb[226] | Any age, ST ↑ or LBBB | Alteplase, 100 mg, 90 min | <12 h | 30 days | 565 | 573 | 114 min‡ | 72 min‡ |
| Garcia et al[227] | Any age, anterior MI | Alteplase, 100 mg, 90 min | <5 h | 30 days | 95 | 94 | 69 min* | 84 min* |
| Ribichini et al[228] | <80 y, inferior MI + anterior ST ↓ | Activase 90 min | <12 h | Hospital discharge | 41 | 42 | 40 min‡ | 33 min‡ |
| Pooled | — | — | — | — | 1290 | 1316 | — | — |

GUSTO, Global Utilization of Streptokinase and Tissue Plasminogen Activator for Occluded Coronary Arteries; LBBB, left bundle branch block; MI, myocardial infarction; PAMI, Primary Angioplasty in Myocardial Infarction; PTCA, percutaneous transluminal coronary angioplasty; SK, streptokinase; ST, ST segment.

↑, elevation; ↓, depression.
*From admission.
†From chest pain onset.
‡From randomization.

**TABLE 11–8. META-ANALYSIS OF PRIMARY PTCA VERSUS THROMBOLYTIC THERAPY: MORTALITY**

| TRIAL | PTCA | THROMBOLYSIS | ODDS RATIO (95% CI) | p |
|---|---|---|---|---|
| Streptokinase trials | | | | |
|   Zjilstra et al[218] and De Boer et al[219] | 2.0% | 7.4% | — | — |
|   Ribeiro et al[220] | 6.0% | 2.0% | — | — |
|   Grinfeld et al[221] | 9.3% | 10.3% | — | — |
|   Zjilstra et al[222] | 2.2% | 0% | — | — |
|   All streptokinase trials | 4.0% | 5.9% | 0.66 (0.29, 1.50) | 0.38 |
| 3- to 4-h tPA trials | | | | |
|   Grines et al[223]: the PAMI trial | 2.6% | 6.5% | — | — |
|   Gibbons et al[224] | 4.3% | 3.6% | — | — |
|   DeWood[225] | 6.5% | 4.6% | — | — |
|   All 3- to 4-h tPA trials | 3.5% | 5.7% | 0.60 (0.24, 1.41) | 0.28 |
| Accelerated tPA trials | | | | |
|   GUSTO-IIb[226] | 5.7% | 7.0% | — | — |
|   Garcia et al[227] | 3.2% | 10.6% | — | – |
|   Ribichini et al[228] | 0% | 2.4% | — | — |
|   All accelerated tPA trials | 5.0% | 7.2% | 0.68 (0.42, 10.8) | 0.10 |
| All trials | 4.4% | 6.6% | 0.66 (0.46, 0.94) | 0.02 |

CI, confidence interval; GUSTO, Global Utilization of Streptokinase and Tissue Plasminogen Activator for Occluded Coronary Arteries; PAMI, Primary Angioplasty in Myocardial Infarction; PTCA, percutaneous transluminal coronary angioplasty; tPA, tissue-type plasminogen activator.

to 4.4% after primary PTCA, corresponding to an odds ratio reduction of 0.66 (95% confidence interval [CI]: 0.46 to 0.94) (Table 11–8). This absolute benefit of saving 2 lives per 100 patients treated with PTCA rather than thrombolysis is similar in magnitude to the survival benefit of thrombolytic therapy in comparison to a medically treated control population (Fig. 11–5).[114] As seen in Table 11–8, the magnitude of the reduction in mortality after primary PTCA in comparison with thrombolytic therapy was similar across the three thrombolytic regimens. The relative reduction in death or nonfatal reinfarction after primary PTCA in comparison with tPA is even more striking (11.9% vs. 7.2%; odds ratio, 0.58 [95% CI: 0.44 to 0.76]; $p = 0.001$)

(Table 11–9). Nonfatal reinfarction alone was reduced from 5.3% after thrombolysis to 2.9% after PTCA ($p = 0.002$).

The findings of the meta-analyses comparing total stroke and intracranial hemorrhage appear in Tables 11–10 and 11–11, respectively. Total stroke rate was reduced from 2.0% after thrombolysis to 0.7% after PTCA, an odds ratio of 0.35 (95% CI: 0.14 to 0.77). As seen in Figure 11–5, this reduction in stroke with primary PTCA is in direct opposition to the excessive rate of stroke with thrombolysis in comparison with placebo. The reduction in total stroke with primary PTCA could be attributed almost completely to the near elimination of the risk of intracranial hemorrhage after PTCA in comparison with

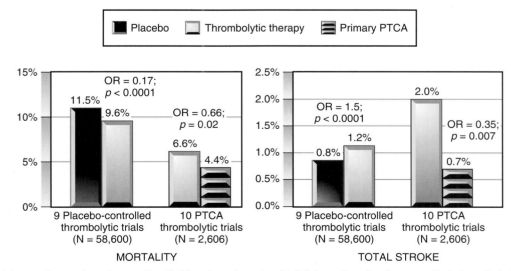

FIGURE 11–5. Meta-analyses of total mortality *(left)* and stroke rates *(right)* from the placebo-controlled thrombolytic therapy trials (adapted from reference 114) and from a 10-study analysis of primary PTCA versus thrombolytic therapy. OR, odds ratio; PTCA, percutaneous transluminal coronary angioplasty.

**TABLE 11–9.    META-ANALYSIS OF PRIMARY PTCA VERSUS THROMBOLYTIC THERAPY: DEATH OR NONFATAL REINFARCTION**

| TRIAL | PTCA | THROMBOLYSIS | ODDS RATIO (95% CI) | p |
|---|---|---|---|---|
| Streptokinase trials | | | | |
| Zjilstra et al[218] and De Boer et al[219] | 3.2% | 15.4% | — | — |
| Ribeiro et al[220] | 10.0% | 4.0% | — | — |
| Grinfeld et al[221] | 11.1% | 12.1% | — | — |
| Zjilstra et al[222] | 2.2% | 16.0% | — | — |
| All streptokinase trials | 5.6% | 13.0% | 0.41 (0.21, 0.75) | 0.003 |
| 3- to 4-h tPA trials | | | | |
| Grines et al[223]: the PAMI trial | 5.1% | 12.0% | — | — |
| Gibbons et al[224] | 6.4% | 8.9% | — | — |
| DeWood[225] | 6.5% | 4.5% | — | — |
| All 3- to 4-h tPA trials | 5.6% | 10.3% | 0.51 (0.26, 0.99) | 0.047 |
| Accelerated tPA trials | | | | |
| GUSTO-IIb[226] | 9.6% | 12.2% | — | — |
| Garcia et al[227] | 7.4% | 14.9% | — | — |
| Ribichini et al[228] | 0% | 2.4% | — | — |
| All accelerated tPA trials | 8.7% | 12.0% | 0.70 (0.48, 1.0) | 0.05 |
| All trials | 7.2% | 11.9% | 0.58 (0.44, 076) | 0.001 |

CI, confidence interval; GUSTO, Global Utilization of Streptokinase and Tissue Plasminogen Activator for Occluded Coronary Arteries; PAMI, Primary Angioplasty in Myocardial Infarction; PTCA, percutaneous transluminal coronary angioplasty; tPA, tissue-type plasminogen activator.

thrombolytic therapy (0.1% vs. 1.1%; odds ratio, 0.07 [95% CI: 0.0 to 0.43]). Indeed, only one hemorrhagic stroke occurred in any of these trials after primary PTCA. Thus, the results of this meta-analysis strongly support the contention that in comparison with thrombolytic therapy, primary PTCA improves survival rates and reduces the rates of reinfarction, total stroke, and hemorrhagic stroke, independently of lytic regimen.

*Lessons from the Randomized PTCA-Thrombolysis Trials*

Three trials (the PAMI trial, the Zwolle trial, and GUSTO-IIb) were sufficiently large to potentially demonstrate differences in the composite end point

of death or reinfarction between primary PTCA and thrombolytic therapy.

**THE PRIMARY ANGIOPLASTY IN MYOCARDIAL INFARCTION (PAMI) TRIAL.**[223, 229–241] The PAMI trial was instrumental in establishing the superiority of primary PTCA as a reperfusion modality in AMI. In the PAMI trial,[223] 395 patients of any age with AMI within 12 hours of AMI onset were prospectively assigned randomly at 12 international centers to undergo primary PTCA or receive a 3-hour, 100-mg tPA infusion, at that time the most widely used thrombolytic regimen in the United States. The trial was powered to demonstrate a reduction in the combined end point of death or nonfatal reinfarction.

**TABLE 11–10.    META-ANALYSIS OF PRIMARY PTCA VERSUS THROMBOLYTIC THERAPY: TOTAL STROKE**

| TRIAL | PTCA | THROMBOLYSIS | ODDS RATIO (95% CI) | p |
|---|---|---|---|---|
| Streptokinase trials | | | | |
| Zjilstra et al[218] and De Boer et al[219] | 0.7% | 2.0% | — | — |
| Ribeiro et al[220] | 0% | 0% | — | — |
| Grinfeld et al[221] | 1.9% | 0% | — | — |
| Zjilstra et al[222] | 2.2% | 4.0% | — | — |
| All streptokinase trials | 1.0% | 1.6% | 0.62 (0.10, 3.22) | 0.77 |
| 3- to 4-h tPA trials | | | | |
| Grines et al[223]: the PAMI trial | 0% | 0% | — | — |
| Gibbons et al[224] | 0% | 3.5% | — | — |
| DeWood[225] | 0% | 0% | — | — |
| All 3- to 4-h tPA trials | 0% | 2.3% | 0.00 (0.00, 0.54) | 0.016 |
| Accelerated tPA trials | | | | |
| GUSTO-IIb[226] | 1.1% | 1.9% | — | — |
| Garcia et al[227] | 0% | 3.2% | — | — |
| Ribichini et al[228] | 0% | 0% | — | — |
| All accelerated tPA trials | 0.9% | 2.0% | 0.43 (0.13, 1.20) | 0.12 |
| All trials | 0.7% | 2.0% | 0.35 (0.14, 0.77) | 0.007 |

CI, confidence interval; GUSTO, Global Utilization of Streptokinase and Tissue Plasminogen Activator for Occluded Coronary Arteries; PAMI, Primary Angioplasty in Myocardial Infarction; PTCA, percutaneous transluminal coronary angioplasty; tPA, tissue-type plasminogen activator.

**TABLE 11–11.  META-ANALYSIS OF PRIMARY PTCA VERSUS THROMBOLYTIC THERAPY: HEMORRHAGIC STROKE**

| TRIAL | PTCA | THROMBOLYSIS | ODDS RATIO (95% CI) | p |
|---|---|---|---|---|
| Streptokinase trials | | | | |
| Zjilstra et al[218] and De Boer et al[219] | 0.7% | 2.0% | — | — |
| Ribeiro et al[220] | 0% | 0% | — | — |
| Grinfeld et al[221] | 0% | 0% | — | — |
| Zjilstra et al[222] | 0% | 4.0% | — | — |
| All streptokinase trials | 0.3% | 0.7% | 0.49 (0.01, 9.47) | 0.99 |
| 3- to 4-h tPA trials | | | | |
| Grines et al[223]: the PAMI trial | 0% | 0% | — | — |
| Gibbons et al[224] | 0% | 3.5% | — | — |
| DeWood[225] | 0% | 0% | — | — |
| All 3- to 4-h tPA trials | 0% | 1.3% | 0.00 (0.00, 1.14) | 0.13 |
| Accelerated tPA trials | | | | |
| GUSTO-IIb[226] | 0% | 1.4% | — | — |
| Garcia et al[227] | 0% | 1.2% | — | — |
| Ribichini et al[228] | 0% | 0% | — | — |
| All accelerated tPA trials | 0% | 1.3% | 0.00 (0.00, 0.40) | 0.004 |
| All trials | 0.1% | 1.1% | 0.07 (0.00, 0.43) | 0.0005 |

CI, confidence interval; GUSTO, Global Utilization of Streptokinase and Tissue Plasminogen Activator for Occluded Coronary Arteries; PAMI, Primary Angioplasty in Myocardial Infarction; PTCA, percutaneous transluminal coronary angioplasty; tPA, tissue-type plasminogen activator.

Among the 195 patients randomly assigned to undergo PTCA, angioplasty was performed in 175 (90%). The other 20 patients either were managed conservatively, spontaneous reperfusion having already occurred ($n = 9$), or underwent urgent or emergency CABG for left main coronary artery disease ($n = 1$) or severe triple-vessel disease with features unfavorable for PTCA ($n = 8$). One patient had a small diagonal branch occlusion, which was also managed medically, and one patient with primary thrombosis was treated with intracoronary urokinase. Core laboratory analysis revealed that among the patients undergoing dilatation, TIMI grade 2 or 3 flow was restored in 99%, 94% achieved TIMI grade 3 flow, and 97% had residual stenosis involving less than 50% of the vessel diameter. Although the tPA infusion was started, on average, 28 minutes earlier than angiography (60 vs. 32

minutes; $p = 0.001$), patients treated with PTCA were free of pain sooner than after tPA ($290 \pm 174$ minutes vs. $354 \pm 241$ minutes; $p = 0.004$). As seen in Figure 11–6, PTCA, in comparison with tPA, resulted in lower rates of death or reinfarction, recurrent ischemia, total stroke, and intracranial hemorrhage and in a reduced need for unplanned (nonprotocol) predischarge angiography and angioplasty.[223] Patients treated with PTCA rather than tPA were also less likely to have a positive result of the predischarge exercise treadmill test (3% vs. 9%; $p = 0.04$) or thallium test (27% vs. 38%; $p = 0.06$). Although the study was not powered to show a reduction in mortality, there was a strong trend for improved survival after PTCA, and multivariate analysis revealed that treatment by PTCA rather than tPA (in addition to younger age) was an independent determinant of reduced mortality (2.6% vs.

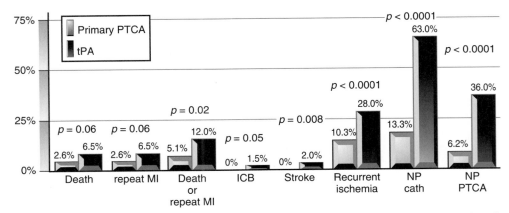

FIGURE 11–6. Major in-hospital outcomes in the first Primary Angioplasty in Myocardial Infarction (PAMI-1) trial. ICB, intracranial bleeding; NP, nonprotocol (i.e., unscheduled); PTCA, percutaneous transluminal coronary angioplasty; ReMI, repeat myocardial infarction; tPA, tissue-type plasminogen activator.

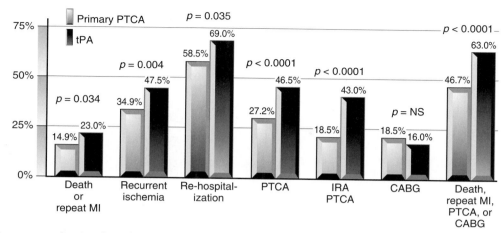

FIGURE 11–7. Occurrence of major clinical end points 2 years after reperfusion therapy in the first Primary Angioplasty in Myocardial Infarction (PAMI-1) trial. CABG, coronary artery bypass grafting; IRA, infarct-related artery; PTCA, percutaneous transluminal coronary angioplasty; ReMI, repeat myocardial infarction; tPA, tissue-type plasminogen activator.

6.5%; $p$ = 0.039).[229] Patients treated with PTCA rather than tPA were also able to be discharged from the hospital a mean of 1 day earlier (7.5 vs. 8.4 days; $p$ = 0.03). Furthermore, the beneficial effects of the invasive approach were sustained after hospital discharge. At 2-year follow-up,[230] patients treated by PTCA rather than tPA had a significantly higher rate of infarct-free survival and freedom from recurrent ischemia or reintervention, and fewer hospital readmissions (Fig. 11–7).

**THE ZWOLLE TRIALS.**[218, 219, 222, 242–245] The advantages of primary PTCA over thrombolytic therapy that were found in PAMI were reinforced and in fact even more striking in two randomized trials from the group in Zwolle, The Netherlands. In the first study, 301 patients of any age presenting within 6 hours of symptom onset (or up to 24 hours if ischemia was continuing) were randomly assigned to undergo primary PTCA or to receive 1.5 MU of intravenous streptokinase over 1 hour. Among the PTCA recipi-

ents, angioplasty was performed in 92%, TIMI grade 3 flow was restored in 94% of infarcted arteries, and patency (TIMI grade 2 or 3 flow) was achieved in 97% of vessels. The benefits of primary PTCA in comparison with thrombolysis were even more compelling in this study than in the PAMI trial; there were markedly fewer in-hospital deaths, reinfarctions, episodes of recurrent ischemia, and unplanned revascularization procedures required after PTCA (Fig. 11–8). As in PAMI, the independent determinants of mortality according to multivariate analysis were advanced age, higher Killip class, and treatment by thrombolytic therapy rather than by primary PTCA. The relative risks of death and reinfarction after streptokinase in comparison with PTCA were 8.5 (95% CI: 1.7 to 41.7) and 9.7 (95% CI: 2.1 to 45.1) respectively. Patients treated with the invasive strategy were discharged, on average, 2.1 days earlier than those treated with streptokinase. At a mean follow-up time of 2.6 years, the PTCA-treated patients continued to demonstrate

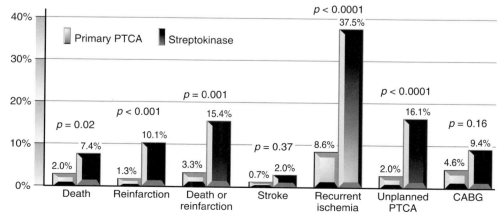

FIGURE 11–8. Major in-hospital adverse events in the Zwolle randomized trial of primary PTCA and streptokinase. CABG, coronary artery bypass grafting; PTCA, percutaneous transluminal coronary angioplasty.

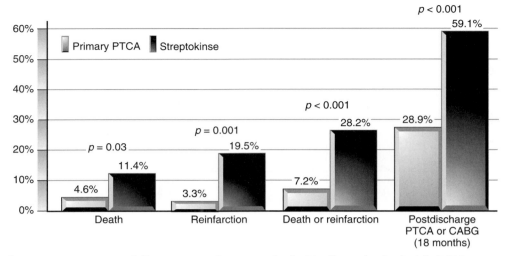

FIGURE 11–9. Adverse events at a mean follow-up time of 2.6 years in the Zwolle randomized trial. CABG, coronary artery bypass grafting; PTCA, percutaneous transluminal coronary angioplasty.

greatly improved survival and infarct-free survival rates in comparison with lytic-treated patients, with a decreased need for late revascularization procedures (Fig. 11–9).

An additional unique aspect of this trial was the completion of routine postdischarge angiographic follow-up in 94% of hospital survivors, at a mean time of $92 \pm 67$ days in 130 PTCA-treated patients, and $22 \pm 38$ days in 139 streptokinase-treated patients. According to quantitative angiographic analysis, patients treated with PTCA rather than streptokinase had a greater minimal luminal diameter of the infarcted vessel ($1.99 \pm 0.83$ mm vs. $0.69 \pm 0.60$ mm; $p < 0.001$), lower residual stenosis ($35\% \pm 22\%$ vs. $77\% \pm 20\%$; $p < 0.001$), and less frequent reocclusion of the infarcted artery (5% vs. 34%; $p < 0.001$), despite the longer duration of follow-up.

Thus, the PAMI and Zwolle trials were consistent in their findings: in comparison with thrombolytic therapy, primary PTCA resulted in improved patency of the infarcted artery with higher rates of in-hospital and long-term infarct-free survival.

THE GUSTO-IIb ANGIOPLASTY SUBSTUDY. The PAMI and Zwolle trials were criticized on four grounds: (1) insufficient size, despite their statistically significant findings; (2) the fact that the "best" thrombolytic regimen, accelerated or front-loaded tPA, was not tested[7]; (3) the fact that the high 2.0% rate of intracerebral hemorrhage after tPA in the PAMI trial was not representative of the outcomes expected from thrombolytic therapy, despite the overall low 6.5% mortality rate among the tPA recipients in the PAMI trial; and (4) the fact that the participating PTCA institutions and physicians were rigorously selected, representing the most skilled and dedicated operators, and that these results could not be achieved in most laboratories.

To address these limitations, the GUSTO-IIb Angioplasty Substudy[226] was performed as part of the primary GUSTO-IIb trial in which heparin and hirudin were compared as adjunctive antithrombin strategies with accelerated tPA.[246] In the GUSTO-IIb Angioplasty Substudy (hereafter referred to as GUSTO-IIb), 1138 patients of any age with AMI at 57 centers in nine countries were randomly assigned to treatment with primary PTCA or accelerated, weight-adjusted tPA. The first 1012 patients were also randomly assigned to heparin or hirudin treatment subsets in a $2 \times 2$ factorial design. Because the outcomes in the heparin- and hirudin-treated patients were not statistically different, they were combined for analysis. The primary, prespecified end point for which the trial was powered was the composite of death, nonfatal reinfarction, and nonfatal disabling stroke after primary PTCA in comparison with tPA. The GUSTO-IIb results appear in Figure 11–10. In comparison with accelerated tPA, primary PTCA resulted in a 30% reduction in major clinical events (death, nonfatal reinfarction, or nonfatal disabling stroke). Of note, intracranial hemorrhage developed in 1.4% of patients after accelerated tPA in this large, age-unrestricted trial; this percentage was similar to the 2.0% rate of intracranial bleeding after a 3-hour tPA course in the PAMI trial. Thus, the rate of intracranial hemorrhage after thrombolytic therapy increases as an elderly population at increasingly high risk is enrolled.[82–93] Conversely, for the rate of intracranial bleeding to be held to only 0.5% (as seen in several earlier thrombolytic trials[3–6]), the use of thrombolytic therapy must be restricted to patients at low risk. Also of note, no patient in GUSTO-IIb sustained an intra-

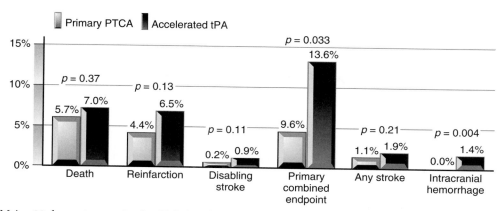

FIGURE 11–10. Major 30-day outcomes in the Global Utilization of Streptokinase and Tissue Plasminogen Activator for Occluded Arteries (GUSTO)–IIb angioplasty substudy. The primary composite end point was the combined incidence of death, nonfatal repeat myocardial infarction, and disabling stroke. PTCA, percutaneous transluminal coronary angioplasty; tPA, tissue-type plasminogen activator.

cranial hemorrhage after primary PTCA, as in previous studies.

Patients treated initially with primary PTCA rather than thrombolytic therapy in GUSTO-IIb also were less likely to suffer medically refractory recurrent ischemia (5.5% vs. 9.0%; $p$ = 0.03) and had a markedly reduced need for unplanned (nonprotocol) in-hospital angiography (7.5% vs. 62.7%; $p$ < 0.0001) and angioplasty (4.4% vs. 36.3%; $p$ < 0.0001); these findings were nearly identical to those in the PAMI and Zwolle trials. In addition, patients treated by primary PTCA rather than tPA in GUSTO-IIb had a 2-day shorter hospital stay, which was also consistent with the earlier trials.

The benefits of primary PTCA in comparison with tPA in GUSTO-IIb first became evident between 5 and 10 days after hospital admission, which suggests that the reduced rates of recurrent ischemia and reinfarction after PTCA (as well as fewer late deaths from ventricular dysfunction and cardiac rupture) are responsible for the improved prognosis with mechanical reperfusion. Indeed, the differences between the two modes of therapy were widening between 10 and 30 days (Fig. 11–11). However, 6 months after admission, there was no longer a statistically significant difference in the occurrence of the composite end point (15.7% after tPA vs. 13.3% after PTCA; $p$ = NS). The 6-month rates of hospital readmissions for recurrent chest pain, myocardial infarction, stroke, and repeat cardiac procedures were also similar between the two groups. Thus, in contrast to the PAMI and Zwolle trials, in which the short-term gains of primary PTCA were maintained or accentuated during follow-up, a partial catch-up phenomenon for thrombolytic therapy was noted in GUSTO-IIb.

Two of the Spanish centers participating in GUSTO-IIb reported long-term angiographic data from 123 patients (61 randomly assigned to receive tPA, and 62 to undergo PTCA).[246a] At 1 year after admission, the composite incidence of death, reinfarction, and target vessel revascularization in these patients was 36.1% after tPA, in comparison with 24.2% after PTCA ($p$ = 0.15). Angiographic follow-up was performed at 1 year after admission in 85% of eligible patients. In comparison with PTCA-assigned patients, patients treated with tPA had greater stenosis of the infarcted vessel (70% ± 34% vs. 31% ± 31%; $p$ < 0.001), were more likely to have stenosis involving 50% or more of the luminal diameter of the infarcted vessel (91% vs. 26%; $p$ < 0.001), were less likely to have TIMI grade 3 flow in the infarcted artery (64% vs. 89%; $p$ = 0.02), and tended to have a lower LVEF (46% ± 25% vs. 53%

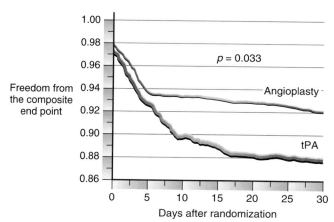

FIGURE 11–11. Freedom from the composite end point in the GUSTO-IIb trial up to 30 days, demonstrating that improved outcomes after primary percutaneous transluminal coronary angioplasty (PTCA) in comparison with accelerated tissue-type plasminogen activator (tPA) became evident in this trial on approximately hospital day 5. (Adapted from The Global Utilization of Streptokinase and Tissue Plasminogen Activator for Occluded Coronary Arteries [GUSTO-IIb] Angioplasty Substudy Investigators: A clinical trial comparing primary coronary angioplasty with tissue plasminogen activator for acute myocardial infarction. N Engl J Med 336:1621–1628, 1997.)

**TABLE 11–12. MAJOR SHORT-TERM CLINICAL OUTCOMES AFTER PRIMARY PTCA AND THROMBOLYTIC THERAPY IN THE GUSTO IIb TRIAL, IN COMPARISON WITH THE PAMI AND ZWOLLE TRIALS**

| THERAPY | N | DEATH No. | p | REINFARCTION No. | p | STROKE No. | p |
|---|---|---|---|---|---|---|---|
| Thrombolytic therapy | | | 0.95 | | 0.37 | | 0.35 |
| PAMI + Zwolle | 349 | 24 (6.9%) | | 28 (8.0%) | | 10 (2.9%) | |
| GUSTO IIb | 573 | 40 (7.0%) | | 37 (6.5%) | | 11 (1.9%) | |
| Primary PTCA | | | 0.016 | | <0.05 | | 0.16 |
| PAMI + Zwolle | 347 | 8 (2.3%) | | 7 (2.0%) | | 1 (0.3%) | |
| GUSTO IIb | 565 | 32 (5.7%) | | 25 (4.4%) | | 6 (1.1%) | |

GUSTO, Global Utilization of Streptokinase and Tissue Plasminogen Activator for Occluded Coronary Arteries; PAMI, Primary Angioplasty in Myocardial Infarction; PTCA, percutaneous transluminal coronary angioplasty.

± 21%; $p = 0.24$). These findings are consistent with the 3-month angiographic data from the randomized Zwolle trial.

### GUSTO-IIb Versus PAMI/Zwolle: Understanding the Differences

Although the short-term outcomes of primary PTCA were superior to those of accelerated tPA in GUSTO-IIb, the relative reductions in death (19% vs. 67%) and reinfarction (31% vs. 75%) were not as great as in the PAMI and Zwolle trials. This disparity cannot be explained by the fact that the patients treated with accelerated tPA in GUSTO-IIb had outcomes superior to those of the patients in the PAMI and Zwolle trials who were treated with 3-hour tPA and streptokinase infusions, respectively. In view of the similar baseline characteristics in the PAMI, Zwolle, and GUSTO-IIb studies, the 7.0% absolute rate of mortality and the 6.5% reinfarction rate after accelerated tPA in GUSTO-IIb were similar to the 6.9% mortality and 8.0% reinfarction rates after the more conventional lytic regimens in PAMI and Zwolle trials (Table 11–12). Furthermore, 63% of patients randomly assigned to receive accelerated tPA in GUSTO-IIb underwent in-hospital angiography (14% on an emergency basis), 36% of the total group underwent PTCA before discharge (17% on an emergency basis), and 8% of the total group underwent bypass surgery in the hospital; these rates were nearly identical to those in the PAMI trial after a 3-hour tPA regimen.

In contrast to the similar interstudy results after thrombolytic therapy, patients treated by primary PTCA had less favorable outcomes in GUSTO-IIb than in the prior studies (see Table 11–12). There may be several explanations for why primary PTCA was less successful in GUSTO-IIb (Fig. 11–12). First, in the PAMI and Zwolle trials, angiography was performed in 100% of patients randomly assigned to undergo primary PTCA, 91% of whom underwent angioplasty. In GUSTO-IIb, in contrast, only 94% of patients randomly assigned to undergo primary PTCA underwent immediate angiography, and angioplasty was performed in only 81% of patients. Also, for unclear reasons, primary PTCA (without thrombolysis) was performed in 1.4% of the patients randomly assigned to receive tPA, and 3.6% of patients assigned to undergo primary PTCA received thrombolytic therapy instead without catheterization or mechanical revascularization. In GUSTO-IIb, patients for whom primary PTCA was intended and performed had markedly better outcomes than if primary PTCA was not performed; among patients assigned to undergo primary PTCA, the likelihood of mortality was 4.1-fold increased if primary PTCA was not performed, and the likelihood of death, reinfarction, or disabling stroke was 3.2-fold increased (Fig. 11–13). Thus, in view of the low per-

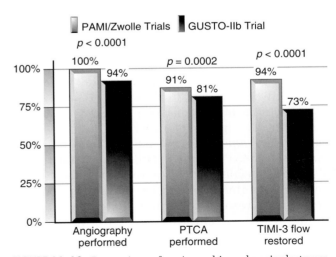

FIGURE 11–12. Comparison of angiographic and angioplasty performance and success in patients randomly assigned to primary percutaneous transluminal coronary angioplasty (PTCA) in the Primary Angioplasty in Myocardial Infarction (PAMI) and Zwolle trials, in comparison with the Global Utilization of Streptokinase and Tissue Plasminogen Activator for Occluded Arteries (GUSTO)–IIb trial. TIMI, Thrombolysis In Myocardial Infarction.

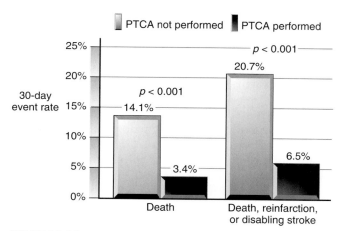

FIGURE 11–13. Implications of not performing PTCA in patients managed with a primary PTCA strategy in the Global Utilization of Streptokinase and Tissue Plasminogen Activator for Occluded Arteries (GUSTO)–IIb trial. PTCA, percutaneous transluminal coronary angioplasty.

centage of patients randomly assigned to undergo PTCA who actually underwent the procedure, the benefits of PTCA in the entire population may have been diluted, especially if the operators were reluctant to perform PTCA in patients at high risk—those who have the most to gain from mechanical reperfusion.[247]

Second, according to core laboratory analysis, TIMI grade 3 flow was restored in 94% of patients undergoing primary PTCA in the PAMI and Zwolle trials and in 97% of patients from the PAR study. In contrast, TIMI grade 3 flow after primary PTCA was restored in only 73% of arteries in GUSTO-IIb, according to core laboratory analysis (85% by clinical site estimation). As discussed later, the establishment of TIMI grade 3 flow is the most critical predictor of survival after reperfusion therapy. It is possible that some of the disparity seen in TIMI grade 3 flow rates after primary PTCA between GUSTO-IIb and the PAMI and Zwolle trials may relate to interstudy core laboratory differences in the manner in which TIMI grade 3 flow was defined or measured. However, in view of the higher-than-expected rates of death and reinfarction after primary PTCA in GUSTO-IIb, it is more likely that the interstudy differences in TIMI grade 3 flow rates after primary PTCA are real and in fact explain much of the differences in outcomes between the trials. The low procedural success rate in GUSTO-IIb also probably explains why the late outcomes between the two reperfusion modalities were attenuated, in contrast to the findings from the PAMI and Zwolle trials, in which the early benefits of primary PTCA in comparison with thrombolysis were maintained or accentuated during follow-up.

Thus, like those of any other surgical technique, the results of primary PTCA may indeed vary with operator experience and technique, the presumption of which was one of the original hypotheses of the GUSTO-IIb investigators. In GUSTO-IIb, participating operators and hospitals had to meet minimum volume standards for the performance of elective PTCA, which were similar to the recommendations of the American College of Cardiology/American Heart Association (ACC/AHA) PTCA Task Force (200 PTCA procedures per year per site, with at least one cardiologist performing more than 50 PTCA procedures per year).[248] No criteria were established, however, for prior site or operator experience with primary PTCA, and it is unclear whether these centers had significant previous experience with primary PTCA on a regular basis. With 1157 patients randomly assigned at 57 sites over an 18-month period, the average GUSTO-IIb site enrolled only 1.1 patients per month, which represents either low-volume programs or significant bias in enrollment selection. In contrast, the 13 centers participating in the PAMI and Zwolle trials were committed primary PTCA sites[249] and randomly assigned an average of 4.9 patients per month.

The mechanism through which greater operator and center experience translates into greater PTCA success is currently undetermined. As discussed later in the section Primary PTCA: Technical Considerations, higher TIMI grade 3 flow rates may result from more optimal balloon sizing or inflation strategy, proper choice of contrast agent, greater attention to anticoagulation status, more appropriate use of adjunctive pharmacotherapy, or better management of the hemodynamic and arrhythmic complications that frequently occur during primary PTCA. For example, in PAMI and PAR, the use of the low osmolar ionic contrast material Ioxaglate, which has been shown to reduce thromboembolic complications after PTCA in patients with acute ischemic syndromes, was mandated.[174–177] However, Ioxaglate was used in only 41% of PTCA-treated patients in GUSTO-IIb.

Furthermore, within both the PAMI 1 and 2 studies,[250] as well as the GUSTO-IIb trial,[226] no relationship was found between the level of operator or hospital experience and clinical outcomes. Thus, excellent primary PTCA results may be obtained at low-volume centers that are dedicated to and skilled in mechanical reperfusion in AMI. Conversely, in view of the unique methodologic considerations of primary PTCA and the somewhat different skill set required in comparison with elective intervention, even the performance of several thousand *elective* PTCAs per year does not guarantee superior results of primary PTCA during AMI.

The differences between the PAMI/Zwolle and GUSTO-IIb randomized trials of primary PTCA versus thrombolytic therapy may be summarized as follows: If primary PTCA is performed in only 81% of the presenting population, and if TIMI grade 3 flow is restored in only 73% of patients (GUSTO-IIb results), significant, important short-term benefits of the invasive approach can still be expected; for every 1000 patients treated by PTCA rather than accelerated tPA, 41 deaths, reinfarctions, and major strokes will be prevented, as seen in GUSTO-IIb. However, if primary PTCA is performed in 90% of patients and TIMI grade 3 flow is obtained in 94%, marked benefits in terms of preventing early death, reinfarction, and stroke may be anticipated: for every 1000 patients treated by primary PTCA rather than thrombolytic therapy, 39 deaths, 59 reinfarctions, and 22 strokes will be prevented, as in the PAMI and Zwolle experiences. In addition, these differences will be maintained or accentuated during long-term follow-up. Furthermore, at all centers, regardless of skill level, withholding thrombolytic therapy to perform primary PTCA will prevent 10 episodes of intracranial bleeding for every 1000 patients treated. For this reason alone, some investigational review boards now consider it unethical to involve patients in trials of thrombolytic therapy if primary PTCA is available.

### Registry Studies of Reperfusion Therapy in AMI: Comparison with Data from Randomized Trials

In contrast to the convincing advantages of primary PTCA demonstrated in the prospective, randomized trials, data from large community registries in which the outcomes of primary PTCA have been retrospectively compared with those of thrombolytic therapy have been more inconclusive. In the Myocardial Infarction, Triage and Intervention (MITI) trial, the outcomes of 3750 consecutive patients with AMI at all 10 hospitals in the metropolitan Seattle area possessing angiographic facilities were tracked over a 3-year period between 1988 and 1990.[251] Treatment was with thrombolytic therapy in 653 patients (17%) and with primary PTCA in 441 (12%). Patients treated with PTCA were more likely to be 75 years of age or older, to be hypotensive or in shock, and not to have ST segment elevation (38% vs. 24%; $p < 0.001$). PTCA was successful in 88% of patients. In-hospital mortality rates among patients treated with PTCA and those treated with thrombolysis were similar. However, patients undergoing primary PTCA had fewer strokes (0.6% vs. 2.1%; $p = 0.12$), shorter hospital stays (7.0 vs. 8.1 days; $p < 0.001$), and lower incidence of recurrent ischemia (20% vs. 30%; $p = .009$).

The MITI registry has been updated to include all 12,331 patients with AMIs admitted between 1988 and 1994 to 19 metropolitan Seattle hospitals, 11 of which had cardiac catheterization facilities.[252] Thrombolytic therapy was administered within 6 hours of symptom onset in 2664 patients (22%), and primary PTCA was performed within 6 hours in 1272 patients (10%). Although most baseline characteristics were similar between the two groups, patients treated with primary PTCA were more likely to have a history of prior gastrointestinal bleeding, of stroke, or of prior CABG. Among patients undergoing emergency catheterization, PTCA was performed in 93%, with an 89% reported success rate. Among the thrombolytic therapy group, 65% were treated with tPA, 32% with streptokinase, and 3% with prourokinase; 8% of patients were treated before hospital admission. After thrombolysis, 74% of patients underwent angiography, 32% required PTCA, and 10% required CABG. As in the randomized trials, patients treated with primary PTCA rather than thrombolytic therapy had lower in-hospital rates of stroke (0.7% vs. 1.5%; $p = 0.04$) and shorter hospital stays (6.8 ± 4.4 days vs. 7.9 ± 5.3 days; $p < 0.01$) as a result of less frequent recurrent ischemia, which necessitated fewer predischarge revascularization procedures. In contrast to the randomized trials, however, rates of in-hospital mortality (5.6% vs. 5.5%; $p =$ NS) and reinfarction (4.3% vs. 3.5%; $p = 0.37$) were similar for the two strategies. There were also no differences in early or late survival after adjustment for baseline variables.

Other registries have found more favorable results after primary PTCA. Primary PTCA without antecedent thrombolysis was performed in 4336 patients between 1990 and 1994 at 40 hospitals contributing to the Society for Cardiac Angiography and Interventions (SCA&I) registry.[253] PTCA was successful in 91.5% of patients, with an overall mortality rate of 2.5%. Neuhaus and associates examined the outcomes of primary PTCA within 24 hours of AMI onset in 758 patients from 60 German community hospitals between October 1992 and June 1995.[254] Despite the fact that cardiogenic shock was present in 17% of patients, PTCA was successful in 93% of patients and TIMI grade 3 flow was restored in 90%. The in-hospital mortality rate was 3.5% among 629 patients without shock and 50% among 129 patients with shock. In the 60 Minutes Myocardial Infarction Project, all 14,980 patients with ST-elevation MI developing within 96 hours of chest pain onset who presented at 136 German hospitals were prospectively entered into a registry between July 1992 and September 1994.[255] Thrombolytic therapy was administered to 7522 patients, whereas only 210 patients were treated with primary PTCA. A 3:1 matching analysis was performed to correct for differences in baseline age, gender, blood pressure, infarction location, history of previous myocardial infarction, and delayed hospital presentation. Other baseline demographic characteristics were similar between the groups. In comparison with the patients treated with thrombolysis, patients managed with primary PTCA had reduced rates of in-hospital mortality (4.3% vs. 10.3%; odds ratio, 0.39 [95% CI: 0.17 to 0.92]) and reinfarction (3.0% vs. 10.6%; odds ratio, 0.26 [95% CI: 0.07 to 1.05]) and a trend toward fewer hemorrhagic complications or allergic reactions (3.2% vs. 5.7%; odds ratio, 0.55 [95% CI: 0.21 to 1.44]).

Some have argued that the MITI data support the position that primary PTCA is less effective (and is associated with a correspondingly higher mortality rate) when performed on a communitywide basis than in controlled studies.[256] In support of this contention, primary PTCA was performed faster, and with higher rates of success and lower rates of in-hospital mortality, at high-volume than at low volume PTCA hospitals in the MITI trial.[252] In the SCA&I registry, laboratory volume (but not operator volume) was also associated with primary PTCA success.[253] Furthermore, between 1990 and 1994, the PTCA success rate among SCA&I hospitals progressively increased from 86.7% to 92.4%,[253] which is consistent with a learning curve.

The SCA&I registry and German studies demonstrated that primary PTCA could be performed with excellent results outside of randomized studies. Ultimately, however, the conclusions that can be drawn from observational registry experiences, whether retrospective (as in MITI) or prospective (as in the SCA&I registry and the 60 Minutes Myocardial Infarction Project), are limited and inherently flawed. There is little quality control in observational studies; charts are not abstracted by study monitors, and the accuracy of the data collected is unverified. Selection bias is inevitable in registry studies and cannot be controlled for, even with the most rigorous statistical adjustments. The reasons for selecting one reperfusion strategy over another can never be known with certainty unless these data are prospectively collected. Patients undergoing primary PTCA in most communities are, in general, more critically ill and more likely to have conditions contraindicating thrombolytic therapy. Physicians regularly delivering thrombolytic therapy tend to refer only the most ill patients for primary PTCA. Randomized trials are performed in order to eliminate selection bias and thus are superior to registries when physicians decide on the relative advantages and disadvantages of different treatment modalities. In this regard, the data from 10 prospective, randomized trials in which a wide variety of patients were studied have convincingly demonstrated that primary PTCA saves lives, reduces the incidence of reinfarction, and prevents life-threatening hemorrhagic complications in comparison with thrombolytic therapy.

### Recurrent Ischemia and Time to Discharge After Primary PTCA Versus Thrombolytic Therapy

Recurrent ischemia after reperfusion therapy is associated with hemodynamic and arrhythmic complications, prolongs the hospital stay, necessitates expensive predischarge catheterization and revascularization procedures, and increases hospital costs. In the PAMI trial, 76 (19%) of 395 randomized patients experienced one or more recurrent ischemic events before discharge.[84] In comparison with patients without recurrent ischemia, patients with recurrent ischemia had higher rates of ventricular tachycardia, atrioventricular block, cardiac arrest, sustained hypotension, congestive heart failure, and need for intubation (Table 11–13). Patients with recurrent ischemia also had a greatly increased need for unscheduled invasive and revascularization procedures, were hospitalized on average 2 days longer, and accrued an additional mean $7800 in hospital charges (see Table 11–13). Five (28%) of the 18 deaths in the PAMI trial occurred after recurrent ischemic events.[84]

The results from the four major randomized trials of primary PTCA vs. thrombolytic therapy (1937 randomized patients) reveal that the incidence of recurrent ischemia was reduced from 16.8% after thrombolysis to 7.1% after primary PTCA ($p < 0.0001$) (Table 11–14). As a result of this clinical stability, a markedly lower percentage of PTCA-treated patients than of lytic-treated patients required predischarge angiography (7.8% vs. 61.9%; $p < 0.0001$) and unplanned PTCA after admission (4.2% vs. 48.8%; $p < 0.0001$) and tended to require CABG less frequently (7.4% vs. 9.4%; $p = 0.11$). Consequently, patients randomly assigned to undergo PTCA were discharged on average 1.7 days earlier than patients who received thrombolytic therapy (8.5 days vs. 10.2 days; $p < 0.05$). Reducing the residual stenosis and stabilizing the ruptured plaque are the most likely explanations for the marked decrease in recurrent ischemia after primary PTCA in comparison with that seen after thrombolytic therapy.[54, 58, 86, 88, 167, 218, 257–260] As discussed later, the beneficial effects of primary PTCA in reducing recurrent ischemia are realized in both patients at high risk and those at low risk with AMI.

### Cost Effectiveness of Primary PTCA in Comparison with Thrombolytic Therapy

In the current era of diminishing health care budgets and increased cost constraint, concern has been expressed that the clinical benefits of primary PTCA

**TABLE 11–13.    RAMIFICATIONS OF RECURRENT ISCHEMIA IN THE PAMI TRIAL**

| IN-HOSPITAL EVENT | RECURRENT ISCHEMIA (N = 76 [19%]) | NO RECURRENT ISCHEMIA (N = 319 [21%]) | p |
|---|---|---|---|
| **Arrhythmic Complications** | | | |
| Atrioventricular block | 11.8% | 4.1% | 0.008 |
| Sustained VT | 5.3% | 2.4% | 0.21 |
| Nonsustained VT | 40.8% | 24.5% | 0.004 |
| Ventricular fibrillation | 7.9% | 3.5% | 0.09 |
| Cardioversion/defibrillation | 10.5% | 4.7% | 0.05 |
| Cardiopulmonary resuscitation | 9.2% | 2.4% | 0.006 |
| **Hemodynamic Complications** | | | |
| Congestive heart failure | 23.7% | 11.9% | 0.008 |
| Pulmonary edema | 10.5% | 1.9% | 0.0002 |
| Sustained hypotension | 21.1% | 9.4% | 0.004 |
| Need for intra-aortic balloon pump | 11.8% | 1.2% | 0.0001 |
| Respiratory failure | 9.2% | 3.8% | 0.046 |
| Need for intubation | 10.5% | 3.1% | 0.006 |
| **Unplanned Catheterization and Revascularization Procedures** | | | |
| Unscheduled catheterization | 75.0% | 29.8% | <0.0001 |
| Unscheduled PTCA | 53.9% | 13.5% | <0.0001 |
| CABG | 23.7% | 6.9% | <0.0001 |
| **Major End Points** | | | |
| Death | 6.6% | 4.1% | 0.35 |
| Reinfarction | 23.7% | 0% | <0.0001 |
| Death or reinfarction | 27.6% | 4.1% | <0.0001 |
| Length of stay (days) | 9.6 ± 4.7 | 7.6 ± 3.8 | 0.0003 |
| Hospital charges (× $1000)* | 36.7 ± 24.8 | 28.9 ± 14.9 | 0.0018 |

CABG, coronary artery bypass grafting; PAMI, Primary Angioplasty in Myocardial Infarction; PTCA, percutaneous transluminal coronary angioplasty; VT, ventricular tachycardia.

*Includes professional fees.

may be eroded by the high up-front costs of cardiac catheterization required in all patients managed with the invasive strategy. Cost analyses were therefore performed both in the PAR registry of primary PTCA in thrombolytic candidates and in the four major studies (Fig. 11–14). In the PAR registry,[261] all hospital and physician bills were summed, including charges for initial hospital care and through 6 months of clinical follow-up. Hospital charges were converted to costs by means of cost/charge ratios and per diem charges derived from each hospital's annual Medicare Cost report.[262] The total mean baseline hospital cost for 270 patients was $13,113; average physician fees (uncorrected) were $5694. These baseline costs were similar to those in the conservatively treated group of the TIMI-II trial, in which average hospital costs (inflated to 1991 dollars) were $14,942 and average physician fees were $3217.[263, 264] Mean follow-up costs in the PAR registry over a 6-month period were $3174, and average physician fees were $1443.

In the PAMI trial, the in-hospital charges and physician fees were summed for all 358 patients enrolled in the United States.[265] Total hospital charges were on average $3436 lower per patient treated with PTCA than per patient treated with tPA ($23,468 ± $13,410 vs. $26,904 ± $18,246; $p =$ 0.04). In-hospital physician fees were higher with PTCA, however ($4185 ± $3183 vs. $3332 ± $2728; $p =$ 0.001), and thus total charges tended to be lower with PTCA by $2574 per patient ($27,653 ± $13,709 vs. $30,227 ± $18,903; $p =$ 0.21). In the Mayo Clinic trial,[224] in-hospital charges and professional fees were roughly converted to costs by multiplying by a ratio of 0.8. In comparison with tPA, PTCA was $4589 less expensive per patient treated ($16,811 ± $8827 vs. $21,400 ± $14,806; $p =$ 0.09). Furthermore, during the 6-month period after hospital discharge, patients treated with PTCA rather than tPA had a significantly lower rate of readmissions (4% vs. 18%; $p =$ 0.04), which was associated with a reduction in follow-up costs ($480 ± $3069 for PTCA vs. $2738 ± $7666 for tPA; $p =$ 0.03). Thus, total 6-month costs were $6387 less with initial PTCA treatment than with tPA ($17,292 ± $8967 vs. $24,129 ± $18,806; $p =$ 0.09).

In the GUSTO-IIb trial, costs were calculated through methods similar to those in the PAR registry.[266] Preliminary analysis of the data showed a similar pattern as that seen in PAMI: lower mean hospital costs with PTCA than with accelerated tPA ($13,337 vs. $14,236; $p =$ 0.004), increased professional fees with the invasive strategy ($3912 vs. $3367; $p =$ 0.002), and a trend toward reduced total

**TABLE 11–14.   IN-HOSPITAL RECURRENT ISCHEMIA, UNSCHEDULED REVASCULARIZATION PROCEDURES, AND LENGTH OF HOSPITAL STAY IN THE FOUR MAJOR RANDOMIZED PRIMARY PTCA/THROMBOLYTIC TRIALS**

| OUTCOME | PTCA | THROMBOLYSIS | p |
|---|---|---|---|
| *Recurrent Ischemia* | | | |
| PAMI | 10.3% | 28.0% | <0.0001 |
| Zwolle | 8.6% | 37.5% | <0.0001 |
| Mayo Clinic* | 14.9% | 35.7% | 0.02 |
| GUSTO-IIb† | 5.5% | 9.0% | 0.03 |
| Pooled | 7.1% | 16.8% | <0.0001 |
| *Unscheduled Cardiac Catheterization* | | | |
| PAMI | 13.3% | 63.0% | <0.0001 |
| Zwolle | NR | NR | NR |
| Mayo Clinic | NR | NR | NR |
| GUSTO-IIb | 7.5% | 61.7% | <0.0001 |
| Pooled | 7.8% | 61.9% | <0.0001 |
| *Unscheduled PTCA* | | | |
| PAMI | 6.2% | 36.0% | <0.0001 |
| Zwolle | 2.0% | 16.1% | <0.0001 |
| Mayo Clinic | 2.1% | 28.6% | 0.0003 |
| GUSTO-IIb | 4.4% | 63.7% | <0.0001 |
| Pooled | 4.2% | 48.8% | <0.0001 |
| *CABG* | | | |
| PAMI | 8.2% | 12.0% | NS |
| Zwolle | 4.6% | 9.4% | NS |
| Mayo Clinic | 12.8% | 12.5% | NS |
| GUSTO-IIb | 7.5% | 8.3% | NS |
| Pooled | 7.4% | 9.4% | 0.11 |
| *Duration of Hospitalization (Days)‡* | | | |
| PAMI | 7.5 | 8.4 | 0.03 |
| Zwolle | 12.0 | 13.5 | <0.001 |
| Mayo Clinic* | 7.7 | 10.6 | 0.01 |
| GUSTO-IIb† | 8 | 10 | <0.05 |
| Pooled | 8.5 | 10.2 | <0.05 |

CABG, coronary artery bypass grafting; GUSTO, Global Utilization of Streptokinase and Tissue Plasminogen Activator for Occluded Coronary Arteries; NR, not reported; NS, nonsignificant; PAMI, Primary Angioplasty in Myocardial Infarction.
*Recurrent ischemia requiring additional revascularization.
†Medically refractory recurrent ischemia.
‡Mean or median, as reported.

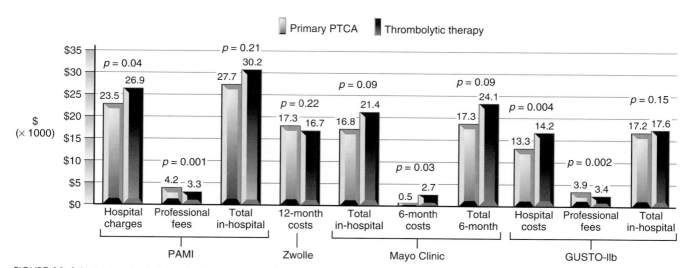

FIGURE 11–14. Cost analysis from the four major randomized trials of thrombolytic therapy versus primary percutaneous transluminal coronary angioplasty (PTCA). GUSTO, Global Utilization of Streptokinase and Tissue Plasminogen Activator for Occluded Arteries; PAMI, Primary Angioplasty in Myocardial Infarction.

costs with PTCA ($17,249 vs. $17,603; $p = 0.15$). The absolute cost differences between the two therapies, however, were less marked than in PAMI, which is consistent with the more equivocal differences in clinical outcomes between PTCA and tPA in GUSTO-IIb, as previously discussed.

Finally, in the Zwolle randomized trial, in which the less expensive agent streptokinase was used,[267] charges were corrected with estimated fixed costs of procedures and converted from Dutch guilders into 1992 U.S. dollars. The total in-hospital plus median physician costs for PTCA were greater than those for streptokinase ($12,723 vs. $11,010; $p < 0.05$). However, in the first 12 months after discharge, patients treated by streptokinase required significantly more revascularization procedures (56% vs. 32%; $p < 0.001$); had greater incidences of death, reinfarction, and stroke (26.2% vs. 7.2%; $p < 0.001$); and were more likely to have recurrent angina (38% vs. 21%; $p < 0.01$) than did PTCA-treated patients. As a result, total 12-month costs were no longer significantly different between the two cohorts ($17,316 for PTCA vs. $16,681 for streptokinase; $p = 0.21$). Furthermore, cost efficacy analysis showed that the average cost for an event-free survivor was $25,431 with PTCA, in contrast to $36,798 with streptokinase ($p < 0.01$).

Thus, in contrast to what otherwise may have been expected, the hospital costs of primary PTCA are actually reduced in comparison with those of thrombolytic therapy, and total costs (when professional fees are included) are similar or reduced. Considering the improved outcomes with primary PTCA in comparison with thrombolysis, PTCA is clearly a cost-effective mode of therapy and thus should be preferred, especially at skilled centers. The explanation for the lower-than-expected relative costs of primary PTCA despite the high up-front costs of cardiac catheterization is directly related to the lower incidence of complications, the lower incidence of recurrent ischemia, and the shorter hospital stays with the invasive approach. In the PAMI trial, the most important determinant of hospital costs was the duration of hospitalization.[265] Other important correlates with increased costs were the development of adverse in-hospital events, including stroke, and of recurrent ischemia, which necessitated unplanned PTCA and CABG procedures. In comparison with thrombolytic therapy, primary PTCA virtually eliminated the risk of intracranial hemorrhage, lowering the total stroke rate, and markedly reduced the rate of recurrent ischemia and subsequent revascularization procedures, thereby facilitating early discharge and reducing costs. Similarly, in the PAR registry, each episode of recurrent ischemia increased costs by a mean of

$8430.[261] Thus, although radiology and cardiac catheterization charges were higher in the PAMI trial with PTCA than with tPA, these up-front expenses were more than recovered by the savings realized from reduced charges for drug and solutions, room and board, and clinical laboratory tests and electrocardiography. Primary PTCA thus represents an emerging mode of therapy that, in comparison with the available alternatives, offers greater efficacy with improved clinical outcomes at similar or reduced costs.

Although actual reimbursements after PTCA and thrombolytic therapy have not been directly measured, average reimbursements may be analyzed for a Medicare population.[265] If a patient with an AMI is treated conservatively (with or without thrombolysis and/or cardiac catheterization) but does not undergo a revascularization procedure, the hospital is reimbursed under the Diagnosis-Related Group (DRG) 122. If PTCA is performed (with or without thrombolysis), the hospital bills the higher reimbursing DRG 112. Finally, if CABG is performed (with or without PTCA or thrombolysis), DRG 106 applies. According to data from the randomized PTCA-thrombolytic trials, as part of the primary PTCA strategy, PTCA alone is typically performed in 85% of patients, bypass surgery is performed with or without PTCA in 10% of patients, and 5% of patients are treated with catheterization only. After thrombolytic therapy, 60% of patients are treated conservatively with or without catheterization, 30% undergo PTCA, and 10% undergo bypass surgery. In fiscal year 1997, the average Medicare reimbursement for DRG 122 was $5050, in comparison with $9106 for DRG 112 and $25,156 for DRG 106. Thus, by simple calculation, the hospital would receive an average of $8178 for every patient treated with thrombolytic therapy, as opposed to $10,408 for every patient treated with primary PTCA, and therefore a $2230 increase in reimbursement would be realized for every patient managed with primary PTCA. Thus, not only is primary PTCA less expensive for the hospital but it also yields greater reimbursement.

### Advantages of Primary PTCA in Patients at High Risk

If primary PTCA reduces mortality in comparison with thrombolytic therapy, as demonstrated in the meta-analysis of the randomized studies (see Table 11–8), it would be reasonable to expect to find a gradient of effect in which the advantages of PTCA over lytic therapy are most pronounced in the patients at highest risk. They are those with the most

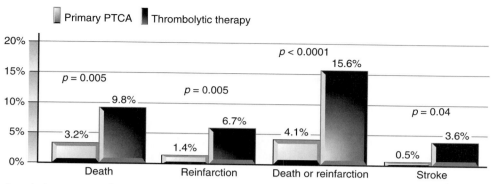

FIGURE 11–15. In-hospital outcomes of patients defined as being at high risk (age >70, anterior myocardial infarction, or admission tachycardia) treated with primary percutaneous transluminal coronary angioplasty (PTCA) in comparison with thrombolytic therapy. Data pooled from the Primary Angioplasty in Myocardial Infarction (PAMI), Zwolle, and Mayo Clinic trials.

to gain from effective reperfusion. This concept has been verified in most of the randomized trials. Many different criteria may be used to stratify patients into high- and low-risk groups. In the early TIMI studies, patients at high risk were defined as those possessing one or more of the following characteristics: age of 70 years or more, occurrence of anterior myocardial infarction, or admission heart rate of more than 100 beats per minute. Pooled results from the PAMI, Zwolle, and Mayo Clinic trials[268] demonstrate that patients at high risk, so defined, have marked reductions in mortality, reinfarction, and stroke when treated with primary PTCA rather than with thrombolytic therapy (Fig. 11–15). Women, nonsmokers, elderly patients, patients with diabetes mellitus, those who have undergone prior bypass surgery, those who present late, and those with congestive heart failure, hypotension, or cardiogenic shock on admission also have historically been at high risk for early and late morbidity and mortality after medical therapy or thrombolysis. Subset analyses from the PAMI trial[123, 269] have shown benefits of primary PTCA in comparison with thrombolytic

therapy in terms of reducing mortality in most of the high-risk patient groups examined (Table 11–15).

Another difference between the GUSTO-IIb and PAMI trials is that patients at high risk in GUSTO-IIb did not have greater relative benefit with PTCA in comparison with tPA than did their lower risk counterparts.[226] This may be another reflection of the fact that interventionalists who participated in GUSTO-IIb were less experienced than those in PAMI; because patients at high risk are inherently more unstable and have more complex problems, greater technical facility is required from the operator (e.g., the ability to rapidly place temporary pacemakers, establish intra-aortic balloon counterpulsation, and quickly manage hemodynamic and electrical instability). Failure of these measures could counteract many of the advantages of primary PTCA. It is also unknown whether the PTCA operators in GUSTO-IIb were particularly reluctant to perform PTCA in patients at high risk; as discussed earlier, withholding the benefits of PTCA from such patients may have especially worsened the outcomes in this group. Although this conjecture is

**TABLE 11–15.    IN-HOSPITAL MORTALITY IN HIGH-RISK PATIENTS TREATED WITH THROMBOLYTIC THERAPY VERSUS PRIMARY PTCA IN THE PAMI TRIAL**

| HIGH-RISK FEATURE | tPA | PTCA | p |
|---|---|---|---|
| Age ≥ 65 y | 15.0% | 5.7% | 0.066 |
| Female gender | 14.0% | 4.0% | 0.07 |
| Diabetes mellitus | 20.8% | 0% | 0.01 |
| Prior bypass surgery | 14.3% | 0% | 0.38 |
| Anterior myocardial infarction | 11.9% | 1.4% | 0.01 |
| Current nonsmokers | 17.9%* | 6.6% | 0.05 |
| Presentation after >4 h | 12.2% | 0% | 0.03 |
| Killip class ≥ 2 | 7.1% | 0% | 0.14 |

PAMI, Primary Angioplasty in Myocardial Infarction; PTCA, percutaneous transluminal coronary angioplasty; tPA, tissue-type plasminogen activator.
*Death or reinfarction.
Adapted from Stone GW: Primary coronary angioplasty in high risk patients with acute myocardial infarction. J Invas Cardiol 7(suppl F):12F–21F, 1995.

unestablished, these factors may have resulted in lower PTCA TIMI flow 3 success rates in patients at high risk in GUSTO-IIb, with worse subsequent outcomes.

### Primary PTCA in the Elderly Patient

Elderly patients with AMI are at particular risk for early mortality, even after reperfusion therapy.[9, 93, 185, 225, 270–273] In both the PAMI and GUSTO-I trials, advanced age was found to be the strongest determinant of early and late mortality in the reperfusion era.[225, 229] Because 80% of all deaths after AMI occur in patients more than 60 years of age,[274] optimal therapy is critical for this subset of patients. The Fibrinolytic Therapy Trialists (FTT) performed a meta-analysis of the nine largest placebo-controlled randomized trials of thrombolytic therapy, comprising 58,600 prospectively randomized patients.[114] Stratifying by age, they found that mortality was reduced in all patients treated with thrombolytic therapy in comparison with placebo except for patients 75 years of age or older, among whom the mortality rate was a startling 24.8% (24.3% after thrombolysis vs. 25.3% with placebo; $p = 0.58$). This was verified in the more recent GUSTO-I trial, wherein the mortality rate among lytic-treated patients 75 years of age or older was 20%.[124] Part of the reason why elderly patients failed to benefit from thrombolysis is the high risk of hemorrhagic stroke after fibrinolytic therapy in this group. The FTT study found an excess of 10 strokes per 1000 patients 75 years of age and older in the first 24 hours after thrombolytic administration in comparison with placebo-treated controls.[114] Other groups have identified advanced age as an independent risk factor for hemorrhagic stroke after thrombolytic therapy.[92–94] As a result of the high risk and marginal benefit, many physicians are reluctant to treat elderly patients with thrombolytic therapy. Krumholz and coworkers found that in 1992 to 1993, of 3093 consecutive patients 65 years of age or older with AMI who presented at all acute care nongovernmental hospitals in Connecticut, only 753 (24%) were even eligible to receive thrombolytic therapy; of those patients, only 334 (44% of those eligible, or 11% of all elderly patients) actually received thrombolysis.[275]

Primary PTCA, by avoiding the risk of intracranial bleeding and restoring patency in a high percentage of patients, may be of particular benefit in elderly patients as an alternative to thrombolytic therapy. In the PAMI trial, 38% of the patients enrolled were 65 years of age or older.[229] The in-hospital mortality rate was markedly higher in this age group than among patients less than 65 years of age (10.7% vs. 0.8%; $p < 0.0001$). Patients 65 years old and older who were treated with PTCA rather than tPA in the PAMI trial had reduced in-hospital rates of death (5.7% vs. 15.0%; $p = 0.066$) and of death or reinfarction (8.6% vs. 20.0%; $p = 0.048$).[229] A pooling of the results of the PAMI, Zwolle, and Mayo Clinic trials reveals that a marked reduction in mortality with primary PTCA in comparison with thrombolytic therapy in elderly patients is clearly seen, and greater relative benefits are apparent for each decile of age (Fig. 11–16).[268] Even in GUSTO-IIb, there was a strong trend for improved survival among patients 70 years of age or older treated with primary PTCA rather than with thrombolysis.[226]

### Primary PTCA in Women

Women with AMI have long been recognized to have reduced survival rates in comparison with men after conservative medical management or thrombolysis.[3–6, 276–281] Although part of the reason may be a greater prevalence of comorbid baseline risk factors in women presenting with AMI (including advanced age, diabetes, hypertension, late presentation, and congestive heart failure), female gender may represent an independent biologic risk factor for mortality after AMI.[276, 278, 279] Female gender has also been identified as a risk factor for intracranial hemorrhage after thrombolytic therapy.[100, 104, 105] In the PAMI trial,[282] in-hospital mortality was increased 3.3-fold among women in comparison with men (9.3% vs. 2.8%; $p = 0.004$). By multivariate analysis, treatment with PTCA rather than tPA was an independent predictor of reduced mortality rate among women (4.0% vs. 14.0%; $p = 0.034$). Part of this difference could be explained by the high incidence of intracranial bleeding after tPA treatment in women in comparison with men (5.3% vs. 0.7%; $p = 0.037$), whereas no patient treated with

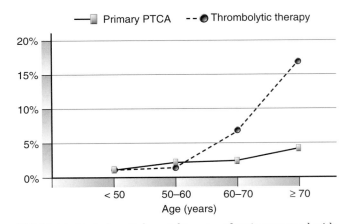

FIGURE 11–16. In-hospital mortality rates of patients treated with primary percutaneous transluminal coronary angioplasty (PTCA), in comparison with thrombolytic therapy, as a function of age. Data pooled from the Primary Angioplasty in Myocardial Infarction (PAMI), Zwolle, and Mayo Clinic trials.

primary PTCA experienced intracranial bleeding. Large single-center series have confirmed that primary PTCA is equally efficacious in women as in men.[141, 154, 158, 160] In the PAMI-2 trial, in which 1100 patients at 34 centers were treated with a primary PTCA strategy (to be discussed), the in-hospital mortality rates (2.8%) and the rates of stroke (1%) among men and women were identical despite the fact that the women were older, were more likely to have diabetes and hypertension, and presented later.[282a] Thus, primary PTCA appears to be especially efficacious in women, offsetting the otherwise increased risk of stroke and death after thrombolytic therapy.

### Primary PTCA in Patients with Anterior AMI

Patients in whom the admitting electrocardiogram demonstrates an anterior myocardial infarction have reduced survival in comparison with those with nonanterior AMI.[3, 4, 283–288] In GUSTO-I, 10% of patients with anterior AMI died after thrombolytic therapy.[7] The randomized trial by Garcia and co-workers was specifically designed to examine whether primary PTCA could improve upon the outcomes of thrombolytic therapy in patients with anterior AMI.[227] In this trial, 189 patients presenting within 5 hours of onset of anterior AMI were prospectively assigned randomly to receive accelerated tPA or to undergo primary PTCA. Patients treated with the invasive approach had lower rates of in-hospital mortality and recurrent ischemia and similar rates of reinfarction and stroke (Fig. 11–17). Predischarge angiography was routinely performed and demonstrated higher rates of TIMI grade 3 flow (88% vs. 58%; $p = 0.0004$) and less severe residual stenosis (34% vs. 69%; $p < 0.0001$) in patients treated by primary PTCA than in tPA-treated patients. In PAMI, patients with anterior AMI treated with primary PTCA as opposed to tPA had lower rates of in-hospital death (1.4% vs. 11.9%; $p = 0.01$), recurrent ischemia (11.3% vs. 24.8%; $p = 0.01$), and stroke (0% vs. 6.0%; $p = 0.037$).[289] Multivariate analysis revealed that treatment of patients with anterior AMI with PTCA was the strongest predictor of survival. At 6 months, the cumulative rate of death or reinfarction among patients with anterior AMI was 7.0% after initial management with PTCA, in contrast to 20.9% after tPA treatment ($p = 0.018$). Thus, patients with anterior AMI who are at high risk because a greater amount of jeopardized myocardium was involved than in patients with nonanterior AMI preferentially benefit from primary PTCA rather than from thrombolysis.

### Primary PTCA in Patients with Diabetes Mellitus

Diabetes mellitus is present in 10% to 25% of patients with AMI[290, 291] and has been shown to be an independent predictor of mortality.[291–294] In addition, patients with diabetes and AMI are usually older, are more likely to be female, have had prior myocardial infarction, present later, and have more severe coronary artery disease and worse left ventricular function than do patients without diabetes.[291–297] Although thrombolytic therapy is undoubtedly more beneficial than placebo in patients with diabetes mellitus,[114] the mortality rate remains high. In the GUSTO-I trial, 5944 (14.5%) of 41,021 patients receiving thrombolytic therapy had diabetes. The mortality rate at 30 days was 6.2% among patients without diabetes, 9.7% among patients with

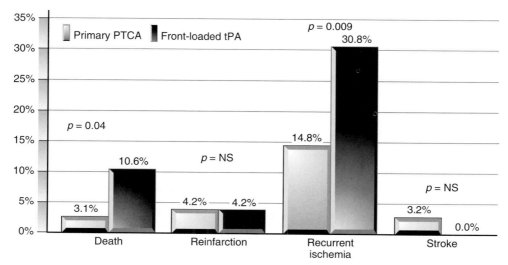

FIGURE 11–17. In-hospital outcomes in patients with anterior acute myocardial infarction who presented within 5 hours of symptom onset; patients were randomly assigned to receive either accelerated tissue-type plasminogen activator (tPA) or primary percutaneous transluminal coronary angioplasty (PTCA). (Data from Garcia E, Elizaga J, Soriano J, et al: Primary angioplasty versus thrombolysis with tPA in anterior myocardial infarction: Results from a single center trial. J Am Coll Cardiol 29:389A, 1997.)

non–insulin-treated diabetes, and 12.5% among patients with insulin-dependent diabetes ($p < 0.001$).[292] The incidence of stroke was also increased among patients with diabetes (1.9% vs. 1.4%; $p < 0.001$).

In the PAMI trial,[298] patients with diabetes were older (65 vs. 59 years old; $p = 0.002$), more often female (40% vs. 25%; $p = 0.03$), more frequently had hypertension (68% vs. 39%; $p = 0.0001$), had a history of prior heart failure (8% vs. 1%; $p = 0.0001$), had multivessel disease (76% vs. 51%; $p = 0.01$), and presented later (3.8 vs. 3.0 hours; $p = 0.03$) than patients without diabetes. The in-hospital mortality rate was 10.0% in patients with diabetes, in contrast to 3.8% in patients without diabetes ($p < 0.05$). Mortality rates among patients treated with tPA were markedly higher among patients with diabetes than among patients without diabetes (20.8% vs. 4.5%; $p < 0.01$). In contrast, the prognosis of patients with diabetes was improved by primary PTCA, in such a way that mortality rates among patients with and without diabetes were similar (0% vs. 3.0%; $p = NS$). The in-hospital mortality among diabetic patients was 20.8% after tPA, in contrast to 0% after primary PTCA ($p = 0.01$). The rate of death or reinfarction was also lower in patients with diabetes treated with PTCA than in those treated with tPA (4% vs. 25%, $p = 0.03$).

Despite these improved results of primary PTCA in comparison with thrombolytic therapy in patients with diabetes mellitus, patients with insulin-dependent diabetes remain at high risk. Stuckey and associates found that patients with diabetes were more likely than AMI patients without diabetes to be female, to have multivessel disease, and to have an infarct vessel diameter of less than 3.0 mm.[299] Primary PTCA had equally high success rates in patients with and without diabetes (both >93%). The rates of 30-day mortality among patients without diabetes and those with non–insulin-dependent diabetes were similar. In contrast, however, patients with insulin-dependent diabetes were more likely to present in cardiogenic shock and had significantly reduced survival rates. After correction for the presence of multivessel disease and shock, patients with insulin-dependent diabetes still had a 2.2-fold increased risk of mortality after primary PTCA.[299]

### Primary PTCA in Patients with Delayed Presentation

Although several placebo-controlled trials have shown improved survival if thrombolytic therapy is given within 12 hours of chest pain onset,[3, 4, 134, 300] thrombolysis is most beneficial if given within the first 4 hours after symptoms begin.[114] As the time from symptom onset to drug administration is prolonged, myocardial salvage is reduced and mortality

increases. This may be partly because patients who present late are more likely to be elderly, to have diabetes, to have hypertension, to have had a prior myocardial infarction, and to have congestive heart failure[301]; however, thrombolytic efficacy also diminishes as the clot ages.[302, 303] In contrast, primary PTCA restores TIMI grade 3 flow in more than 90% of patients, independently of the time to reperfusion. In the 1100-patient PAMI-2 study, primary PTCA restored TIMI grade 3 flow in 93% of patients; stratified by hourly time intervals from chest pain onset to treatment, the results showed that TIMI grade 3 flow rates varied from 89% to 95% ($p = NS$).[304] Pooling of the results of the PAMI, Zwolle, and Mayo Clinic randomized trials[268] reveals that although primary PTCA, in comparison with thrombolysis, was associated with improved survival at all treatment intervals, the invasive approach yielded relatively greater survival rates among patients presenting late (Fig. 11–18). Another way to interpret these data is that the observed increase in mortality after thrombolytic therapy with later treatment did not occur after primary PTCA. The relative advantages of primary PTCA over tPA were also more marked in patients presenting more than 4 hours after symptom onset in the GUSTO-IIb study.[226] Patients presenting late thus appear to benefit from preferential management with PTCA to ensure reperfusion success. The implications of these findings regarding myocardial salvage and transfer of patients to tertiary centers are explored in further detail in the section Expanding the Reach of Primary PTCA.

### Primary PTCA in Patients with Prior Bypass Surgery

Approximately 3% to 5% of saphenous vein grafts fail per year, and 3% of CABG-treated patients expe-

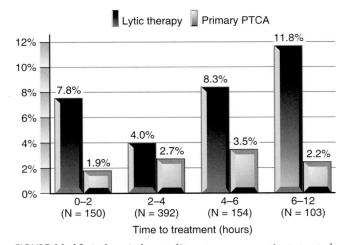

FIGURE 11–18. In-hospital mortality rates among patients treated with primary percutaneous transluminal coronary angioplasty (PTCA) versus thrombolytic therapy as a function of time to treatment after symptom onset. Data pooled from the Primary Angioplasty in Myocardial Infarction (PAMI), Zwolle, and Mayo Clinic trials.

rience AMI per year.[305–307] Among patients who have undergone previous CABG mortality rates are similar or increased after AMI, in comparison with patients without prior surgery, despite the fact that the infarction size tends to be smaller in patients with prior surgery; this finding possibly reflects the coexistence of other high-risk features such as prior myocardial infarction, left ventricular dysfunction, and multivessel disease.[308–312] In prior studies, 5% to 15% of all AMIs have occurred in patients who have undergone prior bypass surgery,[141, 311, 313] a percentage that is likely to increase. Patients who have undergone prior bypass surgery, however, have been excluded from many prior thrombolytic trials because of perceived lack of efficacy.[5, 6, 142, 314, 315] The most frequent cause of AMI in CABG-treated patients is saphenous vein graft occlusion, often with extensive thrombus burden. As a result, reperfusion rates of occluded saphenous vein grafts after thrombolysis are lower than in native vessels, and the mortality rate has remained high.[312, 313] In the GUSTO angiographic substudy, 48 patients (2.5%) had saphenous vein graft occlusion.[246] TIMI grade 2 or 3 flow was established in 48% of patients with vein graft AMI, in contrast to 69% with native coronary occlusion ($p < 0.01$). TIMI grade 3 flow was restored in only 34% of vein grafts after thrombolytic therapy. Saphenous vein graft occlusion was an independent determinant of thrombolytic failure.[316] Similarly, in the Duke University experience, thrombolytic therapy resulted in TIMI grade 2 or 3 flow in only 47% of patients who had previously undergone CABG, as opposed to 65% of those who had not.[312]

The results of primary PTCA in 229 patients who had undergone prior CABG have been reported.[123, 141, 154, 313, 317, 318] (Table 11–16). TIMI grade 2 or 3 flow was restored in 87% of patients; the in-hospital mortality rate was 10%. In the series of 1000 consecutive patients with AMI from the Mid America Heart Institute, 13% had undergone prior CABG.[141] The acute PTCA success rate (TIMI grade 2 or 3 flow

and stenosis of <50% of the vessel diameter) was lower in occluded vein grafts than in native coronary arteries (86% vs. 95%; $p < .0001$). In-hospital survival rates among patients who had and had not undergone prior CABG were similar (90% vs. 92%; $p = NS$), however, and in CABG-treated patients, serial LVEF increased from 44% on admission to 51% before discharge.[141] Repeat predischarge angiography in 34 of these patients showed continued patency in 94%, although 15% required repeat PTCA for early restenosis, dissection, or recoil.[319]

In the combined experience from the first two PAMI trials, 63 of 1295 patients assigned to primary PTCA had undergone prior CABG.[318] These patients were older (65 ± 10 years vs. 60 ± 12 years; $p = 0.001$), more likely to have had prior myocardial infarction (57% vs. 15%; $p < 0.0001$), more likely to have had prior congestive heart failure (9% vs. 2%; $p = 0.003$), and more likely to have triple-vessel disease (65% vs. 18%; $p < 0.0001$). Also in comparison to patients who had not undergone prior CABG, PTCA was less likely to be performed (81% vs. 90%; $p = 0.04$) and, when performed, resulted in lower rates of TIMI grade 3 flow (82% vs. 93%; $p = 0.01$) and a residual stenosis involving less than 50% of the vessel diameter (86% vs. 96%; $p = 0.007$). In the PAMI-1 trial,[123] the only randomized trial in which the outcomes in CABG-treated patients have been stratified by reperfusion modality, PTCA was successful in all 5 CABG-treated patients, none of whom experienced recurrent ischemia or reinfarction or died. In contrast, 3 (43%) of 7 patients treated with tPA had recurrent ischemia ($p = 0.09$ in comparison to PTCA); 2 of these 3 died or experienced reinfarction. Thus, from the available data, primary PTCA appears to be the treatment of choice for CABG-treated patients, although the results are less optimal in occluded saphenous vein grafts than in native coronary arteries. As discussed in the following chapter, the results of primary PTCA in patients with occluded vein grafts are likely to be further improved with the adjunctive use of thrombectomy before PTCA, stent implantation after PTCA, and administration of glycoprotein IIb/IIIa inhibitors in conjunction with PTCA.

## TABLE 11–16. RESULTS OF PRIMARY PTCA IN PATIENTS WITH PRIOR BYPASS GRAFTING

| STUDY | N | PTCA SUCCESS | IN-HOSPITAL MORTALITY RATE |
|---|---|---|---|
| Brodie et al[154] | 12 | 75% | 25% |
| Kavanaugh and Topol[317] | 9 | 78% | 11% |
| O'Keefe et al[141] | 130 | 90% | 10% |
| Grines et al[313] | 15 | 80% | 13% |
| Stone[123] | 5 | 100% | 0% |
| Stone et al[315] | 58 | 84% | 7% |
| Pooled | 229 | 87% | 10% |

PAMI, Primary Angioplasty in Myocardial Infarction; PTCA, percutaneous transluminal coronary angioplasty.

### Primary PTCA Versus Thrombolytic Therapy in Patients Historically Excluded from Thrombolysis Treatment

As previously reviewed, many patients at high risk have been excluded from prior trials of thrombolytic therapy because of concerns about lack of efficacy or hemorrhagic complications.[3–9, 132, 133] With the demonstration that thrombolytic therapy does improve survival and salvage myocardium in comparison with placebo treatment and that these benefits may extend to patients at high risk, it has been widely recommended that the indications for thrombolytic therapy be expanded, with acceptance of the increased risks of hemorrhagic complications. An alternative means of reperfusion for these patients, however, is primary PTCA, which can be applied to nearly all patients with AMI.[141, 183] Himbert and associates found that of 45 consecutive patients with AMI and contraindications to thrombolytic therapy, all were eligible for primary PTCA.[320] The PTCA success rate in this group was 93%; reperfusion was established 52 ± 27 minutes after admission. O'Keefe and Brodie and colleagues examined their single-center experiences with primary PTCA in patients with absolute or relative contraindications to thrombolysis.[141, 154] Pooling of these studies revealed that of 1383 consecutive patients undergoing primary PTCA, 39% would have been ineligible to receive thrombolysis at these two centers. In comparison with patients eligible for thrombolytic therapy, patients who would have been ineligible had only slightly lower rates of PTCA success (90% vs. 94%) but significantly higher rates of in-hospital mortality (16% vs. 3%). Of the patients excluded from thrombolytic therapy, however, 12% were in cardiogenic shock, and the remainder had multiple other high-risk conditions. Similarly, in a report from the Zwolle group,[321] 29% of 486 consecutive primary PTCA patients would have been ineligible for thrombolytic therapy on the basis of hemorrhagic contraindications (73%), cardiogenic shock (19%), or a nondiagnostic electrocardiogram (15%). At 6 months, the mortality rate was 10.6% among lytic-ineligible patients, in contrast to 4.9% among lytic-eligible patients ($p < 0.03$), and the incidence of death and reinfarction or of stroke was similarly increased (14.1% vs. 6.0%; $p < 0.01$).[321]

Thus, although mortality is increased in patients with contraindications for thrombolytic therapy and who are undergoing primary PTCA, reperfusion is achieved in approximately 90% of patients, and the survival rate is greater than reported from historical controls. For these reasons, it has been very difficult to perform a randomized trial of medicine versus PTCA in patients with contraindications for thrombolysis. The preliminary results of one such study, the Study of Medicine vs. Angioplasty Reperfusion Trial (SMART), have been presented.[322] In this small pilot study, 50 patients were randomly assigned to undergo angiography, followed, if appropriate, by revascularization, or to receive medical therapy. PTCA was actually performed in only 60% of patients receiving invasive treatment. Despite the limited power of this study, patients treated with the invasive strategy rather than with medical therapy had lower rates of severe recurrent ischemia (12% vs. 36%; $p = 0.04$) and reinfarction (0% vs. 12%; $p = 0.07$); had less severe residual stenosis of the infarcted artery at discharge (37% ± 19% vs. 77% ± 14%; $p < 0.0001$); and exhibited trends toward improved mean LVEF (57% ± 15% vs. 51% ± 14%) and infarcted artery patency (88% vs. 77%).

A second randomized trial of an early invasive approach versus conservative care in patients with contraindications to thrombolysis, the Medicine versus Angiography in Thrombolytic Exclusion (MATE) trial, has been completed.[322a] In this larger study, 201 patients with suspected AMI and conditions contraindicating thrombolytic therapy at four centers were randomly assigned to undergo early angiography, followed, if appropriate, by revascularization, or to receive conservative medical management. Myocardial infarction was confirmed in 53% of patients. In the invasively treated group 109 (98%) of 111 patients underwent early angiography. As in the SMART trial, revascularization was performed in 64 patients (59%) with thrombolytic exclusions, including PTCA in 48 patients and CABG in 16 patients. In the conservatively treated group angiography was ultimately performed in 54 (60%) of 90 patients before hospital discharge ($p < 0.0001$ in comparison with the invasively treated group), in 27 patients for recurrent ischemia, and in 27 patients as part of routine care without ischemia. Of the patients in whom angiography was performed in the conservative arm, 33 (61%) underwent revascularization, including PTCA in 27 and CABG in 6. Patients treated with the early invasive strategy rather than with the conservative approach were revascularized significantly earlier (27 ± 23 hours vs. 88 ± 98 hours; $p = 0.0001$) and had lower incidences of in-hospital recurrent ischemia (3% vs. 13%; $p = 0.004$) and recurrent nonischemic chest pain (8% vs. 23%; $p = 0.003$). Major adverse end points in this trial occurred infrequently in both arms; no differences in the rates of in-hospital death (1% vs. 3%) or reinfarction (2% vs. 0%) were noted, which suggests that a cohort of patients at low risk was enrolled. It is most likely that patients truly at high risk who had conditions contraindicating thrombolytic therapy were not randomly assigned by the centers participating in MATE and were instead selectively treated with angiography and PTCA or CABG.

The benefits of reperfusion by PTCA in patients with exclusions for thrombolytic therapy have clearly been demonstrated in terms of myocardial recovery. Brodie and coworkers[154] reported that although noncandidates for thrombolytic therapy had a lower acute mean LVEF than did thrombolytic candidates (47.8% vs. 53.3%; $p = 0.03$), paired acute and predischarge studies demonstrated that their serial improvement in LVEF was significantly greater (+10.5% vs. +4.4%; $p = 0.002$), which was consistent with marked myocardial salvage in this high-risk group. As a result, the final predischarge LVEFs of the lytic-eligible and lytic-ineligible groups were similar (57.7% vs. 58.3%; $p$ = NS).

To examine whether patients historically excluded from thrombolytic therapy should now be treated with thrombolysis or should instead preferentially undergo reperfusion by PTCA, a subset analysis from the PAMI trial was performed.[323] Patients were defined as being historically excluded from thrombolysis if they were more than 70 years old, presented more than 4 hours after symptom onset, or had undergone prior bypass surgery. Because thrombolytic therapy is now used routinely in all these patient subsets, however, they were included in PAMI. (Other subsets of patients in whom thrombolysis is still contraindicated, including patients with cardiogenic shock, a nondiagnostic electrocardiogram, and hemorrhagic predisposition, were also excluded from PAMI). Of the 395 patients randomly assigned, 151 (38%) had one or more conditions that previously would have rendered them ineligible for thrombolysis. In comparison with patients without prior lytic exclusions, patients with these conditions had increased rates of in-hospital mortality (8.6% vs. 2.0%; $p$ = 0.002), stroke (3.3% vs. 0.8%; $p$ = 0.02), and 6-month mortality (10.0% vs. 2.9%, $p$ = 0.003). Patients with former contraindications to thrombolytic therapy who were treated with primary PTCA rather than thrombolytic therapy, however, had lower in-hospital rates of death or reinfarction, recurrent ischemia, and stroke; these benefits were maintained at 6 months (Fig. 11–19). Thus, patients with relative contraindications to thrombolytic therapy constitute a group at high risk for increased early and late mortality and stroke. Although the outcomes in these patients after thrombolytic therapy may be improved in comparison with outcomes after conservative medical management, their prognosis may be further enhanced if thrombolytic therapy is withheld in lieu of the preferential performance of primary PTCA, thereby ensuring higher initial patency rates while minimizing hemorrhagic complications.

## Primary PTCA in Patients in Cardiogenic Shock

The development of cardiogenic shock is the most powerful predictor of mortality in AMI.[125, 126, 324–328] Cardiogenic shock may be present when the patient presents to the emergency room with AMI, or it may develop during the course of conservative management or reperfusion therapy. The incidence of cardiogenic shock among patients with AMI, 5% to 15% in most prior reports, has not changed significantly since 1980.[125, 126, 329] Goldberg and colleagues reviewed the Worcester, Massachusetts, community-wide experience with cardiogenic shock in 4762 patients with AMI at 16 hospitals between 1975 and 1988.[329] The yearly incidence of cardiogenic shock varied between 7% and 9%; the mortality rate among these patients ranged from 72% in 1975 to 81% in 1988. Thrombolytic therapy was used in only 8% of patients, however, and PTCA was used in only 2% and CABG in 1%. The authors recognized that more aggressive modes of therapy would be needed to improve the prognosis in shock.

Unfortunately, intensive supportive therapy—including monitoring in the coronary care unit, aggressive arrhythmia prophylaxis and treatment, and hemodynamic support with vasopressor agents and the use of intra-aortic balloon counterpulsation—has not improved outcomes in patients with shock.[324–330] Similarly, as discussed earlier, the dismal prognosis when cardiogenic shock develops is also not materially affected by thrombolytic therapy[3, 127–131] (see Fig. 11–4).

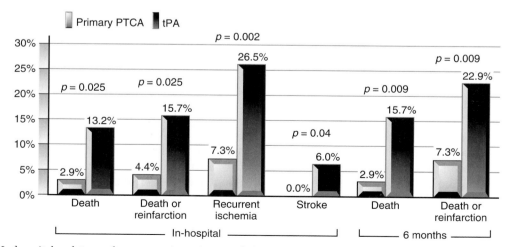

FIGURE 11–19. In-hospital and 6-month outcomes in patients with former contraindications to thrombolytic therapy, randomly assigned to primary percutaneous transluminal coronary angioplasty (PTCA) or to tissue-type plasminogen activator (tPA) in the first Primary Angioplasty in Myocardial Infarction (PAMI-1) trial.

It was only from a thorough appreciation of the pathophysiology of cardiogenic shock that rational strategies were developed to combat this lethal condition. Cardiogenic shock is present when the heart is unable to deliver sufficient blood flow to meet the resting metabolic needs of the body.[331] From the pioneering studies of Forrester and coworkers, a hemodynamic definition of cardiogenic shock has become widely accepted: a systolic blood pressure of less than 80 mm Hg in association with a cardiac index of less than 2.0 L/minute/m$^2$ and a pulmonary capillary wedge pressure of more than 12 mm Hg.[332, 333] The underlying substrate for cardiogenic shock is extensive myocardial necrosis. Most pathologic studies have shown that more than 40% of the left ventricular myocardium is infarcted in patients dying from shock (either from a single massive infarction, usually involving occlusion of the proximal left anterior descending artery, or from new infarction superimposed on one or more prior infarctions).[334, 335]

Of importance is that infarction extension or reinfarction, often clinically silent, is frequently present as well.[335, 336] Alonso and associates documented infarction extension, averaging 6% of the left ventricular mass in 18 (82%) of 22 patients dying of shock.[336] Angiographic studies have documented multivessel disease in approximately 60% to 75% of patients with cardiogenic shock.[337–339] Grines and colleagues demonstrated that an important correlate with mortality in patients with cardiogenic shock is hypokinesis, or the lack of compensatory hyperkinesis, in the noninfarcted myocardial zones.[340] Finally, although left ventricular failure from acute coronary occlusion is the most common etiology of cardiogenic shock, other important causes that must be considered are right ventricular failure, the development of mechanical complications of transmural infarction (including papillary muscle rupture, ventricular septal defect, and free wall rupture), and nonischemic conditions (including myocarditis, cardiomyopathy, myocardial contusion, aortic or mitral stenosis, and left atrial myxoma).[341]

From this understanding, a rational approach to the treatment of cardiogenic shock has evolved. Urgent angiography and left ventriculography have been proved to be safe for use in patients with cardiogenic shock who are hemodynamically supported by pressors and intra-aortic balloon counterpulsation.[342–345] These studies are performed to establish the underlying etiology of shock, assess myocardial and valvular function, and evaluate the status of the coronary arteries, thereby setting the stage for mechanical reperfusion therapy. If catheterization demonstrates papillary muscle rupture, ventricular septal defect or ventricular rupture, or severe left main artery or triple-vessel disease with features unfavorable for PTCA, emergency or urgent surgery should be performed. When the predominant etiology of shock is left ventricular failure from acute coronary occlusion, PTCA of the culprit artery is performed to halt myocardial necrosis, prevent infarction extension and expansion, and enhance electrical stability. If severe multivessel disease is present and the left ventriculogram does not demonstrate compensatory hyperkinesis of the noninfarcted zones, PTCA of multiple noninfarcted vessels may be performed to improve regional wall motion in the noninfarcted zone and relieve ischemia.

The prognosis of patients in cardiogenic shock appears to be improved to a greater extent after primary PTCA than with more conservative approaches.[324, 341, 346] Meyer and associates initially reported the use of angioplasty to reverse cardiogenic shock in 1982.[347] The publication of the University of Michigan experience of PTCA in 27 patients with cardiogenic shock, however, was the first major report to demonstrate the applicability of PTCA in cardiogenic shock.[348] The PTCA success rate was 88% in this series; 70% of patients survived to hospital discharge, and 75% of patients with successful PTCA were discharged alive, in contrast to 33% after unsuccessful PTCA. Other predictors of mortality in patients with shock who underwent PTCA were anterior AMI location, symptom duration of more than 12 hours, multivessel disease, and age of more than 60 years.[348]

The outcomes of primary PTCA without thrombolytic therapy in 739 patients with cardiogenic shock from 18 studies have now been reported[131, 141, 154, 324, 338, 339, 348–364] (Table 11–17). Pooling of the data revealed that PTCA restored patency in 73% of patients, and 54% of patients survived to hospital discharge. The in-hospital mortality rate was 30% after successful PTCA, in contrast to 77% after unsuccessful PTCA, which was similar to the expected outcome with conservative medical management. A real-world demonstration of the beneficial effects of primary PTCA in patients with cardiogenic shock may be appreciated from the William Beaumont Hospital experience between 1982 and 1992 (Fig. 11–20). Before 1989, patients in shock at this institution were treated conservatively, and yearly mortality rates ranged from 78% to 89%. In 1989, an aggressive interventional approach to these patients was initiated, and yearly mortality rates subsequently declined to approximately 50%.

The invasive approach to cardiogenic shock may also benefit patients who have received thrombolytic therapy. In the GUSTO-I trial, cardiogenic shock was present in 2972 (7.2%) of 41,021 enrolled patients who received one of four different thrombolytic regimens.[130] Only 315 patients (11%) presented

## TABLE 11–17. REPORTED RESULTS OF PTCA IN PATIENTS WITH CARDIOGENIC SHOCK

| STUDY | N | PTCA SUCCESS | OVERALL SURVIVAL | SURVIVAL WITH REPERFUSION | SURVIVAL WITHOUT REPERFUSION |
|---|---|---|---|---|---|
| Kaplan et al[349] | 88 | 61% | 42% | 65% | 29% |
| O'Keefe et al[141] | 79 | 82% | 56% | 63% | 21% |
| Lee et al[338] | 69 | 71% | 55% | 69% | 20% |
| Hochman et al[131] | 55 | 69%* | 40% | 39%* | 27%* |
| Gacioch et al[350] | 48 | 73% | 46% | 61% | 7% |
| Bengtson et al[324] | 46 | 85% | 54% | NR | NR |
| Hibbard et al[339] | 45 | 62% | 56% | 71% | 29% |
| Moosvi et al[351] | 38 | 76% | 53% | 62% | 22% |
| Eltchaninoff et al[352] | 33 | 76% | 64% | 76% | 25% |
| Brown et al[353] | 28 | 61% | 43% | 58% | 18% |
| O'Neill et al[348] | 27 | 88% | 70% | 75% | 33% |
| Yamamoto et al[354] | 26 | 62% | 38% | 56% | 10% |
| Meyer et al[355] | 25 | 88% | 53% | 59% | 0% |
| Lee et al[356] | 24 | 54% | 50% | 77% | 18% |
| Brodie et al[154] | 22 | 68% | 50% | NR | NR |
| Seydoux et al[357] | 21 | 85% | 57% | 67% | 0% |
| Himbert et al[358] | 18 | 89% | 22% | 19% | 50% |
| Stomel et al[359] | 12 | NR | 75% | NR | NR |
| Heuser et al[360] | 10 | 60% | 70% | 100% | 25% |
| Shani et al[361] | 9 | 67% | 67% | 83% | 0% |
| Disler et al[362] | 7 | 71% | 43% | 60% | 0% |
| Verna et al[363] | 7 | 100% | 86% | 86% | NR |
| Shawl et al[364] | 5 | 100% | 100% | 100% | NR |
| Pooled | 739 | 73% | 54% | 70% | 23% |

NR, not reported; PTCA, percutaneous transluminal coronary angioplasty.
*Data available for 48 patients.

in shock, whereas 2657 patients (89%) went into shock after thrombolytic treatment. In comparison with patients without shock, patients with shock were older, were more likely to be female, and had higher rates of prior myocardial infarction, anterior AMI location, and diabetes mellitus. The mortality rate was markedly higher among patients who presented with or went into shock (57% and 55%, respectively) than among patients in whom shock did not develop (3%) ($p < 0.001$). Reinfarction also occurred significantly more commonly among patients in shock than among patients not in shock (11% vs. 3%; $p < 0.001$), as did recurrent ischemia (28% vs. 19%; $p < 0.001$). Among patients in shock, intra-aortic balloon counterpulsation was estab-

lished in only 25%, cardiac catheterization was performed in only 45%, and PTCA and CABG were performed in only 19% and 11%, respectively. However, the 30-day mortality rate among patients in shock was strikingly lower when PTCA was performed than when it was not performed (34% vs. 61%; $p < 0.001$).

In the TIMI-IIB study, cardiogenic shock developed in 196 (6%) of 3309 tPA-treated patients.[365] As in GUSTO-I, participating TIMI-IIB physicians were allowed to manage patients in shock at their discretion, either conservatively or with catheterization and, if appropriate, subsequent revascularization by PTCA or CABG. Striking differences in hospital survival rates were also noted on the basis of the ther-

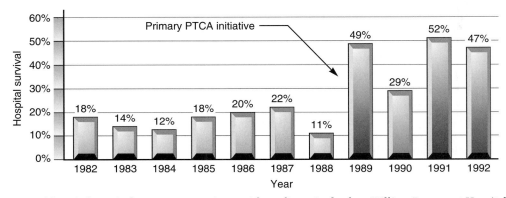

FIGURE 11–20. Improved hospital survival rates among patients with cardiogenic shock at William Beaumont Hospital after 1989 with institution of a primary percutaneous transluminal coronary angioplasty (PTCA) approach.

apy selected; mortality occurred in 29% of patients in shock managed aggressively, as opposed to 79% who were managed with conservative treatment. Finally, in the series by Stomel and coworkers of 64 consecutive patients with cardiogenic shock who presented at a community hospital without PTCA facilities, survival rates were 75% among patients transferred to a tertiary center where PTCA was performed but 17% among patients treated conservatively with thrombolytic therapy and/or intra-aortic balloon counterpulsation alone.[359]

Similarly, in the Second National Registry of Myocardial Infarction (NRMI-2), 1.3% of 29,908 patients with AMI of 12 hours' duration or longer who were treated with tPA and 4.2% of 4939 such patients treated with primary PTCA presented in shock ($p <$ 0.001).[365a] The in-hospital mortality rates were 52.3% among patients in shock treated with tPA and 32.4% among those after primary PTCA ($p < 0.001$).

Thus, primary PTCA appears to reduce the approximately 80% rate of mortality from cardiogenic shock after conservative treatment to approximately 45%. The dramatic clinical improvement that often occurs after PTCA in cardiogenic shock may be related to early myocardial recovery or the prevention of infarction extension and expansion, enhanced electrical stability with fewer lethal arrhythmic events, or resolution of ischemic mitral regurgitation.[364] However, although the pooled data from these observational series are encouraging, several caveats must be borne in mind when the effectiveness of primary PTCA in cardiogenic shock is considered. Most of the reports to date have been nonrandomized, retrospective chart review studies. Only two studies have even compared the outcomes to historical control groups.[338, 351] Furthermore, it has been suggested that patients in shock who undergo catheterization and PTCA may be a highly selected subset with a generally improved prognosis in comparison with patients in shock who are too ill to undergo angiography or PTCA or in whom the decision for conservative terminal care has been made. In the SHould we revascularize Occluded coronaries for Cardiogenic shocK (SHOCK) registry, 251 patients with cardiogenic shock at 19 centers were prospectively entered into a clinical database.[131] Cardiac catheterization was performed in 58% of patients, PTCA in 26% of patients, and CABG in 8% of patients. Patients undergoing catheterization were on average 6.2 years younger than those not studied and had markedly lower rates of mortality (51% vs. 85%; $p < 0.001$). Performance of cardiac catheterization was independently correlated with survival even after adjustments for age, use of thrombolytic therapy, electrocardiographic changes, and AMI location. However, the mortality rate was lower among patients undergoing catheterization

who did not undergo PTCA or CABG than among those not catheterized (58% vs. 85%; $p < .001$), which demonstrates the probable operation of selection bias in determining the eligibility of patients with shock for an invasive approach. In this study, the mortality rate among patients catheterized who were revascularized with PTCA or CABG was only marginally lower than the rate among those catheterized but not revascularized (51% vs. 58%).

As in the SHOCK registry, thrombolytic-treated patients in the GUSTO-I trial with cardiogenic shock who underwent an early aggressive strategy of angiography followed, if appropriate, by PTCA or CABG also were younger, were less likely to have had prior myocardial infarction, and were treated earlier than patients with shock who were managed conservatively without catheterization.[366] However, after adjustments for differences in baseline variables with multiple logistic regression analysis, the aggressive revascularization strategy was still independently associated with a reduction in 30-day mortality (odds ratio, 0.43 [95% CI: 0.34 to 0.54], $p = 0.0001$).[131]

Cardiac catheterization may also enable physicians to identify patients with cardiogenic shock who are likely to benefit from emergency CABG. Despite the inherent delays in performing CABG and the adverse effects of general anesthesia and cardiopulmonary bypass in elderly and critically ill patients, emergency CABG is undoubtedly effective in selected patients with cardiogenic shock. The rate of survival among 323 shock patients from 19 surgical series has averaged 68%.[367] The ability of surgery to provide complete revascularization may be beneficial particularly in patients with cardiogenic shock and underlying severe multivessel disease. CABG is unlikely to be an option for the majority of patients with shock, however; in both the series by DeWood and by Mundth and colleagues, fewer than 50% of patients with shock were found to have operable conditions.[344, 345] At most centers, the percentage of patients with shock who are eligible for emergency CABG is likely to be far lower, in view of logistic constraints and surgeon reluctance. Nonetheless, the relative effectiveness of CABG in cardiogenic shock confirms the importance of revascularization for survival. Results of ongoing randomized studies from the SHOCK investigators and the Swiss Multicenter study of Angioplasty for SHock (SMASH) trial will define the appropriate roles of primary PTCA and CABG in cardiogenic shock.

Despite the improved outcomes with primary PTCA, cardiogenic shock continues to be the most powerful determinant of early mortality in the interventional era.[130, 141, 154, 158, 167, 341] The 73% rate of patency achieved by PTCA in patients with shock, although greater than the 43% reperfusion rate after thrombolysis,[127] is lower than the rate of patency after PTCA in patients without shock (95% to 99%). Low coronary perfusion pressure, diffuse coronary disease, refractory ventricular arrhythmias, and cardiac arrest may contribute to the relatively high failure rate of PTCA in patients with shock. Anecdotal reports from small series of patients suggest that coronary stents, possibly in conjunction with more potent antiplatelet agents, may improve the patency rate in shock and possibly prevent recurrent ischemia and reinfarction.[368, 369] The PAMI investigators are examining the utility of stent implantation with the Johnson and Johnson heparin-coated stent in patients with AMI complicated by shock in a registry experience from 65 centers.[370, 371] Transmyocardial or percutaneous myocardial revascularization (TMR or PMR) with holmium laser may offer an alternative means of restoring myocardial perfusion in patients with shock and poor arterial targets for bypass surgery or PTCA.[372] Other strategies are being directed toward the limitation of reperfusion injury or promotion of myocardial recovery with agents such as adenosine, L-carnitine, P-selectin inhibitors, and fructose diphosphate.[373–375] Newer circulatory support devices—including percutaneous cardiopulmonary bypass,[376, 377] coronary sinus diastolic retroperfusion,[378] and the hemopump[376, 379, 380]—may, in selected cases, maintain hemodynamic stability to allow complete percutaneous revascularization. As a last resort, a left ventricular assist device or a total artificial heart may serve as a bridge to cardiac transplantation.[376, 381–383]

### Advantages of Primary PTCA in Low-Risk Patients

In contrast to the reduction in mortality when patients with AMI and at high risk are managed with primary PTCA instead of thrombolytic therapy, patients at low risk (those without any high-risk characteristics) have excellent survival rates with both reperfusion modalities.[123, 223] Patients at low risk may benefit from primary PTCA as opposed to lytic therapy because of a reduction in recurrent ischemia and reinfarction, a shorter hospital stay, and lower costs that occur with PTCA therapy. In the PAMI trial,[223] patients defined as having low risk (age <70, heart rate <100 beats per minute, and nonanterior AMI location) had similar mortality rates with PTCA and tPA (3.1% vs. 2.2%; $p$ = NS). Patients at low risk who were treated with PTCA rather than tPA, however, had markedly lower rates of reinfarction or recurrent ischemia (10.0% vs. 29.7%; $p$ = 0.0007) and, as a result, required fewer unscheduled cardiac catheterization (7.8% vs. 60.4%; $p$ < 0.0001) and PTCA procedures (4.4% vs. 36.3%; $p$ <

0.0001) before discharge. This allowed PTCA-treated patients at low risk to be discharged earlier than tPA-treated patients (7.0 ± 3.1 days vs. 8.3 ± 4.5 days; $p$ = 0.03) and resulted in a mean reduction in hospital charges of $4365 per patient ($22,038 ± $12,896 after PTCA vs. $26,403 ± $16,104 after tPA; $p$ = 0.025).[265]

Zijlstra and coworkers performed a prospective, randomized trial specifically designed to determine whether primary PTCA offers any advantages in patients at low risk.[222] In this study, 95 (40%) of 240 consecutive patients with AMI were classified as being at low risk (lytic eligible, Killip class I, and nonextensive nonanterior AMI) and were randomly assigned to undergo primary PTCA or receive intravenous streptokinase. The 6-month rate of death, reinfarction, or stroke, which constituted the primary end point, was markedly lower in patients treated with primary PTCA than in those treated with streptokinase (20.0% vs. 4.4%; $p$ < 0.02), as a result of a greatly reduced rate of reinfarction (Fig. 11–21). As in the PAMI trial, patients at low risk assigned to undergo PTCA also had lower rates of recurrent ischemia, which resulted in fewer unscheduled angioplasty procedures after admission (see Fig. 11–21). The LVEF measured at 6 months tended to be higher after primary PTCA than after streptokinase treatment (51% ± 9% vs. 48% ± 10%; $p$ = 0.11). Finally, whereas total 6-month costs (in Dutch guilders) were similar after PTCA and streptokinase treatment the total costs per event-free survivor were lower after primary PTCA than with thrombolysis (mean Fl 23,869 vs. Fl 27,765; $p$ < 0.05). Thus, even in patients at low risk, by reducing recurrent ischemia, reinfarction, and repeat revascularization procedures and facilitating earlier discharge, primary PTCA is cost effective in comparison with thrombolytic therapy. In addition, in patients at low risk, among whom the survival rate is excellent with either reperfusion modality, primary PTCA is especially warranted to avoid the risk of intracranial hemorrhage inherent in thrombolytic therapy.

## Optimizing the Results of Primary PTCA: The PAMI-2 Trial

Primary PTCA has been demonstrated to be the best reperfusion option currently available for most patients with evolving AMI. The PAMI-2 trial was designed to explore ways to further enhance the outcomes and cost effectiveness of primary PTCA in patients with AMI who are at low and high risk. Patients with high-risk features continue to have significant rates of morbidity and mortality despite primary PTCA and, if identified early, might benefit from methods to improve myocardial recovery, en-

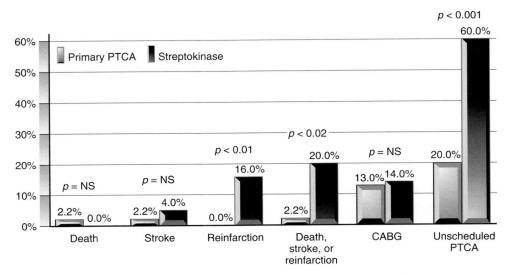

FIGURE 11–21. Six-month outcomes in low-risk patients randomly assigned to receive streptokinase (SK) or primary percutaneous transluminal coronary angioplasty (PTCA). CABG, coronary artery bypass grafting. (Data from Zjilstra F, Beukema W, Van't Hof AWJ, et al: Randomized comparison of primary coronary angioplasty with thrombolytic therapy in low risk patients with acute myocardial infarction. J Am Coll Cardiol 29:980–991, 1997.)

hance hemodynamics and electrical stability, and prevent reinfarction and reocclusion of the infarcted artery. Patients at low risk, on the other hand, are extremely stable after PTCA and may not require monitoring in the coronary care unit, prolonged anticoagulation, predischarge exercise testing, and the extended hospital stay, which are considered routine for patients with AMI.

### The PAMI-2 Hypotheses

In the PAMI-2 trial,[384, 385] three hypotheses were therefore tested. First, in patients with AMI who undergo primary PTCA, the combination of clinical and angiographic variables readily available at the time of immediate cardiac catheterization can be used for risk stratification to identify patients at high and low risk for subsequent morbidity and mortality. Most adverse outcomes after AMI, including death, usually occur within the first 48 hours of coronary occlusion.[3–7, 114, 124, 229, 386–388] Therefore, risk stratification must occur early in the course of AMI in order to be useful. Variables derived during cardiac catheterization, including the number of diseased vessels, LVEF and regional wall motion, presence of collateral vessels, and TIMI flow grades are of powerful prognostic value.[9–20, 91, 141–152, 154, 192, 340, 389–391] Up to 70% of patients treated with thrombolytic therapy undergo catheterization before hospital discharge,[226, 312, 393] but it is usually performed late in their hospital course. Because most deaths have occurred before this point, delayed catheterization data cannot be used to identify which patients are likely to be stable and which will require more

intensive intervention. Therefore, in PAMI-2, after acute angiography and left ventriculography, *early* risk stratification was performed with the variables present at the time of acute cardiac catheterization and reperfusion.

Second, patients identified as being at high risk will benefit from the prophylactic use of intra-aortic balloon counterpulsation for 48 hours. Routine intra-aortic balloon pump (IABP) use, by augmenting proximal coronary blood flow velocity and reducing afterload and preload,[394–397] might decrease the rate of infarcted vessel reocclusion after primary PTCA, thus promoting myocardial recovery, and may reduce the incidences of reinfarction and, possibly, mortality. Beneficial effects of prophylactic IABP use had previously been observed in two observational studies.[398, 399] Ohman and coworkers therefore organized a prospective, multicenter, randomized trial involving 182 patients who, within 24 hours of onset of AMI, achieved successful reperfusion by primary PTCA, by rescue PTCA after failed thrombolysis, or by intracoronary thrombolysis or who had documented triple-vessel disease with a patent infarction-related vessel. These patients were randomly assigned to undergo routine IABP counterpulsation for 48 hours or to receive traditional care.[400] Patients undergoing IABP counterpulsation had lower rates of recurrent ischemia (4% vs. 21%; $p = 0.001$), infarcted artery reocclusion (8% vs. 21%; $p < 0.03$), and need for emergency PTCA (2% vs. 11%, $p < 0.02$). The beneficial effect of the IABP strategy in reducing infarcted artery reocclusion was particularly pronounced in the subgroup of patients undergoing primary PTCA without antecedent thrombolysis (4% vs. 18%).[401] The role of prophylactic IABP use in patients with AMI at high risk was therefore examined in PAMI-2, with the expectation that outcomes would be significantly improved with routine intra-aortic balloon counterpulsation.

Third, patients at low risk may be monitored after primary PTCA in the standard elective PTCA unit (bypassing the coronary care unit entirely), treated with an abbreviated heparin course, and safely discharged on the third hospital day without predischarge exercise testing; this would result in significant cost savings in comparison with standard care. Current guidelines recommend that patients with AMI undergo extensive observation, monitoring, and predischarge testing.[402] These measures are prudent after reperfusion with thrombolytic therapy, in few of the frequent occurrence and unpredictable timing of recurrent ischemia after fibrinolysis.[60, 84, 89] In contrast, in the PAMI trial, recurrent ischemia after successful primary PTCA occurred in only 1 (0.6%) of 170 patients after the second hospital day[84] (Fig. 11–22). The safety and cost savings of an accelerated discharge strategy was therefore tested in patients at low risk in PAMI-2.

### PAMI-2 Trial Design, Overall Results, and Effectiveness of Acute Risk Stratification

Entry criteria for the PAMI-2 trial were deliberately nonrestrictive. Patients of any age were enrolled with symptom duration of less than 12 hours, with any electrocardiographic pattern of AMI, and with acute infarction related to disease in either a native coronary artery or a bypass graft conduit. The major exclusion criteria were cardiogenic shock and contraindications to aspirin or heparin.

The study algorithm of the PAMI-2 trial appears in Figure 11–23. For risk stratification purposes, patients were considered to be at high risk if one or more of the following conditions were present: age of more than 70 years, LVEF of 45% or less, triple-vessel disease, saphenous vein graft occlusion, persistent postreperfusion malignant ventricular arrhythmias, or a suboptimal PTCA result. If none of these criteria was present, the patient was stratified as being at low risk. Patients at high risk in whom PTCA was performed and who had no absolute requirement for or contraindications to IABP insertion were randomly assigned to undergo 48 hours of prophylactic IABP counterpulsation or standard conservative care. Protocol predischarge angiography was performed in patients at high risk to assess patency of the infarcted artery. After primary PTCA, patients at low risk were randomly assigned to receive standard care (initial observation in the coronary care unit, 3 to 5 days of intravenous heparin, followed by discharge on days 5 to 7, after a negative result of a predischarge exercise test) or to receive accelerated care (observation in the standard PTCA stepdown unit, with an abbreviated 60-hour heparin course, and targeted day 3 discharge for stable patients, without predischarge exercise testing).

Between September 1993 and January 1995, 1100 patients were enrolled at 34 clinical centers in North America, South America, Europe, and Japan, making PAMI-2 the largest prospective, multicenter primary PTCA study to date.[384, 385] Study sites were quite diverse and included academic and community hospitals in urban and rural settings, with a wide range in annual total PTCA volume for the hospitals (60 to 3318 procedures/year) and for individual operators (22 to 507 procedures/year). The liberal entry criteria resulted in the enrollment of many patients with high-risk characteristics: The mean age was 60 ± 12 years (range, 26 to 90 years), 26% were female, 16% had diabetes mellitus, 17% had had a prior myocardial infarction, 5% had undergone prior CABG, and 37% presented with an anterior AMI. In addition, 23% of patients were

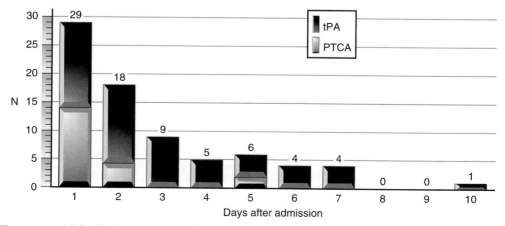

FIGURE 11–22. Time course of developing recurrent ischemia after reperfusion with either tissue-type plasminogen activator (tPA) or primary percutaneous transluminal coronary angioplasty (PTCA) in the Primary Angioplasty in Myocardial Infarction (PAMI)–1 trial.

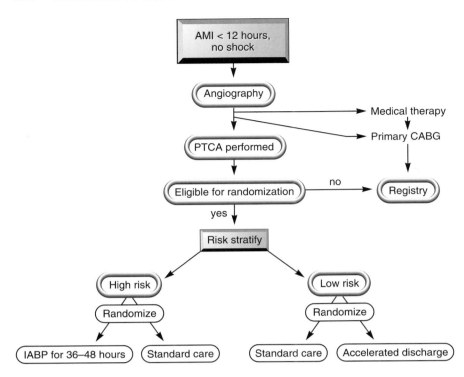

FIGURE 11–23. Study algorithm of the Primary Angioplasty in Myocardial Infarction (PAMI)–2 trial. AMI, acute myocardial infarction; CABG, coronary artery bypass grafting; IABP, intra-aortic balloon pump; PTCA, percutaneous transluminal coronary angioplasty.

tachycardic on admission, 32% had a systolic blood pressure reading of less than 100 mm Hg, and 30% would have been considered ineligible for thrombolysis because of excessive hemorrhagic risk, advanced age, late presentation, severe hypertension or hypotension, or a nonqualifying electrocardiogram. The mean time from symptom onset to emergency room presentation was 150 ± 175 minutes, the mean time from symptom onset to angiography was 260 ± 167 minutes, and the mean time from symptom onset to PTCA was 276 ± 165 minutes.

Of the 1100 enrolled patients, 982 (89%) underwent PTCA, whereas 53 (5%) underwent CABG, and 65 (6%) were treated with medical therapy alone. Among patients undergoing primary PTCA, angioplasty was successful in 96% of patients and re-

stored TIMI grade 3 flow in 93% of vessels. Emergency bypass surgery was required for failed PTCA in only 0.5% of cases. The overall in-hospital mortality rate among the entire 1100-patient population (including randomized and registry patients) was 2.9% (2.8% of patients undergoing primary PTCA, 5.7% of patients treated with CABG, and 1.5% of medically managed patients), the lowest mortality rate ever reported in a reperfusion AMI trial with no age restriction. This is even more remarkable in view of the high-risk nature of the population. Reinfarction occurred in 1.8% of patients before hospital discharge, and stroke occurred in only 0.8% (including 2 patients [0.2%] with hemorrhagic stroke and 7 patients [0.6%] with nonhemorrhagic stroke). In accordance with prior primary PTCA

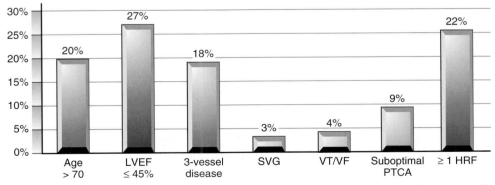

FIGURE 11–24. Prevalence of high-risk features in the Primary Angioplasty in Myocardial Infarction (PAMI)–2 study population. HRF, high risk features; LVEF, left ventricular ejection fraction; PICA, percutaneous transluminal coronary angioplasty; subopt., suboptimal; SVG, saphenous vein graft (culprit vessel); 3VD, triple-vessel disease; VT/VF, refractory malignant ventricular arrhythmias.

studies, recurrent ischemia occurred in only 11.8% of patients, repeat angiography after admission was performed in 13.5% of patients, and repeat PTCA was required in 8.1% of patients. The mean duration of hospital stay was 7.9 ± 6.4 days.

The risk stratification process classified 596 (54%) of 1100 patients as being at high risk (Fig. 11–24). Patients so identified were at markedly increased risk for short-term mortality and morbidity in comparison with patients at low risk, including 12.5-fold increased rate of mortality (Table 11–18). The mean duration of hospitalization was also 4.4 days longer for patients stratified as being at high risk than for those at low risk (10.0 ± 5.6 days vs. 5.6 ± 4.0 days; $p < 0.0001$). Particularly striking is the observation that the risk stratification process was able to isolate approximately half of an AMI population in whom the mortality rate after PTCA during AMI (0.4%) was similar to that expected after PTCA in the elective setting. Of note is that of the six variables used in the risk stratification score, four were angiographic measures (presence or absence of left ventricular dysfunction and triple-vessel disease, whether the infarct vessel was a vein graft or not and whether an optimal acute PTCA result was obtained or not). After all the clinical variables were accounted for by logistic regression analysis, the information derived from acute cardiac catheterization independently identified patients with a 3.8-fold increased rate of mortality.[403]

Of the 982 patients in whom primary PTCA was performed, 908 patients were eligible for random assignment. Of these patients, 437 patients (48.1%) were stratified as being at high risk after primary PTCA, and 471 patients (51.9%) were classified as low risk. Among randomly assigned patients, the mortality rates were 3.7% among patients at high risk and 0.4% among patients at low risk ($p = 0.0002$). Patients at high risk were randomly assigned to undergo 48 hours of IABP (N = 211) or to receive standard care without IABP (N = 226);

patients at low risk were randomly assigned to receive accelerated care (management in the PTCA stepdown unit, with a 60-hour tapering heparin course and targeted day 3 discharge without noninvasive testing; N = 237) or to receive standard care (monitoring in the coronary care unit, 72 hours or more of heparin administration, and predischarge exercise testing before discharge on hospital day 5 or later; N = 234).

## Utility of Intra-aortic Counterpulsation in Patients at High Risk After Primary PTCA[384]

Aortic counterpulsation was established in 86.3% of patients randomly assigned to receive an IABP after primary PTCA for a mean duration of 47.9 ± 28.0 hours. An IABP was required in 11.5% of patients assigned to conservative care because of hemodynamic instability, persistent ischemia, abrupt reocclusion of the vessel, or severe dissection or thrombosis. Unfortunately, in contrast to the earlier smaller studies that had demonstrated significant advantages of a routine IABP strategy,[398–401] in the PAMI-2 trial no major benefits were found for prophylactic IABP use in patients at high risk undergoing primary PTCA. By intention-to-treat analysis, the primary, prespecified composite end point of death, reinfarction, reocclusion of the infarcted vessel, stroke, or the development of new-onset heart failure or sustained hypotension was reached in 28.9% of patients who received IABP treatment and 29.2% of patients managed conservatively ($p = 0.95$) (Fig. 11–25). Intra-aortic counterpulsation did confer modest benefits in reducing recurrent ischemia (13.3% vs. 19.6%; $p = 0.08$) and reducing the need for subsequent unplanned predischarge angiography (7.6% vs. 13.3%; $p = 0.05$). However, the appropriate management of recurrent ischemia resulted in equivalent low rates of both death (4.3% vs. 3.1%; $p = 0.64$) and reinfarction (6.2% vs. 8.0%; $p = 0.64$) in the IABP and no-IABP groups, respectively. Furthermore, there was no evidence of enhanced myocardial recovery in patients treated with or without a prophylactic IABP (Table 11–19). The use of the IABP was surprisingly safe, however; patients treated with IABP, in comparison with those who received standard care, had similar rates of requirement for blood transfusion (20% vs. 18%; $p = 0.56$), pseudoaneurysm or arteriovenous fistula (1.4% vs. 1.3%; $p = 1.0$), sepsis (0.9% vs. 0.9%; $p = 1.0$), and vascular surgical repair (0.5% vs. 0.4%; $p = 1.0$), although minor hematomas were more common in the IABP group (20.9% vs. 13.3%; $p = 0.03$). There was, however, a statistically significant excess number of strokes associated with IABP use (Fig. 11–25). Chance may have been responsible for this finding; one stroke was present at admission,

**TABLE 11–18.    OUTCOMES IN PATIENTS STRATIFIED AS HIGH RISK VERSUS LOW RISK IN THE PAMI-2 STUDY**

| OUTCOME | HIGH RISK (N = 596) | LOW RISK (N = 504) | p |
|---|---|---|---|
| Death | 5.0% | 0.4% | <0.0001 |
| Reinfarction or reocclusion of infarcted artery | 6.0% | 2.7% | 0.007 |
| Recurrent ischemia | 15.3% | 7.7% | <0.0001 |
| New-onset heart failure or hypotension | 23.8% | 5.4% | <0.0001 |
| Stroke | 0.9% | 0.8% | NS |

PAMI, Primary Angioplasty in Myocardial Infarction.

## TABLE 11–19. INDICES OF MYOCARDIAL RECOVERY IN HIGH-RISK PATIENTS IN THE PAMI-2 TRIAL

| INDEX | IABP (N = 211) | No IABP (N = 226) | p |
|---|---|---|---|
| **Analysis of Paired Admission and Predischarge Contrast Ventriculograms** | | | |
| Mean change in LVEF | +2.6% | +2.2% | 0.75 |
| Mean change in infarcted zone wall motion (SD/chord) | +0.24 SD | +0.27 SD | 0.73 |
| Mean change in noninfarcted zone wall motion (SD/chord) | −0.12 SD | −0.11 SD | 0.96 |
| **Analysis of 6-Week Rest and Exercise Radionuclide Ventriculography** | | | |
| Resting LVEF | 47.6% | 46.6% | 0.60 |
| Exercise LVEF | 50.9% | 50.5% | 0.93 |

IABP, intra-aortic balloon pump; LVEF, left ventricular ejection fraction; PAMI, Primary Angioplasty in Myocardial Infarction; SD, standard deviation.

one occurred postoperatively, one occurred after new-onset atrial fibrillation, one occurred after prolonged hypotension, and one episode of intracranial bleeding occurred after the patient received a head wound. Nonetheless, the possibility that the presence of the large-bore pulsatile IABP in the central circulation contributed to the increased stroke rate cannot be totally discounted.

The lack of relative effectiveness of the routine IABP strategy in patients at high risk in PAMI-2 in comparison to prior reports may be explained by the observation that the patients who received standard care in PAMI-2 had better than expected outcomes. Both the in-hospital mortality rate of only 3.1% and the 5.5% rate of reocclusion in the infarcted artery among the conservatively treated patients were significantly lower than in the prior studies (e.g., 18%

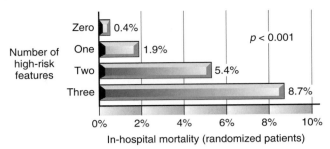

FIGURE 11–26. Prognostic ability of simple clinical and angiographic variables, readily obtainable within the first several hours of admission, to risk-stratify patients for subsequent in-hospital mortality after primary percutaneous transluminal coronary angioplasty (PTCA) in acute myocardial infarction. (Data from the Primary Angioplasty in Myocardial Infarction [PAMI]–2 study.[384, 385])

rate of reocclusion in the infarcted artery after primary PTCA in the Duke randomized trial[400, 401]). In PAMI-2, post hoc analysis did show that as the risk profile of patients in the high-risk group increased, so did the relative benefit of intra-aortic balloon counterpulsation. As the number of high-risk features present increased, so did the in-hospital mortality rate (Fig. 11–26). Whereas patients with only one high-risk feature experienced no gains with routine IABP use, patients with two or more high-risk features experienced a reduction in the primary composite end point with IABP use (Table 11–20).[404]

Thus, routine establishment of intra-aortic counterpulsation for 48 hours may be of benefit in patients at very high risk with AMI who are treated with primary PTCA. Furthermore, the randomly assigned patients in PAMI-2 were hemodynamically stable, with no absolute requirement for an IABP. The IABP is undoubtedly useful in patients who are hemodynamically unstable, have refractory ischemia or heart failure, or develop cardiogenic shock,[247] all of whom were excluded from the PAMI-2 trial.

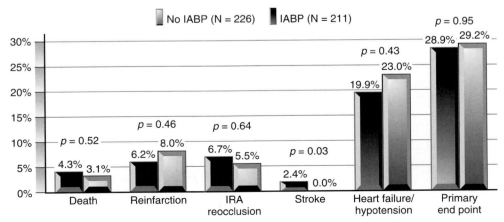

FIGURE 11–25. Major in-hospital adverse outcomes in the high-risk randomized group of the Primary Angioplasty in Myocardial Infarction (PAMI)–2 trial. The primary composite end point was the combined incidence of death, repeat myocardial infarction, infarct-related artery (IRA) reocclusion, or new-onset or progressive heart failure or sustained hypotension. IABP, intra-aortic balloon pump.

**TABLE 11–20.    Benefits of Routine Intra-Aortic Balloon Counterpulsation (IABP) in High-Risk Patients with AMI Undergoing Primary PTCA, Stratified by the Number of High-Risk Features Present (PAMI-2)**

| | ONE HIGH-RISK FEATURE | | | TWO OR MORE HIGH-RISK FEATURES | | |
|---|---|---|---|---|---|---|
| OUTCOME | IABP (N = 120) | No IABP (N = 139) | p | IABP (N = 91) | No IABP (N = 87) | p |
| Death | 2.5% | 1.4% | 0.67 | 6.7% | 5.8% | 0.82 |
| Composite without stroke | 20.0% | 18.7% | 0.79 | 18.9% | 32.6% | 0.04 |
| Composite with stroke | 20.8% | 18.7% | 0.67 | 21.1% | 32.6% | 0.09 |
| Recurrent ischemia | 22.5% | 29.5% | 0.20 | 23.3% | 40.7% | 0.01 |
| Vascular complications | 0.8% | 1.4% | 0.90 | 2.2% | 4.7% | 0.44 |
| Transfusion | 9.6% | 10.3% | 0.86 | 18.5% | 18.9% | 0.95 |

Composite consists of death, reinfarction, infarcted artery reocclusion, hypotension or heart failure, with or without stroke.
AMI, acute myocardial infarction; PAMI, Primary Angioplasty in Myocardial Infarction; PTCA, percutaneous transluminal coronary angioplasty.

Brodie and colleagues also reported that prophylactic IABP placement, when inserted before rather than after mechanical reperfusion, prevents hemodynamic deterioration in patients at high risk.[405] Finally, routine IABP use may have a role for patients undergoing rescue PTCA after failed thrombolysis, a situation in which infarcted artery reocclusion rates are known to be increased.[406]

### Safety, Feasibility, and Cost Effectiveness of Accelerated Discharge in Patients at Low Risk After Primary PTCA[385]

TIMI grade 3 flow was restored in 98% of patients at low risk. As a result, patients at low risk treated by primary PTCA were extremely stable, with low rates of in-hospital mortality (0.4%), reinfarction (0.4%), recurrent ischemia (6.8%), stroke (0.8%), and heart failure or hypotension (4.2%). Of the 237 patients assigned to accelerated discharge, 59 (25%) had medical conditions necessitating hospitalization beyond the third day (the target discharge date), such as heart failure or recurrent chest pain. Of the 178 remaining patients eligible for day 3 discharge, 142 (80%) were discharged on day 3 (including 92%

of eligible patients in the United States vs. 17% in non-U.S. sites). The mean duration of hospitalization was 3 days less with an accelerated discharge strategy than with standard care (Fig. 11–27).

Omission of the coronary care unit phase, prolonged heparinization, and predischarge exercise testing in patients at low risk after successful primary PTCA proved to be safe. The in-hospital, 1-week, and 6-month outcomes were similar for the standard care and accelerated discharge groups (Table 11–21). The 3-day-shorter length of hospitalization in patients randomly assigned to receive accelerated care, in comparison with those receiving standard care, resulted in markedly reduced hospital costs and charges (see Fig. 11–27), attributable to reduced expenses for room and board, pharmaceuticals, laboratory testing, and cardiac testing. By withholding thrombolytic therapy and instead treating lytic-eligible patients with primary PTCA, this early discharge strategy could reduce U.S. health care expenditures by approximately $293,000,000 per year.[385]

Even earlier discharge may be possible in selected patients with AMI treated by primary PTCA.[407] In PAMI-2, 150 patients were identified as being at

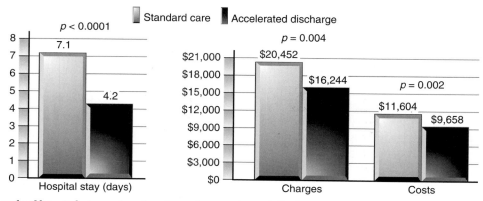

FIGURE 11–27. Length of hospital stay and cost savings of an accelerated discharge strategy in patients prospectively identified as low risk after primary percutaneous transluminal coronary angioplasty (PTCA). (Data from the Primary Angioplasty in Myocardial Infarction [PAMI]–2 study.[385])

**TABLE 11–21.** **IN-HOSPITAL AND LATE OUTCOMES IN LOW-RISK PATIENTS WITH AMI AFTER SUCCESSFUL PRIMARY PTCA RANDOMLY ASSIGNED TO ACCELERATED DISCHARGE VERSUS STANDARD CARE**

| OUTCOME | ACCELERATED CARE (N = 237) | STANDARD CARE (N = 234) | p |
|---|---|---|---|
| **In-Hospital Outcomes** | | | |
| Death | 0.4% | 0.4% | 0.99 |
| Reinfarction | 0.4% | 0.4% | 0.99 |
| Recurrent ischemia | 5.9% | 7.7% | 0.33 |
| Reocclusion of infarcted artery | 1.7% | 3.0% | 0.57 |
| Stroke | 0% | 1.7% | 0.06 |
| Heart failure or hypotension | 4.2% | 4.3% | 0.98 |
| Combined primary end point | 9.7% | 12.4% | 0.35 |
| Duration of hospitalization (days) | 4.2 ± 2.3 | 7.1 ± 4.7 | 0.0001 |
| **Events Within 1 Week of Discharge** | | | |
| Death | 0% | 0% | 1.0 |
| Reinfarction | 0% | 0% | 1.0 |
| Recurrent chest pain | 1.5% | 1.1% | 0.92 |
| Symptoms necessitating readmission | 2.1% | 1.1% | 0.53 |
| Target vessel revascularization | 0% | 0% | 1.0 |
| **Cumulative 6-Month Events** | | | |
| Death | 0.8% | 0.4% | 1.0 |
| Unstable ischemia | 10.1% | 11.1% | 0.73 |
| Reinfarction | 1.3% | 0.4% | 0.62 |
| Stroke | 0.4% | 2.6% | 0.08 |
| Heart failure or hypotension | 4.6% | 4.3% | 0.85 |
| Combined primary end point | 15.6% | 17.5% | 0.58 |
| Readmission for unstable ischemia | 5.1% | 3.8% | 0.52 |
| Target vessel revascularization | 8.5% | 10.3% | 0.50 |

AMI, acute myocardial infarction; PTCA, percutaneous transluminal coronary angioplasty.

"ultra–low risk"; this group consisted of patients at low risk with additional characteristics: age of less than 60, single-vessel disease, and post-PTCA TIMI grade 3 flow with residual stenosis affecting less than 30% of the vessel diameter, and no thrombus or dissection. Among patients stratified as being at ultra–low risk, the in-hospital survival rate was 100%, reinfarction or infarct artery reocclusion occurred in only 1 patient, new or progressive heart failure or hypotension occurred in only 1 patient, and no patient suffered a stroke; 98.7% of patients at ultra–low risk were discharged without experiencing any major in-hospital end point.[407]

### Clinical Implications of the PAMI-2 Trial

The PAMI-2 trial has demonstrated that primary PTCA is capable of restoring TIMI grade 3 flow in more than 90% of patients, many of whom are at high risk and otherwise ineligible for thrombolytic treatment. As a result, 97% of patients managed with a primary PTCA strategy survive to hospital discharge and have extremely low rates of reinfarction and stroke. Of importance is that these results were obtained without the use of costly glycoprotein IIb/IIIa receptor blocking agents and, in 99% of patients, without stents. These outcomes were achieved in a wide variety of practice settings and by operators with varying experience levels. From

the knowledge of baseline clinical features and variables derived from immediate cardiac catheterization, a powerful prognostic instrument may be constructed and used to prospectively stratify patients into high- and low-risk groups. In the approximately 50% of patients who are identified as being at low risk, management may consist of monitoring in the standard PTCA stepdown unit, early ambulation after an abbreviated heparin course, and accelerated discharge on day 3 for stable patients, without noninvasive functional testing. As a result, the adverse psychosocial effects of AMI are minimized, more rapid and complete return to work is facilitated, and hospital costs are markedly reduced (with similar reimbursement), which will further enhance the cost effectiveness of primary PTCA in comparison with other reperfusion modalities.

Patients at high risk are also prospectively identified during cardiac catheterization. In these patients, the outcomes after primary PTCA are still excellent in comparison with those in thrombolytic-treated controls, although rates of absolute mortality remain increased in comparison to patients without adverse features. The number of adverse baseline features may be used to further stratify patients at high risk. Although a routine IABP strategy was not found to be of major benefit, the patients at highest risk appeared to benefit in terms of reduced rates of

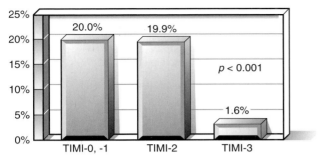

FIGURE 11–28. Relationship between final Thrombolysis In Myocardial Infarction (TIMI) flow on the 90-minute angiogram and 30-day mortality in the primary percutaneous transluminal coronary angioplasty (PTCA) recipients in the Global Utilization of Streptokinase and Tissue Plasminogen Activator for Occluded Arteries (GUSTO)–IIb trial.[226]

recurrent ischemia and freedom from hemodynamic deterioration. Further studies are necessary to identify adjunctive pharmacologic and mechanical measures to improve the prognosis of patients at high risk with AMI.

## Understanding the Mortality Benefit of Primary PTCA

Primary PTCA, in comparison with thrombolytic therapy, may improve survival in patients with AMI through two major mechanisms: (1) by more frequently restoring patency of the infarcted artery and effective myocardial perfusion and (2) by avoiding iatrogenic complications.

### Central Unifying Concept of TIMI Grade 3 Flow After Reperfusion Therapy

As previously discussed, it has been conclusively demonstrated that the early restoration of TIMI grade 3 flow is a primary determinant of survival after thrombolytic administration. Data have confirmed that a similar relationship is valid after primary PTCA. In the GUSTO-IIb trial, although primary PTCA restored TIMI grade 3 flow in only 73%

of patients, the 30-day mortality rate was $\frac{1}{12}$ that among patients in whom TIMI grade 3 flow was restored than among those in whom it was not restored (Fig. 11–28).[226] Survival was no better with TIMI grade 2 flow than with TIMI grade 0 or 1 flow.

In the combined PAMI-1 and PAMI-2 trials, among the 1157 patients in whom primary PTCA was performed, TIMI grade 3 flow was restored after PTCA in 93% of patients, TIMI grade 2 flow was restored in 5% of patients, and TIMI grade 0 or 1 flow was present in 2% of patients.[408] In comparison with patients in whom TIMI grade 0 to 2 flow occurred, patients with TIMI grade 3 flow had lower rates of mortality, reinfarction, recurrent ischemia, postadmission heart failure or hypotension, and need for CABG and shorter hospital stays (Table 11–22). In general, the outcomes of patients in the PAMI trials in whom TIMI grade 2 flow was present were intermediate between those with TIMI grade 0 or 1 flow and TIMI grade 3 flow. According to multivariate analysis, the three factors independently related to survival after primary PTCA in PAMI-1 and PAMI-2 were the absence of triple-vessel disease (odds ratio, 4.9), younger age (odds ratio, 4.2), and restoration of TIMI grade 3 flow (odds ratio, 4.8).[408]

The data from all reported studies of thrombolytic therapy and primary PTCA indicate that the central unifying role of TIMI grade 3 flow after reperfusion therapy may be further appreciated by plotting the percentage of patients achieving TIMI grade 3 flow 90 minutes after reperfusion versus the short-term mortality rate (Fig. 11–29).[10, 11, 12, 19, 192, 226, 229, 244, 408, 409] Despite the differing inclusion criteria among these studies (i.e., many of the primary PTCA studies included thrombolytic-ineligible patients), an extremely tight linear relationship is seen to link restoration of TIMI grade 3 flow to early survival. After thrombolytic therapy, TIMI grade 3 flow was restored in these studies in 33% to 62% of patients, with corresponding mortality rates of 4.6% to 7.4%. In contrast, after primary PTCA, TIMI grade 3 flow

**TABLE 11–22.    RELATIONSHIP OF TIMI FLOW AFTER PRIMARY PTCA TO IN-HOSPITAL OUTCOMES IN THE PAMI-1 AND PAMI-2 TRIALS**

| OUTCOME | TIMI GRADE 0 TO 1 | TIMI GRADE 2 | TIMI GRADE 3 | p |
|---|---|---|---|---|
| Death | 17.2% | 7.6% | 2.1% | <0.0001 |
| Reinfarction | 13.8% | 7.6% | 4.0% | 0.01 |
| Death or reinfarction | 31.0% | 13.2% | 6.0% | <0.0001 |
| Recurrent ischemia | 13.8% | 7.6% | 4.0% | 0.01 |
| Postadmission heart failure or hypotension | 44.8% | 28.3% | 15.9% | 0.01 |
| Coronary artery bypass surgery | 17.2% | 9.4% | 5.9% | 0.03 |
| Mean length of hospitalization (days) | 9.2 ± 5.8 | 9.6 ± 6.0 | 7.7 ± 5.2 | 0.06 |

PAMI, Primary Angioplasty in Myocardial Infarction; PTCA, percutaneous transluminal coronary angioplasty; TIMI, Thrombolysis In Myocardial Infarction (flow).

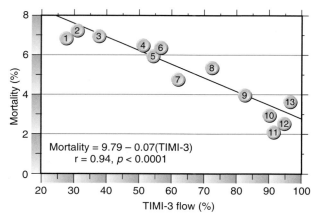

**Thrombolytic therapy**

1. GUSTO-1 SK/SQ heparin (10)
2. GUSTO-1 SK/IV heparin (10)
3. GUSTO-1 SK/tPA (10)
4. GUSTO-1 accelerated tPA (10)
5. TAMI-1 to -3, -5, -7 (19)
7. Four German studies (11)

**Primary PTCA**

8. GUSTO-IIb (226)
9. Mayo Clinic (409)
10. PAMI-2 (408)
11. Zwolle (244)
12. PAMI-1 (229)
13. PAR (192)

FIGURE 11–29. The central unifying concept of the acute restoration of TIMI-3 flow and mortality after reperfusion therapy in acute myocardial infarction. See text for details. GUSTO, Global Utilization of Streptokinase and Tissue Plasminogen Activator for Occluded Arteries; IV, intravenous; PAMI, Primary Angioplasty in Myocardial Infarction; PAR, Primary Angioplasty Revascularization; SK, streptokinase; SQ, subcutaneous; TAMI, Thrombolysis and Angioplasty in Myocardial Infarction; TEAM, Thrombolysis Eminase Acute Myocardial Infarction; TIMI, Thrombolysis In Myocardial Infarction; tPA, tissue-type plasminogen activator.

in higher percentages (73% to 97%) resulted in lower mortality rates (2.0% to 5.7%). Furthermore, as can be seen, the PTCA results from the GUSTO-IIb trial were intermediate between those of most of the thrombolytic trials and those of the other primary PTCA studies, clarifying the reason for the modest benefits of primary PTCA in GUSTO-IIb in comparison with the other primary PTCA trials. Thus, the greater the likelihood that TIMI grade 3 flow can be restored by a given reperfusion modality, the lower the short-term mortality rate will be; patients without cardiogenic shock would have a theoretical survival rate of 97% if TIMI grade 3 flow were restored. With thrombolytic therapy, there is a pharmacologic plateau of restoration of TIMI grade 3 flow, in approximately 55% to 60% of patients, which limits the ultimate efficacy of thrombolysis in reducing mortality. In contrast, TIMI grade 3 flow may be restored in more than 90% of patients by primary PTCA, which is directly responsible for much of the survival benefit of the mechanical approach in comparison with thrombolytic therapy. Furthermore, the early survival benefit of restoring TIMI grade 3 flow is maintained during 5 years of clinical follow-up.[17]

The mechanisms through which restoration of patency of the infarcted artery and of TIMI grade 3 flow is translated into improved survival rate are more complex than was originally thought, and can be separated into two general categories: those dependent on myocardial salvage and those independent of myocardial salvage.

### Myocardial Salvage After Reperfusion Therapy

It is well established that left ventricular function is a major determinant of survival after AMI.[410] Early myocardial reperfusion both in experimental prepa-

rations and in clinical studies has unequivocally been shown to limit myocardial damage.[411–414] Large-scale trials of thrombolytic therapy have clearly demonstrated that earlier treatment results in greater relative survival benefit; for each hour earlier that treatment is initiated, approximately 1.6 additional lives per 1000 patients treated are saved.[114] It is therefore logical to conclude that the major mechanism through which reperfusion therapy results in enhanced survival is myocardial salvage and, by extension, that the improved survival rates among patients treated with primary PTCA rather than thrombolytic therapy may be attributable to greater myocardial recovery, as suggested by early observational studies.[117]

However, the data from the randomized trials conflict with regard to whether primary PTCA does indeed salvage significantly more myocardium than does thrombolytic therapy. In the small early pilot trial of primary PTCA versus intracoronary streptokinase performed by O'Neill and coworkers,[167] myocardial recovery, as assessed by serial admission and paired contrast ventriculograms, was markedly increased after primary PTCA in comparison with thrombolysis (mean change in LVEF, +8% vs. +1%; $p < 0.001$). Similarly, the randomized Zwolle trial demonstrated greater myocardial salvage and late improvement in left ventricular function in patients treated with PTCA than in those treated with tPA.[218, 219, 242] In this study, the infarction size estimated by lactate dehydrogenase analysis was 23% smaller after PTCA than after streptokinase treatment (1003 ± 784 IU vs. 1310 ± 1198 IU; $p = 0.01$). The mean predischarge LVEF was also significantly greater in the PTCA-treated patients (50% ± 11% vs. 44% ± 11%; $p = 0.001$). An improvement in LVEF after primary PTCA was demonstrated in patients with anterior and nonanterior AMI, in patients with single-vessel and multivessel disease, and in those treated 2 hours before and 2 hours after onset of AMI.

In contrast to these positive studies, in the PAMI trial, the 6-week resting LVEF (53% ± 13% vs. 53% ± 13%) and exercise LVEF (56% ± 14% vs. 57% ± 13%) were similar in patients treated by primary PTCA and those treated with tPA.[223] Furthermore, in the Mayo Clinic study,[224] in which myocardial recovery was meticulously assessed by paired acute and predischarge technetium-99m sestamibi imaging,[415–417] no significant difference in myocardial salvage was demonstrated between the PTCA- and tPA-treated patients, although there was a weak trend for more myocardial salvage after PTCA in anterior AMI. There were also weak trends toward an improvement in resting LVEF in patients treated with PTCA rather than tPA, both at discharge (53% ± 12% vs. 50% ± 11%; $p = 0.22$) and at 6 weeks (53% ± 11% vs. 50% ± 10%; $p = 0.22$).

Thus, it is unlikely that myocardial salvage alone can explain the striking 33% reduction in mortality after reperfusion by primary PTCA in comparison with thrombolytic therapy (see Table 11–8). This finding should, in retrospect, not be surprising. Many prior studies have, in fact, failed to demonstrate a substantial relationship between myocardial salvage and improved survival after reperfusion therapy.[418–422] Most of the placebo-controlled studies of thrombolytic therapy have found only modest, if any, gains in left ventricular function,[117, 423–425] despite impressive reductions in mortality.

Furthermore, the time to reperfusion in most prior clinical studies is inconsistent with the attainment of a significant amount of myocardial recovery. For significant myocardial salvage to occur, the infarcted artery must be recanalized within 2 hours of occlusion. Reimer and coworkers first described the "wavefront" of myocardial necrosis that spreads from the endocardium to the epicardium after experimental canine coronary occlusion.[411] If the coronary constriction was released within 1 hour, minimal necrosis was seen. Up to 2 hours, the amount of myocardial damage was proportional to the duration of occlusion. After 2 hours, little myocardium was viable. These observations were confirmed in an experimental model of thrombotic occlusion followed by thrombolytic reperfusion.[426]

In view of the results of human studies, it must be recognized that reperfusion is not instantaneous after thrombolytic administration; the average time for recanalization of the infarcted artery to occur after thrombolytic infusion initiation is 45 to 60 minutes.[8, 427] In accordance with this finding, most clinical studies have found that thrombolytic therapy must be given within 1 hour after symptom onset (to restore patency of the infarcted artery

within 2 hours of occlusion) for substantial myocardial recovery to be realized. In The Netherlands Inter-University Cardiology Trial, the mean reduction in enzymatic infarction size after thrombolysis was 51% in patients treated within the first hour of symptom onset, 31% for those treated between 1 and 2 hours after symptom onset, and only 13% for those treated after the second hour.[428] In the TIMI-II trial, the percentage of patients having LVEF of more than 55% at 6 weeks was 38% if tPA was administered within 1 hour of symptom onset, as opposed to 28% between 1 and 2 hours later, 28% between 2 and 3 hours later, and 27% between 3 and 4 hours later ($p = 0.04$).[429] The MITI investigators found that patients treated within 70 minutes of symptom onset had a smaller infarct size as measured by thallium scintigraphy (4.9% vs. 11.2%; $p < 0.001$), greater mean LVEF at 30 days (53% vs. 49%; $p = 0.03$), and reduced 30-day mortality rates (1.2% vs. 8.7%; $p = 0.04$) than did patients treated more than 70 minutes after AMI onset.[430] These findings have been confirmed by other thrombolytic studies.[431, 432]

Similarly, for primary PTCA to effectively salvage myocardium, the infarcted vessel must be recanalized within 2 hours of occlusion. In a study of 59 patients with AMI who underwent primary PTCA and in whom paired acute and predischarge technetium-99m sestamibi scans were obtained,[415–417] a mean of 41% ± 21% of the left ventricular myocardium was salvaged if the infarcted artery was opened within 2 hours, in contrast to 17% ± 17% at 2 to 4 hours and 12% ± 14% at 4 to 6 hours.[433]

For substantial myocardial salvage to occur, thrombolysis must therefore be initiated within approximately 1 hour of symptom onset, and primary PTCA must be performed within approximately 2 hours. Unfortunately, the median time from AMI symptom onset to emergency room arrival in the United States is close to 4 hours.[137, 302, 434] In the 41,021-patient GUSTO-I trial, fewer than 4% of patients with AMI who were receiving thrombolytic therapy were treated within 1 hour of symptom onset. Thus, most patients with AMI present after the optimal time period for significant myocardial salvage.

It has been argued that in comparison with the speed with which thrombolytic therapy may be initiated, the inherent delay in performing primary PTCA may adversely affect myocardial recovery, especially in patients presenting early after coronary occlusion. In general, thrombolytic therapy may be begun 30 to 60 minutes before the first PTCA balloon inflation.[218, 223, 226, 409] However, after patient presentation, it takes on average 60 minutes for thrombolysis to be initiated,[302, 434] which, when added to the 45 to 60 minutes required for lytic-mediated reperfusion,[8, 427] takes most patients beyond the optimal time period for significant myocardial salvage. In addition, myocardial recovery is affected by factors other than time to reperfusion, including the amount of myocardium at risk,[141, 416, 433, 435–437] the presence of some degree of baseline antegrade flow or collateral vessels before reperfusion,[141, 153, 433, 435, 438–440] TIMI flow grade after reperfusion,[10, 12, 16, 441] and the post-reperfusion residual stenosis.[153, 442] The dependence of myocardial salvage on post-reperfusion establishment of TIMI grade 3 flow and less severe residual stenosis would favor greater myocardial recovery after primary PTCA than after thrombolysis. In the GUSTO-I trial,[10] the mean LVEF was 62% if TIMI grade 3 flow was present at 90 minutes, as opposed to 55% with TIMI grades 0 and 1 flow ($p < 0.001$). Patients with TIMI grade 2 flow had a mean LVEF of 56%, similar to that seen with TIMI grades 0 and 1 flow. Similarly, in the Thrombolysis EMINASE Acute Myocardial Infarction (TEAM)–2 and TEAM-3 studies, only TIMI grade 3 flow correlated with a smaller enzyme rise and with enhanced global and regional left ventricular function.[12, 16] After primary PTCA, restoration of TIMI grade 3 flow also results in greater myocardial salvage and smaller final infarction size than if only TIMI grade 2 flow is present.[441] Furthermore, after thrombolysis, approximately 70% to 85% of patients have high-grade residual stenosis at the infarction site.[73–76] Sheehan and associates found appreciable regional wall motion recovery only if the area of residual stenosis after reperfusion was more than 0.4 mm.[153] Leung and Lau found that an area of residual stenosis of more than 1.5 mm was necessary to prevent left ventricular dilatation in the first year after reperfusion.[442] The more frequent restoration of TIMI grade 3 flow after primary PTCA than after thrombolysis (see Fig. 11–29), in concert with less severe residual stenosis,[167, 218] is probably responsible for the demonstration of superior myocardial salvage in some of the randomized reperfusion trials, despite the relatively late time of patient enrollment in these studies.

### TIMI Grade 3 Flow Improves Survival Independently of Myocardial Salvage

Despite the fact that relatively little myocardium is salvaged when reperfusion occurs more than 2 hours after coronary occlusion, significant improvements in survival have been documented when patients undergo reperfusion as late as 12 hours after symptom onset,[3, 4, 114, 134, 443] which suggests the possibility that recanalization of the infarcted artery may reduce mortality independently of myocardial salvage; this is the so-called open-artery hypothesis.[444] The Western Washington Intracoronary Streptokinase trial was the first study to demonstrate

improved survival at 30 days and at 1 year in patients with a patent infarcted vessel, independently of myocardial salvage.[314, 445, 446] In the Second International Study of Infarct Survival (ISIS-2), thrombolytic therapy improved survival even when given 13 to 24 hours after chest pain onset, clearly beyond the optimal time period for significant myocardial salvage.[4] Other trials have since found that a patent infarcted vessel is predictive of early and late survival after reperfusion with thrombolytic therapy.[447–450] Brodie and coworkers showed that sustained patency of the infarcted artery after primary PTCA is a predictor of 5-year survival in patients with anterior AMI and reduced LVEF, independently of myocardial salvage.[451]

The mechanisms through which the early establishment of TIMI grade 3 flow, with sustained late patency of the infarcted artery, results in enhanced early and late survival are diverse and most likely multifactorial (Table 11–23).[419–422, 444, 452–455] After transmural AMI, geometric remodeling of the left ventricle with infarcted artery expansion may result in aneurysm formation and increased end-systolic volume, which adversely affects prognosis independent of LVEF.[410] Experimental[412, 456] and clinical[457–465] studies have convincingly demonstrated that even late reperfusion may prevent infarcted artery expansion and left ventricular dilatation, independently of absolute infarction size. The mechanism through which late reperfusion prevents left ventricular dilatation and aneurysm formation may relate to the preservation of a rim of viable myocardium in the subepicardium.[411, 419, 466–469] The subsequent reduction of the extent of peri-infarction myocardial edema or hemorrhage, scar thickness, and altered myocardial contracture patterns may preserve left ventricular cavity size. Increased turgor in the reper-

### TABLE 11–23. THE OPEN ARTERY HYPOTHESIS: MECHANISMS OF MORTALITY REDUCTION WITH EARLY AND SUSTAINED VESSEL PATENCY INDEPENDENT OF MYOCARDIAL SALVAGE

Improved geometric remodeling
  Prevention of infarct expansion
  Prevention of left ventricular dilatation and
    aneurysm formation
  Scaffolding
  Improved diastolic function
  Prevention of myocardial rupture
Reversal of hibernating myocardium
Decreased arrhythmogenesis
  Less frequent postinfarction ventricular ectopy
  Fewer late potentials
  Raised threshold for electrophysiologic inducibility
Preservation of collateral flow

fused vasculature, by increasing tensile strength, may also act as a myocardial baffle. In addition, transmural infarction is necessary for aneurysm formation.[456] By preserving a layer of functional myocardium, late reperfusion may decrease the likelihood of aneurysm formation, resulting in reduced mural thrombus deposition and arrhythmic potential, as discussed later.

Myocardial rupture occurs in approximately 4% to 8% of patients after AMI[470, 471] and may be responsible for 20% of all deaths after thrombolytic therapy.[425, 472–474] Because transmural infarction is necessary for myocardial rupture,[470, 475, 476] late reperfusion may limit this catastrophic complication. Paradoxically, however, late reperfusion after thrombolysis has actually been found to increase the likelihood of myocardial rupture by promoting myocardial hemorrhage.[3, 209, 210, 477–480] In contrast, primary PTCA results in bland infarction, and as a result, myocardial rupture is rare, even after late reperfusion.[158, 187, 209, 210, 405] Late reperfusion may also reduce diastolic dysfunction of the left ventricle.[481, 482] Finally, there is accumulating evidence that delayed PTCA of occluded or severely stenosed coronary arteries days to weeks after AMI may result in late improvement of regional wall motion and LVEF, as long as infarcted artery patency is sustained, possibly by restoring function to viable "hibernating" myocardium at the watershed zones of infarction.[50, 465, 483–488]

An additional benefit of restoring myocardial perfusion is improved electrical stability. Sudden cardiac death, often precipitated by ischemia, is the most common cause of late mortality after hospital discharge for AMI.[489–492] After both early and delayed reperfusion with either thrombolytic therapy or primary PTCA, reduced postinfarction ventricu-

lar ectopy, less frequent late potentials, and a heightened threshold for electrophysiologic inducibility of ventricular tachycardia have been noted, independently of myocardial salvage.[493–499] The presence of late potentials after reperfusion therapy has been shown to be an independent adverse prognostic risk factor for late mortality, even after infarcted artery patency and LVEF are accounted for.[500] In this regard, Karam and colleagues, in a retrospective analysis of 109 patients with AMI, found that late potentials after successful reperfusion were more frequently present after thrombotic therapy than after either primary or rescue PTCA (35% vs. 17% and 8%, respectively; $p < 0.05$), which suggests that late electrical stability may be enhanced with mechanical rather than pharmacologic reperfusion.[499]

A final benefit of late reperfusion may be the provision of collateral flow to the noninfarcted zones, which may prevent future ischemia, infarction, or arrhythmias in patients with multivessel disease. Multiple studies have demonstrated the importance of collateral vessels in preserving myocardium and improving long-term prognosis after AMI.[153, 433, 435, 438, 439, 501–503]

### Effect of Treatment Delay on Mortality After Reperfusion: Primary PTCA Versus Thrombolytic Therapy

Further evidence that the salutary effects of primary PTCA in reducing mortality are largely independent of time to reperfusion (and by extension, myocardial salvage) is seen in Figure 11–30, in which rate of the in-hospital mortality from 4432 primary PTCA procedures from the Mid America Heart Institute, Moses Cone Hospital, and the PAMI-2 trial are pre-

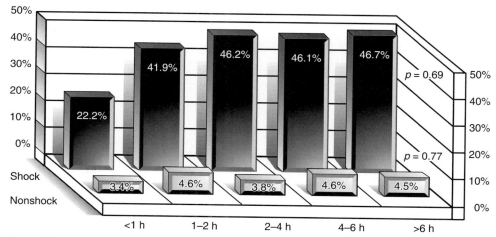

FIGURE 11–30. In-hospital mortality after 4432 primary percutaneous transluminal coronary angioplasty (PTCA) procedures, stratified by the time from symptom onset to reperfusion, in patients with cardiogenic shock (N = 284) and those without shock (N = 4148). Data were pooled from the Primary Angioplasty in Myocardial Infarction (PAMI)–2 study and from the individual databases from all primary PTCA procedures at the Mid America Heart Institute in Kansas City, Missouri, and at the Moses Cone Hospital in Greensboro, North Carolina, through April 1997.

sented in relation to the time from symptom onset to dilatation.[504] As demonstrated, the rate of survival after primary PTCA in patients without shock is excellent at all time intervals. Even in patients with cardiogenic shock, no definite relationship between the time to reperfusion and survival was noted (except possibly for patients undergoing dilation within the first hour, although the numbers were too small for firm conclusions). In contrast, in both the TIMI-II and GUSTO-I trials, in-hospital mortality steadily increased as time to treatment was delayed (Fig. 11–31).[301, 428]

There are several possible reasons why mortality after primary PTCA may be less dependent on the time to reperfusion than is mortality after thrombolysis. First, TIMI grade 3 flow is restored after primary PTCA in more than 90% of patients, independently of the time to reperfusion.[304, 504] In contrast, the efficacy of thrombolytic therapy declines as the clot ages. In an analysis of the 90-minute angiographic data from the combined TIMI-I and European Cooperative Study Group (ECSG) trials,[37, 302, 505] TIMI grade 2 or 3 flow was present after tPA in 81% of 42 patients treated within 3 hours of symptom onset, in contrast to 67% of 162 patients treated between 3 and 6 hours after symptom onset ($p = 0.08$). Similarly, after streptokinase, 90-minute patency was restored in 55% of 56 patients treated within 3 hours, in contrast to 42% of 151 patients treated after 3 to 6 hours ($p = 0.09$). In the GUSTO-I angiographic substudy, TIMI grade 3 flow after accelerated tPA was restored in 62% of patients treated within 2 hours of symptom onset, in 54% of patients treated between 2 and 4 hours after symptom onset, and in 50% of patients treated between 4 and 6 hours after symptom onset ($p = 0.17$ for <2 hours vs. ≥2 hours).[303] In the RAPID-2 trial, the likelihood of restoring TIMI grade 3 flow 90 minutes after thrombolytic therapy was notably greater if the time from symptom onset to treatment was 6 hours or less, in comparison with more than 6 hours (47%

vs. 35% for tPA [N = 147, $p < 0.04$] and 63% vs. 40% for rPA [N = 156, $p = 0.09$]).[506]

Second, patients who present late in the course of their AMI are more likely to have coexisting adverse risk factors—including advanced age, female gender, diabetes, hypertension, and tachycardia, heart failure, or hypotension on admission—than are those who present early.[137, 301, 434, 507] As previously discussed, patients with most of these comorbid risk factors fare better with primary PTCA than with thrombolytic therapy, because of enhanced reperfusion rates or avoidance of life-threatening hemorrhagic complications. Third, in the GUSTO-I trial, it was noted that the rate of intracranial bleeding steadily increased from 0.5% of patients treated with thrombolysis within 2 hours of symptom onset to 1.0% of patients treated after 6 hours.[301] The total stroke rate increased from 1.3% to 2.0% over the same time period. This relationship disappeared, however, after correction by multivariate analysis, which signifies that other comorbid risk factors associated with treatment delay (such as advanced age) are responsible for the increased stroke and intracranial bleeding rates observed.[100] Finally, thrombolytic therapy given late in the course of a transmural AMI may result in hemorrhagic transformation of an otherwise bland infarction, thereby increasing the rate of myocardial rupture.[3, 209, 210, 477–480] In contrast, reperfusion injury with myocardial hemorrhage and rupture is much less frequent after primary PTCA, even with late reperfusion.[158, 187, 209, 210, 211, 216, 405]

The data in Figure 11–30 should not be misinterpreted to imply that unnecessary delays in either presentation or treatment before primary PTCA are permissible or acceptable. This mortality analysis does not take into account indices of morbidity such as the development of hypotension, heart failure, or myocardial salvage. As previously discussed, early treatment in selected patients may reduce infarction size, especially in patients at high risk with a large

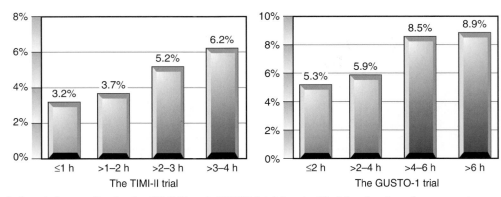

FIGURE 11–31. In-hospital mortality in the TIMI-II and GUSTO-I trials, stratified by the time from symptom onset to treatment. GUSTO, Global Utilization of Streptokinase and Tissue Plasminogen Activator for Occluded Arteries; TIMI, Thrombolysis In Myocardial Infarction.

amount of myocardium at risk. The optimal time period for substantial myocardial salvage may extend well beyond 1 to 2 hours in patients with dynamic obstruction of the infarcted vessel and when collateral flow is present. The critical time interval for myocardial recovery is therefore unpredictable for the individual patient. Needless delays may also permit the emergence of serious ventricular arrhythmias or heart block, allow heart failure to become clinically evident, and decrease the likelihood that the patient will be hemodynamically stable before and during catheterization. Patients in whom excessive delays result in death before reperfusion would not have been accounted for by the analysis in Figure 11–30, inasmuch as these data represent the outcomes of patients surviving to undergo primary PTCA. All efforts must be taken to ensure that reperfusion is restored as quickly as possible in patients with AMI.

### Avoidance of Hemorrhagic Complications by Primary PTCA

As demonstrated in the meta-analysis of the PTCA-thrombolysis randomized trials, the incidences of intracranial hemorrhage and total stroke are significantly reduced by withholding thrombolytic therapy (see Tables 11–10 and 11–11). In view of the high mortality rate after intracranial bleeding,[92–103] approximately 1 life per 100 patients treated would be saved by the primary PTCA strategy solely by avoiding thrombolytic-induced iatrogenic intracranial hemorrhage. Avoidance of intracranial hemorrhage in patients at increased risk for this life-threatening complication, such as women and the elderly, also partly explains the favorable outcomes of primary PTCA in high-risk subsets.

The near elimination of intracranial hemorrhage may also partly explain the observation that the short-term mortality rate among patients achieving TIMI grade 3 flow after primary PTCA may be lower than if TIMI grade 3 flow had been restored by thrombolytic therapy. Pooling of the results of five TAMI trials, four German studies, and the TEAM-2 and GUSTO-I trials[10–12, 19] reveals that patients with TIMI grade 3 flow 90 minutes after thrombolysis had a 4.0% mortality rate (range, 2.7% to 4.5%). In contrast, the short-term mortality rate among patients achieving TIMI grade 3 flow after primary PTCA in the PAMI-1, PAMI-2, and GUSTO-IIb trials[226, 229, 408] was only 1.9% (range, 1.6% to 2.1%; p = 0.001).

## Primary PTCA: Technical Considerations

From the preceding analysis, it is clear that the major factor determining survival after primary PTCA is whether the interventional cardiologist is able to restore TIMI grade 3 flow in the infarcted vessel. It is not surprising that, as with the effect of operator experience on outcomes after CABG surgery[508–510] or elective angioplasty,[511–515] the results of primary PTCA in AMI may vary from operator to operator (see Fig. 11–12). Because the variability in reported PTCA reperfusion success (TIMI grade 3 flow achieved in 73% to 95% of patients) may translate to an absolute mortality difference of approximately 3 to 4 lives per 100 patients treated (see Table 11–12 and Fig. 11–29), a detailed understanding of the technical considerations that increase the likelihood of primary PTCA success is of paramount importance. Although no studies have been performed to address this issue directly, insight may be gained from inspection of the primary PTCA methodology and rationale employed in the PAMI trials (Table 11–24). This topic has been reviewed in depth[516] and is summarized here.

**TABLE 11–24. PRIMARY PTCA: THE PAMI WAY**

Establish a primary PTCA orientation
  All patients with confirmed or suspected AMI undergo emergency angiography; thrombolytic therapy is withheld
  The referring physicians (emergency room physicians, internists, noninvasive cardiologists) and catheterization laboratory staff are educated about invasive treatment
PTCA should be performed as rapidly as possible
  The catheterization laboratory team is called in as soon as notice is received that a patient with myocardial infarction is being transported to or has arrived at the emergency room
  An abbreviated history is taken and a physical examination is performed in the emergency room, laboratory samples are drawn, medications are given (chewable aspirin, ticlopidine, intravenous heparin, and intravenous β blockade in the absence of contraindications), and the patient is urgently transferred to the catheterization laboratory
  Guidelines for "bumping" elective cases are established
After angiography and left ventriculography, perform triage care appropriate for PTCA, CABG, or conservative therapy
Primary PTCA: technical imperatives
  Use only low osmolar, ionic contrast (ioxaglate)
  Ensure ACT of >350 seconds before PTCA (200–300 seconds if abciximab is used)
  Low threshold for intra-aortic balloon counterpulsation for hemodynamic instability (mandatory for cardiogenic shock)
  Gentle wire reperfusion: prepare for reperfusion arrhythmias
  Gradual, low-pressure inflation; balloon:artery ratio ~1:1 (increase balloon size as the artery expands)
  Some degree of residual dissection and thrombus is common; avoid thrombolytics
  The goal is TIMI grade 3 flow, with residual stenosis of <30% of vessel diameter; use prolonged inflations with a low-pressure, slightly oversized balloon if necessary; consider perfusion balloons; consider stent implantation for stenosis of >30% of luminal diameter or severe dissection
  Postprocedural care: PAMI-2 guidelines (see text)

ACT, activated clotting time; AMI, acute myocardial infarction; CABG, coronary artery bypass grafting; PAMI, Primary Angioplasty in Myocardial Infarction; PTCA, percutaneous transluminal coronary angioplasty; TIMI, Thrombolysis In Myocardial Infarction.

### *Primary PTCA: the PAMI Way* (see Table 11–24)

A high volume of primary PTCA procedures neither is required for a successful primary PTCA program nor guarantees success. More crucial is a thorough knowledge of the principles through which primary PTCA improves outcomes (discussed throughout this chapter), technical considerations of the procedure, and establishing a primary PTCA mindset, which means that primary PTCA must be the reperfusion modality of choice for nearly all patients with AMI, high risk or low risk, day or night. It is only through this commitment and experience that the excellent results that are achieved in dedicated centers may be duplicated. In order for this approach to work, it is not sufficient that just the interventional cardiologist, or even a group of cardiologists, commit to primary PTCA. Rather, all physicians and health care providers who interact with the AMI patient must be involved, including the emergency room physician, internist, family practitioner, and noninvasive cardiologist. The hospital nursing staff and the catheterization laboratory staff must also be well-informed, because a team approach is required for optimal efficiency and outcomes. An ongoing program of education must be initiated at the parent institution, outside referring hospitals, urgent care centers, and even ambulance transport units. One of the most difficult lessons to be taught is that thrombolytic therapy must be withheld, because it worsens the outcomes of primary PTCA and markedly increases bleeding risk after an invasive strategy. Furthermore, efforts must continue to educate the lay public about coronary artery disease, risk factor modification, recognition of the symptoms of angina and AMI, and the importance of early presentation to allow for effective reperfusion therapy.

### Time Issues

As previously emphasized, despite the possible lack of relationship between time to reperfusion after primary PTCA and mortality (see Fig. 11–30), it is imperative that all efforts be made to treat the patient as rapidly as possible. The patient should be in the catheterization laboratory within 60 to 90 minutes after presentation at the emergency room, and reperfusion should be established within an additional 30 minutes. The leading programs have been able to institute efficient procedures so that the median time from emergency room arrival to first balloon inflation is approximately 60 to 90 minutes. To streamline the process, all participating caregivers (physicians and catheterization laboratory staff) should live within 30 minutes of the hospital. The catheterization laboratory staff should be called in as soon as a patient with probable myocardial infarction is identified. This determination may be made in the field by a paramedic or in the emergency room after the emergency room physician or fellow quickly assesses the patient. We have found that although this policy results in the catheterization laboratory staff's being sent home because of a "false alarm" in approximately 5% of cases, this rare inconvenience is well accepted. It is critical that the interventional cardiologist is contacted directly as soon as a probable AMI is identified. No delays should occur while the internist or noninvasive cardiologist is called in to examine the patient. Elective cases should be bumped from the schedule and, at times, even removed from the table for the benefit of a patient in whom an AMI is strongly suspected.

Each hospital should institute a regular quality assurance program that tracks the times from presentation in the emergency room to arrival in the cardiac catheterization laboratory and to reperfusion (as well as in-hospital mortality and morbidity). Caputo and coworkers showed that a continuous quality assurance program helped reduce the time between arrival in the emergency room and PTCA from 205 minutes in 1994 to 119 minutes in the first 6 months of 1995 to 97 minutes by the end of 1995 ($p < 0.001$), as a result of shortening both the times from arrival to lidocaine (Xylocaine) administration in the catheterization laboratory and from lidocaine administration to first balloon inflation.[517] As the time from arrival to PTCA shortened between 1994 and 1995, parallel decreases in mortality rates (26.0% vs. 0%; $p = 0.004$), the composite of death, reinfarction, or repeat revascularization (47% vs. 18%; $p = 0.05$) and a shorter duration of hospitalization (13.3 ± 13.7 days vs. 8.4 ± 4.4 days; $p =$ NS) were achieved.

### Emergency Room Care

In the emergency room, an electrocardiogram is performed as soon as a patient with chest pain or hemodynamic instability arrives, and an abbreviated history is taken and a physical examination is performed. Standard blood work is performed (including cardiac enzyme measurement), but awaiting test results does not delay transfer to the catheterization laboratory. Specifically, catheterization should proceed if AMI is strongly suspected, even before indices of renal function and blood cell counts are established. Similarly, a portable chest radiograph is desirable, but waiting for it should never slow transfer to the catheterization suite.

In the emergency room, the patient receives a 5000- to 10,000-U heparin bolus intravenously, four 81-mg tablets (total dose of 324 mg) of chewable non–enteric-coated aspirin,[172, 173] and intravenous β-blocking agent in the absence of contraindications (asthma or bronchospasm, second- or third-degree heart block, or Killip classification of ≥2), which may lessen reperfusion arrhythmias and recurrent ischemia. Clopidogrel, 300 mg, may also be given at the operator's discretion for further antiplatelet effect and as a prequel to possible intracoronary stent placement.[513–523] Oxygen delivery by nasal cannula is a prudent measure, as is administration of topical or intravenous nitrates if the blood pressure is elevated (hypotension should be avoided, however). After giving written consent, the patient is given premedication for sedation and is transferred to the catheterization laboratory without further delay.

### Catheterization Laboratory Procedures

In the catheterization laboratory, femoral arterial access is obtained with an 8-French sheath.u Brachial or radial entry is also feasible but is in general more time consuming, except at selected centers where the technique is regularly performed, and restricts active guide manipulation and upsizing to larger sheath sizes if required. Femoral venous catheter placement increases the risk of bleeding and arteriovenous fistula formation and is generally not required if one or two good peripheral intravenous catheters are in place, unless the patient is hemodynamically unstable or has refractory arrhythmias or heart block. A femoral venous catheter may also be placed before the recanalization of an occluded right coronary artery (or dominant left circumflex artery) in anticipation of the need for rapid treatment of reperfusion arrhythmias. However, many centers do not routinely establish femoral venous access for otherwise uncomplicated inferior myocardial infarctions and have equally favorable outcomes.

After arterial access, left ventriculography is performed to assess ventricular and valvular function, measure hemodynamic parameters, localize the infarction (e.g., left circumflex artery or right coronary artery), and identify mechanical complications of myocardial infarction such as ventricular septal defect, papillary muscle rupture, or, in rare cases, left ventricular free wall rupture. Alternatively, left ventriculography may be performed after coronary arteriography and PTCA; however, the time required for performing left ventriculography (usually <5 minutes) is trivial, and the 35 to 45 mL of low-osmolar contrast material necessary to opacify the left ventricle will not result in hemodynamic deterioration (except possibly in patients with severe cardiogenic shock). Coronary arteriography is then performed first, in the noninfarcted vessel, to assess the extent of disease and collateral flow, and then in the infarcted artery with the use of a guide catheter. Usually, only two orthogonal projections of the right coronary artery and two to four angulated views of the left coronary artery are required.

Low-osmolar contrast agents should be used in order to minimize hemodynamic and arrhythmic disturbance. The contrast agent of choice is ioxaglate (Hexabrix) (Mallinkrodt; St. Louis MO), which is the only ionic, low-osmolar agent currently available. The importance of ioxaglate during AMI angiography and intervention is strongly emphasized. Numerous experimental and in vivo studies have documented the reduced thromboembolic potential of ionic contrast material in comparison with nonionic contrast material,[174–177, 524–537] which is particularly critical in patients with active thrombosis in situ (i.e., AMI). In the largest of the clinical studies,[174] 211 patients with AMI or unstable angina undergoing PTCA were prospectively assigned randomly to receive either low-osmolar nonionic (iohexol) or ionic (ioxaglate) contrast media. In comparison with patients receiving nonionic media, those receiving the ionic preparation were less likely to experience decreased blood flow during the procedure (8.1% vs. 17.8%; $p = 0.04$) and had had fewer postprocedure recurrent ischemic events requiring repeat catheterization (3.0% vs. 11.4%; $p = 0.02$) and repeat PTCA (1.0% vs. 5.8%; $p = 0.06$) during the index hospitalization. One month after the procedure, patients treated with ionic rather than nonionic contrast continued to benefit, with fewer symptoms of any angina (8.5% vs. 20.0%; $p = 0.04$) or rest angina (1.4% vs. 11.8%; $p = 0.01$), and had a lower subsequent need for CABG (0% vs. 5.9%; $p = 0.04$). Furthermore, in the Evaluation of 7E3 for the Prevention of Ischemic Complications (EPIC) trial, although the selection of contrast agents was not prespecified, patients in whom ionic contrast agents were administered had significantly reduced rates of death (odds ratio, 0.27; $p = 0.016$) and Q-wave myocardial infarction (odds ratio, 0.32; $p = 0.012$), after abciximab use was controlled for by logistic regression analysis.[177] The in vitro documentation of greater inhibition of coagulation and platelet function with ionic contrast than with nonionic contrast may underlie the mechanism of the reduced thromboembolic potential in patients with acute ischemic syndromes who undergo PTCA.[524–531]

After arteriography, the patient is assigned by triage to receive conservative medical therapy, CABG, or PTCA. Conservative therapy is typically indicated for approximately 5% of patients, including cases of spontaneous reperfusion when the infarcted vessel contains stenosis involving less than 70% of the vessel diameter with TIMI grade 3 flow, when a small artery supplying a limited amount of myocardium is identified as the culprit vessel or if the infarcted artery cannot be identified. Approximately 5% of patients are best served by urgent or emergency CABG. These patients have significant left main artery disease, severe triple-vessel disease, or features otherwise unfavorable for PTCA. Intra-aortic balloon counterpulsation is often established to reduce ischemia and provide hemodynamic support before surgery. Primary PTCA is performed in approximately 90% of patients, including most patients with triple-vessel disease. In many patients who ultimately require CABG for extensive multivessel disease, PTCA is performed first to abort the infarction, after which surgery may be accomplished in several days or weeks when the patient is more stable.

Before PTCA, additional heparin is given to achieve an activated clotting time (ACT) of more than 350 seconds. Investing the time and effort to verify this degree of anticoagulation may be particularly important, because lower ACT levels have been associated with increased abrupt closure and ischemic complications in patients undergoing high-risk PTCA.[178–180] Two studies have suggested that the optimal ACT may be as long as 400 to 500 seconds.[538, 539] The ACT should be rechecked every 30 minutes throughout the procedure and additional heparin given as necessary to maintain an ACT of longer than 350 seconds.

PTCA is performed with the use of standard large-lumen guide catheters and over-the-wire balloon catheters. Most acute infarction lesions can be crossed with a floppy-tipped guide wire; in rare cases, a wire of intermediate or standard stiffness is required. After wire recanalization of the vessel, the operator should wait a few moments to let reperfusion arrhythmias resolve. If passage of the wire does not restore flow, the balloon may be passed distally and withdrawn (without being inflated) to achieve some distal perfusion.

The balloon should be sized at a 1:1 ratio to the reference segment. It is normal for the artery to expand as flow is established and myogenic vasoconstriction resolves. Intracoronary nitrates should be administered liberally (100- to 400-μg boluses), and the balloon upsized as necessary to maintain the 1:1 balloon-to-artery ratio. The goals are residual stenosis involving less than 30% of the vessel diameter and TIMI grade 3 flow. To achieve this result, prolonged inflations with a perfusion balloon, low-pressure inflations with a slightly oversized balloon, or both may be helpful. Underdilating the vessel, which may predispose to recurrent ischemia and reocclusion of the infarcted artery, should be avoided.[185, 540, 541]

### Intra-aortic Balloon Counterpulsation

Although there is no indication for the routine prophylactic use of intra-aortic balloon counterpulsa-

tion in most patients,[384] IABP insertion should be considered for patients with multiple high-risk features[404] and for patients with continued ischemia after reperfusion, refractory heart failure, hypotension, severe left ventricular dysfunction with multivessel disease, and instability of the infarcted lesion after PTCA. An IABP is also clinically useful for providing hemodynamic support before surgery and in patients with mechanical defects such as ventricular septal defect or papillary muscle rupture with severe mitral regurgitation. Finally, for patients with shock, intra-aortic balloon counterpulsation is mandatory for hemodynamic support,[548–550] and should be established before arteriography or PTCA. Intra-aortic balloon counterpulsation as sole therapy, however, does not improve survival in shock without revascularization.[551–553]

### Adverse Events After Primary PTCA

Although all the same complications can occur after primary PTCA as after elective PTCA, the operator must be knowledgeable about and ready to manage two adverse events in particular that occur more frequently after angioplasty in the AMI setting: reperfusion arrhythmias and the no-reflow phenomenon.

#### Reperfusion Arrhythmias

Gacioch and Topol described the fact that abrupt and profound hypotension, bradycardia, and ventricular fibrillation can occur within minutes after PTCA-mediated reperfusion, especially of the right coronary artery (RCA).[554] In this study, PTCA of the RCA in comparison with the left anterior descending artery (LAD) more frequently resulted in sustained hypotension, necessitating treatment with inotropic agents or an IABP (11% vs. 3%; $p = 0.16$), and in a greater need for cardiopulmonary resuscitation (16% vs. 2%; $p = 0.02$). However, 84% of the patients in this report underwent dilation after failed thrombolysis; thus they represented a highly selected group of patients with ongoing ischemia resistant to reperfusion who are prone to myocardial hemorrhage and reperfusion injury.[209, 210, 216] Similar complications have been noted by other authors after rescue PTCA for failed thrombolysis.[555, 556] The mechanism of deterioration after sudden PTCA-mediated reperfusion of an occluded RCA may relate to stimulation of vagal afferent fibers, which are heavily represented in the inferior wall, resulting in the Bezold-Jarisch reflex.[557–560]

In contrast to rescue PTCA after failed thrombolytic therapy, studies of primary PTCA without antecedent thrombolysis have found that reperfusion-related arrhythmias, although definitely a real phenomenon, usually do not result in major morbidity. In a series of 250 consecutive patients at the Mid America Heart Institute,[190] minor events in the catheterization laboratory were more frequent in patients undergoing primary PTCA of the RCA than of the LAD or left circumflex artery (LCX). Major events, defined as death, need for cardiopulmonary resuscitation, defibrillation, cardioversion, and need for intra-aortic balloon pumping or urgent surgery, were uncommon and unrelated to the infarcted artery dilated, occurring in 8% of RCA infarctions, 10% of LAD infarctions, and 8% of LCX infarctions. Major adverse events occurred primarily in patients with cardiogenic shock (100% of patients in shock vs. 3% of patients not in shock; $p < 0.0001$). From a series of 459 consecutive patients undergoing PTCA in AMI (7.4% of whom experienced thrombolysis failure), Kaplan and associates found a higher incidence of procedural bradyarrhythmias (8.4% vs. 0.8%; $p < 0.0001$), need for defibrillation (5.7% vs. 1.7%; $p < 0.02$), and persistent angiographic thrombus or no-reflow (8.8% vs. 4.3%; $p < 0.05$) after RCA reperfusion than after LAD reperfusion.[561] Hospital outcomes were worse in the LAD group, however; these outcomes primarily represented increased mortality among patients presenting with cardiogenic shock with LAD occlusion as opposed to RCA occlusion (58% vs. 23%; $p < 0.005$). Among patients not in shock, mortality was infrequent after primary PTCA when the culprit artery was either the LAD or RCA (3.0% vs. 1.5%; $p$ = NS). The authors concluded that case selection and shock, and not the development of reperfusion-related arrhythmias, are the primary determinants of adverse outcomes after primary PTCA.

In the PAMI trial,[562, 563] PTCA was successful in 97% of patients who underwent primary PTCA (without antecedent thrombolysis) but in only 82% of those who underwent PTCA procedures after tPA administration, performed for either lytic failure or recurrent ischemia ($p$ = 0.0001). Major adverse events in the catheterization laboratory occurred during primary PTCA in 7% of 175 patients, in 9% of 58 tPA recipients who underwent dilatation for recurrent ischemia, and in 43% of 14 patients who underwent rescue PTCA ($p < 0.0001$). Major adverse events were more common with RCA than LAD or LCX dilatation (13% vs. 6%; $p$ = 0.04). However, only 39% of the adverse events in the catheterization laboratory occurred during or after PTCA, the majority actually occurring before dilatation; thus, fewer than 4% of patients experienced a true reperfusion-related arrhythmia directly after PTCA. No patient died in the catheterization laboratory.

Thus, reperfusion-related arrhythmias are less common after primary PTCA than after rescue PTCA for failed thrombolysis and, with appropriate man-

agement, do not result in adverse sequelae. Although it is unproven, reperfusion-related arrhythmias may be diminished in frequency by gentle wire or balloon recanalization of the infarcted vessel for 1 to 2 minutes before balloon expansion, allowing gradual distal perfusion. Intravenous β-blockade before PTCA may reduce the occurrence of sudden ventricular fibrillation, whereas prophylactic lidocaine is ineffectual in this setting. The regular use of intravenous β-blocking agents before PTCA in PAMI-2, as opposed to PAMI-1, in which β blockers were not used prophylactically, was associated with a reduction in ventricular fibrillation from 6.7% to 3.5% ($p$ = 0.01). Intravenous atropine infusion before RCA recanalization is also prudent, although not always sufficient to prevent bradycardia. Prophylactic transvenous pacemaker insertion before recanalization of a large, occluded RCA may also be considered but is not considered mandatory by many authorities. Idioventricular rhythm is common after reperfusion, usually lasts only several minutes, and does not necessitate treatment. Most reperfusion arrhythmias are short-lived, and once they abate, they rarely recur. The operator must be attentive, however, to the development of reperfusion-related arrhythmias and be ready to manage them with temporary pacing, pharmacologic intervention, cardioversion, or defibrillation as necessary.

### The No-Reflow Phenomenon

*No-reflow* after primary PTCA may be strictly defined as the occurrence of TIMI grade 0 or 1 flow in the infarcted vessel after PTCA in the absence of significant residual epicardial coronary stenosis at the infarcted site or downstream in the vessel. *Slow-reflow* (TIMI grade 2 flow after PTCA without mechanical obstruction) is defined also as no-reflow. The cause of the no-reflow phenomenon is unknown and is most likely multifactorial; in certain instances, it is caused by microvascular spasm, capillary block from distal thromboemboli or myocardial edema, or reperfusion injury with loss of microvascular integrity.[564–574] The development of no-reflow during primary PTCA results in greater myocardial loss with diminished regional left ventricular function and an increase in cardiac rupture and death.[575, 576] In several reports, the incidence of no-reflow or slow-reflow after primary PTCA has ranged from 17% to 34%,[575–578] although in the PAMI trials, true no-reflow has occurred in fewer than 5% of patients. The lower incidence of no-reflow in the PAMI trials in comparison with other series may relate to the routine use of ionic contrast.[174–177, 524–537] In the randomized iohexol-ioxaglate trial,[174] patients with acute ischemic syndromes who underwent PTCA had a significantly lower incidence of slow- or no-reflow when ioxaglate was used than when the nonionic contrast media was used (8.1% vs. 17.8%; $p = 0.04$). The practice of obtaining an ACT of more than 350 seconds before PTCA in the PAMI trials may also have reduced the occurrence of the no-reflow phenomenon.[178–180, 539, 540]

If no-reflow occurs after PTCA, a mechanical cause such as dissection or macroemboli must be excluded. In the absence of visible causes for diminished antegrade flow, treatment of no-reflow consists of ensuring adequate hydration, administration of intracoronary vasodilators (including nitrates, verapamil, diltiazem, adenosine, or papaverine[574, 576, 579]), and possibly use of intra-aortic balloon counterpulsation.[576] In three studies, intracoronary verapamil, 50 to 300 μg, has been particularly effective in improving antegrade flow, although transient hypotension, bradyarrhythmias, and high-degree atrioventricular block occasionally occur after its use, especially in the RCA.[574, 576, 580] In contrast, no benefits have been seen after treatment with intracoronary streptokinase, urokinase, or tPA.[576, 581, 582] Although few data are yet available, the use of full-dose intravenous or reduced-dose intracoronary abciximab for the prevention or treatment of no-reflow is promising and deserves further study.[583] Finally, intracoronary administration of sodium nitroprusside (50 to 200 μg) or epinephrine (100 to 200 μg) may be used in refractory cases.

### Post-PTCA Care

After primary PTCA, patients are assigned by triage on the basis of simple clinical and angiographic variables into low-risk and high-risk groups, as in the PAMI-2 trial.[384, 385] Patients at low risk (aged <70 years, with single- or double-vessel disease, having undergone successful PTCA of a native coronary artery, and with the absence of refractory malignant ventricular arrhythmias after reperfusion) may be managed in the usual post-PTCA ward or stepdown unit. Sheaths are removed 4 to 6 hours after the procedure; next, heparin is reinstituted for 48 hours at full dose (to achieve an activated partial thromboplastin time of 1.5 to 2.0 times that of control levels or an ACT of 180 to 240 seconds), then reduced to half dose for 12 hours, and discontinued afterward. This gradual tapering may prevent a rebound hypercoagulable state.[584–589] The patient is progressively ambulated and is discharged on the third hospital day if pain free and hemodynamically stable without significant arrhythmias. Patients with one or more high-risk features are monitored in the coronary care unit for 24 hours or longer, typically receive maintenance-level heparin for 3 to 7 days, and then are discharged when stable. In the absence of recurrent chest pain, predischarge exercise testing is

**TABLE 11–25.  MEDICATION USE AFTER PRIMARY PTCA**

Enteric-coated aspirin, 325 mg PO qd indefinitely
Clopidogrel, 75 mg PO qd, if a stent was implanted (optional after PTCA alone; no data)
β blockers in the absence of contraindications
  Examples:
    Metoprolol, 50 mg PO bid for 2 days, then 100 mg PO bid
    Atenolol, 100 mg PO qd
    Propranolol, 60 mg PO tid
    Timolol, 20 mg PO qd
Angiotensin-converting enzyme inhibitors for hypertension, heart failure, or LVEF of ≤40% should be initiated within 24 hours of the infarction started at low doses and then titrated up to maximal tolerated doses
  Examples:
    Captopril, 100 mg PO tid
    Lisinopril, 20 mg PO qd
    Enalapril, 10 mg PO bid
Warfarin is indicated for atrial fibrillation, severe cardiomyopathy, mural thrombus, and other specific indications such as prosthetic valves or deep venous thrombosis or pulmonary embolus
Other agents, such as calcium channel blockers and nitrates, are not routinely recommended but are reserved for specific indications

LVEF, left ventricular ejection fraction; PTCA, percutaneous transluminal coronary angioplasty.

not required after primary PTCA. Patients in whom recurrent ischemic symptoms with electrocardiographic changes, a new loud murmur, hypotension, or heart failure develops should undergo urgent repeat catheterization and treatment as appropriate. Recommended medication use after primary PTCA is summarized in Table 11–25.

## Expanding the Reach of Primary PTCA

For primary PTCA to be feasible, cardiac catheterization facilities (at a minimum) are required; they currently exist in fewer than 20% of hospitals in the United States.[590, 591] Even fewer hospitals have the additional capability for surgical standby. Current registries have estimated that primary PTCA is being performed in approximately 10% to 12% of eligible patients with AMI.[251, 592]

Several strategies can be envisioned to expand the reach of primary PTCA (Table 11–26). One possible solution is to equip more hospitals with cardiac catheterization laboratories. Unfortunately, this may

**TABLE 11–26.  STRATEGIES TO EXPAND THE REACH OF PRIMARY PTCA**

Build more cardiac catheterization laboratories
Eliminate the requirement for on-site coronary artery bypass surgery
Modify ambulance triage strtegies, and transfer patients to AMI centers of excellence (with qualified primary PTCA programs)

AMI, acute myocardial infarction; PTCA, percutaneous transluminal coronary angioplasty.

be prohibitively costly. Assuming that 200 patients with AMIs present to a hospital per year, Lieu and colleagues constructed a mathematical model showing that the cost per primary PTCA patient to a hospital with existing catheterization laboratories, surgical facilities, and night call already in place is $1597 per procedure.[593] If, however, a new cardiac catheterization laboratory were to be built, and if a new cardiac surgical program were also required, the cost per primary PTCA procedure (amortized over 10 years) would rise to $14,339, which would far outstrip reimbursement. If on-site surgery were not required (as discussed later), the cost would still be $7387 per primary PTCA procedure. However, if the new catheterization laboratory also performed 800 angiographic and elective PTCA procedures per year, the cost would fall further to $3866 per primary PTCA procedure, making this a potentially viable option at current reimbursement rates.

### Are On-Site Cardiac Surgical Facilities Required for Primary PTCA?

A second strategy to broaden the application of primary PTCA is to eliminate the requirement for on-site surgical capability. However, current American College of Cardiology/American Heart Association (ACC/AHA) Task Force recommendations state that on-site cardiac surgery must be available during the performance of all percutaneous interventional procedures.[594] Despite this position, there is increasing evidence that an on-site surgery program is not required in order to obtain excellent results with primary PTCA. First, in most prior large series, emergency CABG for failed primary PTCA has been performed in fewer than 1% of patients.[141, 154, 192, 219, 223, 244, 251] An additional 4% to 5% of patients undergoing acute arteriography have severe triple-vessel disease, left main artery disease, or features highly unfavorable for angioplasty; for these patients, PTCA is withheld and urgent CABG is performed. Most of these patients, however, may, if unstable, be stabilized with an intra-aortic balloon pump and transferred to a tertiary-care hospital for surgery.

Several reports have focused on the outcomes of primary PTCA at centers with and without on-site cardiac surgery. According to the MITI registry, primary PTCA was performed in 1062 patients with AMI at 10 hospitals in the metropolitan Seattle area, 4 of which had angiographic facilities without cardiac surgery.[595] Approximately half of the primary PTCA procedures (470, or 44%) took place at centers without surgical facilities. Baseline characteristics were similar for patients in whom primary PTCA was performed at hospitals with and without on-site surgery. Both the PTCA success rates (88%) and times to PTCA (78 minutes) were nearly identi-

cal at both hospital types. Patients presenting at hospitals with surgical facilities were more likely to undergo emergency CABG within 6 hours of angioplasty (3.8% vs. 0.7%; $p < 0.01$), urgent CABG within 24 hours of admission (5.1% vs. 2.6%; $p = 0.03$), or CABG at any time during their hospitalization (12.0% vs. 8.5%; $p = 0.07$). Of most importance, however, was that both the in-hospital and 1-year mortality rates were identical for patients treated with primary PTCA at centers with and without on-site cardiac surgery (7% vs. 7% and 11% vs. 11%, respectively; boths $p = NS$).

From an earlier, more detailed MITI report on 441 patients,[251] of 55 patients in whom PTCA was unsuccessful, only 6 patients underwent emergency CABG (including 5 patients from hospitals with on-site surgery, in whom the mean time from the catheterization laboratory to surgery was 45 minutes [range, 23 to 120 minutes] and 1 in-patient from a hospital without on-site surgery after transfer to a tertiary-care center [for whom the time to surgery was 45 minutes]). In an additional 49 patients with failure of reperfusion after primary PTCA, surgery was not performed because of either a small amount of myocardium at risk or mild persistent symptoms. Ten deaths (2.5%) occurred in the catheterization laboratory, 6 at centers with and 4 at centers without on-site surgery; of these 10 patients, 9 presented in cardiogenic shock. The MITI investigators stressed that the sites at which primary PTCA was performed without cardiac surgery were (and must be) staffed by operators and catheterization laboratory personnel skilled in elective as well as emergency PTCA and that a ready means for urgent transport to a tertiary-care center be present.[251, 594]

Multiple other institutions in the United States, Europe, and Canada have documented excellent outcomes of both elective and primary PTCA at centers without on-site surgery.[596–605a] The need for emergency surgery is also likely to decline with the availability of stents as a bail-out option for failed PTCA.[606–613] Thus, excellent results of primary PTCA may be obtained regardless of whether surgical facilities are present, as long as the patient is cared for by a team skilled in primary PTCA (implying prior experience at tertiary-care hospitals) and the logistics for transfer to a surgical center are in place, if CABG becomes necessary. Although patients may in rare cases be disadvantaged by primary PTCA at a hospital without on-site surgery if emergency CABG is truly required, most patients will benefit by this approach through the prevention of intracranial hemorrhage, by withholding thrombolysis, and through the reduction of overall death and reinfarction rates by performing primary PTCA.

### Transferring the Patient for Primary PTCA

Although the minority of patients with AMI in the United States present at centers with angiographic facilities, zip code analysis suggests that 63% and 83% of the U.S. population live within 30 and 60 minutes, respectively, of a cardiac catheterization laboratory.[614] Thus, by instituting routine ambulance or air triage of patients with chest pain to a tertiary-care AMI center, or by transferring on an emergency basis patients with AMI who present at hospitals without invasive capabilities to hospitals with primary PTCA facilities (similar to the selective routing of trauma patients to qualified trauma centers), virtually all patients with AMI could be managed with primary PTCA. Such a strategy is tenable (and in fact warranted) if the disadvantages of a 1- to 2-hour delay to reperfusion are outweighed by the advantages of withholding thrombolysis and performing primary PTCA.

Accumulating evidence indicates that such an approach may indeed be feasible and effective. As previously discussed, there appears to be little correlation between time to reperfusion and mortality after primary PTCA in an unselected AMI population (see Fig. 11–30); mortality rates, even in high-risk subgroups, remain low when reperfusion is achieved between 1 and 12 hours after symptom onset. Over a 5-year period, Zjilstra and colleagues performed primary PTCA in 520 patients, 104 of whom had been transferred from a community hospital before reperfusion.[615] In comparison with nontransferred patients, transferred patients were more likely to have anterior AMI, to have thrombolytic contraindications, and to present in Killip class 3 or 4. The mean time required for transfer was 70 ± 27 minutes. However, because transferred patients were sent directly to the cardiac catheterization suite, bypassing the emergency room, the mean time from admission to the tertiary-care center to PTCA was actually 28 minutes *shorter* for them than for nontransferred patients (39 ± 31 minutes vs. 67 ± 28 minutes). The transfer strategy therefore delayed reperfusion by an average of only 42 minutes. One patient (1%) in profound cardiogenic shock died during transportation. Despite the greater prevalence of high-risk baseline features in transferred patients, at 6 months the rates of death, reinfarction, and revascularization were similar for the transferred and nontransferred groups.

The ongoing Air PAMI trial is directly testing the hypothesis that the outcomes of primary PTCA will be superior to thrombolytic therapy even if a 1- to 2-hour delay is required before angioplasty.[268] In this multicenter study, thrombolytic-eligible patients at high risk who present at hospitals without PTCA facilities are being prospectively assigned randomly to treatment with accelerated tPA, as opposed to withholding thrombolytic therapy and urgently transferring the patient by ground or air to a tertiary-care center, accepting up to a 2-hour delay. Patients at high risk are defined as possessing one or more of the following characteristics: age of more than 70 years, anterior AMI location or left bundle branch block, tachycardia on admission, systolic blood pressure of less than 100 mm Hg, or Killip class 2 or 3. Patients transferred for primary PTCA receive, before transport, chewable aspirin, which was responsible for half of the reduction in mortality present after thrombolysis in the ISIS-2 trial.[4] High-dose intravenous heparin (300 U/kg) will also be given before transfer; this is usually well tolerated and is the standard dosing regimen before cardiopulmonary bypass. In the Heparin in Early Patency (HEAP) study, a 300-U/kg bolus of heparin restored TIMI grades 2 and 3 flow in 56% of patients within 90 minutes,[616] which compares favorably with the 20% reperfusion rate in the PAMI-1 and -2 trials after 70 to 150 U/kg of intravenous heparin.[192, 617] In addition, the results of primary PTCA in lytic-eligible patients at high risk who undergo primary PTCA at hospitals without on-site surgery will be tracked in the No Surgery On Site (NO SOS) registry of the Air PAMI study, in accordance with the hypothesis that patients so treated will have favorable outcomes at least equal to those of the group transferred to full-range tertiary-care centers and with more rapid reperfusion. The results of the Air PAMI study, if strongly positive, may revolutionize the management of patients with acute coronary syndromes and may mandate the creation of AMI centers of excellence.

# REFERENCES

1. DeWood MA, Spores J, Notske R, et al: Prevalence of total coronary occlusion during the early hours of transmural myocardial infarction. N Engl J Med 303:897–902, 1980.
2. Davies MJ, Thomas AC: Plaque fissuring—The cause of acute myocardial infarction, sudden ischemic death, and crescendo angina. Br Heart J 53:363–373, 1985.
3. Gruppo Italiano per lo Studio della Streptochinasi nell'Infarto Miocardico (GISSI): Effectiveness of intravenous thrombolytic treatment in acute myocardial infarction. Lancet 1:397–402, 1986.
4. ISIS-2 (Second International Study Group of Infarct Survival) Collaborative Group: Randomised trial of intravenous streptokinase, oral aspirin, both, or neither among 17,187 cases of suspected acute myocardial infarction. Lancet 2:349–360, 1988.
5. Wilcox RG, Olsson CG, Skene AM, et al: Trial of tissue plasminogen activator for mortality reduction in acute myocardial infarction. Anglo-Scandinavian Study of Early Thrombolysis (ASSET). Lancet 2:525–530, 1988.
6. AIMS Trial Study Group: Effect of intravenous APSAC on mortality after acute myocardial infarction: Preliminary report of a placebo-controlled clinical trial. Lancet 1:545–549, 1988.
7. The GUSTO Investigators: An international randomized trial comparing four thrombolytic regimens consisting of tissue plasminogen activator, streptokinase, or both for acute myocardial infarction. N Engl J Med 329:673–682, 1993.
8. The TIMI Study Group: The Thrombolysis in Myocardial Infarction (TIMI) trial: Phase 1 findings. N Engl J Med 312:932–936, 1985.

9. Topol EJ, Califf RM, George BS, et al: Insights derived from the Thrombolysis and Angioplasty in Myocardial Infarction (TAMI) trials. J Am Coll Cardiol 12:24A–31A, 1988.

10. The GUSTO Angiographic Investigators: The effects of tissue plasminogen activator, streptokinase, or both on coronary artery patency, ventricular function, and survival after acute myocardial infarction. N Engl J Med 329:1615–1622, 1993.

11. Vogt A, von Essen R, Tebbe U, et al: Impact of early perfusion status of the infarct-related artery on short-term mortality after thrombolysis for acute myocardial infarction: Retrospective analysis of four German multicenter studies. J Am Coll Cardiol 21:1391–1395, 1993.

12. Karagounis L, Sorensen SG, Menlove RL, et al, for the TEAM-2 Investigators: Does Thrombolysis in Myocardial Infarction (TIMI) perfusion grade 2 represent a mostly patent artery or a mostly occluded artery? Enzymatic and electrocardiographic evidence from the TEAM-2 study. J Am Coll Cardiol 19:1–10, 1992.

13. Ishihara M, Sato H, Tateishi H, et al: Comparison of thrombolysis in myocardial infarction perfusion grades 2 and 3 after anterior wall infarction. Am J Cardiol 71:428–430, 1993.

14. Clemmensen P, Ohman EM, Sevilla D, et al: Importance of early and complete reperfusion to achieve myocardial salvage after thrombolysis in acute myocardial infarction. Am J Cardiol 70:1391–1396, 1992.

15. Simes RJ, Topol EJ, Holmes DR, et al: Link between the angiographic substudy and mortality outcomes in a large randomized trial of myocardial reperfusion. Circulation 91:1923–1928, 1995.

16. Anderson JL, Karagounis LA, Becker LC, et al: TIMI perfusion grade 3 but not grade 2 results in improved outcome after thrombolysis for myocardial infarction. Ventriculographic, enzymatic, and electrocardiographic evidence from the TEAM-3 study. Circulation 87:1829–1839, 1993.

17. Lenderink T, Simoons ML, Van Es G-A, et al: Benefit of thrombolytic therapy is sustained throughout five years and is related to TIMI perfusion grade 3 but not grade 2 flow at discharge. Circulation 92:1110–1116, 1995.

18. Vogt A, von Essen R, Tebbe U, et al: Frequency of achieving optimal reperfusion with thrombolysis in acute myocardial infarction (analysis of four German multicenter studies). Am J Cardiol 74:1–4, 1994.

19. Lincoff MA, Topol EJ, Califf RM, et al: Significance of a coronary artery with thrombolysis in myocardial infarction grade 2 flow "patency" (Outcome in the Thrombolysis and Angioplasty in Myocardial Infarction Trials). Am J Cardiol 75:871–876, 1995.

20. Anderson JL, Karagounis LA, Califf RM: Metaanalysis of five reported studies on the relation of early coronary patency grades with mortality and outcomes after acute myocardial infarction. Am J Cardiol 78:1–8, 1996.

21. Neuhaus K-L, Feurer W, Jeep-Tebbe S, et al: Improved thrombolysis with a modified dose regimen of recombinant tissue-type plasminogen activator. J Am Coll Cardiol 14:1566–1599, 1989.

22. Neuhaus K-L, von Essen R, Tebbe U, et al: Improved thrombolysis in acute myocardial infarction with front-loaded administration of alteplase: Results of the rt-PA–APSAC patency study (TAPS). J Am Coll Cardiol 19:885–891, 1992.

23. Smalling RW, Bode C, Kalbfleisch J, et al: More rapid, complete, and stable coronary thrombolysis with bolus administration of reteplase compared with alteplase infusion in acute myocardial infarction. Circulation 91:2725–2732, 1995.

24. Bode C, Smalling RW, Berg G, et al: Randomized comparison of coronary thrombolysis achieved with double bolus reteplase (r-PA) and front-loaded "accelerated" alteplase (rt-PA) in patients with acute myocardial infarction. Circulation 94:891–898, 1996.

25. Bode C, Nordt T, Peter K, et al: Patency trials with reteplase (r-PA): What do they tell us? Am J Cardiol 78(suppl 12A):16–19, 1996.

26. Maes A, Van de Werf F, Nuyts J, et al: Impaired myocardial tissue perfusion early after successful thrombolysis: Impact on myocardial blood flow, metabolism, and function at late follow-up. Circulation 92:2072–2078, 1995.

27. Ito H, Tomooka T, Sakai N, et al: Lack of myocardial perfusion immediately after successful thrombolysis. A predictor of poor recovery of left ventricular function in anterior myocardial infarction. Circulation 85:1699–1705, 1992.

28. Ito H, Okamura A, Iwakura K, et al: Myocardial perfusion patterns related to thrombolysis in myocardial infarction perfusion grades after coronary angioplasty in patients with acute anterior myocardial infarction. Circulation 93:1993–1999, 1996.

29. Kern MJ, Moore JA, Aguirre FV, et al: Determination of angiographic (TIMI grade) blood flow by intracoronary Doppler flow velocity during acute myocardial infarction. Circulation 94:1545–1552, 1996.

30. Verheugt FWA, Meijer A, Lagrand WK, et al: Reocclusion: The flip side of coronary thrombolysis. J Am Coll Cardiol 27:766–773, 1996.

31. Lincoff MA, Topol EJ: Illusion of reperfusion: Does anyone achieve optimal reperfusion during acute myocardial infarction? Circulation 88:1361–1374, 1993.

32. Brouwer MA, Bohncke JR, Veen G, et al: Adverse long-term effects of reocclusion after coronary thrombolysis. J Am Coll Cardiol 26:1440–1444, 1995.

33. Ohman EM, Califf RM, Topol EJ, et al: Consequences of reocclusion after successful reperfusion therapy in acute myocardial infarction. Circulation 82:781–791, 1990.

34. Ellis SG, Gallison L, Grines CL, et al: Incidence and predictors of early recurrent ischemia after successful percutaneous transluminal coronary angioplasty for acute myocardial infarction. Am J Cardiol 64:263–268, 1989.

35. Serruys PW, Simoons ML, Suryapranata H, et al: Preservation of global and regional left ventricular function after early thrombolysis in acute myocardial infarction. J Am Coll Cardiol 7:729–742, 1986.

36. Timmis GC, Mammen EF, Ramos RG, et al: Hemorrhage vs. rethrombosis after thrombolysis for acute myocardial infarction. Arch Intern Med 146:667–672, 1986.

37. Chesebro JH, Knatterud G, Roberts R, et al: Thrombolysis in myocardial infarction (TIMI) trial, phase 1: A comparison between intravenous tissue plasminogen activator and intravenous streptokinase. Circulation 76:142–154, 1987.

38. Topol EJ, Califf RM, George BS, et al: A randomized trial of immediate versus delayed elective angioplasty after intravenous tissue plasminogen activator in acute myocardial infarction. N Engl J Med 317:197–202, 1987.

39. Abbottsmith CW, Topol EJ, George BS, et al: Fate of patients with acute myocardial infarction with patency of the infarct-related vessel achieved with successful thrombolysis versus rescue angioplasty. J Am Coll Cardiol 16:770–778, 1990.

40. Wall TC, Califf RM, George BS, et al: Accelerated plasminogen activator dose regimens for coronary thrombolysis. J Am Coll Cardiol 19:482–489, 1992.

41. Hsia J, Hamilton WP, Kleiman N, et al: A comparison between heparin and low-dose aspirin as adjunctive therapy with tissue plasminogen activator for acute myocardial infarction. N Engl J Med 323:1433–1437, 1990.

42. Califf RM, Topol EJ, Stack RS, et al: Evaluation of combination thrombolytic therapy and timing of cardiac catheterization in acute myocardial infarction: Results of Thrombolysis and Angioplasty in Myocardial Infarction—Phase 5 randomized trial. Circulation 83:1543–1556, 1991.

43. Neuhaus K, Tebbe U, Gottwik M, et al: Intravenous recombinant tissue plasminogen activator (rt-PA) and urokinase in acute myocardial infarction: Results of the German Activator Urokinase Study (GAUS). J Am Coll Cardiol 12:581–587, 1988.

44. Reiner JS, Lundergan CF, Rohrbeck SC, et al: The impact of left ventricular function of coronary reocclusion after successful thrombolysis for acute myocardial infarction [Abstract]. J Am Coll Cardiol 23:13A, 1994.

45. White HD, French JK, Hamer AW, et al: Frequent reocclusion of patent infarct-related arteries between four weeks and one year: Effects of antiplatelet therapy. J Am Coll Cardiol 25:218–223, 1995.

46. Topol EJ, Califf RM, Vandormael M, et al, and the Thrombolysis and Angioplasty in Myocardial Infarction (TAMI-6) Study Group: A randomized trial of late reperfusion therapy for acute myocardial infarction. Circulation 85:2090–2099, 1992.

47. Meijer A, Verheugt FWA, Werter CPJP, et al: Aspirin versus Coumadin in the prevention of reocclusion and recurrent ischemia after successful thrombolysis: A prospective placebo-controlled angiographic study. Circulation 87:1524–1530, 1993.

48. Jang I-K, Vanhaecke J, de Geest H, et al: Coronary thrombolysis with recombinant tissue-type plasminogen activator: Patency rate and regional wall motion after 3 months. J Am Coll Cardiol 8:1455–1460, 1986.

49. Takens BH, Brugemann J, van der Meer J, et al: Reocclusion three months after successful thrombolytic treatment of acute myocardial infarction with anisoylated plasminogen streptokinase activating complex. Am J Cardiol 65:1422–1424, 1990.

50. Meijer A, Verheugt FWA, Eenige MJ, et al: Left ventricular function at 3 months after successful thrombolysis: Impact of reocclusion without reinfarction on ejection fraction, regional function, and remodeling. Circulation 90:1706–1714, 1994.

51. The Multicenter Postinfarct Research Group: Risk stratification and survival after myocardial infarction. N Engl J Med 309:331–336, 1983.

52. White HD, Norris RM, Brown MA, et al: Left ventricular end-systolic volume as the major determinant of survival after recovery from myocardial infarction. Circulation 76(suppl I):I-44–I-51, 1987.

53. Grines CL, Topol EJ, Bates ER, et al: Infarct vessel status after tissue plasminogen activator and acute coronary angioplasty: Prediction of clinical outcome. Am J Cardiol 115:1–7, 1988.

54. Wall T, Mark DB, Califf RM, et al: Prediction of early recurrent myocardial ischemia and coronary occlusion after successful thrombolysis: A qualitative and quantitative angiographic study. Am J Cardiol 63:423–428, 1989.

55. Gibson CM, Cannon CP, Piana RN, et al: Angiographic predictors of reocclusion after thrombolysis: Results from the Thrombolysis in Myocardial Infarction (TIMI) 4 Trial. J Am Coll Cardiol 25:582–589, 1995.

56. Veen G, Meyer A, Verheugt FWA, et al: Culprit lesion morphology and stenosis severity in the prediction of reocclusion after coronary thrombolysis: Angiographic results of the APRICOT study. J Am Coll Cardiol 22:1755–1762, 1993.

57. Harrison DG, Furguson DW, Collins SM, et al: Rethrombosis after reperfusion with streptokinase: Importance of geometry of residual lesions. Circulation 69:991–999, 1984.

58. Gash AK, Spann JF, Sherry S, et al: Factors influencing reocclusion after thrombolysis for acute myocardial infarction. Am J Cardiol 57:175–177, 1986.

59. Badger RS, Brown BG, Kennedy JW, et al: Usefulness of recanalization to lumen diameter of 0.6 mm or more with intracoronary streptokinase during acute myocardial infarction in predicting "normal" perfusion status, continued arterial patency and survival at one year. Am J Cardiol 59:519–522, 1987.

60. Ellis SG, Topol EJ, George BS, et al: Recurrent ischemia without warning: Analysis of risk factors for in-hospital ischemic events following successful thrombolysis with intravenous tissue plasminogen activator. Circulation 80:1159–1165, 1989.

61. Reiner JS, Lundergan CF, Van den Brand M, et al: Early angiography cannot predict postthrombolytic coronary reocclusion: Observations from the GUSTO angiographic study. J Am Coll Cardiol 24:1439–1444, 1994.

62. Ellis SG, Van de Werf F, Riberio-DaSilva E, et al: Present status of rescue coronary angioplasty: Current polarization of opinion and randomized trials. J Am Coll Cardiol 19:681–686, 1992.

63. Califf RM, Topol EJ, Stack RS, et al: Evaluation of combination thrombolytic therapy and timing of cardiac catheterization in acute myocardial infarction: The TAMI-5 randomized trial. Circulation 83:1543–1556, 1991.

64. Ellis SG, da Silva ER, Heyndrickx G, et al: Randomized comparison of rescue angioplasty with conservative management of patients with early failure of thrombolysis for acute anterior myocardial infarction. Circulation 90:2280–2284, 1994.

65. Kircher BJ, Topol EJ, O'Neill WW, et al: Prediction of infarct coronary artery recanalization after intravenous thrombolytic therapy. Am J Cardiol 59:513–519, 1987.

66. Krucoff MW, Jackson YR, Burdette DL, et al: Digital real-time 12-lead ST segment trends: A bedside noninvasive monitor of infarct vessel patency. Circulation 80:II-353, 1989.

67. Laperche T, Steg PG, Benessiano J, et al: Patterns of myoglobin and MM creatine kinase isoforms release early after intravenous thrombolysis or direct percutaneous transluminal coronary angioplasty for acute myocardial infarction, and implications for the early noninvasive diagnosis of reperfusion. Am J Cardiol 70:1129–1134, 1992.

68. Adams JE, Bodor GS, Davila-Roman VG, et al: Cardiac troponin-I: A marker with high specificity for cardiac injury. Circulation 88:101–106, 1993.

69. Adams JE, Sicard GA, Allen BT, et al: Diagnosis of perioperative myocardial infarction with measurement of cardiac troponin I. N Engl J Med 330:670–674, 1994.

70. Katus HA, Looser S, Hallermayer K, et al: Development and in vitro characterization of a new immunoassay of cardiac troponin T. Clin Chem 38:386–393, 1992.

71. Hamm CW, Ravkilde J, Gerhardt W, et al: The prognostic value of serum troponin T in unstable angina. N Engl J Med 339:1380–1382, 1992.

72. Ellis AK, Little T, Masud ARZ, et al: Early noninvasive detection of successful reperfusion in patients with acute myocardial infarction. Circulation 78:1352–1357, 1988.

73. Serruys PW, Wijns W, van den Brand M, et al: Is transluminal angioplasty mandatory after successful thrombolysis? Br Heart J 50:257–265, 1983.

74. Lee G, Row RI, Takeda P, et al: Importance of follow-up medical and surgical approaches to prevent reinfarction, reocclusion, and recurrent angina following intracoronary thrombolysis with streptokinase in acute myocardial infarction. Am Heart J 66:914–916, 1982.

75. Satler LF, Pallas RS, Bond OB, et al: Assessment of residual coronary arterial stenosis after thrombolytic therapy during acute myocardial infarction. Am J Cardiol 59:1231–1233, 1987.

76. Kereiakes DJ, Topol EJ, George BS, et al: Myocardial infarction with minimal coronary atherosclerosis in the era of reperfusion. J Am Coll Cardiol 17:304–312, 1991.

77. Schroder R, Neuhaus K-L, Leizorovicz A, et al: A prospective placebo-controlled double-blind multicenter trial of Intravenous Streptokinase in Acute Myocardial Infarction (ISAM): Long-term mortality and morbidity. J Am Coll Cardiol 9:197–203, 1987.

78. Schroder R, Neuhaus K-L, Linderer T, et al: Risk of death from recurrent ischemic events after intravenous streptokinase in acute myocardial infarction: Results from the Intravenous Streptokinase in Acute Myocardial Infarction (ISAM) study. Circulation 76(suppl II):II-44–II-51, 1987.

79. Simoons ML, Serruys PW, Van den Brand M, et al: Early thrombolysis in acute myocardial infarction: Limitation of infarct size and improved survival. J Am Coll Cardiol 7:717–728, 1986.

80. Mueller HS, Forman SA, Menegus MA, et al: Prognostic significance of nonfatal reinfarction during 3-year follow-up: Results of the Thrombolysis in Myocardial Infarction (TIMI) phase II clinical trial. J Am Coll Cardiol 26:900–907, 1995.

81. Kornowski R, Goldbourt U, Zion M, et al, for the SPRINT Study Group: Predictors and long-term prognostic significance of recurrent infarction in the year after a first acute myocardial infarction [Abstract]. Am J Cardiol 72:883–888, 1993.

82. Califf RM, Topol EJ, Ohman M, et al: Isolated recurrent ischemia after thrombolytic therapy is a frequent, important and expensive adverse clinical outcome. J Am Coll Cardiol 19:301A, 1992.

83. Schroder R, Neuhaus K-L, Linderer T, et al: Risk of death from recurrent ischemic events after intravenous streptokinase in acute myocardial infarction: Results from the Intravenous Streptokinase in Acute Myocardial Infarction (ISAM) Study. Circulation 76(suppl II):II-44–II-51, 1987.

84. Stone GW, Grines CL, Browne KF, et al: Implications of recurrent ischemia after reperfusion therapy in acute myocardial infarction: A comparison of thrombolytic therapy and primary angioplasty. J Am Coll Cardiol 26:66–72, 1995.

85. White CW: Recurrent ischemic events after successful thrombolysis in acute myocardial infarction. Circulation 80:1482–1485, 1989.

86. Ellis SG, Gallison L, Grines CL, et al: Incidence and predictors of early recurrent ischemia after successful percutaneous transluminal coronary angioplasty for acute myocardial infarction. Am J Cardiol 63:263–268, 1989.

87. Ellis SG, Debowey D, Bates ER, et al: Treatment of recurrent ischemia after thrombolysis and successful reperfusion for acute myocardial infarction: Effect on in-hospital mortality and left ventricular function. J Am Coll Cardiol 17:752–757, 1991.

88. Barbagelata A, Granger CB, Topol EJ, et al: Frequency, significance and cost of recurrent ischemia after thrombolytic therapy for acute myocardial infarction. Am J Cardiol 76:1007–1013, 1995.

89. Newby LK, Califf RM, Guerci A, et al, for the GUSTO Investigators: Early discharge in the thrombolytic era: An analysis of criteria for uncomplicated infarction from the Global Utilization of Streptokinase and t-PA for Occluded Coronary Arteries (GUSTO) trial. J Am Coll Cardiol 27:625–632, 1996.

90. Topol EJ, Burek K, O'Neill WW, et al: A randomized controlled trial of hospital discharge three days after myocardial infarction in the era of reperfusion. N Engl J Med 318:1083–1088, 1988.

91. Mark DB, Sigmon K, Topol EJ, et al: Identification of acute myocardial infarction patients suitable for early hospital discharge after aggressive interventional therapy. Circulation 83:1186–1193, 1991.

92. O'Connor CM, Califf RM, Massey EW, et al: Stroke and acute myocardial infarction in the thrombolytic era: Clinical correlates and long-term prognosis. J Am Coll Cardiol 16:533–540, 1990.

93. Lew AS, Hod H, Cercek B, et al: Mortality and morbidity rates of patients older and younger than 75 years with acute myocardial infarction treated with intravenous streptokinase. Am J Cardiol 59:1–5, 1987.

94. Gore JM, Sloan M, Price TR, et al: Intracerebral hemorrhage, cerebral infarction, and subdural hematoma after acute myocardial infarction and thrombolytic therapy in the Thrombolysis in Myocardial Infarction trial. Circulation 83:448–459, 1991.

95. Kase CS, O'Neal AM, Fisher M, et al: Intracranial hemorrhage after use of tissue plasminogen activator for coronary thrombolysis. Ann Intern Med 112:17–21, 1990.

96. Bovill EG, Terrin ML, Stump DC, et al, for the TIMI Investigators: Hemorrhagic events during therapy with recombinant tissue-type plasminogen activator, heparin, and aspirin for acute myocardial infarction. Ann Intern Med 115:256–265, 1991.

97. Sobel BE: Intracranial bleeding, fibrinolysis, and anticoagulation: Causal connections and clinical implications. Circulation 90:2147–2152, 1994.

98. deJaegere PP, Arnold AA, Balk AH, et al: Intracranial hemorrhage in association with thrombolytic therapy: Incidence and clinical predictive factors. J Am Coll Cardiol 19:289–294, 1992.

99. Sane DC, Califf RM, Topol EJ, et al: Bleeding during thrombolytic therapy for acute myocardial infarction: Mechanisms and management. Ann Intern Med 111:1010–1022, 1989.

100. Gore JM, Granger CB, Simoons ML, et al: Stroke after thrombolysis: Mortality and functional outcomes in the GUSTO-I trial. Circulation 2:2811–2818, 1995.

101. Carlson S, Aldrich MS, Greenberg HS, et al: Intracerebral hemorrhage complicating intravenous tissue plasminogen activator treatment. Arch Neurol 45:1070–1073, 1988.

102. Simoons ML, Maggioni AP, Knatterud G, et al: Individual risk assessment for intracranial hemorrhage during thrombolytic therapy. Lancet 342:1523–1528, 1993.

103. Bovill EG, Tracy RP, Knatterud GL, et al: Hemorrhagic events during therapy with recombinant tissue plasminogen activator, heparin, and aspirin for unstable angina (Thrombolysis in Myocardial Ischemia, phase IIIB trial). Am J Cardiol 79:391–396, 1997.

104. White HD, Barbash GI, Modan M, et al: After correcting for worse baseline characteristics, women treated with thrombolytic therapy for acute myocardial infarction have the same mortality and morbidity as men except for a higher incidence of hemorrhagic stroke. Circulation 88(pt 1):2097–2103, 1993.

105. Gruppo Italiano per lo Studio Della Sopravvivenza Nell'Infarto Miocardico: GISSI-2: A factorial randomised trial of alteplase versus streptokinase and heparin versus no heparin among 12,490 patients with acute myocardial infarction. Lancet 336(suppl B):65–71, 1990.

106. Passamani E, Hodges M, Herman M, et al: The Thrombolysis in Myocardial Infarction (TIMI) phase II pilot study: Tissue plasminogen activator followed by percutaneous transluminal coronary angioplasty. J Am Coll Cardiol 10:51B–64B, 1987.

107. Sobel BE: Intracranial bleeding, fibrinolysis, and anticoagulation. Causal connections and clinical implications. Circulation 90:2147–2152, 1994.

108. Antman EM: Hirudin in acute myocardial infarction. Safety report from the Thrombolysis in Myocardial Infarction (TIMI) 9A trial. Circulation 90:1624–1630, 1994.

109. The Global Use of Strategies to Open Occluded Coronary Arteries (GUSTO) IIa Investigators: GUSTO IIa: Randomized trial of intravenous heparin versus recombinant hirudin for acute coronary syndromes. Circulation 90:1631–1637, 1994.

110. Neuhaus K-L, von Essen R, Tebbe U, et al: Safety observations from the pilot phase of the randomized r-Hirudin for Improvement of Thrombolysis (HIT-III) study. A study of the Arbeitsgemeinschaft Leitender Kardiologischer Krankenhausarzte (ALKK). Circulation 90:1638–1642, 1994.

111. Rao AK, Pratt C, Berke A, et al, for the TIMI Investigators: Thrombolysis in Myocardial Infarction (TIMI) Trial—phase I: Hemorrhagic manifestations and changes in plasma fibrinogen and the fibrinolytic system in patients treated with recombinant tissue plasminogen activator and streptokinase. J Am Coll Cardiol 11:1–11, 1988.

112. Topol EJ: The GUSTO-III Trial. Plenary session presentation, 46th Annual Scientific Sessions of the American College of Cardiology, Anaheim CA, March 1997.

113. Braunwald E, Kloner RA: Myocardial reperfusion: A double-edged sword? J Clin Invest 76:1713–1719, 1985.

114. The Fibrinolytic Therapy Trialists (FTT) Collaborative Group: Indications for fibrinolytic therapy in suspected acute myocardial infarction: Collaborative overview of early mortality and major morbidity results from all randomised trials of more than 1000 patients. Lancet 343:311–322, 1994.

115. Honan NB, Harrell FE, Reimer KA, et al: Cardiac rupture, mortality, and the timing of thrombolytic therapy: A meta-analysis. J Am Coll Cardiol 16:359–367, 1990.

116. Loukinen KL, O'Neill W, Laufer N, et al: Myocardial rupture complicating tissue plasminogen activator therapy of acute myocardial infarction [Abstract]. J Am Coll Cardiol 13:94A, 1989.

117. Levine MN, Goldhaber SZ, Gore JM, et al: Hemorrhagic complications of thrombolytic therapy in the treatment of myocardial infarction and venous thromboembolism. Chest 108(suppl S):291S–301S, 1995.

118. Sane DC, Califf RM, Topol EJ, et al: Bleeding during thrombolytic therapy for acute myocardial infarction: mechanisms and management. Ann Intern Med 111:1010–1022, 1989.

119. Rao AK, Pratt C, Berke A, et al, for the TIMI Investigators: Thrombolysis in Myocardial Infarction (TIMI) trial—phase I: Hemorrhagic manifestations and changes in plasma fibrinogen and the fibrinolytic system in patients treated with

recombinant tissue plasminogen activator and streptokinase. J Am Coll Cardiol 11:1–11, 1988.

120. Bovill EG, Terrin ML, Stump DC, et al, for the TIMI Investigators: Hemorrhagic events during therapy with recombinant tissue-type plasminogen activator, heparin and aspirin for acute myocardial infarction. Ann Intern Med 115:256–265, 1991.

121. Califf RM, Topol EJ, George BS, et al, for the Thrombolysis and Angioplasty in Myocardial Infarction study group: Hemorrhagic complications associated with the use of intravenous tissue plasminogen activator in treatment of acute myocardial infarction. Am J Med 885:353–359, 1988.

122. Berkowitz SD, Granger CB, Pieper KS, et al, for the GUSTO Investigators: Incidence and predictors of bleeding after contemporary thrombolytic therapy for myocardial infarction. Circulation 95:2508–2516, 1997.

123. Stone GW: Primary PTCA in high risk patients with acute myocardial infarction. J Invasive Cardiol 7(suppl F):12F–21F, 1995.

124. Lee KL, Woodlief LH, Topol EJ, et al: Predictors of 30-day mortality in the era of reperfusion for acute myocardial infarction. Results from an international trial of 41,021 patients. Circulation 91:1659–1668, 1995.

125. Rackley CE, Russell RP, Mantle JA, et al: Cardiogenic shock. Cardiovasc Clin 11:15–24, 1981.

126. Hands ME, Rutherford JD, Muller JE, et al: The in-hospital development of cardiogenic shock after acute myocardial infarction: Incidence, predictors of occurrence, outcome and prognostic factors. J Am Coll Cardiol 14:40–46, 1989.

127. Kennedy JW, Gensini GG, Timmis GC, et al: Acute myocardial infarction treated with intracoronary streptokinase: A report of the Society for Cardiac Angiography. Am J Cardiol 55:871–877, 1985.

128. Bates ER, Topol EJ: Limitations of thrombolytic therapy for acute myocardial infarction complicated by congestive heart failure and cardiogenic shock. J Am Coll Cardiol 18:1077–1084, 1991.

129. GISSI-2: The International Study Group: In-hospital mortality and clinical course of 20,891 patients with suspected acute myocardial infarction randomised between alteplase and streptokinase with or without heparin. Lancet 336:71–75, 1990.

130. Holmes DR, Bates ER, Kleiman NS, et al: Contemporary reperfusion therapy for cardiogenic shock: The GUSTO-I trial experience. J Am Coll Cardiol 26:668–674, 1995.

131. Hochman JS, Boland J, Sleeper LA, et al: Current spectrum of cardiogenic shock and effect of early revascularization on mortality. Results of an international registry. Circulation 91:873–881, 1995.

132. Grines CL, DeMaria AN: Optimal utilization of thrombolytic therapy for acute myocardial infarction: Concepts and controversies. J Am Coll Cardiol 16:223–231, 1990.

133. Cragg DR, Friedman HZ, Bonema JD, et al: Outcome of patients with acute myocardial infarction who are ineligible for thrombolytic therapy. Ann Intern Med 115:173–177, 1991.

134. LATE Study Group: Late Assessment of Thrombolytic Efficacy (LATE) study with alteplase 6–24 hours after onset of acute myocardial infarction. Lancet 342:759–766, 1993.

135. Jha P, DeBoer D, Sykora K, et al: Characteristics and mortality outcomes of thrombolysis trial participants and nonparticipants: A population-based comparison. J Am Coll Cardiol 27:1335–1342, 1996.

136. Rosamund WD, Shahar E, McGovern PG, et al: Trends in coronary thrombolytic therapy for acute myocardial infarction (The Minnesota Heart Survey Registry, 1990 to 1993). Am J Cardiol 78:271–277, 1996.

137. Rogers WJ, Bowlby LJ, Chandra NC, for the Participants in the National Registry of Myocardial Infarction: Treatment of myocardial infarction in the United States (1990–1993). Observations from the National Registry of Myocardial Infarction. Circulation 90:2103–2114, 1994.

138. McGovern PG, Pankow JS, Shahar E, et al: Recent trends in acute coronary heart disease. Mortality, morbidity, medical care and risk factors. N Engl J Med 334:884–890, 1996.

139. Every NR, Parsons LS, Hlatky M, et al: A comparison of thrombolytic therapy with primary coronary angioplasty for acute myocardial infarction. N Engl J Med 335:1253–1260, 1996.

140. Blankenship JC, Almquist AK: Cardiovascular complications of thrombolytic therapy in patients with a mistaken diagnosis of acute myocardial infarction. J Am Coll Cardiol 14:1579–1582, 1989.

141. O'Keefe JO, Bailey WL, Rutherford BD, et al: Primary angioplasty for acute myocardial infarction in 1000 consecutive patients. Am J Cardiol 72(suppl G):107G–115G, 1993.

142. Taylor GJ, Humprites JO, Mellits ED, et al: Predictors of clinical course, coronary anatomy, and left ventricular function after recovery from acute myocardial infarction. Circulation 62:960–970, 1980.

143. Lee KL, Sigmon KN, Califf RM, et al: How much prognostic information does catheterization after thrombolytic therapy add to noninvasive clinical factors? J Am Coll Cardiol 19:80, 1992.

144. Schulman SP, Achuff SC, Griffith LS, et al: Prognostic cardiac catheterization variables in survivors of acute myocardial infarction. J Am Coll Cardiol 11:1164–1172, 1988.

145. Turner JD, Rogers WJ, Mantle JA, et al: Coronary angiography soon after myocardial infarction. Chest 77:58–64, 1980.

146. Harris PJ, Lee KL, Harrell FE, et al: Outcome in medically treated coronary artery disease: Ischemic events, nonfatal infarction and death. Circulation 62:718–726, 1980.

147. Kulick DL, Rahimtoola SH: Risk stratification in survivors of acute myocardial infarction: Routine cardiac catheterization and angiography is a reasonable approach in most patients. Am Heart J 121:641–656, 1991.

148. Califf RM, Phillips HR, Hindman MC, et al: Prognostic value of a coronary artery jeopardy score. J Am Coll Cardiol 5:1055–1063, 1985.

149. Simoons ML, Vos J, Tijssen JG, et al: Long-term benefit of early thrombolytic therapy in patients with acute myocardial infarction: 5-Year follow-up of a trial conducted by the Interuniversity Cardiology Institute of The Netherlands. J Am Coll Cardiol 14:1609–1615, 1989.

150. White HD, Norris RM, Brown M, et al: Left ventricular end-systolic volume as the major determinant of survival after recovery from myocardial infarction. Circulation 76:44–51, 1987.

151. Bertrand ME, Lefebvre JM, Laisne CL, et al: Coronary arteriography in acute transmural myocardial infarction. Am Heart J 97:61–69, 1979.

152. Turner JD, Rogers WJ, Mantle JA, et al: Coronary angiography soon after myocardial infarction. Chest 77:58–64, 1980.

153. Sheehan FH, Mathey DG, Schoffer J, et al: Factors that determine recovery of left ventricular function after thrombolysis in patients with acute myocardial infarction. Circulation 71:1121–1128, 1985.

154. Brodie BR, Weintraub RA, Stuckey TD, et al: Outcomes of direct coronary angioplasty for acute myocardial infarction in candidates and non-candidates for thrombolytic therapy. Am J Cardiol 67:7–12, 1991.

155. Beauchamp GD, Vacek JL, Robuck W: Management comparison for acute myocardial infarction: Direct angioplasty versus sequential thrombolysis-angioplasty. Am Heart J 120:237–242, 1990.

156. Hanlon JT, Combs DT, McLellan BA, et al: Early hospital discharge after direct angioplasty for acute myocardial infarction. Catheter Cardiovasc Diagn 35:187–190, 1995.

157. Nakagawa Y, Iwasaki Y, Takeshi T, et al: Serial angiographic follow-up after successful direct angioplasty for acute myocardial infarction; single center experience [Abstract]. Circulation 88(suppl I):I-106A, 1993.

158. Rothbaum DA, Linnemeier TJ, Landin RJ, et al: Emergency percutaneous transluminal coronary angioplasty in acute myocardial infarction: A 3 year experience. J Am Coll Cardiol 10:264–272, 1987.

159. Zimarino M, Corcos T, Favereau X, et al: Predictors of short term clinical and angiographic outcome after coronary angioplasty for acute myocardial infarction. Catheter Cardiovasc Diagn 36:203–208, 1995.

160. Miller PF, Brodie BR, Weintraub RA, et al: Emergency coro-

nary angioplasty for acute myocardial infarction. Arch Intern Med 147:1565–1570, 1987.

161. Dageford DA, Genovely HC, Goodin RR, et al: Emergency percutaneous transluminal coronary angioplasty in acute myocardial infarction. J Ky Med Assoc 85:368–372, 1987.

162. O'Neill WW, Weintraub R, Grines CL, et al: A prospective, placebo-controlled, randomized trial of intravenous streptokinase and angioplasty versus lone angioplasty therapy of acute myocardial infarction. Circulation 86:1710–1717, 1992.

163. Brush JE, Thompson S, Ciuffo AA, et al: Retrospective comparison of a strategy of primary coronary angioplasty versus intravenous thrombolytic therapy for acute myocardial infarction in a community hospital without cardiac surgical backup. J Invasive Cardiol 8:91–98, 1996.

164. Kimura T, Nosaka H, Ueno K, et al: Role of coronary angioplasty in acute myocardial infarction. Circulation 74(suppl II):II-22, 1986.

165. Topol EJ: Direct or sequential PTCA. In Topol EJ (ed): Acute Coronary Intervention, pp 79–94. New York: Alan R. Liss, 1988.

166. Marco J, Caster L, Szatmary LJ, et al: Emergency percutaneous transluminal coronary angioplasty without thrombolysis as initial therapy in acute myocardial infarction. Int J Cardiol 15:55–63, 1987.

167. O'Neill W, Timmis GC, Bourdillon PD, et al: A prospective randomized clinical trial of intracoronary streptokinase versus coronary angioplasty for acute myocardial infarction. N Engl J Med 314:812–818, 1986.

168. Grines CL, Nissen SE, Booth DC, et al: A prospective, randomized trial comparing half-dose tissue-type plasminogen activator with streptokinase to full-dose tissue-type plasminogen activator. Circulation 84:540–549, 1991.

169. Carney RJ, Murphy GA, Brandt TR, et al: Randomized angiographic trial of recombinant tissue-type plasminogen activator (alteplase) in myocardial infarction. J Am Coll Cardiol 20:17–23, 1992.

170. Granger CB, Ohman EM, Bates E: Pooled analysis of angiographic patency rates from thrombolytic therapy trials. Circulation 86(suppl I):I-269, 1992.

171. O'Neill WW: Impact of different reperfusion modalities on ventricular function after acute myocardial infarction. Am J Cardiol 61(suppl G):45G–53G, 1988.

172. Dabaghi SF, Damat S, Hendricks O, et al: Low dose aspirin inhibits in vitro platelet aggregation within minutes after ingestion [Abstract]. Circulation 86(suppl I):I-126, 1992.

173. Lacoste L, Lam JUT, Letchacovski G: Comparative antithrombotic efficacy of aspirin: 80 mg vs. 325 mg daily [Abstract]. Circulation 90(suppl I):I-552, 1994.

174. Grines CL, Schreiber TL, Savas V, et al: A randomized trial of low osmolar ionic versus nonionic contrast media in patients with myocardial infarction or unstable angina undergoing percutaneous transluminal coronary angioplasty. J Am Coll Cardiol 27:1381–1386, 1996.

175. Piessens JH, Stammen F, Vrolix MC, et al: Effects of an ionic versus a nonionic low osmolar contrast agent on the thrombotic complications of coronary angioplasty. Catheter Cardiovasc Diagn 28:99–105, 1993.

176. Royer T, Berrocal D, Rosenblat E, et al: Acute thrombosis in coronary angioplasty: Effect of ionic versus nonionic contrast media. Eur Heart J 11:1999–2005, 1990.

177. Aguirre F, Topol EJ, Donohue T: Impact of ionic and nonionic contrast agent on the thrombotic complications of coronary angioplasty [Abstract]. J Am Coll Cardiol 25:8A, 1995.

178. Ferguson J, Dougherty K, Gaos C, et al: Relation between procedural activated coagulation time and outcome after percutaneous transluminal coronary angioplasty. J Am Coll Cardiol 23:1061–1065, 1994.

179. Winters K, Oltrona L, Hiremath Y, et al: Heparin-resistant thrombin activity is associated with acute ischemic events during high-risk coronary interventions [Abstract]. Circulation 92(suppl I):I-608, 1995.

180. Harrington RA, Leimberer JD, Berdan L, et al: The ACT Index: A method for stratifying likelihood of success and risk of acute complications in coronary intervention [Abstract]. Circulation 88(suppl I):I-208, 1993.

181. Naqvi T, Ivy P, Linn P, et al: Low dose heparin enhances and high dose heparin suppresses platelet P-selectin expression and platelet aggregation [Abstract]. Circulation 9(suppl I):I-673, 1995.

182. Ahmed W, Meckel C, Grines CL, et al: Relation between ischemic complications and activated clotting time during angioplasty and abrupt closure [Abstract]. J Am Coll Cardiol 23:470A, 1994.

183. Stone GW, Rutherford BD, McConahay DR, et al: Direct coronary angioplasty in acute myocardial infarction: Outcome in patients with single vessel disease. J Am Coll Cardiol 15:534–543, 1990.

184. Kahn JK, Rutherford BD, McConahay DR, et al: Results of primary angioplasty for acute myocardial infarction in patients with multivessel coronary artery disease. J Am Coll Cardiol 16:1089–1096, 1990.

185. O'Keefe JH, Rutherford BD, McConahay DR, et al: Early and late results of coronary angioplasty without antecedent thrombolytic therapy for acute myocardial infarction. Am J Cardiol 64:1221–1230, 1989.

186. Bedotto JB, Kahn JK, Rutherford BD, et al: Failed direct coronary angioplasty for acute myocardial infarction: In-hospital outcome and predictors of death. J Am Coll Cardiol 22:690–694, 1993.

187. Kahn JK, O'Keefe JH, Rutherford BD, et al: Timing and mechanism of in-hospital and late death after primary coronary angioplasty during acute myocardial infarction. Am J Cardiol 66:1045–1048, 1990.

188. Lee TC, Laramee LA, Rutherford BD, et al: Emergency percutaneous transluminal coronary angioplasty for acute myocardial infarction in patients 70 years of age and older. Am J Cardiol 66:663–667, 1990.

189. Kahn JK, Rutherford BD, McConahay DR, et al: Usefulness of angioplasty during acute myocardial infarction in patients with prior coronary artery bypass grafting. Am J Cardiol 65:698–702, 1990.

190. Kahn JK, Rutherford BD, McConahay DR, et al: Catheterization laboratory events and hospital outcome with direct angioplasty for acute myocardial infarction. Circulation 82:1910–1915, 1990.

191. O'Keefe JH, Sayed-Taha K, Gibson W, et al: Do patients with left circumflex coronary artery–related acute myocardial infarction without ST-segment elevation benefit from reperfusion therapy? Am J Cardiol 75:718–720, 1995.

192. O'Neill WW, Brodie BR, Ivanhoe R, et al: Primary coronary angioplasty for myocardial infarction (the Primary Angioplasty Registry). Am J Cardiol 73:627–634, 1994.

193. Brodie BR, Grines CL, Ivanhoe R: Six-month clinical and angiographic follow-up after direct angioplasty for acute myocardial infarction. Final results from the Primary Angioplasty Registry. Circulation 25:156–162, 1994.

194. Topol EJ, Califf RM, George BS, et al: A randomized trial of immediate versus delayed elective angioplasty after intravenous tissue plasminogen activator in acute myocardial infarction. N Engl J Med 317:197–202, 1987.

195. The TIMI Research Group: Immediate vs. delayed catheterization and angioplasty following thrombolytic therapy for acute myocardial infarction. JAMA 260:2849–2858, 1988.

196. Simoons ML, Arnold AER, Betric A, et al: Thrombolysis with tissue plasminogen activator in acute myocardial infarction: No additional benefit from immediate percutaneous transluminal coronary angioplasty. Lancet 1:197–202, 1988.

197. The TIMI Study Group: Comparison of invasive and conservative strategies after treatment with intravenous tissue plasminogen activator in acute myocardial infarction. Results of the Thrombolysis in Myocardial Infarction (TIMI) phase II trial. N Engl J Med 320:618–627, 1989.

198. SWIFT (Should We Intervene Following Thrombolysis?) Trial Study Group: SWIFT trial of delayed elective intervention vs. conservative treatment after thrombolysis with anistreplase in acute myocardial infarction. BMJ 302:555–560, 1991.

199. Barbash GI, Roth A, Hod H, et al: Randomized controlled

trial of late in-hospital angiography and angioplasty versus conservative management after treatment with recombinant tissue-type plasminogen activator in acute myocardial infarction. Am J Cardiol 66:538–545, 1990.

200. Van den Brand MJ, Betrui A, Bescos LL, et al: Randomized trial of deferred angioplasty after thrombolysis for acute myocardial infarction. Coron Artery Dis 3:393–401, 1992.

201. Ozbek C, Dyckmans J, Sen S, et al: Comparison of invasive and conservative strategies after treatment with streptokinase in acute myocardial infarction: Results of a randomized trial (SIAM) [Abstract]. J Am Coll Cardiol 15:63A, 1990.

202. Ellis SG, Van de Weft F, Riberio-DaSilva E, et al: Present status of rescue coronary angioplasty: Current polarization of opinion and randomized trials. J Am Coll Cardiol 19:681–686, 1992.

203. O'Neill WW, Weintraub R, Grines CL, et al: A prospective, placebo-controlled, randomized trial of intravenous streptokinase and angioplasty versus lone angioplasty therapy of acute myocardial infarction. Circulation 86:1710–1717, 1992.

204. Ambrose JA, Almeida OD, Sharma SK, et al: Adjunctive thrombolytic therapy during angioplasty for ischemic rest pain. Results of the TAUSA trial. Circulation 90:69–77, 1994.

205. Mehran R, Ambrose JA, Bongu RM, et al: Angioplasty of complex lesions in ischemic rest angina. Results of the Thrombolysis and Angioplasty in UnStable Angina (TAUSA) trial. J Am Coll Cardiol 26:961–966, 1995.

206. Spielberg C, Schnitzer L, Linderer T, et al: Influence of catheter technology and adjuvant medication on acute complications in percutaneous coronary angioplasty. Catheter Cardiovasc Diagn 21:72, 1990.

207. The TIMI-3B Investigators: Effects of tissue plasminogen activator and a comparison of early invasive and conservative strategies in unstable angina and non Q-wave myocardial infarction. Circulation 89:1545–1556, 1994.

208. Anderson H, Cannon C, Stone P, et al: One year results of the Thrombolysis in Myocardial Infarction (TIMI) 3B clinical trial. J Am Coll Cardiol 26:1643–1650, 1995.

209. Waller BF, Rothbaum DA, Pinkerton CA, et al: Status of the myocardium and infarct-related coronary artery in 19 necropsy patients with acute recanalization using pharmacologic (streptokinase, r-tissue plasminogen activator), mechanical (percutaneous transluminal coronary angioplasty) or combined types of reperfusion therapy. J Am Coll Cardiol 9:785–801, 1987.

210. Colavita PG, Ideker RE, Reimer KA, et al: The spectrum of pathology associated with percutaneous transluminal coronary angioplasty during acute myocardial infarction. J Am Coll Cardiol 8:855–860, 1986.

211. Ambrose JA, Almeida OD, Sharma SK, et al: Angiographic evolution of intracoronary thrombus and dissection following percutaneous transluminal coronary angioplasty (the Thrombolysis and Angioplasty in UnStable Angina [TAUSA] Trial). Am J Cardiol 79:559–563, 1997.

212. Kerins DM, Roy L, Fitzgerald GA, et al: Platelet and vascular function during coronary thrombolysis with tissue-type plasminogen activator. Circulation 80:1718–1725, 1989.

213. Bennett WR, Yawn DH, Migliore PJ, et al: Activation of the complement system by recombination tissue plasminogen activator. J Am Coll Cardiol 10:627–632, 1987.

214. Merlini PA, Cattaneo M, Spinola A, et al: Activation of the hemostatic system during thrombolytic therapy. Am J Cardiol 72(suppl G):59G–65G, 1993.

215. Coller BS: Platelets and thrombolytic therapy. N Engl J Med 322:33–42, 1990.

216. Ohnishi Y, Butterfeld MC, Saffitz JE, et al: Deleterious effects of a systemic lytic state on reperfused myocardium. Minimalization of reperfusion injury and enhanced recovery of myocardial function by direct angioplasty. Circulation 92:500–510, 1995.

217. Fung AY, Lai P, Juni JE, et al: Prevention of subsequent exercise-induced periinfarct ischemia by emergency coronary angioplasty in acute myocardial infarction: Compari-

son with intracoronary streptokinase. J Am Coll Cardiol 8:496–503, 1986.

218. Zijlstra F, DeBoer MJ, Hoorntje JCA, et al: A comparison of immediate coronary angioplasty with intravenous streptokinase in acute myocardial infarction. N Engl J Med 328:680–684, 1993.

219. De Boer MJ, Hoorntje JCA, Ottervanger JP, et al: Immediate coronary angioplasty versus intravenous streptokinase in acute myocardial infarction: Left ventricular ejection fraction, hospital mortality and reinfarction. J Am Coll Cardiol 23:1004–1008, 1994.

220. Ribeiro EE, Silva LA, Cardeiro R, et al: Randomized trial of direct coronary angioplasty versus intravenous streptokinase in acute myocardial infarction. J Am Coll Cardiol 22:376–380, 1993.

221. Grinfeld L, Berrocal D, Belardi J, et al: Fibrinolytics vs. primary angioplasty in acute myocardial infarction (FAP): A randomized trial in a community hospital in Argentina [Abstract]. J Am Coll Cardiol 27:222A, 1996.

222. Zijlstra F, Beukema W, Van't Hof AWJ, et al: Randomized comparison of primary coronary angioplasty with thrombolytic therapy in low risk patients with acute myocardial infarction. J Am Coll Cardiol 29:908–912, 1997.

223. Grines CL, Browne KR, Marco J, et al: A comparison of primary angioplasty with thrombolytic therapy for acute myocardial infarction. N Engl J Med 328:673–679, 1993.

224. Gibbons RJ, Holmes DR, Reeder GS, et al: Immediate angioplasty compared with the administration of a thrombolytic agent followed by conservative treatment for myocardial infarction. N Engl J Med 328:685–691, 1993.

225. DeWood MA: Direct PTCA vs. intravenous t-PA in acute myocardial infarction: Results from a prospective, randomized trial. Presented at the Thrombolysis and Interventional Therapy in Acute Myocardial Infarction Symposium VI. Washington DC: George Washington University, 1990, pp 28–29.

226. The Global Use of Strategies to Open Occluded Coronary Arteries in Acute Coronary Syndromes (GUSTO-IIb) Angioplasty Substudy Investigators: A clinical trial comparing primary coronary angioplasty with tissue plasminogen activator for acute myocardial infarction. N Engl J Med 336:1621–1628, 1997.

227. Garcia E, Elizaga J, Soriano J, et al: Primary angioplasty versus thrombolysis with tPA in anterior myocardial infarction: Results from a single center trial [Abstract]. J Am Coll Cardiol 29:389A, 1997.

228. Ribichini F, Steffenino G, Dellavalle A, et al: Primary angioplasty versus thrombolysis in inferior acute myocardial infarction with anterior ST-segment depression: A single center randomized trial. J Am Coll Cardiol 27:221A, 1996.

229. Stone GW, Grines CL, Browne KF, et al: Predictors of in-hospital and 6 month outcome after acute myocardial infarction in the reperfusion era: The Primary Angioplasty in Myocardial Infarction (PAMI) Trial. J Am Coll Cardiol 25:370–377, 1995.

230. Nunn C, O'Neill WW, Rothbaum D, et al: Long-term outcome following primary angioplasty. Report from the Primary Angioplasty in Myocardial Infarction (PAMI) Trial. J Am Coll Cardiol 33:640–646, 1999.

231. Stone GW, Grines CL, Browne KF, et al: Implications of recurrent ischemia after reperfusion therapy in acute myocardial infarction: A comparison of thrombolytic therapy and primary coronary angioplasty. J Am Coll Cardiol 26:66–72, 1995.

232. Stone GW, Grines CL, Browne KF, et al: Comparison of in-hospital outcome in men versus women treated by either thrombolytic therapy or primary coronary angioplasty for acute myocardial infarction. Am J Cardiol 75:987–992, 1995.

233. Stone GW, Grines CL, Browne KF, et al: Outcome of different reperfusion strategies in patients with former contraindications to thrombolytic therapy: A comparison of primary angioplasty and tissue plasminogen activator. Catheter Cardiovasc Diagn 39:333–339, 1996.

234. Stone GW, Grines CL, Browne KF, et al: Influence of acute myocardial infarction location on in-hospital and late out-

come after primary percutaneous transluminal coronary angioplasty versus tissue plasminogen activator. Am J Cardiol 78:19–25, 1996.

235. Stone GW, Grines CL, Browne KF, et al: Does primary angioplasty improve the prognosis of patients with diabetes and acute myocardial infarction? [Abstract]. J Am Coll Cardiol 25:401A, 1995.

236. Stone GW: Primary PTCA in high risk patients with acute myocardial infarction. J Invasive Cardiol 7(suppl F):12F–21F, 1995.

237. Stone GW, Grines CL, Browne KF, et al: Acute outcome after primary angioplasty in myocardial infarction—The Primary Angioplasty in Myocardial Infarction (PAMI) trial [Abstract]. J Am Coll Cardiol 21:331A, 1993.

238. Stone GW, Grines CL, Browne KF, et al: Adverse catheterization laboratory events after primary PTCA vs. PTCA following thrombolytic therapy—A report from the Primary Angioplasty in Myocardial Infarction (PAMI) trial [Abstract]. J Am Coll Cardiol 23:244A, 1994.

239. Bernard ST, Grines CL, Browne K, et al: Does antecedent angina predict whether reperfusion by thrombolysis or primary angioplasty will be most beneficial? [Abstract]. J Am Coll Cardiol 23:244A, 1994.

240. Stone GW, Grines CL, Browne KF, et al: Is primary angioplasty less effective in patients presenting in the early morning hours? A report from the Primary Angioplasty in Myocardial Infarction (PAMI) trial. J Am Coll Cardiol 25:295A, 1995.

241. Krikorian R, Puchrowicz S, O'Keefe J, et al: Differential effects of long-term beta-blocker therapy following thrombolysis versus primary angioplasty [Abstract]. J Am Coll Cardiol 25:402A, 1995.

242. De Boer MJ, Suryapranata H, Hoorntje JCA, et al: Limitation of infarct size and preservation of left ventricular function after primary coronary angioplasty compared with intravenous streptokinase in acute myocardial infarction [Abstract]. Circulation 90:753–761, 1994.

243. Ziljstra F, De Boer MJ, Ottervanger JP, et al: Primary coronary angioplasty versus intravenous streptokinase in acute myocardial infarction: Differences in outcome during a mean follow-up of 18 months. Coron Artery Dis 5:707–712, 1994.

244. De Boer MJ, Reiber JHC, Suryapranata H, et al: Angiographic findings and catheterization laboratory events in patients with primary coronary angioplasty or streptokinase therapy for acute myocardial infarction. Eur Heart J 16:1347–1355, 1995.

245. Zijlstra F, de Boer MJ, Beukema WP, et al: Mortality, reinfarction, left ventricular ejection fraction and costs following reperfusion therapies for acute myocardial infarction. Eur Heart J 17:382–387, 1996.

246. The Global Use of Strategies to Open Occluded Coronary Arteries (GUSTO) IIb Investigators: A comparison of recombinant hirudin with heparin for the treatment of acute coronary syndromes. N Engl J Med 335:775–782, 1996.

246a. Masotti M, Fernandez-Aviles F, Alonso J, et al: Primary angioplasty and thrombolysis in acute myocardial infarction. One year angiographic follow-up. Eur Heart J 18:126, 1997.

247. Stone GW: Primary PTCA in high risk patients with acute myocardial infarction. J Invasive Cardiol 7(suppl F):12F–21F, 1995.

248. Ryan T, Bauman WB, Kennedy JW, et al: Guidelines for percutaneous transluminal coronary angioplasty. A report of the American College of Cardiology and American Task Force, an assessment of diagnostic and therapeutic cardiovascular procedures (Committee on Percutaneous Transluminal Coronary Angioplasty). J Am Coll Cardiol 22:2033–2054, 1993.

249. Grines CL, Stone GW, O'Neill WW: Establishing a program and performance of primary PTCA—The PAMI way. J Invasive Cardiol 9:44B–52B, 1996.

250. O'Neill W, Griffin J, Stone GW, et al: Operator and institutional volume do not affect the procedural outcome of primary angioplasty therapy. J Am Coll Cardiol 27(suppl A):13A, 1996.

251. Weaver WD, Litwin PE, Martin JS: Use of direct angioplasty for treatment of patients with acute myocardial infarction in hospitals with and without on-site cardiac surgery. Circulation 88:2067–2075, 1993.

252. Every NR, Parsons LS, Hlatky M, et al: A comparison of thrombolytic therapy with primary coronary angioplasty for acute myocardial infarction. N Engl J Med 335:1253–1260, 1996.

253. Grassman ED, Johnson SA, Krone RJ: Predictors of success and major complications for primary percutaneous transluminal coronary angioplasty in acute myocardial infarction: An analysis of the 1990 to 1994 Society for Cardiac Angiography and Interventions Registry. J Am Coll Cardiol 30:201–208, 1997.

254. Neuhaus K-L, Vogt A, Harmjanz D, et al: Primary PTCA in acute myocardial infarction: Results from a German multicenter registry [Abstract]. J Am Coll Cardiol 27:62A, 1996.

255. Zahn R, Koch A, Rustige J, et al: Primary angioplasty versus thrombolysis in the treatment of acute myocardial infarction. Am J Cardiol 79:264–269, 1997.

256. Lange RA, Hillis LD: Thrombolysis—The preferred therapy (clinical debate). N Engl J Med 335:1311–1312, 1996.

257. Schweiger MJ, McMahon RP, Terrin M, et al, for the TIMI Investigators: Comparison of patients with <60% to ≥60% diameter narrowing of the myocardial infarct-related artery after thrombolysis. Am J Cardiol 74:105–110, 1994.

258. Kereiakes DJ, Topol EJ, George BS, et al: Myocardial infarction with minimal coronary atherosclerosis in the era of thrombolytic therapy. J Am Coll Cardiol 17:304–312, 1991.

259. Gohlke H, Heim E, Roskamm H: Prognostic importance of collateral flow and residual coronary stenosis of the myocardial infarction artery after anterior wall Q-wave acute myocardial infarction. Am J Cardiol 67:1165–1169, 1991.

260. Veen G, Meyer A, Verheugt FWA, et al: Culprit lesion morphology and stenosis severity in the prediction of reocclusion after coronary thrombolysis: Angiographic results of the APRICOT study. J Am Coll Cardiol 22:1755–1762, 1993.

261. Mark DB, O'Neill WW, Brodie BR, et al: Baseline and 6-month costs of primary angioplasty for acute myocardial infarction: Results from the Primary Angioplasty Registry. J Am Coll Cardiol 26:688–695, 1995.

262. Mark DB: Medical economics and health policy issues for interventional cardiology. In Topol EJ (ed): Textbook of Interventional Cardiology, 2nd ed, pp 1323–1325. Philadelphia: WB Saunders, 1993.

263. Charles E, Mark DB: The economics of percutaneous intervention. In Roubin GS, Califf RM, O'Neill WW, et al (eds): Interventional Cardiovascular Medicine: Principles and Practice, pp 373–384. New York: Churchill Livingstone, 1994.

264. Mark DB, Jollis J: Economic aspects of therapy for acute myocardial infarction. In Bates ER (ed): Adjunctive Therapy for Acute Myocardial Infarction, pp 471–496. New York: Marcel Dekker, 1991.

265. Stone GW, Grines CL, Rothbaum D, et al: Analysis of the relative costs and effectiveness of primary angioplasty compared to tissue plasminogen activator: The Primary Angioplasty in Myocardial Infarction trial. J Am Coll Cardiol 29:901–907, 1997.

266. Mark DB, Granger CB, Ellis SB, et al: Costs of direct angioplasty versus thrombolysis for acute myocardial infarction: Results from the GUSTO II randomized trial [Abstract]. Circulation 94:I-168, 1997.

267. de Boer MJ, van Hout BA, Liem AL, et al: A cost-effective analysis of primary coronary angioplasty versus thrombolysis for acute myocardial infarction. Am J Cardiol 76:830–833, 1995.

268. Grines CL: Transfer of high-risk myocardial infarction patients for primary PTCA. J Invasive Cardiol 9(suppl B):13B–19B, 1997.

269. Bowers TR, Terrien EF, O'Neill WW, et al: Effect of reperfusion modality on outcome in nonsmokers and smokers with acute myocardial infarction (a Primary Angioplasty in Myocardial Infarction [PAMI] substudy). Am J Cardiol 78:511–515, 1996.

270. Mueller HS, Cohen LS, Braunwald E, et al: Predictors of early morbidity and mortality after thrombolytic therapy of acute myocardial infarction: Analysis of patient subgroups in the Thrombolysis in Myocardial Infarction (TIMI) trial, phase II. Circulation 85:1254–1264, 1992.

271. Eckman MH, Wong JB, Salem DN, et al: Direct angioplasty for acute myocardial infarction: A review of outcomes in clinical subsets. Ann Intern Med 117:667–676, 1992.

272. Rich MW, Bosner MS, Chung MK, et al: Is age an independent predictor of early and late mortality in patients with acute myocardial infarction? Am J Med 92:7–13, 1992.

273. Weaver WD, Litwin PE, Martin JS, et al: Effect of age on thrombolytic therapy and mortality in acute myocardial infarction. J Am Coll Cardiol 18:657–662, 1991.

274. Gurwitz JH, Osganian V, Goldberg RJ, et al: Diagnostic testing in acute myocardial infarction: Does patient age influence utilization patterns? Am J Epidemiol 134:948–957, 1991.

275. Krumholz HM, Murillo JE, Chen J, et al: Thrombolytic therapy for eligible elderly patients with acute myocardial infarction. JAMA 277:1683–1688, 1997.

276. Woodfield SL, Lundergan CF, Reiner JS, et al: Gender and acute myocardial infarction: Is there a different response to thrombolysis? J Am Coll Cardiol 29:35–42, 1997.

277. Lincoff AM, Califf RM, Ellis SG, et al, for the Thrombolysis and Angioplasty in Myocardial Infarction Study Group: Thrombolytic therapy for women with myocardial infarction: Is there a gender gap? J Am Coll Cardiol 22:1780–1787, 1993.

278. Puletti M, Sunseri L, Curione M, et al: Acute myocardial infarction: Sex related differences in prognosis. Am Heart J 108:63–66, 1984.

279. Tofler GH, Stone PH, Muller JE, et al, for the MILIS Study Group: Effects of gender and race on prognosis after myocardial infarction: Adverse prognosis for women, particularly black women. J Am Coll Cardiol 9:473–482, 1987.

280. Lerner DJ, Kannel WB: Patterns of coronary heart disease morbidity and mortality in the sexes: A 26 year follow-up of the Framingham population. Am Heart J 111:383–390, 1986.

281. Dittrich H, Gilpin E, Nicod P, et al: Acute myocardial infarction in women: Influence of gender on mortality and prognostic variables. Am J Cardiol 62:1–7, 1988.

282. Stone GW, Grines CL, Browne KF, et al: Comparison of in-hospital outcome in men versus women treated by either thrombolytic therapy or primary coronary angioplasty for acute myocardial infarction. Am J Cardiol 75:987–992, 1995.

282a. Griffin J, O'Neill W, Brodie B, et al: Primary PTCA results in similar in-hospital outcomes in females and males presenting with acute MI [Abstract]. J Am Coll Cardiol 27:154A, 1996.

283. Maisel AS, Gilpin E, Hoit B, et al: Survival after hospital discharge in matched populations with inferior or anterior myocardial infarction. J Am Coll Cardiol 6:731–736, 1985.

284. Stone PH, Raabe DS, Jaffe AS, et al: Prognostic significance of location and type of myocardial infarction: Independent adverse outcome associated with anterior location. J Am Coll Cardiol 11:453–463, 1988.

285. Thanavaro S, Kleiger RE, Province MA, et al: Effect of infarct location on the in-hospital prognosis of patients with first transmural myocardial infarction. Circulation 66:742–747, 1982.

286. Hands ME, Lloyd BL, Robinson JS, et al: Prognostic significance of electrocardiographic site of infarction after correction for enzymatic size of infarction. Circulation 73:885–891, 1986.

287. Fukui S, Tani A, Hamano Y, et al: Immediate and long-term prognoses of acute myocardial infarction: Analysis of determinants of prognosis. Jpn Circ J 51:344–351, 1987.

288. Dubois C, Pierard LA, Albert A, et al: Short-term risk stratification at admission based on simple clinical data in acute myocardial infarction. Am J Cardiol 61:216–219, 1988.

289. Stone GW, Grines CL, Browne KF, et al: Influence of acute myocardial infarction location on in-hospital and late outcome after primary percutaneous transluminal coronary angioplasty versus tissue plasminogen activator. Am J Cardiol 78:19–25, 1996.

290. Abbud ZA, Shindler DM, Wilson AC, et al: Effect of diabetes mellitus on short- and long-term mortality rates in patients with acute myocardial infarction: A statewide study. Am Heart J 130:51–59, 1995.

291. Malmberg K, Ryden L: Myocardial infarction in patients with diabetes mellitus. Eur Heart J 9:259–264, 1988.

292. Mak K-H, Moliterno DJ, Granger CB, et al: Influence of diabetes mellitus on clinical outcome in the thrombolytic era of acute myocardial infarction. J Am Coll Cardiol 30:171–179, 1997.

293. Stone PH, Muller JE, Hartwell T, et al: The effect of diabetes mellitus on prognosis and serial left ventricular function after acute myocardial infarction: Contribution of both coronary artery disease and diastolic left ventricular dysfunction to the adverse prognosis. J Am Coll Cardiol 14:49–57, 1989.

294. Singer DE, Moulton AW, Nathan DM: Diabetic myocardial infarction: Interaction with other preinfarction risk factors. Diabetes 38:350–357, 1989.

295. Granger CB, Califf RM, Young S, et al: Outcome of patients with diabetes mellitus and acute myocardial infarction treated with thrombolytic agents. J Am Coll Cardiol 22:707–713, 1993.

296. Molstad P, Nustad M: Acute myocardial infarction in diabetic patients. Acta Med Scand 222:433–437, 1987.

297. Rytter L, Troelsen S, Beck-Nielsen H: Prevalence and mortality of acute myocardial infarction in patients with diabetes. Diabetes Care 8:230–234, 1985.

298. Stone GW, Grines CL, Browne KF, et al: Does primary angioplasty improve prognosis of patients with diabetes and acute myocardial infarction? [Abstract]. J Am Coll Cardiol 25:401A, 1995.

299. Stuckey TD, Brodie BR, Wall TC, et al: Significance of diabetes mellitus in patients with acute myocardial infarction receiving primary angioplasty [Abstract]. Circulation 94:I-330, 1996.

300. EMERAS (Estudio Multicentrico Estreptoquinasa Republicas de America del Sur) Collaborative Group: Randomised trial of late thrombolysis in patients with suspected acute myocardial infarction. Lancet 342:767–772, 1993.

301. Newby LK, Rutsch WR, Califf RM, et al: Time from symptom onset to testament and outcomes after thrombolytic therapy. J Am Coll Cardiol 27:1646–1655, 1996.

302. Collen D: Coronary thrombolysis: Streptokinase or recombinant tissue-type plasminogen activator. Ann Intern Med 112:529–538, 1990.

303. The GUSTO trial. Data on file, Genentech Inc., San Francisco, CA.

304. Stone GW, Brodie B, Griffin J, et al: Should the risk of delaying reperfusion prohibit inter-hospital transfer to perform primary PTCA in acute myocardial infarction? [Abstract]. Circulation 94:I-331, 1996.

305. Campeau L, Lesperance J, Bourassa MG: Natural history of saphenous vein aortocoronary bypass grafts. Mod Concepts Cardiovasc Dis 53:59–63, 1984.

306. Davis KB, Alderman EL, Kosinski AS, et al: Early mortality of acute myocardial infarction in patients with and without prior coronary revascularization therapy. Circulation 85:2100–2109, 1992.

307. Coronary Artery Surgical Study (CASS) Principal Investigators and Their Associates: A randomized trial of coronary artery bypass. Quality of life in patients randomly assigned to treatment groups. Circulation 68:951–956, 1983.

308. Maynard C, Weaver WD, Litwin P, et al: Prior coronary artery surgery and acute myocardial infarction: Patient characteristics, treatment and outcome [Abstract]. J Am Coll Cardiol 17:65A, 1991.

309. Wiseman A, Waters DD, Walling A, et al: Long-term prognosis after myocardial infarction in patients with previous coronary artery bypass surgery. J Am Coll Cardiol 12:873–880, 1988.

310. Waters DD, Pelletier GB, Hache M, et al: Myocardial infarction in patients with previous coronary artery bypass surgery. J Am Coll Cardiol 3:909–915, 1984.

311. Dittrich HC, Gilpin E, Nicod P, et al: Outcome after acute myocardial infarction in patients with prior coronary artery bypass surgery. Am J Cardiol 72:507–513, 1993.

312. Nathan PE, Sketch MH, Fortin DF, et al: Acute myocardial infarction in patients with previous coronary artery bypass surgery: Association of complex anatomy and lower reperfusion rates with poor long-term survival [Abstract]. J Am Coll Cardiol 21:349A, 1993.

313. Grines CL, Booth DC, Nissen SE, et al: Mechanism of acute myocardial infarction in patients with prior coronary artery bypass grafting and therapeutic implications. Am J Cardiol 65:1292–1296, 1990.

314. Kennedy JW, Ritchie JL, Davis KB, et al: The Western Washington randomized trial of intracoronary streptokinase in acute myocardial infarction: A 12 month follow-up report. N Engl J Med 312:1073–1092, 1985.

315. Van de Werf F, Arnold AER: Intravenous tissue plasminogen activator and size of infarct, left ventricular function, and survival in acute myocardial infarction. BMJ 297:1374–1379, 1988.

316. Reiner JS, Lundergan CF, Kopecky SL, et al: Ineffectiveness of thrombolysis for acute MI following vein graft occlusion [Abstract]. Circulation 94:I-570, 1996.

317. Kavanaugh KM, Topol EJ: Acute intervention during myocardial infarction in patients with prior coronary artery bypass surgery. Am J Cardiol 65:924–926, 1990.

318. Stone GW, Brodie BR, Griffin J, et al: Primary angioplasty in patients with prior bypass surgery [Abstract]. Circulation 94:I-243, 1996.

319. Kahn JK, Rutherford BD, McConahay DR, et al: Usefulness of angioplasty during acute myocardial infarction in patients with prior coronary artery bypass grafting. Am J Cardiol 65:698–702, 1990.

320. Himbert DH, Juliard J-M, Steg G, et al: Primary coronary angioplasty for acute myocardial infarction with contraindication to thrombolysis. Am J Cardiol 71:377–381, 1993.

321. Liem A, Van't Hof AW, Suryapranata H, et al: Primary angioplasty for acute myocardial infarction in candidates and non-candidates for thrombolytic therapy [Abstract]. Circulation 94:I-329, 1996.

322. McKendall GR, Drew TM, Kelsey SF, et al: What is the optimal treatment for thrombolytic ineligible AMI? Preliminary results of the Study of Medicine vs. Angioplasty Reperfusion Trial (SMART) [Abstract]. J Am Coll Cardiol 23:225A, 1994.

322a. McCullough PA, O'Neill WW, Graham M, et al: A prospective, randomized trial of triage angiography in acute coronary syndromes ineligible for thrombolytic therapy: Results of the Medicine Versus Angiography in Thrombolytic Exclusion (MATE) trial. J Am Coll Cardiol 32:596–605, 1998.

323. Stone GW, Grines CL, Browne KF, et al: Outcome of different reperfusion strategies in patients with former contraindications to thrombolytic therapy: A comparison of primary angioplasty and tissue plasminogen activator. Catheter Cardiovasc Diagn 39:333–339, 1996.

324. Bengston JR, Kaplin AJ, Pieper KS, et al: Prognosis in cardiogenic shock after acute myocardial infarction in the interventional era. J Am Coll Cardiol 20:1482–1489, 1992.

325. Binder MJ, Ryan JA, Marcus S, et al: Evaluation of therapy in shock following acute myocardial infarction. Am J Med 18:622–632, 1955.

326. Swan HJC, Forrester JS, Danzig R, et al: Power failure in acute myocardial infarction. Prog Cardiovasc Dis 12:568–600, 1970.

327. Scheidt S, Ascheim R, Killip T: Shock after acute myocardial infarction: A clinical and hemodynamic profile. Am J Cardiol 26:556–564, 1970.

328. Killip T, Kimball JT: Treatment of myocardial infarction in a coronary care unit: A two year experience with 250 patients. Am J Cardiol 20:457–464, 1967.

329. Goldberg RJ, Gore JM, Alpert JS, et al: Cardiogenic shock after acute myocardial infarction: Incidence and mortality from a community-wide perspective, 1975–1988. N Engl J Med 325:1117–1122, 1991.

330. Griffith GC, Wallace WB, Chochran B, et al: The treatment of shock associated with myocardial infarction. Circulation 9:527–535, 1954.

331. Dole WP, O'Rourke RA: Pathophysiology and management of cardiogenic shock. Curr Probl Cardiol 8:1–72, 1983.

332. Forrester JS, Diamond G, Chatterjee K, et al: Medical therapy of acute myocardial infarction by application of hemodynamic subsets (first of two parts). N Engl J Med 295:1356–1361, 1976.

333. Forrester JS, Diamond G, Chatterjee K, et al: Medical therapy of acute myocardial infarction by application of hemodynamic subsets (second of two parts). N Engl J Med 295:1404–1410, 1976.

334. Page DL, Caulfield JB, Kastor JA, et al: Myocardial changes associated with cardiogenic shock. N Engl J Med 285:133–137, 1971.

335. Hornorayan C, Bennett MA, Pentecost BC, et al: Quantitative study of infarcted myocardium in cardiogenic shock. Br Heart J 32:728–732, 1970.

336. Alonso DR, Schiedt S, Post M, et al: Pathophysiology of cardiogenic shock: Quantification of myocardial necrosis, clinical, pathological and electrocardiographic correlations. Circulation 48:588–596, 1973.

337. Wackers FJ, Lie KI, Becker AE, et al: Coronary artery disease in patients dying from cardiogenic shock or congestive heart failure in the setting of acute myocardial infarction. Br Heart J 38:906–912, 1976.

338. Lee L, Erbel R, Brown TM, et al: Multicenter registry of angioplasty therapy of cardiogenic shock: Initial and long-term survival. J Am Coll Cardiol 17:599–603, 1991.

339. Hibbard MD, Holmes DR, Bailey KR, et al: Percutaneous transluminal coronary angioplasty in patients with cardiogenic shock. J Am Coll Cardiol 19:639–646, 1992.

340. Grines CL, Topol EJ, Califf RM et al: Prognostic implications and predictors of enhanced regional wall motion of the noninfarct zone after thrombolysis and angioplasty therapy of acute myocardial infarction. Circulation 80:245–251, 1989.

341. Califf RM, Bengston JR: Cardiogenic shock. N Engl J Med 330:1724–1730, 1994.

342. Leinbach RC, Dinsmore RE, Mundth ER, et al: Selective coronary and left ventricular cineangiography during intraaortic balloon pumping for cardiogenic shock. Circulation 45:845–851, 1972.

343. Johnson SA, Scanlon PJ, Loeb HS, et al: Treatment of cardiogenic shock in myocardial infarction by intraaortic balloon counterpulsation and surgery. Am J Med 62:672–687, 1977.

344. Mundth ED: Surgical treatment of cardiogenic shock and of mechanical complications following myocardial infarction. Cardiovasc Clin 8:241–261, 1977.

345. DeWood MA, Notske RN, Hensley GR, et al: Intraaortic balloon counterpulsation with and without reperfusion for myocardial infarction shock. Circulation 61:1105–1112, 1980.

346. O'Neill WW: Angioplasty therapy of cardiogenic shock: Are randomized trials necessary? Am J Cardiol 19:915–917, 1992.

347. Meyer J, Merx W, Dorr R, et al: Successful treatment of acute myocardial infarction shock by combined percutaneous transluminal coronary recanalization (PTCR) and percutaneous transluminal coronary angioplasty. Am Heart J 103:132, 1982.

348. O'Neill WW, Erbel R, Laufer N, et al: Coronary angioplasty therapy of cardiogenic shock complicating acute myocardial infarction [Abstract]. Circulation 72:III-309, 1985.

349. Kaplan AJ, Bengtson JR, Aronson LG, et al: Reperfusion improves survival in patients with cardiogenic shock after acute myocardial infarction. J Am Coll Cardiol 15:155, 1990.

350. Gacioch GM, Ellis SG, Lee L, et al: Cardiogenic shock complicating acute myocardial infarction: The use of coronary angioplasty and the integration of the new support devices into patient management. J Am Coll Cardiol 19:647–653, 1992.

351. Moosvi AR, Villaneuva L, Gheorghiade M, et al: Early revascularization improves survival in cardiogenic shock. Circulation 82(suppl III):III-308, 1990.

352. Eltchaninoff H, Simpendorfer C, Whitlow PL: Coronary an-

gioplasty improves both early and 1-year survival in acute myocardial infarction complicated by cardiogenic shock. J Am Coll Cardiol 17:167, 1991.

353. Brown TM, Iannone LA, Gordon DF, et al: Percutaneous myocardial reperfusion reduces mortality in acute myocardial infarction complicated by cardiogenic shock [Abstract]. Circulation 72:III-309, 1985.

354. Yamamoto H, Hayashi Y, Oka Y, et al: Efficacy of percutaneous transluminal coronary angioplasty in patients with acute myocardial infarction complicated by cardiogenic shock. Jpn Circ J 56:815–821, 1992.

355. Meyer P, Blanc P, Badouy M, et al: Treatment de choc cardiogenique primaire par angioplastie transluminale coronarienne à la phase aigue de l'infarctus. Arch Mal Coeur 83:329–334, 1990.

356. Lee L, Bates ER, Pitt B, et al: Percutaneous transluminal coronary angioplasty improves survival in acute myocardial infarction complicated by cardiogenic shock. Circulation 78:145–151, 1988.

357. Seydoux C, Goy J-J, Beuret P, et al: Effectiveness of percutaneous transluminal coronary angioplasty in cardiogenic shock during acute myocardial infarction. Am J Cardiol 68:968–969, 1992.

358. Himbert D, Juliard J-M, Steg G, et al: Limits of reperfusion therapy for immediate cardiogenic shock complicating acute myocardial infarction. Am J Cardiol 74:492–494, 1994.

359. Stomel RJ, Rasak M, Bates ER: Treatment strategies for acute myocardial infarction complicated by cardiogenic shock in a community hospital. Chest 105:997–1002, 1994.

360. Heuser RR, Maddoux GL, Goss JE, et al: Coronary angioplasty in the treatment of cardiogenic shock: The therapy of choice. J Am Coll Cardiol 7:219, 1986.

361. Shani J, Rivera M, Geengart A, et al: Percutaneous transluminal coronary angioplasty in cardiogenic shock. J Am Coll Cardiol 7:149, 1986.

362. Disler L, Haitas B, Benjamin J, et al: Cardiogenic shock in evolving myocardial infarction: Treatment by angioplasty and streptokinase. Heart Lung 16:649, 1987.

363. Verna E, Repetto S, Boscarina M, et al: Emergency coronary angioplasty in patients with severe left ventricular dysfunction of cardiogenic shock after acute myocardial infarction. Eur Heart J 10:958–966, 1989.

364. Shawl FA, Forman MB, Punja S, et al: Emergent coronary angioplasty in the treatment of acute ischemic mitral regurgitation: Long-term results in five cases. J Am Coll Cardiol 14:986–991, 1989.

365. Garrahy PJ, Henzlova MJ, Forman S, et al: Has thrombolytic therapy improved survival from cardiogenic shock? Thrombolysis in Myocardial Infarction (TIMI II) results [Abstract]. Circulation 80:II-623, 1989.

365a. Tiefenbrunn AJ, Chandra NC, French WJ, et al, for the Second National Registry of Myocardial Infarction Investigators: Experience with primary angioplasty in 4939 patients with myocardial infarction: Comparison with alteplase. Eur Heart J 17:515, 1996.

366. Berger PB, Holmes DR, Stebbens AL, et al: Impact of an aggressive invasive catheterization and revascularization strategy on mortality in patients with cardiogenic shock in the Global Utilization of Streptokinase and Tissue Plasminogen Activator for Occluded Coronary Arteries (GUSTO-I) Trial. Circulation 96:122–127, 1997.

367. Hochman JS: Cardiogenic shock: Can we save the patient? ACC Educational Highlights 12:1–5, 1996.

368. Webb JG, Carere RG, Hilton JD, et al: Usefulness of coronary stenting for cardiogenic shock. Am J Cardiol 79:81–84, 1997.

369. Schultz RD, Heuser RR, Hatler C, et al: Use of c7E3 Fab in conjunction with primary coronary stenting for acute myocardial infarctions complicated by cardiogenic shock. Catheter Cardiovasc Diagn 39:143–148, 1996.

370. Serruys PW, Emanuelsson HU, van der Giessen W, et al: Heparin-coated Palmaz-Schatz stents in human coronary arteries. Circulation 93:412–422, 1996.

371. Grines CL, Morice MC, Mattos L, et al: A prospective, multicenter trial using the JJIS heparin-coated stent for primary reperfusion of acute myocardial infarction. J Am Coll Cardiol 29:389A, 1997.

372. Brown T, Gordon D, Wheeler W, et al: Percutaneous myocardial reperfusion (PMR) reduces mortality in acute myocardial infarction (MI) complicated by cardiogenic shock [Abstract]. Circulation 72:III-309, 1985.

373. Garratt KN, Gibbons RG, Reeder GS, et al: Intravenous adenosine and lidocaine in humans with myocardial infarction: Preliminary safety data. Drug Dev Res 31:273, 1994.

374. Corbucci GG, Locke F: L-Carnitine in cardiogenic shock therapy—Pharmacodynamic aspects and clinical data. Int J Clin Pharm Res 13:87–91, 1993.

375. Corbucci GG, Lettieri B: Cardiogenic shock and L-carnitine: Clinical data and therapeutic perspectives. Int J Clin Pharm Res 11:283–293, 1991.

376. Gacioch GM, Ellis SG, Lee L, et al: Cardiogenic shock complicating acute myocardial infarction: The use of coronary angioplasty and the integration of the new support devices into patient management. J Am Coll Cardiol 19:647–653, 1992.

377. Shawl FA, Domanski MJ, Hernandez TJ, et al: Emergency percutaneous cardiopulmonary bypass support in cardiogenic shock from acute myocardial infarction. Am J Cardiol 64:967–970, 1989.

378. Jacobs AK, Faxon DP: Retroperfusion and PTCA. In Topol EJ (ed): Textbook of Interventional Cardiology, pp 477–495. Philadelphia: WB Saunders, 1990.

379. Lincoff AM, Popma JJ, Bates ER, et al: Successful coronary angioplasty in two patients with cardiogenic shock using the Nimbus Hemopump support device. Am Heart J 120:970–972, 1990.

380. Zumbro GL, Kitchens WR, Shearer G, et al: Mechanical assistance for cardiogenic shock following cardiac surgery, myocardial infarction and cardiac transplantation. Ann Thorac Surg 44:11–13, 1987.

381. Adamson RM, Dembitsky WP, Peichman RT, et al: Mechanical support: Assist or nemesis? J Thorac Cardiovasc Surg 98:915–921, 1989.

382. Smedira NG, Patel AN, Vargo R, et al: Cardiogenic shock after acute myocardial infarction: Successful bridge to transplantation with the implantable left ventricular assist device [Abstract]. J Am Coll Cardiol 27:250A, 1996.

383. Joyce LD, Johnson KE, Toninato CJ, et al: Results of the first 100 patients who received Symbion total artificial hearts as a bridge to cardiac transplantation. Circulation 80(suppl III):III-192–III-201, 1989.

384. Stone GW, Marsalese D, Brodie BR, et al: A prospective, randomized evaluation of prophylactic intraaortic balloon counterpulsation in high risk patients with acute myocardial infarction treated with primary angioplasty. J Am Coll Cardiol 29:1459–1467, 1997.

385. Grines CL, Marsalese D, Brodie B, et al: Safety and cost effectiveness of early discharge after primary angioplasty in low risk patients with acute myocardial infarction. J Am Coll Cardiol 31:967–972, 1998.

386. Maggioni AP, Maseri A, Fresco C, et al, on Behalf of the Investigators of the Gruppo Italiano per lo Studio della Streptochinasi nell'Infarto Miocardico (GISSI-2): Age related increase in mortality among patients with first myocardial infarctions treated with thrombolysis. N Engl J Med 329:1442–1448, 1993.

387. Volpi A, De Vita C, Franzosi MG, et al: Determinants of 6-month mortality in survivors of myocardial infarction after thrombolysis. Results of the GISSI-2 database. Circulation 88:416–429, 1993.

388. The TIMI Study Group: Comparison of invasive and conservative strategies after treatment with intravenous tissue plasminogen activator in acute myocardial infarction: Results of the Thrombolysis in Myocardial Infarction (TIMI) trial: Phase 1 findings. N Engl J Med 320:618–627, 1989.

389. Simoons ML, Vos J, Tijssen JG, et al: Long-term benefit of early thrombolytic therapy in patients with acute myocardial infarction: 5-Year follow-up of a trial conducted by the Interuniversity Cardiology Institute of The Netherlands. J Am Coll Cardiol 14:1609–1615, 1989.

390. Boehrer JD, Lange RA, Willar JE, et al: Influence of collateral

filling of the occluded infarct-related coronary artery on prognosis after acute myocardial infarction. Am J Cardiol 69:10–12, 1992.

391. Muller DWM, Topol EJ, Ellis SG, et al: Multivessel coronary artery disease: A key predictor of short-term prognosis after reperfusion therapy for acute myocardial infarction. Am Heart J 121:1042–1049, 1991.

392. Rogers WJ, Chandra NC, Gore JM, for the NRMI Investigators: National Registry of Myocardial Infarction (NRMI): What have we learned from the first 100,000 patients? [Abstract]. J Am Coll Cardiol 21:349A, 1993.

393. Ross J Jr, Gilpin EA, Madsen EB, et al: A decision scheme for coronary angiography after acute myocardial infarction. Circulation 79:292–303, 1989.

394. Kern MJ, Aguirre F, Bach R, et al: Augmentation of coronary blood flow by intra-aortic balloon pumping in patients after coronary angioplasty. Circulation 87:500–511, 1993.

395. Gurbel PA, Anderson RD, MacCord CS, et al: Arterial diastolic pressure augmentation by intra-aortic balloon counterpulsation enhances the onset of coronary reperfusion by thrombolytic therapy. Circulation 89:361–365, 1994.

396. Kern MJ, Aguirre FV, Tatineni S, et al: Enhanced coronary blood flow velocity during intraaortic balloon counterpulsation in critically ill patients. J Am Coll Cardiol 21:359–368, 1993.

397. Smalling RW, Cassidy DB, Barrett R, et al: Improved regional myocardial blood flow, left ventricular unloading, and infarct salvage using an axial-flow, transvalvular left ventricular assist device. Circulation 85:1152–1159, 1992.

398. Ishihara M, Sato H, Tateishi H, et al: Intraaortic balloon pumping as the post angioplasty strategy in acute myocardial infarction. Am Heart J 122:385–389, 1991.

399. Ohman EM, Califf RM, George BS, et al, and the Thrombolysis and Angioplasty in Myocardial Infarction (TAMI) Study Group: The use of intraaortic balloon counterpulsation as an adjunct to reperfusion therapy in acute myocardial infarction. Am Heart J 191:895–901, 1991.

400. Ohman EM, George BS, White CJ, et al, for the Randomized IABP Study Group: Use of aortic counterpulsation to improve sustained coronary artery patency during acute myocardial infarction. Results of a randomized trial. Circulation 90:792–799, 1994.

401. Ohman EM, George BS, White CJ, et al: Reocclusion of the infarct-related artery after primary or rescue angioplasty: Effect of aortic counterpulsation [Abstract]. Circulation 88:I-107, 1993.

402. ACC/AHA Task Force on Assessment of Diagnostic and Therapeutic Cardiovascular Procedures: Guidelines for the early management of patients with acute myocardial infarction. J Am Coll Cardiol 16:249–292, 1990.

403. Grines C, Marsalese D, Brodie B, et al: Acute catheterization provides the best method of risk stratifying MI patients [Abstract]. Circulation 92:I-531, 1995.

404. Stone GW, Marsalese D, Brodie B, et al: The routine use of intra-aortic balloon pumping after primary PTCA improves clinical outcomes in very high risk patients with acute myocardial infarction—Results of the PAMI-2 Trial [Abstract]. Circulation 92:I-139, 1995.

405. Brodie B, Stuckey T, Weintraub R, et al: Timing and mechanism of death after direct angioplasty for acute myocardial infarction [Abstract]. J Am Coll Cardiol 25:47A, 1995.

406. Ellis SG, Van de Weft F, Riberio-DaSilva E, et al: Present status of rescue coronary angioplasty: Current polarization of opinion and randomized trials [Abstract]. J Am Coll Cardiol 19:681–686, 1992.

407. Schreiber T, Marsalese D, Donohue B, et al: Identification of ultra low-risk patients following primary angioplasty for acute myocardial infarction [Abstract]. J Am Coll Cardiol 27:83A, 1996.

408. Stone GW, O'Neill WW, Jones D, et al: The central unifying concept of TIMI-3 flow after primary PTCA and thrombolytic therapy in acute myocardial infarction [Abstract]. Circulation 94:I-515, 1996.

409. Berger PB, Bell MR, Holmes DR, et al: Time to reperfusion with direct coronary angioplasty and thrombolytic therapy in acute myocardial infarction. Am J Cardiol 73:231–236, 1994.

410. White HD, Norris RM, Brown MA, et al: Left ventricular end-systolic volume as the major determinant of survival after recovery from myocardial infarction. Circulation 76:44–51, 1987.

411. Reimer KA, Lowe JE, Rasmussen MM, et al: The wavefront phenomenon of ischemic cell death: Myocardial infarct size versus duration of coronary occlusion in dogs. Circulation 56:786–794, 1977.

412. Hochman JS, Choo H: Limitation of infarct expansion by reperfusion independent of myocardial salvage. Circulation 75:299–306, 1987.

413. Koren G, Weiss AT, Hasin Y, et al: Prevention of myocardial damage in acute myocardial ischemia by early treatment with intravenous streptokinase. N Engl J Med 313:1384–1389, 1985.

414. O'Rourke M, Baron O, Keogh A, et al: Limitation of myocardial infarction by early infusion of recombinant tissue-type plasminogen activator. Circulation 77:1311–1315, 1988.

415. De Coster PM, Wijns W, Cauwe F, et al: Area-at-risk determination by technetium-99m-hexakis-2-methoxyisobutyl isonitrile in experimental reperfused acute myocardial infarction. Circulation 82:2152–2162, 1990.

416. Gibbons RJ, Christian TF, Hopfenspirger M, et al: Myocardium at risk and infarct size after thrombolytic therapy for acute myocardial infarction: Implications for the design of randomized trials of acute intervention. J Am Coll Cardiol 24:616–623, 1994.

417. O'Connor MK, Gibbons RJ, Juni JE, et al: Quantitative myocardial SPECT for infarct sizing: Feasibility of a multicenter trial evaluated using a cardiac phantom. J Nucl Med 36:1130–1136, 1995.

418. Dalen JE, Gore JM, Braunwald E, et al: Six and twelve month follow-up of the phase I Thrombolysis in Myocardial Infarction (TIMI) trial. Am J Cardiol 62:179–185, 1988.

419. Ambrose JA: The open artery: Beyond myocardial salvage. Am J Cardiol 72(suppl G):85G–90G, 1993.

420. Van de Werf F: Discrepancies between the effects of coronary reperfusion on survival and left ventricular function. Lancet 1:1367–1369, 1989.

421. Gersh BJ, Anderson JL: Thrombolysis and myocardial salvage. Results of clinical trials and the animal paradigm—Paradoxic or predictable? Circulation 88:296–306, 1993.

422. Califf RM, Harrelson-Woodlief L, Topol EJ: Left ventricular ejection fraction may not be useful as an endpoint of thrombolytic comparative trials. Circulation 82:1847–1853, 1990.

423. The I.S.A.M. Study Group: A prospective trial of intravenous streptokinase in acute myocardial infarction. N Engl J Med 314:1471–1476, 1986.

424. Meinertz T, Kasper W, Schumacher M, et al: The German multicenter trial of anisoylated plasminogen streptokinase activator complex versus heparin for acute myocardial infarction. Am J Cardiol 62:347–351, 1988.

425. National Heart Foundation of Australia Coronary Thrombolysis Group: Coronary thrombosis and myocardial salvage by tissue plasminogen activator given up to 4 hours after onset of myocardial infarction. Lancet 1:203–208, 1988.

426. Bergman SR, Lerch RA, Fox KAA, et al: Temporal dependence of beneficial effects of coronary thrombolysis characterized by positron tomography. Am J Med 73:573–581, 1982.

427. Langer A, Krucoff MW, Klootwijk P, et al, for the GUSTO Investigators: Noninvasive assessment of speed and stability of infarct-related artery reperfusion: Results of the GUSTO ST-segment monitoring study. J Am Coll Cardiol 25:1552–1557, 1995.

428. Simoons ML, Serruys PW, van den Brand M, et al, for the Working Group on Thrombolytic Therapy in Acute Myocardial Infarction of The Netherlands Interuniversity Cardiology Institute: Early thrombolysis in acute myocardial infarction: Limitation of infarct size and improved survival. J Am Coll Cardiol 7:717–728, 1986.

429. Timm TC, Ross R, McKendall GR, et al, and the TIMI Investigators: Left ventricular function and early cardiac events

as a function of time to treatment with t-PA: A report from TIMI II [Abstract]. Circulation 84:II-230, 1991.

430. Weaver WD, Cerqueira M, Hallstrom AP, et al: Prehospital-initiated vs. hospital-initiated thrombolytic therapy. The Myocardial Infarction Triage and Intervention Trial. JAMA 270:1211–1216, 1993.

431. Hermans WT, Willems GM, Nijssen KM, et al, for the European Cooperative Study Group: Effect of thrombolytic treatment delay on myocardial infarct size. Lancet 340:1297–1303, 1992.

432. Koren G, Weiss AT, Hasin Y, et al: Prevention of myocardial damage in acute myocardial ischemia by early treatment with intravenous streptokinase. N Engl J Med 313:1384–1389, 1985.

433. O'Keefe JH, Grines CL, DeWood MA, et al: Factors influencing myocardial salvage with primary angioplasty. J Nucl Cardiol 2:35–41, 1995.

434. Weaver WD: Time to thrombolytic treatment: Factors affecting delay and their influence on outcome. J Am Coll Cardiol 25(suppl):3S–9S, 1995.

435. Brodie BR, Weintraub RA, Hansen CJ, et al: Factors that predict improvement in left ventricular ejection fraction after coronary angioplasty for acute myocardial infarction. Catheter Cardiovasc Diagn 13:372–380, 1987.

436. O'Keefe JH, Rutherford BD, McConahay DR, et al: Myocardial salvage with direct coronary angioplasty for acute infarction. Am Heart J 123:1–6, 1992.

437. Marzoll U, Kleiman NS, Dunn JK, et al: Factors determining improvement in left ventricular function after reperfusion therapy for acute myocardial infarction: Primacy of the baseline ejection fraction. J Am Coll Cardiol 17:613–620, 1991.

438. Habib GN, Heibig J, Forman SA, et al: Influence of coronary collateral vessels on myocardial infarct size in humans. Results of phase 1 Thrombolysis in Myocardial Infarction (TIMI) trial. Circulation 83:739–746, 1991.

439. Rogers WJ, Hood WP, Mantle JA, et al: Return of left ventricular function after reperfusion in patients with myocardial infarction: Importance of subtotal stenoses or intact collaterals. Circulation 69:338–349, 1984.

440. Sheehan FH, Braunwald E, Canner P, et al: The effect of intravenous thrombolytic therapy on left ventricular function: A report on tissue-type plasminogen activator and streptokinase from the Thrombolysis in Myocardial Infarction (TIMI) phase I trial. Circulation 75:817–829, 1987.

441. Laster SB, O'Keefe JH, Gibbons RJ: Incidence and importance of Thrombolysis in Myocardial Infarction grade 3 flow after primary percutaneous transluminal coronary angioplasty for acute myocardial infarction. Am J Cardiol 78:623–626, 1996.

442. Leung WH, Lau CP: Effects of severity of the residual stenosis of the infarct-related coronary artery on left ventricular dilation and function after acute myocardial infarction. J Am Coll Cardiol 20:307–313, 1992.

443. EMERAS (Estudio Multicentrico Estreptoquinasa Republicas de America del Sur) Collaborative Group: Randomised trial of late thrombolysis in patients with suspected acute myocardial infarction. Lancet 342:767–772, 1993.

444. Braunwald E: Myocardial reperfusion, limitation of infarct size, reduction of left ventricular dysfunction, and improved survival: Should the paradigm be expanded? Circulation 79:441–444, 1989.

445. Kennedy JW, Ritchie JL, Davis KB, et al: The Western Washington randomized trial of intracoronary streptokinase in acute myocardial infarction. N Engl J Med 309:1477–1482, 1983.

446. Stadius ML, Davis K, Maynard C: Risk stratification for 1 year survival based on characteristics identified in the early hours of acute myocardial infarction. Circulation 74:703–710, 1986.

447. Galvani M, Ottani F, Ferrini D: Patency of the infarct-related artery and left ventricular function as the major determinants of survival after Q-wave acute myocardial infarction. Am J Cardiol 71:1–7, 1993.

448. Cigarroa RG, Lange RA, Hillis LD: Prognosis after acute myocardial infarction in patients with and without residual antegrade coronary blood flow. Am J Cardiol 64:155–160, 1989.

449. White HD, Cross DB, Elliott JM, et al: Long-term prognostic importance of the infarct-related coronary artery after thrombolytic therapy for acute myocardial infarction. Circulation 89:61–67, 1994.

450. Lamas GA, Flaker GC, Mitchell G, et al: Effect of infarct artery patency on prognosis after acute myocardial infarction. Circulation 27:1327–1332, 1995.

451. Brodie BR, Stuckey TD, Kissling G, et al: Importance of infarct-related artery patency for recovery of left ventricular function and late survival after primary angioplasty for acute myocardial infarction. J Am Coll Cardiol 28:319–325, 1996.

452. Anderson JL: Overview of patency as an endpoint of thrombolytic therapy. Am J Cardiol 67(suppl E):11E–16E, 1991.

453. Califf RM, Topol EJ, Gersh BJ: From myocardial salvage to patient salvage in acute myocardial infarction: The role of reperfusion therapy. J Am Coll Cardiol 14:1382–1388, 1989.

454. Fortin DF, Califf RM: Long-term survival from acute myocardial infarction: Salutary effect of an open coronary vessel. Am J Med 88(suppl N):9N–15N, 1990.

455. Kim CB, Braunwald E: Potential benefits of late reperfusion of infarcted myocardium. Circulation 88:2425–2436, 1993.

456. Hochman JS, Bulkley BH: Expansion of acute myocardial infarction: An experimental study. Circulation 65:1446–1450, 1982.

457. Touchstone DA, Beller GA, Nygaard TW, et al: Effects of successful reperfusion therapy on regional myocardial function and geometry in humans: A tomographic assessment using two-dimensional echocardiography. J Am Coll Cardiol 13:1506–1513, 1989.

458. Popovic A, Neskovic AN, Marinkovic J, et al: Acute and long-term effects of thrombolysis after anterior wall acute myocardial infarction with serial assessment of infarct expansion and late ventricular remodeling. Am J Cardiol 77:446–450, 1996.

459. Hirayama A, Adachi T, Asada S, et al: Late reperfusion for acute myocardial infarction limits the dilatation of the left ventricle without the reduction of infarct size. Circulation 88:2565–2574, 1993.

460. Marino P, Zanolla L, Zardini P: Effect of streptokinase on left ventricular modeling and function after myocardial infarction: The GISSI trial. J Am Coll Cardiol 14:1149–1158, 1989.

461. Lavie CJ, O'Keefe JH, Chesebro JA, et al: Prevention of late ventricular dilatation after acute myocardial infarction by successful thrombolytic reperfusion. Am J Cardiol 66:31–36, 1990.

462. Jeremy RW, Hackworthy RA, Bautovich G, et al: Infarct artery perfusion and changes in left ventricular volume in the month after acute myocardial infarction. J Am Coll Cardiol 9:989–995, 1987.

463. Pfeffer MA, Lamas GA, Vaughan DE: Effect of captopril on progressive dilatation after anterior myocardial infarction. N Engl J Med 319:80–86, 1988.

464. Topol EJ, Califf RM, Vandormael M, and the Thrombolysis and Angioplasty in Myocardial Infarction (TAMI-6) Study Group: A randomized trial of late reperfusion therapy for acute myocardial infarction. Circulation 85:2090–2099, 1992.

465. Garot J, Sherrer-Crosbie M, Monin JL, et al: Effect of delayed percutaneous transluminal coronary angioplasty of occluded coronary arteries after acute myocardial infarction. Am J Cardiol 77:915–921, 1996.

466. Hale SL, Kloner RA: Left ventricular topographic alterations in the completely healed rat infarct caused by early and late coronary artery reperfusion. Am Heart J 116:1508–1513, 1988.

467. Connelly CM, Vogel WM, Wiegner AW, et al: Effects of reperfusion after coronary artery occlusion on post-infarction scar tissue. Circ Res 57:562–577, 1985.

468. Kloner RA: Coronary angioplasty: A treatment option for left ventricular remodeling after myocardial infarction? J Am Coll Cardiol 20:314–316, 1992.

469. Gaasch WH, Bing OHL, Pine MB, et al: Myocardial con-

tracture during prolonged ischemic arrest and reperfusion. Am J Physiol 235(suppl H):H619–H623, 1978.

470. Rasmussen S, Leth A, Kjoller E, et al: Cardiac rupture in acute myocardial infarction: A review of 72 consecutive cases. Acta Med Scand 205:11–16, 1979.

471. Bates RJ, Beutler S, Resnekov L, et al: Cardiac rupture—Challenge in diagnosis and management. Am J Cardiol 40:429–437, 1977.

472. The I.S.A.M. Study Group: A prospective trial of intravenous streptokinase in acute myocardial infarction: Mortality, morbidity, and infarct size at 21 days. N Engl J Med 314:1465–1471, 1986.

473. White HD, Rivers JT, Maslowski AH, et al: Effect of intravenous streptokinase as compared with that of tissue plasminogen activator on left ventricular function after first myocardial infarction. N Engl J Med 320:17–21, 1989.

474. Gertz SD, Kalan JM, Kragel AH, et al: Quantitative histopathologic observations in patients treated with recombinant tissue plasminogen activator during acute myocardial infarction [Abstract]. Circulation 80:II-350, 1989.

475. Wessler S, Zoll PM, Schlesinger MJ: The pathogenesis of spontaneous cardiac rupture. Circulation 6:334–351, 1952.

476. Lewis AJ, Burchell HB, Titus JL: Clinical and pathologic features of post infarction cardiac rupture. Am J Cardiol 23:43–53, 1969.

477. Mauri F, BeBiase AM, Franzosi MG, et al: Analisi delle cause di morte intraospedaliera. G Ital Cardiol 17:37–44, 1987.

478. Honan MB, Harrell FE, Reimer KA, et al: Cardiac rupture, mortality and the timing of thrombolytic therapy: A meta-analysis. J Am Coll Cardiol 16:359–367, 1990.

479. Berry CL: Thrombolytic therapy and myocardial infarction. J Clin Pathol 28:352–356, 1975.

480. Mathey DE, Shofer J, Kuck K, et al: Transmural hemorrhagic myocardial infarction after intracoronary streptokinase: Clinical, angiographic, and necropsy findings. Br Heart J 48:546–551, 1982.

481. Force T, Kemper A, Leavitt M, et al: Acute reduction in functional infarct expansion with late coronary reperfusion: Assessment with quantitative two-dimensional echocardiography. J Am Coll Cardiol 11:192–200, 1988.

482. Kurnik PB, Courtois MR, Ludbrook PA: Diastolic stiffening induced by acute myocardial infarction is reduced by early reperfusion. J Am Coll Cardiol 12:1029–1036, 1988.

483. Miketic S, Carlsson J, Tebbe U: Improvement of global and regional left ventricular function by percutaneous transluminal coronary angioplasty after myocardial infarction. J Am Coll Cardiol 25:843–847, 1995.

484. Linderer T, Guhl B, Spielberg C, et al: Effect on global and regional left ventricular functions by percutaneous transluminal coronary angioplasty in the chronic stage after myocardial infarction. Am J Cardiol 69:997–1002, 1992.

485. Dzavik V, Beanlands DS, Davies RF, et al: Effects of late percutaneous transluminal coronary angioplasty of an occluded infarct-related coronary artery on left ventricular function in patients with a recent (<6 weeks) Q-wave acute myocardial infarction (total occlusion post-myocardial infarction intervention study (TOOMIS)—A pilot study. Am J Cardiol 73:856–861, 1994.

486. Guerci AD, Gerstenblith G, Brinker JA, et al: A randomized trial of intravenous tissue plasminogen activator for acute myocardial infarction with subsequent randomization to elective coronary angioplasty. N Engl J Med 317:1613–1618, 1987.

487. Montalescot G, Faraggi M, Drobinski G, et al: Myocardial viability in patients with Q-wave myocardial infarction and no residual ischemia. Circulation 86:47–55, 1992.

488. Sabia PJ, Powers ER, Ragosta M, et al: An association between collateral blood flow and myocardial viability in patients with recent myocardial infarction. N Engl J Med 327:1825–1831, 1992.

489. Bigger JT, Fleiss JF, Kliger R, et al, and the Multicenter Post-Infarction Research Group: The relationship among ventricular arrhythmias, left ventricular dysfunction and mortality in the 2 years after myocardial infarction. Circulation 69:250–258, 1984.

490. Denniss AR, Richards DA, Cody DV, et al: Prognostic significance of ventricular tachycardia and fibrillation induced at programmed stimulation and delayed potentials detected on the signal-averaged electrocardiograms of survivors of acute myocardial infarction. Circulation 74:731–745, 1986.

491. Kuchar DL, Thornburn CW, Sammel NL: Late potentials detected after myocardial infarction: Natural history and prognostic significance. Circulation 74:1280–1289, 1986.

492. Davies MJ, Thomas A: Thrombosis and acute coronary artery lesions in sudden cardiac ischemic death. N Engl J Med 310:1137–1140, 1984.

493. Aguirre FV, Kern MJ, Hsia J, et al: Importance of myocardial infarct artery patency on the prevalence of ventricular arrhythmia and late potentials after thrombolysis in acute myocardial infarction. Am J Cardiol 68:1410–1416, 1991.

494. Brugada P, Waldecker B, Kersschot Y, et al: Ventricular arrhythmias initiated by programmed stimulation in four groups of patients with healed myocardial infarction. J Am Coll Cardiol 8:1035–1040, 1986.

495. Sager PT, Perlmutter RA, Rosenfeld LE, et al: Electrophysiologic effects of thrombolytic therapy in patients with a transmural anterior myocardial infarction complicated by left ventricular aneurysm formation. J Am Coll Cardiol 12:19–24, 1988.

496. Kersschot IE, Brugada P, Ramentol M, et al: Effect of early reperfusion in acute myocardial infarction on arrhythmias induced by programmed stimulation: A prospective, randomized study. J Am Coll Cardiol 7:1234–1242, 1986.

497. Gang ES, Lew AS, Hong M, et al: Decreased incidence of ventricular late potentials after successful thrombolytic therapy for acute myocardial infarction. N Engl J Med 321:712–716, 1998.

498. de Chillou C, Rodriguez LM, Doevendans P, et al: Effects of the signal averaged electrocardiogram of opening the coronary artery by thrombolytic therapy or percutaneous transluminal coronary angioplasty during acute myocardial infarction. Am J Cardiol 71:805–809, 1993.

499. Karam C, Golmard JL, Steg PG: Decreased prevalence of late potentials with mechanical versus thrombolysis-induced reperfusion in acute myocardial infarction. J Am Coll Cardiol 27:1343–1348, 1996.

500. Hohloser SH, Franck P, Klingenheben T, et al: Open infarct artery, late potentials and other prognostic factors in patients after acute myocardial infarction in the thrombolytic era. A prospective trial. Circulation 90:1747–1756, 1994.

501. Ambrose JA, Tannenbaum MA, Alexopoulos D, et al: Angiographic progression of coronary artery disease and the development of myocardial infarction. J Am Coll Cardiol 12:56–62, 1988.

502. Gohlke H, Heim E, Roskamm H: Prognostic importance of collateral flow and residual coronary stenosis of the myocardial infarct artery after anterior wall Q-wave acute myocardial infarction. Am J Cardiol 67:1165–1169, 1991.

503. Christian TF, Gibbons RJ, Gersh BJ: Effect of infarct location on myocardial salvage assessed by technetium-99m isonitrile. J Am Coll Cardiol 17:1303–1308, 1991.

504. Stone GW, O'Keefe J, Brodie BR, et al: Lack of relationship between the time to reperfusion and short-term mortality after primary infarct angioplasty [Abstract]. J Am Coll Cardiol 32:271A, 1998.

505. Verstraete M, Bernard J, Bory M, et al: Randomised trial of intravenous recombinant tissue-type plasminogen activator versus streptokinase in acute myocardial infarction. Report from the European Cooperative Study Group for Recombinant Tissue-Type Plasminogen Activator. Lancet 1:842–847, 1985.

506. Bode C, Smalling RW, Berg G, et al, and the RAPID Investigators: Randomized comparison of coronary thrombolysis achieved with double bolus reteplase (r-PA) and front-loaded "accelerated" alteplase (rt-PA) in patients with acute myocardial infarction. Circulation 94:891–898, 1996.

507. Maynard C, Weaver WD, Lambrew C, et al: Factors influencing the time to administration of thrombolytic therapy with recombinant tissue plasminogen activator (data from the national Registry of Myocardial Infarction). Am J Cardiol 76:548–552, 1995.

508. Hannan EL, Kilburn H, O'Donnell JF, et al: Coronary artery bypass surgery: The relationship between in hospital mortality rate and surgical volume after controlling for clinical risk factors. Med Care 29:1094–1107, 1991.

509. Luft HS, Bunker JP, Enthoven AC: Should operations be regionalized? The empirical relation between surgical volume and mortality. N Engl J Med 301:1364–1369, 1979.

510. Showstack JA, Rosenfeld KE, Garnick DW, et al: Association of volume with outcome of coronary artery bypass graft surgery: Scheduled vs. nonscheduled operations. JAMA 257:785–789, 1987 [published erratum, JAMA 257:2438, 1987].

511. Jollis JG, Peterson ED, Delong ER, et al: Relationship between physician angioplasty volume and outcome in 97,000 elderly Americans. Circulation 95:2485–2491, 1997.

512. Ellis SG, Weintraub W, Holmes D, et al: Relation of operator volume and experience to procedural outcome of percutaneous coronary revascularization at hospitals with high interventional volume. Circulation 95:2479–2484, 1997.

513. Hannan EL, Racz M, Ryan TJ, et al: Coronary angioplasty volume-outcome relationships for hospitals and cardiologists in New York State, 1991–1994. JAMA 277:892–898, 1997.

514. Ritchie JL, Phillips KA, Luft HS: Coronary angioplasty: Statewide experience in California. Circulation 88:2735–2743, 1993.

515. Kimmel SE, Berlin JA, Laskey WK: The relationship between coronary angioplasty volume and major complications. JAMA 274:1137–1142, 1995.

516. Grines CL, Stone GW, O'Neill WW: Establishing a program and performance of primary PTCA—The PAMI way. J Invasive Cardiol 9:44B–52B, 1996.

517. Caputo RP, Ho KKL, Stoler RC, et al: Effect of continuous quality improvement analysis on the delivery of primary percutaneous coronary angioplasty for acute myocardial infarction. Am J Cardiol 79:1159–1164, 1997.

518. Khurana S, Westley S, Maltson JC, et al: Is it possible to expedite the antiplatelet effect of ticlopidine? J Invasive Cardiol 8:65, 1996.

519. Jeong M, Owen W, Staabon G, et al: Does ticlopidine effect platelet deposition and acute stent thrombosis? [Abstract]. Circulation 92:I-489, 1995.

520. Gregorini L, Marco J, Fajadet J, et al: Ticlopidine attenuates post-angioplasty thrombin generation [Abstract]. Circulation 92:I-608, 1995.

521. Schomig A, Neumann FJ, Kastrati A, et al: A randomized comparison of antiplatelet and anticoagulant therapy after the placement of coronary-artery stents. N Engl J Med 334:1084–1089, 1996.

522. Jordan C, Carvalho H, Fajadet J, et al: Reduction of subacute thrombosis rate after coronary stenting using a new anticoagulant protocol [Abstract]. Circulation 90:I-125, 1994.

523. Leon MB, Baim DS, Gordon P, et al: Clinical and angiographic results from the stent anticoagulation regimen study (STARS) [Abstract]. Circulation 95:I-685, 1996.

524. Dawson P, Hewitt P, Mackie JJ, et al: Contrast, coagulation and fibrinolysis. Invest Radiol 21:248–252, 1986.

525. Grabowski EF: Effects of contrast media on endothelial cell monolayers under controlled flow conditions. Am J Cardiol 64(suppl E):10E–15E, 1989.

526. Stormorken H, Skalpe IO, Testart MC: Effect of various contrast media on coagulation, fibrinolysis, and platelet function in an in vivo and in vitro study. Invest Radiol 21:348–354, 1986.

527. Zir LM, Carvahlo AC, Hawthorne JW, et al: Effects of contrast agents on platelet aggregation and $^{14}$C-serotonin release. Lancet 1:134–135, 1974.

528. Shapiro GA, Loeb PM, Berk RN, et al: Influence of cholografin and renografin 76 on platelet function. Radiology 124:641–643, 1977.

529. Rao AK, Rao VM, Willis J, et al: Inhibition of platelet function by contrast media: Iopamidol and ioxaglate versus iothalamate. Radiology 156:311–313, 1985.

530. Greenbaum RA, Barrados MA, Mikhailidis DP, et al: Effect of heparin and contrast medium on platelet function during routine cardiac catheterization. Cardiovasc Res 21:878–885, 1987.

531. Chronos NAF, Goodall AH, Wilson DJ, et al: Profound platelet degranulation is an important side effect of some types of contrast media used in interventional cardiology. Circulation 88:2035–2044, 1993.

532. Belleville J, Baquet J, Paul J, et al: In vitro study of the inhibition of the coagulation induced by different radiocontrast molecules. Thromb Res 38:149–162, 1985.

533. Dehmer GJ, Gresalfdi N, Daly D, et al: Impairment of fibrinolysis by streptokinase, urokinase and recombinant tissue-type plasminogen activator in the presence of radiographic contrast agents. J Am Coll Cardiol 25:1069–1075, 1995.

534. Grines CL, Mickelson JK, Diaz CM, et al: Acute thrombosis in a canine model of arterial injury: Effect of ionic versus nonionic contrast media. J Invasive Cardiol 3(suppl B):18B–23B, 1991.

535. Grollman JH, Liu CK, Astone RA, et al: Thromboembolic complications in coronary angiography associated with the use of nonionic contrast medium. Catheter Cardiovasc Diagn 14:159–164, 1988.

536. Dorey AJ, Stillabower ME, Gale N, et al: Catastrophic thrombus development despite systemic heparinization during coronary angioplasty: Possible relationship to nonionic contrast. Clin Cardiol 15:117–120, 1992.

537. Lembo NJ, King SB, Roubin GS, et al: Effects of non-ionic versus ionic contrast media on complications of percutaneous transluminal coronary angioplasty. Am J Cardiol 67:1046–1050, 1991.

538. Ahmed W, Meckel C, Grines CL, et al: Relation between ischemic complications and activated clotting times during coronary angioplasty: Different profiles for heparin and hirulog [Abstract]. Circulation 92:I-608, 1995.

539. Narins CR, Hillegass WG, Nelson CL, et al: Relation between activated clotting time during angioplasty and abrupt closure. J Am Coll Cardiol 80:1718, 1989.

540. Grines C, Brodie B, Griffin J, et al: Which primary PTCA patients may benefit from new technologies? Circulation 92:I-146, 1995.

541. Benzuly KH, O'Neill WW, Brodie B, et al: Predictors of maintained infarct artery patency after primary angioplasty in high risk patients in PAMI-2 [Abstract]. J Am Coll Cardiol 27:279A, 1996.

542. Walton AS, Osterle S, Yeung AC: Coronary artery stenting for acute closure complicating primary angioplasty for acute myocardial infarction. Catheter Cardiovasc Diagn 34:142–146, 1995.

543. Wong SW, Franklin M, Teirstein PS, et al: Stenting in acute myocardial infarction secondary to delayed vessel closure following balloon angioplasty. J Invasive Cardiol 4:331–334, 1992.

544. Wong PHC, Wong CM: Intracoronary stenting in acute myocardial infarction. Catheter Cardiovasc Diagn 33:39–45, 1994.

545. Repetto S, Onofri M, Castiglioni B, et al: Stenting of the infarct related artery during complicated angioplasty in acute myocardial infarction. J Invasive Cardiol 8:177–183, 1996.

546. Setiha ME, El Gamal M, Koolen J, et al: Coronary stenting for failed angioplasty in acute myocardial infarction. Catheter Cardiovasc Diagn 39:149–154, 1996.

547. The EPIC Investigators: Use of a monoclonal antibody directed against the platelet glycoprotein IIb/IIIa receptor in high-risk coronary angioplasty. N Engl J Med 330:956–961, 1994.

548. Mueller H, Ayres SM, Gianelli S, et al: Effect of isoproterenol, L-norepinephrine, and intraaortic counterpulsation on hemodynamics and myocardial metabolism in shock following acute myocardial infarction. Circulation 45:339–340, 1972.

549. Weiss AT, Engle S, Gotsman CJ: Regional and global left ventricular function during intra-aortic balloon counterpulsation in patients with acute myocardial infarction shock. Am Heart J 108:249–255, 1984.

550. Ehrich DA, Biddle TL, Kronenberg MW, et al: The hemodynamic response to intra-aortic balloon counterpulsation in

patients with cardiogenic shock complicating acute myocardial infarction. Am Heart J 93:274–279, 1977.
551. Scheidt S, Wilner G, Mueller H, et al: Intra-aortic balloon counterpulsation in cardiogenic shock: Report of a co-operative clinical trial. N Engl J Med 288:979–984, 1973.
552. O'Rourke MF, Norris RM, Campbell TJ, et al: Randomized controlled trial of intraaortic balloon counterpulsation in early myocardial infarction with acute heart failure. Am J Cardiol 47:815–820, 1981.
553. Bengston JR, Kaplin AJ, Pieper KS, et al: Prognosis in cardiogenic shock after acute myocardial infarction in the intervention era. J Am Coll Cardiol 20:1482–1489, 1992.
554. Gacioch GM, Topol EJ: Sudden paradoxic clinical deterioration during angioplasty of the occluded right coronary artery in acute myocardial infarction. J Am Coll Cardiol 14:1202–1209, 1989.
555. Reiner JS, Lundergan CF, Varghese PJ, et al: Complications following angioplasty for failed thrombolysis in GUSTO: Further evidence for the "rescue right" syndrome [Abstract]. J Am Coll Cardiol 23:454A, 1994.
556. Abbottsmith CW, Topol EJ, George BS, et al: Fate of patients with acute myocardial infarction with patency of the infarct-related vessel achieved with successful thrombolysis versus rescue angioplasty. J Am Coll Cardiol 16:770–778, 1990.
557. Frink RJ, James TN: Intracardiac route of the Bezold-Jarisch reflex. Am J Physiol 221:1464–1469, 1971.
558. Thames JD, Klopfenstein HS, Abboud FM, et al: Preferential distribution of inhibitory cardiac receptors with vagal afferents to the inferoposterior wall of the left ventricle activated during coronary occlusion in the dog. Circ Res 43:512–519, 1978.
559. Mark AL: The Bezold-Jarisch reflex revisited: Clinical implication of inhibitor reflexes originating in the heart. J Am Coll Cardiol 1:90–102, 1983.
560. Wei JY, Markis JE, Malagold M, et al: Cardiovascular reflexes stimulated by reperfusion of ischemic myocardium in acute myocardial infarction. Circulation 67:796–801, 1983.
561. Kaplan BM, Safian RD, Grines CL, et al: Differences in outcome after angioplasty for acute myocardial infarction: The left anterior descending artery vs. the right coronary artery [Abstract]. J Am Coll Cardiol 27:166A, 1996.
562. Stone GW, Grines CL, Browne KF, et al: Acute outcome after primary angioplasty in myocardial infarction—The Primary Angioplasty in Myocardial Infarction (PAMI) Trial [Abstract]. J Am Coll Cardiol 21:331A, 1993.
563. Stone GW, Grines CL, Browne KF, et al: Adverse catheterization laboratory events after primary PTCA vs. PTCA following thrombolytic therapy—A report from the Primary Angioplasty in Myocardial Infarction (PAMI) trial. J Am Coll Cardiol 23:244A, 1994.
564. Kloner RA, Gantone CE, Jennings RB: The "no-reflow" phenomenon after temporary coronary occlusion in the dog. J Clin Invest 54:1496–1508, 1974.
565. Kloner RA, Rude RE, Carlson N, et al: Ultrastructural evidence of microvascular damage and myocardial cell injury after coronary artery occlusion: Which comes first? Circulation 62:945–952, 1980.
566. Kloner RA: No-reflow revisited. J Am Coll Cardiol 14:1814–1815, 1989.
567. Kloner RA: Does reperfusion injury exist in humans? J Am Coll Cardiol 21:537–545, 1993.
568. Feld H, Lichstein E, Schacter J, et al: Early and late angiographic findings of "no-reflow" phenomenon following direct angioplasty as primary treatment for acute myocardial infarction. Am Heart J 123:782–784, 1992.
569. Lefer DJ, Shandelya SML, Serrano CV, et al: Cardioprotective actions of a monoclonal antibody against CD-18 in myocardial ischemia-reperfusion injury. Circulation 80:1846–1861, 1989.
570. Armiger LC, Gavin JB: Changes in the microvasculature of ischemic and infarcted myocardium. Lab Invest 33:51–56, 1975.
571. Engler RE, Schmid-Schonhein GW, Pavelee RS: Leukocyte capillary plugging in myocardial ischemia and reperfusion in the dog. Am J Pathol 111:98–111, 1983.
572. Folts JD, Crowell EB, Rowe GG: Platelet aggregation in partially obstructed vessels and its elimination with aspirin. Circulation 54:365–370, 1976.
573. Wilson RF, Laxton DD, Lesser JR, et al: Intense microvascular constriction after angioplasty of acute thrombotic coronary arterial lesions. Lancet 1:807–811, 1989.
574. Piana RN, Paik GY, Moscucci M, et al: Incidence and treatment of "no-reflow" after percutaneous coronary intervention. Circulation 89:2514–2518, 1994.
575. Morishima I, Sone T, Mokuno S, et al: Clinical significance of no-reflow phenomenon observed on angiography after successful treatment of acute myocardial infarction with percutaneous transluminal coronary angioplasty. Am Heart J 130:239–243, 1995.
576. Abbo KM, Dooris M, Glazier S, et al: Features and outcome of no-reflow after percutaneous coronary intervention. Am J Cardiol 75:778–782, 1995.
577. Mercho N, Eldin AM, Shareef B, et al: Angiographic complications of primary angioplasty [Abstract]. J Am Coll Cardiol 27:61A, 1996.
578. Marzilli M, Gliozheni E, Fedele S, et al: Prevalence and prediction of no-reflow after direct angioplasty in acute myocardial infarction [Abstract]. J Am Coll Cardiol 29:90A, 1997.
579. Ishihara M, Sato H, Tateishi H, et al: Attenuation of the no-reflow phenomenon after coronary angioplasty for acute myocardial infarction with intracoronary papaverine. Am Heart J 132:959–963, 1996.
580. Pomerantz RM, Kuntz RE, Diver DJ, et al: Intracoronary verapamil for the treatment of distal microvascular coronary artery spasm following PTCA. Catheter Cardiovasc Diagn 24:283–285, 1991.
581. Kloner RA, Alker KJ: The effect of streptokinase on intramyocardial hemorrhage, infarct size and the "no-reflow" phenomenon during coronary reperfusion. Circulation 70:513–521, 1984.
582. Kloner RA, Alker KJ, Campbell C, et al: Does tissue-type plasminogen activator have direct beneficial effects on the myocardium independent of its ability to lyse intracoronary thrombi? Circulation 79:1125–1136, 1989.
583. Muhlestein J, Gomez M, Karagounish L: Rescue ReoPro: Acute utilization of abciximab for the dissolution of coronary thrombus developing as a complication of coronary angioplasty [Abstract]. Circulation 92:I-607, 1995.
584. Smith AJC, Holt RE, Fitzpatrick K, et al: Transient thrombotic state after abrupt discontinuation of heparin in percutaneous coronary angioplasty. Am Heart J 131:434–439, 1996.
585. Granger C, Armstrong P, for the GUSTO-IIa Investigators: Reinfarction following discontinuation of intravenous heparin or hirudin for unstable angina and acute myocardial infarction [Abstract]. Circulation 92:I-460, 1995.
586. Granger C, Miller J, Bovill E, et al: Rebound increase in thrombin generation and activity after cessation of intravenous heparin in patients with acute coronary syndromes. Circulation 91:1929–1935, 1995.
587. Flather M, Weitz J, Campeau J, et al: Evidence for rebound activation of the coagulation system after cessation of intravenous anticoagulant therapy for acute MI [Abstract]. Circulation 92:I-485, 1995.
588. Stony J, Ahmed W, Meckel C, et al: Clinical evidence for thrombin rebound after stopping heparin but not Hirulog [Abstract]. Circulation 92:I-609, 1995.
589. Khan M, Sepulveda J, Jeroudi M, et al: Rebound increase in thrombin activity with associated decrease in antithrombin III levels after PTCA [Abstract]. Circulation 92:I-785, 1995.
590. Lange RA, Hillis LD: Immediate angioplasty for acute myocardial infarction [Editorial]. N Engl J Med 328:726–728, 1993.
591. Facilities and services in the United States. In Hospital Statistics, 1992–1993 ed, pp 208–209. Chicago: American Hospital Association, 1992.
592. Rogers WJ, Chandra NC, French WJ, et al: Trends in the use of reperfusion therapy: Experience from the second National Registry of Myocardial Infarction (NRMI 2) [Abstract]. Circulation 94:I-196, 1996.

593. Lieu TA, Lundstrom RJ, Ray GT, et al: Initial cost of primary angioplasty for acute myocardial infarction. J Am Coll Cardiol 28:882–889, 1996.

594. Ryan T, Bauman WB, Kennedy JW, et al: Guidelines for percutaneous transluminal coronary angioplasty. A report of the American College of Cardiology and American Task Force, an assessment of diagnostic and therapeutic cardiovascular procedures (Committee on Percutaneous Transluminal Coronary Angioplasty.). J Am Coll Cardiol 22:2033–2054, 1993.

595. Weaver WD, Parsons L, Every N, for the MITI Project Investigators: Primary coronary angioplasty in hospitals with and without surgery backup. J Invasive Cardiol 7(suppl F):34F–39F, 1995.

596. Vogel JHK: Changing trends for surgical standby in patients undergoing percutaneous transluminal coronary angioplasty. Am J Cardiol 70:1520–1525, 1992.

597. Vogel JHK: Guidelines for surgical standby in patients undergoing percutaneous transluminal coronary angioplasty. *In* Vogel JHK, King SB III (eds): The Practice of Interventional Cardiology, 2nd ed, pp 415–423. St. Louis: Mosby–Year Book, 1993.

598. Iannone LA, Anderson SM, Phillips SJ: Coronary angioplasty for acute myocardial infarction in a hospital without cardiac surgery. Tex Heart Inst J 20:99–104, 1993.

599. Meier B, Urban P, Doraz PA, et al: Surgical standby for coronary balloon angioplasty. JAMA 268:741–745, 1992.

600. Richardson SG, Morton P, Murtagh SG, et al: Management of acute coronary occlusion during percutaneous transluminal coronary angioplasty: Experience of complications in a hospital without on-site facilities for cardiac surgery. BMJ 300:355–358, 1990.

601. Reifart N, Schwarz F, Preusler H, et al: Results of PTCA in more than 5000 patients without surgical standby in the same center [Abstract]. J Am Coll Cardiol 19:229A, 1992.

602. Iniguez A, Macaya C, Hernandez R, et al: Comparison of results of percutaneous transluminal coronary angioplasty with and without selective requirements of surgical standby. Am J Cardiol 70:1161–1165, 1992.

603. Klinke WP, Hui WK: Percutaneous transluminal coronary angioplasty without on-site surgical facilities. Am J Cardiol 70:1520–1525, 1992.

604. Wharton T, McNamara N, Schmitz J, et al: The value of immediate coronary angiography with primary PTCA standby in the triage and treatment of acute myocardial infarction at community hospitals without heart surgery: Experience in 305 cases [Abstract]. J Am Coll Cardiol 27:205A, 1996.

605. McNamara NS, Hiett D, Allen B, et al: Can community hospitals provide effective primary PTCA coverage at all hours? [Abstract]. J Am Coll Cardiol 29:91A, 1997.

605a. Smyth DW, Richards AM, Elliott JM: Direct angioplasty for myocardial infarction: One-year experience in a center with surgical backup 220 miles away. J Invasive Cardiol 9:324–332, 1997.

606. Roubin GS, Cannon AD, Agrawal SK, et al: Intracoronary stenting for acute and threatened closure complicating percutaneous transluminal coronary angioplasty. Circulation 85:916–927, 1992.

607. George BS, Voorhees WD, Roubin GS, et al: Multicenter investigation of coronary stenting to treat acute or threatened closure after percutaneous transluminal coronary angioplasty: Clinical and angiographic outcomes. J Am Coll Cardiol 22:135–143, 1993.

608. Hearn JA, King SB, Douglas JS, et al: Clinical and angiographic outcomes after coronary artery stenting for acute and threatened closure after percutaneous transluminal coronary angioplasty. Initial results with a balloon-expandable, stainless steel design. Circulation 88:2086–2096, 1993.

609. Hermann HC, Buchbinder M, Clemen MW, et al: Emergent use of balloon-expandable coronary artery stenting for failed percutaneous transluminal coronary angioplasty. Circulation 86:812–819, 1992.

610. Lincoff AM, Topol EJ, Chepekis AT, et al: Intracoronary stenting compared with conventional therapy for abrupt vessel closure complicating coronary angioplasty: A matched case-control study. J Am Coll Cardiol 21:866–875, 1993.

611. Thomas CN, Weintraub WS, Shen Y, et al: "Bailout" coronary stenting in patients with a recent myocardial infarction. Am J Cardiol 77:653–655, 1996.

612. Lindsay J, Hong MK, Pinnow EE, et al: Effects of endoluminal coronary stents on the frequency of coronary artery bypass grafting after unsuccessful percutaneous transluminal coronary revascularization. Am J Cardiol 77:647–649, 1996.

613. Altmann DB, Racz M, Battleman D, et al: Reduction in complications after the introduction of coronary stents: Results from a consecutive series of 2242 patients. Am Heart J 132:503–507, 1996.

614. ZS Associates: Methodology of the PTCA analysis. Angioplasty Today 3:3, 1989.

615. Zjilstra F, van't Hof AWJ, Liem AL, et al: Transferring patients for primary angioplasty. Heart, in press.

616. Verheugt FWA, Marsh RC, Veen G, et al: Megadose bolus heparin as reperfusion therapy for acute myocardial infarction: Results of the HEAP pilot study [Abstract]. Circulation 92:I-415, 1995.

617. Wharton T, Marsalese D, Brodie B, et al: How often do infarct-related arteries show early perfusion without prior thrombolytic therapy, and should these vessels be dilated acutely? Results from PAMI-2 [Abstract]. Circulation 92:I-530, 1995.

# 12

# Beyond Primary PTCA: New Approaches to Mechanical Reperfusion Therapy in Acute Myocardial Infarction

*Gregg W. Stone*     *Cindy L. Grines*

## LIMITATIONS OF PRIMARY PTCA

Primary percutaneous transluminal coronary angioplasty (PTCA), when performed by experienced operators at well-organized centers, has emerged as the reperfusion modality of choice for the treatment of evolving acute myocardial infarction (AMI).[1-5] There exist, however, several limitations of primary PTCA that have yet to be overcome with traditional balloon techniques (Table 12–1). It is well recognized that AMI is caused by thrombus formation superimposed on a fissured atherosclerotic plaque.[6, 7] Although balloon angioplasty is successful in restoring patency in the infarcted artery in more than 90% of patients, a residual stenosis involving more than 30% of the luminal diameter is present in approximately one third of lesions (caused by bulky

## TABLE 12–1.    LIMITATIONS OF PRIMARY PTCA FOR ACUTE MYOCARDIAL INFARCTION

**Procedural Limitations**
TIMI grade 3 flow is not restored in 5%–10% of patients
Residual stenosis involving >30% luminal diameter is common
Some degree of arterial dissection is frequently present
Post-PTCA dissection and residual stenosis involving >30% luminal diameter correlate with recurrent ischemia and reocclusion of the infarcted artery
**In-hospital Adverse Events**
Recurrent ischemia in 10%–15% of patients
Reinfarction in 3%–5% of patients
Reocclusion infarcted artery in 5%–10% of patients
Vascular complications and blood transfusion in ~10% of patients
**Postdischarge Adverse Events**
6-month restenosis rates of 37%–49%
Late reocclusion of infarcted artery in 9%–14% of vessels
6-month target vessel revascularization in 20% of patients

PTCA, percutaneous transluminal coronary angioplasty; TIMI, Thrombolysis In Myocardial Infarction.

underlying plaque, inadequate dilatation, or elastic recoil), typically with some degree of arterial dissection and residual thrombus.[8, 9] As a result, spontaneous recurrent ischemia develops in approximately 10% to 15% of patients after successful primary PTCA and before hospital discharge.[1-5, 10] This development typically necessitates recatheterization and frequent target vessel revascularization with either repeat PTCA or coronary artery bypass grafting (CABG).[1-5, 10] The development and necessary management of recurrent ischemia prolong the hospital stay and increase costs markedly.[10] Furthermore, reocclusion of the infarcted artery before hospital discharge, which results in blunted myocardial recovery, occurs in 5% to 10% of patients.[1, 3, 4, 8, 9] In about half of patients with reocclusion of the infarcted artery, clinically manifest reinfarction develops (reported in 3% to 5% of patients after primary PTCA in most prior series); this limits myocardial recovery and increases early mortality.[1-5, 8-19] Finally, the most common adverse outcome of primary PTCA is the occurrence of restenosis within 6 months of the procedure, which has been documented in 37% to 49% of patients in five studies with high rates of angiographic follow-up (Fig. 12–1).[11, 20-23] Furthermore, 9% to 14% of infarcted arteries have become occluded by late follow-up; this too results in decreased myocardial recovery and increased late mortality.[24] As a result, approximately 20% of patients who have undergone primary PTCA require repeat revascularization procedures within the first 6 months after hospital discharge (Fig. 12–2).[21, 25, 26]

To further enhance the acute and late results of mechanical reperfusion in AMI, investigation since the mid-1990s has shifted to the adjunctive use of powerful new pharmacologic agents during primary PTCA and to alternative percutaneous interventional strategies, including stent implantation, ath-

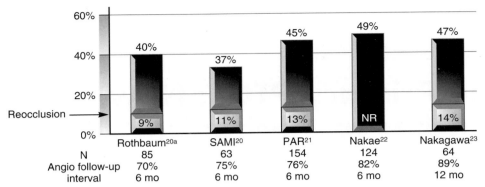

FIGURE 12–1. Incidence of restenosis after primary PTCA from five published reports in which angiographic follow-up was performed in 70% or more of patients at 6 months or later. *Black bars* represent restenosis (including reocclusion); *speckled bars* represent reocclusion of infarcted arteries. The reocclusion rate was not reported (NR) in the study by Nakae et al.[22] %angio follow-up, percentage of patients in whom angiographic follow-up was completed; interval, time to angiographic follow-up; PAR, Primary Angioplasty Registry; SAMI, Streptokinase Angioplasty in Myocardial Infarction (trial).

erectomy, laser use, and the use of a variety of new devices. This chapter considers these new approaches to mechanical reperfusion in AMI. Only the studies reporting significant data with these agents and devices in patients with AMI are detailed. However, because there has been little published direct experience with several of these novel drugs or devices in patients with AMI, their utility for thrombotic lesions and acute ischemic syndromes (e.g., unstable angina and postinfarction angina) is reviewed, in view of the commonality of the origin of these conditions with AMI.

## ADJUNCTIVE PHARMACOTHERAPY DURING MECHANICAL REPERFUSION

The occlusive thrombus in AMI is composed of a dense platelet-fibrin mesh, upon which erythrocytes

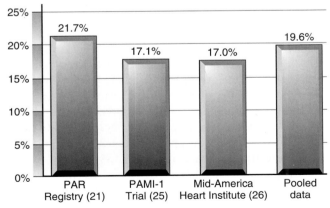

FIGURE 12–2. Target vessel revascularization—percutaneous transluminal coronary angioplasty (PTCA) or coronary artery bypass grafting (CABG)—in the first 6 months after hospital discharge in patients undergoing successful primary PTCA without in-hospital CABG. Numbers in parentheses are references. PAMI, Primary Angioplasty in Myocardial Infarction; PAR, Primary Angioplasty Registry.

later adhere and become trapped, resulting in a leading and trailing tail of red blood cells.[27, 28] Platelet activation is enhanced in patients with acute ischemic syndromes, as evidenced by increased urinary excretion of platelet metabolites such as thromboxane $B_2$ shortly after coronary occlusion.[29] Plaque disruption with thrombus formation is also associated with activation of the factor XII–kallikrein–kinin system and, secondarily, endogenous fibrinolytic pathways.[30] Increased markers of thrombin generation and activity, including prothrombin fragment $1 + 2$ ($F1 + 2$), thrombin-antithrombin complex, fibrin monomer, D-dimer, and fibrinopeptide A, are also present during the acute phase of unstable angina and AMI and are predictors associated with subsequent mortality.[31–33] The platelet and thrombin cascades are tightly linked; thrombin is an intense stimulus for platelet activation,[34] which results in further thrombus growth and thrombin internalization into the growing lesion.[35, 36]

Furthermore, balloon angioplasty exposes the basement submembrane containing highly thrombogenic components such as collagen and von Willebrand factor, as well as the lipid-rich core of the atherosclerotic plaque, all of which are intense stimuli for platelet adherence, activation, and aggregation.[37–40] Platelet deposition at the site of medial disruption markedly increases within minutes after balloon deflation.[41, 42] Thus, in patients with AMI undergoing primary PTCA, the angioplasty procedure itself induces further platelet activation and thrombin generation, in excess of the heightened baseline level of platelet metabolism.[43, 44] As a result, recurrent ischemia and infarcted artery reocclusion resulting from recurrent thrombosis occur significantly more frequently in patients with AMI and acute ischemic syndromes undergoing PTCA than in patients with stable angina during percutaneous intervention. Finally, heightened platelet activity may contribute to reperfusion injury by direct effects on the microcirculation.[45, 46] Studies have therefore focused on the role of antiplatelet and antithrombotic agents as an adjunct to primary PTCA.

## Antiplatelet Agents

Since the mid-1990s, a more thorough understanding of platelet metabolism and activation pathways has been attained, which has resulted in a more complete appreciation of the central role of the platelet in both AMI and PTCA.[47–49] Platelets are activated either after direct adhesion to the PTCA-induced injury site or through one of several mediators, including thrombin, epinephrine, adenosine diphosphate (ADP), and thromboxane $A_2$.[50, 51] The net effect of platelet activation is to result in a conformational change in the glycoprotein (GP) IIb/IIIa receptor, an integrin molecule which is expressed as approximately 50,000 to 100,000 copies in the cell membrane of each platelet.[52, 53] The activated GPIIb/IIIa receptor is then able to crosslink circulating von Willebrand's factor, fibronectin, fibrinogen, and subsequently numerous other platelets, the end result of which is a platelet-fibrin plug. The GPIIb/IIIa receptor is thus termed the *common final pathway* of platelet aggregation.[50–53]

### Aspirin and Ticlopidine

Agents such as aspirin and ticlopidine are relatively weak platelet antagonists, inasmuch as they interfere with only one or a few of the modes of GPIIb/IIIa activation. Aspirin irreversibly blocks platelet prostaglandin cyclooxygenase activity, thereby interfering with the thromboxane $A_2$ limb of platelet activation.[54] The mechanism of ticlopidine action, in contrast, is not as well understood. Ticlopidine blocks ADP-induced platelet potentiation,[55] decreases the exposure of activated GPIIb/IIIa receptors on the platelet membrane, and inhibits platelet serotonin release.[56] Despite the modest activities of these agents, they have turned out to be quite effective in improving outcomes in patients with acute ischemic syndromes, and in those undergoing PTCA.

The Second International Study of Infarct Survival (ISIS-2) demonstrated that aspirin alone, when given in the early hours of AMI, is as effective as streptokinase alone in reducing the 30-day mortality rate.[57] Furthermore, reinfarction rates were reduced 50% with aspirin therapy, but they increased with the thrombolytic agent alone. The combination of aspirin and streptokinase was synergistic in reducing rates of early mortality and in preventing reinfarction (Fig. 12–3). The utility of chronic aspirin (or ticlopidine) use in preventing late death and reinfarction after stabilization of unstable angina[58–63] or AMI[62–64] has been well described. Furthermore, both aspirin and ticlopidine have well-documented efficacy in preventing ischemic complications after PTCA.[65–68] The combination of aspirin and ticlopidine has also been found to be more effective than aspirin alone or aspirin plus warfarin in the prevention of subacute thrombosis after stent implantation.[69, 70] These studies highlight the key role of the platelet in the pathogenesis of AMI and PTCA/stent-related complications and suggest that even more potent platelet blockade could further improve outcomes in patients with AMI who undergo percutaneous intervention.

### Glycoprotein IIb/IIIa Receptor Antagonists

With the development of a class of pharmacologic agents that has direct activity against the GPIIb/IIIa receptor, it has become possible to selectively inhibit 80% to 90% of platelet function in vitro and in vivo. The GPIIb/IIIa receptor inhibitors include antibody derivatives (e.g., abciximab), synthetic heptapeptides (e.g., eptifibatide), and synthetic nonpeptides (e.g., tirofiban and lamifiban). These drugs have been extensively investigated, primarily in patients undergoing PTCA and more recently in patients with unstable angina and AMI. Three studies have investigated the role of GPIIb/IIIa receptor blockade as an adjunct to primary PTCA in patients with AMI (Table 12–2).

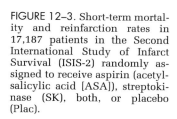

FIGURE 12–3. Short-term mortality and reinfarction rates in 17,187 patients in the Second International Study of Infarct Survival (ISIS-2) randomly assigned to receive aspirin (acetylsalicylic acid [ASA]), streptokinase (SK), both, or placebo (Plac).

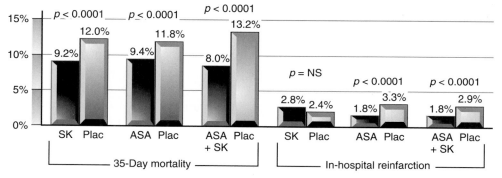

**TABLE 12–2. RANDOMIZED STUDIES OF GLYCOPROTEIN IIb/IIIa RECEPTOR BLOCKADE DURING PRIMARY PTCA IN ACUTE MYOCARDIAL INFARCTION**

| TRIAL | DRUG | N | KEY FINDINGS | COMMENTS |
|---|---|---|---|---|
| EPIC | Abciximab | 66 | Strong trend toward reduced 30-day rates of death, reinfarction, and TVR with abciximab; strongly significant at 6 months | Subset of 2099 randomly assigned patients; rescue PTCA in 33% |
| RAPPORT | Abciximab | 483 | Intention to treat: decreased 30-day and 6-month rates of urgent TVR with abciximab; no differences in rates of death, reinfarction, or total TVR at 6 months | Only 72% of patients had PTCA + 12-hour drug; results more positive in analysis of treatment received |
| RESTORE | Tirofiban | 134 | 56% reduction in death, myocardial infarction, and total TVR at 7 days with tirofiban; 22% reduction at 30 days (both $p = $ NS) | Subset of 2141 patients randomly assigned |

EPIC, Evaluation of 7E3 for the Prevention of Ischemic Complications; NS, nonsignificant; PTCA, percutaneous transluminal coronary angioplasty; RAPPORT, ReoPro in AMI Primary PTCA Organization and Randomized Trial; RESTORE, Randomized Efficacy Study of Tirofiban for Outcomes and Restenosis; TVR, target vessel revascularization.

## The EPIC Trial

The best studied of these drugs is c7E3, or abciximab (ReoPro), a chimeric molecule containing the variable region antibody fragments (Fab) of the murine monoclonal antibody 7E3 directed against the GPIIb/IIIa receptor, joined to the human constant region immunoglobulin G (IgG) Fab fragment (Centocor; Malvern PA, and Lilly and Co.; Indianapolis IN). At clinically useful doses, abciximab reduces platelet aggregation to less than 20% of baseline levels.[71] In addition to blocking the GPIIb/IIIa receptor, abciximab has multiple other effects, including anti-inflammatory properties (by blocking the MAC-1 receptor on macrophages and monocytes) and antiproliferative properties (through inhibition of the vitronectin receptor—the integrin $a_v b_3$—which is involved in the regulation of smooth muscle cell proliferation and migration).[72–74] Abciximab can also cause clot "de-thrombosis" (fragmentation), by inhibiting factor XIII and plasminogen activator inhibitor-1 (PAI-1) and by directly displacing fibrinogen from the GPIIb/IIIa receptor.[74, 75] These features theoretically should make abciximab very useful as an adjunct to PTCA in patients with acute ischemic syndromes who are undergoing intervention.

In the Evaluation of 7E3 for the Prevention of Ischemic Complications (EPIC) trial, 2099 patients at high risk for needing either PTCA or directional coronary atherectomy (DCA) were randomly assigned prospectively to receive one of three regimens: (1) abciximab, 0.25 mg/kg in an intravenous (IV) bolus plus 10 μg/minute infusion for 12 hours; (2) abciximab bolus plus placebo infusion; or (3) placebo bolus plus infusion.[76, 77] Patients were classified in three subgroups in this study: patients with high-risk clinical and/or anatomic features ($N = 1544$ [73% of the study]); those with unstable angina or recent non–Q-wave myocardial infarction (MI) ($N = 489$ [23%]); and patients undergoing primary PTCA or rescue PTCA after failed thrombolysis within 12 hours of AMI ($N = 66$ [3%]). PTCA was performed in 90% of patients; 10% underwent DCA. All patients received aspirin at least 2 hours before the procedure, and 10,000 to 20,000 U of IV heparin during the intervention, with a heparin drip maintained for 12 hours or more afterward. Vascular sheaths were left in place for at least 6 hours after the procedure.

In comparison with placebo, the abciximab bolus plus infusion reduced the occurrence of the primary composite end point (death, MI, and urgent target vessel revascularization [TVR]) at 30 days (12.8% of placebo recipients vs. 8.4% of abciximab recipients; $p = 0.008$).[76, 77] Examination of the separate components of the composite end point revealed no difference in mortality rates with abciximab treatment but a reduction in both periprocedural MI (8.6% vs. 5.2%; $p = 0.01$) and urgent repeat TVR (7.8% vs. 4.0%; $p = 0.003$). At 3 years, the composite incidence of death, MI, and TVR was still reduced (47.2% vs. 41.1%; $p = 0.009$).[77] Of note, in a post hoc analysis, the 3-year rate of mortality in the combined subgroup with unstable angina, recent MI, or AMI was reduced (12.7% vs. 5.1%; $p = 0.01$).[78] The patients who received abciximab only in a bolus experienced minimal early efficacy and no late benefit, and therefore this protocol is no longer in use. The utility of abciximab in reducing periprocedural MI and cardiac enzyme release and in reducing the need for urgent repeat TVR was also demonstrated in patients with unstable angina undergoing PTCA and DCA in the Evaluation of PTCA to Improve Long-term Outcome by c7E3 GP IIb/IIIa Receptor Blockade (EPILOG) and c7E3 (ab) Anti Platelet Therapy in Unstable Refractory Angina (CAPTURE) trials.[79, 80]

Although only 66 patients in EPIC undergoing PTCA during AMI were randomly assigned to treatment, the results were strikingly positive and thus bear detailed inspection.[76] Of 64 patients for whom detailed data were reported, 42 underwent primary PTCA for AMI and 22 underwent rescue PTCA for failed thrombolysis.[81] The outcomes of the EPIC trial in the AMI subgroup are presented in Table 12–3. At 30 days, the proportion of patients reaching primary composite end point was 26.1% of the placebo recipients, in contrast to only 4.5% of those receiving abciximab bolus plus infusion ($p = 0.06$). At 6 months, event rates were further reduced with the active therapy (47.8% vs. 4.5%; $p = 0.002$). Although only a small number of patients were studied, it is noteworthy that no patient in the abciximab cohort experienced clinical restenosis during 30 days and 6 months of follow-up. Furthermore, the reduction in the 6-month end point with the GPIIb/IIIa blocker was much more marked in the AMI subset than in the rest of the trial (Fig. 12–4).

The mechanism by which GPIIb/IIIa inhibition improved clinical outcomes in this trial could not be attributed to more favorable acute angiographic results of the PTCA procedure. As seen in Table 12–4 and Figure 12–5, there were no differences in stenotic luminal diameter, post-PTCA dissection or residual thrombus, or improvement in Thrombolysis In Myocardial Infarction (TIMI) flow grade between patients treated with abciximab and those who received placebo. It is therefore likely that ab-

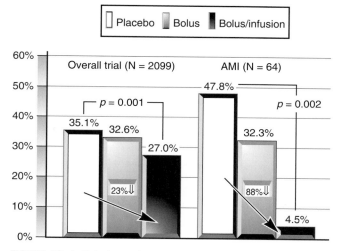

FIGURE 12–4. Relative reductions in the primary 6-month composite end point of death, reinfarction, repeat percutaneous transluminal coronary angioplasty (PTCA), or coronary artery bypass grafting (CABG) in the entire Evaluation of 7E3 for the Prevention of Ischemic Complications (EPIC) trial *(left)* vs. the subset with acute myocardial infarction (AMI) only *(right)*.

ciximab reduced the rate of reinfarction and the need for TVR after primary PTCA during AMI by stabilizing the inherently unstable ruptured plaque and ameliorating the adverse effects of PTCA-induced vascular injury on platelet activation and subsequent thrombosis.

The major problem for patients taking abciximab in EPIC was a significant increase in hemorrhagic complications, both in the overall population and in the AMI subset (see Table 12–3). This was subsequently shown to be a reflection of the high doses of heparin used in this study, as well as the prolonged sheath dwell times. In the subsequent EPILOG trial, reducing the heparin dose to achieve a target acti-

**TABLE 12–3.   OUTCOMES OF PATIENTS WITH ACUTE MYOCARDIAL INFARCTION IN THE EPIC TRIAL**

| EVENT | PLACEBO (N = 23) | BOLUS (N = 19) | BOLUS + INFUSION (N = 22) | $p^*$ |
|---|---|---|---|---|
| ***30-Day Outcomes*** | | | | |
| Death | 0% | 10.5% | 4.5% | 0.31 |
| Reinfarction | 8.7% | 5.6% | 0% | 0.17 |
| Urgent TVR | 17.4% | 5.3% | 0% | 0.05 |
| Composite† | 26.1% | 21.1% | 4.5% | 0.06 |
| Major bleeding | 13.0% | 31.6% | 18.2% | 0.63 |
| Intracranial bleed | 0% | 5.3% | 0% | 0.99 |
| Blood transfusion | 8.7% | 31.6% | 22.7% | 0.19 |
| ***6-Month Outcomes*** | | | | |
| Death | 0% | 15.8% | 4.5% | 0.31 |
| Reinfarction | 17.4% | 5.6% | 0% | 0.05 |
| Repeat PTCA | 34.8% | 11.6% | 0% | 0.003 |
| CABG | 4.3% | 0% | 0% | 0.82 |
| Composite | 47.8% | 32.2% | 4.5% | 0.002 |

CABG, coronary artery bypass grafting; EPIC, Evaluation of 7E3 for the Prevention of Ischemic Complications; PTCA, percutaneous transluminal coronary angioplasty; TVR, target vessel revascularization.
*Placebo vs. bolus + infusion groups.
†Death, reinfarction, or urgent TVR at 30 days.

**TABLE 12–4. ANGIOGRAPHIC OUTCOMES IN THE ACUTE MYOCARDIAL INFARCTION SUBSET OF THE EPIC TRIAL**

| OUTCOME | PLACEBO (N = 23) | BOLUS (N = 19) | BOLUS + INFUSION (N = 22) |
|---|---|---|---|
| Percentage undergoing PTCA | 73% | 58% | 68% |
| Mean diameter stenosis before PTCA | 96% | 97% | 98% |
| Mean diameter stenosis after PTCA | 28% | 24% | 30% |
| Major dissection after PTCA | 4.5% | 10.5% | 13.6% |
| Thrombus present after PTCA | 9.1% | 10.5% | 13.6% |
| Distal emboli after PTCA | 4.5% | 5.3% | 4.5% |
| Intracoronary thrombolysis | 9.1% | 15.8% | 13.6% |

$p$ = NS for all comparisons.
EPIC, Evaluation of 7E3 for the Prevention of Ischemic Complications; PTCA, percutaneous transluminal coronary angioplasty.

vated clotting time (ACT) of 200 to 300 seconds before PTCA, eliminating postprocedural heparin use, and early sheath removal reduced bleeding complications to the degree seen in the control group.[79]

### The RAPPORT Study

Despite the small number of primary PTCA patients enrolled in EPIC, the results were sufficiently compelling to organize a larger trial specifically designed to test the efficacy of abciximab in AMI patients undergoing a primary PTCA strategy. In the ReoPro in AMI Primary PTCA Organization and Randomized Trial (RAPPORT), 483 patients with AMI and symptoms of less than 12 hours' duration in whom primary PTCA was intended were enrolled in a placebo-controlled, double-blind trial at 39 U.S. centers (Fig. 12–6).[82] Stent use was strongly discouraged in this study. After enrollment, drug initiation (placebo or abciximab) began in the emergency room or the catheterization laboratory, either before or after coronary angiography. PTCA was then performed if the coronary anatomy was appropriate. No patients had received thrombolytic therapy before enrollment in this trial. All patients were treated with aspirin. Of note, however, is that because this trial was organized before the EPILOG results, relatively high doses of heparin were mandated in the protocol (100-U/kg bolus initially plus infusion, with target ACT of >300 seconds). As discussed later, sheath dwell times were also prolonged.

In order to accurately interpret the RAPPORT results, it is necessary to understand the patient treatment strategy in this study (Fig. 12–7). In accordance with the prior Primary Angioplasty in Myocardial Infarction (PAMI) trials,[1, 83, 84] primary PTCA was performed in only 89% of patients. As a consequence, only 91% of patients received any study drug. Furthermore, because of bleeding complications, administration of the drug was terminated early in 21% of patients (however, in equal proportions of patients receiving abciximab and placebo). Thus, only 85% of patients actually under-

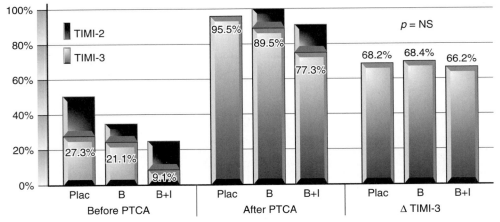

FIGURE 12–5. TIMI flow grades in the AMI subset of the EPIC trial. TIMI grade 3 flow tended to be more common at baseline in the subjects receiving placebo (Plac) than in those receiving bolus (B) and those receiving bolus and infusion (B+I); as a result, relatively more placebo recipients achieved TIMI-3 flow after percutaneous transluminal coronary angioplasty (PTCA). Among the patients achieving TIMI-3 flow in whom TIMI-3 flow was not present at baseline (Δ TIMI-3), TIMI-3 flow after PTCA was restored in approximately the same percentages of patients in the three groups, irrespective of IIb/IIIa receptor blockade. Percentages in the graph refer to patients achieving TIMI-3 flow. AMI, acute myocardial infarction; EPIC, Evaluation of 7E3 for the Prevention of Ischemic Complications; TIMI, Thrombolysis In Myocardial Infarction.

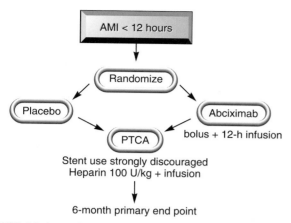

FIGURE 12–6. Study algorithm of the ReoPro in AMI Primary PTCA Organization and Randomized Trial (RAPPORT). AMI, acute myocardial infarction; PTCA, percutaneous transluminal coronary angioplasty.

went primary PTCA and received at least some study drug, and only 72% of patients undergoing primary PTCA received the entire 12-hour infusion. Although the primary analysis of the trial is by intention to treat, any beneficial effects of the active drug as an adjunct to primary PTCA in this analysis may be diluted by including the outcomes in the 11% of patients in whom PTCA was not performed and the 21% of patients not able to tolerate the entire 12-hour infusion (but early discontinuation of the study drug was not increased by abciximab use in relation to control).

The final adjudicated outcomes of the RAPPORT trial are presented in Figure 12–8. Intention-to-treat analysis revealed that the composite end point of death, reinfarction, and TVR at 30 days occurred at a rate of 11.1% among patients receiving primary

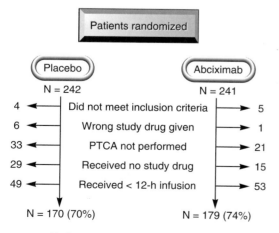

FIGURE 12–7. Patient recruitment in the ReoPro in AMI Primary PTCA Organization and Randomized Trial (RAPPORT). PTCA, percutaneous transluminal coronary angioplasty.

PTCA plus placebo but only 5.8% among those receiving primary PTCA plus abciximab ($p = 0.04$). As seen in Table 12–5, the improved early outcomes were attributable primarily to fewer TVRs. In addition, fewer abciximab-treated patients required stent implantation for a true "bail-out" indication (17.4% vs. 11.6%; $p = 0.06$, by intention-to-treat analysis). Analysis of the subsets of patients who underwent primary PTCA and/or received any study drug yielded more striking results (see Table 12–5). Indeed, in the patients who underwent primary PTCA and tolerated the full dose of study drug, the 30-day rate of reinfarction was also decreased (5.3% vs. 0.6%; $p = 0.02$). Because of selection bias and cohort effects in analysis of treatment-received subset data, however, these results cannot be considered definitive. As in EPIC, there were no differences in restoration of normal antegrade blood flow in the patients treated with abciximab; TIMI grade 3 flow after primary PTCA was present in 85.2% of patients treated with placebo and in 86.6% after abciximab ($p = $ NS).

Thus, these data suggest that abciximab, when used as an adjunct to primary PTCA, is able to stabilize the freshly dilated unstable plaque, resulting acutely in a lower need for salvage stent implantation and reduced need for urgent TVR to treat recurrent ischemia within 30 days. Unfortunately, as in EPIC, hemorrhagic complications were significantly increased with the use of abciximab in RAPPORT. According to intention-to-treat analysis, abciximab-treated patients had a higher rate of major bleeding (16.6%) than did placebo recipients (9.5%; $p = 0.02$), and their use of blood product transfusion (13.7%) was also higher (7.9%; $p = 0.04$). Most of the bleeding was related to access site; no patient in the RAPPORT trial experienced intracranial bleeding.

The likely causes of the excess bleeding with abciximab were the high doses of heparin used and prolonged sheath dwell times. The median maximal ACT within the first 48 hours of the study was 367 seconds in the abciximab recipients and 339 seconds in the placebo recipients, significantly higher than the 250-second median currently recommended. Similarly, median sheath duration was 17 hours with abciximab and 19 hours with placebo, also longer than the 4 to 6 hours as is currently standard. Theoretically, the use of lower heparin doses and earlier sheath removal should reduce hemorrhagic complications without affecting the protective anti-ischemic effect of this class of agents, as was seen in EPILOG.[79]

Finally, the primary end point in RAPPORT was prespecified to be the combination of death, reinfarction, and any TVR at 6 months. With this composite end point, there was no difference in

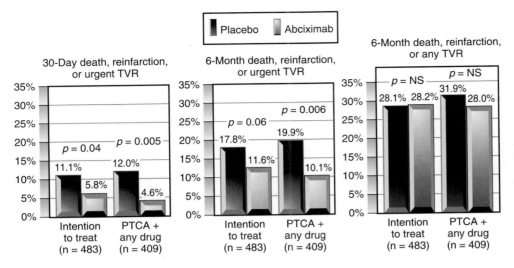

FIGURE 12–8. Final 30-day and 6-month outcomes in the ReoPro in AMI Primary PTCA Organization and Randomized Trial (RAPPORT). Data are presented in an intention-to-treat analysis ($N = 483$), and in the subset of 409 patients in whom primary percutaneous transluminal coronary angioplasty (PTCA) was performed and some or all of the study drug administered in a bolus and/or an infusion (whether placebo or abciximab). TVR, target vessel revascularization.

outcomes between the abciximab and placebo recipients, either according to intention-to-treat analysis or in the subgroup of patients who actually underwent primary PTCA and received abciximab (Table 12–6; see also Fig. 12–8, right graph). If only the necessity for the repeat urgent TVR events were considered, however, the 6-month composite outcome was improved with abciximab both according to intention-to-treat analysis (11.6% vs. 17.8%; $p = 0.06$) and, even more strongly, in the group of primary PTCA patients receiving abciximab (10.1% vs. 19.9%; $p = 0.006$) (see Fig. 12–8). The improvement in the incidence of late composite events was attributable mostly to a reduction in the need for urgent TVR. The greater use of bail-out stent implantation in the placebo recipients may have artifactually reduced the rates of restenosis and elective late TVR

in these patients in comparison with the abciximab recipients. However, the absence of any abciximab effect on late elective TVR (e.g., clinical restenosis) is in agreement with the findings from EPILOG[79] and is consistent with the angiographic and intravascular ultrasound results from the ERASER trial, in which no evidence for reduced neointimal proliferation was seen with abciximab use after coronary stent implantation.[85]

### The RESTORE Trial

The second GPIIb/IIIa receptor antagonist that has been studied as an adjunct to primary PTCA in AMI is MK-383, or tirofiban (Aggrastat). In contrast to abciximab, tirofiban is a potent, nonpeptide tyrosine derivative with a short half-life (1.5 to 2.0 hours)

### TABLE 12–5.   30-DAY OUTCOMES IN THE RAPPORT TRIAL

| OUTCOME | PLACEBO | ABCIXIMAB | p |
|---|---|---|---|
| ***Intention to Treat*** ($N = 483$) | | | |
| Death | 2.1% | 2.5% | NS |
| Reinfarction | 4.1% | 3.3% | NS |
| Urgent TVR | 6.6% | 1.7% | 0.006 |
| Composite | 11.1% | 5.8% | 0.04 |
| ***Any Study Drug Given*** ($N = 439$) | | | |
| Death | 1.9% | 1.8% | NS |
| Reinfarction | 4.7% | 2.7% | NS |
| Urgent TVR | 5.6% | 1.8% | 0.04 |
| Composite | 10.3% | 4.9% | 0.03 |
| ***Primary PTCA Performed + Any Drug Received*** ($N = 409$) | | | |
| Death or reinfarction | 5.8% | 3.2% | 0.03 |
| Urgent TVR | 7.9% | 1.8% | 0.003 |
| Composite | 12.0% | 4.6% | 0.008 |
| ***Primary PTCA Performed + 12-Hour Infusion Received*** ($N = 349$) | | | |
| Death | 1.8% | 1.1% | NS |
| Reinfarction | 5.3% | 0.6% | 0.02 |
| Urgent TVR | 7.0% | 1.7% | 0.01 |
| Composite | 11.8% | 2.8% | 0.001 |

NS, nonsignificant; PTCA, percutaneous transluminal coronary angioplasty; RAPPORT, ReoPro in AMI Primary PTCA Organization and Randomized Trial; TVR, target vessel revascularization.

## TABLE 12–6.  6-MONTH OUTCOMES IN THE RAPPORT TRIAL

| OUTCOME | PLACEBO | ABCIXIMAB | p |
|---|---|---|---|
| **Intention to Treat** (N = 483) | | | |
| Death or reinfarction | 11.2% | 8.7% | NS |
| Death, reinfarction, or urgent TVR | 17.8% | 11.6% | 0.06 |
| Death, reinfarction, or any TVR | 28.1% | 28.2% | NS |
| **Primary PTCA Performed + Any Drug Received** (N = 409) | | | |
| Death or reinfarction | 12.0% | 6.9% | 0.06 |
| Death, reinfarction, or urgent TVR | 19.9% | 10.1% | 0.006 |
| Death, reinfarction, or any TVR | 31.9% | 28.0% | NS |

NS, nonsignificant; PTCA, percutaneous transluminal coronary angioplasty; RAPPORT, ReoPro in AMI Primary PTCA Organization and Randomized Trial; TVR, target vessel revascularization.

and is a selective inhibitor of the GPIIb/IIIa receptor.[86, 87] Because of these properties, tirofiban theoretically could have an improved safety profile in comparison with longer acting, less selective noncompetitive GPIIb/IIIa inhibitors such as abciximab.

The safety and efficacy of tirofiban during PTCA in patients with acute ischemic syndromes were evaluated in the Randomized Efficacy Study of Tirofiban for Outcomes and Restenosis (RESTORE).[88] In this large, multicenter prospective study, 2141 patients with unstable angina (69%), MI within the previous 72 hours (28%), or acute MI within the previous 12 hours (3%) undergoing PTCA (93%) or DCA (7%) were randomly assigned to receive either IV tirofiban (10-μg/kg bolus plus 0.15-μg/kg/minute infusion for 36 hours) or placebo (bolus plus infusion). All patients received aspirin. Patients were randomly assigned after the wire successfully crossed the lesion during PTCA or DCA. Stent use was discouraged except for a true bail-out indication. The ACT was targeted during the procedure to 300 to 400 seconds, but in contrast to EPIC, no postprocedural heparin was used, and the sheaths were removed as soon as the ACT fell below 180 seconds.

The primary end point in RESTORE was the composite end point of death, MI or reinfarction, any TVR, or the necessity of stent implantation for bailout. By the second postprocedure day, a significant decrease in adverse events was noted in the tirofiban-treated patients versus those taking placebo (5.4% vs. 8.7%; $p = 0.005$), which was maintained by day 7 (7.6% vs. 10.4%; $p = 0.02$). By day 30, however, the difference between the two groups was no longer significant (10.3% vs. 12.2%; $p = 0.16$).

Of the 2141 patients, 134 had AMI and underwent primary PTCA. The results of this subgroup analysis are shown in Figure 12–9; the breakdown of the composite end point into its components is shown in Table 12–7. The outcomes in the patients undergoing primary PTCA mirrored those in the entire trial. The tirofiban-treated patients experienced a 56% reduction in adverse events within the first

week, the magnitude of which diminished over the next 3 weeks so that by 30 days, only a weak trend existed for a 22% reduction in adverse events. All the differences were statistically insignificant given the sample size.

Thus, the results of RESTORE in both the overall study population and the AMI primary PTCA cohort are consistent with those of EPIC and RAPPORT in demonstrating improved early clinical outcomes in patients with acute ischemic syndromes undergoing PTCA with GPIIb/IIIa receptor blockade. In contrast to abciximab use, however, the improved early outcomes with tirofiban in RESTORE were attenuated over the next several weeks. There may be several explanations for this discrepancy. First, the very different biologic effects of the two molecules may explain the differences: the longer half-life and lack of specificity of abciximab may confer distinct clinical advantages over shorter acting agents that have greater specificity for the GPIIb/IIIa receptor, in view of the time required for plaque stabilization after PTCA in acute ischemic syndromes, and the complex nature of thrombus generation and dissolution. Second, however, differences in trial design may

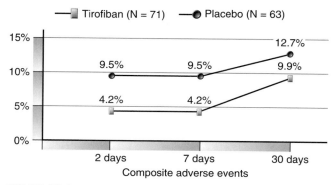

FIGURE 12–9. Incidence of the primary composite end point (death, reinfarction, repeat percutaneous transluminal coronary angioplasty [PTCA], coronary artery bypass grafting [CABG], or stent for acute closure) at different time intervals in the primary PTCA for the subset of patients with acute myocardial infarction in the Randomized Efficacy Study of Tirofiban for Outcomes and Restenosis (RESTORE).

**TABLE 12–7.  SHORT-TERM OUTCOMES IN PATIENTS WITH ACUTE MYOCARDIAL INFARCTION RANDOMLY ASSIGNED IN THE RESTORE TRIAL**

| OUTCOME | 2-DAY ADVERSE EVENTS | | | 30-DAY ADVERSE EVENTS | | |
|---|---|---|---|---|---|---|
| | PLACEBO | TIROFIBAN | p | PLACEBO | TIROFIBAN | p |
| Death | 0% | 2.8% | NS | 1.6% | 2.8% | NS |
| Reinfarction | 3.2% | 1.4% | NS | 4.8% | 1.4% | NS |
| Repeat PTCA | 1.6% | 0% | NS | 4.8% | 1.4% | NS |
| CABG | 3.2% | 1.4% | NS | 4.8% | 4.2% | NS |
| Stent implantation for acute closure | 3.2% | 2.8% | NS | 3.2% | 2.8% | NS |
| Composite | 9.5% | 4.2% | NS | 12.7% | 9.9% | NS |

CABG, coronary artery bypass grafting; NS, nonsignificant; PTCA, percutaneous transluminal coronary angioplasty; RESTORE, Randomized Efficacy Study of Tirofiban for Outcomes and Restenosis.
Data from Merck.

partly explain the disparity in results between the two trials. Specifically, the primary end point in RESTORE included both urgent and elective TVR, whereas in EPIC and RAPPORT, the 30-day end points included only urgent TVR. In a post hoc manner, when the results of RESTORE were readjudicated in accordance with the EPIC 30-day composite end point (death, MI, or urgent TVR), the differences between the two groups retained borderline statistical significance at 30 days (8.0% with tirofiban vs. 10.5% with placebo; $p = 0.052$).[88] Second, creatine-phosphokinase (CPK) values were obtained only at 36 hours and then on an as-needed basis in RESTORE, whereas they were obtained at regular, repeated intervals in EPIC and RAPPORT. As a result, some episodes of periprocedural MI and reinfarction may have been missed in RESTORE. Finally, the use of bail-out stent implantation was somewhat more frequent in RESTORE than EPIC (2.5% vs. 0.6%), which may have slightly narrowed the differences in outcomes between the groups. Because of these issues, it cannot be stated with certainty whether abciximab is more effective than tirofiban in the setting of primary PTCA. The recently completed TARGET study suggests a superiority for abciximab in patients with acute coronary syndromes.

### The Use of GPIIb/IIIa Receptor Antagonists as a Primary Reperfusion Agent

Another drawback of primary PTCA is the inherent delay before reperfusion that exists during patient evaluation in the emergency room, transfer to the cardiac catheterization laboratory, and performance of pre-PTCA angiography. Reported time intervals from emergency room arrival to reperfusion by PTCA range from 60 minutes at the most coordinated centers[2] to 90 to 120 minutes at other institutions reporting excellent outcomes,[83, 84] to more than 150 minutes at novice centers starting up a primary PTCA program.[89] AMI trials with thrombolytic therapy have demonstrated that earlier reperfusion can

result in greater myocardial salvage and reduced rates of mortality, especially if treatment is given within the first hour.[90, 91]

Thrombolytic administration before catheterization, either administered before hospitalization or in the emergency room, could theoretically enhance reperfusion before PTCA. Such an approach, however, exposes the patient to a greater risk of intracranial hemorrhage and increases the likelihood of reocclusion of the infarcted artery and access site hemorrhagic complications after catheter-based reperfusion in comparison with primary PTCA alone.[92] Furthermore, relatively few patients achieve reperfusion within 30 minutes after thrombolytic administration; the majority require 60 to 90 minutes for maximal restoration of antegrade flow.[93] The use of high-dose heparin therapy to restore early patency was evaluated in the Heparin in Early Patency (HEAP) pilot trial; a 300-U/kg IV bolus of heparin was found to result in TIMI grade 2 or 3 flow in 56% of patients.[94] However, the HEAP randomized trial subsequently found no difference in early reperfusion rates with high-dose compared to lower-dose heparin.[95]

For these reasons, consideration has been given to the potential use of GPIIb/IIIa receptor blockers either as primary reperfusion agents or to more rapidly restore partial or complete reperfusion before primary PTCA. The attractiveness of this approach is twofold. First, the hemorrhagic risk with GPIIb/IIIa receptor inhibition is less than that with thrombolysis (intracranial bleeding is very infrequent with proper case selection,[96] and rates of access site bleeding are similar to those of controls with proper use of heparin and sheath management[79]). Second, as discussed earlier, the use of these agents in concert with primary PTCA may reduce early recurrent ischemia and the need for urgent TVR.[82]

The efficacy of abciximab as a stand-alone reperfusion agent was initially explored by Gold and associates.[97] In 13 patients with AMI undergoing primary PTCA in this study, IV abciximab improved

TIMI flow grade by at least one flow grade in 11 patients (85%) within 10 minutes of the bolus. TIMI grade 2 or 3 flow was achieved in 7 patients (54%). After this pilot study, the ability of abciximab to enhance the rate and extent of early patency in larger numbers of patients was investigated in the TIMI-14b study,[98] in the GRAPE pilot study,[99] and, in more depth, by the Boston group.[100] These studies found that within 45 to 90 minutes of abciximab infusion, 24% to 33% of infarcted vessels attained TIMI grade 3 flow, and approximately 50% had TIMI grade 2 or 3 flow. These preliminary data therefore suggest that abciximab is approximately as effective as streptokinase as a reperfusion agent, although less potent than tissue-type plasminogen activator (tPA).[101] However, in the Boston trial, a crossover design study in which 42 patients with ST segment elevation and chest pain of less than 6 hours' duration were randomly assigned to receive abciximab or placebo, the rates of TIMI grades 2 and 3 flow on the first angiogram (mean time, 45 minutes) were similar for abciximab and placebo recipients (47% vs. 43%; $p$ = NS).[100] Thus, it is unlikely that abciximab has sufficient efficacy as a stand-alone reperfusion agent. Whether its use before primary PTCA could result in enhanced myocardial salvage and improved survival in selected patients remains speculative; proof would require large randomized trials.

## Conclusions: GPIIb/IIIa Receptor Blockade in Acute Myocardial Infarction

The current data suggest that GPIIb/IIIa receptor inhibition in AMI, as an adjunct to primary PTCA, may offer short-term clinical benefits by stabilizing the plaque, thereby reducing the need for urgent repeat TVR procedures. Post hoc subset data from RAPPORT further suggest that the rate of reinfarction may be reduced in patients undergoing primary PTCA who are able to tolerate the entire 12-hour dose of IV abciximab. However, in view of the hazard of selection bias and cohort effects in such retrospective analyses, this finding cannot be considered certain, and a reduced rate of reinfarction was not present in the intention-to-treat analysis of the entire population. Furthermore, with the anticoagulation and sheath management strategies employed in EPIC and RAPPORT, hemorrhagic complications were increased with active drug therapy. Although it is logical to assume that the efficacy of GPIIb/IIIa receptor inhibition with primary PTCA in AMI would be maintained or even enhanced with lower heparin dosages, while at the same time reducing access site bleeding (as in EPILOG), this hypothesis has not yet been proved.

Several additional questions must be answered before IV GPIIb/IIIa receptor blockade can be unequivocally recommended as a routine part of primary PTCA. First, the benefits shown to date have been relatively modest: reduced urgent TVR rates at 30 days, with no overall difference in death, reinfarction, or total TVR at 6 months according to intention-to-treat analysis. Similar in-hospital quantitative benefits were demonstrated with the use of routine intra-aortic balloon counterpulsation (IABP) after primary PTCA in AMI, without excessive major hemorrhagic or vascular complications; however, this advantage has not been deemed sufficiently compelling to result in widespread adoption of routine IABP use after PTCA.[84] Studies of GPIIb/IIIa receptor blockers, in which larger numbers of patients are randomly assigned to treatment and heparin dosing and sheath dwell times are restricted, may be necessary to demonstrate early and late improvements in reinfarction and TVR rates in an intention-to-treat analysis. The important issue of enhanced myocardial salvage with GPIIb/IIIa inhibition before primary PTCA—possible through decreased distal embolization, platelet plugging or transient slow flow, or improved tissue metabolism—has not been proved. The adjunctive role of abciximab or other GPIIb/IIIa receptor antagonists as part of a primary stent strategy in AMI is also unestablished, as discussed later. It is further undetermined whether agents such as tirofiban that have shorter half-lives and more selectively target the GPIIb/IIIa receptor are as effective as abciximab. Other GPIIb/IIIa receptor antagonists, such as eptifibatide (Integrilin), have not been studied at all in AMI patients undergoing mechanical reperfusion.[107, 108] Finally, the cost effectiveness of GPIIb/IIIa receptor inhibition in AMI has not been established; this is a critical concern in the current health care environment. Some of these issues will be addressed in large, multicenter studies that are under way, including the CADILLAC trial (discussed later at the conclusion of the stent section).

## Low Molecular Weight Heparins and Direct Antithrombin Agents

Proper anticoagulation with intravenous heparin during and for several days after primary PTCA has an integral role in ensuring high procedural success with low rates of recurrent ischemia. It is well established that inadequate anticoagulation with heparin during PTCA is correlated with acute vessel thrombosis and ischemic complications[109–113]: this relationship is critical especially during primary PTCA when thrombus is already present before vessel injury. Moreover, adequate inhibition of thrombin formation is complementary to effective platelet blockade in acute ischemic syndromes. Aspirin, for example, blocks only the thromboxane $A_2$ pathway of platelet activation and leaves the thrombin-dependent pathways unaffected. Thus, as expected from these considerations, the combination of aspirin and heparin has been shown to be superior to either alone in patients with unstable angina.[114]

As previously discussed, despite the use of aspirin and heparin during primary PTCA, acute ischemic complications occur in approximately 10% of patients during the procedure, including acute vessel thrombosis, distal thromboemboli, and transient or sustained no-reflow or slow reflow.[115–121] More effective antithrombotic agents (as well as more potent platelet inhibition) may therefore be necessary to improve immediate outcomes. Furthermore, recurrent ischemia during the in-hospital phase occurs in approximately 10% of patients after primary PTCA.[1, 3, 4, 8, 9] Part of the explanation for recurrent ischemia after primary PTCA may be the presence of a clinically relevant rebound hypercoagulable state after heparin discontinuation.[122–127] In two trials examining the role of heparin in the treatment of unstable angina, a transient increase in adverse ischemic events, not present in patients treated with aspirin only, was found shortly after heparin discontinuation.[58, 128] The explanation for this temporary hypercoagulable state may relate to the release of thrombin from residual thrombotic material as heparin is cleared, as well as consumption of antithrombin and release of tissue factor pathway inhibitor during heparin treatment.[129, 130] Thus, alternative antithrombotic approaches that avert this rebound state may reduce rates of recurrent ischemia after primary mechanical reperfusion in AMI.

Heparin is a glycosaminoglycan composed of a mixture of polysaccharides of varying molecular weights. Heparin has little direct anticoagulant effect; rather, it works by complexing with antithrombin III (AT-III), increasing the latter's anticoagulant activities greater than 1000-fold.[131] The heparin–AT-III complex is able to inhibit thrombin directly and has secondary anti–factor Xa activity. Heparin, at high concentrations, can also interfere with thrombin directly by combining with heparin cofactor II and can inhibit platelet aggregation.

Heparin has several drawbacks as an antithrombotic agent. First, the efficacy of heparin requires AT-III as a cofactor. Second, activated platelets secrete a number of proteins, including platelet factor 4, that block the interaction between heparin and AT-III.[132] Thus, states characterized by heightened platelet activity and platelet-rich thrombi, such as acute ischemic syndromes and the post-PTCA condition, are inherently resistant to the effects of heparin.[133] Furthermore, thrombin bound to fibrin within the clot surface is also relatively protected from the heparin–AT-III complex.[134] Factor Xa is also not

susceptible to heparin when complexed with factor Va and calcium on the platelet surface.[135] Third, heparin can also increase blood vessel wall permeability, which contributes to its tendency to cause hemorrhagic complications. Fourth, the bioavailability of heparin and its anticoagulant activity varies widely depending on the state of acute-phase reactant plasma proteins and other conditions, such as the degree of platelet activation. Fifth, clinically significant thrombocytopenia develops in approximately 3% of patients treated with heparin.[136] Additional inherent limitations of heparin also include the necessity of intravenous administration, as well as the necessity for frequent monitoring with the activated partial thromboplastin time (APTT) or ACT. Finally, the clinical significance of the rebound hypercoagulable state seen after heparin withdrawal in patients with acute ischemic syndromes has already been discussed.

To overcome the limitations of traditional unfractionated heparin, two alternative classes of antithrombotic agents have been studied as adjuncts during PTCA and in the treatment of patients with acute ischemic syndromes: the low molecular weight heparins and the direct antithrombin agents.

### Low Molecular Weight Heparins

In contrast to unfractionated heparin, which consists of polysaccharides whose molecular weights range from approximately 2000 to 30,000 daltons, low molecular weight (LMW) heparins consists only of the shorter chain fragments (<6000 D).[137] There are many preparations of LMW heparins, including enoxaparin, dalteparin, reviparin, and nadroparin, that vary somewhat in formulation. LMW heparins have greater specificity and activity against factor Xa than does heparin, but they have less direct thrombin activity.[131] Thus, LMW heparin has predominant anti–factor Xa activity, whereas unfractionated heparin has primarily anti–factor IIa activity. Furthermore, the lower molecular weight fractions contain most of the anticoagulant properties of heparin and fewer of the properties that tend to cause hemorrhage,[138] and therefore the LMW heparins are potentially safer at any given level of anticoagulation.

Because of differences in plasma clearance and metabolism (LMW heparins do not bind plasma proteins or endothelium), LMW heparin has significantly less person-to-person biologic variability than does unfractionated heparin, and its activity does not vary with disease states.[137] All of these features result in a stable dose-response relationship, which reduces the risk-benefit ratio of these agents in comparison with standard heparin. LMW heparins also reduce the generation of antiheparin antibodies by 70% in comparison with standard heparin,[139] which may lower the incidence of heparin-induced thrombocytopenia. LMW heparins also have good bioavailability when given subcutaneously, which may facilitate prolonged use. Another important difference with heparin is that the LMW heparins have little effect on the global tests of coagulation, such as the ACT or APTT; therefore, clinical monitoring is not routinely performed.

No studies have directly compared the use of unfractionated heparin with that of LMW heparin in patients undergoing mechanical reperfusion for AMI. However, insights into the potential utility of these agents may be gleaned from studies of LMW heparins used as an adjunct to PTCA and in patients with unstable angina or recent MI as an alternative to standard IV heparin.

Two trials have examined the utility of LMW heparin in patients with acute ischemic syndromes. In the Efficacy and Safety of Subcutaneous Enoxaparin in Non–Q-wave Coronary Events (ESSENCE) trial, a double-blind, placebo-controlled study, 3171 patients with at-rest angina or recent non–Q-wave MI were treated with aspirin and randomly assigned to receive either subcutaneous (SC) enoxaparin or IV unfractionated heparin for 2 to 8 days.[140] At 30 days, the incidences of death, MI, and recurrent angina were significantly lower in the enoxaparin recipients than in the patients receiving unfractionated heparin (19.8% vs. 23.3%; $p = 0.016$), as was the need for revascularization procedures (27.0% vs. 32.2%; $p = 0.001$). The incidence of any hemorrhagic complication was somewhat increased in the enoxaparin group (18.4% vs. 14.2%; $p = 0.001$), primarily because of injection site ecchymoses, although major bleeding occurred at similar rates in the two groups (6.5% vs. 7.0%, respectively; $p = NS$).

In the Fragmin in Unstable Coronary Artery Disease (FRIC) study, 1482 patients with unstable angina or recent non–Q-wave MI were randomly assigned in an open-label format to receive either dalteparin or unfractionated heparin for 5 days.[141] In this study, in contrast to ESSENCE, there was no difference in the rates of death, MI, or angina recurrence between the dalteparin and unfractionated heparin recipients (9.3% vs. 7.6%, respectively; $p = NS$), nor were there differences in this period in revascularization procedures (4.8% vs. 5.3%; $p = NS$) or major or minor bleeding. It is undetermined whether the disparity in results of the ESSENCE and FRIC studies is attributable to differences in study design or to the use of enoxaparin in ESSENCE, which has relatively greater activity against factor Xa than does dalteparin.

There are limited data regarding the utility of LMW heparins in ameliorating procedural complications in patients with acute ischemic syndromes

who undergo PTCA. In the Reduction of Restenosis After PTCA, Early Administration of Reviparin in a Double-Blind, Unfractionated Heparin and Placebo-Controlled Evaluation (REDUCE) trial 625 patients at 26 Canadian centers undergoing single-lesion PTCA were randomly assigned to receive either reviparin or unfractionated heparin.[142] Reviparin was given as a 7000-U IV bolus before PTCA, followed by a 24-hour infusion and then SC application for 28 days. The control group received 10,000 U of unfractionated heparin intravenously followed by 1000 U/hour intravenously for 24 hours. Of note, patients who had had an MI within 14 days before PTCA were excluded from the study, and only 18.3% of patients enrolled in this study had NYHA class IV angina. At 24 hours, the composite incidence of death, MI, unplanned stent use, CABG, or repeat PTCA was 3.9% in the reviparin group, in contrast to 8.2% in the control group ($p = 0.027$), primarily as a result of a reduced need for emergency stent implantation (2.0% vs. 6.9%; $p = 0.003$). There were no differences in major bleeding complications between the two cohorts. By 30 weeks, there were no differences in the incidences of the primary composite end point between the reviparin and standard heparin recipients (33.3% vs. 32.0%; $p = NS$).

In contrast to the findings of the REDUCE study, no acute benefits during PTCA were seen with pre-PTCA administration of the LMW heparin nadroparin in the Fraxiparine Angioplastie Coronaire Transluminale (FACT) study.[143] In this prospective, double-blind, multicenter trial, 354 patients undergoing elective PTCA were randomly assigned to receive either SC nadroparin daily for 3 days before PTCA and for 3 months thereafter or placebo. All patients, however, received unfractionated heparin during the angioplasty procedure. Unstable angina was present in 36% of patients. No differences were seen in the rates of periprocedural complications between the nadroparin recipients and the control group; rates of death (0.6% vs. 0%), AMI (1.1% vs. 1.1%), emergency bypass surgery (3.4% vs. 1.7%), and repeat PTCA (2.9% vs. 4.5%; all $p = NS$) were similar. It is unknown whether the difference between the REDUCE and FACT studies was a result of study design, enrollment criteria, chance, or the fact that the LMW heparin was not used during the PTCA procedure itself in the latter study.

It was hoped that use of the LMW heparins might abolish the rebound hypercoagulable state present after heparin discontinuation. Unfortunately, this has not been borne out in clinical studies. In the Fragmin During Instability in Coronary Artery Disease (FRISC) trial, 1506 patients with unstable angina or recent non–Q-wave MI were randomly assigned in a double-blind, placebo-controlled study to receive either dalteparin plus aspirin or aspirin alone for 6 days.[144] A significant risk reduction of 63% in the combined end point of death or reinfarction was present with dalteparin at 6 days (1.7% vs. 4.7%, $p = 0.001$), confirming the activity of LMW heparin in acute ischemic syndromes. However, within 3 to 5 days after discontinuation of the SC administration of dalteparin, there was a relative increase in adverse ischemic events in this group that continued for at least 5 weeks.[145] As a result, there was no long-term statistically significant reduction in death or reinfarction with LMW heparin treatment (plus aspirin) in comparison with aspirin alone (14.0% vs. 15.5%; $p = 0.41$ at 150 days). Thus, it is likely that antithrombotic treatment would have to be continued for 3 to 6 months after plaque disruption to avoid a rebound hypercoagulable state after drug discontinuation.

Finally, it had also been anticipated that both unfractionated and LMW heparins might reduce restenosis after PTCA. In this regard, although heparin has significant antiproliferative properties in vitro,[146–148] the ability of LMW heparins to inhibit smooth muscle cells is even greater and independent of their ability to bind AT-III.[148–150] Clinical studies have not, however, shown reduced restenosis with either IV or SC unfractionated heparin use after PTCA.[151, 152] In one small study of dalteparin, a trend toward reduced restenosis was seen in comparison with conventional treatment.[153] However, in the larger REDUCE study, there was no difference in angiographically documented restenosis between patients treated with extended subcutaneous reviparin and those treated with heparin (33.0% vs. 34.4%; $p = $ NS).[142] Two other studies with extended-use SC enoxaparin[154, 155] and one study with nadroparin[156] also failed to show any reduction in restenosis with LMW heparin after PTCA, even when given for 3 to 6 months. Thus, there is, unfortunately, no reliable evidence to suggest that either unfractionated or LMW heparin, when given systemically, has any significant salutary effect on restenosis after PTCA.

### Conclusions: Low Molecular Weight Heparin Use During Primary PTCA

Together, the results of the studies just discussed are inadequate for concluding whether LMW heparins are likely to have significant beneficial effects in patients undergoing percutaneous intervention as primary reperfusion therapy for AMI. The studies of LMW heparin use in patients with unstable angina suggest that early event rates may be somewhat reduced in comparison with IV unfractionated heparin, primarily because of a slightly reduced rate of recurrent angina. Bleeding complications are not increased with the use of these agents, except for local injection site ecchymoses. However, PTCA was rarely performed during the drug phase of these studies. Although the REDUCE study suggests that IV followed by SC reviparin may improve the acute safety profile of PTCA, this finding (a secondary end point of the trial) needs to be confirmed both in larger studies of patients with acute ischemic syndromes and with other agents. Unfortunately, there is no reported experience with enoxaparin and dalteparin (the two formulations currently available in the United States) during PTCA. Finally, there are no data regarding the use of these agents as an adjunct to primary PTCA or stent implantation in AMI, either acutely during the procedure or afterwards, as a replacement for the standard 48- to 72-hour post-PTCA course of IV heparin.

On the other hand, the SC route of administration and the lack of necessity for clinical monitoring make the LMW heparins easy to use for extended periods. Therefore, at present, it may be most rational to reserve the use of this category of compounds for suboptimal results after primary PTCA (or stent implantation: see later discussion), such as in patients with major residual dissection, thrombus, persistent filling defects, or TIMI grade 2 flow. Enoxaparin in a dosage of 1 mg/kg subcutaneously twice a day for 5 to 14 days, for example, might be used in this setting. However, the use of LMW heparin in these applications has not been studied, and it is unknown whether the benefits will outweigh the small but definite hemorrhagic risk that accrues with their use.

The Aspirin/Ticlopidine vs. Low–Molecular Weight Heparin/Aspirin/Ticlopidine High-Risk Stent Trial (ATLAST) is an ongoing double-blind, placebo-controlled investigation in which 2000 patients undergoing high-risk stent implantation (including acute and recent MI) treated with a standard antiplatelet regimen are randomly assigned to receive 14 days of SC enoxaparin or placebo.[157] The results of this trial will determine whether there are routine benefits of LMW heparin in any subset of patients who have received stents for stabilization of acute ischemic syndromes.

### Direct Thrombin Inhibitors

The direct thrombin inhibitors constitute a second novel class of drugs distinct from heparin; they work directly against thrombin, not requiring AT-III as a cofactor.[158–161] In addition, unlike heparin, which inhibits only circulating, unbound thrombin, the direct thrombin inhibitors are active against free and clot-bound thrombin.[160] This was thought to represent a major advantage of these agents over heparin, inasmuch as residual thrombus is a potent thrombogenic stimulus.[160] Finally, the direct thrombin inhibitors are not antagonized by plasma proteins or platelet factor 4. These agents appear to have an important role for patients with known heparin-induced thrombocytopenia undergoing percutaneous intervention, because there seems to be even less cross-reactivity in this regard than with the LMW heparins.[162, 163]

Two groups of direct thrombin inhibitors have been identified: those that occur naturally as derivatives from the saliva of the medicinal leech *(Hirudo medicinalis)* and those that have been synthetically produced.[159] Examples of the direct thrombin inhibitors are hirudin, bivalirudin (Hirulog), argatroban, efegatran, and inogatran.

In contrast to the LMW heparins, the direct thrombin inhibitors have been extensively evaluated in patients undergoing elective PTCA, those with unstable angina and those with AMI. The direct thrombin inhibitors have been shown to decrease platelet deposition at the site of balloon-mediated vascular disruption and, in animal models, to reduce restenosis after PTCA.[164–166] The initial use of the direct thrombin inhibitors as an adjunct to thrombolysis, however, was halted in three large pilot trials because of excessive hemorrhagic complications (especially intracranial bleeding).[167–169] As a result, the dosing regimens of these agents were modified to limit the total dose administered. This has, unfortunately, resulted in lowered efficacy of these drugs, although their safety profile is now similar to that of IV unfractionated heparin.

Results of completed studies suggest that the direct thrombin inhibitors may improve short-term outcomes in patients with acute ischemic syndromes, managed either medically (without thrombolysis) or with PTCA. In the Organization to Assess Strategies for Ischemic Syndromes (OASIS) Trial, 909 patients with unstable angina (82%) or AMI without ST elevation (18%) were treated with aspirin and randomly assigned to receive 72 hours of either IV heparin or low- or medium-dose hirudin.[170] In comparison with the heparin recipients, the patients treated with medium-dose hirudin had a lower rate of the composite of death, new MI, or refractory angina at 7 days (6.5% vs. 3.0%; $p = 0.47$), the primary end point of the study. The development of new MI was also decreased in the medium-dose hirudin recipients in comparison with the heparin recipients (1.9% vs. 4.9%; $p = 0.046$), as was the need for bypass surgery (1.1% vs. 4.0%; $p = 0.02$). PTCA was performed in only 5% of patients during the index hospitalization. Major bleeding occurred in only 1% of patients and was independent of anticoagulant strategy. Minor bleeding was more common with hirudin than with heparin, however (21.3% vs. 10.5%; $p = 0.001$). Further-

more, after discontinuation of hirudin, there was a significant increase in occurrence of adverse cardiac events in relation to the heparin recipients, so that at 180 days, there was only a weak trend for improved outcomes (death, new MI, or refractory angina) in the medium-dose hirudin recipients in comparison with the heparin recipients (13.6% vs. 9.4%; $p = 0.15$). The results of OASIS may not be applicable in the United States, in view of the infrequent use of angiography and revascularization procedures in the acute phase.

The results of direct thrombin inhibition were less impressive in the Global Utilization of Streptokinase and Tissue Plasminogen Activator for Occluded Coronary Arteries (GUSTO) IIb study.[171] In this large trial, 12,412 patients at 373 hospitals with transmural AMI and ST segment elevation (34%) or unstable angina or recent non–Q-wave MI (66%) received aspirin and were randomly assigned to receive 3 to 5 days of either IV heparin or hirudin in a double-blind manner.[171] Thrombolytic therapy was also administered to 74% of the patients with ST segment elevation. At 24 hours, the risk of death or MI was lower in the patients treated with hirudin than in those treated with heparin (1.3% vs. 2.1%; $p = 0.001$). At 30 days, however, the primary end point of death or new MI was reached in 8.9% of the hirudin recipients and in 9.8% of the heparin recipients ($p = 0.06$). The 30-day incidence of MI was decreased with hirudin in comparison with heparin (5.4% vs. 6.3%; $p = 0.04$); mortality rates in the two groups were identical. Whereas the rates of overall major bleeding complications were similar in the two anticoagulant regimens (12% with hirudin vs. 11% with heparin; $p = $ NS), intracranial hemorrhage was more common with hirudin treatment in patients without ST segment elevation (0.2% vs. 0.02%; $p = 0.06$), and moderate bleeding and the need for blood transfusions were more common with hirudin.

Several multicenter, prospective trials have used the direct thrombin inhibitors as an alternative to IV heparin during PTCA. In the Hirudin in a European Trial versus Heparin in the Prevention of Restenosis after PTCA (HELVETICA) study, 1141 patients with unstable angina undergoing PTCA were randomly assigned to receive either heparin or hirudin, administered intraprocedurally and for 24 hours afterward.[172] In comparison with heparin, hirudin was associated with a decreased incidence of the composite end point of death, MI, CABG, bailout procedure, or repeat PTCA within 96 hours (11.0% vs. 6.7%; $p < 0.01$). There were no excessive major (6.2% vs. 6.1%; $p = $ NS) or minor (11.3% vs. 14.1%; $p = $ NS) bleeding events with either drug. By 3 months after the procedure, however, a catch-up phenomenon was noted in the hirudin-treated patients, in that there was no difference in incidence of the primary composite end point (32.7% with heparin vs. 34.2% with hirudin; $p$ = NS). This late catch-up phenomenon is consistent with the demonstration that discontinuation of the direct thrombin inhibitors does not prevent the development of a hypercoagulable state, because of continuing new thrombin generation.[31, 173] Furthermore, at routine 7-month follow-up angiography, no difference was noted in late lumen loss or angiographic restenosis between the heparin and hirudin recipients.

In the larger Hirulog Angioplasty Study,[174] 4098 patients with unstable angina (83%) or postinfarction angina (17%) undergoing PTCA were randomly assigned to receive either heparin or bivalirudin immediately before dilatation. In contrast to the results from the HELVETICA study, which demonstrated fewer adverse post-PTCA events with direct thrombin inhibition than with heparin, there was no difference in the occurrence of the in-hospital composite end point of death, MI, acute vessel closure, or rapid cardiac deterioration in patients treated in this study with bivalirudin or heparin (11.4% vs. 12.2%; $p$ = NS). The incidence of the primary end point was, however, reduced with bivalirudin treatment among the 704 patients with postinfarction angina (9.1% vs. 14.2%; $p$ = 0.04). Overall bleeding complications were fewer in the bivalirudin recipients than in the heparin recipients (3.8% vs. 9.8%; $p$ < 0.001). At 6 months, the composite incidences of death, MI, or need for repeat revascularization procedures were similar in the patients treated with bivalirudin and those treated with heparin, both in the overall cohort (25.7% vs. 26.6%; $p$ = 0.54) and in the patients with only postinfarction angina (20.5% vs. 25.1%; $p$ = 0.17), further evidence of a catch-up phenomenon.

Only one study has directly investigated the value of a direct thrombin inhibitor as an adjunct to primary PTCA in AMI. In the GUSTO IIb Angioplasty Substudy,[175] 565 patients who had experienced AMI underwent a primary PTCA strategy within 12 hours of onset as part of a randomized trial; other participants received accelerated tPA. Of the patients assigned to undergo PTCA, the first 503 patients (89%) were subrandomly assigned to receive either heparin or hirudin for 3 to 5 days to keep the APTT 60 to 85 seconds. As seen in Table 12–8, there were no significant differences in the 30-day rates of death, reinfarction, or disabling stroke in patients undergoing primary PTCA assigned to receive heparin or hirudin, although the wide confidence intervals make it difficult to draw firm conclusions. A weak trend was present, in fact, the number of 30-day events was 24% lower in the hirudin-treated patients. The ability to demonstrate the efficacy of hirudin in patients undergoing primary PTCA may have been further limited in this study because angioplasty was performed in only 82% of the patients assigned to undergo primary PTCA. Other important clinical and angiographic end points, such as achievement of TIMI grade 3 flow, the development of recurrent ischemia, and the 6-month outcomes in the two groups were not reported. Nonetheless, on the basis of this trial, it appears that there is no marked advantage to using a direct thrombin inhibitor rather than heparin in patients with AMI undergoing primary PTCA.

### Conclusions: Direct Thrombin Inhibitors During Primary PTCA

The trials of direct thrombin inhibitors suggest that this class of agents possesses at most a small benefit (in relation to heparin) in reducing the periprocedural complications of patients with acute ischemic syndromes undergoing PTCA. In addition, the toxic-therapeutic window of this class of agents appears to be quite narrow. Heparin, by interfering with the coagulation cascade at a higher level, may actually have an advantage over the direct thrombin inhibitors by inhibiting thrombin generation as well as thrombin activity.[176, 177] Moreover, as a class effect, the relative efficacy of the direct thrombin inhibitors (as well as the LMW heparins) as an adjunct to

**TABLE 12–8.** **OUTCOMES OF PATIENTS WITH ACUTE MYOCARDIAL INFARCTION UNDERGOING PRIMARY PTCA IN THE GUSTO-IIb TRIAL, RANDOMLY ASSIGNED TO HEPARIN VERSUS HIRUDIN TREATMENT**

| 30-DAY OUTCOMES | PTCA + HIRUDIN (N = 256) | PTCA + HEPARIN (N = 247) | ODDS RATIO (95% CONFIDENCE INTERVAL) | $p$ |
|---|---|---|---|---|
| Death | 4.7% | 6.1% | 0.77 (0.34, 1.67) | 0.50 |
| Reinfarction | 4.3% | 4.5% | 0.97 (0.41, 2.27) | 0.94 |
| Disabling stroke | 0% | 0.4% | — | — |
| Any event | 8.2% | 10.6% | 0.76 (0.42, 1.39) | 0.37 |

GUSTO, Global Use of Strategies to Open Occluded Coronary Arteries in Acute Coronary Syndromes; PTCA, percutaneous transluminal coronary angioplasty.

improve the acute safety profile of PTCA in acute ischemic syndromes appears to be significantly less than that of the GPIIb/IIIa receptor inhibitors. In addition, a significant rebound phenomenon in adverse clinical events was present in all the studies after discontinuation of the antithrombotic agent, whether heparin, LMW heparin, or a direct thrombin inhibitors. As a result, much or all of the early benefit of the anticoagulant present during its acute administration is lost by 30 days, and the benefits of the direct thrombin inhibitors are not sustained at 6 months. In contrast, the sustained long-term reduction in death, MI, or need for urgent TVR after GPIIb/IIIa receptor inhibition suggests a more durable effect of marked platelet inhibition.

Finally, there is no evidence to suggest that the direct thrombin inhibitors or LMW heparins reduce clinical or angiographic restenosis after PTCA in patients with acute ischemic syndromes. In this regard, with the exception of the EPIC study, which demonstrated evidence of a late reduction in clinical restenosis,[77, 78] the lack of a long-term effect of TVR is concordant with the findings from the trials of the GPIIb/IIIa receptor antagonists, including RAPPORT, EPILOG, CAPTURE, and ERASER.[79, 80, 82, 85] Additional studies with the GPIIb/IIIa receptor blockers, LMW heparins, and direct thrombin inhibitors, are necessary, however, for a comprehensive understanding of the effects and utility of these agents in patients with AMI undergoing mechanical reperfusion.

## NEW CATHETER-BASED APPROACHES TO ACUTE MYOCARDIAL INFARCTION

There is accumulating evidence that the major limitations of primary PTCA (i.e., recurrent ischemia, reinfarction, and late restenosis) may be diminished by new catheter-based solutions. "New" devices (as distinguished from balloon angioplasty), particularly coronary stents, by alleviating the moderate residual stenosis that often remains after PTCA and by preventing or resolving post-PTCA dissection, offer the potential for improving early and late outcomes after mechanical reperfusion therapy in AMI. Primary PTCA is also complicated by the occasional occurrence of no-reflow and distal thromboemboli. In this regard, researchers have become interested in the use of thrombectomy devices in selected patients with AMI, either in a stand-alone mode or before definitive percutaneous intervention.

## Implantation in Acute Myocardial Infarction

Investigation during the 1990s firmly established that the routine implantation of coronary stents has

improved the safety of percutaneous intervention in comparison with balloon angioplasty alone in stable angina pectoris. Because stents create a round regular lumen free of dissection planes, the rates of acute closure and need for emergency bypass surgery are lower after stent implantation than after PTCA.[179–181] Furthermore, the recognized ability of stents to produce a larger postprocedural lumen than PTCA[182, 183] has translated into improved clinical and angiographic late outcomes in the elective setting.[178, 179, 184–186] However, implanting a permanent metallic endoprosthesis in an obviously thrombotic environment was, until the late 1990s, strictly avoided because of concerns of unacceptably high rates of subacute thrombosis[187, 188]; patients with AMI, recent MI, unstable angina, or angiographically visible filling defects were therefore excluded from all of the initial stent studies.

It is only since the late 1990s that stents have cautiously been implanted in patients with an evolving AMI. Stent use in AMI was first reported for individual patients for failed primary PTCA, then in small single-center retrospective series of bail-out use after failed primary or rescue PTCA, and later in single-center and multicenter prospective registry studies of routine (primary) stent implantation. The results of these reports were sufficiently positive that small single-center or multicenter prospective randomized trials were then performed and, more recently, large international multicenter trials compared results of a routine stent strategy with primary PTCA. A growing body of data is beginning to indicate that stent implantation in patients with AMI may be the most significant breakthrough in reperfusion therapy since the advent of primary PTCA. In view of the dominant role that stent implantation for AMI is likely to have, this subject is reviewed in detail.

### *Rationale for the Safety and Efficacy of Stent Implantation in Acute Myocardial Infarction*

Rather than being hazardous, the direct implantation of metallic stents in an acutely ulcerated and thrombosed atherosclerotic plaque may actually be safer than PTCA alone, for several reasons. First, stent implantation may reduce the frequency of post-PTCA complications that result in recurrent ischemia. In the PAMI-2 trial, in which primary PTCA was performed in 982 patients at 34 centers, the only predictors of recurrent ischemia and reocclusion of infarcted arteries after primary PTCA were a reduced left ventricular ejection fraction (LVEF) during the acute study and the presence of either post-PTCA residual stenosis affecting more than 30% of the luminal diameter or the appearance of any angiographic dissection[189, 190] (Fig. 12–10).

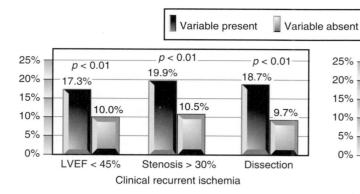

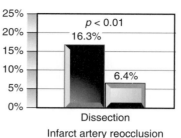

FIGURE 12–10. Correlates of in-hospital recurrent ischemia and reocclusion of infarcted arteries in the Second Primary Angioplasty in Myocardial Infarction (PAMI-2) trial. LVEF, left ventricular ejection fraction.

Stents, by sealing dissection planes and markedly reducing the post-PTCA residual stenosis, may therefore be expected to reduce the occurrence of these adverse events even if subacute stent thrombosis does, in rare cases, occur. By reducing recurrent ischemia, stent implantation may even facilitate early discharge after AMI and therefore may be cost effective or at least cost neutral.

Second, although in PAMI-2 residual stenosis affecting less than 50% of the luminal diameter with TIMI grades 2 to 3 flow could be restored in 98% of patients by PTCA and only 1.3% of patients required bail-out stent implantation, other series have reported significantly worse procedural results with primary PTCA, with correspondingly higher early rates of death and reinfarction.[175, 191] Stent implantation may therefore be useful in improving suboptimal results of PTCA at less experienced centers. In this regard, stent implantation may serve as the "great equalizer" to improve upon the results of operators unable to recreate the results in the PAMI and Zwolle trials.

### Studies of "Bail-Out" Stent Implantation in Acute Myocardial Infarction

Randomized trials of bail-out stent implantation in AMI after failed PTCA (e.g., in comparison with perfusion PTCA, conservative care, or surgery) have not been performed and are not likely to be in the future. The utility and safety of stent implantation in AMI after failed PTCA can be assessed, however, by a careful analysis of reported observational series, in which bail-out stent implantation after "failed" primary or rescue PTCA was performed in at least 70% of patients in each report (Tables 12–9, 12–10).[192–203]

A total of 1150 patients received stents in these studies, 90% of which were for a bail-out indication after unsuccessful PTCA. The Palmaz-Schatz stent with the sheath delivery system was the stent most frequently used in these series. Stents were implanted after failed rescue PTCA that followed unsuccessful thrombolysis in 9% of patients; the re-

mainder were for suboptimal results of primary PTCA without antecedent lytic therapy. Of note, after stent implantation, most patients were treated with aspirin indefinitely, ticlopidine for 4 weeks, and IV or LMW heparin for 3 to 7 days.

The rate of success of stent implantation for failed or suboptimal PTCA in these series was high, averaging 96%; subacute thrombosis developed in only 3.4% of patients (see Table 12–10). Because failure of PTCA during AMI portends an extremely poor prognosis (with mortality rates reported as high as 40%),[108–110] the 5.4% rate of early mortality, 1.2% reinfarction rate, and approximate 7.0% need for predischarge TVR in these studies after bail-out stent implantation are extremely favorable. Most of the deaths occurred in patients presenting with cardiogenic shock.

In the study by Schomig and colleagues,[199] half the patients who received stents were randomly assigned to receive treatment with aspirin and IV heparin, until full anticoagulation with warfarin; the other half were assigned to receive antiplatelet agents alone. The aspirin/warfarin regimen, in comparison with aspirin/ticlopidine use, was associated with a significantly higher incidence of stent thrombosis (9.7% vs. 0%) and with correspondingly increased rates of reinfarction and repeat target vessel PTCA (see Tables 12–9, 12–10).[199] Thus, aspirin, ticlopidine (4 weeks), and several days of either IV or SC heparin or enoxaparin should be considered standard treatment after stent implantation for AMI. It is unknown whether the postprocedure heparin course may be abandoned in patients with an optimal angiographic result.

There is less available information on long-term follow-up after a bail-out PTCA strategy in AMI. Data have been reported from 338 patients monitored for a mean time of 8.5 months after bail-out stent implantation for failed PTCA in seven studies (Table 12–11).[196, 198, 199, 202, 207–209] Although long-term outcomes have not been described in patients in whom primary PTCA failed and who were treated conservatively, the 10.8% rate of TVR and the com-

**TABLE 12–9.** **REPORTS OF BAIL-OUT STENT IMPLANTATION IN ACUTE MYOCARDIAL INFARCTION (TRIALS WITH 50 OR MORE PATIENTS)**

| AUTHOR/STUDY | NO. PATIENTS | NO. SITES | INDICATION | | POST-LYTICS‡ | STENT TYPE | ANTICOAGULATION AFTER STENT PLACEMENT | | | |
| | | | PRIMARY* | BAIL-OUT† | | | ASA | TICLOPIDINE | HEPARIN | WARFARIN |
|---|---|---|---|---|---|---|---|---|---|---|
| **Multicenter Trials** | | | | | | | | | | |
| Steffenino et al[192] | 150 | 6 | 17% | 83% | 13% | — | Yes | 78% | — | 7% |
| Monassier et al[193] | 134 | 20 | 18% | 92% | 19% | 83% PS | Yes | Yes | IVH × 72 h + LMWH × 7–14 days | No |
| Steinhubl et al[194] | 44 | 6 | 5% | 95% | 32% | — | Yes | 19% | — | — |
| **Single-Center Registries** | | | | | | | | | | |
| Glatt et al[195] | 266 | 1 | 27% | 73% | 0% | Multiple | Yes | Yes | IVH × 72 h | No |
| Spaulding et al[196] | 124 | 1 | 0% | 100% | — | PS | Yes | Yes | IVH × 3 days | No |
| Neumann et al[197] | 80 | 1 | 0% | 100% | 0% | PS | Yes | 37% | 63% IVH × 5–10 days | 63% |
| Repetto et al[198] | 66 | 1 | 0% | 100% | 29% | 91% PS | Yes | 85% | 15% IVH × 3–7 days | 15% |
| Schomig et al[199] | 62 | 1 | 0% | 100% | 0% | PS | Yes | No | IVH × 5–10 days | 100% |
| Schomig et al[199] | 61 | 1 | 0% | 100% | 0% | PS | Yes | Yes | IVH × 12 h | No |
| Levy et al[200] | 54 | 1 | 0% | 100% | 0% | — | Yes | Yes | LMWH | No |
| Horstkotte et al[201] | 53 | 1 | 0% | 100% | 0% | — | Yes | Yes | — | No |
| Hans-Jurgen et al[202] | 50 | 1 | 0% | 100% | — | PS | — | — | — | — |
| Himbert et al[203] | 50 | 1 | 0% | 100% | 18% | 50% PS | Yes | Yes | IVH × ≥5 days | No |
| **Pooled** | 1194 | 42 | 10% | 90% | 9% | — | — | — | — | — |

ASA, acetylsalicylic acid (aspirin); IVH, intravenous heparin; LMWH, subcutaneous low-molecular-weight heparin; PS, Palmaz-Schatz; RAI, Italian Angioplasty Registry; STENTIM, Stent in Myocardial Infarction. Dashes indicate not reported.
*Primary stent strategy intended regardless of PTCA result.
†Post-PTCA lesion is stent-implanted only if major dissection or residual stenosis.
‡Percentage of patients receiving stents as part of a rescue PTCA strategy after failed thrombolysis.

**TABLE 12–10.** **SHORT-TERM RESULTS OF BAIL-OUT STENT IMPLANTATION IN ACUTE MYOCARDIAL INFARCTION (TRIALS WITH 50 OR MORE PATIENTS)**

| AUTHOR/STUDY | PRIMARY SUCCESS RATE | STENT THROMBOSIS | SHORT-TERM OUTCOMES | | | | COMMENTS |
| | | | DEATH | REPEAT MYOCARDIAL INFARCTION | CABG | REPEAT PTCA | |
|---|---|---|---|---|---|---|---|
| **Multicenter Trials** | | | | | | | |
| RAI Registry[192]* | 95% | 6.6% | 5.3% | — | 2.7% | — | All high-risk acute myocardial infarction |
| STENTIM I[193]* | 96% | 3.0% | 4.5% | — | 1.5%‡ | — | 8.2% in cardiogenic shock |
| Steinhubl et al[194]* | 95% | 4.5% | 6.8% | 4.5% | 4.5% | 2.3% | |
| **Single-Center Registries** | | | | | | | |
| Glatt et al[195]† | 97% | 2.3% | 4.9% | 0.8% | 1.1% | — | 85% of the deaths were in patients in shock |
| Spaulding et al[196]* | — | 0.8% | 6.5% | 0% | 3.2% | — | 75% of the deaths were in patients in shock |
| Neumann et al[197]* | 99% | 2.5% | 8.8% | 1.3% | — | — | Mortality, 28.6% with shock vs. 4.5% without shock |
| Repetto et al[198]* | 97% | 4.7% | 1.5% | — | 4.7% | 1.5% | |
| Schomig et al[199]† | 100%¶ | 9.7% | 1.6% | 6.5% | 1.6% | 6.5% | Shock excluded; 21% received abciximab |
| Shomig et al[199]† | 100%¶ | 0% | 0% | 0% | 0% | 1.6% | Shock excluded; 20% received abciximab |
| Levy et al[200]* | 89% | 1.8% | 5.5% | — | 0%† | — | |
| Horstkotte et al[201]* | — | 0% | 5.3% | — | — | 7.9% | |
| Hans-Jurgen et al[202]* | 92% | 8.0% | 2.0% | 2.0% | — | 6.0% | |
| Himbert et al[203]* | 98% | 4.0% | 12.0% | — | — | — | 67% of the deaths were in patients in shock |
| **Pooled** | 96% | 3.4% | 5.4% | 1.2% | 1.9% | 5.1% | |

CABG, coronary artery bypass grafting; PTCA, percutaneous transluminal coronary angioplasty; RAI, Italian Angioplasty Registry; STENTIM, Stent in Myocardial Infarction. Dashes indicate not reported.
*In-hospital outcomes.
†30-day outcomes.
‡Emergency CABG only.
¶Unsuccessful stents (3.3%) excluded from this randomized trial.

**TABLE 12–11. LATE RESULTS OF BAIL-OUT STENT IMPLANTATION IN ACUTE MYOCARDIAL INFARCTION (TRIALS WITH 10 OR MORE PATIENTS)**

| AUTHOR/STUDY | NO. PATIENTS | FOLLOW-UP DURATION | LATE CLINICAL OUTCOMES | | | | | | PROTOCOL ANGIOGRAPHIC FOLLOW-UP | | | | |
|---|---|---|---|---|---|---|---|---|---|---|---|---|---|
| | | | DEATH | REPEAT MYOCARDIAL INFARCTION | CABG | REPEAT PTCA | TVR | COMPOSITE | N | FOLLOW-UP | DURATION | RESTENOSIS RATE | LATE REOCCLUSION RATE |
| Schomig et al[199] | 62 | 8 months | — | — | — | — | — | 24.2% | 52 | 83% | 6 months | 26.5% | 14.5% |
| Schomig et al[199] | 61 | 8 months | — | — | — | — | — | 18.0% | 49 | 90% | 6 months | 26.9% | 1.6% |
| Repetto et al[198] | 59 | 6 months | 1.7% | 0% | 3.4 | 0% | 3.4% | 5.1% | — | — | — | — | — |
| Spaulding et al[196] | 55 | 12 months | 10.9% | — | — | — | 10.9% | — | 95 | 82% | 7 months | 18.9% | 1.1% |
| Hans-Jurgen et al[202] | 50 | 4–6 months | 0% | 0% | — | — | 26.0% | — | 50 | 100% | 4–6 months | 40.0% | — |
| Rodriguez et al[207] | 29 | 12 months | 0% | 0% | 3.5% | 0% | 3.5% | 3.5% | — | — | — | — | — |
| Setiha et al[208] | 12 | 1.5 years | 0% | 0% | 0% | 0% | 0% | 0% | — | — | — | — | — |
| Ahmad et al[209] | 10 | 7 months | 10.0% | 0% | 0% | 0% | 0% | 10.0% | — | — | — | — | — |
| Pooled | 338 | 8.5 months | 4.8% | 0% | 3.0% | 0% | 10.8% | 13.3% | 246 | 87% | 6.2 months | 26.4% | 5.1% |

CABG, coronary artery bypass grafting; PTCA, percutaneous transluminal coronary angioplasty; TVR, target vessel revascularization. Dashes indicate not reported.

posite rate of 13.3% for death, reinfarction, or TVR at 8 months appears again to be improved over what would have been expected after suboptimal PTCA alone. In a subset of 246 patients undergoing angiographic follow-up at 6 months, restenosis was found in only 26% of patients; this rate was not significantly greater than that of restenosis after primary stent implantation (see later discussion). Late patency of infarcted vessels was documented in 98.7% of patients treated with aspirin and ticlopidine, as opposed to 85.5% treated with aspirin and warfarin.[199] The high rate of late patency of infarcted arteries in patients with stents who were treated with aspirin and ticlopidine compares well with those of historical controls of primary PTCA alone, in which 9% to 14% of infarcted vessels have been occluded at 6-month angiographic follow-up.[11, 20, 21, 23] As sustained late vessel patency after primary infarct intervention is a major determinant of myocardial recovery,[205, 210] stent implantation after failed primary PTCA would be expected to improve late left ventricular function.

Several caveats must be kept in mind when these data are considered. Most of these studies were retrospective; nine of the series represent a single-center experience, whereas three were multicenter; the data are incomplete in most cases, especially with regard to angiographic follow-up; and there was no uniformity in the post–stent implantation anticoagulation regimens. Of most importance is that the criteria required for bail-out stent implantation varied widely among the studies, ranging from a suboptimal post-PTCA result (stenosis involving >30% of the luminal diameter) to failed PTCA (stenosis involving >50% of the luminal diameter) to true acute or threatened vessel closure. In some of these series, minimal attempts were made to optimize the results of PTCA (e.g., with oversized balloons or with a perfusion catheter) before stent implantation. Nonetheless, this compilation provides a reasonably accurate picture of what may be expected after bail-out stent implantation in AMI as currently practiced.

### Current Recommendations for Bail-Out Stent Implantation

From these studies, reasonable recommendations for bail-out stent implantation in AMI may be formulated. It may be concluded that bail-out stent implantation has a high success rate with favorable short- and long-term outcomes when used after PTCA yields suboptimal results. Thus, bail-out stent implantation may unequivocally be recommended for most situations in which primary (or rescue) PTCA results in recoil or a severe dissection that compromises more than 50% of the luminal diameter. No firm recommendations can currently be made for stent implantation in the setting of successful but suboptimal PTCA results (e.g., stenosis affecting ≥30% but <50% of the luminal diameter, or any successful result with an NHLBI type B or worse dissection). However, some degree of dissection and recoil is almost always present after PTCA, often responds well to gentle balloon oversizing or perfusion dilatation, and is of no consequence in most patients.

Furthermore, data available from these studies are inadequate support for generalized recommendations for stent use after suboptimal PTCA in all circumstances. In view of the absence of prospective, randomized trials comparing bail-out stent implantation with other strategies, it is unknown whether this approach is cost effective if an acceptable primary PTCA result can be otherwise achieved or whether late outcomes are improved. Whether perfusion PTCA should be performed before stent implantation in stable patients with unsuccessful primary PTCA (i.e., without true acute or threatened closure, in which case expeditious stent implantation may be more preferable) is undetermined. In the elective setting, stent use after suboptimal PTCA results in improved outcomes in comparison with salvage balloon angioplasty[211]; it is unknown whether the same holds for stent implantation in AMI. Thus, stent implantation for stenoses affecting 30% to 50% of the vessel diameter and for mild, non–flow-limiting dissections cannot currently be routinely recommended until the results of the large multicenter studies of primary stent implantation versus primary PTCA are known and a positive effect is demonstrated in this regard.

Finally, on the basis of the available data, if bail-out stent implantation is performed, the recommended anticoagulation regimen is non–enteric-coated aspirin (enteric-coated aspirin after discharge); ticlopidine, 250 mg orally twice a day for 4 weeks, or clopidogrel, 75 g orally once daily for 4 weeks; and either IV or LMW heparin for at least 3 days. As discussed later, in comparison with a primary stent strategy, the rate of subacute thrombosis may be somewhat increased after bail-out stent implantation for primary PTCA (which argues for close follow-up of these patients), although the late outcomes appear equally favorable.

### Studies of Primary Stent Implantation in Acute Myocardial Infarction: Observational Series and Registry Studies

*Primary stent implantation* refers to the strategy of routine stent implantation in all patients in whom the infarcted artery contains one or more lesions eligible for and capable of receiving one or more stents, regardless of the adequacy of the initial primary PTCA result. Such a population therefore necessarily includes patients with a suboptimal angiographic PTCA result, as well as those with acceptable and even excellent outcomes after balloon dilatation alone. In this approach, the patient is brought to the cardiac catheterization laboratory and, after angiography, undergoes primary PTCA, if appropriate, to arrest the infarction process. The PTCA result is not intended to be optimal; rather, balloon dilatation is used to quickly halt the infarction process, thereby stabilizing the patient, and to permit visualization of the downstream vessel so that a decision regarding the appropriateness of stent implantation can be made. The principal goal of the primary stent approach is to improve late outcomes in comparison with PTCA alone, although, as discussed later, preliminary data from observational and randomized trials are beginning to indicate that in-hospital and 30-day results may also be enhanced over those of primary PTCA alone.

A comprehensive literature review revealed only six studies to date (each reporting 10 or more patients) in which the outcomes of a primary stent approach have been reported in a total of 544 patients (Tables 12–12 and 12–13).[212-217] Patients with cardiogenic shock were excluded from most of these series. Of note is that only one of these studies was a true prospective, controlled, multicenter investigation.[212] The Palmaz-Schatz stent was, again, the device most frequently used in these series, although the AVE Microstent predominated at one center.[215] As in the bail-out stent series, the antiplatelet/anticoagulant regimen most often used was aspirin, ticlopidine, and IV heparin for 2 days or more after stent implantation.

The average reported primary stent success rate was high (98%), and the low 1.8% rate of subacute thrombosis is similar to that reported for elective stent implantation when complex lesion subsets are routinely included (see Table 12–13).[218, 219] The reported short-term rates of death (0.9%), reinfarction (1.3%), need for CABG (1.8%), and repeat TVR (2.1%) are extremely favorable in comparison with those expected after primary PTCA alone, which suggests (1) a major early clinical benefit of primary stent implantation in comparison with primary PTCA, (2) significant patient selection, or (3) reporting bias.

There are few data describing late clinical and angiographic events after primary stent implantation. In the 18-patient series reported by Turi and associates,[217] the composite rate of death, reinfarction, or TVR at 6 months was only 11.1% among patients after primary stent implantation. In the small series by Saito and coworkers,[214] angiographic follow-up at a mean time of only 3 months in 48 (67%) of 72 patients demonstrated a restenosis rate of 17% with no vessel reocclusion. In the report by Medina and colleagues,[216] of 27 patients who underwent primary stent implantation, 15% developed restenosis by 6 months.

In the study by Siegel and associates,[220] the acute and late outcomes of 79 patients with AMI who underwent stent implantation between January 1995 and March 1997 (for either a bail-out or primary indication) were compared with the outcomes of 300 patients undergoing primary PTCA alone during the same period. There were no differences in the in-hospital rates of death (0.3% after primary PTCA vs. 0% after stent implantation) or emergency CABG (1.8% vs. 2.5%). With follow-up 95% complete at a mean time of 7.5 ± 4.5 months, patients treated with PTCA and those receiving stents had similar rates of mortality (2.0% vs. 1.3%), reinfarction (1.7% vs. 0%), repeat PTCA (6.0% vs. 6.3%), and late CABG (2.0% vs. 3.8%; all $p$ = NS). In view of differing patient baseline characteristics between the two populations and the retrospective nonrandomized nature of this study, no definitive conclusions can be drawn regarding the early and late

**TABLE 12–12.  REPORTS OF PRIMARY STENT IMPLANTATION IN ACUTE MYOCARDIAL INFARCTION (NONRANDOMIZED TRIALS WITH 10 OR MORE PATIENTS)**

| AUTHOR/STUDY | NO. PATIENTS | NO. SITES | POSTLYTICS* | STENT TYPE | ANTICOAGULATION AFTER STENT IMPLANTATION | | | |
|---|---|---|---|---|---|---|---|---|
| | | | | | ASA | TICLOPIDINE | HEPARIN | WARFARIN |
| *Multicenter Trials* | | | | | | | | |
| PAMI Stent Pilot[212] | 240 | 9 | 0% | 97% PS | Yes | Yes | IVH × 60 hours | No |
| *Single Center Registries* | | | | | | | | |
| Delcan et al[213] | 86 | 1 | 10% | PS or Wiktor | Yes | Most | IVH × >48 hrs | — |
| Saito et al[214] | 74 | 1 | 0% | PS | Yes | Yes | IVH × 48 hrs in 39% | No |
| Valeix et al[215] | 67 | 1 | 11% | 94% Microstent | Yes | Yes | — | No |
| Medina et al[216] | 59 | 1 | 0% | PS | — | — | — | — |
| Turi et al[217] | 18 | 1 | 0% | PS | Yes | 78% | IVH until warfarin | 94% |
| *Pooled* | 544 | 14 | 3% | — | — | — | — | — |

ASA, aspirin; IVH, intravenous heparin; PAMI, Primary Angioplasty in Myocardial Infarction; PS, Palmaz-Schatz. Dashes indicate not reported.
*Percentage of patients receiving stents as part of a rescue percutaneous transluminal coronary angioplasty strategy after failed thrombolysis.

**TABLE 12–13.     EARLY RESULTS OF PRIMARY STENT IMPLANTATION IN ACUTE MYOCARDIAL INFARCTION (NONRANDOMIZED TRIALS WITH 10 OR MORE PATIENTS)**

| AUTHOR/STUDY | PRIMARY SUCCESS RATE | STENT THROMBOSIS | SHORT-TERM OUTCOMES | | | | COMMENTS |
|---|---|---|---|---|---|---|---|
| | | | DEATH | REPEAT MYOCARDIAL INFARCTION | CABG | REPEAT PTCA | |
| **Multicenter Trials** | | | | | | | |
| PAMI Stent[212]* | 98% | 1.3% | 0.8% | 1.7% | 2.9% | 2.5% | Shock excluded; 5% received abciximab |
| **Single-Center Registries** | | | | | | | |
| Delcan et al[213]† | — | 3.5% | 1.2% | 0% | — | — | Patients in shock and bail-out recipients excluded |
| Saito et al[214]† | 97% | 1.4% | 1.4% | 1.4% | 0% | 1.4% | |
| Valeix et al[215]† | 96% | 3.0% | 1.5% | 1.5% | — | — | |
| Medina et al[216]† | — | 0% | 0% | 0% | 0% | 1.7% | |
| Turi et al[217]† | 100% | 5.6% | 0% | 5.6% | 0% | 0% | Patients in shock and with arteries with thrombus excluded |
| **Pooled** | 98% | 1.8% | 0.9% | 1.3% | 1.8% | 2.1% | |

CABG, coronary artery bypass grafting; PAMI, Primary Angioplasty in Myocardial Infarction; PTCA, percutaneous transluminal coronary angioplasty. Dashes indicate not reported.

*30-day outcomes.

†In-hospital outcomes.

efficacy of primary stent implantation versus primary PTCA from this report. This study does attest, however, to the excellent outcomes that can be obtained with primary PTCA alone and reinforces the necessity for prospective, multicenter, randomized trials comparing primary stent implantation with primary PTCA.

*The PAMI Stent Pilot Trial*

In the PAMI Stent Pilot Trial,[212] the feasibility, safety, and efficacy of primary stenting were studied in 312 consecutive patients with AMI who presented less than 12 hours after chest pain onset and who underwent primary PTCA at nine centers in the United States, France, and Brazil. This study represents the largest experience with primary stent implantation to date, and it was organized as a true prospective, multicenter trial incorporating an independent core angiographic laboratory; therefore, significant lessons can be learned from a detailed review of the reported results. Patients of any age with any electrocardiographic pattern of AMI were enrolled. The only major exclusion criteria were cardiogenic shock; absolute contraindications to aspirin, ticlopidine, or heparin; and inability to give informed consent. The algorithm for the PAMI Stent Pilot trial appears in Figure 12–11. After coronary arteriography and left ventriculography, PTCA was performed, if appropriate, to halt the infarction. All patients in whom PTCA was performed were formally entered into the study. After PTCA, the angiographic eligibility for stent implantation was determined. For this pilot trial, the target lesion was considered eligible for stent implantation if the reference vessel diameter was 2.75 mm or more (i.e., large enough to accommodate a ≥3.0-mm-diameter

sheathed Palmaz-Schatz stent), if the lesion could be covered by one or two 15-mm stents, if the lesion did not involve a major side branch (≥3.0 mm in diameter), if the lesion was not a true stenosis of the ostial left anterior descending artery (LAD) or ostial left circumflex artery (LCX), and if there was an absence of excessive proximal tortuosity or lesion calcification so that the operator was confident that the stent or stents could be successfully delivered to and deployed at the target lesion. No patient was excluded from stent implantation because of the presence of thrombus before PTCA or a small to moderate amount of thrombus after PTCA. However, if a large or gigantic amount of thrombus (length

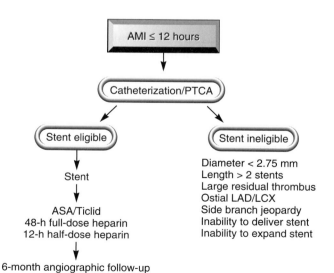

FIGURE 12–11. The study algorithm for the Primary Angioplasty in Myocardial Infarction (PAMI) Stent Pilot Trial. AMI, acute myocardial infarction; ASA, acetylsalicylic acid; LAD, left anterior descending artery; LCX, left circumflex artery; PTCA, percutaneous transluminal coronary angioplasty.

greater than twice the diameter of the infarcted artery) was present after PTCA and was refractory to repeated dilatation or adjunctive anticoagulant or antiplatelet agents, stents were not implanted. As described later, this situation occurred in only a small percentage of patients.

If the lesion was judged eligible for stent implantation, a stent or stents were implanted, regardless of the initial post-PTCA result. The Palmaz-Schatz stent was the stent predominantly used in this study, in view of its proven ability to reduce clinical and angiographic restenosis in prior randomized trials.[178, 179, 184] After deployment, the stent was, per protocol, dilated at 18 atm of pressure with a noncompliant balloon, because it had been demonstrated that the Palmaz-Schatz stent continues to expand as the pressure is raised from 12 to 18 atm.[221] All peristent edge dissections were to be treated by implanting additional stents. Furthermore, any lesion causing severe stenosis (involving ≥70% of the luminal diameter of the infarcted vessel) that constituted a potential inflow or outflow stenosis was also treated with stents if possible. Only the infarcted vessel was treated, however, in the acute phase. The goal of stent implantation was to obtain residual stenosis affecting less than 10% of the luminal diameter (visual assessment) with TIMI grade 3 flow, with no edge dissections or residual filling defects within or adjacent to the stent.

After stent implantation, patients were treated with aspirin indefinitely, ticlopidine for 4 weeks, and a 60-hour tapering IV heparin regimen to avoid a rebound hypercoagulable state.[222, 223] Sheaths were pulled before the heparin drip was started, however, if an excellent angiographic result was obtained without residual thrombus or dissection. Patients were discharged when stable, according to the PAMI-2 high- and low-risk guidelines[83, 84] and monitored for at least 6 months. Follow-up angiography was planned at 9 months in all patients with stents. All films were read by an independent angiographic core laboratory (at the Washington Hospital Center, Washington DC).

Stent implantation was considered feasible and was attempted in 240 (77%) of the 312 consecutive patients with AMI in whom primary PTCA was performed. In 236 (98%) of these patients, the stent was successfully deployed; in 4 patients, the relatively large-profile sheathed delivery system could not reach the lesion and was removed without stent loss. The predominant clinical reason for not attempting stent implantation was vessel size of 2.5 mm or less, which was present in 10% of patients. Only 5 patients (1.6%) did not undergo the procedure because of excessive thrombus burden. In comparison with patients in whom stents were not implanted, patients with stents were more likely to

have an infarcted vessel with a larger diameter and with a more proximal occlusion that affected blood supply to a greater amount of myocardium, with lower acute LVEF.[212]

The Palmaz-Schatz stent was used in 97% of lesions; Cook, Schneider, and AVE stents were implanted in the other 3%. A mean of 1.4 ± 0.7 stents were implanted per patient (range, 1 to 7) at 17.3 ± 2.4 atm. The median stent size was 3.5 mm. Intravascular ultrasound guidance was used in 20% of patients with stents. Core laboratory quantitative angiographic analysis revealed that the mean percentage of luminal diameter affected by stenosis was 12.1% ± 16.2% after stent implantation, in contrast to 33.3% ± 14.3% after PTCA only ($p < 0.0001$). TIMI grade 3 flow was restored in 94% of patients with stents. As seen in Figure 12–12, in-hospital events were uncommon after primary stent implantation. Subacute thrombosis occurred in 3 (1.3%) patients with stents, all within the hospital period.

A comparison of the in-hospital outcomes of all 312 patients in the PAMI Stent Pilot (76% of whom received stents) with those of the 982 patients undergoing primary PTCA in PAMI-2 (1% of whom received stents), the strategy of implanting stents in all eligible lesions resulted in lower rates of death, reinfarction, recurrent ischemia, and repeat PTCA of the infarcted vessel before hospital discharge (Fig. 12–13), despite the fact that the PAMI Stent Pilot patients presented later and were more likely to have triple-vessel disease.[224] Of note is that these results were obtained with the infrequent use of abciximab (in 5% of patients with stents) and intracoronary thrombolytics (in 1% of patients with stents). Within 30 days after hospital discharge, no patient with stents died, developed subacute thrombosis, or experienced a reinfarction, and only 1 patient (0.4%) required TVR. Thus, despite the well-known limitations of comparing registry expe-

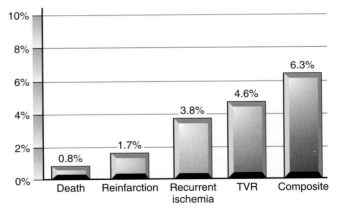

FIGURE 12–12. In-hospital events in 240 patients with acute myocardial infarction undergoing a primary stent strategy in the Primary Angioplasty in Myocardial Infarction (PAMI) Stent Pilot Trial. TVR, target vessel revascularization.

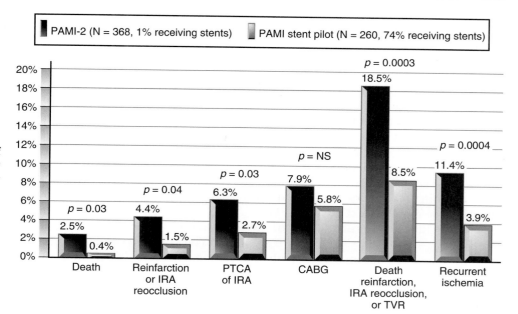

FIGURE 12–13. Comparison of the in-hospital outcomes in the Second Primary Angioplasty in Myocardial Infarction (PAMI-2) trial, in which only 1% of patients received stents, with those of the PAMI Stent Pilot trial, in which stents were implanted in 76% of patients. CABG, coronary artery bypass grafting; IRA, infarct-related artery; PTCA, percutaneous transluminal coronary angioplasty; TVR, target vessel revascularization.

riences to historical controls, these data suggest that rather than being dangerous, stent implantation in AMI may actually improve the acute safety profile of mechanical reperfusion therapy in comparison with primary PTCA.

An enlightening observation from this study was that stent implantation is an extremely effective approach to treating the thrombotic lesion. In the PAMI Stent Pilot,[225] thrombus was identified by the core laboratory as being present in 22.3% of lesions before PTCA and in 17.5% after PTCA ($p$ = NS). After stent implantation, however, angiographic thrombus was seen in only 3.0% of lesions ($p$ < 0.0001 vs. post-PTCA). Thus, considering only angiographic resolution of thrombus, stent implantation appears to compare favorably with intervention with other thrombectomy devices, such as the transluminal extraction catheter[226, 227] and the Angio-Jet.[228, 229] Furthermore, angiographic in-hospital clin-

ical outcomes were equally favorable in patients with and without thrombus (Table 12–14).

During a mean follow-up period of 7.4 ± 2.6 months after hospital discharge of the patients with stents, 1.7% died, reinfarction occurred in 2.1%, and TVR was required in 11.1%. The postdischarge 6-month TVR rate of 11.1% after primary stent implantation in this study compares favorably with the approximate 20% 6-month rate of TVR reported after primary PTCA (see Fig. 12–2) and is similar to that reported after elective stent implantation in the noninfarction setting.[178, 179, 184, 186, 230–232] Cox regression analysis revealed that the strongest determinants for the occurrence of TVR after hospital discharge were small reference vessel diameter (odds ratio [OR] = 2.2, confidence interval [CI] = 1.1, 4.6; $p$ = 0.03) and the number of stents implanted (OR = 2.0, CI = 0.9, 4.8; $p$ = 0.08).

Angiographic follow-up was completed in 76% of

**TABLE 12–14.  ANGIOGRAPHIC AND IN-HOSPITAL CLINICAL OUTCOMES AFTER STENT IMPLANTATION IN LESIONS WITH VERSUS WITHOUT ANGIOGRAPHICALLY EVIDENT THROMBUS (CORE LABORATORY DETERMINATION) IN PATIENTS WITH ACUTE MYOCARDIAL INFARCTION IN THE PAMI STENT PILOT TRIAL**

| OUTCOME | THROMBUS | NO THROMBUS | $p$ |
| --- | --- | --- | --- |
| TIMI grade 3 flow restored | 96.3% | 93.5% | 0.44 |
| Final diameter stenosis | 14% ± 14% | 12% ± 17% | 0.34 |
| No-reflow development | 0% | 0.6% | 0.99 |
| Distal thromboemboli development | 1.9% | 1.2% | 0.56 |
| Death | 1.9% | 1.7% | 0.42 |
| Reinfarction | 3.7% | 1.2% | 0.24 |
| Death or reinfarction | 3.7% | 1.7% | 0.34 |
| TVR | 5.6% | 4.6% | 0.78 |
| Death, reinfarction, or TVR | 5.6% | 4.6% | 0.78 |

PAMI, Primary Angioplasty in Myocardial Infarction; TIMI, Thrombolysis In Myocardial Infarction; TVR, target vessel revascularization.

eligible patients at a mean time of 7.8 months. Binary restenosis (defined as >50% of the luminal diameter affected by stenosis on any follow-up angiogram) was present in 27.5% of vessels with stents in this relatively unselected population, including reocclusion of the infarcted artery in 6.4%. This therefore appears to represent an approximate 40% reduction in restenosis and reocclusion of the infarcted artery after primary stent implantation in comparison with primary PTCA in historical controls (see Fig. 12–1).[11, 19–23] The independent predictors of binary restenosis included the absence of thrombus before PTCA (OR = 4.3, CI = 1.4, 19.0; $p$ = 0.02) and the implantation of two or more stents (OR = 2.2, CI = 1.0, 4.9; $p$ = 0.05). The relationship of the absence of thrombus to freedom from restenosis after stent implantation has not previously been described, possibly because thrombotic lesions have been excluded from most prior stent studies. In addition, however, the presence of angiographically evident thrombus may be a marker of less underlying plaque burden, which has been shown to be predictive of freedom from restenosis after stent implantation.[233, 234]

### The PAMI Heparin-Coated Stent Trial

One way to potentially improve the safety profile of stent implantation during AMI is to add a thrombus-resistant coating to the stainless steel surface.[239] In this regard, the agent that has received the most extensive study is heparin.[240–245] Heparin may be coated onto the stainless steel surface of a stent either passively or actively. In the Carmeda Bioactive Surface (CBAS) process, the longitudinal heparin molecules are covalently bonded to the stent surface in such a way that the active AT-III binding site is exposed to the blood stream, which contains circulating inactive AT-III. Activated AT-III, locally bound to the heparin molecule, is then able to complex and inactivate ambient thrombin. The inactivated AT-III/thrombin moiety then dissociates from the heparin molecule, which reexposes the active binding sites, allowing the process to continue.

The heparin-coated Palmaz-Schatz stent has been demonstrated, in a baboon arteriovenous shunt model, to be highly resistant to platelet and thrombus deposition in comparison with a noncoated Palmaz-Schatz stent.[240] In this experiment, the heparin-coated stent remained thrombus-resistant even when incompletely expanded or apposed to the vessel wall, two conditions in which the risk of subacute stent thrombosis is increased.[241, 242] The addition of heparin coating may therefore provide an extra level of protection against stent thrombosis if stent implantation technique is less than optimal (e.g., for low-volume operators).

Significant clinical experience with the heparin-coated stent suggests that the thrombus-resistant coating may indeed translate into lower rates of subacute thrombosis. The heparin-coated Palmaz-Schatz stent has been implanted in 616 patients in the Second Belgian-Netherlands Stent (BENESTENT-II) Pilot and randomized trials; only 1 case of subacute thrombosis (0.16%) was documented—a rate approximately one tenth of that expected.[245, 246] The utility of this device has also been tested in patients with recanalized chronic total occlusions and demonstrated a significant improvement in sustained arterial patency and a decrease in restenosis[246a] (results from the Total Occlusion Study of Canada [TOSCA] trial) and may be studied in patients undergoing stent implantation in small vessels (≤2.5 mm in diameter), both situations in which subacute or late vessel reocclusion rates have been reported to be increased.[218, 247]

The safety and efficacy of the sheathed heparin-coated Palmaz-Schatz stent system were prospectively examined in 101 consecutive patients undergoing primary stent implantation for AMI at 18 European centers in the PAMI Heparin-Coated Stent Pilot trial.[248, 249] In this study it was hypothesized that the heparin-coated stent, by virtue of its local anticoagulant effect, would obviate the need for systemic IV heparin. This, in turn, should reduce bleeding and vascular complications and facilitate earlier discharge. Thus, after successful stent implantation for AMI, patients were treated only with aspirin and ticlopidine.

The inclusion and exclusion criteria in the PAMI Heparin-Coated Stent Pilot trial were similar to those in the PAMI (non–heparin-coated) Stent Pilot trial, except for additional exclusion criteria—age more than 75 years, the absence of ST segment elevation, the infarcted vessel's being a saphenous vein graft, and acute LVEF of less than 35%. Otherwise, the baseline characteristics of the enrolled patients were typical; the mean age of the study population was 59 years, 14% of patients were female, 14% had diabetes mellitus, the mean time from chest pain onset to emergency room presentation was 3.2 hours, and the LAD constituted 54% of the infarcted vessels. One patient was excluded from analysis because of stent placement in a saphenous vein graft. The stent was successfully delivered in 98 of the remaining 100 patients. Independent core laboratory analysis (Cardialysis, The Netherlands) revealed that TIMI grade 3 flow was restored in 96% of patients; the remaining 4% had TIMI grade 2 flow. Of note is that abciximab was used in only 3% of patients, and no patient received intracoronary thrombolytic therapy.

The early and 6-month results are shown in Table 12–15. There were two in-hospital deaths (2%); one patient died from a nonhemorrhagic stroke, and the other from a severe gastrointestinal hemorrhage after

**TABLE 12–15.   SHORT- AND LONG-TERM OUTCOMES IN 100 PATIENTS RECEIVING HEPARIN-COATED PALMAZ-SCHATZ STENTS IN THE PAMI HEPARIN-COATED STENT PILOT TRIAL**

| OUTCOME | IN-HOSPITAL RATE | 30-DAY CUMULATIVE RATE | 7-MONTH CUMULATIVE RATE |
|---|---|---|---|
| Death | 2.0% | 3.0% | 4.0% |
| Reinfarction | 0% | 1.0% | 4.0% |
| Q-wave | 0% | 0% | 1.0% |
| Non–Q-wave | 0% | 1.0% | 3.0% |
| CABG | 0% | 0% | 2.0% |
| Repeat PTCA | 0% | 0% | 13.9% |

CABG, coronary artery bypass grafting; PAMI, Primary Angioplasty in Myocardial Infarction; PTCA, percutaneous transluminal coronary angioplasty.

renal failure necessitating dialysis developed. There were two deaths after the initial hospitalization (2%): One patient, who signed out against medical advice and refused to take aspirin and ticlopidine, died of recurrent MI and shock 2 days after discharge. The other patient developed ventricular fibrillation during exercise 4 months after discharge, and was resuscitated; repeat arteriography demonstrated no evidence of stent occlusion, but he subsequently died of noncardiac causes (pneumonia and sepsis).

The 6-month rate of TVR was 12.0% (see Table 12–15), which was similar to the rate of TVR in the PAMI (non–heparin-coated) Stent Pilot trial. At the end of the 6-month follow-up period, 96% of patients were alive; 93% were, in addition, free of reinfarction; and 81% of patients survived without reinfarction or need for TVR. At 6 months, 85% of patients were free of angina, 14% had stable angina, and 1% had unstable angina. The acute and follow-up angiographic results appear in Table 12–16. With angiographic follow-up completed in 88 patients to date, restenosis was present in only 16 patients (18.2%), and reocclusion of infarcted arteries was documented in only 3 patients (4.4%).

## Studies of Primary Stent Implantation in Acute Myocardial Infarction: Randomized Trials

The encouraging single-center and multicenter observational and registry experience with primary stent implantation in AMI has generated global interest in directly comparing the primary stent approach with primary PTCA. Eight prospective, randomized trials either are under way or have been completed (Table 12–17).

### The Zwolle Randomized Trial 5 (Principal Investigators: H. Suryapranata and F. Zijlstra)[252, 253]

In this single-center study from the Weezenlanden Hospital in The Netherlands, 227 patients with AMI and chest pain duration of less than 6 hours (<24 hours if symptoms were persistent) were randomly assigned to undergo either primary stent implantation with the bare mounted Palmaz-Schatz stent or primary PTCA. Recruitment began in June 1995 and concluded in March 1997. The post–stent implantation anticoagulation regimen included aspirin and warfarin in 1995; an aspirin/ticlopidine regimen was initiated in 1996. Of note is that no randomly assigned patient received IV abciximab or intracoronary thrombolysis.

The mean age of the patients was 58 years, 16% of patients were female, 20% presented in Killip class 2 or worse, 44% had multivessel disease, and the infarcted vessel was the LAD in 60% of patients; baseline attributes were well matched between the two treatment groups. There were also no differences in mean balloon size (3.4 vs. 3.3 mm) or pressure (13 vs. 12 atm) between the 112 patients receiving stents and the 115 undergoing primary

**TABLE 12–16.   ANGIOGRAPHIC OUTCOMES IN 100 PATIENTS RECEIVING HEPARIN-COATED PALMAZ-SCHATZ STENTS IN THE PAMI HEPARIN-COATED STENT PILOT TRIAL**

| CORE LABORATORY ANGIOGRAPHIC MEASURES | BEFORE PTCA | AFTER STENT IMPLANTATION | FOLLOW-UP (N = 88) |
|---|---|---|---|
| Reference diameter (mm) | 2.78 ± 0.46 | 3.05 ± 0.46 | 2.86 ± 0.61 |
| Minimal luminal diameter (mm) | 0.27 ± 0.45 | 2.52 ± 0.39 | 1.93 ± 0.71 |
| Diameter stenosis (%) | 90 ± 16 | 17 ± 8 | 33 ± 19 |
| TIMI flow grade | | | |
| 0/1 | 75% | 1% | 3% |
| 2 | 12% | 4% | 1% |
| 3 | 13% | 95% | 96% |

PAMI, Primary Angioplasty in Myocardial Infarction; PTCA, percutaneous transluminal coronary angioplasty; TIMI, Thrombolysis In Myocardial Infarction.

**TABLE 12–17.** **RANDOMIZED TRIALS OF PRIMARY STENT IMPLANTATION VERSUS PRIMARY PTCA**

| STUDY | ORIGIN | N | STENT | CROSSOVER* | COMMENTS |
|---|---|---|---|---|---|
| Zwolle Randomized Trial 5 | The Netherlands; single center | 227 | PS | 13% | Enrolled 50% of screened patients with acute myocardial infarctions |
| PASTA | Japan; 6 centers | 136 | PS | 10% | Only randomized TIMI grades 0–2 + RS > 50% after initial PTCA |
| STENTIM 2 | France; 17 sites | 211 | Wiktor | 37% | Randomization after angiography, before PTCA |
| PRISAM | Japan; multicenter | 300 | Wiktor | Not reported | Patients with TIMI grades 2–3 flow excluded |
| GRAMI | South America; 8 centers | 104 | GR-II | 25% | Randomization after wire crossing |
| FRESCO | Florence, Italy; single center | 150 | GR-II | 0% | Randomization after optimal PTCA only |
| PAMI randomized stent trial | USA/International | 900 | PS-H | ~16% | ~63% screened patients randomly assigned |
| CADILLAC trial | USA/International | 2600 | Multi-Link | Unknown | 2 × 2 randomization: PTCA ± abciximab vs. stent ± abciximab |

CADILLAC, Controlled Abciximab and Device Investigation to Lower Late Angioplasty Complications; FRESCO, Florence Randomized Elective Stenting in Acute Coronary Occlusion; GR-II, Gianturco-Roubin II stent; GRAMI, Gianturco-Roubin II Stent in Acute Myocardial Infarction; PASTA, Primary Angioplasty vs. Stent Implantation in AMI; PRISAM, Primary Stenting for AMI; PTCA, percutaneous transluminal coronary angioplasty; PS, Palmaz-Schatz stent; PS-H, heparin-coated Palmaz-Schatz stent; RS, residual stenosis; STENTIM 2, Stent in Myocardial Infarction; TIMI, Thrombolysis In Myocardial Infarction.

*Crossover from PTCA to stent implantation in patients initially assigned to undergo PTCA.

PTCA. Angiographic success rates were high in both groups (98% after stent implantation and 96% after PTCA; $p$ = NS), although 13% of the PTCA group "crossed over" to receive stents for treatment of dissection or threatened vessel closure. Subacute occlusion occurred in five PTCA patients (4.3%), in contrast to one stent recipient (0.9%; $p$ = 0.21). Thirty-day mortality was rare, occurring in three PTCA patients and one stent recipient ($p$ = NS). Reinfarction by 30 days also developed in three PTCA patients and one stent recipient ($p$ = NS). TVR, however, was performed in significantly fewer stent recipients than PTCA patients (2% vs. 10%; $p$ = 0.03), and thus the 30-day composite incidence of freedom from death, reinfarction, and TVR was higher among patients who received stents than among those who underwent PTCA (97% vs. 87%; $p$ = 0.02). There were no differences between the two groups in infarct size as measured by enzyme analysis (mean peak CPK levels, 1880 vs. 1743) and radionuclide LVEF (mean 44% vs. 45%) or in length of hospital stay (mean 5.3 vs. 4.8 days). Hemorrhagic complications tended to be slightly increased among the stent recipients (6.3% vs. 2.6%, $p$ = 0.18), largely because of the early use of warfarin in those patients in 1995.

At 9-month follow-up, there were no differences in the rates of death (3% vs. 4%) and CABG (6% vs. 13%) between the stent recipients and the patients who underwent PTCA. However, the stent recipients had lower rates of reinfarction (1% vs.

9%; $p$ = 0.02), need for repeat PTCA (4% vs. 16%; $p$ = 0.009), and TVR (PTCA or CABG, 10% vs. 29%; $p$ = 0.01). Thus, the combined 9-month primary end point of death, reinfarction, or TVR was reduced with the stent strategy in comparison with primary PTCA in this study (12% vs. 30%; $p$ = 0.001).

The improved freedom from TVR was mirrored by reduced rates of restenosis with stent implantation in this trial. Data from complete 6-month follow-up in 188 (83%) of patients revealed that patients with stents had a larger mean minimal luminal diameter than did the PTCA patients both immediately after the procedure (2.57 vs. 2.17 mm; $p$ < 0.0001) and at 6 months (2.07 vs. 1.82 mm; $p$ < 0.0002). The corresponding binary angiographic restenosis rates were 11% after primary stent implantation and 34% after primary PTCA ($p$ = 0.0009).

The 227 patients randomly assigned in this trial represented 50% of the 452 patients with AMI who were screened at this institution during this period; approximately half the patients not randomly assigned were excluded because of the presence of diffuse disease or because a vessel was too small for a stent. Of note were the outcomes reported from the 225 registry patients who were not randomly assigned. In comparison with those randomly assigned, the registry patients were older, more frequently presented in cardiogenic shock and required IABP, and were more likely to have multivessel disease. The rate of primary angiographic success was lower in registry patients than in randomly assigned patients (89% vs. 97%; $p = 0.0003$); this lower rate was associated with higher rates of in-hospital mortality (7% vs. 2%; $p = 0.01$), reinfarction (7% vs. 3%; $p = 0.05$), and TVR (14% vs. 4%; $p = 0.0001$) and with a longer hospital stay (mean, 8.9 vs. 5.1 days; $p = 0.0001$) in the registry patients.

### The Primary Angioplasty vs. Stent Implantation in AMI (PASTA) Trial (Principal Investigator: S. Saito)[254, 255]

The PASTA trial is a six-center Japanese prospective trial in which 142 patients with AMI of less than 12 hours' duration and initial TIMI grades 0 to 2 flow were randomly assigned to undergo primary stent implantation or primary PTCA. The randomly assigned study population represented 68% of the 230 patients with AMI enrolled at these centers during the study period. If residual stenosis affecting more than 50% of the luminal diameter or TIMI grades 0 to 2 flow was present after the first attempt at PTCA, an effort to obtain an acceptable PTCA result with a perfusion balloon had to be attempted before random assignment. Patients requiring bail-out stent implantation were excluded. Six patients (three from each group) were excluded because of failure to cross the lesion with a guide wire or a balloon, the presence of TIMI grade 3 flow, or crossover stenting despite an optimal PTCA result; this left 136 patients who could be randomly assigned. Patients with cardiogenic shock were not excluded. Patients were treated with aspirin, ticlopidine, and 48 hours of IV heparin after stent implantation.

Of the 136 patients, 69 were assigned to undergo primary PTCA and 67 to receive stents with the bare mounted Palmaz-Schatz stent implanted at 14 atm. Multiple high-risk features were present in the patients enrolled in this study; the mean age was 67 years, 28% of the patients were female, 20% had diabetes mellitus, 23% presented in Killip class 3 or 4, and TIMI grade 0 or 1 flow was present in 93%. Angiographic success was high in both groups (97.1% after stent implantation and 98.5% after PTCA; $p = $ NS), although bail-out stent implantation was required in 10% of patients who underwent PTCA. Comparison of the in-hospital outcomes in the two groups revealed that the composite incidence of death, reinfarction, and TVR was reduced in patients who received stents (6.0% vs. 18.8%; $p = 0.008$). The two groups had similar rates of mortality (3.0% vs. 7.2%; $p = $ NS) and nonfatal reinfarction (0% vs. 4.4%; $p = $ NS), although the composite rate of death and reinfarction was also lower in the stent recipients (3.0% vs. 11.6%; $p = 0.05$). Major bleeding was observed in

fewer than 2% of patients in each group. At 9-month follow-up, there was again no difference in the rates of death between the two groups (4.5% vs. 7.2%), although the combined incidences of death and reinfarction (4.5% vs. 13.0%) and of death, reinfarction, and TVR (20.9% vs. 46.4%) were lower in the stent recipients.

In-hospital angiography was performed immediately, at the time of hospital discharge, and 3 to 6 months later. Stent implantation acutely resulted in a greater minimal luminal diameter and a lower percentage of luminal diameter affected by stenosis in comparison with PTCA. At the time of discharge, significant recoil of the target lesion was present in patients treated with PTCA only, whereas no deterioration of the immediate poststent result occurred. Follow-up angiography demonstrates a significantly greater late minimal luminal diameter (mean, $2.24 \pm 0.64$ mm vs. $1.72 \pm 0.70$ mm; $p = 0.002$) and a correspondingly lower binary restenosis rate (17.0% vs. 37.5%; $p = 0.02$) in the patients with stents than in the patients who underwent PTCA.

### The Second Stent in Acute Myocardial Infarction (STENTIM 2) Trial (Principal Investigator: J. P. Monassier)[256]

In the STENTIM 2 randomized trial, which followed the STENTIM 1 pilot study,[193] 211 patients with AMI of less than 12 hours' duration were randomly assigned to undergo either primary stent implantation with the Medtronic Wiktor stent or primary PTCA; 17 sites in France participated. Patients with cardiogenic shock were excluded, as were those who had undergone prior PTCA or CABG within the previous 6 months. The primary end point in this trial was the incidence of angiographic restenosis and reocclusion of the infarcted artery at 6 months. Of note is that in contrast to the other trials, patients were randomly assigned after angiography but before PTCA was performed. The infarcted vessel had to be larger than 3.0 mm in diameter, and TIMI grades 0 to 2 flow had to be present before random assignment. Stents were implanted at 10 atm by protocol. The post–stent implantation anticoagulation regimen consisted of aspirin, ticlopidine for 30 days, and LMW heparin for 48 hours.

Baseline characteristics were well matched between the two groups; the mean age was 58 years, 19% of patients were female, 15% had diabetes mellitus, and the infarcted artery was the LAD in 51% of patients. Of 211 randomly assigned patients, 101 were assigned to receive stents which were successful in 99 (98%) of patients. Of the 110 patients assigned to undergo primary PTCA, 40 (36%) crossed over to receive one of a variety of stents.

The results, including the effects of this liberal bail-out strategy, were that TIMI grade 2 or 3 flow with residual stenosis affecting less than 50% of the luminal diameter was achieved in 97% of both groups, and TIMI grade 3 flow with residual stenosis affecting less than 50% of the luminal diameter was achieved in 89% of patients who underwent PTCA and in 93% of stent recipients.

Intention-to-treat analysis revealed no significant differences in the in-hospital rates of death (1.0% vs. 0%), reinfarction (4.0% vs. 3.7%), recurrent ischemia (5.1% vs. 5.6%), or TVR (5.1% vs. 5.6%) between patients who received stents and those who underwent PTCA, respectively. The composite incidences of in-hospital death, reinfarction, repeat angiography, and TVR were identical (6%) in the two groups. No patient in this trial suffered a stroke. The durations of hospitalization were also reported to be similar in the two groups (10.2 vs. 9.9 days; $p =$ NS). Core laboratory angiographic analysis (performed at Cardialysis) and late clinical follow-up are pending.

### The Primary Stenting for AMI (PRISAM) Study (Principal Investigator: H. Tamai)[257, 258]

In the PRISAM study, 300 patients aged 40 to 79 years with AMI are enrolled, within 24 hours of onset, at multiple Japanese centers and randomly assigned to undergo either primary PTCA or implantation with the Wiktor stent. Patients are randomly assigned after primary PTCA if the lesion is less than 20 mm in length, more than 2.5 mm in diameter, and nonostial. Patients with cardiogenic shock and those in whom TIMI grade 2 or 3 flow is shown in the infarcted vessel on the first angiogram are excluded. Preliminary data from the first 130 patients have been released. With 65 patients treated in each group, the procedural success rate was reported to be 100% after both stent implantation and PTCA, and no patient died, required emergency CABG, or had a major bleeding complication after either treatment. Subacute vessel closure developed in 1.5% of stent recipients, in contrast to 6.2% of PTCA patients ($p =$ NS). At 6 months, TVR was required in 10 patients with stents, in contrast to 22 who had undergone primary PTCA alone (15.4% vs. 33.8%; $p < 0.05$).

Preliminary angiographic analysis demonstrated that the immediate postprocedure minimal luminal diameter was larger in the stent recipients (mean, 2.66 vs. 2.27 mm; $p < 0.0005$), which resulted in a lower binary rate of restenosis in the stent recipients, of the initial 70 patients in whom 6-month angiographic follow-up is completed (32.3% vs. 59.0%; $p < 0.05$). There was a trend for a reduced rate of late reocclusion of the infarcted artery among stent recipients in comparison with those treated with PTCA alone (9.7% vs. 18.0%; $p =$ NS).

### The Gianturco-Roubin II Stent in Acute Myocardial Infarction (GRAMI) Trial (Principal Investigator: A. Rodriguez)[259]

In the GRAMI trial, 104 patients aged 75 years or younger who had suffered AMI within the previous 24 hours were randomly assigned to undergo either primary stent implantation with the Cook-Gianturco-Roubin II stent or primary PTCA at eight centers in Argentina, Chile, and Uruguay. Random assignment occurred after successful wire crossing of the lesion. After stent implantation, patients were chronically treated with aspirin and ticlopidine. IV heparin was administered for 48 hours. Of note is that 16% of patients enrolled in this study were in Killip class 3 or 4.

Angiographic success (which required residual stenosis affecting less than 30% of the luminal diameter with dissection score of less severity than NHLBI type B) before crossover was present in 98.1% of stent recipients, in contrast to only 69.5% of PTCA patients ($p < 0.0001$); bail-out stent implantation was performed in 25.0% of patients who had undergone PTCA. Rates of final angiographic success, determined after the outcomes of crossover stent implantation, were similar in patients who received stents and those who underwent PTCA (98.1% vs. 94.2%; $p =$ NS). The composite incidence of death, reinfarction, TVR, and recurrent ischemia was significantly lower in stent recipients than in patients who underwent PTCA, both in hospital (4% vs. 19%; $p = 0.03$) and 1 year later (17% vs. 35%; $p = 0.002$), primarily because the rates of death or reinfarction were lower after stent implantation in the patients who presented in Killip class 3 or 4. At 30 days, there were no statistically significant differences after stent implantation and after PTCA in the rates of death (2.0% vs. 4.0%), reinfarction (0% vs. 7.7%), or repeat PTCA of the infarcted vessel (0% vs. 5.8%); most of the difference in the prespecified 30-day end point was attributable to reduced recurrent ischemia in the stent recipients (0% vs. 11.5%; $p = 0.02$). Furthermore, by 1 year there were no significant differences in the rates of TVR (11.5% vs. 15.4%; $p =$ NS), or in angiographic restenosis (determined in 51% of patients) (17.4% vs. 21.1%; $p =$ NS) after primary stent implantation and after primary PTCA in this trial.

### The Florence Randomized Elective Stenting in Acute Coronary Occlusion (FRESCO) Study (Principal Investigator: D. Antoniucci)[260, 261]

The study design of the FRESCO trial differs from that of the others in that patients were not randomly assigned to undergo stent implantation or PTCA unless an optimal primary PTCA result had been achieved (defined as TIMI grade 3 flow with residual stenosis affecting <30% of the luminal diameter). This trial was therefore a test of a "provisional stent strategy" after successful primary PTCA. As in the GRAMI trial, the Cook-Gianturco-Roubin II was the stent of choice in this investigation. Of note is that 9% of patients were in cardiogenic shock when enrolled. The only angiographic exclusion criterion was reference vessel diameter of less than 2.5 mm. Repeat catheterization was planned at 48 to 72 hours, 1 month, and 6 months after the index procedure.

Of 223 patients enrolled who underwent primary PTCA, 150 (67%) met the criterion of optimal PTCA; 75 were subsequently randomly assigned to undergo stent implantation and 75 to undergo PTCA only. Stents (88% of which were Gianturco-Roubin II) were implanted successfully in all patients randomly assigned to receive stents. By study design, stents were implanted in none of the patients assigned to PTCA only. An optimal result was obtained in 100% of PTCA patients and 99% of stent recipients (1 stent recipient developed persistent TIMI grade 2 flow after stent implantation). At 30 days, the combined end point of death, reinfarction, and ischemia-driven TVR was reached in 11 primary PTCA patients (15%), as opposed to 2 stent recipients (3%) ($p < 0.01$). There were no statistically significant differences in the individual components of cardiac death (0% in both groups), reinfarction (2.7% vs. 1.3%), or TVR (12.0% vs. 1.3%; $p = 0.08$) between the PTCA patients and the stent recipients, respectively.

Six-month follow-up has been completed for 115 patients. The primary composite end point was reached in a significantly greater proportion of patients who underwent only PTCA than of those who received stents (26% vs. 10%; $p = 0.03$). Again, there were no differences in rates of mortality (0% vs. 1.7%) or reinfarction (1.7% in both groups); the primary end point was driven by a significantly greater need for TVR in the PTCA-only patients than in the patients who received stents (25% vs. 7%; $p = 0.009$). Angiographic follow-up is ongoing; interim restenosis rates are reported to be 33% after primary PTCA only, in contrast to 15% after stent implantation ($p = 0.036$).

## Lessons from the Completed Randomized Trials of Primary PTCA Versus Stent Implantation

On the basis of the results from these six studies, it appears that primary stent implantation and primary PTCA achieve similar rates of acute angio-

graphic success (although as expected, the acute and predischarge luminal dimensions are greater after stent implantation than after PTCA). However, 10% to 40% of patients randomly assigned to undergo PTCA in these trials "crossed over" and received stents (except in FRESCO, by design). This finding is in striking contrast to PAMI-2, wherein only 1.3% of 982 patients undergoing primary PTCA later received stents, and demonstrates the readiness of present-day operators to rely on stents. Thus, rather than being studies of pure primary PTCA versus primary stent implantation, these trials more accurately compared a strategy of primary PTCA, accompanied by variable degrees of provisional stent implantation for suboptimal results, with primary stent implantation. With this proviso, no overall differences were present in the short-term rates of death or reinfarction after stent implantation and after PTCA (except possibly in high-risk patients in GRAMI), although the numbers of patients enrolled were singly and collectively too few to reliably demonstrate such differences. Primary stent implantation did, however, seem to lower the necessity for repeat urgent TVR before hospital discharge in these trials, in comparison with primary PTCA.

## The PAMI Heparin-Coated Stent Randomized Trial

After the promising results of the PAMI Stent Pilot Trial and the PAMI Heparin-Coated Stent Trial were analyzed, it was concluded that stent deployment could be safely performed in patients with AMI. Whether immediate or long-term outcomes could be enhanced compared with PTCA was uncertain; therefore, the PAMI Heparin-Coated Stent Randomized Trial was conducted. Over an 11-month period, 1458 patients presenting within 12 hours of symptom onset of AMI were screened in 69 centers. Of these patients, 900 met inclusion criteria and were randomized to PTCA therapy or routine stent implantation. Patients were excluded because of surgical anatomy, infarcted vessels unsuitable for stent implantation, or severe flow-limiting dissections mandating bail-out stenting. This study should therefore be viewed as testing the strategy of PTCA alone with stent bail-out versus routine stent implantation after an acceptable PTCA result.

The overall clinical and angiographic results are depicted in Table 12–18. The primary end point of this trial was event-free survival at 7 months (Fig. 12–14). Some interesting and surprising findings occurred. As expected, event-free survival (largely driven by TVR) was significantly improved by routine stent implantation. A surprising lower rate of TIMI grade 3 flow occurred in the stent group, which was associated with a worrisome trend to-

**TABLE 12–18.  CLINICAL AND ANGIOGRAPHIC RESULTS OF THE PAMI HEPARIN-COATED STENT RANDOMIZED TRIAL**

|  | STENT | PTCA | p VALUE |
|---|---|---|---|
| N | 452 | 448 | |
| Angio. restenosis (6.5 mon) | 23.5% | 35.4% | <0.0001 |
| Ischemic TVR (6 mon) | 10.6% | 21.0% | <0.0001 |
| TIMI-3 flow final (operator) | 92.9% | 96.4% | 0.02 |
| TIMI-3 flow final (core lab) | 89.5% | 92.7% | 0.046 |
| Mortality (12 mon) | 5.4% | 3.0% | 0.054 |
| Stent | | Heparin-coated PS-153 | |
| Abciximab | 5.8% | 4.5% | NS |

wards a higher mortality at 12 months in the stent group. It is speculated that the bulky delivery sheath and rigid stent as well as the mandatory high-pressure implantation all contributed to distal embolization decrease in microvascular flow and to increased mortality. Thus, the randomized PAMI trial validated the benefit of stent implantation but raised a flag of caution concerning distal embolization.

### The Controlled Abciximab and Device Investigation to Lower Late Angioplasty Complications (CADILLAC) Trial

The PAMI Stent Trial has allowed important conclusions to be drawn regarding the clinical and angiographic outcomes, and cost effectiveness, of a heparin-coated stent strategy in comparison with primary PTCA. The PAMI Stent Trial has suggested a disturbing higher late mortality after stent implantation that may be due in part to stent design. Furthermore, the final major piece of the AMI interven-

tion puzzle unaddressed by this trial is the possible role of GPIIb/IIIa receptor blockade as an adjunct to primary PTCA or primary stent implantation. As discussed earlier, GPIIb/IIIa receptor blockade holds promise of improving the early outcomes after primary PTCA, although the high doses of heparin and prolonged sheath dwell times in most of the early trials resulted in excessive bleeding rates with the active antiplatelet agent.

Furthermore, until 1997, no study had examined the possible role of GPIIb/IIIa blockade during AMI stent implantation. Indeed, with the low rates of recurrent ischemia and of the need for TVR seen with primary stent implantation even with a non–heparin-coated stent, the utility of combining these two approaches may be questioned. A provocative study by Neumann and coworkers suggests that GPIIb/IIIa receptor antagonism during AMI stent implantation may in fact have value.[262] In this trial, 200 patients who underwent coronary stent implantation within 48 hours of AMI at a single center were treated with aspirin and heparin and then were prospectively assigned randomly to receive either abciximab in a bolus plus a 12-hour infusion ($N = 102$) or placebo ($N = 98$) before stent implantation. Although the primary success rates were 99% in both groups, 10 placebo patients "crossed over" and received abciximab during the procedure for complications. The overall incidence of major adverse cardiac complications (death, reinfarction, or TVR) was 2.0% in the abciximab recipients, as opposed to 9.2% in the placebo recipients ($p = 0.03$), mostly as a result of a lower need for repeat PTCA in the abciximab-treated patients. Furthermore, at repeat catheterization, the abciximab recipients had greater global and regional left ventricular function and greater peak coronary flow velocity (Fig. 12–15).

These data suggest that abciximab, as an adjunct to stent implantation during AMI or after recent MI, may reduce recurrent ischemia and result in greater myocardial recovery. In view of the single center nature of this study, however, and the relatively high failure rate among the placebo recipients that necessitated bail-out abciximab. Firm conclusions

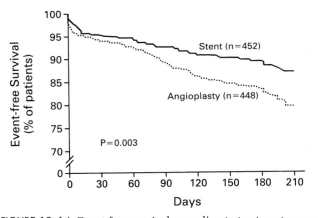

FIGURE 12–14. Event-free survival according to treatment group. Event-free survival was greater in the group of patients assigned to implantation of a heparin-coated stent than in the group assigned to primary angioplasty alone ($p = 0.003$ by the log-rank test). This difference was due to the lower proportion of patients in the stent group who underwent target-vessel revascularization for ischemia. Events (other than death) included reinfarction, disabling stroke, and target-vessel revascularization for ischemia. (From Grines CL, Cox DA, Stone GW, et al: Coronary angioplasty with or without stent implantation for acute myocardial infarction. N Engl J Med 341:1949–1956, 1999.)

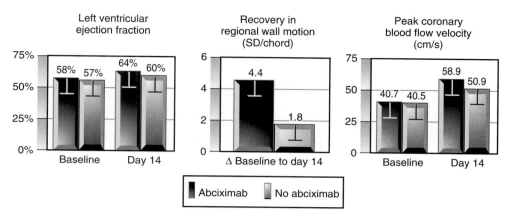

FIGURE 12–15. Changes in left ventricular ejection fraction, regional wall motion, and peak coronary flow velocity in patients receiving stents during acute myocardial infarction who were randomly assigned to receive abciximab or no abciximab; comparisons of the baseline and 14 day follow-up angiograms.[262] See text for details.

regarding the role of GPIIb/IIIa receptor inhibition during stent implantation for AMI must await the results of larger, multicenter trials.

In addition, by blocking the vitronectin receptor, which is involved in the regulation of smooth muscle cell proliferation and migration,[73, 74] abciximab has been postulated to possess anti-restenotic properties.[263] Results of the completed trials of PTCA with abciximab in acute ischemic syndromes, however, have not supported the presence of a clinically significant anti-restenosis property of abciximab. However, whereas the restenosis process after PTCA is complex, involving variable degrees of vessel recoil, remodeling, and neointimal proliferation, restenosis after stent implantation is caused solely by neointimal ingrowth within the stent.[264] Furthermore, organization of the platelet-rich thrombus, as well as thrombus-mediated stimulation of smooth muscle cell proliferation and migration, has also been implicated in the development of restenosis.[265] Thus, if an agent such as abciximab does indeed have anti-restenosis properties, the ideal model for demonstrating this effect would be stent implantation during AMI, in which thrombus is invariably present to some degree.

The CADILLAC trial was formulated (1) to examine the ability of a new stent with enhanced design features to improve outcomes in AMI intervention in relation to primary PTCA and (2) to investigate the role of GPIIb/IIIa receptor blocking agents as an adjunct to both primary PTCA and primary stent implantation to improve short- and long-term outcomes. In the CADILLAC trial, 2665 patients with AMI onset within the past 12 hours (patients with cardiogenic shock excluded) were randomly assigned at 76 international centers to undergo one of four protocols: primary PTCA alone, primary PTCA with IV abciximab (standard bolus plus 12-hour infusion), primary stent implantation with the Multi-Link stent, or primary Multi-Link stent implantation with abciximab (bolus plus a 12-hour infusion). The algorithm of the CADILLAC trial is shown in Figure

12–16. Random assignment is performed after angiography but before PTCA. The Multi-Link stent was available in sizes to treat vessels ranging from 2.5 to 4.0 mm in diameter, and the enhanced flexibility of this stent allows inclusion of lesions up to 65 mm in length. Patients assigned to either of the abciximab protocols received no additional postprocedure heparin; in these patients, the peak ACT was meticulously limited to 200 to 300 seconds, and sheaths were removed 4 to 6 hours after the procedure. These approaches should minimize bleeding complications as in the EPILOG trial.[79] Furthermore, because abciximab has an extended antiplatelet biologic effect that lasts for several days after discontinuation of the IV infusion,[266] this agent has the potential to stabilize the freshly dilated or stent-implanted infarcted lesion, which should prevent recurrent ischemia and closure of the infarcted vessel after mechanical reperfusion. Thus, postprocedure heparin was used in abciximab-treated patients, and all abciximab-treated patients with an optimal angiographic result (stent or PTCA) were targeted for accelerated discharge on day 2 (day 3 in high-risk patients). In this way, CADILLAC is the most ambitious early discharge study yet attempted. In non–abciximab-treated patients, the standard 60-hour tapering heparin regimen is recommended, followed by discharge of stable patients shortly thereafter. Clinical follow-up will continue for 12 months, with protocol-driven angiographic restudy planned at 7 months in a subset of 700 patients. Core laboratory analysis of all films will be performed at the Washington Hospital Center.

The primary composite end point in CADILLAC is the 6-month composite incidence of death, reinfarction, disabling stroke, or ischemia-driven TVR. Detailed cost-effectiveness analysis is also an integral part of this study. As in PAMI, blinded intravascular ultrasound study will be performed at selected centers at the completion of PTCA and stent implantation to evaluate the potential prognostic role of ultrasonography after AMI intervention. Further-

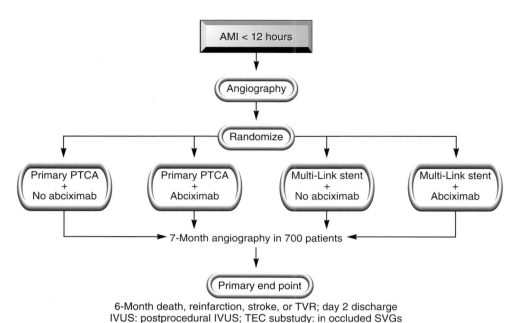

FIGURE 12–16. The study algorithm for the Controlled Abciximab and Device Investigation to Lower Late Angioplasty Complications (CADILLAC) trial. Abciximab-treated patients with an optimal result (stent or percutaneous transluminal coronary angioplasty [PTCA]) receive no postprocedural heparin and are scheduled for discharge on day 2 or 3, the safety of which is a major secondary end point. AMI, acute myocardial infarction; IVUS, intravascular ultrasound; SVG, saphenous vein graft; TEC, transluminal extraction catheter; TVR, target vessel revascularization.

more, a thrombectomy substudy is being performed with patients with AMI caused by saphenous vein graft disease (excluded from the primary random assignment), in whom the results of primary PTCA are known to be less successful than in patients with native coronary artery occlusion. At sites qualified for thrombectomy, patients will undergo thrombectomy with the transluminal extraction catheter, followed by PTCA or stent implantation, whereas at other sites, abciximab will be used at an adjunct to percutaneous intervention.

The preliminary results of the CADILLAC Trial have now been reported (Table 12–19).[266a–266d] Unlike in PAMI, no decrement in TIMI grade 3 flow occurred with stent implantation. In-hospital mortality was less than 2% in all subgroups, and 6-month mortality did not differ between these groups. Like PAMI, CADILLAC demonstrated a significant reduction in angiographic restenosis and TVR for stent therapy. The major advantage of additional abciximab therapy after routine stent placement was a reduction in subacute stent thrombosis.

No decrease in restenosis or TVR occurred with the addition of abciximab to stent therapy. Abciximab did appear to improve clinical outcome after PTCA therapy. A trend towards decreased mortality (4.3% vs. 2.3%) and decrease in major adverse cardiac events (18.4% vs. 14.2%, $p = 0.06$) occurred when abciximab was added to PTCA treatment. Finally, unlike the Neumann study,[262] no additional benefit with respect to improved ventricular function occurred with the addition of abciximab. This study thus demonstrated that routine stent implantation with modern lower profile devices is safe and results in decreased angiographic and clinical restenosis. Only marginal benefit is conferred to stent therapy by addition of abciximab. In contrast, abciximab does improve initial and long-term outcome after PTCA therapy alone.

### Conclusions and Recommendations for Stent Implantation in Acute Myocardial Infarction

Currently, on the basis of the data available from single-center registries and PAMI Stent and CADIL-

**TABLE 12–19.    END POINT RESULTS OF CADILLAC TRIAL**

|  | PTCA | PTCA/ABCIXIMAB | STENT | STENT/ABCIXIMAB |
|---|---|---|---|---|
| N | 516 | 529 | 512 | 525 |
| TIMI-3 flow (%) | 95.3 | 96.3 | 94.6 | 96.1 |
| 6-month events |  |  |  |  |
| Death (%) | 4.3 | 2.3 | 2.7 | 3.8 |
| Stroke (%) | 0.2 | 0 | 0.2 | 0.6 |
| Re MI (%) | 1.6 | 2.1 | 1.2 | 2.3 |
| TVR | 14.0 | 11.9 | 7.2 | 5.0 |
| MACE | 18.4 | 14.2 | 10.4 | 9.5* |

*$p = 0.0001$.

LAC studies, stent implantation for AMI can be unequivocally recommended for patients undergoing primary PTCA of vessels 3.0 to 4.0 mm in diameter that is unsuccessful (residual stenosis affecting ≥50% of the luminal diameter) because of either significant dissection or elastic recoil. Primary stent implantation can also be recommended for acceptable but suboptimal results of primary PTCA. Results of the studies reported to date are sufficient for concluding that a stent should be implanted if an optimal PTCA result is obtained (residual stenosis affecting <30% of the luminal diameter) because long-term adverse clinical events are reduced by this therapy. Further studies are necessary to evaluate the results of primary stent implantation in smaller vessels and in complex lesion subsets and to establish the cost effectiveness of primary stent implantation in relation to primary PTCA. GPIIb/IIIa receptor antagonists do not appear to further improve the short- or long-term outcomes of primary stent implantation, although the CADILLAC study suggests early subacute closure is reduced.

In summary, routine stent placement can be performed safely during AMI and decreases long-term adverse events. Certain anatomic subsets still must be approached with extreme caution, such as ostial lesions, lesions involving major bifurcations, and lesions with extensive intraluminal thrombus. Stent therapy appears to impart an equal level of predictability and long-term efficacy to acute therapy and elective PTCA.

### Stent Implantation in Acute Myocardial Infarction: Technical Considerations

By sealing dissection planes and reducing the residual stenosis in relation to PTCA, stent implantation in the AMI setting has the potential to improve the early safety profile of mechanical reperfusion. In comparison with PTCA, however, coronary stent implantation is inherently more complex, with even greater potential to harm rather than benefit the patient unless meticulous attention to detail is considered. Some of the important technical advice for stenting in AMI are summarized in Table 12–20.

Although much of the technical approach to primary stent implantation in AMI is similar to that of primary PTCA (as reviewed in the previous chapter), there are several unique aspects to AMI stent implantation with which the operator must be familiar. In comparison with balloon catheters, stents are bulkier, less trackable, and less deliverable and require greater guide support and more supportive guide wires; the likelihood for trauma to the infarcted vessel or the left main coronary artery is therefore greater. In the PAMI Stent Pilot Trial,[212] stent implantation was unsuccessful in four patients

**TABLE 12–20. STENT IMPLANTATION IN ACUTE MYOCARDIAL INFARCTION: USEFUL TECHNICAL INFORMATION\***

Femoral approach is standard for rapidity and maximal flexibility, including access for intra-aortic balloon pump, temporary pacemaker, or right-sided heart catheterization if necessary
Use ionic, low osmolar contrast material to minimize thromboembolic complications
Ensure activated clotting time (ACT) of >350 seconds before predilatation (200–300 seconds if abciximab is used)
Predilate with balloon same size as or slightly larger than the reference vessel diameter:
  Same size balloon as the stent
  Upsize the balloon if the vessel "grows" as flow improves
  Ensure complete balloon expansion before stent implantation
Assess lesion for stent eligibility:
  The PAMI Stent Pilot guidelines are a good starting place, but this may be liberalized in selected cases
Excellent guide support and extra-support guide wires are strongly recommended
Balloon-expandable corrugated ring or multicellular stents are recommended
Implant stents at ≥16 atm pressure, sized ≥1:1 to ensure complete expansion
If possible, implant stent from one normal reference segment to another
Implant stents for all edge dissections more severe than NHLBI type B
Implant stents for all significant inflow and outflow stenoses (stenosis affecting ≥70% of vessel diameter)
Goal is complete lesion coverage, stenosis affecting <10% of luminal diameter, with no dissections or filling defects left without stents
Standard poststent pharmacologic regimen is currently aspirin indefinitely, ticlopidine 250 mg PO bid for 4 weeks or clopidogrel 300 mg load and 75 mg PO for 4 weeks, and IV (or SQ) heparin (or enoxaparin) for ≥48 hours

PAMI, Primary Angioplasty in Myocardial Infarction; PTCA, percutaneous transluminal coronary angioplasty.
\*In addition, all the technical information suggested for optimal primary PTCA should be followed, as reviewed in Table 11–24 and the text of Chapter 11.

because of inability to deliver the sheathed Palmaz-Schatz stent system to the lesion. Although all four stents were successfully withdrawn, PTCA alone was unsuccessful in one of the remaining patients, and two required CABG. In the randomized PAMI Stent trial, one patient assigned to undergo stent implantation died because a guide catheter iatrogenically induced dissection of the left main coronary artery. The new generation of stents have dramatically improved flexibility and profile. As a result, lesion selection is rapidly expanding.

Still, proper case selection is critical. Stent implantation should not be attempted in heavily calcified or extremely tortuous vessels, in which it is unlikely that the stent can be delivered or completely expanded. Most experience to date has been with implantation of stents into vessels 3.0 to 4.0 mm in diameter. Although larger vessels (including saphenous vein grafts) do not pose a dilemma for stents (as long as appropriate stents that can expand sufficiently without deforming are used), there are minimal data to suggest that stents placed in 2.5-mm and smaller vessels offer any benefit in addition to routine PTCA. Similarly, there is little experience thus far with the newer, more flexible long stents, and the advantages of stent placement in long lesions (e.g., >30 mm) in relation to PTCA alone is unknown. If long stents are used, especially in small vessels, to maximize lumen dimensions and minimize acute complications, the balloon-expandable corrugated ring or multicellular designs, such as the Multi-Link (Guidant), Nir (Boston Scientific), or GFX (AVE), which have optimal expansion characteristics with minimal elastic recoil, are recommended. The heparin-coated stent may also have particular utility in small vessels, long lesions, and other complex lesion subsets, although no comparative data are available in this regard.

Placement of stents into ostial LAD and ostial LCX lesions has generally been avoided in the AMI setting as well, to prevent left main coronary artery complications or retrograde extrusion of clots. It may be necessary and desirable, however, in such lesions that demonstrate significant elastic recoil after PTCA, which is not an uncommon occurrence. Stent placement for complex bifurcation is also best not practiced in the AMI setting; a more prudent approach is to temporize with primary PTCA.

Finally, the initial concerns that stent implantation in thrombus-laden lesions would be excessively hazardous[187, 188] have proved unfounded when proper technique is applied. Direct stent implantation resulted in angiographic resolution of thrombus in more than 80% of patients who received stents in the PAMI Stent Pilot trial; clinical outcomes were identical to those of patients without thrombus. Furthermore, a provocative observation from the PAMI Stent Pilot trial was that the presence of thrombus was predictive of freedom from long-term restenosis after primary stent implantation in AMI; restenosis developed in 9.7% of patients with thrombus, in contrast to 32.4% of patients without thrombus ($p = 0.007$). Thus, not only should stent implantation with thrombus not be contraindicated, but it may actually be considered the treatment of choice for moderate amounts of clot burden. In lesions with extensive thrombosis, stent may be implanted in conjunction with GPIIb/IIIa receptor blockade or, as discussed later, after mechanical thrombectomy.

Before stent implantation, primary PTCA is performed to stop the infarction and stabilize the patient. An adequate PTCA result should be obtained; a perfect or optimal result is not necessary. In general, a PTCA balloon sized in an approximate 1.1:1 ratio to the reference vessel size, identical to the final stent diameter, is chosen to ensure that complete balloon expansion and adequate predilatation are achieved before stent delivery.

Minimizing the risk of stent thrombosis, which is inherently increased by stent placement into thrombotic occlusions, requires attention to detail, including selection of the proper anticoagulant and antiplatelet regimens during and after the procedure, the use of appropriate contrast agents, and optimal deployment technique. Specifically, the use of low osmolar, ionic contrast (Ioxaglate) is strongly recommended because of its inherent anticoagulant properties, which have been shown to reduce thromboembolic complications after primary PTCA.[267–270] A regimen of aspirin indefinitely and ticlopidine or clopidogrel for 4 weeks after stent implantation is an integral part of the stent protocol and has been shown to reduce the rates of subacute thrombosis in comparison with other anticoagulant and antiplatelet regimens.[271, 272] Ticlopidine may be given as a loading dose of 500 mg orally twice a day for 48 hours, which significantly decreases the time delay for its antiplatelet effect to become manifest.[273] Similarly, clopidogrel may be given as a 300-mg load with 75 mg orally daily thereafter. In higher-risk cases, abciximab may be used before stent implantation to achieve profound platelet inhibition. Abciximab may also be administered intravenously in the setting of residual thrombus after stent implantation to "dissolve" the clot,[75] thereby theoretically lowering the risk of subacute thrombosis.

Optimal stent implantation technique is critical if subacute stent thrombosis is to be avoided and restenosis minimized.[274, 275] The stent should be sized in an approximate 1.1:1 ratio to the vessel and implanted at high pressure (16 to 18 atm) to ensure adequate apposition against the vessel wall. Both the Palmaz-Schatz and Multi-Link stents have been shown to continue to expand as pressure is raised from 8 to 12 atm to 16 to 18 atm,[221, 276] and thus the latter range is typically chosen. Achieving maximal stent dimensions results in lower rates of clinical and angiographic restenosis.[277, 278] At the same time, however, overly aggressive stent implantation can result in perforation, which must be avoided.[274, 275] The edges of the stent should be implanted in normal- or nearly normal-appearing reference segments; this will minimize the likelihood of margin dissections.[279] Single, longer stents may be preferable in this application to multiple, overlapping stents, from the perspectives of both reduced cost and avoidance of vascular injury at the site of stent overlap.

The role of intravascular ultrasound (IVUS) guidance in AMI stent implantation is currently undetermined. IVUS guidance was used in 20% of stent recipients in the PAMI Stent Pilot trial; the outcomes in these patients were similar to those in whom IVUS guidance was not used. Currently, IVUS guidance is not considered mandatory for AMI stent implantation but may be helpful in complex anatomy or if complications arise during the procedure. If IVUS guidance is used, the goals should be to facilitate maximal stent expansion, to ensure adequate strut apposition against the vessel wall, and to exclude large angiographically unsuspected edge dissections. Small edge dissections, however, and small amounts of residual thrombus are probably of no consequence, and their recognition on IVUS study should not necessarily prompt extensive reintervention. The utility of IVUS guidance to predict adverse ischemic complications and restenosis is being investigated with blinded pullback studies after successful stent implantation in both the PAMI Heparin Coated Stent trial and the CADILLAC trial.

Peristent dissections are common and, if untreated (with additional stents), may resurface as extensive propagating dissections culminating in recurrent ischemia or reinfarction. In the PAMI Stent Pilot trial,[212] dissections were present in 45 (19%) of 236 patients after PTCA before stent implantation. Although stent implantation led to the complete angiographic resolution of 39 (87%) of these dissections, 11 new peristent dissections (5%) developed after stent implantation. Seven of these dissections were treated by the implantation of additional stents. In two patients in whom a peristent dissection was treated conservatively, without additional stents, recurrent ischemia caused by a distal propagating dissection developed several days later. Moreover, in one patient with an excellent result after PTCA alone, an extensive dissection developed after stent implantation, and emergency CABG was required; this is a rare complication with primary PTCA alone.

Although adverse events after primary stent implantation for AMI are rare, their occurrence may be prevented by proper stent technique. In the PAMI Stent Pilot trial,[280] adverse in-hospital events (death, reinfarction, or recurrent ischemia necessitating repeat TVR) occurred in only 15 stent recipients (6.3%). Of 51 clinical, angiographic, and procedural variables examined for their relationship to ischemic complications after primary stent implantation, only two—implantation of stents at less than 18 atm of pressure and the appearance of an NHLBI type B or worse dissection after stent implantation (according to core laboratory determination)—were correlated with the development of an adverse outcome (Fig. 12–17). Complications occurred in only 2.9% of patients in whom neither of these two variables was present, in contrast to 11.5% of patients in whom one or both variables were present. Because both of these factors are, for the most part, under the control of the operator, the acute proce-

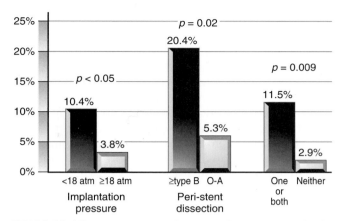

FIGURE 12–17. Correlates or in-hospital adverse events (death, reinfarction, recurrent ischemia, or target vessel revascularization) after primary stent implantation in 240 patients with acute myocardial infarction in the Primary Angioplasty in Myocardial Infarction (PAMI) Stent Pilot trial.

dural success rate of primary stent implantation for AMI should approach 99%; subsequent in-hospital major complications would occur in fewer than 5% of patients.

## Thrombectomy and Atherectomy Devices in Acute Myocardial Infarction

With the excellent results of primary PTCA and the emerging role of primary stent implantation, the need for adjunctive devices can be questioned. There may, however, be a role for devices that can ablate thrombus in selected patients with AMI, especially in patients with large amounts of angiographic thrombus, occluded saphenous vein grafts, and cardiogenic shock.

Large thrombus burden is a harbinger of complications after PTCA in patients with acute ischemic syndromes.[281–288] By reducing the thrombus burden before PTCA or stent implantation, thrombectomy devices have the potential to reduce the incidence of no-reflow or slow-reflow after mechanical intervention and to decrease the occurrence of distal thromboemboli, thereby increasing ultimate vessel patency rates and myocardial salvage. No-reflow, defined as the presence of TIMI grade 0 or 1 flow in the infarcted vessel after PTCA in the absence of a significant residual epicardial coronary stenosis at the infarction site or downstream in the vessel, has been reported in 5% to 34% of patients after primary PTCA.[289–295] The wide variability of its occurrence may reflect differences in operator technique, including selection of contrast agent[267–270] and degree of heparinization before angioplasty.[109–112] Regardless, the occurrence of no-reflow (or slow-reflow, TIMI grade 2 flow in the vessel) results in blunted myocardial recovery and increased rates of myocardial rupture and mortality.[289, 290] Distal thromboemboli may have the same effects if a large branch is occluded (macroemboli) or if diffuse microemboli result in capillary block. Because microemboli typically are angiographically unappreciated, the true incidence of distal thromboemboli is likely underreported, and these complications may retard myocardial recovery in a greater proportion of patients than is realized. These complications contribute to the inability to restore TIMI grade 3 flow in approximately 5% to 10% of patients undergoing primary PTCA, which results in increased rates of death, reinfarction, recurrent ischemia, heart failure, and a longer, more complex, and more expensive hospital stay.[175, 296] Furthermore, although the occurrence of transient no-reflow or small distal thromboemboli may be acceptable if the infarcted vessel is totally occluded at baseline, the development of these complications after angioplasty of an initially patent vessel can significantly worsen the patient's acute condition.

No-reflow, distal thromboemboli, and the inability to restore TIMI grade 3 flow after primary PTCA for AMI are more likely to occur with mechanical intervention of occluded vein grafts, in which the occurrence of grumous degeneration as saphenous vein grafts age, along with stasis of blood after distal graft occlusion, results in a larger occlusive thrombus and atheroma burden than in native coronary arteries.[205, 297–301] Distal thromboemboli and no-reflow are also more common after PTCA in vein grafts if thrombus is angiographically present.[302, 303] The overall success rate of primary PTCA is lower for saphenous vein grafts than for native coronary arteries. In a series of 1000 consecutive patients undergoing primary PTCA at the Mid America Heart Institute, 13% had undergone prior CABG.[12] The acute PTCA success rate was lower for occluded vein grafts than for native vessels (86% vs. 95%; $p < 0.0001$). In two smaller series, the PTCA success rate with vein graft occlusion was 75% to 80%.[298, 304] In the combined PAMI-1 and PAMI-2 trials,[301] TIMI grade 3 flow was restored in 79% of occluded vein grafts, in contrast to 93% of native arteries ($p < 0.001$), and a residual stenosis affecting less than 50% of the luminal diameter was obtained in 83% of vein graft occlusions, in contrast to 96% of native artery occlusions ($p < 0.001$). Residual thrombus was also present after PTCA in a greater proportion of patients with vein graft disease than in those with native vessel disease (30% vs. 18%). Mortality rates also tended to be higher in patients with vein graft disease than in those with native vessel disease undergoing primary PTCA (9.1% vs. 2.6%; $p = 0.06$).

Reperfusion rates are also lower in patients with cardiogenic shock, because of greater clot burden, more diffuse disease, and lower perfusion pressure.[205, 305] Therefore, strategies to reduce thrombus burden before mechanical intervention may be of particular benefit in patients with shock and vein graft disease. Most pharmacologic approaches to thrombus, including intracoronary thrombolysis, have been unsuccessful in patients with angiographic evidence of thrombus.[306, 307] Although the use of GPIIb/IIIa receptor blockers as an adjunct to PTCA to reduce complications in patients with thrombus is promising,[283] there are few reports of their efficacy in patients with occluded vein grafts or cardiogenic shock. It is therefore probable that thrombectomy devices will be most useful in these patient subgroups, as well as in patients with failed primary PTCA because of extensive thrombosis or no-reflow. It is also possible that by debulking plaque before stent implantation, atherectomy devices may reduce long-term restenosis rates and improve late outcomes,[234] although this hypothesis requires prospective validation.

Several devices possessing the ability to remove thrombus and/or atheroma have been developed and tested in limited numbers of patients with AMI and acute ischemic syndromes (Table 12–21).

### The Transluminal Extraction Catheter (TEC) Device

The TEC device consists of a closed system containing a flexible hypotube with three attached stainless steel blades at the distal tip, a drive unit, and a collection vacuum bottle. The cutter sizes

**TABLE 12–21.    THROMBECTOMY CATHETERS AND STRATEGIES**

Transluminal extration catheter (Interventional Technologies, San Diego, California [IVT])
Directional coronary atherectomy (Advanced Cardiovascular System, Sunnyvale, California [ACS])
AngioJet (Possis Medical)
Hydrolyser (Cordis)
Ultrasound thrombolysis
    ACULYSIS system (Angiosonics)
    ACS system
Laser angioplasty
    Thermal balloon (ACS)
    Contact lasers
        Excimer (Spectranetics)
        Holmium (Eclipse)
Local drug delivery
    Passive diffusion or pressure-driven systems
    Hydrogel coated balloons
    Iontophoresis
    Direct intramural injection
    Microspheres
Aspiration thrombectomy
    Through diagnostic or guide catheters
    Rescue Percutaneous Thrombectomy (RPT) catheter (Scimed)
Miscellaneous approaches
    Pulse spray thrombolysis (Scimed)
    Autologous vein graft–coated stents

vary from 5.5- to 7.5-French. Rotating at 750 rpm, these blades excise and aspirate soft plaque (including friable, grumous saphenous vein graft material) and thrombi. This device may be useful in patients with AMI and large thrombus burden or totally occluded vein grafts.[308] Thrombus is present in almost all patients with acute ischemic syndromes, even if it is recognized angiographically in only a minority of patients.[226, 227] Using angioscopy, several studies have demonstrated that the TEC device removes thrombus either partially or completely in 75% to 100% of these vessels.[226, 227] The TEC device has been reported to have high success rates in older, diffusely diseased saphenous vein grafts, especially when combined with stent implantation, in comparison with historical controls with PTCA only.[227, 303, 309–312] In a retrospective comparison of the TEC device with PTCA in 76 diseased vein grafts with angiographic evidence of thrombus,[303] distal thromboemboli occurred in only 5.6% of patients after TEC use plus PTCA, in contrast to 31.8% of patients after PTCA alone ($p = 0.005$); this low incidence was associated with a reduced incidence of non–Q-wave MI in the TEC-treated patients. Similarly, in a separate study of 124 patients undergoing the TEC procedure ($N = 65$) or PTCA ($N = 59$) for diseased vein grafts at the University of Alabama, the frequency of creatine-kinase with muscle and brain subunits (CK-MB) rise above the level of 25 ng/mL was significantly reduced in the TEC-treated patients (7% vs. 22%; $p < 0.02$), despite a greater prevalence of thrombus and longer lesion length in the TEC-treated vein grafts; this reduction was consistent with decreased distal thromboembolism.[313]

In contrast, the use of the TEC device in the U.S. TEC registry was associated with a high complication rate.[314] In the New Approaches to Coronary Intervention (NACI) registry, the outcomes of TEC use in 385 lesions in 331 patients were studied.[315] Thrombus was present in 38.4% of lesions, 15% were total occlusions, and 76% of treated lesions were in saphenous vein grafts. Distal embolization was not infrequent, occurring in 8.3% of patients and 7.4% of lesions,[316] and was noted in 5.1% of arteries after TEC use and 4.6% after adjunctive PTCA. Univariate analysis showed that distal embolization was more likely to occur in TEC-treated vein grafts than in TEC-treated native vessels (9.1% vs. 2.2%; $p < 0.01$), in thrombotic lesions (11.9% vs. 4.8%; $p < 0.01$), and in patients who had suffered MI within the previous 6 weeks (14.0% vs. 6.3%; $p < 0.05$). Abrupt closure occurred in 5.9% of vessels after TEC treatment and in 2.7% of vessels after PTCA and was persistent at the completion of the procedure in 2.8% of patients. In-hospital death, Q-wave MI, or repeat TVR (CABG or PTCA) oc-

curred in 3.4% of patients undergoing TEC treatment of native coronary vessels and in 8.2% of patients after TEC treatment of saphenous vein grafts ($p < 0.05$).

Several case reports have demonstrated the utility of TEC treatment in patients with AMI and extensive clot burden in whom thrombolysis or PTCA has failed.[317, 318] The possible utility of the TEC device during AMI has been reported from several single-center and multicenter experiences. Larkin and associates found that the TEC procedure was feasible in 17 of 19 patients with AMI in whom thrombolysis had failed or was contraindicated, and it was successfully performed in 16 patients (94%).[319] One patient (6%) suffered in-hospital reocclusion.

The largest registry report of the use of TEC in patients with AMI was that of the combined experience from William Beaumont Hospital and Northwestern University.[320] At these two centers, TEC treatment was prospectively evaluated in 100 patients with either AMI ($N = 72$) or postinfarction angina ($N = 28$). High-risk features included thrombolytic failure in 40% of patients, cardiogenic shock in 11%, saphenous vein graft occlusion in 29%, and presence of angiographically documented thrombus in 66%. PTCA was performed after TEC treatment in 94% of patients. In occluded vessels, TEC improved TIMI flow by two or more grades in 72% of lesions. Final procedural success after PTCA (defined as TIMI grade 2 or 3 flow with residual stenosis affecting less than 50% of the luminal diameter) was achieved in 94% of patients. Distal embolization, no-reflow, or both occurred in only 6% of patients, usually after adjunctive PTCA. Major flow-limiting dissections occurred in 8% of patients after TEC treatment, however, and contained perforations occurred in two patients after TEC treatment; most of these episodes were managed with prolonged balloon inflations, and there were no procedural deaths or emergency bypass procedures performed. In-hospital death occurred in 5.0% of patients (including 3 [27.3%] of 11 patients initially in cardiogenic shock and 2 [2.2%] of 89 patients not in shock). Considering the high proportion of patients with shock or failed thrombolysis in this series, this mortality rate is quite encouraging and compares favorably with those of prior reports of PTCA alone in these settings.[205, 305, 321–326] Recurrent ischemia with vessel renarrowing occurred in only 2% of patients (both treated with repeat PTCA and stents), and no patient developed reinfarction. Within 6 months, however, clinical restenosis (repeat TVR) occurred in 38% of patients, and 10% died.

Only one prospective, randomized trial has examined the role of TEC treatment in patients as an adjunct to PTCA with acute ischemic syndromes. In the TEC or PTCA in Thrombus (TOPIT) study, 245 patients at high risk with AMI, failed thrombolysis, post-MI angina, unstable angina, or thrombotic lesions in native coronary arteries were randomly assigned to TEC treatment or PTCA at 17 U.S. centers.[326] Stents were also implanted in 25% of patients in both groups; abciximab was used in only 3.5% of patients. In comparison with those who underwent PTCA, patients who underwent TEC treatment showed a strong trend toward a reduction in the primary combined end point of death, Q-wave MI, abrupt closure, or TVR (2.7% vs. 8.2%; $p$ = 0.06) (Fig. 12–18, top graph). The incidence of periprocedural MI (CPK levels more than three times normal) was significantly reduced in the patients with unstable angina and those with post-MI angina (4.5% vs. 15.4%; $p < 0.04$). The relative degree of reduction in adverse events with TEC treatment in TOPIT is similar to that in the EPIC trial with GPIIb/IIIa inhibition in patients with acute ischemic syndromes,[76] although the smaller number of patients enrolled in TOPIT precluded statistical significance. Among the 98 TOPIT patients undergoing PTCA either for primary reperfusion of AMI or acutely after failed thrombolysis, a similar trend was apparent (2.6% adverse events after TEC treatment vs. 6.8% after PTCA; $p$ = NS) (see Fig. 12–18, bottom graph). No angiographic differences were seen, however, in the occurrence of no-reflow, distal thromboemboli, final TIMI flow grades, or residual stenosis between patients treated with the TEC device plus PTCA and those who underwent PTCA alone, either in the entire study or in the AMI cohort.

Limitations of TEC atherectomy include its inability to cut hard plaque, its unsuitability for vessels less than 3.0 mm in diameter, the necessity for 9- or 10-French guide catheters and a dedicated unibody steel guide wire with ball tip (which steers poorly), its large size and poor trackability, the cost and time to prepare, and the frequent presence of dissections and significant residual stenosis after its use. Distal thromboemboli has still been reported in 7% to 12% of patients after TEC treatment of saphenous vein grafts, and restenosis rates have been high.[312, 327–329] As a result, PTCA, stent implantation, or both are frequently required after TEC treatment; this can result in additional distal thromboembolism. In the NACI registry, perforation from the TEC device occurred in 2.9% of 385 patients; perforation is a complication rarely seen with PTCA alone.[315]

Ongoing studies such as TEC Before Stent (TEC-BEST-II) will help establish the role of this device (and abciximab) in the treatment of diseased saphenous vein grafts in patients with stable and unstable ischemic syndromes (AMIs are excluded from TECBEST-II, unfortunately). In the CADILLAC trial, AMI patients with occluded vein grafts are excluded from the primary four-way randomization. These grafts will be treated either by the TEC device before PTCA or stent implantation (without abciximab) by operators who are qualified in TEC use or with PTCA or stents alone, plus abciximab, by operators unfamiliar with TEC use. The primary end point of this nonrandomized comparison is angiographically documented (TIMI grade 3 flow and complications such as distal emboli). The results of this CADILLAC substudy in occluded vein grafts, when compared to historical controls treated with primary PTCA alone, should afford insight into selection of the best therapy for patients with AMI secondary to diseased vein grafts. Until that time, on the basis of favorable trends in the TOPIT trial, TEC can be recommended for patients with AMI and large clot

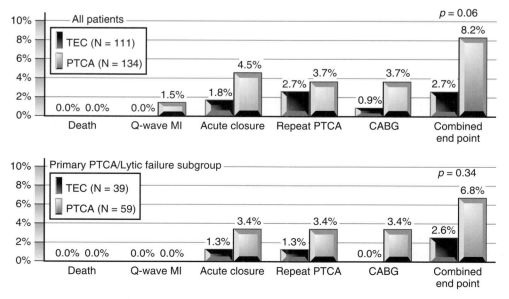

FIGURE 12–18. Adverse events in patients with acute ischemic syndromes undergoing percutaneous transluminal coronary angioplasty (PTCA) alone or PTCA after a transluminal extraction catheter (TEC) procedure. Top graph represents entire study population; bottom graph represents primary subgroup of patients experiencing PTCA/lytic failure. CABG, coronary artery bypass grafting; MI, myocardial infarction.

burden, especially in diffusely diseased saphenous vein grafts, as an adjunct to primary PTCA and stent implantation. If the TEC device is used in this manner, the operator and catheterization laboratory must be skilled in its use, and undue delays to reperfusion must not be tolerated. At times, in complex cases, this may necessitate establishing distal perfusion with a small balloon catheter (e.g., 1.5 to 2.0 mm in diameter) before TEC thrombectomy.

## Directional Coronary Atherectomy (DCA)

DCA has also been used in patients with AMI. In comparison with PTCA in patients undergoing elective intervention, DCA results in less residual stenosis with an equal number of or fewer dissections.[330–332] Optimal DCA, in comparison with PTCA, was shown to lower the rate of restenosis in the Balloon versus Optimal Atherectomy (BOAT) trial by virtue of creating a larger initial lumen.[333] DCA is also effective in salvaging selected cases of PTCA failure, including acute occlusions,[334] although its use in this regard has greatly diminished since the advent of stents.

Several studies have described the outcome of DCA in patients with thrombus, with mixed results. In a multicenter series of 400 lesions in 378 patients treated by DCA, Holmes and coworkers reported a higher procedural success rate with fewer major complications in 30 patients with thrombus (21% of whom had had a recent MI) than in 348 patients without thrombus.[335] In contrast, in a study of 418 lesions by Emmi and associates, the procedural success rate of DCA in patients with thrombus was similar to that in patients without thrombus (76% vs. 80%; $p$ = NS), but major complications (16% vs. 8%; $p$ = 0.06), including need for emergency CABG (10% vs. 4%; $p$ = 0.03), were increased in patients with thrombus.[336] In a NACI registry report, the outcomes of DCA in 147 lesions in 170 patients with recent MI (occurring within the previous 30 days) were compared with those in 490 lesions in 438 patients without prior MI.[337] Thrombus was more frequently present in patients with recent MI than in those without recent MI (19% vs. 6%). In comparison to patients without recent MI, the clinical success rate was lower in patients with recent MI (83% vs. 88%; $p$ < 0.01), and the rates of dissection (7% vs. 3%; $p$ < 0.05), abrupt closure (5% vs. 1%; $p$ < 0.05), and major procedural complications (3.4% vs. 1.1%; $p$ < 0.07) were higher. The clinical success rate increased from 77% for DCA attempted 1 to 9 days after MI to 90% and 95% for DCA attempted 10 to 19 and 20 to 30 days after MI, respectively ($p$ = 0.07).

Several investigators published initially encouraging individual case reports of DCA during AMI.[338, 339]

including those of patients rescued from cardiogenic shock with DCA after PTCA failure.[340] The outcomes of primary DCA for AMI have been reported in several small series of patients. Baldwin and colleagues performed DCA during AMI in 11 patients, 6 of whom had received thrombolytic therapy.[341] Adjunctive PTCA was used in 8 patients, and 5 patients also received intracoronary thrombolysis. DCA was successful (decreasing stenosis severity by ≥20% and reducing thrombus burden) in 10 patients (91%). In one patient, however, acute reocclusion of the LAD developed in the catheterization laboratory, and emergency CABG was required. The in-hospital survival rate was 100%, and no other patient experienced recurrent ischemia.

Kurisu and coworkers performed DCA in 32 patients with AMI who had undergone successful reperfusion by intracoronary tPA and in whom high-grade residual stenosis persisted.[342] DCA was successful in 31 patients (97%). No patient experienced coronary perforation or distal embolization, although in one patient (3%) abrupt closure developed with reinfarction; this was treated successfully with repeat PTCA. Repeat angiography before discharge was performed in all 32 patients and demonstrated no reocclusions. However, restenosis was present in 12 (41%) of 29 patients undergoing angiographic follow-up at a mean time of 4.5 ± 1.5 months. Kurisu and coworkers reported the in-hospital outcomes after successful DCA of the LAD in 24 patients with anterior MI (unsuccessful procedures were excluded from this report).[343] No patient experienced reinfarction, and predischarge angiography demonstrated patent vessels in all cases.

In comparison with PTCA, primary DCA in AMI is technically more demanding, requires greater operator expertise, and cannot be performed as expeditiously. Randomized studies of patients undergoing elective intervention have demonstrated greater rates of periprocedural cardiac enzyme release after DCA than after PTCA, which is consistent with increased distal microembolization.[332, 344–347] Like PTCA, DCA is associated with more complications in patients with thrombus. In view of the excellent results reported thus far with primary stent implantation, which is a much simpler technique than atherectomy for achieving a large immediate postprocedure lumen, it is unlikely that DCA will be commonly used as a primary reperfusion modality in AMI. DCA may nonetheless be useful in selected patients with AMI who have ostial LAD or LCX stenoses or complex bifurcation lesions, for which treatment with both PTCA and stents still has significant deficiencies.

## The AngioJet

The AngioJet is a rheolytic thrombectomy system.[348] A hydraulic pump delivers heparinized saline to the distal catheter at a pressure of 2500 psi, with flow rates of 50 to 60 mL/minute. The saline exits the catheter from small holes in the distal tip at 500 km/hour and courses in a retrograde direction and inward, toward the centerline, in such a way that the jet does not contact the vessel wall. This high-velocity jet generates a low-pressure zone near the catheter tip (the Bernoulli principle), which is close to a perfect vacuum. This in turn creates a vortex (the Venturi effect) that breaks up and aspirates thrombi in a process called *entrainment.* The effluent is delivered down the catheter shaft, driven by the jet pressure, and is deposited into a collection bag. The system is isovolumetric; the amount of fluid (saline) that enters the body is the same as the amount removed (saline plus blood).

The catheter is a 5-French double-lumen design that travels over standard 0.014-inch guide wires and passes easily through 8-French guide catheters. The AngioJet may be used in vessels as small as 2.0 mm in diameter and as large as 8 mm. The system is activated by a foot switch. Thrombi may be partially aspirated before the catheter tip is passed into the clot. The tip is then passed through the clot for maximal thrombus extraction. During in vitro embolization tests with a coronary flow model, 99.4% of thrombi was extracted, 0.5% embolized distally, and 0.1% embolized proximally (data on file, Possis Medical, Minneapolis MN). Almost all embolized material was smaller than the diameter of a red blood cell and therefore capable of passing through the capillary system. Activation of the device can, like high-speed rotational atherectomy, occasionally cause transient bradycardia or asystole, especially in the right coronary artery, which occasionally necessitates temporary pacemaker usage.

The AngioJet has been used successfully to treat acutely occluded lower limb vessels, dialysis grafts, intrahepatic portosystemic shunts, and diseased native coronary arteries and saphenous vein grafts.[228, 229, 349, 350] In a preliminary report from the Euro-ART (European AngioJet Rapid Thrombectomy) study, 35 patients with angiographic thrombus present in native coronary arteries or saphenous vein grafts, including 10 patients with AMI, underwent thrombectomy with the AngioJet.[228] Thrombus removal was complete in 54% of vessels and partial in 26% of vessels. Temporary pacing for asystole was required in 26% of patients. The AngioJet resulted in significant dissection in 17% of vessels. IV abciximab was also given to 26% of patients, and 69% received stents. Device success was obtained in 80% of patients, and the final procedural success rate was 86%. No patient died, experienced reinfarction, or required CABG or repeat PTCA during the hospital stay.

In the VeGAS I Pilot study,[229] 90 patients at high risk with angiographic evidence of thrombus and either unstable angina ($N = 60$) or AMI ($N = 30$) underwent rheolytic thrombectomy of 91 vessels. Cardiogenic shock was present in 10% of patients. The target vessel was a native coronary artery in 39 patients (43%) and a saphenous vein graft in 52 patients (57%). Thrombus burden measured by the core angiographic laboratory was 81.80 mm$^2$ before the procedure, 21.37 mm$^2$ after AngioJet use, and 11.39 mm$^2$ after adjunctive PTCA or stent implantation. TIMI grade 3 flow was present in 49% of arteries before intervention, in 69% after AngioJet use, and in 88% at the completion of the procedure. TIMI grade 3 flow with residual stenosis affecting less than 50% of the luminal diameter was achieved in 39% of patients with the AngioJet alone (including 52% of patients with AMI and 33% with unstable angina) and in 88% of patients at the end of the procedure (including 90% of patients with AMI and 87% with unstable angina). In-hospital complications included death in 4 patients (4.4%) and Q-wave MI in 4 patients (4.4%). In patients with unstable angina, 25% of patients had a Q-wave MI or a non–Q-wave MI, evidenced by a CPK rise to more than three times normal levels and an additional 12% had a smaller CPK rise. By the 30-day follow-up in 81 patients, 2 patients (2.5%) had required repeat TVR, and 12 patients (15%) had recurrent angina.

Thus, these studies have demonstrated that the AngioJet removes thrombi in native coronary arteries and in saphenous vein grafts both in patients with AMI and in those with unstable angina. There is little evidence, however, that this device removes friable, grumous vein graft material or older, organized thrombi, which is a significant limitation. Although it is easier to use than other atherectomy devices (the AngioJet is compatible with 8-French guide catheters and standard guide wires and offers enhanced flexibility), temporary pacemaker insertion is frequently required, dissections are not uncommon, distal embolization can still occur, and the rate of periprocedural enzyme rise is not insignificant. Randomized trials will be necessary to determine whether this device offers significant advantages to alternative thrombectomy devices (such as the TEC device, which also performs limited atherectomy), GPIIb/IIIa receptor antagonists, or stand-alone PTCA or stent implantation in patients with thrombotic lesions and acute ischemic syndromes. One such trial, the VeGAS II study, has been performed in 540 patients with diseased saphenous vein grafts containing angiographic thrombus, with random assignment to undergo AngioJet treatment or a prolonged intragraft urokinase infusion. AngioJet studies are also being performed in patients with

AMI and in patients with conditions contraindicating thrombolytic therapy.

### The Hydrolyser

The Hydrolyser is a double-lumen, over-the-wire (0.014- or 0.018-inch) thrombectomy catheter that aspirates thrombi also by means of the Venturi principle.[351, 352] Saline solution is delivered to the distal catheter at 9 mL/second through a conventional contrast injector. A high-velocity (150 km/hour) saline jet is directed out a side hole at a 180-degree bend at the tip of the catheter, creating a vortex. As a result, thrombus is aspirated into the side hole, fragmented, and deposited into a distal collection bag.

The initial 7-French version of this device was successfully used in peripheral arteries, bypass grafts, and dialysis shunts.[352–355] Van Ommen and coworkers evaluated the efficacy of a 6-French version of the Hydrolyser in 31 thrombotic lesions in 31 patients with coronary artery disease, including 20 saphenous vein bypass grafts and 11 native coronary arteries.[356] Five patients were treated during AMI; the other 26 patients had NYHA class III or IV angina. The Hydrolyser reached the lesion in 30 (97%) of 31 patients, although PTCA was required first in five lesions. After Hydrolyser treatment, adjunctive PTCA was performed in 28 patients (90%); 9 of these patients also underwent stent placement. Thrombi were extracted by the Hydrolyser in 29 patients (94%). Less than 150 mL of saline was retained as a result of the procedure, and hemolysis did not occur. Before the Hydrolyser treatment, TIMI grade 0 or 1 flow was present in 24 patients (77%); the Hydrolyser restored TIMI grade 2 or 3 flow in 14 (58%) of these patients, who accounted for 7 (47%) of 15 grafts and 7 (78%) of 9 native coronary vessels. After adjunctive PTCA (and intracoronary thrombolytic therapy in four patients), TIMI grade 2 or 3 flow was present in 25 (81%) of 31 patients (with TIMI grade 3 flow in all but 1 patient). Distal embolization was noted in 2 patients (6%) after Hydrolyser use, both instances in venous bypass grafts, one of which resulted in a non–Q-wave myocardial infarction. Two patients died in the hospital: one with an AMI secondary to an occluded vein graft in which both thrombectomy and adjunctive PTCA were unsuccessful in restoring reperfusion, and one in whom subacute stent thrombosis developed 1 day after a successful procedure, culminating in AMI and shock. In a separate report, restenosis was present in three of the first six patients treated with this device.[357]

Thus, the Hydrolyser effectively and safely removes thrombi in a majority of patients with acute ischemic syndromes. One advantage of this system over the AngioJet is that the Hydrolyser establishes the Venturi effect at substantially lower pressures (500 to 600 psi vs. 10,000 psi), affording the use of a standard contrast injector for saline injection, whereas the AngioJet requires a specialized high-pressure delivery device. Limitations of the Hydrolyser include its large size, necessitating large guide catheters (8-French or larger) and restriction of use to vessels 3.0 mm or more in diameter; its relative inflexibility and lack of steerability, resulting in failure to track to the lesion in tortuous vessels; its failure to remove organized thrombi, friable graft material, and underlying atherosclerotic plaque, necessitating definitive angioplasty in most patients; and the continued propensity for distal embolization (especially in venous bypass grafts), although this may possibly occur more frequently if this device was not used. As with all the thrombectomy devices, randomized comparisons with stand-alone PTCA or stent implantation are necessary to determine whether a niche role exists for the Hydrolyser in patients undergoing mechanical intervention for AMI and thrombus-containing lesions.

### Ultrasound Thrombolysis

An emerging technique for the dissolution of thrombus is the application of high-intensity therapeutic ultrasound energy.[358–361] In vitro studies have demonstrated that therapeutic ultrasound lyses clot rapidly by selective disruption of the fibrin matrix of the thrombus, creating mostly sub–capillary-sized particles.[361, 362] Both red and white thrombi are ablated.[363] Thrombolysis is effected mostly by cavitation, the production and subsequent collapse of microbubbles by an alternating pressure field.[364] High-intensity, low-frequency ultrasound thrombolysis (~20 kHz) has been shown to be more effective in ablating thrombi than are lower intensity and higher frequency (>120 kHz).[365] The characteristics of therapeutic ultrasound thrombolysis make it inherently safe.[361, 362, 366, 367] The degree of ablation is inversely related to the elasticity of the tissue; because thrombus is more than 20 times as elastic as the vessel, the ultrasound power level required to lyse thrombus is only approximately 5% of that required for arterial wall damage. Ultrasound energy as applied induces vasodilatation, which facilitates particulate clearance, and does not generate heat.[368] In comparison with thrombolytic therapy alone, the addition of ultrasound energy has been shown to significantly accelerate clot dissolution[369] and effectively ablates thrombus that is resistant to thrombolysis.[370, 371]

Several ultrasonic angioplasty devices have been developed and tested clinically. The ACULYSIS system has undergone the most in-depth testing for thrombus dissolution. This device consists of a 140-cm-long solid metal probe housed within a plastic catheter, connected proximally to a piezoelectric transducer that operates at 20 W. The catheter ends distally in a 1.6-mm ball tip. The transducer delivers 10-μm-long longitudinal pulses of ultrasound energy from the distal tip at 45 kHz. The distal catheter tip is placed in the thrombus and activated for 60 to 180 seconds. A computer controls the power output and frequency and maintains constant energy output at the distal tip under variable loading conditions. The device is a monorail system that accepts a 0.014-inch guide wire and requires a 10-French guide catheter.

The use of the ACULYSIS system for thrombus dissolution as an adjunct to PTCA in AMI has been tested in the Analysis of Coronary Ultrasound Thrombolysis Endpoints in Acute Myocardial Infarction (ACUTE) trial. Rosenschein and associates published the results of this study for the first 15 consecutive enrolled patients with anterior AMI and angiographically documented TIMI grade 0 or 1 flow.[372] Ultrasound treatment restored TIMI grade 3 flow in 13 (87%) of the patients. In one patient, reocclusion at the treated site developed within 10 minutes. Quantitative coronary analysis revealed that the mean amount of luminal diameter affected by stenosis was 100% at baseline, 48% after ultrasound thrombolysis, and 20% after adjunctive PTCA (performed in 14 patients). Distal thromboemboli and no-reflow did not occur. One patient experienced recurrent ischemia during the hospital phase with angiographic documentation of reocclusion without reinfarction. This was treated successfully with repeat PTCA. One other patient required CABG for diffuse disease.

The interim multicenter experience with this device (including the first 15 patients), 33 patients with anterior MI and TIMI grade 0 or 1 flow, has been reported.[373] After ultrasound treatment, TIMI grade 3 flow was restored in 25 patients (76%), and TIMI grade 2 flow was present in 6 patients (18%). No patient developed dissection, perforation, distal emboli, or no-reflow after therapeutic ultrasound thrombolysis. After adjunctive PTCA, all patients had TIMI grade 2 or 3 flow; TIMI grade 3 flow was present in 29 patients (88%). The amount of luminal diameter affected by residual stenosis was 48% ± 24% after ultrasound treatment and 20% ± 12% after PTCA (patients included four who received stents). Of the first 26 patients treated, 2 (8%) developed reinfarction and none suffered in-hospital death or stroke. At 6-month follow-up of the first 15 patients successfully treated,[374] there had been no deaths; 1 patient (7%) had experienced reinfarction resulting from a new lesion. Of 9 patients undergoing angiographic follow-up, 2 had reocclusion of the infarcted artery and 3 had restenosis. The other 6 patients, who refused angiographic follow-up, were asymptomatic with no evidence of inducible ischemia.

The Advanced Cardiovascular Systems (ACS) therapeutic ultrasound device has also been tested in patients with AMI. This device consists of a 145-cm-long 4.2-French catheter enclosing a titanium wire probe that transmits ultrasound energy at 19.5 kHz to a distal ball tip from a proximal piezoelectric transducer operating at 16 to 20 W. The longitudinal pulses are delivered with an amplitude of 15 to 30 μm. The ball tip is either 1.2 or 1.7 mm in diameter, and the catheter fits through a standard 8-French guide catheter. It is an over-the-wire design (0.014 inch) and contains a distal infusion port. The catheter is flushed with normal saline at 10 mL/minute during ultrasound generation to prevent it from overheating.

Hamm and coworkers[375] performed ultrasound thrombolysis with the ACS device in 14 patients with AMI and TIMI grade 0 to 1 flow in the three native coronary arteries: LAD (8 patients), RCA (4 patients), and LCX (2 patients). The ultrasound catheter reached the lesion in 14 patients (93%). Ultrasound thrombolysis applied for 1.5 to 10 minutes, after which TIMI grade 2 or 3 flow was present in 11 patients (73%); only 3 patients, however, had TIMI grade 3 flow. After adjunctive PTCA, TIMI grade 3 flow was restored in 13 patients (87%); one patient had TIMI grade 0 flow and another had TIMI grade 2 flow. Percentage of luminal diameter affected by stenosis was reduced from 98% ± 3% at baseline to 71% ± 14% after ultrasound thrombolysis and to 37% ± 13% after PTCA. Minor distal thromboemboli were noted in two patients (13%), and one patient developed transient sinus bradycardia during ultrasound treatment. Major complications consisted of death in one patient (7%), in whom an occluded dominant right coronary artery could not be recanalized with either ultrasound treatment or PTCA; he died of cardiogenic shock 3 days after the procedure. Control angiography at 24 hours in 10 patients demonstrated no reocclusions and one case of asymptomatic restenosis, for which the vessel was redilated. No patient experienced recurrent ischemia. Follow-up angiography was performed at 6 months in 10 patients with a successful procedure; restenosis was found in 3 patients (30%).

Thus, catheter-based ultrasound treatment has been demonstrated to effectively lyse thrombi and has several advantages over other thrombectomy devices, including ease of use, lack of heat generation, and minimal trauma to the vessel wall. The rarity of distal thromboemboli and reduced antegrade flow thus far reported is possibly a function of the intrinsic vasodilation produced by ultrasound treatment, which facilitates clearance of distal debris. As with the other thrombectomy devices, however, adjunctive PTCA or stent implantation is required, and reocclusion of infarcted arteries and restenosis are not infrequent. The efficacy of ultrasound thrombolysis may be enhanced by adding microbubbles to the perfusate or low-dose intracoronary urokinase.[376, 377] Ultimately, randomized trials will be necessary to demonstrate whether this device truly has utility in patients with AMI and acute ischemic syndromes and whether it is cost effective.

## Laser Angioplasty

The interaction of laser light energy with thrombotic lesions has been investigated with two distinct methods: the thermal (laser) balloon and the laser catheter.

### The Thermal Balloon

Laser, radiofrequency, and ultrasonic and chemical methods of locally administering heat to the thrombus or atherosclerotic plaque during balloon angioplasty have been developed. In the thermal balloon angioplasty system, a continuous-wave neodymium:yttrium-aluminum-garnet (Nd:YAG) laser is used as an energy source within a balloon to perform controlled photothermal warming. The judicious application of heat to complex plaque during or after PTCA has been demonstrated with this system to "weld" or seal dissections, diminish elastic recoil, and reduce the thrombogenicity at the PTCA site by desiccating thrombi and thermally denaturing or crosslinking thrombogenic proteins, which may reduce platelet adhesion.[378–380] The thermal balloon was extensively tested and was found to be effective in treating abrupt closure after PTCA.[378–383] These attributes triggered interest in its potential use during AMI intervention. Unfortunately, restenosis rates of more than 50% were documented after thermal balloon angioplasty, possibly as a result of the relatively high local temperatures achieved with this device, which led to the termination of the testing.[383, 384] Preliminary reports with radiofrequency pyroplasty systems also demonstrated high restenosis rates, despite generation of lower temperatures.[385, 386] It is therefore unlikely that thermal balloon angioplasty will be resurrected for coronary use.

### Direct Laser Ablation

Laser light energy may be transmitted through optical fibers and directly applied to atherosclerotic plaque or thrombus. The direct atheroablative effect of laser light energy originates from the generation of photoacoustic trauma by the creation, rapid expansion, and dispersion of vapor gas bubbles.[387, 388] Laser catheters have been used to successfully treat many lesion subtypes that typically respond poorly to standard PTCA,[389] resulting in optimism that lasers could be used to ablate or desiccate thrombus. In a porcine model, the ultraviolet xenon chloride excimer laser has been shown to ablate thrombus.[390] In contrast, clinical experience with this laser in thrombotic lesions has suggested a lower success rate and an increase in complications in comparison with nonthrombotic lesions. In a report from the Excimer Laser Coronary Angioplasty Registry,[391] the procedural success rate was 81% in 127 lesions with thrombus, as opposed to 90% in 1406 "simple" stenoses ($p = 0.002$). Embolic complications occurred in 5.7% of patients with thrombotic lesions treated with the excimer laser; this percentage was greater than that for all other subgroups except friable vein grafts. Estella and associates[392] also found that the clinical success of excimer laser angioplasty was lower for lesions with thrombus than for those without thrombus (58% vs. 95%; $p = 0.0001$). In this study, the strongest independent determinant of procedural failure according to multivariate analysis was the presence of thrombus. As a result, the excimer laser is avoided when thrombus is present, and its use in treating AMI has not been reported. This device is partially effective in ablating friable vein graft material, however, and thus may have a role in the treatment of acute ischemic syndromes secondary to high-grade stenoses in degenerated vein grafts without large thrombus burden. In this regard, however, the TEC device has the advantage of aspirating both thrombus as well as atherosclerotic graft material.

In contrast to the disappointing clinical results of the excimer laser in thrombus, the mid-infrared holmium:YAG laser may have a particular niche role in this application. Thrombi possess a high water content that avidly absorbs light in the mid-infrared region, which may facilitate thrombolysis.[393] As a result, the holmium:YAG laser has been found to be particularly effective in treating thrombus-containing lesions and acute ischemic syndromes, and it has been used extensively at several institutions in patients with AMI.[394–399] In these observational reports, thrombus ablation was achieved in more than 90% of patients, procedural success rates were higher than 95%, and the incidences of recurrent ischemia and reocclusion of infarcted arteries were low. Distal thromboemboli have been infrequently noted after mid-infrared laser thrombolysis. Furthermore, the holmium:YAG laser has been shown to be effective in recanalizing occluded arteries in AMI that are resistant to pharmacologic thrombolytic therapy.[397]

Other advantages of the holmium:YAG laser over

the excimer laser include short warm-up times, minimal maintenance, a smaller console, no toxic gases to vent, and lower cost. The necessity for adjunctive balloon angioplasty in all patients after holmium:YAG laser angioplasty is a limitation, however.[397, 399] Moreover, although the solid-state nature of the holmium:YAG laser system facilitates rapid setup and deployment, some delay is inevitable, and "blind" laser deployment across a total occlusion without visualization of the distal vessel is potentially hazardous. Finally, in the prospective, multicenter, randomized Laser Angioplasty Versus Angioplasty (LAVA) trial, which compared the acute and 1-year outcomes of holmium:YAG laser–assisted balloon angioplasty with those of stand-alone PTCA in 215 patients with stable and unstable angina, use of the laser resulted in more frequent complications, including spasm, acute occlusion, MI, and a trend toward more frequent new thrombus formation, and in no benefits in long-term outcome.[400] Although the procedural results obtained with the laser were relatively improved in thrombotic lesions in comparison with nonthrombotic lesions, clinical outcomes were still superior to those of PTCA alone (Fig. 12–19). As a result of this trial, the Eclipse holmium:YAG laser will not be marketed in the United States. This study confirms the hazards of relying on observational registry data and the essential importance of performing well-designed randomized trials before the acceptance of new technologies or new applications of existing drugs and devices.

### Local Drug Delivery

Systemic side effects of pharmacologic agents, when administered intravenously at high doses, limit their ultimate efficacy. The appeal of a drug delivery catheter is that by confining a therapeutic substance to a specific location, extremely high concentrations of antithrombotic or antiproliferative drugs may be directly applied to thrombi or atherosclerotic plaque, while simultaneously eliminating systemic toxicity.[401–403] Such devices may also be used to achieve intramural penetration of pharmacologically active compounds or genetic material into the coronary arterial wall.

A comprehensive review of local drug delivery catheters and agents is beyond the scope of this chapter. Numerous catheter-based systems have been developed for local drug delivery via passive diffusion or pressure-driven drug transfer, including the double-balloon catheter,[404] the Wolinsky perforated balloon,[405, 406] microporous balloons,[407, 408] the channel catheter,[409–411] the double-balloon Transport catheter,[412, 413] the Dispatch catheter,[414–418] and the infusion sleeve.[419, 420] An alternative way to deliver an agent locally is accomplished by the hydrogel-coated balloon. Hydrogel is a hydrophilic polyacrylic acid polymer that acts as a drug-absorbing sponge. The drug (or genetic material) is loaded onto a standard balloon simply by dipping the catheter into aqueous solution and letting it dry. When the balloon is then expanded against the wall of the artery, the agent is deposited.[421–425] Local drug delivery has also been achieved by iontophoresis, in which an electric field is used to force an agent into the blood vessel wall.[426, 427] The iontophoretic balloon catheter can result in local concentrations of drug 80 to 100 times greater than those achieved by passive diffusion alone. An additional novel device for achieving intramural drug delivery is the

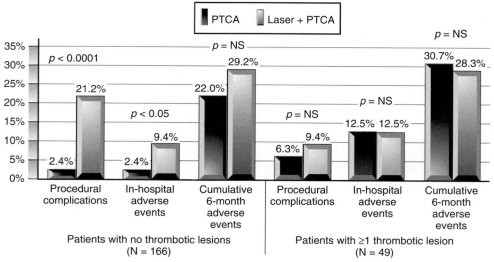

FIGURE 12–19. In-hospital and 6-month events in patients with and without thrombotic lesions randomly assigned to undergo either laser-facilitated percutaneous transluminal coronary angioplasty (PTCA) or stand-alone PTCA in the Laser Angioplasty Versus Angioplasty (LAVA) trial. Procedural complications included acute closure, death, need for emergency coronary artery bypass grafting (CABG), distal thromboemboli, new thrombus formation, spasm, perforation, neurologic event, and side branch occlusion. In-hospital and 6-month adverse events included death, Q-wave or non–Q-wave myocardial infarction, need for repeat PTCA, and need for CABG.

Infiltrator angioplasty balloon catheter. Balloon inflation with this catheter introduces multiple "infiltrator nipples" into the media through which drug may be infused.[428, 429] Finally, a unique way to prolong the retention of drugs or genetic material in the vessel wall may be to load the desired agent into microspheres or nanoparticles, which are then locally deposited and slowly biodegraded.[430, 431]

These different catheter systems vary in the type, amount, and concentration of agent that can be delivered; in flexibility and ease of use; in the capacity to provide antegrade blood perfusion during drug delivery; in the ability to perform PTCA during drug delivery; in the degree and depth to which the agent is delivered into the vessel wall; in the duration of retention of the agent (i.e., rapidity of washout); and in the degree of vascular damage or inflammation resulting directly from their use. All the catheters suffer from low efficiency of drug delivery and poor intramural drug retention, although to varying degrees. These complex issues, which are interrelated, must be resolved before it can be established which delivery system is optimal for coronary use. Furthermore, competing technologies that can locally deliver drugs include coated or polymeric stents, endothelial paving, and stent seeding of genetically modified endothelial cells that can locally produce antithrombotic or thrombolytic compounds such as tPA.[432–436]

The interest in local drug delivery as an adjunct to PTCA has been focused in two clinical arenas: (1) the delivery of site-specific anti-inflammatory, antiproliferative, antineoplastic, or DNA-based agents and vectors to reduce restenosis (this topic is not addressed further in this chapter; see Chapter 45) and (2) antithrombotic drug infusion to prevent or treat the thrombotic complications of PTCA, especially in patients with acute coronary syndromes (including AMI) and thrombotic lesions. By achieving a high concentration of an antithrombotic or antiplatelet agent at the site of thrombus, the performance of PTCA with the use of a local drug delivery catheter has the potential to enhance primary procedural success rates in acute coronary syndromes and reduce the risk of transient or sustained no-reflow and distal thromboemboli, while simultaneously avoiding systemic hemorrhagic toxicity. A variety of site-specific drug delivery catheters have been used successfully for the local intracoronary delivery of unfractionated heparin,[405, 408, 416, 417, 419, 420, 423] LMW heparins,[406, 411, 428] thrombolytic agents such as urokinase,[410, 413, 418, 424, 425] and newer antithrombins.[426, 437] Animal studies also suggest that locally delivered GPIIb/IIIa receptor inhibitors may have potent site-specific antiplatelet effects.[438, 439] The optimal agent for local drug delivery to afford the maximal antithrombotic or antiplatelet effect during PTCA in acute ischemic syndromes has not yet been determined, however, and the efficacy of any of these agents has not been convincingly demonstrated in relation to PTCA alone.

Data are too limited to determine the effectiveness of local antithrombotic drug delivery in comparison with PTCA alone in patients undergoing primary mechanical reperfusion for AMI. Mercho and associates reported their retrospective experience with 143 consecutive patients with AMI undergoing primary PTCA; 73 were treated in a nonrandomized manner with conventional PTCA, and 70 were treated with urokinase-coated hydrogel balloons.[440] TIMI grade 3 flow was restored in similar percentages of both groups (84% after standard PTCA vs. 89% after PTCA with urokinase; $p = 0.36$). However, despite starting with greater thrombus burden (thrombus score, $1.6 \pm 1.0$ vs. $1.3 \pm 1.0$; $p = 0017$), patients undergoing primary PTCA with urokinase-coated hydrogel balloons had lower rates of distal embolization (7.1% vs. 17.8%; $p = 0.076$), no-reflow (10.0% vs. 24.6%; $p = 0.027$), and residual thrombus present (0% vs. 8.2%; $p = 0.028$) than did the patients undergoing standard primary PTCA. In the Cohort of Rescue Angioplasty in Myocardial Infarction (CORAMI-2) study, 108 patients who had suffered AMI within the previous 12 hours were prospectively assigned randomly, in a double-blind manner, to undergo primary PTCA with a hydrogel balloon dipped either in saline or in urokinase.[441] There were no statistically significant differences between the saline- and urokinase-treated patients in the rates of PTCA success or the occurrence of distal thromboemboli, although no-reflow occurred less frequently in the urokinase recipients (Fig. 12–20). Residual thrombus also tended to be present more frequently in the saline recipients than in the urokinase recipients. Predischarge angiography demonstrated reocclusion of the infarcted artery in 3.8% of the patients who underwent standard primary PTCA and in 3.6% of the urokinase-treated patients ($p = $ NS). There were no differences in bleeding complications or access site hematomas between the two groups.

Thus, these data suggest that the performance of primary PTCA with urokinase-coated hydrogel balloons is safe and may decrease angiographic complications of the procedure. However, it remains to be demonstrated that major clinical events are improved with this approach. Because outcomes are worsened when PTCA is performed in the presence of systemic thrombolytic therapy,[20, 306, 307] well-designed trials will have to be performed to clearly demonstrate the value of adjunctive local thrombolysis in patients undergoing primary PTCA with hydrogel balloons before this approach can be recommended.

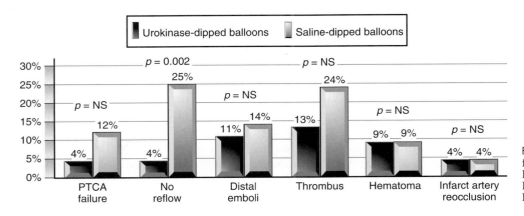

FIGURE 12–20. Clinical outcomes for patients randomized to saline- or urokinase-dipped balloons. PTCA, percutaneous transluminal coronary angioplasty.

The PAMI investigators studied the effects of adjunctive local heparin delivery during primary PTCA for AMI. High-concentration heparin achieved locally by a variety of drug delivery catheters has been shown to persist for 12 to 90 hours at the PTCA site and to decrease local platelet deposition by up to 81% without a systemic anticoagulant effect.[415, 416, 420, 423, 442] The hypotheses of the local PAMI study group were that (1) local heparin infusion during angioplasty could reduce the incidence of recurrent ischemia and reinfarction after primary PTCA; (2) local intracoronary heparin delivery would obviate the need for postprocedure IV heparin, reducing hemorrhagic and vascular complications and facilitating early discharge, without increasing recurrent ischemic events; and (3) by inhibiting neointimal proliferation,[423] local heparin infusion would result in a low rate of late TVR. The local PAMI study was a pilot study in which 120 patients with AMI were treated at nine centers by primary PTCA with standard techniques, after which 4000 U of heparin was delivered by an infusion sleeve drug delivery catheter into the coronary arterial wall.[419, 420] Final procedural success (TIMI grade 2 or 3 flow with residual stenosis affecting <50% of the luminal diameter) was obtained in 99% of patients, although two patients experienced decreased TIMI flow immediately after heparin infusion as a result of dissection, which was treated with repeat PTCA and stents. Overall, stents were placed in 24% of patients with suboptimal results. In-hospital complications, which were infrequent, included death (1.7%), abrupt closure (1.7%), reinfarction (0.9%), recurrent ischemia (6.7%), and TVR (1.7%); the composite of one or more of these adverse events occurred in 12.0% of patients. In the final phase of the study, no additional heparin was given to 20 patients at low risk. One patient (5%) in this group developed recurrent ischemia that was treated medically, but no patient died, experienced reinfarction, or required TVR before hospital discharge. The mean length of hospital stay was 4.1 days. By 6-month follow-up, TVR had been performed in only 7.5% of patients. This pilot study has therefore demonstrated that local heparin delivery, as an adjunct during primary PTCA for AMI, is safe and is associated with a low incidence of in-hospital and postdischarge adverse events. Local heparin so delivered in patients at low risk may eliminate the need for systemic heparin, thereby reducing hemorrhagic and vascular complications and facilitating early discharge.

The field of local drug delivery as an adjunct during primary PTCA is in its infancy and is currently limited by lack of knowledge or efficacy regarding drug dosing, retention, and even the selection of the optimal catheter or agent for a given clinical setting. With the excellent outcomes that are currently achieved routinely with primary PTCA alone, the value and cost effectiveness of adjunctive local drug delivery during primary PTCA must be shown in large-scale, randomized trials with a primary clinical (rather than angiographic) end point. The desirability of local drug infusion during primary PTCA must also be assessed in relation to the superior clinical results reported thus far with primary stent implantation, as well as to the potentially enhanced safety profile and ease of administration of the GPIIb/IIIa receptor blocking agents.

## Aspiration Thrombectomy

The mechanical aspiration of thrombus is no doubt of benefit in selected patients with AMI. Several case reports have demonstrated that large amounts of thrombus may be aspirated by applying suction through the guide catheter (which may need to be intubated deeply down a coronary artery), which has in individual patients restored patency in infarcted vessels and hemodynamic stability (including rescue of patients in cardiogenic shock) when all other measures have failed.[443–450] New thrombectomy catheters, including active aspiration devices, are being developed for this purpose. The Rescue Percutaneous Thrombectomy (RPT) catheter (also known as the Aspiration Thrombectomy catheter) is a 4.5-French dual-lumen tubular device that travels over a 0.014-inch guide wire and is compatible with a 7-French guide catheter.[451, 452] When it is passed into a thrombus, distal suction of 550 to 690 mm Hg can be generated, resulting in thrombus fragmentation and aspiration into a proximal collection bottle. In a series of 11 patients with AMI in whom thrombolytic therapy failed,[453] Michels and coworkers found that thrombus could be aspirated by the RPT catheter in 10 patients (91%), restoring TIMI grade 3 flow and reducing the mean residual stenosis from 93% of the luminal diameter at baseline to 46% after thrombectomy. After adjunctive PTCA, TIMI grade 3 flow was present in all patients. Distal thromboembolization occurred in one patient during device use; the embolism was then aspirated successfully by passing the catheter distally.

### Other Thrombectomy Devices and Novel Pharmacologic Approaches

Other unique methods have been developed to deal with complex thrombotic lesions. The pulse spray thrombolysis system is a 3.6-French catheter through which a thrombolytic agent is actively delivered distally through eight side holes located 4 cm from the distal catheter tip. The lytic spray results in mechanical maceration and fragmentation of the thrombus, while pharmacologic thrombolysis occurs simultaneously.[454] This device has been shown to accelerate thrombolysis experimentally and has been used successfully in obstructed hemodialysis shunts and occluded peripheral vessels.[455–460] Saito and associates demonstrated marked clot reduction in three patients with complex thrombotic coronary lesions treated with this device, including one patient with AMI and an occluded LAD after IV tPA, one patient with thrombotic stent thrombosis, and one patient with thrombotic left main coronary artery occlusion and cardiogenic shock who was undergoing cardiopulmonary resuscitation.[454]

A second novel approach to complex lesion morphology is the autologous vein graft–coated stent, the goal of which is to exclude large thrombi and friable bypass graft atherosclerosis from the general circulation, thereby preventing distal embolization, increasing patency rates, and improving late outcomes.[461] This coated stent also can be used to treat coronary artery aneurysm or rupture.[462–464] Stefanadis and colleagues treated 10 patients with AMI and native coronary occlusion with a Palmaz or Palmaz-Schatz stent with an external autologous cephalic vein graft lining.[465] TIMI grade 3 flow was restored in all 10 patients after implantation of the coated stent. All vessels were patent at follow-up angiography on day 10. In one patient (10%), recur-

rent infarction developed during follow-up with stent occlusion. The time and technical expertise required for the manufacture of this endoprosthesis (including the need for a surgeon to harvest the vein) limits its application to the most experienced centers and unique circumstances, until a commercially produced biocompatible coated stent becomes available (one such device is now marketed in Europe). Whether this approach is superior to implantation with a standard stent or a heparin-coated stent in acute ischemic syndromes is also conjectural.

Finally, pharmacologic adjuncts to primary PTCA are being sought to reduce infarction size and enhance myocardial salvage. One such agent that has been extensively studied is RheothRx (a formulation of poloxamer 188), a surfactant that reduces whole blood viscosity, platelet and red blood cell aggregation, and clot adherence; facilitates thrombolysis; and reduces leukocyte chemotaxis and migration into ischemic tissue.[466] In a small randomized study of 114 patients with AMI treated with thrombolysis, RheothRx reduced infarction size and the rate of reinfarction.[467] In contrast, in the subsequent large multicenter Collaborative Organization for RheothRx Evaluation (CORE) study in which 2948 patients were randomized, RheothRx had no effect on mortality or reinfarction and resulted in worsened LVEF, an increased rate of congestive heart failure, and a 2% to 3% excess rate of renal failure.[468] Similarly, in a phase II study evaluating the efficacy of this agent as an adjunct to primary PTCA in 150 patients with AMI,[469] RheothRx did not salvage myocardium or improve the rates of death or reinfarction; renal failure, however, was increased sixfold in the RheothRx recipients (12% vs. 2%; $p = 0.048$). This agent is therefore no longer being used.

An alternative means to potentially reduce infarction size is the prevention of reperfusion injury, the accelerated tissue damage that occurs when ischemic myocardium is reperfused with unmodified whole blood.[470–472] The causes of reperfusion injury are complex and multifactorial but are thought to involve the activation and accumulation of neutrophils in damaged tissue and the subsequent generation of free radicals, proteolytic enzymes, and metabolites, including leukotrienes. Restoration of vessel patency by primary PTCA for AMI has been demonstrated to markedly increase free radical production,[473] which suggests that white blood cell inhibitors or free radical scavengers may enhance myocardial salvage after PTCA. A randomized trial, however, in which the free radical scavenger superoxide dismutase was administered to patients undergoing primary PTCA for AMI failed to show evidence of enhanced myocardial salvage.[474]

The addition of adenosine or lidocaine to the reperfusate solution has been shown to reduce reperfusion injury in animals.[475–478] Furthermore, left ventricular dysfunction in humans after CABG has been reduced when adenosine was added to cardioplegic solutions.[479–481] In a pilot study in 45 patients with AMI performed at the Mayo Clinic, IV adenosine and lidocaine were administered before reperfusion by primary PTCA.[482] Indices of late myocardial salvage were improved in comparison to historical controls. As a result, the AMISTAD trial, a multicenter double-blind randomized trial, is under way in which AMI patients undergoing primary PTCA are being assigned to pretreatment with either adenosine and lidocaine or placebo; serial technetium-99m scans are used to detect myocardial salvage.

Now that sustained arterial patency and TIMI grade 3 flow can be assured in greater than 90% of patients with AMI, future research direction must shift to myocardial protection. In addition to the novel techniques just described, microcirculatory preservation, protection from distal embolization, and metabolic protection strategies are all being explored. These strategies, in combination with aggressive and well-organized triage and transport community programs, have the promise to further expand the availability and impact of mechanical reperfusion. The major challenge facing clinicians will be how to incorporate these dramatic technical advances into widespread daily treatment of large numbers of patients facing this potentially lethal disease.

# REFERENCES

1. Grines CL, Browne KR, Marco J, et al: A comparison of primary angioplasty with thrombolytic therapy for acute myocardial infarction. N Engl J Med 328:673–679, 1993.
2. Stone GW, Grines CL, Browne KF, et al: Predictors of in-hospital and 6 month outcome after acute myocardial infarction in the reperfusion era: The Primary Angioplasty in Myocardial Infarction (PAMI) Trial. J Am Coll Cardiol 25:370–377, 1995.
3. Zijlstra F, DeBoer MJ, Hoorntje JCA, et al: A comparison of immediate coronary angioplasty with intravenous streptokinase in acute myocardial infarction. N Engl J Med 328:680–684, 1993.
4. Gibbons RJ, Holmes DR, Reeder GS, et al: Immediate angioplasty compared with the administration of a thrombolytic agent followed by conservative treatment for myocardial infarction. N Engl J Med 328:685–691, 1993.
5. Michels KB, Yusuf S: Does PTCA in acute myocardial infarction affect mortality and reinfarction rates? A quantitative (meta-analysis) of the randomized clinical trials. Circulation 91:476–485, 1995.
6. DeWood MA, Spores J, Notske R, et al: Prevalence of total coronary occlusion during the early hours of transmural myocardial infarction. N Engl J Med 303:897–902, 1980.
7. Davies MJ, Thomas AC: Plaque fissuring—The cause of acute myocardial infarction, sudden ischaemic death, and crescendo angina. Br Heart J 53:363–373, 1985.
8. O'Neill WW, Brodie BR, Ivanhoe R, et al: Primary coronary angioplasty for acute myocardial infarction (The Primary Angioplasty Registry). Am J Cardiol 73:627–634, 1994.
9. Stone GW, Rutherford BD, McConahay DR, et al: Direct coronary angioplasty in acute myocardial infarction: Outcome in patients with single vessel disease. J Am Coll Cardiol 15:534–543, 1990.
10. Stone GW, Grines CL, Browne KF, et al: Implications of recurrent ischemia after reperfusion therapy in acute myocardial infarction: A comparison of thrombolytic therapy and primary coronary angioplasty. J Am Coll Cardiol 26:66–72, 1995.
11. Rothbaum DA, Linnemeier TJ, Landin RJ, et al: Emergency percutaneous transluminal coronary angioplasty in acute myocardial infarction: A 3 year experience. J Am Coll Cardiol 10:264–272, 1987.
12. O'Keefe JH, Bailey WL, Rutherford BD, et al: Primary angioplasty for acute myocardial infarction in 1000 consecutive patients. Am J Cardiol 72(suppl G):107G–115G, 1993.
13. Miller PF, Brodie BR, Weintraub RA, et al: Emergency coronary angioplasty for acute myocardial infarction. Arch Intern Med 147:1565–1570, 1987.
14. Grines CL, Marsalese DL, Brodie BR, et al: Safety and cost effectiveness of early discharge after primary angioplasty in low risk patients with acute myocardial infarction. J Am Coll Cardiol 31:967–972, 1998.
15. Stone GW, Marsalese D, Brodie BR, et al: A prospective, randomized evaluation of prophylactic intraaortic balloon counterpulsation in high risk patients with acute myocardial infarction treated with primary angioplasty. J Am Coll Cardiol 29:1459–1467, 1997.
16. Ishihara M, Sato H, Tateishi H, et al: Intraaortic balloon pumping as the post angioplasty strategy in acute myocardial infarction. Am Heart J 122:385–389, 1991.
17. Ohman EM, Califf RM, George BS, et al, and the Thrombolysis and Angioplasty in Myocardial Infarction (TAMI) Study Group: The use of intraaortic balloon counterpulsation as an adjunct to reperfusion therapy in acute myocardial infarction. Am Heart J 191:895–901, 1991.
18. Ohman EM, George BS, White CJ, et al, for the Randomized IABP Study Group: Use of aortic counterpulsation to improve sustained coronary artery patency during acute myocardial infarction. Results of a randomized trial. Circulation 90:792–799, 1994.
19. Ohman EM, Califf RM, Topol EJ, et al: Consequences of reocclusion after successful reperfusion therapy in acute myocardial infarction. Circulation 82:781–791, 1990.
20. O'Neill WW, Weintraub R, Grines CL, et al: A prospective, placebo-controlled, randomized trial of intravenous streptokinase and angioplasty versus lone angioplasty therapy of acute myocardial infarction. Circulation 86:1710–1717, 1992.
21. Brodie BR, Grines CL, Ivanhoe R, et al: Six-month clinical and angiographic follow-up after direct angioplasty for acute myocardial infarction. Circulation 90:156–162, 1994.
22. Nakae I, Fujita M, Fudo T, et al: Relation between preexistent coronary collateral circulation and the incidence of restenosis after successful primary coronary angioplasty for acute myocardial infarction. J Am Coll Cardiol 27:1688–1692, 1996.
23. Nakagawa Y, Iwasaki Y, Kimura T, et al: Serial angiographic follow-up after successful direct angioplasty for acute myocardial infarction. Am J Cardiol 78:980–984, 1996.
24. Brodie BR, Stuckey TD, Kissling G, et al: Importance of infarct-related artery patency for recovery of left ventricular function and late survival after primary angioplasty for acute myocardial infarction. J Am Coll Cardiol 28:319–325, 1996.
25. Nunn C, O'Neill W, Rothbaum D, et al: Primary angioplasty for myocardial infarction improves long-term survival: PAMI-1 follow-up. J Am Coll Cardiol 33:640–646, 1999.
26. Hartzler GO, Rutherford BD, McConahay DR: Percutaneous transluminal coronary angioplasty: Application for acute myocardial infarction. Am J Cardiol 53(suppl C):117C–121C, 1984.
27. Friedman MF, Van der Bovenkamp EJ: The pathogenesis of a coronary thrombus. Am J Pathol 48:19–44, 1966.
28. Chandler AB: The anatomy of a thrombus. In Sherry S,

Brinkhous K, Genton E, et al (eds): Thrombosis. Washington, DC: National Academy of Sciences, 1969, pp 279–299.

29. Hamm CW, Lorenz RL, Bleifeld W, et al: Biochemical evidence of platelet activation in patients with persistent unstable angina. J Am Coll Cardiol 10:988–1006, 1987.

30. Hoffmeister HM, Jur M, Wendel HP, et al: Alterations of coagulation and fibrinolytic and kallekrein-kinin systems in acute and post acute phases in patients with unstable angina pectoris. Circulation 91:2520–2527, 1995.

31. Kontny F: Reactivation of the coagulation system: Rationale for long-term antithrombotic treatment. Am J Cardiol 80(suppl E):55E–60E, 1997.

32. Merlini PA, Bauer KA, Oltrona L, et al: Persistent activation of coagulation mechanism in unstable angina and myocardial infarction. Circulation 90:61–68, 1994.

33. Ardissino D, Merlini P, Gamba G, et al: Thrombin activity and early outcome in unstable angina pectoris. Circulation 93:1634–1639, 1996.

34. Coughlin SR, Vu TK, Hung DT, et al: Characterization of a functional thrombin receptor: Issues and opportunities. J Clin Invest 89:351–355, 1992.

35. Chesebro JH, Webster MW, Zoldhelyi P, et al: Antithrombotic therapy and progression of coronary artery disease. Antiplatelet versus antithrombins. Circulation 86:100–111, 1992.

36. Francis CW, Markham RE, Barlow GH, et al: Thrombin activity of fibrin thrombi and soluble plasma derivatives. J Lab Clin Med 102:220–230, 1983.

37. Pope CF, Ezekowitz MD, Smith EO, et al: Detection of platelet deposition at the site of peripheral balloon angioplasty using indium-111 platelet scintigraphy. Am J Cardiol 55:495–497, 1985.

38. Gasperetti CM, Gonias SL, Gimple LW, et al: Platelet activation during coronary angioplasty in humans. Circulation 88:2728–2734, 1993.

39. Steele PM, Chesebro JH, Stanson AW, et al: Balloon angioplasty: Natural history of the pathophysiologic response in a pig model. Circ Res 57:105–112, 1985.

40. Minar E, Ehringer H, Ahmadi R, et al: Platelet deposition at angioplasty sites and platelet survival time after PTA in iliac and femoral arteries: Investigations with indium-111–oxide labeled platelets in patients with ASA (1.0 g/D) therapy. Thromb Haemost 58:718–723, 1987.

41. Badimon L, Badimon JJ, Galvez A, et al: Influence of arterial wall damage and wall shear rate on platelet deposition: Ex vivo study in a swine model. Arteriosclerosis 6:312–320, 1986.

42. Wilentz JR, Sanborn TA, Haudenschild CC, et al: Platelet accumulation in experimental angioplasty: Time course in relation to cardiovascular injury. Circulation 75:636–642, 1987.

43. Gawaz M, Neumann FJ, Ott I, et al: Platelet function in acute myocardial infarction treated with direct angioplasty. Circulation 93:229–237, 1996.

44. Marmur JD, Merlini PA, Sharma SK, et al: Thrombin generation in human coronary arteries after percutaneous transluminal coronary angioplasty. J Am Coll Cardiol 24:1484–1491, 1994.

45. Uren NG, Crake T, Lefroy DC, et al: Reduced coronary vasodilator function in infarcted and normal myocardium after myocardial infarction. N Engl J Med 331:222–227, 1994.

46. Chen LY, Nichols WW, Hendricks JB, et al: Monoclonal antibody to P-selectin (PB1.3) protects against myocardial reperfusion injury in the dog. Cardiovasc Res 28:1414–1422, 1994.

47. Frink RJ, Rooney PAJ, Trowbridge JO, et al: Coronary thrombosis and platelet/fibrin microemboli in death associated with acute myocardial infarction. Br Heart J 59:196–200, 1988.

48. Weinberger I, Fuchs J, Davidson E, et al: Circulating aggregated platelets, number of platelets per aggregate, and platelet size during acute myocardial infarction. Am J Cardiol 70:981–983, 1992.

49. Patrono C, Renda G: Platelet activation and inhibition in unstable coronary syndromes [Abstract]. Am J Cardiol 80(5A):17E–20E, 1997.

50. Fuster V, Jang IK: Role of platelet-inhibitor agents in coronary artery disease. In Topol EJ (ed): Textbook of Interventional Cardiology, 2nd ed, vol 1. Philadelphia: WB Saunders, 1994, pp 3–22.

51. Leung L, Nachman R: Molecular mechanisms of platelet aggregation. Annu Rev Med 37:179–186, 1986.

52. Phillips DR, Charo IF, Parise LV, et al: The platelet membrane glycoprotein IIb-IIIa complex. Blood 71:831–843, 1988.

53. Lefkovits J, Plow EF, Topol EJ: Platelet glycoprotein IIb/IIIa receptors in cardiovascular medicine. N Engl J Med 332:1553–1559, 1995.

54. Roth GJ, Stanford N, Majerus PW: Acetylation of prostaglandin synthase by aspirin. Proc Natl Acad Sci U S A 72:3073–3076, 1975.

55. Cattaneo M, Akkawat B, Lecchi A, et al: Ticlopidine selectively inhibits human platelet response to adenosine diphosphate. Thromb Haemost 66:694–699, 1991.

56. Harker LA, Bruno JJ: Ticlopidine's mechanism of action on human platelets. In Hass WK, Eastgon JD (eds): Ticlopidine, Platelets and Vascular Disease. New York: Springer-Verlag, 1991, pp 41–51.

57. ISIS-2 (Second International Study Group of Infarct Survival) Collaborative Group: Randomized trial of intravenous streptokinase, oral aspirin, both, or neither among 17,187 cases of suspected acute myocardial infarction. Lancet 2:349–360, 1988.

58. The RISC Group: Risk of myocardial infarction and death during treatment with low dose aspirin and intravenous heparin in men with unstable coronary artery disease. Lancet 336:827–830, 1990.

59. Lewis HD, Davis JW, Archibald DG, et al: Protective effects of aspirin against myocardial infarction and death in men with unstable angina. Results of a Veterans Administration Cooperative Study. N Engl J Med 309:396–403, 1983.

60. Cairns JA, Gent M, Singer J: Aspirin, sulfinpyrazone, or both in unstable angina. Results of a Canadian multicenter trial. N Engl J Med 313:1369–1375, 1985.

61. Balsano F, Rizzon P, Violi F, et al: Antiplatelet treatment with ticlopidine in unstable angina. A controlled multicenter clinical trial. The Studio della Ticlopidina nell'Angina Instabile Group. Circulation 82:17–26, 1990.

62. Antiplatelet Trialists' Collaboration: Collaborative overview of randomized trial of antiplatelet therapy I: Prevention of death, myocardial infarction, and stroke by prolonged antiplatelet therapy in various categories of patients. BMJ 308:81–106, 1994.

63. Patrono C: Unstable coronary artery disease: Need for long-term antithrombotic treatment? Aspirin alone may not be the ideal antithrombotic strategy, but that's what we have adequate trial data for. Cardiovasc Res 33:295–296, 1997.

64. Garcia-Dorado D, Theroux P, Tornos P, et al: Previous aspirin use may attenuate the severity of the manifestation of acute ischemic syndromes. Circulation 92:1743–1748, 1995.

65. Schwartz L, Bourassa MG, Lesperance J, et al: Aspirin and dipyridamole in the prevention of restenosis after percutaneous transluminal coronary angioplasty. N Engl J Med 318:1714–1719, 1988.

66. White CW, Chairman B, Knudtson ML, et al: Antiplatelet agents are effective in reducing the acute ischemic complications of angioplasty but do not prevent restenosis: Results from the ticlopidine trial. Coron Artery Dis 2:757–767, 1991.

67. Bertrand ME, Allain H, Lablanche JM, et al: Results of a randomized trial of ticlopidine versus placebo for prevention of acute closure and restenosis after coronary angioplasty: The TACT study [Abstract]. Eur Heart J 11:368, 1990.

68. Barry WL, Sarembock IJ: Antiplatelet and anticoagulant therapy in patients undergoing percutaneous transluminal coronary angioplasty. Cardiol Clin 12:517–535, 1994.

69. Schomig A, Neumann FJ, Kastrati A, et al: A randomized comparison of antiplatelet and anticoagulant therapy after the placement of coronary artery stents. N Engl J Med 334:1084–1089, 1996.

70. Leon MB, Baim DS, Popma JJ, et al: A clinical trial comparing three antithrombotic drug regimens after coronary-artery stenting. N Engl J Med 339:1665, 1998.

71. Tcheng JE, Ellis SG, George BS, et al: Pharmacodynamics of chimeric glycoprotein IIb/IIIa antiplatelet antibody Fab 7E3 in high-risk coronary angioplasty. Circulation 90:1757–1764, 1994.

72. Charo IF, Bekeart LS, Phillips DR: Platelet glycoprotein IIb-IIIa–like proteins mediate endothelial cell attachment to adhesive proteins and the extracellular matrix. J Biol Chem 262:9935–9938, 1987.

73. Choi ET, Engel L, Callow AD, et al: Inhibition of neointimal hyperplasia by blocking the $a_vb_3$ integrin with a small peptide antagonist GpenGRGDSPCA. J Vasc Surg 19:125–134, 1994.

74. Deng G, Royle G, Seiffert D, et al: The PAI-1/vitronectin interaction: Two cats in a bag? Thromb Haemost 74:66–70, 1995.

75. Muhlestein JB, Karagounis LA, Treehan S, et al: "Rescue" utilization of abciximab for the dissolution of coronary thrombus developing as a complication of coronary angioplasty. J Am Coll Cardiol 30:1729–1734, 1997.

76. The EPIC Investigators: Use of a monoclonal antibody directed against the platelet glycoprotein IIb/IIIa receptor in high-risk coronary angioplasty. N Engl J Med 330:956–961, 1994.

77. Topol EJ, Califf RM, Weisman HF, et al: Randomised trial of coronary intervention with antibody against platelet IIb/IIIa integrin for reduction of clinical restenosis: Results at 6 months. Lancet 343:881–886, 1994.

78. Topol EJ, Ferguson JJ, Weisman HF, et al: Long-term protection from myocardial ischemic events in a randomized trial of brief integrin B3 blockade with percutaneous coronary intervention. JAMA 278:479–484, 1997.

79. The EPILOG Investigators: Platelet glycoprotein IIb/IIIa receptor blockade and low-dose heparin during percutaneous coronary revascularization. N Engl J Med 336:1689–1696, 1997.

80. The CAPTURE Investigators: Randomised placebo-controlled trial of abciximab before and during coronary intervention in refractory unstable angina: The CAPTURE study. Lancet 349:1429–1435, 1997.

81. Lefkovits J, Ivanhoe RJ, Califf RM, et al: Effects of platelet glycoprotein IIb/IIIa receptor blockade by a chimeric monoclonal antibody (abciximab) on acute and six-month outcomes after percutaneous transluminal coronary angioplasty for acute myocardial infarction. Am J Cardiol 77:1045–1051, 1996.

82. Brener SJ, Barr LA, Burchenal J, et al: A randomized, placebo-controlled trial of abciximab with primary angioplasty for acute MI. The RAPPORT trial. Circulation 96:I-473, 1997.

83. Brodie B, Grines CL, Spain M, et al: A prospective, randomized trial evaluating early discharge (day 3) without non-invasive risk stratification in low risk patients with acute myocardial infarction [Abstract]. J Am Coll Cardiol 25:5, 1995.

84. Stone GW, Marsalese D, Brodie BR, et al: A prospective, randomized evaluation of prophylactic intraaortic balloon counterpulsation in high risk patients with acute myocardial infarction treated with primary angioplasty. J Am Coll Cardiol 29:1459–1467, 1997.

85. Ellis SG, Serruys PW, Popma JJ, et al: Can abciximab prevent neointimal proliferation in Palmaz-Schatz stents? The final ERASER results [Abstract]. Circulation 96:I-87, 1997.

86. Peerlinck K, De Lepeleire I, Goldberg M, et al: MK-383 (L-700,462), a selective nonpeptide platelet glycoprotein IIb/IIIa antagonist, is active in man. Circulation 88:1512–1517, 1993.

87. Egbertson MS, Chang CT, Duggan ME, et al: Non peptide fibrinogen receptor antagonists: 2. Optimization of a tyrosine template as a mimic for Arg-Gly-Asp. J Med Chem 37:2537–2551, 1994.

88. The RESTORE Investigators: Effect of platelet glycoprotein IIb/IIIa blockade with tirofiban on adverse cardiac events in patients with unstable angina or acute myocardial infarction undergoing coronary angioplasty. Circulation 96:1445–1453, 1997.

89. Caputo RP, Ho KKL, Stoler RC, et al: Effect of continuous quality improvement analysis on the delivery of primary percutaneous coronary angioplasty for acute myocardial infarction. Am J Cardiol 79:1159–1164, 1997.

90. Gruppo Italiano per lo Studio della Streptochinasi nell'Infarto Miocardico (GISSI): Effectiveness of intravenous thrombolytic treatment in acute myocardial infarction. Lancet 1:397–402, 1986.

91. The Fibrinolytic Therapy Trialists (FTT) Collaborative Group: Indications for fibrinolytic therapy in suspected acute myocardial infarction: Collaborative overview of early mortality and major morbidity results from all randomised trials of more than 1000 patients. Lancet 343:311–322, 1994.

92. O'Neill WW, Weintraub R, Grines CL, et al: A prospective, placebo-controlled, randomized trial of intravenous streptokinase and angioplasty versus lone angioplasty therapy of acute myocardial infarction. Circulation 86:1710–1717, 1992.

93. Chesebro JH, Knatterud G, Roberts R, et al: Thrombolysis in Myocardial Infarction (TIMI) Trial, phase I: A comparison between intravenous tissue plasminogen activator and intravenous streptokinase. Circulation 76:142–154, 1987.

94. Verheugt FWA, Marsh RC, Veen G, et al: Megadose bolus heparin as reperfusion therapy for acute myocardial infarction: Results of the HEAP pilot study [Abstract]. Circulation 92:I-415, 1995.

95. Liem A, Zijlstra F, Ottervanger JR, et al: High dose heparin as pretreatment for primary angioplasty in acute myocardial infarction: The Heparin in Early Patency (HEAP) randomized trial. J Am Coll Cardiol 35:600, 2000.

96. Deckers J, Califf RM, Topol EJ, et al: Use of abciximab (ReoPro) is not associated with an increase in the risk of stroke: Overview of three randomized trials [Abstract]. J Am Coll Cardiol 29:241, 1997.

97. Gold HK, Garabedian HD, Dinsmore RE, et al: Restoration of coronary flow in myocardial infarction by intravenous chimeric 7E3 antibody without exogenous plasminogen activators. Circulation 95:1755–1759, 1997.

98. Antman EM: TIMI-14: Abciximab plus thrombolytic therapy. Presented at the George Washington University 13th International Workshop: Thrombolysis and Interventional Therapy in Acute Myocardial Infarction, Orlando FL, November 8, 1997.

99. Merkhof-Van Den LFM, Liem A, Olsson H, et al: Early coronary patency evaluation of a platelet glycoprotein receptor antagonist (abciximab) in primary PTCA: The GRAPE-pilot study [Abstract]. Circulation 96:I-474, 1997.

100. Gold HK, Kereiakes DJ, Dinsmore RE, et al: A randomized, placebo-controlled crossover trial of ReoPro alone or combined with low-dose plasminogen activator for coronary reperfusion in patients with acute myocardial infarction: Preliminary results [Abstract]. Circulation 96:I-474, 1997.

101. The GUSTO Angiographic Investigators: The effects of tissue plasminogen activator, streptokinase, or both on coronary-artery patency, ventricular function, and survival after acute myocardial infarction. N Engl J Med 329:1615–1622, 1993.

102. Coller BS, Anderson K, Weisman HF, et al: New antiplatelet agents: Platelet GPIIb/IIIa antagonists. Thromb Haemost 74:302–308, 1995.

103. Coutre S, Leung L: Novel antithrombotic therapeutics targeted against platelet glycoprotein IIb/IIIa. Annu Rev Med 46:257–265, 1995.

104. TIMI 12 Trial Investigators: Evaluation of the oral glycoprotein IIb/IIIa antagonist R0 48-3657 in patients post acute coronary syndromes: Primary results of the TIMI 12 trial [Abstract]. Circulation 94:I-552, 1996.

105. Kereiakes DJ, Kleiman N, Ferguson JJ, et al: Sustained platelet glycoprotein IIb/IIIa blockade with oral xemilofiban in 170 patients after coronary stent deployment. Circulation 96:1117–1121, 1997.

106. Simpfendorfer C, Kottke-Marchant K, Mowrie M, et al: First chronic platelet glycoprotein IIb/IIIa integrin blockade. A randomized, placebo-controlled pilot study of xemilofiban

in unstable angina with percutaneous coronary interventions. Circulation 96:76–81, 1997.

107. Phillips DR, Scarborough RM: Clinical pharmacology of eptifibatide [Abstract]. Am J Cardiol 80(4A):11B–20B, 1997.

108. The IMPACT-II Investigators: Randomised placebo-controlled trial of effect of eptifibatide on complications of percutaneous coronary intervention: IMPACT-II. Lancet 349:1422–1428, 1997.

109. Ferguson J, Dougherty K, Gaos C, et al: Relation between procedural activated coagulation time and outcome after percutaneous transluminal coronary angioplasty. J Am Coll Cardiol 23:1061–1065, 1994.

110. Winters K, Oltrona L, Hiremath Y, et al: Heparin-resistant thrombin activity is associated with acute ischemic events during high-risk coronary interventions [Abstract]. Circulation 92:I-608, 1995.

111. Harrington RA, Leimberer JD, Berdan L, et al: The ACT Index: A method for stratifying likelihood of success and risk of acute complications in coronary intervention. Circulation 88:I-208, 1993.

112. Ahmed W, Meckel C, Grines CL, et al: Relation between ischemic complications and activated clotting times during coronary angioplasty: Different profiles for heparin and hirulog [Abstract]. Circulation 92:I-608, 1995.

113. Narins CR, Hillegass WG, Nelson CL, et al: Relation between activated clotting time during angioplasty and abrupt closure. J Am Coll Cardiol 80:1718, 1989.

114. Theroux P, Ouimet H, McCans J, et al: Aspirin, heparin, or both to treat acute unstable angina. N Engl J Med 319:1105–1111, 1988.

115. Grines CL, Stone GW, O'Neill WW: Establishing a program and performance of primary PTCA—The PAMI way. J Invas Cardiol 9(suppl B):44B–52B, 1996.

116. Morishima I, Sone T, Mokuno S, et al: Clinical significance of no-reflow phenomenon observed on angiography after successful treatment of acute myocardial infarction with percutaneous transluminal coronary angioplasty. Am Heart J 130:239–243, 1995.

117. Abbo KM, Dooris M, Glazier S, et al: Features and outcome of no-reflow after percutaneous coronary intervention. Am J Cardiol 75:778–782, 1995.

118. Mercho N, Eldin AM, Shareef B, et al: Angiographic complications of primary angioplasty. J Am Coll Cardiol 27:61A, 1996.

119. Marzilli M, Gliozheni E, Fedele S, et al: Prevalence and prediction of no-reflow after direct angioplasty in acute myocardial infarction [Abstract]. J Am Coll Cardiol 29:90, 1997.

120. Stone GW, Grines CL, Browne KF, et al: Adverse catheterization laboratory events after primary PTCA vs. PTCA following thrombolytic therapy—A report from the Primary Angioplasty in Myocardial Infarction (PAMI) trial [Abstract]. J Am Coll Cardiol 23:244, 1994.

121. De Boer MJ, Reiber JHC, Suryapranata H, et al: Angiographic findings and catheterization laboratory events in patients with primary coronary angioplasty or streptokinase therapy for acute myocardial infarction. Eur Heart J 16:1347–1355, 1995.

122. Smith AJC, Holt RE, Fitzpatrick K, et al: Transient thrombotic state after abrupt discontinuation of heparin in percutaneous coronary angioplasty. Am Heart J 131:434–439, 1996.

123. Granger C, Armstrong P, for the GUSTO-IIa Investigators: Reinfarction following discontinuation of intravenous heparin or hirudin for unstable angina and acute myocardial infarction [Abstract]. Circulation 92:I-460, 1995.

124. Granger C, Miller J, Bovill E, et al: Rebound increase in thrombin generation and activity after cessation of intravenous heparin in patients with acute coronary syndromes. Circulation 91:1929–1935, 1995.

125. Flather M, Weitz J, Campeau J, et al: Evidence for rebound activation of the coagulation system after cessation of intravenous anticoagulant therapy for acute MI. Circulation 92:I-485, 1995.

126. Stony J, Ahmed W, Meckel C, et al: Clinical evidence for

127. Khan M, Sepulveda J, Jeroudi M, et al: Rebound increase in thrombin activity with associated decrease in antithrombin III levels after PTCA. Circulation 92:I-785, 1995.

128. Theroux P, Waters D, Lam J, et al: Reactivation of unstable angina after the discontinuation of angina. N Engl J Med 327:141–145, 1992.

129. Marciniak E, Gockerman JP: Heparin-induced decrease in circulating antithrombin-III. Lancet 2:581–584, 1977.

130. Iverson N, Abildgaard U: Role of antithrombin and tissue factor pathway inhibitor in the control of thrombosis and mediation of heparin action. Clin Appl Thromb Haemost 2:1–6, 1996.

131. Fiore L, Deykin D: Anticoagulant therapy. In Beutler E, Lichtman MA, Coller BS, et al (eds): Williams Hematology, 5th ed. New York: McGraw-Hill, 1995, pp 1562–1584.

132. Ware JA, Coller BS: Platelet morphology, biochemistry, and function. In Beutler E, Lichtman MA, Coller BS, et al (eds): Williams Hematology, 5th ed. New York: McGraw-Hill, 1995, pp 1161–1201.

133. Hirsh J, Fuster V: Guide to anticoagulant therapy: I. Heparin. Circulation 89:1449–1468, 1994.

134. Weitz J: New anticoagulant strategies. Current status and future potential. Drugs 48:485–497, 1994.

135. Jesty J, Nemerson Y: The pathways of blood coagulation. In Beutler E, Lichtman MA, Coller BS, et al (eds): Williams Hematology, 5th ed. New York: McGraw-Hill, 1995, pp 1227–1338.

136. Hirsh J, Raschke R, Warkentin TE, et al: Heparin: Mechanism of action, pharmacokinetics, dosing considerations, monitoring, efficacy, and safety. Chest 108(suppl S):258S–275S, 1995.

137. Hirsh J, Levine MN: Low-molecular-weight heparin. Blood 79:1–17, 1992.

138. Cade JF, Buchanan MR, Boneu B, et al: A comparison of the antithrombotic and hemorrhagic effects of low-molecular-weight heparin fractions: The influence of the method of preparation. Thromb Res 35:613–625, 1984.

139. Warkentin TE, Levine MN, Hirsh J, et al: Heparin-induced thrombocytopenia in patients treated with low-molecular-weight heparin or unfractionated heparin. N Engl J Med 332:1330–1335, 1995.

140. Cohen M, Demers C, Gurfinkel EP, et al: A comparison of low-molecular-weight heparin with unfractionated heparin for unstable coronary artery disease. N Engl J Med 337:447–452, 1997.

141. Klein W, Buchwald A, Hillis SE, et al: Comparison of low-molecular-weight heparin with unfractionated heparin acutely and with placebo for 6 weeks in the management of unstable coronary artery disease. Fragmin in Unstable Coronary Artery Disease Study (FRIC). Circulation 96:61–68, 1997.

142. Karsh KR, Preisack MB, Baildon R, et al: Low molecular weight heparin (reviparin) in percutaneous transluminal coronary angioplasty. Results of a randomized, double-blind, unfractionated heparin and placebo-controlled, multicenter (REDUCE) Trial. J Am Coll Cardiol 1996; 28:1437–1443, 1996.

143. Lablanche JM, McFadden EP, Meneveau N, et al: Effect of nadroparin, a low-molecular-weight heparin, on clinical and angiographic restenosis after coronary balloon angioplasty. The FACT study. Circulation 96:3396–3402, 1997.

144. Fragmin during Instability in Coronary Artery Disease (FRISC) Study Group: Low-molecular-weight heparin during instability in coronary artery disease. Lancet 347:561–568, 1996.

145. Swahn E, Wallentin L, for the FRISC Study Group: Low-molecular-weight heparin (Fragmin) during instability in coronary artery disease (FRISC). Am J Cardiol 80(suppl E):25E–29E, 1997.

146. Clowes AW, Karnowsky MJ: Suppression by heparin of smooth muscle cell proliferation in injured arteries. Nature 265:625–626, 1977.

147. Castello J, Cochran D, Karnowsky M: Effect of heparin on

vascular smooth muscle cell: I. Cell metabolism. J Cell Physiol 124:21–28, 1985.

148. Guyton J, Rosenberg R, Clowes A, et al: Inhibition of rat arterial smooth muscle cell proliferation by heparin: In vitro studies with anticoagulant heparin. Circ Res 46:625–634, 1980.

149. Buchwald AB, Unterberg C, Nebendahl K, et al: Low-molecular-weight heparin (enoxaparin) reduces neointimal proliferation after coronary stent implantation in hypercholesterolemic minipigs. Circulation 86:531–537, 1992.

150. Hanke H, Oberhoff M, Hanke S, et al: Inhibition of cellular proliferation after experimental balloon angioplasty by low molecular weight heparin. Circulation 85:1548–1556, 1992.

151. Ellis SG, Roubin GS, Wilentz J, et al: Effect of 18 to 24 hour heparin administration for prevention of restenosis after uncomplicated coronary angioplasty. Am Heart J 117:777–782, 1989.

152. Brack MJ, Ray S, Chauhan A, et al: The Subcutaneous Heparin and Angioplasty Restenosis Prevention (SHARP) trial. J Am Coll Cardiol 26:947–954, 1995.

153. Schmidt T, Tebbe U, Brune SS, et al: Pharmacologic therapy after coronary angioplasty: Early experience with low molecular weight heparin for prophylaxis of reocclusion. Klin Wochenschr 68:294–295, 1990.

154. Faxon DP, Spiro TE, Minor S, et al: Low molecular weight heparin in prevention of restenosis after angioplasty. Results of the Enoxaparin Restenosis (ERA) trial. Circulation 90:908–914, 1994.

155. Cairns JA, Gill J, Morton B, et al: Fish oils and low-molecular-weight heparin for the reduction of restenosis after percutaneous transluminal coronary angioplasty. The EMPAR study. Circulation 94:1553–1560, 1996.

156. Lablanche JM, McFadden EP, Meneveau N, et al: Effect of nadroparin, a low-molecular-weight heparin, on clinical and angiographic restenosis after coronary balloon angioplasty. The FACT study. Circulation 96:3396–3402, 1997.

157. Zidar JP: Rationale for low-molecular weight heparin in coronary stenting. Am Heart J 134(suppl S):S81–S87, 1997.

158. Lefkovits J, Topol EJ: Direct thrombin inhibitors in cardiovascular medicine. Circulation 90:1522–1536, 1994.

159. Turpie AGG, Weitz JI, Hirsh J: Advances in antithrombotic therapy: Novel agents. Thromb Haemost 74:565–571, 1995.

160. Weitz JI, Hirsh J: New antithrombotic strategies. J Lab Clin Med 122:364–373, 1993.

161. Kaiser B: Anticoagulant and antithrombotic action of recombinant hirudin. Semin Thromb Hemost 17:130–135, 1991.

162. Lewis BE, Ferguson JJ, Grassman ED, et al: Successful coronary interventions performed with argatroban anticoagulation in patients with heparin-induced thrombocytopenia and thrombosis syndrome. J Invas Cardiol 8:410–417, 1996.

163. Schiele F, Villemenot A, Kramarz P, et al: Use of recombinant hirudin as antithrombotic treatment in patients with heparin-induced thrombocytopenia. Am J Hematol 50:20–25, 1995.

164. Heras M, Chesebro JH, Webster MWI, et al: Hirudin, heparin and placebo during deep arterial injury in the pig: The in vivo role of thrombin in platelet-mediated thrombosis. Circulation 82:1476–1484, 1990.

165. Heras M, Chesebro JH, Penny WJ, et al: Effects of thrombin inhibition on the development of acute platelet-thrombus deposition during angioplasty in pigs. Heparin versus recombinant hirudin, a specific thrombin inhibitor. Circulation 79:657–665, 1989.

166. Sarembock IJ, Gertz SD, Gimple LW, et al: Effectiveness of recombinant desulphatohirudin in reducing restenosis after balloon angioplasty of atherosclerotic femoral arteries in rabbits. Circulation 84:232–243, 1991.

167. Antman EM: Hirudin in acute myocardial infarction. Safety report from the Thrombolysis and Thrombin Inhibition in Myocardial Infarction (TIMI) 9A Trial. Circulation 90:1624–1630, 1994.

168. The Global Use of Strategies to Open Occluded Coronary Arteries (GUSTO) IIa Investigators: GUSTO IIA: Randomized trial of intravenous heparin versus recombinant hirudin for acute coronary syndromes. Circulation 90:1631–1637, 1994.

169. Neuhaus KL, von Essen R, Tebbe U, et al: Safety observations from the pilot phase of the randomized r-Hirudin for Improvement of Thrombolysis (HIT-III) study. A study of the Arbeitsgemeinschaft Leitender Kardiologischer Krankenhausarzte (ALKK). Circulation 90:1638–1642, 1994.

170. Organization to Assess Strategies for Ischemic Syndromes (OASIS) Investigators: Comparison of the effects of two doses of recombinant hirudin compared with heparin in patients with acute myocardial ischemia without ST elevation. Circulation 96:769–777, 1997.

171. The Global Use of Strategies to Open Occluded Coronary Arteries (GUSTO) IIb Investigators: A comparison of recombinant hirudin with heparin for the treatment of acute coronary syndromes. N Engl J Med 335:775–782, 1996.

172. Serruys PW, Herman JPR, Simon R, et al: A comparison of hirudin with heparin in the prevention of restenosis after coronary angioplasty. N Engl J Med 333:757–763, 1995.

173. Gold HK, Torres FW, Garabedian HD, et al: Evidence for a rebound coagulation phenomenon after cessation of a 4-hour infusion of a specific thrombin inhibitor in patients with unstable angina pectoris. J Am Coll Cardiol 21:1039–1047, 1993.

174. Bittl JA, Strony J, Brinker JA, et al: Treatment with bivalirudin (Hirulog) as compared with heparin during coronary angioplasty for unstable or postinfarction angina. N Engl J Med 333:764–769, 1995.

175. The Global Use of Strategies to Open Occluded Coronary Arteries in Acute Coronary Syndromes (GUSTO-IIb) Angioplasty Substudy Investigators: A clinical trial comparing primary coronary angioplasty with tissue plasminogen activator for acute myocardial infarction. N Engl J Med 336:1621–1628, 1997.

176. Zoldhelyi P, Janssens S, Lefevre G, et al: Effects of heparin and hirudin (CGP 39393) on thrombin generation during thrombolysis for acute myocardial infarction [Abstract]. Circulation 92:I-740, 1995.

177. Merlini PA, Ardissino D, Bauer K, et al: Persistent thrombin generation during heparin treatment in patients with acute coronary syndromes [Abstract]. Circulation 92:I-623, 1995.

178. Serruys PW, de Jaegere P, Kiemeneij F, et al: A comparison of balloon-expandable-stent implantation with balloon angioplasty in patients with coronary artery disease. N Engl J Med 331:489–495, 1994.

179. Fischman DL, Leon MB, Baim DS, et al: A randomized comparison of coronary-stent placement and balloon angioplasty in the treatment of coronary artery disease. N Engl J Med 331:496–501, 1994.

180. Lindsay J, Hong MK, Pinnow EE, et al: Effects of endoluminal coronary stents on the frequency of coronary artery bypass grafting after unsuccessful percutaneous transluminal coronary revascularization. Am J Cardiol 77:647–649, 1996.

181. Altmann DB, Racz M, Battleman DS, et al: Reduction in angioplasty complications after the introduction of coronary stents: Results from a consecutive series of 2242 patients. Am Heart J 132:503–507, 1996.

182. Kuntz RE, Safian RD, Carrozza JP, et al: The importance of acute luminal diameter in determining restenosis after coronary atherectomy or stenting. Circulation 86:1827–1835, 1992.

183. Kuntz RE, Gibson CM, Nobuyoshi M, et al: Generalized model of restenosis after conventional balloon angioplasty, stenting and directional atherectomy. J Am Coll Cardiol 21:15–25, 1993.

184. Versaci F, Gaspardone A, Tomai F, et al: A comparison of coronary-artery stenting with angioplasty for isolated stenosis of the proximal left anterior descending artery. N Engl J Med 336:817–822, 1997.

185. Legrand V, Serruys PW, Emanuelsson H, et al: BENESTENT-II Trial—Final results of visit I: A 15-day follow-up. J Am Coll Cardiol 29:170A, 1997.

186. Garcia E, Serruys PW, Dawkins K, et al: BENESTENT-II trial: Final results of visit II & III: A 7 month follow-up [Abstract]. Eur Heart J 1997;18:350, 1997.

187. Schatz RA, Baim DS, Leon M, et al: Clinical experience with the Palmaz-Schatz coronary stent: Initial results of a multicenter trial. Circulation 83:148–161, 1991.

188. Agrawal SK, Ho DSV, Liu MW, et al: Predictors of thrombotic complications after placement of a flexible coil stent. Am J Cardiol 73:1216–1219, 1994.

189. Grines C, Brodie B, Griffin J, et al: Which primary PTCA patients may benefit from new technologies [Abstract]? Circulation 92:I-146, 1995.

190. Benzuly KH, O'Neill WW, Brodie B, et al: Predictors of maintained infarct artery patency after primary angioplasty in high risk patients in PAMI-2 [Abstract]. J Am Coll Cardiol 27:279A, 1996.

191. Ribeiro EE, Silva LA, Cardeiro R, et al: Randomized trial of direct coronary angioplasty versus intravenous streptokinase in acute myocardial infarction. J Am Coll Cardiol 22:376–380, 1993.

192. Steffenino G, Chierchia S, Fontanelli A, et al: Use of stents during emergency coronary angioplasty in patients with high-risk acute myocardial infarction: In-hospital results from the Italian Multicenter Registry (RAI). Eur Heart J 18:272, 1997.

193. Monassier JP, Hamon M, Elias J, et al: STENTIM I: Early versus late coronary stenting following acute myocardial infarction: Results of the STENTIM I study (French registry of stenting in acute myocardial infarction). Catheter Cardiovasc Diagn 42:243–248, 1997.

194. Steinhubl SR, Moliterno DJ, Teirstein PS, et al: Stenting for acute myocardial infarction; the early United States experience [Abstract]. J Am Coll Cardiol 27:279A, 1996.

195. Glatt B, Stratiev V, Guyon B, et al: Two years' experience of primary stenting in unselected acute myocardial infarction: One month follow-up. Eur Heart J 18:274, 1997.

196. Spaulding C, Cador R, Benhamda K, et al: One-week and six-month angiographic controls of stent implantation after occlusive and nonocclusive dissection during primary balloon angioplasty for acute myocardial infarction. Am J Cardiol 79:1592–1595, 1997.

197. Neumann FJ, Walter H, Richardt G, et al: Coronary Palmaz-Schatz stent implantation in acute myocardial infarction. Heart 75:121–126, 1996.

198. Repetto S, Onofri M, Castiglioni B, et al: Stenting of the infarct related artery during complicated angioplasty in acute myocardial infarction. J Invas Cardiol 8:177–183, 1996.

199. Schomig A, Neumann FJ, Kastrati A, et al: A randomized comparison of antiplatelet and anticoagulant therapy after the placement of coronary-artery stents. N Engl J Med 334:1084–1089, 1996.

200. Levy G, de Boisgelin R, Volpiliere R, et al: Intracoronary stenting in direct infarct angioplasty: Is it dangerous [Abstract]? Circulation 92:I-139, 1995.

201. Horstkotte D, Piper C, Anderson D, et al: Stent implantation in acute myocardial infarction: Results of a pilot study with 80 consecutive patients. Eur Heart J 17:297, 1996.

202. Hans-Jurgen R, Thomas V, Jurgen T, et al: Short- and long-term results of stent implantation within 12 hours after failed PTCA in acute myocardial infarction. Circulation 94:I-577, 1996.

203. Himbert D, Juliard JM, Benamer H, et al: Hospital outcomes after bail-out coronary stenting in patients with acute myocardial infarction. Eur Heart J 18:125, 1997.

204. Abbottsmith CW, Topol EJ, George BS, et al: Fate of patients with acute myocardial infarction with patency of the infarct-related vessel achieved with successful thrombolysis versus rescue angioplasty. J Am Coll Cardiol 16:770–778, 1990.

205. O'Keefe JO, Bailey WL, Rutherford BD et al: Primary angioplasty for acute myocardial infarction in 1000 consecutive patients. Am J Cardiol 72:107G–115G, 1993.

206. Brodie BR, Weintraub RA, Stuckey TD, et al: Outcomes of direct coronary angioplasty for acute myocardial infarction in candidates and non-candidates for thrombolytic therapy. Am J Cardiol 67:7–12, 1991.

207. Rodriguez AE, Fernandez M, Santaera O, et al: Coronary stenting in patients undergoing percutaneous transluminal coronary angioplasty during acute myocardial infarction. Am J Cardiol 77:685–689, 1996.

208. Setiha ME, El Gamal M, Koolen J, et al: Coronary stenting for failed angioplasty in acute myocardial infarction. Catheter Cardiovasc Diagn 39:149–154, 1996.

209. Ahmad T, Webb JG, Carere R, et al: Coronary stenting for acute myocardial infarction. Am J Cardiol 76:77–80, 1995.

210. Brodie BR, Stuckey TD, Kissling G, et al: Importance of infarct-related artery patency for recovery of left ventricular function and late survival after primary angioplasty for acute myocardial infarction. J Am Coll Cardiol 28:319–325, 1996.

211. Lincoff AM, Topol EJ, Chapekis AT, et al: Intracoronary stenting compared with conventional therapy for abrupt vessel closure complicating coronary angioplasty: A matched case-control study. J Am Coll Cardiol 21:866–875, 1993.

212. Stone GW, Brodie BR, Griffin JJ, et al: A prospective, multicenter study of the safety and feasibility of primary stenting in acute myocardial infarction: In-hospital and 30 day results of the PAMI Stent Pilot Trial. J Am Coll Cardiol 31:23–30, 1998.

213. Delcan JL, Garcia E, Soriano J, et al: Primary coronary stenting in acute myocardial infarction: In-hospital results. Eur Heart J 18:275, 1997.

214. Saito S, Hosokawa G, Kim K, et al: Primary stent implantation in acute myocardial infarction. J Am Coll Cardiol 28:74–81, 1996.

215. Valeix BH, Labrunie PJ, Massiani PF: Systemic coronary stenting in the first eight hours of acute myocardial infarction [Abstract]. Circulation 94:I-577, 1996.

216. Medina A, Hernandez E, Suarez de Lezo J, et al: Primary stent treatment for acute evolving myocardial infarction [Abstract]. Circulation 94:I-576, 1996.

217. Turi ZG, McGinnity JG, Fischman D, et al: Retrospective comparative study of primary intracoronary stenting versus balloon angioplasty for acute myocardial infarction. Catheter Cardiovasc Diagn 40:235–239, 1997.

218. Karrillon GJ, Morice MC, Benveniste E, et al: Intracoronary stent implantation without ultrasound guidance and with replacement of conventional anticoagulation by antiplatelet therapy: 30-day clinical outcome of the French multicenter registry. Circulation 94:1519–1527, 1996.

219. Moussa I, Di Mario C, Reimers B, et al: Subacute stent thrombosis in the era of intravascular ultrasound-guided coronary stenting without anticoagulation: Frequency, predictors and clinical outcome. J Am Coll Cardiol 29:6–12, 1997.

220. Siegel RM, Bhaskaran A, Underwood PL, et al: Stenting or balloon angioplasty in direct infarct intervention: Does it make a difference [Abstract]? Circulation 96:I-327, 1997.

221. Stone GW, St. Goar F, Fitzgerald P, et al: The Optimal Stent Implantation Trial—Final core lab angiographic and ultrasound analysis [Abstract]. J Am Coll Cardiol 29:369A, 1997.

222. Smith AJC, Holt RE, Fitzpatrick K, et al: Transient thrombotic state after abrupt discontinuation of heparin in percutaneous coronary angioplasty. Am Heart J 131:434–439, 1996.

223. Granger C, Miller J, Bovill E, et al: Rebound increase in thrombin generation and activity after cessation of intravenous heparin in patients with acute coronary syndromes. Circulation 91:1929–1935, 1995.

224. Stone GW, Brodie BR, Griffin JJ, et al: Improved short-term outcomes of primary stenting compared to primary angioplasty in acute myocardial infarction—The PAMI Stent Pilot Trial [Abstract]. Circulation 96:I-594, 1997.

225. Stone GW, Brodie BR, Griffin JJ, et al: Is stenting the treatment of choice for thrombus containing lesions? Core lab analysis from the PAMI Stent Pilot Trial [Abstract]. Circulation 96:I-397, 1997.

226. Annex B, Larkin TJ, O'Neill WW, et al: Evaluation of thrombus removal by transluminal extraction atherectomy by percutaneous coronary angioscopy. Am J Cardiol 74:606–609, 1994.

227. Kaplan BM, Safian RS, Grines CL, et al: Usefulness of ad-

junctive angioscopy and extraction atherectomy before stent implantation in high risk narrowings in aorto-coronary artery saphenous vein grafts. Am J Cardiol 76:822–824, 1995.

228. Hamburger J, Brekke M, di Mario C, et al: The Euro-ART study: An analysis of the initial European experience with the AngioJet rapid thrombectomy catheter [Abstract]. J Am Coll Cardiol 29:186, 1997.

229. Ramee SR, Schatz RA, Carrozza JP, et al: Results of the VeGAS I pilot study of the Possis AngioJet thrombectomy catheter [Abstract]. Circulation 94:I-3622, 1996.

230. Carrozza JP, Kuntz RE, Levine MJ, et al: Angiographic and clinical outcome of intracoronary stenting: Immediate and long-term results from a large single-center experience. J Am Coll Cardiol 20:328–337, 1992.

231. Kimura T, Yokoi H, Nakagawa Y, et al: Three-year follow-up after implantation of metallic coronary-artery stents. N Engl J Med 334:561–566, 1996.

232. Serruys PW, Emanuelsson H, van der Giessen W, et al: Heparin-coated Palmaz-Schatz stents in human coronary arteries. Early outcome of the BENESTENT-II pilot study. Circulation 93:412–422, 1996.

233. Moussa I, Moses JW, Strain JE, et al: Angiographic and clinical outcome of patients undergoing "stenting after optimal lesion debulking": The "SOLD" pilot study [Abstract]. Circulation 96:I-81, 1997.

234. Hoffman R, Mintz GS, Mehran R, et al: Intravascular ultrasound predictors of angiographic restenosis in lesions treated with Palmaz-Schatz stents. J Am Coll Cardiol 31:43–49, 1988.

235. Stone GW, Grines CL, Rothbaum D, et al: Analysis of the relative costs and effectiveness of primary angioplasty versus tissue-type plasminogen activator: The Primary Angioplasty in Myocardial Infarction (PAMI) Trial. J Am Coll Cardiol 29:901–907, 1997.

236. Leon MB, Popma JJ, O'Shaughnessy C, et al: Quantitative angiographic outcomes after Gianturco-Roubin II stent implantation in complex lesion subsets [Abstract]. Circulation 96:I-653, 1997.

237. Dussaillant GR, Mintz GS, Pichard AD, et al: Small stent size and intimal hyperplasia contribute to restenosis: A volumetric intravascular ultrasound study. J Am Coll Cardiol 26:720–724, 1995.

238. Baim DS, Cutlip DE, Midei M, et al: Acute 30-day and late clinical events in the randomized parallel-group comparison of the ACS multi-link coronary stent system and the Palmaz-Schatz stent [Abstract]. Circulation 96:I-593, 1997.

239. Rogers C, Edelman ER: Endovascular stent design dictates experimental restenosis and thrombosis. Circulation 91:2995–3001, 1995.

240. Chronos NAF, Robinson KA, King SB, et al: Heparin coated Palmaz-Schatz stents are highly thrombo-resistant: A baboon A-V shunt study [Abstract]. J Am Coll Cardiol 27:84, 1996.

241. Chronos NAF, Robinson KA, White D, et al: Heparin coating dramatically reduces platelet deposition on incompletely deployed Palmaz-Schatz stent in the baboon A-V shunt [Abstract]. J Am Coll Cardiol 27:84, 1996.

242. Kocsis JF, Lunn AC, Mohammad SF: Incomplete expansion of coronary stents: Risk of thrombogenesis and protection provided by a heparin coating [Abstract]. J Am Coll Cardiol 27:84, 1996.

243. Hardhammar PA, van Beusekom HMM, Emanuelsson HU, et al: Reduction in thrombotic events with heparin-coated Palmaz-Schatz stents in normal porcine coronary arteries. Circulation 93:423–430, 1996.

244. Serruys PW, Emanuelsson HU, van der Giessen W, et al: Heparin-coated Palmaz-Schatz stents in human coronary arteries. Circulation 93:412–422, 1996.

245. Serruys PW, Emanuelsson H, van der Giessen W, et al: Heparin-coated Palmaz-Schatz stents in human coronary arteries. Early outcome of the BENESTENT-II Pilot Study. Circulation 93:412–422, 1996.

246. Legrand V, Serruys PW, Emanuelsson H, et al: BENESTENT-II Trial—Final results of visit I: A 15-day follow-up [Abstract]. J Am Coll Cardiol 29:170, 1997.

246a. Buller CE, Dzavik V, Carere RG, et al: Primary stenting plus balloon angioplasty in occluded coronary arteries: The Total Occlusion Study of Canada (TOSCA). Circulation 100:236–242, 1999.

247. Mak HK, Belli G, Ellis SG, et al: Subacute stent thrombosis: Evolving issues and current concepts. J Am Coll Cardiol 27:494–503, 1996.

248. Grines CL, Morice MC, Mattos L, et al: A prospective, multicenter trial using the JJIS heparin-coated stent for primary reperfusion of acute myocardial infarction [Abstract]. J Am Coll Cardiol 29:389, 1997.

249. Serruys PW, Garcia-Fernandez E, Kiemeney F, et al: Stenting in acute MI: A pilot study as preamble to a randomized trial comparing balloon angioplasty and stenting [Abstract]. Circulation 96:I-326, 1997.

250. Kuiper KK, Robinson KA, Chronos NAF, et al: Implantation of metal phosphorylcholine coated stents in rabbit iliac and porcine coronary arteries [Abstract]. Circulation 96:I-289, 1997.

251. Aggarwal RK, Ireland DS, Azrin MA, et al: Antithrombotic potential of polymer-coated stents eluting platelet glycoprotein IIb/IIIa receptor antibody [Abstract]. Circulation 94:3311–3317, 1996.

252. Hoorntje JC, Suryapranata H, de Boer MJ, et al: ESCOBAR: Primary stenting for acute myocardial infarction: Preliminary results of a randomized trial [Abstract]. Circulation 94:I-570, 1996.

253. Suryapranata H, Hoorntje JC, de Boer MJ, et al: Randomized comparison of primary stenting with primary balloon angioplasty in acute myocardial infarction [Abstract]. Circulation 96:I-327, 1997.

254. Saito S, Hosokawa G, Suzuki S, et al: Primary stent implantation is superior to balloon angioplasty in acute myocardial infarction—The result of the Japanese PASTA (Primary Angioplasty versus Stent Implantation in Acute Myocardial Infarction) trial [Abstract]. J Am Coll Cardiol 29:390, 1997.

255. Saito S: Primary Palmaz-Schatz stent implantation for acute myocardial infarction: The final results of the Japanese PASTA (Primary Angioplasty vs. Stent Implantation in AMI in Japan) trial [Abstract]. Circulation 96;I-595, 1997.

256. Monassier JP: The STENTIM-2 Trial: Presentation at the 4th Annual Thoraxcenter course on Coronary Stenting, Rotterdam, The Netherlands, December 1997.

257. Nishida Y, Ueda K, Iwase T, et al: In-hospital outcome of primary stenting for acute myocardial infarction using the Wiktor coil stent: Results from a multicenter randomized PRISAM study [Abstract]. Circulation 1997;96:I-531, 1997.

258. Ueda K, Nishida Y, Iwase T, et al: Quantitative angiographic restenosis of primary stenting using Wiktor coil stent for acute myocardial infarction: Results from a multicenter, randomized PRISAM study [Abstract]. Circulation 96:I-531, 1997.

259. Rodriguez A, Fernandez M, Bernardi V, et al: Coronary stents improved hospital results during coronary angioplasty in acute myocardial infarction: Preliminary results of a randomized controlled study (GRAMI Trial) [Abstract]. J Am Coll Cardiol 29:221, 1997.

260. Antoniucci D, Santoro GM, Bolognese L, et al: Elective stenting in acute myocardial infarction: Preliminary results of the Florence Randomized Elective Stenting in Acute Coronary Occlusion (FRESCO) study [Abstract]. J Am Coll Cardiol 29:456, 1997.

261. Antoniucci D, Santoro GM, Bolognese L, et al: A prospective, randomized trial of elective stenting in acute myocardial infarction—Preliminary results of the FRESCO study (Florence Randomized Elective Stenting in Acute Coronary Occlusion) [Abstract]. Circulation 96:I-327, 1997.

262. Neumann FJJ, Blasini R, Dirschinger J, et al: Intracoronary stent implantation and antithrombotic regimen in acute myocardial infarction: Randomized placebo-controlled trial of the fibrinogen receptor antagonist abciximab [Abstract]. Circulation 96:I-398, 1997.

263. Ellis SG, Bates ER, Schaible T, et al: Prospects for the use of antagonists to the platelet glycoprotein IIb/IIIA receptor to prevent post-angioplasty restenosis and thrombosis. J Am Coll Cardiol 17(suppl B):89B–95B, 1991.

264. Painter JA, Mintz GS, Wong SC, et al: Serial intravascular

ultrasound studies fail to show evidence of chronic Palmaz-Schatz stent recoil. Am J Cardiol 75:398–400, 1995.

265. Ip JH, Fuster V, Israel D, et al: The role of platelets, thrombin and hyperplasia in restenosis after coronary angioplasty. J Am Coll Cardiol 17(suppl B):77B–88B, 1991.

266. Jordan RE, Mascelli MA, Nakada MT, et al: Abciximab causes profound, immediate inhibition of platelet function that recovers gradually after PTCA [Abstract]. Circulation 96:I-721, 1997.

266a. Stone GW, Grines CL, Cox DA, et al: A prospective, multicenter, international randomized trial comparing four reperfusion strategies in acute myocardial infarction: Principal report of the Controlled Abciximab and Device Investigation to Lower Late Angioplasty Complications (CADILLAC) trial [Abstract]. J Am Coll Cardiol 37:342, 2001.

266b. Stuckey T, Grines CL, Cox DA, et al: Does stenting and glycoprotein IIb/IIIa receptor blockade improve the prognosis of diabetics undergoing primary angioplasty in acute myocardial infarction [Abstract]? The CADILLAC trial. J Am Coll Cardiol 37:342, 2001.

266c. Grines CL, Cox DA, Tcheng JE, et al: Effect of stent implantation and glycoprotein IIb/IIIa receptor blockade on TIMI flow and mortality after primary PTCA in acute myocardial infarction: Final results of the CADILLAC trial [Abstract]. J Am Coll Cardiol 37:342, 2001.

266d. Tcheng JE, Effron M, Grines CL, et al: Abciximab use during percutaneous intervention in patients with acute myocardial infarction improves early and late clinical outcomes: Final results of the CADILLAC trial [Abstract]. J Am Coll Cardiol 37:343, 2001.

267. Grines CL, Schreiber TL, Savas V, et al: A randomized trial of low osmolar ionic versus nonionic contrast media in patients with myocardial infarction or unstable angina undergoing percutaneous transluminal coronary angioplasty. J Am Coll Cardiol 27:1381–1386, 1996.

268. Piessens JH, Stammen F, Vrolix MC, et al: Effects of an ionic versus a nonionic low osmolar contrast agent on the thrombotic complications of coronary angioplasty. Catheter Cardiovasc Diagn 28:99–105, 1993.

269. Royer T, Berrocal D, Rosenblat E, et al: Acute thrombosis in coronary angioplasty: Effect of ionic versus nonionic contrast media. Eur Heart J 11:1999–2005, 1990.

270. Aguirre F, Topol EJ, Donohue T: Impact of ionic and nonionic contrast agent on the thrombotic complications of coronary angioplasty [Abstract]. J Am Coll Cardiol 25:8, 1995.

271. Schomig A, Neumann FJ, Kastrati A, et al: A randomized comparison of antiplatelet and anticoagulant therapy after the placement of coronary-artery stents. N Engl J Med 334:1084–1089, 1996.

272. Leon MB, Baim DS, Gordon P, et al: Clinical and angiographic results form the Stent Anticoagulation Regimen Study (STARS). Circulation 95:I-685, 1996.

273. Khurana S, Westley S, Maltson JC, et al: Is it possible to expedite the antiplatelet effect of ticlopidine? J Invas Cardiol 8:65, 1996.

274. Nakamura S, Colombo A, Gaglione A, et al: Intracoronary ultrasound observations during stent implantation. Circulation 89:2026–2034, 1994.

275. Goldberg SL, Colombo A, Nakamura S, et al: Benefit of ultrasound in the deployment of Palmaz-Schatz stents. J Am Coll Cardiol 24:996–1003, 1994.

276. Carrozza JP, Hermiller JB, Linnemeier TJ, et al: Quantitative coronary angiographic and intravascular ultrasound assessment of a new nonarticulated stent: Report from the Advanced Cardiovascular Systems MultiLink stent pilot study. J Am Coll Cardiol 31:50–56, 1998.

277. Kuntz RE, Gibson CM, Nobuyoshi M, et al: Generalized model of restenosis after conventional balloon angioplasty, stenting and directional atherectomy. J Am Coll Cardiol 21:15–25, 1993.

278. Ziada KM, Kim MH, Potts W, et al: Predictors of target vessel revascularization following coronary stent deployment [Abstract]. J Am Coll Cardiol 29:239, 1997.

279. Schwarzacher SP, Metz JA, Yock PG, et al: Vessel tearing at the edge of intracoronary stents detected with intravascular ultrasound imaging. Catheter Cardiovasc Diagn 40:152–155, 1997.

280. Stone GW, Brodie B, Griffin J, et al: In-hospital and late outcomes following primary stenting in acute myocardial infarction—Comparison with primary PTCA [Abstract]. J Am Coll Cardiol, in press.

281. Deligonul V, Gabliani GI, Caroles DG, et al: PTCA in patients with intracoronary thrombus. Am J Cardiol 62:474–476, 1988.

282. Mabin TA, Holmes DR, Smith HC, et al: Coronary artery thrombus as a risk factor for acute vessel occlusion complicating PTCA. J Am Coll Cardiol 5:198–202, 1985.

283. Khan MM, Ellis SG, Aguirre FV, et al: Does intracoronary thrombus influence the outcome of high risk percutaneous transluminal coronary angioplasty? Clinical and angiographic outcomes in a large multicenter trial. J Am Coll Cardiol 31:31–36, 1998.

284. Lincoff AM, Popma JJ, Ellis SG, et al: Abrupt vessel closure complicating coronary angioplasty: Clinical, angiographic and therapeutic profile. J Am Coll Cardiol 19:26–35, 1992.

285. Mooney MR, Mooney JF, Goldenberg IF, et al: Percutaneous transluminal coronary angioplasty in the setting of large intracoronary thrombi. Am J Cardiol 65:427–431, 1990.

286. Vaitkus PT, Herrman HC, Laskey WK: Management and immediate outcome of patients with intracoronary thrombus during percutaneous transluminal coronary angioplasty. Am Heart J 4:1–8, 1992.

287. Ellis SG, Roubin GS, King SB III, et al: Angiographic and clinical predictors of acute closure after native vessel coronary angioplasty. Circulation 77:372–379, 1988.

288. Sugrue DD, Holmes DR, Smith HC, et al: Coronary artery thrombus as a risk factor for acute vessel occlusion during percutaneous transluminal coronary angioplasty. Br Heart J 56:62–66, 1986.

289. Morishima I, Sone T, Mokuno S, et al: Clinical significance of no-reflow phenomenon observed on angiography after successful treatment of acute myocardial infarction with percutaneous transluminal coronary angioplasty. Am Heart J 130:239–243, 1995.

290. Abbo KM, Dooris M, Glazier S, et al: Features and outcome of no-reflow after percutaneous coronary intervention. Am J Cardiol 75:778–782, 1995.

291. Mercho N, Eldin AM, Shareef B, et al: Angiographic complications of primary angioplasty [Abstract]. J Am Coll Cardiol 27:61, 1996.

292. Marzilli M, Gliozheni E, Fedele S, et al: Prevalence and prediction of no-reflow after direct angioplasty in acute myocardial infarction [Abstract]. J Am Coll Cardiol 29:90, 1997.

293. Gacioch GM, Topol EJ: Sudden paradoxic clinical deterioration during angioplasty of the occluded right coronary artery in acute myocardial infarction. J Am Coll Cardiol 14:1202–1209, 1989.

294. Kahn JK, Rutherford BD, McConahay DR, et al: Usefulness of angioplasty during acute myocardial infarction in patients with prior coronary artery bypass grafting. Am J Cardiol 65:698–702, 1990.

295. Kahn JK, Rutherford BD, McConahay DR, et al: Catheterization laboratory events and hospital outcome with direct angioplasty for acute myocardial infarction. Circulation 82:1910–1915, 1990.

296. Stone GW, O'Neill WW, Jones D, et al: The central unifying concept of TIMI-3 flow after primary PTCA and thrombolytic therapy in acute myocardial infarction [Abstract]. Circulation 94:I-515, 1996.

297. Nathan PE, Sketch MH, Fortin DF, et al: Acute myocardial infarction in patients with previous coronary artery bypass surgery: Association of complex anatomy and lower reperfusion rates with poor long-term survival [Abstract]. J Am Coll Cardiol 21:349, 1993.

298. Grines CL, Booth DC, Nissen SE, et al: Mechanism of acute myocardial infarction in patients with prior coronary artery bypass grafting and therapeutic implications. Am J Cardiol 65:1292–1296, 1990.

299. Kavanaugh KM, Topol EJ: Acute intervention during myo-

cardial infarction in patients with prior coronary bypass surgery. Am J Cardiol 65:924–926, 1990.

300. Kahn JK, Rutherford BD, McConahay DR, et al: Usefulness of angioplasty during acute myocardial infarction in patients with prior coronary artery bypass grafting. Am J Cardiol 65:698–702, 1990.

301. Stone GW, Brodie BR, Griffin J, et al: Primary angioplasty in patients with prior bypass surgery [Abstract]. Circulation 94:I-243, 1996.

302. Liu MW, Douglas JS, Lembo NJ, et al: Angiographic predictors of a rise in serum creatine kinase (distal embolization) after balloon angioplasty of saphenous vein coronary artery bypass grafts. Am J Cardiol 72:514–517, 1993.

303. Misumi K, Matthews R, Sun GW, et al: Reduced distal embolization with transluminal extraction atherectomy compared to balloon angioplasty for saphenous vein graft disease. Catheter Cardiovasc Diagn 39:246–251, 1996.

304. Brodie BR, Weintraub RA, Stuckey TD, et al: Outcomes of direct coronary angioplasty for acute myocardial infarction in candidates and non-candidates for thrombolytic therapy. Am J Cardiol 67:7–12, 1991.

305. Califf RM, Bengston JR: Cardiogenic shock. N Engl J Med 330:1724–1730, 1994.

306. Ambrose JA, Almeida OD, Sharma SK, et al: Adjunctive thrombolytic therapy during angioplasty for ischemic rest pain. Results of the TAUSA Trial. Circulation 90:69–77, 1994.

307. Mehran R, Ambrose JA, Bongu RM, et al: Angioplasty of complex lesions in ischemic rest angina. Results of the Thrombolysis and Angioplasty in UnStable Angina (TAUSA) Trial. J Am Coll Cardiol 26:961–966, 1995.

308. O'Neill WW: Mechanical alternatives to thrombolytics and PTCA in acute ischemic syndromes. J Invas Cardiol 8(suppl C):28C–33C, 1996.

309. Twidale N, Barth C, Kipperman RM, et al: Acute results and long-term outcome of transluminal extraction atherectomy for saphenous vein graft stenoses. Catheter Cardiovasc Diagn 31:187–191, 1994.

310. Braden GA, Xenopoulos NP, Young T, et al: Transluminal extraction catheter atherectomy followed by immediate stenting in treatment of saphenous vein grafts. J Am Coll Cardiol 30:657–663, 1997.

311. Dorris M, Hoffmann M, Glazier S, et al: Comparative results of transluminal extraction coronary atherectomy in saphenous vein graft lesions with and without thrombus. J Am Coll Cardiol 25:1700–1705, 1995.

312. Hong MK, Wong SC, Popma JJ, et al: Favorable results of debulking followed by immediate adjunct stent therapy for high-risk saphenous vein graft lesions [Abstract]. J Am Coll Cardiol 27:179, 1996.

313. Al-Shaibi KF, Goods CM, Jain SP, et al: Does transluminal extraction atherectomy reduce distal embolization in saphenous vein grafts [Abstract]? Circulation 92:I-329, 1995.

314. Gitlin JB, Sutton JM, Casale PN, et al: Transluminal extraction catheter atherectomy in bypass grafts vs. native vessels: Are there significant differences [Abstract]? J Am Coll Cardiol 23:22, 1994.

315. Sketch MH, Davidson CJ, Yeh W, et al: Predictors of acute and long-term outcome with transluminal extraction atherectomy: The New Approaches to Coronary Intervention (NACI) registry [Abstract]. Am J Cardiol 80(10A):68K–77K, 1997.

316. Moses JW, Yeh W, Popma JJ, et al: Predictors of distal embolization with the TEC catheter: A NACI registry report [Abstract]. Circulation 92:I-329, 1995.

317. Lasorda DM, Incorvati DL, Randall RR: Extraction atherectomy during myocardial infarction in a patient with prior coronary artery bypass surgery. Catheter Cardiovasc Diagn 26:117–121, 1992.

318. Topaz O: Transluminal extraction atherectomy for acute myocardial infarction. Catheter Cardiovasc Diagn 40:291–296, 1997.

319. Larkin TJ, Niemyski PR, Parker MA, et al: Primary and rescue extraction atherectomy in patients with acute myocardial infarction [Abstract]. Circulation 84:II-537, 1991.

320. Kaplan BM, Larkin T, Safian RD, et al: Prospective study of

extraction atherectomy in patients with acute myocardial infarction. Am J Cardiol 78:383–388, 1996.

321. Ellis SG, da Silva ER, Heyndrickx G, et al: Randomized comparison of rescue angioplasty with conservative management of patients with early failure of thrombolysis for acute anterior myocardial infarction. Circulation 90:2280–2284, 1994.

322. Ellis SG, Van de Weft F, Riberio-DaSilva E, et al: Present status of rescue coronary angioplasty: Current polarization of opinion and randomized trials. J Am Coll Cardiol 19:681–686, 1992.

323. Lee L, Erbel R, Brown TM, et al: Multicenter registry of angioplasty therapy of cardiogenic shock: Initial and long-term survival. J Am Coll Cardiol 17:599–603, 1991.

324. Hibbard MD, Holmes DR, Bailey KR, et al: Percutaneous transluminal coronary angioplasty in patients with cardiogenic shock. J Am Coll Cardiol 19:639–646, 1992.

325. Holmes DR, Bates ER, Kleiman NS, et al: Contemporary reperfusion therapy for cardiogenic shock: The GUSTO-I trial experience. J Am Coll Cardiol 26:668–674, 1995.

326. Schreiber TL, Kaplan BM, Brown CL, et al: Transluminal extraction atherectomy vs. balloon angioplasty in acute ischemic syndromes (TOPIT): Hospital outcomes and 6 month status [Abstract]. J Am Coll Cardiol 29:132, 1997.

327. Safian RD, Grines CL, May MA, et al: Clinical and angiographic results of transluminal extraction coronary atherectomy in saphenous vein bypass grafts. Circulation 89:302–312, 1994.

328. Popma JJ, Leon MB, Mintz GS, et al: Results of coronary angioplasty using the transluminal extraction catheter. Am J Cardiol 70:1526–1532, 1992.

329. Hong MK, Popma JJ, Leon MB, et al: Distal embolization after transluminal catheter treatment of saphenous vein graft lesions [Abstract]. J Am Coll Cardiol 21:228, 1993.

330. Rowe MH, Tomoaki H, White NW, et al: Comparison of dissection rates and angiographic results following directional coronary atherectomy and coronary angioplasty. Am J Cardiol 66:49–53, 1990.

331. Umans VA, Beatt KJ, Rensing BJWM, et al: Comparative quantitative angiographic analysis of directional coronary atherectomy and balloon coronary angioplasty. Am J Cardiol 68:1556–1563, 1991.

332. Topol EJ, Leya F, Pinkerton CA, et al: A comparison of directional atherectomy with coronary angioplasty in patients with coronary artery disease. N Engl J Med 329:221–227, 1993.

333. Baim DS, Popma JJ, Sharma SK, et al: Final results of the Balloon versus Optimal Atherectomy Trial (BOAT): 6 month angiography and 1 year clinical follow-up [Abstract]. Circulation 94:I-436, 1996.

334. McCloskey ER, Cowley MJ, Raymond RE: Rescue atherectomy (DCA) for acutely failed angioplasty [Abstract]. Circulation 88:I-586, 1993.

335. Holmes DR, Ellis SG, Garratt KN: Directional coronary atherectomy for thrombus containing lesions: Improved outcome [Abstract]. Circulation 84:II-26, 1991.

336. Emmi R, Movsowitz H, Manginas A, et al: Directional coronary atherectomy in lesions with coexisting thrombus [Abstract]. Circulation 88:I-596, 1993.

337. Kramer B, Larkin T, Niemyski P, et al: Coronary atherectomy in acute ischemic syndromes: Implications of thrombus on treatment outcome [Abstract]. J Am Coll Cardiol 17:385, 1991.

338. Arie S, Serrano CV, Ramires JAF: Successful coronary atherectomy during acute myocardial infarction. Int J Cardiol 36:236–239, 1992.

339. Saito S, Arai H, Kim K, et al: Primary directional coronary atherectomy for acute myocardial infarction. Catheter Cardiovasc Diagn 32:44–48, 1994.

340. Smucker ML, Sarnat WS, Kil D, et al: Salvage from cardiogenic shock by atherectomy after failed emergency coronary artery angioplasty. Catheter Cardiovasc Diagn 21:23–25, 1990.

341. Baldwin TF, Lash RE, Whitfield SS, et al: Directional coronary atherectomy in acute myocardial infarction. J Invas Cardiol 5:288–294, 1993.

342. Kurisu S, Sato H, Tateishi H, et al: Directional coronary atherectomy for the treatment of acute myocardial infarction. Am Heart J 134:345–350, 1997.

343. Kurisu S, Sato H, Tateishi H, et al: Usefulness of directional coronary atherectomy in patients with acute anterior myocardial infarction. Am J Cardiol 79:1392–1394, 1997.

344. Holmes DR, Topol EJ, Califf RM, et al: A multicenter, randomized trial of coronary angioplasty versus directional atherectomy for patients with saphenous vein bypass graft lesions. Circulation 91:1966–1974, 1995.

345. Lefkovits J, Holmes DR, Califf RM, et al: Predictors and sequelae of distal embolization during saphenous vein graft intervention from the CAVEAT-II trial. Circulation 92:734–740, 1995.

346. Harrington RA, Lincoff AM, Califf RM, et al: Characteristics and consequences of myocardial infarction after percutaneous coronary intervention: Insights from the coronary angioplasty versus excisional atherectomy trial (CAVEAT). J Am Coll Cardiol 25:1693–1699, 1995.

347. Cutlip DE, Baim DS, Senerchia C, et al: Clinical consequences of myocardial infarction following balloon angioplasty or directional coronary atherectomy: Acute and 1 year results of the balloon versus optimal atherectomy trial (BOAT) [Abstract]. J Am Coll Cardiol 29:187, 1997.

348. Drasler W, Jenson M, Wislon G, et al: Rheolytic catheter for percutaneous removal of thrombus. Radiology 1992; 182:263–267, 1992.

349. Ramee SR, Lansky AJ, Money SR, et al: A randomized trial comparing rheolytic thrombectomy to surgical embolectomy for thrombosed hemodialysis grafts and peripheral arteries: An interim report [Abstract]. Circulation 92:I-57, 1995.

350. Muller-Hulsbeck S, Link J, Hopfner M, et al: Rheolytic thrombectomy of an acutely thrombosed transjugular intrahepatic portosystemic stent shunt. Cardiovasc Intervent Radiol 19:294–297, 1996.

351. van Ommen V, van der Veen F, Daemen M, et al: In vivo evaluation of the hydrolyser hydrodynamic thrombectomy catheter. J Vasc Intervent Radiol 5:823–826, 1994.

352. Reekers J, Kromhout J, van der Waal K, et al: Catheter for percutaneous thrombectomy: First clinical experience. Radiology 188:871–874, 1993.

353. Reekers J, Kromhout J, Spithoven H, et al: Arterial thrombosis below the inguinal ligament: Percutaneous treatment with a thrombosuction catheter. Radiology 198:49–53, 1996.

354. Vorwerk D, Sohn M, Schurmann K, et al: Hydrodynamic thrombectomy of hemodialysis fistulas: First clinical results. J Vasc Intervent Radiol 5:813–821, 1994.

355. Henry M, Amor M, Henry I, et al: Percutaneous hydrodynamic thrombectomy with the use of the hydrolyser system [Abstract]. J Am Coll Cardiol 29:308, 1997.

356. van Ommen VG, van den Bos A, Pieper M, et al: Removal of thrombus from aortocoronary bypass grafts and coronary arteries using the 6F hydrolyser. Am J Cardiol 79:1012–1016, 1997.

357. van den Bos AA, van Ommen V, Corbeij MA: A new thrombosuction catheter for coronary use: Initial results with clinical and angiographic follow-up in 7 patients. Catheter Cardiovasc Diagn 40:192–197, 1997.

358. Rosenschein U, Rozenszajn LA, Kraus L, et al: Ultrasonic angioplasty in totally occluded peripheral arteries: Initial clinical, histologic and angiographic results. Circulation 83:1876–1986, 1991.

359. Ariani M, Fishbein MC, Chae JS, et al: Dissolution of peripheral arterial thrombi by ultrasound. Circulation 84:1680–1688, 1991.

360. Hong AS, Chae JS, Dubin SB, et al: Ultrasonic clot disruption: An in vitro study. Am Heart J 120:418–422, 1990.

361. Rosenschein U, Bernstein J, DiSegni E, et al: Experimental ultrasonic angioplasty: Disruption of atherosclerotic plaques and thrombi in vitro and arterial recanalization in vivo. J Am Coll Cardiol 15:711–717, 1990.

362. Rosenschein U, Frimerman A, Laniado S, et al: Study of the mechanism of ultrasound angioplasty from human thrombi and bovine aorta. Am J Cardiol 74:1263–1266, 1994.

363. Phillipe F, Drobinski G, Bucherer C, et al: Effects of ultrasound energy on thrombi in vitro. Catheter Cardiovasc Diagn 28:173–178, 1993.

364. Neppiras EA: Acoustic cavitation. Phys Rep 61:159–201, 1980.

365. Siegel RJ, Luo DY, Steffen W, et al: Ultrasound dissolution of thrombus: Studies using three different types of ultrasound devices. Presented at the VIIth International Congress of Endovascular Interventions, Phoenix AZ, 1993.

366. Hartnell GG, Saxton JM, Friedl SE, et al: Coronary ultrasonic thrombus ablation: In vitro assessment of a novel device for intracoronary use. J Intervent Cardiol 6:69–76, 1993.

367. Siegel RJ, Gunn J, Absan A, et al: Use of therapeutic ultrasound in percutaneous coronary angioplasty: Experimental in vitro studies and initial clinical experience. Circulation 89:1587–1592, 1994.

368. Siegel RJ, Gaines P, Procter A, et al: Clinical demonstration that catheter-delivered ultrasound energy reverses arterial vasoconstriction. J Am Coll Cardiol 20:732–735, 1992.

369. Tachibana K, Tachibana S: Accelerated thrombolysis using a new intravascular therapeutic ultrasound catheter [Abstract]. J Am Coll Cardiol 27:274, 1996.

370. Manzelle J, Combe S, Mirashahi M, et al: Catheter delivered ultrasound dissolves organized thrombi resistant to tissue plasminogen activator (tPA) [Abstract]. Circulation 84:468, 1991.

371. Steffen W, Luo H, Fishbein MC, et al: Ultrasound induced thrombolysis is more effective than streptokinase induced thrombolysis in vitro [Abstract]. J Am Coll Cardiol 27:392, 1996.

372. Rosenschein U, Roth A, Rassin T, et al: Analysis of coronary ultrasound thrombolysis endpoints in acute myocardial infarction. Results of the feasibility phase. Circulation 95:1411–1416, 1997.

373. Rosenschein U, Thuesen L, Anderson HR, et al: Coronary ultrasound thrombolysis in acute myocardial infarction: Results from the ACUTE study [Abstract]. Circulation 96:I-206, 1997.

374. Agmon Y, Miller HA, Roth A, et al: Coronary Ultrasound Thrombolysis in Acute Myocardial Infarction (ACUTE study): 6 month follow-up of the feasibility phase patients. [Abstract]. Eur Heart J 18:271, 1997.

375. Hamm CW, Steffen W, Terres W, et al: Intravascular therapeutic ultrasound thrombolysis in acute myocardial infarction. Am J Cardiol 80:200–204, 1997.

376. Nishioka T, Luo H, Bond G, et al: Microbubbles markedly enhance ultrasound clot dissolution [Abstract]. Circulation 92:I-260, 1995.

377. Mitchel JF, Kirkman TR, Alberghini TV: Ultrasound catheter enhanced thrombolysis with urokinase: In vivo studies [Abstract]. Circulation 96:I-288, 1997.

378. Jenkins DR, Spears JR: Laser balloon angioplasty: A new approach to abrupt coronary occlusion and chronic restenosis. Circulation 81(suppl IV):IV:101–IV-108, 1990.

380. Spears JR: Percutaneous transluminal coronary angioplasty restenosis: Potential prevention with laser balloon angioplasty. Am J Cardiol 60(suppl B):61B–64B, 1987.

381. Spears JR, Kundu SK, McMath LP: Laser balloon angioplasty: Potential for the reduction of the thrombogenicity of the injured arterial wall and for local application of bioprotective materials. J Am Coll Cardiol 17:179B–188B, 1991.

382. Sanborn TA, Faxon DP, Kellett MA, et al: Percutaneous coronary laser thermal angioplasty. J Am Coll Cardiol 8:1437–1440, 1986.

383. Spears JR, Safian RD, Douglas JS, et al: Multicenter acute and chronic results of laser balloon angioplasty for refractory abrupt closure after PTCA [Abstract]. Circulation 84:II-517, 1991.

384. Reis GJ, Pomerantz RM, Jenkins RD, et al: Laser balloon angioplasty: Clinical, angiographic and histologic results. J Am Coll Cardiol 18:193–202, 1991.

385. Schwartz L, Andrus S, Sinclair IN, et al: Restenosis following laser balloon angioplasty—A randomized pilot multicenter trial [Abstract]. Circulation 84:II-361, 1991.

386. Makowski S, O'Neill B, Sarkis A, et al: Physiological low stress angioplasty at 60°C. Initial results and 6 month follow-up [Abstract]. J Am Coll Cardiol 21:440, 1993.

387. van Leeuwen TG, Meertens JH, Velema E, et al: Intraluminal vapor bubble induced by excimer laser causes microsecond arterial dilatation and invagination leading to extensive wall damage in the rabbit. Circulation 87:1258–1263, 1993.

388. van Leeuwen TG, van Erven L, Meertens JH, et al: Origin of arterial wall dissection induced by pulsed excimer and mid-infrared laser ablation in the pig. J Am Coll Cardiol 19:1610–1618, 1992.

389. Cook SL, Eigler NL, Shefer A, et al: Percutaneous excimer laser coronary angioplasty of lesions not ideal for balloon angioplasty. Circulation 84:632–643, 1991.

390. Shefer A, Forrester JS, Litvack F: Recanalization of acute thrombus: Comparison of acute success and short-term patency after excimer laser coronary angioplasty, balloon angioplasty and intracoronary thrombolysis in pigs [Abstract]. J Am Coll Cardiol 17:205, 1991.

391. Klein LW, Litvack F, Holmes D, et al: Prospective multicenter analysis of excimer laser coronary angioplasty (ELCA) in stenoses with complex morphology [Abstract]. J Am Coll Cardiol 21:448, 1991.

392. Estella P, Ryan T, Landzberg JS, et al: Excimer laser–assisted coronary angioplasty for lesions containing thrombus. J Am Coll Cardiol 21:1550–1556, 1993.

393. van Leeuwen TG, Borst C: Fundamental laser-tissue interactions. Semin Intervent Cardiol 1:121–128, 1996.

394. Topaz O: Holmium laser angioplasty. Semin Intervent Cardiol 1:1461–1491, 1996.

395. De Marchena E, Larrain G, Posada JD, et al: Holmium laser–assisted coronary angioplasty in acute ischemic syndromes. Clin Cardiol 19:315–319, 1996.

396. Topaz O, Vetrovec G: Laser for optical thrombolysis and facilitation of balloon angioplasty in acute myocardial infarction following failed pharmacologic thrombolysis. Catheter Cardiovasc Diagn 36:38–42, 1995.

397. Topaz O, Rozenbaum EA, Battista S, et al: Laser facilitated angioplasty and thrombolysis in acute myocardial infarction complicated by prolonged or recurrent chest pain. Catheter Cardiovasc Diagn 28:7–16, 1993.

398. Topaz O: Holmium laser coronary thrombolysis—A new treatment modality for revascularization in acute myocardial infarction: Review. J Clin Laser Med Surg 10:427–431, 1992.

399. de Marchena E, Mallon S, Posada JD, et al: Direct holmium laser–assisted balloon angioplasty in acute myocardial infarction. Am J Cardiol 71:1223–1225, 1993.

400. Stone GW, de Marchena E, Dageforde D, et al: Prospective, randomized, multicenter comparison of laser-facilitated balloon angioplasty versus stand-alone balloon angioplasty in patients with obstructive coronary artery disease. J Am Coll Cardiol 30:1714–1721, 1997.

401. Lincoff AM, Topol EJ, Ellis SG: Local drug delivery for the prevention of restenosis. Circulation 90:2070–2084, 1994.

402. Riessen R, Isner JM: Prospects for site-specific delivery of pharmacologic and molecular therapies. J Am Coll Cardiol 23:1234–1244, 1994.

403. Wolinsky H: Local delivery: Let's keep our eyes on the wall. J Am Coll Cardiol 24:825–827, 1994.

404. Goldman B, Blanke H, Wolinsky H: Influence of pressure on permeability of normal and diseased muscular arteries to horseradish peroxidase. Atherosclerosis 65:215–225, 1987.

405. Wolinsky H, Thung SN: Use of a perforated balloon catheter to deliver concentrated heparin into the wall of the normal canine artery. J Am Coll Cardiol 15:475–481, 1990.

406. Oberhoff M, Herdeg C, Baumbach A, et al: Time course of smooth muscle cell proliferation after local drug delivery of low molecular weight heparin using a porous balloon catheter. Catheter Cardiovasc Diagn 41:268–274, 1997.

407. Lambert CR, Leone JE, Rowland SM: Local drug delivery catheters: Functional comparison of porous and microporous designs. Coron Artery Dis 126:47–56, 1993.

408. Thomas CN, Robinson KA, Cipolla GD, et al: Local intracoronary heparin delivery with a microporous balloon catheter. Am Heart J 132:969–972, 1996.

409. Hong MK, Wong SC, Farb A, et al: Feasibility and drug delivery efficiency of a new balloon angioplasty catheter capable of performing simultaneous local drug delivery. Coron Artery Dis 4:1023–1027, 1993.

410. Mitchel JF, Barry JJ, Bow L, et al: Local urokinase delivery with the channel balloon: Device safety, pharmacokinetics of intracoronary drug delivery, and efficacy of thrombolysis. Catheter Cardiovasc Diagn 41:254–260, 1997.

411. Hong MK, Wong SC, Barry JJ, et al: Feasibility and efficacy of locally delivered enoxaparin via the channeled balloon catheter on smooth muscle cell proliferation following balloon injury in rabbits. Catheter Cardiovasc Diagn 41:241–245, 1997.

412. Cumberland DC, Gunn J, Tsikaderis D, et al: Initial clinical experience of local drug delivery via a porous balloon during percutaneous coronary angioplasty [Abstract]. J Am Coll Cardiol 23:186, 1994.

413. Hong MK, Wong SC, Popma JJ, et al: A dual purpose angioplasty-drug infusion catheter for the treatment of intragraft thrombus. Catheter Cardiovasc Diagn 32:193–195, 1994.

414. Groh WC, Kurnik PB, Matthai WH, et al: Initial experience with an intracoronary flow support device providing localized drug infusion: The SciMed Dispatch catheter. Catheter Cardiovasc Diagn 36:67–73, 1995.

415. Fram DB, Mitchel JF, Azrin MA, et al: Local delivery of heparin to balloon angioplasty sites with a new angiotherapy catheter: Pharmacokinetics and effect on platelet deposition in the porcine model. Catheter Cardiovasc Diagn 41:275–286, 1997.

416. Camenzind E, Bakker WH, Reijs A, et al: Site-specific intracoronary heparin delivery in humans after balloon angioplasty. Circulation 96:154–165, 1997.

417. Camenzind E, Kint PP, Di Mario C, et al: Intracoronary heparin delivery in humans. Acute feasibility and long-term results. Circulation 92:2463–2472, 1995.

418. Glazier JJ, Kiernan FJ, Bauer HH, et al: Treatment of thrombotic saphenous vein bypass grafts using local urokinase infusion therapy with the Dispatch catheter. Catheter Cardiovasc Diagn 41:261–267, 1997.

419. Kaplan AV, Vandormael M, Hofmann M, et al: Heparin delivery at the site of angioplasty with a novel drug delivery sleeve. Am J Cardiol 77:307–310, 1996.

420. Moura A, Lam JYT, Hebert D, et al: Intramural delivery of agent via a novel drug-delivery sleeve. Histologic and functional evaluation. Circulation 92:2299–2305, 1995.

421. Fram DB, Aretz T, Azrin MA, et al: Localized intramural drug delivery during balloon angioplasty using hydrogel-coated balloons and pressure augmented diffusion. J Am Coll Cardiol 23:1570–1577, 1994.

422. Riessen R, Rahimizadeh H, Takeshita S, et al: Successful vascular gene transfer using a hydrogel coated balloon angioplasty catheter [Abstract]. J Am Coll Cardiol 21:74, 1993.

423. Azrin MA, Mitchel JF, Fram DB, et al: Decreased platelet deposition and smooth muscle cell proliferation after intramural heparin delivery with hydrogel-coated balloons. Circulation 90:433–441, 1994.

424. Glazier JJ, Hirst JA, Kiernan FJ, et al: Site-specific intracoronary thrombolysis with urokinase-coated hydrogel balloons: Acute and follow-up studies in 95 patients. Catheter Cardiovasc Diagn 41:246–253, 1997.

425. Mitchel JF, Azrin MA, Fram DB, et al: Inhibition of platelet deposition and lysis of intracoronary thrombus during balloon angioplasty using urokinase-coated hydrogel balloons. Circulation 90:1979–1988, 1994.

426. Fernandez-Ortiz A, Meyer BJ, Mailhae A, et al: A new approach for local intravascular drug delivery. The iontophoretic balloon. Circulation 89:1518–1522, 1994.

427. Mitchel JF, Azrin MA, Fram DB, et al: Localized delivery of heparin to angioplasty sites with iontophoresis. Catheter Cardiovasc Diagn 41:315–323, 1997.

428. Barath P, Popov A, Dillehay GL, et al: Infiltrator angioplasty balloon catheter: A device for combined angioplasty and intramural site-specific treatment. Catheter Cardiovasc Diagn 41:333–341, 1997.

429. Pavlides GS, Barath P, Maginas A, et al: Intramural drug delivery by direct injection within the arterial wall: First

clinical experience with a novel intracoronary delivery-infiltrator system. Catheter Cardiovasc Diagn 41:287–292, 1997.

430. Guzman LA, Labhassetwar V, Song C, et al: Local intraluminal infusion of biodegradable polymeric nanoparticles. A novel approach for prolonged drug delivery after balloon angioplasty. Circulation 94:1441–1448, 1996.

431. Dev V, Eigler N, Fishbein MC, et al: Sustained local drug delivery to the arterial wall via biodegradable microspheres. Catheter Cardiovasc Diagn 41:324–332, 1997.

432. Langer R: New methods of drug delivery. Science 249:1527–1533, 1990.

433. Schwartz RS, Murphy JG, Edwards WD, et al: Bioabsorbable, drug eluting, intracoronary stents: Design and future applications. *In* Sigwart U, Frank GI (eds): Coronary Stents. Berlin: Springer-Verlag, 1992, pp 135–153.

434. Dichek DA, Neville RF, Zwiebel JA, et al: Seeding of intravascular stents with genetically engineered endothelial cells. Circulation 80:1347–1353, 1989.

435. Zidar JP, Lincoff AM, Stack RS: Biodegradable stents. *In* Topol EJ (ed): Textbook of Interventional Cardiology, 2nd ed. Philadelphia: WB Saunders, 1994, pp 787–802.

436. Murphy JG, Schwartz RS, Huber KC, et al: Polymeric stents: Modern alchemy or the future? J Invas Cardiol 3:144–148, 1991.

437. Meyer BJ, Fernandez-Ortiz A, Mailhac A, et al: Local delivery of r-hirudin by a double-balloon perfusion catheter prevents mural thrombosis and minimizes platelet deposition after angioplasty. Circulation 90:2474–2480, 1994.

438. Mitchel JF, Azrin MA, Alberghini TV, et al: Local delivery of ReoPro: Pharmacokinetics and effect on platelet deposition following balloon angioplasty [Abstract]. Circulation 94:I-615, 1996.

439. Hebert NL, Kaplan AV, Grant G, et al: Local intramural delivery of MK-383, a platelet GPIIb/IIIa receptor blocker, reduces platelet deposition at the site of arterial injury [Abstract]. J Am Coll Cardiol 29:187, 1997.

440. Mercho N, Lynch K, Shareef B, et al: Use of urokinase-coated hydrogel balloons for primary angioplasty in patients with acute myocardial infarction [Abstract]. J Am Coll Cardiol 27:221, 1996.

441. Steg PG, Spaulding CM, Makowski S, et al, for the CORAMI-2 Study Group: Final results of CORAMI-2: A double blind randomized trial of local delivery of urokinase during primary angioplasty [Abstract]. Circulation 96:I-532, 1997.

442. Mitchel JF, Azrin MA, Fram DB, et al: Localized delivery of heparin to angioplasty sites with iontophoresis. Catheter Cardiovasc Diagn 41:315–323, 1997.

443. Kahn JK, Hartzler GO: Thrombus aspiration in acute myocardial infarction. Catheter Cardiovasc Diagn 20:54–57, 1990.

444. Lablanche JM, Fourrier JL, Gommeaux A, et al: Percutaneous aspiration of a coronary thrombus. Catheter Cardiovasc Diagn 17:97–98, 1989.

445. Kipperman RM, Feit AS, Einhorn AM, et al: Intracoronary thrombectomy: A new approach to total occlusion. Catheter Cardiovasc Diagn 18:244–248, 1989.

446. Dooris M, Grines CL: Successful reversal of cardiogenic shock precipitated by saphenous vein graft distal embolization using aspiration thrombectomy. Catheter Cardiovasc Diagn 33:267–271, 1994.

447. Brown SE, Segar DS, Weinberg BA, et al: Transcatheter aspiration of intracoronary thrombus after myocardial infarction. Am Heart J 90:688–690, 1990.

448. Cohen HM, Kleiman JH: Aspiration of a mobile thromboembolus from saphenous vein graft. Catheter Cardiovasc Diagn 27:49–51, 1992.

449. Shani J, Abittan M, Gallarello F, et al: Mechanical manipulation of thrombus: Coronary thrombectomy, intracoronary clot displacement, and transcatheter aspiration. Am J Cardiol 72(suppl G):116G–118G, 1993.

450. Reeder GS, Lapeyre AC, Edwards WD, et al: Aspiration thrombectomy for removal of coronary thrombus. Am J Cardiol 70:107–110, 1992.

451. Reisman M, Dewhurst TA, DeVore LJ, et al: A new percutaneous thrombectomy catheter: An early investigational report [Abstract]. J Am Coll Cardiol 27:392, 1996.

452. Dow CJ, Devour L, Gordon L, et al: Successful use of a novel percutaneous aspiration thrombectomy catheter in coronary arteries [Abstract]. Circulation 94:I-618, 1996.

453. Michels RH, van Ommen V, Heijmen EP, et al: Thrombectomy after failure of fibrinolytic drug therapy in acute myocardial infarction [Abstract]. Circulation 96:I-647, 1997.

454. Saito T, Taniguchi I, Nakamura S, et al: Pulse spray thrombolysis in acutely obstructed coronary artery in critical situations. Catheter Cardiovasc Diagn 40:101–108, 1997.

455. Kandrapa K, Drinker PA, Singer SJ, et al: Forceful pulsatile local infusion of enzymes accelerates thrombolysis: In vitro evaluation of a new delivery system. Radiology 168:739–744, 1988.

456. Bookstein JJ, Fellmeth B, Roberts AC, et al: Pulsed-spray pharmacomechanical thrombolysis: Preliminary clinical results. 152:1097–1100, 1989.

457. Valji K, Bookstein JJ, Roberts AC, et al: Pulse-spray pharmacomechanical thrombolysis of thrombosed hemodialysis access grafts: Long-term experience and comparison of original and current techniques. Am J Radiol 164:1495–1500, 1995.

458. Mewissen MW, Minor PL, Beyer GA, et al: Symptomatic native arterial occlusions: Early experience with "over-the-wire" thrombolysis. J Vasc Intervent Radiol 1:43–47, 1990.

459. Valji K, Bookstein JJ, Roberts AC, et al: Occluded peripheral arteries and bypass grafts: Lytic stagnation as an end point for pulse-spray pharmacomechanical thrombolysis. Radiology 188:343–389, 1993.

460. Yusuf SW, Whitaker SC, Gregson RH, et al: Immediate and early follow-up results of pulse-spray thrombolysis in patients with peripheral ischemia. Br J Surg 82:338–340, 1995.

461. Stefanadis C, Toutouzas P, Vlachopoulos C, et al: Autologous vein graft–coated stent for treatment of coronary artery disease. Catheter Cardiovasc Diagn 38:148–154, 1996.

462. Dooros G, Jain A, Kumar K: Management of coronary artery rupture: Covered stent of microcoil embolization. Catheter Cardiovasc Diagn 36:148–154, 1995.

463. Wong SC, Kent KM, Mintz GS, et al: Percutaneous transcatheter repair of a coronary aneurysm using a composite autologous cephalic vein-coated Palmaz-Schatz biliary stent. Am J Cardiol 76:990–991, 1995.

464. Kaplan BM, Stewart RE, Sakwa MP, et al: Repair of a coronary pseudoaneurysm with percutaneous placement of a saphenous vein graft allograft attached to a biliary stent. Catheter Cardiovasc Diagn 37:208–212, 1996.

465. Stefanadis C, Tsiamis E, Vlachopoulos C, et al: Autologous vein graft–coated stents for the treatment of thrombus-containing coronary artery lesions. Catheter Cardiovasc Diagn 40:217–222, 1997.

466. Carter C, Fisher TC, Hamai H, et al: Haemorheological effects of a nonionic copolymer surfactant (poloxamer 188). Clin Hemorheol 12:109–120, 1992.

467. Schaer GL, Spaccavento LJ, Browne KF, et al: Beneficial effects of RheothRx injection in patients receiving thrombolytic therapy for acute myocardial infarction: Results of a randomized, double blind, placebo controlled trial. Circulation 94:298–307, 1996.

468. The Collaborative Organization for RheothRx Evaluation (CORE) Investigators: Effects of RheothRx on mortality, morbidity, left ventricular function, and infarct size in patients with acute myocardial infarction. Circulation 96:192–201, 1997.

469. O'Keefe JH, Grines CL, DeWood MA, et al: Poloxamer-188 as an adjunct to primary percutaneous transluminal coronary angioplasty for acute myocardial infarction. Am J Cardiol 78:747–750, 1996.

470. Grech ED, Jackson MJ, Ramsdale DR: Reperfusion injury after acute myocardial infarction. BMJ 310:477–488, 1995.

471. Jennings R, Yellon D: Reperfusion injury: Definitions and historical background. *In* Yellon DM, Jennings RB (eds): Myocardial Protection: The Pathophysiology of Reperfusion and Reperfusion Injury. New York: Raven Press, 1992, pp 1–11.

472. Forman MB, Perry JM, Wilson BH, et al: Demonstration of

myocardial reperfusion injury in humans: Results of a pilot study utilizing acute coronary angioplasty with perfluorochemical in anterior myocardial infarction. J Am Coll Cardiol 18:911–918, 1991.

473. Grech ED, Dodd NJF, Jackson MJ, et al: Evidence for free radical generation after primary percutaneous transluminal coronary angioplasty in acute myocardial infarction. Am J Cardiol 77:122–127, 1996.

474. Werns SW, Brinker J, Graber J, et al: A randomized, double blind trial of recombinant human superoxide dismutase (SOD) in patients undergoing PTCA for acute MI [Abstract]. Circulation 80:II-213, 1989.

475. Ely SW, Berne RM: Protective effects of adenosine in myocardial ischemia. Circulation 85:893–904, 1992.

476. Forman M, Velasco C, Jackson E: Adenosine attenuates reperfusion injury following regional myocardial ischemia. Cardiovasc Res 27:9–17, 1993.

477. Pitarys C, Virmani R, Vildibill H, et al: Reduction of myocardial reperfusion injury by intravenous adenosine administration during the early reperfusion period. Circulation 83:237–247, 1991.

478. Lesnefsky E, Van Benthuysen K, McMurtry I, et al: Lidocaine reduces canine infarct size and decreases release of a lipid peroxidation product. J Cardiovasc Pharmacol 13:895–901, 1989.

479. Vinten-Johansen J, Zhao ZQ, Sato H: Reduction in surgical ischemic reperfusion injury with adenosine and nitric oxide therapy. Ann Thorac Surg 60:852–857, 1995.

480. van der Lee C, Huizer T, Janssen M, et al: Adenosine, added to St. Thomas' Hospital cardioplegic solution, improves functional recovery and reduces irreversible myocardial damage. Cardioscience 5:269–275, 1994.

481. Hudspeth DA, Nakanishi K, Vinten-Johansen J, et al: Adenosine in blood cardioplegia prevents post ischemic dysfunction in ischemically injured hearts. Ann Thorac Surg 58:1637–1644, 1994.

482. Garratt KN, Holmes DR, Molina-Viamonte V, et al: Intravenous adenosine and lidocaine in patients with acute myocardial infarction. Am Heart J 136:196–204, 1998.

# 13

# Interventional Therapy of Cardiogenic Shock

*William W. O'Neill*

Cardiogenic shock caused by myocardial infarction (MI) continues to carry an ominous prognosis despite the enormous advances in treatment of MI that have occurred over the last 50 years. A resurgence of interest in interventional therapy of cardiogenic shock has occurred. Angioplasty is now a preferred reperfusion strategy when logistics allow. As cardiologists increasingly use a catheterization-based reperfusion strategy, they must be prepared to deal with the daunting challenge that is presented by a patient in shock. Without question, such patients provide an enormous opportunity for both therapeutic benefit and misadventure. The near-miraculous resuscitation that can occur with successful reperfusion may provide interventionalists with some of the most rewarding clinical experiences they encounter. Alternatively, the demise of such patients may provide the most haunting and frustrating experiences of their careers. As reperfusion therapy drops MI mortality into the single digits, future mortality reductions can only occur by decreasing shock mortality.

This chapter provides a historical overview of therapy for cardiogenic shock. It also provides a review of current interventional therapy of cardiogenic shock. I hope that it will provide interventionalists with the understanding of pathophysiology and pathoanatomy that is required in order to have a comprehensive treatment plan outlined before taking these high-risk patients to the catheterization laboratory. Pathophysiology and coronary pathoanatomy are discussed first. Subsequently, reperfusion trials are reviewed. With this information, a rationally planned therapeutic approach to cardiogenic shock patients can be developed.

## HISTORICAL OVERVIEW

The fact that MI was not immediately, invariably fatal was first discussed by Herrick in 1912.[1] Before this time, MI was considered a sudden catastrophic and invariably lethal consequence of coronary thrombosis. At the same time Herrick published his clinical series, development of the electrocardiogram (ECG) finally provided a concrete premortem tool for MI diagnosis. Pardee demonstrated ECG findings of acute epicardial injury in 1920.[2] With this background, natural history studies of MI could commence. Fishberg first described the syndrome of profound circulatory collapse after acute MI in 1934.[3] He incorrectly attributed the condition to peripheral circulatory collapse. Stead and Ebert ultimately attributed the profound systemic consequence of cardiogenic shock to profound myocardial dysfunction.[4]

*A clinical picture that is similar in certain respects to that observed in surgical shock or hemorrhage is sometimes seen in patients with chronic congestive heart failure or with acute myocardial infarction.... when patients with chronic congestive heart failure or myocardial infarction present the clinical picture considered characteristic of shock, the heart rather than the peripheral circulation is primarily at fault.*

EUGENE STEAD[4]

During World War II, the entity of MI became more recognized, and these patients were congregated in special areas of the hospital. The overall MI mortality was 45% to 50% at that time. Patients in cardiogenic shock were recognized to have an especially lethal outcome. Because morphine and nitrates were the only therapy available, the prognosis for these patients seemed hopeless. Great hope occurred in the 1950s with the introduction of the potent vasopressor L-norepinephrine.

The first therapeutic norepinephrine trial in shock was conducted by Griffith and colleagues and reported in 1954.[5] Although norepinephrine did augment systolic pressure, the mortality rate was 80%. Friedberg reviewed the cumulative experience in shock for studies conducted in the 1950s and found a pooled mortality of 79%.[6] This distressingly low survival probability was persistent over the next 3 decades.

The 1960s ushered in dramatic advances in cardiology. Thrombolytic therapy first underwent extensive testing. Electrocardioversion and transvenous pacing were invented. Cardiac care units (CCUs) were organized. In fact, Norris and Sammel reported a reduction of mortality from 21% to 13% after CCU care was organized.[7] Of note, the mortality reduction was almost entirely related to decreases in lethal arrhythmias. No decline in mortality from congestive heart failure (CHF) or cardiogenic shock occurred. At this time, the clinical presentation, hemodynamic profile, and clinical course of shock were carefully described. Killip and Kimball defined shock on the basis of hypotension and end-organ hypoperfusion and found an 81% hospital mortality.[8] Scheidt and associates described the extreme emergency that this condition poses by demonstrating that 50% of patients expire within 12 hours of the onset of shock.[9] Forrester and coworkers greatly advanced the management of MI patients by applying data derived from flotation pulmonary artery catheters.[10] They defined four hemodynamic subsets. These investigators and others[11] defined the low output and high pulmonary capillary wedge pressure that in association with systemic hypotension became the modern definition of cardiogenic shock.

## Definition of Shock

When clinical series are reviewed and outcomes from various treatment modalities are compared, difficulty is encountered because of the various definitions of cardiogenic shock that have been proposed. Killip and Kimball first proposed a clinical definition.[8] Patients in Killip class IV were patients with systemic hypotension and evidence of end-organ hypoperfusion (mental obtundation, oliguria, cold, mottled extremities). Forrester and coworkers proposed a definition of class IV patients based on hemodynamic profile including elevated pulmonary wedge pressure and low cardiac index.[10] Currently, some authors require a strict hemodynamic definition with pulmonary wedge pressure of 12 mm Hg or greater (to exclude hypovolemia) and cardiac index of 2.2 L/minute/m² or less to exclude high-output shock. Other authors employ only clinical criteria. Other authors only require a substantial decline in systolic blood pressure (BP) from a baseline value. For the purposes of clinical research, a standard definition of shock is required. Currently, the Should We Emergently Revascularize Occluded Coronaries for Cardiogenic Shock (SHOCK) investigators accept hypotension (systolic BP ≦90 mm Hg) that persists for at least 1 hour in the absence of hypovolemia.[11] Systemic hypotension must be associated with signs of end-organ hypoperfusion (e.g., oliguria, mental obtundation, cold extremities). For practical purposes, this definition can easily be ap-

plied. It does not require invasive confirmation and would only misclassify a small number of patients with occult hypovolemia. In the future, it is hoped that this definition will be uniformly applied so that outcomes can be compared across clinical trials.

One final point to emphasize is the variation in the level of systolic BP that has been described as a definition of shock. Thrombolytic studies have demonstrated that the prognosis dramatically declines when the systolic BP drops below 100 mm Hg.[12] The GUSTO (Global Utilization of Streptokinase and Tissue Plasminogen Activator for Occluded Arteries) investigators define shock based on a systolic BP less than 90 mm Hg. Previous angioplasty trials have used a more severe criterion of a systolic BP less than 80 mm Hg.[13] There is a clear gradient in mortality based on the systolic BP that is employed (Fig. 13–1). Suffice to say that once systolic BP drops below 90 mm Hg, a dramatic increase in mortality occurs. Griffith and colleagues demonstrated that a lack of response of systolic BP to vasopressors implies an invariably lethal outcome.[5] It is imperative to standardize the definition of shock when assessing the results of various therapeutic interventions.

## Current Incidence and Outcome

Cardiogenic shock has been largely excluded from modern reperfusion trials, and so characterizing its current incidence and outcome is difficult. However, some general inferences can be gleaned from the literature. Friedberg pooled the large series gathered in the 1950s and found an incidence of 14% and a mortality of 79%.[6] Killip and Kimball de-

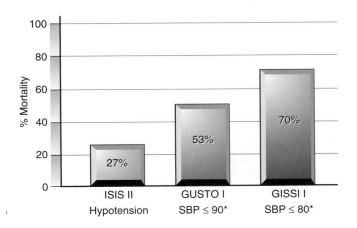

* Systolic blood pressure in mm Hg

FIGURE 13–1. Mortality based on admission blood pressure in thrombolytic trials. GISSI, Gruppo Italiano per lo Studio della Streptochinasi nell'Infarto Miocardico; GUSTO, Global Utilization of Streptokinase and Tissue Plasminogen Activator for Occluded Arteries; ISIS, International Study of Infarct Survival; SBP, systolic blood pressure in millimeters of mercury.

scribed a 19% incidence and an 81% mortality for patients admitted to the New York Hospital in the mid-1960s.[8] In 1978, Mirowski and coworkers described a large community-based series.[14] They found that 12% of patients developed shock and had an 81% mortality. Goldberg and associates described a community-wide experience from 1975 to 1988.[15] The incidence of shock in this study averaged 7.5%. Gheorghiade and colleagues described a decline in the incidence of shock from 11% in 1981–1984 to 6% in 1990–1992 for all MI patients admitted to the Henry Ford Hospital CCU.[16] A final clue to the current incidence of shock is obtained from the GUSTO experience. In this study, unlike other reperfusion trials, shock was not an exclusion and was present overall in 7.2% of patients. In this trial, 1% of patients presented in shock and 6.2% developed shock during hospitalization. One can cautiously infer that the incidence of shock has declined in the last 40 years and may in part explain the improved prognosis for MI patients. Once shock develops, the outcome is grim and appears unchanged. Griffith and colleagues reported an 80% mortality in 1954, Friedberg a 79% mortality in 1961, Killip and Kimball an 81% mortality in 1967, Mirowski and associates an 81% mortality in 1978, and Goldberg and coworkers a 70% mortality in 1991. As other causes of death during MI decline and as thrombolytic therapy becomes a more widely used modality, deaths related to shock will take on increasing importance. Before CCU care, Friedberg found that 11% of all MI deaths were related to shock. After CCU care, Norris and Sammel found that 60% of all MI deaths were related to shock or CHF. Mirowski and associates found that 73% of all MI deaths were related to shock in 1978. In the post-thrombolytic era, the overall mortality in the GUSTO trial was 7%. Although cardiogenic shock occurred in only 7.4% of patients, it accounted for 1682 of 3159 (59%) of the deaths that occurred. Similarly, shock accounted for 75% of all MI deaths in the TIMI (Thrombosis In Myocardial Infarction) IIB trial.[17] Ultimately, the best therapy for shock will be the prevention of its occurrence (Fig. 13–2). Once it develops, altering the prognosis is problematic.

## Pathophysiology of Shock

Extensive myocardial dysfunction with subsequent end-organ failure is the sine qua non of this entity (Fig. 13–3). Myocardial dysfunction may be reversible or irreversible. In the setting of viral myocarditis, some patients may develop such extreme dysfunction that death seems imminent, only to recover completely. The more typical substrate for this condition is related to myocardial infarction in patients with thrombotic occlusion. Page and associates re-

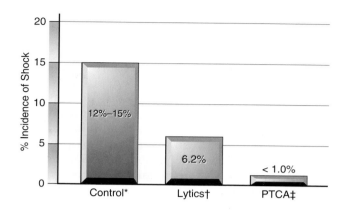

\* data derived from pre–thrombolytic era studies
† data derived from GUSTO I experience
‡ data derived from PAMI II registry

FIGURE 13–2. Development of shock after admission based on reperfusion strategy. PAMI, Primary Angioplasty in Myocardial Infarction; PTCA, percutaneous transluminal coronary angioplasty.

viewed histologic findings in patients who expired after MI and found that greater than 40% of myocardial necrosis was required for shock to develop.[18] This necrosis could be related to one massive infarction or be cumulative after more than one MI. They also found evidence of extensive patchy infarction at the border zone of the infarct. Alonso and colleagues demonstrated that infarct extension or reinfarction commonly occurred after shock developed.[19] In this series, reinfarction was rarely detected before death. Gutovitz and associates provided premortem confirmation of the active ongoing myonecrosis inferred in postmortem studies.[20] They carefully timed cardiac isoenzyme determination in a series of cardiogenic shock patients and found a

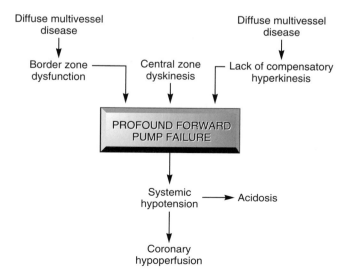

FIGURE 13–3. Pathogenesis of myocardial dysfunction during cardiogenic shock.

markedly delayed time to peak creatinine kinase MB level in the 15 patients who developed shock. These pathologic and laboratory studies quantified the extensive necrosis that occurs. They also suggest that a therapeutic window of opportunity exists, because prevention of reinfarction, prevention of infarct extension, and decreasing border zone ischemic necrosis can be realistically accomplished. It must be recognized, however, that some patients may present with such profound, extensive, irreversible myonecrosis that only organ transplantation would be lifesaving.

In addition to extensive myonecrosis, extensive coronary artery disease has been described in the postmortem studies. Hornorayan and colleagues found occlusive thrombi in 95% of infarct arteries.[21] Wackers and associates found severe diffuse triple-vessel disease in 68% of patients.[22] The presence of such diffuse extensive disease may explain the lower percutaneous transluminal coronary angioplasty (PTCA) success rates that are subsequently described.

Because postmortem studies are skewed toward lethal cases, more balanced data concerning the coronary anatomy may be derived from coronary angiography. Leinbach and associates first courageously attempted angiography in shock patients as a prelude to bypass.[23] They found that angiography could be performed with relative safety if balloon counterpulsation was used as support. They also found that multivessel disease was present in 9 of 11 cases and that the left anterior descending (LAD) artery was invariably occluded or severely stenosed. Johnson and coworkers reported that if patients could be stabilized enough to undergo catheterization, 50% to 60% were technically suited for bypass.[24] More recently, DeWood and colleague reported the Spokane experience and found that 19 of 40 patients in shock who underwent early catheterization were technically suitable for bypass.[25] Williams and associates first systematically catheterized a consecutive group of MI patients.[26] In this study, patients who developed shock had a higher incidence of multivessel disease, greater prevalence of total occlusion of the infarct artery, and less frequent occurrence of angiographic collaterals. Schafer has compared the angiographic anatomy of two contemporaneous reperfusion trials.[27] The Primary Angioplasty in Myocardial Infarction (PAMI) I trial excluded shock,[28] whereas the National Shock Registry prospectively collected data on patients treated with PTCA in shock.[27] In the Registry, they found a significantly higher rate of multivessel disease and lower rate of collateral formation in the shock patients (Table 13–1).

The extent and complexity of coronary disease may have been underestimated by early angiographic studies. Hochman and colleagues have demonstrated that a selection bias exists in the performance of catheterization.[11] In a large prospective registry, 40% of patients did not undergo catheterization. Those not undergoing catheterization were older, presented later, were less likely to be eligible for thrombolytic therapy, and had a higher mortality. When these data are taken into account, it is quite likely that the large majority of patients in cardiogenic shock have severe multivessel disease. The importance of multivessel disease in the development of cardiogenic shock has been further defined by angioplasty trials. The Mid-America Heart Group has demonstrated that shock occurs in 2% of patients with single-vessel disease and 12% of patients with multivessel disease who present for infarct angioplasty.[29, 30] The PAMI II trial excluded patients in cardiogenic shock from recruitment.[31] In this study, one-vessel disease occurred in 59%, two-vessel disease in 22%, and three-vessel disease in 19%. In contradistinction, the National Shock Registry has found single-vessel disease in only 36% of patients, whereas three-vessel disease was present in 32%. Lee and associates reported that 61% of patients in their series had multivessel disease.[32] Similarly Hibbard and colleagues found multivessel disease in 31 of 45 (69%) of patients and left main disease in 5 of 45 (11%) of patients.[33]

Important clues indicating why multivessel disease is so important in the development of cardiogenic shock have been provided by Grines and coworkers.[34] These investigators demonstrated that regional myocardial function of a noninfarct zone is normal or exhibits compensatory hyperkinesis for most stable MI patients undergoing early catheterization. Hypokinesis of the noninfarct zone did occur and was prevalent only in patients with multivessel disease. Because hyperkinesis is a compensatory mechanism to attenuate the loss of contractile function that occurs in the infarct zone, profound global dysfunction develops when hyperkinesis cannot occur. Ross and the GUSTO Angiographic Substudy Investigators have corroborated the observation that a lack of non–infarct zone hyperkinesis is associated with an increase in mortal-

**TABLE 13–1.  INFARCT-RELATED ARTERY**

|  | PAMI I | SHOCK REGISTRY |
|---|---|---|
| Single-vessel CAD (%) | 46.9 | 36.3 |
| Double-vessel CAD (%) | 33.1 | 27.4 |
| Triple-vessel CAD (%) | 19.4 | 31.8 |
| Left main CAD (%) | 0.6 | 4.5 |
| Collaterals (%) | 28.4 | 18.5 |

CAD, coronary artery disease; PAMI, Primary Angioplasty in Myocardial Infarction.

ity.[35] These studies explain why most patients in cardiogenic shock have multivessel disease. Not only are the extensive areas of myocardium at the central ischemic zone dysfunctional, but normal viable myocardium remote to the infarct is also unable to compensate normally because of limited coronary reserve. In addition, once the shock state develops, the presence of multivessel disease enhances the risk of reinfarction and reinfarct extension. This may further aggravate the critical situation and results in the patient's demise. An important mechanism by which revascularization stabilizes myocardial function relates to the immediate impact of reperfusion on infarct zone function. Experimental studies have demonstrated that immediately after coronary occlusion, myocardial segments become akinetic, then dyskinetic. Clinical studies demonstrate akinesis and dyskinesis of the infarct zone before reperfusion. Although reperfusion rarely allows immediate return of contractile function, dyskinesis is often ameliorated. Reperfusion often causes hemorrhage and edema that stiffens the injured myocardium and retards dyskinesis. If dyskinesis improves, global myocardial function and forward cardiac output are greatly enhanced even without a change in noninvolved myocardial segments.

These pathologic and angiographic studies provide a rational basis for aggressive resuscitative measures, coupled with revascularization. Both experimental[36] and clinical[37] studies had suggested that most myocardial salvage with reperfusion occurs within less than 2 hours after the onset of symptoms. Very early reperfusion appears critical to the salvage of the central ischemic zone, especially in cardiogenic shock patients because they tend to have poor collateral flow and multivessel disease. The decline in the incidence of shock in the thrombolytic era is presumably attributable to early, successful reperfusion that prevents massive infarction and thus prevents shock from developing. Therapeutic benefit may still be derived from delayed intervention. Once the shock state has developed, marked decreases in arterial pressure and elevation of left ventricular end-diastolic pressure occurs. Thus, the transmural gradient for coronary blood flow is greatly diminished. As coronary blood flow diminishes, further profound myocardial dysfunction occurs in the border zone myocardium and myocardium distant to the infarct zone. This diminished blood flow may predispose to infarct extension or reinfarction. A vicious, lethal cycle develops in which hypotension causes hypoperfusion, which causes worsening myocardial dysfunction, which in turn causes worsening hypotension, which causes worsening myocardial dysfunction.

Because non–ischemic zone dysfunction appears to be so crucial for the development of cardiogenic shock, complete revascularization may be warranted. Revascularization of the central ischemic zone is unlikely to augment myocardial function immediately, especially if delayed revascularization occurs. On the other hand, revascularization of non–ischemic zones should allow immediate compensatory hyperkinesis to develop. This augments myocardial function immediately and helps reverse the shock state. Morrison and coworkers have demonstrated that an immediate improvement in systolic pressure occurs in survivors of PTCA therapy of shock.[38] This immediate augmentation could result only from improved non–infarct zone function.

In summary, pathologic and angiographic studies suggest that two therapeutic windows of opportunity exist. First, rapid reperfusion may salvage central ischemic zone function and abort the shock state altogether. Once shock develops, a second therapeutic widow occurs. Intervening late may prevent reinfarction or infarct extension. Intervening late may also salvage some central ischemic function that is protected by collaterals. Most importantly, delayed intervention may salvage border-zone jeopardized myocardium and cause immediate preservation or enhancement of myocardial function distant to the infarct zone.

## Rationale for Aggressive Intervention

The understanding of the pathophysiology and pathoanatomy of cardiogenic shock provides a rationale for intervention. Balloon counterpulsation, PTCA, and bypass all appear to improve the prognosis compared with historical controls (Fig. 13–4). Hochman, however, has elegantly demonstrated that case selection bias alone may explain the implied improved outcome.[11] The field is lacking in prospective randomized trials of an aggressive versus a conservative approach to this entity.[39] Many investigators have been unable to enroll such patients because of ethical concerns and logistic difficulty in the informed consent process. The SHOCK trial has answered many questions concerning the scientific merit of an aggressive approach. Pending complete publication of this trial, clinicians must rely on reports of a systematic aggressive strategy. Goldberg, in fact, demonstrated that aggressive treatment of shock is rarely employed in a community setting.[15] During the Worchester survey, less than 10% of patients underwent catheterization, 1% underwent coronary bypass, 2% underwent PTCA, and only 7.6% were treated with thrombolytic therapy. In this setting, 80% of patients died (Fig. 13–5), and the mortality rate was unchanged from 1975 to 1989.

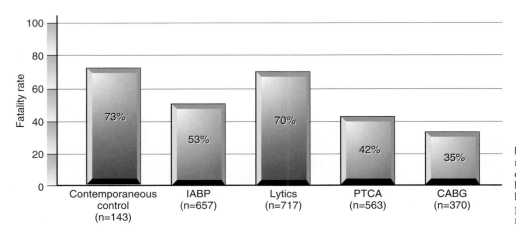

FIGURE 13–4. Pooled analysis of mortality based on therapy received. CABG, coronary artery bypass graft; IABP, intra-aortic balloon counterpulsation; PTCA, percutaneous transluminal coronary angioplasty.

Gheorghiade inferred that shock occurs less frequently with increasing interventions.[16] In the 1981–1984 era, 17.7% of MI patients underwent catheterization and 6.4% had revascularization, whereas among patients treated in 1990–1992, 51.4% had catheterization and 32% had revascularization. In association with this increased use of revascularization, shock declined from 11% to 6% and hospital mortality decreased from 9.4% to 4.8%. The same group (Moosvi and associates) demonstrated an improved survival for PTCA-treated patients compared with the historical control of cardiogenic shock treated medically at Henry Ford Hospital.[40] During the thrombolytic era, the outcome of an aggressive strategy has been reported for the Thrombolysis In Myocardial Infarction (TIMI) II trial[41] and the Duke Medical Center experience.[42] In both instances, survival was greater for patients undergoing catheterization and revascularization (if technically feasible).

The strongest argument for an aggressive approach comes from the GUSTO trial. Worldwide patient recruitment occurred, and marked disparity in aggressiveness occurred among countries (Table 13–2). Patients treated in the United States were far more likely to be treated with intra-aortic balloon counterpulsation (IABP), undergo catheterization, and undergo revascularization. Mortality was lower (50% vs. 66%, $p < 0.001$) for U.S. patients in shock. Logistic regression analysis furthermore demonstrated that revascularization independently improved 30-day and 1-year mortality (Fig. 13–6). Because so few patients underwent revascularization in non-U.S. countries, these patients serve as excellent contemporaneous controls. Even more impressive is the 73% survival for shock patients undergoing coronary artery bypass graft (CABG) and 70% survival for shock patients undergoing PTCA in the United States.

At the conclusion of the TIMI II trial, we reviewed the outcome for cardiogenic shock at William Beaumont Hospital, Royal Oak, Michigan. At this time, a very conservative approach to these patients was employed (Fig. 13–7). Because of this poor outcome, in 1988 our institution embarked on a systematic effort to more aggressively treat cardiogenic shock

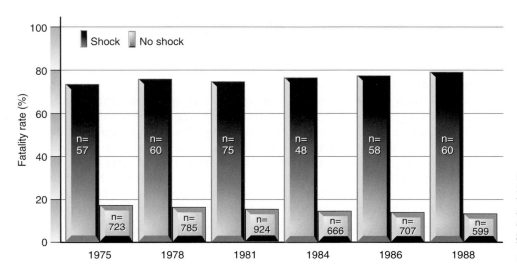

FIGURE 13–5. In-hospital case-fatality rates among patients with acute myocardial infarction according to the year studied and the occurrence of cardiogenic shock. Data derived from Worchester experience in cardiogenic shock.

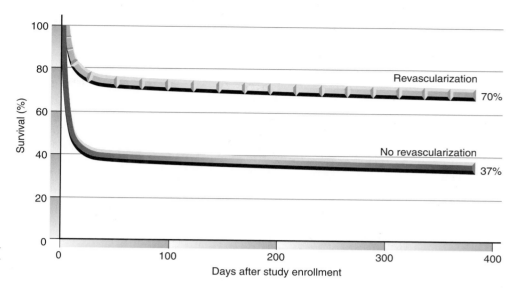

FIGURE 13–6. GUSTO experience with the survival of patients in cardiogenic shock.

## TABLE 13–2.   GUSTO EXPERIENCE WITH TREATMENT OF SHOCK

| INTERVENTION | U.S.A. (N = 1891) | OTHER COUNTRIES (N = 1081) | $p^*$ |
|---|---|---|---|
| Cardiac catheterization | 1092 (58%) | 253 (23%) | <0.001 |
| IABP | 652 (35%) | 80 (7%) | <0.001 |
| Right heart catheterization | 1074 (57%) | 236 (22%) | <0.001 |
| Ventilatory support | 1021 (54%) | 405 (38%) | <0.001 |
| CABG | 295 (16%) | 43 (4%) | <0.001 |
| PTCA | 483 (26%) | 82 (8%) | <0.001 |
| Inotropic agent | 1850 (98%) | 998 (93%) | <0.001 |
| ß Blocker | 1024 (54%) | 410 (38%) | <0.001 |
| Aspirin | 1768 (94%) | 1016 (94%) | 0.6120 |
| Mortality | 50 | 66 | <0.001 |

CABG, coronary artery bypass graft; GUSTO, Global Utilization of Streptokinase and Tissue Plasminogen Activator for Occluded Coronary Arteries; IABP, intra-aortic balloon pump; PTCA, percutaneous transluminal coronary angioplasty.

*Data on types of interventions used for some patients were not available; differences between geographic locations were assessed only for patients whose data were available.

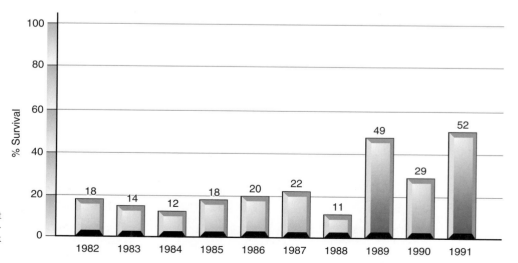

FIGURE 13–7. William Beaumont Hospital experience with survival after cardiogenic shock from 1982 through 1991.

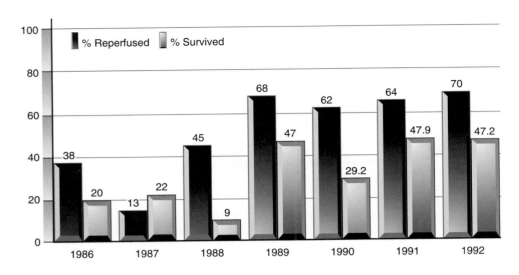

FIGURE 13–8. William Beaumont Hospital experience, depicting the percentage of patients reperfused and hospital survival after cardiogenic shock from 1986 through 1992.

patients. Catheterization, PTCA, and surgery became much more frequently employed. In association with this more aggressive intervention, a markedly higher survival occurred for patients presenting in shock to our institution (Fig. 13–8). These historical studies, the GUSTO experience, and the William Beaumont Hospital experience provide a compelling argument for a systematic, aggressive approach to management of cardiogenic shock. Ultimately, the most compelling argument for aggressive revascularization is provided by the SHOCK trial. This study has been completed and the 1-year follow-up has been presented.[42a, 42b] Although only a trend to improved 1-month survival occurred for the revascularization arm, at 6 months significant improvement in survival was present for patients treated aggressively (Fig. 13–9). It is likely that this will be the last controlled trial without a revascularization arm. Thus, at present, an ethical imperative will drive clinicians to refer SHOCK trial–eligible patients for revascularization.

## MODERN INTERVENTIONS IN CARDIOGENIC SHOCK
### Intra-aortic Balloon Counterpulsation
Soon after development of CCUs in the 1960s, it became apparent that cardiogenic shock persisted as the major cause of death after acute MI. The first therapeutic intervention in the CCU era was the use of IABP. Scheidt and coworkers prospectively treated 87 patients in shock with IABP.[43] Although systemic pressure and cardiac output were increased and lactate metabolism was improved, only 15% of patients survived hospitalization, and of these 13 patients, only 8 survived for 1 year. Rourke and associates randomized 50 Killip class III and class IV patients to balloon pump or control and found no difference in the enzymatic infarct size and no difference in the hospital mortality for treated and control patients.[44] Based on these initial trials, IABP is currently used in only a minority of shock patients. In the Worchester survey, IABP was used in only 7.5% of patients in shock.[15] Because of the concern for increased hemorrhagic risk after thrombolytics,[45] IABP is used only infrequently in this setting. In the GUSTO I trial, 2657 patients presented with or developed cardiogenic shock; only 25% of these patients were treated with IABP.[46] Of interest, a marked worldwide heterogeneity of use exists. In the United States, 35% of patients with shock have IABP use, whereas only 7% usage of IABP occurs in the non-U.S. GUSTO sites. At the present time, no data validate IABP alone as a therapeutic strategy. Its main use is as a bridge for

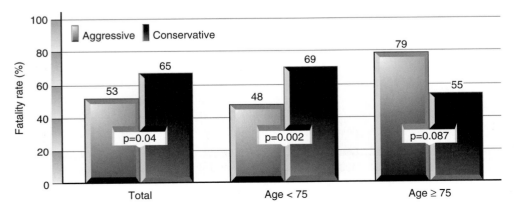

FIGURE 13–9. Six-month fatality rate for Should We Emergently Revascularize Occluded Coronaries for Cardiogenic Shock (SHOCK) trial patients, based on treatment strategy and age.

safe catheterization and percutaneous or surgical revascularization. The intriguing potential for potentiation of thrombolytic efficacy in these patients by the use of IABP is subsequently addressed.

## Thrombolytic Therapy

Pathologic and angiographic studies have demonstrated the high prevalence of occlusive coronary thrombi in shock patients. The timely administration of thrombolytic therapy should be particularly useful in this setting. Mathey and associates first demonstrated that shock could be reversed with intracoronary thrombolytic therapy.[47] Unfortunately, a large series including the Society for Cardiac Angiography Registry showed a disappointing rate of survival for patients in shock.[48] Additionally, this registry provided insight into the reason for this low survival. Although the overall rate of reperfusion was 71%, only 43% of shock patients had successful reperfusion. Survival, in fact, was 58% for those successfully reperfused shock patients.

Intravenous thrombolytic therapy has proved disappointing in this population (Table 13–3). The only placebo-controlled trial (GISSI [Gruppo Italiano per lo Studio della Streptochinasi nell'Infarto Miocardico] I) randomized 280 patients to intravenous streptokinase or placebo and found a 70% mortality rate for both treatment arms.[49] The comparative efficacy of streptokinase and recombinant tissue-type plasminogen activator (r-tPA) was initially studied in the GISSI II[50] and ISIS (International Study of Infarct Survival) II[51] trials. In addition, the GUSTO study enrolled a small proportion of patients in cardiogenic shock. These studies suggest the marginal benefit of streptokinase over tPA. Both groups still have a disappointingly high mortality.

Stomel and Bates have explored the adjunctive use of IABP after thrombolytic therapy of cardiogenic shock.[52] This therapy is based on the experimental observation that tPA-induced reperfusion is enhanced when hypotension is treated with counterpulsation.[53] Doppler studies have corroborated enhancement of flow velocity with balloon counterpulsation.[54] In fact, Ohman and associates have demonstrated that IABP therapy enhances sustained patency after interventional therapy of acute MI.[55] These original studies led Stomel and Bates to treat a cohort of shock patients with IABP and thrombolytic therapy before tertiary care transfer. When they compared the 22 patients treated in this manner with a cohort of patients treated with thrombolytics alone, they found a marked improvement in survival (32% vs. 7% mortality, $p < 0.005$). In addition to this mechanical approach, future studies must be conducted with combined thrombolytic and antiplatelet therapies. It is apparent that currently available intravenous thrombolytic regimens have poor rates of sustained patency and thus are associated with a high mortality. Furthermore, Hochman has demonstrated that only 50% of shock patients are eligible for thrombolytic therapy.[11] For all these reasons, intravenous therapy alone is unlikely to enhance the improvement and outcome for these patients, and more comprehensive mechanical or surgical approaches will require further extensive clinical testing.

## Role of Percutaneous Transluminal Coronary Angioplasty

Guide wire mechanical coronary recanalization was initially employed by Rentrop to facilitate reperfusion.[56] After intracoronary thrombolytic therapy became commonly used, Meyer and colleagues demonstrated the ability of PTCA to enhance reperfusion and eliminate the underlying residual stenotic lesion.[57] At the same time, Meyer and associates described in a case report the use of PTCA to successfully treat cardiogenic shock.[58] We reported our initial experience with PTCA therapy of shock at

**TABLE 13–3.** **THROMBOLYTIC THERAPY FOR CARDIOGENIC SHOCK COMPLICATING ACUTE MYOCARDIAL INFARCTION**

| TRIAL | THERAPY | N | SHOCK AT ENTRY N (%) | IN-HOSPITAL MORTALITY (%) |
|---|---|---|---|---|
| GISSI-I | SK vs. control | 11,806 | 80 (2.4) | SK-70 Control-70 |
| International Study Group | SK vs. tPA | 20,768 | 322 (1.6) | SK-65 tPA-78 |
| GUSTO-I | SK vs. tPA | 41,021 | 315 (0.8) | SK-55 tPA-59 |

GISSI, Gruppo Italiano per lo Studio della Streptochinasi nell'Infarto Miocardico; GUSTO, Global Utilization of Streptokinasae and Tissue Plasminogen Activator for Occluded Coronary Arteries; SK, streptokinase; tPA, tissue-type plasminogen activator.

**TABLE 13–4.    SURVIVAL FROM CARDIOGENIC SHOCK**

| PATIENT CONDITION | >48 N (%) | HOSPITAL DISCHARGE N (%) |
| --- | --- | --- |
| Successful PTCA | 23/24 (96) | 18/24 (75) |
| Unsuccessful PTCA | 1/3 (33) | 1/3 (33) |
| Anterior | 15/17 (88) | 10/17 (62) |
| Inferior | 9/10 (90) | 8/10 (80) |
| Symptoms <12 h | 16/18 (89) | 14/18 (77) |
| Symptoms >12 h | 8/9 (88) | 5/9 (55) |
| Single vessel | 11/12 (92) | 11/12 (92) |
| Multivessel | 13/15 (86) | 8/15 (53) |
| Age <60 y | 12/13 (92) | 11/13 (92) |
| Age >60 y | 12/14 (85) | 8/14 (57) |

PTCA, percutaneous transluminal coronary angioplasty.
From O'Neill WW, Topol EJ, Fung A, et al: Coronary angioplasty as therapy for acute myocardial infarction: University of Michigan experience. Circulation 76 (suppl II): II-79, 1987.

the University of Michigan in 1985 (Table 13–4), demonstrating the promise of PTCA for this condition.[59, 60] A 70% in-hospital survival rate occurred overall, and 75% of successfully reperfused patients survived. Patients with inferior MI, those presenting less than 12 hours after the onset of symptoms, those with one-vessel disease, and patients younger than 60 years had a higher survival rate, whereas patients with multivessel disease had a lower survival. These patients had attempts at infarct artery angioplasty only.

Lee and associates attempted to define subgroups with different survival rates further in a multicenter registry experience.[32] The most important finding of this study was that patients with multivessel disease had a 62% mortality and patients with unsuccessful reperfusion had an 80% mortality. Angioplasty achieved successful reperfusion in 71% of cases. The GUSTO reports have now confirmed these initial observations.[61] Moosvi and coworkers found a 56% survival for patients revascularized with PTCA or bypass, and a 77% survival for patients treated within 24 hours of symptom onset.[40] Hibbard and colleagues reviewed the Mayo Clinic experience with 45 patients in shock treated with PTCA.[33] They reported a 56% survival. Most recently, Eltchaninoff and associates reported a 64% survival in the Cleveland Clinic experience with 33 patients in cardiogenic shock.[62] An overview of the outcomes with this approach confirms the excellent survival of patients having successful angioplasty therapy. Although these small clinical series have been consistently encouraging, caution must be used in making definitive conclusions about angioplasty therapy. All reports have been small retrospective chart review studies. Only the studies by Moosvi and coworkers and by Lee and colleagues have historical control groups. A high mortality occurs for extremely aged patients who have PTCA. A strong concern exists that a case selection bias and publica-

tion of only positive results have occurred. In spite of these reservations, this form of therapy is the only therapy that offers any hope of altering the grim outlook for these patients. Even more importantly, the SHOCK trial has provided the necessary scientific underpinning for mechanical reperfusion therapy. For these reasons, patients in cardiogenic shock presenting early after MI who have no terminal comorbidities and who are not older than 75 years should be considered for percutaneous coronary revascularization.

## Role of Coronary Bypass

Coronary revascularization employing surgical revascularization must also be considered. As a sole treatment strategy, coronary bypass is unlikely to alter overall shock mortality. Mundth reviewed the Massachusetts General Experience with surgical revascularization.[63] He found that survival was 46% for patients deemed operable. Unfortunately, only 51 of 120 patients could be operated on. The mortality for inoperable patients was so high that overall survival was only 34 of 120 (28%) in this series. Similarly, DeWood and associates reported an extremely favorable (58%) survival for shock patients operated on within 6 hours of symptom onset.[25] Only 19 of 40 patients were deemed operable. In spite of these limitations, surgical revascularization has great promise. Buckberg and colleagues demonstrated that controlled reperfusion and myocardial rest may significantly preserve jeopardized myocardial function.[64] In addition, surgical revascularization may provide more complete revascularization if chronic total artery occlusion is present. Finally, coronary lesions that are technically high risk (American Heart Association/American College of Cardiology [AHA/ACC] type C) may be more safely treated with coronary bypass. Our own philosophy has been to offer surgical revascularization to patients with severe multivessel disease who are anatomically unsuitable for PTCA and who present within 6 hours of the onset of symptoms. The comparative efficacy of PTCA and bypass has not been prospectively evaluated in this setting. Moscucci and Bates have summarized the published angioplasty and surgical experience in cardiogenic shock. They summarized 19 angioplasty trials and reported on a total of 563 patients. The overall survival rate was 58%. Overall, PTCA was successful in 81% of cases. Of importance is that the survival rate was 71% among patients with successful PTCA. Similarly, among 370 bypass patients reported in another study, the survival rate was 65%.

## RESUSCITATIVE MEASURES
## General Supportive Measures

Once a patient in cardiogenic shock has been identified as a candidate for potential intervention, a systematic and comprehensive treatment regimen is essential. These patients represent the most challenging, most dangerous, and most rewarding cases for coronary intervention. Although successful revascularization improves the likelihood for survival, a great risk of iatrogenic complications exists. Patients present in extreme distress. They are profoundly hypotensive, which makes percutaneous arterial access problematic. They are often mentally obtunded and confused, leading to difficulty following instructions. Often they have been sedated with narcotics, putting them at risk of respiratory arrest, vomiting, and aspiration. Often, bradyarrhythmia or complete heart block is present, and frequently recurrent ventricular fibrillation and ventricular tachycardia occur, requiring frequent electric cardioversion. These complications represent an enormous logistic challenge to just complete a catheterization procedure safely, further magnifying the difficulty in performing safe and adequate PTCA. We have demonstrated that PTCA is successful in 95% of patients undergoing angioplasty therapy for MI who are clinically stable.[66] Conversely, studies have demonstrated success rates varying from 40% to 70% for patients in cardiogenic shock. No doubt, the lower success rate for cardiogenic shock patients is largely related to these technical difficulties. To ensure a safe and successful coronary intervention, a predefined treatment algorithm by an experienced interventional team is mandatory (Fig. 13–10).

## General Resuscitation

As a first step, general resuscitative measures are immediately required after patient presentation. A brief cardiovascular examination should be performed. Noncardiac causes of hypotension must be ruled out (e.g., massive pulmonary embolism, tension pneumothorax, dissecting aortic aneurysm, ruptured viscus). Mechanical complications of MI must be excluded (e.g., acute ventricular septal defect, acute papillary muscle rupture). Pericardial tamponade or myocardial rupture must be considered. The peripheral vasculature must be evaluated because multiple-site vascular access will be needed for arterial access, IABP, and possibly cardiopulmonary support (CPS). If a history of peripheral vascular disease is present, this must be taken into account in planning the coronary intervention. The iliofemoral artery with least disease should be saved for balloon counterpulsation or CPS. Occasionally, iliofemoral peripheral angioplasty may be required to improve vascular access.

Optimal oxygenation and airway stability is essential. A low threshold for intubation should exist. (The oral route is preferred for intubation if the patient has received thrombolytic therapy because of the risk of hemorrhage into the lungs with nasal intubation.) Patients are combative, especially in the face of ongoing chest pain or when frequent cardioversions are required. To ensure a safe and effective procedure, intubation, sedation, and muscular paralysis may be required. It is essential, however, that impediments to a thorough catheterization study and a complete PTCA procedure be eliminated.

If physical examination fails to demonstrate pulmonary edema, rapid volume challenge should be accomplished to exclude hypovolemia as a cause of hypotension. Loeb and coworkers demonstrated that

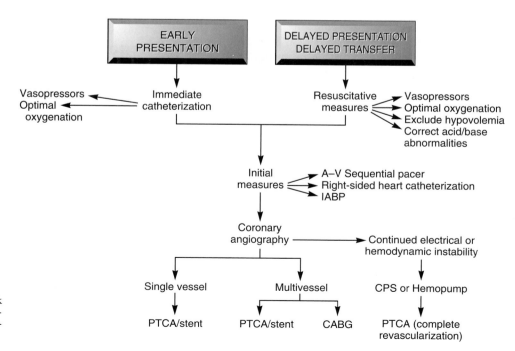

FIGURE 13–10. Cardiogenic shock treatment algorithm. A-V, atrioventricular; CPS, cardiopulmonary support.

volume expansion can in fact reverse the shock state in many patients.[67] This is especially critical when a history of diuretic use or persistent vomiting is present. Relative hypotension related to right ventricular infarction must be considered in patients with inferior MI and ST-segment elevation in the right precordial ECG leads.[68] Acidosis secondary to respiratory insufficiency or secondary lactic acidosis may exist. The presence of lactic acidosis is an extremely grave sign. Acidosis must be corrected to improve the efficacy of inotropic agents. Hypokalemia or hypomagnesemia may also be present and need to be corrected to reduce the likelihood of recurrent refractory arrhythmias. All these resuscitative measures should be rapidly initiated while arrangement for catheterization occurs.

## Support of Systemic Arterial Pressure

The most critical and initial resuscitative measure is BP support with vasopressor therapy. This therapy has been extensively evaluated during the past decade. Clearly no long-term, prognostic benefit has been derived from this therapy. Mortality has remained unchanged for patients treated with L-norepinephrine,[5] dopamine,[69] dobutamine,[70] or salbutamol.[71] In part, this is related to the great increase in myocardial oxygen demand caused by inotropic agents, as first demonstrated by Mueller and colleagues in their comparative studies of isoproterenol and L-norepinephrine for cardiogenic shock patients.[72] Conversely, coronary blood flow may be greatly augmented by improving coronary perfusion pressure, and ischemic myocardial zones may improve function. Occasionally, vasopressors will reverse the cardiogenic shock state (presumably related to augmented perfusion of jeopardized ischemic myocardial segments). A BP response to inotropic agents is in fact a good prognostic sign. Patients with hypotension who are refractory to vasopressors have an extremely poor prognosis. Because total occlusion of the infarct artery is invariably present, inotropic agents alone could never correct the fundamental central zone ischemia. Therefore, vasopressors should be used as adjuncts to coronary revascularization. The transient increase in oxygen demand will be greatly offset by the improved blood flow directly through stenotic, patent noninfarct arteries. Furthermore, after successful recanalization of occluded vessels, improved blood flow to the central ischemic zone may greatly decrease the size of the infarct. For these reasons, vasopressors should be used aggressively before coronary intervention. With successful recanalization, the patient can often be weaned from vasopressors within hours of the procedure. Currently, norepinephrine or, less optimally, high-dose (>30 μg/kg/minute) dopamine is preferred as an initial resuscitative vasopressor.

When prolonged need for vasopressor therapy exists after coronary revascularization, a combination of dopamine and dobutamine (7 to 10 μg/kg/minute) appears to be optimal.[73] Long-term use of norepinephrine is deleterious because of the profound systemic vasoconstriction that occurs. Dobutamine alone augments myocardial oxygen demand and may worsen hypotension because of its peripheral vasodilatory effects. Dopamine alone also increases myocardial oxygen consumption; in addition, it increases pulmonary resistance and pulmonary wedge pressure, which worsens oxygenation. Low to moderate doses of dopamine and dobutamine appear to provide optimal myocardial inotropic effects without profound systemic vasoconstriction or vasodilation and without pulmonary congestion. Amrinone alone or in combination with other inotropes has not been extensively evaluated in cardiogenic shock.

The clinical presentation frequently includes bradycardia or complete heart block, especially during inferior MI. Initial pharmacologic therapy, including atropine therapy, should be initiated. Attempts to increase the heart rate may include the need for temporary pacemaker insertion. It is critical to maintain atrioventricular (AV) synchrony in this setting. Cardiac output may be augmented as much as 30% when dual-chamber pacing is initiated.[74] AV synchronous pacing is especially crucial in massive inferior MI with right ventricular (RV) involvement.[75] In this setting, blood flow to the right side of the heart is almost entirely related to right atrial contraction. For this reason, AV synchrony is essential to maintain forward blood flow.

## Mechanical Support

If these initial resuscitative measures are unsuccessful, more extensive mechanical support may be required. Mueller and associates elegantly demonstrated the favorable hemodynamic effects and improvement in myocardial metabolism associated with IABP.[72] Balloon counterpulsation alone increased mean aortic pressure 15 mm Hg and improved coronary blood flow 23 mL per 100 g/minute without increasing myocardial oxygen consumption and with a 15% improvement in lactate extraction. Ehrich and associates demonstrated that balloon pump therapy raised the cardiac index, improved the stroke work index, lowered the systemic resistance, lowered the wedge pressure, and greatly augmented the mean aortic pressure.[76] Weiss and coworkers observed global and regional myocardial function in shock patients treated with balloon counterpulsation.[77] These investigators found that the global ejection fraction increased from 27% to 36%, entirely related to improved function of the infarct zone. Furthermore, the most improvement in infarct zone function occurred in dyskinetic infarct zones. Regional wall motion of hypokinetic ischemic zones and motion of adjacent noninfarct zones did not improve. These results suggest that the beneficial effect on ventricular function was primarily related to an afterload reduction effect. Unfortunately, marginal ischemic zone function and nonischemic zone function were not improved. Port and colleagues studied coronary blood flow in patients with highly stenotic coronary arteries and found no improvement in flow through these stenotic vessels after the initiation of balloon pump therapy.[78] These physiologic observations suggest that balloon counterpulsation has useful beneficial effects on systemic hemodynamics but no effect on central ischemic zone function or noninfarct zone function. Thus, it is unlikely that IABP therapy alone will alter the prognosis for myocardial infarction patients in shock.

Although balloon pump therapy is not proved to have prognostic benefit as a sole therapy, important advantages of the use of balloon pump therapy occur. Currently, this therapy is seen strictly as a supportive measure. The chief role of balloon counterpulsation is to permit the performance of a safe catheterization procedure in shock patients. All shock patients should routinely have balloon pump therapy with one-to-one augmentation initiated before contrast angiography, to enhance the likelihood of a safe procedure.

The Duke experience with balloon counterpulsation after thrombolytic therapy reported by Ohman and coworkers suggested significant beneficial effects.[55] Patients treated with balloon counterpulsation after thrombolytic therapy had a significant decrease in coronary reocclusion rates. Furthermore, Ishihara and associates demonstrated an improvement of myocardial function in patients treated with IABP after thrombolytic therapy.[79] For these reasons, the use of balloon pump therapy should be considered mandatory for patients in cardiogenic shock.

## Cardiopulmonary Support

In some patients, even vasopressor therapy and balloon counterpulsation fail to stabilize hemodynamics. Attempting PTCA in this setting is futile and may simply hasten the patient's demise. Instability is related either to refractory hypotension or to recurrent refractory ventricular tachycardia/fibrillation. In this situation, percutaneous CPS[80] or Hemopump therapy,[81] if available, are indicated. CPS at 3 to 5 L flow per minute will greatly augment the mean systemic pressure. Once patients are on full

bypass, mean aortic pressures of 60 to 70 mm Hg are possible even when myocardial contractility has totally ceased. Furthermore, CPS improves the electric stability in this setting. At our institution, 20 patients with catheterization laboratory cardiac arrest were treated with emergency CPS. All these patients were refractory to standard Advanced Cardiac Life Support resuscitative measures. In all 20 patients, the baseline cardiac rhythm could be restored after the initiation of CPS. Of these patients, 16 of 20 underwent revascularization with PTCA or surgery, and 8 of 16 patients survived the hospital discharge. Shawl and colleagues reported the use of CPS as a supportive measure for patients in shock who were undergoing emergency PTCA.[82] These workers stabilized 10 patients with CPS and found that 8 of 10 patients were suitable for PTCA. All 8 patients were successfully revascularized with PTCA, and all 8 patients survived with 1-year follow-up. Smalling and associates treated cardiogenic shock patients with Hemopump therapy.[83] Nine patients in cardiogenic shock were treated with insertion of the Hemopump. The hemodynamics were measured before and 72 hours after the initiation of therapy. The cardiac output was enhanced from 3.4 to 5.8 L/minute. The wedge pressure declined from 26 to 17 mm Hg, and the mean arterial pressure increased from 54 to 86 mm Hg. Survival occurred in four of nine patients. Gacioch and coworkers have reported 20% survival for cardiogenic shock patients treated with the Hemopump at the University of Michigan.[84] The largest multicenter experience was reported by Wampler and associates.[85] In this study, 41% of the patients treated with Hemopump therapy who had refractory cardiogenic shock survived. These patients with refractory shock were treated primarily with Hemopump therapy and were not revascularized.

These small clinical studies have demonstrated that mechanical support with CPS or Hemopump is highly effective in stabilizing shock patients. However, these supportive measures alone do not improve long-term survival. Pavlides and colleagues in fact reported a deleterious metabolic effect of CPS therapy on myocardial lactate metabolism.[86] Accordingly, these devices must be used strictly as measures to support patients through percutaneous or surgical revascularization. Perhaps the chief benefit of CPS is the outstanding support that can be provided, allowing a complete revascularization to be attempted. In addition to CPS, percutaneous left ventricular assist employing a left atrial cannula is being developed.

## Revascularization

Once patients have been sedated and stabilized, a safe catheterization study can occur. Rapid evaluation for mechanical problems (ventricular septal defect [VSD], acute mitral regurgitation, myocardial rupture) should now occur. Complete instrumentation including temporary pacing, pulmonary artery monitoring lines, and balloon pump must all be in place. Our practice has been to defer contrast ventriculography until after coronary angiography because of the dye load that is necessary. Coronary angiography of the noninfarct artery is first performed to permit the identification of collateral flow to the infarct artery and critical lesions of the noninfarct artery. One or at most two coronary angiograms should be obtained. Biplane angiography may in fact be very useful in this setting. Angiograms of the infarct artery should next be obtained. At all times, meticulous attention to the patient's response to contrast injections must occur. Profound hypotension that persists for minutes after contrast ejection is an ominous sign that must be countered immediately with more extensive supportive measures. If hemodynamics cannot be maintained during coronary angiography, they will never be maintained during coronary intervention.

Once coronary angiography is completed, a decision about surgical or percutaneous revascularization must be made. If percutaneous revascularization is chosen, infarct artery angioplasty should be performed first. When the infarct artery is in the left coronary distribution, extreme caution must be used regarding subsequent contrast injections. Further contrast injections may critically depress myocardial function of the noninfarct zone. Although as a general rule we prefer to perform only infarct artery angioplasty during PTCA of acute MI (AMI), cardiogenic shock is an exception. In this setting, complete revascularization may be beneficial. If critically stenosed noninfarct vessels exist and they are technically suited for PTCA, immediate dilation should be performed. Obtaining an optimal angioplasty result is more critical in this setting than in any other setting facing an interventionist. Patients usually do not survive coronary reocclusion. For this reason, a careful procedure with optimal balloon sizing, prolonged balloon inflation, and judicious use of intracoronary stent therapy is mandated.

Because a stable, optimal angioplasty result is so critical in cardiogenic shock patients, the role of stenting must be discussed. As with other patient subsets, stent usage has become widespread for infarct angioplasty. The Stent–Primary Angioplasty in Myocardial Infarction (Stent-PAMI) trial has demonstrated the comparison with primary angioplasty with bailout stenting for suboptimal results; routine stent implantation results in less recurrent ischemia and less target vessel revascularization at 6 months.[87] These modest benefits must be counterbalanced by the possible catastrophic consequences of stent thrombosis, which is known to be more frequent in patients with impaired left ventricular function.

Antoniucci and coworkers have described an experience with stent implantation in cardiogenic shock.[88] In this noncontrolled series, the overall hospital mortality was 24%. Patients were treated with angioplasty and stenting if feasible. Only 47% of patients could have stents deployed. Stent implantation resulted in less recurrent ischemia. Two cases of stent thrombosis occurred, and stent implantation was less feasible than in patients without shock. Patients in shock had more severe, extensive diffuse disease and often could not be treated by stent implantation. Future randomized trials of stent therapy of shock are required. At the present time, there is a suggestion that modest additional benefit will occur over PTCA therapy.

Once angioplasty is completed, contrast ventriculography should be performed. This provides prognostic data and a baseline for future evaluation of ventricular function. Additionally, these data may permit triage data with regard to temporary ventricular assist or emergency cardiac transplantation. Careful hemodynamic monitoring after coronary intervention also provides extremely useful prognostic data. Raneses and coworkers showed that cardiac output improves systolic arterial pressure increases, and wedge pressure decreases within 8 to 12 hours in survivors of cardiogenic shock.[89] Conversely, persistence of the shock state 8 to 12 hours after intervention carries an invariably lethal outcome. If shock persists at this time frame, referral for ventricular assist or emergency transplantation is the only remaining treatment option to achieve survival.

## CONCLUSION: THE FUTURE OF TREATMENT OF SHOCK

Angioplasty appears to have a fundamental role in the management of shock. Unfortunately, many deficiencies of this approach exist. A reocclusion rate of 10% to 15% occurs for primary PTCA in the nonshock setting. The main predictor of reocclusion is the presence of an occlusive dissection. Stent implantation may enhance the stability of the PTCA result. Because reocclusion is likely to be catastrophic for shock patients, the value of stenting may be particularly strong in this setting. Although no published experience exists for the use of glycoprotein receptor blockers, these agents may have an important role as adjunctive therapy because of their ability to prevent reocclusion and enhance left ventricular function. Schafer has compared the result of PTCA in a shock and a nonshock setting.[27] PTCA resulted in TIMI-3 flow rates in 95% of cases not in shock, whereas only 73% of shock patients had TIMI-3 flow reestablished. Again, stent implantation may improve these results. Webb and associates treated 15 patients in shock with stent implantation.[90] They were able to reestablish TIMI-3 flow in all cases and achieved a 73% 1-month survival. In spite of the improved stability of the culprit artery, further research must be conducted on methods to enhance myocardial salvage. Regardless of how pristine the arterial patency is rendered, if irreversibly injured muscle is revascularized, survival still may not occur. In these cases patients without other comorbidities may be considered for left ventricular assist devices.[91, 92] Adjuncts to reperfusion such as adenosine, leukofiltration, or even glucose/insulin/potassium[93] should be studied. Finally, aggressive myocardial support with ventricular assist devices needs further prospective investigation. A final note of caution must be sounded. A certain proportion of patients presenting in shock will be too far gone to survive. Aggressive intervention is futile and expensive and now carries the penalty of report card medicine. Identifying these patients and treating them with comfort measures only may in the end be the greatest challenge facing a coronary interventionalist.

## REFERENCES

1. Herrick JB: Clinical features of sudden obstruction of the coronary arteries. *In* Willius FA, Keys TE (eds): Cardiac Classics, p 817. St. Louis: CV Mosby, 1941.
2. Pardee HEB: An electrocardiographic sign of coronary artery obstruction. Arch Intern Med 26:244, 1920.
3. Fishberg AM, Hitzig WM, King FH: Circulatory dynamics in myocardial infarction. Arch Intern Med 54:997, 1934.
4. Stead EA, Ebert RV: Shock syndrome produced by failure of the heart. Arch Intern Med 69:369, 1942.
5. Griffith GC, Wallace WB, Chochran B, et al: The treatment of shock associated with myocardial infarction. Circulation 9:527, 1954.
6. Friedberg CK: Cardiogenic shock in acute myocardial infarction. Circulation 23:325, 1961.
7. Norris RM, Sammel NL: Predictors of late hospital death in acute myocardial infarction [Abstract]. Prog Cardiovasc Dis 23:129, 1980.
8. Killip T, Kimball T: Treatment of myocardial infarction in a coronary care unit. Am J Cardiol 20:457, 1967.
9. Scheidt S, Ascheim R, Killip T: Shock after acute myocardial infarction. Am J Cardiol 26:556, 1970.
10. Forrester JS, Diamond G, Chatterjee K, et al: Medical therapy of acute myocardial infarction by application of hemodynamic subsets (first of two parts). N Engl J Med 295:1356, 1976.
11. Hochman JS, Boland J, Sleeper LA, et al: Current spectrum of cardiogenic shock and effect of early revascularization on mortality. Circulation 91:873, 1995.
12. ISIS-2 (Second International Study of Infarct Survival) Collaborative Group: Randomized trial of intravenous streptokinase, oral aspirin, both, or neither among 17,187 cases of suspected acute myocardial infarction. Lancet 2:349, 1988.
13. Lee L, Bates ER, Pitt B, et al: Percutaneous transluminal coronary angioplasty improves survival in acute myocardial infarction complicated by cardiogenic shock. Circulation 78:1345, 1988.
14. Mirowski M, Israel W, Antonopoulos A, et al: Treatment of myocardial infarction in a community hospital coronary care unit. Arch Intern Med 138:210, 1978.
15. Goldberg RJ, Gore JM, Alpert JS, et al: Cardiogenic shock after acute myocardial infarction: Incidence and mortality from a community-wide perspective, 1975 to 1988. N Engl J Med 325:1117, 1991.
16. Gheorghiade M, Ruzumna A, Borzak S: Decline of the rate of hospital mortality from acute myocardial infarction: Impact of changing management strategies. Am Heart J 131:250, 1996.
17. Kleiman NS, Terrin M, Mueller H, et al: Mechanisms of early death despite thrombolytic therapy: Experience from the thrombolysis in myocardial infarction phase II (TIMI II) study. J Am Coll Cardiol 19:1129, 1992.
18. Page DL, Caulfield JB, Kastor JA, et al: Myocardial changes associated with cardiogenic shock. N Engl J Med 285:133, 1971.
19. Alonso DR, Schiedt S, Post M, Killiip T: Pathophysiology of cardiogenic shock: Quantification of myocardial necrosis, clinical, pathologic and electrocardiographic correlations. Circulation 48:588, 1973.
20. Gutovitz AL, Sobel BE, Roberts R: Progressive nature of myocardial injury in selected patients with cardiogenic shock. Am J Cardiol 41:469, 1978.
21. Hornorayan C, Bennett MA, Pentecost BC, et al: Quantitative study of infarcted myocardium in cardiogenic shock. Br Heart J 32:728, 1970.
22. Wackers FJ, Lie KI, Becker AE, et al: Coronary artery disease in patients dying from cardiogenic shock or congestive heart failure in the setting of acute myocardial infarction. Br Heart J 38:906, 1976.
23. Leinbach RC, Dinsmore RE, Mundth ED, et al: Selective coronary and left ventricular cineangiography during intraaortic balloon pumping for cardiogenic shock. Circulation 45:845, 1972.
24. Johnson SA, Scanlon PJ, Loeb HS, et al: Treatment of cardiogenic shock in myocardial infarction by intraaortic balloon counterpulsation and surgery. Am J Med 62:687, 1977.
25. DeWood MA, Notske RN, Hensley GR, et al: Intraaortic balloon counterpulsation with and without reperfusion for myocardial infarction shock. Circulation 61:1105, 1980.
26. Williams DO, Amsterdam EZ, Miller RR, et al: Functional significance of coronary collateral vessels in patients with acute myocardial infarction: Relation to pump performance, cardiogenic shock and survival. Am J Cardiol 37:345, 1976.
27. Schafer JA: Comparison of angioplasty for acute myocardial infarction in patients with and without cardiogenic shock. Personal communication.
28. Grines CL, Brown KF, Marco J, et al: A comparison of immediate angioplasty with thrombolytic therapy for acute myocardial infarction. N Engl J Med 328:673, 1993.
29. Stone GW, Rutherford BD, McConahay DR, et al: Direct coronary angioplasty in acute myocardial infarction: Outcome in patients with single vessel disease. J Am Coll Cardiol 15:534, 1990.
30. Kahn JK, Rutherford BD, McConahay DR, et al: Results of primary angioplasty for acute myocardial infarction in patients with multivessel coronary artery disease. J Am Coll Cardiol 16:1089, 1990.
31. Stone GW, Marsalese D, Brodie BR, et al: A prospective, randomized evaluation of prophylactic intraaortic balloon counterpulsation in high risk patients with acute myocardial infarction treated with primary angioplasty. J Am Coll Cardiol 29:1459, 1997.
32. Lee L, Erbel R, Brown TM, et al: Multicenter registry of angioplasty therapy of cardiogenic shock: Initial and long-term survival. J Am Coll Cardiol 17:599, 1991.
33. Hibbard MD, Holmes DR, Bailey KR, et al: Percutaneous transluminal coronary angioplasty in patients with cardiogenic shock. J Am Coll Cardiol 19:639, 1992.
34. Grines, CL, Topol EJ, Califf RM, et al: Prognostic implications and predictors of enhanced regional wall motion of the non-infarct zone after thrombolysis and angioplasty therapy of acute myocardial infarction. Circulation 80:245, 1989.
35. The GUSTO Angiographic Investigators: The effects of tissue plasminogen activator, streptokinase, or both on coronary-artery patency, ventricular function, and survival after acute myocardial infarction. N Engl J Med 329:1615, 1993.
36. Reimer KA, Jennings RB: The "wavefront phenomenon" of

myocardial ischemic cell death. II. Transmural progression of necrosis within the framework of ischemic bed size (myocardium at risk) and collateral flow. Lab Invest 40:633, 1979.

37. Koren G, Weiss A, Hasin Y, et al: Prevention of myocardial damage in acute myocardial ischemia by early treatment with intravenous streptokinase. N Engl J Med 313:1384, 1985.

38. Morrison D, Crowley ST, Bies R, et al: Systolic blood pressure response to percutaneous transluminal coronary angioplasty for cardiogenic shock. Am J Cardiol 76:313, 1995.

39. O'Neill WW: Angioplasty therapy of cardiogenic shock: Are randomized trials necessary? J Am Coll Cardiol 19:915, 1992.

40. Moosvi AR, Khaja F, Villanueva L, et al: Early revascularization improves survival in cardiogenic shock complicating acute myocardial infarction. J Am Coll Cardiol 19:907, 1992.

41. Garrahy PJ, Henzlova MJ, Forman S, et al: Has thrombolytic therapy improved survival from cardiogenic shock? Thrombolysis in myocardial infarction; (TIMI II) results [Abstract]. Circulation 80(suppl):II-623 1989.

42. Bengtson JR, Kaplan AJ, Pieper KS, et al: Prognosis in cardiogenic shock after acute myocardial infarction in the interventional era. J Am Coll Cardiol 20:1482, 1992.

42a. Hochman JS, Sleeper LA, Webb JG, et al: Early revascularization in acute myocardial infarction complicated by cardiogenic shock. SHOCK Investigators. Should We Emergently Revascularize Occluded Coronaries for Cardiogenic Shock. N Engl J Med 341:625–634, 1999.

42b. Hochman JS, Sleeper LA, White HD, et al: One-year survival following early revascularization for cardiogenic shock. JAMA 285:190–192, 2001.

43. Scheidt S, Wilner G, Mueller H, et al: Intra-aortic balloon counterpulsation in cardiogenic shock: Report of a co-operative clinical trial. N Engl J Med 288:979, 1973.

44. O'Rourke MF, Norris RM, Campbell TJ, et al: Randomized controlled trial of intraaortic balloon counterpulsation in early myocardial infarction with acute heart failure. Am J Cardiol 47:815, 1981.

45. Califf RM, Topol EJ, George BS, et al for the TAMI Study Group: Hemorrhagic complications associated with the use of intravenous tissue plasminogen activator in treatment of acute myocardial infarction. Am J Med 85:353, 1988.

46. Holmes DR Jr, Califf RM, Van de Werf F, et al: Difference in countries' use of resources and clinical outcome for patients with cardiogenic shock after myocardial infarction: Results from the GUSTO trial. Lancet 349:75, 1997.

47. Mathey D, Kuck KH, Remmecke J, et al: Transluminal recanalization of coronary artery thrombosis: A preliminary report of its application in cardiogenic shock. Eur Heart J I:207, 1980.

48. Kennedy J, Gensini G, Timmis G, et al: Acute myocardial infarction treated with intracoronary streptokinase: A report of the Society for Cardiac Angiography. Am J Cardiol 55:871, 1985.

49. Gruppo Italiano per lo Studio della Streptochinasi nell'Infarto Miocardico (GISSI): Effectiveness of intravenous thrombolytic treatment in acute myocardial infarction. Lancet I:397, 1986.

50. GISSI-2: A factorial randomized trial of alteplase versus streptokinase and heparin versus no heparin among 12,490 patients with acute myocardial infarction. Lancet I:65, 1990.

51. ISIS-3: A randomized comparison of streptokinase vs tissue plasminogen activator vs anistreplase and of aspirin plus heparin vs aspirin alone among 41,299 cases of suspected acute myocardial infarction. Lancet I:753, 1992.

52. Stomel RJ, Rasak M, Bates ER: Treatment strategies for acute myocardial infarction complicated by cardiogenic shock in a community hospital. Chest 105:997, 1994.

53. Prewitt RM, Gu S, Schick U, Ducas J: Intraaortic balloon counterpulsation enhances coronary thrombolysis induced by intravenous administration of a thrombolytic agent. J Am Coll Cardiol 23:794, 1994.

54. Kern MJ, Aguirre FV, Tatineni S, et al: Enhanced coronary blood flow velocity during intraaortic balloon counterpulsation in critically ill patients. J Am Coll Cardiol 21:359, 1993.

55. Ohman EM, Califf RM, George BS, et al: The use of intraaortic balloon pumping as an adjunct to reperfusion therapy in acute myocardial infarction. Am Heart J 121:895, 1991.

56. Rentrop KP: Thrombolytic therapy in patients with acute myocardial infarction. Circulation 71:627, 1985.

57. Meyer J, Merx W, Schmitz H, et al: Percutaneous transluminal coronary angioplasty immediately after intracoronary streptolysis of transmural myocardial infarction. Circulation 66:905, 1982.

58. Meyer J, Merx W, Dorr R, et al: Successful treatment of acute myocardial infarction shock by combined percutaneous transluminal coronary recanalization (PTCR) and percutaneous transluminal coronary angioplasty (PTCA). Am Heart J 103:132, 1982.

59. O'Neill WW, Erbel R, Laufer N, et al: Coronary angioplasty therapy of cardiogenic shock complicating acute myocardial infarction [Abstract]. Circulation 72(suppl III):III-309, 1985.

60. O'Neill WW, Topol EJ, Fung A, et al: Coronary angioplasty as therapy for acute myocardial infarction: University of Michigan experience. Circulation 76(suppl II):II-79, 1987.

61. Holmes DR Jr, Kleiman NS, Horgan JHS, et al: Contemporary reperfusion therapy for cardiogenic shock: The GUSTO-I trial experience. J Am Coll Cardiol 26:668, 1995.

62. Eltchaninoff H, Simpfendorfer C, Franco I: Early and 1-year survival rates in acute myocardial infarction complicated by cardiogenic shock: A retrospective study comparing coronary angioplasty with medical treatment. Am Heart J 130:459, 1995.

63. Mundth ED: Surgical treatment of cardiogenic shock and of acute mechanical complications following myocardial infarction. Cardiovasc Clin 8:241, 1977.

64. Rosenkranz ER, Buckberg GD, Laks H, et al: Warm induction of cardioplegia with glutamate-enriched blood in coronary patients with cardiogenic shock who are dependent on inotropic drugs and intra-aortic balloon support: Initial experience and operative strategy. J Thorac Cardiovasc Surg 86:507, 1983.

65. Moscucci M, Bates ER: Cardiogenic shock. Cardiol Clin 13:391, 1995.

66. O'Neill WW, Brodie BR, Ivanhoe R, et al: Primary coronary angioplasty for acute myocardial infarction (the Primary Angioplasty Registry). Am J Cardiol 73:627, 1994.

67. Loeb HS, Pietras RJ, Tobin JR, et al: Hypovolemia in shock due to acute myocardial infarction. Circulation 40:653, 1969.

68. Correale E, Battista R, Martone A, et al: Electrocardiographic patterns in acute inferior myocardial infarction with and without right ventricle involvement: Classification, diagnostic and prognostic value, masking effect. Clin Cardiol 22:37, 1999.

69. Holzer J, Karliner JS, O'Rourke RA, et al: Effectiveness of dopamine in patients with cardiogenic shock. Am J Cardiol 32:79, 1973.

70. Fowler MB, Timmis AD, Crick JP, et al: Comparison of haemodynamic responses to dobutamine and salbutamol in cardiogenic shock after acute myocardial infarction. BMJ 284:73, 1982.

71. Dawson JR, Poole-Wilson PA, Sutton GC: Salbutamol in cardiogenic shock complicating acute myocardial infarction. Br Heart J 43:523, 1980.

72. Mueller H, Ayres SM, Giannelli S, et al: Effect of isoproterenol, L-norepinephrine, and intraaortic counterpulsation on hemodynamics and myocardial metabolism in shock following acute myocardial infarction. Circulation 45:335, 1972.

73. Richard C, Ricome JL, Rimaiho A, et al: Combined hemodynamic effects of dopamine and dobutamine in cardiogenic shock. Circulation 67:620, 1983.

74. Love JC, Haffajee CI, Gore JM, et al: Reversibility of hypotension and shock by atrial or atrioventricular sequential pacing in patients with right ventricular infarction. Am Heart J 108:5, 1984.

75. Bowers TR, O'Neill WW, Grines CL, et al: Effect of reperfusion on biventricular function and survival after right ventricular infarction. N Engl J Med 338:933, 1998.

76. Ehrich DA, Biddle TL, Kronenberg MW, et al: The hemodynamic response to intra-aortic balloon counterpulsation in patients with cardiogenic shock complicating acute myocardial infarction. Am Heart J 93:274, 1977.

77. Weiss AT, Engle S, Gotsman CJ: Regional and global left ventricular function during intra-aortic balloon counterpulsation in patients with acute myocardial infarction shock. Am Heart J 108:249, 1984.

78. Port SC, Shantilah P, Schmidt DM: Effects of intraaortic balloon counterpulsation on myocardial blood flow in patients with severe coronary artery disease. J Am Coll Cardiol 3:1367, 1984.

79. Ishihara M, Sato H, Tateishi H, et al: Intraaortic balloon pumping as the postangioplasty strategy in acute myocardial infarction. Am Heart J 122:385, 1991.

80. Vogel RA, Shawl F, Tommaso C, et al. Initial report of the national registry of elective cardiopulmonary bypass supported coronary angioplasty. J Am Coll Cardiol 15:23, 1990.

81. Scholz KH, Figulla HR, Schweda F, et al: Mechanical left ventricular unloading during high risk coronary angioplasty: First use of a new percutaneous transvalvular left ventricular assist device. Cathet Cardiovasc Diagn 31:61, 1994.

82. Shawl FA, Domanski MJ, Hernandez TJ, et al: Emergency percutaneous cardiopulmonary bypass support in cardiogenic shock from acute myocardial infarction. Am J Cardiol 64:967, 1989.

83. Smalling RW, Sweeney MJ, Cassidy DB, et al: Hemodynamics in cardiogenic shock after acute myocardial infarction with the Hemopump assist device [Abstract]. Circulation 80(suppl II):II-624, 1989.

84. Gacioch GM, Ellis SG, Lee L, et al: Cardiogenic shock complicating acute myocardial infarction: The use of coronary angioplasty and the integration of the new support devices into patient management. J Am Coll Cardiol 19:647, 1992.

85. Wampler RK, Frazier OH, Lansing AM, et al: Treatment of cardiogenic shock with the Hemopump left ventricular assist device. Ann Thorac Surg 52:506, 1991.

86. Pavlides G, Hauser A, Stack R, et al: Effect of peripheral cardiopulmonary bypass on left ventricular size, afterload and myocardial function during supported coronary angioplasty. J Am Coll Cardiol 18:499, 1991.

87. Grines CL, Stone GW, Cox DA, et al: Stent PAMI 6 month angiographic follow-up: Incidence and predictors of reocclusion following primary PTCA or stenting. J Am Coll Cardiol 33(suppl A):397A, 1999.

88. Antoniucci D, Valenti R, Santoro GM, et al: Systematic direct angioplasty and stent-supported direct angioplasty therapy for cardiogenic shock complicating acute myocardial infarction: In-hospital and long-term survival. J Am Coll Cardiol 31:294, 1998.

89. Raneses R, Grines C, Almany S, et al: Hemodynamic parameters 12-hours after onset of cardiogenic can predict survival [Abstract]. J Am Coll Cardiol 19:362, 1992.

90. Webb JG, Carere RG, Hilton JD: Usefulness of coronary stenting for cardiogenic shock. Am J Cardiol 79:81, 1997.

91. Chua TP, Pepper JR, Fox KM: The use of an implantable left ventricular assist device in a patient with cardiogenic shock following acute myocardial infarction. Int J Cardiol 66:55, 1998.

92. Lewis CT, Graham TR, Marrinan MT: The use of an implantable left ventricular assist device following irreversible ventricular fibrillation secondary to massive myocardial infarction. Eur J Cardiothorac Surg 4:54, 1990.

93. Díaz R, Paoloasso EA, Leopoldo S, et al: Metabolic modulation of acute myocardial infarction. The ECLA glucose-insulin-potassium pilot trial. Circulation 98:2227, 1998.

# 14

# Interventional Strategy in Patients with Previous Coronary Bypass Surgery

*Mina Madan*  *Michael H. Sketch, Jr.*

Since the introduction of direct internal mammary–coronary artery anastomosis by Kolessov[1] in 1967 and the use of saphenous vein–coronary artery grafts by Favaloro[2] in 1968, these conduits have been widely utilized in the treatment of ischemic heart disease. Over the past three decades, there has been a trend toward greater utilization of these vessels. In 1997, more than 607,000 coronary artery bypass operations were performed in the United States, and it is estimated that the worldwide annual rate easily exceeds 800,000.[3] Low operative mortality, immediate symptomatic benefit, and improved longevity have fostered this greater utilization.

With the growing pool of post-bypass patients, there has been a subsequent increase in the number of patients with recurrent or worsening symptoms, at an annual rate of 5% to 10%.[4, 5] The deterioration in symptomatic status after surgery is due to progression of atherosclerotic disease in the native coronary arteries, attrition of saphenous vein or internal mammary artery (IMA) grafts, or both. Progression of coronary artery disease (CAD) in native arteries (worsening of a preexisting lesion or the appearance of a new diameter narrowing greater than 49%) occurs at an approximate annual rate of 5%. The rate of disease progression appears highest in arterial segments already showing evidence of disease.[6] Saphenous vein graft occlusion occurs in up to 10% of patients during the first month after surgery, in an additional 10% during the remainder of the first year, in 1% to 2% per year between the 1st and 6th years, and in 5% per year between the 6th and 12th years. With this occlusion rate, only 30% to 40% of saphenous vein grafts are without significant (>50% luminal reduction) atherosclerotic narrowing 12 years after surgery.[7–10] This attrition rate is presumably responsible for the reduction in survival benefit that occurs approximately 7 years after surgery.

In contrast, the attrition rate for the IMA graft is only 10% to 15% at 10 years after surgery.[9, 11, 12] The use of this conduit has had a substantial beneficial effect on long-term patient survival.[13] Thus, the IMA has become the conduit of choice for coronary artery bypass grafting (CABG). However, the routine use of the right IMA is often not practical, and vein grafts are still needed in most patients with multivessel disease.

The high attrition rate for saphenous vein grafts poses a discouraging and difficult management problem. This chapter focuses on (1) the mechanism of closure of vein grafts and IMA grafts, (2) the role of a second bypass procedure, (3) the role of percutaneous transluminal coronary angioplasty (PTCA), (4) the role of new interventional technologies, including thrombolytic agents, and (5) the management of special situations, such as acute myocardial infarction (MI) and the coronary-subclavian steal syndrome.

## MECHANISMS OF GRAFT CLOSURE

An understanding of the mechanisms of graft closure is important in the management of patients who have undergone CABG. The three mechanisms that play a role in graft closure are thrombosis, intimal hyperplasia, and atherosclerosis.[14] Each mechanism is operative at a different time after surgery (Fig. 14–1).

## Thrombosis

Thrombosis is the usual cause of graft closure in the perioperative and early postoperative period (up to 1 month). Both platelet deposition and the coagulation system play an important role in this process. Platelet deposition begins at the time of graft implantation.[15] The most common site of thrombosis is the distal anastomosis.[16]

A multitude of factors may predispose to saphe-

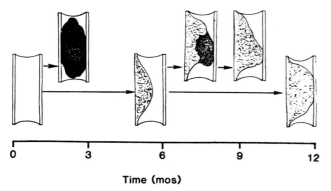

**Time (mos)**

FIGURE 14–1. The phases of vein graft disease leading to occlusion within the first postoperative year: (1) early thrombotic occlusion *(high in panel, left)*, (2) intermediate phase of intimal hyperplasia *(low in panel, middle)*, and (3) late phase of occlusion related to intimal hyperplasia *(low in panel, right)* or to thrombus superimposed on the intimal hyperplasia and fibrotic organization of thrombus *(high in panel, right)*. The phase of atherosclerotic disease, after the first postoperative year, is not depicted in this scheme. (From Fuster V, Chesebro JH: Role of platelets and platelet inhibitors in aortocoronary artery vein-graft disease. Circulation 73:227–232, 1986.)

nous vein graft thrombosis during the early postoperative period. Damage to the venous endothelium may lead to platelet deposition and stimulation of the coagulation cascade. This damage may be produced by the sudden exposure of the vein to the high-pressure arterial system, impaired nutrition of the venous wall, and injury secondary to the venotomy and arteriotomy.[14, 16] Technical factors that may stimulate thrombus formation include twisting of the graft and implantation of the graft under tension.[17, 18] Low blood flow in the vein graft and small luminal size of the grafted artery may predispose to early occlusion of bypass grafts. The highest graft patency rates are observed when the lumina of the vessels distal to the graft insertion (1) are greater than 1.5 mm in diameter, (2) perfuse a large vascular bed, and (3) are no more than 25% occluded by atheroma.[19, 20]

Perioperative platelet inhibitor therapy, with both low-dose and high-dose aspirin and dipyridamole, appears to diminish the rate of early occlusion.[20, 21] In addition, both in greater surgical and technical experience and increased use of IMA grafts may reduce early postoperative occlusion rates.

## Intimal Hyperplasia

All patent vein grafts develop intimal hyperplasia between the 1st and 12th postoperative months.[22] This hyperplasia is stimulated by the aggregation of platelets and the secretion of growth factors, such as platelet-derived growth factor (PDGF), epidermal growth factor, and transforming growth factor β.[23, 24] Intimal hyperplasia produces a diffuse reduction in graft caliber of 25% to 30%. By the 12th postoperative month, approximately 10% of patent vein grafts

have a minimum of a 50% segmental luminal diameter narrowing.[19, 25] This narrowing is most common at the distal anastomosis. The most common mechanism of graft closure during this time is the development of occlusive thrombi superimposed upon intimal hyperplasia.[14]

In contrast to that in saphenous vein grafts, the development of intimal hyperplasia in IMA grafts is rare. When fibrointimal proliferation does occur in IMA grafts, it is most common at the distal anastomosis and occurs predominantly within the first year after bypass surgery.[26, 27]

Platelet inhibitor therapy does not prevent intimal hyperplasia; however, it may reduce the incidence of superimposed thrombosis.[28]

## Atherosclerosis

Atherosclerotic lesions in vein grafts are usually not apparent until 3 years after graft insertion. These lesions appear similar to the native coronary lesion, in that they contain foam cells, blood product debris, cholesterol clefts, fibrocollagenous tissue, and calcific deposits. In contrast to native coronary lesions, the predominant cell type in vein graft lesions is the foam cell; thus, there is less fibrocollagenous tissue and fewer calcific deposits in vein graft lesions. The foam cells appear to erode the intima and predispose to plaque fissure or rupture. These characteristics account for the fragility of vein graft lesions and the frequent presence of blood in the atheroma (Fig. 14–2).[29, 30]

## MANAGEMENT OPTIONS

As the number of patients with prior CABG requiring second revascularization procedures grows, clinicians are faced with the challenge of recommending either a percutaneous or second surgical approach to revascularization. A thorough under-

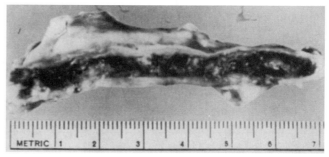

FIGURE 14–2. A segment of an old saphenous vein graft that reveals friable atheromatous material and recent and old thrombus. (From Cote G, Myler RK, Stertzer SH, et al: Percutaneous transluminal angioplasty of stenotic coronary artery bypass grafts: 5 years' experience. J Am Coll Cardiol 9:8, 1987, with permission from the American College of Cardiology.)

standing of the success, morbidity, and mortality associated with each strategy is essential to the management of such patients.

## Reoperation

Reoperations account for 5% to 10% of all CABG procedures.[31, 32] The clinical indication for reoperation is recurrent angina not responsive to medical management or percutaneous revascularization. The angiographic indications for reoperation are primary graft failure alone (~50% of patients), graft failure and progression of CAD in native arteries (20% to 30%), progression of CAD in native arteries (10% to 20%), and incomplete revascularization (5% to 10%).[31–33]

Despite improvements in myocardial protection and greater surgical experience, the risks of reoperation still exceed those for the initial revascularization. The operative morbidity and mortality rates depend significantly on institutional experience (Table 14–1).[31, 33–40] The perioperative mortality rate for the first reoperation varies from 2.0% to 7.5%, and that for a second reoperation has been reported to be 9.0%.[40] Perioperative MI occurred in 2.0% to 9.2% of patients undergoing a reoperation, and postoperative bleeding, that required reexploration in 2.4% to 6.8%. In an analysis of the Coronary Artery Surgery Study (CASS) registry, the operative mortality rate for reoperation, 5.3%, was significantly higher than the 3.1% rate observed for the initial revascularization procedure.[31]

In addition to the higher operative mortality rate associated with reoperation, there is less relief of angina in the first year after the reoperation than after the initial operation. The annual increases in recurrence of angina after the first postoperative year are similar for the reoperation and the initial operation (Fig. 14–3).[32] Despite less early relief of angina, late survival with reoperations is excellent. The 5-year survival rate has been reported to be as high as 94%, and the 10-year survival rate to be as high as 82%. These rates are similar to those seen after the initial operation.[32, 33, 38, 39]

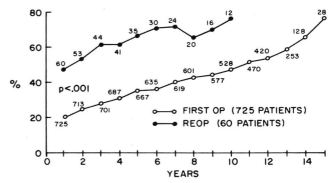

FIGURE 14–3. Plot of annual recurrence of angina (%) and time (years) after initial operation (First Op, O—O) and reoperation (Reop, ●—●). The absolute numbers of patients at risk in each year are indicated. (From Cameron A, Kemp HG, Green GE: Reoperation for coronary artery disease: 10 years of clinical follow-up. Circulation [suppl I]:I-78, 1988. By permission of the American Heart Association, Inc.)

The higher rates of perioperative morbidity and mortality and lower rates of early relief of angina associated with reoperations may be related to a multitude of factors. The effective myocardial protection obtained during the initial operation may not have been reproduced during the reoperation. The time between the induction of anesthesia and the initiation of cardiopulmonary bypass is longer for reoperations, and ischemia occurring during that interval may lead to perioperative myocardial damage. The complex anatomy of the myocardial blood supply in patients undergoing reoperation can make delivery of cardioplegic solution and myocardial protection difficult.[38] Atherosclerotic embolization from patent atherosclerotic vein grafts is a well-documented cause of MI during reoperation.[41, 42] Diffuse coronary disease and limitations in available bypass conduits contribute to a higher likelihood of incomplete revascularization during reoperation.

## Percutaneous Transluminal Coronary Angioplasty

Since the introduction of PTCA by Gruentzig and associates[43] in 1979, this alternative to reoperation

## TABLE 14–1.    COMPLICATION RATES OF SECOND CORONARY ARTERY BYPASS PROCEDURES

| STUDY (YEAR) | NO. OF PATIENTS | OPERATIVE MORTALITY (%) | RATE OF PERIOPERATIVE MYOCARDIAL INFARCTION (%) | RATE OF REEXPLORATION DUE TO POSTOPERATIVE BLEEDING (%) |
|---|---|---|---|---|
| Reul et al (1979)[34] | 168 | 4.8 | 2.0 | 2.4 |
| Schaff et al (1983)[35] | 106 | 2.8 | 7.5 | 4.7 |
| Foster et al (1984)[31] | 283 | 5.3 | 6.4 | 4.6 |
| Pidgeon et al (1985)[36] | 102 | 2.0* | 7.8 | 2.9 |
| Lytle et al (1987)[38] | 1500 | 3.4 | 7.8 | 6.8 |
| Osaka et al (1988)[33] | 119 | 2.5 | 9.2 | 3.4 |
| Verheul et al (1991)[39] | 200 | 7.5 | 4.0 | 5.5 |

*Within 24 hours of operation, versus 30 days for all other studies.

has evolved for selected stenotic saphenous vein and IMA grafts in patients with angina that is relatively refractory to medical management.[43]

### Saphenous Vein Grafts

#### Success and Complication Rates

In carefully selected patients and lesions, balloon angioplasty of stenotic vein grafts can be performed with a high procedural success rate and a low complication rate. The exact mechanisms by which angioplasty improves vessel patency are unclear; however, they may be related to the morphologic characteristics of the graft stenoses (Fig. 14–4).[30] Because early vein graft stenoses (occurring in the first postoperative year) are composed predominantly of fibrocollagenous tissue, the mechanism probably involves graft stretching. In contrast, late vein graft stenoses (occurring later than 1 year and generally 3 years after graft insertion) contain atherosclerotic plaque, and thus, the mechanism probably involves plaque fracture.

There is a remarkable congruence among the multiple series of patients undergoing saphenous vein graft angioplasty (Table 14–2).[44–65] The primary success rate in these series ranges from 78% to 97%. MI, emergency CABG, and death were reported in up to 8.3%, 3.5%, and 5.3% of patients, respectively. Successful saphenous vein graft angioplasty with a low incidence of complications depends strongly on lesion-specific characteristics. These characteristics include vein graft age, lesion location, and lesion length.

The age of a vein graft at the time of angioplasty may influence the likelihood of primary success. As discussed earlier, lesions appearing within the first year after graft insertion usually represent intimal hyperplasia. These lesions tend to dilate well in response to PTCA, with a low incidence of complications. In contrast, lesions appearing 3 years after graft insertion are atherosclerotic and demonstrate a lower success rate for PTCA with a higher incidence of complications. Platko and associates[55] reported on a series of patients who underwent vein graft

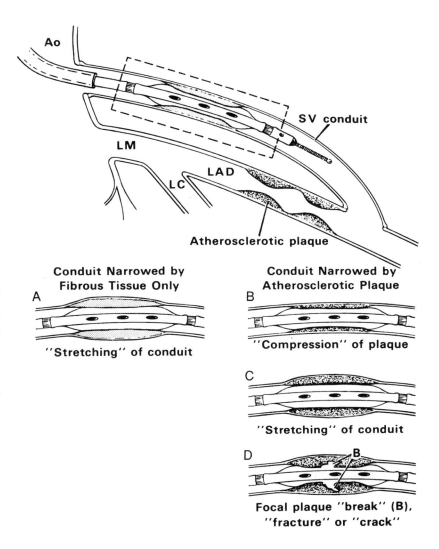

FIGURE 14–4. Diagram illustrating possible mechanism of angioplasty in stenotic saphenous vein (SV) bypass grafts. Two types of lesions characterize saphenous vein stenoses, depending on graft age. Early vein graft lesions (≤1 year) contain intimal thickening composed primarily of fibrocollagenous tissue without calcium, and dilatation is probably accomplished by graft stretching (A, left). Late vein graft lesions (>1 year) contain intimal thickening composed of atherosclerotic plaque and calcium, and dilation probably involves one of three mechanisms (B, C, and D, right). Ao, aorta; LAD, left anterior descending coronary artery; LC, left circumflex coronary artery; LM, left main coronary artery. (From Waller BF, Rothbaum DA, Gorfinkel HJ, et al: Morphologic observations after percutaneous transluminal balloon angioplasty of early and late aortocoronary saphenous vein bypass grafts. J Am Coll Cardiol 4:784–792, 1984, with permission from the American College of Cardiology.)

**TABLE 14–2. PERCUTANEOUS TRANSLUMINAL CORONARY ANGIOPLASTY OF SAPHENOUS VEIN GRAFTS**

| STUDY (YEAR) | LESIONS (n) | SUCCESS (%) | COMPLICATION RATES (%) | | |
| --- | --- | --- | --- | --- | --- |
| | | | DEATH | MI | CABG |
| Douglas et al (1983)[44] | 62 | 94 | 0 | 2 | 2 |
| Dorros et al (1984)[45] | 33 | 79 | 0 | — | — |
| El Gamal et al (1984)[46] | 44 | 93 | 0 | 6 | 0 |
| Block et al (1984)[47] | 40 | 78 | 0 | 0 | 2.5 |
| Corbelli et al (1985)[48] | 47 | 92 | — | — | 2 |
| Douglas et al (1986)[49] | 235 | 92 | 0 | 8 | 1.3 |
| Reeder et al (1986)[50] | 19 | 84 | 5.3 | 5.3 | 0 |
| Cote et al (1987)[53] | 83 | 86 | 0 | 0 | 0 |
| Cole et al (1987)[51] | 96 | 84 | 0 | 3.6 | 1.2 |
| Ernst et al (1987)[52] | 33 | 97 | 0 | 0 | 0 |
| Pinkerton et al (1988)[54] | 100 | 93 | — | — | — |
| Platko et al (1989)[55] | 107 | 94 | 2 | 5.9 | 2 |
| Dorros et al (1989)[56] | 241 | 91 | 2.3 | 5.2 | 1.4 |
| Webb et al (1990)[57] | 168 | 85 | 0 | 4 | 1 |
| Meester et al (1991)[58] | 93 | 84 | 1.2 | 8.3 | 2.4 |
| Jost et al (1991)[61] | 49 | 94 | 0 | 0 | 0 |
| Plokker et al (1991)[59] | 454* | 90† | 0.7 | 1.3 | 1.3 |
| Douglas et al (1991)[61] | 672 | 90 | 1.2 | 2.3 | 3.5 |
| Miranda et al (1992)[63] | 409 | 94 | — | — | — |
| Unterberg et al (1992)[62] | 55 | 89 | — | — | — |
| Tan et al (1994)[65] | 50 | 86 | — | — | — |
| Morrison et al (1994)[64] | 89 | 93 | 3 | 3 | 1 |

CABG, coronary artery bypass grafting; MI, myocardial infarction.
*Number of patients.
†Clinical success.

angioplasty and were classified into two groups according to the age of the graft (≤36 months since graft insertion and >36 months since graft insertion).[55] There was a significant difference in rates of major cardiac complications between the groups. The patients with late vein graft stenosis had a 12.5% incidence of MI, a 4% incidence of emergency bypass surgery, and a 4% mortality rate, whereas there were no major cardiac complications in patients with early vein graft stenosis. The incidence of distal embolization after angioplasty is higher in older vein grafts because the lesions are very friable and have a thin fibrous cap.[49] The risk of distal embolization during passage of the balloon catheter is probably higher in older vein grafts. Emergency bypass surgery may be ineffective in salvaging myocardium after embolization during vein-graft angioplasty.

The specific location of a lesion within a vein graft is an important determinant of outcome (Fig. 14–5). The success of angioplasty is highest with lesions at the distal anastomosis, intermediate with lesions in the body of the graft, and least favorable with lesions at the proximal anastomosis. In the series reported by Webb and associates,[57] the success rate was 89% for distal anastomotic lesions, 86% for lesions in the body of the graft, and 80% for lesions at the proximal anastomosis. The less favorable outcome associated with proximal anastomotic lesions may be related to the thick elastic

aortic wall and thus may be comparable to the less favorable outcome associated with angioplasty of ostial right coronary and renal artery lesions.

Antecdotal experience suggests that long saphenous vein graft lesions (>15 to 20 mm) frequently are technically more difficult to dilate and may be associated with a lower primary success rate than shorter lesions.

The experience with PTCA of totally occluded vein grafts has been limited and discouraging.[66–69] Because success rates range from 27% to 73%, de Feyter and coworkers have suggested that angioplasty of occluded vein grafts is a "challenge that should be resisted." In the series reported by de Feyter and coworkers,[66] an initial success rate of 54% was achieved in 13 patients; however, in only 1 of 13 patients was there long-term success. The incidence of distal embolization in these patients was 38%. Margolis and colleagues[67] reported a 31% incidence of distal embolization complicating PTCA of totally occluded vein grafts. Kahn and associates[68] reported a favorable initial experience in 83 patients after PTCA of totally occluded bypass grafts. The initial success rate was 73%; death, Q-wave MI, and distal embolization occurred in 2%, 2%, and 11% of patients, respectively. However, follow-up catheterization in 37 patients with initially successful results showed that 27 patients (72%) either had restenosis at the treated site or experienced graft occlusion. Berger and coworkers[69] studied the effect

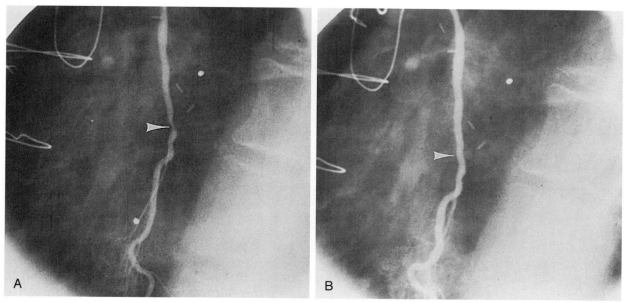

FIGURE 14–5. *A*, An angiogram demonstrating a subtotal occlusion *(arrow)* at the distal anastomosis of a saphenous vein graft to the left anterior descending coronary artery in a left anterior oblique projection. *B*, Final result after angioplasty, revealing a residual minor irregularity *(arrow)*.

of procedural success on immediate and long-term outcomes in 77 patients undergoing PTCA of occluded vein grafts. Patients with MI in the previous 24 hours were excluded from the study. Angioplasty was successful in 55 patients (71%). The 30-day incidences of death, Q-wave MI, and second bypass surgery were 5.2%, 1.3% and 7.8%, respectively. These events occurred with similar frequency in patients in whom angiographically demonstrated success was and was not achieved. No differences in rates of 3-year survival or freedom from recurrent ischemic events were revealed between the patients with successful and unsuccessful PTCA.

Despite the less favorable results of intervention noted for occluded saphenous vein grafts, reports of better success with new interventional devices or prolonged infusions of intragraft thrombolytic agents have provided the impetus for continuing to attempt these difficult procedures.[70, 71] At this time, it appears unlikely that patients with occluded vein grafts in whom PTCA is initially successful derive long-term benefit from the procedure. It is important to note that all of the studies mentioned here involve older occluded vein grafts. The results may be different for occlusions in grafts not older than 1 month, because in such cases, the occlusion is due to thrombosis and is usually related to technical factors of graft implantation.

Additional complications associated with saphenous vein graft angioplasty include abrupt closure and vein graft rupture. Abrupt closure occurs in approximately 1% to 2% of patients undergoing vein graft angioplasty,[46–49, 51] a rate that appears to be lower than the 3% to 5% incidence associated with native coronary angioplasty. Vein graft rupture is an extremely rare complication of balloon angioplasty and can be treated conservatively in most cases.[72–74] Cardiac tamponade is unusual after graft rupture because of the extrapericardial course of vein grafts and postpericardiotomy fibrosis.

### Restenosis

A major limitation of saphenous vein graft angioplasty is restenosis. The precise incidence of restenosis after vein graft angioplasty is unknown because of the relatively small number of patients reported, incomplete angiographic follow-up, the different definitions used, and the varying intervals between angioplasty and follow-up angiography.

The reported restenosis rates vary from 31% to 73% in patients undergoing angiographic follow-up (Table 14–3).[44, 47, 48, 50, 52, 55, 57, 65, 75] Higher rates of angiographic follow-up appear to correlate with higher rates of restenosis. Angiographic follow-up is essential to document the true restenosis rate in this patient population, in which symptoms of restenosis may be particularly unreliable because of either progression of native coronary artery and vein graft disease or ungraftable vessels. Factors predictive of restenosis include the location of the vein graft lesion and the age of the vein graft.

Stenosis recurrence appears to be lower with distal anastomotic lesions, intermediate with graft body lesions, and least favorable with proximal anastomotic lesions. In 599 cases of saphenous vein graft angioplasty reported by Douglas and associates,[60] restenosis occurred in 68% of proximal anastomotic

**TABLE 14–3.  RESTENOSIS AFTER PERCUTANEOUS TRANSLUMINAL CORONARY ANGIOPLASTY OF SAPHENOUS VEIN GRAFTS**

| STUDY (YEAR) | NO. OF PATIENTS | ANGIOGRAPHIC FOLLOW-UP | RESTENOSIS |
|---|---|---|---|
| Douglas et al (1983)[44] | 62 | 34/58 (50%) | 13/34 (38%) |
| Block et al (1984)[47] | 40 | 22/31 (71%) | 12/22 (55%) |
| Marquis et al (1985)[75] | 18 | 12/14 (86%) | 7/12 (58%) |
| Corbelli et al (1985)[48] | 35 | 18/31 (58%) | 6/18 (33%) |
| Reeder et al (1986)[50] | 19 | 11/16 (69%) | 8/11 (73%) |
| Ernst et al (1987)[52] | 33 | — | (31%) |
| Platko et al (1989)[55] | 101 | 49/90 (54%) | 30/49 (61%) |
| Webb et al (1990)[57] | 158 | 76/143 (53%) | 38/76 (50%) |
| Tan et al (1994)[65] | 50 | 28/50 (56%) | 11/28 (39%) |

lesions, 61% of graft body lesions, and 45% of distal anastomotic lesions. Webb and associates[57] made a similar observation about rates of saphenous vein graft restenosis. This site variation may be related to various pathologic phenomena at different sites in the graft. The proximal anastomotic stenosis involves the thick, elastic wall of the thoracic aorta. Distal graft anastomotic lesions may be associated with plaque in the recipient coronary artery or fibrointimal hyperplasia, whereas the graft body lesions are often composed of friable atherosclerotic plaque.

The age of a vein graft at the time of angioplasty may influence the incidence of restenosis. In the aforementioned series reported by Douglas and associates,[60] restenosis occurred in 32% of lesions dilated within 6 months after surgery, in 43% dilated 6 months to 1 year after surgery, in 61% dilated 1 to 5 years after surgery, and in 64% dilated more than 5 years after surgery.[60] In another series of 101 patients undergoing saphenous vein graft angioplasty, the patients were classified into two groups on the basis of age of the graft (surgery ≤ 36 months before angioplasty versus surgery > 36 months before angioplasty).[55] Both groups were evaluated for clinical and angiographic recurrence. Clinical recurrence, defined as a cardiac event (i.e., MI, second angioplasty or bypass procedure, or death) or progression to Canadian Cardiovascular Society (CCS) functional class III or IV, was significantly higher for the older vein-graft group, at 64.1%, than for the younger vein graft group, at 33.3% ($p < 0.01$). Also, 42% of the younger vein graft group had angiographic evidence of restenosis, compared with 83% of the older vein graft group ($p < 0.01$).

## IMA Grafts

### Success and Complication Rates

The IMA is the conduit of choice for the surgical revascularization in ischemic heart disease. This vessel has been shown to have a low incidence of atherosclerotic narrowing, a high long-term patency rate, and a substantial beneficial effect on the survival of patients undergoing CABG.[13, 76–80] Because the patency of the IMA graft is critical to long-term patient survival, postoperative stenosis of this graft is a major clinical problem. However, the low attrition rate of IMA grafts has limited our knowledge of the role of PTCA in the treatment of stenoses in them.

Documentation of the safety and efficacy of IMA graft angioplasty has been limited to isolated case reports and series involving small numbers of patients (Table 14–4).[27, 53, 54, 81–88] The majority of the stenoses in these studies were situated at the distal anastomotic site (Fig. 14–6). The initial success rate varied from 80% to 100%. The failures in these series were attributed to an inability either to cross the lesion or dilate it, rather than to elastic recoil or the development of periprocedural complications. Inability to cross the lesion with the guide wire was due to severe tortuosity of the IMA. None of these studies reported any major complications or evidence of distal embolization. Successful stent placement in both right and left IMA grafts after unsuccessful balloon angioplasty has been reported.[89–91]

### Restenosis

In the majority of studies of IMA angioplasty, long-term follow-up has been primarily limited to clinical profiles. In the largest series reported to date, Hearne and associates[88] conducted follow-up coronary angiography in 47 of 60 eligible patients (78%), 9 of whom (19%) had restenosis.

In comparison with the reported restenosis rates of 31% to 73% for saphenous vein graft angioplasty, IMA graft angioplasty appears to have a significantly better long-term outcome. Part of this discrepancy may be related to location of the lesion, because the majority of IMA lesions involve the distal anastomosis. Thus, it appears that lesions involving the distal anastomosis, whether in saphenous vein or IMA grafts, are less susceptible to restenosis. As mentioned, the explanation for this difference is unclear;

**TABLE 14–4.    PERCUTANEOUS TRANSLUMINAL CORONARY ANGIOPLASTY OF INTERNAL MAMMARY ARTERY GRAFTS**

| STUDY (YEAR) | NO. OF PATIENTS | INITIAL SUCCESS | ANGIOGRAPHIC FOLLOW-UP | ANGIOGRAPHIC RESTENOSIS |
|---|---|---|---|---|
| Pinkerton et al (1987)[81] | 5 | 5 (100%) | — | — |
| Cote et al (1987)[53] | 5 | 5 (100%) | — | — |
| Pinkerton et al (1988)[54] | 13 | 12 (92%) | — | — |
| Shimshak et al (1988)[82] | 26 | 24 (92%) | 8 (335) | 1/8 (13%) |
| Hill et al (1989)[83] | 11 | 9 (82%) | — | — |
| Bell et al (1989)[84] | 7 | 7 (100%) | 2 (29%) | 0/2 (0%) |
| Dimas et al (1991)[85] | 31* | 28 (90%) | 7 (25%) | 1/7 (14%) |
| Popma et al (1992)[86] | 20 | 16 (80%) | — | — |
| Sketch et al (1992)[27] | 14 | 13 (93%) | 12 (92%) | 1/12 (8%) |
| Hearne et al (1995)[88] | 68 | 68 (88%) | 47 (78%) | 9/47 (17%) |
| Najm et al (1995)[87] | 29 | 26 (90%) | 14 (54%) | 4/14 (29%) |

*Includes three patients who underwent dilation of the native vessel through the internal mammary artery.

however, it may be related to vessel injury during mobilization of the graft, faulty anastomotic technique, or differing tissue plasticity and healing characteristics at anastomoses versus other sites.[92]

## Choosing a Revascularization Strategy

Limited data exist to guide clinicians in choosing the optimal revascularization strategy for patients with previous bypass surgery. Comparative studies are available for CABG versus medical therapy and for CABG versus PTCA; however, patients with prior CABG have generally been excluded from such comparisons thus far.[93–100] The publication of two large nonrandomized trials provides important insights regarding the outcome of either percutaneous or surgical revascularization in patients with prior CABG.[101, 102]

In a retrospective analysis, Stephan and associates[101] reported data from 632 patients with prior CABG who required either elective second CABG (N = 164) or PTCA (N = 468).[101] Although complete revascularization was achieved more frequently in the patients undergoing second CABG (92% vs. 38%; $p < 0.0001$), these patients had significantly higher rates of in-hospital mortality (7.3% vs. 0.3%; $p < 0.0001$) and Q-wave MI (6.1% vs. 0.9%; $p < 0.0001$) than patients undergoing PTCA. Actuarial survival was equivalent in the two groups at 1 year and 6 years of follow-up, and the two procedures resulted in similar rates of event-free survival (freedom from death or Q-wave MI) and relief of angina. However, the need for second PTCA, surgery, or both by 6 years was significantly higher in the PTCA group (64% vs. 8%; $p < 0.0001$). Through multivariate analysis, age greater than 70 years, left ventricular ejection fraction less than 40%, unstable angina, number of diseased vessels, and diabetes were identified as being independent predictors of higher overall mortality.

In a larger series reported by Weintraub and co-

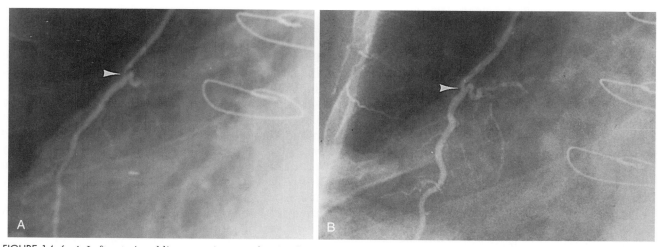

FIGURE 14–6. *A*, Left anterior oblique arteriogram of a significant internal mammary artery anastomosis lesion *(arrow)*. *B*, Left anterior oblique arteriogram of internal mammary artery anastomosis *(arrow)* after a successful angioplasty procedure. (From Sketch MH, Quigley PJ, Perez JA, et al: Angiographic follow-up after internal mammary artery graft angioplasty. Am J Cardiol 70:401, 1992.)

workers,[102] the immediate and long-term outcomes of second CABG (n = 1561) and PTCA (n = 2613) were compared in patients with prior CABG. Although in-hospital mortality rates were 1.2% after PTCA and 6.8% after CABG ($p < 0.0001$), long-term survival rates (10-year follow-up) did not vary with choice of procedure. Patients who underwent PTCA suffered more frequently from recurrent angina and had more additional procedures after PTCA.

These two revascularization strategies appear to provide equivalent overall survival and event-free survival. PTCA offers lower periprocedural morbidity and mortality rates; however, it is associated with less complete revascularization and a greater need for further procedures. Angiographic data and the presence of other comorbidities will indicate that some patients are candidates only for PTCA and that some should undergo CABG as the best alternative. Still other patients will be found candidates for either strategy. The ultimate decision regarding choice of revascularization must be made through the use of a combination of variables, including clinical criteria, angiographic evidence, and, finally, patient preference.

## New Interventional Technologies

The attempt to overcome the major limitations of saphenous vein graft angioplasty (i.e., distal embolization, restenosis) has led to the development of an array of new devices and approaches for percutaneous revascularization, including atherectomy, lasers, intravascular stents, and distal protection devices. The roles of these devices in the management of saphenous vein graft disease have evolved now that many of them have been evaluated in large clinical trials. Only directional atherectomy and intravascular stents have been formally compared with conventional balloon angioplasty in prospective randomized trials.

### Atherectomy

The concept of atherectomy centers on the hypothesis that excising and removing plaque achieves a better local rheologic environment in the treated vessel segment with less trauma to the vessel wall, in comparison to balloon angioplasty, thereby reducing the potential for acute occlusion and restenosis. At present, three atherectomy devices are available for clinical use. They are (1) a directional coronary atherectomy (DCA) catheter (Guidant Corporation; Temecula, CA), (2) a transluminal extraction catheter, or TEC, (Interventional Technologies, Inc.; San Diego, CA), and (3) a rotational atherectomy catheter, or Rotablator (Scimed, Boston Scientific Corporation; Maple Grove, MN).

### DCA

The DCA catheter consists of a catheter-mounted, cylindrical metallic housing with a central rotating blade. The housing has a longitudinal opening on one side through which an enclosed, cup-shaped cutter can gain access to atheromatous plaque.

Use of DCA for the treatment of focal lesions in the ostium and body of vein grafts has revealed primary success rates of 85% to 97% (Table 14–5).[103–111] However, the incidence of postprocedural MI (Q wave and non–Q wave) may be as high as 17.4%. Restenosis rates in patients in whom angiographic follow-up was performed have also remained high (23% to 76%) and are comparable to rates observed with conventional angioplasty techniques. Several studies have described significantly higher restenosis rates when DCA is performed in restenosis lesions versus de novo lesions.[104, 109, 110]

The second Coronary Angioplasty Versus Excisional Atherectomy Trial (CAVEAT II) was a multicenter randomized trial comparing DCA with PTCA in 305 patients with de novo vein graft lesions.[111] Atherectomy was associated with improved rates of initial angiographically demonstrated success (89.2% vs. 79%; $p = 0.019$) and better luminal enlargement than with PTCA (% diameter stenosis 31.5 vs. 37.6; $p < 0.001$). However, the combined incidence of death, MI, emergency CABG, and acute closure was higher in the atherectomy group (20.1% vs. 12.2%; $p = 0.059$), largely related to a higher incidence of non–Q-wave MI in these patients. At 6 months, restenosis occurred at similar proportions of patients who received DCA (45.6%) and PTCA (50.5%; $p = 0.491$). Although the immediate outcome of DCA is favorable in selected cases, the occurrence of distal embolization and restenosis, particularly after treatment of restenosis lesions, has prevented this device from gaining superiority over conventional balloon angioplasty.

### Transluminal Extraction Atherectomy

Because balloon angioplasty of aged and diffusely diseased vein grafts is associated with problems such as distal embolization, no-reflow phenomenon, thrombosis, and high restenosis rates, the TEC may have utility in this situation. The TEC is a wire-based, motor-driven, rotating flexible torque tube with two stainless steel blades at the conical head of the catheter (Chapter 32). The TEC device is able to extract debris from saphenous vein grafts by means of vacuum aspiration during rotational cutting, thus theoretically lessening the possibility of distal embolization (Fig. 14–7).

Primary success with TEC atherectomy has ranged from 81% to 93% (Table 14–6).[112–117] In the largest series of patients (n = 538) with saphenous vein graft disease undergoing a TEC procedure, the lesion

## TABLE 14-5.  DIRECTIONAL CORONARY ATHERECTOMY OF SAPHENOUS VEIN GRAFTS

| STUDY (YEAR) | LESIONS (n) | SUCCESS RATE (%) | COMPLICATION RATES (%) | | | RESTENOSIS RATE (%) |
| | | | DEATH | MI* | CABG‡ | |
|---|---|---|---|---|---|---|
| Kaufman et al (1990)[103] | 15 | 93 | 0 | 7 | 0 | 63 |
| Selmon et al (1991)[104] | 87 | 91 | 0 | 9.2 | 1.3 | 60 |
| Ghazzal et al (1991)[105] | 162 | 88 | | 1.2† | | 58 |
| DiScasio et al (1992)[106] | 69 | 98 | 0 | 8 | 0 | 23 |
| Pomerantz et al (1992)[107] | 35 | 94 | 0 | 0 | 0 | 28 |
| Garatt et al (1992)[108] | 26 | 96 | 4 | 0 | 4 | 76 |
| Cowley et al (1993)[109] | 363 | 86 | 0.9 | 5.7 | 0.9 | 57 |
| Stephan et al (1995)[110] | 57 | 86 | 0 | 11 | 0 | 65 |
| CAVEAT II (1995)[111] | 149 | 89 | 2 | 17.4 | 0.6 | 46 |

*Represents both Q-wave and non–Q-wave myocardial infarctions.
†Overall complication rate for the cohort.
‡Emergency coronary artery bypass grafting (CABG) procedures represented.

success rate was 93%.[116] A subanalysis of data in these patients revealed success rates of 94% for vein grafts more than 3 years of age and 90% for vein graft lesions with thrombus. The overall mortality rate was 3.2%, and the rate of emergency bypass surgery was 0.4%. The mortality rate for patients not experiencing an acute MI was lower, at 2.4%. The incidence of distal embolization in the multicenter TEC atherectomy registry was 3.7%, whereas other studies have reported rates as high as 23%.[112, 113, 116] Angiographically determined restenosis rates for TEC atherectomy have ranged from 52% to 69%.[113–116]

Some comparative data for TEC atherectomy and PTCA have also been reported. Misumi and coworkers[117] compared clinical outcomes in 103 patients who underwent TEC atherectomy (with or without adjunctive PTCA) with those in 60 patients who had PTCA alone. The success rates were comparable in the two groups (TEC 90.3% vs. PTCA 83.3%; *p* = NS); however, the incidences of distal embolization (3.9% vs. 16.7%) and non–Q-wave MI (3.9% vs. 15%) were significantly higher in the PTCA group. As would be expected, thrombus-containing lesions had a higher incidence of embolization than lesions without thrombus, regardless of treatment strategy. Several researchers have noted that embolization

during TEC procedures often occurs with adjunctive balloon angioplasty.[117, 119] A marked increase in morbidity and mortality rates has been observed in patients who experience distal embolization, whether it occurs after TEC atherectomy or after PTCA.[117–120] Although the risk of distal embolization is potentially reduced by use of the TEC, it is not eliminated, especially in lesions with superimposed thrombus. The lack of restenosis benefit over PTCA has limited the current use of TEC atherectomy in the management of post-bypass patients. Further work on the combination of TEC atherectomy and stent implantation is required. Braden and associates[120a] suggested that a significant decrease in risk of distal embolization and CPK-MB isoenzyme elevation is conferred when TEC atherectomy is employed, rather than PTCA, before stent implantation.

### Rotational Atherectomy

The rotational atherectomy catheter, or Rotablator, consists of a high-speed rotary, oblong metal burr that is embedded with fine diamond abrasive particles (30 to 40 mm). The burr and drive shaft track over a central coaxial 0.009-inch guide wire and rotate at approximately 180,000 rpm.

The Rotablator has been used successfully in

## TABLE 14-6.  TRANSLUMINAL EXTRACTION CATHETER ATHERECTOMY IN SAPHENOUS VEIN GRAFTS

| STUDY (YEAR) | LESIONS (n) | RATE OF PTCA* (%) | SUCCESS RATE (%) | COMPLICATION RATES (%) | | | | | RATE OF ANGIOGRAPHIC RESTENOSIS (%) |
| | | | | DEATH | MI | CABG | AC | DE | |
|---|---|---|---|---|---|---|---|---|---|
| Popma et al (1992)[112] | 22 | 86 | 82 | 13.6 | — | — | — | 22.7 | — |
| Safian et al (1994)[113] | 154 | 91 | 84 | 2 | 8.8 | 0.7 | 5 | 11.9 | 69 |
| Twidale et al (1994)[114] | 88 | 95 | 86 | 0 | 4.1 | 1.3 | 5 | 5 | 52 |
| Dooris et al (1999)[115] | 183 | 92 | 81 | 2 | 4 | 0.5 | 4 | 7 | 58 |
| Meany et al (1995)[116] | 650 | 74 | 93 | 3.2 | 0.7 | 0.4 | 3.2 | 3.7 | 60 |
| Misumi et al (1996)[117] | 103 | — | 90 | 0 | 3.9 | 1 | — | 3.9 | — |

AC, abrupt closure; CABG, coronary artery bypass grafting; D, death; DE, distal embolization; MI, Q-wave and non–Q-wave myocardial infarction; PTCA, adjunctive percutaneous transluminal coronary angioplasty.

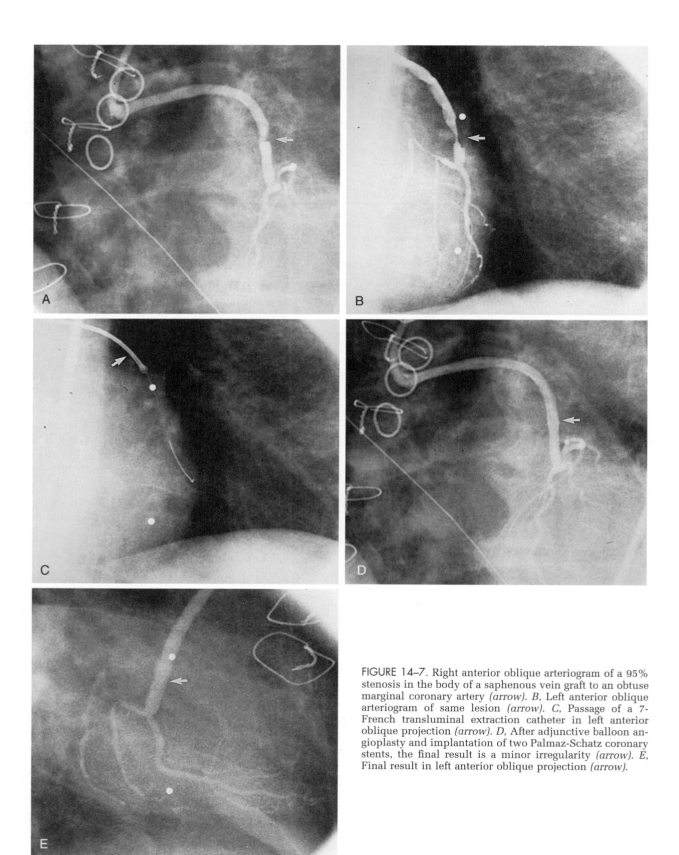

FIGURE 14–7. Right anterior oblique arteriogram of a 95% stenosis in the body of a saphenous vein graft to an obtuse marginal coronary artery *(arrow)*. B, Left anterior oblique arteriogram of same lesion *(arrow)*. C, Passage of a 7-French transluminal extraction catheter in left anterior oblique projection *(arrow)*. D, After adjunctive balloon angioplasty and implantation of two Palmaz-Schatz coronary stents, the final result is a minor irregularity *(arrow)*. E, Final result in left anterior oblique projection *(arrow)*.

some aorto-ostial and distal anastomotic vein graft lesions; however, the use of this device in the body of friable degenerated grafts or thrombus-containing lesions is contraindicated because the risk of distal embolization, no-reflow phenomenon, abrupt closure, and MI.[121–123] In the William Beaumont Hospital saphenous vein graft experience, 4 patients were treated with the device, and subsequent acute closure occurred in 3, of whom 2 required emergency bypass surgery and the third suffered an MI.[121] In a rotational atherectomy registry of more than 1400 patients, only 17 patients had rotational atherectomy of a vein graft.[122] In this subgroup, the procedural success rate was 100% without any major complications, but the restenosis rate was 89%.

### Other Atherectomy Devices

Other atherectomy devices are currently under investigation. The Possis AngioJet catheter removes intravascular thrombus bodies via rheolytic thrombectomy: A Venturi effect is created by precisely directed high-pressure saline jets located at the tip of a 5-French over-the-wire catheter.[124, 125] Successful removal of thrombus appears to prepare the vessel for subsequent coronary intervention.

The Vein Graft AngioJet Study (VeGAS) I pilot study evaluated the AngioJet catheter in 52 saphenous vein grafts and 35 native coronary lesions containing thrombus.[125] As the initial therapy, use of the AngioJet catheter was successful in reducing mean thrombus area (from 79 mm$^2$ to 21 mm$^2$) and improving minimal luminal diameter (from 0.81 mm to 1.70 mm). More definitive therapy was required in 97% of patients. Angiographically detected complications comprised no-reflow phenomenon in 11%, abrupt closure in 4%, and transient heart block requiring temporary pacing in 20% of patients. In-hospital complications were three deaths, one Q-wave MI, and one elective CABG. The benefits of AngioJet catheterization over intragraft urokinase will be evaluated in the VeGAS II trial.

The Cordis Hydrolyser, a device similar to the AngioJet, has been evaluated in a small number of patients.[126, 127] Further investigation is required to confirm the efficacy of these new devices.

### Excimer Laser Angioplasty

The largest experience with laser ablation of atheromatous tissue in vein grafts has been accumulated with the excimer laser, particularly the Spectranetics laser (Spectranetics Corporation; Colorado Springs, CO) (Fig. 14–8) (Table 14–7).[128–131]

In the Percutaneous Excimer Laser Coronary Angioplasty (PELCA) Registry, excimer laser angioplasty was used to treat 545 saphenous vein graft lesions in 495 patients.[128] The mean graft age was 8.0 ± 2.0 years, and 24% of lesions were more than 10 mm long. Clinical success was achieved in 92% of patients. At least one complication occurred in 6.1% of patients (n = 30) as follows: death, 1%; CABG, 0.6%; Q-wave MI, 2.4%; and non–Q-wave MI, 2.2%. Embolization occurred in 3.3% of cases, and abrupt closure and vessel perforation occurred in 4.0% and 1.3%, respectively. Lesion length greater than 10 mm was an independent predictor of procedural failure and restenosis, whereas ostial location and vessel diameter smaller than 3 mm were associated with fewer major complications. In a substudy evaluating the treatment of aorto-ostial disease with PELCA, a total of 64 ostial saphenous vein graft lesions were treated, with a 100% procedural success rate.[131]

PELCA with adjunctive PTCA can be successfully performed in older diseased vein grafts; however, late restenosis and abrupt closure mitigate the early procedural benefits.

### Intravascular Stents

Coronary stenting has become an accepted treatment for acute or threatened arterial closure complicating PTCA.[132–134] In addition, compared with PTCA, elective stent placement is associated with a lower rate

## TABLE 14–7.   EXCIMER LASER ANGIOPLASTY IN SAPHENOUS VEIN GRAFTS

| STUDY (YEAR) | LESIONS (n) | RATE OF PTCA (%) | SUCCESS RATE (%) | COMPLICATION RATES (%) | | | RESTENOSIS RATE (%) |
|---|---|---|---|---|---|---|---|
| | | | | DEATH | MI | CABG | |
| Tcheng et al (1992)[131] | 64* | — | 100 | — | — | — | — |
| Litvack et al (1994)[129] | 480 | — | 92 | — | — | — | — |
| Bittl et al (1994)[128] | 545 | 91 | 92 | 1 | 4.6 | 0.6 | 55 |
| Strauss et al (1995)[130] | 125 | 83 | 89 | 0.9 | 4.5 | 0.9 | 52 |

CABG, emergency coronary artery bypass grafting; MI, Q-wave and non–Q-wave myocardial infarction; PTCA, adjunctive percutaneous transluminal coronary angioplasty.
*These were all aorto-ostial lesions.

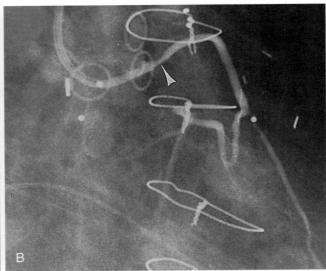

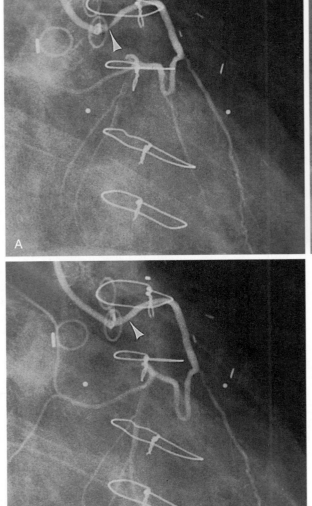

FIGURE 14–8. *A*, Right anterior oblique arteriogram of a subtotal stenosis *(arrow)* at the ostium of saphenous vein graft to an obtuse marginal coronary artery. *B*, Significant improvement in lumen diameter *(arrow)* after passage of a 1.7-mm eccentric monorail excimer laser catheter. *C*, Final result after adjunctive balloon angioplasty revealing a residual minor irregularity *(arrow)*.

of restenosis in de novo native coronary lesions.[135, 136] Several different stent designs have been evaluated for the treatment of saphenous vein graft lesions.[137] They include the Wallstent (Schneider, Inc.; Minneapolis, MN), the Gianturco-Roubin stent (Cook, Inc.; Bloomington, IN), the Palmaz-Schatz stent, coronary and biliary (Johnson & Johnson Interventional Systems; Warren, NJ), and the Wiktor stent (Medtronic, Inc.; Minneapolis, MN) (Table 14–8). In the last decade, numerous observational trials with different stent designs have shown that stent implantation in patients with vein graft lesions can be undertaken with high rates of angiographically verified success (90% to 100%), an acceptable major complication rate (2% to 3%), and, potentially, a lower rate of restenosis (<30% in some studies) than observed with other new technologies.[70, 138–154]

The Palmaz-Schatz coronary stent has been the stent design most extensively studied in vein grafts (Fig. 14–9). Wong and associates[152] reported on the U.S. multicenter experience evaluating the safety and efficacy of the Palmaz-Schatz stent in the treatment of saphenous vein graft lesions. In 589 patients, 624 lesions were treated. Stent delivery was successful in 98.8% of cases, and the procedural success rate was 97.1%. Major in-hospital complications occurred in 17 patients (2.9%). Death occurred in 1.7% of cases, MI (Q wave and non–Q wave) in 5.1%, and CABG in 0.9%. Stent thrombosis occurred in 1.4% of lesions, and distal embolization was noted in 1.9%. Major vascular or bleeding complications were observed in 14.3% of patients. Angiographic follow-up was obtained in 357 patients (61%). The overall 6-month angiographically detected restenosis rate was 30%. Restenosis was significantly lower in patients with de novo versus restenotic lesions (18.3% vs. 46.1%; $p < 0.0001$), and in patients with larger (≥3 mm) versus smaller vein grafts (26% vs. 47.5%, $p < 0.001$).

The significant incidence of bleeding and vascular

## TABLE 14–8. STENTS IN SAPHENOUS VEIN GRAFTS

| STUDY (YEAR) | STENT USED | LESIONS (n) | SUCCESS RATE (%) | COMPLICATION RATES (%) | | | | RESTENOSIS RATE (%) |
| --- | --- | --- | --- | --- | --- | --- | --- | --- |
| | | | | DEATH | MI | CABG | AC | |
| Urban et al (1986)[138] | W | 14 | 100 | 0 | 0 | 0 | 0 | 20 |
| de Scheerder et al (1992)[139] | W | 95 | 91 | 1.4 | 4.3 | 2.8 | 10 | 47 |
| Strauss et al (1992)[140] | W | 145 | — | 0 | 0 | 0 | 8 | 39 |
| Bilodeau et al (1992)[141] | GR | 37 | — | 0 | 13.5 | — | — | 35 |
| Pomerantz et al (1992)[142] | PS | 84 | 99 | 0 | 0 | 0 | 0 | 25 |
| Fortuna et al (1993)[143] | WK | 101 | 95 | 1 | 3 | 1 | 2 | — |
| Dorros et al (1994)[144] | GR | 100 | 99 | 3 | 8 | 0 | 1 | — |
| Fenton et al (1994)[145] | PS | 209 | 98 | 0.5 | 0.5 | 0.5 | 0.5 | 34 |
| Keane et al (1994)[146] | W | 29 | 97 | 0 | 0 | 0 | 3.4 | 32 |
| Eeckhout et al (1994)[147] | W/WK | 58 | 97 | 0 | 2 | 2 | 2 | 33 |
| Piana et al (1994)[148] | PS/B | 200 | 98 | 0.6 | 0 | 0 | 0.6 | 17 |
| Wong et al (1994)[150] | PS/B | 104 | 97 | 1 | 0 | 1 | 0 | 62 |
| Denardo et al (1995)[70] | PS/B | 30 | 93 | 0 | 20 | 0 | 6.7 | — |
| Wong et al (1995)[150] | PS/B | 305 | 95 | 1.3 | 0.9 | 0.4 | 0.9 | — |
| Rechavia et al (1995)[151] | PS/B | 29* | 100 | 0 | 0 | 0 | 0 | — |
| Wong et al (1995)[152] | PS | 624 | 97 | 1.7 | 5.1 | 0.9 | 1.4 | 30 |
| de Jaegere et al (1995)[153] | W/PS | 62 | 89 | 3 | 5 | 5 | 5 | 53 |

AC, abrupt closure; B, Palmaz-Schatz biliary stent; CABG, emergency coronary artery bypass grafting; GR, Gianturco-Roubin stent; MI, α-wave and non–α-wave myocardial infarction; PS, Palmaz-Schatz coronary; W, Wallstent; WK, Wiktor stent.
*These were all aorto-ostial lesions.

complications noted in this multicenter experience is worrisome. During the early experience with coronary stents, concerns about stent thrombosis led to the institution of intensive warfarin-based anticoagulation protocols. Accordingly, several trials reported higher rates of peripheral vascular and hemorrhagic complications and longer hospital stays among receiving stents patients.[135, 136] Thus, antiplatelet therapy alone (aspirin and ticlopidine), with adjunctive high-pressure (12 to 20 atm) balloon dilation and intravascular ultrasound (IVUS), has been advocated.[155, 156] This strategy is undergoing investigation for the treatment of saphenous vein graft stenoses.

Investigators for the Reduced Anticoagulation VEin graft Stent (RAVES) study reported on the first 140 patients enrolled in this prospective multicenter registry.[157] The study was designed to assess the safety and efficacy of a reduced anticoagulation regimen (aspirin and ticlopidine) in patients with simple and complex saphenous vein graft disease who were treated with Palmaz-Schatz coronary stents. All stents were implanted with post-stent high-pressure (>16 atm) balloon dilations and appropriate balloon sizes to achieve a final angiographically detected residual stenosis rate of less than 10%. IVUS was performed after each stent procedure to document results but not to guide stent implantation. Adverse in-hospital events occurred in only 3 patients (2.1%). Distal embolization was noted in 3.1% of cases. Stent thrombosis did not occur in this initial cohort of patients. These observations in the management of complex saphenous vein graft disease are encouraging and may lead to reduced

rates of vascular and hemorrhagic complications, shorter hospital stays, and lower costs.[158]

Savage and associates[159] reported a comparison of stenting with PTCA for vein graft disease. In the Saphenous Vein De Novo (SAVED) trial, 220 symptomatic patients with focal de novo vein graft stenoses were randomly assigned to placement of Palmaz-Schatz stents or standard balloon angioplasty.[159] In this group of patients, Palmaz-Schatz stent placement resulted in higher procedural success rates (92% vs. 69%; $p < 0.001$) and better luminal enlargement than PTCA. The outcome, expressed in terms of freedom from death, MI, second bypass procedure, or revascularization of the target lesion, was significantly better in the stent group (73% vs. 58%; $p = 0.03$). At 6-month follow-up however, there was no significant difference in the rate of angiographically detected restenosis (37% vs. 46%; $p = 0.24$).

Although the challenge of limiting restenosis remains, the intravascular stent is the first device to demonstrate procedural success superior to that of PTCA, with favorable clinical outcomes. Several high-risk types of lesions continue to be problematic. They include the aorto-ostial lesion, the restenotic lesion, the occluded vein graft, and the thrombus-containing lesion. A promising approach will be the "synergistic" use of new technologies, such as the performance of atherectomy, laser angioplasty, or prolonged intragraft thrombolytic therapy, to debulk vein graft lesions prior to stent placement.[70, 160, 161] This strategy will require further study.

Despite high rates of procedural success for stent placement in vein grafts, the long-term outlook for

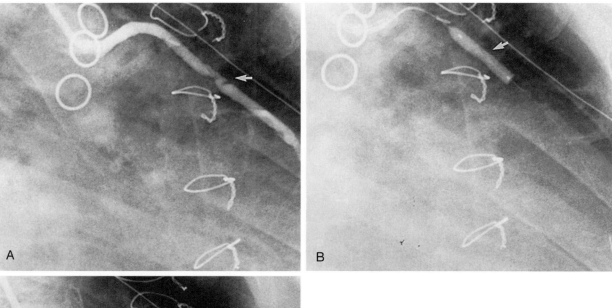

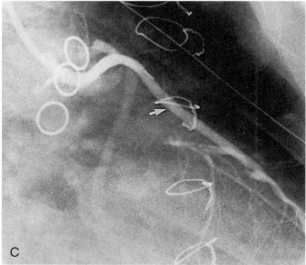

FIGURE 14–9. *A*, Right anterior oblique arteriogram of a 95% stenosis in body of saphenous vein graft to left anterior descending artery *(arrow)*. *B*, After predilation with balloon angioplasty, a 3.0-mm–15-mm Palmaz-Schatz coronary stent is being deployed *(arrow)*. *C*, After adjunctive balloon angioplasty, final result is a minor irregularity *(arrow)*.

patients undergoing the procedure is somewhat discouraging. It appears that at least 50% of such patients require further revascularization procedures in the following 2 years, mainly owing to progression of disease at other sites.[140, 148, 162]

Waksman and coworkers[162a] reported that gamma radiation decreases recurrences of in-stent restenosis. It is possible that lesion restenosis may therefore be decreased. Unfortunately, graft degeneration at sites distant from the stent site will still remain a problem.

### Thrombolysis for Chronically Occluded Saphenous Vein Grafts

The etiology of saphenous vein graft occlusion depends on the time since bypass surgery. Early graft occlusion is predominantly due to thrombosis, whereas late graft occlusion believed to be secondary to an atherosclerosis-like lesion, with or without associated thrombus. The management of the acutely occluded venous graft is discussed later in this chapter.

The management of chronic total vein graft occlusions is a difficult issue, given the large associated thrombus burden. Hartmann and coworkers[163] described a method of administering a prolonged, low-dose infusion of intragraft thrombolytic therapy in an attempt to reduce the likelihood of distal embolization, thrombotic reocclusion, and restenosis associated with PTCA alone. Since this early report, several investigative teams have published acceptable results for this technique (Table 14–9).[70, 71, 164–168] In the largest series, 107 patients with occluded vein grafts were treated with a urokinase infusion, at a dose of 100,000 to 360,000 U/hour over a mean duration of 25.4 hours.[71] Successful recanalization was achieved in 69% of the grafts. Adverse events consisted of acute MI in 5 patients (5%), creatinine kinase enzyme elevation in 18 (17%), emergency CABG in 4 (4%), stroke in 3 (3%), and death in 7 (6.5%). Six-month angiographic follow-up was obtained in 40 patients (54%), only 16 of whom (40%) were found to have a patent graft.

**TABLE 14–9.    INTRAGRAFT THROMBOLYSIS FOR CHRONICALLY OCCLUDED VEIN GRAFTS**

| STUDY (YEAR) | NO. OF PATIENTS | ADJUVANT THERAPY | SUCCESS RATE (%) | COMPLICATION RATES (%) | | | RESTENOSIS RATE (%) |
|---|---|---|---|---|---|---|---|
| | | | | DEATH | MI | CABG | |
| Hartmann et al (1991)[164] | 47 | PTCA | 79 | 0 | 13 | 0 | 35 |
| Sabri et al (1992)[166] | 3 | DCA | 100 | 0 | 0 | 0 | — |
| Levine et al (1992)[165] | 10 | PTCA | 60 | 2 | 2 | 0 | 100 |
| Eagan et al (1993)[167] | 3 | PTCA/stent | 100 | 0 | 0 | 0 | 33 |
| Lotan et al (1994)[168] | 21 | PTCA | 76 | 0 | 19 | 0 | 69 |
| Denardo et al (1995)[70] | 30 | PTCA/stent | 93 | 0 | 20 | 4 | 29 |
| Hartmann et al (1996)[71] | 107 | PTCA | 69 | 6.5 | 17 | 4 | 60 |

CABG, emergency coronary artery bypass grafting; DCA, directional coronary atherectomy; MI, Q-wave and non–Q-wave myocardial infarction; PTCA, percutaneous transluminal coronary angioplasty.

Although early patency of occluded vein grafts can be achieved in many patients with prolonged thrombolytic therapy, the risk of embolic MI, estimated to be 13% to 20% in larger series, remains a significant concern.[70, 71, 164] In addition, the initial rates of recanalization in these occluded grafts do not appear to be sustained at long-term follow-up (see Table 14–9).

The overall value of this strategy remains uncertain. It may represent an effective alternative to reoperation in carefully selected patients. This strategy should be considered only after rigorous medical therapy has failed to control symptoms. The physician must carefully weigh the risks of this percutaneous intervention with those of a second bypass procedure.

## Special Situations

### Management of Acute MI

Since the 1980s, there has been a progressive rise in the number of patients with prior bypass surgery who present with acute MI. Few data exist regarding the appropriate reperfusion strategy for such patients. Patients with previous CABG were usually excluded from reperfusion trials using early angiography, primarily because of difficulty in identifying the infarct-related artery. In these patients, acute MI may potentially result from occlusion of a graft to an artery that has already closed, occlusion of an artery whose graft was already closed, or occlusion of an ungrafted native coronary artery. The existing data would indicate that acute MI in the post-bypass patient usually results from occlusion of a saphenous vein graft and that conventional intravenous thrombolytic therapy may be inadequate to restore flow.[169, 170]

Little and associates[171] reported on 40 patients with acute MI occurring more than 1 month after CABG.[171] Angiography performed at a mean of 16 ± 14 days from acute MI revealed that graft occlusion was responsible for the infarct in 66% of cases and that closure of an unbypassed native vessel was responsible in 34% of cases. In a retrospective analysis conducted by Grines and coworkers[169] of 50 post-bypass patients with acute MI, the infarct-related vessel was identified as a vein graft in 38 patients (76%) and as a native vessel in 8 (16%). The infarct-related vessel could not be accurately determined in 4 patients (8%). Interestingly, intravenous thrombolytic therapy was successful at recanalizing grafts in 2 of 8 patients (25%), whereas intragraft thrombolysis, with or without additional angioplasty, was successful in restoring flow in 8 of 10 patients (80%).

The first Global Utilization of Streptokinase and Tissue Plasminogen Activator for Occluded Coronary Arteries (GUSTO-I) trial has provided further insights into the management of these patients.[172] In this study of 41,021 patients with acute MI, 4% of patients had previous bypass surgery. These patients were significantly older, had a higher incidence of prior MI, and had significantly more risk factors for coronary disease than the group without prior CABG. These significant differences probably account for the higher 30-day mortality rate (10.6% vs. 6.7%) and higher reinfarction rate (5.4% vs. 3.7%) seen in the patients with prior CABG.[173] Reiner and associates[174] reported on the angiographic findings in 48 patients with saphenous vein graft occlusion in the angiographic substudy of the GUSTO-I trial.[174] At angiography, performed 90 or 180 minutes after thrombolytic therapy, the patency rate was significantly higher in native vessels than in vein grafts (69% vs. 48%; $p = 0.01$). Furthermore, these investigators demonstrated that saphenous vein graft occlusion is a potent and independent predictor of thrombolytic failure.

Although intravenous thrombolytic therapy continues to be the "first-line" therapy for all patients with acute MI, alternative strategies in post-bypass patients warrant consideration, given the suboptimal outcome of thrombolysis.

Several small series have examined the use of direct PTCA for post-CABG patients with acute MI. Kahn and coworkers[170] reported on 72 patients with previous bypass surgery who underwent direct PTCA. PTCA was successful in 41 of 48 vein grafts (85%) and 2 of 24 native arteries (100%). Santiago and associates[175] reported a 97% success rate for direct PTCA in 35 post-CABG patients with acute MI, compared with a 92% success rate for direct PTCA in 258 patients who had not undergone CABG.

Stone and colleagues[176] examined combined data from the first and second Primary Angioplasty in Myocardial Infarction (PAMI-1 and PAMI-2) trials, in which direct PTCA was performed in 1103 patients at 40 centers.[176] Forty-two patients with prior CABG were enrolled in these studies. Patients with prior CABG were older and were more likely to have multivessel disease and prior MI than enrolled patients who had not undergone CABG. The infarct-related vessel in patients with prior CABG was the bypass graft in 19 patients (45%) and a native coronary artery in 22 patients (53%). These investigators reported no significant difference in procedural success rate of direct PTCA in patients with or without prior CABG. In the patients with prior CABG, the achievement of TIMI-3 (Thrombosis in Myocardial Infarction scale grade 3) flow grade (84% and 91% respectively; $p = 0.65$) and rates of death or reinfarction were similar in patients in whom infarct vessel was a bypass graft and those in whom it was a native coronary artery. Despite the frequent presence of adverse comorbid factors in patients with prior CABG, high rates of reperfusion may be achieved with primary PTCA in the setting of acute MI.

Although these initial reports are encouraging, the long-term outcomes of percutaneous revascularization in patients with acute MI has not been formally compared to thrombolytic therapy. The same risk of distal embolization present with elective procedures is greater with acute MI intervention. New strategies employing thrombectomy devices, laser, and distal protection are required.

### Coronary-Subclavian Steal Syndrome

The coronary-subclavian steal syndrome is an entity occasionally encountered in patients who have received IMA grafts. This disorder is due to a stenosis in the subclavian artery proximal to the origin of an IMA that is serving as a coronary bypass conduit. The subclavian stenosis causes ischemia to, or even frank reversal of blood flow from, the territory of myocardium supplied. Clinical manifestations include angina pectoris, arm claudication, vertebrobasilar insufficiency, cervical or subclavian bruit, blood pressure difference (20 mm Hg or greater) in the arms, and diminished upper extremity pulses. Traditional therapy for this problem was carotid-subclavian bypass; however, percutaneous therapies such as subclavian artery angioplasty, stent placement, and directional atherectomy have been shown to yield favorable results.[177–181]

Rarely, coronary-subclavian steal syndrome result from an unligated large intercostal branch of the IMA. In this situation, microcoil embolization of the side branch has been successful in relieving myocardial ischemia.[182, 183]

For information on distal protection, see Chapter 38.

## CONCLUSIONS

The management of patients with saphenous vein graft disease is one of the most complex and challenging areas in cardiology. The current standard approach to managing such patients consists of either percutaneous coronary intervention or a second bypass procedure. This approach is associated with high rates of acute complications and low rates of long-term success. The development of an individual strategy for each patient requires an understanding of the natural history of saphenous vein and IMA grafts, the role of risk factor modification, and the risks and benefits of the various mechanical revascularization procedures.

The key to understanding the natural history of saphenous vein and internal mammary artery grafts involves the duration of time since bypass surgery. The primary cause of graft failure in the early postoperative period (up to 1 month) is thrombosis, and between the postoperative 1st and 12th months it is the development of occlusive thrombi superimposed upon intimal hyperplasia. Atherosclerotic lesions usually do not become apparent until 3 years after graft insertion. The development of thrombus, intimal hyperplasia, and atherosclerosis in IMA grafts is rare.

Understanding the natural history of these grafts allows one to comprehend the important role of risk factor modification. Antiplatelet agents have been shown to effectively reduce early graft thrombosis. Their use should be mandatory during the first year after surgery. The efficacy of these agents in preventing late graft thrombosis has not been adequately documented. The development and progression of atherosclerosis beyond the first year after the operation may be related to the usual coronary risk factors, and adequate control of these factors is important. Successful lowering of total and low density lipoprotein cholesterol levels and raising of the high density lipoprotein cholesterol level have been shown to have beneficial effect on the progression and regression of atherosclerotic lesions in vein grafts.[184, 185] Smoking cessation is important in the inhibition of vein graft atherosclerosis.[186]

Important anatomic factors that the cardiologist must understand before attempting mechanical revascularization include the length of time since surgery and location of the lesion. Revascularization of lesions appearing 3 years after surgery has a lower success rate, a higher incidence of complications, and a higher restenosis rate with angioplasty than that of lesions appearing within the first 3 years of surgery. Success rates for angioplasty are highest and restenosis rates are lowest for lesions at the distal anastomosis.

A myriad of new interventional technologies have been employed to overcome the difficulties encountered with vein graft angioplasty. However, the role of new technologies has been limited, largely because none of these new procedures seems to reduce the restenosis rate in these difficult lesions. The use of intravascular stents for these lesions does appear to be promising. Studies of stent placement in vein grafts have demonstrated higher procedural success rates and, possibly, lower rates of restenosis than are seen with conventional balloon angioplasty. Perhaps a combined strategy of stent placement with "debulking" techniques may yield the most favorable results, but this issue is being investigated. A major breakthrough has been development of distal protection devices such as the PercuSurge Guardwire distal protection device (Abbott Corporation; Chicago, IL). This device appears to significantly decrease the risk of distal embolization and thus improve procedural safety.[186a]

The future management of these complex cases may be dramatically altered by the development of more powerful platelet inhibitors, inhibitors of smooth muscle cell proliferation, more potent antithrombotic agents, and radiation treatment. The success of platelet glycoprotein IIb/IIIa inhibitors, such as abciximab, in improving outcomes after native coronary artery intervention, has not been successful in the post-bypass setting.[187–190] It is to be hoped that refinements in current device technologies and development of new technologies will improve the long-term outcome for these patients.

# REFERENCES

1. Kolessov VI: Mammary artery–coronary artery anastomosis as method of treatment for angina pectoris. J Thorac Cardiovasc Surg 54:535, 1967.
2. Favaloro RG: Saphenous vein autograft replacement of severe segmental coronary artery occlusion: Operative technique. Ann Thorac Surg 5:334, 1968.
3. Open Heart Surgery Statistics. http://www.americanheart.org/Heart_and_Stroke_A_Z_Guide/openh.html
4. Campeau L, Lesperance J, Hermann J, et al: Loss of the improvement of angina between 1 and 7 years after aorto-coronary bypass surgery. Circulation 60(suppl I):I-1, 1979.
5. Seides SF, Borer JS, Kent KM, et al: Long-term anatomic fate of coronary artery bypass grafts and functional status of patients five years after operation. N Engl J Med 298:1213, 1978.
6. Hwang MH, Meadows WR, Palac RT, et al: Progression of native coronary artery disease at 10 years: Insights from a randomized study of medical versus surgical therapy for angina. J Am Coll Cardiol 16:1066, 1990.
7. Fitzgibbon GM, Leach AJ, Kafka HP, et al: Coronary bypass graft fate: Long-term angiographic study. J Am Coll Cardiol 17:1075, 1991.
8. Campeau L, Enjalbert M, Lespérance J, et al: Atherosclerosis and late closure of aortocoronary saphenous vein grafts: Sequential angiographic studies at 2 weeks, 1 year, 5 to 7 years, and 10 to 12 years after surgery. Circulation 68(suppl II):I-1, 1983.
9. Lytle BW, Loop FD, Cosgrove DM, et al: Long-term (5 to 12 years) serial studies of internal mammary artery and saphenous vein coronary bypass grafts. J Thorac Cardiovasc Surg 89:248, 1985.
10. Frey RR, Bruschke AVG, Vermeulen FEE: Serial angiographic evaluation 1 year and 9 years after aorta-coronary bypass: A study of 55 patients chosen at random. J Thorac Cardiovasc Surg 87:167, 1984.
11. Barner HB, Standeven JW, Reese J: Twelve-year experience with internal mammary artery for coronary artery bypass. J Thorac Cardiovasc Surg 90:668, 1985.
12. Grondin CM, Campeau L, Lespérance J, et al: Comparison of late changes in internal mammary artery and saphenous vein grafts in 2 consecutive series of patients 10 years after operation. Circulation 70(suppl I):I-208, 1984.
13. Loop FD, Lytle BW, Cosgrove DM, et al: Influence of the internal-mammary-artery graft on 10-year survival and other cardiac events. N Engl J Med 314:1, 1986.
14. Israel DH, Adam PC, Stein B, et al: Antithrombotic therapy in the coronary vein graft patient. Clin Cardiol 14:283, 1991.
15. Fuster V, Dewanjee MK, Kaye MP, et al: Noninvasive radioisotopic technique for detection of platelet deposition in coronary artery bypass grafts in dogs and its reduction with platelet inhibitors. Circulation 60:1508, 1979.
16. Bulkley BH, Hutchins GM: Pathology of coronary artery bypass graft surgery. Arch Pathol Lab Med 102:273, 1978.
17. Spray TL, Roberts WC: Tension of coronary bypass conduits: A neglected cause of real or potential obstruction of saphenous vein grafts. J Thorac Cardiovasc Surg 72:282, 1976.
18. Roberts WC, Lachman AS, Virmani R: Twisting of aortocoronary bypass conduits, a complication of coronary surgery. J Thorac Cardiovasc Surg 75:772, 1978.
19. Fuster V, Chesebro JH: Role of platelets and platelet inhibitors in aortocoronary artery vein-graft disease. Circulation 73:227, 1986.
20. Chesebro JH, Clements IP, Foster V, et al: A platelet-inhibitor drug trial in coronary-artery bypass operations: Benefit of perioperative dipyridamole and aspirin therapy on early postoperative vein-graft patency. N Engl J Med 307:73, 1982.
21. Sanz G, Pajafon A, Coello I, et al, and the Grupo Espanol para el Seguimiento del Injerto Coronario: Prevention of early aortocoronary bypass occlusion by low-dose aspirin and dipyridamole. Circulation 82:765, 1990.
22. Campeau L, Enjalbert M, Lespérance J, et al: The relation of risk factors to the development of atherosclerosis in saphenous-vein bypass grafts and the progression of disease in the native circulation. N Engl J Med 311:1329, 1984.
23. Assoian RK, Grotendorst GR, Miller DM, et al: Cellular transformation by coordinated action of three peptide growth factors from human platelets. Nature 309: 804, 1984.
24. Assoian RK, Komoriya A, Meyers CA, et al: Transforming growth factor-beta in human platelets. J Biol Chem 258:7155, 1983.
25. Lawrie GM, Lie JT, Morris GC, et al: Vein graft patency and intimal proliferation after aortocoronary bypass: Early and long-term angiographic correlations. Am J Cardiol 38:856, 1976.
26. Shelton ME, Forman MB, Virmani R, et al: A comparison of morphologic and angiographic findings in long-term internal mammary artery and saphenous vein bypass grafts. J Am Coll Cardiol 11:297, 1988.
27. Sketch MH Jr, Quigley PJ, Perez JA, et al: Angiographic follow-up after internal mammary artery graft angioplasty. Am J Cardiol 70:401, 1992.
28. Chesebro JH, Foster V, Elveback LR, et al: Does dipyridamole plus aspirin affect aortocoronary vein graft narrowing over the first postoperative year? Circulation 65(suppl II): II-105, 1984.
29. Smith SH, Geer JC: Morphology of saphenous vein-coronary artery bypass grafts. Arch Pathol Lab Med 107:13, 1983.

30. Waller BF, Rothbaum DA, Gorfinkel HJ, et al: Morphologic observations after percutaneous transluminal balloon angioplasty of early and late aortocoronary saphenous vein bypass grafts. J Am Coll Cardiol 4:784, 1984.

31. Foster ED, Fisher LD, Kaiser GC, et al: Comparison of operative mortality and morbidity for initial and repeat coronary artery bypass grafting: The Coronary Artery Surgery Study (CASS) Registry experience. Ann Thorac Surg 38:563, 1984.

32. Cameron A, Kemp HG, Green GE: Reoperation for coronary artery disease: 10 years of clinical follow-up. Circulation 78(suppl I):I-158, 1988.

33. Osaka S, Barratt-Boyes BG, Brandt PW, et al: Early and late results of reoperation for coronary artery disease: A 13-year experience. Aust N Z J Surg 58:537, 1988.

34. Reul GJ Jr, Cooley DA, Ott DA, et al: Reoperation for recurrent coronary artery disease: Causes, indications and results in 168 patients. Arch Surg 114:1269, 1979.

35. Schaff HV, Orszulah TA, Gersh BJ, et al: The morbidity or mortality of reoperation for coronary artery disease and analysis of late results with use of actuarial estimate of event-free interval. J Thorac Cardiovasc Surg 85:508, 1983.

36. Pidgeon J, Brooks N, Magee P, et al: Reoperation for angina after previous aortocoronary bypass surgery. Br Heart J 53:269, 1985.

37. Laird-Meeter K, Vandomburg R, Vanden Brand MJBM, et al: Incidence, risk, and outcome of reintervention after aortocoronary bypass surgery. Br Heart J 57:427, 1987.

38. Lytle BW, Loop FD, Cosgrove DM, et al: Fifteen hundred coronary reoperations: Results and determinants of early and late survival. J Thorac Cardiovasc Surg 93:847, 1987.

39. Verheul HA, Moulijn AC, Hondema S, et al: Late results of 200 repeat coronary artery bypass operations. Am J Cardiol 67:24, 1991.

40. Lytle BW, Cosgrove DM, Taylor PC, et al: Multiple coronary reoperations: Early and late results. Circulation 80(suppl II):II-626, 1989.

41. Keon WJ, Heggtrait HA, Ledue J: Perioperative myocardial infarction caused by atheroembolism. J Thorac Cardiovasc Surg 84:849, 1982.

42. Grondin CM, Pomar JL, Hébert Y, et al: Reoperation in patients with patent atherosclerotic coronary vein grafts. J Thorac Cardiovasc Surg 87:379, 1984.

43. Gruentzig AR, Senning A, Siegenthaler WE. Nonoperative dilatation of coronary-artery stenosis: Percutaneous transluminal coronary angioplasty. N Engl J Med 301:61, 1979.

44. Douglas JS, Gruentzig AR, King SB, et al: Percutaneous transluminal coronary angioplasty in patients with prior coronary bypass surgery. J Am Coll Cardiol 4:745, 1983.

45. Dorros G, Johnson WD, Tector AJ, et al: Percutaneous transluminal coronary angioplasty in patients with prior coronary artery bypass grafting. J Thorac Cardiovasc Surg 87:17, 1984.

46. El Gamal ME, Bonnier H, Michels R, et al: Percutaneous transluminal angioplasty of stenosed aortocoronary bypass grafts. Br Heart J 52:617, 1984.

47. Block PC, Cowley MJ, Kaltenbach M, et al: Percutaneous angioplasty of stenoses of bypass grafts or of bypass graft anastomotic sites. Am J Cardiol 53:666, 1984.

48. Corbelli J, Franco I, Hollman J, et al: Percutaneous transluminal coronary angioplasty after previous coronary artery bypass surgery. Am J Cardiol 56:398, 1985.

49. Douglas J, Robinson K, Schlumpf M: Percutaneous transluminal angioplasty in aortocoronary venous graft stenoses: Immediate results and complications. Circulation 74(suppl II):II-363, 1986.

50. Reeder GS, Bresnahan JF, Holmes DR, et al: Angioplasty for aortocoronary bypass graft stenosis. Mayo Clin Proc 61:14, 1986.

51. Cole G, Myler RK, Stertzer SH, et al: Percutaneous transluminal angioplasty of stenotic coronary artery bypass grafts: 5 years experience. J Am Coll Cardiol 9:8, 1987.

52. Ernst S, van der Feltz T, Ascoop C, et al: Percutaneous transluminal coronary angioplasty in patients with prior coronary artery bypass grafting. J Thorac Cardiovasc Surg 93:268, 1987.

53. Cote GC, Myler RK, Stertzer SH, et al: Percutaneous transluminal angioplasty of stenotic coronary artery bypass grafts: 5 years experience. J Am Coll Cardiol 9:8, 1987.

54. Pinkerton CA, Slack JD, Orr CM, et al: Percutaneous transluminal angioplasty in patients with prior myocardial revascularization surgery. Am J Cardiol 61:156, 1988.

55. Platko WP, Hollman J, Whitlow PL, et al: Percutaneous transluminal angioplasty at saphenous vein graft: Long-term follow-up. J Am Coll Cardiol 14:1645, 1989.

56. Dorros G, Lewin RF, Mathiak LM: Coronary angioplasty in patients with prior coronary bypass surgery: All prior coronary artery bypass surgery patients and patients more than 5 years after coronary bypass surgery. Cardiol Clin 9:791, 1989.

57. Webb JG, Myler RK, Shaw RE, et al: Coronary angioplasty after coronary bypass surgery: Initial results and late outcome in 422 patients. J Am Coll Cardiol 16:812, 1990.

58. Meester BJ, Samson M, Suryapranata H, et al: Long-term follow-up after attempted angioplasty of saphenous vein grafts: The Thoraxcenter experience 1981–1988. Eur Heart J 12:648, 1991.

59. Plokker HWT, Meester BH, Serruys PW: The Dutch experience in percutaneous transluminal angioplasty of narrowed saphenous veins used for aortocoronary arterial bypass. Am J Cardiol 67:361, 1991.

60. Douglas JS, Weintraub WS, Liberman HA, et al: Update of saphenous graft angioplasty: Restenosis and long-term outcome. Circulation 84(suppl II):II-249A, 1991.

61. Jost S, Gulba D, Daniel WG, et al: Percutaneous transluminal angioplasty of aortocoronary venous bypass grafts and the effect of the caliber of the grafted coronary artery on graft stenosis. Am J Cardiol 68:27, 1991.

62. Unterberg C, Buchwald A, Wiegand V, et al: Coronary angioplasty in patients with previous coronary artery bypass grafting. Angiology 43:653, 1992.

63. Miranda CP, Rutherford BD, McConahay DR, et al: Angioplasty of older saphenous vein grafts continues to be a sound therapeutic option. J Am Coll Cardiol 19:350A, 1992.

64. Morrison DA, Crowley ST, Veerakul G, et al: Percutaneous transluminal angioplasty of saphenous vein grafts for medically refractory unstable angina. J Am Coll Cardiol 23:1066, 1994.

65. Tan K, Henderson R, Sulke N, et al: Percutaneous transluminal coronary angioplasty in patients with prior coronary artery bypass grafting: Ten years' experience. Cathet Cardiovasc Diagn 31:11, 1994.

66. de Feyter PJ, Serruys P, Van Den Brand M, et al: Percutaneous transluminal angioplasty of a totally occluded venous bypass graft: A challenge that should be resisted. Am J Cardiol 64:88, 1989.

67. Margolis JR, Mogensen L, Mehta S, et al: Diffuse embolization following percutaneous transluminal coronary angioplasty of occluded vein grafts: The blush phenomenon. Clin Cardiol 14:489, 1991.

68. Kahn JK, Rutherford BD, McConahay DR, et al: Initial and long-term outcome of 83 patients after balloon angioplasty of totally occluded bypass grafts. J Am Coll Cardiol 23:1038, 1994.

69. Berger PB, Bell MR, Grill DE, et al: Influence of procedural success on immediate and long-term clinical outcome of patients undergoing percutaneous revascularization of occluded coronary artery bypass vein grafts. J Am Coll Cardiol 28:1732, 1996.

70. Denardo SJ, Morris NB, Rocha-Singh KJ, et al: Safety and efficacy of extended urokinase infusion plus stent deployment for the treatment of obstructed older saphenous vein grafts. Am J Cardiol 76:776, 1995.

71. Hartmann JR, McKeever LS, O'Neill WW, et al: Recanalization of chronically occluded aortocoronary saphenous vein bypass grafts with long-term low dose direct infusion of urokinase (ROBUST): A serial trial. J Am Coll Cardiol 27:60, 1996.

72. Drummer E, Furey K, Hollman J: Rupture of a saphenous vein bypass graft during coronary angioplasty. Br Heart J 58:78, 1987.

73. Namay DL, Roubin GS, Tommaso CL, et al: Saphenous vein

graft rapture during percutaneous transluminal angioplasty. Cathet Cardiovasc Diagn 14:258, 1988.

74. Teirstein PS, Hartzler GO: Nonoperative management of aortocoronary saphenous vein graft rapture during percutaneous transluminal coronary angioplasty. Am J Cardiol 60:377, 1987.

75. Marquis JF, Schwartz L, Brown R, et al: Percutaneous transluminal angioplasty of coronary saphenous vein bypass grafts. Can J Surg 28:335, 1985.

76. Lytle BW, Loop FD, Thurer RL, et al: Isolated left anterior descending coronary atherosclerosis: Long-term comparison of internal mammary artery and venous autografts. Circulation 61:869, 1980.

77. Singh RN, Sosa JA, Green GE: Long-term fate of the internal mammary artery and saphenous vein grafts. J Thorac Cardiovasc Surg 86:359, 1983.

78. Barner HB, Mudd JG, Mark AL, et al: Patency of internal mammary–coronary grafts. Circulation 54(suppl III):III-70, 1976.

79. Barbour DJ, Roberts WC: Additional evidence for relative resistance to atherosclerosis of the internal mammary artery compared to saphenous vein when used to increase myocardial blood supply. Am J Cardiol 56:488, 1985.

80. Kay HR, Korns ME, Flemma RJ, et al: Atherosclerosis of the internal mammary artery. Ann Thorac Surg 21:504, 1976.

81. Pinkerton CA, Slack JD, Orr CM, et al: Percutaneous transluminal angioplasty involving internal mammary artery bypass grafts: A femoral approach. Cathet Cardiovasc Diagn 13:414, 1987.

82. Shimshak TM, Giorgi LV, Johnson WL, et al: Application of percutaneous transluminal coronary angioplasty to the internal mammary artery graft. J Am Coll Cardiol 12:1205, 1988.

83. Hill DM, McAuley BJ, Sheehan DJ, et al: Percutaneous transluminal angioplasty of internal mammary artery bypass grafts. J Am Coll Cardiol 13:221A, 1989.

84. Bell MR, Holmes DR, Vliestra RE, et al: Percutaneous transluminal angioplasty of left internal mammary artery grafts: Two years experience with a femoral approach. Br Heart J 61:417, 1989.

85. Dimas AP, Arora RR, Whitlow PL, et al: Percutaneous transluminal angioplasty involving internal mammary artery grafts. Am Heart J 122:423, 1991.

86. Popma JJ, Cooke RH, Leon MB, et al: Immediate procedural and long-term clinical results in internal mammary artery angioplasty. Am J Cardiol 69:1237, 1992.

87. Najm HK, Leddy D, Hendry PJ, et al: Postoperative symptomatic internal thoracic artery stenosis and successful treatment with PTCA. Ann Thorac Surg 59:323, 1995.

88. Hearne SE, Wilson JS, Harrington J, et al: Angiographic and clinical follow-up after internal mammary artery graft angioplasty: A 9-year experience. J Am Coll Cardiol 25:139A, 1995.

89. Hadjimiltiades S, Gourassas J, Louridas G, et al: Stenting the distal anastomotic site of the left internal mammary artery graft: A case report. Cathet Cardiovasc Diagn 32:157, 1994.

90. Almagor Y, Thomas J, Colombo A: A balloon expandable stent at the origin of the left internal mammary artery graft. Cathet Cardiovasc Diagn 24:256, 1991.

91. Bajaj RK, Roubin GS: Intravascular stenting of the right internal mammary artery. Cathet Cardiovasc Diagn 24:252, 1991.

92. Tector AJ, Schmahl TM, Janson B, et al: The internal mammary artery graft: Its longevity after coronary bypass. JAMA 246:2181, 1981.

93. The Veterans Administration Coronary Artery Bypass Surgery Cooperative Group: Eighteen-year follow-up in the Veterans Affairs cooperative study of coronary artery bypass surgery for stable angina. Circulation 86:121, 1992.

94. Varnauskas E and the European Coronary Surgery Study Group: Twelve-year follow-up of survival in the randomized European coronary surgery study. N Engl J Med 319:332, 1988.

95. Alderman EL, Bourassa MG, Cohen LS, et al: Ten-year follow-up of survival and myocardial infarction in the ran-

domized Coronary Artery Surgery Study (CASS). Circulation 82:1629, 1990.

96. RITA Trial Participants: Coronary angioplasty versus coronary artery bypass surgery: The Randomized Intervention Treatment of Angina (RITA) trial. Lancet 341:573, 1993.

97. Hamm CW, Reimers J, Ischinger T, et al, for the German Angioplasty Bypass Surgery Investigation: A randomized study of coronary angioplasty compared with bypass surgery in patients with symptomatic multivessel coronary disease. N Engl J Med 331:1037, 1994.

98. King SB III, Lembo NJ, Weintraub WS, et al, for the Emory Angioplasty versus Surgery Trial (EAST): A randomized trial comparing coronary angioplasty with coronary artery bypass surgery. N Engl J Med 331:1044, 1994.

99. Rodriguez A, Boullon F, Perez-Balino N, et al: Argentine randomized trial of percutaneous transluminal coronary angioplasty versus coronary artery bypass surgery in multivessel disease (ERACI): In-hospital results and 1 year follow-up. J Am Coll Cardiol 22:1060, 1993.

100. The BARI Investigators: Comparison of coronary bypass surgery with angioplasty in patients with multivessel disease. N Engl J Med 335:217, 1996.

101. Stephan WJ, O'Keefe JH, Piehler JM, et al: Coronary angioplasty versus repeat coronary artery bypass grafting for patients with previous bypass surgery. J Am Coll Cardiol 28:1140, 1996.

102. Weintraub WS, Jones EL, Morris DC, et al: Outcome of reoperative surgery versus coronary angioplasty after bypass surgery. Circulation 95:868, 1997.

103. Kaufmann UP, Garratt KN, Vlietstra RE, et al: Transluminal atherectomy of saphenous vein aortocoronary bypass grafts. Am J Cardiol 65:1430, 1990.

104. Selmon MR, Hinohara T, Robertson GC, et al: Directional coronary atherectomy for saphenous vein graft stenoses. J Am Coll Cardiol 17:23A, 1991.

105. Ghazzal ZMB, Douglas JS, Holmes DR, and the Directional Atherectomy Multicenter Investigational Group: Directional coronary atherectomy of saphenous vein grafts: Recent multicenter experience. J Am Coll Cardiol 17:23A, 1991.

106. DiScasio G, Cowley MJ, Vetrovec CW, et al: Directional coronary atherectomy of saphenous vein graft lesions unfavorable for balloon angioplasty: Results of a single center experience. Cathet Cardiovasc Diagn 26:75, 1992.

107. Pomerantz RM, Kuntz E, Carozza JP, et al: Acute and long-term outcome of narrowed saphenous venous grafts treated by endoluminal stenting and directional atherectomy. Am J Cardiol 70:161, 1992.

108. Garratt KN, Holmes DR Jr, Bell MR, et al: Results of directional atherectomy of primary atheromatous and restenosis lesions in coronary arteries and saphenous vein grafts. Am J Cardiol 70:449, 1992.

109. Cowley MJ, Whitlow PL, Baim DS, et al: Directional coronary atherectomy of saphenous vein graft narrowings: Multicenter investigational experience. Am J Cardiol 72:30E, 1993.

110. Stephan WJ, Bates ER, Garratt KN, et al: Directional atherectomy of coronary and saphenous vein graft ostial stenoses. Am J Cardiol 75:1015, 1995.

111. Holmes DR Jr, Topol EJ, Califf RM, et al: A multicenter randomized trial of coronary angioplasty versus directional atherectomy for patients with saphenous vein graft lesions. Circulation 91:1966, 1995.

112. Popma JJ, Leon MB, Mintz GS, et al: Results of coronary angioplasty using the transluminal extraction catheter. Am J Cardiol 70:1526, 1992.

113. Safian RD, Grines CL, May MA, et al: Clinical and angiographic results of transluminal extraction coronary atherectomy in saphenous vein bypass grafts. Circulation 89:302, 1994.

114. Twidale N, Barth CW III, Kipperman RM, et al: Acute results and long-term outcome of transluminal extraction atherectomy for saphenous vein graft stenoses. Cathet Cardiovasc Diagn 31:187, 1994.

115. Dooris M, Hoffman M, Glazier S, et al: Comparative results of transluminal extraction coronary atherectomy in saphe-

nous vein graft lesions with and without thrombus. J Am Coll Cardiol 25:1700, 1995.

116. Meany TB, Leon MB, Kramer BL, et al: Transluminal extraction catheter for the treatment of diseased saphenous vein grafts: A multicenter experience. Cathet Cardiovasc Diagn 34:112, 1995.

117. Misumi K, Matthews RV, Guo-Wen S, et al: Reduced distal embolization with transluminal extraction atherectomy compared to balloon angioplasty for saphenous vein graft disease. Cathet Cardiovasc Diagn 39:246, 1996.

118. Al-Shaibi KF, Goods CM, Jain SP, et al: Does transluminal extraction atherectomy reduce distal embolization in saphenous vein grafts? Circulation 92:1, 1995.

119. Hong MK, Popma JJ, Pichard AD, et al: Clinical significance of distal embolization after transluminal extraction atherectomy in diffusely diseased saphenous vein grafts. Am Heart J 127:1496, 1994.

120. Moses JW, Teirstein PS, Sketch MH Jr, et al: Angiographic determinants of risk and outcome of coronary embolus and myocardial infarction (MI) with the transluminal extraction catheter (TEC): A report from the New Approaches to Coronary Intervention (NACI) registry. J Am Coll Cardiol 23(special issue): 220A, 1994.

120a. Braden GA, Xenopoulos NP, Young T, et al: Transluminal extraction catheter atherectomy followed by immediate stenting in treatment of saphenous vein grafts. J Am Coll Cardiol 30:657–663, 1997.

121. Dooris M, Safian RD: Coronary artery bypass grafts. In Freed M, Grines C, Safian RD (eds): The New Manual of Interventional Cardiology, p 334. Birmingham, MI: Physicians Press, 1996.

122. Freed M, Niazi K, O'Neill W: Percutaneous coronary rotational atherectomy: The William Beaumont hospital experience. In Restenosis after Intervention with New Mechanical Devices, p 297. Dordrecht, The Netherlands: Kluwer Academic, 1992.

123. Bass TA, Gilmore PS, Buchbinder M, et al: Coronary rotational atherectomy (PTCRA) in patients with prior coronary revascularization: A registry report. Circulation 86(suppl I):I-653, 1992.

124. Ramee SR, Kuntz RE, Schatz RA, et al: Preliminary experience with the Possis coronary AngioJet rheolytic thrombectomy catheter in the VeGAS I pilot study. J Am Coll Cardiol 25:69A, 1996.

125. Ramee SR, Schatz RA, Carrozza JP, et al: Results of the VeGAS I pilot study of the Possis coronary AngioJet thrombectomy catheter. Circulation 94(suppl I):I-619, 1996.

126. Fajadet J, Olivier R, Jordan C, et al: Human percutaneous thrombectomy using the new Hydrolyser catheter: Preliminary results in saphenous vein grafts. J Am Coll Cardiol 23:22A, 1994.

127. van Ommen V, van der Veen E, Daemen M, et al: In vivo evaluation of the safety to the vessel wall of the Hydrolyser (a hydrodynamic thrombectomy catheter). J Am Coll Cardiol 23:406A, 1994.

128. Bittl JA, Sanborn TA, Yardley DE, et al, for the Percutaneous Excimer Laser Coronary Angioplasty Registry: Predictors of outcome of percutaneous excimer laser coronary angioplasty of saphenous vein bypass graft lesions. Am J Cardiol 74:144, 1994.

129. Litvack F, Eigler N, Margolis J, et al: Percutaneous excimer laser coronary angioplasty: Results in the first consecutive 3,000 patients. J Am Coll Cardiol 23:323, 1994.

130. Strauss BH, Natarajan MK, Batchelor WB, et al: Early and late quantitative angiographic results of vein graft lesions treated by excimer laser with adjunctive balloon angioplasty. Circulation 92:348, 1995.

131. Tcheng JE, Bittl JA, Sanborn TA, et al, for the PELCA Registry: Treatment of aorto-ostial disease with percutaneous excimer laser coronary angioplasty. Circulation 86(suppl I):I-513, 1992.

132. Roubin GS, Cannon AD, Agrawal SK, et al: Intracoronary stenting for acute and threatened closure complicating percutaneous transluminal coronary angioplasty. Circulation 85:916, 1992.

133. George BS, Voorhees WD III, Roubin GS, et al: Multicenter investigation of coronary stenting to treat acute or threatened closure after percutaneous transluminal coronary angioplasty. J Am Coll Cardiol 22:135, 1993.

134. Maiello L, Colombo A, Gianrossi R, et al: Coronary stenting for the treatment of acute or threatened closure following dissection after balloon angioplasty. Am Heart J 125:1570, 1993.

135. Serruys PW, de Jaegere P, Kiemeneij F, et al: A comparison of balloon-expandable stent implantation with balloon angioplasty in patients with coronary artery disease. N Engl J Med 331:489, 1994.

136. Fischman DL, Leon MB, Baim DS, et al: A randomized comparison of coronary-stent placement and balloon angioplasty in the treatment of coronary artery disease. N Engl J Med 331:496, 1994.

137. Wong SC, Leon MB: Stent implantation in saphenous vein grafts. Coron Artery Dis 5:575, 1994.

138. Urban P, Sigwart U, Golf S, et al: Intravascular stenting for stenosis of aortocoronary venous bypass grafts. J Am Coll Cardiol 13:1085, 1989.

139. de Scheerder IK, Strauss BH, de Feyter PJ, et al: Stenting of venous bypass grafts: A new treatment modality for patients who are poor candidates for reintervention. Am Heart J 123:1046, 1992.

140. Strauss BH, Serruys PW, Bertrand ME, et al: Quantitative angiographic follow-up of the coronary Wallstent in native vessels and bypass grafts (European experience—March 1986 to March 1990). Am J Cardiol 69:475, 1992.

141. Bilodeau L, Iyer S, Cannon AD, et al: Flexible coil stent (Cook, Inc.) in saphenous vein grafts: Clinical and angiographic follow-up. J Am Coll Cardiol 19:264A, 1992.

142. Pomerantz RM, Kuntz E, Carozza JP, et al: Acute and long-term outcome of narrowed saphenous venous grafts treated by endoluminal stenting and directional atherectomy. Am J Cardiol 70:161, 1992.

143. Fortuna R, Heuser RR, Garratt KN, et al: Wiktor intracoronary stent: Experience in the first 101 vein graft patients. Circulation 88(suppl I):I-309, 1993.

144. Dorros G, Bates MC, Kumar IK, et al: The use of Gianturco-Roubin flexible metallic coronary stents on old saphenous vein grafts: In-hospital outcome and 7 day angiographic patency. Eur Heart J 15:1456, 1994.

145. Fenton SH, Fischman DL, Savage MP, et al: Long-term angiographic and clinical outcome after implantation of balloon-expandable stents in aortocoronary saphenous vein grafts. Am J Cardiol 74:1187, 1994.

146. Keane D, Buis B, Reifart N, et al: Clinical and angiographic outcome following implantation of the new less shortening Wallstent in aortocoronary vein grafts: Introduction of a second generation stent in the clinical arena. J Interven Cardiol 7:557, 1994.

147. Eeckhout E, Goy J-J, Stauffer J-C, et al: Endoluminal stenting of narrowed saphenous vein grafts: Long-term clinical and angiographic follow-up. Cathet Cardiovasc Diagn 32:139, 1994.

148. Piana RN, Moscucci M, Cohen DJ, et al: Palmaz-Schatz stenting for treatment of focal vein graft stenosis: Immediate results and long-term outcome. J Am Coll Cardiol 23:1296, 1994.

149. Hardigan KR, Strumpf RK, Eagan JT Jr, et al: Single center Palmaz biliary stent experience in coronary arteries and saphenous vein grafts. Circulation 88(suppl I):I-308, 1993.

150. Wong SC, Popma JJ, Pichard AD, et al: Comparison of clinical and angiographic outcomes after saphenous vein graft angioplasty using coronary versus biliary tubular slotted stents. Circulation 91:339, 1995.

151. Rechavia E, Litvack F, Macko G, et al: Stent implantation of saphenous vein graft aorto-ostial lesions in patients with unstable ischemic syndromes: Immediate angiographic results and long-term clinical outcome. J Am Coll Cardiol 25:866, 1995.

152. Wong SC, Baim DS, Schatz RA, et al: Immediate results and late outcomes after stent implantation in saphenous vein graft lesions: The multi-center U.S. Palmaz-Schatz stent experience. J Am Coll Cardiol 26:704, 1995.

153. de Jaegere PP, van Domburg RT, de Feyter PJ, et al: Long-

term clinical outcome after stent implantation in saphenous vein grafts. J Am Coll Cardiol 28:89, 1996.

154. Wong SC, Hong MK, Popma JJ, et al: Stent placement for the treatment of aorto-ostial saphenous vein graft lesions. J Am Coll Cardiol 23:118A, 1994.

155. Colombo A, Hall P, Nakamura S, et al: Intracoronary stenting without anticoagulation accomplished with intravascular ultrasound guidance. Circulation 91:1676, 1995.

156. Schomig A, Neumann F-J, Kastrati A, et al: A randomized comparison of antiplatelet and anticoagulant therapy after the placement of coronary-artery stents. N Engl J Med 334:1084, 1996.

157. Leon MB, Ellis SG, Moses J, et al: Interim report from the reduced anticoagulation vein graft stent (RAVES) study. Circulation 94(suppl I):I-683, 1996.

158. Wong SC, Popma JJ, Chuang YC, et al: Economic impact of reduced anticoagulation after saphenous vein graft intervention. J Am Coll Cardiol 25:80A, 1995.

159. Savage MP, Douglas JS, Fischman DL, et al: Stent placement compared with balloon angioplasty for obstructed coronary bypass grafts. N Engl J Med 337:740 1997.

160. Hong MK, Pichard AD, Kent KM, et al: Assessing a strategy of stand-alone extraction atherectomy followed by staged stent placement in degenerated saphenous vein graft lesions. J Am Coll Cardiol 125:394A, 1995.

161. Hong MK, Wong SC, Popma JJ, et al: Favorable results of debulking followed by immediate adjunct stent therapy for high risk saphenous vein graft lesions J Am Coll Cardiol 27:179A, 1996.

162. Sketch MH Jr, Wong SC, Chuang YC, et al: Progressive deterioration in late (2 year) clinical outcomes after stent implantation in saphenous vein grafts: The multicenter JJIS experience. J Am Coll Cardiol 25:79A, 1995.

162a. Waksman R, White RL, Chan RC, et al: Intracoronary gamma-radiation therapy after angioplasty inhibits recurrence in patients with in-stent restenosis. Circulation 101:2165–2171, 2000.

163. Hartmann J, McKeever L, Teran J, et al: Prolonged infusion of urokinase for recanalization of chronically occluded aortocoronary bypass grafts. Am J Cardiol 61:189, 1988.

164. Hartmann JR, McKeever LS, Stamato NJ, et al: Recanalization of chronically occluded aortocoronary saphenous vein bypass grafts by extended infusion of urokinase: initial results and short-term clinical follow-up. J Am Coll Cardiol 18:1517, 1991.

165. Levine DJ, Sharaf BL, Williams DO: Late follow-up of patients with totally occluded saphenous vein grafts treated by prolonged selective urokinase infusion. J Am Coll Cardiol 19:292A, 1992.

166. Sabri MN, Johnson D, Warner M, et al: Intracoronary thrombolysis followed by directional atherectomy: A combined approach for thrombotic vein graft lesions considered unsuitable for angioplasty. Cathet Cardiovasc Diagn 26:15, 1992.

167. Eagan JT, Strumpf, Heuser RR, et al: New treatment approach for chronic total occlusions of saphenous vein grafts. Cathet Cardiovasc Diagn 29:62, 1993.

168. Lotan C, Mosseri M, Rosenman Y, et al: Combined mechanical and thrombolytic treatment for totally occluded bypass grafts. Br Heart J 74:455, 1994.

169. Grines CL, Booth DC, Nissen SE, et al: Mechanism of acute myocardial infarction in patients with prior coronary artery bypass grafting and therapeutic implications. Am J Cardiol 65:1292, 1990.

170. Kahn JK, Rutherford BD, McConahay DR, et al: Usefulness of angioplasty during acute myocardial infarction in patients with prior coronary artery bypass grafting. Am J Cardiol 65:698, 1990.

171. Little WC, Gwinn NS, Burrows MT, et al: Cause of acute myocardial infarction late after successful coronary artery bypass grafting. Am J Cardiol 65:808, 1990.

172. The GUSTO Investigators: An international randomized trial comparing four thrombolytic strategies for acute myocardial infarction. N Engl J Med 329:673, 1993.

173. Sketch MH Jr, Labinaz M, Nathan PE, et al: Acute care of the patient with previous bypass surgery. In Califf RM, Mark DB, Wagner GS (eds): Acute Coronary Care, 2nd ed, p 668. St. Louis: CV Mosby, 1995.

174. Reiner JS, Lundergan CF, Kopecky SL, et al: Ineffectiveness of thrombolysis for acute MI following vein graft occlusion. Circulation 94(suppl I):I-570 , 1996.

175. Santiago P, Vacek JL, Rosmond TL, et al: Comparison of results of coronary angioplasty during acute myocardial infarction with and without previous coronary bypass surgery. Am J Cardiol 72:1348, 1993.

176. Stone GW, Brodie B, Griffen I, et al: Primary angioplasty in patients with previous bypass surgery. Circulation 94(suppl I):I-243, 1996.

177. Perrault LP, Carrier M, Hudson G, et al: Transluminal angioplasty of the subclavian artery in patients with internal mammary grafts. Ann Thorac Surg 56:927, 1993.

178. Holmes JR, Crane R. Coronary steal through a patent internal mammary artery graft: Treatment by subclavian angioplasty. Am Heart J 125:1166, 1993.

179. Breall JA, Kim D, Baim DS, et al: Coronary-subclavian steal: An unusual case of angina pectoris after successful internal mammary-coronary artery bypass grafting. Cathet Cardiovasc Diagn 24:274, 1991.

180. Breall JA, Grossman W, Stillman IE, et al: Atherectomy of the subclavian artery for patients with symptomatic coronary-subclavian steal syndrome. J Am Coll Cardiol 21:1564, 1993.

181. Dooris M, Safian RD: Coronary artery bypass grafts. In Freed M, Grines C, Safian RD (eds): The New Manual of Interventional Cardiology, p 340. Birmingham, MI: Physician's Press, 1996.

182. Mishkel GJ, Willinsky R: Combined PTCA and microcoil embolization of a left internal mammary artery graft. Cathet Cardiovasc Diagn 27:141, 1992.

183. Sbarouni E, Corr L, Fenech A:. Microcoil embolization of large intercostal branches of internal mammary artery grafts. Cathet Cardiovasc Diagn 31:334, 1994.

184. Blankenhorn DH, Nessini SA, Johnson Rl, et al: Beneficial effects of combined colestipol-niacin therapy on coronary atherosclerosis and coronary venous bypass grafts. JAMA 257:3233, 1987.

185. The Post Coronary Artery Bypass Trial Investigators: The effect of aggressive lowering of low-density lipoprotein cholesterol levels and low-dose anticoagulation on obstructive changes in saphenous-vein coronary-artery bypass grafts. N Engl J Med 336:153, 1997.

186. Solymoss BC, Nadeau P, Millette D, et al: Late thrombosis of saphenous vein bypass grafts related to risk factors. Circulation 78:140, 1988.

186a. Carlino M, De Gregorio D, Di Mario C, et al: Prevention of distal embolization during saphenous vein graft lesion angioplasty. Experience with a new temporary occlusion and aspiration system. Circulation 99:3221–3223, 1999.

187. The EPIC Investigators: Use of a monoclonal antibody directed against the platelet glycoprotein IIb/IIIa receptor in high risk coronary intervention. N Engl J Med 330:956, 1994.

188. Ward SR, Lincoff AM, Miller DP, et al: Clinical outcome is improved at 30 days regardless of pre-treatment clinical and angiographic risk in patients receiving abciximab for angioplasty: Results from the EPILOG study. Circulation 94(suppl I):I-198, 1996.

189. Challapalli RM, Eisenberg MJ, Sigmon K, et al: Platelet glycoprotein IIb/IIIa monoclonal antibody (c7E3) reduces distal embolization during percutaneous intervention of saphenous vein grafts. Circulation 94(suppl I):I-60, 1996.

190. Tcheng JE, Anderson K, Tardiff BE, et al: Reducing the risk of percutaneous intervention after coronary bypass surgery: Beneficial effects of abciximab treatment. J Am Coll Cardiol 29:187A, 1996.

# 15

# The Economics of Percutaneous Coronary Intervention

*David J. Cohen*    *Craig A. Sukin*

Since 1990, discussions and concerns about medical costs have moved from the esoteric domain of the economist and the health service researcher to the center stage of public attention. Medical costs now receive more attention in the national lay press than they do in major journals. Unfortunately, much of this coverage is negative and repeats a single troublesome question: Is the United States spending too much for health care and getting too little in return? One area that has received particular scrutiny and is likely to remain under close watch in the future is percutaneous coronary revascularization.

Since its original description by Gruentzig and coworkers,[1] percutaneous transluminal coronary angioplasty (PTCA) has undergone tremendous growth and development. More than 300,000 procedures are performed each year in the United States alone, and coronary angioplasty is now performed more commonly than coronary artery bypass grafting (CABG). The technical aspects of coronary intervention have evolved rapidly. Devices available to the interventional cardiologist now include stents, lasers, and atherectomy catheters, and many other new devices are under clinical investigation. Moreover, coronary interventionalists are beginning to reap the benefits of the biotechnology revolution with the development of important medical adjuncts to angioplasty, such as the platelet glycoprotein IIb/IIIa receptor antagonists.

As these procedures have developed and proliferated, their contribution to medical costs has grown as well. The cost of percutaneous coronary intervention is currently estimated at $3 billion per year and the cost of all forms of coronary revascularization at between $15 and $20 billion in the United States alone. Because the field is rapidly evolving, there is clearly a need for understanding the impact of each component of the interventional armamentarium on clinical outcomes and costs relative to other available therapies, including medical therapy and CABG. The purpose of this chapter is to provide an overview of the current knowledge regarding the economic aspects of percutaneous coronary revascularization.

## MEDICAL CARE COST CONCEPTS

The financial terminology used in the health care industry is complex and often confusing. Part of the reason for this is that health care economists, health service researchers, hospital accountants, and administrators are each involved in the arena of medical costs, but each has a different perspective and, consequently, different disciplines. The economist attempts to understand the human behavior of production and consumption of societal resources through the development and testing of theories and through empirical data analysis. To an economist, "costs" are a convenient numerical metric that can be used to assign a common scale value to the consumption of resources. A key assumption of economics is that resources are limited and that a person or a society must choose among alternative resources, as in Paul Samuelson's classic example of a society considering "guns versus butter": With more resources diverted to the production of weapons, less will be available to produce food.

Resources are usually subsumed under broad generic categories, such as labor and equipment. In the pricing of goods or services, accountants determine prices on the basis of the cost of purchasing these resources, plus an adequate markup for profit. Purchasers make rational decisions on the basis of knowledge of the product and available alternatives. In the typical free market economies, providers of goods or services compete on the basis of price.

However, the health care market meets almost none of the classical criteria for a competitive free market. Traditionally, prices have not been an accurate reflection of resource cost, and hospitals and doctors have not competed on the basis of price.[2] Consumers have not been well informed and do not have adequate information to make purchasing decisions; in some cases, they are not in a physical or mental state to make such decisions. Much more commonly, doctors and hospitals have competed on the basis of technologic advances—not price. Price competition has not been deemed necessary by most Americans, because they are exempted from paying for care directly at the point of purchase. Third-party payers (the insurance carriers and the governmental agencies) pay the bills.

This lack of traditional market forces in the medical arena is one major reason for the substantial distortions in the prices assigned to medical goods and services. In a practice called *cost-shifting*, hospitals inflate or deflate various prices to maximize the reimbursement to the hospital. Hospitals justify these techniques by pointing to problems affecting the cost of health care delivery.[3] First, most hospitals treat a good number of patients from whom they do not receive reimbursement equal to the cost of the treatment. Care for other paying patients must therefore cover the cost of care for these patients. Second, some key hospital departments may not have a sufficient volume of patients or services to generate adequate revenues; therefore, the departments that generate strong revenues must cover the weak ones. For example, to help cover the costs of an obstetrics unit that loses money, the hospital administration may price cardiac catheterization substantially above its true costs. Thus, hospital charges are not an accurate reflection of true hospital resource costs.[4]

The first major terminologic distinction exists between medical charges and medical costs. Because of the aforementioned distortion in the market forces affecting the production and consumption of health care, both hospitals and physicians tend to inflate their charges above a true market price and above the costs of the resources involved in producing a given health care product or service. In this chapter, the term *cost* is synonymous with the dollar value of the resources consumed in the production of a particularly medical commodity.

Several other cost terms are worth mentioning because they appear in the medical economics literature with some regularity. Accountants originated the concept of direct versus indirect cost to be able to classify costs according to whether they could be traced to a particular object or service.[5,6] *Direct costs* are those that can be linked directly to a given medical care service or product. For example, in a coronary angioplasty procedure, the disposable supplies (e.g., angiographic catheters, tubing, and contrast dye) and the personnel time (e.g., physician, nurse, technician) required for the procedure would all be classified as direct. *Indirect costs*, on the other hand, are not attributable to a specific service or product. Commonly referred to as *overhead*, indirect costs include the depreciation or rent

on the catheterization laboratory rooms and equipment as well as laundry service, electricity, maintenance, billing, and medical records. Accountants are interested in distinguishing direct versus indirect costs so that they can ensure that all expenditures are accounted for and matched up against appropriate revenues in the overall hospital or clinic budget.

A different set of cost terms relates to the behavior of costs as the amounts of medical goods and services produced are either increased or decreased relative to some initial level. *Variable costs* are those that change with unit changes in volume. For example, in the catheterization laboratory, disposable supplies (e.g., catheters, intravenous tubing, contrast dye) would all be variable costs because the amount of these items needed is directly related to the number of catheterization procedures performed each day. *Fixed costs*, alternatively, do not change with small changes in production volume. For example, the facility cost of the catheterization laboratory is fixed because it is not necessary to build a new laboratory each time a catheterization procedure is performed. Once the laboratory exists, the costs associated with having that laboratory are the same, regardless of how frequently it is used. Such costs are often expressed in terms of depreciation over a fixed period of time, such as the useful life span of the building or equipment. Many costs do not fit comfortably into the fixed and variable distinction, and several hybrid categories have been created. A more complete discussion of this issue is provided elsewhere.[5-7]

Two additional terms that are frequently used in medical economics are *marginal cost* and *incremental cost*. Marginal cost is the cost of producing one more or one less unit of product, such as cardiac catheterization and coronary angioplasty, per unit of time. Thus, marginal cost is synonymous with variable cost. In contrast, incremental cost is commonly used to indicate the cost differences incurred by shifting groups of patients from one diagnostic or therapeutic strategy to another. The distinction between marginal and incremental costs is thus one of degree, and some health economists use the terms synonymously.

## TYPES OF MEDICAL ECONOMIC STUDIES

One of the major objectives of an economic analysis of a new drug, device, or strategy is to discover the ways in which the new strategy will alter costs for the patients so treated. Fundamentally, this requires an understanding of the resource consumption patterns and associated variable costs of the new strategy versus the reference strategy (often referred to as *usual* or *standard* care). For a new interventional procedure, this would include equipment and supply costs as well as personnel costs required for the performance of the procedure. It is also critical to determine whether additional diagnostic or therapeutic procedures or complications are added or averted as a consequence of implementing the new strategy and the cost effects of these changes in practice and outcome.[8]

In any comparison of new medical strategies with conventional care, there are three main possibilities: (1) the new strategy may provide better outcomes than the old, (2) the outcomes may be the same, or (3) the new strategy may prove to be inferior. In general, inferior strategies would be considered for adoption only if they were accompanied by substantial cost savings and only if the health care system were forced by external constraints to accept inferior outcomes because of a need to control costs through rationing of care. With equivalent effectiveness, cost may end up being the deciding point in the choice between the new strategy and the old. If the new strategy is more costly but provides no better outcomes, there is no reason to employ it. If, however, the new strategy is able to provide the equivalent outcome at a lower total cost, then it may rapidly become the preferred approach. Most commonly, however, a new strategy is shown to have some increase in effectiveness relative to conventional care but is also significantly more costly.

Empirical studies of medical cost outcomes serve two important functions. First, they provide an empirical basis for understanding how the new technology or strategy affects resource use and cost relative to the reference strategy. Second, in the common situation in which effectiveness is improved but costs are also increased, empirical cost studies provide the database for cost-effectiveness models to examine the question of whether the new technology or strategy is sufficiently worthwhile for it to be adopted by the medical community. Thus, it is important to recognize the technical distinction between a cost study, which seeks to determine how much a new method of percutaneous revascularization costs relative to standard revascularization techniques, and a cost-effectiveness analysis, which seeks to answer the question of whether the new technique represents a worthwhile investment of societal health care dollars given that the total amount of dollars available for spending on health care is fixed.

## Cost-Effectiveness Analysis

Cost effectiveness is a frequently misunderstood concept in medical economics. Although most clinicians assume that *cost effective* is synonymous with *worthwhile* in a broad sense, the term actually refers to a specific comparison of incremental costs and medical outcomes among two or more alternative management strategies for a particular disease or clinical problem that is expressed in ratio form.[7, 8] It is critical to understand that cost-effectiveness analysis always involves a comparison with some explicit alternative investment of dollars, so that it is impossible to pronounce some treatment or strategy as cost effective in isolation. In addition, there is no level of the cost-effectiveness ratio that is universally agreed to represent the dividing point between those investments that are worthwhile and those that are not. The assessment of what is economically attractive falls primarily in the domain of health policy. Cost-effectiveness data may contribute to that assessment but not to the exclusion of other considerations. Thus, the role of cost-effectiveness analysis is to define in a structured format how a given health care expenditure will improve the overall health of a specific population relative to other potential uses for the same health care dollars.

Cost-effectiveness analysis involves measurement or estimation of two quantities that are then expressed as an *incremental cost-effectiveness ratio:* the difference in costs between one strategy and the other divided by the difference in health outcomes (Table 15–1). The notion of incremental costs is critical to an understanding of cost-effectiveness analysis. In a comparison of two treatment strategies for coronary disease patients, for example, those resources or costs that both strategies incur in equal amounts do not contribute to the incremental cost figure and hence can be ignored.

On the effectiveness side, there are several different ways of proceeding (see Table 15–1). Most commonly, analysts choose to express the denominator of the ratio in terms of incremental life expectancy, and the resulting cost-effectiveness ratios are framed in terms of dollars per additional life year saved. However, one of the major problems in this type of analysis is that it is very difficult to obtain empirical life expectancy data for diseases that are not rapidly fatal. In addition, even when such data are available, they usually do not pertain exactly to the population of interest, or they necessarily describe the outcome of that population from an earlier era when available treatments were not as effective as they currently are. For all these reasons, life expectancy in cost-effectiveness analysis is almost always based on a pooled analysis of the available empirical survival data plus an extrapolation for the remaining years of life obtained by use of some form of parametric survival function. Most commonly, the assumption is made that the mortality rate from the disease of interest remains constant for these remaining years of life and thus can be described by a simple expo-

**TABLE 15–1.  EXAMPLES OF CALCULATIONS FOR COST-EFFECTIVENESS AND COST-UTILITY ANALYSIS**

| STRATEGY | TREATMENT COSTS | EFFECTIVENESS (LIFE EXPECTANCY) | QUALITY-OF-LIFE WEIGHT (UTILITY) | QUALITY-ADJUSTED LIFE EXPECTANCY |
|---|---|---|---|---|
| Treatment A | $20,000 | 4.5 years | 0.80 | 3.6 QALYs |
| Treatment B | $10,000 | 3.5 years | 0.90 | 3.15 QALYs |
| Incremental cost-effectiveness ratio | $\frac{\$20,000 - \$10,000}{4.5 - 3.5 \text{ years}}$ | = $10,000/life year saved | | |
| Incremental cost-utility ratio | $\frac{\$20,000 - \$10,000}{3.6 - 3.15 \text{ QALYs}}$ | = $22,222/QALY gained | | |

QALY, quality-adjusted life year.

nential survival function.[8] It is not obligatory in cost-effectiveness analysis to use life expectancy in the denominator, and some analysts have chosen to express the ratio in terms of additional life years saved over a 5-year follow-up period or some other arbitrary period. In addition, it is possible to express the ratio in terms of an intermediate outcome, such as change in functional status. The main drawback of using a denominator other than life expectancy is that it becomes very difficult to judge the resulting cost-effectiveness ratio against reference standards that reflect other economic choices. For this reason, despite all the approximations required, most analysts still use estimated changes in life expectancy in their cost-effectiveness calculations.

If the new therapy under study changes life expectancy without any effect on quality of life, then the type of cost-effectiveness analysis described earlier is most appropriate. However, if both the quantity and the quality of life are changed (either in the same direction or in opposite directions), then expressing the cost-effectiveness ratio in terms of additional life years saved may be insufficient. In

such situations, net health benefits are generally measured in terms of *quality-adjusted life years* (QALYs). In this framework, each year of life expectancy is weighted by a *utility* factor that reflects an individual's preference for his or her state of health relative to perfect health (utility = 1) and death (utility = 0).[8]

Once the cost-effectiveness ratio is constructed, it is typically compared with other ratios in what is commonly referred to as a *league table*[10–15] (Table 15–2). This final step in the analytic process is designed to allow health policy researchers and decision makers to judge how the new therapy or strategy compares with alternative expenditures of health care dollars. Although there is no absolute standard for cost effectiveness, rough thresholds may be established by such comparisons. In general, cost-effectiveness ratios of less than $20,000 per quality-adjusted year of life gained—such as those for the treatment of severe diastolic hypertension[10–15] and cholesterol lowering in patients with established coronary heart disease[11, 14]—are viewed as highly favorable.[17] Incremental cost-effectiveness

**TABLE 15–2.  LEAGUE TABLE OF COMPARATIVE COST-EFFECTIVENESS RATIOS**

| TARGET POPULATION (REFERENCE) | TREATMENT | COMPARISON TREATMENT | C/E RATIO ($ PER LIFE YEAR SAVED) |
|---|---|---|---|
| CAD secondary prevention[10] | Aspirin | No aspirin | $0–$500 |
| Hypercholesterolemia, secondary prevention (CHL = 261)[11] | Simvastatin | Diet alone | $5000–$10,000 |
| Left main disease[12] | CABG | Medical treatment | $9200 |
| Severe hypertension[13] | Propranolol | No medication | $18,000 |
| Chronic renal failure[17] | Outpatient hemodialysis | No dialysis | $35,000 |
| Mild hypertension[13] | Medication | No medication | $41,900 |
| Hypercholesterolemia, primary prevention (men aged 55–64 years, CHL > 300 mg/dL, 2 additional risk factors)[14] | Lovastatin, 20 mg/d | No medication | $41,800 |
| Hypercholesterolemia, primary prevention (men aged 55–64 years, CHL > 300 mg/dL, no additional risk factors)[14] | Lovastatin, 20 mg/d | No medication | $58,000 |
| Acute renal failure, ICU patient[15] | Hospital hemodialysis | No dialysis | $128,000 |
| Low-risk patients undergoing cardiac catheterization[16] | Nonionic contrast | Ionic contrast | $220,000 |

C/E, cost-effectiveness; CABG, coronary artery bypass grafting; CAD, coronary artery disease; CHL, serum cholesterol level (mg/dL); ICU, intensive care unit.

ratios between $20,000 and $40,000 per QALY are also consistent with many accepted medical treatments and may be viewed as reasonably cost effective as well. Conversely, cost-effectiveness ratios greater than $80,000 to $100,000 are higher than most generally accepted medical treatments and are thus viewed as relatively unattractive in most medical systems.[17]

## COST STUDIES OF INTERVENTIONAL THERAPIES IN NON–MYOCARDIAL INFARCTION PATIENTS

### PTCA for Single-Vessel Disease

Two important issues must be addressed in any evaluation of the costs and other economic implications of coronary angioplasty: the appropriate reference strategy (e.g., medicine, CABG) and the major determinants of cost outcomes. Coronary angioplasty was initially proposed as a less invasive, low-cost alternative to coronary bypass surgery. Over the past decade, however, the cumulative experience with this technology would suggest that more often it represents a more invasive, high-cost alternative to medical therapy. Any economic evaluation of coronary angioplasty must therefore be placed in an appropriate clinical context, as discussed in other sections of this book. In any economic comparison of PTCA with CABG or medication, for example, the percentage of the coronary artery disease population for whom the comparison is relevant must be kept in mind.

Although it is common for clinicians and others to wonder what a coronary angioplasty costs, it is important to recognize that one dollar figure cannot appropriately represent the cost of PTCA any more than one mortality rate can represent the true mortality rate for all acute myocardial infarction (MI) patients. Costs vary in complex and as yet incompletely defined ways, and medical costs do not always relate to medical outcomes in easily predictable ways. We have found it convenient to analyze cost determinants in four general categories: (1) patient-specific, (2) provider-specific, (3) treatment-specific, and (4) geographic-economic factors. The patient-specific (e.g., age, sex, disease severity) and treatment-specific factors are analogous to the determinants of medical outcomes that are traditionally evaluated. However, provider-specific and geographic-economic factors can have an important influence on medical costs independent of any baseline characteristic or medical outcome factors and are often what distinguish the ideal cost situation from the actual one.

With these caveats in mind, it is possible to cite some representative figures for PTCA costs from the literature. Topol and coworkers[18] studied a private insurance claims database of 2100 PTCA patients and found an average hospital charge of approximately $10,000 for the baseline hospitalization, with an additional $4000 for physician fees and $4000 to $5000 more in charges during the first year after the procedure. Similar hospital charges were found in a series of 119 elective PTCA patients treated at Duke during 1986.[19] As suggested by the preceding section, both of these charge figures would be expected to overestimate substantially the true marginal cost of providing PTCA.

Cohen and colleagues,[20] from the Beth Israel Hospital in Boston, calculated total hospital costs from hospital charges in 113 elective PTCA patients and obtained an average direct cost of $5400 (excluding the diagnostic catheterization); the procedural laboratory cost accounted for $2940 of this total. In the multicenter Coronary Angioplasty Versus Excisional Atherectomy Trial (CAVEAT), mean hospital costs (calculated from charges) for the PTCA arm were $8300.[21] More recently, the average initial hospital cost for patients treated with conventional balloon angioplasty in the Balloon vs. Optimal Atherectomy Trial (BOAT) was $8600, including procedural costs of nearly $3400.[22] Thus, it seems that a representative hospitalization for coronary angioplasty in 1997 would likely cost from $5500 to $8500, without taking into account the cost of the preceding diagnostic catheterization.

Understanding whether angioplasty is economically attractive requires more than a simple grasp of the procedural and hospital costs. This determination requires comparison of the costs and the clinical benefits of PTCA with alternative management strategies. For most patients currently undergoing PTCA, the appropriate strategy for comparison is medical therapy. Unfortunately, to date, there have not been any published empirical cost comparisons of PTCA and medical therapy. Initial results in a large consecutive cohort of patients with coronary artery disease from the Duke cardiovascular database have shown that the initial costs of PTCA are at least twice those of initial medical therapy.[23] In the only randomized trial to compare PTCA with medical therapy, the Angioplasty Compared to Medicine (ACME) investigators found that medical resource utilization was considerably higher for patients assigned to initial PTCA than for those assigned to initial medical therapy. Specifically, PTCA patients were hospitalized for a mean of 3.8 days during the 6-month study period, compared with 2.4 days on average for medically treated patients.[24] Moreover, 7% of patients assigned to PTCA underwent bypass surgery (emergent or elective) during follow-up, compared with none of the medical therapy patients ($p < 0.01$). Unfortunately, because the ACME trial was performed in the Veterans

Administration system, no direct medical care cost comparison was performed. Nonetheless, the ACME trial clearly demonstrates that compared with medical therapy, balloon angioplasty increases short- and intermediate-term medical care costs.

Given the higher cost of interventional therapy for most patients, the cost effectiveness of PTCA for patients with single-vessel disease depends on whether the benefits of such therapy are worth the cost. In the case of PTCA for single-vessel disease, no study to date has demonstrated that percutaneous coronary revascularization prolongs life expectancy. In fact, given the generally excellent long-term prognosis of such patients with medical therapy,[25] it is difficult to imagine that any form of revascularization therapy would offer a significant survival advantage.

To date, only one study has formally examined the cost effectiveness of balloon angioplasty for patients with single-vessel coronary disease.[26] In 1989, Wong and colleagues[26] developed a computer simulation model to estimate the relative cost effectiveness of angioplasty, bypass surgery, and conservative (i.e., medical) therapy for patients with chronic stable angina. For the purposes of analysis, patients were grouped by age, gender, coronary anatomy, ventricular function, and severity of angina. For each group, lifetime medical care costs and quality-adjusted life expectancy were estimated by the model, and cost-effectiveness ratios were calculated.

The investigators found that compared with medical therapy, angioplasty increased quality-adjusted life expectancy in all patient subgroups, regardless of the severity of angina, the ventricular function, or the number of diseased vessels. In general, angioplasty appeared to be reasonably cost effective compared with medical therapy for all patients with single-vessel disease, except those with very mild angina. For example, in patients with severe angina, normal ventricular function, and single-vessel left anterior descending coronary artery disease, the quality-adjusted life expectancy with angioplasty as initial therapy was 18.3 QALYs, compared with 17.4 QALYs with initial conservative therapy, with an estimated cost-effectiveness ratio of $6000 per QALY gained. Moreover, their model predicted that PTCA was highly cost effective compared with medical therapy for all subgroups of patients with single-vessel disease and severe angina (incremental cost-effectiveness ratios <$10,000/QALY). For patients with only mild angina, however, initial PTCA was projected to be significantly less cost effective, with incremental cost-effectiveness ratios on the order of $80,000 to $100,000/QALY.

Although these analyses are based on data from the late 1980s, it is unlikely that incorporation of more recent data would change their findings appreciably. If anything, one would suspect that the cost effectiveness of PTCA for single-vessel coronary artery disease has improved since the late 1980s. Since then, the development of new devices—particularly intracoronary stents—and adjunctive antiplatelet therapy has led to significant improvements in the outcomes of percutaneous coronary revascularization.[27-30] Concurrently, the hospital costs of balloon angioplasty have decreased as a result of reductions in resource costs as well as improved efficiency of practice (e.g., combined diagnostic angiography and percutaneous revascularization, routine same-day sheath removal).[31, 32] For example, at Boston's Beth Israel Hospital, the typical length of stay for uncomplicated PTCA has fallen from 3 days to 1 since the early 1990s. Thus, although ideal data are not available (and rarely are), the best available data suggest that balloon angioplasty is reasonably cost effective for patients with single-vessel coronary disease and severe angina but is only marginally cost effective for patients with mild angina or no symptoms. If studies suggesting that PTCA may improve survival in patients with chronic stable angina and silent myocardial ischemia can be confirmed,[33] the cost effectiveness of PTCA compared with medical therapy would improve even further.

## Percutaneous Versus Surgical Revascularization for Multivessel Disease

As alternative means of mechanical revascularization, considerable attention has been focused on the relative economic impacts of balloon angioplasty and coronary bypass surgery on patients with multivessel coronary disease. To date, at least nine studies have compared PTCA costs with those of CABG (Table 15–3). In contrast to single-vessel disease, in which observational data and simulation models provide the only insight into the cost effectiveness of PTCA, in the case of multivessel disease, at least five randomized clinical trials have been performed that have compared conventional PTCA with bypass surgery.

Although each of these studies has specific inclusion and exclusion criteria and have used different time frames and cost measurement techniques, several general observations can still be made. First, the initial hospital cost of PTCA is approximately 30% to 50% lower than that of bypass surgery, and these cost savings persist for the first year of follow-up. The absolute magnitude of this cost difference is highly dependent on the cost accounting methodology used. In a 1986 study, Hlatky and colleagues,[19] at Duke University, found that hospital charges for bypass surgery were more than $10,000 higher than

## TABLE 15–3.    COST STUDIES COMPARING BALLOON ANGIOPLASTY WITH BYPASS SURGERY

| STUDY | DATE | METHOD | N | NO. OF DISEASED VESSELS | COST MEASURE | TIME PERIOD | PTCA COST | CABG COST |
|---|---|---|---|---|---|---|---|---|
| Reeder et al[34] | 1979–1981 | OBS | 168 | 1, 2, 3 | Medical charges | Initial hospitalization<br>1 year | $7571<br>$11,384 | $12,154<br>$13,387 |
| Kelly et al[35] | | OBS | 163 | 1, 2, 3 | Hospital and MD charges | 1 year | $7689 | $13,559 |
| Hlatky et al[19] | 1986–1987 | OBS | 389 | 1, 2, 3 | Hospital charges | Initial hospitalization | $9556 | $19,644 |
| Cohen et al[20] | 1990–1991 | OBS | 202 | 1 (PTCA) 1, 2, 3 (CABG) | Hospital and procedural costs | Initial hospitalization | $5396 | $20,937 |
| Weintraub et al[36] | 1984–1985 | OBS | | 2 | Hospital charges, cost model | 5-year cumulative | $19,305 | $24,182 |
| RITA[37] | 1993–1994 | RCT | 999 | 2, 3 | Hospital costs | Initial hospitalization<br>London center<br>Non-London center | <br>£3753<br>£3024 | <br>£7319<br>£5722 |
| | | | | | Hospital, procedural, medication costs | 2-year total costs<br>London center<br>Non-London center | <br>£6916<br>£5448 | <br>£8739<br>£6498 |
| EAST[38] | 1987–1990 | RCT | 384 | 2, 3 | Hospital costs and MD charges | Initial hospitalization<br>3-year total costs | $16,223<br>$23,734 | $24,005<br>$25,310 |
| BARI[39] | 1988–1995 | RCT | 952 | 2, 3 | Hospital and outpatient costs, MD fees | Initial revascularization<br>5-year total cost | $21,113<br>$56,225 | $32,347<br>$58,889 |

BARI, Bypass Angioplasty Revascularization Investigation; CABG, coronary artery bypass grafting; EAST, Emory Angioplasty vs. Surgery Trial; MD, physician; OBS, observational study; PTCA, percutaneous transluminal coronary angioplasty; RCT, randomized controlled trial; RITA, Randomized Intervention Treatment of Angina.

those for PTCA ($19,644 vs. $9556). However, the estimated difference in hospital cost narrowed considerably when charges were converted to costs. For example, when only the costs of supplies were considered to be variable, the cost difference between balloon angioplasty and bypass surgery was estimated to be only $1900. When it was assumed that the costs of both supplies and personnel were variable, the difference increased to $4600. Finally, when all costs were assumed to be variable (as they would be in the long run), the cost difference was approximately $7800. Regardless of the accounting methodology used, however, the initial cost of PTCA remained about half that of bypass surgery in this study.

Second, despite the substantial initial cost savings with multivessel PTCA, over a 3- to 5-year follow-up period, much of these initial cost savings is lost because of the need for repeat PTCA or bypass surgery in approximately 50% of patients. Weintraub and colleagues[38] recently reported 3-year economic data for 384 patients randomly assigned to balloon angioplasty or bypass surgery in the Emory Angioplasty vs. Surgery Trial (EAST). Initial hospital costs and professional charges for the PTCA group were an average of $16,223, compared with $24,005 for the CABG group (see Table 15–3). By the end of 3 years of follow-up, however, mean PTCA costs had

increased to 93% of those for bypass surgery, and the difference was no longer statistically significant. In patients with focal two-vessel disease, however, the 3-year cost of PTCA remained significantly lower than that of bypass surgery ($20,875 ± 13,533 vs. $23,639 ± 6848, $p < 0.001$). Similarly, in the Randomized Intervention Treatment of Angina (RITA) study, initial hospital costs in the PTCA arm were 52% of those in the CABG group.[37] This difference narrowed considerably during follow-up, and by 2 years after initial treatment, aggregate costs in the PTCA group were 80% of those initially treated with coronary bypass surgery.

Finally, results of a 5-year economic substudy of the Bypass Angioplasty Revascularization Investigation (BARI) have been reported.[39] To date, this study represents the largest and most comprehensive economic evaluation of alternative revascularization strategies for patients with multivessel coronary disease. Among 934 patients randomly assigned to initial PTCA or bypass surgery, initial medical care costs were 35% lower with PTCA ($21,113 vs. $32,347). Over the first 3 years of follow-up, this cost difference narrowed progressively, such that by the end of 5 years of follow-up, aggregate costs with PTCA remained slightly (5%) but significantly lower than those with bypass surgery ($56,225 vs. $58,889, $p = 0.047$). Subgroup analysis demonstrated that

PTCA remained approximately $6000 less expensive than CABG for patients with two-vessel disease, but 5-year costs were no different for patients with three-vessel disease. Because bypass surgery was associated with a trend toward improved survival in BARI, formal cost-effectiveness analysis was performed to determine whether routine CABG would be economically attractive for such patients. The BARI investigators found the overall cost-effectiveness ratio for bypass surgery in comparison with angioplasty to be $26,000 per year of life gained. Although this analysis suggests that CABG may be an economically attractive initial revascularization strategy for patients with multivessel disease, the confidence limits around this cost-effectiveness ratio were wide and included a 13% probability that the cost-effectiveness ratio was greater than $100,000/life year gained. Further analyses will be required to identify patient- and treatment-specific determinants of long-term cost and cost effectiveness in these populations.

Published studies on cost effectiveness to date have compared only conventional balloon angioplasty with coronary bypass surgery. It is possible that advances in adjunctive pharmacotherapy and newer percutaneous interventions—particularly coronary stenting—might eventually affect clinical outcomes sufficiently to achieve meaningful long-term cost savings compared with bypass surgery in patients with multivessel disease. Two major randomized clinical trials comparing multivessel stenting with bypass surgery are currently being planned (Arterial Revascularization Therapies Study [ARTS], Surgery or Stent [SOS]) and will include prospective evaluations of both health care costs and quality of life.

In summary, both observational studies and randomized trials have consistently demonstrated that multivessel PTCA is considerably less resource intensive and less costly than bypass surgery during initial hospitalization. However, because of the need for more frequent repeat revascularization procedures, the initial economic advantage of multivessel PTCA diminishes over time. Because bypass surgery does not appear to confer a survival benefit compared with multivessel PTCA (except possibly for diabetics),[40, 41] quality-of-life outcomes should play an important role in determining the relative cost effectiveness of these procedures. In general, the randomized trials have shown that initial recovery is quicker after PTCA, but at 1 to 3 years of follow-up, patients treated with initial PTCA have more frequent angina and require more antianginal medications.[38, 39, 42] Beyond 3 years of follow-up, however, these modest advantages of bypass surgery are largely attenuated. In BARI, for example, there were no major differences in quality of life between the PTCA and CABG groups at 5-year follow-up.[39] Because the current evidence suggests that most of the clinical and economic differences between PTCA and CABG for the treatment of multivessel coronary disease are minor and transient, neither procedure is clearly superior on the grounds of cost effectiveness. Thus, the choice of a revascularization procedure for multivessel coronary disease remains a complex decision that must be made on the basis of multiple factors, including clinical judgment, anatomic considerations, and individual patient preference.

## Newer Percutaneous Interventional Devices

As described in detail elsewhere in this book, coronary angioplasty represents a significant addition to the therapeutic armamentarium of the cardiologist, but it is far from perfect. Despite considerable technical advances from its earliest days, conventional PTCA remains limited by short-term complications, including abrupt vessel closure (often resulting in acute myocardial infarction or emergent bypass surgery) in 4% to 8% of patients and symptomatic restenosis requiring additional revascularization procedures in 25% to 40% of initially successful interventions. In addition, a substantial proportion of patients with significant obstructive coronary disease are technically unsuitable for coronary angioplasty. These limitations of conventional PTCA have prompted the development of new devices, including atherectomy catheters (directional, rotational, extraction), excimer laser angioplasty, and coronary stents. Although economic analyses of these devices have generally lagged behind their proliferation in clinical practice, numerous single-center observational studies and controlled clinical trials have been performed for these devices. Because most of the clinical studies have addressed the issue of whether these new techniques are truly superior to balloon angioplasty, the primary focus of economic studies is the incremental cost difference between the new technique and conventional PTCA.

CORONARY STENTS. Of the new interventional techniques, coronary stenting has undergone the closest economic scrutiny. Several factors have contributed to this intense interest. First, coronary stenting is expensive. In 1997, the price of a single Palmaz-Schatz coronary stent was $1650—more than four times the cost of a typical angioplasty balloon. Moreover, coronary stents are the only non-reusable interventional device. Thus, stenting of lesions longer than 15 or 20 mm (the lengths of the approved coronary stents available in the United States today) or of multiple vessels requires the use of multiple stents. However, intracoronary stenting is also the first new coronary intervention to demonstrate improved angiographic[43–45] and clinical[44, 45] outcomes over those of conventional balloon angioplasty. As a result, the use of stents has grown rapidly, raising concerns that their overuse might have undesirable economic consequences.[46–48]

Three observational studies have examined the relative costs of stenting and balloon angioplasty (Table 15–4). In 1991, Dick and colleagues[49] examined hospital *charges* for patients undergoing elective stenting or PTCA at the University of Michigan. They found that catheterization laboratory charges (including devices) were $2600 higher for stenting and that overall hospital charges were nearly $6300 higher ($12,574 vs. $6220). This study was limited by the small number of stent patients included (N = 27) as well as by the use of charges as a surrogate for costs. Cohen and colleagues[20] studied in-hospital costs of 211 patients undergoing elective single-vessel coronary revascularization at Boston's Beth Israel Hospital in 1990 and 1991. They found that elective stenting increased overall *costs* by approximately $2500 compared with conventional PTCA. Only

30% of the higher cost of stenting was due to procedural costs, however. The increased length of stay required for initiation of oral anticoagulation after stenting was associated with substantial increases in room/nursing costs and other ancillary services. Moreover, the higher incidence of major vascular complications (transfusion, surgical repair) in stent patients (9% vs. 1%) accounted for approximately 20% of the higher cost of stenting in this study. Finally, in 1993, Ellis and colleagues[52] at the Cleveland Clinic found that stenting increased median hospital costs by more than $6000. During the time period of this study, many of their patients underwent stenting emergently to treat PTCA-induced complications, however, and in a model controlling for preprocedural and procedural variables, use of a coronary stent itself was associated with only a 25% increase in cost.

To date, the Stent Restenosis Study (STRESS) trial is the only published randomized trial to directly compare the costs of elective stenting with those of conventional PTCA. The STRESS trial randomly

## TABLE 15–4. COST STUDIES COMPARING NEW DEVICES WITH CONVENTIONAL PTCA

| STUDY | DATE | METHOD | N | COST MEASURE | TIME FRAME | DEVICE | LOS | COST ($) |
|-------|------|--------|---|--------------|------------|--------|-----|----------|
| Dick et al[49] | 1989–1990 | OBS | 149 | Hospital charges | Initial hospitalization | PTCA | 1.5 ± 1.3 | 6220 ± 5716 |
| | | | | | | DCA | 2.2 ± 3.9 | 8329 ± 8588 |
| | | | | | | Stent | 4.9 ± 2.4 | 12,574 ± 4564 |
| Guzman et al[50] | 1991 | OBS—native and SVG | 252 | Adjusted hospital charges | Initial hospitalization | PTCA—native | | 7059 ± 4765 |
| | | | | | | DCA—native | | 7420 ± 3780 |
| | | | | | | PTCRA—native | | 8855 ± 4144 |
| | | | | | | TEC-SVG | | 15,168 ± 20,817 |
| Cohen et al[20] | 1990–1991 | OBS | 211 | Hospital costs and itemized procedural costs | Initial hospitalization | PTCA | 2.6 ± 1.7 | 5396 ± 2829 |
| | | | | | | DCA | 2.3 ± 1.5 | 5726 ± 2716 |
| | | | | | | Stent | 5.5 ± 2.6 | 7878 ± 3270 |
| Nino et al[51] | 1989–1992 | OBS | 384 | Equipment at hospital purchase price (exclusive of capital costs) | Initial procedure | PTCA | | 1337 ± 643 |
| | | | | | | PTCRA | | 2145 ± 794 |
| | | | | | | TEC | | 2924 ± 869 |
| | | | | | | Laser | | 3053 ± 1179 |
| CAVEAT[21] | 1991–1992 | RCT | 605 | Hospital costs | Initial hospitalization | PTCA | 5.8 | 10,637 |
| | | | | | | DCA | 5.7 | 11,904 |
| Ellis et al[52] | 1992–1993 | OBS | 1258 | Hospital accounting system costs and MD fees | Initial hospitalization | PTCA | | 8520 |
| | | | | | | DCA | | 9360 |
| | | | | | | Laser | | 9243 |
| | | | | | | PTCRA | | 10,343 |
| | | | | | | Stent | | 14,631 |
| | | | | | | TEC | | 18,891 |
| STRESS[53] | 1991–1993 | RCT | 207 | Hospital costs and itemized procedure costs | Initial hospitalization | PTCA | 4.8 ± 3.6 | 7505 ± 5015 |
| | | | | | | Stent | 7.5 ± 3.4 | 9738 ± 3248 |
| | | | | | 1-year medical care costs | PTCA | | 10,865 ± 9073 |
| | | | | | | Stent | | 11,656 ± 5674 |
| BOAT[22] | 1994–1996 | RCT | 714 | Hospital costs, itemized procedure costs, MD fees | Initial hospitalization | PTCA | 1.9 ± 1.5 | 8628 ± 5058 |
| | | | | | | DCA | 2.2 ± 2.9 | 10,449 ± 5822 |
| | | | | | 6-month total | PTCA | | 11,501 ± 7848 |
| | | | | | | DCA | | 12,568 ± 7669 |
| Peterson et al[54] | 1995–1996 | OBS | 496 | Hospital costs (RCC method) and MD fees | Initial hospitalization | PTCA | 3.4 | 10,076 |
| | | | | | | Stent/warf | 7.4 | 15,926 |
| | | | | | | Stent/ticlid | 3.7 | 13,294 |

BOAT, Balloon vs. Optimal Atherectomy Trial; CAVEAT, Coronary Angioplasty Versus Excisional Atherectomy Trial; DCA, directional atherectomy; LOS, length of stay; MD, physician; OBS, observational study; RCT, randomized controlled trial; PTCA, percutaneous transluminal coronary angioplasty; PTCRA, percutaneous transluminal rotational ablation; RCC, ratio of cost to charges; Stent/warf, stenting with oral anticoagulation; Stent/ticlid, stenting with combined antiplatelet therapy; STRESS, Stent Restenosis Study; SVG, saphenous vein graft; TEC, transluminal extraction catheter.

assigned 410 patients undergoing elective revascularization of a single, discrete coronary stenosis to balloon angioplasty or Palmaz-Schatz coronary stent implantation. At 6-month follow-up, patients assigned to initial stenting had less angiographic restenosis (31% vs. 42%, $p < 0.05$) and required less frequent clinically driven target vessel revascularization (10% vs. 15%, $p = 0.06$) than patients assigned to initial PTCA.[43]

The STRESS Economic Substudy included 207 consecutive patients randomly assigned to stenting or PTCA at 8 of 13 U.S. clinical sites.[53] The results of this study are summarized in Tables 15–5 and 15–6. During the index procedure, cardiac catheterization laboratory resource utilization and costs were significantly higher for patients who underwent coronary stenting. Specifically, stent patients required more contrast volume, more angioplasty balloons, and more stents per procedure than patients who underwent conventional PTCA. As a result, catheterization laboratory costs were $1200 higher for stenting than for balloon angioplasty. In addition, the use of high-dose oral anticoagulation after stenting in the STRESS trial led to significant increases in major vascular complications with stenting (10% vs. 4%) and a 2-day longer hospital stay. Thus, mean initial hospital costs were $2200 higher for stenting than for PTCA ($9738 vs. $7505).

Over the first year of follow-up, patients treated with initial stenting required fewer subsequent hos-

**TABLE 15–5.   INITIAL PROCEDURAL RESOURCE UTILIZATION AND COST IN THE STRESS ECONOMIC SUBSTUDY**

|  | PTCA (N = 105) | STENT (N = 102) |
|---|---|---|
| **Resource utilization** | | |
| Procedure duration (min) | 89 ± 47 | 86 ± 35 |
| Contrast volume (mL) | 234 ± 123 | 165 ± 110 |
| Balloon catheters (excluding delivery system) (N) | 1.7 ± 1.0 | 2.0 ± 0.9 |
| Stents (N) | 0.1 ± 0.4 | 1.1 ± 0.4 |
| Postprocedure length of stay (d) | 3.5 ± 3.3 | 5.5 ± 3.2 |
| **Initial hospital costs ($)** | | |
| Catheterization laboratory | 3643 ± 1570 | 4705 ± 1164 |
| Room/nursing | 1512 ± 1586 | 2232 ± 1393 |
| Laboratory | 531 ± 485 | 721 ± 407 |
| Professional | 1118 ± 598 | 1053 ± 339 |
| Other | 701 ± 362 | 1027 ± 496 |
| Total cost | 7505 ± 5015 | 9738 ± 3248 |

Adapted from Cohen DJ, Krumholz HM, Sukin CA, et al: In-hospital and one-year economic outcomes after coronary stenting or balloon angioplasty: Results from a randomized clinical trial. Circulation 92:2480–2487, 1995. By permission of the American Heart Association, Inc.
PTCA, percutaneous transluminal coronary angioplasty; STRESS, Stent Restenosis Study.

**TABLE 15–6.   ONE-YEAR OUTCOMES, MEDICAL RESOURCE UTILIZATION AND COSTS IN THE STRESS ECONOMIC SUBSTUDY**

|  | PTCA (N = 105) | STENT (N = 102) |
|---|---|---|
| **Late events (%)** | | |
| Repeat revascularization | 21 | 15 |
| Repeat hospitalization | 33 | 28 |
| **Repeat revascularizations (N)** | | |
| Bypass surgery | 11 | 6 |
| PTCA | 24 | 13 |
| Total | 35 | 19 |
| **Repeat hospital admissions (N)** | | |
| Cardiac | 43 | 28 |
| Noncardiac | 5 | 11 |
| Total | 48 | 39 |
| **One-year medical costs ($)** | | |
| Index hospitalization | 7505 ± 5015 | 9738 ± 3248 |
| Follow-up | 3359 ± 7100 | 1918 ± 4841 |
| Total | 10,865 ± 9073 | 11,656 ± 5674 |

Adapted from Cohen DJ, Krumholz HM, Sukin CA, et al: In-hospital and one-year economic outcomes after coronary stenting or balloon angioplasty: Results from a randomized clinical trial. Circulation 92:2480–2487, 1995. By permission of the American Heart Association, Inc.
PTCA, percutaneous transluminal coronary angioplasty; STRESS, Stent Restenosis Study.

pital admissions and fewer repeat revascularization procedures (see Table 15–6). As a result, follow-up medical care costs (not including outpatient or indirect costs) were, on average, $1400 lower after stenting. These "downstream" cost savings were insufficient to fully offset the higher initial cost of stenting, however. Over the full 1-year study period, cumulative medical care costs were thus $800 higher with stenting than with PTCA ($11,656 ± 5674 vs. $10,865 ± 9073, $p < 0.001$).

Although advances in stent deployment techniques (routine high-pressure postdilation, aspirin plus ticlopidine anticoagulation) have both significantly improved the safety of stenting and reduced the length of stay, studies of stenting during the reduced anticoagulation era suggest that the net economic impact of stenting remains essentially unchanged. Sukin and colleagues[55] at Beth Israel Hospital reported on 78 patients who underwent elective stenting of a single discrete coronary lesion in 1995 and compared their procedural resource utilization and costs with those of STRESS PTCA and stenting. They found that "optimal stenting" required significantly more angioplasty balloons (2.5 vs. 2.0, $p < 0.01$) and more stents (1.3 vs. 1.1, $p < 0.01$) per patient than stenting as performed in the STRESS trial. As a result, optimal stenting increased average catheterization laboratory costs by approximately $600 compared with stenting in the STRESS trial and by more than $2200 compared with PTCA. Peterson and colleagues[54] studied hospital costs in 496 patients who underwent Palmaz-Schatz coronary stenting (elective or unplanned) or conventional PTCA between 1994 and 1996. They found that the initial hospital cost for stenting with aspirin/ticlopidine anticoagulation was more than $3000 higher than that for simple balloon angioplasty. Long-term clinical and economic follow-up is planned in this observational study. If late medical outcomes and follow-up costs with modern-day stent techniques remain similar to those observed in the earlier clinical trials—as suggested by some studies[56, 57]—it is likely that overall 1-year costs will remain $500 to $1000 higher with stenting than with balloon angioplasty.

Nonetheless, it remains possible that stenting, at least for discrete coronary stenoses, will eventually become cost saving relative to balloon angioplasty. Such cost savings may be achieved through several mechanisms. First and foremost, the maturation of the stent market should produce significant reductions in the price of stents. Development of longer stents and stents without articulation defects will ultimately reduce procedural resource consumption as well. Finally, it is possible that optimization of poststent geometry or second-generation stent designs will lead to further reductions in clinical restenosis and thus additional cost savings compared with those observed in the STRESS trial. Preliminary studies suggest that current stent techniques may result in clinical restenosis rates as low as 13%.[58, 59] If these findings are confirmed in large clinical trials, the additional procedural resource utilization and costs would certainly be justified.

Until such clinical benefits or additional in-hospital cost savings are demonstrated, however, the cost effectiveness of elective coronary stenting depends on whether its proven clinical benefits—namely a reduction in recurrent angina and the need for repeat revascularization procedures—are sufficient to justify the additional long-term costs of the procedure. To formally address the issue, we have developed an analytic decision model to study the long-term costs and clinical effectiveness of alternative strategies for treating patients with symptomatic single-vessel coronary disease. A detailed description of the model is beyond the scope of this chapter but is available elsewhere.[60] Although it was originally based largely on observational data, the model has been updated to incorporate the pooled clinical results of the STRESS and Belgium-Netherlands Stent Trial (BENESTENT) trials as well as 1996 cost data from the Beth Israel Hospital experience.[55] Thus, the model reflects the best available data on the results of PTCA and stenting, current as of March 1997. Based on this model, we estimate that stenting for single-vessel coronary disease has an incremental cost-effectiveness ratio of $33,700 per quality-adjusted year of life gained—similar to the cost effectiveness of treating mild diastolic hypertension.[13] Thus, although coronary stenting remains more expensive than conventional PTCA, even in the long run, its cost effectiveness appears to compare favorably with that of other medical practices.

It is overly simplistic to define the cost effectiveness of coronary stenting in terms of a single cost-effectiveness ratio, however. Just as the overall effectiveness of coronary stenting depends on a variety of patient and lesion-specific characteristics, the cost effectiveness of elective coronary stenting depends on these factors as well. Figure 15–1 demonstrates the impact of simultaneous variations in the PTCA abrupt closure and restenosis rates on the cost effectiveness of elective stenting. If one were willing to spend up to $40,000/QALY—similar to the cost effectiveness of treating mild hypertension—our model suggests that stenting would be cost effective as long as the PTCA restenosis rate were greater than 31% and the PTCA abrupt closure rate were greater than 5%. Alternatively, if the probabilities of both abrupt closure and restenosis with conventional PTCA were significantly lower than the average results from the randomized clinical trials, then stenting would be significantly less cost effective. For example, for a type A midright coronary stenosis, data suggest that the abrupt closure rate might be as low as 3% and the angiographic restenosis rate might be 25% to 30%. For such a lesion, our model projects a cost-effectiveness ratio for elective stenting of $200,000/QALY—much higher than most accepted medical interventions. These findings suggest that although stenting may be reasonably cost effective for most suitable lesions, there are other lesions for which PTCA remains the preferred initial treatment—at least on economic grounds.

**DIRECTIONAL ATHERECTOMY.** Directional coronary atherectomy (DCA) was the first new device to receive approval from the U.S. Food and Drug Administration for percutaneous treatment of coronary stenoses. Several single-center and small multicenter series have demonstrated that DCA can be performed safely, with residual stenoses of 10% to 15% and with angiographic restenosis rates of 28% to 31%.[61–63] Until 1996, however, controlled clinical trials had failed to replicate the results of these selected series or to demonstrate sustained angiographic or clinical benefits compared with PTCA.[21, 64] In the randomized BOAT study, however, DCA was associated with a lower 6-month angiographic restenosis rate and a trend toward less repeat revascularization of the target vessel in comparison with conventional balloon angioplasty.[65]

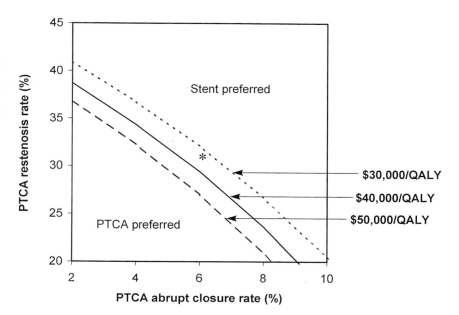

FIGURE 15–1. Plot of the relation between angiographic restenosis and abrupt closure rates, level of acceptable cost effectiveness, and optimal revascularization strategy. For combinations of percutaneous transluminal coronary angioplasty (PTCA) abrupt closure and restenosis rates above each threshold line, initial stenting would be preferred at that cost-effectiveness threshold, whereas angioplasty would be preferred for those combinations below the line. The *star* indicates the baseline values for this analysis based on the BENESTENT and STRESS trials (probability of angiographic restenosis = 31%; probability of abrupt vessel closure = 6%). QALY, quality-adjusted life year. (Adapted from Sukin CA, Cohen DJ: Percutaneous revascularization of coronary artery disease. *In* Talley JD, Maulkin PD, Becker ER [eds]: Cost Effective Diagnosis and Treatment of Coronary Artery Disease. Baltimore: Williams & Wilkins, 1997.)

In the early 1990s, 3 observational studies compared initial hospital costs for these two procedures (see Table 15–4). In 1991, Dick and colleagues[49] reported that directional atherectomy increased catheterization laboratory charges by $600 and overall hospital charges by $2100 compared with conventional PTCA. Cohen and colleagues[20] compared the variable costs of 34 patients undergoing elective DCA with those of 113 patients undergoing elective PTCA at Beth Israel Hospital in 1990 and 1991. They found that DCA increased procedural costs by approximately $500. Finally, Guzman and colleagues[50] reported similar results for age- and gender-matched patients undergoing single-vessel DCA or PTCA at the Cleveland Clinic. Directional atherectomy increased hospital costs by approximately $700 compared with PTCA—primarily because of additional catheterization laboratory supplies.

Two randomized trials have compared the costs of DCA with those of PTCA. CAVEAT was the first randomized trial to compared directional coronary atherectomy with conventional PTCA. In an economic substudy that included 605 patients enrolled at 19 of 32 clinical sites, the CAVEAT investigators found that DCA increased cardiac catheterization laboratory costs by $700 (see Table 15–4).[21] Although mean length of stay was identical for DCA and PTCA in this trial, DCA also increased nonprocedural hospital costs by an additional $600, so that the overall cost difference in initial hospital costs was $1300. Given the lack of additional clinical benefit seen with DCA in CAVEAT, this cost difference persisted at 6-month follow-up.[66]

In the BOAT study, detailed health economic data were collected for 714 of 989 randomly assigned patients, and preliminary findings have been re-

ported.[22] Similar to CAVEAT, the BOAT investigators found that DCA increased procedural costs by approximately $1300 and other hospital costs by an additional $500, such that initial hospital costs were $1800 higher with DCA than with conventional PTCA. Although 6-month resource utilization tended to be somewhat less in patients randomly assigned to DCA, the resulting downstream cost savings were insufficient to fully offset the higher initial costs of DCA. Thus, aggregate 6-month medical care costs remained $1000 higher with DCA than with PTCA. Whether these additional costs are warranted given the relatively modest clinical benefits of DCA is open to debate.

**ROTATIONAL ATHERECTOMY.** Three observational studies have compared the costs of rotational atherectomy with balloon angioplasty (see Table 15–4). Guzman and colleagues[50] compared 44 patients undergoing rotational atherectomy with 126 age- and gender-matched patients undergoing single-lesion PTCA in 1991. Catheterization laboratory resource utilization was significantly greater for rotational atherectomy, resulting in an $1800 increase in total hospital costs compared with PTCA. Ellis and colleagues[52] found that rotational atherectomy increased hospital costs by 25% compared with balloon angioplasty, even after controlling for patient characteristics and lesion complexity. Finally, in a study of 384 patients undergoing single-vessel revascularization at William Beaumont Hospital, Nino and colleagues[51] found that rotational atherectomy increased procedural equipment costs by $800. This study tended to underestimate the current procedural cost difference, however, because it assumed a Rotablator device cost of $450 (low relative to current pricing) and PTCA balloon cost of $700 (high relative to current pricing). If current device cost estimates were used, the difference in equipment cost would increase to $1400.

The available data thus suggest that rotational atherectomy increases procedural costs by $1400 to $1800 compared with conventional PTCA. In the absence of studies demonstrating clear clinical benefits (i.e., fewer ischemic complications and/or reduced restenosis), the cost effectiveness of rotational atherectomy for lesions amenable to standard PTCA remains in question. Both the efficacy and the cost effectiveness of the device for type A and B1 coronary stenoses are currently being evaluated in the randomized Dilation and Rotational Ablation Trial (DRAT).

## Adjunctive Pharmacotherapy

In addition to new mechanical devices, the 1990s has witnessed the development of new pharmacologic agents that can be used as adjuncts to percutaneous coronary revascularization. Although several of these agents remain investigational (e.g., hirudin, bivalirudin [Hirulog]), c7E3 Fab (abciximab), a monoclonal antibody directed against the platelet glycoprotein IIb/IIIa receptor, has been shown to significantly reduce ischemic complications in patients undergoing PTCA or DCA. In the Evaluation of 7E3 for the Prevention of Ischemic Complications (EPIC) trial, patients treated with abciximab at the time of "high-risk" PTCA were found to have a 33% reduction in the combined end point of death, nonfatal myocardial infarction, emergency repeat PTCA, emergency bypass surgery, stent placement, and balloon pump insertion.[29] The Evaluation of PTCA to Improve Long-term Outcome by c7E3 GP IIb/IIIa Receptor Blockade (EPILOG) trial reported similar benefits in a less selected patient population.[30] Consequently, despite concerns about the high "up-front" cost of abciximab, its use has become commonplace at many institutions.

Mark and colleagues[67] performed a prospective economic analysis in conjunction with the EPIC trial. They found that exclusive of drug costs, total in-hospital costs were similar among the three treatment groups. However, during the 6-month period after hospital discharge, medical care costs were significantly lower for patients treated with abciximab bolus and infusion than those for patients treated with placebo ($2881 ± 8983 vs. $3998 ± 10,602, $p < 0.02$). This difference was mainly due to less frequent rehospitalization and fewer repeat revascularization procedures in the treatment group. Thus, total 6-month medical care costs exclusive of drug costs were $1270 lower for the abciximab bolus and infusion group than those for placebo. When the average drug cost ($1407 per patient) was included in the analysis, total 6-month costs were $300 higher for the bolus and infusion groups in comparison with placebo ($18,269 vs. $17,999, $p = $ not significant).

The EPIC results suggest that despite its higher initial cost, use of abciximab has a relatively minor impact on long-term medical care costs, at least in high-risk PTCA patients. Moreover, multivariable analysis of the EPIC results suggests that abciximab could be cost saving if the excess bleeding complications associated with its use could be substantially reduced or eliminated.[67] In the EPILOG trial, use of low-dose heparin in conjunction with abciximab effectively eliminated any excess bleeding complications while preserving the initial clinical benefits seen in EPIC. Nonetheless, it does not appear that abciximab will be cost saving compared with conventional therapy in EPILOG. In contrast to EPIC, in EPILOG, there was no additional benefit with abciximab beyond the initial hospitalization—thus eliminating much of the economic benefit seen in the earlier trial. Preliminary data from an economic analysis of the EPILOG results suggest that 6-month costs with abciximab will be $800 to $1000 higher than those with placebo.[68] Whether this difference in the two trials reflects the different heparin doses, the higher frequency of bailout stenting in EPILOG, or simple random variation is unclear. If these results are confirmed in the final study results, formal cost-effectiveness analysis will be required to determine whether routine abciximab therapy is economically attractive and to identify the most appropriate candidates for such therapy.

## ECONOMIC EVALUATION OF INTERVENTIONAL THERAPIES IN ACUTE MI PATIENTS

### Direct PTCA

Several major randomized clinical trials have shown a consistent trend toward improved clinical outcomes with direct PTCA in comparison with thrombolytic therapy in patients presenting with acute MI.[69-71] As a result, there has been considerable revival of interest in direct infarct angioplasty. At least five major studies have examined the economic impact of direct PTCA on acute MI patients (Table 15-7). In general, these studies have shown direct angioplasty to be at least no more costly than thrombolytic therapy with tissue-type plasminogen activator, the most common thrombolytic agent used in the United States.[73, 74, 77] Only two studies have shown direct PTCA to be more costly than thrombolytic therapy. In the Zwolle (Netherlands) trial, initial hospital costs were approximately $2000 lower

**TABLE 15–7.** **COST STUDIES OF DIRECT PTCA VERSUS THROMBOLYTIC THERAPY IN ACUTE MYOCARDIAL INFARCTION**

| STUDY | YEARS | TYPE | N | COST MEASURE | TIME FRAME | MEAN COSTS ($) | |
|---|---|---|---|---|---|---|---|
| | | | | | | PTCA | Lytic Rx |
| O'Neill et al[72] | 1988–1990 | RCT (vs. SK) | 122 | Hosp charges | Initial hospitalization | 19,643 ± 7250 | 25,191 ± 15,368 |
| Gibbons et al[73] | 1989–1991 | RCT (vs. tPA) | 103 | Hosp charges, global RCC, MD fees | Initial hospitalization | 16,811 ± 8827 | 21,400 ± 14,806 |
| | | | | | 6-mon f/u | 480 ± 3069 | 2738 ± 7666 |
| | | | | | Total 6-mon | 17,292 ± 89,667 | 24,129 ± 18,806 |
| PAMI 1[74] | 1990–1992 | RCT (vs. tPA) | 358 | Hosp charges, MD fees | Initial hospitalization | 27,653 ± 13,709 | 30,227 ± 18,903 |
| Zwolle[75] | 1990–1992 | RCT (vs. SK) | 301 | Hosp costs, MD fees | Initial hospitalization | 12,722 | 11,099 |
| | | | | | 1-y f/u | 4592 | 5671 |
| | | | | | Total 1-y | 17,316 | 16,681 |
| MITI[76] | 1988–1994 | OBS | 3145 | Hosp costs (RCC method) | Initial hospitalization | 19,702 ± 12,175 | 16,838 ± 12,480 |
| | | | | | Total 3-y | 23,882 ± 15,768 | 21,760 ± 17,438 |
| GUSTO IIb[77] | 1994–1996 | RCT (vs. tPA) | 386 | Hosp costs (RCC method), MD fees | Initial hospitalization | 17,753 | 17,398 |

f/u, follow-up; GUSTO, Global Utilization of Streptokinase and Tissue Plasminogen Activator for Occluded Coronary Arteries; Hosp, hospital; MD, physician; MITI, Myocardial Infarction Triage and Intervention; OBS, observational study; PAMI, Primary Angioplasty in Myocardial Infarction; PTCA, percutaneous transluminal coronary angioplasty; RCC, ratio of cost to charges; RCT, randomized clinical trial; SK, streptokinase; tPA, tissue-type plasminogen activator.

with thrombolytic therapy than with direct PTCA.[75] In this study, however, the thrombolytic agent was streptokinase rather than tissue-type plasminogen activator. Substitution of tissue-type plasminogen activator for streptokinase in this trial would have completely negated the initial cost advantage of the thrombolytic group. Moreover, in this study, follow-up costs were significantly lower for the direct PTCA group, such that by the end of 1-year follow-up, the absolute cost difference was less than $500 (see Table 15–7). In a formal cost-effectiveness analysis, the Zwolle investigators found that the incremental cost per additional event-free survivor at 1 year was only $3010.[75] Although this value lacks a clear external reference for comparison, comparison with the average cost-effectiveness ratio for streptokinase in this trial ($37,000 per event-free survivor) suggests that direct PTCA is reasonably cost effective, even compared with the least expensive thrombolytic agent.

The Myocardial Infarction Triage and Intervention (MITI) investigators reported initial and 3-year follow-up costs for 3145 patients presenting within 6 hours of acute MI and treated with direct PTCA or thrombolytic therapy.[76] In this observational study, the investigators found that initial hospital costs (excluding physician fees) were approximately $3000 higher for patients treated with direct PTCA compared with thrombolytic therapy (65% tissue-type plasminogen activator, 32% streptokinase). This striking cost difference was somewhat surprising given the high rates of coronary angiography (74%) and PTCA (32%) in the thrombolytic group as well as the shorter length of stay in the direct PTCA group (6.8 ± 4.4 vs. 7.9 ± 5.3 days, $p < 0.001$). Moreover, in contrast to the randomized tri-

als, there was no difference in late medical care costs over the 3-year follow-up period. As a result, aggregate 3-year medical care costs remained more than $3000 higher with direct PTCA in this study ($25,459 ± 17,543 vs. $22,163 ± 18,118, $p < 0.001$).

There are several potential explanations for the discrepant results between the MITI registry data and the randomized trials. First, as a nonrandomized comparison, it is possible that patients treated with direct PTCA in MITI were generally "sicker" than thrombolytic patients. Although the MITI investigators attempted to adjust for such differences in multivariate analyses, the possibility of unmeasured confounding cannot be excluded. A second possibility is that the clinical and economic outcomes with direct PTCA in the randomized trials were produced by a highly dedicated group of selected PTCA operators and cannot be generalized beyond such operators and institutions. The relatively modest clinical benefits seen with direct PTCA in the Global Use of Strategies to Open Occluded Arteries in Acute Coronary Syndromes (GUSTO IIb) "megatrial" provide further support to this hypothesis.[71] However, the most likely explanation is that the observed cost differences in MITI reflect *cross-hospital* cost differences rather than true differences between the treatment strategies.

The available data thus suggest that in expert hands, a strategy of direct PTCA for acute MI is at least no less efficacious and no more costly than thrombolytic therapy. Nonetheless, because direct PTCA cannot be performed on many acute MI patients in a timely fashion, it is unlikely that direct PTCA will supplant thrombolytic therapy for most acute MI patients in the foreseeable future. Simulation models suggest that the option of building additional catheterization laboratories and PTCA programs would impose prohibitive costs on the health care system that would probably outweigh any modest advantages of extending a direct PTCA strategy to additional patients.[78]

## Adjunctive PTCA

The use of adjunctive procedures in combination with thrombolytic therapy to improve early coronary patency rates and to ensure long-term patency after acute MI has been the subject of vigorous debate over the past decade. There have been two major studies of different catheterization/revascularization strategies in conjunction with thrombolytic therapy that have included economic substudies: the Thrombolysis in Myocardial Infarction study (TIMI-II) and the Thrombolysis and Angioplasty in Myocardial Infarction (TAMI-5) study. The TIMI-II trial randomly assigned 3262 patients with acute MI who were treated with tissue-type plasminogen activator to an "invasive" strategy of cardiac catheterization in all patients versus a "conservative strategy" of catheterization only in the presence of recurrent ischemia. The invasive strategy was further subdivided into an "immediate invasive" strategy of immediate catheterization after thrombolysis or a "delayed invasive" strategy of catheterization 18 to 48 hours after presentation. The TIMI-II cost substudy was performed on the 376 patients who were enrolled in this multicenter trial at the University of Alabama and at the Mayo Clinic.[79] The major results are presented in Table 15–8. In this substudy, there was a modest difference in hospital costs between the immediate invasive strategy and the conservative strategy plus a twofold difference in professional fees, so that total costs were approximately $2000 lower for the conservative strategy arm. After the baseline hospitalization, cardiac catheterization and coronary angioplasty were more common in the delayed invasive and the conservative arms than in the immediate invasive arm. Cumulative 1-year costs for this study have not been reported.

The TAMI-5 randomized trial tested two angiographic strategies: immediate angiography followed by emergency revascularization if the infarct artery was occluded or if the patient had severe ongoing ischemia with reduced flow in the infarct vessel and (2) deferred revascularization management for the remaining patients. This was contrasted with a deferred angiography strategy at 5 to 10 days that allowed early crossover to angiography in the case of severe ischemia. The results of the economic substudy for these two arms were similar to those of the TIMI-II trial.[80] Repeat catheterization (17% vs. 53%) and revascularization (65% vs. 75%) were significantly less common in the deferred angiography arm than in the immediate angiography arm. As a result, mean hospital costs were approximately $2600 less with the deferred catheterization strategy ($18,028 ± 9640 vs. $20,630 ± 14,027).

Although empirical data clearly indicate that routine coronary angiography after acute MI increases medical care costs, no empirical data are available to determine whether such a strategy is cost effective. The possibility that routine post-MI catheterization might be cost effective is suggested by the observed trend toward improved 1-year survival with an aggressive catheterization and intervention strategy in both the TIMI-II and the TIMI-IIIB studies.[81, 82] Kuntz and colleagues[83] used a decision-analytic model to evaluate the cost effectiveness of cor-

## TABLE 15–8.   RESULTS OF THE TIMI-II COST SUBSTUDY

| | MANAGEMENT STRATEGY | | |
| --- | --- | --- | --- |
| | IMMEDIATE INVASIVE (N = 66) | DELAYED INVASIVE (N = 160) | CONSERVATIVE (N = 150) |
| Initial hospitalization | | | |
| Hospital days | 10 | 9 | 9 |
| PTCA performed (%) | 67 | 58 | 21 |
| CABG performed (%) | 26 | 16 | 16 |
| Hospital costs* | $10,739 ± 5039 | $11,571 ± 6685 | $10,601 ± 6622 |
| Professional fees | $4548 ± 3068 | $3754 ± 2346 | $2698 ± 2649 |
| Total costs | $15,287 | $15,325 | $13,299 |
| One-year follow-up | | | |
| Cardiac catheterization (%) | 3.0 | 13.6 | 15.4 |
| PTCA (%) | 1.5 | 7.2 | 5.1 |
| CABG (%) | 6.6 | 6.4 | 6.8 |
| Cardiac rehospitalization (%) | 21.2 | 27.2 | 30.7 |

CABG, coronary artery bypass grafting; PTCA, percutaneous transluminal coronary angioplasty; TIMI-2, Thrombolysis in Myocardial Infarction study; tPA, tissue-type plasminogen activator.

*Excludes cost of tPA.

Adapted from Charles ED, Rogers WJ, Reeder GS, et al: Economic advantages of a conservative strategy for AMI management: rt-PA without obligatory PTCA [Abstract]. J Am Coll Cardiol 13:152A, 1989. Reprinted with permission from the American College of Cardiology.

onary angiography in the postinfarction setting.[83] They found that coronary angiography (and subsequent revascularization based on coronary anatomy) was reasonably cost effective (i.e., cost-effectiveness ratio <$50,000 per QALY gained) in patients with severe postinfarction angina or a strongly positive exercise tolerance test result. In addition, cost-effectiveness ratios were favorable for patients with a prior MI, even in the absence of recurrent myocardial ischemia. On the other hand, the cost effectiveness of postinfarct coronary angiography was estimated to be less favorable for patients with preserved left ventricular function, no prior MI, and no evidence of recurrent ischemia (cost-effectiveness ratio, $60,000 to $250,000/QALY).

## CONCLUSIONS

In today's health care climate, decisions about medical interventions need to reflect measures of cost as well as clinical benefit. With more than 300,000 procedures performed in the United States each year at a direct cost of more than 3 billion, percutaneous coronary revascularization is clearly a "big ticket" item and a prime target for cost-reduction measures. Although the field of economic technology assessment is still in its infancy, many high-quality economic studies have been performed to evaluate new techniques or treatment strategies in interventional cardiology.

As in most medical studies, economic evaluations of percutaneous coronary revascularization techniques have generally found that newer and more aggressive treatments tend to increase costs compared with the established alternatives. Nonetheless, cost-effectiveness analyses incorporating the results of such studies suggest that most treatments that have been shown to improve clinical outcomes are probably cost effective. For example, despite increasing medical care costs, balloon angioplasty appears to be reasonably cost effective compared with medical therapy for patients with moderate-to-severe angina and one- or two-vessel coronary disease. Similarly, coronary stenting increases long-term costs for most patients but is associated with improved outcomes compared with conventional PTCA. Formal cost-effectiveness analysis suggests that these benefits are worth the cost, at least for patients with single, discrete lesions treatable by a single stent. A few advances—such as abciximab in high-risk patients undergoing balloon angioplasty and direct infarct angioplasty in experienced centers—may even improve outcomes without increasing overall health care costs. Conversely, many new coronary interventions have yet to be shown to improve clinical outcomes compared with conven-

tional PTCA. Given the higher procedural and hospital costs associated with these devices, it is difficult to justify their use at present, except for very specific lesions where angioplasty is unlikely to be successful, or in ongoing clinical investigations.

## REFERENCES

1. Gruentzig AR, Stenning A, Siegenthaler WE: Nonoperative dilatation of coronary artery stenosis: Percutaneous transluminal angioplasty. N Engl J Med 391:61–68, 1979.
2. Robinson JC, Luft HS: Competition and the cost of hospital care, 1972 to 1982. JAMA 257:3241, 1987.
3. Mark DB, Jollis J: Economic aspects of therapy for acute myocardial infarction. In Bates ER (ed): Adjunctive Therapy for Acute Myocardial Infarction, p 471. New York: Marcel Dekker, 1991.
4. Finkler SA: The distinction between costs and charges. Ann Intern Med 96:102–109, 1982.
5. Cleverley WO: Essentials of Health Care Finance, 3rd ed. Gaithersburg, MD: Aspen Publishers, 1992.
6. Stewart RD: Cost Estimating, 2nd ed. New York: John Wiley & Sons, 1991.
7. Mark DB: Medical economics and health policy issues for interventional cardiology. In Topol EJ (ed): Textbook of Interventional Cardiology, 2nd ed. Philadelphia: WB Saunders, 1993.
8. Beck JR, Kassirer JP, Pauker SG: A convenient approximation of life expectancy (the DEALE): I. Validation of the method. Am J Med 73:883, 1982.
9. Weinstein MC, Stason WB: Foundations of cost-effectiveness analysis for health and medical practices. N Engl J Med 296:716–721, 1977.
10. Gaspoz JM, Goldman P, Williams L, et al: Cost-effectiveness of aspirin in secondary prevention of coronary heart disease [Abstract]. Circulation 92(suppl):I-47, 1995.
11. Johannesson M, Jönsson B, Kjekshus J, et al: Cost effectiveness of simvastatin treatment to lower cholesterol levels in patients with coronary heart disease. N Engl J Med 336:332–336, 1997.
12. Weinstein MC, Stason WB: Cost-effectiveness of coronary artery bypass surgery. Circulation 66(suppl III):III-56–III-66, 1982.
13. Stason WB, Weinstein MC: Allocation of resources to manage hypertension. N Engl J Med 296:732–739, 1977.
14. Goldman L, Weinstein MC, Goldman PA, et al: Cost-effectiveness of HMG-CoA reductase inhibition for primary and secondary prevention of coronary heart disease. JAMA 265:1145–1151, 1991.
15. Hamel MB, Phillips RS, Davis RB, et al: Outcomes and cost-effectiveness of initiating dialysis and continuing aggressive care in seriously ill hospitalized adults. Ann Intern Med 127:195–202, 1997.
16. Goel V, Deber RB, Detsky AS: Nonionic contrast media: A bargain for some, a burden for many. Can Med Assoc J 143:480, 1990.
17. Goldman L, Gordon DJ, Rifkind BM, et al: Cost and health implications of cholesterol lowering. Circulation 85:1960–1968, 1992.
18. Topol EJ, Ellis SG, Cosgrove DM, et al: Analysis of coronary angioplasty practice in the United States with an insurance-claims data base. Circulation 87:1489, 1993.
19. Hlatky MA, Lipscomb J, Nelson C, et al: Resource use and cost of initial coronary revascularization: Coronary angioplasty versus coronary bypass surgery. Circulation 82(suppl IV):IV-208–IV-213, 1990.
20. Cohen DJ, Breall JA, Ho KKL, et al: Economics of coronary revascularization: Comparison of costs and charges for conventional angioplasty, directional atherectomy, stenting and bypass surgery. J Am Coll Cardiol 22:1052–1059, 1993.
21. Topol EJ, Leya F, Pinkerton CA, et al: A comparison of directional coronary atherectomy with coronary angioplasty in patients with coronary artery disease. The CAVEAT Study Group. N Engl J Med 329:221–227, 1993.

22. Cohen DJ, Sukin CA, Berezin RH, et al: In-hospital and follow-up costs of balloon angioplasty and directional atherectomy: Results from the randomized BOAT trial [Abstract]. Circulation 94:I-324, 1996.

23. Mark DB: Personal communication, November 1997.

24. Parisi AF, Folland ED, Hartigan P: A comparison of angioplasty with medical therapy in the treatment of single-vessel coronary artery disease. N Engl J Med 326:10–16, 1992.

25. Hlatky MA, Califf RM, Kong Y, et al: Natural history of patients with single-vessel disease suitable for percutaneous transluminal coronary angioplasty. Am J Cardiol 52:225–229, 1983.

26. Wong JB, Sonnenberg FA, Salem DN, et al: Myocardial revascularization for chronic stable angina: Analysis of the role of percutaneous transluminal coronary angioplasty based on data available in 1989. Ann Intern Med 113:852–871, 1990.

27. Detre K, Holubkov R, Kelsey S, et al: Percutaneous transluminal coronary angioplasty in 1985–1986 and 1977–1981: The National Heart, Lung, and Blood Institute Registry. N Engl J Med 318:265–270, 1988.

28. Lindsay J, Hong MK, Pnoow EE, et al: Effects of endoluminal coronary stents on the frequency of coronary bypass grafting after unsuccessful percutaneous coronary revascularization. Am J Cardiol 77:647–649, 1996.

29. The EPIC Investigators: Use of a monoclonal antibody directed against the platelet glycoprotein IIb/IIIa receptor in high-risk coronary angioplasty. N Engl J Med 330:956–961, 1994.

30. The EPILOG Investigators: Platelet glycoprotein IIb/IIIa receptor blockade and low-dose heparin during percutaneous coronary revascularization. N Engl J Med 336:1689–1696, 1997.

31. O'Keefe JH, Gernon C, McCallister BD, et al: Safety and cost effectiveness of combined coronary angiography and angioplasty. Am Heart J 122:50–54, 1991.

32. Friedman HZ, Cragg DR, Glazier SM: Randomized prospective evaluation of prolonged versus abbreviated intravenous heparin therapy after coronary angioplasty. J Am Coll Cardiol 24:1214–1219, 1994.

33. Davies RF, Goldber AD, Forman S, et al: Asymptomatic Cardiac Ischemia Pilot (ACIP) study two-year follow-up: Outcomes of patients randomized to initial strategies of medical therapy versus revascularization. Circulation 95:2037–2043, 1997.

34. Reeder GS, Krishan I, Norbrega FT, et al: Is percutaneous coronary revascularization less expensive than bypass surgery? N Engl J Med 311:1157–1162, 1984.

35. Kelly ME, Taylor GJ, Moses HW, et al: Comparative cost of myocardial revascularization: Percutaneous transluminal coronary angioplasty and coronary bypass surgery. J Am Coll Cardiol 5:16–20, 1985.

36. Weintraub WS, Mauldin P, Gilbert S, et al: Comparison of resource utilization and estimated cumulative cost over 5 years after coronary surgery or coronary angioplasty in patients with two vessel coronary disease [Abstract]. J Am Coll Cardiol 21:132A, 1993.

37. Sculpher MJ, Seed P, Henderson RA, et al: Health service costs of coronary angioplasty and coronary artery bypass surgery: The Randomised Intervention Treatment of Angina. Lancet 344:927–930, 1994.

38. Weintraub WS, Mauldin PD, Becker E, et al: A comparison of the costs and quality of life after coronary angioplasty or coronary surgery for multi-vessel coronary artery disease: Results from the Emory Angioplasty Versus Surgery Trial (EAST). Circulation 92:2831–2840, 1995.

39. Hlatky MA, Rogers WJ, Johnstone I, et al: Medical care costs and quality of life after randomization to coronary angioplasty or coronary bypass surgery. N Engl J Med 336:92–99, 1997.

40. Pocock SJ, Henderson RA, Rickards AF, et al: Meta-analysis of randomized trials comparing coronary angioplasty with bypass surgery. Lancet 346:1184–1189, 1995.

41. The Bypass Angioplasty Revascularization Investigation (BARI) Investigators: Comparison of coronary bypass surgery with angioplasty in patients with multivessel disease. N Engl J Med 335:217–225, 1996.

42. RITA Trial Participants: Coronary angioplasty versus coronary artery bypass surgery: The Randomised Intervention Treatment of Angina (RITA) trial. Lancet 341:573–580, 1993.

43. Fischman DL, Leon MB, Baim DS, et al: A randomized comparison of coronary stent placement and balloon angioplasty in the treatment of coronary artery disease. N Engl J Med 331:496–501, 1994.

44. Serruys PW, de Jaegere P, Kiemeneij F, et al: A comparison of balloon expandable stent implantation with balloon angioplasty in patients with coronary artery disease. N Engl J Med 331:489–495, 1994.

45. Versaci F, Gaspardone A, Tomai F, et al: A comparison of coronary artery stenting with angioplasty for isolated stenosis of the proximal left anterior descending coronary artery. N Engl J Med 336:817–822, 1997.

46. Serruys PW, Strauss BH, van Beusekom HM, et al: Stenting of coronary arteries: Has a modern Pandora's box been opened? J Am Coll Cardiol 17:143B–154B, 1991.

47. Topol EJ: Caveats about elective coronary stenting. N Engl J Med 331:539–541, 1994.

48. Topol EJ: The stentor and the sea change. Am J Cardiol 76:307–308, 1995.

49. Dick RJ, Popma JJ, Muller DWM, et al: In-hospital costs associated with new percutaneous coronary devices. Am J Cardiol 68:879–885, 1991.

50. Guzman LA, Simpfendorfer C, Fix J, et al: Comparison of costs of new atherectomy devices and balloon angioplasty for coronary artery disease. Am J Cardiol 74:22–25, 1994.

51. Nino CL, Freed M, Blankenship L, et al: Procedural cost of new interventional devices. Am J Cardiol 74:1165–1166, 1994.

52. Ellis SG, Miller DP, Brown KG, et al: In-hospital cost of percutaneous coronary revascularization: Critical determinants and implications. Circulation 92:741–747, 1995.

53. Cohen DJ, Krumholz HM, Sukin CA, et al: In-hospital and one-year economic outcomes after coronary stenting or balloon angioplasty: Results from a randomized clinical trial. Circulation 92:2480–2487, 1995.

54. Peterson ED, Cowper PA, Zidar JP, et al: In-hospital costs of coronary stenting (with or without Coumadin) compared with angioplasty [Abstract]. Circulation 94:I-325, 1996.

55. Sukin CA, Baim DS, Caputo RP, et al: The impact of optimal stenting techniques on cardiac catheterization laboratory resource utilization and costs. Am J Cardiol 79:275–280, 1997.

56. Fischman DL, Savage MP, Penn I, et al: High pressure inflation in conjunction with ticlopidine and aspirin following coronary stent placement: Results of the STRESS III trial [Abstract]. J Am Coll Cardiol 29:171A, 1997.

57. Legrand V, Serruys PW, Emanuelsson H, et al: BENESTENT II trial: Final results of visit I: A 15-day follow-up [Abstract]. J Am Coll Cardiol 29:170A, 1997.

58. Colombo A, Hall P, Nakamura S, et al: Intracoronary stenting without anticoagulation accomplished with intravascular ultrasound guidance. Circulation 91:1676–1688, 1995.

59. Serruys PW, Emanuelsson H, van der Giessen W, et al: Heparin-coated Palmaz-Schatz stents in human coronary arteries: Early outcome of the Benestent-II Pilot Study. Circulation 93:412–422, 1996.

60. Cohen DJ, Breall JA, Ho KKL, et al: Evaluating the potential cost-effectiveness of stenting as a treatment for symptomatic single-vessel coronary disease: Use of a decision-analytic model. Circulation 89:1859–1874, 1994.

61. Hinohara T, Robertson GC, Selmon MR, et al: Restenosis after directional coronary atherectomy. J Am Coll Cardiol 20:623–632, 1992.

62. Fishman RF, Kuntz RE, Carrozza JP Jr, et al: Long-term results of coronary atherectomy: Predictors of restenosis. J Am Coll Cardiol 20:1101–1110, 1992.

63. Simonton CA, Leon MB, Kuntz RE, et al: Acute and late clinical and angiographic results of directional atherectomy in the Optimal Atherectomy Restenosis Study (OARS) [Abstract]. Circulation 92:I-545, 1995.

64. Adelman AG, Cohen EA, Kimball BP, et al: A comparison of directional atherectomy with balloon angioplasty for lesions of the left anterior descending coronary artery. N Engl J Med 329:228–233, 1993.

65. Baim DS, Popma JJ, Sharma SK, et al: Final results of the Balloon vs. Optimal Atherectomy Trial (BOAT): 6 month angiography and year clinical follow-up [Abstract]. Circulation. 94:I-436, 1996.

66. Mark DB, Talley JD, Lam LC, et al: Economic outcomes following coronary angioplasty versus coronary atherectomy: Results from the CAVEAT randomized trial [Abstract]. J Am Coll Cardiol 1994;23:284A.

67. Mark DB, Talley JD, Topol EJ, et al: Economic assessment or platelet glycoprotein IIb/IIIa inhibition for prevention of ischemic complications of high risk coronary angioplasty. Circulation 94:629–635, 1996.

68. Lincoff AM, Mark DB, Califf RM, et al: Economic assessment of platelet glycoprotein IIb/IIIa receptor blockade during coronary intervention in the EPILOG trial [Abstract]. J Am Coll Cardiol 29:240A, 1997.

69. Grines CL, Browne KF, Marco J, et al: A comparison of immediate angioplasty with thrombolytic therapy for acute myocardial infarction. N Engl J Med 328:673–679, 1993.

70. De Boer MJ, Hoorntje JCA, Ottervanger JP, et al: Immediate coronary angioplasty versus intravenous streptokinase in acute myocardial infarction: Left ventricular ejection fraction, hospital mortality, and reinfarction. J Am Coll Cardiol 23:1004–1008, 1994.

71. The Global Use of Strategies to Open Occluded Coronary Arteries in Acute Coronary Syndromes (GUSTO IIB) Angioplasty Substudy Investigators: A clinical trial comparing primary coronary angioplasty with tissue plasminogen activator for acute myocardial infarction. N Engl J Med 336:1621–1628, 1997.

72. O'Neill WW, Weintraub R, Grines CL, et al: A prospective, placebo-controlled, randomized trial of intravenous streptokinase and angioplasty versus lone angioplasty therapy of acute myocardial infarction. Circulation 86:1710–1717, 1992.

73. Gibbons RJ, Holmes DR, Reeder GS, et al: Immediate angioplasty compared with the administration of a thrombolytic agent followed by conservative treatment for myocardial infarction. N Engl J Med 328:685–691, 1993.

74. Stone GW, Grines CL, Rothbaum D, et al: Analysis of the relative costs and effectiveness of primary angioplasty versus tissue-type plasminogen activator: The Primary Angioplasty in Myocardial Infarction (PAMI) trial. J Am Coll Cardiol 299:901–907, 1997.

75. De Boer MJ, van Hout BA, Liem AL, et al: A cost-effective analysis of primary coronary angioplasty versus thrombolysis for acute myocardial infarction. Am J Cardiol 76:830–833, 1995.

76. Every NR, Parsons LS, Hlatky M, et al: A comparison of thrombolytic therapy with primary coronary angioplasty for acute myocardial infarction. N Engl J Med 335:1253–1260, 1996.

77. Mark DB, Granger CB, Ellis SG, et al: Costs of direct angioplasty versus thrombolysis for acute myocardial infarction: Results from the GUSTO II randomized trial [Abstract]. Circulation 94:I-168, 1996.

78. Lieu TA, Lundstrom RJ, Ray GT, et al: Initial cost of primary angioplasty for acute myocardial infarction. J Am Coll Cardiol 28:882–889, 1996.

79. Charles ED, Rogers WJ, Reeder GS, et al: Economic advantages of a conservative strategy for AMI management: rt-PA without obligatory PTCA [Abstract]. J Am Coll Cardiol 13:152A, 1989.

80. Mark DB, Lam LC, Hlatky MA, et al: Effects of three thrombolytic regimens and two interventional strategies on acute MI costs: Results from a prospective randomized trial [Abstract]. Circulation 84:I-22, 1991.

81. Williams DO, Braunwald E, Knatterud G, et al: One-year results of the Thrombolysis in Myocardial Infarction Investigation (TIMI) Phase II Trial. Circulation 85:533–542, 1992.

82. Anderson HV, Cannon CP, Stone PH, et al: One-year results of the Thrombolysis in Myocardial Infarction (TIMI) IIIB clinical trials: A randomized comparison of tissue-type plasminogen activator versus placebo and early invasive versus early conservative strategies in unstable angina and non-Q wave myocardial infarction. J Am Coll Cardiol 26:1643–1650, 1995.

83. Kuntz KM, Tsevat J, Goldman L, et al: Cost-effectiveness of routine coronary angiography after acute myocardial infarction. Circulation 94:957–965, 1996.

84. Sukin CA, Cohen DJ: Percutaneous revascularization of coronary artery disease. In Talley JD, Maulkin PD, Becker ER (eds): Cost Effective Diagnosis and Treatment of Coronary Artery Disease. Baltimore: Williams & Wilkins, 1997.

# 16

# Medicolegal Issues in Interventional Cardiology

*M. Lee Cheney*

Today, more than ever, each encounter between a physician (now depersonalized as "provider") and patient (or "consumer" of health care services) is a potential basis for a medical malpractice suit. Regardless of whether these suits reflect only a small portion of the number and magnitude of medical errors, as some commentators maintain,[1] or are the result of a conspiracy of greed among plaintiffs, plaintiffs' attorneys, and insurance companies, as others charge,[2, 3] the risks of being sued and the costs related to those risks are substantial and increasing.[4, 5] A number of factors, including practice specialty (specialties in which invasive medical procedures having higher risk are often performed),[4–6] affect the statistical likelihood that a physician will be sued. A history of small claims against a physician has been associated with the occurrence of future large claims, and the risk of malpractice liability is greater when the number of claims against a physician is high in relation to the number of years in practice. Moreover, it appears that attitude and poor communication contribute more to the likelihood of a claim than does lack of medical/technical expertise.[7, 8] As the movement toward managed delivery of health care expands, physicians can expect a concomitant increase in patient dissatisfaction and professional liability claims.

Today, in an environment in which all parties (insurers, patients, physicians, and government) demand both lower costs for health care and improvements in a system designed to lower those costs, the economic cost of malpractice continues to rise.[7] The direct costs related to the risk of malpractice are reflected in amounts paid for malpractice suits, now estimated to be as high as $7 billion.[6] In the 1980s, malpractice premiums for the average physician almost tripled, climbing at an average annual rate of 19.5%.[7] According to data collected by the Physician Insurers Association of America (PIAA), the average cost of defending against a malpractice claim more than doubled between 1985 and 1995.[6] One element of these increasing defense costs is the medical expert witness, whose fees for the expert testimony required in medical malpractice cases have nearly tripled. During the same decade, despite the occasional "runaway" jury verdict, average payouts in jury verdicts, although rising, have not yet doubled.

Defensive medicine, defined as actions taken by a physician or other health care provider for the purpose of deterring legal claims rather than primarily for the promotion of the patient's health, cost the nation an estimated $40 billion in 1990.[7] The practice of defensive medicine is in direct conflict with the cost containment requirements that are increasingly imposed on the medical profession. Not only do such defensive practices increase costs, but they also increase the total number of risks to which the individual patient is subjected, which may further increase costs related to adverse outcomes that would not otherwise have occurred. Ironically, the practice of defensive medicine, even when not beneficial and perhaps even detrimental to the patient, is often cited by medical expert witnesses as the legal standard of care to which the average physician must adhere.

In addition to these economic costs, there are societal costs associated with the increasing risk of medical liability as well. Societal costs include the adversarial elements introduced into the physician-patient relationship; the psychologic impact of malpractice suits on physicians; the migration of many physicians, particularly specialists, away from smaller communities; and the growing disparity between patient expectations and what their insurance companies will pay for. Managed care can be expected to distance physicians from their patients further and to contribute to patients' distrust of the medical profession.

Until workable solutions to the problems with the malpractice system are found, physicians must realize that compliance with acceptable medical practices alone is no longer sufficient protection against a suit. Although plaintiffs still have the burden of proving that medical negligence occurred, this burden is increasingly met more easily because of the growing number of physicians in all specialties willing to provide the necessary expert testimony. As a result, the legal burden has shifted to physicians to prove that they complied with the applicable standard of care. As discussed in this chapter, it is considerably more difficult to prove affirmatively that medical care was appropriate and acceptable than many clinicians suspect. Therefore, physicians must learn to practice in a way that is both medically appropriate and legally defensible; that is, instead of *defensive* medicine, physicians must practice *defensible* medicine.

The purpose of this chapter is to explain the general law of medical malpractice, as well as discuss some of the specific areas of concern to the interventional practitioner. It also presents some recommendations both for minimizing the risk of being sued and for maximizing a successful defense in the event of a malpractice suit.

## OVERVIEW OF MEDICAL MALPRACTICE LAW

### Tort Law Background and Theory

Tort law is based on the premise that a person who is injured by the negligence of another is entitled to recover compensation for the losses sustained as a result of that injury. Negligence, or fault, is central to most tort actions, including medical malpractice. *Negligence* is generally defined as the failure to exercise the degree of care and skill ordinarily exercised by a reasonably prudent person under similar circumstances. Within the context of medical malpractice, a physician's care and treatment of a patient are measured (theoretically) against the degree of care and skill ordinarily exercised by an average physician in similar circumstances. The specific standard of care must be proved in each case.

### Elements of a Medical Malpractice Case

Fortunately for all people who, regardless of how competent and careful they are, make mistakes from time to time, negligence alone does not mean professional liability. A plaintiff in a medical malpractice action must be able to demonstrate the following four elements in order to establish a legally sufficient case of medical negligence:

1. A duty on the part of the physician to comply with an applicable standard of care and
2. a breach of that duty of care, or failure to comply with the applicable standard of care, which is

3. a proximate cause
4. of damage to the patient.

In addition, a suit must be brought within the relevant state's statutory time limit, known as the statute of limitations.

If the plaintiff's evidence (e.g., medical records, testimony of fact, and expert witnesses) presumptively "proves" each of these four essential elements, the plaintiff is said to have met the burden of proof, and the burden then shifts to the defendant to try to rebut or explain the plaintiff's evidence. If the plaintiff fails to present sufficient evidence of each element, the defendant is entitled to ask the court for summary judgment, which means dismissing the case as a matter of law without submitting to a jury trial.

### Duty Arises from Doctor-Patient Relationship

A threshold requirement for any medical malpractice case, a duty of care arises out of and is dependent on the existence of a doctor-patient relationship at the time of the alleged negligence. The duty begins when the doctor-patient relationship is established for a particular medical problem or purpose and ends when the care has ceased for that problem or purpose. Unless and until a doctor-patient relationship has been established with a given patient, the physician has no duty of care with regard to that patient. If a duty capable of being breached does not exist, there can be no negligence and thus no medical malpractice case. So-called "curbside consults" are examples of situations in which a doctor-patient relationship may not exist and therefore cannot alone serve as the basis for a malpractice action.[9] However, managed care and technologic innovations may be changing this principle, as discussed later.

Termination of an established doctor-patient relationship is usually by mutual assent after the problem for which the patient initially sought treatment has been resolved, unless the physician has meanwhile undertaken to diagnose, treat, or care for an additional problem. Furthermore, patients may unilaterally terminate the doctor-patient relationship either expressly (telling the physician that his or her services are no longer required) or by implication (failure to keep appointments). Although the law defines the doctor-patient relationship as contractual and physicians are considered to be free to choose with whom they will contract, a physician may not *unilaterally* stop caring for a patient without sufficient advance notice to allow the patient to find another physician to continue the care.[10] Otherwise, the physician may incur liability for abandonment (i.e., breach of duty of care).

## Duty Is to Exercise Standard of Care

Once a doctor-patient relationship has been established, a physician has a duty to exercise that degree of care and skill ordinarily exercised by the average physician under similar circumstances. The conduct of a specialist is judged with reference to the average member of the physician's specialty under similar circumstances.

As a practical matter, the standard of care applied to any physician being sued for medical malpractice is usually established by so-called expert witnesses. An expert witness is not necessarily a physician practicing within the defendant's own specialty[11] or even another physician. Courts have allowed nurses, chiropractors, and other health care providers to testify as experts against physicians.[12]

Although the trend toward raising standards of care has resulted in widespread abandonment of the so-called "locality rule," a local standard of care still prevails in some states.[13] Under a local standard of care, the defendant physician is held to the degree of care and skill ordinarily exercised by other physicians in the defendant's specialty in the same (or sometimes a similar) community as it existed at the time the care was rendered. In these states, expert witnesses must usually be able to testify that they are familiar with the local standard of care[14]; however, out-of-state experts may be permitted to express their opinions by testifying that they are familiar with the standard of care prevailing in similar communities[15] or that there are universal minimal standards.[16] A small minority of states, however, has passed legislation prohibiting expert witnesses from testifying in medical malpractice trials unless they are licensed in the state in question or in a bordering state.[17]

In most states, a national standard of care has been adopted,[18] especially with regard to specialists. The rationale for the national standard lies with the nationalization of medical education and training, certification of most specialists by national boards, their attendance at national meetings, and the fact that they subscribe to national professional specialty journals.[19] Therefore, the professional knowledge and information available within a given specialty, if not the level of technology, should not differ substantially from place to place.

A "common knowledge" exception to the requirement for expert testimony in medical malpractice cases is recognized when the act of alleged negligence relates to noncomplex matters that are within the knowledge and understanding of the average juror and do not need to be explained by an expert.[20]

## Proximate Cause Must Be Established

Once the plaintiff has one or more expert witnesses to testify as to the applicable standard of care and the defendant physician's breach of that standard, the plaintiff must show that the negligence caused an injury. Even in cases in which medical negligence is clearly shown, there is no viable malpractice case if there is no injury (damages) to the plaintiff. Furthermore, if the physician made an error and the plaintiff suffered an injury but the physician's error was not a substantial factor in producing the injury, the physician is not liable. Causation, within the legal context, is a less exacting standard than it is in medicine. In most cases, the physician's negligence need only be more likely than not (i.e., 51% or greater probability) a cause of the plaintiff's injuries in order to satisfy the proximate cause element. In general, this element is also established by expert testimony.

## Damages

Proximately caused medical injuries suffered by a patient plaintiff may lead to compensatory damages and, in cases of gross negligence, punitive damages. Compensatory damages involve compensation for economic losses, such as medical expenses, lost wages if a patient's injury interfered with the ability to work, and costs of rehabilitating or maintaining a patient with an injury-related disability. Compensatory damages also involve noneconomic losses, such as the loss of a chance for a cure (resulting from delay in diagnosis or treatment), pain and suffering, inconvenience, mental suffering, severe emotional distress, loss of society and companionship, and loss of enjoyment of life (hedonic damages). Punitive damages are monetary awards unrelated to compensation issues; they are designed to punish errant defendants.

Persons other than the patient may also recover for their own injuries as a result of the negligence to the patient. For example, all states allow spouses or parents to recover compensation for medical expenses paid on behalf of the injured patient. In addition, the spouse of an injured patient may be entitled to recover on a claim for loss of consortium. A growing number of states allow persons other than the injured patient to recover damages for the severe emotional distress arising out of the negligent treatment of a patient.

## SOME APPLICATIONS OF MEDICAL MALPRACTICE LAW TO INTERVENTIONAL CARDIOLOGY

Some of the major areas in which the interventional cardiologist may confront medicolegal problems include complications of and adverse outcomes related to invasive procedures, informed consent, consultations, withholding and withdrawing treatment, acquired immunodeficiency syndrome (AIDS), diagnosis-related issues, telemedicine, and documentation. Each of these areas is discussed, and steps for risk minimization are suggested. It is important to appreciate that the details of various malpractice cases may vary according to patient diagnosis, physician specialty, and state law, but ultimately all cases must adhere to the framework outlined earlier.

## Complications and Adverse Outcomes

Surgical issues and those related to invasive procedures—including coronary catheterization; angioplasty; implantation of pacemakers, defibrillators, or other devices; and Swan-Ganz catheterization—tend to generate the greatest number of malpractice claims. Legal accountability may attach not only for the misuse of medical technology but also for undue delay in using, or failure to use, a new or accepted technology when indicated. Therefore, physicians are expected to familiarize themselves with new technology and understand its applications in daily practice.

For example, in 1986 a Connecticut court addressed the issue of a defendant physician's failure to use a Swan-Ganz catheter in a patient who subsequently died.[21] The plaintiff's expert witness, a cardiologist, testified that the Swan-Ganz catheter would have helped establish the diagnosis of hypovolemia. However, there was no evidence that the physician's failure to use the Swan-Ganz catheter caused or contributed to the patient's death; that is, the patient did not die from problems related to hypovolemia. Thus, the patient's case lacked an essential element (causation), and the court concluded as a matter of law that there was no evidence of malpractice.

Suits have also arisen out of the inappropriate use of medical technology. In one case, a Swan-Ganz catheter perforated a patient's pulmonary artery, resulting in his death.[22] In another case, a physician was found liable when a patient died after a bilateral pneumothorax developed as a result of the improper insertion of a chest tube.[23]

A valid malpractice case arises when a physician's negligent failure to use, or negligent performance of, a procedure results in injury to or death of the patient. Although physicians must keep abreast of evolving technologic methods and changes in medical practice, this does not mean that every physician must or should offer the latest technology. The association between high-volume rates of procedures and outcome suggests that some physicians should refer certain types of patients. For example, the American College of Physicians/American College of Cardiology/American Heart Association (ACP/ACC/AHA) Task Force on Clinical Privileges in Cardiology estimated that in order to perform or offer angioplasty procedures, an individual physician must perform at least 75 percutaneous transluminal coronary angioplasty (PTCA) procedures per year as the primary operator, and an institution must provide at least 200 PTCA procedures annually.[24] Similar considerations apply to coronary bypass surgery.[25] With the proliferation of catheterization and PTCA facilities at community hospitals and in mobile laboratories, this issue remains controversial, and problems in this area can be expected to increase.

In addition to suits based on failure to use or on misuse of a given device or technology, physicians may also be sued when complications occur despite the absence of any identifiable negligence by the physician. The law recognizes that there are certain risks inherent in every medical procedure. For example, all cardiac catheterizations carry a risk of bleeding. Infection (both local and systemic), vascular complications, thrombosis, and dysrhythmias are also recognized risks of the procedure. The mere occurrence of a complication does not in and of itself establish negligence. Nevertheless, physicians often find themselves defending against charges of medical negligence when a known risk of a particular procedure or device occurs. Such suits are usually subject to summary dismissal if the plaintiff is unable to produce an expert witness to testify that the particular complication did in fact occur as the result of some identifiable act of negligence on the part of the defendant physician. Increasingly, however, plaintiffs are able to find such expert witnesses willing to sell the necessary testimony. Therefore, physicians who perform invasive procedures must be prepared to defend themselves in court by showing a thorough knowledge of the procedure or device and its indicated uses, how its use complied with standards of accepted practice, that the benefits outweighed the potential risks for the particular patient, and that the patient's informed consent was obtained. Such a defense requires the physician to carefully and thoroughly document the patient's course in his or her chart.

## Informed Consent

Informed consent is the process through which a patient decides whether to undergo a selected procedure or therapy on the basis of information from the health care provider.[26] First articulated in 1957, the Doctrine of Informed Consent has its roots in certain fundamental rights recognized in this country, including the constitutional right of privacy[27] and the common-law right of bodily integrity and self-determination.[28]

In recognition that the human body is not to be

touched by others without authorization, the goal of the informed consent process is to provide for the clear, understandable disclosure of information necessary for the patient to make a decision. A physician violates a patient's fundamental rights, as well as state statutes that codify them, when performing a procedure or operation on a patient without first obtaining the informed consent of the patient or of the patient's legally authorized representative.

A physician's performance of an unauthorized procedure, the performance of an unauthorized extension of an authorized procedure, or the performance of an authorized procedure by an unauthorized person can constitute a civil battery for which the patient may recover monetary damages. Liability for battery may attach even when there was no negligence in the actual performance of the procedure at issue. For example, a surgeon was held liable for the nonnegligent but unauthorized removal of a mole during the course of an otherwise consented-to procedure.[29]

Informed consent issues may also arise when the patient's consent was not truly "informed." Although lack of consent cases can give rise to liability for battery, cases involving the quality of the disclosure underlying a patient's consent, which are the most common medicolegal cases, give rise to liability for negligence. Negligence cases usually involve allegations of failure to inform of a particular risk or hazard known to be inherent in the procedure. In addition, cases have established that physicians have a duty to inform patients of relevant financial incentives present in the particular plan under which a patient is being treated.

In general, physicians are not required to inform patients of a procedure's every conceivable risk, but they must advise patients of the most frequent risks and hazards. Some states require that the most serious risks be discussed, even though they may be rare. Depending on state law, one of two standards is usually used in judging the quality of a physician's disclosure of information to a patient. In most states, the test is whether the physician's actions in obtaining the consent of the patient (or of another person authorized to consent for the patient) were in accordance with the standards of practice of members of the same health care profession under similar circumstances. Commonly referred to as the "professional test," it usually requires expert testimony to prove the physician liable.[30, 31]

A minority of jurisdictions apply the "material risk" or "lay standard," which measures the appropriateness of a physician's disclosure by what a reasonably prudent person in the patient's position would have considered material in making a decision about whether to accept or reject the proposed medical intervention. In states using this test, expert testimony is still necessary to prove the existence and magnitude of risks but not to prove the standard of disclosure.[32] The lay standard is almost universally applied as an objective rather than a subjective test[33]; that is, the jury is usually instructed to consider whether the information about a certain risk would have been material to a reasonable person, irrespective of whether it would have been material to the plaintiff.

As in all negligence cases, when the quality of the physician's disclosure is challenged, the plaintiff must be able to show proximate cause. Thus, if a patient experiences a complication about which he or she was not informed and if it can be shown that the patient would have consented to the procedure even if the risk had been disclosed, the physician is not liable because there is no causal link between the failure to inform and the patient's injury. In addition, claims made by patients that they did not understand what the physician told them are ordinarily not enough for a successful suit if the jury or other trier of fact determines that a reasonable person would have understood the disclosed information.

Physicians whose practices involve the use of invasive procedures must understand and consistently follow the informed consent requirements. Many physicians incorrectly believe that informed consent is a mere formality, the goal of which is to obtain a signed consent form from the patient. A signed consent form alone, even though it may expressly state that the risks of and alternatives to the procedure have been explained by the physician, almost never conclusively establishes that the process of informed consent took place. As evidence, the form can be rebutted by testimony from the plaintiff that all or some of the requisite information was not provided, especially if the consent contains only a general statement that "all the risks and benefits have been explained to me." For this reason, the consent process should be separately documented in the patient's chart. In the absence of such documentation, the plaintiff's experts will be able to testify that "If it wasn't documented, it wasn't done."

Separate documentation of the informed consent *process,* as contrasted with the informed consent *document,* should record that the patient was informed of the diagnosis or differential diagnoses, the nature and purpose of the proposed procedure, and the expected benefits and potential risks of the proposed procedure. It should also ideally include any alternatives to the procedure (including nontreatment) together with their expected benefits and potential risks (including the possible consequences of nontreatment), the physician's rationale for recommending a particular procedure over other alternatives, an assertion that the procedure was described in reasonable detail, and an assertion that the patient appeared to understand and voluntarily consented.

The law recognizes some exceptions to the informed consent requirement, the most important ones being emergency and patient incompetence. In an emergency setting, when the patient is unconscious or when obtaining informed consent is otherwise not feasible or realistic, a physician may perform a necessary procedure or operation without first obtaining informed consent. In such cases, the requirements of informed consent are suspended because the time necessary to make an adequate disclosure and obtain consent would delay treatment to the patient's detriment.[30] Accordingly, the patient's consent in an emergency is implied by law as a matter of public policy, unless the physician has some particular reason to know that the patient would have withheld authorization. It is pertinent to note that the emergency exception applies only when a patient's life or health is in immediate, not future, danger.[30]

When dealing with a competent patient, consent must be obtained. As long as the physician has explained the possible adverse consequences of refusing a recommended procedure or treatment, the right of a competent patient to refuse treatment must be respected, even if the physician strongly believes the refusal is not in the patient's best interests. Of course, the fact that the patient refused treatment after full disclosure should be carefully documented.

In contrast, consent by an incompetent patient is invalid; that is, an incompetent person's decision is not a legally sufficient consent to treatment, and a physician is not protected if he or she renders treatment on the basis of the invalid consent of an incompetent patient. Furthermore, a physician may be liable for failure to treat an incompetent patient who has refused treatment.[30]

Patients may be generally incompetent by virtue of unconsciousness, intoxication, senility, psychosis, or severe retardation or incompetent specifically for the purpose of making the relevant health care decision. Patients may also be incompetent as a matter of law, as, for example, when a patient is an unemancipated minor or has been adjudicated by the courts to be incompetent. In addition, an otherwise competent patient's decision-making capacity may be intermittently impaired (e.g., by medication or depression).

Decision-making capacity should not be confused with ability to communicate decisions. A competent patient may be prevented from voicing preferences by intubation and similar measures, and care must be taken in judging competency in such patients. When a patient is clearly incompetent, consent must be obtained from a guardian or some other person recognized by law to consent to treatment on the patient's behalf. If no person is authorized to give consent for the incompetent patient, however, the incompetency exception permits physicians to go forward with the necessary treatment without first obtaining consent.

There are no standard tests to determine a patient's competence to consent to treatment. Although recourse to formal legal procedures exists for this purpose, the President's Commission for the Study of Ethical Problems in Medicine and Biomedical and Behavioral Research has recommended that these determinations be made by the attending physician with regulation and review at the institutional level but without routine involvement of the courts.[34] When making these assessments, the President's Commission recommended that attending physicians evaluate "the patient's capacity to understand information relevant to the decision; to communicate with caregivers about the decision; and to reason about relative alternatives against a background of sound, stable personal values and life goals."[34] In some cases, it may be useful to obtain a psychiatric consultation so that these elements can be assessed (and documented) by a neutral physician not directly involved in the performance of any procedures at issue.

Informed consent does not mean that physicians are obliged to force detailed information upon every patient, regardless of how the patient feels about this disclosure. Actually, the reverse is true. Just as patients have a right to give consent on the basis of full disclosure, they also have a right to give consent on the basis of no disclosure.[29] If a patient does not wish a detailed discussion of the possible risk before giving consent, the physician need merely document that the attempt was made and the patient waived this right. Another possible exception to informed consent requirements, known as *therapeutic privilege,* involves situations in which disclosure is likely to have a detrimental effect on the patient's condition. A great deal of controversy exists in this area, and the existence and extent of the privilege varies considerably among states.

Consent may be express or implied. Express consent may be given orally, in writing, or by actions (e.g., sign language, nodding the head). Consent may be implied by law, by a patient's inaction, or by custom. It must be voluntary and free from threats, coercion, unfair persuasion, or fraudulent inducements. Once full disclosure has been made and the patient's consent conveyed by whatever means, it must be documented in the patient's chart. As important as the documentation is, however, it is nothing more than a written record that the process actually took place. Although documentation is important for evidentiary purposes, it is the process that is legally required. Studies show that patients rarely weigh the risks and benefits of a recommended procedure or other form of treatment and that they do not pay serious attention to unrecommended alternatives.[34-36] Perhaps this is why many physicians place form over substance, believing that informed consent is merely the formality of getting the patient's signature on a preprinted form. In addition, studies of patients from whom fully informed consent was obtained have shown that after 1 day after the explanation, only 50% of patients understood the nature of the procedure and only 55% could correctly list even one major risk or complication.[37]

With this in mind, a physician's practices in connection with giving the required information when obtaining a patient's consent should be unvarying. A physician should have a standard practice of disclosing the required information about coronary angioplasty or any other procedure to competent patients, who are then given a chance to discuss this information, ask questions, and make voluntary decisions. The physician should then faithfully document this process. This additional documentation will bolster the physician's later testimony that he or she informed the plaintiff of a particular risk even when the physician may not specifically remember the discussions of 2 or more years ago. An unvarying practice in combination with specific documentation can be very strong evidence of informed consent. By contrast, poor documentation and physician acknowledgment of a lack of specific memory concerning the discussion can be quite damaging.

## Consultations

Traditionally, cardiologists who are formally consulted about a patient's diagnosis and/or treatment both examine the patient and review the pertinent portions of the patient's medical record. Such involvement in a patient's care will give rise to a physician-patient relationship, which in turn creates a duty of care on the part of the cardiologist. Typically, malpractice liability is shared between the attending physician and the consulting cardiologist.

Issues may arise between the physicians in terms of which physician bears the responsibility for the missed diagnosis, improper treatment, or failure to obtain informed consent (to name a few possible causes of negligence actions). For example, in a case in which the consulting cardiologist examined the patient with unstable angina and made a recommendation for cardiac catheterization about which the cardiologist wrote, "I have discussed this with the patient and indicated I would also advise [the attending physician]," the cardiologist took the position that the documentation notified the attending physician that the latter should implement the recommended treatment. However, the attending physician asserted that the documentation suggested that the cardiologist had put the recommended treatment into effect, especially in light of the fact that the cardiologist never "advised" the attending physician other than in the foregoing documentation. Such confusion when more than one physician is involved in a patient's care is not unusual. Other issues arising from consultations may involve an attending physician who claims to have relied on the erroneous advice of a consultant, each physician believing that the other would obtain informed consent, or a consultant who argues that the attending physician did not give accurate or complete information on which to base a proper opinion or recommendation. For these reasons, it is crucial that the physicians communicate directly with one another and document their involvement unambiguously. Finally, the attending physician should make specific inquiry about the consultation if either the consultant fails to make direct contact or the consultant's documentation is in any way unclear.

Even in the absence of a traditional physician-patient relationship, plaintiffs have argued that a specialist giving a so-called curbside (informal) consultation knows or should know that his or her colleague will rely on the advice that the specialist gives in treating the specific situation being discussed. Thus, the consultant owed a duty of care in that situation to give proper advice. The financial incentives of managed care organizations can be expected to result in an increase in informal, inexpensive curbside consultations. As this occurs, it seems almost inevitable that grounds for legal liability in this regard will be recognized. To date, curbside consultations generally have not been the basis of malpractice liability. As traditional paradigms of health care delivery are being altered by managed care and as courts continue to expand the accountability of health care providers, however, this can be expected to change.

### Telemedicine

Technology and cost concerns have given rise to a new type of consultation—telemedicine, which includes videoconferencing and transmission of radiologic images, electrocardiographic tracings, and other such data. A survey by the Office of Rural Health Policy found that more than 400 U.S. hospitals have implemented some form of telemedicine. Managed care organizations and other large providers use videoconferencing to link outlying hospitals and clinics with urban specialists, particularly cardiologists. Numerous hospitals have also established links to their radiologists, who can receive and interpret transmitted images from their homes.

The courts have not yet addressed the issue of whether telemedical consultations form a physician-patient relationship or give rise to some other basis for liability. Standards of care are not well defined, and to date, only the American College of Radiology and the American Electroencephalograph Society have adopted specific telemedicine standards. Other questions are also unanswered in the wake of high-technology health care, such as telemedicine. For example, although physicians are licensed on a state-by-state basis, telemedical consultations frequently cross state lines. Is a physician who provides telemedicine consultations practicing in his or her location or in the location of the patient? Many states allow an out-of-state physician to consult with a locally licensed physician. Some of those states limit such consultations to "occasional" or "infrequent," and not all states have this exception to the requirement that physicians be licensed to practice medicine (typically defined as any attempt to diagnose or treat a person for any physical or mental illness) in their state. Only 10 states have so far enacted laws to accommodate telemedicine practices, including requiring out-of-state physicians to become licensed by any state in which patients being treated by telemedicine are located.

The Federal Office of State Medical Boards has developed a model act that states can adopt to establish a registry for physicians who practice telemedicine. Under the model act, a telemedicine practitioner could submit an application to each state in which he or she wishes to practice (and which has enacted the model legislation), along with a fee and a certified copy of his or her medical license. At the present time, however, most physicians who regularly practice in different states obtain licenses in each state. The safe assumption for the time being is that a physician practicing telemedicine across state lines should obtain a license to practice in the patient's state. The American Medical Association (AMA) officially recommended this approach in 1999. Hospital credentialing procedures also need to be overhauled to accommodate telemedicine practices.

Technologic advances must be required to meet certain standards, including security. Liability for compromised patient care as a result of inability to access computerized information is foreseeable, and physicians should refuse to participate in consultations in which standards are not met. Some type of record of every telemedicine consultation should be kept. Videotaping has been suggested as the best way to provide an incontrovertible record of telemedicine treatment. Physicians may even face suits for not using telemedicine or for applying the raw technology inappropriately. In addition, it is crucial for physicians practicing any form of high-technology medicine to ascertain that such practices, including practice in other states, are covered by their professional liability insurance.

## Withdrawing and Withholding Medical Intervention

The Doctrine of Informed Consent, based on the fundamental right of patients to control the decisions relating to their medical care, includes not only the right to give consent after being fully informed but also the right to refuse any type of medical treatment. The law therefore recognizes a competent person's right to refuse any form of medical intervention, including life-saving measures, artificial nutrition and hydration, and use of a respirator.[38] The fundamental rights of autonomy and privacy extend to incompetent patients as well, but these rights are exercised in a distinctly different manner.[38]

What is the physician's responsibility when, as frequently happens, patients are not competent to make or communicate decisions relating to their health care? Must everything possible be done to forestall death merely because these patients have been unable to request otherwise? May such a patient's attending physician make such decisions independently, guided by the ethical obligation to do the least harm? May the patient's health care providers lawfully carry out the wishes of the patient's family? What if family members disagree? What if there is no family? May close friends make these decisions?

In Indiana, a physician was held liable for issuing a Do Not Resuscitate (DNR) order for a seriously ill patient upon the request of the patient's sister.[39] The patient was a 65-year-old alcoholic suffering from numerous ailments, including malnutrition, uremia, hypertensive cardiovascular disease, and chronic obstructive lung disease. His condition deteriorated during his hospitalization, but he remained awake and alert. The patient's sister visited and requested his physician to issue a DNR order. The physician complied, and the patient died several hours later. Cardiopulmonary resuscitation was not attempted. When the physician later sued the patient's estate for nonpayment of medical bills, he brought upon himself a countersuit for malpractice, alleging a failure to obtain the patient's informed consent for the DNR order.

In deciding this case, the appellate court observed that there were no reported decisions addressing the liability of a physician for entering a no code order.

It referred to an unpublished opinion from a New York court upholding an award of punitive damages for assigning DNR status to and failing to prevent the death of an 87-year-old patient without the knowledge of the patient's family or personal physician.

Many state legislatures have now passed natural death legislation to provide some guidance to health care providers. Attorneys preparing wills for their clients are now routinely being asked to prepare living wills as well. Many people have prepared their own declarations. It is certain that physicians in the future will be dealing with an increasing number of patients who have prior written directions concerning their health care should they become incompetent. Accordingly, it is recommended that physicians familiarize themselves with the specific statutory requirements for living wills, as well as other provisions of natural death legislation, in the states where they practice.

Natural death legislation typically provides guidelines for physicians when there is no written declaration by the patient concerning withholding or withdrawing medical interventions. For persons who are comatose with no reasonable probability of returning to a cognitive, sapient state or who are otherwise mentally incapacitated and whose condition has been determined by their attending physician to be "terminal, incurable, and irreversible," the statutes generally establish a hierarchy of authorized decision makers on the issue of withholding or withdrawing extraordinary means. Usually, the attending physician may withhold or discontinue extraordinary means with the concurrence of (1) the patient's spouse, (2) the patient's guardian, or (3) a majority of the relatives of the first degree, in that order. If none of the foregoing persons is available, the decision is left to the discretion of the attending physician alone or in combination with other designated decision makers.

There arises the question of whether a physician may be liable for deciding to withhold or withdraw treatment over, for example, the objection of a minority of first-degree relatives, a close friend, or a relative not of the first degree. In most states, statutory protection is provided to any physician against whom criminal or civil liability is asserted because of conduct in compliance with these provisions.

## AIDS

Human immunodeficiency virus (HIV), the virus identified as the cause of AIDS and of AIDS-related complex (ARC), is transmitted by contact with contaminated bodily fluids. While the predominant mode of transmission is sexual contact, health care workers are also at risk of infection through exposure to HIV-infected blood or other bodily fluids and body tissues. The Centers for Disease Control and Prevention (CDC) have identified three ways in which health care workers may be exposed to HIV infection: parenteral contact, entry through the mucous membranes, and cutaneous routes.[38]

Although HIV is not easily transmitted—indeed, 1988 data from the Presidential Commission on AIDS and the CDC indicate that much fewer than 1% of health care workers had acquired HIV infection in the course of their work—AIDS remains incurable and fatal. Fear of infection has caused many health care workers to refuse to provide care to known AIDS patients and to call for routine screening of all hospitalized patients. Many patients are being refused treatment simply for being members of groups that are at high risk of acquiring AIDS, such as homosexual men and intravenous drug users. One case involved a cardiothoracic surgeon who refused to operate on carriers of HIV.[40]

Federal law proscribes discrimination against handicapped persons, including HIV-positive patients. The Rehabilitation Act of 1973 applies to any hospital, nursing home, or other facility that receives federal funds. Whether individual physicians and health care providers have legal duty under the Rehabilitation Act to treat AIDS patients is a separate issue. The Thirteenth Amendment to the United States Constitution guarantees that no person can be forced to serve another against his or her will, and freedom-of-contract principles have governed in this area (exceptions being the emergency on-call situation and abandonment considerations once a physician-patient relationship has been formed). For example, a Massachusetts staff physician refused to perform elective surgery on a patient who was found to be HIV-positive. The court held that the hospital but not the individual surgeon was subject to liability under the federal antidiscrimination laws.[41]

With the enactment of the Americans with Disabilities Act, individual practitioners who own, lease (or lease to), or operate professional offices, clinics, hospitals, and other health care facilities may not discriminate against patients who are HIV-positive, with the following exceptions: (1) A physician is not required to accept patients outside his or her specialty; (2) a physician is not prohibited from referring a patient with a disability to another physician if the disability itself creates specialized complications for the patient's health that the physician lacks the experience or knowledge to address; and (3) a physician is not required to treat a patient whose disability poses a direct threat to the health and safety of others, according to an individualized assessment informed by objective medical evidence. Because this sweeping civil rights legislation is so new, litigation has not yet begun to construe and define the parameters of its coverage.

Legalities aside, the AMA Council on Ethical and Judicial Affairs proclaimed in 1987 that a physician "may not ethically refuse to treat a patient whose condition is within the physician's current realm of competence based solely on the fact that the patient has AIDS or is infected with HIV."[42]

A related basis for liability is a physician's failure to inform patients receiving blood transfusions of the risk of HIV-contaminated blood. To date, all these cases have involved plaintiffs who have actually contracted transfusion-related AIDS. It is conceivable, however, that liability could attach irrespective of whether the patient ultimately develops AIDS, solely on the basis of the patient's knowledge that contaminated blood was infused and the allegation of severe emotional distress arising out of the increased risk of contracting AIDS.

In a recent Maryland case, for example, an HIV-infected surgeon operated on a patient whose subsequent HIV test yielded negative results.[43] She filed an action against the surgeon's estate, seeking to recover damages for her fear of contracting AIDS. The court dismissed the plaintiff's action for failure to state a viable claim, holding that the plaintiff had not suffered a compensable injury. Not only had there never been a documented case of AIDS transmission from a surgeon to a patient, but also the plaintiff had not alleged that the surgeon failed to use proper barrier techniques or that there occurred an intraoperative incident that would have caused the surgeon's blood to enter the patient's body. The court recognized, however, that damages for fear of contracting a disease might be recoverable in a case that involved actual exposure to a disease-causing agent.

Moreover, in keeping with the requirements of informed consent, physicians have a duty to advise their patients of the alternatives to a transfusion with blood from an anonymous donor; these alternatives could include no transfusion, directed transfusion, and autologous transfusion. Patients for whom the risks of no transfusion could be serious but not life-threatening may well decide, and will certainly swear that they would have if they later become infected plaintiffs, to refuse a transfusion. Autologous transfusion is an option that must now be explained to every patient for elective surgery.

In another case, a patient with severe coronary disease underwent a five-vessel coronary artery bypass graft procedure in 1984.[44] During the surgery, the patient received blood that was contaminated with HIV. In the subsequent malpractice action, the court ruled that the patient failed to establish a case for lack of informed consent, not because his surgeon had no duty to inform him of the risk of transfusion-related AIDS but because a reasonably prudent person in the plaintiff's position would not have refused such necessary surgery on the basis of the remote risk of AIDS. Moreover, the court found that the surgeon's failure to inform the plaintiff patient of the option of autologous blood donations was not actionable because the patient's condition would have prevented him from exercising that option. Finally, there was no duty to disclose the option of directed blood because (1) there was no evidence that a directed blood program was available at the hospital in 1984 and (2) there was doubt as to whether directed donations would have lowered the risk of contamination.

## Diagnosis-Related Issues

Whereas surgery or procedure-related claims tend to be the most common, claims involving misdiagnosis tend to be the most costly. Diagnostic errors are the leading cause of loss in suits against cardiologists.[45] A delayed diagnosis or failure to recognize a diagnosis altogether can lead not only to costly delays in administering necessary treatment but also to consequent mistreatment. In addition, the misdiagnosis of a disease state that the patient does not have can result in unnecessary treatment and patient anxiety. Rather than being relieved upon learning that a particularly serious disease did not exist, some patients have actually sued for the unnecessary treatment and anxiety caused by the mistaken diagnosis.

In general patient care, a physician may rely on an adequate history elicited from the patient or other reliable sources, on the results of an adequate physical examination, on appropriate laboratory and other diagnostic test results, and on indicated consultations and referrals. The plaintiff's medical experts often testify that one or more serious conditions possibly suggested by the plaintiff's clinical presentation must first be ruled out before a less serious diagnosis is made, and it has been suggested that physicians could reduce loss from diagnostic errors by ruling out conditions carrying the greatest risk.[45] The distinction between appropriate testing based on a set of differential diagnoses and testing for unlikely diagnoses because of concerns about malpractice (defensive medicine) is not clear at this time. The development of practice guidelines by professional organizations and research groups may provide clinicians with a more secure basis for decision making in the future.

Indeed, partly because of their ambiguity and the inherent problems with the "cookbook" approach to medicine, guidelines are proving to benefit malpractice plaintiffs more than defendants. Moreover, the guidelines have not reduced litigation costs, but they have given rise to a number of questions that tend to increase rather than decrease the need for medical experts. Medical experts still have to testify, for example, whether the guidelines establish the applicable standard of care; whether they really apply to the case in question; whether the physician should or should not have followed the guidelines; whether the physician adequately interpreted, implemented, and complied with the guidelines; whether deviations can be justified; whether guidelines should have been followed until the appearance of an exceptional circumstance and then abandoned; and whether the physician correctly identified an exceptional circumstance.

## Documentation

The importance of good documentation cannot be overemphasized. Medical liability experts estimate that 35% to 40% of all medical malpractice suits are rendered indefensible by problems with the medical record.[2] Regardless of the facts and standards exercised, a bad result combined with a bad record almost inevitably results in money for plaintiffs.

One reason why good medical records in malpractice litigation are so important lies in the fact that most cases come to trial anywhere from 2 to 10 years after the challenged care was rendered. By this time, the defendant physician has little independent recollection of the events that transpired in the care of any single patient, and the plaintiff patient's knowledge, which may have been incomplete or inaccurate to begin with, has most likely been colored by the subsequent course of his or her condition.

The importance of good documentation also lies in the fact that some of the more unconscionable physicians who testify as medical expert witnesses for plaintiffs are willing to swear to the jury to a reasonable degree of medical certainty that if something was not documented, that means it was not done. For example, the following testimony was given by a plaintiff's medical expert witness in a medical malpractice case in which the defendant physician made the mistake of recording only his abnormal findings.[46]

*Question* (*by attorney*): "...What was your criticism in connection with that?"

*Answer* (*by physician*): "In a patient with this kind of trouble you should put down what you did. He should have tested...and he didn't do that."

*Question:* "...So, again, the problem was the documentation, not necessarily the examination that he performed; would you agree with that?"

*Answer:* "I have the same answer to that that I had to all the other questions. If he didn't record it, he didn't do it."

A third reason why it is so important to maintain good medical records is that poorly maintained records, rightly or wrongly, reflect adversely on the record keeper's quality of practice and can suggest medical negligence, even when there was none.

A medical record is maintained for the purpose of preserving a factual and objective record of the patient's course of treatment. It should document, in a legible and understandable way, the patient's medical history and presenting complaints, physical examination and findings, laboratory or other diagnostic testing and the results, differential diagnoses, and the ultimate diagnosis, including an explanation of how the diagnosis was established and how the other diagnoses were excluded. In addition, all important conversations, including telephone conversations, with the patient and the patient's family should be summarized. All informed consent discussions, as well as the patient's refusal to undergo recommended tests or therapies and failure to keep appointments, must be documented.

In one case, a patient who refused to undergo myelography and discontinued seeing her neurosurgeon ultimately developed spastic quadriparesis and sued the neurosurgeon.[47] She alleged that the neurosurgeon had not adequately explained the consequences of her failure to undergo the myelography. Unfortunately, the neurosurgeon had failed to document explicitly his discussions with the patient, leaving him vulnerable to the charge of expert witnesses that he should have done more to cause her to change her mind.

An important aspect of proper documentation is knowing what not to write. A patient's medical record is not the place for subjective, critical observations by health care providers concerning patients or their families or such observations of the care provided by other physicians or health care providers. Although it is important to make the record understandable, medical terminology such as "Alzheimer's disease" is always preferable to nontechnical observations, such as "patient's head is off with the birds," no matter how accurate such descriptions may be. Cases such as the one involving the comment just mentioned must sometimes be settled for a great deal more than they might otherwise have been because of such comments in the medical record and the fear of their impact on a jury verdict.

In addition, the medical record is never the place to express open criticism of another physician's judgment. This contributes nothing toward creating a factual, objective record of the patient's course of care and treatment, and it certainly does not help the patient. Such improper entries in the medical record, which are seen more frequently in the medical records of the patients cared for at academic medical centers than at community hospitals, undermine and discredit the writer and demonstrate unprofessional conduct and poor judgement.

Consider the following example from the medical record of a patient hospitalized at a major university hospital:

This seems to be our window of opportunity for operative intervention and repair, and this is what should be done because he is likely to continue to bleed and he cannot stand any more instability. He is relatively stable now and [I] doubt will be more stable. However, cardiology *refuses* to allow surgery. I have notified Dr. [name deleted] to get another general surgery attending involved because I cannot see that he will be [a] surgical candidate any later than now.

The author of this note created a medical malpractice case that almost any plaintiff's lawyer would readily agree to take. Moreover, he created possible legal problems not only for the attending physician with whom he disagreed but also for himself. The consultant was vulnerable to charges of medical negligence and patient abandonment by virtue of unilaterally taking himself off the case without making any meaningful effort, short of writing an angry note in the medical record, to see that the patient received the treatment that the consultant evidently believed to be essential.

Practicing good medicine alone does not protect health care providers from liability for medical practice. In addition to practicing good medicine, one of the best ways for physicians to minimize the risk of a malpractice suit and maximize their chances for a successful defense is to develop and consistently use good record-keeping skills. Even though physicians who are *not* sued may never become aware of the occasions on which they were saved by their records, physicians who are or would have been sued will certainly agree that good medical records are well worth the extra time and effort they require.

## MANAGED CARE

The legal system, steeped in and very fond of its tradition, has been cautious and exceedingly slow to adapt to the rapid and dramatic changes in the health care system. A new paradigm for health care delivery, central to which is cost control, continues to be governed by a body of law that evolved over many years to fit the now-outdated modes of fee-for-service care. As physicians increasingly become employees of large businesses or accept the financial risks of capitation, resulting tradeoffs between cost and quality set the scene for significant legal battles in the coming years.

The California courts have led the way in defining some of the issues that arise when physicians are discouraged or prevented from exercising their best clinical judgment. For example, *Wickline v. State of California* was the "first attempt to tie a health care payor into the medical malpractice causation chain."[48] In *Wickline,* a patient's third-party payor refused to authorize an extension of her hospitalization as recommended by her attending physician. As a result, she suffered a vascular injury that resulted in amputation of her leg. After she prevailed in her suit against Medi-Cal, a California appellate court reversed under the rationale that her physician breached his duty to appeal Medi-Cal's decision. He could not avoid the ultimate responsibility for his patient's care by merely complying because his medical judgment dictated otherwise. Although this case acknowledged the new physician-patient relationship, the court resorted to the traditional paradigm in deciding the case.

A later California case, *Fox v. Healthnet,*[49] also involved a denial of recommended care by a patient's health maintenance organization (HMO). As in the *Wickline* case, Mrs. Fox's physician protested her HMO's denial of coverage for an expensive autologous bone marrow transplant to treat her advanced breast cancer. The treatment was delayed until Mrs. Fox's family was able to raise the necessary funds—a delay that ultimately may have cost Mrs. Fox's life. At the trial of the family's wrongful death suit against Healthnet, the evidence showed that the HMO awarded generous bonuses to executives who successfully reduced overall plan costs, reductions that often involved denying costly treatment. A jury awarded $12.1 million in compensatory damages and $77 million in punitive damages, displaying the outrage that the jurors felt when potentially life-saving treatment was denied to a dying woman for financial reasons.

Another California case, *Puna v. Rale,* involved a surgeon who was found liable for failure to convey the urgency of an operation for which he sought authorization from the patient's HMO and for failing to follow up when the HMO did not respond in a few days.

These cases suggest that physicians must become advocates for their patients, often placing them in a direct conflict with a managed care organization (MCO) or another health insurer. Such organizations, many of which have a corporate philosophy that is strongly focused on the generation of profit, may have little tolerance for physicians who frequently recommend diagnostic tests that are not strongly indicated and even less tolerance for physicians who repeatedly contest the health plan decisions. In all these situations, it is advisable for physicians to inform patients of their financial arrangements with the organization.

## CONCLUSION

As Congress and state legislatures debate issues concerning managed care standards, health care cost containment, and tort reform, the future direction of medical malpractice law is uncertain. Many specialty boards have adopted practice guidelines in the hopes of setting practice standards, adherence to which would (theoretically) constitute a defense against malpractice claims. The legal system itself has been experimenting with alternative forms of resolving malpractice actions, such as arbitration, but no superior means have yet emerged. For the time being, physicians must rely on lay juries to decide often complicated medical issues that are almost always described by the conflicting testimony of medical experts.

To date, tort reform at the national level has been nonexistent. Unfortunately, when the health care reform efforts that would have included relevant malpractice system reforms failed, business interests seized the opportunity to assume the authority, with the short-sighted cooperation of the medical profession, to create a system wherein physicians have traded their autonomy and, some people might argue, status as professionals for the security of a paycheck. No longer the owners of the product they sell, physicians are allowing business interests to control almost all aspects of production, including receipt of profits, with health care becoming largely indistinguishable from other large industries. This private restructuring of the so-called health care delivery system has not created new laws to reflect the changing paradigms of delivery. Tort reform has proceeded slowly at the state level; only seven states—California, Colorado, Florida, Illinois, Kansas, Missouri, and Oregon—have enacted significant reforms. The problem, nevertheless, remains monumental and costly. In 1995, the Congressional Budget Office estimated that $200 million could be saved over a 7-year period as a result of medical liability reforms.

In providing a general overview of the principles of medical malpractice, I have intentionally avoided dealing with the significant variations among states in the details and applications of the principles outlined here. Moreover, it is pertinent to note that malpractice law in each state is constantly evolving as new cases are decided and new legislation is passed. It is therefore impossible to provide, particularly in a single chapter, an exhaustive survey of the law or definitive practices that will entirely eliminate the possibility of malpractice liability. The information contained in this chapter, however, should enable prudent physicians to incorporate into their clinical practices measures that will lessen both the risk of being sued and the risk of potential malpractice liability.

## ACKNOWLEDGMENT

I am grateful for the exceptional editorial support provided by Tracey Simons.

## REFERENCES

1. Localio AR, Lawthers AG, Brennan TA, et al: Relation between malpractice claims and adverse events due to negligence: results of the Harvard Medical Practice Study III. N Engl J Med 325:245–251, 1991.
2. Curran WJ: Medical malpractice claims since the crisis of 1975: Some good news and some bad. N Engl J Med 309:1107–1108, 1983.
3. Blackman NS: Medical malpractice and the contingent legal fee. N Y State J Med 75:1295–1298, 1975.
4. Campion FX: Grand Rounds on Medical Malpractice. Milwaukee: American Medical Association, 1990.
5. Prager LO: Tort reform still possible. American Medical Association News 40:1, 1997.
6. Garnick DW, Hendricks AM, Brennan TA: Can practice guidelines reduce the number and costs of malpractice claims? JAMA 266:2856–2860, 1991.
7. Comerford JD: Rescuing tort reform. J Med Assoc Ga 81:31–32, 1992.
8. Hickson GB, Clayton EW, Entman SS, et al: Obstetricians' prior malpractice experience and patients' satisfaction with care. JAMA 272:1583–1587, 1994.
9. Glynn v. Bausch, 469 NW2d 125, Neb. 1991.
10. American Medical Association: Neglect of the patient. *In* Principles of Medical Ethics: Current Opinions on Ethical and Judicial Affairs. Chicago: American Medical Association, 1986.
11. Melville v. Southward, 791 P2d 383, Colo. 1990.
12. Wozny v. Godsil, 474 So2d 1078, Ala. 1985.
13. Shuffler v. Blue Ridge Radiology Associates, 326 SE2d 96, NC App. 1985.
14. Raitt v. Johns Hopkins Hospital, 336 A2d 90, MD App. 1975.
15. Yang v. Stafford, 515 NE 1157, Ind. App. 1987.
16. Duvall v. Laidlaw, 490 NE2d 1004, Ill. App. 1986.
17. Ralph v. Nagy, 950 F2d 326, 6th Cir. 1991.
18. Capitol Hill Hospital v. Jones, 532 A2d 89, DC App. 1987.
19. Thomas v. McPherson Community Health Center, 400 NW2d 629, Mich. App. 1986.
20. Totten v. Adongay, 337 SE2d 2, W.Va. 1985.
21. Sochard v. St. Vincent's Medical Center, 510 A2d 1367, Conn. App. 1986.
22. Taylor v. Security Industrial Insurance Co., 454 So2d 1260, Ct. App. La. 1984.
23. Jones v. City of New York, 395 NYS2d 10, N.Y. App. Div., 1st Dept., 1977.
24. ACP/ACC/AHA Task Force on Clinical Privileges in Cardiology: Clinical competence in percutaneous transluminal coronary angioplasty. J Am Coll Cardiol 15:1469–1474, 1990.
25. Jacobs HB: The Spectre of Malpractice. Pueblo CO: Nationwide Press, 1978.
26. Salgo v. Leland Stanford Jr., University Board of Trustees, 317 P2d 170, Cal. App. 1957.
27. Public Health Trust of Dade County v. Wons, 541 So2d 96, Fla. 1989.
28. Fosmire v. Nicoleau, 551 NE2d 77, NY App. 1990.
29. Cheney ML, Mark DB: Medico-legal principles of emergency and intensive medical care. *In* Califf RM, Wagner GS (eds): Acute Coronary Care 1987, pp 37–48. Boston: Martinus Nijhoff, 1987.
30. Nyman DJ, Sprung CL: Ensuring informed consent: Essentials and specific exceptions. J Crit Illness 6:891–906, 1991.
31. Pardy v. United States, 783 F2d 710, 7th Circ. 1986.
32. Pauscher v. Iowa Methodist Medical Center, 408 NW2d 355, Iowa 1987.
33. Goodreau v. State, 514 NYS2d 291, N.Y. App. Div. 4th Dept., 1985.
34. President's Commission for the Study of Ethical Problems in Medicine and Biomedical and Behavioral Research: Making health care decisions: A report on the ethical and legal implications of informed consent in the patient-provider relationship. *In* The Ethical and Legal Implications of Informed Consent in the Patient-Practitioner Relationship, pp 17–410. Washington DC: U.S. Government Printing Office, 1982.
35. Lidz C, Meisel A, Zerubavel E: Informed Consent: A Study of Decision-Making in Psychiatry. New York: Guildford, 1984.

36. Lankton JW, Batchelder BM, Ominsky AJ: Emotional responses to detailed risk disclosure for anesthesia: A prospective randomized study. Anesthesiology 46:294–296, 1977.
37. Cassileth BR, Zupkis RV, Suton-Smith K, et al: Informed consent—Why are its goals imperfectly realized? N Engl J Med 302:896–900, 1980.
38. Annas GJ, Law SA, Rosenblatt RE, et al: American Health Law. Boston: Little Brown, 1990.
39. Payne v. Marion General Hospital, 549 NE2d 1043, Ind. App. 1990.
40. New York Times, Sunday, July 11, 1987, p 1.
41. Glanz v. Vernick, 756 F. Supp. 632, D. Mass. 1991.
42. Council on Ethical and Judicial Affairs: Ethical issues involved in the growing AIDS crisis. JAMA 259:1360–1361, 1988.
43. Rossi v. Estate of Almaraz, 1991 Westlaw 166924, Md. Circuit Court, 1991.
44. Knight v. Department of the Army, 757 F. Supp. 790, W.D. Tex. 1991.
45. Kuehm SL, Abraham E: Medical malpractice claims in cardiology. N J Med 87:393–398, 1990.
46. Deposition of plaintiff's expert witness, Case No. 90-CVS-1257, General Court of Justice, Superior Court Division, State of North Carolina, County of Robeson, 1990, p 173.
47. Lewis v. Satler et al, Case No. 90-CVS-1257, General Court of Justice, Superior Court Division, State of North Carolina, County of Robeson, 1990.
48. Wickline v. State of California, 228 Cal. Rptr 661, App. 2nd Dist. 1986.
49. Fox v. HealthNet, 219 Ca. Sup. Ct. 1993.

# IV

# Practice and Techniques of Coronary Intervention

# 17

# Design of the Interventional Cardiac Catheterization Laboratory

*James E. Tcheng*    *Richard P. Wawrzynski*    *Michael H. Sketch, Jr.*

Design and construction of the interventional cardiac catheterization laboratory presents special challenges unique even for the hospital environment. One must:

- Consider the needs of patient, family, staff, and physicians
- Accommodate radiographic equipment, power conditioners, computers, and specialty equipment
- Allow for adequate storage space
- Provide for electrical and radiation safety
- Maximize space and time efficiency

For those fortunate enough to have a "clean slate" when designing a laboratory, overestimation of the potential space requirements is a good starting point. In general, the more space the better. In the setting of significant space constraints, careful planning becomes even more critical. Benefits of the well-designed laboratory are a pleasant and efficient work environment conducive to the best possible patient care and avoidance of the additional expense and downtime associated with retrofitting a preexisting structure.

This chapter describes practical considerations important in the design and construction of the modern interventional cardiac catheterization laboratory. Floor plans from construction projects at two institutions are shown to illustrate the design concepts.

## GENERAL CONSIDERATIONS

### Laboratory Volume

One cardiac catheterization laboratory can be expected to support 7 to 10 diagnostic (left heart) catheterization procedures per 8-hour day. Because interventional procedures require somewhat more time per procedure, a more typical laboratory (performing simple and complex diagnostic procedures as well as coronary interventions) should be able to perform 5 or 6 procedures per day. Simple extrapolation would suggest that such a laboratory could handle 1500 procedures per year; however, because of laboratory downtime and schedule fluctuations, a more realistic number is 1000 to 1200 procedures per year per laboratory. This number is reduced further if the laboratory is dedicated to interventional work. Because only 4 or 5 interventional procedures can be performed in a routine day, each laboratory should probably be expected to perform only 750 interventional procedures or so per year.

Facility design and function are keys to optimizing laboratory efficiency and maximizing throughput in the cardiology suite. Locating the catheterization suite on the same floor as and adjacent to the majority of in-patient cardiology beds increases efficiency. Reducing operational bottlenecks, such as patient elevators, also improves overall laboratory efficiency.

Other variables directly affect the daily capacity of the department. Innovative methods of scheduling personnel work time, such as multiple shifts, 10-hour days, and staggered shifts, permit extension of the workday beyond the traditional 8 hours and the accommodation of additional procedures. Although these approaches allow for a greater volume of cases, such scheduling can occur only through the cooperation and mutual agreement of the nursing, technical, medical, and surgical personnel who care for the angioplasty patient.

### "Patient-Centric" Design

The design of the modern interventional cardiac catheterization laboratory must consider traffic patterns typical of the anticipated functions of the laboratory. The ideal laboratory design optimizes efficiency in all areas; however, first and foremost, the laboratory should be designed with the patient (and family) in mind. As the proportion of outpatient procedures increases, the interface between the outside world and the catheterization laboratory becomes more and more important. Central to this concept is incorporation of a family waiting room, ideally with a separate, adjacent private conference room for consultation. Also adjacent to the waiting room should be a patient receiving office for patients scheduled for same-day procedures. This area serves the important functions of patient registration and insurance verification and can provide liaison services for family members in the patient waiting area. The receiving office can also be the hub for centralized scheduling of future procedures. Such a function is essential in large referral centers, in particular those with competing cardiology groups, to manage the scheduled capacity in order to satisfy the demand for service. Scheduling a procedure for an evening block on a Friday can often disappoint the patient and family. Hence, there is an added incentive for institutions to encourage maximum efficiency during peak demand hours of operation.

Designing traffic flow patterns to accommodate the needs of patient and family substantially reduces anxiety and improves public relations. From the perspective of patient flow, the optimal design should facilitate the movement of both in-patients (ingress and egress via private patient transport corridors) and outpatients (dressing facility, lavatory, and holding area adjacent to both a public corridor and the patient corridor). Accommodation of all these features may be difficult, especially in the remodeling of an existing space, but awareness of the needs of the patient and family can make what is typically a stressful and difficult situation less taxing.

A second primary consideration deserving of special attention is the function of scheduling. Because of the volatile flux of a typical schedule, scheduling generally requires a person dedicated to management of laboratory flow, with a telephone and erasable board nearby. Ideally, this function should be centrally located in an area adjacent to the patient corridor (to monitor patient flow) as well as the family waiting area. Management of the daily schedule by the charge person must be tightly integrated with the rest of the department and involves not only timely coordination but exemplary communication skills. Because there remains a fair amount of unpredictability even on the best of days, a capable charge person must manage the schedule. Some charge nurses work well at minimizing gaps between procedures. Doing so is essential to keep the flow smooth and to decrease the probability of late days. Suggestions for minimizing gaps between procedures include (1) having patients queued outside the door of a catheterization laboratory room while the preceding procedure is being completed, (2) making sure all blood work is checked, (3) allocating personnel assignments on the basis of workload, and (4) practicing early notification of the physician responsible for a patient's procedure.

## Other Design Elements

Several other elements are central to a good design; they are:

- The needs of support (technical and nursing) personnel
- Supply receiving and distribution
- Physician functions
- Procedure archiving and review
- Infection control considerations

A comprehensive list of facilities, along with space estimates, is provided in Table 17–1.

### Needs of Support Personnel

The success of a catheterization facility depends on the staff. Because of the potential for 24-hour

**TABLE 17–1.    FACILITIES LIST FOR CARDIAC CATHETERIZATION LABORATORY**

Ambulatory patient and visitor area
    Family waiting room, with broadcast television, vending machines, and telephones
    Private conference room
    Patient and visitor lavatories
    Public corridor access
    Examination/preparation/holding rooms, with broadcast televisions and video cassette recorders
    Controlled access to patient corridor
Catheterization laboratories
    Diagnostic catheterization
    Interventional catheterization
    Electrophysiology studies
    Pediatric catheterization
    Central viewing area for observation
    Radiographic subsystems
Central facilities
    Central supply receiving and storage
    Cine radiography review and reporting room
    Cine radiography archiving room
    Equipment/gurney storage room
    Physician work office
    "Soiled" utility room
    Offices (physician director, supervisor, assistant supervisor)
    Hallway access to patient and service corridors
    Controlled access to public corridor
Patient holding and recovery area
    Holding/recovery room, including hemodynamic monitoring capabilities
    Nursing station
    Hallway access to operating rooms
    Hallway access to nursing units
Support space
    Staff lounge (lockers, showers, refreshment facilities)
    Physician lounge
    Physician assistant/nurse practitioner/fellows office
    Research nurse office
    Conference room

operation, it is critical to provide adequate support space, in the form of a personnel lounge suitable for breaks, as well as lockers, dressing areas, lavatories, and showers. Administrative offices for the supervisor and assistant supervisory staff are also critical for personnel management, instruction, and counseling. Although at first blush it might seem advisable to have personnel facilities in close proximity to the family waiting area, the repetitive routine of the catheterization laboratory may make staff indifferent to the emotional and psychological needs of the patient and family. For this reason, some distancing between staff support facilities (especially the personnel lounge) and patient and family corridors is suggested to minimize the potential for inadvertent miscommunication.

### Supply Receiving and Distribution

Effective inventory management remains the hallmark of an efficient operation. With the advent of overnight delivery, emulation of the "just-in-time" model common in manufacturing becomes feasible in the catheterization laboratory. With this approach, inventory can be kept at a minimum, with resupply performed on an as-needed basis. True replication of the model is not possible in the catheterization laboratory owing to the lack of complete predictability of equipment utilization. Inventory control can nonetheless substantially decrease stockpiles and space requirements while permitting expansion in the range of equipment that can be stocked. The best approach to inventory control is a centralized receiving facility for equipment accession and inventory, from which items are dispensed as needed. The alternative is to stock duplicate sets of equipment in each catheterization laboratory. Inventory distributed to individual laboratories does have the advantage of convenience and ready accessibility. This distributed inventory approach may therefore improve care and support of the critically ill patient. However, the cost of this model derives from duplication of stock and concomitant loss of control over inventory flow. The ultimate decision regarding implementation of inventory management and control must consider space constraints and personal preferences; the higher the number of laboratories, the greater the advantages of a centralized distribution system.

The use of integrated information systems for inventory control provides several benefits that are worth recognizing. A reasonable estimate is a cost of savings between 5% and 20% with the use of a computerized inventory management system. Integrating the inventory system with the clinical database, which should also be interfaced with the hemodynamic computer system, improves data ac-

curacy, reduces labor support, and saves time in stocking the rooms, generating clinical reports, and producing billing summaries. Such automation promotes operational efficiencies and provides an important service to the patients and practicing cardiologists. The laboratory design must include the space and network requirements for the various servers of such integrated computer systems.

### Physician Functions

Dedicated space for physicians should also be included in any catheterization laboratory design. This support space serves as the physician's "home away from home," particularly when the physician's office is not adjacent to the catheterization laboratory. Functions that should be anticipated for this area are (1) the writing of orders, history, and procedure notes, (2) transcription and dictation, (3) impromptu consultation, and (4) telephone communication with other physicians, staff, patients, and family. An office-size room equipped with a desk, file space for forms, telephone, and computer link should be part of the design.

### Procedure Archiving and Review

The design of the facility must also accommodate procedure archiving, retrieval, and review. Space is needed for the processing and development of cineradiographic film, library storage (film and digital media), and cineradiography film and digital projectors. It is recommended that sufficient space be allotted for the storage of at least 1 year's procedures on site, because of the propensity for restenosis and need for second catheterization procedures in patients undergoing interventional revascularization procedures. Although digital storage promises to reduce overall operational costs significantly, its effect on square footage requirements will be more modest. Even with condensed archiving media, physical space is required for the archiving function.

### Infection Control

One should also involve the infection control department in the design of the cardiac catheterization suite. A number of standards related to infection control should be incorporated into the modern catheterization laboratory. Interventional practice has evolved beyond treatment merely with removable devices (such as balloons) to the implantation of permanent devices (in particular, stents). Adequate air exchange must be planned, and scrub sinks adjacent to the procedure rooms must be incorporated for proper infection control. Both "clean" and "dirty" sinks and counters should be identified, and infection control boundaries should be provided for biohazard waste and blood sampling.

## DESIGN SPECIFICS

### Configuration of the Catheterization Laboratory

There are two basic cardiac catheterization laboratory configurations: the traditional single-table room and the newer "swing" laboratory design. The conventional laboratory is a more or less rectangular room, with a single patient table oriented along the long axis of the room and a control room nearby. A minimum working area is 500 square feet or so, with 600 square feet or larger being optimal. When

two laboratories are adjacent, a design incorporating a centralized control room facilitates the observation of simultaneous procedures (Fig. 17–1). This traditional design augments controlled ingress and egress by patients and staff, as it is generally easy to separate patient and family corridors from the staff facilities.

The swing laboratory is a newer design innovation. In this configuration, the base of the C-arm is positioned at the apex of a V, with a separate patient table located on each leg of the V (Fig. 17–2). In general, space efficiency is greatest when the arms of the V are at a 90 degree angle; however, the legs of the V can be opened up to as much as 180 degrees if the room is longer than it is wide. The primary advantage of the swing laboratory is greater patient

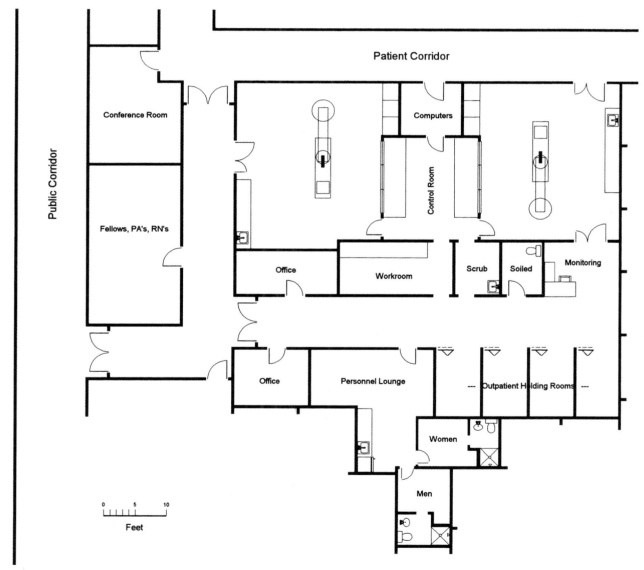

FIGURE 17–1. Partial floor plan of the Cardiac Catheterization Laboratory at Duke University Medical Center. The design concepts incorporated in this plan are (1) a single-patient table per laboratory, (2) a control room between the two laboratories, permitting simultaneous observation of two procedures, (3) a patient holding area with centralized monitoring, and (4) controlled access via dedicated patient and public corridors. (Courtesy of Duke University Medical Center, Durham, NC, and Isley Architects, Durham, NC.)

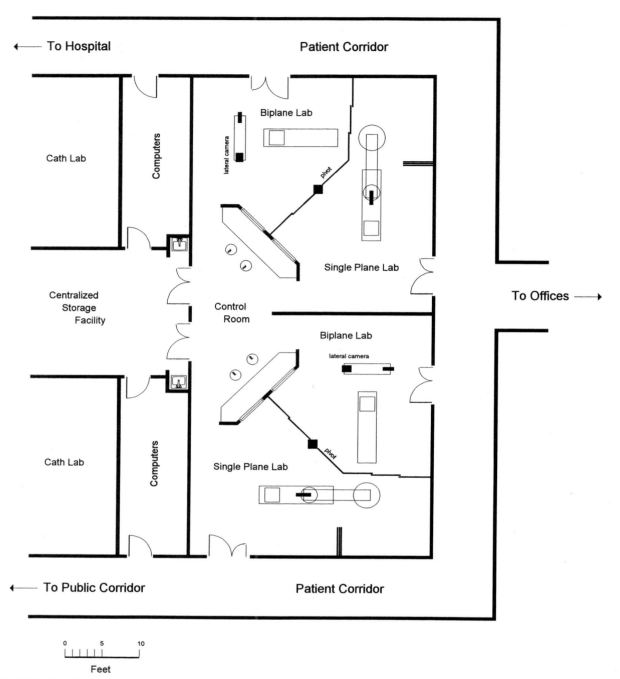

FIGURE 17–2. Partial floor plan of the Cardiac Catheterization Laboratory at Washington Hospital Center. The design concepts incorporated in this plan are (1) a "racetrack" surrounding the entire laboratory facility that serves as the primary corridor for all traffic, with a supply distribution area central to all the laboratories, (2) two "swing" catheterization laboratories, (3) controlled public access with a family waiting area, and (4) a command post for case scheduling and traffic control (not shown). (Courtesy of Washington Hospital Center, Washington, DC, and Philips Medical Systems North America, Springfield, VA.)

throughput. For a minimal additional investment (mostly the cost of a second patient table and set of monitors), throughput can be increased by 25% to 40%. This increase is achieved by a reduction in the effective laboratory turnover time spent in patient preparation. While one procedure is being performed, the next patient can be placed on the other table and prepared. Then, for the second procedure,

the divider between the two areas is opened and the C-arm swung into place over the second patient. Also, for diagnostic catheterization procedures, the arterial sheath can be removed following the catheterization with the patient still on one table while a procedure is being performed at the other table. The primary drawbacks of the swing room configuration are that (1) the room, generally square, requires patient access via two corridors (along the two back walls of the laboratory) and (2) the room itself must be larger than a standard, single-table laboratory.

The control room should be configured so as to enable staff to easily observe the patient and procedure directly while allowing ready and unencumbered access to physiologic monitors, radiographic controls, and recording devices. Ideally, this room should be 150 square feet or more; 120 square feet should be considered the minimum.

## Ancillary Radiographic Equipment

Regardless of the laboratory configuration, there must be space for ancillary radiographic equipment. Depending on the vendor, 10 to 15 linear feet of wall space within the laboratory proper plus a separate, environmentally controlled cold room measuring 100 to 200 square feet must be allocated for the housing of electronic subsystems. Certain items with less restrictive environmental requirements, such as the power conditioner, may be placed in the interstitial space above or below the laboratory (if such space exists). Cooperation between the vendor of the radiographic equipment and the project architect ensures that these requirements are incorporated into the design in the best manner possible.

## Additional Procedural Equipment

The design plan should allocate sufficient space to accommodate the additional equipment necessary to perform complex interventional procedures in critically ill patients. Because both the complexity of the coronary interventional techniques and the acuity of patient illness continue to increase, space allocation for this equipment in the laboratory should probably be designed along the lines of a mini–operating room. There should be sufficient room for an emergency code cart, respirator, anesthesia machine, intra-aortic balloon pump, and percutaneous cardiopulmonary bypass machine. For laboratories in which laser angioplasty or transmyocardial revascularization is performed, additional space should be allotted for the laser system. Also, because many of the newer interventional techniques are designed for device exchanges over 300-cm guide wires, it is suggested that a 10-foot patient table be ordered instead of the standard 7-foot table. A comprehensive list of equipment and facilities for a contemporary "percutaneous operating room" is provided in Table 17–2.

## Patient Holding Area

The patient holding facility is another area deserving of special mention. This area is used by patients both before and after procedures; thus, it is im-

**TABLE 17–2. CONTEMPORARY "PERCUTANEOUS OPERATING ROOM" FACILITIES AND EQUIPMENT**

Biplane x-ray angiography system with digital acquisition and playback
Pivoting table (to facilitate peripheral vascular procedures)
Hemodynamic monitoring equipment
Oxygen, vacuum ports (built in)
Ventilator (maintained by respiratory therapy personnel)
General anesthesia cart (maintained by anesthesia personnel)
Intra-aortic balloon pump
Percutaneous cardiopulmonary bypass equipment
Resuscitation cart
Activated clotting time analyzer
Blood gas analyzer
Intravenous infusion pumps
Transthoracic, transesophageal echocardiography equipment
Intravascular ultrasound
Laser system

portant to include sufficient space and privacy for functions ranging from undressing to invasive hemodynamic monitoring and emergency resuscitation. Walls separating individual rooms provide the greatest level of privacy; if walls (rather than curtains) are used to separate patients, care must be taken to provide adequate space in each room for both the stretcher and emergency equipment. For the acutely ill patient transferred directly to the interventional catheterization laboratory for treatment, this area is often used for preprocedure assessment and preparation. Postprocedure monitoring must also be available in this area, because the holding room often becomes a postintervention recovery room.

A well-designed holding area also permits more efficient use of hospital beds, allowing patients to be held and monitored while waiting for other hospitalized patients to be discharged. As hospitals have tried to reduce or optimize the number of staffed hospital beds, the operational impact is often experienced further upstream; holding areas in the catheterization laboratory now have become patient staging areas that relieve the patient discharge bottleneck. Preparing this area for operational adaptability and staff flexibility yields significant returns.

Ideally, the holding area should be on the same floor as the catheterization suite and adjacent to the scheduling charge nurse office. Designing the space so it can be used as a preintervention staging area provides a safe environment (compared with a hallway) to hold patients just before the start of an intervention. This staging arrangement establishes some functional overlap to buffer variable patient transport times and and to minimize costly procedure room turnaround time. Like other areas, the holding area must contain communications equipment, such as telephone, intercom, and emergency call system. Finally, commercially connected television may be included as a way to help occupy the patient awaiting a procedure, with videocassette tape playback capabilities being of potential educational value.

## Wiring

A design detail that is often overlooked is electrical and electronic wiring. In general, electrical requirements should be overestimated; for example, in the catheterization room proper, four-socket "quad" 120 V outlets should be placed wherever one might ordinarily place a duplex outlet. In addition, a 120 V quad outlet near or on the base of the patient table will prove invaluable. Some equipment, particularly laser systems, may have special electrical requirements. Computer cabling should be run to every location where there is a desk telephone or an angiographic (cineradiographic or digital) viewing station and to the hemodynamic monitoring equipment in the control room. Even if a local area network is beyond the scope of the construction project, installation of this extra wire during construction adds only minimal cost to the project while potentially saving the much greater expense of retrofitting the laboratory for a computer network at a later date. It is recommended that either Category 5 (or better) wire be used to support the computer network standards of today and position the laboratory for the new high-speed standards currently being introduced.

Several other electronic subsystems should be specified in the planning phase. Careful placement of an integrated telephone and intercom system facilitates point-to-point as well as external communications. Emergency call buttons must be strategically placed to summon help rapidly. A music system, with speakers positioned above the patient table to provide the patient with stereo sound, may make the patient's experience more tolerable and allow music to be played in the laboratory for the staff during downtime. Wiring for cable television to the patient holding rooms and to the family waiting room should also be incorporated. Finally, a broadband radiofrequency (RF) antenna should be placed outside the hospital, with the amplified signal sent to a broadcast antenna located within the confines of the laboratory. This maneuver (1) circumvents the problems of poor RF reception typical of the catheterization laboratory and (2) improves the reliability of beeper paging systems.

## Room Dimensions

Suggested dimensions for the various rooms are listed in Table 17–3. In general, individual rooms, such as offices and personnel lounges, should be

**TABLE 17–3.  SUGGESTED ROOM DIMENSIONS FOR CARDIAC CATHETERIZATION LABORATORY (SUPPORTS 2–4 CATHETERIZATION LABORATORIES)**

| ROOM | DIMENSIONS (FEET) |
| --- | --- |
| Catheterization laboratory | |
|     Procedure room (single laboratory) | 25 × 25 |
|     Procedure room ("swing" laboratory) | 35 × 35 |
|     Control room (single laboratory) | 12 × 15 |
|     Radiographic electronics | 10 × 15 |
|     Patient holding/recovery room | 10 × 12 |
|     Supply room | 20 × 30 |
|     Film darkroom/processing room | 10 × 10 |
|     Media storage | 10 × 10 |
| Personnel | |
|     Lounge, locker, lavatory | 25 × 25 |
|     Office (single) | 10 × 10 |
|     Office (shared) | 10 × 15 |
|     Nursing/scheduling area | 15 × 20 |
|     Conference room | 20 × 20 |
| Physician | |
|     Office (single) | 12 × 15 |
|     Work area | 15 × 15 |
| Family | |
|     Waiting room | 20 × 20 |

designed with careful attention to functionality, efficiency, and traffic patterns. The supply receiving and distribution area should be easily accessible to delivery services as well as centralized within the confines of the laboratory.

## REGULATORY REQUIREMENTS

This chapter was not meant to be a treatise on the architectural design of catheterization laboratory facilities; rather, the emphasis has been on practical considerations that are often overlooked in the design and planning phase. One should also be aware of the numerous design and code requirements imposed by local, state, and federal agencies, which are well beyond the scope of this short chapter. These requirements, which are specified in great detail in code and regulatory documents, are designed to protect staff and patient alike. The best resources for this information remain the architectural and engineering firms employed to assist in the planning, design, and construction of a new or a remodeled facility.

## CONCLUSION

Effective planning, design, and construction of a catheterization laboratory facility requires the cooperative efforts of physicians, hospital administrators, laboratory staff, architects, contractors, and subcontractors. Physicians continue to have the primary responsibility for defining the scope of such a project, including specific items that affect patient care. Hospital administrators, who in general are responsible for the funding of such projects, must balance the needs identified by the physicians with space and budgetary constraints. The laboratory administrative staff must consider not only the needs of the patient but also the requirements placed on laboratory staff in this high-stress setting. Efficiency coupled with a pleasant working environment will serve all parties well; incorporation of the many varied needs in the planning and design of the cardiac catheterization laboratory will make the working environment conducive to the delivery of the best possible patient care.

# Physical Principles of Radiographic and Digital Imaging in the Cardiac Catheterization Laboratory

*Steven E. Nissen*

Successful performance of diagnostic and interventional procedures requires a fundamental working knowledge of the operational principles of imaging in the catheterization laboratory. Optimal radiographic imaging enhances the technical quality of the procedure and the safety of the operator and patient. During the initial decade of coronary angiography, many catheterization laboratories were configured and medically directed by radiologists; however, since the 1980s, this role has shifted largely to cardiologists. Unfortunately, most cardiovascular specialists receive little formal training in the principles and practice of radiography.

Interventional cardiologists must determine the optimal configuration for the catheterization laboratory. The choice of vendor and equipment for an interventional room typically involves expenditures of more than $1 million. The rapid shift toward digital acquisition and archiving since the mid-1990s requires invasive cardiologists to learn a whole new vocabulary. Suboptimal choices in equipment can significantly impede success during interventional procedures. Inadequate maintenance of radiographic equipment can quickly reduce image quality to below acceptable standards. Accordingly, the knowledgeable interventionist must be reasonably familiar with the operational principles of radiographic systems. This chapter introduces the practitioner to the physical principles of radiographic imaging in the catheterization laboratory. It also better prepares the reader to choose a vendor and equipment for interventional practice.

The importance of optimal radiographic technique is amplified by the fundamental limitations of cineangiography in the diagnosis and therapy of coronary disease. Even under ideal circumstances, coronary angiography provides marginally adequate image quality for clinical decision making. The re-solving power of the best current equipment is less than 5 line pairs per millimeter—a capability severely taxed by the need to image vessels of 1 mm or smaller. The imaging requirements for increasingly sophisticated interventional devices will likely continue to challenge radiographic imaging technology. New interventional techniques with major implications for imaging include the use of 0.009-inch guide wires, angioplasty of distal lesions, intracoronary stent placement, intravascular ultrasound, atherectomy, and radiation therapy.

## GENERATION OF X-RAYS
### Components of Radiographic Systems

The radiographic equipment required for optimal cardiac imaging is complex, involving many electrical and mechanical components. Although many different vendors provide catheterization laboratories, the design and components of the laboratories are generally quite similar. Figure 18–1 illustrates the principal elements of the modern catheterization laboratory, which include a generator, an x-ray tube, an image intensifier, a light distribution system, a video camera and recording system, a positioner, and a cine camera. Nearly all recently installed laboratories also include a digital imaging system, and many laboratories include a device for archiving digital images. The design and operation of each of these components represent significant tradeoffs between image quality, versatility, durability, and cost. An understanding of these choices requires familiarity with the physical principles underlying the generation of x-rays.

### Production of Radiation

Diagnostic x-ray equipment produces radiation by the method originally discovered by Röntgen in the

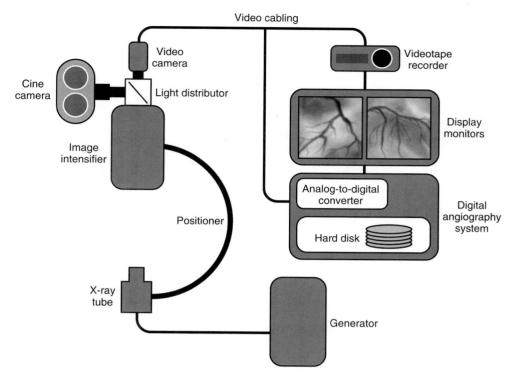

FIGURE 18–1. Components of a typical catheterization laboratory.

early 1900s. An *x-ray tube* consists of a positively charged tungsten metal target (anode) that is bombarded by electrons produced at a negatively charged cathode (Fig. 18–2). These electrons are accelerated across a very high-voltage, electrically charged gap between the cathode and the anode. This high voltage accelerates electrons to high energy levels (high velocity); the electrons then strike the target and interact with the tungsten atoms to produce x-rays. The most important interaction is known by the original German word *bremsstrahlung,* which is translated into English as "braking radiation." When the electrons pass close to tungsten atoms, the dense, positively charged tungsten nuclei alter the path of the electron, causing the

particle to decelerate. The energy lost in this braking action is emitted as a single x-ray photon, whose energy is determined by the degree of velocity change.

The maximum energy level of the electrons striking the tungsten is determined by the difference in voltage between the cathode and anode. For diagnostic x-ray systems employed in the catheterization laboratory, this voltage difference is typically 60 to 120 thousands of volts, abbreviated as kVp (kilovolts potential). The spectrum of energy levels of x-ray photons produced by the bremsstrahlung reaction is determined by the kVp and is measured in thousands of electron volts (keV). The peak kVp determines the maximum keV of x-ray photons in

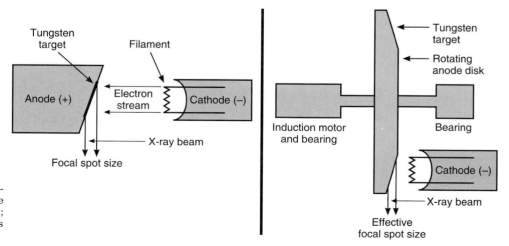

FIGURE 18–2. Fixed versus rotating anode x-ray system. On the left, the tungsten target is fixed; on the right, the tungsten target is located on a rotating disk.

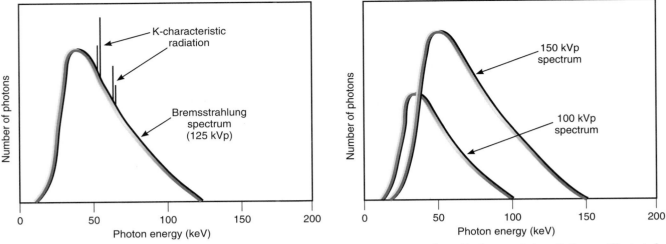

FIGURE 18–3. Energy spectra for typical x-ray angiography. On the left, the distinctive spikes of k-characteristic radiation are illustrated. On the right, the effect of changing the kilovolts potential (kVp) is illustrated.

the beam (Fig. 18–3, *left*). The higher the kVp, the greater the mean keV energy level and the more heterogeneous the pattern of photon energies (see Fig. 18–3, *right*). The spectrum of energy values strongly influences how the x-ray interacts with human tissue during radiographic examination.

A second, less important source of radiation arises within the tungsten target when an incident electron of sufficient energy displaces an electron from the inner shell of the tungsten atom. The inner "k-shell" electron is ejected from the tungsten atom and the vacant position is filled by an electron from an outer shell. This decay generates an x-ray photon with a keV level determined by the energy difference between the two shells and is known as *k-characteristic radiation*. The possible energy levels for x-ray photons are limited by the available energy differences for the particular target material and appear as a narrow but potentially important peak in the radiation spectrum (see Fig. 18–3, *left*).

The size of the electrical current between the cathode and anode, typically measured in milliamperes (mA), determines the quantity of x-ray photons produced. In cineangiography, x-rays are generated in short pulses and last a few milliseconds (ms) to coincide with the opening of a mechanical shutter that exposes individual frames of film. One important measure of the total quantity of radiation produced by the x-ray system consists of the current (mA) multiplied by the total duration of exposure (seconds). This value, expressed in milliampere-seconds (mAs), reflects the total number of photons generated by the x-ray source during a period of exposure.

## The X-ray Tube

The simplest construction of an x-ray tube is schematically illustrated in the left panel of Figure 18–2.

This type of arrangement is typical of an x-ray tube employed in a portable C-arm fluoroscopy unit. The electron beam is focused to strike a relatively small area of the tungsten target. The physical dimensions of this *focal spot* represent the size of the area from which photons emerge from the x-ray tube. The importance of the focal spot size is illustrated in Figure 18–4. The larger the focal spot size, the greater the "unsharpness" of the borders of any object placed in the x-ray beam (penumbra). This phenomenon, known as *focal spot unsharpness*, is one of several major factors that limit image quality in

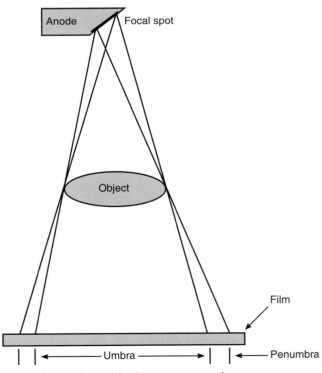

FIGURE 18–4. Effect of focal spot on image sharpness.

coronary cineangiography. An ideal x-ray source generates radiation from an infinitely small source. If other radiographic factors are held constant, reduction in focal spot size usually yields a slightly sharper film or video image.

Unfortunately, there are significant engineering constraints that preclude reduction in the focal spot size. X-ray tubes are highly inefficient for converting electrical energy to x-rays; they release more than 99% of the energy as waste heat. Although tungsten has a high melting point, there are significant limits on the ability to concentrate all the energy within a small focal spot. X-ray tubes take advantage of geometry to improve the *effective focal spot size* by focusing the electron beam on a beveled surface of the tungsten (see Fig. 18–2). In cineangiography, the requirement of 30 frames per second results in heat production so large that a bombardment of a constant small area of the anode would destroy the tungsten. Accordingly, cineangiographic x-ray tubes employ a high-speed rotating anode, typically turning at about 10,000 revolutions per minute (see Fig. 18–2, *right*). Each pulse of electrons strikes a different location on the anode, permitting a relatively small focal spot without overheating. For typical cineangiographic x-ray tubes, the operator can select from two different focal spot sizes, usually labeled "large" and "small," with typical effective sizes of approximately 0.6 and 0.9 mm.

X-ray tubes are rated in kilowatts (kW) for their ability to sustain high power operation (high kVp and mAs). This rating depends on the focal spot size selected, typically about 40 kW for the small focal spot and 80 kW for the large one. X-ray tubes are also rated in *heat units* for their ability to store and dissipate heat. A heat unit is defined as kVp multiplied by mAs, a crude but useful measurement of heat produced during the generation of x-rays. The x-ray tube is typically rated for its capacity to store heat (up to 1 million heat units or more) and by the ability to dissipate heat (typically 100,000 units per minute or more). All other technical factors being equal, a tube with a high heat capacity and better dissipation characteristics can provide a larger number of exposures (more acquisitions) before requiring temporary suspension of imaging.

## X-Ray Generators

The x-ray *generator* serves a number of important functions, including transformation of the electrical supply current to the high voltage levels required for generation of x-rays. Because x-ray tubes require one-way electron flow, the generator also *rectifies* the electrical current from alternating current (AC) to direct current (DC). Oscillations in output voltage appear as variations in kVp, a phenomenon some-times referred to as *ripple*. Because a constant kVp is desirable for exposure consistency, the quality of rectification is often measured by the consistency of the kVp produced by the generator. Most modern generators exhibit very little oscillation in their output, although small differences in design still exist. The output capacity of the generator is also measured in kW and should match or exceed the maximum capability of the x-ray tube. Thus, an 80-kW tube (large focal spot) should be used with a 80- to 125-kW generator.

Because x-rays produced during cineangiography must be generated in short pulses, the generator must rapidly switch on and off the current to the x-ray tube. The most sophisticated modern generators switch the current directly at the x-ray tube, a process known as *grid control*. A grid control tube generates a nearly perfect square wave x-ray pulse even at low output levels. The ability to pulse at low exposure levels is useful in pediatric catheterization and facilitates pulsed fluoroscopy, a feature with distinct advantages for imaging during interventional procedures. Systems lacking grid control produce less sharply controlled x-ray pulses because the cables between the generator and the x-ray tube store energy (capacitance), resulting in low-level but significant pre-exposure and postexposure radiation.

## Regulation of Exposure

In cineangiography, regulation of the radiographic acquisition parameters represents an extremely important function of the generator control circuit. This *automatic exposure control* typically involves an electronic feedback loop in which a light-sensitive detector observes the brightness of the radiographic image and signals this value to the generator. The generator circuitry must continuously adjust the kVp, mA, or duration of the x-ray pulse (ms) to keep brightness values within the optimal range for recording on film. The radiographic technique strongly influences the quality of the film image. Accordingly, generator *programming* represents an important issue in the design of an x-ray system for coronary angiography. It is customary for the automatic exposure control to continuously regulate the radiographic technique during cineangiography. Thus, film density is constantly adjusted during panning or following a large bolus of iodinated contrast material. Occasionally, a fixed radiographic technique is preferred, and most generator systems have a "hold" feature that keeps technique constant during an imaging sequence.

The method used for generator control of exposure is extremely important. The earliest cineangiographic systems regulated only the kVp while holding mA and pulse width constant. Regulation of kVp alone was acceptable in an earlier era of catheterization, primarily because cradle systems rarely resulted in highly angulated hemiaxial views. In the interventional era, systems that exclusively regulate kVp are undesirable because high kVp levels are common during steeply angulated views and the high kVp degrades image quality (discussed later). Alternatively, the programming of the automatic exposure control can regulate the pulse width, thereby increasing or decreasing the duration of exposure to maintain constant film density. This approach has some advantages, primarily the ability to keep kVp in the range that yields optimal image contrast. However, coronary artery motion during cineangiography is also an important variable affecting image quality. During rapid coronary artery motion, a pulse width greater than 7 to 8 ms results in unacceptable motion blur.

The most sophisticated modern generators regulate both pulse width and kVp in an intelligent fashion. For example, the system might begin with a kVp of 70 (for optimal contrast) and a pulse width of 4 ms (for motion stopping). If the detected light output is insufficient, the pulse width is gradually increased until 7 ms is reached. If image brightness is still insufficient, the system gradually increases kVp until 100 kVp is attained. If the image is still too dark, pulse width is again increased until 9 ms is reached, and finally, if needed, kVp is increased to the maximum of 120 to 150. This complex regulatory process optimizes radiographic technique for the greatly varying patient sizes and angles of view encountered in current interventional practice.

## INTERACTION OF X-RAYS WITH MATTER

## Radiation Exposure: Dosimetry

X-rays behave in a manner similar to that noted for all other electromagnetic radiation. The radiation intensity is measured in units of energy striking a unit of area during a unit of time. As distance from the x-ray source increases, radiation intensity decreases by the *inverse square law*—a doubling of distance produces one fourth of the radiation intensity. During diagnostic x-ray production, little or no radiation is absorbed by air. However, when x-ray photons strike solid materials, a complex set of interactions is initiated, including both *absorption* and *scattering*. These interactions determine the ability of x-rays to form an image and the biologic effects of the radiation.

The unit of radiation exposure from x-rays is the *roentgen* (R), defined as the amount of radiation that will produce $2.1 \times 10^9$ ion pairs in 1 cm$^3$ of air. For diagnostic imaging, the exposure rate is typically

reported in units of R per minute. The absorbed dose of radiation is the *rad*, a unit that represents absorption by the subject of 100 ergs ($10^{-5}$ J) of energy per gram. An alternative unit, the *rem* (rad equivalent man), takes into account differences in the *biologic* effects of exposure to different types of radiation. Total annual radiation burden from background sources for individuals without occupational exposure to x-ray typically averages about 125 mrem.

Any exposure to ionizing radiation is injurious to human tissue—there is no known safe exposure level for radiation. The primary adverse effect of low doses is neoplastic disease, particularly leukemia, with a long latent period of 5 to 30 years following exposure. This recognition has led to a steep reduction in the permissible occupational dose over the last 60 years. In 1931, the maximum permissible dose (MPD) was 50 rem per year. In 1936, the MPD was reduced to 30 rem. It was reduced in 1948 to 15 rem and again in 1958 to 5 rem annually. These values can be exceeded during short periods, but the long-term exposure must not average more than 5 rems for each year of age older than 18. The 5-rem limit refers to *whole body* radiation; for a given tissue, the limits are higher or lower depending on the sensitivity to ionizing radiation. For example, a dose of 75 rem annually is permitted for the hands and 30 rem annually for the forearms.

Cardiac catheterization generates a significant radiation burden to the patient and operator. Accordingly, federal regulations limit maximum exposure rates for both fluoroscopy and cineangiography. The actual regulations are complex, but several restrictions are important in the design of x-ray equipment. For example, fluoroscopy is limited to 10 R per minute measured at the table top unless the images are also recorded. For the safety of the patient and operator, careful and regular maintenance of x-ray equipment must ensure that these regulations are observed.

## Radiation Protection

In the earliest days of catheterization, the image intensifier was viewed directly by the operator. The close proximity to the radiation source and high ocular dose resulted in a high incidence of cataract formation among pioneers of catheterization. Improvements in radiographic equipment during the 1960s and 1970s significantly reduced average operator exposure, particularly with the introduction of indirect viewing of the image intensifier via television systems. However, during the 1990s, the complexity and duration of interventional catheterization procedures have again increased total radiation burden.

Other than increasing distance from the source, the only practical method for reduction in radiation exposure is *shielding*. The ability of material to absorb x-rays is measured by the *half-value layer* (HVL), defined as the thickness of the material that will reduce the exposure rate by one half. Absorption of x-rays is not linear with respect to the thickness of shielding. Instead, the relationship between thickness and the attenuation of x-rays is an exponential function (precisely correct only for monochromatic radiation). For typical diagnostic x-rays, the HVL might be several centimeters for water and only one tenth of a millimeter for lead. The HVL is dependent on the energy spectrum of the x-ray beam. For example, a beam formed at a peak kVp of 70 has an HVL of approximately 0.15 mm for lead, whereas a beam produced at 125 kVp typically requires twice the thickness of lead for similar protection.

Current protective lead aprons offer greatly improved comfort and performance in comparison to earlier designs. The most sophisticated aprons use a mixture of lead and tin compounds, primarily because tin is lighter and more efficient at absorbing low-energy radiation. A prudent practitioner takes every possible measure to reduce the occupational exposure of personnel. For example, a ceiling or table-mounted transparent leaded glass screen can be highly effective at reducing radiation exposure. Because of increased radiation sensitivity, special attention to the eyes and thyroid are important. Protective glasses and a thyroid shield should be worn by all participants during catheterization procedures. Lead aprons should be examined radiographically every 3 months and repaired or discarded when leakage is evident. The angiographer should recognize the potential for steep caudally angulated views to increase radiation burden. This increased exposure reflects two phenomena, the redirection of scatter radiation toward the operator and the increased scatter produced by the higher kVp levels required for hemiaxial angulation.

Reduction in patient exposure is more difficult to achieve. Good radiation safety practices in the catheterization laboratory are of inestimable value. Restriction of the radiation beam by movable lead shields, commonly known as *collimation,* is highly effective for reducing radiation scatter and may also significantly improve image quality. Collimation is frequently underused in poorly supervised catheterization laboratories. Because radiation dose is directly proportional to length of exposure, fluoroscopy should be performed only while the operator is actually viewing the video monitor. Often, a short-duration burst of fluoroscopy suffices for confirming balloon or catheter position. The duration of each cineangiographic imaging sequence should be care-fully modulated by the operator to obtain the optimal balance of image content and radiation safety.

## Interaction with Matter

When incident radiation strikes solid matter, a complex series of high-energy interactions is initiated. One important process is called *Compton scattering*, an interaction in which an incident photon collides with an electron of the target. This collision imparts kinetic energy to the electron and yields a new x-ray photon of lesser energy traveling in a different direction. For any material, Compton scattering attenuates radiation in proportion to the electron density of the absorbing substance. Another important interaction between x-rays and matter is known as the *photoelectric effect*. This process is observed as a sudden increase in the absorption of radiation for a given material whenever a fixed threshold of keV energy is exceeded (Fig. 18–5). This threshold is known as the *k-edge* and is determined by the atomic number of the absorbing material.

Whenever an x-ray photon with an energy level greater than the k-edge strikes a target, there is an increased likelihood that the photon will eject a k-shell electron. For photon energies of less than the k-edge, interaction consists mostly of Compton scatter, whereas for photons with energies slightly greater than the k-edge binding energy, the interaction often results in the ejection of a k-shell electron (the photoelectric effect). The k-edge absorption phenomenon has important implications for production of radiographic images. Iodine and barium (with k-edges of 33.2 and 37.4 keV, respectively) are most useful as contrast agents because their k-shell binding energies occur at levels that allow photoelectric absorption of a significant proportion of photons produced at typical radiographic kVp values.

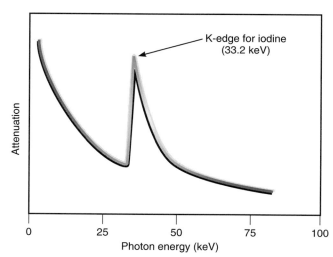

FIGURE 18–5. The effect of the k-edge of iodine on attenuation of an x-ray beam.

## Contrast Formation

The term *radiographic contrast* is used to describe the differences in image brightness between various areas of density in the subject. In diagnostic coronary angiography, a low kVp generally produces an image with excellent contrast as long as most photons have energy levels sufficient to penetrate the chest structures of greatest density (i.e., sternum, ribs). For coronary angiography, iodine is a nearly ideal contrast agent because the high atomic number results in many Compton interactions, and the k-edge of 33.2 keV results in absorption of many other photons. For coronary angiography, an optimal range of photon energies to take advantage of Compton interactions and the k-edge of iodine is typically produced by kVp levels of 70 to 90. Heavy patients or highly angulated views may require high kVp levels to effectively penetrate the subject, resulting in a high proportion of photons not attenuated by Compton interactions or k-edge absorption.

Although iodine is an excellent angiographic contrast agent, radiation scatter can significantly reduce the radiographic contrast of a coronary image. X-rays interact with patient tissues to produce many secondary x-ray photons by Compton scatter. The x-rays are randomly directed, and some of the scattered photons strike the input phosphor of the image intensifier, thus reducing contrast (Fig. 18–6). The ratio of scattered to primary radiation is directly

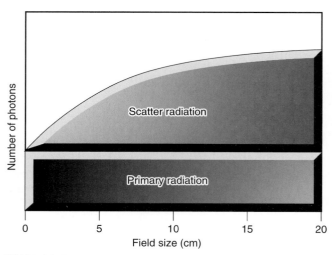

FIGURE 18–7. Relationship between field size and the proportion of primary versus scatter radiation.

proportional to the field size (Fig. 18–7). For large fields of view, the quantity of scattered photons in the image may actually exceed the primary transmitted photons. Because scatter radiation reduces contrast, reduction of field size by collimation represents a highly effective technique for improving image contrast.

Virtually all cineangiographic equipment also employs a radiographic "grid" to reduce the effect of scatter radiation. The grid consists of finely structured lead strips designed to obstruct incident x-ray photons traveling at oblique angles (see Fig. 18–6). Because the obliquely angled radiation contains almost exclusively scattered photons, the grid increases the proportion of primary to secondary radiation, thereby improving contrast. A related phenomenon, *veiling glare,* represents the scattering of light photons in the optics of the video or cine camera. An overall measure of the combined effects of scatter and veiling glare determines how much radiographic contrast is lost during actual imaging.

## DETECTION OF X-RAYS

## Image Intensifiers

The two primary functions of the image intensifier are conversion of the x-ray image to a visible wavelength and amplification of the weak fluoroscopic image produced during exposure. Figure 18–8 illustrates the components of a typical image intensifier. An *input fluorescent screen* absorbs each x-ray photon and converts its energy into many light photons (typically >1000). The input phosphor is mounted in close proximity to a *photocathode* composed of a metal screen that emits photoelectrons when illuminated by light. The electrons produced by the photocathode are focused by *electrostatic lenses*

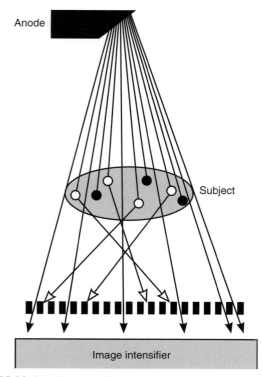

FIGURE 18–6. Influence of Compton scattering on image contrast and the beneficial effect of the x-ray grid.

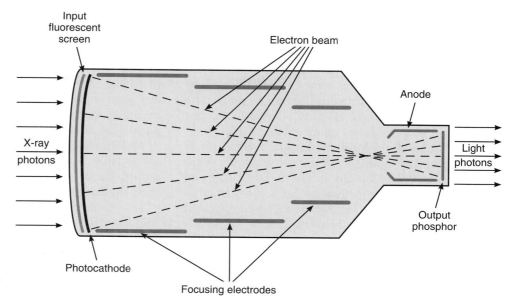

FIGURE 18–8. Typical construction of an image intensifier.

consisting of positively charged electrodes located in the main body of the image intensifier. These electrons produced in the image intensifier are accelerated by an anode near the output side of the image intensifier

The output phosphor consists of a fluorescent screen that emits light photons when struck by the highly accelerated electrons. The resulting visible image is greatly amplified by several phenomena. At the input phosphor, each x-ray photon produces many light photons. The electrons produced by the photocathode are accelerated to high velocities by the anode, which thus results in production of many photons at the output phosphor. In addition, the output phosphor is much smaller than the input phosphor, resulting in concentration of photons into a small but bright field (minification gain). The output phosphor image is sufficiently bright to enable filming (cineangiography) or video display (fluoroscopy). Typical modern image intensifiers distribute the light at the output phosphor into two separate identical images using a semisilvered mirror (see Fig. 18–1). Thus, the image can be simultaneously recorded on film and displayed on a video monitor.

The optimal size for an image intensifier for cardiac examination presents a series of choices and tradeoffs. Nearly all currently manufactured cardiac angiography systems use image intensifiers with switchable field sizes, although the exact field dimensions often vary among different vendors. In typical diagnostic and interventional coronary angiography, an image intensifier with a field size of about 6 inches (15 to 17 cm) is considered to be optimal. Most current equipment also provides a magnification mode of 4 to 4.5 inches (10 to 12 cm).

The inherent spatial resolution for the magnification mode is virtually always better than the larger field of view. Many current image intensifier designs employ a third option, a 9- to 10-inch field of view (22 to 25 cm). This larger field size is generally considered to be optimal for adult ventriculography, but it is suboptimal for coronary angiography.

Although the multiple field sizes of a *triple-focus* image intensifier provide versatility, the triple-mode intensifier generally offers lower image quality than that provided by a single- or dual-field size design. Some current laboratories take advantage of this principle to provide optimal image quality for interventional procedures. A dual-mode image intensifier (10- to 12- and 15- to 17-cm fields) should be considered in centers with adequate catheterization volume to enable a dedicated interventional room. The physical size of this dual-mode image intensifier is smaller, thus allowing easier positioning to achieve compound and highly angulated views. In addition, the dual-mode intensifier almost always outperforms a triple-mode design.

For cardiologists who perform peripheral vascular diagnostic studies and interventions, the opposite principle may apply. A large field size is often helpful, and a 15-inch or larger image intensifier may be required. However, it must be recognized that large-field image intensifiers are definitely inferior for coronary angiography. The careful practitioner resists the economic temptation to configure a single room for both coronary and peripheral vascular interventions. In most designs, the image size can be adjusted to some extent (±10%) in the field by a technician. This often is useful for fine-tuning the laboratory characteristics to meet the needs of a particular site.

The image intensifier and x-ray tube are mounted on a heavy steel *positioner* used to obtain oblique and hemiaxial views (see Fig. 18–1). In an earlier era of catheterization, the image intensifier was fixed in position, and angulated views were obtained by rotation of the patient in a cradle. Some cradle-type systems are still in use in older laboratories, but they should be considered unacceptable for an interventional laboratory. Modern designs typically use an L-, C-, or U-shaped positioner to achieve angulated views. There are no inherent advantages to any of the positioning systems, and most current equipment can achieve similar views when operated by an experienced interventionist.

## Quantum Statistical Noise

One of the most important principles in radiography is a difficult concept known as *quantum statistical noise* or *quantum mottle*. Quantum noise arises because of statistical fluctuations in density produced by the small number of photons used to generate the image. Imagine a radiographic image generated by a single x-ray photon. This photon is absorbed, scattered, or transmitted by the subject, resulting in a single black or white spot in the image. With a single photon, no structure is discernible. Now imagine a radiographic image constructed from 100 x-ray photons. Some photons are absorbed or scattered and some are transmitted, resulting in a very coarse but distinctly structured image. Finally, imagine an image produced by 10,000 photons. The transmitted and absorbed photons result in a definite pattern of light and dark, thus giving significant structure and detail to the image.

Accordingly, the quality of the final image varies with the number of x-ray photons employed to produce the image. The amount of quantum noise is inversely proportional to x-ray exposure dose. Images constructed from few photons have a grainy appearance known as quantum mottle, whereas images constructed from many photons are smooth and detailed. Quantum noise limits the maximal quality of all radiographic studies, but it is particularly evident during low-dose exposure methods such as with fluoroscopy and cineangiography. The grainy appearance of many catheterization films is most often a reflection of quantum mottle, not film grain. No matter how precise the design of each component of the x-ray system, the ultimate image quality is limited by the quantum noise phenomenon.

Currently, there are only two ways to reduce quantum noise in fluoroscopic and cineangiographic imaging. Either the x-ray system must produce more photons (increased exposure) or the image intensifier must detect a higher proportion of the x-ray photons (increased *quantum detection efficiency*). The limits on safe exposure rates and heat loading of x-ray tubes preclude significant increases in x-ray exposure. The quantum detection efficiency of image intensifiers has gradually increased over the last decade, resulting in significant improvements in image quality. There remains only a little additional room for improvement in future designs. A system designed with a nearly perfect generator, x-ray tube, image intensifier, and video camera would yield a definite but not unlimited improvement in image quality.

The limitations imposed by quantum mottle have important implications for clinical practice. Under certain circumstances, costly improvements in the performance of a particular component of the radiographic imaging chain may result in little visible improvement in the image quality. Conversely, an increase in the exposure can make up for deficiencies in the design of x-ray equipment, but it results in greater radiation doses to patient and operator. *Of great importance to the selection of equipment from different vendors, representative images can be compared only if the x-ray exposures are very similar.*

For most current practice, an exposure of approximately 20 to 25 μR per frame (9-inch image field) is required to adequately reduce quantum statistical noise. If higher exposure rates are used, the radiation dose to the patient and operator may be unacceptable and may require a longer x-ray pulse width, thus resulting in significant motion blur. Higher exposure rates also increase heat loading to the x-ray tube and may require a large focal spot size to avoid very shortened tube life. Thus, the current use of 20 to 25 μR per frame represents an optimal balance of suppression of quantum mottle, acceptable radiation doses, reasonably small focal spot sizes, and pulse widths short enough to stop coronary artery motion.

An individual laboratory may wish to customize radiographic technique for a variety of reasons. An older or aging image intensifier may suffer from inadequate contrast and quantum detection efficiency. Accordingly, the laboratory may wish to slightly increase exposure rates to compensate for the reduced image quality while proceeding to purchase new equipment. Conversely, a new laboratory with excellent equipment might wish to gradually reduce the dose while monitoring image quality. As a general principle, a prudent laboratory employs the lowest x-ray dose consistent with adequate diagnostic image quality. However, major reductions in dose are not likely to benefit patient care, primarily because coronary angiography is a technique that barely achieves adequate image quality under optimal circumstances.

## RECORDING AND VIEWING EQUIPMENT

### Film and Cine Cameras

For several decades, 35 mm film has been the principal recording medium for coronary angiography and ventriculography. The actual surface area exposed during cineangiography is 18 × 24 mm, exactly one half of the frame size used for 35 mm photography (Fig. 18–9). Because the conventional shape of the output phosphor of the image intensifier is round, there is a mismatch with the rectangular shape of the film frame. Accordingly, several options exist for controlling the framing size to account for these differences, including *exact framing, partial overframing,* and *total overframing.* All overframing techniques discard some of the image displayed on the output phosphor, but they have the advantage of enlarging the x-ray image, which theoretically may improve resolution. In current practice, the excellent quality of modern films and image intensifiers makes overframing much less desirable, although the technique is still commonly employed in older laboratories.

There is a wide range of cineangiographic films available from several different manufacturers. The response of film to light exposure is curvilinear, conforming to a shape known as a Hurter and Driffield (H & D) curve, named after the early photographic experimenters who first described the exposure-development characteristics of film. Figure 18–10 shows typical H & D curves for cineangiographic film. There is a short "toe" section at low brightness levels, a long linear curve segment, and a short "shoulder" segment where the curve flattens. The steepness of this curve determines the *contrast* of the film. Two different measures of contrast are commonly used: *gamma,* the steepest slope of the H & D curve, and *average gradient,* the mean slope of the curve over its useful range.

The gamma and average gradient are functions of the film design, manufacture, and subsequent chemical development. Thus, one film may have inherently more contrast than another, although changes in development time can increase or decrease the contrast of any film (see Fig. 18–10, *right*). Within certain limits, longer duration of development increases gamma and average gradient, whereas shorter development time reduces contrast. The choice of film type and degree of development are significant variables affecting the appearance of cineangiograms. The optimal contrast level is generally considered a matter of personal preference; some practitioners favor a low-contrast technique with a long gradual gray scale and others prefer films with higher inherent contrast. Regardless of preference, it should be understood that contrast can be precisely controlled by well-trained radiographic technicians.

Many image quality problems in cineangiography are a result of poor quality control in film development. Variation in the temperature of the film developer of more than 0.3°C (0.5°F) can significantly affect contrast. Insufficient agitation of the developer can result in uneven mottling or streaking of the film. Lack of cleanliness can result in spots or other flaws in the film. Good results require a continuous quality assurance program, including weekly *sensitometry,* a procedure in which the laboratory processes a pre-exposed film containing known steps in exposure. The resulting density values are measured with a *densitometer,* and film development subsequently is adjusted to maintain proper overall density and contrast. In any particular laboratory, the final contrast of the image recorded on film is influenced by many different components, including the contrast characteristics of the image intensifier, the amount of light scatter in the camera optics, and even the characteristics of the viewing projector. Accordingly, the final decision regarding film choice and development must be determined by knowledgeable clinicians after careful review of representative films.

### Video Systems and Fluoroscopy

In modern interventional practice, video systems and fluoroscopy have assumed an increasingly important role in safe and effective procedures. Accordingly, video and fluoroscopy systems have

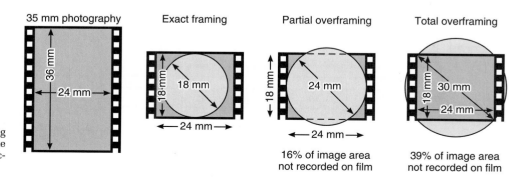

FIGURE 18–9. Different framing techniques for converting the circular x-ray image to the rectangular film format.

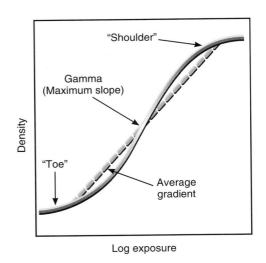

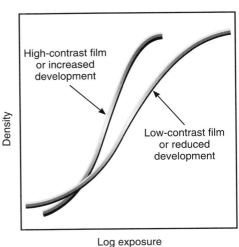

FIGURE 18–10. Hurter and Driffield curves showing the relationship between film density and development.

evolved more rapidly during the 1990s than has any other component of the x-ray system. Figure 18–11 illustrates the construction of a typical video camera used for fluoroscopy. A lens focuses light from the output phosphor of the image intensifier and the incident light strikes a *target* in the video camera composed of small globules of photoconductive material. Each small globule of material is insulated from surrounding areas. All other factors being equal, the larger the target area, the better the image quality.

The light-sensitive photoconductive material emits free electrons in quantities proportional to the intensity of the incident light. The free electrons are attracted to an anode in the video camera, and each globule of photoconductive material thus becomes positively charged, acting as a small capacitor. An electron beam subsequently scans the photoconductive material progressively discharging each tiny globule of material. The resulting current flows through a conductive signal plate and following appropriate amplification constitutes the video signal emerging from the camera. The voltage of the video output signal is proportional to the intensity of light that struck each point in the target.

A television monitor works in an opposite but analogous fashion. An electron beam scans a fluorescent screen that emits light in proportion to the number of electrons striking the phosphor. A *control grid* modulates the current of the scanning beam

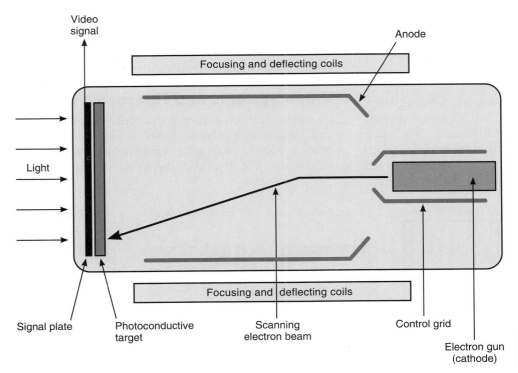

FIGURE 18–11. Typical construction of a video camera used for fluoroscopy.

according to the voltage of the incoming video signal. The resulting television image varies in brightness at each point in the image in proportion to the amount of light that originally illuminated the video camera. The accuracy of video reproduction is determined by the precision with which the video camera converts light into an electrical signal and the accuracy with which the monitor converts the video signal into a fluorescent image.

Television monitors and video cameras use two radically different scanning methods. Traditional broadcast television monitors scan 525 lines in an interlaced fashion (Fig. 18–12), so that one half of the lines are scanned every 1/60 second. This interlaced approach results in two *fields* and one *frame* every 1/30 second (30 frames per second). Interlacing is employed in broadcast television to accommodate the *flicker fusion frequency* of the human eye. If a full frame were reproduced every 1/30 second, the image would exhibit annoying flicker. Because of interlacing, part of each frame is updated each 1/60 second, a frequency perceived by the human eye without noticeable flicker. The interlaced technique was originally chosen by the National Television Standards Committee (NTSC) in the 1940s. Accordingly, NTSC video is quite limited in quality, reflecting the limitations in technology that were prevalent at that time.

In the early era of fluoroscopy in the catheterization laboratory, all systems used 525-line interlaced NTSC video. Such systems employed continuous radiation during fluoroscopy, rather than the pulse-mode x-ray used for cineangiography. In these crude systems, the video camera scanned the target in an interlaced fashion and the monitor displayed an interlaced image. Such interlaced systems offer two significant disadvantages for interventional procedures. The 525-line display is coarse and exhibits highly visible *raster lines*, the horizontal scan lines that are evident in commercial television. Furthermore, the interlaced approach requires that every frame of the image be composed of two fields separated in time by a 1/60-second interval. During 1/60 of a second (approximately 16 ms), a rapidly moving coronary artery can travel a considerable distance, resulting in unacceptable motion blur.

Accordingly, most (but not all) video systems in the modern catheterization laboratory employ several improvements. These improvements commonly include video cameras and monitors with 1024-line capability (high-line-rate video). The most advanced systems also make use of *progressive-scan video*

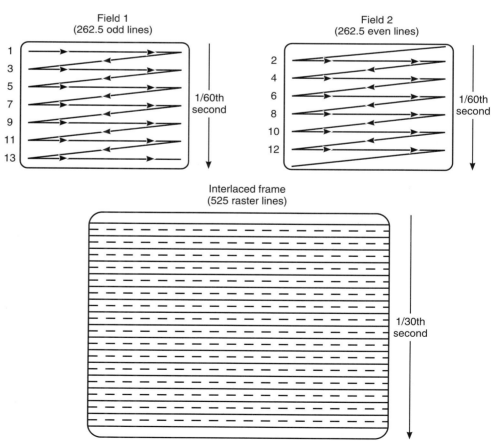

FIGURE 18–12. Interlaced video. Two fields combine to form a single interlaced frame for which half of the scan lines are derived from the first field and the other half are derived from the second field.

rather than the interlaced NTSC approach (Fig. 18–13). The progressive-scan systems employ a video camera that scans all 1024 lines of the image every $\frac{1}{60}$ second. Because the image is updated that frequently, annoying flicker is avoided. Because there are 1024 scan lines, not 525, the unpleasant effects of raster lines are significantly reduced. Despite several important advantages, 1024-line video does not yield images with twice the spatial resolution of 525-line systems. This disparity occurs because the low x-ray doses used for fluoroscopy result in an image significantly impaired by quantum mottle. In addition, high-line-rate video cameras often generate more electronic noise than do 525-line systems. Despite these limitations, nearly all observers prefer a high-line-rate fluoroscopic image, and such systems should be the standard in interventional laboratories.

The finest video systems have one further enhancement, *pulsed fluoroscopy*. Instead of continuous x-ray exposure, these fluoroscopic systems use short pulses of x-radiation in a fashion similar to that for cineangiography. Pulsed fluoroscopy reduces or eliminates motion blur, which may improve image quality, particularly in imaging rapidly moving coronary arteries. Pulsed fluoroscopy also may yield some reduction in x-ray dose, primarily because this approach can potentially use radiation more efficiently than continuous fluoroscopy. However, pulsed fluoroscopy systems generally require a grid control x-ray tube, and not all vendors have chosen to undertake this expensive development. Alternatively, one vendor provides pulsed fluoroscopy by modifying the electronic controls used for cineangiography. This practice results in pulsed fluoroscopy with very high radiation doses. Although image quality is excellent, the radiation doses are unacceptable.

Several important characteristics of the video cameras are controlled by the designers of x-ray systems, and these choices significantly affect the performance of the laboratory. One important feature is *lag,* defined as the degree of persistence of the image on the target of the video camera. During fluoroscopy, because low radiation exposure is employed, images contain considerable quantum statistical noise. Cameras with longer lag characteristics take advantage of a longer image persistence to smooth the appearance during fluoroscopy, which produces a less "noisy" image. However, too much lag results in objectionable motion blur, a problem not often evident in real-time fluoroscopy because moving images are typically viewed. However, following acquisitions to a digital imaging system, still-frame images are commonly reviewed, and excessive lag results in motion blur or even double or "ghost" images.

The most sophisticated television systems in catheterization suites intelligently control camera lag according to the application. During fluoroscopy, moderate lag smoothes the noise, but for recording video images during digital angiography, the camera is electronically altered to yield low lag characteristics. Several vendors also have introduced digital image processing techniques to improve the appearance of fluoroscopy. A variety of approaches have been employed The most prevalent technique uses an electronic edge-enhancing filter to increase the apparent sharpness of the image. A slightly different technique known as *unsharp masking* enhances both image sharpness and contrast. The most sophisticated image filters used for fluoroscopy are *adaptive*, changing their characteristics according to the requirements of the image. It seems likely that digital image filtration techniques will continue to evolve rapidly and will be incorporated in most cardiac x-ray systems in the near future.

## Video Recording

Although video recording systems have undergone continuous development, in the most recent vintage

### Progressive-scan video

Progressive scan
(525 lines)

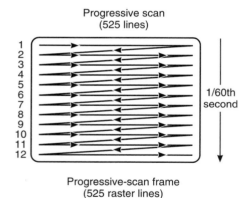

1/60th second

Progressive-scan frame
(525 raster lines)

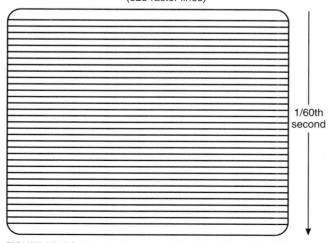

1/60th second

FIGURE 18–13. Progressive-scan video. In this mode, all the scan lines of the video image are derived from a single field.

laboratories, videotape recorders have assumed a less important role. Essentially, digital angiographic systems have completely replaced video recorders as the principal means used to review images during procedures. Analog videotape recording provides marginal image quality even under ideal circumstances. The finest recording devices (1-inch reel-to-reel) can faithfully reproduce less spatial resolution than is available using top quality image intensifiers. A few laboratories have adopted the improved half-inch super-VHS format to store images in a "cine-less" laboratory. This practice results in suboptimal image quality and poor archival properties; it is not recommended.

## Modulation Transfer Function

The components in an angiographic system must work together to produce an image suitable for diagnosis. *Modulation transfer function* (MTF) is a complex but important measure of the contrast and resolution of each component. Imagine a metal wire mesh placed in an x-ray beam in a catheterization laboratory. If the wire mesh is coarse, each strand is registered on the film as a discrete object with a large density difference between the wire and the background. However, if the wire mesh is infinitely fine, the final image is unable to resolve individual strands, and there is no density difference between the wire mesh and the background. Such an image has very low contrast, because there is no apparent pattern of light and dark produced by the infinitely fine wire mesh. Finally, imagine a wire mesh with an intermediate degree of coarseness. The contrast of the image also is intermediate, showing a mesh pattern with small density differences between the wire and background.

MTF uses a complex mathematic approach (Fourier analysis) to provide a graphic measure of the contrast retained by an imaging component for increasingly fine structural details (Fig. 18–14). Contrast is assigned to the vertical axis, with an MTF value of 1.0 representing maximum contrast and a value of zero representing no contrast. Increasingly fine structural detail is graphed on the horizontal axis in units of frequency, typically line pairs per millimeter. MTF curves for a series of radiographic components are shown in Figure 18–14. The MTF values of each component can be multiplied together to yield an overall measure of the resolution characteristics of a particular laboratory (see Fig. 18–14*D*). The ability to retain image contrast for fine (high-frequency) structural details is the most important measure of image quality.

## PRINCIPLES OF DIGITAL ANGIOGRAPHY

Digital angiography has grown steadily in importance following its introduction to the cardiac cathe-

terization laboratory in 1982. The expanding role of digital angiography reflects several inherent advantages provided by this imaging modality. Digital angiography is unsurpassed as a means for immediate access to high-quality images during diagnostic or therapeutic catheterization, a feature that unquestionably improves the speed and efficiency of the operator. Accordingly, virtually all interventional laboratories currently have digital angiographic equipment, and only a few diagnostic-only suites still lack this capability. Although digital imaging was initially used only for review of angiograms during catheterization procedures, its role has expanded in recent years to encompass both long-term archiving and network communication of angiographic studies.[1–4]

## Image Acquisition Configuration

Current digital imaging systems employ a conventional television camera for image acquisition. Many laboratories currently record both cinefilm and digital angiography, employing the digital images primarily for "in-room" guidance of the procedure. Film, on the other hand, is used principally as a long-term archive, but it also still functions as an exchange medium to allow other practitioners to review catheterization images. Simultaneous digital imaging and cineangiography is made possible through the use of a semisilvered mirror that divides the visible image formed on the output phosphor of the image intensifier into two parallel pathways (see Fig. 18–1). Digital angiography systems usually provide 80% to 90% of the light output to cinefilm and 10% to 20% to the video camera. This unequal division is necessary because of the relative insensitivity of the cinefilm emulsions to visible light in comparison with modern video cameras. Although it is commonly believed otherwise, this unequal light distribution does not materially influence image quality for either film- or video-based techniques, because each device operates efficiently within its normal range of sensitivity. During coronary digital imaging, *pulse-mode* x-ray is employed to freeze vessel motion. Digital systems must electronically synchronize camera scanning with film transport to permit each x-ray pulse to simultaneously expose both cineangiography and digital frames.

## Analog-to-Digital Conversion

The principles underlying digital recording of images are relatively simple. The voltage of analog video signal produced during image acquisition is proportional to the brightness in the original image. An analog-to-digital converter in the computer samples the video signal and converts the voltage levels

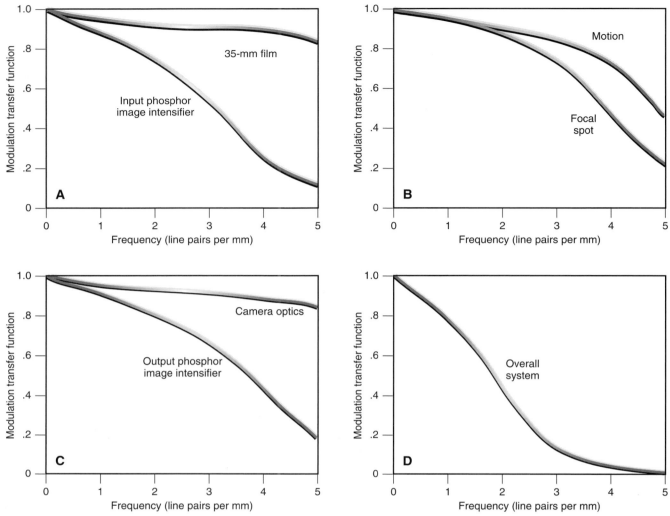

FIGURE 18–14. Modulation transfer function curves for the different components of an x-ray system.

into a series of discrete numbers (Fig. 18–15). Because computers work in binary numbers, the number of possible gray levels for each pixel is determined by the number of *bits* available for analog-to-digital conversion. In cardiac digital angiography, this number is typically 8 bits (1 byte), which in binary numbers corresponds to 256 possible gray levels. No matter how many discrete levels are assigned, the digital representation does not exactly reproduce the original signal and contains a series of discrete steps known as *quantization error* (Fig. 18–16, *right*). Mathematic calculations regarding the anticipated quantum statistical noise indicate that an 8-bit gray scale (256 levels) should be adequate for the typical exposures of 20 to 25 μR per frame used for coronary angiography. Thus, for coronary angiography, 256 gray levels are sufficient to render quantization error clinically negligible. However, during certain critical imaging procedures, particularly the high-exposure techniques employed for peripheral vascular angiography, 10 or more bits of gray scale may be required to maintain image fidelity.

## Resolution Considerations

The horizontal and vertical sampling rates of the digital-to-analog converter determine the *matrix size* of the digital image (see Fig. 18–13, *bottom*). Most current systems for cardiac angiography generate 512 horizontal and 512 vertical samples, each referred to as a picture element, or *pixel*. The *resolution* of the digital image is determined by the number of pixels, typically ranging from 256 rows by 256 columns (64,000 pixels) to 1024 × 1024 (1 million pixels). Coronary angiography is most commonly digitized using 8 bits per pixel (256 gray levels). Thus, cardiac digital angiography most often consists of a 512 × 512 pixel acquisition with 8 bits gray scale per pixel.

It should be noted that this 512 × 512 matrix size is slightly below the optimal size necessary to

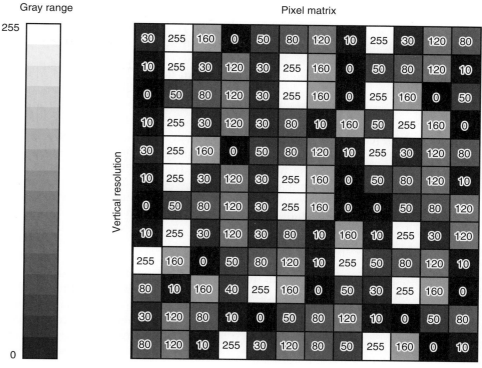

FIGURE 18–15. The process of converting a continuous analog image into a series of digital gray values, each representing a single picture element, or pixel, within the image.

capture all the spatial information available from the best image intensifiers. At a 512 × 512 matrix, the digital system generates 3.4 pixels per millimeter for a 15-cm (6-inch) field of view. However, a top-quality intensifier may resolve 4 to 5 line pairs per millimeter, and technically, at least 2 pixels are required to reproduce each line pair. Thus, a 512 × 512 digital image probably slightly undersamples the available diagnostic information. Accordingly, a strong and growing trend in system design has re-

sulted in the replacement of 512 × 512 matrix acquisition with 1024 × 512 or 1024 × 1024 matrix acquisition for digital coronary angiography.

## Data Storage Requirements

The quantities of data generated by cardiac digital angiography are enormous. A single image at a 512 × 512 pixel matrix with an 8-bit gray scale represents 262,144 bytes of data (262 *kilobytes* [KB]) that

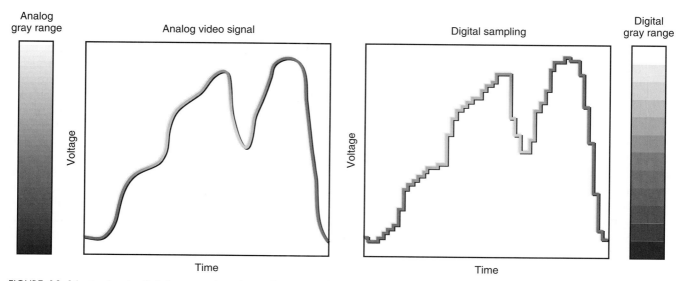

FIGURE 18–16. Analog-to-digital conversion. A continuous analog image *(left)* is converted into a series of discrete digital values, which results in a steplike noncontinuous relationship *(right)*. The distortion produced by this process is known as digitization error.

must be stored in the computer. Because full-motion imaging is typically performed at 30 frames per second, digital coronary angiography generates 30 × 262 KB per second or about 7.5 million bytes of data per second (7.5 *megabytes* [MB]). Thus, an 8-second coronary artery injection study requires about 60 MB, and a full angiographic study in a single patient may require up to 1 billion bytes of data (1 *gigabyte* [GB]).

For a laboratory performing 1000 cases annually, complete archiving of all angiographic studies would require storing approximately 1000 gigabytes (1 *terabyte* [TB]) of data. Because of these requirements, in current practice, digital angiographic images are often stored temporarily on a computer hard disk to enable immediate replay and review. In this application, the size of the hard disk determines the capacity of the digital imaging system, typically 2500 to 25,000 images (2 to 14 complete patient studies). Unless digital long-term archiving is intended, the images recorded on the computer hard disk are erased within hours or days to make room for subsequent patient studies. In laboratories employing digital long-term storage, images recorded on the hard disk are transferred to another medium for archiving, a function usually performed between cases or at the end of the working day.

As noted previously, some digital imaging systems now employ video cameras and monitors with 1024-line capability (high-line-rate video) and digitize the video signal at 1024 × 1024 × 8-bit resolution. Because the output monitor displays 1024 scan lines, not 525, the unpleasant effect of visible raster lines is significantly reduced. Despite several important advantages, 1024-line digital systems do not yield images with twice the spatial resolution of 525-line systems. This disparity occurs because the low radiation doses used for cardiac imaging result in an image significantly degraded by quantum statistical noise. Accordingly, not all the potential for increased resolution (at 1024 matrix) translates into a usable improvement in image quality.

Several factors have limited application of 1024-matrix digital imaging, most notably the increased storage requirements. Digital angiography performed at 1024 matrix increases data capacity requirements by a factor of four over those for a 512 matrix. A compromise strategy for improving image quality is employed by several equipment vendors—the image is stored at a 512 matrix but displayed in the laboratory on a 1024-line monitor (*interpolated upscanning*). The visible effect of raster lines is suppressed, but the data storage requirements are identical to those for 512-matrix imaging. As computer storage technologies evolve, it is likely that true 1024-matrix acquisition will eventually re-place upscanning techniques, although the improvement in image quality will be modest.

## Data Compression Techniques

The large amount of data storage required for digital angiography limits the number of images that can be stored cost-effectively using available computer hard disks or archival media. However, the numeric format of digital angiography represents an ideal setting for application of data compression techniques. Nearly all current digital angiographic systems employ one or another compression algorithm, most commonly a method known as *Huffman encoding*. Huffman compression relies upon the principle that many pixels will have certain common gray values and that the gray value of a pixel is often similar to that of neighboring pixels. Hence, there is some redundancy produced by storing a full 8-bit number to represent the gray value for each pixel. Huffman techniques reduce the number of stored bits by coding these common, redundant values using only a few bits of data. Huffman encoding is *lossless*; that is, images compressed and decompressed using this method are visually identical. Although the data storage required for each image is reduced, the numeric value for each pixel in the decompressed image is unchanged. The major limitation of Huffman encoding is the modest degree of compression produced, which is typically not more than about 2.6 to 1.

Recent advances in computer technology have enabled much higher degrees of data compression with good to excellent image quality. These techniques are *lossy*; that is, there is a measurable difference when the original image is compared with an image that has been compressed and decompressed. The most important lossy compression technique was developed by an international committee known as the Joint Photographic Experts Group (JPEG). The JPEG compression algorithm has been adopted for many computer and imaging applications outside of medicine and is beginning to achieve some popularity in medical imaging. Although lossy, JPEG encoding produces a greater degree of compression than does the Huffman method, with minimal visible reduction of image quality at low compression ratios.

The precise mathematics of JPEG compression are beyond the scope of this chapter, but it is important to understand that this method does not reduce the sharpness or contrast of compressed images. Importantly, the most critical compression step is performed on a subunit of the image consisting of small blocks of pixels, typically an 8 × 8 matrix. At low compression ratios (<4:1), most observers cannot detect differences between compressed and uncompressed images, even in side-by-side comparisons (see Fig. 18–14). At moderate compression ratios (<10:1), the only change in image content is a subtle shifting of gray values and, occasionally, a more objectionable artifact in which the 8 × 8 blocks become visible. At much higher compression ratios, visible deterioration in image quality is often evident.

A multicenter study organized by the American College of Cardiology (ACC) and European Society of Cardiology (ESC) is currently evaluating whether the JPEG compression approach is suitable for recording digital angiography, network transmission, or long-term archiving of images. If lossy compression is clinically acceptable, this approach would probably accelerate the transition to filmless angiography (and 1024-matrix recording) by reducing the storage requirement by eightfold or more, enabling large savings in the cost and bulk of storage media. Furthermore, compressed images could be transmitted to nearby or remote locations at greater speeds than are required for full, uncompressed images.

## Digital Image Filtration

Current digital angiographic equipment commonly employs digital image spatial *filtration* to improve image quality. The mathematic concepts underlying filtration algorithms can be quite complex, although the results are easy to visualize. Filtration involves the modification of numeric pixel values using a predefined mathematic formula to generate a new image with improved visual characteristics. Digital filtration is commonly used to increase image contrast or enhance edge definition or both. This approach is generally sensible, because video-based methods typically produce images with lower contrast and reduced edge resolution in comparison with cinefilm. Although edge-enhancement filtration often produces visually appealing results, the process does not necessarily result in improved diagnostic accuracy. Indeed, the potential exists for a strong edge-enhancement filter to introduce imaging artifacts that might alter diagnostic interpretation. Most equipment vendors have not performed extensive clinical studies to examine the diagnostic impact of their filtration algorithms.

Additional image processing enhancements are commonly available on digital systems designed for the cardiac catheterization laboratory. These features include real-time magnification (*zoom*) of a selected region with the ability to dynamically move the zoomed window during replay (*roam*). Because the pixel size during image acquisition is unchanged, magnification does not change actual resolution. However, the zoomed image can be more readily examined, an advantage most observers find

helpful in evaluating lesion morphology. Some digital systems magnify the image using *pixel replication,* a technique in which every pixel in the original image is cloned to yield 4 pixels in the zoomed image. Zoom by pixel replication generates a magnified image with a coarse texture in which pixels are readily visualized. A more sophisticated approach uses an *interpolated zoom*, a technique in which the transitions between pixels are smoothed, thereby yielding a less *pixelated* image. A further evolution is *acquisition zoom,* a technique in which the system records a 512 × 512 window from a 1024 × 1024 acquisition. Acquisition zoom increases actual pixel density and thereby improves resolution, but it records only one quarter of the image field.

## Film Replacement

During the 1990s, advances in computer storage technology have made feasible the replacement of cinefilm by digital imaging for recording angiographic studies. To understand contemporary trends in filmless catheterization studies, it is essential to consider the various traditional roles played by 35-mm film since 1970. These roles include the functions of a *review* medium, an *archive* medium, and an *exchange* medium. A review medium is used locally to replay catheterization images for clinical decision making. An archive medium is used for semipermanent storage of angiographic studies for subsequent review during future patient encounters. An exchange medium is used to convey images to other practitioners, locally or at more distant centers.

Since 1970, cinefilm has served all three functions: review, archiving, and exchange. As laboratories make the transition to all-digital angiography, various technical approaches to digital image storage may or may not serve all three functions. For example, a laboratory may choose to review digital images immediately after a catheterization study from a computer hard disk but eventually archive these images on a slower digital tape recorder for long-term storage. The computer technology enabling digital storage of images continues to evolve rapidly, a phenomenon that makes it difficult to predict the exact devices most suitable for transition to filmless archiving.

Despite significant uncertainties, it seems most likely that hospitals will adopt one of two strategies for long-term digital storage of angiograms. One approach employs a large digital storage device (much like a tape jukebox) for long-term archiving of digital angiographic images, providing perhaps trillions of bytes of capacity. An alternative strategy would archive each angiographic study as a "unit patient record" on a single piece of medium (such as a compact disk [CD]). For jukebox-based systems, the response time might require several minutes to retrieve a particular study; therefore, most authorities envision a *hierarchical* structure in which a slower tape system is complemented by a faster array of hard disks encompassing several hundred gigabytes. Ideally, these systems would function automatically, so that admission of a patient or scheduling of an outpatient visit would trigger retrieval ("pre-fetching") of relevant digital imaging studies from archival storage.

## Advantages of Digital Archiving

Why the accelerating trend toward digital archiving of catheterization studies? Digital angiography offers many attractive features as the preferred medium for long-term storage of cardiac catheterization studies. For coronary angiography, the typical media costs for film and development approach $100 per patient, not including long-term storage costs such as maintenance of film libraries. Digital image archiving offers the opportunity for substantial cost reduction while potentially improving physician access to clinical studies. Digital technologies currently enable storage of a single angiographic procedure (approximately 1 GB) for as little as $5 per patient, representing a 20-fold cost reduction in comparison with film.

Since 1970, the computer industry has witnessed a doubling of storage density and a halving of cost for such storage every 18 months, a trend known as Moore's law. Given the continued improvements predicted by Moore's law, computer storage technologies will become progressively more economical with each passing year, eventually overwhelming film storage by sheer economic advantages alone. In the first decade of the 21st century, technologic developments may allow holographic storage of terabyte quantities of imaging data on a single small piece of medium. Such devices would enable virtually instantaneous access to a large bank of angiographic studies.

There are many other important advantages provided by digital archiving of catheterization images. Cinefilm is not easily copied—the original angiographic record must be physically conveyed to a consulting physician or to a new physician. However, digital storage media can be readily duplicated, and the numeric nature of the digital image guarantees that each copy is identical to the original. Thus, several identical duplicates of an individual patient's angiograms can be stored concurrently in different locations throughout a hospital (e.g., in the catheterization laboratory, cardiac surgery, or the physician's office).

## Network Transmission

Theoretically, digital angiograms can be transmitted electronically over long distances for remote diagnosis and consultation. Although current transmission schemes are too slow to be practical, more rapid digital networks are planned in the beginning of the 21st century. To deliver digital images throughout a hospital requires evolution from the current Ethernet standard (10 MB per second [MBps]) to *Fast Ethernet* speeds (100 MBps) or the even more rapid *asynchronous transfer mode* (ATM) (155 to >500 MBps). Governments and private companies are currently making large investments to ensure that such high-speed links are widely available for commercial and medical applications. Development of the necessary software to track the location of the thousands of examinations performed annually is required to enable digital archiving in large hospitals.

## Conversion to "Filmless" Angiography

Most experts in radiographic imaging expect an accelerating transition from film to digital image storage during the first years of the 21st century.[3, 4] A few laboratories have already abandoned cinefilm, sometimes employing super-VHS videotape as an archiving medium. Although transfer of digital images to analog videotape is simple and inexpensive, the loss of image quality is substantial and clinically unacceptable. Under ideal circumstances, super-VHS videotape can record only about 50% of the spatial resolution available from modern digital angiographic acquisition systems. This visible reduction in image quality precludes use of videotape for critical applications, such as deciding the suitability of coronary anatomy for surgery or angioplasty. In addition, the long-term storage properties of analog video tapes are poor, resulting in steady degradation of image quality over time. Thus, application of analog videotape for cinefilm replacement is clearly suboptimal and clinically unsupportable. Videotape may be useful to provide referring physicians with a "personal copy" of their patient's catheterization procedure, but it should not be used for primary decision making.

## The DICOM Standard

In the early 1990s, archival devices lacked the one critical feature supplied by cinefilm—worldwide standardization. Under such circumstances, an angiogram performed and archived in one laboratory could not be reviewed in another, a phenomenon the ACC termed a "Tower of Babel in the catheterization laboratory" in a position paper.[4] Under such conditions, referral of the patient to an external institution for surgery, angioplasty, or a second opinion often required a repeat catheterization. The absence of an accepted standard also began to impair clinical investigations that required image analysis at a single core laboratory.

The obvious solution was the development of an interchange standard to enable facile exchange of digital angiographic studies. In 1981, a radiology digital standards group began to develop an industry-wide protocol for the image format and communication between devices. Initially, the effort was jointly sponsored by the American College of Radiology (ACR) and the National Electrical Manufacturers Association (NEMA). In 1992, the ACC assembled interested parties to attempt to coordinate a cardiac angiographic standard. These working groups included representatives appointed by the ESC. Initial meetings led to an agreement by manufacturers, through NEMA, and all three medical organizations (ACC, ACR, and ESC) to work cooperatively toward the development of suitable standards. Eventually, this effort was renamed the Digital Imaging and Communication for Medicine (DICOM) standard to reflect the broader composition of the committee.

Because of the multiplicity of roles served by cineangiographic film, the angiographic committee focused on solving the one critical problem facing digital cardiac catheterization—development of a format and medium for *interchange* of angiographic studies. The committee deliberately avoided any attempt to standardize the *acquisition, display,* or *archiving* of angiographic images. This approach allows vendors to develop a range of products to support the needs of hospitals and laboratories regardless of size. Because the interchange record is standardized, the only requirement for a laboratory to maintain compatibility is the ability to read and write images in a well-defined data format.

## Adoption of the Writable Optical Compact Disk (CD-R)

Since 1992, the DICOM angiographic committee has met for two days each month in Washington, DC, to work out details of an interchange standard. After lengthy discussion and debate, the recordable 5.25-inch optical compact disk (CD-R) emerged as the optimal interchange medium for angiography. The medium is physically similar to the CD-ROM used in popular multimedia applications and has a capacity of approximately 680 MB. The exchange standard for cardiac angiography is nearly completed and was first demonstrated in 1995 at both the ACC scientific sessions and the annual meeting of the ESC. The DICOM format has now been adopted by all major catheterization laboratory vendors and is appearing in many end-user products.

The CD-R storage capacity of 680 MB permits recording of approximately 2400 frames ($512 \times 512 \times 8$-bit gray scale) per disk. This capacity is insufficient to record all cardiovascular examinations on a single piece of medium, which can reach 4000 images or more. Accordingly, the Ad Hoc Standards Committee specified use of digital data compression to increase the storage capacity of the CD-R. The compression scheme adopted by the committee is the lossless Huffman method previously described, resulting in an approximately twofold reduction in the amount of storage space required for each image frame. This increases the CD capacity to about 4800 angiographic frames, sufficient to store more than 98% of all studies on a single piece of medium. The Ad Hoc Angiographic Committee did not include lossy compression for image exchange on CD-R, because the clinical usefulness of a suitable compression scheme and acceptable compression ratio had not been sufficiently determined.

## Transfer Rates and Compression

Data transfer rates available in 1995 when the DICOM angiographic standard was introduced limited the performance of the CD-R medium in the initial clinical applications. This technical limitation allowed display of angiographic images directly from the CD-R at no more than 7.5 frames per second. Thus, full-motion display and review of DICOM images using available CD drives required "uploading" of images from the exchange medium to the computer workstation. Although future developments will gradually increase recording and playback performance of CD-R, drive speeds sufficient for viewing at 30 frames per second directly from the medium are unlikely in the immediate future. Because of the performance limits of CD-R, several equipment vendors have demonstrated an alternative approach to image exchange that uses lossy compression. By applying greater compression ratios on this proprietary CD, the retrieval speed is increased to 30 frames per second, with some degree of image degradation. It is important for readers to understand that this lossy approach to image compression is not yet a part of the official DICOM angiographic standard.

In evaluating appropriate methods for data compression, the Ad Hoc Angiographic Working Group did not rule out the use of lossy compression, if clinical studies demonstrated no significant loss of diagnostic image quality. Therefore, as previously mentioned, the ACC, the ESC, and the industry initiated a clinical study of lossy compression to determine if this approach is suitable for inclusion as a part of the DICOM standard. This study demonstrated that lossy-compressed JPEG at 76:1 compression was not equivalent to uncompressed images.

## Conversion Strategy: Conformance

In developing a conversion strategy, practitioners must realize that DICOM standard is specialized for many different modalities, and support for all of them will not be expected in most equipment (e.g., a computed tomography scanner would have little need to display echocardiograms). To specify precisely which aspects of DICOM are supported, vendors publish *conformance claims,* which should be studied carefully (preferably in consultation with a trusted advisor) to assure that a given piece of equipment will meet the customer's need. An open architecture is critical to taking advantage of the ongoing computer revolution. One cannot expect any computer device to remain state of the art for very long. Accordingly, an upgrade path—without being locked into a single vendor's proprietary hardware—is important to ensure continuing cost competitiveness.

## Transition to Digital Archiving

Although the successful development of an exchange medium ensures the ability to exchange images, there remain important obstacles to the development of a suitable replacement for cinefilm for long-term archiving. Ideally, a cine-replacement medium should permit rapid and *random access* review of any recorded digital angiographic injection sequence. Random access archiving would enable review of imaging sequences in any order and permit viewing of individual injection studies in continuous cine-loop. However, the density and speed of random access computer storage technologies have lagged behind those of *sequential access* devices, such as digital tape. Accordingly, the staggering quantities of digital imaging data currently cannot be stored economically using a medium capable of random access. Nevertheless, the maturation of computer storage devices and the evolution of new storage technologies will almost certainly overcome these limitations within the next few years.

The optimal format for the digital angiographic archiving remains controversial. Some uncertainty exists whether $512 \times 512$ digital angiography offers comparable image quality to that of cinefilm. One early report described some systematic differences in lesion severity as assessed by digital and cinefilm angiography.[2] However, technical developments have continuously improved digital image quality, and recent studies indicate that the two modalities provide comparable assessments. Despite this consensus, some authorities still find digital angiographic images to be suboptimal for critical clinical applications.

Several additional issues must be resolved to enable development of an optimal strategy for replacement of cineangiography. Should the digital archive include nonimaging information, such as hemodynamic data and written reports? The standards committee has begun work on including these data as part of the interchange record, but some current systems may have difficulty adding this capability. Is it clinically acceptable to employ any degree of lossy data compression, such as JPEG compression? Should the archiving approach of a particular hospital support nonradiographic images, such as echocardiography? Given the uncertainties, adopting a prudent course of action requires close monitoring of DICOM standardization process as the group further defines the format, devices, and media for digital archiving. Despite these obstacles, few expert observers doubt that digital angiography will be the dominant archiving method for cardiac catheterization images by the end of the decade.

## REFERENCES

1. Kruger RA, Mistretta CA, Houk TL, et al: Computerized fluoroscopy in real time for noninvasive visualization of the cardiovascular system. Preliminary studies. Radiology 130:49–57, 1979.
2. Gurley JC, Nissen SE, Booth DC, et al: Comparison of simultaneously performed digital and film-based angiography in the assessment of coronary artery disease. Circulation 78:1411–1420, 1988.
3. Gurley JC, Nissen SE: Digital coronary angiography: Is it ready to replace cine film? Cardiology 8:82, 1991.
4. Nissen SE, Pepine CJ, Block PC, et al: Cardiac angiography without cine film: Erecting a "Tower of Babel" in the catheterization laboratory. J Am Coll Cardiol 24:834–837, 1994.

# 19

# Angiographic Views and Techniques for Coronary Intervention

*Gary S. Roubin*

Advanced coronary angiographic technique is important in the practice of percutaneous transluminal coronary angioplasty (PTCA). Whereas diagnostic coronary angiography aims to identify the extent and severity of coronary stenoses and perhaps the suitability of distal vessels for bypass grafting, angiography for PTCA requires the acquisition of much additional information. At this point, it must be said that digital angiographic equipment is the minimal standard that should be expected in contemporary interventional cardiac catheterization laboratories. Such equipment must include high-quality digital replay and freeze frame capacity, zoom and edge enhancement capacity, and, where possible, quantitative edge detection stenosis and vessel size measurement programs. Whereas diagnostic angiography allows the operator the luxury of reviewing the angiographic results at a later time, interventional techniques require immediate, on-line decision making; therefore, high-quality images must be available on-line during the interventional procedure. The expression "You cannot do what you cannot see" applies most accurately to the practice of PTCA. In addition to requiring expertise in general contrast angiographic technique, angiography for PTCA must provide information on

1. Access to the vessel ostium
2. The nature of the proximal coronary vessel conduit to the lesion
3. Lesion morphology
4. The presence and disposition of side branches and the anatomy of the vessels distal to the lesion

Finally, and most importantly, the angiography must allow the operator to make on-line and considered decisions as to the adequacy of the dilatation or interventional result in the target lesion.

In this chapter we discuss in detail the angiographic views found most useful for treating lesions involving the left anterior descending artery (LAD),

the left circumflex artery, the right coronary artery, saphenous vein bypass grafts, and internal mammary artery conduits. However, certain principles apply to good angiographic imaging for the purpose of coronary intervention. First, scrupulous angiographic technique must be mastered to ensure good-quality imaging. Magnification should be set to optimize the information being sought, for example, low magnification when examining branching structures, the course of long saphenous vein grafts, or the presence of collaterals. Alternatively, high magnification is essential when examining the morphology of individual lesions. Depending on the x-ray equipment being used, the filters and shutters should be set to concentrate the x-ray beam on the regions of greatest interest. Panning should be slow and controlled, making sure that the regions of greatest interest are focused in the center of the field of view for an adequate number of cardiac cycles. Because lesions and vessels may move considerably with the cardiac cycle, it is important to be able to examine an adequate number of systolic and diastolic frames. The image intensifiers should always be as close to the patient as panning permits, and the table as low as possible and as close to the x-ray tube as the angulated views being taken permit. It is important to record the lesion to be treated in orthogonal views (at least two and sometimes three) and to include one that shows the least amount of foreshortening possible, and a view that is free of crossing side branches. The patient should be coached with respect to deep breathing for those views in which it is important to lower the diaphragm. This is especially true when imaging the right coronary artery in the left anterior oblique (LAO) view and the proximal LAD in the LAO cranial view. Finally, the patient's comfort must be taken into consideration, and if the patient is asked to hold the arms above the head for the sake of achieving excellent image quality, it is important to

**465**

allow for arm rest during those times in the procedure when critical imaging of the lesion is not important.

## USING GUIDING CATHETERS

Because guiding catheters deliver a large concentration of contrast material to the coronary arteries, they are useful in obtaining high-quality images of the lesion to be treated. It is important, however, to remember that the guiding catheters can decrease flow in the vessel by up to two thirds, even in the presence of a good aortic pressure tracing. This is particularly important when treating left coronary artery lesions, when the guiding catheter may be placed in the origin of the left main stem. It is important to remember that the guiding catheter should be backed out of the left main stem at all times when it is not required in this position, either for contrast injections or for placement of coronary guide wires or interventional devices. When the guiding catheter damps in the coronary ostium, guiding catheters with side holes can be extremely useful. This is most important in the right coronary artery. It must be remembered, however, that side holes can provide the operator with a false sense of security, because once the balloon has passed the segment of the catheter with side holes, then the aortic pressure tracing may appear normal, while flow down the coronary artery may be severely reduced by the combination of the guiding catheter intubated in the vessel and the balloon catheter at the tip of the guiding catheter or the proximal part of the coronary artery. In other words, the pressure tracing seen through the side holes does not reflect the perfusion pressure to the coronary artery. It is my view that guiding catheters with side holes are rarely indicated for use in the left coronary system.

Visualization of the coronary artery to be treated requires angiographic views that offer the operator the following information. First, the image should provide the operator with an assessment of ostial anatomy, including the direction of vessel takeoff and the presence of tortuosity and proximal side branches, and access to the proximal vessel for coronary guide wire placement. Second, the angiogram should include a clear image of the guiding catheter tip; to avoid image magnification distortion, this should be taken as close to the center of the field of the view as possible before panning proceeds down to the lesion in question and then on to the distal vessel. Ideally, there should be at least a number of frames that show the segments of the vessel proximal and distal to the lesion and the guiding catheter tip in the same frame so that accurate estimates of vessel size can be undertaken by comparing the angiographic diameter of the vessel segment to be treated to the known diameter of the guiding catheter tip. Third, the image should focus on the lesion in the center of the field of vision for a number of systolic and diastolic frames, and the projection chosen should delineate the takeoff of the side branches, particularly those proximal to the lesion and in close proximity to the lesion. Finally, the initial angiographic image should clearly display distal vessels so that damage to the distal vessels caused by guide wire placement or occlusion of distal vessels due to embolization can be distinguished should these mishaps occur.

## OPTIMAL ANGIOGRAPHIC PROJECTIONS

### Left Main Stem and Left Anterior Descending Arteries

The greatest degree of variation from individual to individual occurs in the length of the left main stem and the branching and tortuosity of the proximal LAD (Fig. 19–1). Depending on the individual anatomy encountered, the straight anteroposterior (AP) projection with some LAO or right anterior oblique (RAO) rotation to remove it from the spine is ideal for imaging the origin of the left main stem. An AP caudal view is ideal for lengthening the left main stem and showing the origin of the LAD and left circumflex artery. The proximal LAD is best viewed in the RAO projection with variable amounts of cranial or caudal angulation depending on the individual anatomy. In addition, an LAO cranial projection with 30 to 40 degrees of LAO rotation and extreme cranial angulation is often extremely useful in delineating lesions in the proximal LAD. It is important to rotate the image intensifier to a point that shifts the proximal part of the vessel just off the spine and over the lung field. It is also important to have the patient take an extremely deep breath to optimize the value of this angiographic view. It is often worthwhile coaching the patient to take in a deep breath by lowering the diaphragm and raising the abdomen toward the operator's hand to achieve the radiographic lowering of the diaphragm required. The midportion of the LAD and the origin of diagonal vessels is frequently best viewed in the LAO cranial projection. Straight lateral views are also useful in imaging this segment of the LAD. In addition, RAO cranial views can often provide surprisingly good images of the proximal to midsection of the LAD. The 30-degree RAO cranial view is often very useful. Finally, the most underutilized view for the mid-LAD is the extreme AP cranial view or "chin shot," which in the presence of a moderate breath often clearly delineates the mid-LAD and the precise takeoff of both septal and diag-

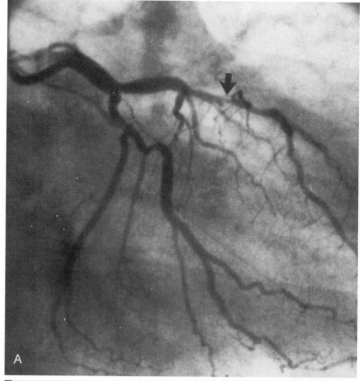

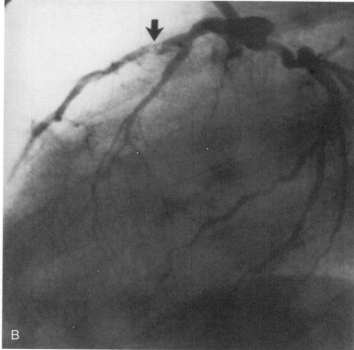

FIGURE 19–1. The left anterior descending artery (LAD) with a proximal stenosis *(arrow)* is shown in four commonly used angiographic views. *A,* The right anterior oblique (RAO) projection shows the origin of the vessel from the left main and the precise location of septal branches. The origins of diagonal branches are usually not seen in this projection. *B,* The left lateral projection opens up the vessel and shows the origin of diagonal branches that septal branches commonly overlap in the LAD in this view.

*Illustration continued on following page*

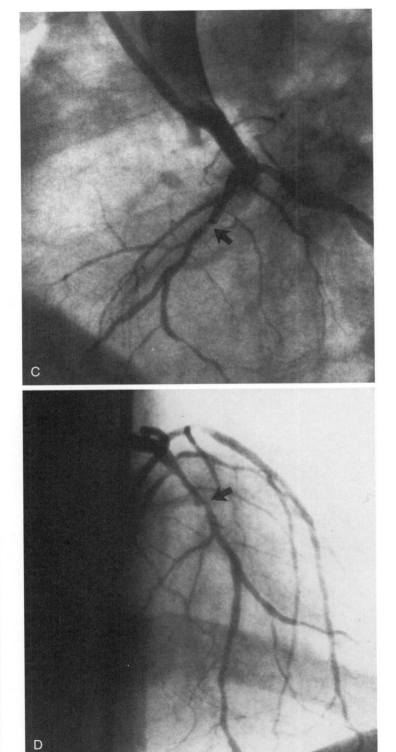

FIGURE 19–1 *Continued. C*, The left anterior oblique (LAO) projection is often necessary for steering the coronary guide wire into the LAD. The origins of diagonal branches are frequently seen well in the projection. *D*, The antero-posterior cranial view in this patient opens out the vessel and clearly demonstrates the origins of all diagonal and septal branches. This angiographic projection is frequently underutilized in dilations involving the LAD.

onal vessels. The distal LAD can be adequately viewed in RAO, lateral, and AP cranial projections. Large septal vessels are best viewed in the straight RAO projection or RAO cranial projection; as previously mentioned, diagonal vessels are usually best viewed in the LAO cranial or AP cranial projections.

## Left Circumflex Artery

The proximal left circumflex artery is frequently best seen in the RAO caudal projection (Fig. 19–2), whereas the LAO caudal or LAO cranial projections also open up this vessel segment, providing good visualization of lesions in this region. The LAO projections are frequently useful when the proximal circumflex artery is extremely tortuous. When the lesion is situated at the origin of the left circumflex artery, then an AP caudal or an LAO caudal view can be useful. Lesions in large ramus intermedius branches can often be seen in the straight RAO or RAO caudal projections, and lesions at the origin of the ramus branch can be seen in the AP caudal projection. In other patients, shallow LAO cranial views with the patient taking a deep breath expose lesions in the proximal portion of the large ramus branch. The obtuse marginal branches of the left circumflex artery are usually best viewed in the RAO caudal projections, and although there is usually some overlap and foreshortening, LAO projections can often be additionally useful. In patients with left dominant systems and posterior descending arteries (PDAs) arising from the left circumflex artery, these vessels can be best imaged in the LAO projection or left lateral projection with or without some cranial angulation.

## Right Coronary Artery

The ostium of the right coronary artery and proximal portions of the right coronary artery are best viewed in the LAO projections with 40 to 60 degrees of rotation depending on the degree of proximal tortuosity. Some caudal or cranial angulation can often be used to decrease foreshortening of the vessel segment around the lesion. In some patients, slight caudal angulation helps remove the shadow of the diaphragm from the image. On occasions, a lateral view of the proximal right coronary artery best delineates the lesion to be treated. When ostial lesions are imaged, it is often useful to place the catheter just under the coronary ostium and inject a large volume of contrast material to define both the extent of the lesion and the precise position of the aortic wall. This is a particularly important maneuver when one is considering placing a stent in an ostial location in the right coronary artery. The mid–right coronary artery can be adequately imaged in LAO, lateral, and RAO projections. Enough RAO rotation should be used to keep the image of the right coronary artery well clear of the shaft of the guiding catheter as it sits in the descending aorta. Occasionally, an AP view is useful in defining a lesion in the mid–right coronary artery. Lesions in the distal right coronary artery beyond the crux of the heart are best shown in the LAO projection. In both the LAO and RAO projections, it is important

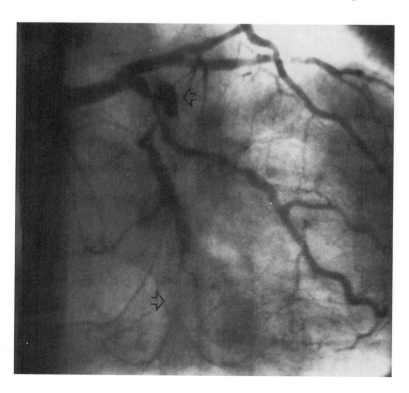

FIGURE 19–2. A diffusely diseased left circumflex artery is shown in the right anterior oblique (RAO) caudal projection. Stenosis in the proximal circumflex is associated with a mushroom-shaped false aneurysm *(upper arrow)* caused by a healed dissection. The distal vessel has severe stenosis *(lower arrow)*. The RAO caudal projection is utilized to provide access to the proximal circumflex artery; it also opens up the obtuse marginal branches.

to have the patient take a deep breath to remove the diaphragmatic shadow from the course of the vessel (Fig. 19–3). The origin of the PDA and takeoff of the posterolateral segment artery (PLSA) is similarly well seen in the LAO projection, but imaging of this branch point can be enhanced by adding cranial angulation to the LAO projection. The PDA itself is best seen in the RAO projection, where there is the least foreshortening of the vessel. The LAO cranial projection is also useful in imaging proximal segments of the PDA (Fig. 19–4). The PLSA branches are best seen in the LAO and lateral projections with variable amounts of cranial angulation depending on the individual anatomy. In some patients, RAO cranial and caudal views also define lesions in these arterial segments (Fig. 19–5).

## Internal Mammary Artery Grafts and Saphenous Vein Bypass Grafts

Guiding catheters should be used with great caution when intubating the ostium of internal mammary

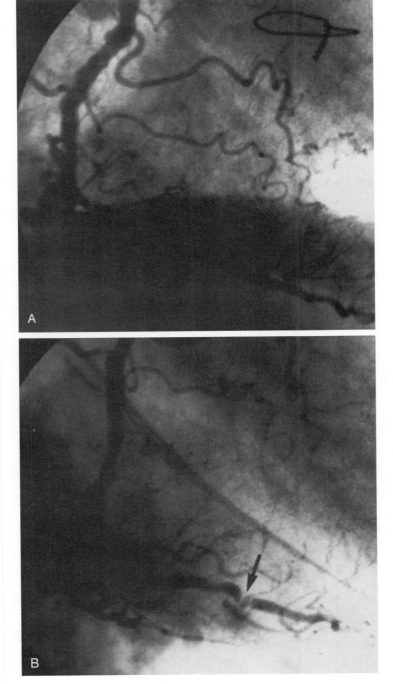

FIGURE 19–3. *A,* The right coronary artery is shown in the RAO projection. The vessel has been injected without the patient's having taken a deep breath, emphasizing the importance of lowering the diaphragm. *B,* The injection is repeated with the patient taking an appropriate deep inspiration. A critical stenosis is now evident *(arrow)* in the posterior decending artery (PDA).

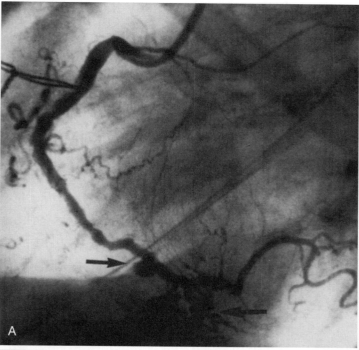

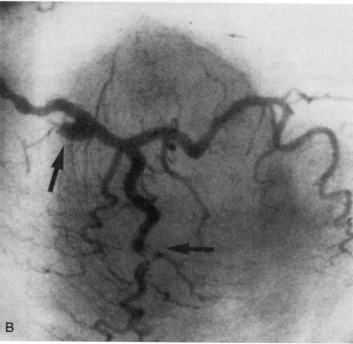

FIGURE 19–4. *A,* The right coronary artery is shown in the left anterior oblique (LAO) (60-degree) projection. The patient has taken a deep inspiration, and the proximal middle and distal vessels are well seen. There is an ectatic, aneurysmal dilation in the distal right coronary artery. In this projection, the posterior descending artery is not seen well. *B,* An LAO cranial projection of the same vessel filmed in deep inspiration and at a higher magnification with the image intensifiers focused on the region of interest. Both the origin and length of the posterior descending artery are seen well, and a critical stenosis *(lower arrow)* is now evident in the midportion of this vessel.

arteries. Injections should be done carefully because dissection of the proximal part of the artery can occur when guiding catheters are not handled with caution. In addition, the internal mammary artery is liable to undergo spasm, and it is advisable to inject 100 to 200 mg of nitroglycerin into the vessel before proceeding with angiography. The courses of the internal mammary artery grafts are well seen in the AP projection, but the anastomosis site (often the site of stenosis) is best seen in RAO, AP cranial, and lateral projections.

Because there is a great deal of variability in the manner in which saphenous vein grafts are sutured to the aortic wall, "creative" views are often required to define ostial anatomy in saphenous vein bypass grafts. I prefer to use Amplatz left 1 or 2 guiding catheters to instrument left saphenous vein bypass grafts. The origins of these grafts are best found by using an LAO projection. The Amplatz catheter is advanced so that the tip can be moved using clockwise rotation anteriorly to the left while it is gently "jiggled" up and down the aortic wall

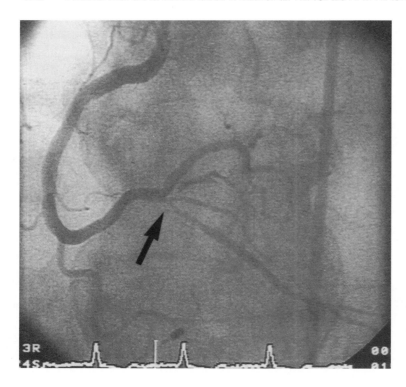

FIGURE 19–5. The right coronary artery shown in an anteroposterior cranial projection. This view is often useful for showing the origin of the posterior descending artery (PDA) *(arrow)*. In this example, the segment of interest is overlying the spine. It can often be better imaged by using shallow left anterior oblique (LAO) projections.

until the operator feels the tip of the guiding catheter encounter the ostium of the graft. LAO projections of saphenous vein bypass grafts to left coronary vessels are useful in defining the tortuosity, particularly in the proximal portions of these grafts. RAO projections are frequently needed to overcome foreshortening encountered in the LAO views. RAO projections are often very useful for defining ostial lesions and lesions close to the ostium of these left grafts (Fig. 19–6). Multiple orthogonal views are usually required to define tortuosity, which may not be obvious in single views. It is important for the angioplasty operator to become familiar with the manner in which saphenous vein bypass grafts to the LAD and left circumflex artery are usually coursed through the mediastinum to the epicardium of the heart. Saphenous vein bypass grafts to the right coronary artery are usually best engaged with the use of a multipurpose catheter. The origin of this graft is usually lower than left grafts and can best be found using, once again, the LAO projection with clockwise rotation of the multipurpose catheter while it is moved gently up and down the aortic wall (Fig. 19–7). Occasionally, right Judkins and left Amplatz shapes are useful for downgoing right coronary artery grafts.

Angiography bypass grafts should focus on the aorto-ostial anatomy, the body of the vein graft, the anastomosis of the vein graft to the distal vessel, and the branches of the distal vessel receiving the graft. This latter aspect of angiographic technique is most important because, should distal embolization occur during treatment of the bypass graft, it is important for the operator to be able to define exactly the distal vessels or branches that have become occluded.

## VISUALIZATION OF THE GUIDING CATHETER TIP, ARTERIAL SEGMENT TO BE DILATED, AND BALLOON SIZING

Choosing the correct angioplasty balloon diameter for treating any given coronary lesion is probably one of the most important aspects of PTCA technique. Choosing the correct balloon size involves many factors, including the type of balloon to be used (compliant vs. noncompliant), the morphology of the lesion, the age of the patient, and the presence of diffuse disease proximal and distal to the target lesion. However, in making a decision about the size of the balloon to be used, adequate images of the guiding catheter tip and the arterial segment that is to be dilated, plus an understanding of any magnification artifacts that may be involved, are of paramount importance. From an angiographic perspective, it is important to define the "normal" vessel segment proximal and distal to the lesion to be dilated and to take into account the presence of any tortuosity present and the degree of tapering of the vessel. It is important for the operator to be aware of "magnification artifacts," particularly when choosing a balloon for the distal right coronary artery and obtuse marginal vessel, where the vessels

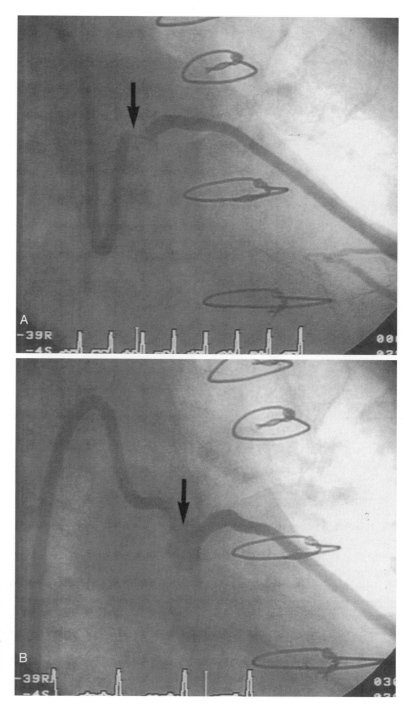

FIGURE 19–6. *A*, A saphenous vein graft to a left anterior descending artery (LAD) engaged with a left Amplatz catheter. Note that there is a severe ostial lesion *(arrow)* and the Amplatz catheter having been placed in the left anterior oblique (LAO) projection is now advanced in the right anterior oblique (RAO) projection to disengage it slightly from the ostium of the graft. *B*, After placement of an ostial stent, the left Amplatz catheter is left in a relaxed position so as not to damage the stent, which is protruding slightly into the aorta.

to be treated are a substantial distance from the tip of the guiding catheter. This is especially true if angulated views are used such that the distance between the structure of interest and the image intensifier is increased. Because of magnification artifacts, in practice the diameters of the distal right coronary artery and obtuse marginal vessels appear larger than they are when compared with the tip of the guiding catheter. Accordingly, care should be taken not to oversize balloons in treating lesions in these vessels.

In practice, the following views are suggested as optimal for balloon sizing when comparing the tip of the guiding catheter with the diameter of the arterial segment to be dilated. In all circumstances, the image intensifier should be as close to the patient's chest as possible. For the LAD, shallow RAO views, with either caudal or cranial angulation, allow the best estimation of arterial size. The mid-LAD can be compared best with the guiding catheter tip in the RAO and left lateral projections. The distal LAD can be viewed in both the RAO cranial and

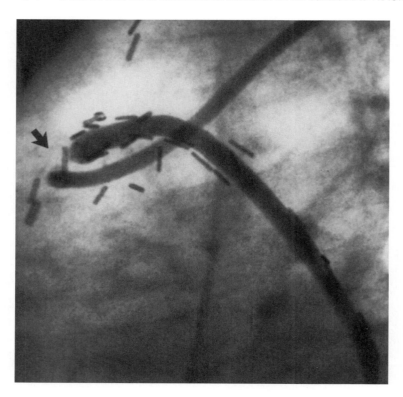

FIGURE 19–7. A saphenous vein graft going toward a circumflex artery has been cannulated in the left anterior oblique (LAO) projection by means of a multipurpose guiding catheter. The LAO projection is usually favored for cannulating both left and right saphenous vein grafts. The multipurpose catheter gives most satisfactory backup support in downgoing right coronary artery grafts. Multipurpose, right Judkins, and left coronary bypass catheters can easily be dislodged from the origin of the graft as a balloon is advanced. Although the left Amplatz catheter is more difficult to engage in left bypass grafts, it provides vastly superior backup support. It should be remembered that in general, the easier it is to engage a bypass graft, the easier it is for the guiding catheter to back out when additional support is required for crossing lesions. *Arrow* shows ostial stenosis.

left lateral projections. Caution should be used when sizing balloons for distal LAD because magnification artifacts will often lead the operator to oversize the balloon in this situation. Balloon sizing for the proximal circumflex can be undertaken in both the RAO caudal and LAO projections. Similarly, caution should be undertaken when sizing balloons for use in distal marginal branches of the left circumflex artery. For the right coronary artery, either RAO, LAO, or left lateral projections allow a good comparison between the guiding catheter tip and the proximal and middle segments of the right coronary artery. Once again, caution should be used when sizing balloons for the distal right coronary artery, PDA, and PLSA branches.

## ANGIOGRAPHIC VIEWS FOR ACCESS TO THE PROXIMAL VESSEL

In practice, a great amount of time can be wasted in attempting to pass a coronary guide wire into the coronary artery to be treated. Although the operator's ability to undertake this maneuver quickly comes with experience, access can be facilitated by the use of the most appropriate angiographic views. The following suggestions are offered to aid the operator in rapidly accessing the proximal coronary vessels. In patients with a relatively long left main stem in which the origin of the LAD is clearly seen in the RAO projection, the RAO view should be the initial one used to instrument this artery. It is

worthwhile to place a little extra angulation routinely on the tip of the coronary guide wire before the instrumentation of any LAD vessel. This is because there is often more angulation to the takeoff of the LAD than is apparent in the RAO projection. If the LAD cannot be accessed in this view, then the operator should switch rapidly to the LAO cranial projection. Biplane imaging systems certainly facilitate this aspect of the PTCA procedure. If the wire is seen to swing widely as it has apparently entered the LAD, then it is usually in a small ramus intermedius branch heading for the lateral wall behind the LAD.

In the LAO cranial projection, the tip of the guide wire should be advanced upward and to the operator's left to encounter the origin of the LAD. If the wire is then advanced, it will be clearly seen whether the wire has in fact entered the LAD or is in the circumflex artery or a ramus branch. Finally, if the operator is unsuccessful in entering the LAD in this view, an LAO caudal or AP caudal view usually provides the operator with a clear delineation of the origin of the LAD and circumflex vessels. If the LAD still cannot be entered, then the guide wire should be withdrawn and the curve increased appropriately. A double "Amplatz-type curve" on the coronary guide wire is often a useful maneuver. Finally, anticlockwise rotation of the guiding catheter directs the guide wire toward the LAD.

In contrast, I find the RAO caudal projection the best for entering the proximal circumflex artery. Some additional angulation on the guide wire and some clockwise rotation on the guiding catheter (particularly if the short-tipped left Judkins guiding catheter is used) facilitates wire movement into the left circumflex artery. When the circumflex artery takes off from the left main stem at an acute angle, the RAO caudal projection provides the operator with a distinct assessment of the amount of prolapse into the LAD that is occurring as the guide wire is manipulated toward the circumflex artery. Deep breaths are helpful in straightening out this angulation and helping passage of the wire. Occasionally, the LAO caudal or AP caudal view is useful in instrumenting the circumflex artery with the coronary guide wire.

The right coronary artery is best instrumented with the coronary guide wire using the LAD projection. In downgoing nontortuous right coronary arteries, it is usually not necessary to have the guiding catheter coaxial with the proximal part of the vessel to place the coronary guide wire. However, if the guiding catheter backs out during advancement of the guide wire, then the operator must "think clockwise rotation" of the guiding catheter and check in the RAO projection to ensure that the guiding catheter is coaxially situated.

## VISUALIZATION AND ASSESSMENT OF SIDE BRANCHES

It is important that the angiographic views used during a coronary interventional procedure provide the operator with an accurate assessment of the presence and position of major and minor side branches. This is essential for rapid access of the coronary guide wire to the lesion and to the distal vessel. For this part of the angioplasty procedure, biplane angiographic equipment is of a distinct advantage. For example, in wiring the LAD, the position of the wire in the septal branch can be easily seen in the RAO projection, and the position of the wire in a diagonal branch can be easily and rapidly seen by "flipping" to the LAO projection. In addition, it is important to understand precisely where the origins of the side branches are in relation to the lesion and the potential for causing ischemia with occlusion of major side branches during balloon inflation. In practice, the following views are helpful in determining the presence of the coronary guide wire and side branches. In the LAD, the RAO projection provides information about the position of septal branches, and the LAO cranial projection provides information about the position of diagonal branches. The RAO view is useful for placing the tip of the coronary wire well around the apex of the left ventricle. The left lateral view provides information about diagonal branches and also allows the

guide wire to be positioned well around the apex of the left ventricle. In the circumflex artery, the obtuse marginal branches are best delineated in the RAO caudal projection, whereas in left dominant circumflex arteries, the LAO or lateral views are useful in placing the guide wire well distally into the circumflex branches. In the right coronary artery, the RAO projection is useful for avoiding septal branches of the PDA and allowing the operator to place the guide wire well distal in the PDA. The LAO projection is useful for placing the guide wire well distal in PLSA branches.

Visualization of the distal vessels in the artery to be dilated is of great importance. Not only does this facilitate distal guide wire placement, but it allows later assessment of distal embolization and dissection, as well as the presence or absence of collateral vessels; in the case of patients with bypass grafting, washout from the presence of bypass grafts can be determined. One of the fundamentally important aspects of safe PTCA practice involves the extreme distal placement of the coronary guide wire. This maneuver, in essence, secures the vessel and the lesion for treatment. It allows flexibility in removing the guiding catheter from the ostium of the vessel, facilitates the movement of the balloon across the lesion, and allows balloon exchanges and other maneuvers to be done safely.

## VISUALIZATION AND ASSESSMENT OF THE LESION

Visualization of the lesion is important for determining not only the dilatation strategy, but also the guiding catheter, guide wire, and type of balloon to be used. The vessel ostium should be assessed with respect to the site of the ostium and the morphology of the vessel immediately distal to the ostium. This is critical for appropriate guiding catheter selection and technique. The proximal vessel should also be assessed for the degree of tortuosity, calcification, and diffuseness of disease. Before contrast material is injected into the vessel, a few frames should be taken to allow the operator to assess the degree of angiographically visible calcium in the vessel and the lesion to be dilated. Assessment of the lesion itself involves finding an angiographic view that defines the precise entry point for wire access to the lesion. This is important if angioplasty is to be a precise and skilled procedure rather than a hit-or-miss "attempt" at gaining access to the lesion. Angiography of the lesion should also clearly define the extent of the lesion, the origin of side branches, and the presence of angiographically visible thrombus in the region of the lesion.

Finally, during and at completion of the procedure, excellent angiography is essential for assessing the final angioplasty result. In general, multiple orthogonal views are required. It is important for the operator to understand the dynamics of vessel wall and plaque recoil after balloon dilation and the role of vessel spasm in determining the angiographic appearance of the vessel after dilation. In my view, liberal amounts of intracoronary nitroglycerin should be used before and after all balloon dilations. It is also important for the angiographic images to delineate the extent and importance of intimal tears and dissections that invariably are associated with balloon dilation. Assessing the angiographic result of an interventional procedure involves a determination of contrast flow through the lesion (as well as assessment of the margins of the lesion), the presence or absence of intimal disruption, the length of the disruption, whether the dissection is spiral or otherwise, whether contrast material is retained in the dilated vessel wall, and the extent of any residual narrowing. It is essential for the operator to take all these factors into account as the clinical status of the patient (including symptoms, hemodynamics, and the presence or absence of electrocardiographic changes) are considered. Finally, angiography during PTCA should include brief imaging of each balloon inflation at the maximal inflation pressure used for the individual inflation. When atherectomy or other devices are used, each passage of the device should be recorded briefly angiographically. Such attention to detail is important for both clinical and medicolegal reasons.

## CONCLUSION

In conclusion, excellent angiographic technique is the most important aspect of excellent PTCA procedural technique. It requires the presence of good angiographic equipment, operator experience, creativity, and, most importantly, scrupulous attention to detail.

# 20

# Coronary Angioplasty: Femoral Approach

*Alan N. Tenaglia*     *James E. Tcheng*     *Harry R. Phillips III*

The percutaneous femoral arterial approach is the most common for performing coronary angioplasty. The femoral approach has the advantage of being relatively safe and straightforward and is the most clinically forgiving. Even so, because the complexity of coronary angioplasty procedures is increasing and the patient population is growing older, the potential for vascular complications is similarly rising, making the femoral approach more and more challenging. Thus, it is critical that the interventional cardiologist become expert in accessing the peripheral vasculature and experienced with the wide variety of guide catheters designed for the femoral approach.

The purpose of this chapter is to provide an overview of practical and technical aspects that should be considered when utilizing the femoral approach. The initial sections discuss the method of accessing the femoral artery and the selection and placement of vascular sheaths. The remainder of the chapter concerns guide catheter technology and reviews the design, construction, configurations, and deployment of guide catheters. Included are practical guidelines and tips that should prove useful in the selection and manipulation of these devices.

## APPROACHES TO CORONARY ANGIOPLASTY

The two standard approaches for performing coronary angioplasty are the brachial and femoral arterial approaches. Access to the brachial artery is usually established through a surgical cutdown, although percutaneous cannulation may be performed when smaller-diameter catheters are used. The brachial arterial approach is discussed in detail elsewhere in this book. The femoral approach is performed percutaneously and is discussed in this chapter. The respective advantages of each approach are listed in Table 20–1. Clinical considerations aside, the primary factors in choosing an approach,

however, remain the operator's training, experience, and comfort with a given approach.

## ACCESS TO THE FEMORAL ARTERY

Successful access to the femoral artery depends on proper identification of anatomic landmarks and palpation of the femoral arterial pulse. In general, the femoral artery should be entered superior to the point where the common femoral bifurcates into the superficial femoral artery and the profunda femoris; a reliable landmark is a point 1 to 2 cm below the inguinal ligament, the ligament that extends from the symphysis pubis to the anterior superior iliac crest. It is important to use the ligament (rather than the inguinal crease) as a landmark as the inguinal crease can be displaced inferiorly, especially in obese patients. When the femoral artery cannot be palpated, as in the patient with severe peripheral vascular disease or multiple previous femoral accesses, the Smart Needle system (Peripheral Systems Group, Mountain View, CA) may be of utility.

**TABLE 20–1.    VASCULAR ACCESS IN CORONARY ANGIOPLASTY**

Advantages of the femoral approach
  Reduced risk of limb ischemia
  Greater margin of safety when using large-diameter guide catheters
  Vascular sheath can remain in place for an extended period of time
  Arterial cutdown, vascular repair not required
  Repeated access less problematic
  Only access route for percutaneous extracorporeal support
  Reduced radiation exposure to operator
Advantages of the brachial approach
  Only access route in the presence of occlusive peripheral vascular disease
  Rapid hemostasis on sheath removal
  Reduced incidence of pseudoaneurysm and arteriovenous fistula
  Augments superselective coronary engagement and active guide catheter support
  More rapid patient mobilization

This device uses ultrasonic guidance to locate the artery.

Once the artery is palpated, several milliliters of 1% to 2% lidocaine (or a substitute in the case of lidocaine allergy) is infiltrated subcutaneously over the artery to provide local anesthesia. Next, a small incision is made in the skin with a No. 11 blade scalpel and a tunnel created through the subcutaneous tissue using blunt dissection. Next, the artery is penetrated with a thin-walled needle in a retrograde fashion at an angle of 30 to 45 degrees from the horizontal. Although the original technique described by Seldinger involved puncture of both the anterior and posterior walls of the femoral artery followed by slow withdrawal of the needle while observing for a flash of blood into the syringe, the currently recommended technique is to puncture only the anterior wall of the femoral artery (Fig. 20–1A). Puncture of the posterior wall, particularly in the setting of the potent anticoagulant and antiplatelet agents of the modern interventional era, increases the risk of bleeding and other vascular complications. Also, thrombolytic therapy may be required during the course of an interventional procedure. Thus, it is critical that the anterior puncture technique be adapted by the practicing interventional cardiologist to reduce the risk of bleeding and concomitant vascular complications.

Once the tip of the needle has been successfully placed into the arterial lumen, signified by a flashback of blood into the syringe, the syringe is disconnected from the needle and a 0.035-inch J-tip guide wire advanced through the needle into the common femoral artery (Fig. 20–1B). If any resistance to advancement is encountered, fluoroscopy should be used to ascertain whether or not there is free movement of the tip of the wire within the arterial lumen and to determine the course of the guide wire in the vasculature. When the guide wire cannot be freely advanced, the needle should be carefully manipulated (usually by slightly retracting the needle) until the guide wire moves freely and without impediment. Otherwise the wire may dissect into the wall of the artery, often with surprisingly little resistance. In the patient with tortuous or diseased peripheral vasculature, a diagnostic right coronary catheter may be placed over the guide wire and advanced to the tip of the wire to help steer the guide wire tip; a gentle injection of contrast material may be invaluable in defining the anatomy. Special guide wires, including the steerable Wholey wire (Peripheral Systems Group) and the coated Terumo Glidewire (Meditech, Watertown, MA) may be of utility in navigating through the tortuous or diseased peripheral artery.

After the guide wire has been successfully advanced into the abdominal aorta, the final step is to

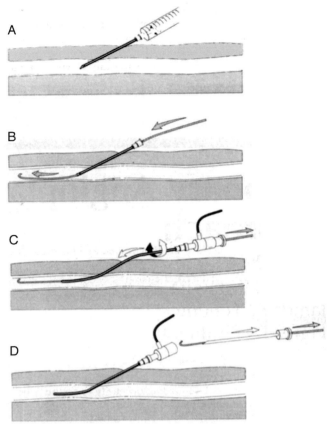

FIGURE 20–1. Modified Seldinger technique for femoral arterial access. *A*, Thin-walled 18-gauge needle inserted through the anterior wall of the femoral artery (without penetration of the posterior wall). *B*, Peripheral guide wire placed through the center of the needle and advanced into the common femoral artery. The guide wire is then advanced into the central circulation, and, with the tip of the wire in the aorta, the needle is removed and manual pressure applied to maintain wire position and hemostasis (not shown). *C*, Sheath with dilator advanced over the guide wire and into the femoral artery with (minimal) rotation of the sheath assembly. *D*, Wire and dilator removed, leaving sheath in artery.

remove the needle from the guide wire, exchanging the needle for a vascular sheath (Fig. 20–1C). Slight retraction of the guide wire assists the advancement of the dilator and sheath assembly into the femoral artery. If there was difficulty with the initial advancement of the guide wire through the iliac or femoral arteries, the guide wire may be left in place in the aorta, the dilator removed, and the guide catheter advanced over the wire and into the ascending aorta. Otherwise, the wire and dilator are removed (Fig. 20–1D) and the guide wire loaded into the guide catheter to facilitate the introduction of the guide.

## FEMORAL SHEATHS

The functions of the vascular sheath are to provide access to the central circulation, maintain a conduit for the insertion of coronary diagnostic and guide catheters, and achieve hemostasis at the puncture site while permitting continued blood flow distal to the sheath insertion site. Sheaths are made of nonthrombogenic materials such as Teflon or polyurethane. The typical sheath is thin walled and pliable while being slightly radiopaque, resistant to compression, and moderately stiff in the axial dimension. The tip of the sheath is tapered to minimize vessel trauma during advancement of the sheath over the dilator. The dilator is less flexible than the sheath and has greater axial stiffness in order to facilitate advancement of the sheath assembly over the peripheral guide wire. One important design feature is the hemostasis valve, which prevents backbleeding when the sheath is in place. From manufacturer to manufacturer, the valve may be more or less competent depending primarily on the match between the rated sheath size and the guide catheter; when using large (10-French or greater) sheaths with smaller catheters (8 French or smaller), placement of an 8- or 9-French sheath into the valve of the 10-French sheath may be used to prevent excessive backbleeding if the valve proves incompetent with a smaller guide catheter in place.

The inner diameters of sheaths for interventional procedures range from 6 to 11 French, with sizes up to 20 French supporting percutaneous cardiopulmonary bypass. New 16-French designs that incorporate a side port have been developed; they may be used either for intra-aortic balloon pumping or for percutaneous cardiopulmonary bypass. The actual sheath chosen for a given case is most dependent on the diameter of the guide catheter used; in general, the smallest possible sheath size should be selected in order to minimize the risk of vascular complications. As a corollary, the thickness of the sheath tubing should be considered when selecting a vascular sheath, because the outer diameter of the sheath is a function of this thickness; the outer diameter in turn determines the ultimate size of the arterial puncture, which may correlate with the incidence of vascular complications.[1]

Sheath lengths may range from 6 to 23 cm. In general, shorter sheaths are recommended for the majority of cases; the less sheath within the femoral and iliac arteries, the lower the potential for vessel occlusion. Longer sheaths may be of particular utility in tortuous peripheral vessels, especially with larger guide catheters.

As with any indwelling device, sheaths should be left in place for the least amount of time possible. Sheath-related complications include oozing around the sheath, vascular occlusion due to thrombosis or occlusion through an area of stenosis, and the morbidity of prolonged sheath insertion, especially when the sheath is left in place overnight. Oozing of blood around the sheath can often be controlled by local external pressure; exchange of the sheath for another 1-French size larger can be performed to control persistent oozing, especially when the insertion has been traumatic. New developments, such as the flexible sheath and the collagen plug[2] may obviate some of these limitations by augmenting more rapid patient mobilization after coronary angioplasty.

## GUIDE CATHETER DESIGN

Guide catheters are designed and engineered to meet four critical functions. First, the guide catheter permits access to the coronary ostium and in this capacity serves as a delivery conduit for the interventional device. Second, the guide catheter provides support for the advancement and deployment of the interventional device to the level of the coronary stenosis. Third, the fluid column within the guide catheter allows measurement of pressure from the tip of the guide catheter by an external transducer. Finally, the catheter provides a conduit for the selective delivery of contrast material into the coronary arterial tree.

The support provided by a guide catheter can be either active or passive. Passive support is that provided by a guide catheter because of the inherent stiffness of the guide catheter combined with the curve configuration of the distal tip and the geometric relationship of the tip to the coronary artery. When a guide that provides a high degree of passive support is used, additional manipulation is generally not required for deployment of interventional devices. Should passive support prove insufficient, however, active support may be required. Active support is typically achieved either by manipulation of the guide catheter into a configuration conforming to the aortic root or by subselective coronary intubation with deep engagement of the guide catheter into the coronary vessel. Techniques for achieving active support are discussed later in this chapter.

Numerous design parameters must be considered when designing a guide catheter. Desirable features include a large-caliber internal lumen, radial strength (to minimize the potential for kinking or collapse), low frictional resistance both internal and external to the guide catheter, columnar and torsional rigidity (to augment transmission of push and torque), flexibility, malleability, and radiodensity. Some compromise is required in order to achieve the proper balance of attributes; for example, increasing the lumen size can only be achieved at the expense of catheter wall thickness, thus compromising radial strength, torsional rigidity, and overall stiffness. Catheters designed to be soft and compli-

**TABLE 20–2. TYPICAL CHARACTERISTICS OF GUIDE AND DIAGNOSTIC CORONARY CATHETERS**

| GUIDE CATHETERS | DIAGNOSTIC CATHETERS |
| --- | --- |
| Three-layer construction | Two-layer construction |
| Thinner wall | Thicker wall |
| Larger internal diameter | Smaller internal diameter |
| Decreased rotational torque transmission | Better rotational torque transmission |
| Coaxial alignment important | Noncoaxial alignment acceptable |
| Radiopaque tip marker present | No tip marker |
| Shorter tip | Longer tip |
| Open final (primary) curve | Angulated final curve |

ant provide an extra margin of safety when active engagement is required for device deployment; conversely, a stiffer catheter may provide better passive support for deployment and thus obviate the potential need for active engagement. One approach taken by several companies is to alter the modulus of the final 8 to 10 cm of a guide catheter so that the final portion of the guide is soft, malleable, and compliant whereas the body of the catheter retains columnar strength and stiffness. The primary differences in characteristics of guide catheters compared with standard diagnostic catheters are listed in Table 20–2.

Table 20–3 provides a list of current guide catheters by vendor and includes manufacturing specifications. To provide the proper balance of characteristics, most guide catheters are constructed of three layers. The inner layer consists of Teflon or another inert, lubricous, biocompatible material, selected to limit the potential for thrombosis and to minimize friction forces. Guide catheters that incorporate a lubricous inner lining such as Teflon have superior performance over unlined guides, especially when deploying larger devices such as intracoronary stents. The middle layer, usually made of a stainless steel or Kevlar weave or braid, provides resistance to deformation, kinking, and collapse. The outer jacket, composed of a lubricous, biocompatible, nonthrombogenic material such as polyethylene or polyurethane, determines to a large extent the degree of intrinsic catheter "memory" and the amount of passive support intrinsic to the guide catheter. Depending on the manufacturer, additional features may be incorporated in the design, including soft tips (to lessen vessel trauma) and radiopaque marker bands. Although soft tips may reduce the potential for trauma, no rigorous clinical data exist to support this contention; indeed, the overall stiffness of the guide and the geometric relationship between the tip of the guide and the coronary ostium probably have at least as important a role in determining the trauma potential of a guide catheter tip. Thus, a greater reduction in the risk of ostial coronary dissection may be achieved by using, whenever possible, less aggressively curved catheters, such as the Judkins configuration guides, in place of catheters that engage and seat the proximal coronary more aggressively.

Most guide catheters are available with preformed side holes. The use of side hole guide catheters

**TABLE 20–3. GUIDE CATHETER SPECIFICATIONS BY MANUFACTURER***

| PRODUCT | CATHETER COMPOSITION | | | CATHETER (FRENCH) INNER DIAMETER (INCHES) | | | | |
| --- | --- | --- | --- | --- | --- | --- | --- | --- |
| | INNER | MIDDLE | OUTER | 6 | 7 | 8 | 9 | 10 |
| ACS ET Hi-Flow | Teflon | Kevlar wind | Polyethylene | | | 0.076 | 0.076 | |
| ACS Powerguide | Teflon | Kevlar braid | Polyurethane | | 0.070 | 0.080 | | |
| Baxter Marathon | Pebax | Stainless steel | Pebax | | 0.070 | 0.078 | | |
| Cordis Brite Tip | Teflon | Stainless steel | Polyurethane | | | 0.074–0.078 | | |
| Cordis Brite Tip/XL Brite Tip | PTFE Teflon | Stainless steel | Duralyn | 0.062 | 0.072 | 0.084 | | |
| Medtronic Safe Tip | Teflon | Stainless steel | Polyurethane | | 0.066 | 0.079 | 0.088 | |
| Medtronic Sherpa | Teflon | Stainless steel | Blended urethane | 0.057 | 0.070 | 0.079 | 0.092 | 0.108 |
| Schneider Softip Standard | Teflon | Stainless steel | Polyurethane | | 0.063 | 0.076 | 0.080 | |
| Schneider Superflow | Teflon | Stainless steel | Polyurethane | | 0.072 | 0.082 | 0.092 | 0.107 |
| Schneider Stamina/Visiguide | Teflon | Stainless steel | Polyurethane | | | 0.079 | | |
| Sci-Med TriGuide | Teflon | Stainless steel | Trilon | | 0.072 | 0.080 | | |
| Intermediate | | | | | | | | |
| Standard | Teflon | Stainless steel | Trilon | | | 0.079 | | |
| USCI DuraGuide | Teflon | Stainless steel | Durathane, urethane | | | 0.078 | | |
| USCI Super 7/Illumen 8 | Teflon | Kevlar braid | Pebax | | 0.070 | 0.080 | | |

*Specifications are courtesy of the respective companies. Product names and some materials are trademarks of the respective companies. ACS, Advanced Cardiovascular Systems, Inc., Santa Clara CA; Baxter, Baxter Healthcare Corporation, LIS Division, Santa Ana CA; Cordis, Cordis Corporation, Miami FL; Medtronic, Medtronic, Inc., Interventional Medical Division, Danvers MA; Schneider, Schneider (USA) Inc., Pfizer Hospital Products Group, Plymouth MN; Sci-Med, SCIMED Life Systems, Inc., Maple Grove MN; USCI, C.R. Bard, Inc., USCI Division, Haverhill MA.

provides an extra margin of safety when the clearance between the outer wall of the guide catheter and the inner lumen of the coronary (or graft) vessel is minimal. The primary disadvantage is a slight reduction in vessel opacification with contrast injection due to loss of contrast material via the side holes. More importantly, however, is the potential for inaccurate pressure transduction; compromised flow into the distal coronary bed may occur even in the presence of a normal pressure tracing because side holes are only marginally capable of supporting normal coronary blood flow rates.

Selection of the guide catheter French diameter is dictated mostly by compatibility with the devices that are to be used during a procedure. With the advent of low-profile balloon catheters and large-lumen guide catheters, balloon angioplasty may now be performed with 7-, and 6-French guide catheters;[3–7] angioplasty with 4-French catheters has been reported.[8] Indeed, the inner diameter of some of the newer 7-French catheters approaches those of the 9-French guides of the 1980s. The primary advantages of smaller-diameter catheters include a smaller femoral arterial puncture, less potential for occlusive intubation of the coronary ostium, easier deep intubation of the coronary artery (for increased active guide catheter support), and greater catheter flexibility. Patients may also be ambulated more quickly. The primary drawback is that only low-profile balloon devices may be used; exchange of catheters for a perfusion balloon may be difficult with a smaller French guide, and stent deployment may be impossible in the case of a failed angioplasty. Smaller French size guide catheters also provide less passive support than their larger-diameter counterparts.

The standard catheter for performing coronary angioplasty remains the 8-French guide catheter. These catheters provide the optimal balance of passive support, guide catheter stability, transmission of axial and rotational force, minimal resistance to contrast injection, pressure transduction fidelity, and a large internal lumen compatible with the broadest range of interventional devices. These are of particular utility in the setting of complex angioplasty as they facilitate the deployment of perfusion balloon catheters and support the use of simultaneous "kissing" balloons. For specialized devices, even larger diameter guide catheters may be required. Stent deployment requires a large-lumen 8-French guide catheter; a 9-French catheter is actually preferable. A 9-French guide catheter is required when performing excimer laser angioplasty with a 2-mm device, although procedures using 1.7-mm or smaller catheters can be performed with large-lumen 8-French catheters. Directional coronary atherectomy requires even larger guides with

modified distal curves to support the deployment of the rigid cutter housing. Drawbacks of the larger guides include the potential for peripheral vascular complications and a greater risk of ostial trauma and occlusive guide catheter engagement.

Guide catheters are available in preformed shapes suitable for specific anatomic situations. As illustrated in Figure 20–2, a guide catheter can be described in terms of the configuration of the primary, secondary, and (when present) tertiary curves of the catheter and the spatial relationship of those curves. In general, the numeric value assigned to each catheter is a measurement of the distance between the primary and secondary curves of the catheter, with a greater number signifying a more open configuration. The most commonly used shapes for both right and left coronary angioplasty are the Judkins configuration catheters (see Fig. 20–2). Judkins catheters are available in different sizes, ranging from 3 to 6 cm. One difference in configuration of standard Judkins guide catheters compared with standard Judkins diagnostic catheters is the use of a shortened final tip with a more open primary curve, a design compromise that improves the coaxial relationship of the distal tip of the guide catheter and reduces the potential for vascular trauma. Of all guide catheter configurations, the modified short-tip Judkins guide catheter, with a tip even shorter and more open than that of the standard (shortened-tip) Judkins guide catheter, typically provides the

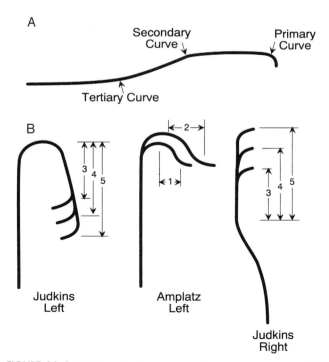

FIGURE 20–2. Guide catheter curves and curve measurement. *A*, Location of the primary, secondary, and tertiary curves of a Judkins right guide catheter. *B*, Comparison of curve sizes for Judkins left. Amplatz left, and Judkins right catheters.

ultimate degree of coaxial alignment and consequently imparts the least resistance to advancement of interventional devices through the end of the guide while providing the greatest margin of safety when active engagement is needed. Thus, provided that guide catheter seating is adequate, the modified short-tip left Judkins guide catheter may be the catheter of choice for angioplasty of the left coronary circulation. Left coronary Judkins configuration guide catheters are also available in which the secondary curve is off center and angled 30 degrees anteriorly (to help select the left anterior descending artery) or posteriorly (for selection of the circumflex artery). Finally, it should be noted that there is significant variability in configuration from one manufacturer to the next for catheters of the same nominal shape and measurement.

Other configurations of guide catheters exist to support angioplasty in those anatomic situations that warrant their use. The Amplatz and Nesto[9] configurations provide a greater degree of passive support when positioned but tend to engage the coronary vessel more aggressively than their Judkins counterparts. Other speciality guides include the multipurpose, hockey stick, Arani,[10] El Gamal, vein bypass, and internal mammary artery guides. The range of available catheter curve configurations is illustrated in Figure 20–3.

## GUIDE CATHETER STRATEGY

With the availability of improved balloon angioplasty catheters, successful coronary intervention is much less dependent today on proper guide catheter selection than in years past. Nonetheless, guide catheter selection remains important for a number of reasons: cost containment, minimizing procedure time, and maximizing the chances of a successful procedural outcome. In selecting a guide catheter, the information of greatest utility is the shape, size, position, and orientation of the diagnostic catheter used during diagnostic angiography. The main problems are that the diagnostic catheter is not entirely predictive of the behavior of a similarly shaped guide catheter, and that a given shape may prove inadequate for device deployment (compared with the minimal support necessary for selective coronary opacification), necessitating use of a more aggressive guide catheter.

For a given stenosis, the three major factors influencing correct guide catheter selection are the size and length of the ascending aorta and aortic arch, the anatomy of the ostium and proximal coronary arterial segments (geometry, vessel diameter, and presence of disease), and lesion-related variables (tortuosity proximal to the lesion, lesion severity, location, and other descriptors). The following sections outline considerations in the selection of guide catheters for stenoses in native coronary arteries, vein grafts, and internal mammary artery grafts.

## Left Coronary Artery

With a normally sized aortic root and horizontal orientation of the origin of the left main coronary artery, the Judkins JL 4 catheters usually fit coaxially

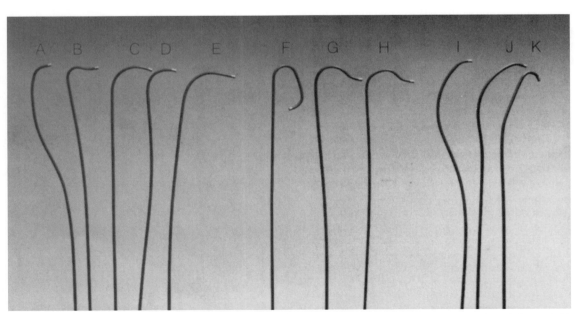

FIGURE 20–3. Shapes of commonly used guide catheters. Right coronary guide catheters: *A,* JR 4. *B,* Amplatz right 2. *C,* El Gamal. *D,* Hockey stick. *E,* Multipurpose BI. Left coronary guide catheters: *F,* JL 4. *G,* Amplatz left 2. *H,* Nesto. Coronary bypass graft guide catheters: *I,* Right coronary bypass. *J,* Left coronary bypass. *K,* Internal mammary artery. (Courtesy of Baxter Healthcare Corporation, LIS Division, Santa Ana, CA.)

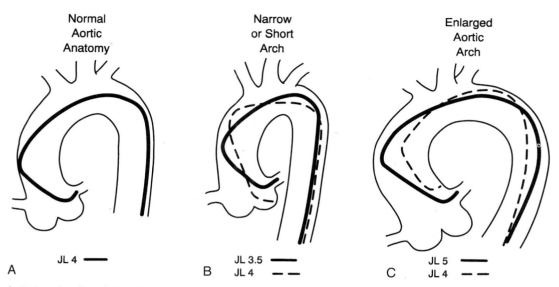

FIGURE 20–4. Sizing of Judkins left catheters based on aortic anatomy. *A,* Typical aortic anatomy. The JL 4 catheter engages adequately in most cases. *B,* Narrow or short aortic arch. Shorter Judkins catheters such as the JL 3 or JL 3.5 provide better fit and coaxial alignment than a JL 4. *C,* Enlarged or elongated aortic arch or widened aortic root. Longer-length curves between 4.5 and 6 provide better alignment and selectivity than a JL 4.

into the left main artery and provide sufficient support (Fig. 20–4). However, when the aortic root is large or the aortic arch wide or elongated, the 4-cm-long curve may not be long enough to reach the ostium of the left main artery or may point superiorly (rather than coaxially) in the left main artery, thus increasing the risk of dissection and reducing support for the deployment of the treatment catheter. In this situation, the use of a longer Judkins curve, up to a JL 6, is needed. Conversely, in the patient with a smaller aortic root or narrower aortic arch, the best fit may be obtained with a JL 3.5 or JL 3 catheter.

In patients with a superior or posterior orientation of the left main artery, left Amplatz catheters often provide better coronary engagement and support. However, the Amplatz catheter requires careful handling. The technique of deployment of this catheter is advancement of the tip into the left aortic cusp followed by rotation and then retraction until the tip enters the coronary ostium. Further retraction often results in deep intubation of the left main artery and so must be done carefully. At the termination of the procedure, removal of the catheter should be performed by first advancing the catheter (to disengage the left main ostium) followed by rotation, rather than simple withdrawal of the catheter. Other options for the superiorly oriented left main coronary artery include the JL 3.5 and El Gamal catheters.

With a short left main coronary artery, the balloon catheter may be directed preferentially into the circumflex artery with the use of a standard JL 4 guide. In order to direct the guide catheter tip into the

left anterior descending artery, a catheter of shorter length curve may be tried, or the guide catheter may be rotated in a counterclockwise direction and advanced (Fig. 20–5*A*). The latter maneuver swings

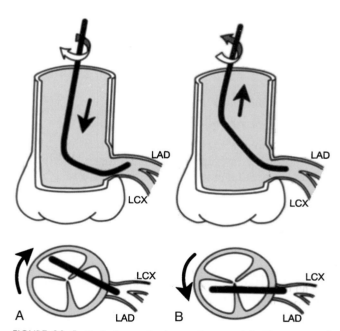

FIGURE 20–5. Techniques for improving coaxial alignment and selective engagement when using Judkins curve guide catheters. *A,* Selective engagement of the left anterior descending artery (LAD) with a Judkins catheter. Counterclockwise rotation with advancement swings the secondary curve more posteriorly and inferiorly, aligning the tip more selectively with the ostium of the LAD. *B,* Selective engagement of the left circumflex artery (LCX) with a Judkins catheter. Clockwise rotation with slight retraction swings the secondary curve more anteriorly and superiorly, improving alignment with the LCX ostium.

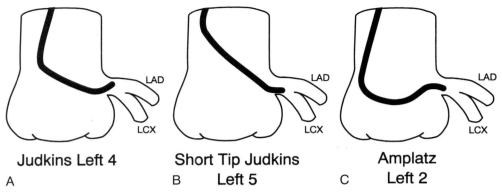

**FIGURE 20–6.** Differences between guide catheter tip geometry when addressing the left circumflex coronary artery (LCX). *A*, The JL 4 catheter may be angled preferentially into the left anterior descending artery (LAD). *B*, A short-tipped JL 4.5 or 5 catheter may provide better coaxial alignment with the *LCX* ostium provided the left main artery may be cannulated with the longer guide catheter. *C*, Amplatz left guide catheters typically point preferentially into the LCX, providing excellent passive support.

the heel more posteriorly and inferiorly in the root of the aorta, resulting in anterior and superior displacement of the tip and improved alignment with the left anterior descending artery.

For more selective intubation of the circumflex, a catheter with a longer secondary curve or a shorter tip may prove advantageous. For example, a short-tip JL 4.5 or JL 5 catheter points more selectively into the circumflex than a JL 4 guide (Fig. 20–6*A*, *B*). Another approach is to use an Amplatz curve guide catheter. When fully engaged, the tip of an Amplatz guide is oriented more inferiorly than a Judkins guide catheter, providing better coaxial alignment with the left circumflex artery (Fig. 20–6*C*). Other options include hockey stick (especially with a narrow root) and multipurpose guide catheters.

## Right Coronary Artery

There is greater variability in the location of the right coronary ostium and the geometric orientation of the proximal segment of the right coronary artery (Fig. 20–7) compared with the left main artery, thus making it more difficult to select a guide catheter that provides optimal engagement and support.[11] In addition, ostial disease is more prevalent in the right coronary artery, adding to the complexity facing the interventionalist.

For the right coronary artery with a horizontal proximal segment, the Judkins right 4 configuration is usually adequate. Smaller and larger curves are available but are usually not required except for extremes in aortic anatomy. Increased support can be attained by active engagement (when using soft guide catheters) or exchange for Amplatz, hockey stick, or Arani guide catheters.

A common variant of proximal right coronary artery geometry is the upward, or "shepherd's crook," configuration. In these cases, the tip of a JR 4 guide

is directed down and away from the coronary ostium (Fig. 20–8*A*). Seating of the guide may be facilitated by having the patient inspire deeply (Fig. 20–8*B*), as this elongates the aorta and results in less severe angulation of the proximal segment. This maneuver should be attempted before proceeding to more aggressive catheters. However, when a Judkins catheter proves inadequate, several other catheters may provide more optimal alignment and support. An Amplatz left guide catheter, because of its supe-

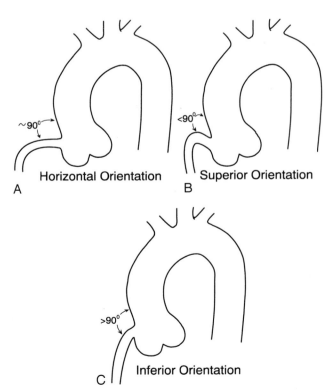

**FIGURE 20–7.** Variants of right coronary ostial orientation and proximal coronary geometry. *A*, Typical horizontal orientation. *B*, Superior angulation. The most extreme variant of this is the "shepherd's crook" right coronary artery. *C*, Inferior angulation.

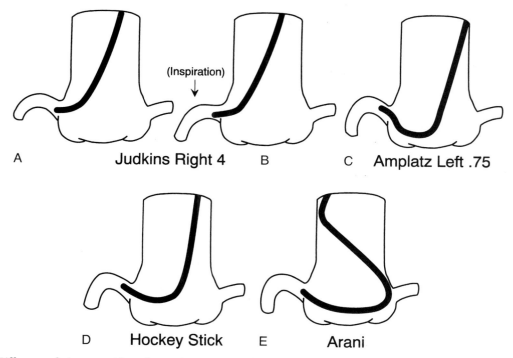

FIGURE 20–8. Differences between guide catheter tip geometry when addressing a right coronary artery with superior orientation of the proximal segment. *A*, Judkins catheters may not cannulate the ostium effectively. *B*, Inspiration pulls the proximal segment inferiorly and may improve coaxial alignment between a Judkins catheter and the proximal right coronary segment. *C*, Seating of a short Amplatz left guide catheter. *D*, Seating of a hockey stick configuration catheter. *E*, Seating of an Arani guide catheter.

rior tip orientation (compared with an Amplatz right), in a 0.5-, 0.75-, or 1-cm-long curve may prove superior in this setting (Fig. 20–8*C*). Other options include shepherd's crook right, hockey stick, and Arani[12] guide catheters (Fig. 20–8*D,E*); care must be exercised with these configurations, however, as there is an increased risk of guide catheter–induced dissection and coronary occlusion. For cases of extreme angulation, a left bypass or internal mammary artery guide[13] may engage adequately for coronary opacification, although often these configurations do not provide firm support.

Severe downward angulation of the right coronary artery is less commonly encountered. Standard Judkins right guide catheters may be less than ideal as the tip tends to point into the wall of the coronary artery (Fig. 20–9*A*). Catheters with a more inferior orientation, including short-tip (modified) Judkins right, hockey stick, multipurpose, Amplatz right, and right bypass guide catheters may prove advantageous in this situation (Fig. 20–9*B–D*).

## Coronary Anomalies

The most common anomaly is the circumflex artery that originates from the proximal right coronary artery or from the right coronary sinus. Techniques that have been described to cannulate the anoma-

lous circumflex artery include clockwise rotation of a JR 4 guide catheter (to orient the tip posteriorly),[14] reshaping the tip of a JR 4 for greater posterior deflection,[15] and use of other catheters including the short-tip JR 4,[16, 17] Amplatz left,[15, 17] Amplatz right,[18] or hockey stick guides (Fig. 20–10*A*). Another method requires the placement of a coronary guide wire through a JR 4 guide into the right coronary artery for stabilization of the guide and then advancement of a second guide wire into the anomalous circumflex for advancement of the balloon.[19]

Another anomaly occasionally encountered is the right coronary artery arising from the left coronary sinus (Fig. 20–10*B*). This may often be successfully cannulated with a left coronary bypass catheter but may require a left Amplatz or multipurpose guide. Other coronary arteries with anomalous origins may be cannulated using the same techniques discussed earlier for normal arteries. Again, the location of the ostium of the anomalous vessel and the geometry of the proximal segment should be the prime determinants dictating selection of a specific guide catheter.

## Vein Grafts

As with native coronary arteries, the key to proper guide catheter selection for vein grafts is selecting the guide that provides coaxial alignment with suf-

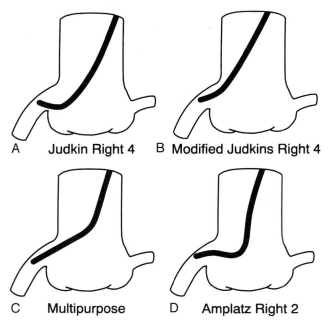

FIGURE 20–9. Differences between guide catheter tip geometry when addressing a right coronary artery with inferior angulation of the proximal segment. *A*, Tip of a Judkins curve catheter may point laterally into the wall of the artery. *B*, The modified (short-tip) Judkins right, with a more open primary curve and a shorter final tip, may provide improved alignment and cannulation. *C*, Seating of a multipurpose catheter. *D*, Seating of an Amplatz right catheter. The Amplatz right catheter tips are oriented more inferiorly than the corresponding Amplatz left guide catheter tips.

ficient guide catheter support. For grafts originating low in the aortic root and on the right side of the aorta (typically grafts to the right coronary artery), catheters that will provide adequate alignment and support include right coronary bypass, Judkins right, multipurpose, and Amplatz right guides (Fig. 20–11*A,B*). For left-sided grafts and grafts originating higher on the ascending aorta (typically grafts to the left anterior descending or the left circumflex artery), choices include the left coronary bypass, Judkins right, hockey stick, multipurpose, El Gamal, Arani,[20] internal mammary artery, Amplatz left, and right venous bypass guides (Fig. 20–11*C,D*). It is often difficult to predict the best catheter for grafts arising very high on the aortic arch, and some degree of trial and error should be anticipated.

## Internal Mammary Artery

In cannulating the internal mammary (internal thoracic) artery, it is important to note that the origin of the artery may be quite friable. The use of smaller guides (6 or 7 French) is therefore recommended as this may reduce the potential for dissection of the origin of the internal mammary artery. The most common catheters used in this setting are the Judkins right coronary and internal mammary graft

guide catheters. On occasion, it may be difficult to cannulate the origin of the internal mammary artery; when this occurs, passage of a soft-tipped, steerable peripheral guide wire (such as the Wholey guide wire) into the internal mammary artery followed by advancement of the guide catheter over the wire may result in successful cannulation.

One other consideration important in performing angioplasty via the internal mammary artery is the distance from the origin of the internal mammary to the anastomosis with the coronary vessel. To compensate for the added length that the use of the internal mammary artery conduit imposes, short (90-cm) guide catheters should be used in place of standard 100-cm guides. Most vendors manufacture the internal mammary guide catheter and the Judkins right guide catheter in 90-cm lengths. When 90-cm guide catheters are not available, the hub of a standard 100-cm-long 8-French guide catheter can be snipped approximately 10 to 15 cm from the end and replaced by a hemostatic 6- or 7-French vascular sheath to achieve the same result.

## Strategies for Increasing Guide Catheter Active Support

The conservative approach to guide catheter use features the selection of guide catheters that cannulate the coronary origins in a coaxial manner and reliance on passive support for the advancement and deployment of the angioplasty device. However, when severe stenoses, calcified lesions, total occlu-

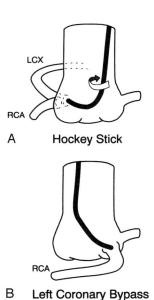

FIGURE 20–10. Common coronary artery anomalies. *A*, Left circumflex artery (LCX) arising from the right coronary sinus. Clockwise rotation of a guide catheter permits cannulation of the anomalous LCX. *B*, Right coronary artery (RCA) arising from the left coronary sinus. The longer reach of the left coronary bypass configuration may be necessary to cannulate the anomalous RCA.

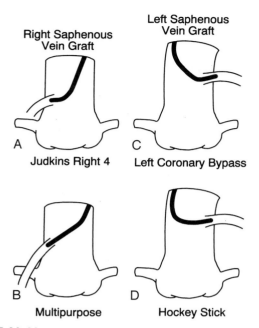

FIGURE 20–11. Approaches for cannulating saphenous vein by-pass grafts. *A*, Seating of a Judkins right coronary catheter in a vein bypass graft to the right coronary artery. *B*, Seating of a multipurpose catheter in a vein bypass graft to the right coronary artery. The multipurpose catheter is of particular utility with the vertically oriented saphenous vein bypass graft. *C*, Seating of left coronary bypass graft catheter in a saphenous vein bypass graft to the left coronary system. *D*, Seating of a hockey stick catheter in a saphenous vein bypass graft to the left coronary system. The hockey stick catheter may need to be advanced and rotated in order to achieve coaxial alignment.

sions, or lesions located distally in a rigid or tortuous artery are treated, guide catheter manipulation to create active support is often required. The two methods for achieving additional active support are manipulation of the guide catheter into a configuration that conforms to the root of the aorta ("Amplatzing") and deep, subselective engagement of the guide into the coronary over a balloon catheter system. Both approaches should be reserved for those situations in which passive support proves insufficient for advancement of the treatment catheter; when there is significant ostial or proximal coronary disease, the Amplatz maneuvers may have a slight advantage by reducing the potential for trauma in the ostium and proximal coronary arterial segments.

For the right coronary artery, the alignment of the guide catheter tip with the proximal vessel segment is best visualized in the right anterior oblique position. Additional clockwise rotation of the guide catheter is usually required for true coaxial alignment. To achieve subselective intubation,[21] advancement of the guide over the balloon catheter shaft is performed, drawing the guide catheter subselectively into the body of the right coronary artery (Fig. 20–12). The operator should feel no resistance when this maneuver is attempted. Once the guide catheter

is deeply seated, the balloon can then be advanced across the lesion and the guide withdrawn from the coronary artery. This technique should be performed only with soft-tip catheters in right coronary arteries large enough to accommodate the guide. There should not be any disease present in the proximal segment of the right coronary artery. A similar technique can be used to augment the degree of active support in left coronary angioplasty. Although mastery of this technique will prove invaluable in the crossing of challenging lesions, potential complications of active subselective engagement include intimal damage, dissection, and occlusion of the artery. In addition, rapid progression of left main artery disease has been described after angioplasty, possibly related to guide catheter trauma.[22]

Conversion of a Judkins guide catheter into an Amplatz configuration can be performed with both right and left guides. With a left Judkins catheter, this maneuver is accomplished by advancing the guide catheter over a deployed balloon catheter while applying counterclockwise torque. The tip then prolapses upward into the left main coronary artery while the secondary curve seats in the coronary cusp (Fig. 20–13). Again, it is critical that this be attempted only by experienced operators using soft catheters with soft tips.

## Guide Catheter Exchange

Although it is best to use the proper guide catheter from the beginning of a procedure, it may become necessary to exchange the guide catheter after a

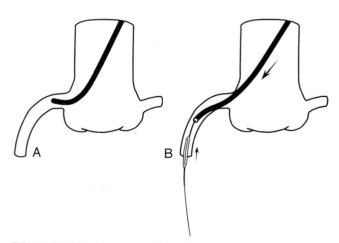

FIGURE 20–12. A technique for achieving active guide catheter support when addressing the right coronary system with a Judkins right catheter. *A*, Normal (passive) support from simple cannulation of the ostium of the right coronary. *B*, Active engagement and support achieved by advancement of the guide catheter over a balloon catheter with simultaneous retraction of the balloon catheter. This should be performed only by experienced interventionalists using soft guide catheters with a balloon catheter in place.

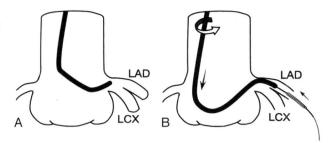

FIGURE 20–13. A technique for achieving the greatest degree of active guide catheter support when addressing the left coronary system with a Judkins left catheter. *A*, Normal (passive) support from simple cannulation of the ostium of the left main coronary artery. *B*, Active engagement of the left anterior descending artery (LAD) with maximal active support achieved by advancement of the guide catheter over a balloon catheter with counterclockwise rotation of the guide and simultaneous retraction of the balloon catheter. Because of the abnormal stress on the tip of the guide catheter, the operator should anticipate sudden disengagement and accommodate accordingly. This technique should be used only by experienced interventionalists using soft guide catheters with a balloon catheter in place. LCX, left circumflex coronary artery.

coronary guide wire has been placed across a lesion while maintaining the position of the coronary guide wire across the target lesion. This may occur when a guide catheter does not provide sufficient passive or active support to permit the crossing of the lesion with the treatment device even after exchange of the catheter for one with the greatest crossing potential. Several techniques for guide catheter exchange have been described. One is to attempt a simple exchange over the coronary guide wire. When this is not possible (because of the flexibility of the coronary guide wire), the guide may be disengaged from the coronary ostium and retracted slightly into the aorta and an 0.035-inch peripheral guide wire placed alongside the coronary guide wire. This may prove sufficient to permit guide catheter withdrawal and exchange.[23] Another technique is to advance the coronary guide wire into the aortic root to create a loop so that there is less chance for withdrawal of the guide wire from the coronary circulation during the guide catheter exchange process.[24]

## CONCLUSION

Successful angioplasty is highly dependent on choosing the proper size and shape guide catheter. Indeed, well-planned guide catheter strategy will benefit both the patient and the interventionalist by saving time, reducing costs, and minimizing the potential for complications.

In the future, further downsizing of balloon and guide catheters will be an important strategy for increasing patient comfort and reducing femoral vascular complications. It may prove to be one of the keys in reducing the length of hospitalization and lowering the overall cost of angioplasty. Continued improvements in guide catheter design, resulting in safer procedures and higher success rates, will also play a role.

## REFERENCES

1. Muller DWM, Shamir KJ, Ellis SG, Topol EJ: Peripheral vascular complications after conventional and complex percutaneous coronary interventional procedures. Am J Cardiol 69:63, 1992.
2. Gibbs S, Gunnes P, Blake J et al: Clinical evaluation of collagen plugs: Single institution experience after coronary angioplasty and diagnostic angiography, abstracted. J Am Coll Cardiol 19:217, 1992.
3. Feldman R, Glemser E, Kaizer J, Standley M: Coronary angioplasty using new 6 French guiding catheters. Cathet Cardiovasc Diagn 23:93, 1991.
4. Kern MJ, Talley JD, Deligonul U, et al: Preliminary experience with 5 and 6 French diagnostic catheters as guiding catheters for coronary angioplasty. Cathet Cardiovasc Diagn 22:60, 1991.
5. Villavicencio R, Urban P, Muller T, et al: Coronary balloon angioplasty through diagnostic 6 French catheters. Cathet Cardiovasc Diagn 22:56, 1991.
6. Panayiotou H, Norris JW, Forman MB: Coronary angioplasty at the time of initial catheterization using small diagnostic catheters. Am Heart J 119:204, 1990.
7. Salinger MH, Kern MJ: First use of a 5 French diagnostic catheter as a guiding catheter for percutaneous transluminal coronary angioplasty. Cathet Cardiovasc Diagn 18:276, 1989.
8. Moles VP, Meier B, Urban P, et al: Percutaneous transluminal coronary angioplasty through 4 French diagnostic catheters. Cathet Cardiovasc Diagn 25:98, 1992.
9. Nesto RW: Performance characteristics of a new shape of guiding catheter for PTCA of the left coronary artery. Cathet Cardiovasc Diagn 24:144, 1991.
10. Arani DT: A new catheter for angioplasty of the right coronary artery. Cathet Cardiovasc Diagn 11:647, 1985.
11. Myler RK, Boucher RA, Cumberland DC, Stertzer SH: Guiding catheter selection for right coronary artery angioplasty. Cathet Cardiovasc Diagn 19:58, 1990.
12. Arani DT, Bunnell IL, Visco JR, Conley JG: Double loop guiding catheter: A primary catheter for angioplasty of the right coronary artery. Cathet Cardiovasc Diagn 15:125, 1988.
13. Kulick DL: Use of the internal mammary artery guiding catheter for percutaneous transluminal coronary angioplasty of the shepherd's crook right coronary artery. Cathet Cardiovasc Diagn 16:190, 1989.
14. Rivitz SM, Garratt KN: Stenotic anomalous circumflex artery causing myocardial infarction following angioplasty of a right coronary artery stenosis. Cathet Cardiovasc Diagn 17:105, 1989.
15. Kimbiris D, Lo E, Iskandrian A: Percutaneous transluminal coronary angioplasty of anomalous left circumflex coronary artery. Cathet Cardiovasc Diagn 13:407, 1987.
16. Schwartz L, Aldridge HE, Szarga C, Ceplo RM: Percutaneous transluminal angioplasty of an anomalous left circumflex coronary artery arising from the right sinus of Valsalva. Cathet Cardiovas Diagn 8:623, 1982.
17. Topaz O, DiSciascio G, Goudreau E, et al: Coronary angioplasty of anomalous coronary arteries: Notes on technical aspects. Cathet Cardiovasc Diagn 21:106, 1990.
18. Bass TA, Miller AB, Rubin MR, et al: Transluminal angioplasty of anomalous coronary arteries. Am Heart J 112:610, 1986.
19. Das GS, Wysham DG: Double wire technique for additional guiding catheter support in anomalous left circumflex coronary artery angioplasty. Cathet Cardiovasc Diagn 24:102, 1991.
20. Arani DT, Visco JP, Conley JG, Bunnell IL: Effectiveness of

the Arani double-loop guiding catheters in angioplasty of aortocoronary vein grafts. Cathet Cardiovasc Diagn 19:136, 1990.

21. Carr ML: The use of the guiding catheter in coronary angioplasty. The technique of manipulating catheters to obtain the necessary power to cross tight coronary stenoses. Cathet Cardiovasc Diagn 12:189, 1986.

22. Vardhan IN, Aharonian VJ, Gordan S, Mahrer PR: A rare complication of percutaneous transluminal coronary angioplasty—left main disease. Am Heart J 121:902, 1991.

23. Newton CM, Lewis SA, Vetrovec GW: Technique for guiding catheter exchange during coronary angioplasty while maintaining guide wire access across a coronary stenosis. Cathet Cardiovasc Diagn 15:173, 1988.

24. Warren SG, Barnett JC: Guiding catheter exchange during coronary angioplasty. Cathet Cardiovasc Diagn 20:212, 1990.

# 21

# Intravascular Ultrasound Imaging in the Evaluation and Interventional Treatment of Coronary Artery Disease

Gary S. Mintz     Kenneth M. Kent      Augusto D. Pichard      Lowell F. Satler
Jeffrey J. Popma     Martin B. Leon

Intravascular ultrasound (IVUS) imaging provides transmural images of coronary arteries in vivo. The normal coronary arterial wall, the major components of the atherosclerotic plaque, accurate lumen dimensions before and after catheter-based therapy, and the serial changes that occur with the atherosclerotic disease process and during catheter-based therapy and that cause restenosis can be studied in humans in a manner previously not possible.

The first true IVUS system was designed by Bom and associates in Rotterdam in 1971[1]; it was conceived as an improved technique for visualizing cardiac chambers and valves. The first transluminal images of human arteries were recorded by Yock and his associates in 1988.[2] Currently, there are two basic technical approaches to catheter-based ultrasound imaging: solid state and mechanical. With solid-state technology, a cylindric array of transducer elements is mounted on the tip of the catheter. By sequentially firing the multielement array, a beam is created and rotated "electronically" in a 360-degree arc to produce the tomographic image. With mechanical technology, a single-element transducer is located within the tip of a polyethylene imaging catheter or sheath; with the use of a flexible drive shaft, the transducer is then rotated "mechanically" to create the tomographic image. (An alternative approach to mechanical IVUS imaging is to attach the transducer to a micromotor and to position this assembly within the tip of the catheter, thereby eliminating the drive shaft.) There are advantages, disadvantages, and qualitative differences in image presentation with each approach; with commercially available systems, however, image quality, measurement accuracy, and catheter handling are all sufficient to be useful in a routine interventional setting. Because of ongoing product development, any technical discussion is likely to become rapidly outdated.

## INTRAVASCULAR ULTRASOUND IMAGING BASICS AND DEFINITIONS

*Transducers* are devices that convert one type of energy into another; IVUS transducers convert electric energy into ultrasound energy and ultrasound energy back into electric energy. An electric impulse triggers the transducer to emit an ultrasound pulse; afterward, the transducer remains silent to detect reflected (or *backscattered*) ultrasound. Assuming that ultrasound travels through all tissues at a fixed speed, then the time that it takes for the transmitted ultrasound impulse to be backscattered and returned to the transducer is a measure of distance. The intensity of the backscattered signal depends on a number of factors. These include (but are not limited to) (1) the intensity of the transmitted signal, (2) the attenuation of the signal as it passes through tissue (tissue attenuates ultrasound energy), (3) the distance from the transducer to the target (intensity is inversely related to distance), (4) the angle of the signal relative to the target (the closer the angle is to 90 degrees, the more intense is the reflected signal),[3, 4] and (5) the density (or reflectivity) of the tissue (which determines how much ultrasound energy passes through the tissue and how much is backscattered). These factors can affect not only the overall appearance of an image slice, but also the relative appearance of different sectors of the image throughout its 360-degree circumference. The backscattered ultrasound is then reconverted into an electric signal; and the reconverted electric signal is sent to the ultrasound system to generate the planar image. (Because the reconverted electric signal is in the *radiofrequency [RF]* range, IVUS is exquisitely sensitive to ambient RF noise; this can appear as alternating spokes or random white dots within the image.)

*Resolution* is the ability to discriminate two closely adjacent objects. Because IVUS creates images in three-dimensional space, there are three resolutions: (1) axial resolution (the ability to discriminate two closely adjacent objects located along the axis of the ultrasound beam), (2) lateral resolution (the ability to discriminate two closely adjacent objects located along the axis of the ultrasound catheter), and (3) angular or circumferential resolution (the ability to discriminate two closely adjacent objects located along the circumferential sweep of the ultrasound beam as it generates the planar image). Because ultrasound beams diverge, the optimal resolution is in the *near field*, the area closest to the transducer. In general, the higher the frequency, the greater the resolution; and for a given frequency, the larger the size of the transducer aperture, the better the resolution. Focusing the transducer also improves resolution within the focused zone; however, the beam then diverges beyond the focal zone, and resolution suffers.

*Penetration* depends on a number of factors including transducer output (which is in part related to transducer design) and imaging frequency (penetration is inversely related to frequency).

*Dynamic range* is the range of gray scales that can be differentiated. The greater the dynamic range, the broader the range of reflected signals (weakest vs. strongest) that can be detected, displayed, and differentiated.

*Ring down* refers to the image area closest to the face of the transducer (contiguous with the surface of the catheter) where the image appears disorganized and has the appearance of a "halo."

*Nonuniform rotational distortion* (NURD) is an artifact unique to mechanical IVUS imaging systems. For optimal imaging, there must be a constant rotational velocity of the transducer. NURD is the consequence of asymmetric friction along any part of the drive shaft mechanism causing the transducer to whip through part of its 360-degree course, resulting in geometric distortion or smearing of the image. Recognizing NURD is especially important in quantifying information from mechanical IVUS imaging systems.[5] (Because there is no drive shaft, NURD is not seen with micromotor technology.)

Appropriate use of system controls can improve an image, whereas misuse of the available controls can degrade an image. Some of these controls are as follows. Increasing overall *gain* increases overall image brightness. Overall gain that is set too low limits the detection of low-amplitude signals. Over-

all gain that is set too high compresses the gray scale (affecting dynamic range) and causes all tissue to appear echoreflective. The *time-gain-compensation* (TGC) curve amplifies parts of the reflected signal and adjusts the image brightness at fixed distances from the catheter. (The term *time-gain compensation* is derived from the fact that *distance* is measured by the *time* that it takes for the signal to be reflected back to the transducer.) Incorrect setting of the TGC curve can introduce significant artifacts into the images. For example, excessive reduction in near-field intensity (in an attempt to reduce blood speckle or ring down) can also blank out echolucent tissue and artificially produce a lumen; this is especially important in assessing in-stent restenosis because neointimal tissue is often echolucent. *Reject* eliminates low-amplitude signals; it is one way of removing noise from an image. However, by increasing the reject, low-amplitude signals are eliminated, the dynamic range is truncated at its lower level, and echolucent tissue can be missed. *Compression* modifies the gray scale to optimize differentiation between different types of tissue. Some systems also have a number of different gray-scale curves that can be selected.

The approximate *axial* position of the images can be determined from the position of the transducer as seen fluoroscopically. However, the precise location and reproducible identification of individual image slices is optimized by the use of a motorized transducer pullback device that withdraws the transducer at a constant speed, especially when combined with careful attention to vascular and perivascular markings. There is no absolute (anterior vs. posterior, left vs. right) *rotational* orientation of the image. Instead, side branches are useful markers during clinical IVUS imaging, and the image is described as if viewing the face of a clock.

## QUANTITATIVE MEASUREMENTS (Fig. 21–1)

The IVUS image is not identical to a histologic image. As with ultrasound imaging in general, cross-sectional images are created when the ultrasound beam encounters an interface between tissues or structures of different density.

The first "structure" that the IVUS beam sees is the blood-filled lumen. At the operational frequency of commercially available systems, blood has a speckled, low-intensity, and continuously changing pattern that is distinct from that of tissue. The intensity of the blood speckle increases exponentially with (1) the frequency of the transducer and (2) stasis. Saline (or contrast) injection through the guiding catheter is useful in clearing the lumen of blood (even static blood), in differentiating blood

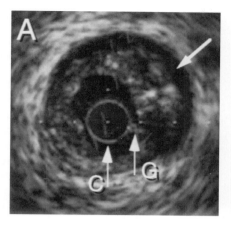
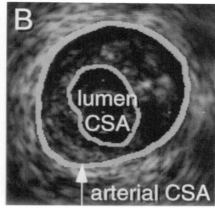
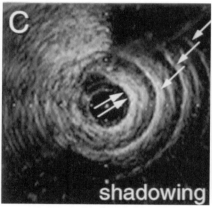
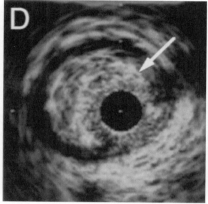
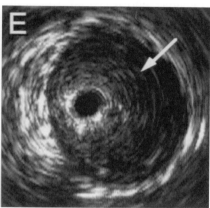

FIGURE 21–1. Basics of image interpretation. *A,* Catheter (C) and guidewire (G) are labeled. The *bold white arrow* indicates the hypoechoic "medial stripe," which is artifactually thick because of the effects of the overlying plaque. *B,* Duplicate of *A* with the media-adventitia and lumen borders outlined in gray; these borders correspond to the measurements of arterial cross-sectional area (CSA) and lumen CSA, respectively. *C,* Example of calcific plaque *(double white arrows)* with reverberations *(single white arrows).* Otherwise, from the 12 o'clock to 8 o'clock positions, there is shadowing. Also notice the faint white sparkles that radiate outward, indicating radiofrequency noise. *D,* Example of echoreflective, noncalcified plaque *(bold arrow).* *E,* Example of echolucent plaque *(bold arrow).* Note that the adventitia is brighter when it is closer to the transducer (7 o'clock to 11 o'clock positions) than when it is farther from the transducer (12 o'clock to 3 o'clock positions).

speckle from tissue, and in defining true lumen borders. Both blood speckle and saline injection are useful for identifying dissection planes.

Although truly normal coronary arteries are rare in the practice of interventional cardiology, only 160 μm of intimal thickening is needed to consistently produce a definitive intimal layer using routine imaging frequencies.[6] (Whether the intimal, medial, and adventitial layers of normal arteries can be distinctly visualized during in vivo IVUS imaging and whether these layers can be measured accurately is the subject of debate.[7, 8]) In normal arteries, the material that most strongly reflects ultrasound is collagen. The reflectivity of collagen is 1000 times that of muscle. The adventitia of coronary arteries has a high collagen content and is echoreflective. Conversely, the media of coronary arteries has a low collagen content, is mostly muscular, and is typically echolucent. Because the ultrasound beam is attenuated as it passes through the overlying plaque, the echolucent zone seen in vivo is almost always

thicker than the true anatomic media. (One indication of a false or "exaggerated" medial thickness is that the media appears to be thicker under a thicker plaque layer than under a thinner plaque layer. Media thickness is less than 200 μm in the absence of atherosclerosis and becomes *thinner* in the presence of severe disease.[9] A study comparing IVUS imaging before and after directional coronary atherectomy showed that cutting into this echolucent zone resulted in media being identified in only 50% of the histologic specimens.[10]) With increasing atherosclerosis, the intima/plaque layer increases in thickness and tends to merge with the internal elastic lamina. The external elastic lamina tends to merge with the adventitia. Because the adventitia and periadventitial structures have similar echoreflectivity, it is not possible to discriminate the adventitia from periadventitial structures.

For these reasons, during clinical IVUS imaging of *nonstented lesions,* there are only two distinct boundaries that have consistent histologic correlates: the lumen-plaque interface and the media-adventitia interface. Thus, there are only two cross-sectional area (CSA) measurements that can be reproducibly performed (arterial CSA and lumen CSA). Because the media cannot be quantified accurately, the cross-sectional measurement of atherosclerotic plaque is usually reported as the plaque-plus-media CSA (calculated as arterial CSA minus lumen CSA). The plaque-plus-media CSA is often divided by the total arterial CSA to generate a measurement called *plaque burden* (which is also sometimes referred to as the *cross-sectional narrowing* or *percentage plaque area* or *cross-sectional area obstruction*).

Because endovascular *stents* are intensely echo-reflective, the metallic prosthesis creates a third IVUS boundary between the lumen and the media-adventitia interface. In stented lesions, the stent CSA can be measured, and the neointimal tissue CSA can be calculated as stent CSA minus lumen CSA. Sometimes, but not always, the media-adventitia border can be seen through stents.

The previously mentioned, cross-sectional IVUS measurements have been validated in vitro (Table 21–1).[11–21] The interobserver variability, intraobserver variability, and reproducibility of these IVUS measurements have been reported by a number of investigators.[21–29] By shadowing deeper arterial structures, significant target lesion calcification can interfere with the measurement of arterial CSA. However, three types of extrapolation/interpolation can be useful. The cross-sectional geometry of the coronary artery is more or less circular; therefore, extrapolation of the circumference of the media-adventitia border is possible provided that each calcific deposit does not shadow more than approximately 60 degrees of the adventitial circumference. Also, real-time axial movement of the transducer just distal and proximal to a calcific deposit (or to find the smallest arc of calcium) may help to unmask and fill in contiguous parts of the adventitia that are otherwise shadowed. The arc of calcium has been shown to vary significantly throughout the length of a lesion.[30] Three-dimensional image reconstruction can identify the media-adventitia border proximal and distal to calcium and therefore allow interpolation.

In addition, motorized transducer pullback through a stationary imaging sheath (as is available with mechanical IVUS systems) permits accurate length measurements. This has been validated in vivo.[31]

## TABLE 21–1. IN VITRO VALIDATION STUDIES OF INTRAVASCULAR ULTRASOUND QUANTIFICATION

| REFERENCE | VESSELS | N | PARAMETER | IVUS | HISTO-MORPHOMETRY | R |
|---|---|---|---|---|---|---|
| Hodgson[11] | Peripheral | | Lumen CSA | | | 0.94 |
| | | | P + M thickness | | | 0.87 |
| Gussenhoven[12] | Peripheral | 11 | Lumen CSA | | | 0.847 |
| | | 577 | Plaque thickness | | | 0.843 |
| Tobis[13] | Mixed | 39 | Lumen CSA | | | 0.88 |
| Mallery[14] | Mixed | 59 | Plaque thickness (mm) | 1.2 ± 0.8 | 0.9 ± 0.8 | 0.91 |
| | | 59 | Media thickness (mm) | 0.5 ± 0.2 | 0.4 ± 0.2 | 0.83 |
| | | 59 | P + M thickness (mm) | 2.4 ± 0.8 | 1.7 ± 0.8 | 0.85 |
| Potkin[15] | Coronary | 54 | EEM CSA (mm²) | 9.43 ± 3.7 | 8.25 ± 3.18 | 0.94 |
| | | 54 | Lumen CSA (mm²) | 2.65 ± 1.19 | 2.86 ± 0.90 | 0.85 |
| | | 216 | P + M thickness (mm) | 0.75 ± 0.38 | 0.61 ± 0.36 | 0.92 |
| Nishimura[16] | Peripheral | 15 | Lumen CSA | | | 0.98 |
| Wenguang[17] | Peripheral | 16 | Lumen CSA | | | 0.977 |
| | | 16 | Plaque CSA | | | 0.968 |
| Yi-qun[18] | Carotid | 17* | Lumen CSA (mm²) | 20.49 ± 5.54 | 19.88 ± 5.73 | 0.96 |
| | | 48† | Lumen CSA (mm²) | 19.56 ± 7.01 | 18.9 ± 6.78 | 0.96 |
| DiMario[19] | Mixed | 112 | Lumen CSA (mm²) | 26.3 ± 21.3 | 21.8 ± 16.6 | 0.96 |
| | | 112 | Plaque area CSA (mm²) | | | 0.87 |
| | | 112 | Media thickness (mm) | | | 0.93 |
| Matar[20] | Coronary | 12 | Lumen volume (mm³) | 166 ± 114 | 162 ± 104 | 0.95 |
| | | 12 | P + M volume (mm³) | 134 ± 95 | 187 ± 129 | 0.96 |
| Von Birgelen[21] | Coronary | 100 | EEM CSA (mm²) | 21.0 ± 4.6‡ | 18.2 ± 3.0 | 0.88 |
| | | 100 | Lumen CSA (mm²) | 13.4 ± 3.6‡ | 10.0 ± 2.4 | 0.94 |
| | | 100 | P + M CSA (mm²) | 7.6 ± 2.0‡ | 8.2 ± 1.9 | 0.80 |
| | | 13 | EEM volume (mm³) | 322.8 ± 92.4‡ | 279.2 ± 71.8 | 0.91 |
| | | 13 | Lumen volume (mm³) | 205.9 ± 70.4‡ | 153.1 ± 46.7 | 0.98 |
| | | 13 | P + M volume (mm³) | 116.8 ± 28.8‡ | 126.1 ± 34.1 | 0.98 |

CSA, cross-sectional area; EEM, external elastic membrane; IVUS, intravascular ultrasound; P + M, plaque plus media.
*Normal carotid arteries.
†Diseased carotid arteries.
‡IVUS measurements performed by automated contour detection; all other IVUS measurements performed by manual border tracing.

Volumetric IVUS calculations can also be performed using Simpson's rule or three-dimensional image reconstruction. Validation has been limited to studies performed using motorized transducer pullback, some of which have even incorporated electrocardiograph-triggered transducer pullback (Table 21–1).

## PLAQUE COMPOSITION

Atherosclerotic lesions are heterogeneous and include varied amounts of calcium, dense fibrous tissue, lipid, smooth muscle cells, and thrombus. In general, although IVUS cannot provide biochemically accurate information regarding plaque composition, IVUS imaging can separate lesions into subtypes according to echodensity (usually using the collagen-rich adventitia as a reference) and the presence or absence of shadowing and reverberations.[12, 15, 16, 32–35] The terminology used to describe specific plaque types is the subject of much debate. Terms that have been used include *calcific, echodense, fibrocalcific, fibrotic, soft, echolucent, fatty,* and *fibrofatty.* Because atherosclerosis is a heterogeneous process, many lesions are mixed, containing more than one plaque type. Regardless of the classification used, it is clear that from the standpoint of therapeutic device response, a calcific, fibrocalcific, or echodense plaque behaves in a much different way than a soft, echolucent, or fibrofatty plaque. True histologic-level plaque composition classification will, perhaps, be possible with IVUS tissue characterization. However, this technology is still experimental.

Calcium (see Fig. 21–1) is a powerful reflector of ultrasound; essentially none of the beam penetrates through or even into the calcium. Thus, calcium casts a shadow over deeper arterial structures, and even calcium thickness cannot be measured. In practice, the signature of calcium is echodense plaque (brighter than the reference adventitia) that shadows; however, dense fibrous tissue without calcium is also echodense and can sometimes cast a shadow. Occasionally, calcium (but not dense fibrous tissue) produces reverberations: one or more equidistantly spaced rings at intervals that are a multiple of the distance from the transducer to the leading edge of the calcium. Detection of lesion-associated calcium by IVUS also depends on the histologic pattern.[36, 37]

Echolucent plaques are less bright compared with the reference adventitia (see Fig. 21–1). Although it has become common to refer to echolucent plaques as "soft" (to differentiate them from echoreflective plaques that are labeled "hard"), it is important to recognize that these plaques are not soft or compli-

ant to the *touch*, but are as firm as "hard" plaques.[38] (Furthermore, the compliance of a lesion—i.e., its response to balloon angioplasty or stent implantation—is dependent on more than just the histologic plaque composition or ultrasound plaque classification. Factors include the patient's age, compliance of the adventitia and periadventitial structures, and the size of the vessel.[39]) Echolucent plaques contain varied amounts of fibrous and fatty tissue. Pure fat is much more echolucent than muscle. A lipid pool, therefore, should appear as a dark or echolucent zone within a lesion; however, in practice, identifying lipid pools (and therefore plaques prone to rupture) in vivo is beyond the limits of current technology. Neointimal hyperplasia within restenotic stents is usually echolucent, especially within the first 6 months after stent implantation.

The identification of thrombus is one of the most difficult aspects of IVUS imaging.[40, 41] Clues to the presence of thrombus include the following: (1) a sparkling "scintillating" appearance, (2) a lobulated mass projection into the lumen, (3) a distinct interface between the suspected thrombus and underlying plaque, (4) identification of blood speckle within the thrombus indicating microchannels through the thrombus, and (5) mobility. It is important to emphasize that although the routine IVUS diagnosis of thrombus in native coronary arteries is difficult, the diagnosis of thrombus in saphenous vein grafts (where degenerated tissue can have many of these same features) is, frankly, unreliable.

## DISCREPANCIES BETWEEN INTRAVASCULAR ULTRASOUND IMAGING AND ANGIOGRAPHY

Although angiography has been the "gold standard" for evaluating coronary artery disease and for guiding catheter-based interventions, it has the following limitations. Atherosclerosis is a disease of the arterial wall; angiography studies the arterial lumen. Coronary arteries are complex three-dimensional structures with branch points, tortuous segments, and bends; angiography is a shadowgraphic technique that visualizes the lumen in multiple projected longitudinal planes. Atherosclerosis is a diffuse process; angiography assesses coronary artery disease by comparing "diseased" segments to supposedly "normal" segments.

## Atherosclerosis in Angiographic Reference Segments

IVUS imaging routinely shows significant atherosclerosis in angiographically "normal" reference segments. In a study of 884 native vessel target lesions and their angiographically "normal" reference segments, only 6.8% of the reference segments were normal and the average plaque burden of the most normal looking reference segment image slice was $51 \pm 13\%$.[42] The independent predictors of the reference segment plaque burden were diabetes mellitus, male gender, advanced patient age, and hypercholesterolemia. The explanation for angiographic "silent" atherosclerosis accumulation is as follows. Adaptive remodeling of the wall of diseased arterial segments (increase in arterial CSA) occurs to compensate for the accumulation of atherosclerotic plaque in direct relationship to the CSA of the accumulated plaque. On average, lumen compromise is delayed until the atherosclerotic lesion occupies more than an estimated 40% to 50% of the potential area within the internal elastic lamina (40% to 50% plaque burden).[43, 44] This compensatory mechanism has been noted in primates with diet-induced atherosclerosis[45] and in human coronary arteries, where it has been seen pathologically[43, 44] and in vivo with high-frequency epicardial echocardiography[46] as well as by IVUS.[41, 42, 47–55]

## Reference Segment Measurements

IVUS imaging routinely measures reference segment dimensions that are different from those of angiography. The IVUS measurements can be used to safely upsize devices. Although IVUS measurement of reference dimensions are usually larger than angiographic measurements, in individual patients this is very variable.

One approach was used in CLOUT (CLinical Outcomes Ultrasound Trial).[52] After percutaneous transluminal coronary angioplasty (PTCA) using conventional (angiographic) balloon sizing, the proximal and distal reference segment *midwall* dimensions (the average of the maximal and minimal arterial and lumen diameters) were measured. Then the smaller of these two measurements was used to select the size of the next PTCA balloon. This permitted upsizing from a nominal balloon size of $2.98 \pm 0.35$ mm to $3.45 \pm 0.40$ mm (a balloon-to-artery ratio of $1.12 \pm 0.15$ to $1.30 \pm 0.17$), resulting in an increase in final IVUS minimal lumen CSA ($3.16 \pm 1.04$ mm$^2$ to $4.56 \pm 1.14$ mm$^2$) and a reduction in angiographic diameter stenosis from $28\% \pm 15\%$ to $18\% \pm 14\%$. There was no increase in complications. Before intervention, the distal reference is typically underperfused (and therefore is artificially small; therefore, this approach to reference segment measurements must be performed after "some" intervention).

Alternatively, we have compared proximal reference lumen dimensions with quantitative angiography (Fig. 21–2). The proximal reference was defined as the most normal looking cross section (largest lumen with the smallest plaque burden) within 10 mm proximal to the lesion but distal to any major size branch; the IVUS reference lumen dimension was measured as the maximal lumen diameter seen in this reference segment image slice. When this

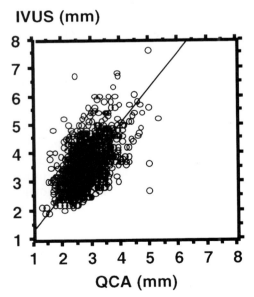

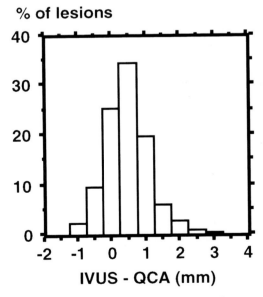

FIGURE 21–2. Comparison of intravascular ultrasound (IVUS) and angiographic measurement of reference lumen dimensions. *A,* Graph showing only a fair correlation between the two measurements ($r = 0.59$). *B,* Distribution of the difference between the two measurements. Although the IVUS reference lumen dimension is most often 0.5 mm larger than the angiographic measurement, there is an important range of differences. Twenty-five percent of the time, the measurements are similar, and 10% of the time (usually in the setting of significant calcium), the IVUS reference lumen dimension is actually smaller than by angiography. QCA, quantitative coronary angiography.

criterion was used, the IVUS reference was 0.45 $\pm$ 0.64 mm larger than the angiographic reference (ratio = 1.16 $\pm$ 0.22), similar to that found in CLOUT.

## Target Lesion Calcium

With the use of IVUS, calcium can be localized to the lesion compared with the reference segment, characterized as superficial (closer to the tissue-lumen interface) compared with deep (closer to the media-adventitia junction), and quantified according to its arc and length.[30, 56]

IVUS routinely detects target lesion calcification that is angiographically "silent." In a study of 1155 native vessel target lesions, IVUS detected calcium in 73%.[56] The mean arc of target lesion calcium measured 115 $\pm$ 110 degrees with a mean arc of superficial calcium of 85 $\pm$ 108 degrees. When present, target lesion calcium was only superficial in 48%, only deep in 28%, and both superficial and deep in 24%. Coronary angiography detected target lesion calcium in 38% ($p < 0.0001$ compared with IVUS), and coronary angiography detected superficial calcium more often than deep calcium ($p < 0.0001$). The sensitivity of angiography was 25% in lesions with one-quadrant calcium, approximately 50% in lesions with two-quadrant calcium, 60% in lesions with three-quadrant calcium, and 85% in lesions with four-quadrant calcium. The overall specificity of angiography was 89% with a false-positive rate of 11%. However, the specificity was 98% for angiographic "severe" lesion calcium (Table 21–2). The presence and classification of angiographic calcium (mild, moderate, or severe) depended on an increasing arc of the target lesion calcium, an increasing arc of the superficial calcium, and the length of the reference segment calcium.

In another study of native vessel lesions in 183 patients, Tuzcu and associates reported that IVUS detected calcium in 138 (75%), whereas angiography detected calcium in 63 (34%).[57] In patients with angiographically visible calcium, the IVUS arc of calcium was greater than in patients without angiographically visible calcium (175 $\pm$ 85 degrees vs. 108 $\pm$ 71 degrees, $p = 0.0001$). In patients without angiographic calcium at the lesion site, IVUS detected calcium in 69%; the only predictor of lesion-associated calcium in these patients was angiographic calcium *elsewhere* in the coronary tree.

Coronary lesion calcium does not correlate with lumen compromise but instead appears to be a marker for plaque burden.[58]

## Eccentricity

IVUS measurement of maximal and minimal plaque-plus-media thicknesses can be used to calculate an eccentricity index. Few lesions are truly concentric (eccentricity index = 1), and although almost all lesions show some degree of eccentric plaque distribution, there is no consensus about the exact IVUS definition of an eccentric plaque. In a large series of 1446 native vessel lesions, the angiographic classification of lesions as eccentric versus concentric was not related to plaque distribution (as measured by the IVUS eccentricity index; Fig. 21–3).[59] Furthermore, when similar criteria (three times as much plaque on one side of the lesion as on the other; e.g., an IVUS eccentricity index of 3) were used, the concordance rate between IVUS and angiography was only 53.8% ($\kappa = 0.086$). The angiographic classification of a lesion as concentric or eccentric was primarily determined by the lesion length (as well as by the absolute measurement of maximal and minimal plaque-plus-media thick-

**TABLE 21–2.   RELATIONSHIP OF ANGIOGRAPHIC CALCIFICATION TO PATTERNS OF IVUS TARGET LESION AND REFERENCE SEGMENT CALCIUM**

| | ANGIOGRAPHIC CALCIUM | | | |
| --- | --- | --- | --- | --- |
| | NONE/MILD* (N = 715) | MODERATE* (N = 306) | SEVERE* (N = 134) | p |
| IVUS calcium | | | | |
| Number of target lesions with calcium (%) | 436 (61%) | 274 (90%) | 141 (98%) | <0.0001 |
| Arc of calcium (degrees) | 71 $\pm$ 83 | 165 $\pm$ 106 | 238 $\pm$ 104 | <0.0001 |
| Length of calcium (mm) | 2.5 $\pm$ 3.2 | 4.5 $\pm$ 3.5 | 6.2 $\pm$ 4.7 | <0.0001 |
| Number with superficial calcium (%) | 261 (37%) | 219 (72%) | 123 (92%) | <0.0001 |
| Arc of superficial calcium (degrees) | 44 $\pm$ 74 | 124 $\pm$ 110 | 215 $\pm$ 119 | <0.0001 |
| Length of superficial calcium (mm) | 1.5 $\pm$ 2.6 | 3.2 $\pm$ 3.1 | 5.7 $\pm$ 5.0 | <0.0001 |
| Reference arc of calcium (degrees) | 25 $\pm$ 63 | 61 $\pm$ 93 | 87 $\pm$ 98 | <0.0001 |
| Length of reference calcium (mm) | 1.0 $\pm$ 2.6 | 2.6 $\pm$ 4.8 | 3.3 $\pm$ 4.1 | <0.0001 |
| Total length of calcium (mm) | 3.6 $\pm$ 4.4 | 7.2 $\pm$ 6.4 | 9.7 $\pm$ 6.4 | <0.0001 |

*Calcification was identified angiographically as readily apparent radiopacities within the vascular wall at the site of the stenosis and was classified as none/mild, moderate (radiopacities only noted during the cardiac cycle before contrast injection), and severe (radiopacities noted without cardiac motion before contrast injection generally compromising both sides of the arterial lumen).

IVUS, intravascular ultrasound.

## # of lesions

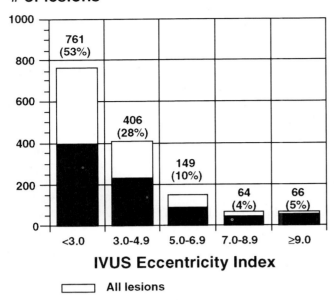

FIGURE 21–3. Using IVUS imaging, lesion eccentricity can be measured as the maximal divided by the minimal plaque-plus-media thickness. This graph was derived from a study of 1446 native vessel lesions. The number (and percentage of lesions) within each range of indices is shown. Angiography classified as eccentric 53% of lesions with an eccentricity index less than 3, 55% of lesions with an eccentricity index of 3 to 4.9, 58% of lesions with an eccentricity index 5 to 6.9, 58% of lesions with an eccentricity index of 7 to 8.9, and 77% of lesions with an eccentricity index of 9.

nesses, but not by their ratio). Angiographic classification requires a visual interpolation of the course of the normal coronary artery and its lumen; interpolation is more difficult in longer lesions and in those with more atherosclerotic plaque.

IVUS studies have also related plaque distribution to side branches and bifurcations. These studies have shown that regardless of the angiographic appearance, plaque is deposited preferentially opposite the major branch. For example, Kimura and colleagues studied lesions located in the very proximal left anterior descending artery and found that these lesions are located opposite the circumflex artery, spare the flow divider, and maintain eccentricity across a wide range of vessel stenoses.[60]

## Lumen Dimensions

Several studies have compared IVUS imaging and quantitative coronary angiography in the measurement of lesion site lumen dimensions before and after intervention. Before intervention, the correlation between the IVUS and angiographic lumen diameters ranged from 0.77 to 0.98.[61–64] However, after PTCA, the correlation fell to 0.28 to 0.42.[65–66] Nakamura and coworkers have indicated that after PTCA,

the discrepancy is greater in the presence of deep vessel injury (N = 39, $r = 0.05$, $p = 0.74$) than in the presence of superficial lesion injury (N = 37, $r = 0.67$, $p = 0.001$).[67]

We compared the measurement of minimal lumen diameters by both IVUS imaging and quantitative coronary angiography in over 2000 patients both before intervention (including IVUS studies performed for diagnostic purposes) (Fig. 21–4) and after intervention (Fig. 21–5). With the exception of stents, the correlation coefficients by device were as follows: post-PTCA, 0.49; after directional coronary atherectomy (DCA), $r = 0.38$; post-DCA plus adjunct PTCA, $r = 0.31$; after rotational atherectomy (RA), $r = 0.21$; post-RA plus adjunct PTCA, $r = 0.55$; after excimer laser coronary angioplasty (ELCA), $r = 0.19$; and post-ELCA plus adjunct PTCA, $r = 0.55$.

## ATHEROGENESIS AND LESION FORMATION

The conventional concept of the development and progression of a focal coronary artery stenosis in "stable" coronary artery disease is that there is a balance between plaque accumulation and adaptive remodeling until plaque accumulation outstrips the ability of the artery to compensate. Several IVUS studies suggest that there is a spectrum in the magnitude of arterial remodeling and that in some lesions inadequate remodeling or perhaps arterial

## IVUS MLD (mm)

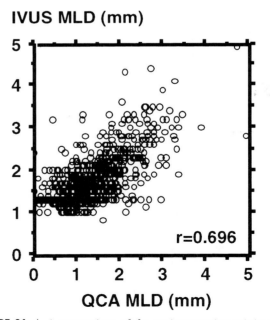

FIGURE 21–4. A comparison of the preintervention minimal lumen diameter (MLD) measured by IVUS imaging and quantitative coronary angiography (N = 1206). The IVUS measurements are truncated at approximately 1 mm because IVUS cannot measure lumen dimensions smaller than the imaging catheter.

# All nonstented lesions

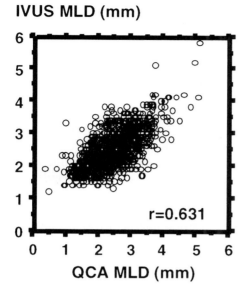

# Stented lesions

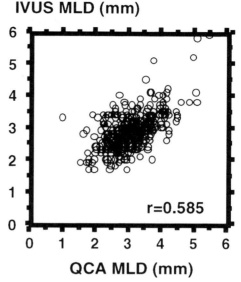

FIGURE 21–5. A comparison of the postintervention MLDs measured by IVUS imaging and quantitative coronary angiography in 1547 nonstented lesions *(A)* and in 616 lesions after Palmaz-Schatz stent placement plus adjunct high-pressure (16 atm) percutaneous transluminal coronary angioplasty *(B)*.

shrinkage may contribute to the development of focal stenoses.[68] Pasterkamp and associates showed that in the majority of diseased femoral arteries, significant arterial remodeling could not be demonstrated; instead, arterial shrinkage accelerated the luminal narrowing caused by plaque accumulation.[69, 70] Nishioka and colleagues studied 35 primary lesions and showed that 54% had compensatory enlargement (lesion arterial CSA greater than that of the proximal reference CSA), 26% had inadequate compensatory remodeling (lesion arterial CSA less than that of the distal reference CSA), and 20% had intermediate compensatory enlargement (lesion arterial CSA intermediate between the proximal and distal reference CSAs).[71] We have found that arterial remodeling appears to be normally distributed. In a study of 603 primary lesions, 15% had inadequate arterial remodeling, a lesion site arterial CSA of 0.78 of the proximal reference arterial CSA (the upper limits of normal arterial tapering[72]).[73] The only predictor of inadequate arterial remodeling was a lesion site arc of superficial calcium, suggesting that "inadequate arterial remodeling" may represent a late response, that is, late arterial shrinkage. Furthermore, a 1997 analysis of primary lesions from our laboratory suggests that insulin use may blunt the adaptive remodeling response to plaque accumulation in diabetic patients; thus, small vessels in diabetic patients may be the result of inadequate remodeling rather than excessive atherosclerotic plaque accumulation.[74]

Although arterial remodeling and its relationship

to lesion formation in native vessels appears to be well established, the existence of remodeling in saphenous vein grafts is the subject of controversy.[75–78]

## MECHANISMS, RESULTS, AND COMPLICATIONS OF CATHETER-BASED INTERVENTIONS

All catheter-based interventions increase acute lumen dimensions by one of the following mechanisms: vessel expansion, plaque dissection, plaque embolization, plaque redistribution, and plaque ablation/removal. When in-stent restenosis is treated, two additional mechanisms can be invoked: neointimal tissue extrusion out of the stent and additional stent expansion. By comparing IVUS images before and after intervention, the mechanisms and results of catheter-based interventions can be delineated.

## Percutaneous Transluminal Coronary Angioplasty

Plaque compression was the mechanism of balloon angioplasty originally proposed by both Dotter and Judkins[79] and Gruentzig[80]; an analogy was drawn to "footprints in the snow." However, IVUS studies have indicated that balloon angioplasty increases lumen dimensions primarily by vessel expansion and plaque dissection.[13, 66, 81–85] Some of these IVUS studies (all performed using single-slice analysis) seemed to confirm the presence of plaque compression because quantitative cross-sectional IVUS analysis after PTCA consistently showed a decrease in the plaque CSA compared with before intervention. Instead, more recent studies have suggested that apparent plaque compression was, in reality, plaque redistribution along the axis of the lesion, analogous to "footprints in the sand."[86] Plaque has liquid and solid elements, and liquids and solids are not compressible. A special case is that of PTCA in the setting of thrombus (acute myocardial infarction, postinfarction angina, unstable angina, and so forth). Thrombus embolization may contribute to the increase in acute lumen dimensions during PTCA of acute myocardial infarction[87]; thrombus embolization can also masquerade as plaque compression on planar or volumetric IVUS analysis.

The most vulnerable sites for plaque dissection are the junctions of focal differences in lesion distensibility (which function as planes of cleavage): the transition from plaque to normal vessel and the junction of calcified and noncalcified plaque elements. In vitro modeling and clinical IVUS studies have indicated that localized calcium deposits, in particular, increase the vulnerability to dissection.[88–91] Typically, a tear is seen to start immediately adjacent to a localized calcium deposit and then extend into the lumen. However, because dissections are one of the mechanisms of successful PTCA, the presence of dissection by IVUS should not automatically be viewed as a complication. Detecting dissections can be enhanced by visualizing blood speckle or microbubbles from injected saline or contrast material in the false lumen. Other unusual complications after PTCA, such as deep wall hematomas, can be detected by IVUS.

Several studies have shown that with the routine use of IVUS-guided balloon sizing, acute results during balloon angioplasty procedures can be optimized,[92] especially in an era of routine "bail-out" stent availability.[93, 94]

## Directional Coronary Atherectomy

Most IVUS studies have indicated that tissue removal accounts for over 75% of the improvement in lumen dimensions after stand-alone DCA.[20, 95] The addition of adjunct PTCA reduces the relative contribution of tissue removal and increases the contribution of vessel expansion to overall lumen improvement.[96, 97] Dissections, especially superficial dissections, are common.[98] Regardless of the mechanism, the amount of plaque removed during DCA (compared with the preintervention plaque mass) is low.[96]

The most important factors affecting delivery of the DCA device are the size, tortuosity, and compliance of the vessel. The most consistent factor affect-

ing vessel compliance is calcium, which magnifies the limits imposed by all other unfavorable lesion and vessel characteristics. Calcium also affects the ability of DCA to cut and remove tissue. One study has indicated that the IVUS arc of target lesion calcium (even angiographically invisible calcium) is the single most powerful predictor of the success of DCA regardless of the end point measured.[99] Other studies have focused on the limitations imposed by superficial calcium (more than deep calcium) and the fact that the diameter of the arc of deep calcium can be used to estimate the CSA of the achievable lumen.[95] Interestingly, pretreatment with rotational atherectomy can alter even a heavily calcified lesion to make it susceptible to tissue removal with the DCA device.[100]

Other lesion characteristics important for optimal performance of the DCA procedure include lesion eccentricity, plaque thickness, and lesion length. For example, plaque thickness defines the margin of safety for performing DCA. IVUS imaging can also be used to exclude potentially unsafe lesions: extensive or spiral dissections outside the confines of the original lesions, dissections in areas of minimal plaque, or guide wires that are in false lumens.

In order to perform IVUS-guided DCA, the first step is to correlate the IVUS with the angiographic images, particularly the relationship of the maximal and minimal plaque thicknesses to major side branches.[101] These side branches can then be used to orient the DCA device toward the maximal plaque thickness and away from the minimal plaque thickness (or, more importantly, away from normal vessel wall in a highly eccentric lesion). In the absence of nearby major side branches, DCA troughs can be used to direct the device.[102] For example, after an initial IVUS run, a single cut can be made with the DCA catheter while carefully noting its fluoroscopic orientation. A repeat IVUS run can be used to locate this single trough, the orientation of the maximal and minimal plaque thicknesses can be noted in relationship to it, and the rest of the DCA cuts can then be directed appropriately. IVUS imaging is also useful in determining whether the target end points (lumen dimension and plaque burden) have been achieved, identifying complications of DCA such as dissection or perforation, and selecting adjunct device use.

The residual plaque burden depends on the aggressiveness of the atherectomy performed; it was 58% in OARS (Optimal Atherectomy Restenosis Study),[96] but 46% in ABACAS (Adjunct Balloon Angioplasty Coronary Atherectomy Study).[97] The integration of IVUS imaging into the DCA device (to perform truly guided DCA) has the theoretic promise of optimizing tissue retrieval and minimizing the residual plaque burden.[103] The residual plaque burden after DCA probably predicts restenosis.[104, 105]

## Rotational Atherectomy

There have been few systematic studies of RA using IVUS imaging, and the ideal IVUS end points after RA are not known. RA effectively ablates calcified atherosclerotic plaque. Stand-alone RA increases lumen dimensions almost exclusively by atheroablation; however, the plaque burden after stand-alone RA is large. Adjunct PTCA increases the lumen almost exclusively by vessel expansion and plaque dissection. Like primary PTCA, dissections typically occur at the junction of calcified and noncalcified plaque.[106] Although initial studies suggested that atheroablation was limited in noncalcified (vs. calcified) plaque,[107] volumetric IVUS analysis indicates that this device is equally effective in the absence of calcium.[108] The final burr/artery ratio measured by IVUS is variable and depends primarily on changes in vascular tone that are greater in noncalcified vessels.[107, 108]

The impact of different strategies for RA device use is being tested in the STRATAS (Study To determine Rotablator And Transluminal Angioplasty Strategy) trial. Preliminary IVUS observations suggest that when a conventional strategy (burr/artery ratio = 0.7 plus adjunct PTCA at 4 to 6 atm) is compared with a "stepped-burr" strategy (burr/artery ratio = 0.8 with or without adjunct PTCA at 1 atm), the latter approach ablates more plaque with fewer dissections (although final lumen dimensions are similar).[109]

The measured arc of calcium has been shown to decrease after RA; however, this decrease is modest.[105] Full-thickness calcium removal is necessary to decrease the arc measured by IVUS, and in heavily calcified plaques, full-thickness calcium removal is unusual.

## Excimer Laser Coronary Angioplasty

Only one report has studied the mechanism of lumen enlargement after ELCA.[110] After primary ELCA, lumen enlargement was found to result from a combination of tissue ablation and vessel expansion with a large residual plaque burden. The lumen CSA was often larger than the CSA of the laser catheter. However, these findings were extremely variable; in some lesions, lumen improvement was entirely due to tissue ablation, whereas in others it was entirely due to vessel expansion. There was no detectable change in calcium. Dissections into superficial calcium had an appearance that was unique to ELCA, consisting of a fragmented or shattered appearance with newly created sharp-edged gaps in a previously solid deposit of superficial cal-

cium. The nonatheroablative (expansion/dissection) IVUS findings after primary ELCA were attributed to laser-induced shock waves and forced expansion of vapor bubbles into tissue.[111–113] As with other devices, adjunct PTCA improved lumen dimensions by a combination of dissection (at the junction of calcified and noncalcified plaque) and vessel expansion.

## Stents

Most IVUS reports have studied tubular slotted stents, primarily for fear of accordioning the first-generation coiled stents. Even with tubular slotted stents, few IVUS studies have attempted to evaluate the mechanism of lumen improvement during stent implantation. One study has indicated that lumen improvement is the result of axial plaque redistribution during stenting.[114] This is similar to what has been observed during PTCA.[86]

There are two potential reasons to advocate routine use of IVUS guidance during stent implantation procedures: avoiding subacute thrombosis and reducing restenosis. Seminal observations by Colombo and his colleagues showed that when conventional stent implantation techniques were used, stents were typically underexpanded, asymmetric, and not fully apposed to the vessel wall.[115] These findings were linked to the occurrence of subacute thrombosis and led to the routine use of aggressive high-pressure adjunct PTCA with IVUS guidance. As a result of IVUS-guided high-pressure adjunct PTCA, lumen CSA increased by an average of 33% to 50%,[116, 117] and subacute thrombosis (with just antiplatelet therapy) became rare.[116, 118]

Since then, the need for routine IVUS use during stent implantation procedures has become a matter of intense debate. A number of studies have shown that with routine high-pressure PTCA, subacute thrombosis is rare even without IVUS guidance, especially if ticlopidine is used after stent implantation.[119–121] However, a 1997 report from the retrospective POST (Prediction of Stent Thrombosis) registry indicates that if subacute thrombosis occurs, there is almost always a reason detectable on IVUS and infrequently a reason detectable on angiography.[122]

Will IVUS guidance decrease restenosis after stenting? Acute tissue prolapse can be angiographically silent and contribute to restenosis.[24] Two concurrent observational studies—both using high-pressure adjunct PTCA, one using IVUS guidance, and one not using IVUS guidance—have reported similarly low restenosis rates (approximately 7%).[123, 124] Nevertheless, numerous studies continue to show that even with routine high-pressure adjunct PTCA, minimal lumen CSA can be further increased with

IVUS guidance in tubular-slotted[125, 126] and, more recently, coiled stents.[127, 128] Three ongoing multicenter studies comparing IVUS-guided versus angiographic-guided stenting are studying this question: AVID (Angiography Versus Intravascular ultrasound-Directed stent placement); OPTICUS (OPTImization with iCUS to reduce stent restenosis); CRUISE (Can Routine Ultrasound Impact Stent Expansion), the IVUS substudy of STARS (Stent Anticoagulation Regimen Study). However, the target end point of aggressive adjunct PTCA stent expansion in these studies is a final lumen CSA that is a percentage (either 80% or 90%) of the final reference lumen CSA. Conversely, two 1997 studies have suggested that stent restenosis is best predicted by the absolute final lumen CSA[129, 130]: the larger the final lumen CSA, the lower the restenosis rate. The impact of IVUS on restenosis may depend on the end points chosen. However, the limits to what can be achieved routinely, practically, and safely (even with IVUS guidance) and the influence of small vessels on these limits are unknown.

Finally, several 1997 reports have suggested that there may be a downside to routine (and automatic) high-pressure adjunct PTCA.[131–135] These reports suggest that although high-pressure adjunct PTCA may be necessary to achieve optimal stent implantation, in some patients it may induce excessive vessel trauma, tissue proliferation both within and surrounding stents, and restenosis. However, not all investigators agree with these findings.[136, 137] The potential negative impact of high-pressure adjunct PTCA may depend on the disease or lesion substrate, whether or not optimal stent expansion has been achieved, and the exact definition of aggressive high-pressure adjunct balloon angioplasty.

## Treatment of In-Stent Restenosis

IVUS studies before and after PTCA of in-stent restenosis showed that tissue extrusion out of the stent contributed 44% to lumen enlargement, and additional stent expansion (even in stents initially implanted using high-pressure adjunctive PTCA) contributed 56%.[138] In that study, (1) PTCA achieved only 85% of the minimal lumen CSA of the original stent implantation procedure, (2) after PTCA, there was significant residual neointimal tissue within the stent (averaging 32% of the stent CSA), and (3) the residual stenosis was relatively high. These IVUS findings have been confirmed by two reports.[139, 140] In-stent dissections may occur because the junction of neointimal tissue and stent metal is an effective plane of cleavage.

More recently, atheroablative techniques have been used (typically followed by adjunct PTCA) in an attempt to improve the acute and long-term results of PTCA for in-stent restenosis.[141–144] Both ELCA and RA increase lumen dimensions through ablation of neointimal tissue (although tissue ablation with RA appears to be greater, in part related to the larger burr sizes available). Adjunct PTCA is needed with both ELCA and RA to optimize final lumen dimensions. Like primary PTCA of in-stent restenosis, (1) the increase in lumen dimensions during adjunct PTCA is a combination of tissue extrusion out of the stent and additional stent expansion, (2) final lumen dimensions do not recover the lumen dimensions achieved during the initial stent implantation procedure, and (3) in-stent dissections can be observed.

## RESTENOSIS

The major contributions of IVUS to the understanding of restenosis have been (1) identifying remodeling (the change in arterial CSA) as a mechanism of restenosis in nonstented lesions, (2) identifying the residual plaque burden as a predictor of restenosis in nonstented lesions, and (3) identifying neointimal hyperplasia (and eliminating chronic stent recoil) as the mechanism of in-stent restenosis.[23, 24, 28, 104, 145]

Certain methodologic issues must be addressed in using IVUS to study restenosis, particularly using planar (single-slice) analysis. (1) The same anatomic slice must be compared on serial studies. If image slices with different axial locations are compared, then the restenosis process cannot be separated from the axial variation in arterial, lumen, and plaque CSA. The axial locations of the image slice with the smallest preintervention, postintervention, and follow-up lumen CSAs are almost always different.[146] (2) The same anatomic slice must be identified on serial studies. This is facilitated by both a standardized image acquisition protocol and by using a motorized transducer pullback device. (3) The axial location of the image slice selected for analysis should be at the smallest follow-up lumen CSA because this is the location of the restenosis process.

In our initial study, the decrease in lumen CSA in nonstented lesions was due more to a decrease in arterial CSA than to an increase in plaque-plus-media CSA.[23] The change in lumen CSA correlated more strongly with the change in arterial CSA ($r = 0.75$, $p < 0.0001$) than with the change in plaque-plus-media CSA ($r = 0.28$, $p < 0.0001$). Restenotic lesions had a greater decrease in arterial CSA ($p < 0.0001$) and lumen CSA ($p < 0.0001$) than nonrestenotic lesions, but only a trend toward a greater increase in plaque-plus-media CSA ($p = 0.0784$). Twenty-two percent of the lesions showed adaptive arterial remodeling (a late *increase* in arterial CSA);

this resulted in a decreased incidence of restenosis and an increased incidence of late lumen gain *despite* a greater increase in plaque-plus-media CSA, analogous to compensatory adaptive arterial remodeling early in the atherosclerotic disease process. These findings have been confirmed in OARS[146] and in the SURE (Serial Ultrasound REstenosis) trial.[28] (The one exception is in diabetic patients; remodeling appears to be similar to that of nondiabetics, but tissue growth, the increase in plaque-plus-media CSA, is exaggerated.[146, 147]) In the SURE trial,[148] patients were treated with PTCA and DCA and studied before and immediately after intervention; 24 hours after intervention; after 1 month of follow-up; and after 6 months of follow-up. There was little change in arterial CSA within the first 24 hours after intervention, an increase in arterial CSA between 24 hours and 1 month, and a decrease in arterial CSA between 1 and 6 months. Thus, the decrease in arterial CSA resulting in restenosis was shown to be a late event, distinct from early passive elastic recoil. Independent volumetric analysis has confirmed these findings. Throughout the duration of the SURE trial, the change in lumen CSA correlated more with the change in arterial CSA ($r = 0.79$) than with the change in plaque-plus- media CSA ($r = 0.18$).

Two studies have shown that the most powerful predictor of restenosis in nonstented lesions (more powerful than clinical or angiographic variables) is the residual plaque burden.[104, 105] It has been suggested that the residual plaque burden acts as an amplifier of the remodeling process.[149] Comparison of the residual plaque burdens (in relationship to the restenosis rates) in the CAVEAT (Coronary Angioplasty Versus Excision Atherectomy Trial), GUIDE (Guidance by Ultrasound Imaging for Decision Endpoints), OARS, and ABACAS studies should further substantiate this finding. The plaque burden (calculated as plaque plus media divided by arterial CSA) is decreased by tissue removal/ablation, but also during PTCA through a combination of axial plaque redistribution and arterial expansion.

Conversely, serial IVUS studies have shown that stents almost never chronically recoil (although they may acutely recoil).[24, 145] In an analysis of stented lesions, the decrease in lumen correlated more strongly with the increase in neointimal tissue than with the change in stent dimensions; this was true whether cross-sectional IVUS analysis was used ($r = 0.98$ vs. $r = 0.20$) or whether volumetric IVUS analysis was used ($r = 0.99$ vs. $r = 0.03$).[24] There was no predilection for tissue accumulation within any one segment of the stent except in the middle, perhaps related to the central articulation.[24] In-stent neointimal tissue proliferation was exaggerated in

diabetic patients.[147] In addition, there appeared to be an increase in persistent tissue that roughly paralleled the in-stent process.[25] Studies reported in 1997 suggest that in stented lesions, the final lumen CSA is the most important IVUS predictor of subsequent restenosis.[129, 130] In addition, the plaque burden at the edge of the stent may be a predictor of stent-margin restenosis.[150] Exaggerated stent-edge plaque burden may occur as the result of plaque extrusion out of the ends of the stents during stent implantation.[114] IVUS assessment (especially volumetric analysis) of in-stent neointimal tissue proliferation may be the most sensitive assay of strategies to reduce in-stent restenosis.[151]

## CLINICAL UTILITY

In general, current imaging catheters fit well into the interventional environment. All IVUS catheters track over 0.014-inch coronary guide wires; some also track over 0.018-inch guide wires. In general, all 8-French guiding catheters will accommodate all IVUS catheter designs. Some large-lumen 7-French guiding catheters can be used as well. Current "solid state" catheters (but no "mechanical" devices) fit inside some 6-French guiding catheters. It is inadvisable to force a mechanical catheter with a rotating transducer into a small guiding catheter; this will introduce excessive NURD and could cause catheter failure.

Imaging should be performed only after the administration of intracoronary nitroglycerin (to minimize catheter-induced spasm) and only after adequate heparinization. Anticoagulation during interventional procedures is usually dictated by the intervention. During diagnostic imaging, we typically administer 5000 to 7500 U of heparin intravenously; when the activated clotting time (ACT) is checked at the end of the diagnostic study, it is usually less than 150 seconds, allowing removal of the sheaths and same-day patient discharge if clinically advisable.

Routine clinical IVUS imaging begins with a careful understanding of coronary angiogram so that the IVUS imaging run can be related to the angiographic anatomy. The imaging run should include careful examination of the vessel: the distal reference, the lesion site, and the proximal reference back to the aorto-ostial junction. It is important to cross the lesion, ideally by at least 10 mm. One common pitfall is that there may be so much plaque in the reference segment proximal to the lesion that the operators may not be aware that they have not crossed the lesion. With current IVUS catheters, pre-intervention imaging can be performed routinely in more than 90% of studies. The major limitations to preintervention imaging are vessel tortuousity (hampering delivery of the imaging catheter) and lesion calcification (impeding crossing of the lesion). Lesion severity does not appear to be a limitation as long as the lesion is not too rigid (usually indicating calcification).

Before intervention, IVUS is useful in assessing the severity of the lesion (lumen compromise and plaque burden), the length of the lesion, the size of the reference vessel, the plaque burden of the reference segment, the composition of the plaque (especially calcium), the eccentricity of the lesion, and unusual morphology (aneurysms, ulcers, dissections, and so forth).[152] Of particular interest is the assessment of angiographically ambiguous, unusual, or intermediate lesions. Common sites for ambiguous or intermediate lesions include vessels with significant tortuousity, kinking, or bending; ostial (especially aorto-ostial) locations; segments of diffuse disease; and bifurcations or trifurcations. Many

"intermediate" or difficult-to-assess lesions are readily shown to contain either insignificant or severe disease. Aneurysms can be differentiated from pseudoaneurysms or ulcerated plaques. Filling defects can occasionally be shown to be calcific "nodules," not thrombi.

Before intervention, IVUS is also useful in assessing restenotic stents to determine whether the stent was implanted correctly (whether it covered the lesion and was full expanded) and whether the restenosis process is within the stent or proximal or distal to the stent. It is also useful in assessing restenosis within intensely radiopaque tantalum stents that are difficult to assess angiographically. Before the atheroablative treatment of in-stent restenosis, IVUS can be used to determine the largest atheroablative device that can be used safely (based on the interstrut stent distance).

During intervention, IVUS is useful in understanding and managing complications, after crossing

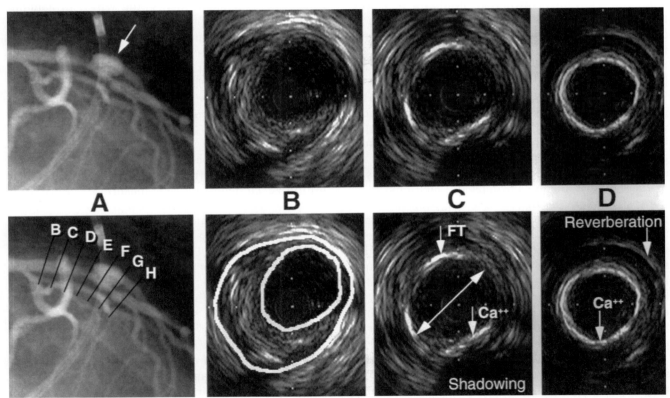

FIGURE 21–6. Example of how IVUS imaging can be used to understand complex coronary anatomy to strategize catheter-based treatment. *A,* An 86-year-old woman was referred for intervention with this de novo lesion in the left anterior descending coronary artery (angiogram, *white arrow*). There was no angiographic calcium. By quantitative coronary angiography, the reference lumen dimensions measured 2.84 mm (with a minimal lumen diameter of 0.76 mm). The angiogram is duplicated to show the location of the IVUS image slices. Although the imaging run was performed from distal to proximal, the images are discussed from proximal (B) to distal (H). The image slices are 3 mm apart, axially, as measured by motorized transducer pullback. B is just distal to the origin of the anterior descending artery; despite being angiographically "normal," the plaque burden measures 65% (the arterial CSA, as outlined by the *outer white line,* measures 18.8 mm²; the lumen CSA, as outlined by the *inner white line,* measures 6.5 mm²; the plaque-plus-media CSA calculates to be 12.3 mm²). *C,* Proximal reference: the most normal looking image slice proximal to the lesion, but distal to any side branches. It contains mixed plaque (note the calcium [Ca⁺⁺] with shadowing and both echolucent and echoreflective [FT, fibrous tissue] plaque elements). The maximal lumen dimension in this reference image slice measures 3.6 mm (*double-headed white arrow*) despite an angiographic reference measurement of 2.84 mm. *D* is at the proximal shoulder of the lesion; it shows circumferential calcium with reverberations.

a total occlusion to determine whether the guide wire is in the true or false lumen, and in evaluating the adequacy of stent placement, especially in adequately covering aorto-ostial lesions.

After intervention, IVUS is useful in determining whether the targeted end points have been reached: if the residual plaque burden (e.g., during DCA procedures) or the final stent or lumen dimensions (e.g., during stent procedures) have been achieved.

An example illustrating the many practical uses of IVUS during a single intervention is shown in Figures 21–6 (before intervention) and 21–7 (after intervention).

## PRACTICAL CONSIDERATIONS

### General

The major resistance to the routine use of IVUS is limited information linking IVUS to improved patient outcomes, procedural costs, physician education (both how to interpret the images and how to use the information), equipment complexity, and difficulties in integrating IVUS into a busy catheterization laboratory. IVUS will be used routinely only if it is quick to set up, is easy to perform, and does not slow down the flow of the clinical cases. Each catheterization laboratory is organized differently. Even tasks performed by the same types of health care professionals vary from laboratory to laboratory. It is possible to integrate clinical IVUS imaging into a busy laboratory, maintain image acquisition standards, and not add significant time to the overall procedure (i.e., more than 5 minutes for an average of three runs: before intervention, at some time during the procedure, and after intervention).

In general, the integration of IVUS will be most successful if it is under the administrative structure of the cardiac catheterization laboratory, not the noninvasive imaging laboratory. The temperament of the two environments is very different; interventional procedures cannot be put "on hold" waiting for equipment or personnel; and the individuals involved in IVUS imaging must have an understanding of interventional procedures.

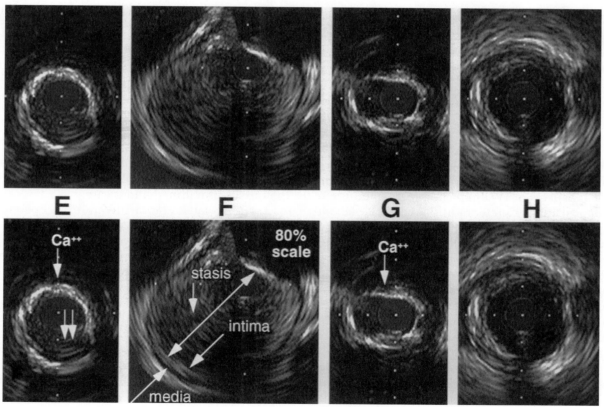

FIGURE 21–6 *Continued. E,* Stenosis just proximal to the aneurysm; it shows circumferential calcium with a small amount of overlying echolucent plaque *(double white arrows). F* is through the aneurysm; it is displayed at an 80% scale relative to the other image slices. Note that the intima, media, and adventitia are intact; therefore, this is a true aneurysm. The "lumen" dimension within the aneurysm *(double-headed white arrows)* measures 6.1 mm. There is evidence of stasis within the aneurysm but nothing to suggest thrombi. *G,* The stenosis just distal to the aneurysm; it shows nearly circumferential calcium. *H* is the distal reference: the most normal-looking image slice distal to the lesion, just proximal to the branch (at the 3 o'clock position). The distance from the proximal to the distal reference *(C to H)* was 15 mm. The therapeutic approach was rotational atherectomy across the aneurysm with a 2 burr (because of the extensive circumferential calcium) followed by placement of a single Palmaz-Schatz stent (the inter-reference distance measured 15 mm) and after dilation with a 3.5-mm balloon to 16 atm (because of the proximal reference lumen measurement). The postintervention angiogram and IVUS study are shown in Figure 21–7.

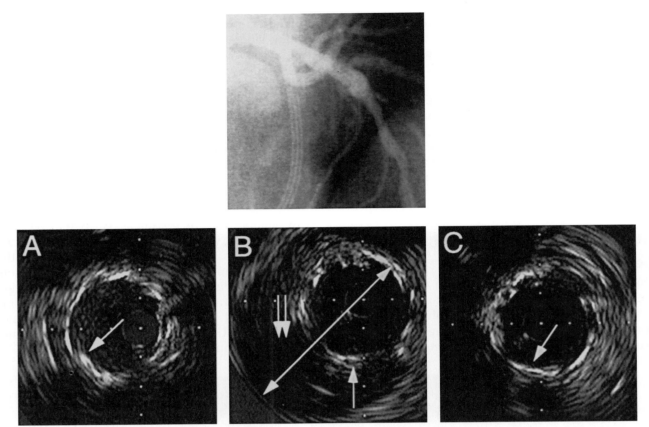

FIGURE 21–7. These are the postintervention angiogram and IVUS study corresponding to Figure 21–6. The IVUS images are proximal to the aneurysm *(A)*, through the aneurysm *(B)*, and distal to the aneurysm *(C)*. The stent is symmetrically expanded throughout *(single white arrows* in all three panels). At the site of the aneurysm, there is lack of apposition *(double white arrows)*. Because it would have taken a 6-mm balloon to fully appose the stent to the aneurysm *(double-headed white arrow)*, no further intervention was performed.

Even in a busy laboratory with constant IVUS use, it is difficult to train all laboratory personnel. Many practical aspects of IVUS imaging (e.g., handling of videotapes) are foreign to traditional catheter laboratory practices. IVUS imaging is facilitated by designating specific IVUS technologists who become responsible for all practical aspects of IVUS imaging: (1) equipment and catheter setup, (2) image optimization, (3) proper recording of IVUS imaging runs, (4) accurate voice and onscreen alphanumeric documentation, (5) patient and procedure logs, (6) equipment maintenance, and so forth. With time, technologists can be trained to interpret images accurately, to provide the iterative feedback necessary for IVUS-based decision making, and to answer questions posed by the primary operators. Measurements should be made off-line (from videotape after the imaging run is complete), not when the catheter is in the vessel; this saves procedure time and minimizes patient ischemia.

The angiographic (e.g., "road map") monitors can be "wired" to display the IVUS images. Angiographic monitors offer superior resolution, are convenient and readily visible to the operator, and allow the IVUS machine to be placed in a position away from the patient table and out of the way of the nurses providing patient care.

In a busy laboratory with multiple operators, it is important to standardize image acquisition and analysis. The use of a motorized transducer pullback device aids (in fact, enforces) discipline and acquisition standards; there is no question whether the transducer is being advanced or withdrawn. (We prefer a pullback speed of 0.5 mm/second. By trial and error, we have found that this is the fastest rate at which the trained eye can assimilate the information. However, with very focal stenoses, especially ostial stenoses, a pullback speed of 0.25 mm/second is preferable. Conversely, we never use a speed of 1 mm/second for fear of missing important information. Motorized transducer pullback also *does not preclude* additional, careful manually controlled interrogation of the lesion.) Standardization of image acquisition facilitates off-line image analysis and comparison of serial (before vs. after intervention or post-intervention vs. follow-up) studies; it is *essential* for multicenter studies.

Accurate procedure information is critical. Even

when verbal commentary is recorded, it is helpful if on-line procedural information is annotated onto the ultrasound system's video screen. The ideal on-screen labeling should contain three elements: (1) the timing of IVUS imaging (e.g., preintervention), (2) the procedure being performed, and (3) the target vessel and location. All IVUS instruments have internal clocks, and the time is automatically recorded onto the videotape. It is helpful to note the "time" that corresponds to the center of the lesion. In the absence of systematic preintervention imaging, voice annotation or recording the "time" corresponding to the lesion may be the only way to identify the target lesion on subsequent review. After some procedures (e.g., DCA with a good result), it may be difficult to identify the target lesion without this information.

Good-quality videotapes are essential. It is recommended that virgin (never-used) broadcast-quality s-VHS tapes be used. There is a quality difference, and the cost differential is minimal. Videotapes should be stored in a secure place. Although they are not expensive, tapes become irresistible targets for petty thieves because they can be used in home or studio videocassette recorders. Backup copies of each tape can be made by hooking two VCRs together; both VCRs should be medical-grade s-VHS units with s-Video turned on. If there is voice annotation information, then the audio circuit must be linked as well. The first-generation copy loses some image quality but is usually acceptable. The second-generation copy (copy of a copy) loses too much image information to be useful. Videotape storage can become unwieldy if each patient has his or her own tape. In general, 20 studies can be recorded on each 120-minute tape. Individual tapes (for each patient) should be reserved for multicenter studies in which the videotape must be sent away to a core laboratory.

Many catheter laboratories have excessive ambient electric or RF noise, which can produce artifacts on the ultrasound image. Offenders include monitoring equipment and intra-aortic balloon pumps. Eliminating these problems requires troubleshooting and working with both the IVUS and non-IVUS equipment vendors. The Doppler FloWire can cause two types of interference. One is electric, but the other is crosstalk between the two signals. Ultrasonic crosstalk is present whenever two sources of ultrasonic signals are used simultaneously. In addition, in some hospitals the paging system generates an RF signal that momentarily "blanks out" the IVUS image. Inexpensive custom filters solve this problem.

## Safety

There have been three large studies of the safety of IVUS. Other than transient spasm, complications appear to be rare. Our experience has been similar to these reports.

Hausmann and associates reported on 2207 patients from 28 centers (including 915 patients studied for diagnostic purposes).[153] There were no complications in 2034 patients (92.2%). In 87 patients (3.9%), complications were judged to be not related to IVUS. In 63 patients (2.9%), transient spasm occurred during imaging. In 9 patients (0.4%), complications were judged to have a "certain" relationship to IVUS (five acute occlusions, two dissections, one embolism, one thrombus). In 14 patients (0.6%), complications were judged to have an "uncertain" relationship to IVUS (five acute occlusions, three dissections, one arrhythmia). Major events (acute myocardial infarction or emergency coronary artery bypass graft [CABG]) occurred in 3 of 9 and 5 of 14 of these patients, respectively. The complication rate was higher in patients with unstable angina or acute myocardial infarction and in patients undergoing intervention.

Batkoff and Linker reported on 718 IVUS "examinations" performed at 12 centers.[154] There were eight events (1.1%) but no adverse clinical consequences; all occurred in patients with unstable angina undergoing PTCA. There were four cases of transient vessel spasm, two cases of dissection, and two cases of wire entrapment.

Gorge and colleagues reported 7085 IVUS studies from 51 centers.[155] Spasm occurred in 3% of all studies. Major complications (dissection, thrombosis, ventricular fibrillation, refractory spasm) occurred in 10 (0.14%). There was only one major event.

## REFERENCES

1. Bom N, Lancee CT, van Egmond FC: An ultrasonic intracardiac scanner. Ultrasonics 10:71–76, 1972.
2. Yock PG, Johnson EL, Linker DT: Intravascular ultrasound: Development and clinical potential. Am J Card Imaging 2:185–193, 1988.
3. Picano E, Landini L, Distante A, et al: Angle dependence of ultrasonic backscatter in arterial tissues: A study in vitro. Circulation 72:572–576, 1985.
4. DiMario C, Madretsma S, Linker D, et al: The angle of incidence of the ultrasonic beam: A critical factor for the image quality in intravascular ultrasonography. Am Heart J 125:442–448, 1993.
5. Kimura BJ, Bhargava V, Palinski W, et al: Distortion of intravascular ultrasound images because of nonuniform angular velocity of mechanical-type transducers. Am Heart J 132:328–336, 1996.
6. Fitzgerald PJ, St. Goar FG, Connolly AJ, et al: Intravascular ultrasound imaging of coronary arteries. Is three layers the norm? Circulation 86:154–158, 1992.
7. Maheswaran B, Leung CY, Gutfinger DE, et al: Intravascular ultrasound appearance of normal and mildly diseased coronary arteries: Correlation with histologic specimens. Am Heart J 130:976–986, 1995.
8. Porter TR, Radio SJ, Anderson JA, et al: Composition of coronary atherosclerotic plaque in the intima and media affects intravascular ultrasound measurements of media thickness. J Am Coll Cardiol 23:1079–1084, 1994.

9. Isner JM, Donaldson RF, Fortin AH, et al: Attenuation of the media of coronary arteries in advanced atherosclerosis. Am J Cardiol 58:937–939, 1986.

10. Takagi A, Sumiyoshi T, Kawaguchi M, et al: Cutting into the sonolucent zone after coronary atherectomy: Correlation between intravascular ultrasound images and histological findings [Abstract]. J Am Coll Cardiol 27:199A, 1996.

11. Hodgson JMcB, Eberle M, Savakus A: Validation of a new real time percutaneous intravascular ultrasound imaging catheter [Abstract]. Circulation 78:II-21, 1988.

12. Gussenhoven EJ, Essed CE, Lancee CT, et al: Arterial wall characteristics determined by intravascular ultrasound imaging: An in vitro study. J Am Coll Cardiol 14:947–952, 1989.

13. Tobis JM, Mallery JA, Gessert J, et al: Intravascular ultrasound cross-sectional arterial imaging before and after balloon angioplasty in vitro. Circulation 80:873–882, 1989.

14. Mallery JA, Tobis JM, Griffith J, et al: Assessment of normal and atherosclerotic arterial wall thickness with an intravascular ultrasound imaging catheter. Am Heart J 119:1392–1400, 1990.

15. Potkin BN, Bartorelli AL, Gessert JM, et al: Coronary artery imaging with intravascular high-frequency ultrasound. Circulation 81:1575–1585, 1990.

16. Nishimura RA, Edwards WD, Warnes CA, et al: Intravascular ultrasound imaging: In vitro validation and pathologic correlation. J Am Coll Cardiol 16:145–154, 1990.

17. Wenguang L, Gussenhoven WJ, Zhong Y, et al: Validation of quantitative analysis of intravascular ultrasound images. In J Card Imaging 6:247–253, 1991.

18. Yi-qun Y, Fang-ling L, Jun T, et al: Assessment of autopsic samples of carotid atherosclerosis in the aged by intravascular ultrasound. Chin Med J 107:750–754, 1994.

19. DiMario C, The SH, Madretsma S, et al: Detection and characterization of vascular lesions by intravascular ultrasound: An in vitro study correlated with histology. J Am Soc Echocardiogr 5:135–146, 1992.

20. Matar FA, Mintz GS, Farb A, et al: The contribution of tissue removal to lumen improvement after directional coronary atherectomy. Am J Cardiol 74:647–650, 1994.

21. Von Birgelen C, van der Lugt A, Nicosia A, et al: Computerized assessment of coronary lumen and atherosclerotic plaque dimensions in three-dimensional intravascular ultrasound correlated with histomorphometry. Am J Cardiol 78:1202–1209, 1996.

22. Hodgson JMcB, Graham SP, Sarakus AD, et al: Clinical percutaneous imaging of coronary anatomy using an over-the-wire ultrasound catheter system. Int J Card Imaging 4:186–193, 1989.

23. Mintz GS, Popma JJ, Pichard AD, et al: Arterial remodeling after coronary angioplasty. A serial intervascular ultrasound study. Circulation 94:35–43, 1996.

24. Hoffmann R, Mintz GS, Dussaillant GR, et al: Patterns and mechanisms of in-stent restenosis: A serial intravascular ultrasound study. Circulation 94:1247–1254, 1996.

25. Hoffmann R, Mintz GS, Popma JJ, et al: Chronic arterial responses to stent implantation: A serial intravascular ultrasound analysis of Palmaz-Schatz stents in native coronary arteries. J Am Coll Cardiol 28:1134–1139, 1996.

26. Mintz GS, Griffin J, Chuang YC, et al: The reproducibility of the intravascular ultrasound assessment of stent implantation in saphenous vein grafts. Am J Cardiol 75:1267–1270, 1995.

27. Hausmann D, Lundkvist AS, Friedrich GU, et al: Intracoronary ultrasound imaging: Intraobserver and interobserver variability of morphometric measurements. Am Heart J 128:674–680, 1994.

28. Kimura T, Kaburagi S, Tamura T, et al: Remodeling responses of human coronary arteries undergoing coronary angioplasty. Circulation 96:475–483, 1997.

29. Blessing E, Hausmann D, Sturm M, et al: Intravascular ultrasound guidance of stent implantation: Intra- and interobserver variability [Abstract]. Circulation 94:I-200, 1996.

30. Mintz GS, Douek P, Pichard AD, et al: Target lesion calcification in coronary artery disease: An intravascular ultrasound study. J Am Coll Cardiol 20:1149–1155, 1992.

31. Fuessl RT, Mintz GS, Pichard AD, et al: In vivo validation of intravascular ultrasound length measurements using a motorized transducer pullback device. Am J Cardiol 77:1115–1118, 1996.

32. Kimura BJ, Bhargava V, De Maria AN: Value and limitations of intravascular ultrasound imaging in characterizing coronary atherosclerotic plaque. Am Heart J 130:386–396, 1995.

33. Hodgson JMcB, Reddy KG, Suneja R, et al: Intracoronary ultrasound imaging: Correlation of plaque morphology with angiography, clinical syndrome and procedural results in patients undergoing coronary angioplasty. J Am Coll Cardiol 21:35–44, 1993.

34. Tobis JM, Mallery J, Mahon D, et al: Intravascular ultrasound imaging of human coronary arteries in vivo. Analysis of tissue characterizations with comparison to in vitro histological specimens. Circulation 83:913–926, 1991.

35. Gussenhoven EJ, Essed CE, Frietman P, et al: Intravascular echographic assessment of vessel wall characteristics: A correlation with histology. Int J Card Imaging 4:105–116, 1989.

36. Friedrich GJ, Moes NY, Muhlberger VA, et al: Detection of intralesional calcium by intracoronary ultrasound depends on the histologic pattern. Am Heart J 128:434–441, 1994.

37. Gutfinger DE, Leung CY, Hiro T, et al: In vitro atherosclerotic plaque and calcium quantitation by intravascular ultrasound and electron-beam computed tomography. Am Heart J 131:899–906, 1996.

38. Hiro T, Leung CY, de Guzman S, et al: Are "soft echoes" really soft?: Ultrasound assessment of mechanical properties in human atherosclerotic tissue [Abstract]. Circulation 92:I-649, 1995.

39. Kok WE, Peters RJ, Prins MH, et al: Contribution of age and intimal lesion morphology to coronary artery wall mechanics in coronary artery disease. Clin Sci (Colch) 89:239–246, 1995.

40. Chemarin-Alibelli MJ, Pieraggi MT, Elbaz M, et al: Identification of coronary thrombus after myocardial infarction by intracoronary ultrasound compared with histology of tissues sampled by atherectomy. Am J Cardiol 77:344–349, 1996.

41. Frimerman A, Miller HI, Hallman M, et al: Intravascular ultrasound characterization of thrombi of different composition. Am J Cardiol 73:1053–1057, 1994.

42. Mintz GS, Painter JA, Pichard AD, et al: Atherosclerosis in angiographically "normal" coronary artery reference segments: An intravascular ultrasound study with clinical correlations. J Am Coll Cardiol 25:1479–1485, 1995.

43. Glagov S, Weisenberg E, Zarins CK, et al: Compensatory enlargement of human atherosclerotic coronary arteries. N Engl J Med 316:1371–1375, 1987.

44. Stiel GM, Stiel LSG, Schofer J, et al: Impact of compensatory enlargement of atherosclerotic coronary arteries on angiographic assessment of coronary heart disease. Circulation 80:1603–1609, 1989.

45. Armstrong ML, Heistad DD, Marcus ML, et al: Structural and hemodynamic responses of peripheral arteries of macaque monkeys to atherogenic diet. Arteriosclerosis 5:336–346, 1985.

46. McPherson DD, Sirna SJ, Hiratzka LF, et al: Coronary arterial remodeling studied by high-frequency epicardial echocardiography: An early compensatory mechanism in patients with obstructive coronary atherosclerosis. J Am Coll Cardiol 17:79–86, 1991.

47. Alfonso F, Macaya C, Goicolea J, et al: Intravascular ultrasound imaging of angiographically normal coronary segments in patients with coronary artery disease. Am Heart J 127:536–544, 1994.

48. Ge J, Erbel R, Zamorano J, et al: Coronary artery remodeling in atherosclerotic disease: An intravascular ultrasound study. Coron Artery Dis 4:981–986, 1993.

49. St. Goar FG, Pinto FJ, Alderman EL, et al: Intravascular ultrasound imaging of angiographically normal coronary arteries: An in vivo comparison with quantitative coronary angiography. J Am Coll Cardiol 18:952–958, 1991.

50. St. Goar FG, Pinto FJ, Alderman EL, et al: Detection of

coronary atherosclerosis in young adult hearts using intravascular ultrasound. Circulation 86:756–763, 1992.

51. Hausmann D, Johnson JA, Sudhir K, et al: Angiographically silent atherosclerosis detected by intravascular ultrasound in patients with familial hypercholesterolemia and familial combined hyperlipidemia: Correlation with high density lipoproteins. J Am Coll Cardiol 27:1562–1570, 1996.

52. Stone GW, Hodgson JMcB, St. Goar FG, et al: Improved procedural results of coronary angioplasty with intravascular ultrasound guided balloon sizing; The CLOUT Trial. Circulation 95:2044–2052, 1997.

53. Hermiller JB, Tenaglia AN, Kisslo KB, et al: In vivo validation of compensatory enlargement of atherosclerotic coronary arteries. Am J Cardiol 71:665–668, 1993.

54. Losordo DW, Rosenfield K, Kaufman J, et al: Focal compensatory enlargement of human arteries in response to progressive atherosclerosis: In vivo documentation using intravascular ultrasound. Circulation 89:2570–2577, 1994.

55. Tuzcu EM, Hobbs RE, Rincon G, et al: Occult and frequent transmission of atherosclerotic coronary disease with cardiac transplantation: Insights from intravascular ultrasound. Circulation 91:1706–1713, 1995.

56. Mintz GS, Popma JJ, Pichard AD, et al: Patterns of calcification in coronary artery disease. A statistical analysis of intravascular ultrasound and coronary angiography in 1155 lesions. Circulation 91:1959–1965, 1995.

57. Tuzcu EM, Berkalp B, De Franco AC, et al: The dilemma of diagnosing coronary calcification: Angiography versus intravascular ultrasound. J Am Coll Cardiol 27:832–838, 1996.

58. Mintz GS, Pichard AD, Popma JJ, et al: Determinants and correlates of target lesion calcium in coronary artery disease: A clinical, angiographic, and intravascular ultrasound study. J Am Coll Cardiol 29:268–274, 1997.

59. Mintz GS, Popma JJ, Pichard AD, et al: Limitation of angiography in the assessment of plaque distribution in coronary artery disease. A systematic study of target lesion eccentricity in 1446 lesions. Circulation 93:924–931, 1996.

60. Kimura BJ, Russo RJ, Bhargava V, et al: Atheroma morphology and distribution in proximal left anterior descending coronary artery: In vivo observations. J Am Coll Cardiol 27:825–831, 1996.

61. Davidson CJ, Sheikh KH, Harrison JK, et al: Intravascular ultrasonography versus digital subtraction angiography: A human in vivo comparison of vessel size and morphology. J Am Coll Cardiol 16:633–636, 1990.

62. Nissen SE, Grines CL, Gurley JC, et al: Application of a new phased-array ultrasound imaging catheter in the assessment of vascular dimensions. In vivo comparison to cineangiography. Circulation 81:660–666, 1990.

63. Nissen SE, Gurley JC, Grines CL, et al: Intravascular ultrasound assessment of lumen size and wall morphology in normal subjects and patients with coronary artery disease. Circulation 84:1087–1099, 1991.

64. De Scheerder I, De Man F, Herregods MC, et al: Intravascular ultrasound versus angiography for measurement of luminal diameters in normal and diseased coronary arteries. Am Heart J 127:243–251, 1994.

65. Tobis JM, Mahon DJ, Honye J, McRae M: Intravascular ultrasound imaging following balloon angioplasty. Int J Card Imaging 6:191–205, 1991.

66. Davidson CJ, Sheikh KH, Kisslo KB, et al: Intracoronary ultrasound evaluation of interventional technologies. Am J Cardiol 68:1305–1309, 1991.

67. Nakamura S, Mahon DJ, Maheswaran B, et al: An explanation for discrepancy between angiographic and intravascular ultrasound measurements after percutaneous transluminal coronary angioplasty. J Am Coll Cardiol 25:633–639, 1995.

68. Wong CB, Porter TR, Xie F, Deligonul U: Segmental analysis of coronary arteries with equivalent plaque burden by intravascular ultrasound in patients with and without angiographically significant coronary artery disease. Am J Cardiol 76:598–601, 1995.

69. Pasterkamp G, Borst C, Post MJ, et al: Atherosclerotic arterial remodeling in the superficial femoral artery. Individual variation in local compensatory enlargement response. Circulation 93:1818–1825, 1996.

70. Pasterkamp G, Wensing PJW, Post MJ, et al: Paradoxical arterial wall shrinkage may contribute to luminal narrowing of human atherosclerotic femoral arteries. Circulation 91:1444–1449, 1995.

71. Nishioka T, Luo H, Eigler NL, et al: Contribution of inadequate compensatory enlargement to development of human coronary artery stenosis: An in vivo intravascular ultrasound study. J Am Coll Cardiol 27:1571–1576, 1996.

72. Javier SP, Mintz GS, Popma JJ, et al: Intravascular ultrasound assessment of the magnitude and mechanism of coronary artery and lumen tapering. Am J Cardiol 75:177–180, 1995.

73. Mintz GS, Kent KM, Pichard AD, et al: The contribution of inadequate arterial remodeling to the development of focal coronary artery stenoses: An intravascular ultrasound study. Circulation 95:1791–1798, 1997.

74. Kornowski R, Mintz GS, Lansky AJ, et al: Insulin dependence blunts the adaptive remodeling response to plaque accumulation in diabetes mellitus: An intravascular ultrasound study [Abstract]. J Am Coll Cardiol 29:365A, 1997.

75. Mintz GS, Popma JJ, Pichard AD, et al: The dimorphic pathology of vein graft lesions effects acute procedural and late angiographic outcomes [Abstract]. J Am Coll Cardiol 25:79A, 1995.

76. Mendelsohn FO, Foster GP, Palacios I, et al: In vivo assessment by intravascular ultrasound of enlargement in saphenous vein bypass grafts. Am J Cardiol 76:1066–1069, 1995.

77. Ge J, Gorge G, Haude M, et al: Doesn't diseased human coronary saphenous vein bypass grafts undergo compensatory enlargement? An intravascular ultrasound study [Abstract]. J Am Coll Cardiol 29:178A, 1997.

78. Nishioka T, Luo H, Berglund H, et al: Absence of focal compensatory enlargement of constriction in diseased human coronary saphenous vein bypass grafts. Circulation 93:683–690, 1996.

79. Dotter CT, Judkins MP: Transluminal treatment of arteriosclerotic obstruction: Description of new technique and a preliminary report of its application. Circulation 30:654–670, 1964.

80. Gruntzig A: Transluminal dilatation of coronary artery stenosis. Lancet 1:263–266, 1978.

81. Potkin BN, Keren G, Mintz GS, et al: Arterial responses to balloon coronary angioplasty: An intravascular ultrasound study. J Am Coll Cardiol 20:942–951, 1992.

82. Tenaglia AN, Buller CE, Kisslo KB, et al: Mechanisms of balloon angioplasty and directional coronary atherectomy as assessed by intracoronary ultrasound. J Am Coll Cardiol 20:685–691, 1992.

83. Braden GA, Herrington DM, Downes TR, et al: Qualitative and quantitative contrasts in the mechanisms of lumen enlargement by coronary balloon angioplasty and directional coronary atherectomy. J Am Coll Cardiol 23:40–48, 1994.

84. Suneja R, Nair RN, Reddy KG, et al: Mechanisms of angiographically successful directional coronary atherectomy: Evaluation by intracoronary ultrasound and comparison with transluminal coronary angioplasty. Am Heart J 126:507–514, 1993.

85. Honye J, Mahon DJ, Jain A, et al: Morphological effects of coronary balloon angioplasty in vivo assessed by intravascular ultrasound imaging. Circulation 85:1012–1025, 1992.

86. Mintz GS, Pichard AD, Kent KM, et al: Axial plaque redistribution as a mechanism of percutaneous transluminal coronary angioplasty. Am J Cardiol 77:427–430, 1996.

87. Boksch WG, Schartl M, Beckmann SH, et al: Intravascular ultrasound imaging in patients with acute myocardial infarction: Comparison with chronic angina pectoris. Coron Artery Dis 5:727–735, 1994.

88. Lee RT, Richardson G, Loree HM, et al: Prediction of mechanical properties of human atherosclerotic tissue by high-frequency ultrasound imaging. An in vitro study. Arterioscler Thromb Vasc Biol 12:1–5, 1992.

89. Lee RT, Loree HM, Cheng GC, et al: Computational structural analysis based on intravascular ultrasound imaging

before in vitro angioplasty: Prediction of plaque fractures. J Am Coll Cardiol 21:777–782, 1993.

90. Fitzgerald PJ, Ports TA, Yock PG: Contribution of localized calcium deposits to dissection after angioplasty. An observational study using intravascular ultrasound. Circulation 86:64–70, 1992.

91. Tenaglia AN, Buller CE, Kisslo KB, et al: Intracoronary ultrasound predictors of adverse outcomes after coronary artery interventions. J Am Coll Cardiol 20:1385–1390, 1992.

92. Abizaid A, Pichard AD, Mintz GS, et al: Acute and long term results of an IVUS-guided/provisional stent implantation strategy. Am J Cardiol 84:1381–1384, 1999.

93. Abizaid A, Mehran R, Pichard AD, et al: Results of high pressure ultrasound-guided "over-sized" balloon PTCA to achieve "stent-like" results [Abstract]. J Am Coll Cardiol 29:280A, 1997.

94. Hodgson JMcB, Muller C, Roskamm H, et al: Ultrasound (ICUS)-guided PTCA and stenting improves acute angiographic results: Acute analysis of the Strategy of IVUS-guided PTCA and Stenting (SIPS) trial [Abstract]. J Am Coll Cardiol 29:96A, 1997.

95. Umans VA, Baptista J, DiMario C, et al: Angiographic, ultrasonic, and angioscopic assessment of the coronary artery wall and lumen area configuration after directional atherectomy: The mechanism revisited. Am Heart J 130:217–227, 1996.

96. Baim DS, Simonton CA, Popma JJ, et al: Mechanism of luminal enlargement by optimal atherectomy: IVUS insights from the OARS Study [Abstract]. J Am Coll Cardiol 27:291A, 1996.

97. Hosokawa H, Kato O, Tamai H, et al: Role of adjunct balloon angioplasty following coronary atherectomy: A serial intravascular ultrasound analysis from the ABACAS Trial [Abstract]. J Am Coll Cardiol 29:281A, 1997.

98. Popma JJ, Mintz GS, Satler LF, et al: Clinical and angiographic outcome after directional coronary atherectomy: A qualitative and quantitative analysis using coronary arteriography and intravascular ultrasound. Am J Cardiol 72:55E–64E, 1993.

99. Matar FA, Mintz GS, Pinnow E, et al: Multivariate predictors of intravascular ultrasound endpoints after directional coronary atherectomy. J Am Coll Cardiol 25:318–324, 1995.

100. Dussaillant GD, Mintz GS, Pichard AD, et al: Mechanisms and acute and long term results of adjunctive directional atherectomy after rotational atherectomy. J Am Coll Cardiol 27:1390–1397, 1996.

101. Yock PG, Fitzgerald PJ, Linker DT, et al: Intravascular ultrasound guidance for catheter-based coronary interventions. J Am Coll Cardiol 17:39B–45B, 1991.

102. Bauman R, Yock PG, Fitzgerald PJ, et al: "Reference cut" method of intracoronary ultrasound guided directional coronary atherectomy: Initial and six months results [Abstract]. Circulation 92:I-546, 1995.

103. Yock PG, Yock CA, Fitzgerald PJ: Ultrasound-guided atherectomy: The vision for the future? Coron Artery Dis 7:299–303, 1996.

104. Mintz GS, Popma JJ, Pichard AD, et al: Intravascular ultrasound predictors of restenosis following percutaneous transcatheter coronary revascularization. J Am Coll Cardiol 27:1678–1687, 1996.

105. The GUIDE Trial Investigators: IVUS-determined predictors of restenosis in PTCA and DCA: Final report from the GUIDE Trial, Phase II [Abstract]. J Am Coll Cardiol 27:156A, 1994.

106. Kovach JA, Mintz GS, Pichard AD, et al: Sequential intravascular ultrasound characterization of the mechanisms of rotational atherectomy and adjunct balloon angioplasty. J Am Coll Cardiol 22:1024–1032, 1993.

107. Fitzgerald PJ, Stertzer SH, Hidalgo BO, et al: Plaque characteristics affect lesion and vessel response to coronary rotational atherectomy: An intravascular ultrasound study. J Am Coll Cardiol 23:353A, 1994.

108. Dussaillant GR, Mintz GS, Pichard AD, et al: Effect of rotational atherectomy in noncalcified atherosclerotic plaque:

A volumetric intravascular ultrasound study. J Am Coll Cardiol 28:856–860, 1996.

109. Feldman T, Bersin RM, Levin TN, et al: IVUS results of the STRATAS Trial: Vessel dimensions after "conventional" vs "stepped burr" rotational atherectomy [Abstract]. Circulation 94:I-317, 1996.

110. Mintz GS, Kovach JA, Javier SP, et al: Mechanisms of lumen enlargement after excimer laser coronary angioplasty: An intravascular ultrasound study. Circulation 92:3408–3414, 1995.

111. Isner JM, Rosenfield K, Losordo DW: Excimer laser atherectomy (the greening of Sisyphus). Circulation 81:2018–2020, 1990.

112. Van Leeuwen TG, van Erven L, Meertens JH, et al: Origin of arterial wall dissections induced by pulsed excimer and mid-infrared laser ablation in the pig. J Am Coll Cardiol 19:1610–1618, 1992.

113. Van Leeuwen TG, Meertens JH, Velema E, et al: Intraluminal vapor bubble induced by excimer laser pulse causes microsecond arterial dilation and invagination leading to extensive wall damage in the rabbit. Circulation 87:1258–1263, 1993.

114. Honda Y, Yock CA, Hermiller JB, et al: Longitudinal redistribution of plaque is an important mechanism for lumen expansion in stenting [abstract]. J Am Coll Cardiol 29:281A, 1997.

115. Nakamura S, Colombo A, Gaglione A, et al: Intracoronary ultrasound observations during stent implantation. Circulation 89:2026–2034, 1994.

116. Colombo A, Hall P, Nakamura S, et al: Intracoronary stenting without anticoagulation accomplished with intravascular ultrasound guidance. Circulation 91:1676–1688, 1995.

117. Garge G, Haude M, Ge J, et al: Intravascular ultrasound after low and high inflation pressure coronary artery stent implantation. J Am Coll Cardiol 26:725–730, 1995.

118. Hall P, Nakamura S, Maiello L, et al: A randomized comparison of combined ticlopidine and aspirin versus aspirin therapy alone after successful intravascular ultrasound-guided stent implantation. Circulation 93:215–222, 1996.

119. Goods CM, Al-Shaibi KF, Yadav SS, et al: Utilization of the coronary balloon expandable coil stent without anticoagulation or intravascular ultrasound. Circulation 93:1803–1808, 1996.

120. Roy PR, Lowe HC, Walker BW, et al: Intracoronary stenting without intravascular ultrasound guidance followed by antiplatelet therapy with aspirin alone in selected patients. Am J Cardiol 77:1105–1107, 1996.

121. Leon MB, Baim DS, Gordon P, et al: Clinical and angiographic results from the Stent Anticoagulation Regimen Study (STARS) [Abstract]. Circulation 94:I-684, 1996.

122. Uren NG, Schwarzacher SP, Metz JA, et al: Intravascular ultrasound prediction of stent thrombosis: Insights from the POST registry [Abstract]. J Am Coll Cardiol 29:60A, 1997.

123. Mudra H, Sunamura M, Figulla H, et al: Six month clinical and angiographic outcome after IVUS-guided stent implantation [Abstract]. J Am Coll Cardiol 29:171A, 1997.

124. Morice MC, Duman P, Voudris V, et al: The MUST Trial. In-hospital and clinical events at six months. Final results [Abstract]. J Am Coll Cardiol 93A:93A, 1997.

125. Akiyama T, DiMario C, Reimers B, et al: Do we need intracoronary ultrasound after high-pressure stent expansion [Abstract]? J Am Coll Cardiol 29:59A, 1997.

126. Roberts DK, Arthur A, Bellinger RL, et al: The impact on coronary stent implantation of intravascular ultrasound guidance following "aggressive" angiographic stent implantation [Abstract]. J Am Coll Cardiol 29:275A, 1997.

127. Werner GS, Schunemann S, Ferrari M, et al: Comparison of slotted-tube and coil stents after high-pressure stent deployment by intravascular ultrasound [Abstract]. J Am Coll Cardiol 29:275A, 1997.

128. Itoh A, Hall P, Moussa I, et al: Comparison of quantitative angiography and intravascular ultrasound after stent implantation with 6 different stents [Abstract]. Circulation 94:I-263, 1996.

129. Ziada KM, Kim MH, Potts W, et al: Predictors of target

vessel revascularization following coronary stent deployment [Abstract]. J Am Coll Cardiol 29:239A, 1997.

130. Moussa I, DiMario C, Moses J, et al: The predictive value of different intravascular ultrasound criteria for restenosis after coronary stenting [Abstract]. J Am Coll Cardiol 29:60A, 1997.

131. Mehran R, Mintz GS, Pichard AD, et al: Morphologic and procedural predictors of diffuse in-stent restenosis [Abstract]. J Am Coll Cardiol 29:76A, 1997.

132. Savage M, Fischman DL, Douglas JS Jr, et al: The dark side of high pressure stent deployment [Abstract]. J Am Coll Cardiol 29:368A, 1997.

133. Hausleiter J, Schuhlen H, Elezi S, et al: Impact of high inflation pressures on six-month angiographic follow-up after coronary stent placement [Abstract]. J Am Coll Cardiol 29:369A, 1997.

134. Fernandez-Aviles F, Alonso JJ, Duran JM, et al: High pressure increases late loss after coronary stenting [Abstract]. J Am Coll Cardiol 29:369A, 1997.

135. Hoffmann R, Mintz GS, Mehran R, et al: Late tissue proliferation *both* within and surrounding Palmaz-Schatz stents is associated with procedural wall injury [Abstract]. J Am Coll Cardiol 29:397A, 1997.

136. Yokoi H, Nosaka H, Kimura T, et al: Influence of high-pressure dilatation on late angiographic and clinical outcome of Palmaz-Schatz stent implantation [Abstract]. J Am Coll Cardiol 29:312A, 1997.

137. Akiyama T, DiMario C, Reimers B, et al: Does high-pressure stent expansion induce more restenosis [Abstract]? J Am Coll Cardiol 29:368A, 1997.

138. Mehran R, Mintz GS, Popma JJ, et al: Mechanisms and results of balloon angioplasty for the treatment of in-stent restenosis. Am J Cardiol 78:618–622, 1966.

139. Schiele F, Meneveau N, Vuillemenot A, et al: Intracoronary ultrasound assessment of balloon angioplasty in intrastent restenosis [Abstract]. J Am Coll Cardiol 29:240A, 1997.

140. Gorge G, Konorza E, Voegle E, et al: Incomplete restoration of luminal dimensions after PTCA in restenotic stented segments: An intravascular ultrasound analysis [Abstract]. J Am Coll Cardiol 29:311A, 1997.

141. Sharma SK, Duvvuri S, Kakarala V, et al: Rotational atherectomy for in-stent restenosis: Intravascular ultrasound and quantitative coronary analysis [Abstract]. Circulation 97:I-454, 1996.

142. Mehran R, Mintz GS, Popma JJ, et al: Treatment of in-stent restenosis: An intravascular ultrasound study in 159 stented lesions [Abstract]. J Am Coll Cardiol 29:77A, 1997.

143. Mehran R, Mintz GS, Popma JJ, et al: Mechanisms of lumen enlargement during atheroablation of in-stent restenosis: A volumetric intravascular ultrasound analysis [Abstract]. J Am Coll Cardiol 29:497A, 1997.

144. Schiele F, Meneveau N, Vuillemenot A, et al: Rotational atherectomy followed by balloon angioplasty for treatment of intra stent restenosis. A pilot study with quantitative angiography and intracoronary ultrasound [Abstract]. J Am Coll Cardiol 29:498A, 1997.

145. Painter JA, Mintz GS, Wong SC, et al: Serial intravascular ultrasound studies fail to show evidence of chronic Palmaz-Schatz stent recoil. Am J Cardiol 75:398–400, 1995.

146. Lansky AJ, Mintz GS, Popma JJ, et al: Remodeling after directional coronary atherectomy (± adjunct PTCA): A serial angiographic and intravascular ultrasound analysis from the Optimal Atherectomy Restenosis Study (OARS). J Am Coll Cardiol 32:329–337, 1998.

147. Kornowski R, Mintz GS, Kent KM, et al: Increased restenosis in diabetes mellitus after coronary interventions is due to exaggerated intimal hyperplasia: A serial intravascular ultrasound study. Circulation 95:1366–1369, 1997.

148. De Vrey E, Mintz GS, Kimura T, et al: Arterial remodeling after directional coronary atherectomy: A *volumetric* analysis from the Serial Ultrasound REstenosis (SURE) Trial [Abstract]. J Am Coll Cardiol 29:280A, 1997.

149. Currier JW, Faxon DP: Restenosis after percutaneous transluminal coronary angioplasty: Have we been aiming at the wrong target? J Am Coll Cardiol 25:516–520, 1995.

150. Hoffmann R, Mintz GS, Kent KM, et al: Serial intravascular ultrasound predictors of restenosis at the margins of Palmaz-Schatz stents. Am J Cardiol 74:951–953, 1997.

151. Mintz GS, Mehran R, Hong MK, et al: A sensitive and cost-effective intravascular ultrasound model to study antirestenosis strategies *in vivo* [Abstract]. J Am Coll Cardiol 27:112A, 1996.

152. Mintz GS, Pichard AD, Kovach JA, et al: Impact of preintervention intravascular ultrasound imaging on transcatheter treatment strategies in coronary artery disease. Am J Cardiol 73:423–430, 1994.

153. Hausmann D, Erbel R, Alibelli-Chemarin M-J, et al: The safety of intracoronary ultrasound: A multicenter survey of 2207 examinations. Circulation 91:623–630, 1995.

154. Batkoff BW, Linker DT: The safety of intracoronary ultrasound: Data from a multicenter European registry [Abstract]. J Am Coll Cardiol 25:143A, 1995.

155. Gorge G, Peters RJG, Pinto F, et al: Intravascular ultrasound: Safety and indications for use in 7085 consecutive patients studied in 32 centers in Europe and Israel [Abstract]. J Am Coll Cardiol 27:155A, 1996.

# 22

# Coronary Doppler Flow Measurements

*Morton J. Kern*   *Frank V. Aguirre*

The use of coronary physiologic data obtained in the catheterization laboratory after diagnostic angiography or before angioplasty can be used to facilitate clinical decisions.[1-9] This chapter reviews the fundamental concepts and clinical applications of intracoronary Doppler flow for interventional procedures.

## CORONARY PHYSIOLOGY IN THE CATHETERIZATION LABORATORY

Although used as the "gold standard," angiography cannot determine the clinical or physiologic importance of coronary stenoses with diameter narrowing between 40% and 80%.[1, 10-17] Because of this limitation, physiologic testing is often performed before deciding whether to proceed with coronary interventions. Although coronary blood flow, coronary flow reserve, and regional perfusion have demonstrated predictable relationships between the anatomic and physiologic parameters in experimental studies,[18-21] clinically reliable physiologic relationships were, in 1980 to 1985, not useful in the catheterization laboratory because of conceptual and technical limitations. Doppler flow velocity was not incorporated into routine procedures for several reasons: (1) relatively large catheters were required, (2) flow data were measured only proximal to a stenosis, and (3) the catheter exchanges were required during interventions. The Doppler guide wire has overcome these limitations. Coronary flow velocity can be measured distal to a coronary stenosis and does not interfere with normal blood flow. Spectral Doppler signal analysis improves the operator confidence of accurate measurements. The Doppler guide wire can be used as a primary interventional guide wire, suitable for continuous flow monitoring after angioplasty. During multivessel angioplasty, secondary lesions can be assessed before additional interventions are undertaken. During diagnostic an-

giography, coronary flow reserve can be used instead of out-of-laboratory stress testing.[5, 7]

The clinical applications of intracoronary flow velocity measurements are summarized in Table 22–1.

## FUNDAMENTAL CONCEPTS

A change in sound frequency can be appreciated as a transmitter moves to or away from a receiver. The change in the sound frequency is proportional to the speed of the target or transmitter, a phenomenon called the *Doppler effect* (Christian Johann Doppler, 1803–1853). For the application of this principle in clinical cardiology, a piezoelectric crystal that both emits and receives high-frequency sounds is mounted on the tip of an intravascular device. The velocity of red blood cells flowing past the device through an artery can be determined.

Coronary flow velocity is calculated from the frequency shift, defined as the difference between the

**TABLE 22–1.    CLINICAL USES OF INTRAVASCULAR DOPPLER CORONARY FLOW VELOCITY**

Intermediate (40%–70%) lesion assessment
Angioplasty
  Determining end point
  Monitoring complications
  Assessing additional lesions
  Determining collateral flow
  Determining stent
  Determining atherectomy
Measuring coronary vasodilatory reserve
  Syndrome X
  Transplant coronary arteriopathy
  Saphenous vein graft, internal mammary artery
Coronary research
  Pharmacologic studies
  Intra-aortic balloon pumping
  Coronary physiology of vascular disease
  Myocardial perfusion imaging correlations

transmitted and returning frequency as described by the Doppler equation:

$$V = (F_1 - F_0) \times (C/2F_0) \times (\cos \theta)$$

Where V = velocity of blood flow

$F_0$ = transmitting (transducer) frequency

$F_1$ = returning frequency

C = constant: speed of sound in blood

$\theta$ = angle of incidence

Volumetric flow can be determined from a velocity value as the product of vessel area (square centimeters) and flow velocity (centimeters per second) yielding a value in cubic centimeters per second. Volumetric flow can also be computed per cardiac cycle by multiplying vessel cross-sectional area times flow area (integral of velocity and time) times heart rate.[22] However, absolute Doppler flow velocities can only be used to represent changes in volumetric coronary flow when the vessel cross-sectional area remains unchanged over the measurement period. Assuming a constant vessel diameter and an interrogating Doppler angle of less than 20%, the flow rate can be calculated from the velocity measurements within 5% of absolute values. For the Doppler-tipped angioplasty guide wire, the velocity integral is readily measured in 3- to 5-mm vessels with an ultrasound beam spread of 30 degrees at 5 mm assuming a parabolic flow profile.

## DOPPLER GUIDE WIRE

The Doppler guide wire (FloWire Endosonics, Inc.; Rancho Cordoba CA) is a 175-cm-long 0.014- to 0.018-inch-diameter flexible, steerable angioplasty guide wire with a piezoelectric ultrasound transducer integrated into the tip (Fig. 22–1).[23] The guide wire is available in extra support configurations to facilitate stent placement. The system is coupled to a real-time spectrum analyzer, videocassette recorder, and thermal page printer. The Doppler signals are continuously displayed on a video monitor.

The cross-sectional area of the Doppler guide wire is 0.164 mm², which is 21% of the cross-sectional area of a 1-mm-diameter catheter. The small diameter of the guide wire does not impair blood flow except in the most severe stenoses. The small cross-sectional area of the Doppler wire would cause only a 15% area reduction in a circular lumen of a 1.2-mm-diameter vessel, whereas a 1-mm-diameter catheter would occlude almost 70% of the same

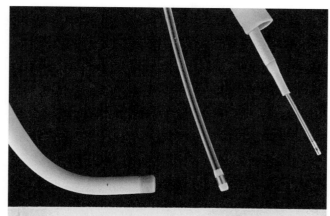

FIGURE 22–1. *Left to right,* A 6-French angiographic catheter; 2.2-French Tracker catheter (Target Therapeutics); and 0.014-inch Doppler FloWire (Endosonics, Inc.; Rancho Cordoba CA) residing within a 2.9-French intravascular ultrasound catheter (CVIS; Mountain View CA) with an 8-French guide catheter. Scale is 1 mm.

cross-sectional area. Substituting a Doppler-tipped guide wire for a standard angioplasty guide wire permits easy incorporation of flow data into procedures without adding unnecessarily complex technical maneuvers.

## Validation Studies

The Doppler guide wire velocity has been validated during intravascular measurement by Doucette and associates[23] and Labovitz and colleagues.[24] The velocity signals, processed on-line by fast Fourier transform, correlated with absolute coronary flow measurements in both in vitro and in vivo validation studies.[23, 24] With pulsatile blood flow, in four straight tubes (internal diameters varying from 0.79 to 4.76 mm), the peak spectral flow velocity was linearly related to the absolute flow velocity measured by in-line electromagnetic flow meters ($r >$ 0.98 for each tube). Quantitative volumetric flow was calculated from the vessel cross-sectional area and mean flow velocity. The average peak velocity was less accurate in larger tubes ($>$7.5 mm in diameter), and a slightly reduced correlation with absolute flow was observed in some tortuous model segments. In four canine circumflex coronary arteries, the electromagnetic flow probe and Doppler flow velocities also demonstrated high correlations in both the proximal and distal segments ($r^2$ = 0.93 to 0.99 in the proximal vessel and 0.86 to 0.99 in the distal vessel) (Fig. 22–2).

## Method of Use

The Doppler guide wire can be used as the primary wire during routine angioplasty in more than 85%

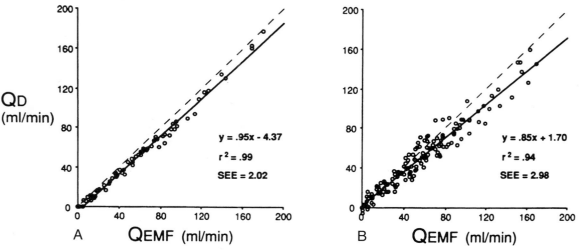

FIGURE 22–2. Validation of Doppler-derived flow ($Q_D$) versus blood flow by electromagnetic flow meter ($Q_{EMF}$) in canine circumflex arteries. *A,* FloWire in coronary cannula. *B,* FloWire in proximal circumflex artery. *Dashed line* is line of identity. *Solid line* is regression line. SEE, standard error of the estimate. (From Doucette JW, Corl PD, Payne HM, et al: Validation of a Doppler guide wire for intravascular measurement of coronary artery flow velocity. Circulation 85:1899–1911, 1992.)

of attempts. After diagnostic angiography or during angioplasty, the Doppler guide wire is passed through an angioplasty Y-connector attached to a small guiding catheter. Intravenous heparin (5000- to 10,000-U bolus) is required. The guide wire is advanced into the artery. If desired, baseline flow velocity data may be obtained at least 1 cm proximal to the lesion. The guide wire is then advanced at least 5 to 10 artery-diameter lengths (>2 cm) beyond the stenosis, and distal flow velocity data are then obtained. Coronary hyperemia is induced by intra-coronary adenosine (12 to 18 μg in the right coronary artery and 18 to 24 μg in the left coronary artery).[24] Coronary flow velocity reserve is computed as the quotient of hyperemic and basal mean flow velocity.

## CLINICAL APPLICATION OF DOPPLER FLOW VELOCITY

Appreciating the normal flow velocity characteristics is useful in the study of the coronary circulation and to facilitate restoration of flow after coronary interventions.

## Normal Phasic Flow Velocity Patterns

Phasic coronary artery flow patterns in animals and humans normally have a diastolic-predominant pattern[25] (Fig. 22–3). With increasing severity of epicardial artery stenoses, diastolic flow is limited, with systolic flow providing an increasing contribution to mean flow. In the left coronary artery, phasic coronary blood flow velocity shows the characteristic predominant diastolic-velocity waveform coupled with a smaller systolic waveform. Using a ratio

of diastolic/systolic flow velocity ratio (DSVR), the normal diastolic-predominant waveform in the left anterior descending and circumflex coronary arteries is greater than in the proximal right coronary artery until flow passes beyond the crux to regions supplying the inferior left ventricle (Table 22–2).[26–28] The average DSVR is normally greater than 1.8 and is maintained in both the proximal and the distal segments (>2 mm in diameter) in patients with normal left ventricles.[27, 29]

Phasic coronary artery blood flow is diminished distal to significant coronary stenoses. Segal and coworkers examined flow velocity in 38 patients undergoing angioplasty and in 12 patients having flow measured in normal vessels as controls.[29] Before angioplasty, the mean DSVR distal to a significant stenosis was decreased compared with that of normal vessels ($1.3 \pm 0.5$ vs. $1.8 \pm 0.5$, $p < 0.01$). After angioplasty, the abnormal phasic velocity pattern generally returned toward normal, increasing from $1.3 \pm 0.5$ to $1.9 \pm 0.6$ ($p < 0.01$). The flow velocity measurements corresponded to angiographic increases in lumen area, despite the fact that coronary reserve did not improve in most patients. The mechanism of improving DSVR appears related to the reduction in diastolic flow resistance compared with that of systolic flow resistance.[20, 21, 30] A decrease in the DSVR with an increasing degree of epicardial stenosis may be explained by the increased stenosis resistance to flow during periods of lowest distal vascular resistance (diastole) compared with that of high distal vascular resistance of systolic ejection.

Ofili and associates also examined coronary flow dynamics before and after angioplasty in patients compared with flow in angiographic normal arter-

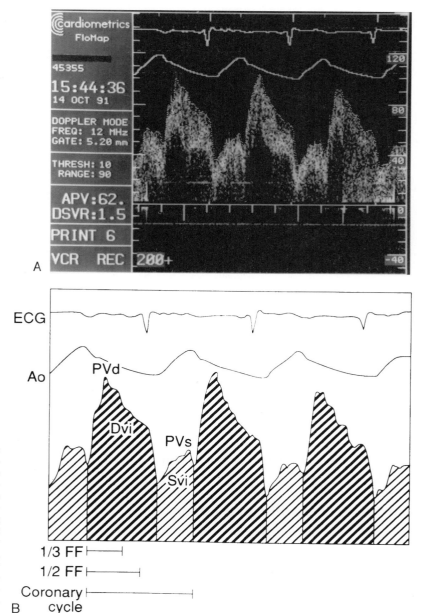

FIGURE 22–3. *A,* Normal coronary spectral flow pattern. The scale is −40 to 140 cm/second. Electrocardiogram and aortic pressure readings are shown above the spectral velocity signal. *B,* Diagram showing measurements obtained from the spectral flow pattern. Ao, aortic pressure; Dvi, diastolic velocity integral; ECG, electrocardiogram; FF, flow fraction; PVd, peak diastolic velocity; PVs, peak systolic velocity; Svi, systolic velocity integral. (From Ofili EO, Kern MJ, Labovitz AJ, et al: Analysis of coronary blood flow velocity dynamics in angiographically normal and stenosed arteries before and after endoluminal enlargement by angioplasty. J Am Coll Cardiol 21:308–316, 1993.)

ies.[27] A significantly lower mean velocity, peak diastolic velocity, and peak systolic velocity were found in the diseased arteries compared with the normal arteries. Phasic velocity showed a significant reduction of diastolic flow with relatively preserved systolic flow velocity. A systolic-predominant pattern was seen in 50% to 70% of diseased arteries and in none of the normal arteries. In proximal arterial segments, a significant overlap of normal and abnormal flow velocity parameters occurs, thus limiting the predictive accuracy of measurements at this location. In 29 patients after angioplasty, the distal average peak hyperemic velocity was significantly increased. Distal mean velocity increased more than proximal velocity, decreasing the proxi-

mal/distal velocity ratio, a marker of lesion severity.[2]

The absolute value of normal flow velocity depends on the size of the vessel. Because of a gradual tapering and branching, velocity, unlike volumetric flow, does not decrease more than 15% along the course of a vessel until the diameter is less than 2 mm. This phenomenon is comparable to normalization of shear stress of coronary flow.[31, 32]

Coronary flow velocity measurements in 55 angiographically normal proximal and distal coronary arteries (right coronary artery = 12, left circumflex artery = 19, left anterior descending artery = 24) demonstrated that the normal average proximal left anterior descending and circumflex time-averaged

**TABLE 22–2.    BASELINE AND HYPEREMIA VELOCITY PARAMETERS IN INDIVIDUAL CORONARY ARTERIES**

| | BASELINE | | | HYPEREMIA* | | |
|---|---|---|---|---|---|---|
| | LAD (N = 24) | LCX (N = 19) | RCA (N = 12) | LAD | LCX | RCA |
| **Proximal** | | | | | | |
| Peak D Vel | 49 ± 20 | 40 ± 15 | 37 ± 12 | 104 ± 28† | 79 ± 20 | 72 ± 13 |
| Mean Vel | 31 ± 15 | 25 ± 8 | 26 ± 7 | 66 ± 18† | 50 ± 14 | 48 ± 13 |
| D Vel Int | 18 ± 11‡ | 13 ± 5 | 11 ± 4 | 37 ± 55† | 27 | 22 ± 9 |
| 1/3 FF (%) | 45 ± 4‡ | 44 ± 5 | 40 ± 5 | 44 ± 5 | 43 ± 6 | 41 ± 4 |
| D/S | 2.0 ± 0.5‡ | 1.8 ± 0.7 | 1.5 ± 0.5 | 2.0 ± 0.5 | 1.9 ± 0.6 | 1.9 ± 0.8 |
| **Distal** | | | | | | |
| Peak D Vel | 35 ± 16 | 35 ± 8 | 28 ± 8 | 70 ± 17 | 71 ± 22 | 67 ± 16 |
| Mean Vel | 23 ± 11 | 21 ± 6 | 21 ± 9 | 45 ± 12 | 45 ± 12 | 42 ± 9 |
| D Vel Int | 13 ± 9 | 10 ± 3 | 8 ± 5 | 9 ± 6 | 11 ± 8 | 9 ± 2 |
| 1/3 FF (%) | 46 ± 2 | 45 ± 9 | 39 ± 6 | 45 ± 3 | 42 ± 7 | 40 ± 9 |
| D/S | 2.4 ± 0.8‡ | 2.1 ± 0.8 | 1.4 ± 0.3 | 2.2 ± 1.0 | 1.9 ± 0.8 | 1.6 ± 0.3 |

Anova: Scheffe F test $p < 0.05$.
*All three coronary arteries had significantly higher absolute velocity parameters during hyperemia ($p < 0.001$).
†LAD vs. LCX and RCA.
‡LAD vs. RCA.
D, diastolic; D/S, peak diastolic/systolic velocity; D Vel Int, diastolic flow velocity integral (units); LAD, left anterior descending artery; LCX, left circumflex artery; RCA, right coronary artery; 1/3 FF, one-third flow fraction; Vel, velocity (cm/sec).
From Miller DD, Donohue TJ, Younis LT, et al: Correlation of pharmacologic 99mTc-sestamibi myocardial perfusion imaging with poststenotic coronary flow reserve in patients with angiographically intermediate coronary artery stenoses. Circulation 89:2150–2160, 1994.

peak velocity range was approximately 25 to 30 cm/second with peak diastolic velocity ranges from 40 to 80 cm/second and peak systolic velocity from 10 to 20 cm/second[27] (Fig. 22–4). Right coronary artery and distal coronary segments (>2 mm in diameter) may show reduced velocity ranges by approximately 15% to 20%.

## Coronary Vasodilatory Reserve

Coronary vasodilatory reserve, the ratio of hyperemia to the basal average peak velocity, responses were measured in 416 coronary arteries in 214 patients in three groups: patients with atypical chest pain syndromes and angiographically normal coronary arteries; those with coronary artery disease and angiographically normal vessels; and those with angiographically normal transplant recipients.[33] Coronary vasodilatory reserve responses were compared by vessel, gender, status after heart transplantation, and the presence of remote coronary artery disease in another artery. In patients with atypical chest pain, the coronary vasodilatory reserve was 2.7 ± 0.6, lower than that in transplant recipients (3 ± 0.6, $p < 0.05$) and higher than that in poststenotic diseased vessel coronary flow reserve (1.8 ± 0.6) (Fig. 22–5). Coronary vasodilatory reserve tended to be higher in men than in women ($p < 0.07$). Coronary vasodilatory reserve was similar among left anterior descending, circumflex, and right coronary

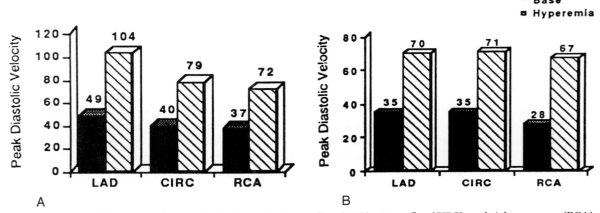

FIGURE 22–4. Normal and hyperemic flows in the left anterior descending (LAD), circumflex (CIRC), and right coronary (RCA) arteries. *A*, Original figure; *B*, diagram of parts of A. (From Ofili EO, Kern MJ, Labovitz AJ, et al: Analysis of coronary blood flow velocity dynamics in angiographically normal and stenosed arteries before and after endoluminal enlargement by angioplasty. J Am Coll Cardiol 21:308–316, 1993.)

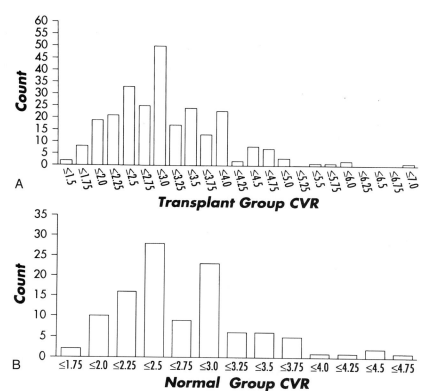

FIGURE 22–5. Histogram showing distribution frequency of coronary vasodilatory reserve (CVR) values for the transplantation *(A)* and angiographically normal *(B)* groups. Each block represents coronary vasodilatory reserve greater than or equal to the value indicated. (From Kern MJ, Bach RG, Mechem C, et al: Variations in normal coronary vasodilatory reserve stratified by artery, gender, heart transplantation and coronary artery disease. J Am Coll Cardiol 28:1154–1160, 1996.)

arteries in patients with atypical chest pain (2.8 ± 0.6, 2.7 ± 0.05, 2.9 ± 0.6, respectively). Regional differences were also not present in the transplantation population. The range of normal coronary vasodilatory reserve should be considered during the assessment of the coronary stenoses and before intervention.

## Reproducibility

The long-term reproducibility of Doppler coronary flow velocity in patients with coronary artery disease has been evaluated by Di Mario and coworkers.[34] Coronary flow velocity was recorded twice in the midvessel location in 31 patients over a 6-month follow-up period. Hemodynamic conditions were similar between the initial and final studies. There were no differences in angiographic or flow parameters.

Baseline velocity was similar (23 ± 8 cm/second) to values at follow-up (22 ± 5 cm/second), but the correlation was weak (slope = 0.3, r = 0.46). The initial coronary flow reserve was 2.9 ± 0.8, and the flow reserve was 3.0 ± 0.8 at follow-up with a larger scatter over the line of identity (slope = 0.22, r = 0.22). The standard deviation of the difference between the initial and follow-up measurements was higher in baseline conditions (±31%) than during hyperemia (±23%). The largest variation was for coronary flow reserve (SD ± 36%). The investigators indicated that the long-term reproducibility

could be improved when the flow velocity was normalized for the cross-sectional area at the site of measurement, thus yielding a volumetric coronary blood flow determination. The coronary vasodilatory reserve variability appeared to be related to the hemodynamic status changes and could be reduced by normalization for volumetric flow and pressure (coronary artery flow resistance).

## Pharmacologic Stimuli for Measuring Coronary Vasodilatory Reserve

The severity of stenosis should always be assessed using flow measurements both at rest and during hyperemia. The most widely used maximal vasodilator agents are dipyridamole, papaverine, and adenosine.[24, 35, 36] The hyperosmolar ionic and low-osmolar nonionic contrast media do not produce maximal vasodilatation.[37] Nitrates increase volumetric flow, but because these agents also dilate epicardial conductance vessels, the increase in coronary flow velocity is less pronounced than with adenosine or papaverine. Intracoronary nitroglycerin should be given before flow velocity reserve measurements to paralyze the vessel and minimize any flow-mediated vasodilatory effects of hyperemia causing an underestimation of flow velocity reserve.

Intracoronary papaverine has been reported to increase coronary blood flow velocity 4 to 6 times over resting values in patients with normal coronary arteries.[36] Papaverine (8 to 12 mg) produces a response equal to that of an intravenous infusion of dipyridamole in a dose of 0.56 to 0.84 mg/kg of body weight[35] but can occasionally cause ventricular tachycardia/ventricular fibrillation.[38] The hyperemic response after intravenous dipyridamole or intravenous/intracoronary adenosine is comparable to that of intracoronary papaverine.

Intracoronary adenosine has a short half-life, with a total duration of the hyperemic response 25% of that of papaverine or dipyridamole (Fig. 22–6).[36] Because bolus intracoronary adenosine does not increase vessel cross-sectional area,[39] the coronary flow velocity reserve can be used as a surrogate for coronary volumetric flow reserve. Intracoronary adenosine has an extremely high safety profile in low doses and has become the pharmacologic stimulus of choice in the catheterization laboratory.

## Practical Points for Coronary Lesion Assessment

Occasionally, it may be difficult to find the maximal distal flow velocity signals, and one may falsely conclude that a significant flow reduction is present because of a significant lesion. Therefore, the Doppler guide wire tip in the distal region should be rotated in several different orientations in all patients to identify the maximal and most intense spectral flow velocity signals that have a complete Doppler envelope. In tortuous segments, stable distal signals can usually be obtained. However, more guide wire manipulation is often needed to achieve

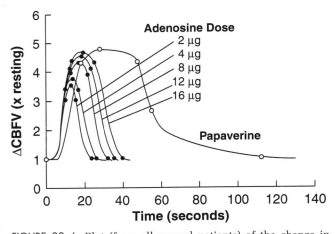

FIGURE 22–6. Plot (from all normal patients) of the change in coronary blood flow velocity (ΔCBFV) after progressively greater doses of intracoronary adenosine. Larger doses caused more prolonged hyperemia. The same figure shows a plot (from all patients) of the change in ΔCBFV after an intracoronary bolus of adenosine (16 μg) or papaverine (maximally vasodilating dose, 10 ± 2 mg). Both agents caused a marked increase in CBFV, but the response to adenosine was much shorter than that elicited by papaverine. (From Wilson RF, Wyche K, Christensen BV, et al: Effects of adenosine on human coronary arterial circulation. Circulation 82:1595–1606, 1990.)

satisfactory signals. In some patients, guide wire manipulation may not be suitable because of tortuosity or lesion complexity. In these instances, the Doppler FloWire can be exchanged for a finer, smaller, and softer guide wire. After the guide wire traverses the lesion, a tracking catheter is placed distally. The FloWire can then be exchanged for the softer guide wire. Both pressure and flow velocity across the lesion can now be measured.

An elevated distal flow velocity and falsely normalized proximal/distal flow velocity ratio, suggesting an insignificant lesion, might be seen if the distal measurements are made in a region with distal disease where there is flow acceleration secondary to distal luminal narrowing. In patients with serial lesions or diffuse distal disease, the proximal/distal flow ratio should not be used. In these cases, confirmation of lesion significance with coronary vasodilatory reserve and translesional pressure gradients at hyperemia is recommended.

## Technical Considerations

Technical factors involved in the accurate acquisition of flow velocity signals include a stable sample volume. Velocity is more accurate in laminar flow regions, undisturbed by turbulence at the lesion site. Maximal flow velocity is more accurately identified with spectral analysis because of the automatic edge detection, wide beam angle, and relative position insensitivity of the signal. The use of a guide wire rather than a catheter allows safe interrogation of smaller, more diffusely diseased arteries. Flow velocity measurements can also be performed continuously during interventional procedures, providing data unavailable by catheter-based techniques.

Problems in the acquisition of coronary flow velocity signal occur in less than 10% of patients within normal arteries and less than 15% of arteries examined in the course of coronary angioplasty.

Guide catheter obstruction to arterial blood inflow at the ostium of the coronary artery may interfere with the interpretation of both pressure and distal velocity signals. For this reason, most lesions can be assessed at the time of diagnostic catheterization with small (6-French) diagnostic or guiding catheters, or with the guiding catheter disengaged from the coronary ostium.

Finally, the translesional resting hemodynamics do not reflect ischemia-producing conditions that could occur during coronary vasoconstriction and exacerbation of lesions as a result of increased myocardial demand during exercise or emotional stimulation. Translesional pressure gradients will be increased to various degrees corresponding to lesion resistance as described by the pressure-velocity relationship. Whether clinical benefit would be conferred by dilating a lesion with a marginal resting pressure gradient, normal fractional flow reserve (see later), and coronary flow reserve compared with medical therapy remains under investigation.

## Translesional Hemodynamics and Ischemic Stress Testing

Excellent correlations with myocardial perfusion imaging and poststenotic coronary flow velocity reserve have been reported by several single-center studies[5, 7, 40] and one multicenter trial.[41] An abnormal distal hyperemic flow velocity reserve (<2) corresponded to reversible myocardial perfusion–imaging defects with high sensitivity (86% to 92%), specificity (89% to 100%), predictive accuracy (89% to 96%), and positive and negative predictive values (94% to 100% and 77% to 95%), respectively. The fractional flow reserve of the myocardium ($FFR_{myo}$; see later) has also been validated against myocardial perfusion using positron-emission tomography,[42] and normal-range values (>0.75) can easily discriminate among stenoses responsible for positive exercise stress testing[43] with excellent (>90%) specificity and sensitivity and high diagnostic accuracy (93% when compared with all noninvasive ischemic stress studies).

Miller and associates studied 33 patients to correlate stress myocardial perfusion imaging with poststenotic coronary flow reserve in patients with angiographically intermediate coronary stenoses.[5] The mean angiographic percentage diameter stenosis by quantitative coronary angiography was 56% ± 14% (range 20% to 84% diameter stenosis). Coronary vasodilatory reserve was obtained with intracoronary adenosine. Intravenous pharmacologic stress imaging was performed with adenosine in 20 patients and dipyridamole in 13 patients with technetium Tc-99m sestamibi tomographic perfusion imaging within 1 week of coronary flow velocity studies. A kappa statistic measuring the strength of correlation among the velocity-imaging and quantitative coronary angiographic variables was computed. The quantitative coronary angiographic stenosis severity (>50% diameter stenosis) and a poststenotic coronary flow velocity reserve of less than 2 were correlated in 20 of 27 patients (74%, kappa = 0.48). Perfusion-imaging abnormalities and the quantitative coronary angiographic stenosis severity were correlated in 28 of 33 patients (85%, kappa = 0.63). Sestamibi imaging results agreed with basal trans-stenotic velocity ratios (normal <1.7, abnormal >1.7) in 48% of patients (kappa = 0.17). The strongest correlation was noted between the hyperemic poststenotic flow velocity reserve and sestamibi perfusion imaging in 24 of 27 patients (89%, kappa = 0.78). Nearly all patients with ab-

normal distal hyperemic flow velocity values had corresponding reversible myocardial perfusion tomographic imaging defects. A similar correlation between poststenotic coronary flow reserve and myocardial perfusion imaging has been described by Joye and coworkers[7] and others.[41, 42]

## Criteria of a Hemodynamically Significant Lesion

The use of flow velocity to assess the hemodynamics of a coronary stenosis is based on the concept that the coronary circulation comprises two major components, a conduit (epicardial arteries) and a microcirculation (capillary and myocardial vascular bed). If the poststenotic vasodilatory flow reserve is normal, then both components are assumed to be normal. If the coronary vasodilatory reserve is abnormal, then examination of lesion-specific indices will separate the conduit obstruction, which can be treated mechanically (angioplasty), from microcirculatory disturbances that are treated medically.

## Lesion-Specific Indices of Coronary Flow Velocity

For a borderline coronary vasodilatory reserve (CVR) value or when the operator has low confidence in an accurate signal, a lesion-specific index should be acquired. The four lesion-specific measurements are (1) the proximal/distal velocity ratio, (2) a DSVR, (3) a translesional pressure gradient at hyperemia, fractional flow reserve of the myocardium (FFR), and (4) the relative coronary vasodilatory reserve ratio ($CVR_{target}/CVR_{normal}$). The accuracy of translesional gradients for fractional flow reserve calculation may be affected when a catheter instead of a guide wire is used (see "Coronary Pressure Measurements").

Because of coronary artery branching, both the volumetric flow and the cross-sectional vessel area diminish from the proximal to the distal myocardial regions. Because both the volume and the cross-sectional area diminish along the course of the vessel, the velocity is relatively unchanged (or only slightly diminished, usually less than 10% to 15% in vessels greater than 2 mm in diameter) from the proximal to the distal locations. The maintenance of flow velocity (but not volume) from the proximal to the distal part of the artery can be used as a marker of lesion-specific disease within the artery. In normal arteries, the proximal/distal flow velocity ratio should be 1.[2, 27] An increase in the proximal/distal mean velocity ratio is related to lesion severity as determined by a resting pressure gradient.[2] Donohue and coworkers[2] demonstrated a strong correlation between translesional pressure gradients and the ratios of the proximal/distal total flow velocity integrals ($r = 0.8$, $p < 0.001$) with a weaker relationship between quantitative angiography and pressure gradients ($r = 0.6$, $p < 0.001$). In angiographically intermediate stenoses (range 50% to 70%), angiography was a poor predictor of translesional gradients ($r = 0.2$, $p = NS$), whereas the flow velocity ratios continued to have a strong correlation ($r = 0.8$, $p < 0.0001$). The proximal/distal flow ratio demonstrated highly significant differences between patients without and with significant stenoses, ranging from $1.1 \pm 0.3$ for the group without gradients to ranges of $2.4 \pm 0.9$ to $2.5 \pm 1.2$ for the group with gradients with regard to diastolic and total velocity integrals and average peak velocity (all $p < 0.001$ vs. the group with gradients) (Fig. 22–7). A proximal/distal flow velocity integral ratio of less than 1.7 was associated with a gradient of less than 30 mm Hg in more than 85% of patients.

Patients with nonbranching right coronary artery lesions had normal proximal/distal flow velocity ratios despite high translesional gradients. The proximal/distal ratio does not apply in single tubes without branches where the continuity equation mandates equality of flow at any point along the circuit. The proximal/distal index is sensitive but not specific for a translesional gradient.

The phasic pattern of coronary flow reflects stenosis resistance and as a stenosis becomes more severe impairs diastolic flow first and then systolic flow. The normal DSVR is less than 1.8, 1.5, and 1.2 for the left anterior descending/circumflex, posterior descending, and proximal right coronary artery, respectively.[26] A reduction of the normal diastolic predominance of the phasic pattern usually indicates an important stenosis. The DSVR relationship with lesion severity requires a normally contracting myocardium in the region of the target stenosis.

## CORONARY PRESSURE MEASUREMENTS

### Pressure Guide Wire Devices

Although translesional pressure measurements are not routinely used in diagnostic or interventional coronary procedures, this information has re-emerged and become important for lesion assessment before or after angioplasty, especially when questionable angiographic results or coronary flow reserve data are obtained. Intracoronary pressure measurements can now be made with two angioplasty guide wire devices. The pressure guide (Radi Medical Systems, Uppsala, Sweden) is a 0.014-inch relatively stiff guide wire with a fiberoptic capability to detect changes in reflected light from a mirror source deformed by pressure changes.[44] The high-fidelity signal produces phasic pressure waveforms equivalent to those of larger high-fidelity catheters. The second device, a fluid-filled 0.014-inch-diameter angioplasty guide wire (Schneider Corporation, Bulag, Switzerland),[45] can be connected to a standard pressure transducer. Because of its small inner lumen, a damped phasic pressure is registered. The accuracy of the mean pressure signals recorded through fluid-filled guide wires has been validated.[46, 47] This device is no longer available. A high-fidelity 0.014-inch-diameter pressure wire is available (from Endosonics, Inc.; Rancho Cordoba CA).

If no guide wire pressure system is available, a small fluid-filled catheter for coronary pressure gradients, a 2.7-French Tracker catheter (Target Therapeutics) with a 2.2-French tip and inner lumen of 0.020 mm, can be used. The following equipment is required to measure pressures across a stenosis: (1) two pressure manifolds, two transducers, and a pressure tubing Y-connector; (2) a hemodynamic monitor and recorder; (3) a small-diameter (<2.7-French, e.g., Tracker, Cook) catheter or pressure guide wire; and (4) a guide catheter, 6-French or greater.

From guide wire pressure measurements, a new

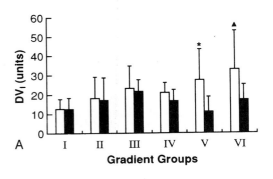

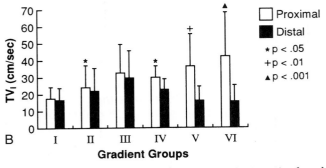

FIGURE 22–7. *A*, Subgroup analysis comparing proximal and distal diastolic velocity integral (DV$_i$). *B*, Subgroup analysis comparing proximal and distal total velocity integral (TV$_i$). See source of figure for the definition of gradient groups. (From Donohue TJ, Kern MJ, Aguirre FV, et al: Assessing the hemodynamic significance of coronary artery stenoses: Analysis of translesional pressure-flow velocity relations in patients. J Am Coll Cardiol 22:449–458, 1993.)

concept for the determination of coronary blood flow, the FFR$_{myo}$, has emerged.[42–47] The FFR$_{myo}$ is defined as the ratio of maximal hyperemic flow in the stenotic artery to the theoretic maximal hyperemic flow in the same artery without a stenosis. FFR$_{myo}$ is computed as the ratio of mean distal coronary pressure and mean aortic pressure during maximal hyperemia and is a specific index to describe the influence of the coronary stenosis on maximal perfusion of the subtended myocardium.

## Technique

With the use of angioplasty technique, the pressure wire signal is matched against guide catheter pressure, and then the guide wire is advanced into the artery and beyond the stenosis (Fig. 22–8). The two pressures are simultaneously recorded at baseline and during hyperemia induced by intracoronary or intravenous adenosine to compute FFR$_{myo}$. The pressure wire can then be pulled back proximal to the stenosis to recheck the signal drift. Any small difference between the two pressures measured proximal to the lesion is called the *intrinsic pressure gradient* and is subtracted from the trans-stenotic pressure gradient, calculated as the difference between aortic (proximal) and distal coronary mean pressures.

## Fractional Flow Reserve Concept

When blood flows from the proximal to the distal part of the normal epicardial coronary artery, the pressure remains constant throughout the conduit. In the case of epicardial coronary narrowing, potential energy is transformed into kinetic energy and heat when blood traverses the lesion. The resultant distal pressure drop reflects the total loss of energy due to stenosis resistance. To maintain resting myo-

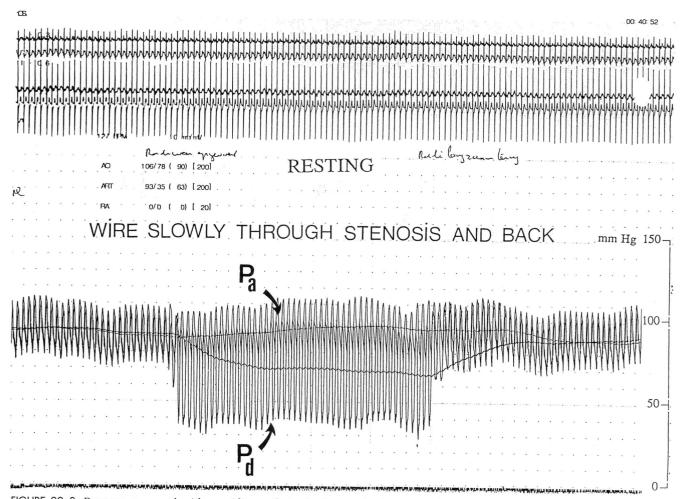

FIGURE 22–8. Pressure measured with a guiding catheter in the proximal coronary location (P$_a$) and pressure measured along the course of a coronary artery with a pressure guide wire. As the pressure guide wire is advanced through the stenosis and pulled back, a pressure drop (P$_d$) in the distal coronary artery can be seen. The scale is 150 mm Hg. Time marks are 1 second. Electrocardiograms are at the *top*. This guide wire pressure can be used to determine the fractional flow reserve measuring P$_d$ during maximal hyperemia. (Courtesy of N. H. J. Pijls, Eindhoven, The Netherlands.)

cardial perfusion at a constant level, myocardial resistance decreases, compensating for the stenosis resistance to flow. The distal pressure at constant maximal flow represents an index of the physiologic consequences of a given coronary narrowing on the myocardium.

As first proposed by Pijls and colleagues,[46] pressure measurements are another means to determine the maximal myocardial blood flow in the presence of a stenosis (Table 22–3). This flow is compared with the expected normal flow in the absence of a stenosis and is expressed as a fraction of the normal expected value. This value, called *fractional flow reserve,* is derived from pressure data alone and identifies flow for the myocardium, the epicardial coronary artery, and the collateral supply based on several assumptions regarding translesional pressure measured during maximal hyperemia. $FFR_{myo}$, the ratio of distal coronary pressure to aortic pressure during maximal hyperemia, has been proposed as a lesion-specific methodology (Fig. 22–9).

Pijls and coworkers compared the myocardial fraction flow reserve with the results of four commonly used noninvasive tests to detect myocardial ischemia.[43] In 45 patients with moderate coronary stenosis and chest pain of uncertain origin, bicycle exercise testing, thallium scintigraphy, and stress dobutamine echocardiography were compared with the results of fractional flow reserve measurements. In all 21 patients with a fractional flow reserve less than 0.75, reversible myocardial ischemia was demonstrated unequivocally on at least one noninvasive test. After coronary revascularization, all positive

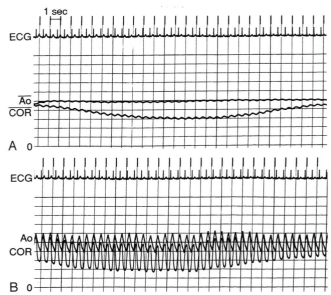

FIGURE 22–9. Pressure gradient measured at rest and during maximal hyperemia demonstrating an increase from the resting gradient of 4 to 40 mm Hg. *A,* Mean aortic pressure (Ao); the lower pressure signal is the distal coronary pressure (COR). *B,* Phasic pressure tracings using the guide catheter and a 2.7-French tracking catheter. The fractional flow reserve is computed from the maximal hyperemic distal pressure and aortic pressure. Aortic pressure equals 100 mm Hg, distal coronary pressure equals 60 mm Hg, and the fractional flow reserve is 0.6, an abnormal value corresponding to a positive stress thallium study in this individual. ECG, electrocardiogram.

results reverted to normal. In 21 of 24 patients with a fractional flow reserve of 0.75 or greater, tests were negative for reversible myocardial ischemia on all tests. No revascularization procedures were performed, and all patients were stable and did not require further intervention over 14 months of follow-up. The sensitivity of fractional flow reserve for reversible ischemia was 88%, specificity 100%, positive and negative predictive value 100% and 88%, respectively, with a predictive accuracy of 93%.

The sole measurement of a pressure gradient alone during hyperemia also has inherent limitations because the pressure-flow curve will remain unknown, thus not differentiating a mild stenosis with impaired microvascular flow from severe stenosis. The absence of a significant trans-stenotic gradient may be related to either the absence of a flow-limiting stenosis or the presence of a low flow across the stenosis due to either an impaired distal vasodilation or a well-developed collateral circulation.

It should be no surprise that coronary velocity reserve responses will not translate into directly measured translesional pressure gradient computations of flow because distal myocardial bed resistance may be variable or impaired and not ac-

### TABLE 22–3. EQUATIONS FOR CALCULATION OF MYOCARDIAL, CORONARY, AND COLLATERAL FRACTIONAL FLOW RESERVE FROM PRESSURE MEASUREMENTS DURING MAXIMAL HYPEREMIA

Myocardial fractional flow reserve ($FFR_{myo}$):

$$FFR_{myo} = 1 - \Delta P/(P_a - P_v)$$
$$= (P_c - P_v)/(P_a - P_v)$$
$$= P_c/P_a$$

Coronary fractional flow reserve ($FFR_{cor}$):

$$FFR_{cor} = 1 - \Delta P(P_a - P_w)$$

Collateral fractional flow reserve ($FFR_{coll}$):

$$FFR_{coll} = FFR_{myo} - FFR_{cor}$$

$\Delta P$, mean translesional pressure gradient; $P_a$, mean aortic pressure; $P_c$, distal coronary pressure; $P_v$, mean right atrial pressure; $P_w$, mean coronary wedge pressure or distal coronary pressure during balloon inflation.

From Pijls NHJ, Van Gelder B, Van der Voort P, et al: Fractional flow reserve: A useful index to evaluate the influence of an epicardial coronary stenosis on myocardial blood flow. Circulation 92:3183–3193, 1995.

counted for in the primary assumptions of this methodology (Fig. 22–10). The use of translesional gradients has important value for determining lesion significance when distal myocardial flow reserve is impaired.

## Clinical Indications for Translesional Physiologic Measurements

There are several major reasons to obtain coronary Doppler flow measurements: (1) for assessment of the angiographically intermediate lesion, (2) for making a decision about performing angioplasty of secondary lesions in multivessel angioplasty, (3) for making an end point determination after angioplasty, and (4) for coronary physiology research.

## Assessment of the Intermediately Severe Stenosis

Approximately 1 million coronary angiograms are performed in the United States each year. In patients having coronary angiography, an intermediate stenosis (40% to 70% diameter narrowing) is encountered in nearly 50%. Intracoronary flow velocity measurements obtained at the time of diagnostic angiography, employing the criteria of lesion significance described earlier, can identify important lesions and assist in decision making (Fig. 22–11).

Deferring angioplasty of intermediate (40% to 70%) lesions with normal translesional hemody-

namics is associated with an excellent long-term clinical outcome.[48] A prospective study of deferring angioplasty based on normal translesional flow reported outcome results in 88 patients with 100 lesions (26 single-vessel, 74 multivessel coronary artery stenoses).[48]

The percentage lumen area reduction, percentage diameter stenosis, and obstruction diameter in the deferred group were 77% ± 8%, 54% ± 7%, and 1.32 ± 0.33 mm, respectively. Translesional pressure gradients were lower for the deferred compared with a reference angioplasty group (10 ± 9 vs. 46 ± 22 mm Hg, $p < 0.01$). Proximal/distal velocity ratios demonstrated similar values for both the normal and the deferred groups with significant differences compared with the angioplasty group (1.1 ± 0.35 for the normal, 1.3 ± 0.55 for the deferred, and 2.3 ± 1.2 for the angioplasty group; $p < 0.05$ vs. both normal and deferred groups).

Clinical follow-up data were available in 84 of 88 (95%) with a mean follow-up of 10 ± 8 months and a minimum follow-up period of 6 months (range 6 to 30 months). In the deferred group, rehospitalization due to both noncardiac and angina-like symptoms occurred in 18 patients, 12 of whom had cardiac events. No patient had a myocardial infarction. One patient died from postangioplasty complications of a nontarget artery. One patient with multivessel coronary artery disease and decreased left ventricular function died suddenly 12 months after assessment of the lesion because of ventricular fibrillation. Ten patients required either coronary artery bypass grafting (N = 6) or coronary angioplasty (N = 4); only six of the procedures involved target arteries. Of the six patients who required bypass surgery, only three had a target artery with previously normal translesional flow velocity involved. There were no complications related to translesional pressure or flow velocity measurements in any patient studied.

This study demonstrated that in patients with angiographically intermediately severe lesions, normal translesional hemodynamic data can be acquired safely and that angioplasty can be deferred with approximately 92% of target arteries evaluated remaining stable without the need for intervention. Translesional flow velocity–pressure measurements can provide objective functional evidence of lesion significance to assist in selecting patients for appropriate coronary interventions.

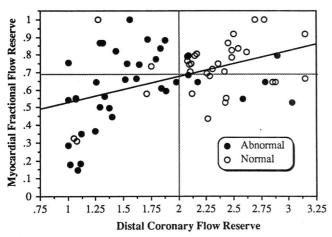

FIGURE 22–10. Poststenotic coronary flow reserve measured with the Doppler flow wire compared with myocardial fractional flow reserve measured with a 2.2-French tracking catheter and pressure during maximal hyperemia. The *black dots* represent abnormal thallium studies; the *open circles* represent normal thallium studies. The correlation between distal coronary flow reserve and positive thallium studies can be demonstrated with the distal coronary flow reserve but not with fractional flow reserve. (From Tron C, Kern MJ, Donahue TJ: Comparison of pressure-derived fractional flow reserve with poststenotic coronary flow velocity reserve for prediction of stress myocardial perfusion imaging results. Am Heart J 130:723–733, 1995.)

## Use During Angioplasty

Angioplasty is performed in a routine manner using the FloWire. During coronary balloon occlusion, the flow velocity rapidly falls to near zero. If persistent antegrade flow occurs, the balloon is undersized or

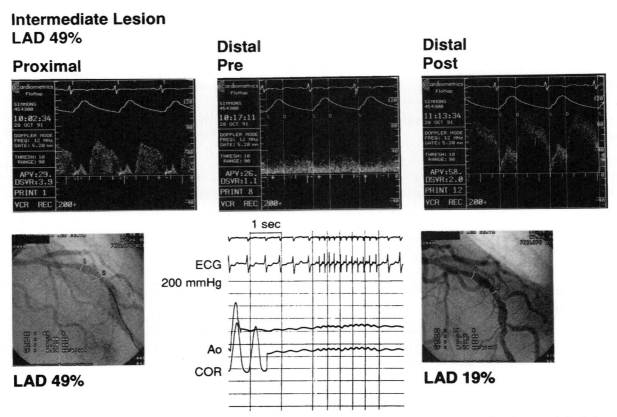

FIGURE 22–11. Angiography of a 53-year-old woman with worsening typical chest pain. Angiographic frames of the left anterior descending (LAD) coronary artery show a moderate (49%) midartery stenosis *(bottom left)*. Proximal flow velocity is normal *(top left)*. Distal flow velocity is diminished *(top middle)* (proximal/distal ratio > 1.7) with a loss of phasic nature to flow (equal systolic and diastolic flow integrals). The translesional gradient shown on both phasic and mean pressure tracings was 40 mm Hg *(bottom middle)*. After angioplasty (Post; 19% final stenosis diameter *[bottom right]*), the distal flow velocity normalized *(top right)* with a residual gradient less than 5 mm Hg. Ao, aortic; COR, distal coronary artery pressure (mm Hg); ECG, electrocardiogram; Pre, before angioplasty. (From Donohue TJ, Kern MJ, Aguirre FV, et al: Assessing the hemodynamic significance of coronary artery stenoses: Analysis of translesional pressure-flow velocity relations in patients. J Am Coll Cardiol 22:449–458, 1993.)

there is collateral input distal to the balloon but proximal to the wire tip. If the flow velocity initially falls to zero and then becomes visible below the baseline (negative), retrograde collateral flow is identified and can be quantitated. The presence of retrograde collateral flow during occlusion occurs in 10% to 15% of cases and may be a useful positive indicator of the patient's potential tolerance for prolonged balloon occlusions.

## Multivessel Angioplasty

Secondary lesions in multivessel coronary artery disease can be addressed at the time of angioplasty of the culprit vessel using flow velocity lesion assessment as described for the intermediate lesion. This approach has the potential to save the costs of addition hospital days, stress testing, angioplasty equipment, and complications. Flow velocity data during coronary angioplasty are shown in Figure 22–12.

## Angioplasty End Point of Treatment

The preliminary results of a European multicenter prospective study (Doppler Endpoint Balloon Angioplasty Trial Europe [DEBATE]) identified the predictive value of coronary flow velocity measurements after angioplasty.[49] In 224 patients after single-vessel angioplasty, poststenotic coronary vasodilatory reserve, proximal/distal flow ratio, and DSVR were determined and compared with early and late clinical events.

After angioplasty, there was no difference in the angiographic minimal lumen diameter between patients with early events (N = 35) and asymptomatic patients (N = 189) (1.81 ± 0.38 mm vs. 1.79 ± 0.29 mm, respectively). However, the poststenotic coronary vasodilatory reserve (2.73 ± 0.93 vs. 2.22 ± 0.65; $p < 0.05$) was higher in asymptomatic patients compared with those experiencing early events. These data indicated that, on average, the symptomatic group could be differentiated but that an isolated coronary vasodilatory reserve value

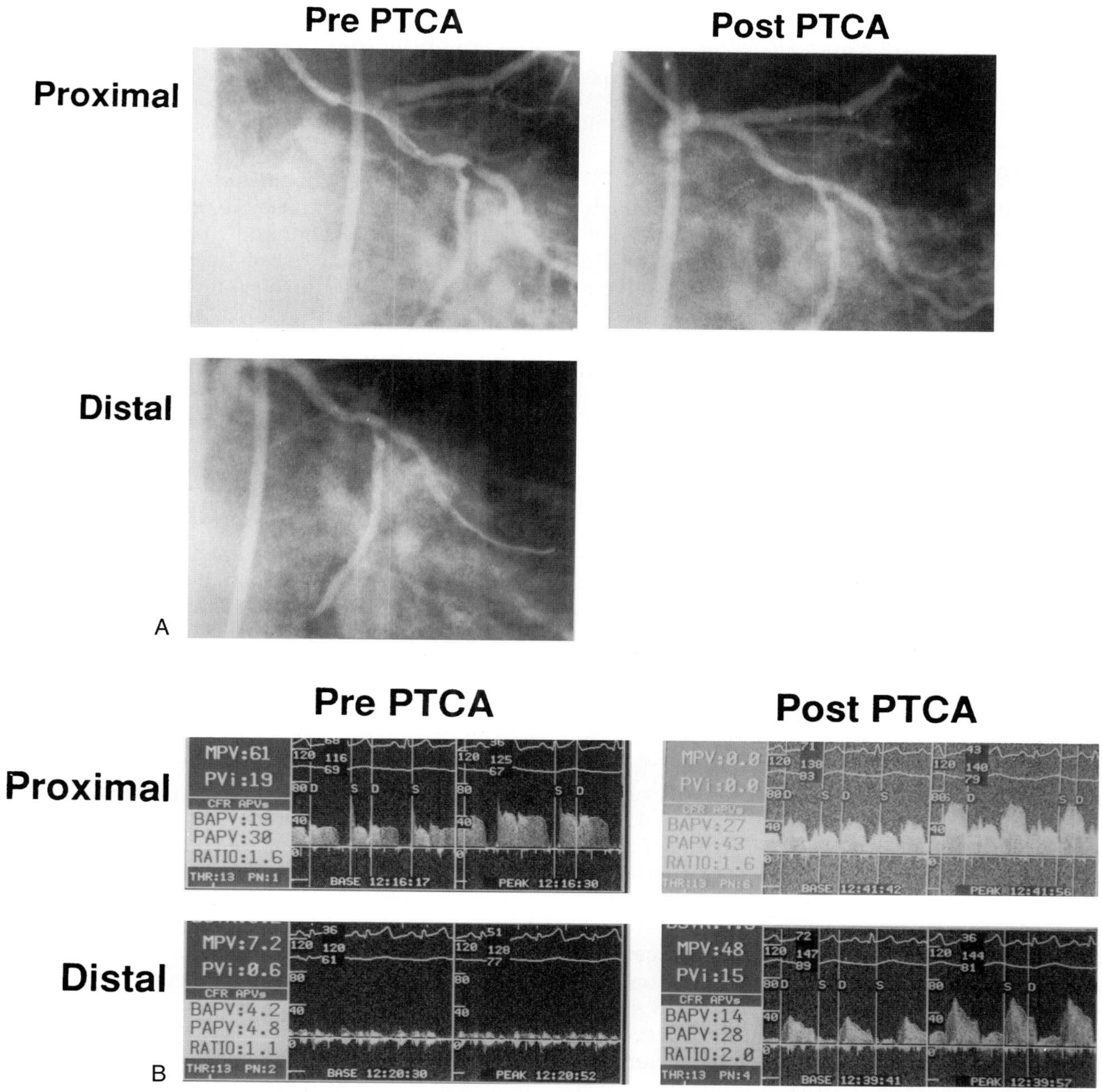

## Pre PTCA        ## Post PTCA

**Proximal**

**Distal**

A

## Pre PTCA        ## Post PTCA

**Proximal**

**Distal**

B

FIGURE 22–12. *A*, Angiograms before and after percutaneous transluminal coronary angioplasty (PTCA) of a circumflex (CFX) obtuse marginal branch lesion. *Top left* panel shows a flow wire in the proximal circumflex artery. *Lower left* panel shows a flow wire in the distal obtuse marginal branch. *Top right* panel shows the angiogram after angioplasty, resulting in conversion of a 95% stenosis to less than 10% residual narrowing. *B*, Coronary flow velocity signals before and after angioplasty in the proximal and distal locations cited in part *A*. Panels are divided into *left* and *right* sections. The *left side* is the basal velocity. The *right side* is the peak hyperemic velocity. Before angioplasty *(left side)*, the proximal coronary flow reserve was 1.6 and the distal flow reserve was 1.1. Note the marked decrease in distal basal average peak velocity (BAPV) relative to the proximal location. After angioplasty *(right side)*, both proximal and distal flow velocities increased. The proximal flow velocity was unchanged. The distal coronary flow reserve increased from 1.1 to 2, corresponding to the improvement in the angiographic findings. PAPV, peak average peak velocity; RATIO, coronary flow reserve.

would not be prognostic except in the extreme ranges. However, further analysis combining post-procedural coronary flow reserve greater than 2.5 with an optimal anatomic result (quantitative angiographic percentage diameter stenosis <35%) identified 44 of 224 patients with a 16% rate of repeat angioplasty at 6 months, a value similar to restenosis rates in some stent trials.

The combined anatomic and functional data were a better prognostic index than either parameter alone, and this combined value was strongly predictive of early and late clinical events. Prospective trials using physiologically guided decisions to assess the need for stenting are ongoing and will further define clinical outcomes in angioplasty patients.

## Physiologically Guided Interventions

The decision to place a stent is commonly made from angiographic data alone, and stent placement is expensive. From intravascular ultrasound (IVUS) imaging and Doppler flow data, traditional balloon angioplasty may not achieve an optimal result for luminal enlargement despite a satisfactory angiographic appearance. If after coronary angioplasty, coronary vasodilatory reserve remains impaired because of unappreciated luminal narrowing, then a coronary stent should normalize the coronary vasodilatory reserve. Decisions for stenting or larger balloon catheters after coronary angioplasty may be facilitated using coronary physiologic data.

A preliminary study examined results in 15 patients undergoing elective angioplasty and stent placement with measurements of coronary flow velocity reserve (0.014 in Doppler FloWire) and IVUS imaging (2.9-French Cardiovascular Interventional System [CVIS]; Mountain View CA) before and after balloon angioplasty and again after stent placement (Fig. 22–13).[50] The percentage diameter stenosis decreased from 71% ± 10% to 37% ± 11% after angioplasty to 7% ± 12% after stent placement. The coronary vasodilatory reserve increased from 1.3 ± 0.6 to 1.6 ± 0.6 after angioplasty to 2.3 ± 0.5 after stent placement. This value was similar to that found in normal adjacent reference vessels (2.5 ± 0.6). There was no relationship between coronary vasodilatory reserve and angiographic percentage diameter stenosis or absolute quantitative coronary angioplasty (QCA) dimensions. The IVUS vessel cross-sectional area was significantly larger after stenting (4.5 mm after percutaneous transluminal coronary angioplasty [PTCA] vs. 7.6 mm after stent placement, $p < 0.01$).

The increase in coronary vasodilatory reserve after stenting, more than angioplasty, suggests that the coronary vasodilatory reserve after angioplasty is related to lumen expansion, which is not always appreciated by angiography. A physiologically guided intervention to achieve an optimal lumen for flow may lead to improved angioplasty techniques and potentially limit unnecessary stent placement.

## Monitoring Coronary Blood Flow During Coronary Interventions

Monitoring flow for variations due to slowly progressive dissection, thrombus formation, or vaso-spasm is easily performed using the velocity trend plot. The flow velocity trend changes often precede angiographic signs of vessel occlusion.[51] Monitoring flow can also reduce the total contrast volume when assessing the stability of angioplasty results and can identify potential unstable flow associated with vessel closure, a benefit that has obvious clinical advantages. Interruption of unstable flow with conversion to a stable postprocedure flow pattern reduces morbidity related to an out-of-laboratory acute vessel closure and reduces the need for a repeat procedure, angioplasty catheters, and/or stent placement. Early warning signs of an adverse outcome derived from flow trend monitoring can potentially save the cost of the repeat angioplasty and/or bypass surgery (Figs. 22–14 and 22–15).

## New Interventional Devices and Flow: Directional Coronary Atherectomy

Deychak and colleagues studied distal coronary artery flow velocities in 18 patients undergoing directional coronary atherectomy using the Simpson AtheroCath system.[52] The significant angiographic improvement after directional atherectomy (76% diameter stenosis before vs. 23% after; $p < 0.001$) was associated with only a modest increase in the mean velocity from 23 ± 19 cm/second to 31 ± 16 cm/second.

The mean DSVR did not increase significantly after atherectomy (1.78 vs. 2.04, $p = 0.18$). The reasons for minimal improvement immediately after directional atherectomy are unclear. Remaining eccentric channels with significant residual plaque burden and thrombus formation have been postulated as the mechanism. As with other techniques that remove tissue in an endovascular approach, the unappreciated release of material that is generally captured by the directional coronary atherectomy catheter may transiently impair the distal circulation and also contribute to the unexpectedly low coronary flow values often observed after directional atherectomy.

## Percutaneous Transluminal Coronary Rotational Atherectomy

Percutaneous transluminal coronary rotational atherectomy (PTCRA) has undergone extensive clinical investigation and established itself as the procedure of choice for coronary stenoses with certain angiographic characteristics, especially lesional calcification. To determine the sequential changes in coronary blood flow occurring after PTCRA and adjunctive coronary angioplasty, flow velocity was measured in 13 patients (10 men, 3 women with a mean age of 62 ± 11 years) undergoing PTCRA

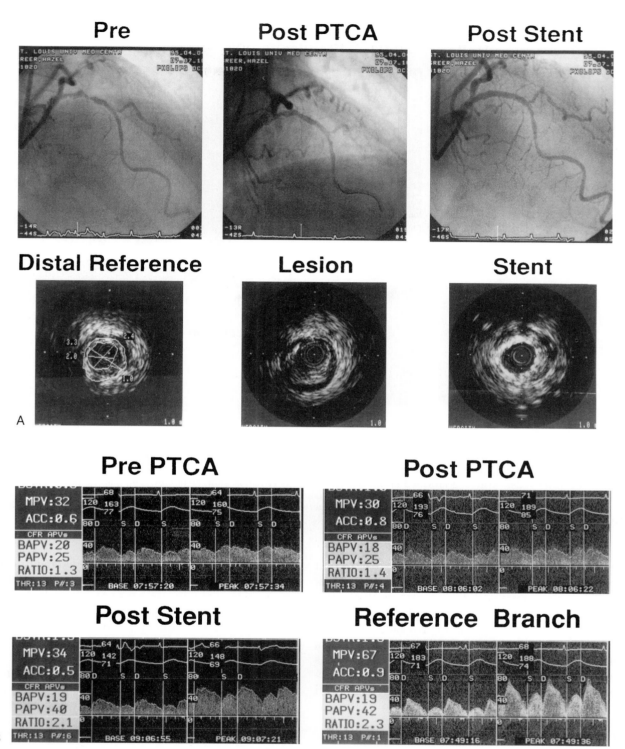

FIGURE 22–13. *A*, Angiography and intravascular ultrasound imaging before and after percutaneous transluminal coronary angioplasty (PTCA) and again after stent placement. Coronary angiography *(top left panel)* demonstrates a severe stenosis. After angioplasty *(top middle panel)*, the 90% stenosis has decreased to 20% narrowing. After stenting *(top right panel)*, residual narrowing is less than 10%. *Lower left panel*, Reference vessel segment. Intravascular ultrasound imaging measures a lumen diameter of 2.4 mm. *Lower middle panel*, Postangioplasty lumen with the irregular configuration. *Lower right panel*, Intravascular ultrasound (IVUS) lumen after stent placement. *B*, Coronary flow reserve (CFR) before and after angioplasty and again after stent placement with comparison with CFR in a reference branch vessel (circumflex artery). The format is similar to that of Figure 22–12*B*. The coronary flow reserve before angioplasty is 1.3; after angioplasty, 1.4; and after stent placement, 2.1. The reference flow reserve is 2.3, similar to that after stent placement. Stenting can normalize the flow reserve in some patients.

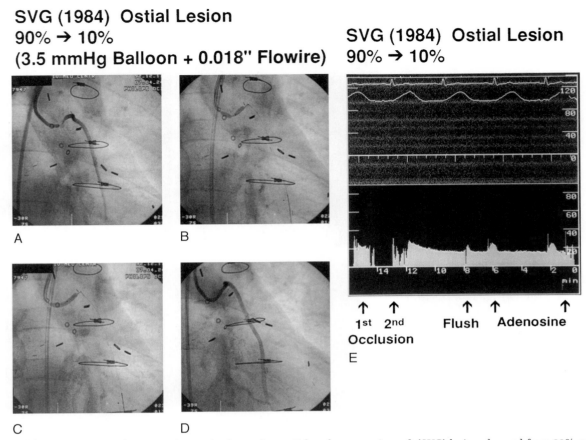

FIGURE 22–14. *A,* Angiograms demonstrating angioplasty of an ostial saphenous vein graft (SVG) lesion changed from 90% narrowing to less than 10% *(A–D).* During the postprocedural period, the flow velocity was continuously monitored. *E,* Flow velocity trend during angioplasty in a saphenous vein graft. Hyperemia after the first and second balloon occlusions can be seen *(arrows).* Coronary flow velocity stabilizes. Contrast injections are identified with a loss of signal and transient hyperemia. Intracoronary adenosine is administered *(arrows)* demonstrating impaired flow reserve with a widely patent graft. Note, however, that the flow velocity is stable for the monitoring periods identified. The scale is zero to 100 cm/second. The average peak velocity time base is 2 minutes for each division. (From Kern MJ, Aguirre FV, Donohue TJ, et al: Coronary flow velocity monitoring after angioplasty associated with abrupt reocclusion. Am Heart J 127:436–438, 1994.)

using standard technique.[53] The arteries treated were the left anterior descending in six patients, right coronary artery in five patients, and circumflex/obtuse marginal in two patients. None of the patients had undergone a prior revascularization procedure in the target vessel. Three patients had a previous myocardial infarction more than 6 months previously. The mean left ventricular ejection fraction was 59% ± 14%, and two patients had wall motion abnormalities in the distribution of the target vessel.

After PTCRA, the minimal luminal diameter increased from 0.7 ± 0.39 mm to 1.9 ± 0.4 mm ($p <$ 0.01 vs. baseline), representing a 1.2-mm gain. After adjunctive balloon angioplasty, the minimal luminal diameter was 2.4 ± 0.5 mm ($p <$ 0.01 vs. PTCRA) with an acute gain of 0.5 mm, a 145% change from baseline, and a 23% change after PTCRA. The no-reflow phenomenon was not encountered in any study patient. Angiographic success was achieved in 13 of 14 lesions.

Before PTCRA, the poststenotic average peak velocity was 15.0 ± 7.2 cm/second with a blunted hyperemic velocity response (17.6 ± 10.5 cm/second) and a coronary flow velocity reserve of 1.1 ± 0.2. Volumetric coronary blood flows at baseline and hyperemia were 47 ± 23 mL/minute and 57 ± 38 mL/minute, respectively ($p =$ NS).

After PTCRA, the average peak velocity increased to 29.5 ± 12.6 cm/second ($p <$ 0.01). Hyperemic average peak velocity was 36.8 ± 13.8 cm/second ($p <$ 0.05 vs. baseline). Coronary blood flow increased to 105 ± 59 mL/minute at baseline and 132 ± 73 mL/minute at hyperemia (both $p <$ 0.05 vs. before PTCRA). The coronary flow reserve, however, remained similar at 1.3 ± 0.2 ($p =$ NS vs. pre-PTCRA coronary flow reserve).

After adjunctive balloon angioplasty, the average peak velocity was 22.8 ± 5.5 cm/second, unchanged from postrotablator flow ($p =$ NS). The hyperemic average peak velocity was 39.7 ± 17.2 cm/second, also unchanged compared with after

**During Flow Monitoring**

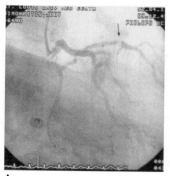 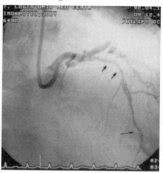

A                    B

**Trend**

FIGURE 22–15. Cineangiographic frames of a lesion in a left anterior descending (LAD) artery stent/stenosis *(A, arrow)* before angioplasty. *B,* After angioplasty, during velocity monitoring, angiographic haziness and mottling *(two arrows)* at the angioplasty site was associated with cyclic flow variations measured at the tip of the Doppler guide wire *(distal arrow)* as shown on the flow velocity trend plot *(C).* The trend plot displays the following signals *(from top to bottom):* electrocardiogram (ECG), aortic pressure, phasic velocity (scale: zero to 200 cm/second), and a continuous plot of the average peak velocity (APV) (scale: zero to 50 cm/second). Events at *arrows* are described in the text. (From Kern MJ, Donohue T, Bach R, et al: Monitoring cyclical coronary blood flow alterations following coronary angioplasty for stent restenosis using a Doppler guidewire. Am Heart J 125:1159–1160, 1993.)

C          **Post dilation**          **Angiogram**          **Heparin bolus**          **Angiogram**

PTCRA. Volumetric coronary blood flow after adjunctive balloon angioplasty was similar to flow velocity values after PTCRA. However, the coronary flow reserve was 1.6 ± 0.3, a statistically significant increase from the baseline value ($p < 0.01$) (Table 22–4).

This study demonstrated a significant improvement in basal and hyperemic coronary blood flow after PTCRA. However, despite the satisfactory post-PTCRA luminal enlargement, the coronary physiology remained compromised as suggested by the persistently impaired coronary flow reserve. Adjunctive coronary balloon angioplasty further increased the angiographic minimal luminal diameter. The calculated coronary flow reserve after adjunctive balloon angioplasty was increased, in large part because of a lower baseline flow value. Prior preliminary studies report similar findings with persistently impaired postprocedural coronary flow reserve.[54, 55]

**TABLE 22–4.    FLOW CHARACTERISTICS AT BASELINE AND AFTER INTERVENTION**

| | AVERAGE PEAK VELOCITY (cm/sec) | | CORONARY BLOOD FLOW (mL/min) | | CORONARY FLOW RESERVE |
|---|---|---|---|---|---|
| | BASELINE | HYPEREMIA | BASELINE | HYPEREMIA | |
| Baseline | 15.0 ± 7.2 | 17.6 ± 10.5 | 46.5 ± 23.0 | 56.5 ± 38.0 | 1.1 ± 0.2 |
| Post-PTCRA | 29.5 ± 12.6 | 36.8 ± 13.8 | 104.9 ± 59.0 | 132.1 ± 73.0 | 1.3 ± 0.2 |
| Post-PTCA | 22.8 ± 5.5 | 39.7 ± 17.2 | 84.0 ± 40.7 | 143.8 ± 81.0 | 1.6 ± 0.3 |
| *p* value base vs. PTCRA | 0.01 | 0.05 | 0.01 | 0.05 | NS |
| *p* value PTCRA vs. PTCA | NS | NS | NS | NS | NS |
| *p* value base vs. PTCA | NS | 0.01 | NS | 0.05 | 0.01 |
| Percentage change base vs. PTCRA | 108 ± 74 | 197 ± 285 | 126 ± 93 | 188 ± 189 | 36 |
| Percentage change PTCRA vs. PTCA | 7 ± 40 | 24 ± 51 | 17 ± 56 | 30 ± 54 | 8 |
| Percentage change baseline vs. PTCA | 110 ± 111 | 325 ± 435 | 122 ± 113 | 342 ± 445 | 64 |

NS, nonsignificant; PTCA, percutaneous transluminal coronary angioplasty; PTCRA, percutaneous transluminal coronary rotational atherectomy.

# Coronary Physiology During Intervention for Acute Myocardial Infarction

In patients with acute myocardial infarction, coronary blood flow can be accurately measured using intracoronary Doppler blood flow velocity. The semiquantitative but clinically predictive TIMI (Thrombosis In Myocardial Infarction) angiographic grade flow, an established standard of reperfusion therapies, was compared with measured flow before and after primary or rescue angioplasty using a 0.014- to 0.018-inch Doppler-tipped angioplasty guide wire in 41 acute myocardial infarct patients.[56] The TIMI angiographic flow grade was assessed by two independent observers and also quantitated by the frames-to-opacification method from cinefilm. Of 41 patients, 33 had primary and 8 had rescue angioplasty, 34 within 24 hours of acute myocardial infarction. Before angioplasty, 34 patients had TIMI grade 0 or 1, 5 patients had TIMI grade 2, and 3 patients had TIMI grade 3 flow in the infarct artery. After angioplasty, the diameter stenosis improved from $95\% \pm 7\%$ to $22\% \pm 10\%$. One patient had TIMI grade 1, 5 patients had TIMI grade 2, and 35 patients had TIMI grade 3 flow. Poststenotic distal flow velocity, mostly in the LAD, increased from $6.6 \pm 6.1$ to $20 \pm 11.1$ cm/second ($p < 0.01$) after angioplasty (Fig. 22–16). Before angioplasty, there were no statistical differences between poststenotic flow velocity values among infarct vessels with TIMI grade 0, 1, or 2 flow; however, those with TIMI grade 3 had higher flow velocity ($9.4 \pm 5$ cm/second vs. $16 \pm 5.4$; $p < 0.05$). After angioplasty, TIMI grade 3 flow increased to $21.8 \pm 10.9$ cm/second ($p$

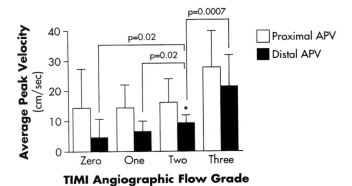

**FIGURE 22–17.** Proximal and distal average peak velocity (APV) and TIMI (Thrombosis In Myocardial Infarction) grade flow in all vessels after angioplasty. *$p < 0.05$ vs. TIMI grade $\leq 2$. (From Kern MJ, Moore JA, Aguirre FV, et al: Determination of angiographic [TIMI grade] blood flow by intracoronary Doppler flow velocity during acute myocardial infarction. Circulation 94:1545–1552, 1996.)

$< 0.05$ vs. preangioplasty distal TIMI grade 3 flow) (Fig. 22–17). After angioplasty, flow velocity correlated with the angiographic frame count ($r = 0.45$; $p < 0.02$). However, for TIMI grade 3 flow, there was a large overlap with low-TIMI ($\leq 2$) flow velocity ($<20$ cm/second), despite frames to opacification of less than 60 (Fig. 22–18). Clinical events in 9 of 11 patients (i.e., death, recurrent myocardial infarction, or a need for repeat coronary revascularization) occurred in the TIMI 3 group with a flow velocity of less than 20 cm/second.

These results indicate that semiquantitative TIMI perfusion grades are distinguished by differences in coronary flow velocity, with a TIMI grade of 2 or less consistently associated with low flow velocity values. On average, the TIMI grade 3 flow velocity is higher than the flow velocity of TIMI grades 2 or

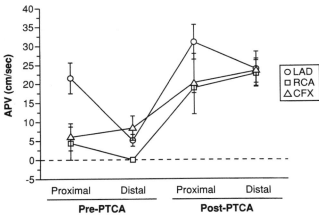

**FIGURE 22–16.** Average peak velocity (APV, cm/sec) before and after angioplasty in proximal and poststenotic (distal) target vessel regions. *Open circles,* left anterior descending (LAD) artery; *open squares,* right coronary artery (RCA); *open triangles,* circumflex artery (CFX); PTCA, percutaneous transluminal coronary angioplasty. (From Kern MJ, Moore JA, Aguirre FV, et al: Determination of angiographic [TIMI grade] blood flow by intracoronary Doppler flow velocity during acute myocardial infarction. Circulation 94:1545–1552, 1996.)

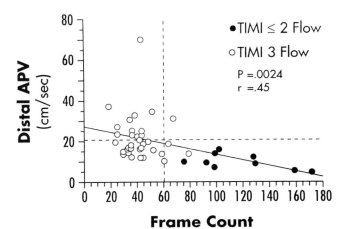

**FIGURE 22–18.** Correlation of poststenotic (distal) average peak velocity (APV) with frames-to-opacification count after angioplasty. (From Kern MJ, Moore JA, Aguirre FV, et al: Determination of angiographic [TIMI grade] blood flow by intracoronary Doppler flow velocity during acute myocardial infarction. Circulation 94:1545–1552, 1996.)

less, but there is a substantial overlap, with low flow values of TIMI 2 flow or less. Quantitative assessment of flow velocity after reperfusion could potentially establish important physiologic correlations among clinical outcomes after various reperfusion therapies.

## Safety and Costs

The Doppler guide wire performs as an angioplasty guide wire and has an excellent safety record. In over 1200 studies performed in our laboratory with normal or mildly diseased vessels, no patient has had a Doppler guide wire complication. Worldwide, only 10 of more than 40,000 uses have resulted in serious artery injury reported to the manufacturer or Food and Drug Administration. This incidence is lower than that of diagnostic angiography alone.

Caution should be employed by operators without guide wire experience. There is no absolute contraindication to the use of appropriate dosages of intracoronary adenosine for coronary vasodilatory reserve measurements. Some cardiac transplantation patients may be sensitive to standard doses of adenosine, which may cause transient heart block lasting less than 2 to 3 seconds. Unlike the situation with papaverine, no complication has been reported with adenosine given for coronary vasodilatory reserve measurements.

Preliminary data from a randomized trial conducted by physicians in Atlanta, GA, using in-laboratory lesion assessment compared with postangiography out-of-laboratory noninvasive thallium testing demonstrate a substantial reduction in hospital days and total expenditures based on thallium cost estimates of $1200 versus Doppler guide wire costs of $500.[57]

## SUMMARY

For coronary angioplasty, intracoronary flow velocity measurements can be used to determine the requirements for success and stability of the angiographic result. Decisions about performing multivessel angioplasty of secondary lesions are based on the same technique as is used for assessing intermediate lesions during diagnostic angiography. The clinical results after interventions appear to be related to both the improved postprocedural anatomy and the coronary flow reserve. Numerous studies have shown that neither thallium testing nor angiography is sufficiently reliable to distinguish the physiologic significance of "marginal" coronary lesions. The incorporation of translesional flow velocity into clinical practice will assist in the identification of appropriate angioplasty candidates and the outcome of interventional procedures. The in-corporation of interventional physiology into routine practice has the potential to improve clinical results for important subsets of these patients.

## REFERENCES

1. White CW, Wright CB, Doty DB, et al: Does visual interpretation of the coronary arteriogram predict the physiologic importance of a coronary stenosis? N Engl J Med 310:819–824, 1984.
2. Donohue TJ, Kern MJ, Aguirre FV, et al: Assessing the hemodynamic significance of coronary artery stenoses: Analysis of translesional pressure-flow velocity relations in patients. J Am Coll Cardiol 22:449–458, 1993.
3. Ofili EO, Kern MJ, Labovitz AJ, et al: Analysis of coronary blood flow velocity dynamics in angiographically normal and stenosed arteries before and after endoluminal enlargement by angioplasty. J Am Coll Cardiol 21:308–316, 1993.
4. Kern MJ, Donohue TJ, Aguirre FV, et al: Clinical outcome of deferring angioplasty in patients with normal translesional pressure-flow velocity measurements. J Am Coll Cardiol 25:178–187, 1995.
5. Miller DD, Donohue TJ, Younis LT, et al: Correlation of pharmacologic 99mTc-sestamibi myocardial perfusion imaging with poststenotic coronary flow reserve in patients with angiographically intermediate coronary artery stenoses. Circulation 89:2150–2160, 1994.
6. Pijls NHJ, van Son AM, Kirkeeide RL, et al: Experimental basis of determining maximum coronary, myocardial, and collateral blood flow by pressure measurements for assessing functional stenosis severity before and after percutaneous transluminal coronary angioplasty. Circulation 87:1354–1367, 1993.
7. Joye JD, Schulman DS, LaSorda D, et al: Intracoronary Doppler guide wire versus stress single-photon emission computed tomographic thallium-201 imaging in assessment of intermediate coronary stenoses. J Am Coll Cardiol 24:940–947, 1994.
8. Kern MJ, Anderson HV (eds): A symposium: The clinical applications of the intracoronary Doppler guidewire flow velocity in patients: Understanding blood flow beyond the coronary stenosis. Am J Cardiol 71:1D–86D, 1993.
9. Serruys PW, Di Mario C, Kern MJ. Intracoronary Doppler. *In* Topol EJ (ed): Textbook of Interventional Cardiology, vol 2, pp 1069–1121. Philadelphia: WB Saunders, 1994.
10. Zijlstra F, van Ommeren J, Reiber JHC, et al: Does the quantitative assessment of coronary artery dimensions predict the physiologic significance of a coronary stenosis? Circulation 75:1154–1161, 1987.
11. Galbraith JE, Murphy ML, DeSoyza N: Coronary angiogram interpretation: Interobserver variability. JAMA 240:2053–2056, 1978.
12. DeRouen TA, Murray JA, Owen W: Variability analysis of coronary arteriograms. Circulation 55:324–328, 1979.
13. Zir LM, Miller SW, Dinsmore RE, et al: Interobserver variability in coronary angiography. Circulation 53:627–632, 1978.
14. Wilson RJ, Marcus ML, White CW: Prediction of the physiologic significance of coronary arterial lesion by quantitative lesion geometry in patients with limited coronary artery disease. Circulation 75:723–732, 1987.
15. Zijlstra F, Fioretti P, Reiber J, et al: Which cineangiographically assessed anatomic variable correlates best with functional measurements of stenoses severity? A comparison of quantitative analysis of the coronary cineangiogram with measured coronary flow reserve and exercise/redistribution thallium-201 scintigraphy. J Am Coll Cardiol 12:686–691, 1988.
16. Wijns W, Serruys PW, Reiber JHC, et al: Quantitative angiography of the left anterior descending coronary artery: Correlations with pressure gradient and results of exercise thallium scintigraphy. Circulation 71:273–279, 1985.
17. Laarman DJ, Serruys PW, Suryapranata H, et al: Inability of coronary blood flow reserve measurements to assess the

efficacy of coronary angioplasty in the first 24 hours in unselected patients. Am Heart J 122:631–639, 1991.

18. De Feyter PJ, Serruys PW, Davies MJ, et al: Quantitative coronary angiography to measure progression and regression of coronary atherosclerosis: Value, limitations, and implications for clinical trials. Circulation 84:412–423, 1991.

19. Harrison DG, White CW, Hiratzka LF, et al: The value of lesion cross-sectional area determined by quantitative coronary angiography in assessing the physiologic significance of proximal left anterior descending coronary arteries stenosis. Circulation 69:1111–1119, 1984.

20. Gould KL, Lipscomb K, Hamilton GW: Physiologic basis for assessing critical coronary stenosis. Am J Cardiol 33:87–94, 1974.

21. Gould KL, Lipscomb K, Hamilton GW: Physiologic basis for assessing critical coronary stenosis: Instantaneous flow response and regional distribution during coronary hyperemia as measures of coronary flow reserve. Am J Cardiol 33:87–94, 1974.

22. Hatle L, Angelsen B: Physics of blood flow. In Hatle L, Angelsen B (eds): Doppler Ultrasound in Cardiology, pp 8–31. Philadelphia: Lea & Febiger, 1982.

23. Doucette JW, Corl PD, Payne HM, et al: Validation of a Doppler guide wire for intravascular measurement of coronary artery flow velocity. Circulation 85:1899–1911, 1992.

24. Labovitz AJ, Anthonis DJ, Craven TL, et al: Validation of volumetric flow measurements by means of a Doppler-tipped coronary angioplasty guide wire. Am Heart J 126:1456–1461, 1993.

24. Wilson RF, Wyche K, Christensen BV, et al: Effects of adenosine on human coronary arterial circulation. Circulation 82:1595–1606, 1990.

25. Spaan JAAE, Breuls NPW, Laird JD: Diastolic-systolic coronary flow differences are caused by intramyocardial pump action in the anesthetized dog. Circ Res 49:584–593, 1981.

26. Ofili EO, Labovitz AJ, Kern MJ: Coronary flow velocity dynamics in normal and diseased arteries. Am J Cardiol 71:3D–9D, 1993.

27. Ofili EO, Kern MJ, Labovitz AJ, et al: Analysis of coronary blood flow velocity dynamics in angiographically normal and stenosed arteries before and after endoluminal enlargement by angioplasty. J Am Coll Cardiol 21:308–316, 1993.

28. Heller LI, Silver KH, Villegas BJ, et al: Blood flow velocity in the right coronary artery: Assessment before and after angioplasty. J Am Coll Cardiol 24:1012–1017, 1994.

29. Segal J, Kern MJ, Scott NA, et al: Alterations of phasic coronary artery flow velocity in man during percutaneous coronary angioplasty. J Am Coll Cardiol 20:276–286, 1992.

30. Furuse A, Klopp EH, Brawley RK, et al: Hemodynamic determinations in the assessment of distal coronary artery disease. J Surg Res 19:25–33, 1974.

31. Murray CD: The physiological principle of minimum work. I. The vascular system and the cost of blood volume. Proc Natl Acad Sci U S A 12:207–214, 1926.

32. Seiler C, Kirkeeide RL, Gould KL: Basic structure-function relations of the epicardial coronary vascular tree. Circulation 85:1987–2003, 1992.

33. Kern MJ, Bach RG, Mechem C, et al: Variations in normal coronary vasodilatory reserve stratified by artery, gender, heart transplantation and coronary artery disease. J Am Coll Cardiol 28:1154–1160, 1996.

34. Di Mario C, Gil R, Serruys PW: Long-term reproducibility of coronary flow velocity measurements in patients with coronary artery disease. Am J Cardiol 75:1177–1180, 1995.

35. Rossen JD, Simonetti I, Marcus ML, et al: Coronary dilation with standard dose dipyridamole and dipyridamole combined with handgrip. Circulation 79:566–572, 1989.

36. Wilson RF, White CW: Intracoronary papaverine: An ideal vasodilator for studies of the coronary circulation in conscious humans. Circulation 73:444–452, 1986.

37. Tatineni S, Kern MJ, Deligonul U, et al: The effects of ionic and non-ionic radiographic contrast media on coronary hyperemia in patients during coronary angiography. Am Heart J 123:621–627, 1992.

38. Kern MJ, Deligonul U, Serota H, et al: Ventricular arrhythmia due to intracoronary papaverine: Analysis of clinical and hemodynamic data with coronary vasodilatory reserve. Cathet Cardiovasc Diagn 19:229–236, 1990.

39. Caracciolo EA, Wolford TL, Underwood RD, et al: Influence of intimal thickening on coronary blood flow responses in orthotopic heart transplant recipients: A combined intravascular Doppler and ultrasound imaging study. Circulation 92(suppl II):II-182–II-190, 1995.

40. Deychak YA, Segal J, Reiner JS, et al: Doppler guide wire flow-velocity indexes measured distal to coronary stenoses associated with reversible thallium perfusion defects. Am Heart J 129:219–227, 1995.

41. Heller LI, Popma J, Cates C, et al: Functional assessment of stenosis severity in the cath lab: A comparison of Doppler and Tl-201 imaging. J Interv Cardiol 7:23A, 1995.

42. De Bruyne B, Baudhuin T, Melin JA, et al: Coronary flow reserve calculated from pressure measurements in humans: Validation with positron emission tomography. Circulation 89:1013–1022, 1994.

43. Pijls NHJ, de Bruyne B, Peels K, et al: Measurement of myocardial fractional flow reserve to assess the functional severity of coronary artery stenosis. N Engl J Med 334:1703–1708, 1996.

44. Emanuelsson H, Dohnal M, Lamm C, et al: Initial experience with a miniaturized pressure transducer during coronary angioplasty. Cathet Cardiovasc Diagn 24:127–143, 1991.

45. De Bruyne B, Pijls NHJ, Paulus WJ, et al: Trans-stenotic coronary pressure gradient measurements in humans: In vitro and in vivo evaluation of a new pressure monitoring angioplasty guidewire. J Am Coll Cardiol 22:119–126, 1993.

46. Pijls NHJ, Van Gelder B, Van der Voort P, et al: Fractional flow reserve: A useful index to evaluate the influence of an epicardial coronary stenosis on myocardial blood flow. Circulation 92:3183–3193, 1995.

47. De Bruyne B, Bartunek J, Sys SU, et al: Relation between myocardial fractional flow reserve calculated from coronary pressure measurements and exercise-induced myocardial ischemia. Circulation 92:39–46, 1995.

48. Kern MJ, Donohue TJ, Aguirre FV, et al: Clinical outcome of deferring angioplasty in patients with normal translesional pressure-flow velocity measurements. J Am Coll Cardiol 25:178–187, 1995.

49. Serruys PW, Di Mario C: Prognostic value of coronary flow velocity and diameter stenosis in assessing the short and long term outcome of balloon angioplasty: The DEBATE study (Doppler Endpoints Balloon Angioplasty Trial Europe) [Abstract]. Circulation 94:I-317, 1996.

50. Kern MJ, Aguirre FV, Donohue TJ, et al: Impact of residual lumen narrowing on coronary flow after angioplasty and stent: Intravascular ultrasound Doppler and imaging data in support of physiologically-guided coronary angioplasty [Abstract]. Circulation 92:I-263, 1995.

51. Kern MJ, Aguirre FV, Donohue TJ, et al: Coronary flow velocity monitoring after angioplasty associated with abrupt reocclusion. Am Heart J 127:436–438, 1994.

52. Deychak YA, Thompson MA, Rohrbeck SC, et al: A Doppler guidewire used to assess coronary flow during directional coronary atherectomy [Abstract]. Circulation 86:I-122, 1992.

53. Khoury AF, Aguirre FV, Bach RG, et al: Influence of percutaneous transluminal coronary rotational atherectomy with adjunctive percutaneous transluminal coronary angioplasty on coronary blood flow. Am Heart J 131:631–638, 1996.

54. Nunez BD, Keelan ET, Lerman A, et al: Coronary hemodynamics after rotational atherectomy [Abstract]. J Am Coll Cardiol (suppl):95A, 1995.

55. Bowers TR, Stewart RE, O'Neill WW, et al: Plaque pulverization during rotablator atherectomy: Does it impair coronary flow dynamics [Abstract]? J Am Coll Cardiol (suppl):96A, 1995.

56. Kern MJ, Moore JA, Aguirre FV, et al: Determination of angiographic (TIMI grade) blood flow by intracoronary Doppler flow velocity during acute myocardial infarction. Circulation 94:1545–1552, 1996.

57. Joye J, Cates C, Farah B, et al: Cost analysis of intracoronary Doppler determination of lesion significance: Preliminary results of the PEACH study. J Invas Cardiol 7:22A, 1995.

# 23

# Coronary Angioscopy

*Frank V. Tilli*

The advent of advanced coronary intervention has mandated the need for advanced imaging modalities for both diagnostic and therapeutic purposes. Although angiography has remained the "gold standard" for imaging the coronary circulation, it provides little insight into the intraluminal pathology that is present in diseased native coronary arteries and bypass grafts. Coronary angioscopy has been used successfully in a variety of clinical scenarios and has been shown to be superior to angiography for the evaluation of plaque morphology and for detection of the presence of both dissection and thrombus. With increased use of new interventional devices and adjunctive pharmacotherapy, the need for precise diagnosis of intraluminal pathology becomes imperative. By employing more precise imaging modalities, physicians can better synthesize a treatment strategy for complex coronary intervention.

## EQUIPMENT

Several percutaneous angioscopes have been manufactured and are commercially available. All of these share essential components required for endoscopic imaging of the coronary arteries. These components include a catheter that is multiluminal and contains a fiberoptic imaging bundle, a guide wire lumen, a flush lumen, and a balloon lumen (Table 23–1). This catheter must then interface with an external high-intensity light source, a video monitor for real-time imaging, and a recording system for image storage and playback. The most extensively used and investigated catheter in the United States has been the Baxter-Edwards coronary angioscope (Fig. 23–1), a 125-cm-long polyethylene catheter that measures 1.5 mm in diameter. The catheter is monorail in design and accepts 0.14-inch guide wires. It is compatible with any 8-French angioplasty guiding catheter. The device itself consists of an inner movable core, which contains the fiberoptic imaging bundle, and an outer sheath, which contains the occlusion balloon. The occlusion balloon is made of a highly compliant synthetic latex material.

## TECHNIQUE

Despite the maneuverability of the angioscope, proper technique requires good guiding catheter support and the use of an extra-support guide wire. Using standard coronary angioplasty technique, the surgeon crosses the stenotic lesion with the angioscopy guide wire. The angioscope is then introduced into the coronary artery through a monorail technique and is positioned under fluoroscopic guidance so that the distal tip marker is proximal to the target vessel. To create a blood-free field, the occlusion balloon is gently inflated to approximately 1 atm in order to occlude blood flow. Because of the extremely soft nature of the synthetic latex balloon material, which can rapidly expand to 5 or 6 mm in size, it is critical that inflation be done gently. Simultaneously with balloon occlusion, heparinized saline or lactated Ringer's solution is infused distally via the irrigation lumen by means of a power injection at a rate of approximately 30 mL/minute. Once a blood-free field is established, the central fiberoptic imaging bundle can be advanced up to and through the lesion, provided there is no evidence of intraluminal adherent thrombus or plaque, which might embolize distally. Imaging is generally performed during pullback with simultaneous video recording and is limited to less than 90 seconds in order to minimize myocardial ischemia. After imaging is complete, the occlusion balloon is

## TABLE 23–1. ESSENTIAL COMPONENTS OF THE CORONARY ANGIOSCOPE

*Catheter*

Fiberoptic imaging bundle
Illumination bundle
Guide wire lumen
Flush lumen
Balloon lumen

*External Connections*

High-intensity light source
Camera system
Television monitor
Video recorder
Power injection irrigation system

**533**

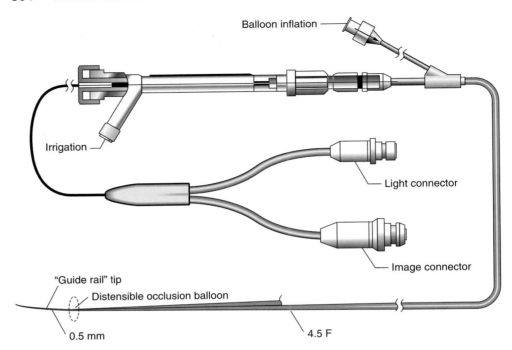

FIGURE 23–1. Baxter-Edwards coronary angioscope.

deflated and the angioscope is pulled back into the guiding catheter.

## EARLY EXPERIENCE

Spears and colleagues first described the use of a fiberoptic endoscope to examine the coronary vasculature in arrested human hearts during coronary artery bypass surgery in 1983.[1] Two years later, this group described the first percutaneous coronary angioscopic procedure during cardiac catheterization.[2] Their initial experience, however, was fraught with difficulties, including geometric distortion of the image, nonlinearities of magnification in light reflex, and lack of adequate angulation of the catheter. With improvement in catheter design, however, subsequent reports by several investigators demonstrated good visualization without major complication.[3–7] Although these initial studies focused on comparison of angioscopic with angiographic findings, it was readily apparent that angioscopy was superior in its ability to detect thrombus, ulceration, and intimal disruption, which were not seen on angiography. In 1989, Ramee and associates reported on the use of percutaneous angioscopy during angioplasty and concluded that high-resolution angioscopy could be performed safely during elective coronary intervention.[6]

Because of the rapidly increasing use of the coronary angioscope as an important diagnostic and scientific tool in interventional cardiology, an angioscopy working team was formed in 1992 in order to create a classification system for angioscopic observations and to evaluate intraobserver and interobserver agreements. In 1994, den Heijer and coworkers reported on the "Ermenonville" classification system.[8] This system divided angioscopic findings into two categories: descriptive items and diagnostic items. Descriptive items included the image quality, the obtained image of the target, the lumen diameter, the shape of the narrowing, the vessel surface description, and the colors of the surface. Diagnostic items included atheroma, dissection, red thrombus, white thrombus, and a mixture of red and white (pink) thrombus. This group found that the intraobserver agreement was satisfactory (kappa statistic ranged from 0.40 to 0.70) but interobserver agreement was poor (kappa statistic ranged from 0.13 to 0.29); for important items, such as red thrombus or dissection, there was good interobserver agreement. Other angioscopic diagnoses, however, should be made with caution.

## CLINICAL APPLICATIONS OF ANGIOSCOPY

### Angioscopy as an Adjunct to Angiography

Despite selective coronary angiography's remaining the "gold standard" for imaging coronary arteries, there are apparent limitations of angiography that are based on the inherent constraint of imaging a three-dimensional structure in two dimensions (Table 23–2). After visual estimation, quantitative coronary angiography is the method most commonly used to assess stenosis severity. This method is

**TABLE 23–2.    CLINICAL APPLICATIONS OF ANGIOSCOPY**

Adjunct to angiography
Detection of intimal dissection
Detection of thrombus
Evaluation of complex plaque
Choice of interventional modality
Assessment of degeneration in vein grafts
Detection of plaque in angiographically "normal" segments

flawed, however, in its ability to assess cross-sectional area from a two-dimensional image. Lee and associates demonstrated the usefulness of angioscopy in providing a topographic view and a quantitative cross-sectional picture of the stenosis that was not observed angiographically.[9] By obtaining a straight, coaxial close-up end-view of the obstruction, luminal cross-sectional area can be measured directly on the basis of the standard relation between the distance from the object to the distal lens of the angioscope and the cross-sectional field of view. With this quantitative technique, angioscopic measurements of cross-sectional stenotic lumina correlate well ($r = 0.90$, $p < 0.001$) with calculations of angiographic lumen narrowings.

Angiography is further limited by its ability to assess complex plaque morphology, intimal disruption, and the presence of thrombus. Meany and associates reported on a series of patients undergoing coronary interventional procedures with adjunctive angioscopy.[10] Angioscopy was more sensitive than angiography in detecting complex plaque morphology both before (31% vs. 8%) and after intervention (39% vs. 22%). Thrombus was the most common unexpected finding before intervention (16%), and intimal disruption was the most common unexpected finding after intervention (31%). These findings were corroborated by other investigators, who found that thrombi and intimal disruption were frequently observed through angioscopy despite a smooth wall appearance seen on angiography.[11]

Using angioscopy as the gold standard, den Heijer and coworkers evaluated the sensitivity and specificity of angiography for the detection of thrombus and dissection.[12] In a series of 52 patients, results of angiography and angioscopy were in agreement in 40% of cases in the absence of thrombus and in 11% of cases in the presence of thrombus. In nearly half of the patients with angioscopically observed thrombi, the thrombi were undetected by angiography. Using angioscopy as the standard, den Heijer and coworkers found the specificity of angiography for thrombus to be 100%; However, the sensitivity was very low, at 19%. Coronary angiography consistently underestimated the presence of intracoronary thrombus. Dissection was detected in 76% of pa-

tients by angioscopy but in only 28% by angiography. With regard to dissection, no correlation was appreciated between the two imaging methods. Rather, it appeared that angioscopy and angiography were complimentary techniques for detecting and grading intimal dissection.

Angiographic detection and characterization of intraluminal filling defects appear to be limited by the size of the defect. Uretsky and colleagues evaluated the sensitivity and specificity of coronary angiography in detecting intraluminal filling defects of varying sizes and characterizing the contents (i.e., thrombus, intimal flap, or both) of such defects, using coronary angioscopy as the gold standard.[13] Again, the overall angiographic sensitivity was poor for thrombus (37%) and for intimal flap (45%), but specificity was high (100% and 96%, respectively). Angioscopically small thrombi were seen less often angiographically (30% of lesions) than were larger ones (75%). Likewise, angioscopically smaller flaps were seen angiographically only 28% of the time, but larger flaps were appreciated 65% of the time by angiography. Angiographic characterizations of filling defects was correct in only 37% of the sites analyzed. This demonstrates that angiography is relatively insensitive in detecting smaller intraluminal filling defects and that angioscopy may be superior in this setting.

Such limitations argue that angiographically normal-appearing coronary segments may not necessarily be free of disease. Alfonso and associates examined 45 patients undergoing coronary angioplasty whose coronary segments appeared normal on angiography proximal to the site of the target lesion.[14] On the basis of angioscopic investigation of these "normal" segments, it was found that these segments were indeed normal angioscopically in only 33% of these patients, whereas 42% of the patients had evidence of plaque, 11% had evidence of thrombus, 9% had evidence of thrombus and plaque, and 4% had evidence of intimal flap. In these patients, angioscopy was performed before angiography in order to avoid any potential abnormalities induced by the angioscope itself. Hence, it cannot be assumed that angiographically "normal" segments are not diseased, particularly in the setting of adjacent disease.

## Detection of Intimal Dissection and Thrombus

On the basis of the earlier experience in the use of intracoronary angioscopy, it quickly became apparent that angioscopy was superior to angiography particularly for the detection of thrombus, as well as for intimal dissection. These clinical findings were confirmed histologically by Johnson and coworkers, who performed angioscopy in the canine model after forceps crush injury, thrombin injection, thrombectomy, and thrombolysis.[15] All arteries were then subjected to angioscopy and cineangiography. Final histologic assessment showed that subintimal flaps or thrombi were present in all cases. Angioscopy detected subintimal dissection in 96% of arteries, whereas cineangiography did not demonstrate flaps in any artery. By angioscopy, thrombus was detected in 100% of observations, whereas only 33% were appreciated by angiography. This simple model provided histologic proof of the superiority of angioscopy over angiography for detection of subintimal dissection and thrombus.

Ramee and associates reported on a series of patients undergoing angioplasty in which a comparison was made among angiography, angioscopy, and ultrasonography for the evaluation of thrombus and dissection.[16] Thrombi were identified in 67% of the patients by angioscopy but in none by angiography or ultrasonography. Likewise, angioscopy was more sensitive than either ultrasonography or angiography for detecting dissection after percutaneous transluminal coronary angioplasty (PTCA). All three diagnostic methods accurately identified atherosclerotic plaque; however, only angioscopy was able to show surface features, pigmentation of lesions, and thrombus. Multiple other studies have confirmed the high specificity but relatively low sensitivity of angiography for detection of thrombus when angioscopy is used as the gold standard[12, 13, 15, 17–19] (Table 23–3).

In an interesting study, Waxman and coworkers used angioscopy to characterize the culprit lesion underlying thrombus.[20, 21] Using coronary angioscopy before PTCA, they imaged the culprit lesion in 69 patients with various coronary syndromes, including stable angina and unstable angina, and after myocardial infarction and correlated the presence or absence of thrombus with plaque color and disruption. Plaques were classified as yellow if all or part of the visible plaque was yellow and as white if the totality of the plaque appeared white. Intracoronary thrombus was likely to be found when the underlying plaque appeared yellow and disrupted angioscopically. White, nondisrupted lesions were infrequently associated with thrombus. These data supported the in vitro observation that lipid-rich plaques may be highly thrombogenic.

## Unstable Angina

As the clinical superiority of angioscopy for the detection of thrombus became more apparent, angioscopy became a valuable research tool for the characterization of acute ischemic syndromes.[22] Perhaps one of the most significant early studies with coronary angioscopy in patients with unstable angina was that published by Sherman and associates in 1986.[23] In this study, fiberoptic angioscopy was used to visualize intracoronary lesions during coronary artery bypass surgery in patients with unstable angina and in patients with stable coronary disease. On angioscopy, none of the arteries in patients with stable coronary disease appeared to have either a complex plaque or thrombus. Alternatively, of the patients with unstable angina, all patients with at-rest angina had thrombi in the culprit vessels, and all patients with accelerated angina had evidence of complex plaque. These landmark observations provided the first in vivo evidence that unstable anginal syndromes were associated with plaque ulceration and that the syndrome of unstable angina at rest was related to the presence of partially occlusive thrombus.

Such observations led Mizuno and colleagues to pursue additional investigation to evaluate the nature of thrombus present in unstable anginal syndromes versus acute myocardial infarction.[24] In 1991, they reported on a series of 84 patients, of whom 14 had acute myocardial infarction and 10 had an unstable anginal syndrome. The remainder of these patients had had recent or nonrecent myocardial infarctions or stable angina. Thrombi were present in most patients with acute coronary syndromes (in all 14 with acute myocardial infarction and in 9 of 10 with unstable angina). Occlusive thrombi were more common in patients with acute myocardial infarction than in those with unstable angina (79% vs. 10%; $p < 0.001$). In contrast, mural thrombi were more common in patients with unstable angina than in those with acute myocardial infarction (80% vs. 21%; $p < 0.001$). Xanthomatous plaques were more common in patients with acute coronary disorders (50%) than in those with stable angina (15%) or those who had had nonrecent myocardial infarction (8%). Conversely, white smooth plaques were seen in patients with stable angina and nonrecent myocardial infarction. These findings reinforced the hypothesis that thrombus overlying a rupture in the lining of the plaque was common in both unstable angina and acute myocardial infarction, that the character of the thrombus could

**TABLE 23–3.   ANGIOGRAPHY FOR THE DETECTION OF THROMBUS USING ANGIOSCOPY AS "GOLD STANDARD"**

| SERIES | N | SENSITIVITY (%) | SPECIFICITY (%) |
|---|---|---|---|
| den Heijer et al[12] | 52 | 19 | 100 |
| Uretsky et al[13] | 40 | 37 | 100 |
| Johnson et al[15] | 15 | 33 | 100 |
| Teirstein et al[18] | 75 | 21 | 94 |
| McFadden et al[19] | 202 | 52 | 89 |

differ between these disorders, and that lipid-rich xanthomatous plaque could precede plaque rupture.

In an effort to further characterize the type of thrombus present in patients with acute coronary syndromes, the same group of investigators examined 31 patients, of whom 15 had unstable angina and 16 had acute myocardial infarction.[25] In the unstable angina population, all imaging was performed within 48 hours after an episode of pain at rest; in patients with acute myocardial infarction, imaging was performed within 8 hours of onset. Coronary thrombi were present in 94% of patients. Of the patients with thrombi, those with unstable angina were frequently observed to have grayish-white thrombi (71%), which were not seen in the patients with acute myocardial infarction. In contrast, reddish thrombi were observed in all patients with acute myocardial infarction who had thrombi present but in only 29% of the patients with unstable angina and thrombi ($p < 0.01$). It was presumed that these differences in color of thrombus probably reflect differences in the composition of the thrombus, which were perhaps related to differences in age of the thrombi or the presence or absence of blood flow in the artery. Pathologic studies have shown that white thrombi are rich in platelets, whereas red thrombi contain an abundance of fibrin mixed with erythrocytes and platelets. Furthermore, when observed after thrombolysis, the white thrombi were found to be older than red thrombi and had a tight fibrin network. Because of the nature of this study, histologic examination of the coronary thrombi could not be performed; however, the investigators hypothesized that the composition of the grayish-white thrombi does in fact differ from that of the red thrombi.

In view of insights provided by angioscopy with regard to the nature of the plaques as well as of thrombi present in acute coronary syndromes, Uchida and colleagues performed a 12-month prospective follow-up study of patients with stable angina pectoris in whom coronary plaques were observed by percutaneous coronary angioscopy, in order to predict the development of such syndromes.[26] These investigators found that acute coronary syndromes occurred more frequently in patients with yellow plaques than in those with white plaques (28% vs. 3%; $p < 0.001$). In addition, these syndromes occurred more frequently in patients with "glistening yellow plaques" than in those with "nonglistening yellow plaques" (69% vs. 8%; $p < 0.001$). Thrombi that arose from the ruptured plaques were confirmed by angioscopy as the culprit lesions of the syndrome. Uchida and colleagues concluded that acute coronary syndromes occur frequently and in a short time frame in patients with glistening yellow plaques and that the use of angioscopy for prediction of such syndromes is feasible.

In a related study, de Feyter and associates performed angiography, angioscopy, and ultrasonography to characterize ischemia-related lesions in patients with stable or unstable angina.[27] Angiographic images were classified as either noncomplex (smooth borders) or complex (irregular borders, multiple lesions, thrombus). An angiographically complex lesion was concordant with unstable angina in 55% of patients, and a noncomplex lesion was concordant with stable angina in 61% of patients. Angioscopic images were classified as either stable (smooth surface) or thrombotic (red thrombus), with strong correlation between the clinical status and the angioscopic findings. An angioscopically thrombotic lesion was concordant with unstable angina in 68% of cases, whereas a stable lesion (i.e., nonthrombotic) was concordant with stable angina in 83% of cases. Ultrasonic characteristics of a lesion, classified as either poorly echoreflective or highly echoreflective, with shadowing or without shadowing, were similar in patients with unstable and stable angina. In summary, angiography and ultrasonography poorly discriminated between lesions in unstable and stable angina. In contrast, angioscopy determined that plaque thrombosis and rupture were present in 17% of patients with stable angina and 68% of patients with unstable angina.

Silva and colleagues used angioscopic findings to evaluate plaque characteristics and the incidence of intracoronary thrombus in patients with diabetes mellitus and unstable angina in comparison with nondiabetic patients with unstable angina.[28] In 55 consecutive patients with unstable angina, 17 of whom were diabetic and 38 of whom were nondiabetic, angioscopy was performed to observe plaque color and texture and the incidence of intracoronary thrombus associated with the culprit lesions of these patients. Ulcerated plaque was present in 94% of the diabetic patients, in contrast to 60% of the nondiabetic patients ($p = 0.01$); intracoronary thrombi were seen in 94% of diabetic patients, in contrast to only 55% of the nondiabetic patients ($p = 0.004$). Hence, diabetic patients with unstable angina have a higher incidence of plaque ulceration and intracoronary thrombus than do nondiabetic patients who had unstable angina, This observation is consistent with the findings that diabetic patients have a disproportionally higher risk for develop of acute coronary syndromes.

## Angioscopy in Acute Myocardial Infarction

The morphology of culprit lesions in acute myocardial infarction has previously been characterized by coronary angiography as well as postmortem histologic examination. Myocardial infarction has been regarded as occurring after plaque disruption and subsequent thrombus formation. With the ability to directly image such culprit lesions by means of the intracoronary angioscope, further insights about the pathogenesis of an acute myocardial infarction can be gleaned. In an attempt to elucidate the composition of thrombus in acute myocardial infarction, Ueda and coworkers performed angioscopic observations of the culprit lesion in patients with acute myocardial infarction.[29] These observations were performed immediately after reperfusion and at 1-month follow-up. Yellow plaque was observed in all patients, both immediately after reperfusion and at 1-month follow-up. Red thrombi were appreciated in 30% and white thrombi in 100% of patients immediately after reperfusion. At 1-month follow-up, red thrombi were observed in 10% and white thrombi in 60%. Intimal flaps were seen in approximately 50% of patients immediately after reperfusion and at 1-month follow-up. During acute myocardial infarction, thrombi were always recognized as formed over yellow plaque. The thrombi that formed directly over the plaque were mainly white thrombi; however, red thrombi might represent thrombi formed after blood flow was obstructed by white thrombi. Of note, at 1-month after infarction, yellow plaques remained in all patients, and over 50% of patients still had evidence of adherent white thrombi.

In a related study, Tabata and associates attempted to characterize coronary thrombi present in patients with postinfarction angina.[30] Fifty-one consecutive patients with the diagnosis of acute myocardial infarction underwent coronary angiography, followed immediately by coronary angioscopy. Of these patients, 17 had postinfarction angina and 34 were without postinfarction angina. The frequency of thrombi as observed by angioscopy was significantly higher in patients with postinfarction angina (100% vs. 15%; $p < 0.01$). No differences were appreciated between the groups with regard to severity of stenosis, multivessel disease, presence of collateral flow, or type of therapy for acute myocardial infarction. Tabata and associates concluded that thrombi are universally present in patients with postinfarction angina.

## ANGIOSCOPY AS AN ADJUNCT TO PTCA

### Balloon Angioplasty

The foregoing discussion demonstrates the importance of angioscopy in the diagnosis of thrombi and complex plaque morphology. To be clinically applicable, however, angioscopy must serve as a useful adjunct to coronary intervention. Much of what is understood about the mechanism of angioplasty has been based on animal studies and human cadaver studies. Significantly less is known about the patho-

physiology of balloon angioplasty in living humans. Several investigators have reported on the feasibility of performing percutaneous coronary angioscopy during coronary angioplasty. One of the earliest reports was by Ramee and associates in 1989.[6] A subsequent larger series from the same group of investigators demonstrated that in patients presenting with stable angina, no thrombus or dissection was seen by angiography or angioscopy before angioplasty. However, in patients with unstable angina, thrombi were detected more frequently by angioscopy both before and after angioplasty.[31] In addition, intimal dissection was also much more frequently seen by angioscopy than by angiography both before and after angioplasty.

In an elegant study published in 1994 by den Heijer and coworkers, serial angioscopic and angiographic observations were performed at 15-minute intervals for up to 60 minutes after balloon angioplasty of a single discrete lesion in a series of 13 patients.[32] Angioscopic findings were classified by the following items: estimated lumen diameter, dissection, thrombus, and color of thrombus. In summary, the interval angiograms that were performed revealed no signs of dissection, although they generally showed some haziness. Only a decrease in mean luminal diameter and an increase in the percentage of stenosis could be demonstrated after 1 hour with quantitative coronary angiography. Conversely, with coronary angioscopy, dramatic signs of vascular wall damage, intimal disruption, and thrombus could be demonstrated. Angioscopic grading of surface disruptions (dissection) increased at each subsequent 15-minute interval, so that large-surface disruptions were present with increasing frequency (from 7.5% immediately after angioplasty to 61.5% at 1 hour). Progressive intracoronary thrombus formation was also observed with increased frequency over the 15-minute intervals after PTCA. Initially, small red mural thrombi were observed immediately after balloon angioplasty; progression in the total amount of observed thrombi was attributable to the emergence of white thrombi and mixed red and white thrombi during the first hour after PTCA. It could be argued that thrombus formation may have been caused by the unusual situation of a guide wire in the artery for such a long period time after balloon angioplasty; however, these thrombi were observed developing only on the vessel wall and not on the guide wire itself. It was speculated that such a thrombotic progress that is too microscopic for angiographic detection could potentially continue for hours or days after PTCA; such a process supports a role for thrombus in restenosis.

Not only was there increasing interest in using the angioscope to predict the development of thrombus, but several operators began using angioscopic evaluation to understand the mechanism of abrupt closure. In 1993, Sassower and colleagues performed angioscopic evaluation in patients who suffered periprocedural and postprocedural abrupt closure.[33] In the case of periprocedural abrupt closure, it was demonstrated that plaque disruption with luminal encroachment of the plaque components was the inciting culprit. In postprocedural abrupt closure, however, the major component of luminal obstruction was a whitish mass consistent with platelet thrombus propagated at the site of an intimal flap.

Such insights into the mechanism of standard balloon angioplasty prompted one group of investigators to compare angioscopic findings using different balloon inflation techniques.[31] In 1995, Cribier and coauthors reported on a series of patients with chronic stable angina who were randomly assigned to undergo either prolonged sequential balloon inflations of 3 to 5 minutes or standard sequential inflations of less than 1 minute each.[34] Percutaneous coronary angioscopy performed immediately after the procedure demonstrated that intimal flaps were seen more commonly in patients who received the standard sequential inflations than in those who received the prolonged inflations (67% vs. 30%; $p < 0.02$). On the basis of den Heijer's study,[32] in which a progression in the severity of small intimal flaps was observed over a period of an hour after angioplasty, it was implied that there may be an advantage of preventing such flaps by using prolonged balloon inflations during PTCA.

Just as the finding of intimal flap progression raised concerns among investigators after balloon angioplasty, so too did the presence of thrombus. White and coworkers set out to determine the clinical importance of thrombi detectable by angioscopy after PTCA.[35] These investigators performed coronary angioscopy in 122 patients undergoing conventional balloon angioplasty at six centers. Unstable angina was present in 78% of the patients. Coronary thrombi were identified in 61% of target lesions by angioscopy but in only 20% by angiography. In this series, major in-hospital complications (i.e., death, myocardial infarction, or need for emergency coronary artery bypass grafting [CABG]) occurred in 14% of patients with angioscopic intracoronary thrombi, in comparison with only 2% of those without thrombi ($p = 0.03$). In-hospital recurrent ischemia, defined as recurrent angina, the need for repeat PTCA, or abrupt occlusion, occurred in 26% of patients with angioscopic intracoronary thrombi, as opposed to only 10% without thrombi ($p = 0.03$). Relative risk analysis demonstrated that the development of angioscopic thrombi was strongly associated with adverse outcome after PTCA and that angiographic filling defects were not associated with these complications.

In order to elucidate the angioscopic findings in totally occluded vessels before and after percutaneous intervention, Alfonso and associates observed 21 consecutive patients undergoing dilation of an occluded vessel by means of coronary angioplasty.[36] In all patients, angioscopy revealed protruding material occluding the coronary lumen where the guide wire was positioned. This material consisted of red thrombi in 90% of the patients and yellow thrombi in 10%. These thrombi were not appreciated by angiography in the majority of patients. After successful dilation, angioscopy was repeated and revealed that 89% of patients had residual thrombi with plaque, and 72% of patients had coronary dissection. Angiography revealed thrombi in only 10% and dissection in only 55% ($p > 0.001$). Hence, an occlusive plaque with thrombus is the most common underlying substrate in occluded coronary vessels, and after successful dilation of this substrate, angiographically silent mural thrombi are still present in most patients.

## Atherectomy

As angioscopy helped to elucidate the mechanism of balloon angioplasty and revealed findings such as the progression of intimal flaps after the procedure, interest developed in elucidating the mechanism of alternative interventional modalities, particularly atherectomy. In most studies evaluating the mechanism of directional atherectomy, intravascular ultrasonography is the primary imaging modality. In one study, Umans and colleagues used angiography, intravascular ultrasonography, and intracoronary angioscopy before and after directional atherectomy, in order to characterize the postatherectomy appearance of the vessel wall contours and the mechanism of lumen enlargement.[37] In this series, patients were investigated by means of quantitative angiography, intravascular ultrasonography, and intracoronary angioscopy before and after atherectomy. It was found that luminal area gain resulted primarily from plaque removal. Intravascular ultrasonography revealed that the atherotome caused a "bite," or crevice, in 85% of the cases, and this finding was corroborated by angioscopy in 74%. As was also evident in this study, both angiography and ultrasound imaging were insensitive to the presence of dissection and new thrombi (10% and 12%, respectively), in comparison with angioscopy (26%). Ultrasonography and angioscopy provided complementary information into the mechanism of directional atherectomy. In particular, Umans and colleagues noted that the postatherectomy luminal lining was not as regular and smooth as suggested by angiography. Although ultrasonography may be useful for guiding atherectomy procedures, angioscopy appears to be more sensitive for the detection of dissection and thrombi.

Rotational atherectomy has gained popularity since 1990, with application particularly in the setting of calcified lesions. Because of the increased risk of distal embolization and no-reflow in the setting of thrombi, rotational atherectomy is generally considered contraindicated with such a lesion. It has previously been suggested in this chapter that adjunctive angioscopy may be used to identify the presence of thrombi and, therefore, minimize such complications. Little has been published on the use of adjunctive angioscopy and rotational atherectomy; however, Eltchaninoff and coworkers used angioscopy in a randomized study of 43 patients with stable angina.[38] The 45 lesions were randomly assigned to treatment with either rotational atherectomy or balloon angioplasty. Angioscopy was performed immediately after each procedure, with particular attention to the presence of flaps, thrombi, and subintimal hemorrhage. Despite compatible angiographic findings in the two groups, angioscopy revealed that flaps were less frequently observed and were less severe in the patients treated with rotational atherectomy (26%) than in those treated with balloon angioplasty (59%). No difference was found in the incidence of angioscopic thrombi or subintimal hemorrhage between the two groups. These findings suggested that rotational atherectomy resulted in less frequent and less severe intraluminal abnormalities than did balloon angioplasty.

## Laser Angioplasty

As interest arose in understanding the mechanism of various interventional techniques, several investigators also became interested in the mechanism of laser angioplasty. In 1992, Nakamura and associates demonstrated that after excimer laser angioplasty, the characteristic angioscopic findings were flaps, fractures of plaques, and abundant tissue remnants.[39] There was no apparent thermal injury to the vessel. The recanalized channels, however, were found to be small and irregular. Nakamura and associates suggested that irregular channels with the presence of abundant tissue remmants may explain the suboptimal results found after laser angioplasty. In a similar study, Itoh and coworkers, using the holmium–yttrium-aluminum-garnet (YAG) laser, revealed similar intimal disruption after laser angioplasty.[40] In 1994, Larrazet and colleagues reported on a series of 44 patients undergoing angioscopy before and after coronary intervention.[41] Balloon angioplasty was performed in 21 patients, and laser angioplasty was performed in the other 23. Tissue remnants were appreciated in all patients after the procedure. More dissections, however, were found in the patients who had undergone balloon angioplasty (47%) than in those who had undergone laser angioplasty (17%). Likewise, subintimal hemor-

rhage was observed more frequently after balloon angioplasty (58%) than after laser angioplasty (17%). On the basis of these findings, Larrazet and colleagues concluded that laser angioplasty resulted in a lower rate of subintimal hemorrhage than did balloon dilation.

## Stent Implantation

One of the earliest reports of angioscopy as an adjunct to coronary stent implantation was published in 1992 by Teirstein and associates.[42] Eight patients underwent stent implantation in native coronary arteries and three in saphenous vein graft lesions. This brief report highlighted some very interesting findings in these early days of stent implantation. The authors found that the stent struts were uniformly expanded, and some of the struts were embedded deep into the intima. Luminal diameter was significantly increased in all the regions with stents except at the stent articulation sites, where stenotic segments bulged into the lumen. Despite attempts to further expand the articulation site with larger balloons, the angioscopic appearance did not improve. Mural tears that were visualized after balloon angioplasty were absent after stent implantation. In saphenous vein grafts, such tears were markedly reduced after stent implantation; or occasion, tissue flaps protruded through the stent into the lumen, or tissue bulged through the diamond-shaped strut spaces, producing a cobblestone appearance. Teirstein and associates used the angioscopic finding of thrombus in one patient to pretreat the patient with a urokinase infusion before stent implantation. Despite the small number of patients in this study, the authors found that (1) thrombus could be treated before stent implantation, (2) stents "tacked up" mural tears, (3) stent struts were occasionally damaged, and (4) persistent stenosis at the articulation site suggested the need for modification in stent design.

In a larger series, Strumpf and coauthors reported on 17 patients undergoing stent implantation.[43] These investigators observed similar results with the Palmar-Schatz stent, as well as with the Strecker stent, in their ability to repair mural tears and "tack up" most tissue flaps. They also reported delicate fronds of tissue, observed infrequently either distal or proximal to the stents, that were not detected by angiography. In addition, angioscopy was useful in detecting pre-stent thrombi, which occurred in 13% of these patients and were successfully treated with urokinase infusion. Of these patients, 2 were reevaluated with angioscopy for in-stent restenosis; under direct visualization, they documented the presence of atheromatous material, which suggested that stent restenosis is caused by tissue overgrowth and not by stent compression. The authors concluded that angioscopy could be safely and successfully performed both in stents placed in native coronary arteries and in stents placed in saphenous vein grafts, providing otherwise unavailable luminal data to (1) guide lesion selection for stenting, (2) monitor initial implantation for optimal deployment, and (3) evaluate the causes of restenosis during follow-up. Angioscopy was particularly valuable in discerning dissection and thrombi that could predispose to early stent failure. On the basis of the angioscopic information obtained, treatment strategies were altered for 53% of these patients.

Angioscopy has been used to determine the time course of neointimal coverage of stents in human coronary arteries.[44] In one study, serial angioscopic observations were performed immediately after, 8 to 45 days after (short-term follow-up), and 65 to 142 days after stent placement (long-term follow-up). Immediately, and even 8 to 18 days after stent placement, the stent was not covered by a neointimal layer. However, by 65 to 142 days after stent placement, the stent was covered by a neointimal layer in all cases. Angioscopically, three types of neointimal layer were appreciated: a white layer with a cotton-like surface, a white layer with a smooth surface, and a transparent layer. This finding suggested that neointimal coverage of stents in human coronary arteries required approximately 3 months. More recently, Asakura and colleagues reported longer term follow-up on the neointima covering stents.[45] They monitored patients with both angioscopy and angiography 1 month, 6 months, and 3 years after implantation of the stents and noted that in the initial 6-month period, the neointimal coverage was either transparent or nontransparent. Mean luminal diameter was noted by quantitative angiography to be smallest at 6 months, with a tendency to be larger at 3 years. The transparent coverage over the stents was not observed angioscopically in any patient at 6 months, but it was observed in 88% of patients at 3 years. Hence, the neointimal coverage over the stent became thick and nontransparent at 6 months and then thinner and transparent 3 years after implantation, which suggests that the proliferative response peaks during the 6-month period after stent implantation and subsequently diminishes.

In a larger series, Teirstein and associates reported on the utility of adjunctive angioscopy in the setting of intracoronary stent placement.[46] They found that the use of angioscopy influenced the clinical management of 38% of patients.[46] Decisions that were directly influenced by the use of angioscopy included intracoronary thrombolytic therapy for thrombi visualized angioscopically but not angiographically; withholding intracoronary thrombolytic therapy for patients with suspected thrombi that were not confirmed by angioscopy; repeat angioplasty in patients in whom the plaque was found

to be bulging into the lumen at the articulation site; and placement of an additional stent when angioscopy revealed significant proximal or distal disease or an unsuspected gap between two tandem stents.

## SPECIAL CONSIDERATIONS

### Saphenous Vein Graft Interventions

The percutaneous treatment of saphenous vein graft disease has long been one of the most challenging problems in the field of interventional cardiology. The risks of periprocedural complications, long-term development of restenosis, and need for revascularization are increased in vein grafts in comparison with native coronary arteries. Although no large-scale studies have addressed the use or potential benefits of adjunctive angioscopy in saphenous vein graft interventions, my institution has found angioscopy highly useful in developing a therapeutic strategy for treatment of vein grafts.

In 1993, White and coauthors published the results of percutaneous angioscopy and angiography for detecting critical elements of surface lesion morphology in 21 patients undergoing balloon angioplasty of saphenous vein bypass grafts.[47] All patients underwent angioscopy and angiography before and after angioplasty of what was deemed the culprit lesion in bypass grafts. The majority of these patients had unstable angina, and the mean age of these grafts was approximately 10 years. As with findings in native coronary arteries, these investigators found that intravascular thrombi were seen more frequently by angioscopy (71%) than by angiography (19%; $p < 0.001$). Likewise, dissection was identified in 66% of patients by angioscopy, in comparison with only 9.5% by angiography ($p < 0.01$). A new finding reported by this group was that friable plaque lining the lumen surface of the vein graft was detected in 52% of patients by angioscopy but in only 19% by angiography ($p < 0.05$). No correlation was found between the age of the saphenous vein graft and the finding of friable plaque.

Annex and associates reported on the use of percutaneous coronary angioscopy to evaluate the extent of thrombus removal by transluminal extraction catheter (TEC) coronary atherectomy.[48, 49] This group reported on a series of 14 consecutive patients undergoing TEC atherectomy, 10 of whom underwent the procedure in saphenous vein grafts. Using adjunctive angioscopy, the authors were able to identify thrombi in 86% of these lesions. Angioscopy confirmed thrombus removal in 75% of those lesions after treatment with TEC atherectomy. In contrast, angiography was of limited value both before and after TEC atherectomy in correctly identifying intraluminal thrombi. This study prompted Kaplan

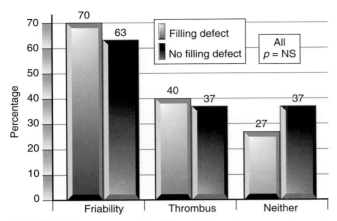

FIGURE 23–2. Angiographic filling defects versus angioscopic findings.

and colleagues to investigate the usefulness of adjunctive angioscopy and TEC atherectomy before stent implantation in saphenous vein grafts.[50] In a series of 20 saphenous vein graft lesions, selected on the basis of high clinical or angiographic suspicion of thrombus and the suitability for stenting, all lesions were subjected to initial angioscopy. If angioscopy demonstrated thrombi, TEC atherectomy was performed before stent implantation. Angioscopy was repeated after TEC atherectomy to assess the degree of thrombus removal. If no thrombus was apparent on initial angioscopy, stent implantation was performed without prior TEC. Through this strategy, complete or partial removal of thrombi was achieved in all patients with preprocedural thrombi. In all lesions with preprocedural thrombus, stent implantation was successful after TEC atherectomy. On the basis of this study, it was recommended that before stent placement in high-risk vein grafts in coronary lesions, angioscopy should be performed carefully to document the presence of thrombus. If no thrombus is identified, stent placement appears to be a reasonable approach without atherectomy because the risk of distal embolization and no-reflow are low. Finally, stent implantation in lesions

with thrombi may be feasible if thrombus removal can first be achieved by TEC atherectomy.

One important finding of Kaplan and colleagues was the suggestion that loose intraluminal debris may be a marker for the development of sustained no-reflow in saphenous vein graft interventions. This prompted me and my colleagues to examine whether the angioscopic appearance of plaque can predict in which grafts atheroembolism and no-reflow are more likely to occur. We examined a series of 33 patients undergoing angioscopy before saphenous vein graft interventions.[51] Angioscopic images were evaluated with special attention to the presence of thrombus, dissection, and plaque friability. All angiographic images were evaluated and graded for the presence or absence of filling defects, the development of transient or sustained no-reflow, and the presence of distal embolization. We discovered that the presence of an angioscopic filling defect did not adequately predict thrombus or plaque friability (Fig. 23–2). Therefore, an angiographic finding defect cannot be assumed to be thrombus. We evaluated the development of no-reflow on the basis of angioscopic findings and found no correlation between the presence of thrombus and the development of transient or sustained no-reflow (Fig. 23–3). Instead, we found that the presence of plaque friability correlated with the development of sustained or transient no-flow and that with increasing plaque friability, there was a trend toward increasing no-reflow (Fig. 23–4). No-reflow did not develop in any of the patients in whom angioscopy detected no plaque friability. We concluded that angioscopic plaque friability is a potent predictor for the development of transient or sustained no-reflow during percutaneous intervention.

## Restenosis

Multiple studies have demonstrated that clinical factors predispose certain patients to the development of restenosis after percutaneous coronary intervention. In contrast, angiographic characteristics

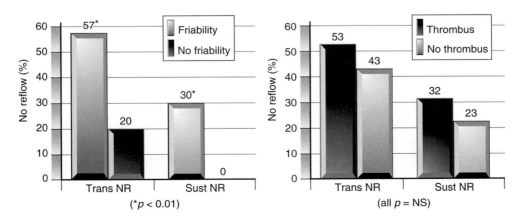

FIGURE 23–3. Angioscopic findings and relationship to no-reflow.

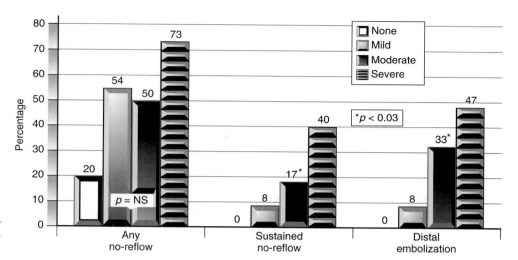

FIGURE 23–4. Plaque friability grade versus procedural complications.

have not been helpful in identifying lesions at high risk of development of restenosis. Discordant results regarding the risk of restenosis after angioplasty for complex lesions have been reported. One study demonstrated that the only angiographic characteristic associated with restenosis was bend location[52]; another study reported that complicated stenosis morphology was a risk factor for restenosis.[53]

Bauters and coauthors suggested that these discrepancies may be related to the limitations of angiography for studying plaque morphology. Therefore, they investigated whether the morphologic characteristics of plaque as assessed by angioscopy were predictive of angiographic restenosis at the 6-month follow-up.[54] They compared the relationship between angioscopic variables at the time of angioplasty and the occurrence of restenosis as assessed by quantitative coronary angiography. There was a trend for high restenosis rates with complex stenoses and with lesions with yellow plaque; however, this trend was not statistically significant. The presence of protruding coronary thrombus, however, was associated with an unfavorable long-term angiographic outcome. Among patients with a protruding thrombus at the PTCA site, restenosis rates were significantly increased (65%) in comparison with mural thrombus (47%) or no thrombus (38%). Despite a high rate of angioscopic dissection (60%), no correlation existed between the occurrence of angioscopically visible dissection and subsequent occurrence of restenosis.

The mechanism by which the presence of intraluminal thrombus might increase the risk of restenosis remains unclear. Results of animal studies have supported a role for the presence of platelet accumulation in determining subsequent neointimal thickening.[55, 56] Other studies have suggested that the volume of intracoronary thrombus at the time of angioplasty may determine subsequent volume of

neointimal formation.[57] This correlation corresponds with the finding that angioplasty performed in an infarction-related lesion is associated with a high rate of total occlusion at follow-up. Plaque morphology, color, or dissection did not portend increased risk of restenosis; only protruding thrombus has been shown to predict subsequent late loss in luminal diameter.

In a more recent study by Guagliumi and coworkers, angioscopic findings before and after stent implantation were analyzed for possible predictors of subsequent stent restenosis.[58] In 90 consecutive patients who underwent successful stent implantation, restenosis—defined by quantitative coronary angiography as a 50% or more reduction in diameter—was not correlated with the presence or absence of yellow plaque, complex plaque, thrombus, or incomplete plaque coverage. The data did indicate that residual plaque protrusion inside the stent was associated with increased angiographic restenosis. A common theme of the studies by Bauters and associates[54] and Guagliumi and colleagues[58] is that protrusion of either thrombus or atheroma into the lumen places patients at increased risk for subsequent restenosis.

## Limitations and Complications

The extent of information that can be gained with angioscopic evaluation of coronary vessels is vast. However, there are limitations inherent in this technique that limit its applicability. Although angioscopy provides a window into the coronary vessels and a wealth of qualitative information, it is difficult to quantitate findings for comparison purposes. At best, angioscopic findings are semiquantitative in nature and have not been useful in the assessment of luminal dimension or flow characteristics. Because of the necessity of a blood-free field, anatomic considerations render angioscopy impossible in certain circumstances. For instance, it is not possible to evaluate either aorto-ostial lesions or lesions in the proximal left anterior descending or circumflex arteries, because of the necessity for transient occlusion of the left main coronary artery. At times, blood flow from adjacent side branches can obscure imaging; therefore, angioscopy is better suited for saphenous vein grafts. Another limitation includes the inability to steer the catheter in angulated or tortuous vessels, which severely limits the field of view.

Inherent risk is associated with the use of a blood-free imaging field; transient occlusion and ischemia are necessary with this imaging modality. Also, injury secondary to use of the occlusion cuff, leading to damage of a potentially normal luminal surface or, in rare cases, perforation, can occur.[59] Advancement of the catheter into the vessel lumen and site of the lesion can likewise damage the arterial intima.[60, 61] The use of a flush solution carries risks of air embolization or, more common, embolization of friable plaque, leading to transient or sustained no-reflow. It has been reported that angioscopy-induced transient or sustained no-reflow can occur in up to 50% of lesions during angioscopy in degenerative saphenous vein grafts.[50] Hence, in the setting in which angioscopy is perhaps most useful, it may be fraught with the most complications. Overall, however, the risk of a serious clinical complication such as death, myocardial infarction, or the need for emergency CABG during this procedure is significantly less than 1%.[21]

## CONCLUSION

Coronary angioscopy provides a view of the coronary architecture that no other available imaging modality can supply. In truth, seeing is believing. Obtained through proper technique, angioscopic images are not vague. Thrombus, dissection, or complex plaque morphology is either present or not. Many of the vagaries seen with angiography can be settled with angioscopic investigation. It is unfortunate, however, that angioscopy has been used primarily as a research tool. Because of the lack of interest from the catheter industry or manufacturers, the lack of enthusiasm to perform the procedure by invasive cardiologists, and the risk, time, and cost factors inherent in the procedure, angioscopy is not routinely performed.

Angioscopy is a technique that is meant not to supplant angiography, intravascular ultrasonography, or Doppler interrogation but rather to complement these modalities. As knowledge of coronary endothelium evolves and an understanding of the mechanisms of coronary intervention, subsequent injury, and healing becomes more complete, angioscopic findings may serve as a more integral tool in developing therapeutic strategies. For instance, the best way to assess thrombus in a coronary vessel is through the use of angioscopy. Likewise, the best way to clearly delineate the characteristics of an angiographic filling defect is to see what the filling defect actually is.

Incredible strides have been achieved in the percutaneous treatment of native coronary artery disease since the early 1980s. Perhaps the last great frontier for the coronary interventionalist is the treatment of saphenous vein graft disease. As a group, these vessels represent the greatest challenge to the interventionalist. It is in this setting that angioscopy will likely serve best. The more information that can be obtained before intervention in these complex vessels, the better prepared interventionalists will be to develop a treatment strategy for minimizing periprocedural complications and optimizing long-term vessel patency.

It is unlikely that angioscopy in its current state will ever become a mainstream imaging modality in clinical practice. It is, however, an important tool for understanding the pathology that is treated on a daily basis and should not be lost from the interventional armory.

## REFERENCES

1. Spears JR, Marais J, Serur J, et al: In vivo coronary angioscopy. J Am Coll Cardiol 5:1311, 1983.
2. Spears JR, Spokojny AM, Marais HJ: Coronary angioscopy during cardiac catheterization. J Am Coll Cardiol 6:93–97, 1985.
3. Uchida Y, Tomaru T, Nakamura F, et al: Percutaneous coronary angioscopy in patients with ischemic heart disease. Am Heart J 114:1216–1222, 1987.
4. Uchida Y: Percutaneous coronary angioscopy by means of a fiberscope with a steerable guidewire. Am Heart J 117:1153–1155, 1989.
5. Mizuno K, Arai T, Satomura K, et al: New percutaneous transluminal coronary angioscope. J Am Coll Cardiol 13:363–368, 1989.
6. Ramee SR, White CJ, McQueen C, et al: Percutaneous coronary angioscopy: Clinical results with a coronary microangioscope. Circulation 80:II-376, 1989.
7. Morice MC, Glatt B, Castillo-Fenoy A, et al: Early clinical results with a new percutaneous coronary angioscope. Circulation 80:II-376, 1989.
8. den Heijer P, Foley DP, Hillege HL, et al: The "Ermenonville" classification of observations at coronary angioscopy—Evaluation of intra- and inter-observer agreement. Eur Heart J 15:815–822, 1994.
9. Lee G, Garcia JM, Corso PJ, et al: Correlation of coronary angioscopic to angiographic findings in coronary artery disease. Am J Cardiol 58:238–241, 1986.
10. Meany TB, Grines CL, Kander NH, et al: Percutaneous coronary angioscopy in the assessment of complex plaque morphology in conjunction with interventional procedures [Abstract]. Eur Heart J 12:99A, 1991.
11. Yanagida S, Mizuno K, Miyamoto A, et al: Comparison of findings between coronary angiography and angioscopy. Circulation 80:II-376, 1989.
12. den Heijer P, Foley DP, Escaned J, et al: Angioscopic versus angiographic detection of intimal dissection and intracoronary thrombus [Abstract]. J Am Coll Cardiol 94:407A, 1994.

13. Uretsky BF, Denys BG, Counihan PC, et al: Angioscopic evaluation of incompletely obstructing coronary intraluminal filling defects: Comparison of angiography. Cathet Cardiovasc Diagn 33:323–329, 1994.

14. Alfonso F, Goicolea J, Hernandez R, et al: Findings of coronary angioscopy in angiographically normal coronary segments of patients with coronary artery disease. Am Heart J 130:987–993, 1995.

15. Johnson C, Hansen D, Vracko R, et al: Angioscopy—more sensitive for identifying thrombus, distal emboli, and subintimal dissection [Abstract]. J Am Coll Cardiol 13:146A, 1989.

16. Ramee SR, White CJ, Jain A, et al: Percutaneous coronary angioscopy versus intravascular ultrasound in patients undergoing coronary angioplasty [Abstract]. J Am Coll Cardiol 17:125A, 1991.

17. den Heijer P, Foley DP, Escaned J, et al: Angioscopic versus angiographic detection of intimal dissection and intracoronary thrombus. J Am Coll Cardiol 24:649–654, 1994.

18. Teirstein PS, Schatz RA, DeNardo SJ, et al: Angioscopic versus angiographic detection of thrombus during coronary interventional procedures. Am J Cardiol 75:1083–1087, 1995.

19. McFadden E, Bauters C, Hamon M, et al: Sensitivity and specificity of angiographic markers for thrombus: A prospective comparison with angioscopy [Abstract]. J Am Coll Cardiol 25:154A, 1995.

20. Waxman S, Sassower M, Mittleman MA, et al: Characterization of the culprit lesion underlying thrombus: Insights from angioscopy. Circulation 92:I-353, 1995.

21. Waxman S, Mittleman MA, Manzo K, et al: Culprit lesion morphology in subtypes of unstable angina as assessed by angioscopy. Circulation 92:I-79, 1995.

22. Forrester JS, Litvack F, Grundfest W, et al: A perspective of coronary disease seen through the arteries of living man. Circulation 75:505–513, 1987.

23. Sherman CT, Litvack F, Grundfest W, et al: Coronary angioscopy in patients with unstable angina pectoris. N Engl J Med 315:913–919, 1986.

24. Mizuno K, Miyamoto A, Satomura K, et al: Angioscopic coronary macromorphology in patients with acute coronary disorders. Lancet 337:809–812, 1991.

25. Mizuno K, Satomura K, Miyamoto A, et al: Angioscopic evaluation of coronary artery thrombi in acute coronary syndromes. N Engl J Med 326:287–291, 1992.

26. Uchida Y, Nakamura F, Tomaru T, et al: Prediction of acute coronary syndromes by percutaneous coronary angioscopy in patients with stable angina. Am Heart J 130:195–203, 1995.

27. de Feyter PJ, Ozaki Y, Baptista J, et al: Ischemia-related lesion characteristics in patients with stable or unstable angina. A study with intracoronary angioscopy and ultrasound. Circulation 92:1408–1413, 1995.

28. Silva JA, Esobar A, Collings TJ, et al: Unstable angina. A comparison of angioscopic findings between diabetic and nondiabetic patients. Circulation 92:1731–1736, 1995.

29. Ueda Y, Asakura M, Hirayama A, et al: Intracoronary morphology of culprit lesions after reperfusion in acute myocardial infarction: Serial angioscopic observations. J Am Coll Cardiol 27:606–610, 1996.

30. Tabata H, Mizuno K, Arakawa K, et al: Angioscopic identification of coronary thrombus in patients with postinfarction angina. J Am Coll Cardiol 25;1282–1285, 1995.

31. Ramee SR, White CH, Collins TJ, et al: Percutaneous angioscopy during coronary angioplasty using a steerable microangioscope. J Am Coll Cardiol 17:100–105, 1991.

32. den Heijer P, van Dijk RB, Hillege HL, et al: Serial angioscopic and angiographic observations during the first hour after successful coronary angioplasty: A preamble to a multicenter trial addressing angioscopic markers for restenosis. Am Heart J 128:656–663, 1994.

33. Sassower MA, Abela GS, Koch JM, et al: Angioscopic evaluation of periprocedural and postprocedural abrupt closure after percutaneous coronary angioplasty. Am Heart J 126:444–450, 1993.

34. Cribier A, Holly N, Eltchaninoff H, et al: Angioscopic evaluation of prolonged vs standard balloon inflations during coronary angioplasty. A randomized study. Eur Heart J 16:930–936, 1995.

35. White CJ, Ramee SR, Collings TJ, et al: Coronary thrombi increase PTCA risk. Angioscopy as a clinical tool. Circulation 93:253–258, 1996.

36. Alfonso F, Goicolea J, Hernandez R, et al: Angioscopic findings during coronary angioplasty of coronary occlusions. J Am Coll Cardiol 26:135–141, 1995.

37. Umans VA, Baptista J, di Mario C, et al: Angiographic, ultrasonic, and angioscopic assessment of the coronary artery wall and lumen area configuration after directional atherectomy: The mechanism revisited. Am Heart J 130:217–227, 1995.

38. Eltchaninoff H, Cribier A, Koning R, et al: Comparative angioscopic findings after rotational atherectomy and balloon angioplasty [Abstract]. J Am Coll Cardiol 25:95A, 1995.

39. Nakamura F, Kvasnicka J, Uchida Y, et al: Percutaneous angioscopic evaluation of luminal changes induced by excimer laser angioplasty. Am Heart J 124:1467–1472, 1992.

40. Itoh A, Miyazaki S, Nonogi H, et al: Angioscopic and intravascular ultrasound imagings before and after percutaneous holmium-YAG laser coronary angioplasty. Am Heart J 125:556–558, 1993.

41. Larrazet FS, Dupouy PJ, Rande JLD, et al: Angioscopy after laser and balloon coronary angioplasty. J Am Coll Cardiol 23:1321–1326, 1994.

42. Teirstein PA, Schatz RA, Rocha-Singh KJ, et al: Coronary stenting with angioscopic guidance [Abstract]. J Am Coll Cardiol 29:223A, 1992.

43. Strumpf RK, Heuser RR, Eagan JT: Angioscopy: A valuable tool in the deployment and evaluation of intracoronary stents. Am Heart J 126:1204–1210, 1993.

44. Ueda Y, Nanto S, Komamura K, et al: Neointimal coverage of stents in human coronary arteries observed by angioscopy. J Am Coll Cardiol 23:341–346, 1994.

45. Asakura M, Ueda Y, Hirayama A, et al: Neointima covering stent became thinner and transparent at 3 years follow-up: Serial angioscopic and angiographic observations. Circulation 94:I-454, 1996.

46. Teirstein PS, Schatz RA, Wong SC, et al: Coronary stenting with angioscopic guidance. Am J Cardiol 75:344–347, 1995.

47. White CJ, Ramee SR, Collins TJ, et al: Percutaneous angioscopy of saphenous vein coronary bypass grafts. J Am Coll Cardiol 21:1181–1185, 1993.

48. Annex BH, Larkin TJ, O'Neill WW, et al: Evaluation of thrombus removal by transluminal extraction coronary atherectomy by percutaneous coronary angioscopy. Am J Cardiol 74:606–609, 1994.

49. Annex BH, Ajluni SC, Larkin TJ, et al: Angioscopic guided interventions in a saphenous vein bypass graft. Cathet Cardiovasc Diagn 31:330–333, 1994.

50. Kaplan BM, Safian RD, Grines CL, et al: Usefulness of adjunctive angioscopy and extraction atherectomy before stent implantation in high-risk aortocoronary saphenous vein grafts. Am J Cardiol 76:822–824, 1995.

51. Tilli FV, Kaplan BM, Safian RD, et al: Angioscopic plaque friability: A new risk factor for procedural complications following saphenous vein graft interventions [Abstract]. J Am Coll Cardiol 27:364A, 1996.

52. Ellis SG, Roubin GS, King SB, et al: Importance of stenosis morphology in the estimation of restenosis risk after elective percutaneous transluminal coronary angioplasty. Am J Cardiol 64:30–34, 1989.

53. Tousoulis D, Kaski JC, Davies G, et al: Preangioplasty complicated coronary stenosis morphology as a predictor of restenosis. Am Heart J 123:15–20, 1992.

54. Bauters C, Lablanche JM, McFadden EP, et al: Relation of coronary angioscopic findings at coronary angioplasty to angiographic restenosis. Circulation 92:2473–2479, 1995.

55. Willerson JT, Yao SK, McNatt J, et al: Frequency and severity of cyclic flow alternations and platelet aggregation predict the severity of neointimal proliferation following experimental coronary stenosis and endothelial injury. Proc Natl Acad Sci U S A 88:10624–10628, 1991.

56. Fingerele J, Johnson R, Clowes AW, et al: Role of platelets in smooth muscle cell proliferation and migration after vascular injury in rat carotid artery. Proc Natl Acad Sci U S A 86:8412–8416, 1989.

57. Schwartz RS, Holmes DR, Topol EJ: The restenosis paradigm revisited: An alternative proposal for cellular mechanisms. J Am Coll Cardiol 20:1284–1293, 1992.

58. Guagliumi G, Tespili M, Valsecchi O, et al: Angioscopic predictors of restenosis in stented coronary vessels [Abstract]. J Am Coll Cardiol 29:77A, 1997.

59. Hamon M, LaBlanche JM, Bauters C, et al: Effect of balloon inflation in angiographically normal coronary segments during coronary angioscopy: A quantitative angiographic study. Cathet Cardiovasc Diagn 31:116–121, 1994.

60. Alfonso F, Hernandez R, Goicolea J, et al: Angiographic deterioration of the previously dilated coronary segment induced by angioscopic examination. Am J Cardiol 74:604–606, 1994.

61. Lee G, Beerline D, Lee MH, et al: Hazards of angioscopic examination: Documentation of damage to the arterial intima. Am Heart H 116:1530–1536, 1988.

# Radial and Brachial Artery–Based Access for Diagnostic and Interventional Procedures

*Steven L. Almany*

## BACKGROUND OF RADIAL ACCESS

The history of radial artery–based intervention appears to date back to 1989, when Campeau performed 100 catheterizations via this approach.[1] He successfully cannulated the coronary arteries in 88 of the patients, although an absent or diminished pulse was documented in 22 patients. The first transradial percutaneous transluminal coronary angioplasty (PTCA) was performed in late 1992 in Amsterdam by Kiemeneij, followed by the first transradial stent in 1993.[2] This type of access has become increasingly popular in many areas of North America and Europe.

## POTENTIAL MARKET FOR RADIAL INTERVENTION

With nearly 850,000 percutaneous coronary interventions and nearly 1.1 million catheterizations being done in the United States alone, the potential market for a superior form of diagnostic and interventional access is large. This does not include the non-U.S. market, which is usually regarded as twice as large. In addition, this type of access is certainly applicable in the field of diagnostic and interventional radiology. The benefits of radial artery–based access lie in the potentially lower direct costs,[3] in patient preference,[4] and in a lower incidence of vascular complications (and their subsequent costs) as well as earlier patient ambulation. Although percutaneous closure devices allow earlier patient ambulation, they are also associated with increased direct costs as well as occasional failure. Collagen devices, though less expensive, often limit access at the same site for weeks or months.

Despite the advantages of radial artery–based access interventions, the incidence of their application has grown slowly in the United States. Such sluggish growth is probably due to physicians' familiarity with the femoral or brachial artery approach and a lack of 6-French–compatible equipment as well as the development of closure devices. However, the development of 6-French–compatible systems, patient preference, and increasing operator experience seem to suggest that more cardiologists and radiologists are willing to learn this procedure.

## BENEFITS

The transfemoral approach for cardiac catheterization and intervention has gained widespread acceptance. Its advantages are well known and include a long history of use and the fact that access is technically easy. In addition, the larger arterial caliber facilitates the use of larger sheaths, catheters, and equipment.[5]

Transfemoral access is plagued, however, with inherent disadvantages. It is the generally accepted practice that patients should remain supine (strict bedrest) for 1 hour for each French sheath size (e.g., 7-French = 7 hours of bedrest).[6] Although closure devices represent a significant technical advancement, they cannot be used in all patients and they are costly. Some devices (e.g., collagen plug–based systems) may prohibit access at the same site for weeks. The incidence of vascular complications, which is reported to be 0.5% to 4.0% (transfusions, fistulas, pseudoaneurysms) with femoral artery–based intervention, is markedly better with radial artery–based access. Femoral artery–based access is more commonly associated with back pain, urinary retention, and neuropathy than is the radial artery approach.[7-9]

The radial artery approach has certain distinct advantages. The dual blood supply (described in length later) limits the potential for limb-threatening ischemia. This benefit is advantageous for patients with severe occlusive aortoiliac disease.[10] Intervention based on radial artery access is desirable for patients with difficulty in lying flat (back pain, obesity, congestive heart failure). The superficial nature of the radial artery makes it easily compressible, and use of this approach is less likely to result in local nerve injury.[11] The radial artery approach allows earlier patient ambulation and will probably cost less, as closure devices are not necessary and interventions can often be accomplished with one guiding catheter. Vascular complications are less frequent.[12] The most important reason for learning the radial artery–based access approach, however, lies in the fact that randomized trials suggest that patients prefer the radial artery approach if they have experienced both a femoral and a radial artery–based intervention.

There are potential disadvantages to a radial approach. The author believes that most of these will be diminished with improved equipment and increasing operator experience.[13, 14] The radial artery is smaller than the femoral artery (approximately 2 to 2.3 mm), which necessitates the use of smaller sheaths, catheters, and interventional devices. Obtaining radial artery access involves a distinct learning curve. Vessel spasm is more common and requires a knowledge of radial artery–based and femoral–based equipment as well as the appropriate adjunctive pharmacologic therapy. Guide catheter placement is more challenging and requires learning new techniques. Many physicians are not familiar with the equipment or the anatomy, or both, and thus are reluctant to try a new approach.[15]

## CONTRAINDICATIONS

Radial artery–based access is not appropriate in all patients. Absolute contraindications include patients who have evidence of an abnormal Allen test result (described later). It has been reported that approximately 10% of the population will have an abnormal Allen test result. The author, in fact, does not advocate the Allen test as the definitive test for assessing the collateral supply of the hand. The author believes that it is quite subjective and questions the reproducibility of the test results. Instead, the author favors the use of oximetry-plethysmography (described later). This modality is thought to be preferable in that it can produce a (legal) record of radial artery competence and is not as subjective

as the Allen test. In addition, the patient can wear a finger oximeter on the hand that is undergoing the intervention, which allows for continuous monitoring of not only overall oxygen saturation but also the integrity of the hand's blood supply. Femoral artery–based intervention should be considered in patients who may require intra-aortic balloon pump counterpulsation (IABP). Patients who may require devices that are not compatible with 7-French or smaller sheaths (transluminal extraction catheter [TEC], larger Rotoblator burs, certain stents) are also better served with femoral artery access. A relatively small subgroup of patients will display significant upper extremity vascular disease. Fewer than 5% of patients will have congenital abnormalities of their upper-extremity arterial system, including extreme tortuosity, anomalous takeoff of the radial artery, and severe atherosclerosis. Radial artery intervention is also contraindicated in patients with Buerger's disease, severe Raynaud's phenomenon, or other forms of upper-extremity peripheral vascular disease.

The relative contraindications include patients with known internal mammary grafts contralateral to the site of entry. It should be noted, however, that catheters specifically designed for internal mammary arteries through a radial or brachial artery contralateral approach are available. Patients in whom the radial artery may be considered as a conduit for coronary artery bypass grafting or for a dialysis graft should be considered for femoral or brachial artery access so as not to damage the potential radial conduit.

## PERTINENT ANATOMY

The aorta trifurcates into the left subclavian, the left common carotid, and the right innominate arteries. Although it is easier to learn the radial artery approach from the left side, as it mimics a transfemoral approach more accurately, a right-sided approach is probably more commonly used because of the current setup in most catheterization laboratories. The innominate artery becomes the subclavian artery after the right common carotid arises. It then becomes the axillary artery as it passes into the shoulder. As the axillary artery passes into the upper arm it becomes the brachial artery. In most patients, the brachial artery divides into the radial and ulnar artery below the elbow. On occasion, the radial artery originates from the upper brachial artery or the axillary artery. It is important for physicians involved in radial artery access to take the time to review not only the pertinent anatomy associated with this procedure but also the anatomic variants that can be found. These are described well in most anatomy books.

## BRACHIAL ARTERY

In most patients, the radial artery (Fig. 24–1) branches off of the brachial artery just below the level of the elbow crease. At this point, it passes on the lateral margin of the forearm until it reaches the level of the wrist. A significant number of patients (reportedly as many as 12%) may have an anatomic variant.[13] The most common involves the radial artery originating just superior to the elbow, although in a few patients it may originate much higher in the arm. In the majority of patients where the artery originates just below the elbow, the vessel is deep to the body of the supinator longus muscle in the upper part of the forearm. In the mid-forearm, down to the level of the wrist, it lies between the tendons of the supinator longus and the flexor carpi radialis.

At the level of the wrist, the radial artery lies atop the scaphoid bone, the trapezium, and the external lateral ligament. Physicians trying to cannulate the artery too distally will encounter the reticulum and find that the artery is diving deep and lateral. In addition, smaller superficial branches of the radial artery exist at this point. It is important therefore to attempt cannulation approximately 2 to 3 cm from the flexion crease of the wrist.

At the level of the hand, the radial artery passes from the space between the metacarpal bones of the thumb and the index finger into the palm of the hand. The vessel then crosses the base of the metacarpal bone of the little finger, where it joins with the deep communicating branch of the ulnar artery and forms the deep palmar arch. The superficialis branch of the radial artery joins with the palmar portion of the ulnar artery to complete the superficial palmar arch.

The ulnar artery also branches off the brachial artery and passes along the inner aspect of the forearm. At the level of the wrist, it divides into two branches, which join the radial artery and its superficial branch to form the deep and superficial palmar arches.

It is not uncommon for a patient to display adequate ulnar and radial artery pulses and have abnormal results on plethysmography, or on an Allen test. Whether these findings represent true radial or ulnar dominance or inadequate or incomplete palmar circulation (reported in as many as 10% to 23% of patients) is difficult to ascertain.[16] Obviously, patients who display radial artery dominance should not undergo radial artery intervention. In addition, patients with ulnar artery dominance have a higher incidence of problems with radial artery–based access, although such problems are not well described in the literature.

## PATIENT PREPARATION

The wrist should be shaved (if necessary) and cleansed in the usual sterile fashion. In addition, the groin should be prepped in case of access failure or the need for urgent IABP or a temporary venous pacemaker. At William Beaumont Hospital, it is the usual practice to perform PTCA using the radial artery access site and an adequate peripheral intravenous line (IV). A central venous line is not routinely placed unless rapid volume or temporary pacing will be necessary. The author and his colleagues prefer that the IV be started in the contralateral arm so as to allow adequate flow even when a hemostasis device is in place. If an IV must be placed in the

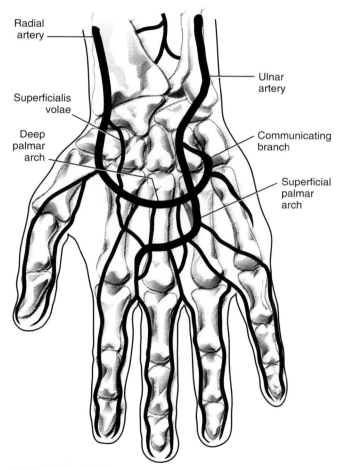

FIGURE 24–1. The brachial artery courses from the level of the shoulder along the inner and anterior aspects of the upper arm. At its origin, it lies medial to the insertion of the humerus and the biceps muscles, but as it approaches the level of the elbow, it lies more anterior. At the level of the elbow, it lies between the two condyles covered by skin and fascia on the medial aspect of the arm and overlapped by the biceps on the other side. At the elbow, the brachial artery travels beneath the supinator longus muscle and the pronator radii teres muscle. At this point, it divides into the radial and ulnar arteries, which extend from the forearm into the hand.

arm on the side of the intervention, it should be placed proximal to the wrist, preferably at the level of the elbow. All potentially constricting clothing, jewelry, and identification (ID) bracelets should be removed prior to the procedure. An Allen test (Fig. 24–2), or preferably oximetry-plethysmography, should be documented by the physician or members of the nursing staff, or both. At William Beaumont Hospital, the author and his associates often place the radial sheath in the holding room, which facilitates catheterization laboratory turnaround.

In patients who require a second procedure through the same radial site, it may be helpful to perform a reverse Allen test. In this situation, the physician releases pressure over the radial artery, rather than the ulnar. This maneuver may detect proximal radial artery disease or occlusion that may be asymptomatic. Patients with an abnormal result on reverse Allen test should not undergo a repeat transradial procedure from this radial artery site.

For patients who require the placement of a Swan-Ganz catheter or an intravenous temporary pacing wire, the author and his colleagues place these in the ipsilateral brachial vein. This access can be achieved in the holding room prior to the intervention, by placing a 16-gauge IV. This size of IV allows

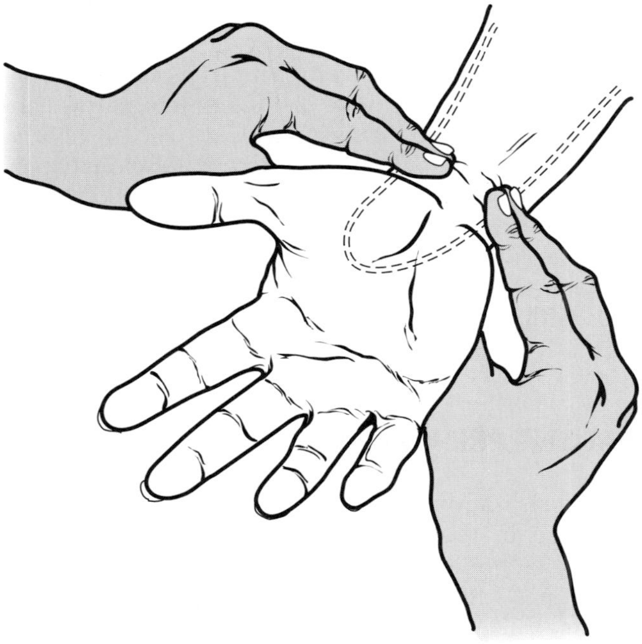

FIGURE 24–2. Allen's test (or modified plethysmography), should be documented in every patient undergoing a radial artery procedure. It is thought by these authors that modified plethysmography allows for more reproducible data and probably serves as a better medical record. To perform an Allen test, both the radial and the ulnar artery should be occluded so as to note obvious pallor of the hand. The operator removes pressure on the ulnar artery while maintaining pressure on the radial site. An abnormal test result occurs when the color of the hand does not return within 8 seconds.

exchange with a .035 J-tip guide wire and placement of a sheath.

## CATHETERIZATION LABORATORY AND STAFF PREPARATION

It is important that the catheterization laboratory staff be educated as to the nuances of radial artery intervention. There are some subtle, but important, differences in the way that staff prepare for an intervention. A pulse oximeter should be placed on the index finger or the thumb of the arm that is undergoing the procedure. This monitoring allows for continuous assessment of the vascular integrity of the radial-ulnar system. The wrist should be adequately "cocked" to facilitate arterial access. This position can be maintained with either a small towel or rolled piece of gauze or a splint-like device (Accumed Systems; Ann Arbor MI). The armboard should allow for access at an angle of approximately 45 degrees from the patient and then allow the arm or wrist to be placed next to the hip. Conventional drapes are often inadequate. Specialized radial drapes are now available. It is often possible to move a femoral drape over, to cover the wrist and the prepped groin, or to use brachial drapes.

## RADIAL ARTERY ACCESS

Various types of equipment are available for radial artery access. The basic components include a needle, wire, and sheath. The specifications of each of these components vary considerably, making it vital to familiarize oneself with the characteristics that allow successful access.

The needle varies in length from approximately 2 to 5 cm and 20 to 21 gauge. The author and his colleagues believe that longer needles allow the operator to pass the needle through the radial artery without seeing the "flash" of blood return (which is quite minimal compared with a femoral approach with a larger-gauge needle). Therefore, shorter needles seem more desirable. The bevel of the needle is important because of the small caliber of the artery. A more gentle bevel angle allows for smoother movement of the wire.

The wires that are supplied are usually 30 to 50 cm and often have a floppy tip and a more rigid shaft. Given the small caliber of the artery, wires with either a small angulation or even a straight tip seem to work better. J-tips often get caught in either the sheath or the proximal artery. If the operator has difficulty with the wire in the kit, successful access is usually obtained with a hydrophilic-coated, angulated wire.

The most common sheath size in radial intervention is 6-French, although both 5-French and 7-French are not uncommon. Experienced operators seem to prefer longer (23-cm) sheaths to limit radial artery spasm. Sheath delivery into the artery can be difficult in cases in which there is a stepup in the transition between the dilator and the sheath. A sidearm on the sheath is preferable, to allow delivery of anticoagulant and antispasmodic medications.

## TRANSRADIAL MEDICATIONS

The medications that are used in transradial access are not yet standardized. Several different combinations are probably effective. The author does not propose a specific combination, but instead offers suggestions for the operator based on his experience and a review of the literature.

**SEDATION.** Sedation in the radial access patient is similar to that in femoral intervention patients with the exception that it is most likely to be uncomfortable for the patient during sheath insertion and removal. Therefore, conscious sedation protocol needs to be particularly addressed during these times. Many operators find fentanyl satisfactory.

**ANTISPASM.** The radial artery can be subject to rather intense spasm that can be painful to the patient and make sheath and catheter movement difficult. A variety of medications have been used to help alleviate this symptom, including nitroglycerin, adenosine, verapamil, lidocaine, and papaverine. These medications are usually given during sheath placement and removal, and when the operator believes that radial spasm is limiting catheter movement. The author usually has syringes of nitroglycerin (200 μg/mL), verapamil (500 μg/mL) and lidocaine 2% (given in 20-mg aliquots) available. Occasionally, the author has used papaverine to wipe the sheath or catheter, as this agent is a short-acting myovascular relaxant. It has a direct paralytic action on the smooth muscle of the blood vessel. Although adenosine appears to have significant arterial dilatation properties, its use seems to be limited by cost.

**ANTICOAGULATION.** Anticoagulation may be the most important aspect of radial artery intervention. Early studies had suggested very high rates of radial artery occlusion or thrombosis, which appeared to be related to insufficient anticoagulation. The author administers a minimum of 5000 U of intra-arterial heparin for diagnostic procedures and a minimum of 10,000 U for interventional procedures. Direct injection of heparin intra-arterially can be quite painful; thus, the author mixes it thoroughly with blood from the sheath. In the author's experience, employment of this method has not resulted in any increased rate of complications with the use of radial artery–based access in patients who had been administered either thrombolytics or intravenous GPIIb/IIIa inhibitors. The author does not reverse anticoagulation before removing the sheath.

## TRANSRADIAL CATHETERS AND GUIDES

### Judkins Left and Right Catheters

One of the limitations of radial artery interventions has been the equipment that we, as interventionists, have available for use. In particular, radial artery–based access has been limited by the diagnostic and guide catheters available. In the last few years, however, several new innovative designs have become available.

Despite these new designs, it is not uncommon to use standard Judkins catheters (Fig. 24–3*A* and *B*). The different orientation in the aorta (from a radial artery approach) makes it necessary to use different

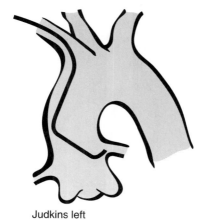

Judkins left

A

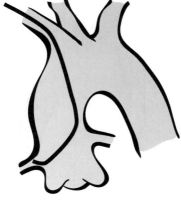

Judkins right

B

FIGURE 24–3. Judkins left *(A)* and Judkins right *(B)* coronary catheters.

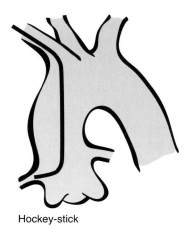

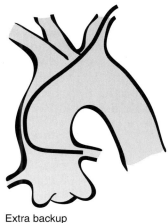

Hockey-stick

A

Extra backup

B

FIGURE 24–4. *A,* Hockey-stick catheter. *B,* Extra backup catheter.

curves. When a Judkins left catheter is used from the right radial artery, the curve should usually be 0.5 cm smaller than would be picked for a femoral artery approach with a similar aortic root. If a 0.5-cm curve is not available, a standard 4-cm curve can be used with a short tip.

When one cannulates the right coronary artery from the right radial artery approach, it is usually helpful to use a curve that is approximately 1 cm larger (i.e., a JR-5 instead of a JR-4). When access is achieved from the left radial artery, conventional curves are usually satisfactory.

## Hockey-Stick and Extra Backup Catheters

Two other catheters that were designed primarily for the femoral artery approach are helpful during radial artery interventions. The hockey-stick (Fig. 24–4*A*) catheter takes advantage of a relatively sharp 90-degree angle and relatively long distal segment (somewhat like a JR-5). This catheter can be used

to cannulate both the right and the left coronary arteries.

The extra-backup (EBU) catheter (see Fig. 24–4*B*), which is similar to the VODA, takes advantage of the support offered by the contralateral wall of the aorta. Although this catheter offers excellent support when used in 6-French sizes, longer stents have some difficulty in traversing the primary and secondary curves. This curve is best suited for a left radial artery approach and is used only for cannulation of the left coronary artery.

## Multipurpose Catheter

The multipurpose catheter (Fig. 24–5*A* and *B*) and its modified version (the Kimny Curve, the Barbeau Curve, and others) can be used from either arm to cannulate both the right and the left coronary arteries as well as vein grafts. The multipurpose A catheter has a more subtle angle and is suited for inferiorly directed takeoffs. The multipurpose B catheter has a right angle curve of approximately 90 degrees

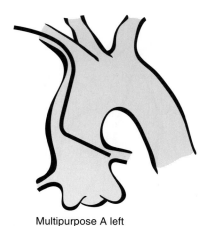

Multipurpose A left

A

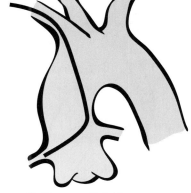

Multipurpose B right

B

FIGURE 24–5. The multipurpose catheter: left *(A)* and right *(B).*

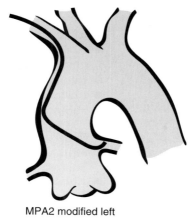
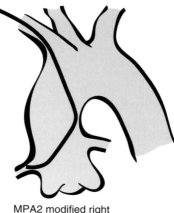

MPA2 modified left

MPA2 modified right

FIGURE 24–6. The MPA2 left *(A)* and MPA2 right *(B)* catheters.

A

B

and is therefore better suited for horizontal or superior takeoffs.

## (Modified) Multipurpose Catheter
### Kimny Curve Catheter

The Kimny Curve catheter (Fig. 24–6*A* and *B*) serves as the workhorse at William Beaumont Hospital for cannulation of both coronary arteries. It is specifically designed for radial artery intervention. The primary curve is 45 degrees, with a secondary curve of 90 degrees that allows it to support itself on the contralateral aortic wall. It is common for the operator to cannulate the left coronary artery from below with this catheter while coming from a horizontal or superior position to cannulate the right.

### Barbeau Curve Catheter

This catheter is a modification of the multipurpose A. It has an additional 135-degree curve at the tip to assist in cannulation. It is best used via a right radial artery approach for the right coronary artery or for vein grafts.

### Others

A number of other catheters and guides suitable for radial artery interventions are not pictured here. These include Sones catheters, Radial catheters, IMA catheters, modified saphenous graft catheters, as well as Castillo curves. The modified saphenous curves and the IMA catheters should be used with caution by experienced operators, as they incorporate very acute angles and could potentially inflict trauma on the patient.

## HEMOSTASIS DEVICES

There are various methods for obtaining hemostasis as well as several hemostasis devices. The optimal

method and device are not known, but operators should probably be familiar with several methods and devices in case they come across a patient in whom it is difficult to achieve hemostasis. The methods and devices include the following:

- Gauze—Hemostasis can be obtained by placing several rolled 4 × 4's over the radial site and securing them with a pressure (elastic adhesive) dressing.
- Hemoband (Access Systems, Inc.)—This was designed to obtain hemostasis in patients with hemodialysis grafts and therefore has a wide-based area that compresses the radial artery. Although usually effective, it causes compression of the venous system, leading to hand engorgement and is uncomfortable.
- Radial Clamp—This device allows for a clamp-like device to put pressure directly on the radial artery site.
- Radistop—A concept similar to the Femstop that allows compression over the site; it is moderately priced.
- Hemostasis Band (Schneider)—A simple elastic strap that allows compression of the entire wrist. It does not allow point compression on the radial artery site and causes some venous engorgement.
- Hemostasis Band (Accumed Systems, Inc.)—This is specifically designed to allow point compression of the radial artery site. Support blocks on the band allow for adequate venous return and therefore minimal patient discomfort.
- Blood Pressure Inflatable Cuff—Although rarely needed, this device can control bleeding if the radial artery site is lacerated.

## SHEATH REMOVAL AND HEMOSTASIS

When the operator prepares to remove the sheath, it is helpful to have several medications and certain equipment available (as noted previously). The medications include the following:

- Verapamil—Although not consistently given by all operators before sheath removal, some believe that it aids in removal by decreasing spasm.
- Nitroglycerin—This agent is not used by all operators. It probably is less successful with regard to arterial vasodilation.
- Lidocaine—This drug is administered by some operators intra-arterially prior to sheath removal to decrease pain. It is given in aliquots up to 20 mg.
- Sedation—The sedation given is similar to the drugs administered during femoral artery line removal. Some operators find fentanyl 50 to 100 μg extremely effective.

## PITFALLS OF RADIAL ARTERY INTERVENTION

### Difficult Access

Hit it on the first try! The radial artery is prone to spasm, and it is not uncommon, after you nick the artery, to notice a diminished, even if transient, pulse. If this occurs and it appears to be related to spasm, you have several options:

- Wait.
- Go to a more proximal site.
- Give nitroglycerin (NTG) intravenously or sublingually.
- Have the patient clench and then open the hand.
- Go to another site.

If, however, there is a good pulse, but no blood flash is noticed in the needle, the physician needs to consider whether the radial artery has potentially closed. If it has, the physician should question whether the pulse represents flow from the ulnar through the palmar system.

On occasion, the artery will be quite palpable, but difficult to stick. This difficulty is often seen in atherosclerotic calcified vessels. The physician usually addresses this by fixing the radial artery with the left thumb while attempting to achieve radial artery access.

### Difficult Guide Wire Movement

After successful access is achieved, it is sometimes difficult to advance the guide wire. The differential diagnosis of this difficulty includes the following:

- Tortuosity
- Spasm
- Occluded radial artery

- Guide wire positioned in a side branch (usually too distal in the artery)
- Abnormal takeoff of the radial artery (off the brachial)
- Radial artery stenosis
- Placement of the guide wire against the wall or subintimally

If this situation occurs, the following options should be tried:

- Rotate the needle to change the angle of the bevel.
- Perform a radial angiogram.
- Use a hydrophilic-coated wire.
- Try a .018 PTCA wire.
- Give vasodilators through the needle and then try to advance wire.

### Difficulty in Removing Sheath

Difficulty in removing the sheath is quite uncommon but can be seen in smaller patients, women, and patients with intense forearm radial spasm. In these cases, the following should be considered:

- Vasodilators and pain medications are given before sheath removal.
- Fix the proximal sheath (near the elbow) with the left hand.
- Gently rotate the sheath on removal.
- Hold the skin distal to the incision to avoid "buckling."

### Difficult Placement of Guide Wire

Although diagnostic and guide catheters are now increasingly suited for radial artery intervention, their placement is still somewhat different from that used for femoral artery access.

Radial artery intervention requires a knowledge of the appropriate catheters and sizes (as detailed earlier in this book). Several other maneuvers facilitate guide wire placement:

- Start the guide wire below the ostium (especially when approaching the left coronary artery). Pushing down on the catheter will bend the tip up toward the left main artery. Pulling the catheter back will then allow the tip to cannulate the ostium. This is different from conventional placement via a femoral artery approach, which usually disengages the ostium from a superior position.
- Always use an exchange-length wire when changing catheters to avoid the need to recross the great vessels.
- The patient can be asked to inspire or change the angle of the arm, or both, to facilitate catheter

movement, although such adjustments are rarely needed.

## Postprocedural Management

It is the current policy at William Beaumont Hospital for operators to pull radial artery lines without waiting for a drop in anticoagulation parameters. Lines are pulled in the setting of thrombolytics and intravenous GPIIb/IIIa inhibitors. Hemostasis is rarely a problem. In general, the authors leave the Accumed hemostasis band on for 30 minutes for diagnostic cases (5000 U of heparin) and for 60 minutes for interventional cases (10,000 or more U of heparin or when GPIIb/IIIa inhibitor was used). The site is then checked for hemostasis. If there is still evidence of bleeding, the band is left intact for another 30 minutes. In cases of profound bleeding where a lacerated artery is suspected, an inflatable blood pressure cuff can be used to control bleeding. Patients who undergo diagnostic radial artery intervention can be discharged within 2 hours. Patients can ambulate when their sedation wears off.

Complications arising from radial artery–based access are extremely rare and seem to be less severe than those from femoral artery–based access, despite the limitations in radial equipment.[7, 17, 18] Pseudoaneurysms may form, but they can be treated with local pressure dressings. If the site is enlarging or quite painful, an ultrasound should be performed and consultation with a surgeon for peripheral vascular surgery obtained.

When patients are discharged, they are instructed to avoid flexion and extension of the wrist for the remainder of the day. Local swelling is treated with ice and analgesics. Rebleeding is treated with hand elevation and local pressure. Rebleeding at a radial artery site is certainly better tolerated by patients and responds better to treatment than is the case with rebleeding at a femoral site.

## ACCESSORIES

A growing number of accessories have become available for helping facilitate radial artery intervention.

## Wrist Splint

The Wrist Splint (Accumed Systems, Inc.) keeps the patient's forearm supinated and facilitates both access and sheath removal and hemostasis. Without the splint, the patients have the tendency to progressively pronate the wrist during the procedure. The splint also reduces flexion of the wrist after hemostasis is obtained, which decreases rebleeding.

## Hemostasis Band

Although there are several satisfactory ways of obtaining hemostasis, the author and his colleagues have found the use of the Hemostasis Band (Accumed Systems, Inc.) to be superior to other available devices and techniques. This band reduces the time needed for the physician, nurse, or technician to achieve hemostasis. In addition, it offers the security of preventing potentially serious rebleeds. Its unique design is comfortable and the foam support pad allows adequate venous return, a problem frequently encountered with bands or tourniquet devices.

## Sheaths

There are a variety of sheaths available on the market that are probably suitable for radial artery access. Some characteristics, however, are desirable in a radial sheath. Although longer sheaths are not utilized by all experienced operators, there is a trend toward the use of these longer sheaths (23 to 25 cm) because of the concern that forearm radial artery spasm may occur. It is not clear whether these devices improve catheter movement, but they are widely used.

The sheaths used often come in a single- or double-dilator setup. The advantage of the double-dilator setup is a more tapered, atraumatic tip, which avoids radial artery laceration. These double-dilator sheaths, however, have a transition between the first and the second dilators, which can often catch on the skin incision. The single-dilator system, while transitionless, is often more traumatic to the skin and radial insertion site.

Several companies are currently engaged in the development of sheaths specifically for radial artery intervention. These prototypes include sheaths that can be dilated up in size; porous sheaths equipped for antispasmodic medication administration; and transitionless systems.

### REFERENCES

Several Websites have been developed that allow the radial artery interventionalist to communicate with colleagues from around the world. The Radial Force at *www.radialforce.org* is an excellent reference site and includes an up-to-date list of radial artery–based interventional literature.

1. Campeau L: Percutaneous radial artery approach for coronary angiography. Catheter Cardiovasc Diagn 16:3–7, 1989.
2. Kiemeneij F, Laarman GJ: Percutaneous transradial artery approach for coronary stent implantation. Catheter Cardiovasc Diagn 30:173–178, 1993.
3. Kiemeneij F, Hofland J, Laarman GJ: Cost comparison between two modes of Palmaz-Schatz coronary stent implantation: Transradial bare stent technique vs. transfemoral

sheath–protected stent technique. Catheter Cardiovasc Diagn 35:301–308, 1995.

4. Cooper C, El-Shiekh R, Cohen D, et al: Effect of transradial access on quality of life and cost of cardiac catheterization: A randomized comparison. Am Heart J 138:430–436, 1999.

5. Noto T, Johnson L, Krone R, et al: Cardiac catheterization 1990: A report of the Registry of the Society for Cardiac Angiography and Interventions. Catheter Cardiovasc Diagn 24:75–86, 1991.

6. Foulger V: Patients' views of day-case cardiac catherisation. Prof Nurse 12:478–480, 1997.

7. Khoury M, Batra S, Berg R, et al: Influence of arterial access sites and interventional procedures on vascular complications after cardiac catheterizations. Am J Surg 164:205–209, 1992.

8. Davis C, Van Riper S, Longstreet J, et al: Vascular complications of coronary interventions. Heart Lung 26:118–127, 1997.

9. Lilly MP, Reichman W, Sarazen AA Jr, et al: Anatomic and clinical factors associated with complications of transfemoral arteriography. Ann Vasc Surg 4:264–269, 1990.

10. Kiemeneij F: Transradial approach for coronary angioplasty and stenting. Stent 1:83–88, 1998.

11. Kent KC, Moscucci M, Gallagher SG, et al: Neuropathy after cardiac catheterization: Incidence, clinical patterns, and long-term outcome. J Vasc Surg 19:1008–1013, 1994.

12. Black A, Cortina R, Aoun A, et al: Efficacy and safety of transradial coronary angioplasty: A report of 5354 consecutive cases [Abstract]. Eur Heart J 20(suppl):268, 1999.

13. Louvard Y, Harvey R, Pezzano M, et al: Transradial complex coronary angioplasty: The influence of a single operator's experience. J Invasive Cardiol 9(suppl C):647–649, 1997.

14. Goldberg SL, Rensio R, Sinow R, et al: Learning curve in the use of the radial artery as vascular access in the performance of percutaneous transluminal coronary angioplasty. Catheter Cardiovasc Diagn 44:147–152, 1998.

15. Barbeau G, Carrier G, Ferland S, et al: Right transradial approach for coronary procedures: Preliminary results. J Invasive Cardiol 8(suppl D):19D–21D, 1996.

16. Slogoff S, Keats AS, Arlund C: On the safety of radial artery cannulation. Anesthesiology 59:42–47, 1983.

17. Kennedy AM, Grocott M, Schwartz MS, et al: Median nerve injury: An underrecognised complication of brachial artery cardiac catheterisation? J Neurol Neurosurg Psychiatry 3:542–546, 1997.

18. Kiemeneij F, Laarman GJ, Odekerken D, et al: A randomized comparison of percutaneous transluminal coronary angioplasty by the radial, brachial and femoral approaches: The Access Study. J Am Coll Cardiol 29:1269–1275, 1997.

# 25

# Chronic Total Occlusions

*Joseph A. Puma*    *James E. Tcheng*

The selection of therapy for patients with coronary artery disease remains a complex process that requires the integration of numerous factors, including patient preference, clinical data, published literature, anatomic variables, clinical experience, and technical expertise. Of the anatomic variables, the presence of a total occlusion, both acute and chronic, remains the greatest challenge to the clinician and the interventional cardiologist. Acute occlusions provide the pathophysiologic substrate for acute myocardial infarction. In this critically ill population, exhaustive research has clearly demonstrated survival benefits of either mechanical or pharmacologic restoration of coronary flow, especially Thrombolysis In Myocardial Infarction (TIMI) grade 3 flow.[1-3] Patients with chronic occlusions ($\geq 1$ month's duration) often have symptoms of stable angina pectoris and do not always have a history of acute infarction. Approximately 10% of patients referred for percutaneous revascularization (PTCA) have a chronic total occlusion as the target lesion.[4] However, this percentage likely underrepresents the true incidence in the coronary artery disease population because patients with chronic total occlusions are often treated medically or with bypass surgery (coronary artery bypass grafting [CABG]).

The purpose of this chapter is to give a broad overview of the literature regarding the percutaneous treatment of patients with chronic total occlusion and to develop an analytic approach based on quantitative methods combining the pragmatic with the clinical literature.

## BACKGROUND

PTCA has been performed for more than 20 years as a treatment for coronary artery disease and now exceeds the annual volume of CABG. The first reported PTCA of a total occlusion was in 1982.[5] Procedural success and restenosis rates have gradually improved since then. Technologic and pharmacologic advances (particularly stent implantation and platelet glycoprotein IIb/IIIa antagonism)[6-8] have improved outcomes and reduced restenosis in patients

with high-grade stenoses who are undergoing PTCA, but it is unclear whether these benefits will be realized in patients with chronic occlusions. Patients with both complete (TIMI-0) and functional (TIMI-1) occlusions have been loosely considered to comprise those with "total" occlusions. The age of an occlusion has been generally estimated by clinical criteria (acute infarction, new Q waves on electrocardiogram, or change in pattern of angina) and has been somewhat arbitrarily defined (Table 25–1).

## PATHOLOGY

Two distinctly different processes lead to total native vessel coronary occlusion. Spontaneous plaque disruption in an atherosclerotic coronary vessel can result in acute thrombus formation, producing a thrombotic acute occlusion and (typically) acute myocardial infarction. Slow progression to occlusion also can occur by repeated injury and vessel repair.[9, 10] The latter process is characterized by an initial platelet/fibrin and arterial wall interaction, followed by smooth muscle proliferation, lipid deposition, fibrosis, ulceration, calcification, and thrombosis. Multiple layers of thrombus can be deposited with the last layer, resulting in complete occlusion. It is also through this last layer that recanalization typically occurs. An autopsy study described age-related histologic correlates of chronic total occlusion.[11] This study observed younger occlusions to be predominantly soft or lipid laden, whereas older lesions were typically hard or fibrocalcific. Fresh clot is associated with a higher percutaneous procedural success rate, whereas older and more fibrocalcific material is less likely to be successfully reopened.[12, 13] Unfortunately, total occlu-

**TABLE 25–1.  DEFINITIONS OF TOTAL OCCLUSIONS**

| | |
|---|---|
| Acute | <12 hours |
| Subacute | $\geq$12 hours and <1 month |
| Early chronic | $\geq$1 month and <3 months |
| Late chronic | >3 months |

sions often have similar angiographic appearances, regardless of age or underlying pathology.

Occlusion of a saphenous vein bypass graft in the first month after surgery is usually due to local or diffuse thrombosis associated with adverse technical factors (narrowing of the anastomosis, vein graft trauma, or inadequate distal runoff). Between the first and 12th month, thrombus superimposed on intimal proliferation is the usual cause of occlusion. While the media undergoes fibrosis and atrophy, the intima develops an admixture of smooth muscle cells, fibroblasts, collagen, and ground substance. Atherosclerosis becomes a significant contributor to occlusion after the first year. As in native coronary arteries, atherosclerotic vein graft plaque is rich in cholesterol, necrotic debris, foam cells, and blood elements.[14]

# PERCUTANEOUS REVASCULARIZATIONS

## Clinical Indications

### Relief of Angina Pectoris

In most series, symptomatic angina is the leading indication for attempted PTCA of a chronic total occlusion.[15–26] Hemodynamically, a chronic occlusion with well-developed collaterals has been shown to be similar to a 90% stenosis without collaterals, which may explain the basis for symptoms in these patients.[27] Successful angioplasty is often associated with relief of symptoms (Table 25–2). Review of the available literature documents that symptom relief is attained in 73% of cases after successful angioplasty, whereas failed attempts are associated with only a 35% incidence of symptom relief. Note that relief may not be due to successful coronary revascularization only; medical therapy in patients with successful procedures may contribute to the improved clinical status. Furthermore, one must question the reason for symptom relief in patients with a failed procedure. Possible explanations include a placebo effect of the attempted intervention, as well as optimization of medical therapy.

## Survival

It is well established that patients presenting with an acute infarction who have an acute coronary occlusion benefit from prompt restoration of flow in the infarct-related artery. Controversy remains over the survival benefit of recanalization of a chronic occlusion in survivors of acute myocardial infarction. Similarly, few data are available to describe outcomes of patients who present with stable or crescendo angina and have a total occlusion.

Lange and coworkers[28] studied retrospective data on acute myocardial infarction survivors with multivessel disease and found a higher mortality in patients with a total occlusion in the infarct-related artery than that in those with antegrade flow in the infarct-related artery (32% vs. 6%, respectively). This relationship was further highlighted in the subgroup with left ventricular ejection fractions less than 50% (49% vs. 9%, respectively). Improved survival with an open infarct-related artery compared with a closed infarct-related artery has been reported by other investigators.[29, 30]

In a 25-year observational analysis of patients with single-vessel chronic occlusions (56% with a history of infarction), treated medically at a single university medical center, 10-year mortality was 25% despite only a 2% death rate at 1 year.[31]

Several investigators have reported better survival

## TABLE 25–2.  RELIEF OF ANGINA PECTORIS AFTER ANGIOPLASTY

| STUDY | FOLLOW-UP (MONTHS) | SUCCESS (NO. OF PATIENTS) | FAILED (NO. OF PATIENTS) |
|---|---|---|---|
| Holmes et al[15] | 7 | 10/13 | 8/11 |
| Kereiakes et al[16] | 7 | 30/40 | NR |
| Serruys et al[17] | 7 | 18/28 | NR |
| DiSciascio et al[18] | 8 | 16/29 | NR |
| Melchior et al[19] | 8 | 40/49 | NR |
| Finci et al[20] | 24 | 58/100 | 26/100 |
| Warren et al[21] | 31 | 16/20 | NR |
| Bell et al[22] | 32 | 178/234 | NR |
| Ruocco et al[23] | 24 | 110/160 | NR |
| Stewart et al[24] | 14 | 31/45 | NR |
| Sathe et al[25] | 4 | 83/116 | 27/62 |
| Berger et al[26] | 6 | 121/139 | NR |
| Total | | 710/973 | 61/173 |
| | | 72% | 42% |
| 95% CI | | 66%–78% | 23%–62% |

CI, confidence interval; NR, not reported.

**TABLE 25–3.    USE OF CORONARY ARTERY BYPASS GRAFT SURGERY AFTER UNSUCCESSFUL ANGIOPLASTY**

| STUDY | SUCCESS (NO. OF PATIENTS) | FAILED (NO. OF PATIENTS) |
|---|---|---|
| Holmes et al[15] | 1/13 | 8/11 |
| Serruys et al[17] | 3/28 | 11/21 |
| Melchior et al[19] | 2/49* | 20/44 |
| Finci et al[20] | 7/100 | 37/100 |
| Warren et al[21] | 3/26 | 7/18 |
| Ivanhoe et al[32] | 10/332 | 33/148 |
| Haine et al[36] | 1/350 | 22/350 |
| Stewart et al[24] | 7/45 | 16/42 |
| Isizaka et al[37] | 0/69 | 5/42 |
| Sathe et al[25] | 8/116 | 15/62 |
| Total | 42/1128 | 174/638 |
|  | 4% | 27% |
| 95% CI | 3%–5% | 24%–31% |

*Seven initial successes lost to follow-up.
CI, confidence interval.

in patients with successful PTCA of a chronic occlusion than in those whose procedure failed.[22, 32] The possibility of harm caused by the failed procedure cannot be excluded as the reason for the survival difference.

### Left Ventricular Function

Englestein and coworkers[33] demonstrated significant improvement in global ejection fraction and regional wall motion in patients with persistent vessel patency after successful PTCA of a chronic occlusion. In their angiographic study of 49 patients before and $10 \pm 6$ weeks after successful PTCA, 37 patients with patent arteries had an increase in ejection fraction from 55.8% at baseline to 62.5% at follow-up ($p < 0.001$) and improved regional wall motion from $-1.7$ to $-0.6$ standard deviations/chord ($p < 0.001$). Similar findings were reported by Danchin and associates,[34] who also found that left ventricular remodeling was reduced in infarct survivors with recanalization of a chronic occlusion. These data are tempered by the study of DiCarli and associates,[35] who found that in patients with chronic occlusions and adequate collateral vessels to the subtended myocardium, viability as assessed by positron emission tomography was found in only 49% of akinetic or dyskinetic regions.

Improvement in global or regional left ventricular function and prevention of remodeling would thus appear to contribute to the improved survival and reduced morbidity in these patients.

### Subsequent Coronary Artery Bypass Graft Surgery

In an analysis of long-term follow-up of 354 patients who underwent angioplasty of a chronic occlusion,

multivariable analysis demonstrated that successful PTCA was the most significant predictor of freedom from CABG.[22] Thus, successful angioplasty of a chronic occlusion may reduce the need for subsequent bypass surgery. Table 25–3 lists the reported experiences and suggests a greater than sixfold increase in the use of CABG after a failed procedure compared who those who underwent a successful PTCA. Whether these data truly mean that successful PTCA reduces the need for CABG or that, alternatively, once the clinician and patient embark on an interventional approach to therapy, failure of one method (PTCA) leads to higher use of another (CABG), regardless of symptom status, is still subject to debate.

## Procedural Outcomes

### Procedural Success and Restenosis

It is generally accepted that a residual stenosis of less than 50% without complications constitutes a successful angioplasty procedure. Despite occasional variations in the literature, most investigators adhere to this definition. Angioplasty of total occlusions has generally been less successful that PTCA of high-grade stenoses. In the early years of occlusion angioplasty, success rates ranged from 53% to 68%.[38, 39] Since then, success rates of greater than 70% have commonly been reported. This most likely reflects a combination of increased operator experience, patient selection bias, and improved equipment. It is now well established that operator experience is directly proportional to improved patient outcomes and is inversely related to complication rates.[42] Several authors have found that the relationship between operator experience, outcomes, and complications also pertains to chronic

**TABLE 25–4.  PROCEDURAL SUCCESS OF PERCUTANEOUS REVASCULARIZATION**

| STUDY | YEAR | NO. OF PATIENTS | % SUCCESS |
|---|---|---|---|
| Holmes et al[15] | 1984 | 24 | 54 |
| Kereiakes et al[16] | 1985 | 76 | 54 |
| Serruys et al[17] | 1985 | 49 | 57 |
| DiSciascio et al[18] | 1986 | 46 | 63 |
| Melchior et al[19] | 1987 | 100 | 56 |
| Safian et al[38] | 1988 | 271 | 69 |
| Ellis et al[39] | 1989 | 484 | 53 |
| Little et al[47] | 1990 | 64 | 73 |
| Hamm et al[40] | 1990 | 154 | 73 |
| Stone et al[41] | 1990 | 905 | 72 |
| Finci et al[20] | 1990 | 200 | 50 |
| Warren et al[21] | 1990 | 44 | 59 |
| Plante et al[48] | 1991 | 90 | 47 |
| Ivanhoe et al[32] | 1992 | 480 | 66 |
| Myler et al[12] | 1992 | 122 | 80 |
| Bell et al[22] | 1992 | 354 | 69 |
| Ruocco et al[23] | 1992 | 271 | 67 |
| Maiello et al[43] | 1992 | 294 | 67 |
| Tan et al[44] | 1993 | 312 | 61 |
| Haine et al[36] | 1993 | 500 | 70 |
| Stewart et al[24] | 1993 | 100 | 47 |
| Sathe et al[25] | 1994 | 178 | 65 |
| Ishizaka et al[37] | 1994 | 110 | 62 |
| Konoshita et al[46] | 1995 | 397 | 81 |
| Herrmann et al[45] | 1996 | 400 | 75 |
| Total | | 6025 | 67% |
| 95% CI | | | 66%–68% |

CI, confidence interval.

occlusion angioplasty.[41, 43] Stone and colleagues[41] reported an improvement in procedural success based on an operator learning curve, and Maiello and associates[43] reported success rates of 41% and 73% in the first and last 6 months, respectively, of a 4-year study ($p < 0.001$).

Table 25–4 reviews the published literature with a point estimate of success of 67%. When these studies were placed in a regression model, a significant association was found between the year of the study and the procedural success rate ($p = 0.002$).

Accurate assessment of restenosis in the general angioplasty population and the chronic occlusion subgroup is difficult because of a lack of controlled studies with 100% angiographic follow-up. Restenosis is probably overstated as a result of symptom-prompted repeat angiography. Restenosis had been reported at between 33% and 75% with a point estimate of 51%.[15–17, 45, 46] Included in the restenosis cohorts are total reocclusion; these usually account for one third of restenosis (Table 25–5).

**TABLE 25–5.  RESTENOSIS AFTER PERCUTANEOUS REVASCULARIZATION***

| STUDY | YEAR | ANGIOGRAPHIC FOLLOW-UP (%) | RESTENOSIS (%) |
|---|---|---|---|
| Holmes et al[15] | 1984 | 92 | 33 |
| Kereiakes et al[16] | 1985 | 30 | 75 |
| Serruys et al[17] | 1985 | 71 | 40 |
| Melchior et al[19] | 1987 | 71 | 58 |
| Finci et al[20] | 1990 | 62 | 45 |
| Hamm et al[40] | 1990 | 46 | 52 |
| Warren et al[21] | 1990 | 96 | 65 |
| Ivanhoe et al[32] | 1992 | 53 | 54 |
| Bell et al[22] | 1992 | 29 | 59 |
| Sathe et al[25] | 1994 | 82 | 63 |
| Ishizaka et al[37] | 1994 | 56 | 55 |
| Konoshita et al[46] | 1995 | 87 | 54 |
| Herrmann et al[45] | 1996 | 88 | 36 |
| Total | | 65 | 61 |

*Restenosis = lesions 51%–99%.

## Predictors of Success

### Functional Versus Absolute Occlusion

With functional occlusions, contrast material can be seen beyond the face of the obstruction in an antegrade manner without opacification of the coronary bed distal to the obstruction (TIMI-1). This finding is associated with an increased likelihood of successful recanalization compared with absolute occlusion (no antegrade flow beyond the point of occlusion [TIMI-0]; Table 25–6). This has been a consistent finding across several studies, with the aggregate evidence demonstrating a significant association between antegrade flow and procedural success ($p < 0.0001$).

### Duration of Occlusion

A strong predictor of procedural success is the duration of occlusion, typically estimated from an index clinical event, such as acute myocardial infarction and change in pattern of angina (Table 25–7). Despite two investigations that did not find this variable significant,[30, 41] the aggregate demonstrate a highly significant inverse relationship between occlusions present for more than 3 months and procedural failure ($p < 0.001$).

### Morphology at Point of Occlusion

**TAPERING VERSUS ABRUPT.** A tapered as opposed to an abrupt morphology at the area of obstruction has been shown to predict a favorable procedure outcome (Fig. 25–1, Table 25–8). Success rates of 68% to 88% have been reported with a tapered morphology ($p < 0.0001$ to $p = 0.01$), versus 43% to 59% with an abrupt occlusion ($p < 0.001$ to $p = 0.001$).[41, 43, 44] Despite one small study that did not find this characteristic to be an important pre-

#### TABLE 25–6. PREDICTORS OF RECANALIZATION SUCCESS: ANTEGRADE FLOW

| STUDY | FUNCTIONAL OCCLUSIONS | ABSOLUTE OCCLUSIONS |
|---|---|---|
| Serruys et al[17] | 13/16 | 15/23 |
| DiSciascio et al[18] | 16/23 | 13/23 |
| Safian et al[38] | 81/102 | 86/169 |
| Stone et al[41] | 35/42 | 46/92 |
| Ivanhoe et al[32] | 90/115 | 84/141 |
| Maiello et al[43] | 78/113 | 171/252 |
| Sathe et al[25] | 31/44 | 70/132 |
| Total | 344/455 | 485/842 |
| | 76% | 58% |
| 95% CI | 71%–80% | 55%–62% |

CI, confidence interval.

#### TABLE 25–7. PREDICTORS OF RECANALIZATION SUCCESS: DURATION OF OCCLUSION

| STUDY | ≤3 MONTHS | >3 MONTHS |
|---|---|---|
| Holmes et al[15] | 13/19 | 0/5 |
| DiSciascio et al[18] | 25/39 | 4/7 |
| Safian et al[38] | 62/97 | 40/72 |
| Hamm et al[40] | 79/97 | 33/57 |
| Stone et al[41] | 26/29 | 29/39 |
| Bell et al[22] | 222/318 | 29/45 |
| Maiello et al[43] | 132/150 | 49/110 |
| Tan et al[44] | 64/87 | 14/194 |
| Herrmann et al[45] | 240/318 | 27/40 |
| Total | 863/1154 | 225/569 |
| | 75% | 40% |
| 95% CI | 72%–77% | 36%–44% |

CI, confidence interval.

dictor,[16] when the studies are combined, the difference is highly significant ($p = 0.0001$).

**BRIDGING COLLATERALS.** A well-developed vasa vasorum that creates a "bridge" from the proximal to the distal vessel around the occlusion creates bridging collaterals (Fig. 25–2). Their presence appears to be directly related to the duration of occlusion and is a strong predictor of procedural failure ($p < 0.001$ in aggregate) (Table 25–8).

**SIDE BRANCH AT POINT OF OCCLUSION.** Although this variable has not been widely studied, there appears to be an inverse relationship between the presence of a side branch at the point of occlusion and procedural success (Fig. 25–3; see also Table 25–8) ($p < 0.001$ in aggregate).

### Lesion Length

The length of a nonvisualized segment of the coronary artery distal to the point of occlusion appears to be an important predictor of success. Shorter lengths of occlusion are associated with higher rates of success (Table 25–9). Although individual studies have reported contradictory results, in aggregate, occlusions less than 1.5 cm have a point estimate of success of 1%, versus 50% for occlusions greater than 1.5 cm.

### Vessel Dilated and Extent of Disease

The target vessel has been shown by several investigators to also be correlated with outcome. Although in aggregate, the confidence intervals overlap for these data, some investigators have observed greater failure rates when the target occlusion is in the right coronary artery.[18, 24, 30, 32] It does appear that there is a better chance of success in patients with single-

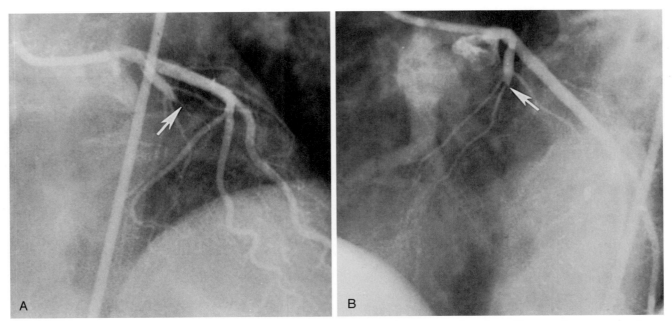

FIGURE 25–1. *A* and *B*, Tapered, rather than abrupt, morphology at area of obstruction predicts favorable procedure outcome. *Arrows* demarcate the "beak" at the entry point of the occlusion.

## TABLE 25–8.    PREDICTORS OF RECANALIZATION SUCCESS: MORPHOLOGIC VARIABLES

| STUDY | TAPERED | ABRUPT | BRIDGING COLLATERALS | | SIDE BRANCH | |
|---|---|---|---|---|---|---|
| | | | PRESENT | ABSENT | PRESENT | ABSENT |
| Stone et al[41] | 59/67 | 22/37 | 2/11 | 79/93 | 15/24 | 66/80 |
| Maiello et al[43] | 108/131 | 119/234 | 9/31 | 224/334 | 107/175 | 131/190 |
| Tan et al[44] | 121/176 | 38/88 | 10/51 | 149/213 | 76/143 | 84/121 |
| Konoshita et al[46] | | | 82/109 | 270/324 | | |
| Total | 288/374 | 179/359 | 103/202 | 722/964 | 198/342 | 291/391 |
| | 77% | 50% | 51% | 75% | 58% | 72% |
| 95% CI | 72%–81% | 45%–55% | 44%–58% | 72%–78% | 53%–63% | 67%–76% |

CI, confidence interval.

## TABLE 25–9.    PREDICTORS OF RECANALIZATION SUCCESS: OTHER DESCRIPTORS

| STUDY | LESION LENGTH (cm) | | VESSEL DILATED | | | EXTENT OF DISEASE | |
|---|---|---|---|---|---|---|---|
| | <1.5 | ≥1.5 | LAD | LCX | RCA | SVD | MVD |
| Kerekiakes et al[16] | 14/18 | 19/45 | 19/32 | 4/12 | 16/30 | NR | NR |
| Serruys et al[17] | | | 19/30 | 3/7 | 5/8 | NR | NR |
| DiSciascio et al[18] | | | 13/20 | 1/3 | 13/21 | NR | NR |
| Stone et al[41] | 36/43 | 137/237 | 25/34 | 24/27 | 27/38 | 22/26 | 59/78 |
| Warren et al[21] | | | 13/24 | 6/11 | 7/9 | NR | NR |
| Ivanhoe et al[32] | | | 156/204 | 78/114 | 98/162 | 272/382 | 60/98 |
| Maiello et al[43] | 113/160 | 123/205 | 107/157 | 52/73 | 90/135 | 103/146 | 131/219 |
| Tan et al[44] | 100/152 | 52/94 | | | | 86/115 | 104/197 |
| Herrmann et al[45] | | | 115/150 | 72/86 | 105/156 | NR | NR |
| Total | 263/373 | 227/393 | 467/651 | 240/333 | 361/559 | 483/669 | 354/592 |
| | 71% | 58% | 72% | 72% | 65% | 72% | 60% |
| 95% CI | 66%–75% | 53%–63% | 68%–75% | 67%–77% | 61%–69% | 69%–76% | 56%–64% |

CI, confidence interval; LAD, left anterior descending; LCX, left circumflex; MVD, multivessel disease; NR, not reported; RCA, right coronary artery; SVD, single-vessel disease.

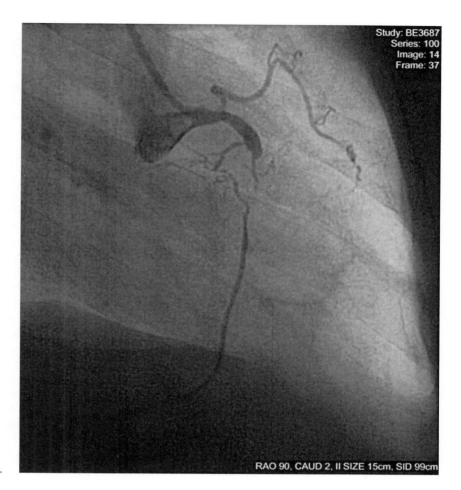

Study: BE3687
Series: 100
Image: 14
Frame: 37

RAO 90, CAUD 2, II SIZE 15cm, SID 99cm

FIGURE 25–2. Bridging collaterals.

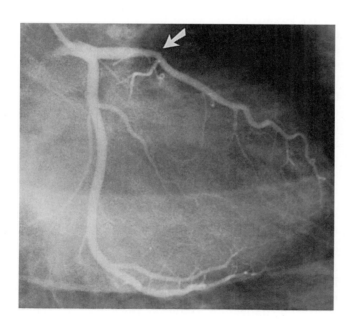

FIGURE 25–3. Side branch at point of occlusion *(arrow).*

vessel disease than in those with multivessel disease[32, 41, 43–45] (Table 25–9).

## Reasons for Procedural Failure

Chronic occlusion angioplasty is often a humbling experience because of its low procedural success rates. Most procedural failures are due to an inability to cross the obstruction with a guide wire.[21, 22, 25, 29] Despite advances in equipment and techniques, inability to cross the lesion with the wire remains the cause of procedural failure in more than two thirds of unsuccessful procedures. The remaining failures are typically due to an inability to cross or dilate the lesion with the balloon.[25, 37] Less common causes of procedural failure include the creation of a false lumen, extravasation, or abrupt reocclusion.

Many new devices have been explored to help improve lesion crossing and have met with variable results. These are discussed later under "New Devices and Techniques."

## Complications

Successful angioplasty of a chronic occlusion can improve the symptom status of patients with angina pectoris; however, its effects on survival are less clear. With this in mind, the interventional cardiologist should adhere to a "do no harm" approach to the patient because even minor complications could adversely affect the "net clinical benefit" philosophy. Although it has previously been believed that complications were less frequent or severe compared with angioplasty of subtotal stenoses,[9] several large investigations have demonstrated similar complication rates between total occlusion and subtotal occlusion angioplasty.[23, 36] It has been believed that abrupt reocclusion would not be detrimental, because it simply returned the vessel to its previous state.[4] However, non–Q-wave myocardial infarction has been reported in 2% to 3% of patients, possibly because of distal embolization or extensive intimal dissection,[24, 36, 45] and is likely underrepresented because cardiac enzyme levels are not generally systematically determined. In other series, the need for emergency bypass surgery has been reported in approximately 1% of patients, and death (usually resulting from left main dissection or ventricular arrhythmia secondary to acute infarction or dissection) in 0.5%.[24, 25, 45]

Other, less frequently encountered complications include coronary artery perforation, guide wire entrapment and fracture, cardiac tamponade, and excessive contrast load sequelae.[47, 48]

## PROCEDURAL AND TECHNICAL CONSIDERATIONS

Percutaneous coronary intervention of the chronic total coronary occlusion is a technically challenging, time-consuming, patience-testing endeavor that requires dedication, skill, and at least some serendipity. Compared with angioplasty of nonocclusive stenoses, occlusion angioplasty takes longer, exposes the operator to more radiation, and utilizes more equipment and contrast.[49] The decision to attempt the chronic total occlusion must take these additional factors into account, along with the more traditional assessment of the benefits and risks of angioplasty.

The importance of the decision-making process (as to whether percutaneous revascularization should even be attempted) cannot be understated. Although superficially one might conclude that technical prowess is the primary determinant of procedural success, careful case selection is of even greater importance. As outlined previously, results of the aggregate experience suggest that the ideal total occlusion has the following properties: limited length, age less than 3 months, absence of side branches arising at the point of occlusion, absence of bridging collaterals, and presence of a tapered funnel leading into the occlusion. Unfortunately, these characteristics describe but a minority of the chronic total occlusions.

Once a decision has been made to attempt percutaneous revascularization, certain preparatory steps should be taken. In describing the procedure to the patient and family, the clinician must acknowledge the unpredictability of the procedure. Depending on the lesion morphology and the expertise of the operator, success rates of 50% to 70% would seem prudent to discuss. (If the expectation is for less than a 50% success rate, perhaps the percutaneous approach should be reconsidered.) Furthermore, the family should be informed that the procedure may take 3 to 4 hours to complete. From a scheduling standpoint, total occlusion cases should be posted at times when the catheterization laboratory schedule is relatively uncluttered; pressure to complete the procedure because of additional pending cases may reduce the chances for success. One approach is to schedule total occlusion cases late in the working day; should the procedure take longer than expected, the interventional cardiologist can still persist without disrupting the flow of the rest of the laboratory.

## Angiography

Optimal visualization is a primary key to success. Although need for visualization should be intuitive, in the fast-paced catheterization laboratory environment, one may not always spend the time to insure optimal visualization. However, the extra time spent in preparation leads to reduced procedural times, contrast consumption, and equipment requirements.

Total occlusion cases should always be performed in a laboratory capable of digital image acquisition, enhancement, and display. The location of the channel through the total occlusion (if one exists) should be clear in the mind of the operator, including the three-dimensional relationships of the channel within the vessel proximal and distal to the total occlusion. At least two scout images in orthogonal views should be obtained. A personal favorite view for angioplasty of the proximal and mid-right coronary segments is the 90-degree right anterior oblique lateral view. Procedures should be performed by use of biplane fluoroscopy to facilitate the rapid moving back and forth between orthogonal views during the critical crossing of the lesion.

Visualization of the vessel distal to the end of the total occlusion is a must. In cases where the collateral supply to the distal vessel is provided by the opposite coronary artery (or via a different graft), a second diagnostic catheter should be placed to perform simultaneous bilateral injections.[50, 51] This obviously necessitates an additional vascular access site, as well as a second hemodynamic monitoring setup, control syringe, manifold, and contrast supply that need to be prepared before the initiation of the case.

## Guide Catheters

In total occlusion angioplasty, the guide catheter needs to provide optimal backup and support for the delivery of both guide wire and treatment devices. Factors to consider in the selection of a guide catheter include the ability of the guide to provide coaxial alignment, safe and consistent ostial engagement, and optimal bracing for the delivery of devices. The ideal guide catheter has a low trauma potential (particularly at the coronary ostium) while providing a stable, nonmoving platform with maximal backup power.

When the left coronary circulation is approached, guide catheters that traverse the root of the aorta to the opposite wall (such as the XB guide from Cordis Corporation, the Voda guide from SciMed, and the DC guide from Medtronics) provide an excellent, stable platform to cannulate the left coronary (Fig. 25–4). Amplatz guides may also provide similar backup power and stability, although the trauma potential of this curve configuration is somewhat higher than that of an XB type of configuration. The more traditional Judkins catheters should be viewed as second-line catheters because they do not "lock in" against the opposite wall of the aorta. When one does use a Judkins guide, several tips may improve the chances of success. Additional support to access the left anterior descending artery can be provided by gentle counterclockwise rotation with advance-

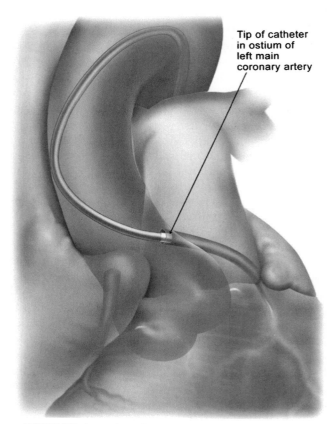

Tip of catheter in ostium of left main coronary artery

FIGURE 25–4. Guide catheter in the aorta.

ment of the guide; similarly, alignment with the left circumflex is often improved by retraction with clockwise rotation of the catheter or by use of a guide with a larger secondary curve (such as a JL 4.5 or 5.0).

For right coronary occlusions, guide catheter selection must take into account the angle of the takeoff of the right coronary artery as well as the width of the aortic root. For horizontal takeoffs, a standard Judkins right catheter often proves adequate; use of a short Amplatz left guide, such as an AL 0.5 and an AL 0.75, may be substituted when additional power is required. For inferior takeoffs, Judkins right guides are again a good starting point. When additional backup is needed, other catheters to consider include Amplatz right guides and (if the root is large) a multipurpose or hockey stick guide. For superior orientations, a short Amplatz left guide or the more aggressive Arani or E1 Gamal configurations, may be needed to provide optimal backup. A note of caution should be raised in regard to the use of Amplatz guides; when disengaging an Amplatz guide catheter, one must be mindful of the increased trauma potential of this configuration. The proper technique for disengagement is to advance the catheter until the tip prolapses out of the artery, and then to rotate the catheter out of plane before withdrawal.

## Support Catheters

The second device to consider is the guide wire support catheter. Unless the operator is absolutely certain that the lesion will be easily crossed, the guide wire should be loaded into a 2.5-French end-hole infusion catheter (rather than a balloon catheter) to attempt the primary crossing. Several vendors market these catheters, including Guidant, Target Therapeutics, and Cordis. It is also recommended that the support catheter be used to cross the lesion first after the guide wire has traversed the lesion. Several advantages of this approach can be enumerated. First, the radiopaque tip marker of support catheters identify the exact location of the distal tip. This permits precise positioning of the catheter and optimization of guide wire backup relative to the origin of the total occlusion. Use of a support catheter facilitates the rapid removal, tip reshaping, and/or exchange of coronary guide wires. Support catheters are extremely low-profile devices; this facilitates both angiographic visualization and (once the occlusion is crossed with the guide wire) passage of the support catheter through the lesion and into the distal coronary bed. It is unusual to find a balloon catheter that crosses a lesion that cannot be crossed with a support catheter. Finally, once the support catheter is across the lesion, contrast can be injected through the catheter to document successful intraluminal placement in the distal vasculature. After making sure that the device is intraluminal in the distal bed, a guide wire with a softer, less traumatic tip can then be exchanged for the primary (crossing) guide wire.

## Guide Wires

There are several philosophical approaches to guide wire selection. The conventional approach is to start with soft, supple wires and move to progressively stiffer devices. A second method is to utilize wires with reduced drag in order to "slip" through total occlusions. A third approach is to use guide wires that incorporate a high-profile tip designed to increase the pushability of the wire and reduce the propensity for subintimal passage. Each approach has advantages and disadvantages, the best approach is the one that works!

With the conventional approach, one often is tempted to begin with the softest, least traumatic guide wire available, typically that used for routine angioplasty cases. However, success with soft guide wires can be expected perhaps only 10% to 20% of the time. A more enlightened approach to the chronic total occlusion, especially with increasing operator experience, is to start with an intermediate-stiffness, 0.014-inch guide wire. Should the intermediate guide wire prove unsuccessful, the operator can then switch to larger-diameter (0.016- or 0.018-inch) and/or stiffer guide wires.

The low-friction/low-profile approach has frequently proved successful when the conventional approach fails. Guide wires in this category include the SciMed Choice PT, the Terumo/MediTech Glidewire, and the 0.010-inch guide wires from Guidant. Although the Choice PT and Glidewire wires are constructed along the lines of more conventional 0.014- to 0.018-inch wires, proprietary hydrophilic coatings reduce their coefficients of friction (when wet) to extremely low levels. These coated devices can then pass through subangiographic channels that would otherwise bind to uncoated guide wires. Case series document successful angioplasty in approximately one half of cases refractory to conventional (uncoated) guide wires.[52, 53] The 0.010-inch guide wire accomplishes the same results as the hydrophilic guide wires by presenting a lower profile. Unfortunately, anecdotes suggest an enhanced propensity for subintimal plaque dissection with any of the aforementioned wires compared with the conventional wires. Therefore, when moderate-to-severe vessel tortuosity proximal to the target lesion is encountered, a soft (conventional) guide wire should be used to approach the lesion, and then a support catheter should be advanced to a point adjacent to the origin of the total occlusion. The soft guide wire is then removed and replaced with the low-friction wire. Also, once the target lesion is crossed and the distal vessel accessed, exchange of the guide wire for a conventional one to perform the remainder of the interventional procedure should be considered.

High-profile, ball-tipped guide wires represent a third approach. The Schneider Magnum-Meier Recanalization Wire is an 0.021-inch guide wire with an olive-shaped ball on the tip, and the Boston Scientific–Mansfield (Walkertown MA) Jag Wire incorporates a similar design on an 0.018-inch nitinol wire with a silicone-coated shaft. In a randomized trial of 91 patients with 94 lesions, Meier and colleagues[54] reported a primary success rate of 71% with the Magnum-Meier system, compared with 45% with conventional guide wires. This included successful recanalization of 10 of 27 (37%) of the conventional guide wire failures. However, contrary results have been published by Haerer and coworkers[55] who had a success rate of only 32% with the Magnum-Meier system versus 59% with either standard guide wires or an Omniflex catheter.

Regardless of the guide wire being used, one critical technical caveat cannot be overemphasized. Crossing of a total occlusion is extremely dependent on the generation of antegrade, coaxial push at the tip of the guide wire. Once the guide wire tip has buckled, more pressure on the guide wire is futile.

Instead, subtle retraction leading to straightening of the tip is the proper maneuver. The greatest axial force is generated when the guide wire is the straightest. The proper technique is to repetitively probe, retract, and turn. Only when all else fails should a "strong-arm" tactic be used. Finally, excessive spinning of the guide wire with the tip embedded in the lesion should be avoided; this has been associated with guide wire tip dislocation and fracture.

## Interventional Devices

Three or four classes of revascularization devices should be in the arsenal of the interventional cardiologist who frequently treats chronic total occlusions. These include a full complement of balloons and stents and one of the debulking devices (excimer laser and/or Rotablator). The final objective, as with all coronary interventions, is to obtain the best possible final angiographic result. Having a selection of devices facilitates attainment of this goal.

In general, the first treatment device should be a low-profile, over-the-wire balloon matched to the nominal reference vessel diameter. We prefer to use over-the-wire balloons instead of monorail catheters because the latter tend to provide less axial push (and crossing potential) than the former. When difficulty is encountered with the primary crossing of the balloon catheter, maneuvers to increase guide catheter support as well as aggressive tapping on the balloon (like a jackhammer) should be employed.

Frequently, the operator is unable to advance the balloon catheter through the lesion. The next step is to consider a 1.5- or 2.0-mm balloon catheter to try to pry the lesion open just enough to pass the definitive treatment device. An alternative approach is to use an ablative device, such as the excimer laser and the Rotablator, to debulk the offending tissue.[56, 57] This ablative strategy should be considered early (or perhaps as the first-line device after guide wire crossing), particularly in the treatment of older occlusions and calcified lesions. When one of these devices is used, the catheter should be sized conservatively because the potential for perforation increases with catheter size. Also, the track of the guide wire through a total occlusion is often unknown. A guide wire that happens to be eccentrically located in the vessel (i.e., near the true lumen wall) provides an unfortunate opportunity for easy perforation with an oversized ablative device.

Once flow has been reestablished through a total occlusion, the next step is to better assess the actual reference vessel diameter. Because of the altered flow dynamics, the distal vessel usually appears smaller than nominal in the scout injections. Once distention pressure has been restored, the vessel should be reimaged (while the patient is given with intracoronary nitroglycerin) to determine the actual reference vessel diameter.

The final stages of a successful procedure are designed to obtain the optimal angiographic result. Balloon sizes should be matched at a 1 to 1.1:1 ratio, and stent implantation should be employed wherever reasonable and technically feasible. In arteries that cannot hold a stent, prolonged balloon inflation (with or without autoperfusion) may improve the angiographic results. Clinical investigations have documented improved short- and long-term outcomes after stent implantation (see "New Devices and Techniques"). The role of adjunctive pharmacology (particularly the platelet glycoprotein IIb/IIIa receptor blockers) is undefined in this application. However, the conventional wisdom is that total occlusion angioplasty provides the ideal milieu for the deposition of platelets, subsequent thrombus formation, restenosis, and reocclusion. Thus, the administration of these agents may be expected to provide additional benefit. The one technical caveat is that profound platelet inhibition is not advisable until such a point in the procedure when vessel perforation becomes unlikely. In general, this means that the lesion should at least have been crossed and dilated (or ablated) before the administration of a parenteral glycoprotein IIb/IIIa antagonist.

In the past, a common therapeutic strategy after successful recanalization of the total occlusion was an overnight infusion of heparin followed by warfarin (Coumadin) therapy. With the introduction of glycoprotein IIb/IIIa inhibition and advances in stent technology, these approaches may no longer be necessary. Our current recommendation is to treat the total occlusion patient in a fashion similar to the patient undergoing successful revascularization of a subtotal stenosis. The patient with the ideal angiographic result remains a candidate for sheath removal on the day of the procedure and discharge home the following day. Aspirin should be prescribed indefinitely as part of the standard medical approach to the patient with known coronary artery disease.

### Adjunct Pharmacology: Intracoronary Thrombolytics

Provocative data suggest that the prolonged administration of intracoronary thrombolytic therapy may improve chronic occlusion recanalization rates.[58–60] Vaska and Whitlow[58] treated 11 uncrossable coronary lesions with an infusion of tissue plasminogen activator via an infusion wire at a rate of 5 to 10 mg/hour for 6 hours, restoring at least TIMI grade 2 flow in 10 of the 11 cases. Of these, angioplasty was subsequently successful in nine. Ruocco and colleagues[59] also gave tissue plasminogen activator via the guide wire lumen of a balloon catheter at a rate of either 0.2 mg/minute for 90 minutes or 0.4 mg/minute for 60 minutes to 17 patients. In their series, flow was improved by at least one TIMI grade in 11 patients, and successful angioplasty result was obtained in 16 of the total cohort. Ajluni and coworkers[60] gave 100,000 to 250,000 units/hour of intracoronary urokinase for 8 to 24 hours to 24 patients. Flow was improved by at least one TIMI grade in 29% of patients, and an ultimately successful angioplasty procedure was obtained in 52%.

Zidar and associates[61] randomly assigned 60 patients with chronic occlusions that were 3 months or older in whom attempts at revascularization with standard percutaneous techniques had failed to one of three 8-hour dosage regimens of intracoronary urokinase (0.8 million units, 1.6 million units, or 3.2 million units). Fifty-three percent of patients had a successful procedure (no significant differences among the three dosages), and major bleeding was lower in the lowest-dose group ($p < 0.05$). Sixty-nine percent of patients underwent 6-month follow-up angiography and had a restenosis rate of 59%.

In summary, consideration should be made for a prolonged infusion of intracoronary thrombolytic therapy to try to convert a refractory chronic total occlusion into a treatable lesion, with a reasonable expectation of success in a limited number of cases.

## NEW DEVICES AND TECHNIQUES

### Crossing the Lesion

Numerous investigational devices have been investigated to address the persistent problem of the uncrossable lesion. Of these, the Spectranetics PRIMA Total Occlusion Guide Wire has been evaluated. This device consists of a 0.018-inch hypotube in which 12 to 13 45-mm silica optical fibers are placed that terminate at the distal tip of the guide wire. Excimer laser energy at 308 nm is delivered through the guide wire to the offending lesion. The guide wire can thus bore through atherosclerotic plaque, creating a new recanalization channel. Schofer and colleagues[62] used the laser wire to successfully recanalize 54% of 68 previous conventional device failure; there were no major complications. Success was independent of the duration of occlusion or the presence of side branches but was inversely related to the length of occlusion ($p < 0.05$) and angulated occlusions. Using the same laser wire system, Steffen and coworkers[63] had similar results, recanalizing 28 of 59 total occlusions that underwent unsuccessful angioplasty with standard wires and techniques.

In the European randomized Total Occlusion Trial with Angioplasty assisted by Laser guide wire (TOTAL) Multicenter Surveillance Study, 345 patients with total occlusions (54 with a previous failed angioplasty attempt) were studied.[64] Overall success was achieved in 205 patients (59%). Vessel perforation occurred in 56 cases (16%), leading to tamponade in four patients. There were no deaths or emergency bypass procedures.

The laser wire experience suggests that it may have a role in managing occlusions that cannot be crossed with conventional guide wires and techniques, but in its current form, it is not superior as a first-line device.

### Revascularization Devices

Newer interventional devices have been studied to determine their usefulness in successfully dilating chronic occlusions and reducing restenosis. These include intracoronary stents, excimer laser, and high-speed rotational atherectomy devices.

### Stents

Mori and associates[65] compared outcomes in 96 patients with total occlusions that were 1 month or older who had undergone PTCA (53 patients before 1994) and Palmaz-Schatz stent placement (43 patients after 1994). This study demonstrated a lower restenosis rate in the stent patients (27.9% vs. 56.6%, $p < 0.005$) than in the angioplasty patients that appeared to be driven by a greater minimal luminal diameter after the procedure. Sirnes and coworkers[66] randomly assigned 117 patients with successfully recanalized chronic occlusions to a strategy of PTCA alone (59 patients) or a Palmaz-Schatz stent (58 patients). Six-month angiographic follow-up was 97% complete and revealed restenosis in 73.7% of the PTCA group and only 31.6% of the stent group ($p < 0.001$). Other investigators have similarly demonstrated markedly lower restenosis rates with the use of Palmaz-Schatz stents and the AVE microstents (20% to 28%) than the rates generally found with balloon angioplasty.[67-69] Improvement in left ventricular ejection fraction at 6-month follow-up has been reported.[67, 68] Use of a Wallstent has been reported to improve postprocedural minimal luminal diameter compared with patients undergoing angioplasty but was not shown to significantly reduce restenosis in a small, single-center report.[70]

On the basis of the promising initial registry reports of the routine use of stent implantation, several randomized trials of stent versus balloon angioplasty treatment of CTO have been completed (Table 25–10). These studies consistently demonstrate a superiority of routine stent implantation. Initial post-

**TABLE 25–10.** **RANDOMIZED TRIALS OF STENT VERSUS PTCA TREATMENT OF CHRONIC TOTAL CORONARY OCCLUSION**

| REFERENCE | STUDY | N | STENT TYPE | INITIAL ANGIOGRAPHIC OUTCOME (MLD/mm) | | ANGIOGRAPHIC RESTENOSIS (%) | | REOCCLUSION (%) | |
|---|---|---|---|---|---|---|---|---|---|
| | | | | PTCA | STENT | PTCA | STENT | PTCA | STENT |
| Mori et al[65] | — | 96 | Palmaz-Schatz | 1.7 ± 0.6 | 2.6 ± 0.4 | 56 | 34 | 11.3 | 7.0 |
| Sirnes et al[66] | SICCO | 117 | Palmaz-Schatz | 2.13 ± 0.57 | 2.78 ± 0.49 | 73.7 | 31.6 | 26.3 | 12.3 |
| Rubartelli et al* | GISSOC | 97 | Palmaz-Schatz | 1.91 ± 0.49 | 2.46 ± 0.5 | 68 | 32 | 34 | 8 |
| Buller et al[71] | TOSCA | 410 | Heparin-coated Palmaz-Schatz | 1.97 ± 0.46 | 2.45 ± 0.59 | 70 | 55 | 20 | 11 |
| Höher et al† | SPACTO | 85 | Wiktor | 1.09 ± 0.53 | 2.51 ± 0.41 | 64 | 32 | 24 | 3 |

*Rubartelli P, Niccoli L, Verna E, et al: Stent implantation versus balloon angioplasty in chronic coronary occlusions: Results from the GISSOC Trial. J Am Coll Cardiol 32:90, 1998.

†Höher M, Wöhrle J, Grebe O, et al: A randomized trial of elective stenting after balloon recanalization of chronic total occlusions. J Am Coll Cardiol 34:722, 1999.

GISSOC, Gruppo Italiano di Studio sullo Stent nelle Occlusioni Coronariche; MLD, minimal lumen diameter; PTCA, percutaneous transluminal coronary angioplasty; SICCO, Stenting in Chronic Coronary Occlusion; TOSCA, Total Occlusion Study of Canada.

procedure minimal lumen diameter is greater after stent implantation, 6-month restenosis rate is lower, and reocclusion rate is lower as well. The largest randomized trial (Total Occlusion Study of Canada [TOSCA][71]) has also demonstrated an important clinical benefit in that target vessel revascularization was reduced by 45% (15.4% vs. 8.4%; $p = 0.03$). Of importance is that no decrease in major adverse cardiac event rates and no differences in mortality have been reported. On the basis of these randomized trials, routine stent implantation is recommended after successful recanalization. This strategy is most likely to provide sustained clinical benefit.

## Excimer Laser

The excimer laser coronary angioplasty (ELCA) registry reported on the feasibility of the use of excimer laser in treating patients with a chronic occlusion.[56] Of the 4625 lesions in this registry 10% were chronic occlusions. Success was achieved in 88% of the lesions, and the mortality rate, was 0.6%. Coronary perforations occurred in 1.3% of patients (60% of which resulted in emergency bypass surgery, myocardial infarction, or death). The excimer laser has had no impact on reducing restenosis.

## High-Speed Rotational Atherectomy

Rotational atherectomy has theoretic advantages in chronic occlusion angioplasty because of its ability to debulk lesions. The early experience is limited and results are mixed. In 1996, Levin and coworkers[57] reported successful rotational atherectomy of 15 occlusions 3 months or older, leaving a mean residual stenosis of 15%. No major complications were reported.[57] However, in 1997, Braden and coworkers[70] reported on their series of 54 consecutive patients; in all 54, their lesions were successfully

crossed with a wire. They reported a 98% success rate with rotational atherectomy, a residual stenosis of 22.6%, and only a 9% repeat revascularization rate at 1-year follow-up. Complication rates were excessive, however, with an event rate of 15% two patients required bypass, five had non–Q-wave myocardial infarctions, and one died).

## SAPHENOUS VEIN GRAFTS

Angioplasty of saphenous vein grafts remains a great challenge to the interventional cardiologist and is discussed in detail in a previous chapter. Vein graft occlusion angioplasty is wrought with technical difficulty, low success rates, and unacceptable complication rates, often associated with intracoronary thromboembolism. Despite various trails of adjunctive intragraft thrombolytic therapy, clinical restenosis and long-term cardiac events are high, and thus occlusion vein graft angioplasty remains a temptation that should be resisted.

## CONCLUSIONS

Percutaneous revascularization of a chronic total coronary occlusion remains a challenge to the interventional cardiologist. Despite advances in device technology and pharmacotherapy that have improved outcomes for patients with subtotal stenoses, occlusion angioplasty continues to have relatively low procedural success rates and high restenosis rates. Complication rates appear to be higher than previously expected and equivalent to high-grade stenosis PTCA, further making the procedure less favorable. Several clinical and angiographic variables can be used to improve case selection and enhance success.

It can be reasonably expected that successful procedures will result in improved anginal status, but if refractory angina is the indication for the procedure, it would be prudent to first optimize the patient's medical regimen. Further analysis regarding the impact on survival and the need for subsequent bypass surgery is required before conclusions can be drawn.

New devices, such as the lase-wire, and new techniques, such as adjunctive intracoronary thrombolytic infusions, appear promising for patients who fail to respond to conventional techniques at recanalization. Intracoronary stents have become mainstay therapy and have produced a decrease in restenosis in comparison with PTCA alone. Future advances such as brachytherapy or implantation of coated stents may further improve long-term outcome.

## REFERENCES

1. Sheehan FK, Braunwald E, Canner P, et al: The effect of intravenous thrombolytic therapy on left ventricular function: A report on tissue-type plasminogen activator and streptokinase from the Thrombolysis in Myocardial Infarction (TIMI phase 1) trial. Circulation 75:817–829, 1987.
2. Gruppo Italiano per lo Studio della Streptochinasi nell'Infaro Miocardico (GISSI): Effectiveness of intravenous thrombolytic treatment in acute myocardial infarction. Lancet 1:397–401, 1986.
3. Grines CL, Browne KF, Marco J, et al: A comparison of immediate angioplasty with thrombolytic therapy for acute myocardial infarction: The Primary Angioplasty in Myocardial Infarction Study Group. N Engl J Med 328:673–679, 1993.
4. Puma JA, Sketch MH Jr, Tcheng JE, et al: Percutaneous revascularization of chronic coronary occlusions: An overview. J Am Coll Cardiol 26:1–11, 1995.
5. Savage R, Holiman J, Gruentzig AR, et al: Can percutaneous transluminal coronary angioplasty be performed in patients with total occlusion? [Abstract] Circulation 66(suppl II): II-330, 1982.
6. Serruys PW, de Jaegere P, Kiemeneij F, et al, for the Benestent Study Group: A comparison of balloon-expandable stent implantation with balloon angioplasty in patients with coronary artery disease. N Engl J Med 331:485–495, 1994.
7. Fishman DL, Leon MB, Baim DS, et al, for the Stent Restenosis Study Investigators: A randomized comparison of coronary stent placement and balloon angioplasty in the treatment of coronary artery disease. N Engl J Med 331:495–501, 1994.
8. EPIC Investigators: Use of a monoclonal antibody directed against the platelet glycoprotein IIb IIIa receptor in high-risk coronary angioplasty. N Engl J Med 330:956–961, 1994.
9. Meier B: Total coronary occlusion: A different animal? J Am Coll Cardiol 17:50B–57B, 1991.
10. Waller BF, Orr CM, Slack JD, et al: Anatomy, histology and pathology of coronary arteries: A review relevant to new interventional and imaging techniques—Part II. Clin Cardiol 15:535–540, 1992.
11. Srivatsa SS, Edwards WD, Boos CM, et al: Histologic correlates of angiographic chronic total coronary artery occlusions. J Am Coll Cardiol 29:955–963, 1997.
12. Myler RK, Shaw RE, Stertzer SK, et al: Lesion morphology and coronary angioplasty: Current experience and analysis. J Am Coll Cardiol 19:1641–1652, 1992.
13. Meier B: Chronic total occlusion. In Topol EJ (ed): Textbook of Interventional Cardiology, pp 300–326. Philadelphia: WB Saunders, 1990.
14. Saber RS, Edward WD, Holmes DR, et al: Balloon angioplasty of aortocoronary saphenous vein bypass grafts: A histopathologic study of six grafts from five patients with emphasis on

15. Holmes DR Jr, Vlietstra RE, Reeder GS, et al: Angioplasty in total coronary artery occlusion. J Am Coll Cardiol 3:845–849, 1984.
16. Kereiakes DJ, Selmon MR, McAuley BJ, et al: Angioplasty in total coronary artery occlusion: Experience in 76 consecutive patients. J Am Coll Cardiol 6:526–533, 1985.
17. Serruys PW, Umans V, Heyndrickx GR, et al: Elective PTCA of totally occluded coronary arteries not associated with acute myocardial infarction: Short-term and long-term results. Eur Heart J 6:2–12, 1985.
18. DiSciascio G, Vetrovec GW, Cowley MJ, et al: Early and late outcome of percutaneous transluminal coronary angioplasty of subacute and chronic total coronary occlusion. Am Heart J 111:833–839, 1986.
19. Melchior JP, Meier B, Urban P, et al: Percutaneous transluminal coronary angioplasty for chronic total coronary arterial occlusion. Am J Cardiol 59:535–538, 1987.
20. Finci L, Meier B, Vavre J, et al: Long-term results of successful and failed angioplasty for chronic total coronary arterial occlusion. Am J Cardiol 66:660–662, 1990.
21. Warren RJ, Black AJ, Valentine PA, et al: Coronary angioplasty for chronic total occlusion reduces the need for subsequent coronary bypass surgery. Am Heart J 120:270–274, 1990.
22. Bell MR, Berger QB, Bresnahan JF, et al: Initial and long-term outcome of 354 patients after coronary balloon angioplasty of total coronary artery occlusions. Circulation 85:1003–1011, 1992.
23. Ruocco NA Jr, Ring ME, Holubkov R, et al: Results of coronary angioplasty of chronic total occlusions: The National Heart, Lung, and Blood Institute 1985–1986 Percutaneous Transluminal Angioplasty Registry. Am J Cardiol 69:69–76, 1992.
24. Stewart JT, Denne L, Bowker TI, et al: Percutaneous transluminal coronary angioplasty chronic coronary artery occlusion. J Am Coll Cardiol 21:1371–1376, 1993.
25. Sathe S, Alt C, Black A, et al: Initial and long-term results of percutaneous transluminal balloon angioplasty for chronic total occlusions: An analysis of 184 procedures. Aust N Z J Med 24:227–281, 1994.
26. Berger PB, Holmes DR Jr, Ohman EM, et al: Restenosis, reocclusion and adverse cardiovascular events after successful balloon angioplasty of occluded versus nonoccluded coronary arteries: Results from the Multicenter American Research Trial with Cilazapril after angioplasty to prevent transluminal coronary obstruction and restenosis (MARCATOR). J Am Coll Cardiol 27:1–7, 1996.
27. Flameng W, Schwarz F, Hehrlein FW: Intraoperative evaluation of the functional significance of coronary collateral vessels in patients with coronary artery disease. Am J Cardiol 42:187–192, 1978.
28. Lange RA, Cigarroa RG, Hillis LD: Influence of residual antegrade coronary blood flow on survival after myocardial infarction in patients with multivessel coronary artery disease. Coron Artery Dis 1:59–63, 1990.
29. Trappe HJ, Lichtlen PR, Klein H, et al: Natural history of single vessel disease: Risk of sudden coronary death in relation to coronary anatomy and arrhythmia profile. Eur Heart J 10:514–524, 1989.
30. Moliterno DJ, Lange RA, Willard JE, et al: Does restoration of antegrade flow in the infarct-related coronary artery days to weeks after myocardial infarction improve long-term survival? Coron Artery Dis 3:299–304, 1992.
31. Puma JA, Sketch MH Jr, Tcheng JE, et al: The natural history of single-vessel chronic coronary occlusion: A 25-year experience. Am Heart J 133:393–399, 1997.
32. Ivanhoe RJ, Weintraub WS, Douglas JS Jr, et al: Percutaneous transluminal coronary angioplasty of chronic total occlusions: Primary success, restenosis, and long-term clinical follow-up. Circulation 85:106–115, 1992.
33. Engelstein E, Terres W, Hofmann D, et al: Improved global and regional left ventricular function after angioplasty for chronic coronary occlusion. Clin Invest 72:442–447, 1994.
34. Danchin N, Angioï M, Cador R, et al: Effect of late percutane-

ous angioplastic recanalization of total coronary artery occlusion on left ventricular remodeling, ejection fraction, and regional wall motion. Am J Cardiol 78:729–735, 1996.

35. DiCarli M, Sherman T, Khanna S, et al: Myocardial viability in asynergic regions subtended by occluded coronary arteries: Relation to the status of collateral flow in patients, chronic coronary artery disease. J Am Coll Cardiol 23:860–868, 1994.

36. Haine E, Urban P, Dorsaz PA, et al: Outcome and complications of 500 consecutive chronic total occlusion coronary angioplasties [Abstract]. J Am Coll Cardiol 21:138A, 1993.

37. Ishizaka N, Issiki T, Saeki F, et al: Angiographic follow-up after successful percutaneous coronary angioplasty for chronic total coronary occlusions: Experience in 110 consecutive patients. Am Heart J 127:8–12, 1994.

38. Safian RD, McCabe CH, Sipperly ME, et al: Initial success and long-term follow-up of percutaneous transluminal coronary angioplasty in chronic total occlusions versus conventional stenoses. Am J Cardiol 61:23G–28G, 1988.

39. Ellis SG, Shaw RE, Gershony G, et al: Risk factors, time course and treatment effect for restenosis after successful percutaneous transluminal coronary angioplasty of chronic total occlusion. Am J Cardiol 63:897–901, 1989.

40. Hamm CW, Kupper W, Kuck KH, et al: Recanalization of chronic, totally occluded coronary arteries by new angioplasty systems. Am J Cardiol 66:1459–1463, 1990.

41. Stone GW, Rutherford BD, McConahay DR, et al: Procedural outcome of angioplasty for total coronary occlusion: An analysis of 971 lesions in 905 patients. J Am Coll Cardiol 15:849–856, 1990.

42. Jollis JG, Petersen ED, DeLong ER, et al: The relationship between the volume of coronary angioplasty procedures at hospitals treating Medicare beneficiaries and short-term mortality. N Engl J Med 331:1625–1629, 1994.

43. Maiello L, Colombo A, Giatuossi R, et al: Coronary angioplasty of chronic occlusions: Factors predictive of procedural success. Am Heart J 124:581–584, 1992.

44. Tan W, Sulke AN, Taub NA, et al: Determinants of success of coronary angioplasty in patients with a chronic total occlusion: A multiple logistic regression model to improve selection of patients. Br Heart J 70:126–131, 1993.

45. Herrmann G, Muurling S, Wille B, et al: Recanalization of chronically occluded coronary arteries: Single-center experience in 400 cases, including long-term angiographic follow-up. J Intervent Cardiol 9:73–79, 1996.

46. Konoshita I, Katou O, Nariyama J, et al: Coronary angioplasty of chronic total occlusions with bridging collateral vessels: Immediate and follow-up outcome in a large single-center experience. J Am Coll Cardiol 26:409–415, 1995.

47. Little T, Rosenbert J, Seides S, et al: Probe angioplasty of total coronary occlusion using the probing catheter technique. Cathet Cardiovasc Diagn 21:124, 1990.

48. Plante S, Laarman GJ, de Feyter PJ, et al: Acute complications of percutaneous transluminal coronary angioplasty for total occlsuion. Am Heart J 121:417, 1991.

49. Bell MR, Berger PB, Menke KK, et al: Balloon angioplasty of chronic total coronary artery occlusions: What does it cost in radiation exposure, time, and materials? Cathet Cardiovasc Diagn 25:10–15, 1992.

50. Sherman CT, Sheehan D, Simpson JB: Simultaneous cannulation: A technique for percutaneous transluminal coronary angioplasty of chronic total occlusions. Cathet Cardiovasc Diagn 13:333, 1987.

51. Grollier G, Commeau P, Foucalt JP, et al: Angioplasty of chronic totally occluded coronary arteries: Usefulness of retrograde opacification of the distal part of the occluded vessel via the contralateral artery. Am Heart J 114:1324, 1987.

52. Rees MR, Sivananthan MV, Verma SP: The use of hydrophilic Terumo glide wires in the treatment of chronic coronary artery occlusions [Abstract]. Circulation 84:II-519, 1991.

53. Freed M, Boatman J, Siegel N, et al: Glide wire treatment of resistant coronary occlusions. Cathet Cardiovasc Diagn 30:201–204, 1993.

54. Meier B, Urban P, Villavicencio R, et al: Magnum/Magnarail versus conventional systems for recanalization of chronic total coronary occlusions: A randomized comparison [Abstract]. Circulation 82:III-678, 1990.

55. Haerer W, Schmidt A, Eggeling T, et al: Angioplasty of chronic total coronary occlusion: Results of a controlled randomized trial [Abstract]. J. Cardiol 17:113A, 1991.

56. Reeder GS: Coronary intervention with the excimer laser: A current prospective. J Intervent Cardiol 9:175–178, 1996.

57. Levin TN, Carroll J, Feldman T: High-speed rotational atherectomy for chronic total coronary occlusions. Cathet Cardiovasc Diagn 3:34–39, 1996.

58. Vaska KJ, Whitlow PL: Selective tissue plasminogen activator infusion for chronic total occlusions of native coronary arteries failing angioplasty. Circulation 84:II-250, 1991.

59. Ruocco NA Jr, Currier JW, Jacobs AK, et al: Experience with low-dose intracoronary recombinant tissue-type plasminogen activator for nonacute total occlusions before percutaneous transluminal coronary angioplasty. Am J Cardiol 68:1609, 1991.

60. Ajluni SC, Jones D, Zidar F, et al: Prolonged urokinase infusion for chronic total native coronary occlusions: Clinical angiographic, and treatment observations. Cathet Cardiovasc Diag 34:106–110, 1995.

61. Zidar FJ, Kaplan BM, O'Neill WW, et al: Prospective, randomized trial of prolonged intracoronary urokinase infusion for chronic total occlusions in native coronary arteries. J Am Coll Cardiol 27:1406–1410, 1996.

62. Schofer J, Rau T, Mathey DG: Laser wire procedures: Determinants for success of recanalization of chronic coronary occlusions—A single center experience [Abstract]. J Am Coll Cardiol 29(suppl A):459A, 1997.

63. Steffen W, Hamm CW, Terres W, et al: Is laserwire recanalization of chronic total occlusions associated with a greater risk than conventional recanalizaton? [Abstract] J Am Coll Cardiol 29(suppl A):459A, 1997.

64. Hamburger JN, Gomes R, Simon R, et al: Recanalization of chronic total coronary occlusions using a laser guidewire: The European TOTAL Multicenter Surveillance Study. J Am Coll Cardiol 29(suppl A):69A, 1997.

65. Mori M, Kurogane H, Hayashi T, et al: Comparison of results of intracoronary implantation of the Palmaz-Schatz stent with conventional balloon angioplasty in chronic total coronary arterial occlusion. Am J Cardiol 78:985–988, 1996.

66. Sirnes A, Golf S, Myreng Y, et al: Stenting in Chronic Coronary Occlusion (SICCO): A randomized controlled trial of adding stent implantation after successful angioplasty. J Am Coll Cardiol 28:1444–1451, 1996.

67. Medina A, Melian F, Suárez de Lezo J, et al: Effectiveness of coronary stenting for the treatment of chronic total occlusion in angina pectoris. Am J Cardiol 73:1222–1224, 1994.

68. Goldberg SC, Colombo A, Maiello L, et al: Intracoronary stent insertion after balloon angioplasty of chronic total occlusions. J Am Coll Cardiol 26:713–719, 1995.

69. Ozaki Y, Violaris A, Hamburger J, et al: Short- and long-term clinical and quantitative angiographic results with the new, less shortening wallstent for vessel reconstruction in chronic total occlusions: A quantitative angiographic study. J Am Coll Cardiol 28:354–60, 1996.

70. Braden GA, Matthews BJ, Love WM et al: Is rotational atherectomy the treatment of choice for chronic total occlusions? [Abstract]. J Am Coll Cardiol 29(suppl A):315A, 1997.

71. Buller CE, Dzavik V, Carere RG, et al: Primary stenting versus balloon angioplasty in occluded arteries. The Total Occlusion Study of Canada. Circulation 100:236, 1999.

# 26

# Support Systems for Percutaneous Cardiac Interventions

*William A. Baxley*   *Gary S. Roubin*   *Johnnie Knobloch*

## SUPPORTED CORONARY ANGIOPLASTY

To many interventional cardiologists, the term "support" is synonymous with intra-aortic balloon pumping. Actually, it is a broad generic concept that can be viewed from various perspectives. The study of this concept reveals important insights into the basis of present-day coronary intervention and provides practical guidelines useful in patient care. Support is the technique of maintaining adequate peripheral and coronary circulation during a procedure as well as before and after it. It can best be understood when approached from three vantage points: historical, physiologic-mechanical, and practical.

## HISTORICAL BACKGROUND

The concept of support actually began with Andreas Gruentzig's concern over the possible detrimental myocardial ischemic effect of transient coronary balloon inflation. Initially, in the late 1970s and early 1980s, the chosen patients had optimal-lesion, single-vessel disease, with good ventricular function and surgical standby. Brief coronary occlusion was generally well tolerated by the patient, although bradycardia was occasionally encountered with right coronary (or circumflex in a left dominant system) angioplasty. For this reason, right ventricular temporary pacing wires were placed prophylactically with this type pathoanatomy.

From the mid-1980s to the early 1990s, angioplasty technology advanced markedly, including new and improved lesion-treatment devices of all types, computerization of data, and greatly enhanced imaging systems. With this better technology came advancement into the realms of multivessel disease, poor ventricular function, and coexisting multiorgan failure. As interventional cardiologists' tools improved, they were embold-

ened into more treacherous terrain. From the earliest angioplasties, one of the major procedural problems was acute or threatened vessel closure. The best treatment for this occurrence, other than a quick trip to the operating room, was prolonged balloon inflation to "tack up" the traumatized vessel. This worked much of the time. However, factors such as a large myocardial segment at risk, multivessel disease, and poor myocardial function could combine with protracted inflation to produce such severe sequelae as progressive hypotension, pulmonary edema, intense angina, or arrhythmias. So during these years, a series of support technologies were devised to lessen these problems, some quite ingenious, as listed in Table 26–1. The intra-aortic balloon pump has been in use since the early 1970s in both cardiology and cardiac surgery settings, and it has continued to be employed throughout all the subsequent eras.[1] A technology of profound importance, it is described in greater detail later. However, because of the vascular trauma associated with the intra-aortic balloon pump and, to a lesser extent, its cost, complexity, and inability to totally support the circulation, other methods were also tried.

One of the earliest methods, which is still occasionally used today, is the autoperfusion coronary angioplasty balloon.[2] This device has luminal side

**TABLE 26–1.   MAJOR TYPES OF SUPPORT SYSTEMS USED IN PERCUTANEOUS CARDIAC INTERVENTIONS**

Intra-aortic balloon pump
Autoperfusion coronary balloon
Corflo distal-perfusion pump
Oxygenated blood-substitute for distal perfusion
Coronary sinus retroperfusion system
Left ventricle–to–aorta Hemopump
General anesthesia
Partial cardiopulmonary bypass

holes proximal and distal to the balloon, allowing downstream coronary flow during prolonged inflation. Flow rates up to 60 mL/min have been reported.[3] However, maximal flows require that the guide wire be withdrawn partially, thus losing its distal position. Although this technique for vessel repair compared favorably with stents in the early 1990s,[4] stent technology has markedly advanced since that time. The autoperfusion balloon concept grew out of the "bail-out catheter," a simple tube with multiple distal side holes, which could be fed over a guide wire across an acute closure.[5] When the guide wire was withdrawn, distal flow could be maintained to some extent, often while the patient was hurriedly transported to the operating room. Indeed, early on, verbal anecdotes abounded of patients rushed to surgery with ongoing angina, while the interventional cardiologist trotted alongside, pumping arterialized blood through such a catheter in conjunction with an improvised stopcock system.

The perfusion balloon is a "passive-flow" device that relies on the patient's arterial pressure. There followed development of several active perfusion devices not so constrained. The Corflo pump is a small, simple electrical piston-pump mounted near the femoral artery area. Oxygenated blood is drafted from any source (a separate femoral artery sheath, or side port of the angioplasty sheath, or from a venous catheter in a renal vein because the kidney extracts very little oxygen). With the balloon inflated at the lesion and the wire removed, active distal coronary artery flows up to 60 mL/min could be maintained extensively through the catheter lumen. Angelini and colleagues[6] utilized this technique in 61 high-risk patients with 96.5% success, although there was a 7.8% hospital mortality.

A variant of the Corflo system that gained some brief popularity involved the use of the "artificial-hemoglobin," or blood-substitute, concept. Perfluorocarbons are not actually hemoglobins, but they do have some milieux-dependent oxygen-binding properties and can be used as such. They could be forced luminally during prolonged balloon inflation to nourish downstream myocardium and attenuate ischemia.[7] Only a pressurized bag or contrast type of power injector was necessary for this procedure.

Another system for myocardial protection during revascularization (terms borrowed from the surgeons) is coronary sinus retroperfusion.[8] This also produces active perfusion but involves somewhat more hardware and technology than do those described earlier. Here, one cannulates the coronary sinus to access the coronary venous drainage system. The catheter has a small, occlusive balloon proximally with oxygenated-blood infusion distally. The device functions rhythmically via an electrocardiogram (ECG)-gated timer. Thus, in diastole, the now-expanded proximal balloon prevents drainage and the distally exiting blood perfuses the myocardium in a retrograde vein-to-capillary manner. During systole, the balloon deflates quickly and normal drainage ensues. Cardiac surgeons have used this technique for regional cardioplegia to areas blocked for antegrade perfusion. However, the difficulty in coannulating the coronary sinus and the general complexity of the technique have prevented its general popularity.

Another more powerful device, unique and intriguing in design, is the Hemopump.[9] Introduced for human use in the late 1980s, it actively enhances left ventricular output and, in so doing, maintains both peripheral and coronary circulation as well as decreases myocardial oxygen demand. The Hemopump is basically a screw pump ("Archimedes screw" or helix) mounted distally inside a catheter with a flexible, high-RPM shaft connected to an external motor. It is inserted into the femoral artery and advanced retrograde across the aortic valve. The screw pump drafts left ventricular chamber blood and discharges it into the ascending aorta. Three sizes are available, a 14-French for percutaneous use and two larger sizes for surgical insertion. Flows up to 4.7 L/min can be achieved. Surprisingly, blood protein damage or red-cell hemolysis have not been problems. Hemodynamic measurements made on 18 patients with the 14-French percutaneous device during high-risk angioplasty revealed a fall from 23.5 mm Hg mean pulmonary artery wedge pressure to 18.6 with pump activation, without a change in heart rate, aortic pressure, cardiac index, or coronary flow velocity.[10] Scholz and associates[11] used this device in 32 high-risk angioplasty cases; mortality was high (4 deaths), and 2 had femoral artery occlusion. However, this was a particularly ill patient group. The size of this device and the vascular complications have thus far limited its widespread popularity, although its ultimate future has yet to be determined.

Pediatric cardiologists have utilized general anesthesia for invasive studies since their origins, for obvious reasons. Adult electrophysiologic procedures likewise often involve this entity to limit patient discomfort and permit complete relaxation. It is also a form of support in certain adult coronary interventional cases, and it has been used sporadically in this context for decades. In the early 1990s, the authors began to intervene in what was then the most complex and riskiest cases of angioplasty utilizing partial cardiopulmonary bypass. Along with bypass, the authors routinely had the services of the Cardiac Anesthesiology Department, with tracheal intubation and the patient asleep.

Partial cardiopulmonary bypass is the most complete form of support that has been utilized in the interventional suite. (This term appears more precise and thus is preferable to "cardiopulmonary support," or CPS. For example, general anesthesia with intra-aortic balloon pumping is "cardiopulmonary support" but does not involve bypass). Historically, this technology was borrowed from the cardiac surgeons, and it involves large-bore percutaneous cannulas in venous and arterial sites, routing blood through the external portable pump–oxygenator–heat exchanger; this is described in greater detail subsequently. The partial bypass technique for high-risk coronary angioplasty was popularized by Shawl and colleagues[12] and can adequately support the circulation, even in the presence of cardiac quiescence. In the early and mid-1990s, the authors utilized this system routinely in ultra-high-risk patients and developed a strict, highly effective protocol.[13] Extracorporeal membrane oxygenator (ECMO) technology is related and is used primarily for more prolonged support in severe but potentially reversible pulmonary disease. However, some cardiac usefulness has been described.[14] In contrast, a system that does not require an oxygenator uses a transvenous and transseptal approach to the left atrium. Blood is then circulated from the left atrium to a femoral arterial cannula to provide hemodynamic support.

In the early and mid 1990s, the continued development and improvement of one particularly important coronary angioplasty device profoundly affected the need for support: the intracoronary stent. Stents, together with improved delivery systems, initial lesion–treatment devices and pharmacologic adjuncts have greatly shortened average procedure time and have markedly improved the treatment of acute or threatened closure. Paralleling the dramatic increase in stent use has been a marked decrease in the need for emergent "bail-out" surgery; in one large multicenter trial, operations were needed in fewer than 0.5% of angioplasty cases.[15] Now the probability of rapid repair of lesions previously considered high risk has made support systems a rarely needed technology, except in a few important areas. Even data as recent as 1996 showing good results in 35 high-risk patients with supported angioplasty (but with 3 deaths in hospital, 5 the first year and 2 the second year)[16] may need reevaluation in the modern stent era. The most common condition currently requiring support is ongoing or threatened myocardial infarction with shock. The intra-aortic balloon pump has stood the test of time and is the device most used in this setting, as will be described later. Even left main coronary lesions, long considered an absolute contraindication to angioplasty, have been safely treated percutaneously. Partial cardiopulmonary bypass still has a rare indication today, as does the simple autoperfusion balloon, and

active coronary perfusion devices may find a place in clinical research.

One other development in coronary disease treatment may alter the future of cardiac or coronary support use, and that is hybrid procedures combining bypass surgery and angioplasty.[17] Also, an example of combined interventional and surgical technology is the percutaneously placed right coronary catheter used in producing temporary electrical quiescence for off-pump surgery.[18] This development of off-pump bypass surgery[19] and the potential for further improvement of hybrid interventions may signal further partnership between surgeons and interventional cardiologists[20] and the need for a change in support system usage in the future. Interventional cardiologists can adapt to these changes best if they understand the history of support technology as well as the physiologic-mechanical properties of the most important devices.

## PHYSIOLOGIC-MECHANICAL CONSIDERATIONS

Of the support devices listed, intra-aortic balloon pumping and partial cardiopulmonary bypass alter the circulation most profoundly and are discussed herein. The intra-aortic balloon pump is the hallmark of cardiac support today, and for the interventional cardiologist it is the most reliable and important adjunct. Its mechanical characteristics have been described in detail,[21] but the functions can be summarized as follows. The intra-aortic balloon, generally 30, 40, or 50 mL in volume (40 mL is the most commonly used) and 9-French to 11-French in size, is inflated and then deflated with helium alternatively and rhythmically, gated to the intrinsic cardiac cycle via either the ECG or aortic pressure wave (as recorded through the balloon-catheter lumen). Precise timing is essential, with inflation adjusted to just after aortic-valve closure, as evidenced by the diacritic notch on the pressure trace. Deflation occurs prior to ejection systole (before the upswing of the pressure curve). The hydraulic effect of this alternating (e.g., 40 mL) aortic volume change is twofold: balloon inflation with the aortic valve closed displaces 40 mL of blood out toward the peripheral (and coronary) arteries, in this way helping the heart "in series" to maintain forward flow. Then in deflation, the balloon lowers the peripheral resistance (or afterload) that the ventricle must eject against, thus enhancing stroke volume. "Creating aortic suction" is too strong a phrase, although it may help the operator in conceptualizing this hydraulic sequence. This phase is also an "in-series" circulatory assist. In contrast, as discussed subsequently, the partial bypass support-form is "in parallel" with the heart, in engineering terms.

As a third benefit, in addition to improving coronary flow and increasing left ventricular contraction (by lowering afterload), left ventricular oxygen requirements tend to decrease with the diminished afterload. This effect can further relieve angina. These physiologic-mechanical events are schematized in Figure 26–1. The resulting physiologic changes in any given patient are predictable only qualitatively, not quantitatively. The reason is that the success of the device depends on multiple factors that involve the individual patient's own circulatory status at the time of pumping. One need only reflect that the clinical effect of the device in the setting of total cardiac-circulatory quiescence would be nil, with blood simply washing back and forth in the vascular system with no net forward flow. Likewise, in a totally normal individual, pumping would undoubtedly not alter the patient's circulation or cardiac status in any clinically important way. The pump best serves the patient who has some, but not total, inefficiency of cardiac function or coronary flow, or both. As pump-induced cardiac output improves, that alone may increase coronary perfusion, and vice versa. This multiparameter interdependency has made it difficult to quantitatively predict its effect, and it has made clinical research in this area tend to be less precise than hoped. Of interest, recall that a left ventricular stroke volume of 40 mL at a heart rate of 100 equals a cardiac output of 4.0 L/min. However, because of the interplay of the multiple physiologic variables previously described, predicting the balloon's effect in this way is incorrect. Furthermore, after 30 years of experience with the balloon pump, cardiologists and surgeons know that this device works well in certain patient subsets; thus, they are reluctant to introduce the concept of "controls" onto these quite ill individuals. So because of the interdependency of pump-result and cardiac function, and the scarcity of controls, much of the physiologic-based research concerning this support form is lacking. However, group-based studies have revealed important insights. Studies have documented a reduction in left ventricular end-diastolic pressure and myocardial oxygen consumption per unit time ($\dot{V}O_2$) during pumping, and cardiac output increases 10% to 40%.[22–24] Coronary flow augmentation is variable, with some studies showing up to a 40% increase.[25–26] Of importance is that studies with a Doppler-tipped guide wire showed that pumping does not augment coronary flow beyond a critical stenosis.[27] Thus, only after angioplasty will this support improve flow to the ischemic zone. Other epidemiology-type investigations are described subsequently, in the section on Cardiogenic Shock.

## Partial Cardiopulmonary Bypass

Although rarely used in today's cardiac interventional procedures, review of the physiologic aspects of partial bypass provides an intriguing foray into an indistinct border between cardiology and surgery. Partial bypass may prove a useful tool in the continuing development of hybrid procedures. The hydraulics of the system are straightforward, with drafting of venous blood from the right atrial cannula via a rotary pump, with circulation through a membrane oxygenator (with air-flow control for carbon dioxide removal). A heat exchanger is required to prevent gradual hypothermia from extracorporeal circuitry. Blood is then returned under pressure to the patient via the femoral artery cannula (Fig. 26–2). This is a closed fluid system, as opposed to the gravity venous drainage used in most open heart operations, and is nonphasic constant flow. At start-up, flow is gradually instituted to allow slow dilution of the approximately 1400-mL nonsanguineous prime, usually Normosol (combined electrolyte solution with dextrose). This results in a hematocrit fall that is generally well tolerated. Flows can achieve approximately 5 L/min with constraints imposed by low right atrial pressure and cannula size.

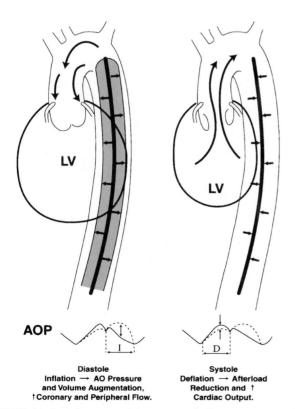

AOP

| Diastole | Systole |
|---|---|
| Inflation → AO Pressure and Volume Augmentation, ↑Coronary and Peripheral Flow. | Deflation → Afterload Reduction and ↑ Cardiac Output. |

FIGURE 26–1. Schematic of intra-aortic balloon pumping; diastolic inflation *(left)* and systolic deflation *(right)*. (AO, aortic; AOP, aorta pressure; D, deflation; I, inflation; LV, left ventricle; -----, effect of pumping.)

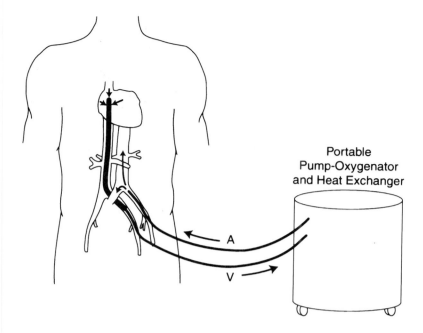

FIGURE 26–2. Schematic of extracorporeal circulation system for partial cardiopulmonary bypass. (A, arterial line; V, venous line.)

A series of interesting physiologic events occurs with bypass. Flow, at least in the lower part of the body, is retrograde up the aorta (Fig. 26–3). The heart's own native cardiac output drops significantly. Figure 26–4 shows blood flow measurements made on a patient undergoing angioplasty with partial bypass. Pulmonary blood flow, as measured by the Fick continuous-monitoring method,[28] is synon-ymous with native left ventricular output. Here, oxygen transport across the lungs, or oxygen consumption as measured transtracheally, represents only part of the total body $\dot{V}O_2$, the oxygenator supplying the remainder. As the measurements show, native cardiac output falls roughly the amount of bypass pump flow, so that total body circulation remains relatively unchanged. Thus, the hydraulic work and

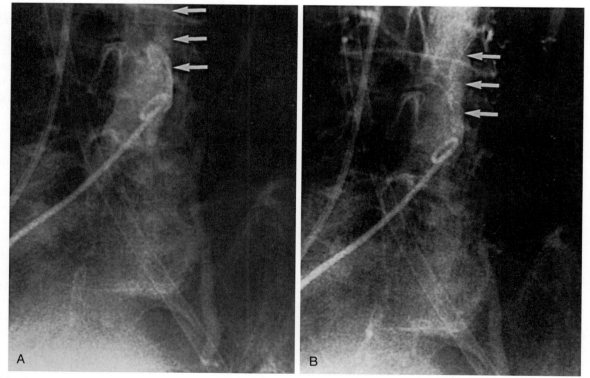

FIGURE 26–3. A descending aortogram during partial bypass. Sequential images (A and B; left to right) reveal the retrograde flow up the aorta (arrows).

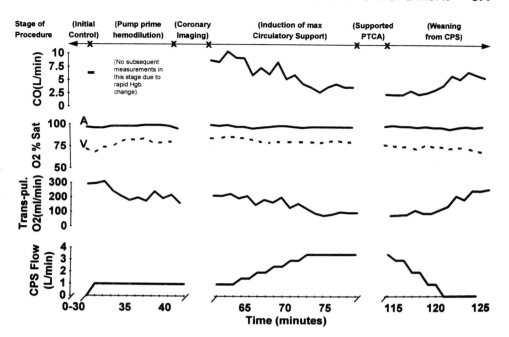

FIGURE 26–4. Continuous monitoring of multiple physiologic parameters before, during, and after coronary angioplasty with partial-bypass support. (CPS, pump oxygenator; transpul, transpulmonary; CO, native cardiac output; max, maximum). Note that as pump flow is increased to about 3 L/min, both native cardiac output (and transpulmonary oxygen extraction) decrease roughly the same amount, as total circulation is basically unchanged. Arterial (A) and mixed venous (V) $O_2$ saturation remain physiologic.

gas exchange functions are shifted partially and temporarily from the heart and lungs to the extracorporeal device.

With partial bypass, cardiac filling pressures and aortic pressure fall dramatically from venous aspiration and preload reduction. One study utilizing simultaneous quantitative echocardiography and hemodynamic monitoring showed that during bypass, left ventricular size and global function remain unchanged.[29] However, regional and global dysfunction still occur with angioplasty balloon inflation.

Cardiac surgeons, more than cardiologists, are aware of the threat of intraprocedure progressive left ventricular distention, with ensuing ischemia and arrhythmias. This condition can be prevented or reversed by temporary ventricular venting and decompression. Figure 26–5 shows a form of venting in a patient undergoing angioplasty with partial bypass. The authors "knuckled" a small catheter across the pulmonic valve to cause incompetence: this results in less forward flow into the left ventricle, higher right atrial pressure, and a greater shift of the circulation to the pump-oxygenator without the need for blood transfusion. That is, when aortic pressure drops below a 65 mm Hg mean or so, transfusion—"addition" is the surgical term—may be necessary if right atrial pressure is also low. Stated another way, if right-sided filling pressure is near zero, pump flow cannot be increased.

An interesting and important phenomenon occurs early after partial bypass. Surgeons have known that extracorporeal circulation causes a transient total body inflammatory reaction.[30] This results in increased capillary permeability, a variable degree of peripheral edema, and fluid "third-spacing." Intra-

vascular volume may drop dramatically, even causing hypotension in the recovery period, which, in turn, may produce limb ischemia if a vascular clamp is in place. Careful attention to pulmonary artery pressures and fluid need are important after the procedure.

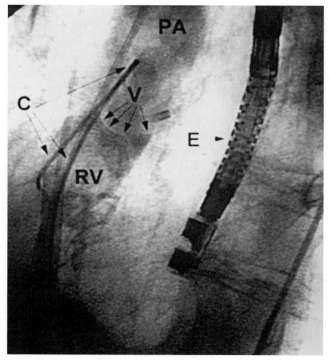

FIGURE 26–5. Pulmonary angiogram during coronary angioplasty with vented partial-bypass support. The right-heart catheter (C) has been knuckled across the pulmonic valve (V) to cause valve incompetence. Dye refluxes from the pulmonary artery (PA) into the right ventricle (RV). (E, transesophageal echo probe.)

## PRACTICAL ASPECTS OF SUPPORT

### Preliminary Evaluation

As the concept of support involves maintaining satisfactory peripheral and coronary circulation during the procedure, every angioplasty patient requires a risk assessment. Angioplasty risk factors, in general, parallel mortality risk factors for coronary surgery, although there are several important differences, and these factors have changed somewhat in recent years, reflecting technologic advances. One large multicenter survey revealed that operative mortality was highest in the aged, in women, with comorbidities, with poor ventricular function or recent or evolving myocardial infarction, or in emergency, hemodynamic-instability settings.[31] Although heart failure is an important risk, recovery is related to the amount of viable myocardium.[32] In another large multicenter study, the risk factors for angioplasty mortality were evaluated[33]: female gender or valve disease was not as important, but increased creatinine, noncardiac vascular disease, and type-C lesions were added to the surgical-risk list. A history of heart failure has been shown to be a risk factor separate from ejection fraction.[34] From a time-related perspective, the risk-predictors of major adverse events in patients scheduled for angioplasty were reported in 1999 by Harrell and colleagues.[35] Historically, with progressive improvements in technology through the years prior to 1999, successful treatment of lesions increased from 91% to 95% and adverse events decreased from 3.6% to 1.6%. In addition to the previously listed factors, this study showed that the total number of lesions treated is a risk factor. Important also is the interventional cardiologist's overall estimate of risk; this proved highly successful in a large European series.[36] Before the procedure, operators should listen to their intuition as well as review the numbers.

In the daily activities of the interventional laboratory, few patients will need a support device, but each is best served by optimal physiologic conditions. Thus, a patient who arrives at the interventional suite lightly sedated and relaxed with normal blood pressure, heart rate and pulmonary capillary wedge pressure (either measured or estimated), and optimal laboratory values has a better chance of coasting through any untoward event than does the patient not well prepared. Routine monitoring of aortic pressure, cardiac rhythm, and arterial oxygenation with a pulse oximeter are further safety measures, though not truly support.

### Pulmonary Artery Monitoring Catheter

This can be considered a simple support device, as its use helps maintain circulatory adequacy in certain patient subsets. This may be inserted before the procedure to optimize fluid and medication management in hemodynamically unstable patients, such as those with overt or impending pulmonary edema, hypotension, renal insufficiency, or severe coexistent pulmonary disease. Likewise, the right ventricular temporary pacing wire is a support device for any patient considered at risk for bradyarrhythmias. Early experience showed occasional right ventricular perforation and pericardial tamponade in this setting, apparently related to the continued slight movement in the femoral artery area associated with the procedure. A good plan is to "park" the pacer tip safely just across the tricuspid valve in standby configuration, where it can be rapidly advanced if needed.

### Intra-aortic Balloon Pump

Most interventional cardiologists receive training in the use of this device and are comfortable with it in the average-build patient with ongoing ischemia or severe heart failure, or both. The principles are simple: percutaneous femoral artery insertion of the long guide wire (contralateral side to the angioplasty site), threading the balloon catheter over it to position the tip distal to the great vessels in the aortic arch, removal of the wire, connecting the balloon-lumen and central lumen appropriately to the console, timing the functions, and commencing augmentation. The interventional cardiologist has the advantage over the surgeon, who cannot visualize the balloon after insertion and must rely on manual sensation for guidance and on markings for proper positioning. Futhermore, fluoroscopic visualization after start-up ensures complete inflation-deflation function.

The judgmental, and more difficult, aspects of balloon-pump support include determining the patients in whom it should be used, dealing with peripheral vascular disease, sizing, anticoagulation, management of complications, weaning to discontinuation, and nursing care (which is not discussed here, except to comment that pump-manufacturers' classes for nurses are excellent for physicians also).

Decision-making regarding pump use in the interventional suite and recovery unit involves three questions:

1. Does the patient's ventricular and coronary status indicate pump use, and if it does, should this device be employed on a functioning or standby basis?
2. What other features of the particular patient, both cardiac and noncardiac, influence this decision?
3. What is the proper balloon size?

Deciding which patient needs balloon-pump support may be primarily judgmental. Table 26–2 lists

## TABLE 26-2.  CONDITIONS CONSIDERED FOR SUPPORT

I. Emergency (support instituted)
   A. Acute myocardial infarction with shock
   B. Acute large-vessel closure not recrossable
   C. Other uncommon cardiac catastrophes (extensive dissection, coronary rupture, cardiac tamponade not quickly corrected)
II. Elective (support may be standby)
   A. Left main coronary angioplasty
   B. Angioplasty with very poor ventricular function
   C. Angioplasty of vessels subtending large myocardial segments
   D. Patients otherwise judged high-risk

some of the clinical situations indicating the possible need for support. Clearly, the individual with ongoing infarction and shock may need this urgently, as discussed in greater detail later. Likewise, the patient with poor ventricular function who has just undergone successful angioplasty of a lesion subtending a large myocardial segment may need this "help" for a few days. Balloon-pump support thus may be anticipatory (placed and functioning before angioplasty) or at procedure completion. If the patient has a high-risk lesion and the operator institutes pump support early but then obtains a fast and perfect result, he or she may have traded off the not-needed support for an increased risk of femoral artery complication from the pump. One popular solution to this dilemma is to utilize the pump on a standby basis. In this configuration, a small-size arterial sheath is inserted into the contralateral femoral artery, pump ECG leads are placed, the console is powered, and the balloon-catheter is kept nearby for quick insertion if needed.

Each potential candidate for balloon-pump support needs a special assessment in addition to that of coronary or ventricular status. Aortic valve insufficiency would increase with diastolic augmentation and is considered a contraindication, as is aortic aneurysm. Femoral artery (and distal vessel) evaluation is important, including bruits and popliteal and pedal pulses. A brief distal aortogram from the angioplasty side, showing the contralateral vessel, may be helpful in this regard. A prior history of femoral-popliteal surgery with its scar formation contraindicates that vessel's use, except in the most urgent circumstances. Monitoring of cardiac rhythm is also germane. Modern pumps can handle atrial fibrillation and paced rhythm reasonably well, although frequent premature ventricular contractions may decrease support. Finally, the patient's ability to tolerate anticoagulation for the duration of anticipated support should be considered in risk assessment.

In anticipation of use, balloon size and type should be selected based on several parameters. Sheathless insertion is less traumatic, but it can lead to oozing at the entry site. The 40-mL balloon size is most popular, although 30 mL is best with smaller arteries and the 50-mL size is best for larger individuals.

Once the pump is functional and the patient is transported to the postprocedure unit, concerns relate to possible pump malfunctions, vascular complications, and the decision for discontinuing support. Pump trouble-shooting is best addressed via a prior knowledge of the individual manufacturer's manual, although in some hospitals this responsibility is shared with nursing, perfusion, or other specially-trained technical staff. Major vascular complications are reported in 5% to 15% of cases[37] and are best minimized by continuous heparin anticoagulation and frequent assessment of entry site and distal perfusion. Balloon pumps have been left operational for weeks, but patient comfort, infection avoidance, and general nursing care become increasing concerns. With the patient optimally medicated and the initial phases of cardiac and coronary recovery progressing, a judgmental decision regarding pump removal is made. Prior to pump discontinuation, the patient is weaned from support. This is done sequentially and gradually by decreasing balloon volume to one half or less, and by shifting augmentation from 1:1 to 1:2 and 1:3. The balloon should not be left totally quiescent, as clots may then form. Tolerance of less support should be assessed periodically by physical examination and, if available, hemodynamic measurements from a pulmonary artery catheter. With weaning, heparin is discontinued and as clotting nears normal, the balloon is fully aspirated and devices withdrawn. Postwithdrawal care is important. A vascular clamp may be needed for several hours, or other artery closure-protocols may need to be followed. Gentle ambulation is often possible the next day.

Of importance here is the emergence of a variety of percutaneous vascular closure devices to limit postprocedure groin complications. These have been developed and tested primarily for earlier ambulation after routine angioplasty, although they clearly have risks as well as benefits.[38] Regarding the larger balloon-pump catheters, one study described 13 patients supported with the use of the Perclose vascular suture device during catheter withdrawal.[39] The balloon catheters were removed in all 13 while they were still anticoagulated at procedure completion, without incident. The ultimate role of these closure-devices in balloon-pump discontinuation awaits further study.

## Partial Cardiopulmonary Bypass

Percutaneous partial cardiopulmonary bypass is rarely used in the interventional suite today because of the current high rate of angioplasty success and short procedure time. There is a learning curve in its use, and cooperation with the cardiac surgical and perfusion teams is required. Also, there is an element of increased procedure expense and duration. However, a small subset of patients with the highest procedural risk may benefit from its use.[40] In general, the qualified interventional cardiologist is able to perform the corrective procedure using partial bypass safely and without hurry in such patients. In 1996, Shawl and colleagues[41] reported 107 high-risk patients having angioplasty with this support form. There was 98% successful treatment of lesions with no procedure-related mortality, Q-wave infarction, or need for surgery, although there was a 4.7% in-hospital mortality. One comparison study of support methods involved 58 patients with partial bypass and 91 with balloon pumping.[42] All had high-risk angioplasty. The bypass group had higher angioplasty success rates (99% vs. 87%) than those in the balloon pumping group but had more peripheral vascular complications, although major cardiac event rates did not differ between the groups.

The protocol the authors developed in more than 90 bypass procedures includes preprocedure coronary unit admission and pulmonary artery catheter monitoring for optimization of hemodynamic variables.[13] Femoral-aortic evaluation may be needed. For the procedure itself, the authors have preferred general anesthesia, with the cardiac anesthesiologist responsible for monitoring and maintaining subsystem function, allowing the interventional cardiologist to concentrate on the angioplasty and circulatory status. Guiding coronary angiograms are taken before bypass to avoid aortic turbulence, and the 17-French to 19-French arterial and 19-French to 20-French venous cannulas are inserted percutaneously into femoral vessels. The venous cannula is advanced to the middle of the right atrium. After full heparinization, pump flow is commenced, pressures are closely monitored, and optimal, supported angioplasty is performed without undue time constraints. With multivessel disease, the most complete revascularization yields the best long-term result in these bypass patients.[43]

Postprocedure management is important. Pump flow is weaned to off, heparin is reversed with protamine, and cannulas are removed. A vascular clamp is carefully applied over the arterial site for 4 hours or more. The patient's blood from the pump is autotransfused, and fluid management is aided by the pulmonary artery pressure measurements. The patient is extubated by the anesthesiologist when appropriate and usually is able to ambulate on postprocedure day 2.

Other uses of partial bypass include the standby mode. In this format, the pump-oxygenator and perfusionist are quickly available and femoral vessel access may be already achieved, but the large cannulas are not introduced unless the support is actually needed. In 1999, the Scripps Clinic Group (La Jolla, CA) reported on the routine use of a form of standby pump-oxygenator support in all angioplasty procedures over a 4 + year period.[44] Eleven patients required the support emergently. Nine were successfully treated, although two died in hospital. Of interest, none of the 11 patients originally fell into a high-risk category.

Finally, partial bypass has been utilized on an emergent basis. For example, the rare patient with sudden irreversible left main coronary artery occlusion may require this support-form as a bridge to urgent surgery. Such patients may require greater support than that with intra-aortic balloon pumping. Interventional centers that plan to use this advanced support system may be advised to embark on a course of instruction, equipment acquisition, and cooperative planning with the other specialists involved.

## Cardiogenic Shock

The practical aspects of circulatory support are most importantly reflected in the management of acute myocardial infarction with cardiogenic shock. In the large multicenter Global Utilization of Streptokinase and Tissue Plasminogen Activator for Occluded Coronary Arteries (GUSTO-1) trial, shock was present in 7.2% of patients with infarction.[45] Shock is a topic of major concern to interventional cardiologists, as it is the most important cause of death in myocardial infarction.[46] There was a mortality rate of 55% among shock patients receiving thrombolytic agents in the GUSTO-1 trial.[45] Modern interventional technology has not improved survival in this patient subset as much as hoped, as discussed subsequently.

A review of the pathophysiology of acute cardiac infarct is past the scope of this text, yet certain features of this important disease bear comment as they relate to balloon pumping, its most popular support entity. Classic cardiogenic shock is basically acute, profound heart failure secondary to pump-function loss involving a large myocardial segment. This loss, in turn, results from gross segmental coronary insufficiency due to the complex interplay of plaque, thrombus, and spasm. The time dimension is important, as the most ischemic segment-center undergoes progression to necrosis, often in a matter of minutes, followed by the more peripheral zones. But there are multiple other factors, different in each patient, that bear on shock development and potential recovery with supported intervention. These factors are summarized in Table 26–3. Without treatment or, unfortunately, even with optimal intervention, a fatal devolutionary spiral often ensues. This may evolve rapidly or slowly, with pro-

## TABLE 26–3. FACTORS CAUSING SHOCK IN ACUTE MYOCARDIAL INFARCTION

I. Necrosing central LV segment and stunned periphery
  A. Large noncontracting segment
  B. Paradoxical systolic expansion
II. Multivessel disease
  A. Limited collateral flow to stunned area
  B. Nonfunctional scar from prior myocardial infarctions
III. Acute mitral regurgitation
  A. 2° to papillary muscle ischemia
  B. 2° to LV dilation
IV. Arrhythmias from ischemic zones
  A. Tachyarrhythmias
  B. Heart block
V. Inadequate LV filling pressure
  A. 2° to right ventricle infarction
  B. 2° to hypovolemia
VI. Hypoxemia 2° to pulmonary edema
VII. Increased total-body $VO_2$ 2° to general adrenergic stress response

LV, left ventricle.

gressive ventricular distention, enlarging infarction, rising end-diastolic pressure, pulmonary edema, and hypoxemia further decreasing myocardial oxygenation, declining cardiac output and aortic pressure with terminal circulatory insufficiency and acidosis. However, some, but not all, of the pathophysiologic events listed in Table 26–3 would appear to be improved by balloon pumping, with its beneficial effect on both coronary flow and ventricular contraction. However, in the subset of GUSTO-1 infarct patients with shock, those treated with balloon pumping showed only a trend toward improved 30-day and 1-year mortality over those without balloon pumping.[47] This study had been designed to test thrombolytic agents. The Second Primary Angioplasty in Myocardial Infarction (PAMI-II) trial provided more focused data: High-risk patients were randomized to balloon pumping 36 to 48 hours or more after angioplasty.[48] Surprisingly, this support did not result in lower mortality or improved measures of myocardial recovery at discharge or 6 weeks. A more recent study of 238 high-risk patients with acute infarction described randomization to balloon pumping or none after primary angioplasty.[49] Similar to the other studies, no differences in enzymatic infarct size or 6-month ejection fraction were found. A partial reason for the less-than-expected improvement in these cases may be reperfusion injury. The first fluid to reach segments of ongoing infarction appears to influence recovery, and blood may not be the optimal medium.[50]

Despite these rather discouraging reports, there do appear to be other factors beneficial to recovery with aggressive management, including support; for instance, zonal myocardium may be stunned and recoverable. In this setting, all interventional cardiologists have seen some sluggish flow through a culprit lesion, or slight collateral from other vessels into the infarct zone. Also, shock may be partially due to low left ventricular filling pressure from right ventricular infarction and, thus, may respond to fluid augmentation. An additional study of the GUSTO-1 data revealed the predictors of death in the cardiogenic shock patients.[51] Interestingly, right-heart catheterization data were predictive of outcome, as well as proving useful in the management of these patients. A cardiac output of 5.1 L/min and wedge pressure of 20 mm Hg were optimal. Also, on a more positive note, balloon pumping appears to improve the effect of thrombolytic agents in cardiogenic shock, apparently by speeding the arrival of the agent to the target lesion. Kovack and colleagues[52] described the improved early outcome of shock patients receiving thrombolytics and, additionally, balloon pumping. Moreover, further analysis of the GUSTO-1 trial data indicates that an aggressive strategy of early angiography in the infarct patients with shock, followed by either angioplasty or surgery if feasible, resulted in a lower 30-day mortality, compared to those not treated aggressively.[53] Within the treatment protocol sequence, the speed with which the balloon-pump support is initiated appears important. In a registry study of patients with infarct-shock, pump support initiated prior to primary angioplasty resulted in fewer adverse catheterization-laboratory events than did support initiated after the revascularization (14.5% vs. 35.1%).[54] Likewise, the speed with which intervention is accomplished is essential in these patients, as would be expected. One study over nearly a 2-year period documented an association between fewer adverse events and progressively shorter time intervals from patient arrival to primary angioplasty; patient mortality in hospital, adverse events, and length of hospitalization all fell in parallel with the increasing speed of institution of patient management.[55]

In recent decades, intracoronary stents have proven to be one of the most important angioplasty innovations. While not "support," they enter the treatment arsenal for acute infarctions and thus are germane to this discussion. The Primary Angioplasty vs. Stent Implantation in Acute Myocardial Infarction trial randomized 136 patients to stent or no stent.[56] The results were impressive, with major cardiac events lower for the stent group in hospital (6% vs. 19%), at 6 months (21% vs. 46%) and 1 year (22% vs. 49%). Furthermore, the minimal lumen diameters were greater before discharge and the 6-month restenosis rates were less.

Current practice patterns in the treatment of ischemic cardiogenic shock reflect all of these described concerns, as well as the principle that an open infarct-related vessel is associated with im-

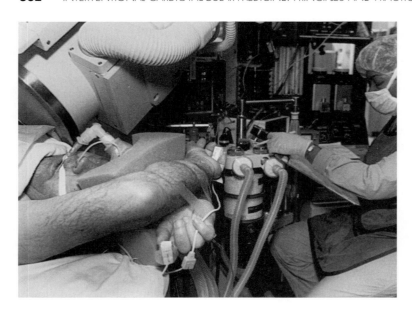

FIGURE 26–6. General endotracheal anesthesia is a support system of major importance during percutaneous intervention in severely ill patients. In addition to the physiologic benefits, the anesthesiologist or anesthetist monitors and controls subsystem function, freeing the interventionalist for a more focused approach to the cardiac problem.

proved short- and long-term survival.[57] They usually dictate an aggressive approach in hospitals so equipped. Early coronary angiography, intra-aortic balloon pumping, and pulmonary artery catheter insertion (along with complex pharmacologic treatment, not discussed here) form the mainstay of this approach. General endotracheal anesthesia may be a consideration in improving oxygenation, retarding pulmonary edema, and lessening the work of breathing (Fig. 26–6). Mechanical revascularization follows quickly and is accomplished usually via angioplasty rather than surgery because of the time frame. Following the procedure, balloon pump assistance for 48 hours or so may be a useful adjunct to initial recovery.

## Treatment of Left Main Coronary Stenoses

The major portion of the left ventricular myocardium is supplied by the left main artery in most patients; thus, its treatment has always been of special concern. Occlusion here, if unprotected by a previously inserted graft, almost always causes death within minutes, and the angina from main artery lesions usually is accompanied by transient heart failure because of its extensive distribution. Only in recent years has percutaneous treatment of this vessel been considered and performed in any significant numbers.[58] Positive in this consideration are its easy access and short length, but negatives, in addition to its life-threatening vulnerability, include its bifurcating configuration, making distal-vessel angioplasty problematic. Earlier left main coronary artery procedures were restricted to inoperable patients and involved support, often with partial bypass; but, more recent reports reflect the

trend to faster, less-supported procedures, even encroaching into the group of patients considered possible surgical candidates. A multicenter registry of 107 patients having unprotected left main coronary artery angioplasty (1994–1996) revealed that both in-hospital and 15 ± 8 month event-free survival strongly correlated with ejection fraction.[59] Of hospital survivors, 10.6% had cardiac death within 6 months. A 1998 report describes 140 elective angioplasty cases, with 97% technical success and 1.4% in-hospital cardiac death.[60] There was a 47% 1-year restenosis rate, but 3-year cardiac survival was 90%. The recent increase in stent usage has affected this unique angioplasty subset: in 1999, Wong and colleagues[61] described 55 patients having elective left main coronary angioplasty with stenting. No support was utilized, technical success was 100%, there were no in-hospital complications, and at 16.1 ± 9.6 months there had been 1 death and 80% of the patients remained asymptomatic. This appears a remarkable achievement. If this trend of success continues, it will significantly impact the treatment plan of this small, but important, subgroup of coronary patients. At present, most cardiologists would recommend bypass surgery routinely in this disease. Poor-surgical-risk patients, however, may well be helped with left main coronary angioplasty, with consideration of stenting and support in the form of intra-aortic balloon pump or partial bypass, at least in the standby mode.

## CONCLUSION

This chapter has outlined the developmental history, physiology, and practicality of circulatory and coronary support devices used by the cardiac interventionalist. This outline serves as a guide for the support aspects of patient care as well as providing a background on the subject; this facilitates the understanding of future developments in both cardiac surgery and percutaneous coronary artery angioplasty.

## REFERENCES

1. Mehlhorn U, Kroner A, de Vivie ER: 30 years clinical intra-aortic balloon pumping: Facts and figures. Thorac Cardiovasc Surgeon 47(suppl 2):298–303, 1999.
2. Timmis SBH, Hermiller JB, Burns WH, et al: Comparison of immediate and in-hospital results of conventional balloon and perfusion balloon angioplasty using intracoronary ultrasound. Am J Cardiol 83:311–316, 1999.
3. Quigley PJ, Hinohara T, Phillips HR, et al: Myocardial protection during coronary angioplasty with an autoperfusion balloon catheter in humans. Circulation 78:1128–1134, 1988.
4. de Munick ED, den Heijer P, van Dijk RB, et al: Autoperfusion balloon versus stent for acute or threatened closure during percutaneous transluminal coronary angioplasty. Am J Cardiol 74:1002–1005, 1994.
5. Ferguson TB, Hinohara T, Simpson J, et al: Catheter reperfusion to allow optimal coronary bypass grafting following failed transluminal coronary angioplasty. Ann Thorac Surg 42:399–405, 1986.
6. Angelini P, Hernandez C, Ferguson JJ III, et al: High-risk coronary angioplasty assisted by active hemoperfusion: A feasibility study. Texas Heart Institute J 23:15–23, 1996.
7. Cowley MJ, Snow FR, DiScascio G, et al: Perfluorochemical perfusion during coronary angioplasty in unstable and high-risk patients. Circulation 81:IV-27, 1990.
8. Costantini C, Sampaolesia A, Serra CM, et al: Coronary venous retroperfusion support during high-risk angioplasty in patients with unstable angina: Preliminary experience. J Am Coll Cardiol 18:283–292, 1991.
9. Merhige ME, Smalling RW, Cassidy D, et al: Effect of hemopump left ventricular assist devices on regional myocardial perfusion and function: Reduction of ischemia during coronary occlusion. Circulation 80:III-158–III-166, 1989.
10. Dubois-Rande JL, Teiger E, Garot J, et al: Effects of the 14F hemopump on coronary hemodynamics in patients undergoing high-risk coronary angioplasty. Am Heart J 135:844–849, 1998.
11. Scholz KH, Dubois-Rande JL, Urban P, et al: Clinical experience with the percutaneous hemopump during high-risk coronary angioplasty. Am J Cardiol 82:1107–1110, 1998.
12. Shawl FA, Quyyumi AA, Bajaj S, et al: Percutaneous cardiopulmonary bypass–supported coronary angioplasty in patients with unstable angina pectoris or myocardial infarction and a left ventricular ejection fraction <25%. Am J Cardiol 77:14–19, 1996.
13. Shawl FA, Baxley WA: Role of percutaneous cardiopulmonary bypass and other support devices in interventional cardiology. Cardiol Clin 12:543–557, 1994.
14. Ricciardi MJ, Moscucci M, Knight BP, et al: Emergency extracorporeal membrane oxygenation (ECMO)–supported percutaneous coronary interventions in the fibrillating heart. Catheter Cardiovasc Interven 48:402–405, 1999.
15. Loubeyre C, Morice MC, Berzin B, et al: Emergency coronary artery bypass surgery following coronary angioplasty and stenting: Results of a French multi-center registry. Catheter Cardiovasc Interven 47:441–448, 1999.
16. Ferrari M, Scholz KH, Figulla HR: PTCA with the use of cardiac assist devices: Risk stratification, short- and long-term results. Catheter Cardiovasc Diagn 38:242–248, 1996.
17. Lewis BS, Porat E, Halon DA, et al: Same-day combined coronary angioplasty and minimally invasive coronary surgery. Am J Cardiol 84:1246–1247, 1999.
18. Timmis SBH, Sakwa MP, Shannon FG, et al: Interventional cardiology techniques utilized to facilitate performance of off-pump coronary artery bypass surgery. Catheter Cardiovasc Diagn 47:126, 1999.
19. Cohen RG, Mack MJ, Fonger JD, Landreneau, RJ (eds): Minimally Invasive Cardiac Surgery. Chapter 23: Combined catheter and minimally invasive direct coronary artery bypass procedures: hybrid revascularization. Quality Medical Publishing, Inc., 1999.
20. Scheidt S: Cardiology and cardiac surgery: A partnership in the new millennium. Am J Cardiol 83:1B–2B, 1999.
21. Bolooki H: Clinical application of the intra-aortic balloon pump, third revised edition. Futura Publishing Company, Inc., 1998.
22. Aroesty JM, Weintraub RM, Paulin S, et al: Medically refractory unstable angina pectoris, II. Hemodynamic and angiographic effects of intra-aortic balloon counterpulsation. Am J Cardiol 43:883–888, 1979.
23. Weber KT, Janicki JS: Intra-aortic balloon counterpulsation: A review of physiological principles, clinical results and device safety. Ann Thorac Surg 17:602–636, 1974.
24. Urschel CW, Eber L, Forrester J, et al: Alteration of mechanical performance of the ventricle by intra-aortic balloon counterpulsation. Am J Cardiol 25:546–551, 1970.
25. Fuchs RM, Brin KP, Brinker JA, et al: Augmentation of regional coronary blood flow by intra-aortic balloon counterpulsation in patients with unstable angina. Circulation 68:117–123, 1983.
26. Williams DO, Korr KS, Gewirtz H, Most AS: The effect of intra-aortic balloon counterpulsation on regional myocardial blood flow and oxygen consumption in the presence of coronary artery stenosis in patients with unstable angina. Circulation 66:593–597, 1982.
27. Kern MJ, Aguirre F, Bach R, et al: Augmentation of coronary blood flow by intra-aortic balloon pumping in patients after coronary angioplasty. Circulation 87:500–511, 1993.
28. Baxley WA, Cavender JB, Knobloch J: Continuous cardiac output monitoring by the Fick method. Catheter Cardiovasc Diagn 28:89–92, 1993.
29. Pavlides GS, Hauser AM, Stack RK, et al: Effect of peripheral cardiopulmonary bypass on left ventricular size, afterload and myocardial function during elective supported coronary angioplasty. J Am Coll Cardiol 18:499–505, 1991.
30. Gulielmos V, Menschikowski M, Thiele S, et al: A prospective randomized analysis of the inflammatory response in coronary artery bypass grafting combining different surgical access and/or the use of cardiopulmonary bypass. J Am Coll Cardiol 35:355A, 2000.
31. Scheidt S: Risk-stratification parameters in patient selection for coronary artery bypass grafting. Am J Cardiol 83:3B–9B, 1999.
32. Pagano D, Townend JN, Littler WA, et al: Coronary artery bypass surgery as treatment for ischemic heart failure: The predictive value of viability assessment with quantitative positron emission tomography for symptomatic and functional outcome. J Thorac Cardiovasc Surg 115:791–799, 1998.
33. O'Connor GT, Malenka DJ, Quinton H, et al: Multivariate prediction of in-hospital mortality after percutaneous coronary interventions in 1994–1996. J Am Coll Cardiol 34:681–691, 1999.
34. Anderson RD, Ohman EM, Holmes DR, et al: Prognostic value of congestive heart failure history in patients undergoing percutaneous coronary interventions. J Am Coll Cardiol 32:936–941, 1998.
35. Harrell L, Schunkert H, Palacios IF: Risk predictors in patients scheduled for percutaneous coronary revascularization. Catheter Cardiovasc Interven 48:253–260, 1999.
36. Brueren BRG, Mast EG, Suttorp MJ, et al: How good are experienced interventional cardiologists in predicting the risk and difficulty of a coronary angioplasty procedure? Catheter Cardiovasc Interven 46:257–262, 1999.
37. Alderman JD, Gabliani GI, McCabe CH, et al: Incidence and management of limb ischemia with percutaneous wire-guided intra-aortic balloon catheters. J Am Coll Cardiol 9:524–530, 1987.
38. Grollman JH: Percutaneous arterial access closure: Now do we have the be all and end all? Not yet! Catheter Cardiovasc Interven 49:148–149, 2000.
39. Rankin KM, Kutcher MA, Applegate RJ, Braden, GA: Removal of intra-aortic balloon pump in the cardiac cath lab

immediately following supported intervention using per-close vascular suture device. J Am Coll Cardiol 35:33A, 2000.

40. Tommaso CL: Current status of percutaneously inserted cardiopulmonary bypass in the cardiac catheterization laboratory. Catheter Cardiovasc Diagn 450:120–121, 1998.

41. Shawl FA, Quyyumi AA, Bajaj S, et al: Percutaneous cardiopulmonary bypass–supported coronary angioplasty in patients with unstable angina pectoris or myocardial infarction and a left ventricular ejection fraction <25%. Am J Cardiol 77:14–19, 1996.

42. Schreiber TL, Kodali UR, O'Neill WW, et al: Comparison of acute results of prophylactic intra-aortic balloon pumping with cardiopulmonary support for percutaneous transluminal coronary angioplasty. Catheter Cardiovasc Diagn 45:115–119, 1998.

43. Aguilar R, Varma V, Baxley WA, et al: Elective PTCA with percutaneous partial cardiopulmonary bypass: Long-term follow-up and determinants of late success. Circulation 90:I-334, 1994.

44. Guarneri EM, Califano JR, Schatz RA, et al: Utility of standby cardiopulmonary support for elective coronary interventions. Catheter Cardiovasc Interven 46: 32–35, 1999.

45. Holmes DR, Bates ER, Kleiman NS, et al: Contemporary reperfusion therapy for cardiogenic shock: The GUSTO-1 trial experience. J Am Coll Cardiol 26:668–674, 1995.

46. Califf RM, Bengtson JR: Cardiogenic shock. N Engl J Med 330: 1724–1731, 1994.

47. Anderson RD, Ohman EM, Holmes DR, et al: Use of intra-aortic balloon counterpulsation in patients presenting with cardiogenic shock: Observations from the GUSTO-I study. J Am Coll Cardiol 30:708–715, 1997.

48. Stone GW, Marsalese D, Brodie BR, et al: A prospective, randomized evaluation of prophylactic intra-aortic balloon counterpulsation in high-risk patients with acute myocardial infarction treated with primary angioplasty. J Am Coll Cardiol 29:1459–1467, 1997.

49. van't Hof AWJ, Liem AL, deBoer MJ, et al: A randomized comparison of intra-aortic balloon pumping after primary coronary angioplasty in high-risk patients with acute myocardial infarction. Eur Heart J 20:659–665, 1999.

50. Forman MR, Perry JM, Wilson RH, et al: Demonstration of myocardial reperfusion injury in humans: Results of a pilot study utilizing acute coronary angioplasty with perfluorochemical in anterior myocardial infarction. J Am Coll Cardiol 18:911–918, 1991.

51. Hasdai D, Holmes DR, Califf RM, et al: Cardiogenic shock complicating acute myocardial infarction: Predictors of death. Am Heart J 138:21–31, 1999.

52. Kovack PJ, Rasak MA, Bates ER, et al: Thrombolysis plus aortic counterpulsation: Improved survival in patients who present to community hospitals with cardiogenic shock. J Am Coll Cardiol 29:1454–1458, 1997.

53. Berger PB, Holmes DR, Stebbins AL, et al: Impact of an aggressive invasive catheterization and revascularization strategy on mortality in patients with cardiogenic shock in the global utilization of streptokinase and tissue plasminogen activator for occluded coronary arteries (GUSTO-I) trial. Circulation 96:122–127, 1997.

54. Brodie BR, Stuckey TD, Hansen C, et al: Intra-aortic balloon counterpulsation before primary transluminal coronary angioplasty reduces catheterization laboratory events in high-risk patients with acute myocardial infarction. Am J Cardiol 84:18–23, 1999.

55. Caputo RP, Ho KKL, Stoler RC, et al: Effect of continuous quality improvement analysis on the delivery of primary percutaneous transluminal coronary angioplasty for acute myocardial infarction. Am J Cardiol 79:1159–1164, 1997.

56. Saito S, Hosokawa G, Tanaka S, Nakamura S: Primary stent implantation is superior to balloon angioplasty in acute myocardial infarction: Final results of the primary angioplasty versus stent implantation in acute myocardial infarction (PASTA) trial. Catheter Cardiovasc Interven 48:262–268, 1999.

57. Bengtson JR, Kaplan AJ, Pieper KS, et al: Prognosis in cardiogenic shock after acute myocardial infarction in the interventional era. J Am Coll Cardiol 20:1482–1489, 1992.

58. Holubkov R, Detre KM, Sopko G, et al: Trends in coronary revascularization 1989 to 1997: The bypass angioplasty revascularization investigation (BARI) survey of procedures. Am J Cardiol 84:157–161, 1999.

59. Ellis SG, Tamai H, Nobuyoshi M, et al: Contemporary percutaneous treatment of unprotected left main coronary stenoses. Circulation 96:3867–3872, 1997.

60. Kosuga K, Tamai H, Hsu YS, et al: Initial and long-term results of elective angioplasty in unprotected left main coronary artery. J Am Coll Cardiol 31:101A, 1998.

61. Wong P, Wong V, Tse KK, et al: A prospective study of elective stenting in unprotected left main coronary disease. Catheter Cardiovascular Interven 46:153–159, 1999.

# 27

# Adjunctive Pharmacologic Support During Percutaneous Coronary Intervention

*Mark C. Thel*    *James E. Tcheng*

In the initial descriptions of percutaneous translu-minal coronary angioplasty (PTCA) by Andreas Gruentzig in 1978, the only medications used were aspirin for 3 days before, heparin and dextran dur-ing, and warfarin (Coumadin) for 6 to 9 months after the procedure.[1, 2] Since then, adjunctive medical support during percutaneous coronary intervention (PCI) has evolved considerably. Medications now used during PCI aim to minimize anxiety and dis-comfort; prevent thrombosis, abrupt closure, and clinical ischemic events; and maintain vessel pat-ency. The purpose of this chapter is to review the pharmacologic strategies for patients undergoing PCI. It must be remembered that pharmacologic therapy is constantly changing and that therapy must be individualized. Indications and contraindi-cations, adverse reactions, and dosage schedules in-cluded on package inserts should always be consid-ered when prescribing a medication.

In this chapter, whenever possible, the primary clinical outcomes of randomized trials are refer-enced.[3–5] Post hoc, subgroup, and retrospective anal-yses, conclusions, and explanations are treated with a fair dose of skepticism.[6–8] Many interventional studies rely on surrogates such as abrupt vessel clo-sure, changes in vessel size, and other angiographic end points. As discussed by Fleming and DeMets, surrogate end points are often misleading because "the disease process could affect the clinical out-come through several causal pathways that are not mediated through the surrogate, with the interven-tion's effect on these pathways differing from its effect on the surrogate. Even more likely, the inter-vention might also affect the clinical outcome by unintended, unanticipated, and unrecognized mechanisms of action that operate independently of the disease process."[9] For agents currently undergo-ing investigation, reference is made to the most re-cent clinical trial, regardless of setting or indication.

## LOCAL ANESTHETICS

Most interventional cardiac procedures can be per-formed with local anesthesia supplemented by con-scious sedation. The ideal local anesthetic has a rapid onset of action, reversibly blocks nerve con-duction, does not induce irreversible neuronal dam-age, and has no toxic systemic effects.[10, 11] As a class, local anesthetics inhibit action potential generation and conduction by blocking membrane sodium per-meability. Therefore, they may also produce neuro-logic and cardiovascular side effects, particularly if the more potent agents are accidentally adminis-tered intravascularly. Commonly used local anes-thetics can be grouped into two classes: amides (including lidocaine, bupivacaine, etidocaine, and mepivacaine) and esters (including procaine, co-caine, and tetracaine). Lidocaine is the most com-monly used agent and is more potent and has a longer duration of action than procaine. Hypersensi-tivity reactions to these drugs are extremely rare; when seen, they more commonly occur with the esters. Alternatives for patients with a history sug-gestive of an allergic reaction include choosing a drug from the other class, using a preservative-free anesthetic (as is used in spinal and epidural anes-thesia), and skin testing.[12] The discomfort associated with local infiltration may be alleviated by warming and buffering.[13]

## CONSCIOUS SEDATION

Despite premedication, patients are frequently dis-satisfied with their level of sedation before and dur-ing cardiac catheterization.[14] Adequate anxiolysis, sedation, and analgesia improve control of tachycar-dia and hypertension and thus reduce myocardial workload and ischemia. The importance of adequate sedation beyond the actual procedure is confirmed by the association of postoperative pain and anxiety with myocardial ischemia and adverse clinical out-comes in patients undergoing more invasive proce-dures.[15] The synergistic combination of lower doses of benzodiazepines and opioids has several advan-tages over higher doses of any single agent and is the currently recommended approach.[16–20]

Benzodiazepines are the most commonly used sedative medication. As a class, these agents produce anxiolysis, sedation, muscle relaxation, and amnesia.[21] They appear to produce their effect by increasing the binding of the inhibitory neurotransmitter γ-aminobutyric acid (GABA) to its receptors.[22] Individual agents differ in pharmacokinetic and pharmacodynamic properties, with the respective characteristics also influenced by the patient's age, hepatic and renal function, and drug interactions. All the benzodiazepines except oxazepam and lorazepam have active metabolites. The plasma half-lives of the most commonly prescribed agents are listed in Table 27–1. In the catheterization suite, midazolam appears particularly useful because of its high potency and ease of titration; this agent has a very rapid onset of action as well as a short half-life and produces a greater degree of hypnosis and amnesia than do other members of this class.[17, 23] However, the potential for deep sedation to the point of respiratory suppression must also be considered when using this agent.

Opioids are effective in preventing and treating moderate to severe pain. However, they produce only minimal amnestic and anxiolytic effects. Morphine is found in immature opium and is the standard against which other narcotics are compared. Narcotics are metabolized by the liver, and many (including morphine and meperidine) have active metabolites excreted by the kidneys. Their pharmacokinetics may therefore be altered by hepatic or renal insufficiency. Hydromorphone and fentanyl are potent synthetic opioids that are frequently used during interventional procedures because of their short half-lives and rapid metabolism by the liver to inactive metabolites.[24, 25] Respiratory depression,

nausea and emesis, altered sensorium, urinary retention, and seizures are the primary adverse effects. Given alone, opioids and benzodiazepines produce minimal hemodynamic depression; however, they may synergistically produce clinically significant hypotension.

Propofol is an intravenous lipophilic anesthetic that is delivered as an emulsion.[26] It has a favorable pharmacokinetic profile compared with the volatile anesthetics, providing a predictable rapid onset and offset of action associated with a "smooth" recovery.[27] Propofol depresses cardiovascular function and produces systemic vasodilation that may result in hypotension, particularly in patients with hemodynamic instability. It also depresses ventilation and must be used only with close respiratory monitoring. Because of its safety, efficacy, and ease of titration, its use during cardiovascular and ambulatory procedures is likely to increase in the near future.

Intravenously administered sedatives reduce alveolar ventilation, hypoxic respiratory drive, and the response to hypercarbia. The administration of sedatives should be delayed until electrocardiographic, blood pressure, and oximetry monitors are in place. Transcutaneous pulse oximeters are generally accurate to within 3% at oxygen saturations between 70% and 100% and have been found to be particularly useful in patients with decreased left ventricular function and those undergoing prolonged procedures.[28–30] Specific recommendations for the monitoring of patients receiving conscious sedation have been advanced by the Joint Commission on the Accreditation of Healthcare Organizations.

Flumazenil is the only approved benzodiazepine antagonist. The standard dosing of flumazenil is 0.2 mg intravenously (IV) repeated every 2 minutes to a maximal dose of 1 mg. Although the effects may be variable, flumazenil generally reverses the anesthetic, sedative, and respiratory depressive effect of the benzodiazepines.[31, 32] Naloxone is the primary opioid antagonist available for parenteral use. The usual initial dose is a 0.4 mg IV; it may need to be repeated every 5 minutes because of its short half-life. The complete reversal of analgesia is its primary limitation.[33]

## MECHANISMS OF THROMBOSIS

Coronary intervention induces an obligate disruption of the vascular endothelium, accompanied by plaque disruption and exposure of subendothelial substrates. This promotes activation of the hemostatic system and the generation of thrombin and platelet aggregates.[34–39] Thrombosis is the fundamen-

**TABLE 27–1. PLASMA HALF-LIVES OF COMMONLY PRESCRIBED BENZODIAZEPINE, NARCOTIC, AND REVERSING AGENTS**

| GENERIC NAME | PROPRIETARY NAME | HALF-LIFE (HOURS) |
|---|---|---|
| Alprazolam | Xanax | 12–15 |
| Diazepam | Valium | 20–80 |
| Lorazepam | Ativan | 10–20 |
| Midazolam | Versed | 1.5–2 |
| Oxazepam | Serax | 5–10 |
| Triazolam | Halcion | 2–4 |
| Fentanyl | Sublimaze | 3–4 |
| Hydromorphone | Dilaudid | 2–3 |
| Meperidine | Demerol | 2–4 |
| Morphine | | 2–4 |
| Flumazenil | Romazicon | 1 |
| Naloxone | Narcan | 1.2 |

From Bailey L, Ward M, Musa N: Clinical pharmacokinetics of benzodiazepines. J Clin Pharmacol 34:804–811, 1994, and manufacturer package inserts.

tal process underlying the acute coronary syndromes and a source of many of the ischemic complications after PCIs. Thrombosis and hemostasis result from the coagulation cascade (Fig. 27–1) and platelet aggregation. Thrombus formation results from the interdependent processes of coagulation and platelet adhesion, activation, and aggregation. Drugs that interrupt these pathways have the potential to improve the clinical outcome of patients after PCI. Fortunately for the field of interventional cardiology, new agents are constantly being evaluated in this setting. In fact, the controlled and predictable events following PCI have provided a convenient and consistent model to test antithrombotic strategies whose results may then be extrapolated to other settings.

The first step in hemostasis and thrombosis is platelet *adhesion* to subendothelial proteins. These proteins, which are exposed to flowing blood when the endothelium is disrupted, attach to platelet integrin receptors. Integrins are a family of heterodimers found on the membranes of essentially all cells that are responsible for cell-cell and cell-matrix interac-

tions.[40] Each integrin is composed of noncovalently bound α and β glycoprotein (GP) transmembrane subunits. Initially described by Hynes in 1987, at least 16 α and 8 β subunits (constituting 22 integrins) have been identified.[40, 41] The extracellular portions determine the receptor affinity and specificity for ligands. The intracellular portions stimulate a cellular response to ligand binding through interactions with cytoplasmic structures. The resting platelets bind to von Willebrand factor (vWF) and collagen through GPIb and GPIa/IIa, respectively, to form a monolayer on the disrupted endothelium.[42] Platelets are *activated* by at least 100 pathways, including shear stress and endogenous ligands such as thrombin, epinephrine, serotonin, adenosine diphosphate (ADP), thromboxane $A_2$ ($TxA_2$), vasopressin, and plasmin.[43] Once activated, the platelet membrane integrin receptor GPIIb/IIIa undergoes conformational changes that permit binding to soluble fibrinogen and vWF.[44, 45] Fibrinogen "bridges" between platelets quickly become the "molecular glue" of platelet *aggregation* because fibrinogen is multivalent and each platelet contains

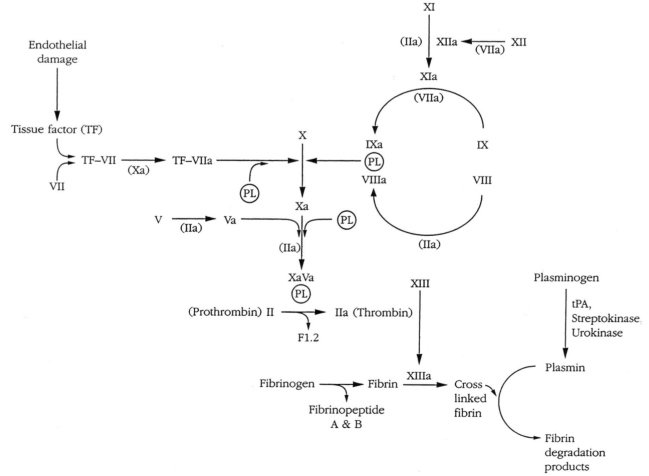

FIGURE 27–1. Coagulation cascade. PL, phospholipid; tPA, tissue-type plasminogen activator.

more than 50,000 GPIIb/IIIa receptors. Activation also increases the absolute number of exposed GPIIb/IIIa receptors as cytoplasmic α granules (which contain additional GPIIb/IIIa receptors) fuse with the outer cell membrane.[45, 46]

The minimal recognition sequence for GPIIb/IIIa binding is Arg-Gly-Asp (RGD). It was identified by Pierschbacher and Ruoslahti on fibronectin in 1984 but is also the obligate sequence in fibrinogen, vWF, collagen, thrombospondin, laminin, and vitronectin.[47, 48] Although the RGD sequence is necessary for ligand binding, the primary GPIIb/IIIa binding sequence in fibrinogen appears to be a Lys-Gln-Ala-Asp-Val sequence on the γ chain.[49]

Tissue factor is another glycoprotein that is normally shielded from the intravascular space.[50] With vascular damage, tissue factor is expressed on activated endothelial and smooth muscle cells and acts with factor VIIa to initiate the extrinsic pathway of coagulation (see Fig. 27–1).[51] The so-called intrinsic pathway amplifies the coagulation cascade through the production of factors IX and VIII. Together, the pathways produce sufficient levels of factor Xa, which catalyzes the transformation of prothrombin to thrombin. Thrombin has two recognition sites and an active (catalytic) site. Through its catalytic site, thrombin plays an integral role in thrombus formation by cleaving fibrinogen to insoluble fibrin and activating factor XIII (which crosslinks and polymerizes fibrin) and factors V and VIII (which produce a positive feedback loop). One recognition site recognizes ligands such as fibrinogen and the thrombin receptor on the platelet surface, which stimulates platelet activation.[52] In clot-bound thrombin, the other recognition site is occupied by fibrin. In this state, the catalytic site is resistant to the antithrombin III–heparin complex but still capable of interacting with its other substrates.[53] Thrombin certainly plays a critical role in thrombus formation through its role in catalyzing fibrin formation and polymerization, vasoconstriction, chemoattraction of neutrophils and monocytes, endothelial cell proliferation, and platelet activation.[54]

## ANTIPLATELET AGENTS

Evidence for immediate platelet *activation, adhesion*, and *aggregation* at the site of vascular intervention includes analysis of biochemical markers, flow cytometry, radiolabeling, histologic examination, and direct visualization by angioscopy.[37, 55–65] The clinical ramifications of platelet aggregation after coronary intervention are expressed as ischemic complications.[66–71] Wilentz and associates demonstrated that platelet accumulation peaked at the site of arterial injury within 2 hours of angioplasty

and returned to baseline by 4 hours and that the extent of platelet aggregation was directly related to histologically graded dissection.[72] In another rabbit model, Groves and colleagues demonstrated that platelets accumulate within 10 minutes of balloon injury and within 1 hour reach a plateau that persists for 24 hours.[73] In humans, Minar and coworkers demonstrated increased platelet activity immediately after peripheral angioplasty.[74] Once platelets accumulate, they further increase thrombus production by stimulating thrombin generation and increasing the shear rate and vasoconstriction.[75–80] The relationship of ischemic complications and platelet aggregation is further established by the marked reduction in ischemic events in patients treated with aspirin, ticlopidine, clopidogrel, and the GPIIb/IIIa antagonists.

The function of platelets can be inhibited at several steps (Table 27–2). Platelet *activation* can be inhibited by the blockade of natural agonists and cytoplasmic enzymes. Platelet *aggregation* can be inhibited by agents that interfere with the binding of endogenous ligands (principally fibrinogen) to the GPIIb/IIIa receptor.

## Aspirin

Aspirin was the first and remains the principal antiplatelet agent. Aspirin irreversibly acetylates cyclooxygenase, producing a biologic effect that persists for the life of the platelet.[81, 82] Cyclooxygenase catalyzes the first step in the synthesis of $TxA_2$ and the prostaglandins through the conversion of arachidonic acid to the endoperoxide prostaglandin $G_2$

### TABLE 27–2.    ANTIPLATELET AGENTS

Cyclooxygenase inhibitors
    Aspirin
Thromboxane synthase inhibitors
Thromboxane $A_2$–receptor antagonists
    Sulotroban
    GR32191B (Vapiprost)
Phosphodiesterase inhibitors
    Dipyridamole
Thienopyridine derivatives
    Ticlopidine
    Clopidogrel
GPIIb/IIIa antagonists
    Monoclonal antibody
        Abciximab
    Cyclic RGD peptides
        Eptifibatide
    Pseudopeptides
        Lamifiban
        Tirofiban
    Orally active drugs
        Xemilofiban
        Orbofiban
        Sibrafiban
        Roxifiban

GP, glycoprotein; RGD, Arg-Gly-Asp.

(PGG$_2$). The nonsteroidal anti-inflammatory agents inhibit cyclooxygenase and prolong the bleeding time only temporarily.[83, 84] The clinical efficacy of aspirin in ischemic heart disease is well recognized; aspirin has been investigated in over 300 randomized trials.[85, 88] Aspirin is effective in the primary prevention of acute myocardial infarction (AMI),[89] in the secondary prevention of AMI,[89] and in the setting of unstable angina[90] and AMI.[91]

Aspirin is the drug of choice for the prevention of ischemic complications after coronary intervention. In 1988, Schwartz and colleagues reported the results of a randomized trial of aspirin and dipyridamole versus placebo in PCI.[92] The incidence of Q-wave infarction was 1.6% in the treatment group and 6.9% in the control group ($p = 0.0113$). In a retrospective analysis of 500 patients, Kent and associates noted a procedural success rate of 92% in patients treated with aspirin versus 80% in patients who did not receive aspirin ($p < 0.01$).[93] In the M-HEART II (Multi-Hospital Eastern Atlantic Restenosis Trial II) experience, patients treated with aspirin had a 27% relative risk reduction ($p = 0.046$) compared with control patients in the incidence of ischemic events at 6 months.[94] Although many of the trials used aspirin in conjunction with dipyridamole in the active treatment groups, Lembo and coworkers demonstrated that dipyridamole does not provide additional benefit to aspirin alone.[95] Finally, in a meta-analysis of over 8000 patients, the Oxford Antiplatelet Trialists' Collaboration demonstrated a 50% relative increase in vessel patency in patients treated with aspirin after coronary artery bypass surgery, PCI, peripheral vascular surgery, and the placement of hemodialysis access shunts.[87]

Notwithstanding these results, aspirin is a relatively weak inhibitor of platelet activity.[96, 97] It inhibits only one pathway of platelet activation, and it does not interfere with platelet adhesion or aggregation. Although the extraordinary cost effectiveness of aspirin and the favorable benefit risk ratio ensure that aspirin will remain the mainstay of antiplatelet agents for the foreseeable future, recognition of the limitations of aspirin have stimulated the development of agents with potentially greater efficacy.

## Thienopyridine Derivatives (Ticlopidine and Clopidogrel)

Although the mechanism is only incompletely understood, ticlopidine and clopidogrel appear to irreversibly inhibit ADP binding to its platelet membrane receptor, thereby preventing ADP-dependent activation of the GPIIb/IIIa receptor.[98–100] Ticlopidine requires hepatic biotransformation to an active metabolite or metabolites, and this delays its maximal effect by about 5 days; the maximal effect of clopi-

dogrel is achieved much more quickly, on the order of several hours.[100] In the Antiplatelet Trialists' meta-analysis of trials comparing aspirin and ticlopidine, there was an insignificant decrease in myocardial infarction, stroke, and vascular death with ticlopidine treatment.[86]

No trial has directly compared ticlopidine with aspirin in the setting of PCI. In the Ticlopidine Multicenter Trial, treatment reduced the incidence of ischemic complications from 14% in the placebo group to 2% ($p < 0.005$) in the ticlopidine group and 5% ($p < 0.005$) in the aspirin and dipyridamole group.[101] In a trial of only 19 patients, Cerisier and associates randomized patients to treatment with aspirin plus ticlopidine or aspirin after PTCA alone of coronary artery occlusions (TIMI [Thrombosis In Myocardial Infarction] flow 0) in vessels less than 3 mm in diameter.[102] At 6 months, the percentage diameter stenosis and reocclusion rates in the aspirin-ticlopidine and aspirin groups were 54% and zero of 10 versus 82% and 6 of 9, respectively ($p < 0.05$ for both comparisons).

A large body of data has accrued about the efficacy of the thienopyridines as adjuncts to coronary stent placement. These data support the recommendation that a thienopyridine should be prescribed to all patients (in the absence of a contraindication) undergoing this procedure. Early observational registries suggested that treatment with ticlopidine and aspirin reduced subacute stent thrombosis compared with either aspirin alone or aspirin treatment combined with oral anticoagulants.[103–106] Hall and colleagues randomized 226 stented patients after intravascular ultrasound interrogation to treatment with aspirin alone or aspirin and ticlopidine.[107] The incidence of major clinical events was 3.9% in the aspirin group and 0.8% in patients treated with both agents. Although the authors concluded that ticlopidine did not add clinical benefit to aspirin alone, the wide confidence intervals indicate that the trial was underpowered. In a nonrandomized comparison using the Cook stent, the combination of aspirin and ticlopidine was clearly superior to aspirin alone.[108] In the ISAR (Intracoronary Stenting and Antithrombotic Regimen) trial, Schömig and coworkers randomly assigned 517 patients who had a single intracoronary stent successfully placed to treatment with ticlopidine and aspirin, or phenprocoumon and aspirin.[109] At 30 days, the incidence of the composite end point (cardiac mortality, myocardial infarction, bypass surgery, or repeat angioplasty) was 6.2% in the anticoagulant arm versus 1.6% in the aspirin and ticlopidine arm. In a separate analysis of the 123 patients who had a single stent placed in the setting of myocardial infarction, those who received the combined antiplatelet regimen had a lower 30-day incidence of clinical events and stent occlusion and at 6 months a lower incidence of recurrent myocardial infarction and stent occlusion compared with those who received the phenprocoumon and aspirin regimen.[110] The French Registry of Stenting in Acute Myocardial Infarction also reported significantly worse outcomes in patients treated with anticoagulation.[111] In the STARS (STent Anticoagulation Regimen Study), 1652 patients who received one or two optimally deployed stents were randomized to receive aspirin and warfarin, aspirin alone, or aspirin and ticlopidine.[112] The incidence of the primary composite end point (death, target vessel revascularization, stent thrombosis, or myocardial infarction) in the three groups was 3.6%, 2.7%, and 0.5% (for aspirin and ticlopidine compared with aspirin and warfarin, $p = 0.001$; for aspirin alone, $p = 0.02$). The overall incidence of any postprocedure creatine kinase MB (CK-MB) elevation was about 20% despite optimal angiographic results. Notably, ticlopidine was not started in these patients until completion of the coronary intervention. The incidence of adverse events in patients who had suboptimal angiographic results ($N = 509$) after stent placement was 13 times higher than in the remainder of the cohort.

The major serious adverse effect of ticlopidine is neutropenia. In two large secondary prevention trials in cerebrovascular disease, the incidence of neutropenia was about 1% and was reversible on discontinuation of ticlopidine.[113, 114] In a review of four randomized trials that enrolled 2048 patients, the incidence of neutropenia was 2.4%, and was severe in 0.85% (absolute neutrophil count $< 0.45 \times 10^9/$L).[115] In several observational studies of ticlopidine given for 1 month after coronary stenting, the incidence of neutropenia was also about 1%.[116, 117]

Clopidogrel is a newer thienopyridine that appears to produce less neutropenia and other adverse side effects. In the CAPRIE (Clopidogrel versus Aspirin in Patients at Risk of Ischemic Events) trial, the incidence of neutropenia (absolute neutrophil count $< 1.2 \times 10^9/$L) was 0.10% in the clopidogrel group and 0.17% in the aspirin group.[118] In this trial, 19,185 patients with a history of recent myocardial infarction, ischemic stroke, or symptomatic peripheral vascular disease were randomized to aspirin or clopidogrel for a mean follow-up of 1.9 years. The incidence of the primary composite end point (ischemic stroke, myocardial infarction, or vascular death) was 5.83% in patients assigned to aspirin and 5.32% in patients assigned to clopidogrel, yielding a relative-risk reduction of 8.7% (95% confidence interval [CI] 0.3 to 16.5).

With direct relevance to the question of thienopyridine use in coronary stenting, the preliminary results of the CLASSICS (CLopidogrel Aspirin Stent International Cooperative Study) trial were an-

nounced in 1999.[119] In this three-arm randomized trial, 1020 patients were randomized to either aspirin with ticlopidine or aspirin with clopidogrel with or without a 300-mg loading dose of clopidogrel. The primary end point of safety and tolerability of the combined clopidogrel treatment groups compared with the ticlopidine cohort favored clopidogrel treatment (4.6% vs. 9.1%, $p = 0.005$). The secondary end point of any major adverse cardiac event was very low (approximately 1%) in all three groups. In addition, single-site registry data that have included over 1600 patients from five clinical centers have also shown clopidogrel to have similar efficacy and safety in this indication compared with ticlopidine.[120–123] On the basis of these data, clopidogrel should be considered the thienopyridine of choice in the stented patient. Our current recommendation is for patients to be given a loading dose of 300 mg of clopidogrel before the initiation of the PCI procedure, and that clopidogrel be continued after stent implantation at a dose of 75 mg/day for 1 month.

## Dipyridamole and Dextran

Dipyridamole and dextran are two agents with questionable antiplatelet activity that until recently were mainstays in the pharmacotherapy of coronary interventions. The mechanism of action of dipyridamole is controversial. Proposed mechanisms include inhibition of platelet phosphodiesterase, inhibition of cellular uptake of adenosine, and stimulation of the synthesis and release of prostacyclin from vascular endothelium.[124] The randomized trial by Lembo and colleagues of aspirin versus aspirin plus dipyridamole in 232 patients undergoing PTCA demonstrated that dipyridamole added no benefit to treatment with aspirin alone.[95] In fact, no randomized clinical trial has demonstrated a therapeutic benefit for dipyridamole when used alone. The use of dextran during coronary interventions was also based more on precedence than scientific evidence.[125] At present, the use of dipyridamole and dextran cannot be recommended.

## GPIIb/IIIa Antagonists

Aspirin and the thienopyridines inhibit selective pathways of platelet *activation*. Because of the multiple pathways leading to platelet activation, these agents cannot completely abolish platelet function. In 1985, Barry Coller identified the GPIIb/IIIa integrin as the receptor mediating platelet *aggregation* and suggested that inhibition of this "final common pathway" would inhibit platelet aggregation irrespective of stimulus.[126]

## Abciximab

The first inhibitor of GPIIb/IIIa to be investigated was the monoclonal antibody 7E3, developed by Coller.[127] The derivative agent abciximab (ReoPro) is the product of molecular reengineering of the original 7E3 antibody. Abciximab is a chimeric monoclonal antibody in which the crystallizable fragment (Fc) portion has been removed; the remaining (Fab) antigen-binding fragment portion is composed of murine-derived variable-region 7E3 Fab with human constant-region Fab to reduce antigenicity. Although the adjunctive use of 7E3 has been studied in the treatment of unstable angina and AMI,[128, 129] most investigations have been in the setting of coronary intervention. In the EPIC (Evaluation of 7E3 for the Prevention of Ischemic Complications) trial, 2099 patients felt to be at high risk for ischemic complications were randomly assigned to treatment with placebo, an abciximab bolus (0.25 mg/kg) followed by a placebo infusion, or abciximab bolus and infusion (0.25 mg/kg followed by 10 µg/minute for 12 hours).[130] In patients treated with both bolus and infusion, there was a 35% relative risk reduction in the incidence of the 30-day primary composite end point (death, nonfatal myocardial infarction, repeat revascularization, and procedural failure identified by the placement of an intra-aortic balloon pump or bailout stent) compared with patients treated with placebo, 12.8% versus 8.3% ($p = 0.008$), respectively. In patients treated with bolus and infusion, there was also a 26% relative risk reduction in the need for repeat angioplasty at 6 months.[131] The price of this reduction in ischemic events was an approximate doubling in rates of bleeding. The vascular access site was the source of bleeding in 71% of patients who bled. Risk factors for bleeding were lighter weight, older age, female gender, higher diastolic pressure, lower platelet count, the use of an intra-aortic balloon pump, and presentation with AMI.[132]

The EPILOG (Evaluation of PTCA to Improve Long-term Outcome by c7E3 GP IIB/IIIA Receptor Blockade) trial was designed to evaluate the efficacy of abciximab in lower-risk patients and to improve the safety profile.[133] Patients were randomly assigned to standard-dose heparin (100 U/kg and a target activated clotting time [ACT] of ≥300 seconds), standard-dose heparin with abciximab (same heparin dosing and ACT target), or abciximab and low-dose heparin (70 U/kg and a target ACT of 200 to 250 seconds). The trial was stopped early because the preliminary analysis of the first 1500 patients enrolled demonstrated a 68% relative risk reduction in the incidence of death and myocardial infarction at 30 days in the active treatment arm ($p = 0.00008$). Analysis of the data from all 2792 patients enrolled documented a 56% relative reduction in the composite end point of death, myocardial infarction, or urgent intervention or bypass surgery (11.7% vs. 5.2% for placebo vs. abciximab with low-dose heparin, $p < 0.0001$). However, the rate of target vessel revascularization at 6 months was not statistically different among the three groups. There was also a 40% reduction in the risk of major bleeding in patients randomized to active treatment (3.1% vs. 1.8%, $p$ nonsignificant [NS]). This strong trend toward reduced bleeding underscores the importance of the practice guidelines followed in EPILOG, namely the removal of vascular sheaths within 4 to 6 hours of intervention, avoiding the placement of venous sheaths, and weight adjustment of heparin targeting an ACT of 200 to 250 seconds.

Another trial of abciximab in PCI, the CAPTURE (c7E3 Fab Antiplatelet Therapy in Unstable Refractory Angina) trial, investigated the utility of pretreatment with abciximab in refractory unstable angina.[134] The CAPTURE trial, like the EPILOG trial, was stopped early because of a 52% relative risk reduction in the incidence of the 30-day composite end point (death, nonfatal myocardial infarction, and urgent reintervention) in patients treated with abciximab (18 to 24 hours before intervention and 1 hour after intervention) compared with patients treated with placebo. However, the primary end point at 6 months showed no advantage to abciximab treatment. This may have been due to the limited (1-hour) post-PCI infusion of abciximab used in the trial.

There is increasing evidence that essentially all patients benefit from treatment with abciximab.[135] The EPIC and CAPTURE trials demonstrated marked reductions in ischemic events at 30 days after coronary intervention in patients felt to be at high risk based on clinical criteria. The results of the EPILOG trial expanded the indication to patients of all risk categories. Ellis and colleagues evaluated the results of both the EPIC and the EPILOG trials with respect to baseline angiographic lesion characteristics.[136] Treatment with abciximab was found to improve outcomes irrespective of angiographic appearance. Examining the EPIC results, they found that patients with type A or B1 lesions actually benefited more from treatment with abciximab than did patients with complex lesions, using the modified American College of Cardiology/American Heart Association (ACC/AHA) definitions. In EPILOG, these investigators found that patients with all lesion types benefited from treatment with abciximab, but those patients with complex lesions appeared to benefit most. In a meta-analysis of the EPIC and EPILOG trials, Tcheng and coworkers found a 41% relative risk reduction in the incidence of the composite end point of death, myocardial infarction, and urgent intervention in patients with a previous coronary artery bypass graft (CABG) who were treated with abciximab.[137] Treatment with abciximab is also cost effective. In the cost-effectiveness analysis of the EPIC results, Mark and associates concluded that routine treatment with abciximab would increase the net cost by $293 per patient.[138] Analysis of the costs in EPILOG confirm that this treatment is likely a cost-effective (although not cost-saving) treatment.[139, 140] Finally, despite its potent antithrombotic effect, treatment with abciximab did not increase the risk of stroke in these three trials.[141]

The clinical trial of GPIIb/IIIa inhibition with perhaps the greatest relevance to contemporary practice is the EPISTENT (Evaluation Platelet of IIb/IIIa Inhibitor for STENTING) trial.[142] This trial was conducted to address the efficacy of abciximab either as an adjunct to coronary stent implantation or to balloon angioplasty with bail-out stenting compared with stent implantation alone. Between July 1996 and September 1997, 2399 patients with anatomy suitable for stent implantation were enrolled into the EPISTENT study. Patients were randomized to one of three approaches: standard stent PCI treatment, stent placement with abciximab and low-dose heparin (70 U/kg, targeting an ACT of 200 to 300 seconds), or balloon angioplasty with abciximab and low-dose heparin, with the provision for bail-out stenting if necessary. High-pressure deployment (to a median pressure of 16 atm) and ticlopidine treatment (used in 92% of patients receiving a stent) were specified in the protocol. In the balloon arm, 19.3% of patients underwent stent placement.

At 30 days, the primary composite end point of death, myocardial infarction, or urgent revascularization was improved in both the abciximab treatment arms compared with stent implantation alone (10.8% with stent treatment; 5.3% in the stent-plus-abciximab arm, $p \leq 0.001$ vs. stent alone; and 6.9% in the balloon-plus-abciximab arm, $p = 0.007$ vs. stent alone). There were consistent approximately 50% reductions in each of the end point components with combination stent-plus-abciximab treatment compared with stenting alone. At 6 months, the absolute difference favoring stent plus abciximab was maintained for the composite of death, myocardial infarction, or target vessel revascularization (18.3% with stent treatment vs. 13% with stent plus abciximab, $p = 0.003$). However, the event rate at 6 months for the balloon approach (20.9%, $p = NS$ vs. stent alone) deteriorated because of repeat target vessel revascularization. Interestingly, efficacy effects were most pronounced in diabetic patients. At 6 months, target vessel revascularization was reduced 51% ($p = 0.021$) in diabetic patients treated with stent plus abciximab compared with stent implantation alone, driving a 49% overall relative re-

duction in the 6-month composite end point of death, myocardial infarction, or target vessel revascularization (25.5% with stent alone vs. 13% with stent plus abciximab, $p = 0.005$). These data suggest that the greatest overall efficacy for PCI procedures in stent-eligible patients is the combination of abciximab with stent implantation. All clinically relevant end points (angiographic and procedural outcomes, periprocedural and subsequent myocardial infarction, urgent and elective repeat revascularization, and death) are improved either by stent implantation, by treatment with a GPIIb/IIIa antagonist, or by the synergy of combined therapy.

### RGD Analogues

Drugs belonging to the second generation of GPIIb/IIIa antagonists share a homologous RGD amino acid sequence that mimics the fibrinogen GPIIb/IIIa recognition sequence.[46] Unlike the monoclonal antibody abciximab, which irreversibly inhibits the receptor, these peptides and peptidomimetics are (reversible) competitive antagonists. As a group, these "designer drugs" have short plasma and biologic half-lives that offer a theoretic advantage in the setting of coronary intervention because of their rapid onset of action and easy reversibility.

#### Eptifibatide

Compared with linear RGD sequences, cyclic RGD analogues are more potent and resistant to enzymatic destruction. Eptifibatide (Integrilin) is a cyclic heptapeptide that incorporates a conservative lysine-for-arginine substitution (producing a KGD sequence) that further enhances its potency and specificity for the GPIIb/IIIa receptor.[143] The IMPACT II (Integrilin to Minimize Platelet Aggregation and Prevent Coronary Thrombosis II) trial enrolled 4010 patients at 82 centers from all risk strata.[144] Patients were randomly assigned to 24-hour treatment with placebo, a 135-μg/kg bolus of eptifibatide followed by a 0.50-μg/kg/minute infusion for 24 hours, or the same bolus followed by a 0.75-μg/kg/minute infusion. At 24 hours, there was an approximately 35% relative risk reduction in the incidence of the composite primary end point (death, myocardial infarction, urgent revascularization, or bail-out stenting) in patients randomized to active treatment. By 30 days, there remained only a statistically insignificant 19% relative risk reduction in the incidence of the primary composite end point. According to the treated patient analysis (including only those who actually received any study drug), those who received low-dose eptifibatide had a 22% relative risk reduction in the composite end point compared with those who received placebo ($p = 0.035$). As predicted, there was no difference in the incidence of bleeding among the groups, regardless of the criteria used. Eptifibatide was approved in April 1998 by the U.S. Food and Drug Administration (FDA) as an adjunct to PCI. However, the possibility that the more modest treatment effects of eptifibatide (compared with the results obtained in trials of abciximab) might be due to inadequate dosing or the duration of treatment[145] still needs to be addressed in additional clinical trials.

### Peptidomimetics

Tirofiban and lamifiban are two peptidomimetics that have been investigated in large phase III clinical trials. These pseudopeptides contain modified peptide bonds and side chains that increase their resistance to enzymatic catabolism. Unlike abciximab and the RGD peptide inhibitors that share sequence homology with naturally occurring ligands, these agents inhibit platelet aggregation by mimicking the three-dimensional structure and charge of the RGD sequence.[146] In the RESTORE (Randomized Efficacy Study of Tirofiban for Outcomes and REstenosis) trial, 2110 patients with unstable angina or AMI before coronary intervention were randomized to placebo or the tyrosine derivative tirofiban (10 $\mu$g/kg bolus and an infusion at the rate of 0.15 $\mu$g/kg/minute for 30 hours).[147, 148] The results were similar to those of the IMPACT II trial of eptifibatide. At 2 days, patients randomized to tirofiban had a 38% relative reduction in the primary composite end point (5.4 % vs. 8.7%, $p=0.005$), but by 30 days the relative risk reduction of 16% was no longer statistically significant ($p=0.16$). Tirofiban has not been approved as adjunctive treatment in PCI, although it is available for use in the early management of patients presenting with an acute coronary syndrome.

Lamifiban is a potent, synthetic nonpeptide with high specificity for the GPIIb/IIIa receptor that has a half-life of about 4 hours.[149] This agent has not been evaluated directly as an adjunct to PCI. Data from trials of lamifiban in unstable angina include the following. In the Canadian Lamifiban Study, Theroux and coworkers randomized 365 patients with unstable angina to an infusion of lamifiban or placebo.[150] At 30 days, the incidence of death or nonfatal myocardial infarction was 8.1% in the placebo group versus 2.5% in patients treated with lamifiban ($p=0.03$). Patients treated with the highest dose of lamifiban also had a reduced need for urgent coronary intervention. The PARAGON (Platelet IIb/IIIa Antagonism for the Reduction of Acute coronary syndrome events in a Global Organization Network) trial also randomized patients with unstable angina to lamifiban or placebo. Of the 306 patients (13.6%) who underwent PTCA, patients treated with lamifi-

ban had a reduced rate of death and nonfatal myocardial infarction.[151]

## ANTICOAGULANTS

Platelet activation and aggregation and the coagulation cascade are fundamentally interdependent pathways. Thrombin, the product of the coagulation cascade, is a potent activator of platelets, whereas platelet $\alpha$ granules contain potent agonists (including factor V and fibrinogen) that activate and accelerate the coagulation cascade. Furthermore, platelet membranes are critical binding sites for the activation of factor X and prothrombin.[152, 153] Prevention of thrombosis thus depends on inhibition of both platelets and the coagulation cascade (Table 27–3).

## Heparin

Heparin is a mixture of sulfated mucopolysaccharides with molecular masses ranging from 3000 to 30,000 D. It is isolated from porcine intestine and bovine lung.[154] The anticoagulant effect of heparin is dependent on binding of heparin to antithrombin III to (indirectly) inactivate thrombin and factor Xa. Only a pentasaccharide chain is required for heparin to bind antithrombin III and inactivate factor Xa.[157] However, heparin chains with at least 18 residues are able to bind antithrombin III and thrombin simultaneously and thus increase the ability of antithrombin III to neutralize thrombin by 1000-fold; the potency of an individual heparin molecule is directly proportional to its chain length.[155, 156] The large heparin–antithrombin III complex inhibits only free thrombin, not clot-bound thrombin.[53] Heparin also inhibits thrombin *generation* chiefly by

**TABLE 27–3.** **SELECTED STUDIES, TRIALS, AND META-ANALYSES OF ANTITHROMBOTIC AGENTS**

| AGENT | REFERENCES |
|---|---|
| Aspirin | 86–88, 92, 95, 109, 112, 175 |
| Ticlopidine | 101, 103–105, 107–109, 112, 175, 192–197 |
| Clopidogrel | 118–123 |
| Eptifibatide | 144, 145 |
| Tirofiban | 147, 148 |
| Abciximab | 128–142 |
| Heparin | 164–168 |
| Low molecular weight heparin | 175 |
| Hirulog | 185 |
| Hirudin | 183 |
| Warfarin | 109, 112, 175, 259, 260 |
| Thrombolytics: native coronary arteries | 209–223, 228–230, 232–234 |
| Thrombolytics: saphenous vein grafts | 211, 236–242 |

inhibiting factors XIIa, XIa, and IXa and the factor V and VIII positive feedback loops.[158, 159]

Precise anticoagulation with heparin is difficult because of its variable pharmacokinetics and pharmacodynamics. Intravenous or subcutaneous delivery is required, and the biologic half-life is approximately 90 minutes. Because heparin binds to plasma proteins, a reproducible dose-response curve cannot be predicted. The potency is nonlinear, increasing rapidly at higher doses. Only free heparin is able to bind antithrombin III and produce anticoagulation. It is deactivated by endothelial cells and platelet factor 4 and eliminated by both renal and hepatic pathways. The heparin–antithrombin III complex is inhibited by fibrin, fibrin degradation products, and the platelet membrane.[160]

The therapeutic use of heparin is limited by a narrow therapeutic index, unpredictable pharmacokinetics and pharmacodynamics, thrombocytopenia, and the need for frequent laboratory monitoring. Bleeding is the most common serious adverse effect and is difficult to prevent because of the unpredictable dose-response relationship. Following a nomogram may help establish a heparin dose that balances the therapeutic effect with bleeding complications.[161, 162] Thrombocytopenia occurs in about 3% of patients and is associated with thrombosis in about 0.4% of patients.[163] This idiosyncratic, immune-mediated thrombocytopenia usually occurs between 3 and 14 days after heparin therapy is started but can occur within hours and is more common with bovine lung than porcine gut preparations.

Although heparin is a mainstay of percutaneous arterial interventions, its use has not been investigated in a randomized trial. Retrospective studies of variable size and design have demonstrated a reduction in abrupt closure and clinical ischemic events in patients treated with heparin and suggest the reduction in events may be proportional to the degree of anticoagulation achieved.[164–168] The optimal ACT for minimizing both ischemic and hemorrhagic complications during PCI in patients not treated with a GPIIb/IIIa antagonist appears to be about 300 seconds using a HemoTec machine and 350 seconds using a Hemochron device.[167–171] The notion that "stabilization" of the unstable plaque (particularly in the presence of angiographic thrombus) using heparin for a few days before coronary intervention to reduce procedural complications cannot be supported presently as this approach appears only to prolong the hospital stay and increase costs.[172]

## Low Molecular Weight Heparin

Low molecular weight heparin (LMWH) is produced from unfractionated heparin by enzymatic or chemical depolymerization into polysaccharide fractions. These heparins have molecular masses between 3000 and 10,000 D.[173, 174] Like standard heparin, LMWH is a heterogeneous mixture. Each proprietary preparation has unique pharmacodynamic and pharmacokinetic properties related to the use of different source material and preparation techniques. The LMWH–antithrombin III complex has minimal direct effect on thrombin activity because of the chain length dependency of this binding. Because binding to factor Xa requires only a pentasaccharide unit, the anti-Xa effect of LMWH is equal to that of unfractionated heparin. Whereas standard heparin has a 1:1 anti-Xa to antithrombin effect, LMWH generally has a 2:1 to 4:1 ratio. Because of a lower affinity for plasma proteins and endothelial cells than standard heparin, the bioavailability of LMWH is greater than that of heparin and the dose-response relationship is more predictable. However, like standard heparin, LMWH does not inhibit clot-bound thrombin.

In the PCI setting, LMWH is most commonly used after intracoronary stenting, particularly in patients felt to be at increased risk for ischemic events. The ENTICES (ENoxaparin, TIClopidine after Elective Stenting) trial (N = 122) demonstrated a reduction in clinical events at 30 days in patients treated with enoxaparin and ticlopidine after elective stent deployment.[175] Surprisingly, there was no statistically significant difference in the primary end point, which evaluated the hematologic markers of thrombin generation and activity. In an observational study of 918 patients, Pan and colleagues compared treatment with aspirin, dipyridamole, and intravenous unfractionated heparin to treatment with ticlopidine, aspirin, and LWMH.[176] Patients treated with the latter regimen had a reduced incidence of thrombotic and hemorrhagic complications; there were no subacute thrombotic events in this group, compared with a 5.8% incidence in the first group ($p < 0.01$). Currently, a clear-cut indication for enoxaparin is the patient who has undergone stent implantation who would ordinarily require warfarin anticoagulation (for example, a patient with a prosthetic valve). Our approach has generally been to defer the reinitiation of warfarin therapy for 2 weeks after stent implantation, with anticoagulation accomplished instead by enoxaparin for 2 weeks after intervention. Recommending enoxaparin (or other LMWH preparations) on a more routine basis will require further validation in large-scale clinical trials.

Heparinoids are a mixture of LMWH and dermatan and chondroitin sulfates. They are used principally as an alternative to heparin in patients with heparin-induced thrombocytopenia (HIT) as they are minimally cross-reactive with sera containing heparin-associated antiplatelet antibodies. In an analysis of 230 patients with HIT, Magnani reported successful use of danaparoid (Orgaran) in 93% of patients and cross-reactivity in 10% of plasma samples.[177] Either an LMWH heparin or a heparinoid preparation should be considered during PCI in the patient with heparin-induced thrombocytopenia or other major contraindications to heparin treatment.

## Direct Thrombin Inhibitors

Thrombin has distinct fibrin-binding and catalytic sites.[53] Despite "therapeutic" treatment with heparin, the inability of heparin to inhibit clot-bound thrombin and thrombin bound to soluble fibrin degradation products leaves a reservoir of thrombin that can continue to cleave fibrinogen to fibrin and activate platelets.[160] This led to the design and evaluation of direct thrombin inhibitors that inactivate free and clot-bound thrombin equally well, independent of antithrombin III.[178–180] As a group, these agents inhibit thrombogenesis, clot production, and thrombin-mediated platelet activation.

Several of the direct thrombin inhibitors have now been studied in clinical trials. Hirudin is the prototypic direct antithrombin and is the most potent and specific antithrombin yet identified.[181] The therapeutic use of hirudin dates back to antiquity. Isolated from a leech salivary peptide, it was cloned in 1986 and is now produced by recombinant DNA technology.[182] In the HELVETICA (Hirudin in a European Trial versus Heparin in the Prevention of Restenosis after PTCA) trial, 1141 patients with unstable angina were randomized to treatment with heparin or hirudin before PTCA.[183] Although there was no difference in the incidence of the primary end point at 30 days or restenosis at 6 months, there was an early 61% relative risk reduction in the primary end point at 96 hours, and hemorrhagic complications were reduced in patients randomized to hirudin. Bivalirudin (Hirulog) is a 20–amino acid synthetic peptide based on the hirudin template.[184] In the Hirulog Angioplasty Study, 4098 patients with unstable or postinfarction angina were randomized to bivalirudin or heparin before PTCA.[185] As with hirudin, there was no difference in the incidence of the 30-day primary end point. Patients randomized to hirulog had a reduced incidence of bleeding, whether measured by the rate of major hemorrhage, retroperitoneal hemorrhage, or need for red blood cell transfusion. Hirugen is a synthetic protein composed of the 12 terminal amino acids that constitute the thrombin binding site on hirudin.[186] Because it does not interfere with the thrombin catalytic site, its antithrombotic effect is much weaker than those of the other compounds in this class. Argatroban is a competitive inhibitor of the thrombin catalytic site that has been evaluated in phase II studies in patients with unstable angina.[187]

In sum, direct thrombin inhibitors may reduce early ischemic events and bleeding after coronary intervention. However, clinical trials data suggest that the benefit is not sustained. Also, their much higher cost compared with that of heparin will likely preclude widespread use. If they become commercially available in the future, these agents may be particularly useful in patients with a history of heparin-induced thrombocytopenia.

## Protamine

The protamines are a family of basic, low molecular weight proteins isolated from the sperm and testes of the fish family Salmonidae that reverse systemic heparinization.[188] Given intravenously, they antagonize platetet function as well as heparin activity. The usual dose is 1 mg protamine for every 100 U of active (remaining) heparin in the body. Although rare, anaphylactoid reactions to protamine typically occur immediately after delivery. Diabetic patients previously treated with neutral protamine Hagedorn (NPH) insulin and patients with previous allergic reactions to fish appear to be predisposed to adverse reactions.[189, 190] Stewart and associates reported that 1.1% of patients (7 of 651) treated with protamine had a major adverse reaction and one patient died.[191] The incidence of severe reactions was 27% (4 of 15) in diabetic patients treated with NPH insulin versus 0.5% (3 of 636) in those without an exposure history to protamine insulin.

## Warfarin

Dicoumarol and warfarin are oral anticoagulants that interfere with the transcarboxylation of factors II, VII, IX, and X by inhibiting the reduction of vitamin K. Treatment with warfarin was standard therapy in the initial trials of coronary stenting and was mandated by the U.S. FDA in this setting. However, three prospective trials demonstrated an increase in cardiac/adverse events in patients randomized to treatment with warfarin compared with antiplatelet therapy alone after coronary stenting.[109, 112, 175] The results from several nonrandomized studies support withholding anticoagulation therapy after coronary stenting with the Palmaz-Schatz device.[103–105, 192–197] Furthermore, treatment with warfarin increases platelet activation, bleeding complication rates, the length of hospitalization, and hospital costs.[109, 110, 198, 199] In summary, these results suggest that warfarin should be avoided after stent implantation. The appropriate medical regimen after optimal and suboptimal stent deployment is discussed further in Chapters 36 to 44.

## FIBRINOLYTIC THERAPY

Each of the currently available thrombolytic agents has distinct pharmacodynamic and pharmacokinetic properties (Table 27–4).[200] Streptokinase is a protein isolated from β-hemolytic streptococcal cultures that undergoes conformational changes on binding to plasminogen. In the bound, activated state, the plasminogen-streptokinase complex cleaves peptide bonds in plasminogen to form plasmin. Urokinase and tissue-type plasminogen activator (tPA) are naturally occurring enzymes that cleave plasminogen directly. Alteplase (recombinant tPA [rtPA]) has a fibrin-binding site that increases its affinity for plasminogen within the thrombus relative to native tPA. Multiple trials of thrombolytic therapy during myocardial infarction have demonstrated improved survival, functional status, and myocardial salvage in patients who present with ST-segment elevation or bundle-branch block.[201] Just as important, these trials and others have also demonstrated that patients (with myocardial infarction) with initial ST-segment depression have a worse prognosis and are harmed by thrombolytic therapy.[201–204]

The initial enthusiasm for adjunctive thrombolytic therapy during coronary intervention is a prime example of the limitations of surrogate end points in clinical trials. It has been well established that pre- and intraprocedural intracoronary thrombus increases the likelihood of abrupt vessel closure, myocardial infarction, the need for emergency bypass surgery, and death after coronary intervention.[205–209] Angiographic improvement, or even resolution of visible thrombus, with treatment with intracoronary thrombolytic therapy in (nonrandomized) studies raised expectations of improved *clinical* outcomes with this approach.[209–214] However, the cumulative data have failed to demonstrate a role for thrombolytic therapy in the setting of PCI. In a prospective trial, O'Neill and associates randomized 122 patients who presented within 4 hours of the onset of myocardial infarction to treatment with streptokinase or placebo before PTCA.[215] The rates of procedural success, arterial patency, restenosis, and ventricular function were equivalent, but hospitalization was longer and more costly and the rate of transfusion was higher in patients pretreated with streptokinase. Two nonrandomized trials also failed to demonstrate an improvement in angioplasty success rate or mortality in patients treated with antecedent thrombolytic therapy.[216, 217]

The efficacy of adjunctive thrombolytic therapy in patients with unstable angina has been investigated in at least six trials. The TAUSA (Thrombolysis and Angioplasty in UnStable Angina) trial demonstrated that improved angiographic outcomes after adjunctive thrombolytic therapy did not translate into improved clinical outcomes.[218] Instead, patients treated with thrombolytic therapy at the time of coronary intervention were at increased risk for cardiac events. In TAUSA, 469 patients with ischemic rest pain were randomized to treatment with intracoronary urokinase or placebo before wire placement and conventional PTCA. Despite the (statistically insignificant) reduction in angiographic thrombus after angioplasty, there was a marked increase in abrupt closure (10.2% vs 4.3%, $p<0.02$) and cardiac events, including ischemia, infarction, and emergency bypass surgery (12.9% vs. 6.3%, $p<0.02$) in the active treatment versus control groups, respectively. A pooled analysis of the six trials that evaluated adjunctive thrombolytic therapy during angioplasty in patients with unstable angina not only failed to reveal improved angiographic success but demonstrated a trend toward increased complications.[211, 218–223] The results from the randomized trials that demonstrated worse outcome in patients with unstable angina treated with *intravenous* thrombolytic therapy support these results.[224–227] Likewise, the pooled analysis by Vaitkus and Laskey of the three studies (including two prospective randomized trials) of 742 patients that evaluated adjunctive fibrinolytic therapy during elective angioplasty also failed to demonstrate improved angiographic or clinical outcomes.[228–230]

In the treatment of the chronic total occlusion, the poor procedural and long-term success rates as-

## TABLE 27–4.    SELECTED PROPERTIES OF THROMBOLYTICS

|  | STREPTOKINASE | UROKINASE | tPA |
|---|---|---|---|
| Half-life (minutes) | 20 | 4 | 6 |
| Typical IC dose | 100–500,000 U | 250,000 U | 10–20 mg |
| Fibrin selective | Minimal | Minimal | Moderate |
| Plasminogen binding | Indirect | Direct | Direct |
| Antigenic | Yes | No | No |
| Fibrinogen degradation | 4+ | 3+ | 1+ |
| Approximate cost | $100/500,000 U | $200/250,000 U | $500/20 mg |

IC, intracoronary; tPA, tissue-type plasminogen activator.
From Gersh BJ, Opie LH: Antithrombotic agents: Platelet inhibitors, anticoagulants, and fibrinolytics. *In* Opie LH (ed): Drugs for the Heart, pp 217–246. Philadelphia: WB Saunders, 1991.

sociated with PCI, coupled with the high postprocedure myocardial infarction rate, have stimulated the use of adjunctive thrombolytic therapy in this setting.[231] In the pooled analysis of three studies that investigated intracoronary thrombolytic treatment of native chronic occlusions, Vaitkus and Laskey reported successful reperfusion in 64% (51 of 80) of patients.[211, 232–234] In a prospective dose-finding study of 60 patients in whom conventional angioplasty failed, Zidar and colleagues demonstrated that an 8-hour intracoronary urokinase infusion improved the angioplasty success rate to 53%, although 91% of patients eventually developed angiographic restenosis.[235] The pooled analysis of seven studies evaluating prolonged urokinase infusions in patients with saphenous vein graft occlusions established an angiographic success rate of 74%.[211, 236–242] Hartmann and associates evaluated the direct infusion of urokinase through an angiographic catheter placed in the ostium of 47 occluded grafts and an infusion wire positioned within the graft.[236] Urokinase was delivered at a rate from 100,000 to 250,000 U/hour, for a mean duration of 31 hours, and a total dose that ranged from 0.7 to 9.8 million U. Recanalization with urokinase alone was successful in 79% of grafts, and after adjunctive angioplasty, 62% of grafts had TIMI-3 flow. Success, however, was achieved at a cost; 13% of patients had evidence of postprocedural myocardial infarction, 22% of patients developed a significant hematoma, and 35% of successful recanalization cases developed subsequent graft reocclusion. In the ROBUST (Recanalization of Chronically Occluded Aortocoronary Saphenous Vein Bypass Grafts with Long-Term, Low Dose Infusion of Urokinase) trial, 107 patients with chronically occluded saphenous vein grafts and refractory angina received urokinase through a 0.035-inch infusion wire for a mean duration of 25.4 hours and mean urokinase infusion of 3.70 million U.[243] The rates of initial recanalization, postprocedural enzyme elevation, in-hospital death, and blood transfusion were 69%, 17%, 6.5%, and 19%, respectively. Angiographic follow-up, available in 54% of successful cases, documented only 40% of grafts to be patent long term.

Based on these results, adjunctive thrombolytic therapy cannot be advocated for any subgroup of patients undergoing mechanical revascularization. The most plausible explanations for the deleterious outcomes observed with adjunctive thrombolytic therapy are increased rates of intramural hemorrhage[244] and platelet activation.[245–249]

## VASODILATORS

Coronary vasoconstriction occurs to some extent in virtually every coronary artery during PCI. Even cannulation with the guide catheter induces spasm.[250] Fischell and associates demonstrated progressive vasoconstriction at the PTCA site and distally in all patients, despite pretreatment with calcium channel antagonists, that was readily prevented with nitroglycerin.[251] Because of the importance of appropriate sizing of vessels before intervention (and particularly before stent implantation), we routinely administer intracoronary nitroglycerin (50 to 300 µg) to all patients before the initial "scout" shots. Quantitative on-line coronary angiography is then used to size the target vessel. Nitroglycerin is given even to patients receiving intravenous nitrates, as these patients remain sensitive to additional intracoronary nitroglycerin. In patients with borderline hypotension, nitroglycerin can be given safely after volume resuscitation.

Vasodilators are also useful in patients with coronary "no-reflow." The etiology of this phenomenon is multifactorial, including occlusive dissection, elastic recoil, distal thromboembolism, and intense microvascular spasm. Of course, therapy must be individualized and other causes evaluated before the administration of medications with the potential to cause hemodynamic embarrassment. Distinct from the epicardial vessels, the microvasculature rarely responds to nitroglycerin.[252–254] But familiarity with its profile and a high therapeutic index make the routine use of nitroglycerin quite practical. Several studies have reported improvement in coronary flow after delivery of calcium channel antagonists. Piana and coworkers reported that the incidence of no-reflow not attributable to dissection, thrombus, discrete distal vessel cutoff, or angiographically visible spasm was 2% in a series of 1919 interventions.[255] In 25 of 37 patients (68%), intracoronary nitroglycerin had no effect. Intracoronary verapamil (mean dose $234 \pm 142$ µg, total dose 50 to 900 µg) increased the TIMI flow grade in 33 of 37 patients (89%). Normal TIMI-3 flow was restored in 30 of 37 patients (81%). One patient developed bradycardia that required a transvenous pacemaker, and none developed systemic hypotension requiring treatment. Verapamil for intracoronary administration was prepared by diluting a 5-mg vial with saline to a total volume of 5 mL, then further dilution of 1 mL of this solution to a total volume of 10 mL for a concentration of 100 µg/mL.

Other agents have been used to treat the no-reflow phenomenon. Weyrens and colleagues reported on the use of diltiazem in 24 patients.[256] Subselective diltiazem improved blood flow in 23 of 24 patients (96%). Diltiazem was diluted to a concentration of 0.5 mg/mL and injected in 0.5- to 2.5-mg increments, for a mean total dose of 3.5 mg (range 0.5 to 8.5 mg). It was delivered through the central lumen of a catheter placed in the artery, rather than through the guide catheter.

The incidence of coronary vasospasm and no-reflow during high-speed rotational atherectomy is perhaps 10% to 20%. Most physicians administer generous amounts of nitroglycerin and verapamil during ablation runs, frequently as a continuous infusion during ablation runs. The CARAFE (Cocktail Attenuation of Rotational Ablation Flow Effects) pilot study treated 27 lesions in 21 patients with a "cocktail" delivered through the 4-French sheath.[257] The cocktail consisted of verapamil 10 μg/mL, nitroglycerin 4 μg/mL, and heparin 20 U/mL delivered at a rate of 10 mL/minute. This approach provides doses of 100 μg of verapamil, 40 μg of nitroglycerin, and 200 U of heparin over a 30-second ablation run. In this small study, spasm occurred in 2 of 27 lesions (7%). Demand pacing was required in 15 of 21 patients, including ablations of all right and circumflex arteries.

## CONCLUSION

Pharmacotherapy during PCI has evolved greatly since the initial description of PTCA by Andreas Gruentzig in 1978. Command and facility with pharmacotherapy as applicable to coronary intervention are requirements for the safe and successful performance of procedures. The synergism produced by the combination of midazolam and hydromorphone provides optimal sedation in most patients. Heparin remains the only anticoagulant in use today because of its effectiveness, low cost, and familiarity. The primary limitations of heparin are high rates of hemorrhage and thrombocytopenia and unpredictable pharmacokinetics. Appreciation of the critical role of the platelet in ischemic events after coronary intervention, and the ability to inhibit these events with targeted GPIIb/IIIa therapy and with the thienopyridines, is the major breakthrough since the previous edition of this book. Conversely, the outcome in patients treated with adjunctive thrombolytics during coronary interventions has been disappointing. The development of new antiplatelet agents will be the focus of clinical research for quite some time. Unfortunately, no pharmacotherapy has proved effective in modulating restenosis. Perhaps gene therapy holds the key as the critical approach to restenosis. This and other pharmacotherapeutics will remain the foci of clinical investigations for years to come.

## REFERENCES

1. Gruentzig A: Transluminal dilation of coronary-artery stenosis (Letter to the Editor). Lancet, 1:263, 1978.
2. Gruentzig AR, Senning A, Siegenthaler WE: Nonoperative dilatation of coronary-artery stenosis: percutaneous transluminal coronary angioplasty. N Engl J Med 301:61–68, 1979.
3. Rosenberg W, Donald A: Evidence based medicine: An approach to clinical problem-solving. BMJ 310:1122–1126, 1995.
4. Califf RM: Why are large-scale trials needed? Coron Artery Dis 3:92–95, 1992.
5. Peto R, Collins R, Gray R: Large-scale randomized evidence: Large, simple trials and overview of trials. J Clin Epidemiol 48:23–40, 1995.
6. Rosati RA, Lee KL, Califf RM, et al: Problems and advantages of an observational data base approach to evaluating the effect of therapy on outcome. Circulation 65(suppl II):II-27–II-32, 1982.
7. Collins R, Gray R, Godwin J, et al: Avoidance of large biases and large random errors in the assessment of moderate treatment effects: The need for systematic overviews. Stat Med 6:245–254, 1987.
8. Peto R, Pike MC, Armitage P, et al: Design and analysis of randomized clinical trials requiring prolonged observation of each patient. II. Analysis and examples. Br J Cancer 35:1–39, 1977.
9. Fleming TR, DeMets DL: Surrogate end points in clinical trials: Are we being misled? Ann Intern Med 125:605–613, 1996.
10. Sklar DP: Local anesthetics. Ann Emerg Med 27:464–465, 1996.
11. Skidmore RA, Patterson JD, Tomsick RS: Local anesthetics. Dermatol Surg 22:511–524, 1996.
12. Feldman T, Moss J, Teplinsky K, et al: Cardiac catheterization in the patient with history of allergy to local anesthetics. Cathet Cardiovasc Diagn 20:165–167, 1990.
13. Mader TJ, Playe SJ, Garb JL: Reducing the pain of local anesthetic infiltration: Warming and buffering have a synergistic effect. Ann Emerg Med 23:550–554, 1994.
14. Bergeron P, Enns J, Delima L, et al: Effects of routine premedication for cardiac catheterization on sedation, level of anxiety and arterial oxygen saturation. Can J Cardiol 11:201–205, 1995.
15. Mangano DT. Perioperative cardiac morbidity. Anesthesiology 72:153–184, 1990.
16. Lau W, Kovoor P, Ross DL: Cardiac electrophysiologic effects of midazolam combined with fentanyl. Am J Cardiol 72:177–182, 1993.
17. Newman M, Reves JG: Pro: Midazolam is the sedative of choice to supplement narcotic anesthesia. J Cardiothorac Vasc Anesth 7:615–619, 1993.
18. Roekaerts P, de Lange S: Con: Midazolam is not the sedative of choice to supplement narcotic anesthesia. J Cardiothorac Vasc Anesth 7:620–623, 1993.
19. Whitwam JG: Co-induction of anaesthesia: Day-case surgery. Eur J Anaesthesiol Suppl 12:25–34, 1995.
20. Shapiro BA, Warren J, Egol AB, et al: Practice parameters for intravenous analgesia and sedation for adult patients in the intensive care unit: An executive summary. Society of Critical Care Medicine. Crit Care Med 23:1596–1600, 1995.
21. Murray MJ, DeRuyter ML, Harrison BA: Opioids and benzodiazepines. Crit Care Clin 11:849–873, 1995.
22. Enna SJ, Mohler H: GABA receptors and their association with benzodiazepines recognition sites. In Meltzer HY (ed): Psychopharmacology: 3rd Generation of Progress, pp. 265–272. New York: Raven Press, 1987.
23. Reves JG, Fragen RJ, Vinik HR, et al: Midazolam: Pharmacology and uses. Anesthesiology 62:310–324, 1985.
24. Willens JS, Myslinski NR: Pharmacodynamics, pharmacokinetics, and clinical uses of fentanyl, sufentanil, and alfentanil [published erratum appears in Heart Lung 22:307, 1993]. Heart Lung 22:239–251, 1993.
25. Lipman AG: Clinically relevant differences among the opioid analgesics. Am J Hosp Pharm 47:S7–S13, 1990.
26. Bryson HM, Fulton BR, Faulds D: Propofol. An update of its use in anaesthesia and conscious sedation. Drugs 50:513–559, 1995.
27. Kanto J, Gepts E: Pharmacokinetic implications for the clinical use of propofol. Clin Pharmacokinet 17:308–326, 1989.

28. Kidd JF, Vickers MD: Pulse oximeters: Essential monitors with limitations. Br J Anaesth 62:355–257, 1989.

29. Dodson SR, Hensley FA Jr, Martin DE, et al: Continuous oxygen saturation monitoring during cardiac catheterization in adults. Chest 94:28–31, 1988.

30. Council on Scientific Affairs AMA: The use of pulse oximetry during conscious sedation. JAMA 270:1463–1468, 1993.

31. Cone AM, Stott SA: Flumazenil. Br J Hosp Med 51:346–348, 1994.

32. Hoffman EJ, Warren EW: Flumazenil: A benzodiazepine antagonist [published erratum appears in Clin Pharm 12:803, 1993]. Clin Pharm 12:641–701, 1993.

33. Chamberlain JM, Klein BL: A comprehensive review of naloxone for the emergency physician. Am J Emerg Med 12:650–660.

34. Fuster V, Badimon L, Badimon JJ, et al: The pathogenesis of coronary artery disease and the acute coronary syndromes (1). N Engl J Med 326:242–250, 1992.

35. Fuster V, Badimon L, Badimon JJ, et al: The pathogenesis of coronary artery disease and the acute coronary syndromes (2). N Engl J Med 326:310–318, 1992.

36. Ip JH, Fuster V, Israel D, et al: The role of platelets, thrombin and hyperplasia in restenosis after coronary angioplasty. J Am Coll Cardiol 17:77B–88B, 1991.

37. Gasperetti CM, Gonias SL, Gimple LW, et al: Platelet activation during coronary angioplasty in humans. Circulation 88:2728–2734, 1993.

38. Landau C, Lange RA, Hillis LD: Percutaneous transluminal coronary angioplasty. N Engl J Med 330:981–993, 1994.

39. Waller BF: "Crackers, breakers, stretchers, drillers, scrapers, shavers, burners, welders and melters"—The future treatment of atherosclerotic coronary artery disease? A clinical-morphologic assessment J Am Coll Cardiol 13:969–987, 1989.

40. Hynes R: Integrins: A family of cell surface receptors. Cell 48:549–554, 1987.

41. Hynes RO: Integrins: Versatility, modulation, and signaling in cell adhesion. Cell 69:11–25, 1992.

42. Kroll MH, Harris TS, Moake JL, Handin RI, Schafer AL, et al: Von Willebrand factor binding to platelet GPIb initiates signals for platelet activation. J Clin Invest 88:1568–1573, 1991.

43. Body SC: Platelet activation and interactions with the microvasculature. J Cardiovasc Pharmacol 27:S13–S25, 1996.

44. Coller BS: The role of platelets in arterial thrombosis and the rationale for blockade of platelet GPIIb/IIIa receptors as antithrombotic therapy. Eur Heart J 16:11–15, 1995.

45. Phillips D, Charo I, Parise L, et al: The platelet membrane glycoprotein IIb/IIIa complex. Blood 71:831–843, 1988.

46. Lefkovits J, Plow E, Topol E: Platelet glycoprotein IIb/IIIa receptors in cardiovascular medicine. N Engl J Med 332:1553–1559, 1995.

47. Pierschbacher MD, Ruoslahti E: Cell attachment activity of fibronectin can be duplicated by small synthetic fragments of the molecule. Nature 309:30–33, 1984.

48. Marguerie GA, Plow EF, Edgington TS: Human platelets possess an inducible and saturable receptor specific for fibrinogen. J Biol Chem 254:5357–5363, 1979.

49. Farrell DH, Thiagarajan P, Chung DW, et al: Role of fibrinogen alpha and gamma chain sites in platelet aggregation. Proc Natl Acad Sci U S A 89:10,729–10,732, 1992.

50. Wilcox JN, Smith KM, Schwartz SM, et al: Localization of tissue factor in the normal vessel wall and in the atherosclerotic plaque. Proc Natl Acad Sci U S A; 86:2839–2843.

51. Jesty J, Nemerson Y: The pathway of blood coagulation. *In* Beutler E, Lichtman Coller BS, et al: (eds): Williams Hematology, vol. 1, pp. 1227–1238. New York: McGraw-Hill, 1995.

52. Vu TK, Wheaton VI, Hung DT, et al: Domains specifying thrombin-receptor interaction. Nature 353:674–677, 1991.

53. Weitz JI, Hudoba M, Massel D, et al: Clot-bound thrombin is protected from inhibition by heparin-antithrombin III but is susceptible to inactivation by antithrombin III–independent inhibitors. J Clin Invest 86:385–391, 1990.

54. Harker LA, Hanson SR, Runge MS: Thrombin hypothesis of thrombus generation and vascular lesion formation. Am J Cardiol 75:12B–17B, 1995.

55. Neumann FJ, Ott I, Gawaz M, et al: Neutrophil and platelet activation at balloon-injured coronary artery plaque in patients undergoing angioplasty. J Am Coll Cardiol 27:819–824, 1996.

56. Tanguay JF, Rodes J, Merhi Y, et al: Differences in coronary platelet deposition after stenting and PTCA. J Am Coll Cardiol 29:94A, 1997.

57. Ueda M, Becker AE, Kasayuki N, et al: In situ detection of platelet-derived growth factor-A and -B chain mRNA in human coronary arteries after percutaneous transluminal coronary angioplasty. Am J Pathol 149:831–843, 1996.

58. Prayson RA, Ratliff NB: An analysis of outcome following percutaneous transluminal coronary artery angioplasty. An autopsy series. Arch Pathol Lab Med 114:1211–1217, 1990.

59. LeBreton H, Topol E, Plow EF: Evidence for a pivotal role of platelets in vascular reocclusion and restenosis [Comment]. Cardiovasc Res 31:235–263, 1996.

60. Nyamekye I, Lui D, Thomas S, et al: The significance of increased $^{111}$indium platelet accumulation at post-angioplasty sites. Clin Radiol 51:507–510, 1996.

61. Inoue T, Hoshi K, Fujito T, et al: Early detection of platelet activation after coronary angioplasty. Coron Artery Dis 7:529–534, 1996.

62. Kutryk MJ, Serruys PW: Platelet activation and coronary interventions [Editorial; Comment]. Eur Heart J 17:1134–1136, 1996.

63. Kolarov P, Tschoepe D, Nieuwenhuis HK, et al: PTCA: Periprocedural platelet activation. Part II of the Duesseldorf PTCA platelet study (DPPS). Eur Heart J 17:1216–1222, 1996.

64. Tanizawa S, Ueda M, van der Loos CM, et al: Expression of platelet derived growth factor B chain and beta receptor in human coronary arteries after percutaneous transluminal coronary angioplasty: An immunohistochemical study. Heart 75:549–556, 1996.

65. Mickelson JK, Lakkis NM, Villarreal-Levy G, et al: Leukocyte activation with platelet adhesion after coronary angioplasty: A mechanism for recurrent disease? J Am Coll Cardiol 28:345–353, 1996.

66. Harker L: Role of platelets and thrombosis in mechanisms of acute occlusion and restenosis after angioplasty. Am J Cardiol 60:20B–28B, 1987.

67. Willerson JT, Golino P, Eidt J, et al: Specific platelet mediators and unstable coronary artery lesions. Experimental evidence and potential clinical implications. Circulation 80:198–205, 1989.

68. Sunamura M, di Mario C, Piek JJ, et al: Cyclic flow variations after angioplasty: A rare phenomenon predictive of immediate complications. DEBATE Investigator's Group. Am Heart J 131:843–848, 1996.

69. Terres W, Lund GK, Hubner A, et al: Endogenous tissue plasminogen activator and platelet reactivity as risk factors for reocclusion after recanalization of chronic total coronary occlusions. Am Heart J 130:711–716, 1995.

70. Tschoepe D, Schultheiss HP, Kolarov P, et al: Platelet membrane activation markers are predictive for increased risk of acute ischemic events after PTCA. Circulation 88:37–42, 1993.

71. Lefkovits J, Blankenship JC, Anderson KM, et al: Increased risk of non-Q wave myocardial infarction after directional atherectomy is platelet dependent: Evidence from the EPIC trial. Evaluation of c7E3 for the Prevention of Ischemic Complications. J Am Coll Cardiol 28:849–855, 1996.

72. Wilentz JR, Sanborn TA, Haudenschild CC, et al: Platelet accumulation in experimental angioplasty: Time course and relation to vascular injury. Circulation 75:636–642, 1987.

73. Groves HM, Kinlough-Rathbone RL, Richardson M, et al: Platelet interaction with damaged rabbit aorta. Lab Invest 40:194–200, 1979.

74. Minar E, Ehringer H, Ahmadi R, et al: Platelet deposition at angioplasty sites and platelet survival time after PTA in iliac and femoral arteries: Investigations with indium-111–oxine labelled platelets in patients with ASA (l.0 g/day)-therapy. Thromb Haemost 58:718–723, 1987.

75. Holme PA, Brosstad F, Solum NO: Platelet-derived microvesicles and activated platelets express factor Xa activity. Blood Coagul Fibrinolysis 6:302–310, 1995.

76. Monroe DM, Roberts HR, Hoffman M: Platelet procoagulant complex assembly in a tissue factor–initiated system. Br J Haematol 88:364–371, 1994.

77. Hoffman M, Monroe DM, Oliver JA, et al: Factors IXa and Xa play distinct roles in tissue factor-dependent initiation of coagulation. Blood 86:1794–1801, 1995.

78. Lam JY, Chesebro JH, Steele PM, et al: Is vasospasm related to platelet deposition? Relationship in a porcine preparation of arterial injury in vivo. Circulation 75:243–8248, 1987.

79. Lam JY, Chesebro JH, Steele PM, et al: Deep arterial injury during experimental angioplasty: Relation to a positive indium-111–labeled platelet scintigram, quantitative platelet deposition and mural thrombosis. J Am Coll Cardiol 8:1380–1386, 1986.

80. Berk BC, Alexander RW, Brock TA, et al: Vasoconstriction: A new activity for platelet-derived growth factor. Science 232:87–90, 1986.

81. Roth GJ, Majeru PW: The mechanism of the effect of aspirin on human platelets. 1. Acetylation of a particulate fraction protein. J Clin Invest 56:624–632, 1975.

82. Roth GJ, Calverley DC: Aspirin, platelets, and thrombosis: Theory and practice. Blood 83:885–898, 1994.

83. Simon LS, Mills JA: Drug therapy: Nonsteroidal antiinflammatory drugs (first of two parts). N Engl J Med 302:1179–1185, 1980.

84. Simon LS, Mills JA: Nonsteroidal antiinflammatory drugs (second of two parts). N Engl J Med 302:1237–1243, 1980.

85. Underwood MJ, More RS: The aspirin papers [Editorial; Comment]. BMJ 308:71–72, 1994.

86. Antiplatelet Trialists' Collaboration: Collaborative overview of randomised trials of antiplatelet therapy—I: Prevention of death, myocardial infarction, and stroke by prolonged antiplatelet therapy in various categories of patients. [published erratum appears in BMJ 308:1540]. BMJ 308:81–106, 1994.

87. Antiplatelet Trialists' Collaboration: Collaborative overview of randomised trials of antiplatelet therapy—II: Maintenance of vascular graft or arterial patency by antiplatelet therapy. Antiplatelet Trialists' Collaboration. BMJ 308:159–168, 1994.

88. Antiplatelet Trialists' Collaboration. Secondary prevention of vascular disease by prolonged antiplatelet treatment. BMJ 296:320–331, 1988.

89. Steering Committee of the Physicians' Health Study Research Group: Final report on the aspirin component of the ongoing Physicians' Health Study. N Engl J Med 321:129–135, 1989.

90. Theroux P, Ouimet H, McCans J, et al: Aspirin, heparin, or both to treat acute unstable angina. N Engl J Med 319:1105–1111, 1988.

91. ISIS-2 (Second International Study of Infarct Survival) Collaborative Group: Randomised trial of intravenous streptokinase, oral aspirin, both, or neither among 17,187 cases of suspected acute myocardial infarction: ISIS-2. ISIS-2 (Second International Study of Infarct Survival) Collaborative Group. Lancet 2:349–360, 1988.

92. Schwartz L, Bourassa MG, Lesperance J, et al: Aspirin and dipyridamole in the prevention of restenosis after percutaneous transluminal coronary angioplasty. N Engl J Med 318:1714–1719, 1988.

93. Kent KM, Ewels CJ, Kehoe MK, et al: Effect of aspirin on complications during transluminal coronary angioplasty [Abstract]. J Am Coll Cardiol 11:132A, 1988.

94. Savage MP, Goldberg S, Bove AA, et al: Effect of thromboxane A2 blockade on clinical outcome and restenosis after successful coronary angioplasty. Multi-Hospital Eastern Atlantic Restenosis Trial (M-HEART II). Circulation 92:3194–200, 1995.

95. Lembo NJ, Black AJ, Roubin GS, et al: Effect of pretreatment with aspirin versus aspirin plus dipyridamole on frequency and type of acute complications of percutaneous transluminal coronary angioplasty. Am J Cardiol 65:422–426, 1990.

96. Chronos NA, Patel DJ, Sigwart U, et al: Intracoronary activation of human platelets following balloon angioplasty despite aspirin and heparin: A flow cytometric study. Circulation 90:I–181, 1994.

97. Terres W, Hamm CW, Ruchelka A, et al: Residual platelet function under acetylsalicylic acid and the risk of restenosis after coronary angioplasty. J Cardiovasc Pharmacol 19:190–193, 1992.

98. Hardisty RM, Powling MJ, Nokes TJ: The action of ticlopidine on human platelets. Studies on aggregation, secretion, calcium mobilization and membrane glycoproteins. Thromb Haemost 64:150–155, 1990.

99. Defreyn G, Bernat A, Delebassee D, et al: Pharmacology of ticlopidine: A review. Semin Thromb Hemost 15:159–166.

100. Sharis PJ, Cannon CP, Loscalzo J: The antiplatelet effects of ticlopidine and clopidogrel. Ann Intern Med 129:394–405, 1998.

101. Bertrand M, Allain H, Lablanche J, on behalf of the investigators of the TACT study: Results of a randomized trial of ticlopidine versus placebo for prevention of acue closure and restenosis after coronary angioplasty (PTCA). The TACT study. Circulation 82:III–190, 1990.

102. Cerisier A, Isaaz K, Dacosta A, et al: Prevention of reocclusion after successful balloon PTCA of totally occluded coronary arteries: A prospective randomized pilot-study comparing ticlopidine-aspirin with aspirin alone. J Am Coll Cardiol 29:395A, 1997.

103. Barragan P, Sainsous J, Silvestri M, et al: Ticlopidine and subcutaneous heparin as an alternative regimen following coronary stenting. Cathet Cardiovasc Diagn 32:133–138, 1994.

104. Morice MC, Bourdonnec C, Lefevre T, et al: Coronary stenting without Coumadin. Circulation 90:I–125, 1994.

105. Colombo A, Hall P, Nakamura S, et al: Intracoronary stenting without anticoagulation accomplished with intravascular ultrasound guidance. Circulation 91:1676–1688, 1995.

106. Nakamura S, Hall P, Gaglione A, et al: High pressure assisted coronary stent implantation accomplished without intravascular ultrasound guidance and subsequent anticoagulation. J Am Coll Cardiol 29:21–27, 1997.

107. Hall P, Nakamura S, Maiello L, et al: A randomized comparison of combined ticlopidine and aspirin therapy versus aspirin therapy alone after successful intravascular ultrasound-guided stent implantation. Circulation 93:215–222, 1996.

108. Goods CM, Al-Shaibi KF, Negus BH, at al: Is ticlopidine a necessary component of antiplatelet regimens following coronary artery stenting? J Am Coll Cardiol 27:137A, 1996.

109. Schömig A, Neumann F, Kastrati A, et al: A randomized comparison of antiplatelet and anticoagulant therapy after the placement of coronary-artery stents. N Engl J Med 334:1084–1089, 1996.

110. Schomig A, Neumann F-J, Walter H, et al. Coronary stent placement in patients with acute myocardial infarction: Comparison of clinical and angiographic outcome after randomization to antiplatelet or anticoagulant therapy. J Am Coll Cardiol 29:28–34, 1997.

111. Monassier JP, Elias J, Meyer P, et al: STENTIM I: The French registry of stenting in acute myocardial infarction. J Am Coll Cardiol 27:68A, 1996.

112. Leon MB, Baim DS, Popma JJ, et al: A clinical trial comparing three antithrombotic-drug regimens after coronary-artery stenting. Stent Anticoagulation Restenosis Study. N Engl J Med 339:1665–1671, 1998.

113. Gent M, Blakely JA, Easton JD, et al: The Canadian American Ticlopidine Study (CATS) in thromboembolic stroke. Lancet 1:1215–1220, 1989.

114. Hass WK, Easton JD, Adams HP Jr, et al: A randomized trial comparing ticlopidine hydrochloride with aspirin for the prevention of stroke in high-risk patients. Ticlopidine Aspirin Stroke Study Group. N Engl J Med 321:501–507, 1989.

115. Haynes RB, Sandler RS, Larson EB, et al: A critical appraisal of ticlopidine, a new antiplatelet agent. Effectiveness and clinical indications for prophylaxis of atherosclerotic events. Arch Intern Med 152:1376–1380, 1992.

116. Szto G, Lewis S, Punamiya S, et el: Incidence of neutro-

penia/fatal thrombocytopenia associated with one month of ticlopidine therapy post coronary stenting. J Am Coll Cardiol 29:343A, 1997.

117. Russo RJ, Stevens KM, Norman SL, et al: Ticlopidine administration after stent placement: Frequency of adverse reactions. J Am Coll Cardiol 29:353A, 1997.

118. CAPRIE Steering Committee: A randomised, blinded, trial of clopidogrel versus aspirin in patients at risk of ischaemic events (CAPRIE). Lancet 348:1329–1339, 1996.

119. Bertrand ME: The CLASSICS trial. American College of Cardiology, 48th Annual Scientific Session, March 7–10, 1999.

120. L'Allier PL, Aronow HD, Yadav JS, et al: Is clopidogrel a safe and effective adjunctive anti-platelet therapy for coronary stenting? J Am Coll Cardiol 33(suppl A):40A, 1999.

121. Berger PB, Bellot V, Melby S, et al: Clopidogrel versus ticlopidine for coronary stents. J Am Coll Cardiol 33(suppl A):34A, 1999.

122. Mishkel GJ, Lucore CL, Ligon RW, et al: Clopidogrel for the prevention of stent thrombosis. J Am Coll Cardiol 33(suppl A):34A, 1999.

123. Jauhar R, Savino S, Deutsch E, et al: Aspirin and clopidogrel combination therapy in coronary stenting: A prospective registry. Am J Cardiol 82(suppl 7A):96S, 1998.

124. Teruya JL, Hart LL: Dipyridamole in angioplasty [published erratum appears in DICP 25:1274, 1991]. DICP 25:747–749, 1991.

125. Swanson KT: Dogs, dextran, and dilatation: A story of empiricism run wild [Editorial]. Cathet Cardiovasc Diagn 32:203–205, 1994.

126. Coller BS: Blockade of platelet GPIIb/IIIa receptors as an antithrombotic strategy. Circulation 92:2373–2380, 1995.

127. Coller BS: A new murine monoclonal antibody reports an activation-dependent change in the conformation and/or microenvironment of the platelet glycoprotein IIb/IIIa complex. J Clin Invest 76:101–108, 1985.

128. Gold HK, Gimple LW, Yasuda T, et al: Pharmacodynamic study of F(ab')2 fragments of murine monoclonal antibody 7E3 directed against human platelet glycoprotein IIb/IIIa in patients with unstable angina pectoris. J Clin Invest 86:651–659, 1990.

129. Kleiman NS, Ohman EM, Califf RM, et al: Profound inhibition of platelet aggregation with monoclonal antibody 7E3 Fab after thrombolytic therapy. Results of the Thrombolysis and Angioplasty in Myocardial Infarction (TAMI) 8 Pilot Study. J Am Coll Cardiol 22:381–389, 1998.

130. The EPIC Investigators: Use of a monoclonal antibody directed against the platelet glycoprotein IIb/IIIa receptor in high-risk coronary angioplasty. The EPIC Investigation. N Engl J Med 330:956–961, 1994.

131. Topol EJ, Califf RM, Weisman HF, et al: Randomised trial of coronary intervention with antibody against platelet IIb/IIIa integrin for reduction of clinical restenosis: Results at six months. The EPIC Investigators. Lancet 343:881–886, 1994.

132. Aguirre FV, Topol EJ, Ferguson JJ, et al: Bleeding complications with the chimeric antibody to platelet glycoprotein IIb/IIIa integrin in patients undergoing percutaneous coronary intervention. EPIC Investigators. Circulation 91:2882–2890, 1995.

133. The EPILOG Investigators: Platelet glycoprotein IIb/IIIa receptor blockade and low-dose heparin during percutaneous coronary revascularization. N Engl J Med 336:1689–1696, 1997.

134. The CAPTURE Investigators: Randomised placebo-controlled trial of abciximab before and during coronary intervention in refractory unstable angina: The CAPTURE Study. Lancet 349:1429–1435, 1997.

135. Tcheng JE, Lincoff AM, Miller DP, et al: Benefits of abciximab accrue in the full spectrum of coronary interventional patients: Insights from the EPILOG trial. J Am Coll Cardiol 29:276A, 1997.

136. Ellis SG, Lincoff AM, Miller D, et al: Reduction in complications of angioplasty with abciximab occurs largely independently of baseline lesion morphology. EPIC and EPILOG Investigators. Evaluation of 7E3 for the Prevention of Ische-

mic Complications. Evaluation of PTCA to Improve Long-term Outcome with abciximab GPIIb/IIIa Receptor Blockade. J Am Coll Cardiol 1998; 32:1619–1623, 1998.

137. Tcheng JE, Anderson K, Tardiff BE, et al: Reducing the risk of percutaneous intervention after coronary bypass surgery: Beneficial effects of abciximab treatment. J Am Coll Cardiol 29:187A, 1997.

138. Mark DB, Talley J, Topol EJ, et al: Economic assessment of platelet glycoprotein IIb/IIIa inhibition for prevention of ischemic complications of high risk coronary angioplasty. Circulation 94:629–635, 1996.

139. Goklaney AK, Murphy JD, Hillegass WB Jr: Abciximab therapy in percutaneous intervention: Economic issues in the United States. Am Heart J 135:S90–S97, 1998.

140. Lincoff AM, Mark DB, Califf RM, et al: Economic assessment of platelet glycoprotein IIb/IIIa receptor blockade during coronary intervention in the EPILOG trial. J Am Coll Cardiol 29:240A, 1997.

141. Deckers J, Califf RM, Topol EJ, et al: Use of abciximab (ReoPro) is not associated with an increase in the risk of stroke: Overview of three randomized trials. J Am Coll Cardiol 29:241A, 1997.

142. The EPISTENT Investigators: Randomised placebo-controlled and balloon-angioplasty-controlled trial to assess safety of coronary stenting with use of platelet glycoprotein-IIb/IIIa blockade. Evaluation of Platelet IIb/IIIa Inhibitor for Stenting. Lancet 352:87–92, 1998.

143. Scarborough RM, Naughton MA, Teng W, et al: Design of potent and specific integrin antagonists. Peptide antagonists with high specificity for glycoprotein IIb-IIIa. J Biol Chem 268:1066–1173, 1993.

144. The IMPACT II Investigators: Randomised placebo-controlled trial of effect of eptifibatide on complications of percutaneous coronary intervention: IMPACT-II. Integrilin to Minimise Platelet Aggregation and Coronary Thrombosis-II. Lancet 349:1422–1428, 1997.

145. Phillips DR, Teng W, Arfsten A, et al: Effect of Ca2+ on GP IIb-IIIa interactions with Integrilin: Enhanced GP IIb-IIIa binding and inhibition of platelet aggregation by reductions in the concentration of ionized calcium in plasma anticoagulated with citrate. Circulation 96:1488–1494, 1997.

146. Egbertson MS, Chang CT, Duggan ME, et al: Non-peptide fibrinogen receptor antagonists. 2. Optimization of a tyrosine template as a mimic for Arg-Gly-Asp. J Med Chem 37:2537–2551, 1994.

147. Gibson CM, Goel M, Cohen DJ, et al: Six-month angiographic and clinical follow-up of patients prospectively randomized to receive either tirofiban or placebo during angioplasty in the RESTORE trial. Randomized Efficacy Study of Tirofiban for Outcomes and Restenosis. J Am Coll Cardiol 32:28–34, 1998.

148. The RESTORE Investigators: Effects of platelet glycoprotein IIb/IIIa blockade with tirofiban on adverse cardiac events in patients with unstable angina or acute myocardial infarction undergoing coronary angioplasty. Randomized Efficacy Study of Tirofiban for Outcomes and REstenosis. Circulation, 96:1445–1453, 1997.

149. Kouns WC, Kirchhofer D, Hadvary P, et al: Reversible conformational changes induced in glycoprotein IIb-IIIa by a potent and selective peptidomimetic inhibitor. Blood 80:2539–2547, 1992.

150. Theroux P, Kouz S, Roy L, et al: Platelet membrane receptor glycoprotein IIb/IIIa antagonism in unstable angina. The Canadian Lamifiban Study. Circulation 94:899–905, 1996.

151. The PARAGON Investigators: International, randomized, controlled trial of lamifiban (a platelet glycoprotein IIb/IIIa inhibitor), heparin, or both in unstable angina. Platelet IIb/IIIa Antagonism for the Reduction of Acute coronary syndrome events in a Global Organization Network. Circulation 97:2386–2395, 1998.

152. Miletich JP, Jackson CM, Majerus PW: Interaction of coagulation factor Xa with human platelets. Proc Natl Acad Sci U S A 74:4033–4036, 1977.

153. Walsh PN, Schmaier AH: Platelet-coagulant protein interactions. *In* Colman RW, Hirsh J, Marder VJ, et al (eds): Hemo-

stasis and Thrombosis: Basic Principles and Clinical Practice, pp 629–651. Philadelphia. JB Lippincott, 1994.

154. Hirsh J: Heparin: N Engl J Med 324:1565–1574, 1991.

155. Rosenberg RD, Damus PS: The purification and mechanism of action of human antithrombin-heparin cofactor. J Biol Chem 248:6490–6505, 1973.

156. Rosenberg RD, Lam L: Correlation between structure and function of heparin. Proc Natl Acad Sci U S A 76:1218–1222, 1979.

157. Casu B, Oreste P, Torri G, et al. The structure of heparin oligosaccharide fragments with high anti-(factor Xa) activity containing the minimal antithrombin III–binding sequence. Chemical and 13C nuclear-magnetic-resonance studies. Biochem J 197:599–609, 1981.

158. Ofosu FA, Sie P, Modi GJ, et al: The inhibition of thrombin-dependent positive-feedback reactions is critical to the expression of the anticoagulant effect of heparin. Biochem J 243:579–588, 1987.

159. Ofosu FA, Gray E: Mechanisms of action of heparin: Applications to the development of derivatives of heparin and heparinoids with antithrombotic properties. Semin Thromb Hemost 14:9–17, 1988.

160. Hogg PJ, Jackson CM: Fibrin monomer protects thrombin from inactivation by heparin–antithrombin III: Implications for heparin efficacy. Proc Natl Acad Sci U S A 86:3619–3623, 1989.

161. Raschke RA, Reill BM, Guidry JR, et al: The weight-based heparin dosing nomogram compared with a "standard care" nomogram. A randomized controlled trial. Ann Intern Med 119:874–881, 1993.

162. Hull RD, Raskob GE, Rosenbloom D, et al: Optimal therapeutic level of heparin therapy in patients with venous thrombosis. Arch Intern Med 152:1589–1595, 1992.

163. Warkentin TE, Levine MN, Hirsh J, et al: Heparin-induced thrombocytopenia in patients treated with low-molecular-weight heparin or unfractionated heparin. N Engl J Med 332:1330–1335, 1995.

164. McGarry TF Jr, Gottlieb RS, Morganroth J, et al: The relationship of anticoagulation level and complications after successful percutaneous transluminal coronary angioplasty. Am Heart J 123:1445–1451, 1992.

165. Dougherty KG, Marsh KC, Edelman SK, et al: Relationship between procedural activated clotting time and in-hospital post-PTCA outcome. Circulation 82:189–III, 1990.

166. Ogilby JD, Kopelman HA, Klein LW, et al: Adequate heparinization during PTCA: Assessment using activated clotting times. Cathet Cardiovasc Diagn 18:206–209, 1989.

167. Ferguson JJ, Dougherty KG, Gaos CM, et al: Relation between procedural activated coagulation time and outcome after percutaneous transluminal coronary angioplasty. J Am Coll Cardiol 23:1061–1065, 1994.

168. Narins CR, Hillegass WB Jr, Nelson CL, et al: Relation between activated clotting time during angioplasty and abrupt closure. Circulation 93:667–671, 1996.

169. Satler LF, Leon MB, Kent KM, et al: Strategies for acute occlusion after coronary angioplasty [Editorial; Comment]. J Am Coll Cardiol 19:936–938, 1992.

170. Popma JJ, Coller BS, Ohman EM, et al: Antithrombotic therapy in patients undergoing coronary angioplasty. Chest 108:486S–501S, 1995.

171. Avendano A, Ferguson JJ: Comparison of Hemochron and HemoTec activated coagulation time target values during percutaneous transluminal coronary angioplasty. J Am Coll Cardiol 23:907–910, 1994.

172. Gangasani SR, Dmuchowski C, Grines CL: Is there a role for IV heparin in unstable angina patients prior to PTCA? J Am Coll Cardiol 29:410A, 1997.

173. Hirsh J, Levine MN: Low molecular weight heparin. Blood 79:1–17, 1992.

174. Wolf H: Low-molecular-weight heparin. Med Clin North Am 78:733–743, 1994

175. Zidar JP: Low-molecular-weight heparins in coronary stenting (the ENTICES trial): ENoxaparin and TIClopidine after Elective Stenting. Am J Cardiol 82:29L, 1998.

176. Pan M, Suarez de Lezo J, Velasco F, et al: Reduction of

thrombotic and hemorrhagic complications after stent implantation. Am Heart J 132:1119–1126, 1996.

177. Magnani HN: Heparin-induced thrombocytopenia (HIT): An overview of 230 patients treated with Orgaran (Org 10172) [published erratum appears in Thromb Haemost 70:1072, 1993]. Thromb Haemost 70:554–561, 1993.

178. Weitz J, Hirsh J: New anticoagulant strategies. J Lab Clin Med 122:364–373, 1993.

179. Lefkovits J, Topol EJ: Direct thrombin inhibitors in cardiovascular medicine. Circulation 90:1522–1536, 1994.

180. Muller TH, Binder K, Guth BD: Pharmacology of current and future antithrombotic therapies. Cardiol Clin 12:411–442, 1994.

181. Adams SL: The medicinal leech: Historical perspectives. Semin Thromb Hemost 15:261–264, 1989.

182. Harvey RP, Degryse E, Stefani L, et al: Cloning and expression of a cDNA coding for the anticoagulant hirudin from the bloodsucking leech, Hirudo medicinalis. Proc Natl Acad Sci U S A 83:1084–1088.

183. Serruys PW, Herrman JP, Simon R, et al: A comparison of hirudin with heparin in the prevention of restenosis after coronary angioplasty. Helvetica Investigators. N Engl J Med:333:757–763, 1995.

184. Maraganore JM, Bourdon P, Jablonski J, et al: Design and characterization of hirulogs: A novel class of bivalent peptide inhibitors of thrombin. Biochemistry 29:7095–9101, 1990.

185. Bittl JA, Strony J, Brinker JA, et al: Treatment with bivalirudin (Hirulog) as compared with heparin during coronary angioplasty for unstable or postinfarction angina. Hirulog Angioplasty Study Investigators. N Engl J Med 333:764–769.

186. Kelly AB, Maraganore JM, Bourdon P, et al: Antithrombotic effects of synthetic peptides targeting various functional domains of thrombin. Proc Natl Acad Sci U S A 89:6040–6044.

187. Gold HK, Torres FW, Garabedian HD, et al: Evidence for a rebound coagulation phenomenon after cessation of a 4-hour infusion of a specific thrombin inhibitor in patients with unstable angina pectoris. J Am Coll Cardiol 21:1039–1047, 1993.

188. O'Reilly RA: Anticoagulant, antithrombotic, and thrombolytic drugs. In Gilman AG, Goodman LS, et al (eds): The Pharmacologic Basis of Therapeutics, pp 1338–1359. New York: Macmillan, 1985.

189. Weiss ME, Adkinson NF Jr: Allergy to protamine. Clin Rev Allergy 9:339–355, 1991.

190. Weiss ME, Nyhan D, Peng ZK, et al: Association of protamine IgE and IgG antibodies with life-threatening reactions to intravenous protamine. N Engl J Med 320:886–892, 1989.

191. Stewart WJ, McSweeney SM, Kellett MA, et al: Increased risk of severe protamine reactions in NPH insulin-dependent diabetics undergoing cardiac catheterization. Circulation 70:788–792, 1984.

192. Albiero R, Hall P, Itoh A, et al: Results of a consecutive series of patients receiving only antiplatelet therapy after optimized stent implantation. Comparison of aspirin alone versus combined ticlopidine and aspirin therapy. Circulation 95:1145–1156, 1997.

193. Karrillon GJ, Morice MC, Benveniste E, et al: Intracoronary stent implantation without ultrasound guidance and with replacement of conventional anticoagulation by antiplatelet therapy. 30-day clinical outcome of the French Multicenter Registry. Circulation 94:1519–1527.

194. Morice MC, Zemour G, Benveniste E, et al: Intracoronary stenting without Coumadin: One month results of a French multicenter study. Cathet Cardiovasc Diagn 35:1–7, 1995.

195. Morice MC, Breton C, Bunouf P, et al: Coronary stenting without anticoagulant, without intravascular ultrasound: Results of the French registry. Circulation 92(suppl I):I-796, 1995.

196. Russo RJ, Schatz RA, Sklar MA, et al: Ultrasound guided coronary stent placement without prolonged systemic anticoagulation. J Am Coll Cardiol 25:50A, 1995.

197. Lablance J-M, Bonnett J-L, Grollier G, et al: Combined antiplatelet therapy without anticoagulation after stent implan-

tation: The Ticlopidine Aspirin Stent Evaluation (TASTE) Study. J Am Coll Cardiol 27:137A, 1996.

198. Cohen DJ, Krumholz HM, Sukin CA, et al: In-hospital and one-year economic outcomes after coronary stenting or balloon angioplasty: Results from a randomized clinical trial. 92:2480–2487, 1995.

199. Goods CM, Liu MW, Iyer SS, et al: A cost analysis of coronary stenting without anticoagulation versus stenting with anticoagulation using warfarin. Am J Cardiol 78:334–336, 1996.

200. Anderson HV, Willerson JT: Thrombolysis in acute myocardial infarction. N Engl J Med 329:703–709, 1993.

201. Fibrinolytic Therapy Trialists' (FTT) Collaborative Group: Indications for fibrinolytic therapy in suspected acute myocardial infarction: Collaborative overview of early mortality and major morbidity results from all randomised trials of more than 1000 patients. 343:311–322, 1994.

202. Krone RJ, Friedman E, Thanavaro S, et al: Long-term prognosis after first Q-wave (transmural) or non-Q-wave (nontransmural) myocardial infarction: Analysis of 593 patients. Am J Cardiol 52:234–239, 1983.

203. Willems JL, Willems RJ, Willems GM, et al: Significance of initial ST segment elevation and depression for the management of thrombolytic therapy in acute myocardial infarction. European Cooperative Study Group for Recombinant Tissue-Type Plasminogen Activator. Circulation 82:1147–1158, 1990.

204. Gruppo Italiano per lo Studio della Streptochinasi nell'Infarto Miocardico (GISSI): Effectiveness of intravenous thrombolytic treatment in acute myocardial infarction. Lancet 1:397–401, 1986.

205. Mooney MR, Mooney JF, Goldenberg IF, et al: Percutaneous transluminal coronary angioplasty in the setting of large intracoronary thrombi. Am J Cardiol 65:427–431, 1990.

206. Deligonul U, Gabliani GI, Caralis DG, et al: Percutaneous transluminal coronary angioplasty in patients with intracoronary thrombus. Am J Cardiol 62:474–476, 1988.

207. Tenaglia AN, Fortin DF, Califf RM, et al: Predicting the risk of abrupt vessel closure after angioplasty in an individual patient. J Am Coll Cardiol 24:1004–1011, 1994.

208. Tan K, Sulke N, Taub N, et al: Clinical and lesion morphologic determination of coronary angioplasty success and complications: Current experience. J Am Coll Cardiol 25:855–865, 1995.

209. Schieman G, Cohen BM, Kozina J, et al: Intracoronary urokinase for intracoronary thrombus accumulation complicating percutaneous transluminal coronary angioplasty in acute ischemic syndromes. 82:2052–2060, 1990.

210. Chapekis AT, George BS, Candela RJ: Rapid thrombus dissolution by continuous infusion of urokinase through an intracoronary perfusion wire prior to and following PTCA: Results in native coronaries and patent saphenous vein grafts. Cathet Cardiovasc Diagn 23:89–92, 1991.

211. Vaitkus PT, Laskey WK: Efficacy of adjunctive thrombolytic therapy in percutaneous transluminal coronary angioplasty. J Am Coll Cardiol 24:1415–1423, 1994.

212. Suryapranata H, de Feyter PJ, Serruys PW. Coronary angioplasty in patients with unstable angina pectoris: Is there a role for thrombolysis? J Am Coll Cardiol 12:69A–77A, 1988.

213. Verna E, Repetto S, Boscarini M, et al: Management of complicated coronary angioplasty by intracoronary urokinase and immediate re-angioplasty. Cathet Cardiovasc Diagn 19:116–122, 1990.

214. The TIMI IIIA Investigators: Early effects of tissue-type plasminogen activator added to conventional therapy on the culprit lesion in patients presenting with ischemic cardiac pain at rest: Results of the Thrombolysis in Myocardial Ischemia (TIMI III) trial. Circulation 87:38–52, 1993.

215. O'Neill WW, Weintraub R, Grines CL, et al: A prospective, placebo-controlled, randomized trial of intravenous streptokinase and angioplasty versus lone angioplasty therapy of acute myocardial infarction. Circulation 86:1710–1717, 1992.

216. Williams DO, Holubkov AL, Detre KM, et al: Impact of pretreatment by thrombolytic therapy upon outcome of

emergent direct coronary angioplasty for patients with acute myocardial infarction. J Am Coll Cardiol: 17:337A, 1991.

217. Beauchamp GD, Vacek JL, Robuck W: Management comparison for acute myocardial infarction: Direct angioplasty versus sequential thrombolysis-angioplasty. Am Heart J 120:237–242, 1990.

218. Ambrose JA, Almeida OD, Sharma SK, et al: Adjunctive thrombolytic therapy during angioplasty for ischemic rest angina. Results of the TAUSA Trial. TAUSA Investigators. Thrombolysis and Angioplasty in Unstable Angina trial. Circulation 90:69–77, 1994.

219. Van den Brand M, van Zijl A, Geuskens R, et al: Tissue plasminogen activator in refractory unstable angina. A randomized double-blind placebo-controlled trial in patients with refractory unstable angina and subsequent angioplasty. Eur Heart J 12:1208–1214, 1991.

220. Ambrose JA, Torre SR, Sharma SK, et al: Adjunctive thrombolytic therapy for angioplasty in ischemic rest angina: Results of a double-blind randomized pilot study. J Am Coll Cardiol 20:1197–1204, 1992.

221. Pavlides GS, Schreiber TL, Gangadharan V, et al: Safety and efficacy of urokinase during elective coronary angioplasty. Am Heart J 121:731–737, 1991.

222. Topol EJ, Nicklas JM, Kander NH, et al: Coronary revascularization after intravenous tissue plasminogen activator for unstable angina pectoris: Results of a randomized, double-blind, placebo-controlled trial. Am J Cardiol 62:368–371, 1988.

223. Haine E, Urban P, Verine V, et al: Lack of immediate benefit of urokinase prior to angioplasty for unstable angina: A double-blind randomized study. J Am Coll Cardiol 21:435A, 1993.

224. Bar FW, Verheugt FW, Col J, et al: Thrombolysis in patients with unstable angina improves the angiographic but not the clinical outcome: Results of UNASEM, a multicenter, randomized, placebo-controlled, clinical trial with anistreplase. Circulation 86:131–137, 1992.

225. The TIMI IIIB Investigators: Effects of tissue plasminogen activator and a comparison of early invasive and conservative strategies in unstable angina and non-Q-wave myocardial infarction: Results of the TIMI IIIB trial. Circulation 89:1545–1556, 1994.

226. Schreiber TL, Rizik D, White C, et al: Randomized trial of thrombolysis versus heparin in unstable angina. Circulation 86:1407–1414, 1992.

227. Freeman MR, Langer A, Wilson RF, et al: Thrombolysis in unstable angina. Randomized double-blind trial of t-PA and placebo. Circulation 85:150–157, 1992.

228. Zeiher AM, Kasper W, Gaissmaier C, et al: Concomitant intracoronary treatment with urokinase during PTCA does not reduce acute complications during PTCA: A double-blind randomized study. Circulation 82 (suppl III):III–189, 1990.

229. Spielberg C, Schnitzer L, Linderer T, et al: Influence of catheter technology and adjuvant medication on acute complications in percutaneous coronary angioplasty. Cathet Cardiovasc Diagn 21:72–76, 1990.

230. Mehan VK, Meier B, Urban P: Influence on early outcome and restenosis of urokinase before elective coronary angioplasty. Am J Cardiol 72:106–108, 1993.

231. Puma JA, Sketch MH Jr, Tcheng JE, et al: Percutaneous revascularization of chronic coronary occlusions: An overview. J Am Coll Cardiol 26:1–11, 1995.

232. Cecena FA: Urokinase infusion after unsuccessful angioplasty in patients with chronic total occlusion of native coronary arteries. Cathet Cardiovasc Diagn 28:214–218, 1993.

233. Grines CL, Ajluni S, Savas V, et al: Prolonged urokinase infusion for chronic total native coronary occlusions. J Am Coll Cardiol 19:33A, 1992.

234. Zidar F, Schreiber T, Jones D, et al: A prospective trial of prolonged urokinase infusion for chronic total occlusion (CTO) in native coronary arteries. Circulation 88:I–505, 1993.

235. Zidar FJ, Kaplan BM, O'Neill WW, et al: Prospective, randomized trial of prolonged intracoronary urokinase infusion

for chronic total occlusions in native coronary arteries. J Am Coll Cardiol 27:1406–1412, 1996.

236. Hartmann JR, McKeever LS, Stamato NJ, et al: Recanalization of chronically occluded aortocoronary saphenous vein bypass grafts by extended infusion of urokinase: Initial results and short-term clinical follow-up. J Am Coll Cardiol 18:1517–1523, 1991.

237. Gurley JC, MacPhail BS: Acute myocardial infarction due to thrombolytic reperfusion of chronically occluded saphenous vein coronary bypass grafts. Am J Cardiol 68:274–275, 1991.

238. Andersen RL, Kemp HG Jr: A complication of prolonged urokinase infusion into a chronically occluded aortocoronary saphenous vein graft. Cathet Cardiovasc Diagn 18:20–22, 1989.

239. Doorey AJ, Rosenbloom MA, Zolnick MR: Successful angioplasty of a chronically occluded saphenous vein graft using a prolonged urokinase infusion from the brachial route. Cathet Cardiovasc Diagn 23:127–129, 1991.

240. Marx M, Armstrong WP, Wack JP, et al: Short-duration, high-dose urokinase infusion for recanalization of occluded saphenous aortocoronary bypass grafts. AJR 153:167–171, 1989.

241. Blankenship JC, Modesto TA, Madigan NP: Acute myocardial infarction complicating urokinase infusion for total saphenous vein graft occlusion. Cathet Cardiovasc Diagn 28:39–43, 1993.

242. Hartmann JR, McKeever LS, Enger EL, et al: Recanalization of chronically occluded bypass grafts with prolonged urokinase infusion site trial. Circulation 88(suppl I):I–504, 1993.

243. Hartmann JR, McKeever LS, O'Neill WW, et al: Recanalization of Chronically Occluded Aortocoronary Saphenous Vein Bypass Grafts With Long-Term, Low Dose Direct Infusion of Urokinase (ROBUST): A serial trial. J Am Coll Cardiol 27:60–66, 1996.

244. Waller BF, Rothbaum DA, Pinkerton CA: Status of the myocardium and infarct-related coronary artery in 19 necropsy patients with acute recanalization using pharmacologic (streptokinase, r-tissue plasminogen activator), mechanical (percutaneous transluminal coronary angioplasty) or combined types of reperfusion therapy. J Am Coll Cardiol 9:785–801, 1987.

245. Fitzgerald DJ, Wright F, FitzGerald GA: Increased thromboxane biosynthesis during coronary thrombolysis. Evidence that platelet activation and thromboxane A2 modulate the response to tissue-type plasminogen activator in vivo. Circ Res 65:83–94, 1989.

246. Rasmanis G, Vesterqvist O, Green K, et al: Evidence of increased platelet activation after thrombolysis in patients with acute myocardial infarction. Br Heart J 68:374–376, 1992.

247. Kerins DM, Roy L, FitzGerald GA, et al: Platelet and vascular function during coronary thrombolysis with tissue-type plasminogen activator. Circulation 80:1718–1725, 1989.

248. Bennett WR, Yawn DH, Migliore PJ, et al: Activation of the complement system by recombinant tissue plasminogen activator. J Am Coll Cardiol 10:627–632, 1987.

249. Fitzgerald DJ, Roy L, Wright F, et al: Functional significance of platelet activation following coronary thrombolysis. Circulation 76(suppl IV):IV-153, 1987.

250. Fischell TA: Coronary artery spasm after percutaneous transluminal coronary angioplasty: Pathophysiology and clinical consequences. Cathet Cardiovasc Diagn 19:1–3, 1990.

251. Fischell TA, Derby G, Tse TM, et al: Coronary artery vasoconstriction routinely occurs after percutaneous transluminal coronary angioplasty. A quantitative arteriographic analysis. Circulation 78:1323–1334, 1988.

252. Abbo KM, Dooris M, Glazier S, et al: Features and outcome of no-reflow after percutaneous coronary intervention. Am J Cardiol 75:778–782, 1995.

253. Winbury MM, Howe BB, Hefner MA: Effect of nitrates and other coronary dilators on large and small coronary vessels: An hypothesis for the mechanism of action of nitrates. J Pharmacol Exp Ther 168:70–95, 1969.

254. Sellke FW, Myers PR, Bates JN, et al: Influence of vessel size on the sensitivity of porcine coronary microvessels to nitroglycerin. Am J Physiol 258:H515–H520, 1990.

255. Piana RN, Paik GY, Moscucci M, et al: Incidence and treatment of "no-reflow" after percutaneous coronary intervention. Circulation 89:2514–2518, 1994.

256. Weyrens FJ, Mooney J, Lesser J, et al: Intracoronary diltiazem for microvascular spasm after interventional therapy. Am J Cardiol 75:849–850, 1995.

257. Cohen BM, Weber VJ, Blum RR, et al: Cocktail attenuation of rotational ablation flow effects (CARAFE) study: Pilot. Cathet Cardiovasc Diagn (suppl 3):69–72, 1996.

258. Fischman DL, Leon MB, Baim DS, et al: A randomized comparison of coronary-stent placement and balloon angioplasty in the treatment of coronary artery disease. Stent Restenosis Study Investigators. N Engl J Med 331:496–501, 1994.

259. Serruys PW, de Jaegere P, Kiemeneij F, et al: A comparison of balloon-expandable-stent implantation with balloon angioplasty in patients with coronary artery disease. Benestent Study Group. N Engl J Med 331:489–495, 331.

# 28

# Acute Closure, Dissection, and Perforation

*David F. Kong    James P. Zidar*

## ACUTE CLOSURE AND DISSECTION

Coronary angioplasty[1] forms the mainstay of interventional therapy, addressing more complex atherosclerotic lesions in a broader patient population than did earlier modalities. The rate of primary success with percutaneous transluminal coronary angioplasty (PTCA) approaches 90%.[2, 3] Although operator experience and equipment continually improve, major dissection, abrupt closure, and arterial perforation remain the primary reasons for failure of angioplasty procedures.[4–9] The following discussion reviews the incidence, recognition, predictors, and treatment of these adverse events. New diagnostic technologies have advanced the understanding of angioplasty mechanisms and extended postintervention assessment of vessels. Ultrasonography and angioscopy now supplement angiographic evaluation of procedural success and complications. A plethora of devices, drugs, and techniques are used in an attempt to reduce or control vascular injury during or after PTCA. Acute closure continues to limit the effectiveness both of newer interventions and of coronary angioplasty. Great enthusiasm surrounds intracoronary stent placement, which has become a successful means of averting closure by "tacking open" dissection flaps. The complication of acute stent thrombosis engenders continuing interest in combination approaches to preserving vessel patency. Although equipment and techniques continue to be refined, there will never be a singular solution to the vexing and persistent curse of acute closure. Rather, efficient management algorithms must identify appropriate interventional actions for individual patients.

## Clinical Significance

The reported incidence of abrupt closure has traditionally ranged between 2% and 14%, depending on investigators' definitions.[2–6, 8–23] For a series of patients studied between 1985 and 1993,[8, 9, 18, 23–25] the closure rate averaged 8.6%. Operator experience and technical improvements have not dramatically decreased the incidence of acute closure.[16, 26] This lack of decrease has been attributed to an increased proportion of patients with complex lesions and acute ischemic syndromes that are associated with a higher likelihood of acute occlusion.[8, 11, 27] Balloon angioplasty has been increasingly applied to patients with multivessel disease, prior bypass surgery, multiple prior PTCA procedures, and diminished ventricular function.[28] For elderly patients with complex coronary anatomy, poor ventricular function, and comorbid disease, the abrupt closure rate may exceed 5%.[29–31] The success of primary infarct angioplasty is limited by an acute reclosure rate approaching 10% of vessels treated.[32]

Abrupt closure is associated with prolonged inpatient stay[26] and major complications, including acute infarction (33% to 40% of patients), need for emergency bypass surgery (23% to 77%), and death (2% to 8%).[6, 8, 9, 13, 16, 26–28, 33] The limited success of nonoperative closure management in early cohorts[8, 9, 13, 23, 34] led to the requirement for immediate surgical backup for angioplasty.[16] Evolving operator experience may account for better reperfusion rates after acute occlusion in later trials[25, 26] with a concurrent reduction in morbidity.

Nonocclusive dissections significantly influence immediate angioplasty outcomes, but their contribution to late restenosis is controversial. Histopathologic studies have associated deep arterial injury with a pronounced neointimal response.[35] In several clinical studies, researchers have examined the relationship between angiographically visible dissections and restenosis. Many found no difference, whereas others have reported a lower incidence of restenosis.[36–38] Hermans and colleagues[39] prospectively monitored patients without obstructive dissections after successful angioplasty. Angiographic follow-up at 6 months was available in 94% of patients. There was no difference in the restenosis rate (29% to 30%) between patient groups with and

**TABLE 28-1.   MORPHOLOGIC CLASSIFICATION OF CORONARY ARTERY DISSECTION**

| TYPE | CLASSIFICATION |
|------|----------------|
| A | Radiolucent areas within the lumen during contrast injection with minimal or no persistent contrast staining after clearance |
| B | Parallel tracts or double lumen separated by radiolucent area during injection with minimal or no persistent contrast staining |
| C | Contrast appearance outside the lumen with persistent contrast staining after clearance of the dye injection |
| D | Spiral luminal filling defects frequently with extensive contrast staining of the coronary artery |
| E | New persistent intraluminal filling defects |
| F | Dissection leading to total occlusion without distal antegrade flow |

Data from Manual of Operations of the NHLBI PTCA Registry 1985 (see ref 130).

without minor dissections. Furthermore, no difference in mortality, infarction, or revascularization rates was detected between the two groups.

## Angiographic Definitions

Many studies have employed clinical and angiographic definitions for abrupt closure and the causative events. The efforts of different investigators to identify patient populations and track interventional outcomes produce sizable variability in these definitions. Classification schemes based on angiographic observations have enabled investigators to associate dissection and closure with adverse events and have allowed comparison between clinical trials. Although the more recent studies have employed newer technologic methods to evaluate the effect of interventions on coronary morphology, angiographic and clinical definitions continue to be essential diagnostic tools for retrospective review and clinical practice.

### Dissection

The modified National Heart, Lung, and Blood Institute (NHLBI) criteria defined dissection as angiographically detectable intimal or medial damage manifesting as a radiolucent area within the vessel or as an extravasation of contrast medium after an interventional procedure.[11, 26] These criteria were refined into a more detailed classification system (Table 28–1). Because dissections may be angiographically apparent after 45% of angioplasty cases, investigators have attempted to distinguish therapeutic minor dissections from detrimental major ones. Major dissections are characterized by numerous morphologic features, including (1) a linear intraluminal filling defect or luminal staining evident in two projections[4] (Fig. 28–1); (2) a linear filling defect extending for greater than one balloon length (20 mm)[40]; and (3) dissection types C to F according to NHLBI criteria.[41] Clinically oriented definitions assert that major dissections produce acute closure or myocardial infarction (MI), necessitate bypass surgery, or cause termination of a procedure before its scheduled completion. Although functional, these definitions only retrospectively recognize major dissections. A more useful definition, applicable during a procedure, integrates morphology and function: Major dissections create intraluminal fill-

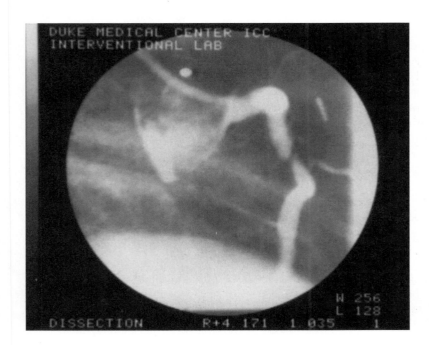

FIGURE 28–1. Angiogram of major transverse dissection of the proximal right coronary artery with intraluminal filling defect.

ing defects of sufficient size to produce a reduction in luminal diameter of at least 50% and/or a reduction in distal coronary flow.[42]

### Thrombosis

Intracoronary thrombus is angiographically defined as (1) an intraluminal filling defect surrounded by contrast material, as seen in multiple projections; (2) absence of calcium within the defect; (3) persistence of contrast material within the lumen; and (4) in the case of total thrombotic occlusion, abrupt vessel cutoff with convex, irregular margins and persistence of luminal contrast material.[43–45] Many studies evaluating therapy for intracoronary thrombus have employed angiographic inclusion criteria. Angiographic studies have attributed 19% to 33% of acute occlusions[16] to intracoronary thrombus formation.

### Acute (Abrupt) Closure

Abrupt vessel closure has been defined as total vessel occlusion during or after a coronary intervention (e.g., PTCA, directional coronary atherectomy, laser, or stent placement). Some authors described abrupt closure as an angioplasty site with absent (Thrombolysis In Myocardial Infarction [TIMI]–0) or critically reduced (TIMI-1 or TIMI-2) coronary blood flow in a previously patent (TIMI-2 or TIMI-3) coronary vessel segment,[23, 45–48] with clinical or electrocardiographic (ECG) evidence of myocardial ischemia.[16, 25, 26] The recurrence of angina previously experienced during PTCA has been a reliable indicator of abrupt coronary artery occlusion. Specific electrocardiographic changes consistent with the ECG during balloon inflation have often confirmed the diagnosis. Unfortunately, nonspecific ECG changes may develop in up to 20% of patients with acute closure.[49]

Some authors limited their definition of abrupt closure events to within 24 hours of the procedure[25] or within the period of hospitalization.[16, 26] Many have distinguished closure occurring within the catheterization laboratory from events outside the laboratory. In-laboratory closure included reclosures of successfully dilated lesions as well as occlusions during attempted interventions. Out-of-laboratory closure occurred in patients who developed symptoms of myocardial ischemia after a successful intervention and in whom repeat catheterization revealed TIMI-0 to TIMI-2 flow. An outcome-oriented definition for abrupt closure identified critical reductions in coronary blood flow leading to MI, emergency repeat coronary angiography, repeated standard or prolonged PTCA within 48 hours, or emergency coronary artery bypass grafting (CABG) within 48 hours.[42]

### Threatened Closure

Although difficult to characterize, threatened closure has been defined as the presence of a large dissection flap at high risk for rapid progression to abrupt closure. Some investigators have identified threatened closure as deterioration in angiographic, ECG, hemodynamic, or clinical indicators after PTCA and a combination of the following criteria: (1) postangioplasty residual stenosis of more than 50%, (2) TIMI-2 flow, (3) significant dissection, or (4) clinical ischemia (angina or ECG changes).[46, 47] Keelan and associates defined threatened closure as worsening stenosis or a decrease of one or more TIMI grades from baseline, with ischemic ECG changes, angina, or both.[48]

## Histologic Observations

Atheromatous plaques are heterogeneous with lipid, fibrous, and calcific components. Early studies of cadaveric arteries[50–53] and animal models[54–60] demonstrated that angioplasty increased luminal diameter by plaque splitting, intimal tearing, and elastic stretching of the media.[10, 56, 59, 61–65] Each of these mechanisms injures the stenosed vessel segment and contributes to acute closure. The degree of injury from PTCA is determined by balloon and arterial size, inflation pressure and duration, morphology of the stenosis, and fragility of the arterial wall.[42] Closure results from intimal and medial dissection, subintimal hemorrhage under plaque, thrombus formation, vasoconstriction, and elastic recoil.[57, 61, 66–68] Occlusion by guide wire–induced invagination of a tortuous vessel wall has also been reported.[69] The incidence of postangioplasty dissection remains uncertain; Potkin and Roberts[63] detected intimal disruption in 98% of angioplasty sites in a postmortem study of 26 PTCA patients.

Waller and coworkers examined 130 necropsy specimens of coronary closure that followed angioplasty.[68] In 55 patients (42%), closure of the angioplasty site occurred within 24 hours of the procedure. Morphologic causes of closure were identified as intimal flaps, intimal-medial flaps, elastic recoil, and thrombi. Large intimal and intimal-medial dissection flaps were the primary cause of abrupt occlusion in 60% of angioplasty sites. In 36% of sites, elastic recoil or spasm was the primary cause; sites occluded as a result of recoil were characterized by eccentric plaques. Plaque hemorrhage with luminal thrombus accounted for two occlusions (4%) and were associated with recent exposure to thrombolytic agents. Mechanisms were similar for 45 patients with closure 1 to 7 days after the procedure (intimal-medial flap in 71%; elastic recoil in 18%). Primary thrombotic closure (11%) was more frequent than plaque hemorrhage (0%) in this group.

In 30 patients with closure 8 to 30 days after the procedure, intimal-medial flaps (59%) and elastic recoil (12%) were also the principal mechanisms of occlusion.

These morphologic causes of acute closure were extensions of successful angioplasty mechanisms. The extent of expected localized medial dissection in successful balloon angioplasty procedures ranged from 0% to 50% of the vessel circumference, whereas procedures complicated by acute closure had tears involving 51% to 100% of the vessel circumference. Larger dissections created mobile flaps that folded or curled to occlude the angioplasty site.[68] In previous angiographic studies, the predominant mechanism of acute closure was thrombus formation in 19% to 33% of patients,[9, 27, 70] dissection in 26%,[16, 27, 70, 71] and a combination in 7%. However, the mechanism was angiographically indeterminate in 42%.[16, 27, 70, 71] The relative insensitivity of angiography to detect thrombus and dissection may account for the difference in these results.[16, 68, 72–74]

## Diagnostic Technologies

In general, angiography underestimates the amount of atherosclerotic plaque present.[72, 75, 76] Most mechanical interventions contribute to luminal eccentricity by fracturing or dissecting the atheroma. Recognition of eccentric plaques and the extent of diffuse coronary disease may be difficult, because the angiogram (a "lumenogram") does not reflect the position of the arterial lumen relative to the external arterial wall.[72] Visual interpretation of angiograms are subject to interobserver variability and to discrepancies between the anatomic severity and physiologic significance of stenoses.[73] New diagnostic adjuncts for coronary intervention (intravascular ultrasound studies, intracoronary Doppler studies, optical interferometry, and angioscopy) attempt to address these issues.

Intravascular ultrasonography (IVUS) precisely measures luminal diameter and cross-sectional area,[73, 74] and its measurements correlate well with coronary anatomy and histology.[72] It has proved useful for quantifying interventional results in clinical trials. IVUS may be more sensitive than angiography or fluoroscopy for detection and localization of calcification. IVUS may help angioplasty operators identify the depth and extent of PTCA-induced dissections and intimal tears.[70, 77] Davidson and associates[78] compared IVUS with angiography in 65 patients undergoing 70 coronary interventions and found that IVUS revealed dissections at 19 sites (27%) not detected by angiography. Tenaglia and colleagues[79] used IVUS to predict adverse outcomes after coronary interventions and found that the incidence of dissection was higher among patients who sustained adverse events than among patients who did not. The severity of the dissection also appeared to correlate with procedural outcome. Other investigators have employed IVUS to ensure adequate intracoronary stent size and deployment[80–82] and to reduce the likelihood of postplacement thrombosis.[83] Despite good angiographic results after deployment, not all stents were found by IVUS to be fully expanded.[84, 85] Current ultrasound devices generate artifacts that can adversely affect image quality. Mechanical transducers may exhibit cyclical oscillations in rotational speed, causing nonuniform rotational distortion (NURD). Interpretation of the images requires caution, because different histologic components of the vessel wall may have similar patterns of echogenicity. Nonetheless, improvements in software algorithms have enabled IVUS to differentiate components of the vessel wall in greater detail than any other diagnostic tool.

Coronary angioscopy provides more vascular surface detail than does angiography and has been increasingly employed for documentation, research, and interventional guidance. A 4.5-French flexible coronary angioscope (Baxter; Edwards LIS Division, Irvine CA) was introduced in 1991. It is currently the most sensitive instrument for detecting coronary thrombus[86–90] and can be used to classify atheromatous plaques.[74, 91] Angioscopy studies have also detected subintimal dissections[65, 77, 88–90] in regions that appeared on contrast angiography to be dissection-free.[92, 93] In 1992, an expert working group created a classification system for angioscopic observations.[91] The system identified and characterized atheroma, dissection, wall hemorrhage, and thrombi. Detailed interpretation of thrombus and dissection was subject to moderate intraobserver variability (uncorrected kappa statistics were 0.57 for dissection and 0.51 to 0.60 for thrombus) and to substantial interobserver variability (uncorrected kappa statistics were 0.27 for dissection and 0.07 to 0.29 for thrombus). There exist several other limitations to angioscopy. Unlike IVUS and interferometry, angioscopy cannot visualize structures beyond the luminal surface. Imaging requires balloon occlusion of the vessel, and there is at present no method for quantifying angioscopic findings.

Intracoronary Doppler imaging addresses the angiographic limitations for determining the physiologic severity of coronary stenoses.[94, 95] Early Doppler systems employed modified Judkins catheters with a distally mounted piezoelectric crystal.[95] Subselective 3-French catheters were later constructed with either end- or side-mounted crystals.[96, 97] The size of these catheters limited Doppler examination to proximal epicardial vessels. A steerable guide wire with a Doppler transducer tip, (Flowire, Cardiometrics Inc.; Mountain View CA) has been developed for use during interventional procedures.[95, 98] These 0.036 and 0.046 guide wires employ 15- and 12-MHz transducers with signals processed by a real-time spectral analyzer by means of on-line fast Fourier transformation. The small size of the wire creates less disturbance of the arterial flow profile and permits Doppler assessment of flow velocity distal to coronary lesions.[95, 98] Physiologically significant coronary stenoses are characterized by reduction of flow velocity in the poststenotic region, loss of diastolic flow velocity, and diminished distal coronary flow reserve. Continuous monitoring during coronary interventions has identified several flow patterns associated with impending vessel occlusion or inadequate results. These include a continuous decline of mean velocity trend,[99] abrupt flow cessation,[95] and cyclic flow variation, which is most likely a result of intermittent thrombus formation and resolution.[98] Abnormal or unstable flow velocity patterns after PTCA may identify postprocedural complications earlier than can angiography.[99]

### Low-Coherence Interferometry

Low-coherence interferometry (optical coherence tomography) is a new investigational imaging technique with spatial resolution 10 to 20 times higher than that of IVUS.[100] The micron-scale resolution of this technology allows cross-sectional visualization of atherosclerotic plaque features, including intimal caps, lipid collections, and fissures. Interferometry can be incorporated into low-profile catheters as small as 0.35 mm in diameter for possible interventional guidance. The device consists of a low-coherence infrared source, which has a wider spectral bandwith than does laser, resulting in a very short coherence time between 30 and 50 $\times 10^{-15}$/second. The light beam is projected onto tissues with a fiberoptic system. The retroreflected signal is collected by a series of photodetectors at different sites along the optical beam. Computerized analysis allows discrimination of reflected signals and their times of flight into a reconstruction of intensity versus spatial depth into tissue, producing an image. Results of in vitro studies[101, 102] have been encouraging for eventual intracoronary applications. Continuing investigations seek to optimize incident source wavelength, reduce image acquisition time, and assess the scattering effect of a blood medium on image quality.

## Predictors of Acute Closure

Although it is difficult to predict acute closure accurately for individual patients, many studies have found that morphologic characteristics of the dilated lesion may identify patients at high risk for abrupt closure.[13, 14, 34, 36, 71, 103–116] Certain angiographic dissection characteristics may predict clinical events. Black and coworkers[7] found that dissection length, residual diameter stenosis, area stenosis, and extraluminal contrast were independent correlates of ischemic complications after PTCA. Huber and associates[41] demonstrated that abrupt closure, MI, and bypass grafting occurred in fewer than 3% of patients with NHLBI type B dissections. In contrast, dissection types C to F were associated with complication rates between 12% and 37% ($p < 0.0005$). Persistent extraluminal contrast, new persistent filling defects, spiral dissection (Fig. 28–2), and occlusive dissections portend adverse clinical outcomes.

Early studies identified other predictors for coronary occlusion, generally with low positive or negative predictive values.[3, 8, 9, 14, 16, 27, 117–121] Predictive factors of acute closure are summarized in Table 28–2; factors predictive of death associated with abrupt occlusion are outlined in Table 28–3. Detre and coworkers[8] analyzed 1801 patients in the 1985–1986 PTCA Registry. Baseline patient factors associated with abrupt closure included three-vessel disease, high-risk status for surgery, and acute coronary insufficiency. In another study, de Feyter and colleagues[9] demonstrated that independent preprocedural variables for abrupt coronary occlusion were unstable angina, multivessel disease, and complex lesions in a cohort of 1423 consecutive patients with attempted PTCA. Periprocedural factors associated with abrupt occlusion included post-PTCA percentage of stenosis, intimal tear or dissection, use of prolonged heparin infusions, and a post-PTCA gradient greater than 20 mm Hg.[3] Absence of any risk factor rendered the probability of acute occlusion very low (2%), whereas presence of one or more risk factors increased the probability of acute occlusion. The presence of three risk factors may contribute to a 25% probability.[9]

The American College of Cardiology/American Heart Association (ACC/AHA) Task Force on Angioplasty developed a lesion classification system in which 12 morphologic characteristics were used to divide individual lesions into three types (A, B, and C).[122] Table 28–4 summarizes this system. Ellis and coworkers[3] modified this system to stratify risk for complications that follow angioplasty: Lesions with a single type B characteristic were designated type B1; those lesions with multiple B characteristics were designated type B2. Success rates were 92% for type A lesions, 84% for type B1 lesions, 76% for type B2 lesions, and 61% for type C lesions. Complication rates were 4% for type A and type B1 lesions, 10% for type B2 lesions, and 21% for type C lesions. Ellis and coworkers[14] reviewed 4772 procedures during their 1986–1987 experience, using a

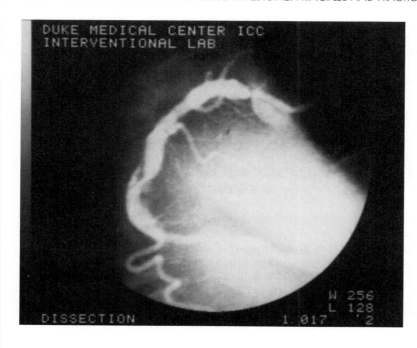

FIGURE 28–2. Angiogram of major spiral dissection of the mid–right coronary artery with significant luminal stenosis and extraluminal contrast staining.

multivariate analysis of 16 clinical variables, and found that female sex was an independent clinical risk factor. Analysis of 35 angiographic variables identified stenosis length of at least twice the luminal diameter, stenosis angulation greater than 45 degrees, stenosis at a branch vessel, stenosis-associated thrombus, other stenoses within the same vessel, and multivessel disease as independent risk factors. However, advances in angioplasty balloons, guide wires, and guiding catheters may limit the current applicability of these classification systems. Myler and associates[18] examined 1000 consecutive lesions from their experience between 1990 and 1991. None of the guiding or dilatation catheters or guide wires used during the study period were clinically available before 1988. Successful angioplasty was accomplished for 99% of type A lesions, 92% of type B lesions, and 90% of type C lesions. Untoward events (Q-wave infarction, emergency CABG, death) associated with target vessel closure occurred in 1.2% of patients with type A lesions, 1.9% of patients with type B lesions, and 2% of patients with type C lesions. The difference between these three groups was not statistically significant, which suggests that the success and complication rates associated with the original morphologic descriptors (A, B, C) are not typical of results achievable with later equipment. Myler and associates'

## TABLE 28–2.  PREDICTORS OF ACUTE CLOSURE

### Clinical Predictors

Female[3]
Unstable angina[8, 9, 117]
Diabetes mellitus[14]
Extreme age[118]
Inadequate platelet therapy[119]
Insufficient anticoagulation[120]

### Lesion Predictors

Intracoronary thrombus[3, 8, 14, 26]
Severe narrowing[8]
Long lesion[3, 14]
Complex lesion[9]
Lesion at branch point[3]
Lesion at bend point >45 degrees[3, 14, 117]
American Heart Association lesion score B2, C[14, 117]
Severe proximal target vessel tortuosity[26]

### Postprocedure Predictors

Dissection[3, 8, 117]
Remaining stenosis gradient >20 mm Hg[3]
Cyclic flow variation by Doppler imaging[98]

### Angiographic Predictors

Multivessel[8, 9, 27]
Multilesion[8, 9, 27]
Collateral flow from target vessel[3, 8, 121]

## TABLE 28–3.  FACTORS PREDICTIVE OF DEATH ASSOCIATED WITH ACUTE CLOSURE

### Clinical Factors

Female sex
Age > 65 years
Congestive heart failure

### Angiographic Factors

Left main coronary artery disease
Three-vessel disease
Left ventricular ejection fraction < 30%

From de Feyter PJ, de Jaegere PT, Murphy ES, et al: Abrupt coronary artery occlusion during percutaneous transluminal coronary angioplasty. Am Heart J 123:1633, 1992.

## TABLE 28–4. AMERICAN COLLEGE OF CARDIOLOGY/AMERICAN HEART ASSOCIATION RISK STRATIFICATION (BASED ON LESION-SPECIFIC CHARACTERISTICS)

### Type A (High Success > 85%, Low Risk)

Discrete (< 10-mm length)
Little or no calcification
Concentric
Readily accessible
Nonangulated segment (45 degrees)
Smooth contour
Less than totally occlusive
Not ostial
No major branch involved
Absence of thrombus

### Type B (Moderate Success 60%–85%, Moderate Risk)

Tubular (10- to 20-mm length)
Moderate to heavy calcium
Eccentric
Total occlusion < 3 months
Moderate tortuosity
Ostial location
Moderately angulated
Bifurcation lesion (double wire)
Irregular contour
Some thrombus present

### Type C (Low Success < 60%, High Risk)

Diffuse (> 2-cm length)
Total occlusion > 3-months
Excessive tortuosity
Inability to protect branch
Extreme angulation
Degenerated vein grafts

From Ryan TJ, Faxon DP, Gunnar RM, et al: Guidelines for percutaneous transluminal coronary angioplasty: A report of the American College of Cardiology/American Heart Association Task Force on Assessment of Diagnostic and Therapeutic Cardiovascular Procedures (Subcommittee on Percutaneous Transluminal Coronary Angioplasty). J Am Coll Cardiol 12:529, 1988.

analysis[18] of morphologic factors associated with angioplasty success included absence of old occlusion and unprotected bifurcation lesion, decreasing lesion length, and absence of thrombus.

The limited applicability of ACC/AHA Task Force guidelines and early broad angioplasty studies[2] to more recent angioplasty risks and outcomes underscores the need for a revised and updated classification scheme. These guidelines have been used as comparative yardsticks of success and risk for new device procedures, evoking considerable concern.[18] Fortunately, the importance of such comparisons diminishes as randomized clinical trials of interventional outcomes supplement registry data.

## Acute Events with Newer Devices

Although newer technologies such as excimer laser angioplasty and atherectomy do not involve direct barotrauma as the major mechanism to increase lu-minal dimension, dissection may also occur during these procedures. Excimer laser energy disrupts molecular bonds, forms vapor bubbles, and generates photoacoustic trauma.[61, 123–127] Atherectomy excises plaque material by means of a cutting system.[61, 128–131] Although atherectomy has been thought to debulk lesions, part of the increase in luminal diameter may result from the low-pressure positioning balloon. Potential mechanisms for the development of dissection during these newer procedures include guide catheter trauma, guide wire trauma, vascular trauma during device delivery or crossing, and barotrauma during adjunctive balloon angioplasty.

### Laser

Excimer-laser coronary angioplasty (ELCA) is a unique method of percutaneous revascularization involving pulsed light energy with a wavelength of 308 nm. Ablation occurs only when the catheter tip is in direct contact with the plaque. In vivo examination[127] with IVUS in 108 patients revealed dissections in 44% of lesions. Dissections were more common in lesions with superficial calcified plaque. The cross-sectional area of the lumen after ELCA was, on average, 30% larger than the cross-sectional area of the laser catheter used. The mechanism of laser angioplasty is more complicated than that of simple photoablation. Rapidly expanding and collapsing vapor bubbles and stress waves may contribute to dissection, creating forced vessel expansion and plaque fragmentation.

Several studies have evaluated ELCA efficacy and closure rates with variable results. Geschwind and colleagues[132] used ELCA in 46 patients; acute closure occurred in 17% and dissections in 7%. Karsch and associates[133] noted a high acute closure rate (20%) among 55 patients after ELCA; most of these lesions were recanalized with conventional PTCA. Ghazzal and coauthors[134] published the results of laser therapy on 220 lesions in 200 patients. The overall procedural success rate was 90.5%. Acute closure occurred in 4.5% of patients, but there were no deaths. Vessel eccentricity was the most important predictor of ELCA complications, including acute closure. Bittl and Sanborn[135] reported a similar 5% incidence of acute closure in 200 consecutive patients undergoing ELCA. All patients were successfully treated with repeat balloon angioplasty, and no patient experienced a Q-wave MI. Lee and Mason's retrospective review[136] of 1893 ELCA patients revealed 123 (6.5%) with acute occlusion. Preisack and colleagues[137] studied 523 patients undergoing PTCA and 83 patients undergoing excimer laser angioplasty in the same laboratory; the acute closure rates were 3.3% after PTCA and 30% after excimer laser angioplasty. Occlusion was associated with severe spasm (without evidence of dissection or thrombus) during laser angioplasty and was responsive to repeat dilatation. In larger series, two ELCA registries reported their clinical and procedural complications.[138, 139] The Spectranectics laser registry reported a 5.5% incidence of abrupt closure, a 2.1% incidence of perforation, and an 18.8% incidence of dissection in 1834 lesions, with a 3.4% risk of MI, a 4.3% incidence of coronary bypass surgery, and a 0.3% incidence of death in 1654 patients.[139, 140] The Advanced Interventional Systems (AIS) registry reported similar rates of procedural complications (abrupt closure, 7.0%; perforation, 1.7%; dissection, 15.0%) for 2803 lesions and clinical events (MI, 4.1%; coronary bypass surgery, 3.6%; death, 0.5%) for 2238 patients. The New Approaches to Coronary Intervention (NACI) device registry[141] reported a 3.6% incidence of in-hospital MI in 850 patients treated with ELCA and a 6.4% incidence of coronary spasm. Baumbach and associates[142] merged U.S. and European registry data to evaluate ELCA in 1521 patients. There was a 22% incidence of dissection and a 6.1% incidence of abrupt closure. Logistic regression analysis revealed a correlation between dissections and larger catheter size, high energy-per-pulse levels, presence of a side branch, and lesion length greater than 10 mm. The presence of intracoronary thrombus also increased the risk of poor clinical outcome after ELCA.[143]

Appelman and colleagues[144] conducted a randomized trial in which 151 patients were assigned to undergo ELCA and 157 patients to undergo PTCA. All patients had lesions longer than 10 mm according to visual assessment of angiograms. Postprocedure intimal dissections occurred in 46.8% of patients treated with ELCA; most (91%) were minor. The total dissection rate was similar for patients treated with balloon angioplasty (54.5%). The incidence of transient occlusions of the randomized segment was significantly higher among patients undergoing ELCA (6.6%) than among patients undergoing PTCA (0.6%). The high incidence of dissections in this study was attributed to patient selection and lesion complexity. In an attempt to minimize arterial wall trauma, Deckelbaum and associates[127] randomly assigned 57 patients to ELCA either in a blood medium or with blood displacement with an intracoronary saline infusion. The incidence of significant dissection was 7% in saline-treated patients, in comparison with 24% of conventionally treated controls.

## Atherectomy

Initial nonrandomized experience with directional coronary atherectomy (DCA) was promising for PTCA failure secondary to elastic recoil, recurrent thrombosis, or limited dissection.[145–149] Some series have suggested that the incidence of dissection after atherectomy is lower than that after balloon angioplasty.[145, 146, 150] However, significantly stiffer and larger catheters may increase the risk of guide-induced dissection and vessel closure in comparison with conventional angioplasty (Fig. 28–3). Occlusion may occur at the atherectomy site, where it is often related to plaque excision. Proximal occlusions secondary to guide catheter trauma at the coronary ostium have been reported, whereas nose cone trauma may produce acute occlusion distal to the treated lesion.

According to historical and registry data, the frequency of acute closure has ranged from 3.6% to 6.9%.[151–153] Popma and coworkers[153] reported that the incidences of abrupt or threatened closure were 3.3% in laboratory and 0.9% out of laboratory for a series of 1020 patients in the U.S. Directional Atherectomy Investigator Group Registry. Abrupt closure was related to thrombosis in 51%, to target-lesion dissection in 30%, and to guide catheter–induced dissection in 9%, and was indeterminate in 9% of cases. The chance of successfully reversing acute closure that was secondary to dissection was only 27%, significantly lower than the rescue rate when angioplasty was performed to treat closures of thrombotic or indeterminate etiology after atherectomy. Balloon angioplasty was attempted in 32 of 43 acute closure episodes, with adequate results in 50%. Of the 16 patients in whom angioplasty was unsuccessful, 15 underwent coronary artery bypass surgery. Hinohara and colleagues[152] noted in-laboratory abrupt closure after DCA in 2.4% of 382 procedures, and out-of-laboratory closure was present in 1.3%. Distal occlusion occurred in 0.8% of patients and tended to occur in tortuous segments distal to the treated segment. In both series,[152, 153] guide catheter–induced dissections occurred exclusively in the right coronary artery, and these dissections may be significantly more common in right coronary arteries that have plaque in the ostium of the vessel or the proximal segment. These dissections may be reduced with the use of shorter tipped and softer guiding catheters.

Other studies suggest that the incidence of acute complications does not appear to be lower for DCA than for angioplasty.[154, 155] Feld and associates[150] evaluated DCA in 116 patients with 125 PTCA-matched controls. Although there were fewer dissections with atherectomy (13%) than with angioplasty (22%), there were more complications (22% vs. 12%) and a trend toward more acute occlusions in the patients who underwent atherectomy (8.5% vs. 4%). There was no advantage with atherectomy in subpopulations with ulcerated or high-risk lesions. The randomized, prospective Coronary An-

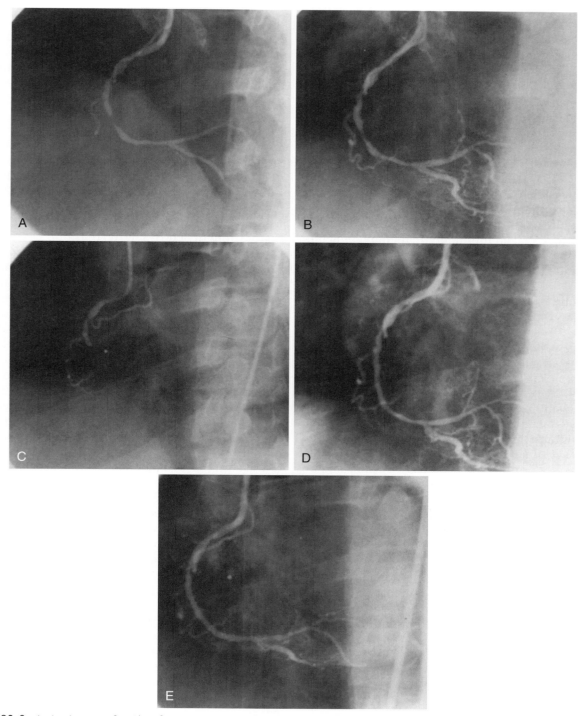

FIGURE 28–3. *A.* Angiogram of 95% right coronary artery lesion. *B,* Post–directional coronary atherectomy result with intraluminal haziness at the site of atherectomy. *C,* Subsequent acute vessel closure. *D,* Angiogram after Gianturco-Roubin stent implantation. *E,* Relook angiogram 24 hours after stent implantation demonstrating maintained vessel patency.

gioplasty versus Excisional Atherectomy Trial (CAVEAT) compared directional atherectomy with PTCA. It revealed a 20% incidence of dissection and a 6.8% incidence of closure among 512 patients treated with atherectomy[26, 154, 156]; among 500 patients treated with PTCA, the incidence of dissection was 24%, whereas closure occurred in 2.8%. In the patients who underwent angioplasty, occlusion usually occurred at the target lesion (91%), whereas the occlusion site was the target lesion for only 58% of the patients who underwent DCA. The remainder of the DCA occlusions were attributed to guide catheter or nose cone trauma. CAVEAT represented atherectomy and PTCA performed in the United States between 1991 and 1992, in which first-generation DCA devices, early guiding catheters, and large residual stenoses were used. The Canadian Coronary Atherectomy Trial (CCAT) showed no distinct superiority of atherectomy over PTCA in patients with lesions restricted to the proximal third of the left anterior descending coronary artery.[155] Abrupt closure occurred in 4.3% of 130 DCA patients, in comparison with 5.1% of 136 patients randomly assigned to undergo PTCA.

The risk of acute vessel closure secondary to DCA may be increased in the peri-infarction period. Potkin and coauthors[157] reported that the incidence of abrupt occlusion after atherectomy in patients who had recently received thrombolytic therapy for acute MI may be higher than for patients without MI. Popma and coworkers' review[153] of the multicenter registry also suggested more frequent abrupt occlusion among post-MI patients. Conversely, Ellis and coworkers[111] found that lesions with thrombus had a higher success rate than did lesions without thrombus, which suggests that DCA may be effective for the treatment of unstable plaque. The role of DCA in unstable angina and recent MI remains unclear.

Further studies continue to evaluate "optimal atherectomy" techniques, which emphasize maximal debulking and minimal residual stenosis of less than 10%. Unlike CAVEAT, post-DCA balloon dilatation has been encouraged to achieve better angiographic results. The Balloon Angioplasty versus Optimal Atherectomy Trial (BOAT) found higher procedural success with optimal atherectomy (93.2%) than with PTCA (86.6%) among 1000 patients.[158] The need for "bail-out" catheter therapy was also lower among the patients who underwent atherectomy (3.8% vs. 9.6%). The Optimal Atherectomy Restenosis Study[159] employed mandatory IVUS to evaluate luminal diameter and as a decision-making tool; dissections were found in 9 of 200 patients.

### Rotational Coronary Ablation

The Rotablator (Heart Technology, Inc.; Bellevue WA), a rotational atherectomy device, consists partly of a brass burr coated with diamond chips to ablate atherosclerotic material. A gas-driven turbine connected by a flexible shaft rotates the burr at up to 190,000 rpm. The Rotablator burr selectively removes rigid atherosclerotic lesions, particularly in heavily calcified sites.[160] Early experience with the Rotablator was favorable in comparison with PTCA and ELCA.[161]

Acute dissection has occurred in approximately 8.2% of cases.[149] Gilmore and colleagues,[162] in a single-site series, documented four infarcts and three emergency CABG complications in a series of 108 patients and 143 lesions. Bertrand and coauthors[163] compiled results from three European centers that used the Rotablator with and without adjunctive angioplasty. In this group of 129 patients, the overall success rate was 86%; the incidence of acute closure was 7.7%.

In a larger study by Warth and coworkers,[164] acute closure was noted in 5.4% (4.3% in-laboratory closure and 1.1% out-of-laboratory closure) of 1403 consecutive patients undergoing rotary ablation. Dissection was visible angiographically in 21% of closures; spasm was evident in 4% of cases. Successful treatment of acute closure, defined as the restoration of TIMI-3 flow without Q-wave MI, CABG, or death, was achieved in 64% of patients. The overall mortality rate, incidence of emergency CABG, and Q-wave MI in patients with acute closure were 6.6%, 13.1%, and 13.1%, respectively. Brown and Buchbinder[165] examined data from the same registry 2 years later and documented a dissection rate of 12.8% in 2303 procedures. Vessel tortuosity, primary rather than restenotic lesions, and ACC/AHA types A and C lesions contributed significantly to dissection. In another study, 224 randomly selected patients (with 286 lesions) undergoing Rotablator therapy at two sites were studied.[166] Among the 5.7% of patients with acute closure, the mortality rate was 6.7%. However, the incidences of Q-wave MI (31%) and emergency CABG (19%) were greater. According to logistic regression analysis, location of the lesion on a hinge point and long lesions were correlated with acute closure, whereas pretreatment with a small burr appeared to reduce the risk. Other features, including gender, degree of lesion calcification, and speed of the burr, were not correlated with acute closure. Aguirre and associates pooled early data that suggested an 8.6% incidence of acute MI among 907 patients, although rotational ablation was used as a stand-alone procedure in 302 cases.[167]

MacIsaac and colleagues[160] analyzed data from the Multicenter Rotablator Registry of 2161 procedures in single lesions, which represented a total of 1078 calcified and 1083 noncalcified lesions. Adjunctive PTCA was performed in 82.9% of calcified lesions and 66.9% of noncalcified lesions. Angiographically apparent coronary dissection occurred in 161 (14.9%) calcified lesions and 122 (11.3%) noncalcified lesions. Abrupt coronary closure occurred in 42 (3.9%) calcified lesions and 36 (3.3%) noncalcified lesions. The randomized multicenter Study to Determine Rotablator and Transluminal Angioplasty Strategy (STRATAS)[168] reported a lower incidence of dissection for a stepped-burr strategy with IVUS evaluation in comparison with conventional Rotablator therapy. An abstract presentation by

Whitlow and associates concluded that significant deceleration of the burr speed was the strongest predictor of adverse clinical outcomes and postprocedural elevations of creatine kinase with muscle and brain subunits (CK-MB), although both aggressive and conventional Rotablator strategies yielded equivalent late clinical outcomes.[168, 169]

### Transluminal Extraction-Endarterectomy Catheter (TEC)

The TEC (Inter Ventional Technologies; San Diego CA) cuts atheroma by means of a conical head rotating at 750 rpm and extracts the excised material through a vacuum system. In the U.S. TEC Multicenter Registry, use of this device in 1147 patients at 29 clinical sites was evaluated.[170–172] Overall success was 89% among 609 patients with native vessel disease who underwent TEC procedures (with or without adjunctive PTCA). Acute closure occurred in 5.5% of patients, resulting in a major complication (acute MI, CABG, or death) in 1.8% of those cases. Late reocclusion occurred in 1.3% of the remaining patients in this cohort. The most common cause of closure in the catheterization laboratory was dissection, followed by spasm and thrombus. Among 538 patients who underwent TEC procedures for saphenous vein graft disease, the success rate was also 89%. In this group, acute closure occurred in 2.8% of patients. In most cases, closure was caused by dissection or thrombus.

Kaplan and colleagues[173] evaluated TEC procedures in 100 patients with acute MI, 66% of whom had angiographically evident thrombus. Procedural success was achieved in 94%, with a 5% need for CABG and a 5% incidence of in-hospital death. Significant flow-limiting lesions occurred after TEC procedures in 8%, and minor dissections occurred in 20%. The randomized, multicenter TEC Or PTCA In Thrombus (TOPIT) trial[174] compared the use of TEC with that of PTCA in clinical situations associated with coronary thrombus. Postprocedure dissections were present in 40% of patients, and 15% required intracoronary stent placement; however, the incidences did not differ between the two treatment groups. The incidence of major in-hospital events was 1.8% for TEC procedures and 6.3% for PTCA.

## Management of Acute Closure
### Coronary Artery Bypass Grafting

During the early angioplasty experience, bypass surgery was the principal therapy for dissection and acute coronary occlusion[4, 6, 8, 11]; up to 20% of patients required CABG.[28] The use of bypass surgery has decreased since the early 1980s.[25, 175, 176] In the pre-stent era, 2% to 4% of PTCA patients required CABG,[2, 9, 13, 177, 178] and the incidence of emergency CABG was similar to that of other interventional technologies (ELCA, DCA, Rotablator, and TEC procedures).[28] Berger and coauthors[179] emphasized that the decline in the proportion of patients treated with CABG (20% in 1982, 5% in 1987, 1% in 1992) is not at the expense of a higher rate of death or MI. Emergency surgery after unsuccessful angioplasty was associated with a 12.5% to 21% incidence of Q-wave MI and a 4.4% to 11% mortality rate in later series.[179–183] Surgical mortality has been higher with emergency CABG than with elective procedures.[176, 177, 184–186] Predictors of poor outcome include ongoing ischemia and hemodynamic instability.[176, 177, 183, 185–189] Although an ACC consensus group noted the potential interference of coronary stents with the creation of distal anastomoses,[190] the incidence of periprocedural MI for CABG after stent placement was comparable to the earlier experience of emergency CABG after PTCA alone.[179] CABG continues to be indicated for patients with adverse events (e.g., acute or threatened closure, perforation, tamponade, arrhythmias, broken guide wire, lost stent) that are refractory to management in the cardiac catheterization laboratory.

### Intra-aortic Balloon Counterpulsation

Intra-aortic balloon counterpulsation (IABP) has been used in patients with acute closure to stabilize them hemodynamically before CABG.[191] Prophylactic IABP placement may be beneficial in maintaining patency of lesions and preventing acute closure in patients who are undergoing PTCA for acute MI.[192] Suneja and Hodgson[193] used IABP in eight consecutive patients (five who underwent PTCA, three who underwent DCA) with refractory acute closure during coronary intervention, who were not hemodynamically compromised. All were treated with prolonged inflations with a perfusion balloon and with intracoronary urokinase and nitroglycerin. When multiple prolonged inflations failed to maintain sustained patency, IABP placement averted closure and the need for emergency CABG, permitting medical management. Intracoronary Doppler flow monitoring has documented insignificant improvement in coronary blood flow velocity from IABP beyond most critical stenoses, followed by balloon pump–mediated augmentation of blood flow after successful revascularization.[95, 194] This finding supported the clinical experience of the beneficial effect of aortic counterpulsation on postangioplasty vessel patency.[195, 196]

### Antithrombotics

ENZYMATIC FIBRINOLYTIC AGENTS. Indications for adjunctive thrombolytic therapy include (1) recently occluded saphenous vein grafts with intracoronary thrombus and (2) acute closure, during PTCA, that is resistant to redilatation alone, presumbly resulting from thrombus formation.[197] Delivery techniques include infusion through the guiding catheter or through infusion catheters with multiple side or end holes or helical inflation coils.[43] Adjunctive thrombolytic therapy increased the average success rate to 65%[16] over balloon inflation alone. Good angiographic outcomes have been observed in limited retrospective reports combining intracoronary streptokinase with repeat PTCA[198, 199] and intracoronary urokinase with repeat PTCA.[198, 200] In a study of 48 patients with intracoronary thrombus complicating angioplasty, investigators noted an angiographic success rate of 90% after the administration of intracoronary urokinase, without procedurally related MI or death.[198] Gulba and coauthors[201] reported reopening of acute occlusions in 22 of 27 patients with intracoronary tissue-type plasminogen activator (tPA) but documented reocclusion in 12 patients 24 to 36 hours later. Lincoff and associates[24] were unable to show benefit from intracoronary thrombolysis in the treatment of abrupt closure complicating PTCA in a retrospective review from two centers. In 43 patients receiving thrombolytic therapy for abrupt closure of presumed thrombotic cause, no benefit was observed at the doses of urokinase (0.5 to 3 million U) or tPA (20 to 100 million U) used. The majority of these patients (81%) also underwent repeat balloon dilatation.

Ambrose and colleagues[197, 202] performed a randomized, multicenter, double-blind trial of 469 patients to examine the role for thrombolysis as prophylaxis during angioplasty in unstable angina. They reported an increased incidence in abrupt closure when adjunctive urokinase was given prophylactically in a setting of PTCA during unstable rest angina (10.2% vs. 4.3% for placebo controls), with concomitant increases in ischemia, MI, and need for emergency CABG. Vaitkus and Laskey[203] observed that adjunctive thrombolysis did not improve angioplasty success or complication rates in elective angioplasty or MI and may be detrimental in rest angina. Coronary patency was usually achieved, but this did not forestall complications in many cases. Selected patients in whom thrombolytic therapy fails may benefit from antiplatelet agents, such as abciximab.

**GLYCOPROTEIN IIb/IIIa INHIBITORS.** Abciximab is a murine monoclonal antibody derivative that specifically antagonizes the glycoprotein IIb/IIIa platelet receptor for fibrinogen.[204–206] Large clinical trials such as Evaluation of 7E3 for the Prevention of Ischemic Complications (EPIC) and Evaluation of PTCA to Improve Long-term Outcome by c7E3 GP IIb/IIIa Receptor Blockade (EPILOG)[207, 208] have shown decreased ischemic complications with abciximab after angioplasty. Muhlestein and coworkers[209] demonstrated dissolution of thrombi and restoration of TIMI-3 flow in 16 consecutive patients who developed intracoronary thrombi after PTCA and were treated with abciximab. In four of these patients, treatment with intracoronary urokinase had failed. Integrelin, a synthetic cyclic peptide antagonist, may also reduce ischemic PTCA complications and the need for repeat revascularization.[210] Investigation continues with other peptide and nonpeptide glycoprotein IIb/IIIa antagonists, some of which are orally active.[206]

**OTHER AGENTS.** Danchin and coauthors,[211] in a single-center retrospective report, described use of adjunctive dipyridamole in 143 consecutive patients in comparison with 171 patients receiving aspirin and heparin alone. The acute closure rate was 2.8% for the dipyridamole recipients, in comparison with 7.5% of the control group. Direct thrombin inhibitors, such as hirudin and bivalirudin (Hirulog), have been examined for their potential in intracoronary thrombosis. Van den Bos and associates[212] showed reduced incidences of MI and of emergency CABG for hirudin-treated patients (1.4%) in comparison with 10.3% of heparin-treated controls. However, Bittl and colleagues' series[213] of 4098 patients undergoing angioplasty revealed no significant reduction in the incidence of death, acute MI, or acute closure in patients randomly assigned to receive Hirulog or heparin.

### Balloon Redilatation

Early experience with balloon reinflation and redilatation[20, 214] showed successful reperfusion in 44% of patients.[8, 9, 13] Successful redilatation was complicated by reocclusion, with a 6% incidence of emergency CABG, 17% risk of MI, and 3.4% rate of mortality.[16] Banka and coauthors[42] reported a reduced rate of acute closure (1.4%) and dissection (1.3%) in 1087 patients in whom predilatation was accomplished with a smaller (2- to 2.5-mm) balloon, followed by maximal dilatation with an optimally sized (3.0- to 4.0-mm) balloon.

Prolonged dilatation has been defined as a single inflation longer than 10 minutes with or without use of a perfusion balloon catheter.[25] Some series have used considerably longer inflations.[215, 216] Prolonged dilatation may "tack up" dissection flaps and may improve vascular remodeling, although it is not always well tolerated by the patient. In a series of 478 patients, primary prolonged balloon inflation reduced the rate of major dissection with less residual stenosis than that produced by standard inflation.[217, 218] Lincoff and associates' acute closure series[24] noted a 48% success for prolonged dilatations, in comparison with 5% for standard dilatations. Perfusion balloon therapy has been employed as bridge to immediate surgery,[219–221] although selected patients have received satisfactory results from autoperfusion catheter alone.[215, 222–224] Jackman and colleagues[215] reported a 65% rate of event-free outcome with prolonged (>20-minute) inflations for major post-PTCA dissections. Balloon inflation for a mean duration of 30 minutes led to procedural success in 80% of the 40 patients studied. Leitschuh and associates[224] compared outcomes of major dissection in 36 patients treated with perfusion balloon catheters with the outcomes in 46 conventionally treated controls. Angiographic success was 84% among patients treated with perfusion balloons, in comparison with 62% among patients treated conventionally ($p < 0.05$). Seventy-four percent of patients receiving prolonged dilatations were discharged event-free, in comparison with 48% treated with standard methods. Stauffer and co-workers[225] employed perfusion balloon therapy in 50 patients with angiographic success in 76%; crossover to stenting (16%) and to CABG (8%) was used in unsuccessful cases. Little and associates[216] performed ultralong dilatations ("coronary splinting") for acute vessel occlusion in 22 patients, with inflations of 4 to 16 (average, 6.3) hours. Success was reported for 91% of patients; one patient required CABG, and another suffered persistent occlusion, which was treated medically. Q-wave MI developed in seven patients after splinting, which was not significantly different from historically matched controls. Although prolonged dilatation was the technique preferred by Danchin and colleagues[25] for vessels less than 2.5 mm in diameter, application of perfusion balloon therapy has been limited in patients with small or tortuous vessels, in patients with angulated lesions, and in the presence of significant thrombi.

## Atherectomy

Directional atherectomy has been attempted for discrete dissection flaps refractory to prolonged inflation.[148, 149, 226] Lee and coauthors[227] reported a case of major dissection in the proximal left anterior descending coronary artery with delayed runoff and ischemic pain. After unsuccessful perfusion balloon inflations of 5 and 20 minutes, directional atherectomy effectively removed four specimens, leaving no residual dissection flap. Histopathologic study revealed atheroma, thrombotic debris, intima, and a small amount of media. Vetter and coworkers[228] noted an 87% success rate in their experience of 30 lesions treated with directional atherectomy for failed angioplasty; complications necessitated surgery in 10% of cases. Whitlow and colleagues[229] found rescue atherectomy for dissection, occlusion, or filling defect successful in 26 of 30 patients. Harris and associates[230] achieved procedural success in 10 of 16 patients after failed angioplasty; one patient suffered a Q-wave MI, and another required emergency CABG. Perforation and delayed coronary rupture from rescue atherectomy have been reported.[11, 220, 231–233] Some authors have avoided atherectomy in cases of acute closure[25] and spiral dissection.[224, 233]

## Balloon Pyroplasty

In thermal balloon angioplasty, a laser, microwave, or radiofrequency energy source is used to produce thermal injury on adjacent plaque.[61, 234, 235] The Spears laser balloon (USCI; Billerica MA), which heats the arterial lumen under several atmospheres of pressure, became available in 1989. Indications for its emergency use were acute or threatened closure or large dissection after PTCA.[236] Technical success was reported in both elective and acute bail-out situations.[237, 238] Initial experience in 154 patients with established or threatened closure demonstrated a clinical success rate of 83%. Ferguson and associates successfully treated 20 of 21 patients with post-PTCA abrupt closure by using neodymium: yttrium-aluminum-garnet (Nd:YAG) laser balloon angioplasty.[239] Scott and colleagues[223] applied the device to 21 patients with dissection refractory to standard balloon reinflation, and they partially attributed improvement in clinical outcomes to use of the device. Yamashita and associates[240] evaluated a radiofrequency thermal balloon device in 32 patients in whom conventional angioplasty failed. Success was obtained with 82% of lesions, and there was one abrupt occlusion. Angiographic restenosis occurred in 14 of 25 lesions at 6 months. Restenosis remains a significant problem,[241] and the use of thermal balloon devices has not become widespread.[25]

## Intracoronary Stent Placement

Intracoronary stent placement has undergone a dramatic increase in use, with promising outcomes for acute closure. Increasing operator experience[25] and advanced antithrombotic regimens have improved stent efficacy for acute closure and dissection. Prompt stent placement is associated with low incidences of MI and emergency CABG.[242] Single-center experience in a New York State registry[178] comparing angioplasty complication rates before and after the availability of stents for acute or threatened closure suggests more than a 50% reduction in angioplasty complications overall and a reduction in need for CABG.[243] A high-volume catheterization laboratory reported a 70% reduction in the need

## TABLE 28–5.  CORONARY WALLSTENT SERIES

| AUTHOR/REFERENCE | YEAR | PATIENTS | | SUCCESS: (%) | THROMBOSIS: N (%) | DEATH: N (%) | Q-AMI: N (%) | CABG: N (%) |
|---|---|---|---|---|---|---|---|---|
| | | Total | Emerg | | | | | |
| Sigwart et al[247] | 1988 | 11 | 11 | 100 | 1 (9.1) | 1 (9.1) | 0 (0) | 0 (0) |
| de Feyter et al[308] | 1990 | 15 | 15 | 100 | 1 (6.7) | 1 (6.7) | 2 (13) | 9 (60) |
| Serruys et al[249] | 1991 | 105 | 14 | 100 | 25 (23.8) | 5 (4.8) | 1 (0.9) | 1 (0.9) |
| Goy et al[309] | 1992 | 17 | 17 | 100 | 1 (5.9) | 0 (0) | 1 (5.9) | 0 (0) |

CABG, coronary artery bypass grafting; Emerg, number of patients receiving emergency stents for acute or threatened closure or suboptimal percutaneous transluminal coronary angioplasty result; Q-AMI, Q-wave acute myocardial infarction.

for emergency revascularization after unsuccessful intervention with the application of stents.[244] Two series[242, 243] have also demonstrated a reduction in need for CABG but no reduction in incidence of Q-wave MI or in-hospital outcome. The Trial of Angioplasty and Stents in Canada (TASC) II trial revealed improved angiographic results after stent placement in comparison with prolonged perfusion balloon therapy in 43 patients.[245] Crossover to stent placement after failed prolonged balloon inflations in 10 patients yielded comparable results at the expense of increased procedural time. Similarly, de Muinck and associates[246] had a higher rate of procedural success with stents (94%) than with perfusion balloons (70%) in a series of 97 patients. Published series of emergency stent placement are summarized in Tables 28–5 to 28–10.

The self-expanding Wallstent was initially used by Sigwart and coworkers[247] with successful restoration of adequate coronary flow. Sigwart and coworkers[248] in 1987 described their initial experience with the stainless steel, multifilament, self-expanding Wallstent (Medinvent-Schneider; Lausanne, Switzerland) in 19 patients. Rigorous postplacement anticoagulation therapy included aspirin, dipyridamole, heparin, urokinase, and warfarin. One thrombotic occlusion was asymptomatic; a second

was treated with thrombolysis. One patient died after suspected but unproven occlusion. Stent thrombosis has been an important limitation of the Wallstent. In a larger cohort by Serruys and associates,[249] early occlusion occurred in 20% of 117 implants within 14 days. In Sigwart and coworkers' series,[250] thrombosis was related to the size of the stent and occurred in only 3% of stents with an average expanded diameter of 4.1 to 0.8 mm, in comparison with 16% in stents with an expanded diameter of 3.5 to 0.5 mm. Table 28–5 summarizes the early Wallstent series.

The prototype coil design is the Gianturco-Roubin stent (Cook, Inc.; Bloomington IN), which has an interdigitating coiled structure of 0.15-mm surgical stainless steel.[15, 251] In 1993, the U.S. Food and Drug Administration (FDA) approved this stent for treatment of acute or threatened closure. Data from the accumulated Gianturco-Roubin stent experience are summarized in Table 28–6.

Procedural complications are more numerous with emergency placement than with elective cases. Sutton and coworkers[252, 253] compared implantation of Gianturco-Roubin stents in 415 patients with acute or threatened closure (emergency cases) with that in 224 patients with restenosis (elective cases). Patients undergoing stent placement for acute clo-

## TABLE 28–6.  GIANTURCO-ROUBIN STENT SERIES

| AUTHOR/REFERENCE | YEAR | PATIENTS | | SUCCESS: % | THROMBOSIS: N (%) | DEATH: N (%) | Q-AMI: N (%) | CABG: N (%) |
|---|---|---|---|---|---|---|---|---|
| | | Total | Emerg | | | | | |
| Roubin et al[15] | 1992 | 115 | 115 | 93 | 9 (8.4) | 2 (1.8) | 8 (7.5) | 5 (4.6) |
| Grinstead et al[254] | 1993 | 500 | 500 | 97 | 44 (8.8) | 18 (3.6) | 37 (7.4) | 81 (16.2) |
| Nath et al[255] | 1993 | 145 | 145 | Retro | 17 (11.7) | 0 (0) | 11 (7.6) | 8 (5.5) |
| Hearn et al[256] | 1993 | 116 | 116 | 89 | 9 (8.7) | 5 (4.8) | 5 (4.8) | 29 (28) |
| George et al[46] | 1993 | 518 | 518 | 95 | 43 (8.7) | 11 (2.2) | 15 (3.0) | 21 (4.3) |
| Lincoff et al[242] | 1993 | 92 | 61 | Retro | 7 (11.5) | 2 (3.3) | 20 (32.8) | 3 (4.9) |
| Sutton et al[253] | 1993 | 639 | 415 | 100 | 28 (6.7) | 12 (2.9) | 21 (5.1) | 51 (12.3) |
| Chan et al[286] | 1995 | 42 | 42 | 95 | 2 (4.9) | 0 (0) | 2 (4.9) | 3 (7.3) |
| Liu et al[47] | 1995 | 1318 | 1318 | Retro | 105 (8.0) | NR | 222 (16.8) | 160 (12.1) |
| Altmann et al[243] | 1996 | 23 | 22 | 96 | 1 (4.3) | 0 (0) | 0 (0) | 0 (0) |
| Thomas et al[307] | 1996 | 187 | 159 | 97 | 11 (7.0) | 6 (3.8) | 16 (10.2) | 17 (10.8) |

CABG, coronary artery bypass grafting; Emerg, number of patients receiving emergency stents for acute or threatened closure or suboptimal percutaneous transluminal coronary angioplasty result; NR, not reported; Q-AMI, Q-wave acute myocardial infarction; Retro, Retrospective analysis.

## TABLE 28–7. PALMAZ-SCHATZ STENT SERIES

| AUTHOR/REFERENCE | YEAR | PATIENTS | | SUCCESS (%) | THROMBOSIS: N (%) | DEATH: N (%) | Q-AMI: N (%) | CABG: N (%) |
|---|---|---|---|---|---|---|---|---|
| | | Total | Emerg | | | | | |
| Haude et al[272] | 1991 | 15 | 15 | 100 | 1 (6.7) | 0 (0) | 0 (0) | 1 (6.7) |
| Herrmann et al[267] | 1992 | 56 | 56 | 98 | 9 (16.4) | 2 (3.6) | 11 (20) | 7 (12.7) |
| Reifart et al[278] | 1991 | 64 | 64 | 95 | 20 (31.2) | 4 (6.3) | 2 (3.1) | 7 (10.9) |
| Fajadet et al[273] | 1992 | 427 | 145 | NR | 18 (12.4) | NR | NR | NR |
| Kimura et al[274] | 1992 | 96 | 23 | 97 | 3 (13) | 0 (0) | 5 (NR) | 0 (0) |
| Colombo et al[83] | 1993 | 56 | 56 | 88 | 1 (1.9) | 2 (3.6) | 2 (3.6) | 3 (5.4) |
| Maiello et al[310] | 1993 | 50 | 50 | 92 | 1 (3.3) | 1 (3.3) | 2 (6.6) | 2 (6.6) |
| de Muinck et al[246] | 1994 | 36 | 36 | 94 | 8 (22.2) | 3 (8.3) | 11 (30.5) | 0 (0) |
| Foley et al[311] | 1994 | 160 | 60 | 100 | 10 (16.7) | 0 (0) | 3 (5.0) | 2 (3.3) |
| Schomig et al[312] | 1994 | 339 | 339 | 96.5 | 21 (7.0) | 5 (1.5) | 14 (4.1) | 3 (0.8) |
| Colombo et al[82] | 1995 | 359 | 98 | 94 | 2 (2.0) | 1 (1.0) | 3 (3.0) | 1 (1.0) |
| Goy et al[313] | 1995 | 32 | 32 | 90.6 | 4 (12.5) | 2 (6.3) | 2 (6.3) | 0 (0) |

CABG, coronary artery bypass grafting; Emerg, number of patients receiving emergency stents for acute or threatened closure or suboptimal percutaneous transluminal coronary angioplasty result; NR, not reported; Q-AMI, Q-wave acute myocardial infarction.

## TABLE 28–8. WIKTOR STENT SERIES

| AUTHOR/REFERENCE | YEAR | PATIENTS | | SUCCESS (%) | THROMBOSIS: N (%) | DEATH: N (%) | Q-AMI: N (%) | CABG: N (%) |
|---|---|---|---|---|---|---|---|---|
| | | Total | Emerg | | | | | |
| Vrolix et al[314] | 1992 | 119 | 119 | 95 | 14 (11.8) | 4 (3.4) | NR | 7 (5.9) |
| Garratt et al[315] | 1993 | 125 | 125 | 95 | 4 (3.2) | 8 (6.4) | 11 (8.8) | 7 (5.6) |
| Vrolix and Piessens[316] | 1994 | 69 | 68 | 95 | 10 (16.9) | 2 (3.4) | NR | 8 (13.5) |
| Goy et al[313] | 1995 | 33 | 33 | 94 | 6 (18.1) | 3 (9.1) | 1 (3.0) | 1 (3.0) |

CABG, coronary artery bypass grafting; Emerg, number of patients receiving emergency stents for acute or threatened closure or suboptimal percutaneous transluminal coronary angioplasty result; NR, not reported; Q-AMI, Q-wave acute myocardial infarction.

## TABLE 28–9. COMBINATION STENT SERIES

| AUTHOR/REFERENCE | YEAR | STENT TYPES | PATIENTS | | SUCCESS: (%) | THROMBOSIS: N (%) | DEATH: N (%) | Q-AMI: N (%) | CABG: N (%) |
|---|---|---|---|---|---|---|---|---|---|
| | | | Total | Emerg | | | | | |
| Eeckhout et al[317] | 1994 | P/S, Wiktor, Wallstent | 123 | 38 | 100 | 6 (15.8) | 1 (2.6) | 10 (26.3) | 3 (7.9) |
| Stauffer et al[225] | 1995 | Wallstent, Wiktor, P/S | 92 | 92 | 98 | 16 (17.3) | 5 (5.4) | 14 (15.2) | 8 (8.7) |
| Van Belle et al[293] | 1995 | Wiktor, P/S, G/R | 45 | 45 | 93 | 0 (0) | 0 (0) | 2 (4.4) | 0 (0) |
| Morice et al[294] | 1995 | P/S, G/R, Wiktor, Strecker | 246 | 123 | 100 | 3 (2.4) | 2 (1.6) | 0 (0) | 2 (1.6) |
| Keelan et al[48] | 1996 | G/R, Wiktor | 271 | 157 | 86.6 | 8 (5.1) | 3 (1.9) | 10 (6.4) | 14 (8.9) |

CABG, coronary artery bypass grafting; Emerg, number of patients receiving emergency stents for acute or threatened closure or suboptimal percutaneous transluminal coronary angioplasty result; G/R, Gianturco-Roubin stent; P/S, Palmaz-Schatz stent: Q-AMI, Q-wave acute myocardial infarction.

## TABLE 28–10. OTHER STENT SERIES

| AUTHOR/REFERENCE | YEAR | STENT TYPES | PATIENTS | | SUCCESS: (%) | THROMBOSIS: N (%) | DEATH: N (%) | Q-AMI: N (%) | CABG: N (%) |
|---|---|---|---|---|---|---|---|---|---|
| | | | Total | Emerg | | | | | |
| Reifart et al[278] | 1991 | Strecker | 48 | 48 | 97 | 10 (20.8) | 5 (10.4) | 1 (2.1) | 3 (6.3) |
| Hamm et al[318] | 1995 | Strecker | 64 | 64 | 98 | 12 (18.8) | 6 (9.4) | 5 (7.8) | 13 (20.3) |
| Ozaki et al[319] | 1995 | Microstent | 20 | 19 | 96 | 0 (0) | 0 (0) | 2 (10) | 1 (5.0) |
| Tresukosol et al[287] | 1996 | Microstent | 85 | 40 | 98 | 4 (10.0) | NR | NR | NR |
| Waigand et al[320] | 1996 | ACS Multilink | 133 | 15 | 98 | 2 (13.3) | 0 (0) | 0 (0) | 0 (0) |
| Leon et al[257] | 1996 | GR II | 83 | 83 | 100 | 2 (2.4) | 0 (0) | 5 (6.0) | 1 (1.2) |

CABG, coronary artery bypass grafting; Emerg, number of patients receiving emergency stents for acute or threatened closure or suboptimal percutaneous transluminal coronary angioplasty result; NR, not reported; Q-AMI, Q-wave acute myocardial infarction.

sure were noted to have higher incidences of MI (5% vs. 1%) and a need for CABG (12% vs. 6%) than did controls. Mortality rates were similar for the two groups. More complex target lesions were associated with more frequent recurrent ischemia within 90 days of the procedure. Lesion characteristics that were associated with early recurrent ischemic events included multiple stenoses, smaller stent/artery diameter ratio, and less lesion expansion.

In a series of 500 patients, Grinstead and colleagues[254] found the risk of preexisting intracoronary thrombus could be controlled with aggressive antithrombotic therapy. All patients received heparin to achieve an activated partial thromboplastin time (APTT) greater than 2.5 times control levels and subsequently received warfarin (Coumadin) and achieved a prothrombin time (PT) greater than 18 seconds. Nath and associates[255] retrospectively examined 145 consecutive patients who underwent Gianturco-Roubin stent implantation, to evaluate the predictors of clinical sequelae after stent thrombosis at two institutions over a 1-year period of time. Multivariate analysis revealed lesion eccentricity, unstable angina, and the indication for stent implantation (abrupt closure vs. restenosis) as predictors for poststent thrombosis. Subsequent studies[46, 256] associated use of the Gianturco-Roubin stent for acute closure with a reduction in the need for emergency CABG. Lincoff and coworkers[242] performed a case-control series to demonstrate that stent placement for abrupt vessel closure resulted in less residual stenosis, a greater likelihood of TIMI-3 flow, and a reduction in the need for CABG. However, the incidences of Q-wave MI in the two groups were not significantly different (32% of stent recipients vs. 20% of controls). The relatively new GR II stent design should expand the use of the Cook stent for nonelective indications with its reduced profile, gold markers, and improved clinical outcomes.[256]

The prototype slotted-tube design is represented by the Palmaz-Schatz stent (Johnson & Johnson Interventional Systems; Warren NJ), constructed of 0.07-mm stainless steel configured into a tube with rectangular slots.[208] Encouraging results in initial small studies[257–261] led to the first multicenter study in the United States by Schatz and associates.[262] Two hundred thirteen stents were successfully implanted as a first-line therapy in 226 native coronary arteries. Eight patients had subacute closure (1 to 14 days later), but seven of these patients did not receive warfarin. Carrozza and colleagues[263] placed 250 elective Palmaz-Schatz stents in 220 patients, with 98% success, no deaths, and no Q-wave MIs. The Palmaz-Schatz stent was approved by the FDA in 1994 for use in native coronary artery lesions. Use of the Palmaz-Schatz stent has expanded to include stenosed vein grafts. Strumpf and coauthors[264] reviewed 30 stent implantations for discrete vein graft lesions; acute closure was not observed in any patient.

Two randomized studies have examined elective placement of single stents at non-restenotic lesion sites 3.0 mm or more in diameter. The Belgium-Netherlands Stent (BENESTENT) study[265, 266] randomly assigned 259 patients to receive the Palmaz-Schatz stent and 257 patients to undergo conventional angioplasty. The Stent Restenosis Study (STRESS)[17] randomly assigned 205 patients to receive the Palmaz-Schatz stent and 202 to undergo PTCA; a significant difference in angiographic outcome (96.1% vs. 89.6%) was demonstrated in favor of the stent. In both trials, stent recipients had a larger lumen diameter after the procedure than did the PTCA controls. No systematic approach to detect MI was used in either of these trials. The observed clinical benefit of the stent largely reflected a reduced need for repeat revascularization.

Table 28–7 summarizes the emergency Palmaz-Schatz stent experience for acute and threatened closure. Using logistic regression analysis, Herrmann and colleagues[267] concluded that the presence of angiographically visible thrombi after stenting was the only significant predictor of subacute stent thrombosis. Other proposed predictors of Palmaz-Schatz stent–related thrombosis include poor flow in the stented vessel, preexisting intraluminal thrombi, small vessel size, increased platelet count, multiple overlapping stents, stent-to-vessel diameter mismatch, and stent length. Patients who received Palmaz-Schatz stents on an emergency basis, especially those with acute closure, were at a higher risk for acute complications and required more careful anticoagulation and clinical follow-up.

The Wiktor stent (Medtronic, Inc.; Minneapolis MN) is an intradigitating, self-expanding tantalum stent. The first 50 patients underwent implantation for restenosis prophylaxis.[268] Five patients experienced acute thrombotic stent occlusion and subsequent nonfatal MI. Major bleeding complications occurred in 11 patients. Subsequent follow-up study in a larger cohort reported in an abstract by Burger and coauthors[269] reviewed the results of the Wiktor stent in 119 patients in native arteries. Implantation was successful in 98%. Anticoagulation therapy consisted of dextran, heparin, aspirin, and warfarin. Acute stent occlusion occurred in 3%, and subacute stent occlusion developed between days 3 and 14 in 8%, resulting in MI in four patients after acute occlusion and in six of nine patients after subacute stent occlusion, necessitating emergency bypass surgery in 2 patients (2%). Six-month angiographic follow-up was performed in 94% of patients and revealed restenosis in 37%. Table 28–8 summarizes the Wiktor stent experience.

**CLOSURE AFTER CORONARY STENT PLACEMENT.** Acute and subacute stent thrombosis accounted for most ischemic complications in early trials,[81, 270, 271] with an incidence of 0.4% to 33%.[15, 47, 83, 247, 249, 262, 263, 267, 268, 270, 272–281] Although redilatation of the stent-implanted segment[15, 255] and local thrombolytic therapy often restored patency, there was an initial learning period with stents during which unsuccessful deployment and stent thrombosis were more common.[262, 282] Important predictors of thrombosis included stent size, presence of post–stent implantation residual dissection, and post–stent implantation residual filling defects.[47, 280, 283] By these criteria, Liu and coworkers[47] categorized 1318 patients receiving Gianturco-Roubin stents into low-risk (no risk factors), intermediate-risk (one risk factor), and high-risk (two or three risk factors) groups; the respective incidences of thrombosis were 5.6%, 9.4%, and 16.7%. Stent composition (stainless steel vs. tantalum) did not affect the thrombogenicity of identical designs.[284] Outcomes improved when stents completely covered dissections[47, 83, 285] and were completely expanded.[285] Risk of stent thrombosis discouraged use of smaller stents (<3.0 mm)[25, 47] in early experience, but later reports have been encouraging.[48, 285–287] Tables 28–9 and 28–10 summarize later clinical data for emergency stent placement.

Early rates of stent thrombosis encouraged the use of aggressive anticoagulation regimens with dextran 40, dipyridamole, aspirin, heparin, and warfarin.[48, 281, 288] Vascular complications were more likely with aggressive anticoagulation[289] and were more common in the early stent experience.[290] Fail and associates[291] noted fewer vascular complications with subcutaneous heparin administration than with intravenous heparin therapy, whereas the incidence of acute closure remained constant.

The incidence of stent thrombosis decreased markedly with improved antiplatelet therapy.[204, 205, 292] Protocols eliminated dextran 40 and dipyridamole and substituted ticlopidine for warfarin,[82, 281, 293, 294] reducing the incidence of stent thrombosis to between 0% and 6% (average 1.3%) in later trials.[281] The Intracoronary and Antithrombotic Regimen (ISAR) trial[295] randomly assigned 517 patients to receive either antiplatelet therapy with aspirin and ticlopidine or anticoagulant therapy with heparin, phenprocoumon, and aspirin. The antiplatelet recipients had a significant 82% risk reduction in MI, a 78% lower need for repeat interventions, and a reduced rate of stent occlusion (0.8% vs. 5.4%). Many operators have subsequently reduced the intensity of anticoagulation in selected patients at low risk for stent thrombosis.[190] Some have used low molecular weight heparin for 1 month in addition to ticlopidine.[294]

Intravascular stent placement remains the focus of considerable ongoing investigation featured elsewhere within this textbook. Stents have been electively deployed for recalcitrant restenotic lesions and placed on an emergency basis for abrupt or threatened closure. The deployment of multiple tandem stents has become common, and several authors have employed dissimilar tandem stents for long dissections.[296, 297] Scott and associates[298] seeded stents with immortalized human dermal microvascular endothelial cells to reduce stent thrombogenic potential, with recovery of human cells from a porcine experimental model. Biodegradable stents have been proposed as an alternative to metallic devices.[299] An adjustable temporary stent catheter has also been described.[300] By 1996, 18 stent patterns, including coils, self-expanding forms, and pharmacologically active stents bonded with heparin or radioactivity, were either approved or under investigation.[190, 208] Further studies will explore combinations of stent therapy with other technologies (atherectomy, ELCA, TEC procedures) to maximize luminal diameter.

## Summary

Limiting the duration of ischemia remains the key to management of abrupt closure. Delay between vessel closure and reperfusion worsens outcome. In the past, management algorithms were poorly defined.[175] Figure 28–4 summarizes one approach to the management of acute and threatened closure from a major dissection; other approaches have been described.[16] Patients with threatened closure often remain asymptomatic and should receive heparin for an additional 24 to 48 hours after sheath removal. Repeat angiography and intervention may be required if symptoms or hemodynamic compromise develops. The therapeutic approach to major coronary dissection and acute closure includes several strategies. Figure 28–4 highlights the expanding role of coronary stents for this situation. Intracoronary nitroglycerin should be initially administered for potentially reversible vasospasm. A coronary guide wire should traverse the lesion if one is not already in place. Redilatation with a standard or perfusion balloon catheter should be considered.[251, 301–306] If an initial 10- to 15-minute inflation improves flow and angiographic lesion appearance, repeat inflation exceeding 15 minutes may be performed. Prolonged inflation results in successful angioplasty in 75% to 80% of major dissections and in a lower complication rate than does standard inflation. Directional atherectomy of dissection flaps has been successful but carries a risk of vessel perforation.

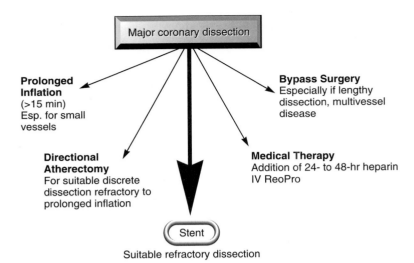

FIGURE 28–4. Management of major dissection complicating percutaneous transluminal coronary angioplasty.

Lesions refractory to prolonged inflation may improve with intracoronary stenting. By displacing large plaques or dissection flaps, stents create a smooth luminal surface without impeding forward flow. Implantation should be considered for refractory acute occlusions in the proximal portion of a vessel, in vessels larger than 2.5 mm in diameter, and in vessels that have adequate distal runoff. Stents should be implanted for dissection only when the limits of the flap can be clearly delineated. Stent placement should be avoided at severe angulation points or in vessels with severe proximal vessel tortuosity. Stent devices should be used with care during acute MI.[80, 307] The initial Wallstent model[247, 249, 308, 309] has been followed by coil[15, 46–48, 242, 243, 253–256, 286, 307] and slotted-tube designs.[82, 83, 225, 246, 267, 272–274, 278, 293, 294, 310–313, 317] Experience with other stent designs continues to accumulate.[278, 287, 314–316, 318–322] Thrombolytic and antiplatelet therapy have significantly improved outcomes after stent implantation. Contraindications to antiplatelet and anticoagulant therapy increase the risk of stenting. These include bleeding diathesis, thrombocytopenia, platelet dysfunction, anemia of unknown origin, active peptic ulcer, menstruation, diabetic retinopathy, disseminated neoplasia, and chronic pulmonary or gastrointestinal inflammatory disease. Long-term outcomes for intracoronary stents will ultimately be determined by further randomized clinical trials.

Intra-aortic balloon counterpulsation and the use of abciximab may also improve outcome. CABG may be needed for patients with lengthy dissections, critical side branches, or hemodynamic instability. Emergency bypass surgery may be required if catheter-based strategies are contraindicated or unsuccessful.

## CORONARY PERFORATION

A potentially catastrophic complication, coronary perforation, may engender localized pseudoaneurysm, perivascular hematoma, arterioventricular fistula, or hemopericardium.[323] Clinical sequelae include cardiac tamponade (17% to 24%), MI (19% to 26%), and death (5% to 9%).[324, 325] Ischemic events arise from either decreased distal perfusion pressure or tamponade of the artery by perivascular hematoma. The degree of contrast extravasation seen on angiography may reflect the likelihood of immediate complications. One proposed classification distinguishes fully contained perforations (type I) from cases with limited (type II) and brisk (type III) extravasation.[325] Types I and II perforations entail a lower incidence of adverse outcomes than do type III perforations. However, delayed cardiac tamponade may present 8 to 24 hours after an angiographically inapparent perforation.[324, 325] Fortunately, coronary perforation is extremely rare after interventional procedures.[324–331] The incidence of perforation is higher for patients treated with newer devices, patients with complex lesions, women, and the elderly.[325] Other characteristics that contribute to perforation risk include extensive dissection, significant vessel angulation, high inflation pressures, and inappropriate size of the interventional device.

## Incidence

The reported rate of coronary perforation complicating PTCA ranges from less than 0.1% to 0.2%.[4, 324, 325] Balloon dilatation infrequently disrupts the adventitia, although intimal and medial injury often occur. Perforation during PTCA usually results from guide wire–induced trauma, balloon rupture, or balloon oversizing.[325] Early experience reported in the NHLBI PTCA Registry showed that perforation occurred in 2 of 3079 patients undergoing balloon angioplasty.[4] Ajluni and coauthors reported perforations in 11 (0.14%) of 7905 PTCA patients treated between 1988 and 1992.[324] Similarly, Ellis and associates[325] reported 14 perforations (0.15%) in 9080

PTCA patients between 1990 and 1991. Increasing lesion complexity and broadening of patient populations over time may explain the higher incidence of perforations in later series.

Newer laser and atherectomy procedures are associated with perforation rates approximately 10 to 100 times higher than those rates with balloon angioplasty.[232, 233, 324, 325, 332] Coronary perforation complicated directional atherectomy in approximately 1.3% of 1041 lesions reviewed by Vetter and colleagues[232] and 0.7% of 1715 patients studied by Ellis and associates[325] Perforation rates were 0.6% in the U.S. Directional Atherectomy Group Registry and 0.4% in the CAVEAT trial and have ranged between 0.5% and 1% in other reports.[148, 241, 333, 334] The cutting mechanism of directional atherectomy often produces deep arterial injury with seemingly high perforation potential[130, 333] (Fig. 28–5). The observed incidence of perforation is remarkably low, in view of the fact that adventitia is recovered in 25% to 30% of procedures.[148, 335] Hemopericardium or tamponade occurred in less than 0.1% of the multicenter participants.[322] Perforation may occur more commonly when directional atherectomy is employed for the treatment of balloon angioplasty–induced flaps or major dissections.[148] A case of coronary perforation from disruption of the cutter drive cable in an angulated lesion was reported.[333] Future devices with improved delivery systems and integrated ultrasound guidance may reduce the risk of perforation by directing cuts away from uninvolved vessel wall and optimizing plaque removal.

Transluminal extraction-endarterectomy with the TEC device was initially associated with less than a 1% incidence of coronary perforation.[149, 336] Lau and Sigwart[241] reported an incidence between 1% and 2% in 1992. More recent estimates suggest a perforation rate between 1.3%[324] and 2.1%.[325] Kaplan and colleagues documented a 2% incidence of contained perforations but no free perforations that necessitated pericardiocentesis.[173]

Rotational ablation does not usually injure deep arterial layers[163] and has rarely been associated with perforation.[241, 324] In a series of 400 stenoses randomly selected from the initial Rotablator experience, the perforation rate was 1.5%.[337] Ellis and associates[325] noted 10 perforations (1.3%) in a series of 771 patients. Analysis of 3717 lesions in 2953 patients listed by the U.S. Multicenter Registry for Rotational Ablation revealed perforations in 0.6% of lesions and 0.7% of patients.[338] Perforation was significantly more common in the right (1.1%) and circumflex (1.2%) coronary arteries than in the left anterior descending (0.06%) or left main coronary (0%) vessels. The risk of perforation was higher in eccentric, tortuous, and long lesions. Using the same multicenter registry data, MacIsaac and colleagues[160] noted that perforation complicated rotational atherectomy in 5 (0.46%) of 1078 calcified lesions and in 11 (1.02%) of 1083 noncalcified lesions.

Estimates of perforation associated with ELCA have ranged from 1% to 7.7%.[241, 339] The most data suggest a rate of approximately 2%.[142, 324, 325] The frequency of perforation may be declining over time with increasing operator experience. Holmes and coworkers noted that coronary artery perforations occurred in 1.6% of 1888 initial patients, in comparison with 0.4% of 1000 subsequent patients in a

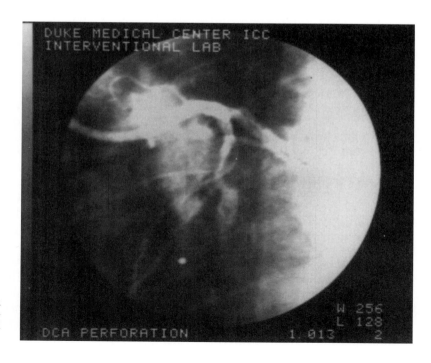

FIGURE 28–5. Angiogram of coronary perforation of the mid–left anterior descending coronary artery after directional atherectomy with pericardial contrast staining.

multicenter registry.[340] The overall risks of needing CABG (41%), MI (16%), and death (6%) were significantly higher for ELCA patients with perforation than for those without.[339] In vitro models of perforation sites have been characterized by extensive calcific deposits and pronounced lesion tortuosity.[341] However, this finding has been difficult to confirm in practice. Two series[140, 340] have been unable to detect statistically significant characteristics in lesion morphology in ELCA patients who experience coronary perforations.

It remains unclear whether coronary stent placement is associated with an increased risk of coronary perforation in comparison with PTCA. An oversized Strecker stent led to coronary perforation in an experimental sheep model.[342] Shammas and coauthors[343] described perforation of a saphenous vein graft after deployment of a Palmaz-Schatz biliary stent. Mendzelevski and Sigwart[344] reported coronary artery perforation during attempted implantation of multiple self-expanding Wallstents. Several reports have highlighted the risk of perforation from the high-pressure balloon inflations used for stent optimization.[329, 345–347] The risk of stent-related perforation can be minimized with appropriate sizing of stent and balloon devices.

## Management

The management of coronary perforation depends on the severity of the perforation and degree of communication with the pericardial space. Some patients have simply needed anticoagulation reversal after perforation from guide wire advancement.[348, 349] Mild pseudoaneurysms can be sealed with prolonged inflations,[325, 346] often by means of perfusion balloon catheters.[323, 343, 348–351] In one series of 36 cases, coronary perforation after ELCA was treated with repeat balloon angioplasty in 26 patients; 15 did not require CABG or develop MI.[340] Expectant therapy requires careful monitoring; the accompanying risk of delayed tamponade may approach 10%.[324, 325] For patients with hemopericardium, percutaneous drainage with or without emergency CABG for treatment of coronary perforation has been widely reported.[330, 331, 350, 352]

Significant pseudoaneurysms found immediately after interventional procedures usually represent contained perforations and warrant early repair. Surgical approaches to coronary perforation have included suture or vein patch closure, ligation of the coronary artery, and CABG.[28, 183, 329, 353–356] A common technique combines ligation of the coronary artery proximal and distal to the perforation with bypass of the perforated segment.[353, 355] Coronary ligation may sacrifice flow to important side branches, prompting some authors to advocate CABG alone.[356]

Alternatively, Dralle and coauthors[355] described plication of a coronary aneurysm in combination with mammary graft placement. Preserved coronary patency and continued antegrade coronary flow may reduce the immediate demands on the distal bypass conduit. Overall, it remains to be determined which of these approaches yields optimal clinical outcomes.

Innovative percutaneous approaches to the management of coronary perforation have included microcoil vessel occlusion and the use of intracoronary stents. Some operators have applied these strategies on an emergency basis, whereas others have performed delayed repair under less urgent circumstances. Dorros and associates[329] described occlusion of ruptured coronary branches with microcoils (Cook; Bloomington IN) in two patients. Finch and Krouse[326] employed small, complex, helical platinum coils (Target Therapeutics; Freemont CA) and absorbable gelatin sponge (Gelfoam, Upjohn; Kalamazoo MI) to embolize a small branch perforated by a guide wire. Both groups of investigators performed pericardiocentesis before addressing the perforation. In a delayed procedure, Saito and colleagues[357] treated an 18 × 13 mm pseudoaneurysm by using microcoil techniques 1 month after an initial coronary rupture.

Several authors have used intracoronary stents to close coronary perforations and pseudoaneurysms. In a patient with intrapericardial hemorrhage after PTCA, Thomas and Wainwright sealed a pinhole coronary rupture with a Palmaz-Schatz stent and averted cardiac surgery.[358] The perforation was thought to be secondary to a transluminal dissection with extension into the pericardial space. Rath and Tripathy[359] implanted a Palmaz-Schatz stent to manage a similar perforation on an emergency basis. Vein-covered stents have attracted interest for percutaneous perforation management.[360] Dorros and associates[329] covered a P104 Palmaz stent (Johnson & Johnson Interventional Systems Co.; Warren NJ) with autologous cephalic vein to close a coronary perforation. Two subsequent reports also described emergency repair of refractory coronary perforation with vein-covered Palmaz stents.[347, 361] Using a Palmaz 154M stent (Johnson & Johnson Interventional Systems Co.; Warren NJ) covered with antecubital vein, Colon and coworkers[362] repaired a saphenous vein graft perforated during a TEC procedure. In separate reports, Kaplan and colleagues[363] and Wong and associates[364] sutured autologous vein to 20-mm articulated PS 204 biliary stents (Johnson & Johnson Interventional Systems Co.; Warren NJ). These devices sealed coronary perforations and pseudoaneurysms during delayed repairs that occurred approximately 1 month after initial atherectomy injury.

Coronary perforation remains a rare but serious

complication of angioplasty and atherectomy. Conservative management and expectant management continue to be successful strategies for selected cases. High-risk patients need prompt therapy. The introduction of new devices with increased perforation rates has spurred development of novel management approaches. IVUS[363, 364] and angioscopy[355] can supplement angiographic determination of vascular injury and adequacy of repair. Refinements to operative and percutaneous techniques may facilitate early, definitive treatment and improve interventional outcomes.

# REFERENCES

1. Gruentzig AR, Senning A, Siegenthaler WE: Nonoperative dilatation of coronary artery stenosis: Percutaneous transluminal coronary angioplasty. N Engl J Med 301:61, 1979.
2. Detre K, Holubkov R, Kelsey S, et al: Percutaneous transluminal coronary angioplasty in 1985–1986 and 1977–1981. N Engl J Med 318:265, 1988.
3. Ellis SG, Roubin GS, King SB III, et al: Angiographic and clinical predictors of acute closure after native vessel coronary angioplasty. Circulation 77:372, 1988.
4. Cowley MJ, Dorros G, Kelsey SF, et al: Acute coronary events associated with percutaneous transluminal coronary angioplasty. Am J Cardiol 53(suppl):12C, 1984.
5. Ischinger T, Gruentzig AR, Meier B, et al: Coronary dissection and total coronary occlusion associated with percutaneous transluminal coronary angioplasty: Significance of initial angiographic morphology of coronary stenoses. Circulation 74:1371, 1986.
6. Simpfendorfer C, Belardi J, Bellamy G, et al: Frequency, management and follow-up of patients with acute coronary occlusions after percutaneous transluminal coronary angioplasty. Am J Cardiol 59:267, 1987.
7. Black AJR, Namay DL, Niederman AL, et al: Tear or dissection after coronary angioplasty: Morphologic correlates of an ischemic complication. Circulation 79:1035, 1989.
8. Detre KM, Holmes DR Jr, Holubkov R, et al: Incidence and consequences of periprocedural occlusion: The 1985–1986 National Heart, Lung, and Blood Institute Percutaneous Transluminal Coronary Angioplasty Registry. Circulation 82:739, 1990.
9. de Feyter PJ, van den Brand M, Jaarman G, et al: Acute coronary artery occlusion during and after percutaneous transluminal coronary angioplasty: Frequency, prediction, clinical course, management, and follow-up. Circulation 83:927, 1991.
10. Waller BF, Orr CM, Pinkerton CA, et al: Coronary balloon angioplasty dissections: "The good, the bad and the ugly." J Am Coll Cardiol 20:701, 1992.
11. Dorros G, Cowley MJ, Simpson J, et al: Percutaneous transluminal coronary angioplasty: Report of complications from the National Heart, Lung, and Blood Institute PTCA Registry. Circulation 67:723, 1983.
12. Goldbaum T, DiSciascio G, Cowie MJ, et al: Early occlusion following successful coronary angioplasty: Clinical and angiographic observations. Catheter Cardiovasc Diagn 17:22, 1989.
13. Sinclair IN, McCabe CH, Sipperly ME, et al: Predictors, therapeutic options and long-term outcome of abrupt reclosure. Am J Cardiol 61(suppl):61G, 1988.
14. Ellis SG, Vandormael MG, Cowley MJ, et al: Coronary morphologic and clinical determinants of procedural outcome with angioplasty for multivessel coronary disease: Implications for patient selection. Circulation 82:1193, 1990.
15. Roubin GS, Cannon AD, Agrawal SK, et al: Intracoronary stenting for acute and threatened closure complicating percutaneous transluminal coronary angioplasty. Circulation 85:916, 1992.
16. de Feyter PJ, de Jaegere PT, Serruys PW: Incidence, predictors, and management of acute coronary occlusion after coronary angioplasty. Am Heart J 127:643, 1994.
17. Fischman DL, Leon MB, Baim DS, et al: A randomized comparison of coronary stent placement and balloon angioplasty in the treatment of coronary artery disease. N Engl J Med 331:489, 1994.
18. Myler RK, Shaw RE, Stertzer SH, et al: Lesion morphology and coronary angioplasty—Current experience and analysis. J Am Coll Cardiol 19:1641, 1992.
19. Ellis SG, Roubin GS, King SB III, et al: In-hospital cardiac mortality of acute coronary angioplasty: Analysis of risk factors from 80 procedures. J Am Coll Cardiol 11:211, 1988.
20. Marquis JF, Schwartz L, Aldridge H, et al: Acute coronary artery occlusion during percutaneous transluminal coronary angioplasty treated by redilatation of the occluded segment. J Am Coll Cardiol 4:1268, 1984.
21. Buccino KR, Brenner AS, Browne KF: Acute reocclusion during percutaneous transluminal coronary angioplasty: Immediate and long-term outcome. Catheter Cardiovasc Diagn 17:75, 1989.
22. Topol EJ: Emerging strategies for failed percutaneous transluminal coronary angioplasty. Am J Cardiol 63:249, 1989.
23. Tenaglia AN, Fortin DF, Frid DJ, et al: Long-term outcome following successful reopening of abrupt closure after coronary angioplasty. Am J Cardiol 72:21, 1993.
24. Lincoff AM, Popma JJ, Ellis SG, et al: Abrupt vessel closure complicating coronary angioplasty: Clinical, angiographic and therapeutic profile. J Am Coll Cardiol 19:926, 1992.
25. Danchin N, Daclin V, Juillière Y, et al: Changes in patient treatment after abrupt closure complicating percutaneous transluminal coronary angioplasty: A historic perspective. Am Heart J 130:1158, 1995.
26. Holmes DR, Simpson JB, Berdan JG, et al: Abrupt closure: The CAVEAT I experience. J Am Coll Cardiol 26:1494, 1995.
27. Holmes DR Jr, Holubkov R, Vlietstra RE, et al: Comparison of complications during percutaneous transluminal coronary angioplasty from 1977 to 1981 and from 1985 to 1986: The National Heart, Lung, and Blood Institute Percutaneous Transluminal Coronary Angioplasty Registry. J Am Coll Cardiol 12:1149, 1988.
28. Topaz O, Salter D, Janin Y, et al: Emergency bypass surgery for failed coronary interventions. Catheter Cardiovasc Diagn 40:55, 1997.
29. Breedlau CE, Roubin GS, Leimgruber PP: In-hospital morbidity and mortality in patients undergoing elective coronary angioplasty. Circulation 72:1044, 1985.
30. O'Keefe JH, Hartzler GO, Rutherford BD: Left main coronary angioplasty: Early and late results of 127 acute and elective procedures. Am J Cardiol 64:144, 1989.
31. Hartzler GO, Rutherford BD, McConahay DR: High risk percutaneous transluminal coronary angioplasty. Am J Cardiol 61:33, 1988.
32. Brodie BR, Grines CL, Ivanhoe R et al: Six-month clinical and angiographic follow-up after direct angioplasty for acute myocardial infarction. Circulation 25:156, 1994.
33. Simpfendorfer C: Acute coronary occlusion after percutaneous transluminal coronary angioplasty. Cleve Clin J Med 55:429, 1988.
34. Gaul G, Holiman J, Simpfendorfer C, et al: Acute occlusion in multiple lesion coronary angioplasty: Frequency and management. J Am Coll Cardiol 13:283, 1989.
35. Nobuyoshi M, Kimura T, Ohishi H, et al: Restenosis after percutaneous transluminal coronary angioplasty: Pathologic observations in 20 patients. J Am Coll Cardiol 17:433, 1991.
36. Quigley PJ, Hlatky MA, Hinohara T, et al: Repeat percutaneous transluminal coronary angioplasty and predictors of recurrent restenosis. Am J Cardiol 63:409, 1989.
37. Leimgruber PP, Roubin GS, Anderson HV, et al: Influence of intimal dissection on restenosis after successful coronary angioplasty. Circulation 72:530, 1985.
38. Black AJR, Anderson HV, Roubin GS, et al: Repeat coronary angioplasty: Correlates of a second restenosis. J Am Coll Cardiol 11:714, 1988.
39. Hermans WRM, Rensing BJ, Foley DP, et al: Therapeutic dissection after successful coronary balloon angioplasty: No

influence on restenosis or on clinical outcome in 693 patients. J Am Coll Cardiol 20:767, 1992.

40. Noveck HD, Klein LW, Kramer B, et al: Balloon dilatation of symptomatic subacute intimal dissection presenting as restenosis. Am J Cardiol 64:980, 1989.

41. Huber MS, Mooney JF, Madison J, et al: Use of a morphologic classification to predict clinical outcome after dissection from coronary angioplasty. Am J Cardiol 68:467, 1991.

42. Banka VS, Kochar GS, Maniet AR, et al: Progressive coronary dilation: An angioplasty technique that creates controlled arterial injury and reduces complications. Am Heart J 125:61, 1993.

43. Boston DR, Malouf A, Barry WH: Management of intracoronary thrombosis complicating percutaneous transluminal coronary angioplasty. Clin Cardiol 19:536, 1996.

44. Rehr R, DiSciascio G, Vetrovec G, et al: Angiographic morphology of coronary artery stenoses in prolonged rest angina: Evidence of intracoronary thrombosis. J Am Coll Cardiol 14:1429, 1989.

45. Mabin TA, Holmes DR Jr, Smith HC, et al: Intracoronary thrombus: Role of coronary occlusion complicating percutaneous transluminal coronary angioplasty. J Am Coll Cardiol 5:198, 1985.

46. George BS, Voorhees WD III, Roubin GS, et al: Multicenter investigation of coronary stenting to treat acute or threatened closure after percutaneous transluminal coronary angioplasty: Clinical and angiographic outcomes. J Am Coll Cardiol 22:135, 1993.

47. Liu MW, Voorhees WD III, Agrawal S, et al: Stratification of the risk of thrombosis after intracoronary stenting for threatened or acute closure complicating coronary balloon angioplasty: A Cook registry study. Am Heart J 130:8, 1995.

48. Keelan ET, Bailey KR, Garratt KN, et al: Impact of stent size and indication for stent placement on immediate outcome. Catheter Cardiovasc Diagn 28:145, 1996.

49. Krucoff MW, Parente AR, Bottner RK, et al: Stability of multilead ST segment fingerprints over time after percutaneous transluminal coronary angioplasty and its usefulness in detecting reocclusion. Am J Cardiol 61:1232, 1988.

50. Baughman KL, Pasternak RC, Fallon JT, et al: Transluminal coronary angioplasty of postmortem human hearts. Am J Cardiol 48:1044, 1981.

51. Kinney TB, Chin AK, Rurick GW, et al: Transluminal angioplasty: A mechanical-pathophysiological correlation of its physical mechanisms. Radiology 153:85, 1984.

52. Saffitz JE, Totty WG, McClennan BL, et al: Percutaneous transluminal angioplasty: Radiological-pathological correlation. Radiology 141:651, 1981.

53. Zafins CK, Lu CT, Gewertz BL, et al: Arterial disruption and remodeling following balloon angioplasty. Surgery 91:1086, 1982.

54. Block PC, Baughman KL, Pasternak RC, et al: Transluminal angioplasty: Correlation of morphologic and angiographic findings in an experimental model. Circulation 61:778, 1980.

55. Pasternak RC, Baughman KL, Fallon JT, et al: Scanning electron microscopy after coronary transluminal angioplasty of normal canine arteries. Am J Cardiol 45:591, 1980.

56. Casteneda-Zuniga WR, Formanek A, Tadavarthy M, et al: The mechanism of balloon angioplasty. Radiology 135:565, 1980.

57. Block PC, Myler RK, Stertzer S, et al: Morphology after transluminal angioplasty in humans. N Engl J Med 305:382, 1981.

58. Faxon DP, Weber VJ, Haudenschild C, et al: Acute effects of transluminal angioplasty in three experimental models of atherosclerosis. Arteriosclerosis 2:125, 1982.

59. Sanborn TA, Faxon DP, Haudenschild C, et al: The mechanism of transluminal angioplasty: Evidence for formation of aneurysms in experimental atherosclerosis. Circulation 68:1136, 1983.

60. Steele PM, Chesbro JH, Stanson AW, et al: Balloon angioplasty: Natural history of the pathophysiological response to injury in a pig model. Circ Res 57:105, 1985.

61. Waller BF: "Crackers, breakers, stretchers, drillers, scrapers, shavers, burners, welders and melters"—The future treatment of atherosclerotic coronary artery disease? A clinical morphologic assessment. J Am Coll Cardiol 13:969, 1989.

62. Waller BF, Pinkerton CA, Orr CM, et al: Restenosis 1 to 24 months after clinically successful coronary balloon angioplasty: A necropsy study of 20 patients. J Am Coll Cardiol 17(suppl):58B, 1991.

63. Potkin BN, Roberts WC: Effects of percutaneous transluminal coronary angioplasty on the atherosclerotic plaque and relation of plaque composition and arterial size to outcome. Am J Cardiol 62:41, 1988.

64. Hokchi K, Takebayashi S, Block PC, et al: Arterial changes after percutaneous transluminal coronary angioplasty: Results at autopsy. J Am Coll Cardiol 10:592, 1987.

65. Uchida Y, Hasegawa K, Kawamure K, et al: Angioscopic observation of coronary luminal changes induced by percutaneous transluminal coronary angioplasty. Am Heart J 117:769, 1989.

66. Fischell TA, Derby G, Tse TM, et al: Coronary artery vasoconstriction routinely occurs after percutaneous transluminal coronary angioplasty. A quantitative arteriographic analysis. Circulation 78:1323, 1988.

67. Rensing BJ, Hermans WRM, Beatt KJ, et al: Quantitative angiographic assessment of elastic recoil after percutaneous transluminal coronary angioplasty. Am J Cardiol 66:1039, 1990.

68. Waller BF, Fry ET, Peters TF, et al: Abrupt (<1 day), acute (<1 week), and early (<1 month) vessel closure at the angioplasty site: Morphologic observations and causes of closure in 130 necropsy patients undergoing coronary angioplasty. Clin Cardiol 19:857, 1996.

69. Shea PJ: Mechanical right coronary artery shortening and vessel wall invagination: A fourth cause of iatrogenic coronary obstruction during coronary angioplasty. Catheter Cardiovasc Diagn 26:136, 1992.

70. Tobis JM, Mallery JA, Gessert J, et al: Intravascular ultrasound cross-sectional arterial imaging before and after balloon angioplasty in vitro. Circulation 80:873, 1989.

71. de Feyter PJ, de Jaegere PT, Murphy ES, et al: Abrupt coronary artery occlusion during percutaneous transluminal coronary angioplasty. Am Heart J 123:1633, 1992.

72. Waller BF, Orr CM, Slack JD, et al: Anatomy, histology, and pathology of coronary arteries: A review relevant to new interventional and imaging techniques—Part III. Clin Cardiol 15:607, 1992.

73. Nissen SE, De Franco AC, Tuzcu EM, et al: Coronary intravascular ultrasound: Diagnostic and interventional applications. Coron Artery Dis 6:355, 1995.

74. Emanuelsson H: Future challenges to coronary angioplasty: Perspectives on intracoronary imaging and physiology. J Intern Med 238:111, 1995.

75. Arnet EN, Isner JM, Redwood DR, et al: Coronary narrowing in coronary heart disease: Comparison of cineangiographic and necropsy findings. Ann Intern Med 91:350, 1979.

76. Vlodaver A, Frech R, Van Tassel RA, et al: Correlation of the antemortem coronary arteriogram and the postmortem specimen. Circulation 47:162, 1973.

77. Baptista J, Umans VA, di Mario C, et al: Mechanisms of luminal enlargement and quantification of vessel wall trauma following balloon coronary angioplasty and directional atherectomy: A study using intracoronary ultrasound, angioscopy, and angiography. Eur Heart J 16:1603, 1995.

78. Davidson CJ, Sheikh KH, Kisslo KB, et al: Intracoronary ultrasound evaluation of interventional technologies. Am J Cardiol 68:1305, 1991.

79. Tenaglia AN, Buller CE, Kisslo KB, et al: Intracoronary ultrasound predictors of adverse outcomes after coronary artery interventions. J Am Coll Cardiol 20:1385, 1992.

80. Walton AS, Oesterle SN, Yeung AC: Coronary artery stenting for acute closure complicating primary angioplasty for acute myocardial infarction. Catheter Cardiovasc Diagn 34:142, 1995.

81. Nakamura S, Colombo A, Gaglione A, et al: Intracoronary ultrasound observations during stent implantation. Circulation 89:2026, 1994.

82. Colombo A, Hall P, Nakamura S, et al: Intracoronary stent-

ing without anticoagulation performed with intravascular ultrasound guidance. Circulation 91:1676, 1995.

83. Colombo A, Goldberg SL, Almagor Y, et al: A novel strategy for stent deployment in the treatment of acute or threatened closure complicating balloon coronary angioplasty. Use of short or standard (or both) single or multiple Palmaz-Schatz stents. J Am Coll Cardiol 22:1887, 1993.

84. Painter JA, Mintz CTS, Wong SC, et al: Intravascular ultrasound assessment of biliary stent implantation in saphenous vein graft lesions. J Am Coll Cardiol 23(suppl):136A, 1994.

85. Colombo A, Hall P, Almagor Y, et al: Results of intravascular ultrasound guided coronary stenting without subsequent anticoagulation [Abstract]. J Am Coll Cardiol 23:335A, 1994.

86. Mizuno K, Miyamoto A, Satomura K, et al: Angioscopic coronary macromorphology in patients with acute coronary disorders. Lancet 337:809, 1991.

87. Mizuno K, Satomura K, Miyamoto A, et al: Angioscopic evaluation of coronary artery thrombi in acute coronary syndromes. N Engl J Med 326:287, 1992.

88. Siegel RJ, Ariani M, Fishbein FC, et al: Histopathologic validation of angioscopy and intravascular ultrasound. Circulation 84:109, 1991.

89. Lee G, Garcia JM, Corso PJ: Correlation of coronary angioscopic to angiographic findings in coronary artery disease. Am J Cardiol 58:238, 1986.

90. Siegel RJ, Chae JS, Forrester JS, et al: Angiography, angioscopy, and ultrasound imaging before and after percutaneous balloon angioplasty. Am Heart J 120:1086, 1990.

91. DenHeijer P, Foley DP, Hillege HL, et al: The Ermenonville classification of observations at coronary angioscopy—Evaluation of intra- and inter-observer agreement. Eur Heart J 15:815, 1994.

92. Johnson C, Hanson DD, Vracko R, et al: Angioscopy is more sensitive for identifying thrombus, distal emboli, and subintimal dissection [Abstract]. J Am Coll Cardiol 13:146A, 1989.

93. Van Stiegmann G, Pearce WH, Bartle EJ, et al: Flexible angioscopy seems faster and more specific than arteriography. Arch Surg 122:279, 1987.

94. White CW, Wright CB, Doty DB, et al: Does visual interpretation of the coronary arteriogram predict the physiologic importance of a coronary stenosis? N Engl J Med, 310:819, 1984.

95. Donohue TJ, Kern MJ: Intracoronary Doppler. Coron Artery Dis 6:381, 1995.

96. Wilson RF, Lauglin DE, Ackell PH, et al: Transluminal subselective measurement of coronary artery blood flow velocity and vasodilator reserve in man. Circulation 72:82, 1985.

97. Sibley DH, Millar HD, Hartley CJ, et al: Subselective measurement of coronary blood flow velocity using a steerable Doppler catheter. J Am Coll Cardiol 8:1332, 1986.

98. Sunamura M, di Mario C, Piek JJ, et al: Cyclic flow variations after angioplasty: A rare phenomenon predictive of immediate complications. DEBATE Investigator's Group. Am Heart J 131:843, 1996.

99. Kern MJ, Aguirre FV, Donohue TJ, et al: Continuous coronary flow velocity monitoring during coronary interventions: Velocity trend patterns associated with adverse events. Am Heart J 128:426, 1994.

100. Chornenky VI: Low-coherence interferometry in coronary arteries. Coron Artery Dis 6:377, 1995.

101. Brezinski ME, Tearney GJ, Bouma BE, et al: Imaging of coronary microstructure (in vitro) with optical coherence tomography. Am J Cardiol 77:92, 1996.

102. Brezinski ME, Tearney GJ, Bouma BE, et al: Optical coherence tomography for optical biopsy: Properties and demonstration of vascular pathology. Circulation 93:1206, 1996.

103. Liu MW, Roubin GS, King SB: Restenosis after coronary angioplasty: Potential biologic determinants and role of intimal hyperplasia. Circulation 79:1374, 1989.

104. Arora RR, Platko WP, Bhadwar K, et al: Role of intracoronary thrombus in acute complications during percutaneous transluminal coronary angioplasty. Catheter Cardiovasc Diagn 16:226, 1989.

105. Kimball BP, Bui S, Dafopoulos N: Angiographic features associated with acute coronary artery occlusion during elective angioplasty. Can J Cardiol 6:327, 1990.

106. Plante S, Laarman G, de Feyter PJ, et al: Acute complications of percutaneous transluminal coronary angioplasty for total occlusion. Am Heart J 121:417, 1991.

107. Cavallini C, Giommi L, Franceschini E, et al: Coronary angioplasty in single-vessel complex lesions: Short- and long-term outcome and factors predicting acute coronary occlusion. Am Heart J 122:44, 1991.

108. Gabliani G, Deligonul U, Kern MJ, et al: Acute coronary occlusion occurring after successful percutaneous transluminal coronary angioplasty: Temporal relationship to discontinuation of anticoagulation. Am Heart J 116:696, 1988.

109. Verna E, Repetto S, Boscarini M, et al: Management of complicated coronary angioplasty by intracoronary urokinase and immediate re-angioplasty. Catheter Cardiovasc Diagn 19:116, 1990.

110. O'Keefe JH Jr, Lapeyre AC III, Holmes DR Jr, et al: Usefulness of early radionuclide angiography for identifying low-risk patients for late restenosis after percutaneous transluminal coronary angioplasty. Am J Cardiol 61:51, 1988.

111. Ellis SG, De Cesare NB, Pinkerton CA, et al: Relation of stenosis morphology and clinical presentation to the procedural results of directional coronary atherectomy. Circulation 84:644, 1991.

112. Matthews BJ, Ewels CJ, Kent KM: Coronary dissection: A predictor of restenosis? Am Heart J 115:547, 1988.

113. Lukas-Laskey MA, Deutsch E, Barnathan E, et al: Influence of heparin therapy on percutaneous transluminal coronary angioplasty outcome in unstable angina pectoris. Am J Cardiol 65:1425, 1990.

114. Goy JJ, Sigwart U, Vogt P, et al: Long-term follow-up of the first 56 patients treated with intracoronary self-expanding stents (the Lausanne experience). Am J Cardiol 67:569, 1991.

115. Bal ET, Plokker HWT, van den Berg EMJ, et al: Predictability and prognosis of PTCA-induced coronary artery aneurysms. Catheter Cardiovasc Diagn 22:85, 1991.

116. Steffenio G, Meyer B, Finci L, et al: Acute complications of elective coronary angioplasty; a review of 500 consecutive procedures. Br Heart J 59:151, 1988.

117. Hermans WRM, Foley DP, Rensing BJ, et al: Usefulness of quantitative and qualitative and angiographic lesion morphology, and clinical characteristics in predicting major adverse cardiac events during and after native coronary balloon angioplasty. Am J Cardiol 72:14, 1993.

118. Kern MJ, Deligonul U, Galan K, et al: Percutaneous transluminal angioplasty in octogenarians. Am J Cardiol 61:457, 1988.

119. Barnathan ES, Schwartz SJ, Taylor L, et al: Aspirin and dipyridamole in the prevention of acute coronary thrombosis complicating coronary angioplasty. Circulation 76:125, 1987.

120. McGarry TF Jr, Gottlieb RS, Morganroth J, et al: The relationship of anticoagulation level and complications after successful percutaneous transluminal coronary angioplasty. Am Heart J 123:1445, 1992.

121. Charney R, Cohen M: The role of the coronary collateral circulation in limiting myocardial ischemia and infarct size. Am Heart J 126:937, 1993.

122. Ryan TJ, Faxon DP, Gunnar RM, et al: Guidelines for percutaneous transluminal coronary angioplasty: A report of the American College of Cardiology/American Heart Association Task Force on Assessment of Diagnostic and Therapeutic Cardiovascular Procedures (Subcommittee on Percutaneous Transluminal Coronary Angioplasty). J Am Coll Cardiol 12:529, 1988.

123. Deckelbaum LI, Isner JM, Donaldson RF, et al: Reduction of laser-induced pathologic tissue injury using pulsed energy delivery. Am J Cardiol 56:662, 1985.

124. Grundfest WS, Litvack F, Forrester JS, et al: Laser ablation of human atherosclerotic plaque without adjacent tissue injury. J Am Coll Cardiol 5:929, 1985.

125. Deckelbaum LI, Isner JM, Donaldson RF, et al: Use of pulsed

energy delivery to minimize tissue injury from carbon dioxide laser irradiation of cardiovascular tissues. J Am Coll Cardiol 7:898, 1986.

126. Mintz GS, Kovach JA, Pichard AD, et al: Intravascular ultrasound findings after excimer laser coronary angioplasty. Catheter Cardiovasc Diagn 37:113, 1996.

127. Deckelbaum LI, Natarajan MK, Bittl JA, et al: Effect of intracoronary saline infusion on dissection during excimer laser coronary angioplasty: A randomized trial. J Am Coll Cardiol 26:1264, 1995.

128. Hinohara T, Robertson GC, Selmon MR, et al: Directional coronary atherectomy. J Invest Cardiol 2:217, 1990.

129. Kaufmann UP, Garratt KN, Vlietstra RE, et al: Coronary atherectomy: First 50 patients at the Mayo Clinic. Mayo Clin Proc 64:747, 1989.

130. Safian RD, Gelbfish JS, Erny RE et al: Coronary atherectomy: Clinical, angiographic, and histologic findings and observations regarding potential mechanisms. Circulation 82:69, 1990.

131. Sketch MH Jr, Phillips HR, Lee MM, et al: Coronary transluminal extraction-endarterectomy. J Invest Cardiol 3:13, 1991.

132. Geschwind HJ, Nakamura F, Kvasnicka J, et al: Excimer and holmium yttrium-aluminum-garnet laser coronary angioplasty. Am Heart J 125:510, 1993.

133. Karsch KR, Haase KK, Voelker W, et al: Percutaneous coronary excimer laser angioplasty in patients with stable and unstable angina pectoris. Circulation 81:1849, 1990.

134. Ghazzal ZMB, Hern JA, Litvack F, et al: Morphologic predictors of acute complications after percutaneous excimer laser coronary angioplasty: Results of a comprehensive angiographic analysis: Importance of the eccentricity index. Circulation 86:820, 1992.

135. Bittl JA, Sanborn TA: Excimer laser-facilitated coronary angioplasty: Relative risk analysis of acute and follow-up results in 200 patients. Circulation 86:71, 1992.

136. Lee G, Mason DT: Excimer coronary laser angioplasty: It's time for a critical evaluation. Am J Cardiol 69:1640, 1991.

137. Preisack MB, Athanasiadis A, Voelker W, et al: Acute closure during coronary excimer laser angioplasty and conventional balloon dilatation: A comparison of management outcome and prediction. Eur Heart J 14:195, 1993.

138. Litvack F, Margolis J, Cummins F, et al: Excimer Laser Coronary Angioplasty (ELCA) registry: Report of the first consecutive 2080 patients [Abstract]. J Am Coll Cardiol 19:276A, 1992.

139. Bittl JA, Sanborn TA, Tcheng JE, et al: Clinical success, complications, and restenosis rates with excimer laser coronary angioplasty. J Am Coll Cardiol 70:1553, 1993.

140. Bittl JA, Ryan TJ Jr, Keaney JF, et al: Coronary artery perforation during excimer laser coronary angioplasty. J Am Coll Cardiol 21:1158, 1993.

141. Waksman R, Ghazzal ZMB, Baim DS, et al: Myocardial infarction as a complication of new interventional devices. Am J Cardiol 78:751, 1996.

142. Baumbach A, Bittl JA, Fleck E, et al: Acute complications of excimer laser angioplasty: A detailed analysis of multicenter results. J Am Coll Cardiol 23:1305, 1994.

143. Estella P, Ryan TJ, Landzberg JS, et al: Excimer laser-assisted coronary angioplasty for lesions containing thrombus. J Am Coll Cardiol 21:1550, 1993.

144. Appelman YEA, Piek JJ, Strikwerda S, et al: Randomized trial of excimer laser angioplasty versus balloon angioplasty for obstructive coronary disease. Lancet 347:79, 1996.

145. Rowe MH, Hinohara T, White NW, et al: Comparison of dissection rates and angiographic results following directional coronary atherectomy and coronary angioplasty. Am J Cardiol 66:49, 1990.

146. Muller DWM, Ellis SG, Debowey DL, et al: Quantitative angiographic comparison of the immediate success of coronary angioplasty, coronary atherectomy and endoluminal stenting. Am J Cardiol 66:938, 1990.

147. Whitlow PL, Franco I: Indications for directional coronary atherectomy: 1993. Am J Cardiol 72(suppl):21E, 1993.

148. Carrozza JP Jr, Baim DS: Complications of directional coronary atherectomy: Incidence, causes, and management. Am J Cardiol 72(suppl):47E, 1993.

149. O'Neill WW: Mechanical rotational atherectomy. Am J Cardiol 69(suppl):12F, 1992.

150. Feld H, Schulhoff N, Lichstein E: Coronary atherectomy versus angioplasty: The CAVA study. Am Heart J 126:31, 1993.

151. Fishman RF, Kuntz RE, Carrozza JP, et al: Long term results of directional coronary atherectomy: Predictors of restenosis. J Am Coll Cardiol 20:1101, 1992.

152. Hinohara T, Rowe MH, Robertson GC, et al: Effect of lesion characteristics on outcome of directional coronary atherectomy. J Am Coll Cardiol 17:1112, 1991.

153. Popma JJ, Topol EJ, Hinohara T, et al: Abrupt vessel closure after directional atherectomy. J Am Coll Cardiol 19:1372, 1992.

154. Topol EJ, Leya F, Pinkerton CA, et al: A comparison of directional atherectomy with coronary angioplasty in patients with coronary artery disease. N Engl J Med 329:221, 1993.

155. Adelman AG, Cohen EA, Kimball BP, et al: A comparison of directional atherectomy with balloon angioplasty for lesions of the left anterior descending coronary artery. N Engl J Med 329:228, 1993.

156. The CAVEAT Investigators: The coronary angioplasty versus excisional atherectomy trial: Preliminary results. Circulation 86(suppl I):I-374, 1992.

157. Potkin BN, Mintz GS, Pichard AD, et al: Late, out of laboratory, abrupt closure after angiographically successful directional atherectomy. Am J Cardiol 69:263, 1992.

158. Baim DS, Popma J, Sharma SK, et al: Final results in the Balloon vs Optimal Atherectomy Trial (BOAT): 6 month angiography and 1 year clinical follow up. Circulation 94(suppl I):I-436, 1996.

159. Dussaillant GR, Mintz GS, Popma JJ, et al: Intravascular ultrasound, directional coronary atherectomy, and the Optimal Atherectomy Restenosis Study (OARS). Coron Artery Dis 7:294, 1996.

160. MacIsaac AI, Bass TA, Buchbinder M, et al: High speed rotational atherectomy: Outcome in calcified and noncalcified coronary lesions. J Am Coll Cardiol 26:731, 1995.

161. Vandormael M, Reifart N, Preusler W, et al: Six months follow-up results following excimer laser angioplasty, rotational atherectomy and balloon angioplasty for complex lesions: ERBAC study. Circulation 90(suppl I):I-213, 1994.

162. Gilmore PS, Bass TA, Conetta DA, et al: Single site experience with high-speed coronary rotational atherectomy. Clin Cardiol 16:311, 1993.

163. Bertrand ME, Lablanche JM, Leroy F, et al: Percutaneous transluminal coronary rotary ablation with Rotablator (European experience). Am J Cardiol 69:470, 1992.

164. Warth D, Spring D, Cohen B, et al: Abrupt vessel closure following PTCA: Clinical and therapeutic profile. Circulation 86(suppl I):I-248, 1992.

165. Brown DL, Buchbinder M: Incidence, predictors, and consequences of coronary dissection following high-speed rotational atherectomy. Am J Cardiol 78:1416, 1996.

166. Ellis SG, Popma JJ, Raymond RE, et al: Abrupt coronary occlusion after Rotablator therapy: Incidence; clinical, angiographic and procedural predictors. Circulation 86(suppl I):I-652, 1992.

167. Aguirre FV, Bach R, Donohue TJ, et al: Rotational coronary ablation: More grist for the interventional mill? J Am Coll Cardiol 21:296, 1993.

168. Whitlow PL, Cowley M, Kuntz RE, et al: Study to determine Rotablator and transluminal angioplasty strategy (STRATAS): Acute results. Circulation 94(suppl I):I-435, 1996.

169. Ferguson JJ: Meeting highlights, 46th Annual Scientific Sessions of the American College of Cardiology. Circulation 96:367, 1997.

170. O'Neill WW, Kramer BL, Sketch MH, et al: Mechanical extraction atherectomy: Report of the U.S. Transluminal Extraction Catheter Investigation. Circulation 86(suppl I):I-779, 1992.

171. Sutton JM, Gitlin JB, Casale PN, for the U.S. Coronary Trans-

luminal Extraction Catheter (TEC) Investigators: Major complications after TEC atherectomy: Preliminary analysis derived from the multicenter registry experience. Circulation 86(suppl I):I-456, 1992.

172. Meany TB, Kramer BL, Knopf WD, et al: Multicenter experience of atherectomy saphenous vein grafts: Immediate results and follow-up. J Am Coll Cardiol 19(suppl):262A, 1992.

173. Kaplan BM, Larkin T, Safian RD, et al: Prospective study of extraction atherectomy in patients with acute myocardial infarction. Am J Cardiol 78:383, 1996.

174. Kaplan BM, Gregory M, Schreiber TL, et al: Transluminal extraction atherectomy versus balloon angioplasty in acute ischemic syndromes: An interim analysis of the TOPIT trial. Circulation 94(suppl I):I-317, 1996.

175. Kulick DL, Rahimtoola SH: Acute coronary occlusion after percutaneous transluminal coronary angioplasty: Evolving strategies and implications. Circulation 82:1039, 1990.

176. Buffet P, Danchin N, Villemot JP: Early and long-term outcome after emergency coronary bypass surgery after failed coronary angioplasty. Circulation 84(suppl III):III-254, 1991.

177. Talley JD, Weintraub WS, Roubin GS, et al: Failed elective percutaneous transluminal coronary angioplasty requiring coronary artery bypass surgery. In-hospital and late clinical outcome at 5 years. Circulation 82:1203, 1990.

178. Hannan EL, Arani DT, Johnson LW, et al: Percutaneous transluminal coronary angioplasty in New York state: Risk factors and outcome. JAMA 268:3092, 1992.

179. Berger PB, Stensrud PE, Doly RC, et al: Time to reperfusion and other procedural characteristics of emergency coronary bypass surgery after unsuccessful coronary angioplasty. Am J Cardiol 76:565, 1995.

180. Craver JM, Justicz AG, Weintraub WS, et al: Coronary artery bypass grafting in patients after failure of intracoronary stenting. Ann Thorac Surg 60:60, 1995.

181. Bartram U, Wahlers TH, Aebert H, et al: Coronary artery bypass grafting after failed percutaneous angioplasty compared to direct coronary bypass grafting in patients with unstable angina. Thorac Cardiovasc Surg 44:31, 1996.

182. Nollert G, Amend J, Detter C, et al: Coronary artery bypass grafting after failed coronary angioplasty: Risk factors and long-term results. J Thorac Cardiovasc Surg 43:35, 1995.

183. Cowley MJ, Dorros G, Kelsey SF, et al: Emergency coronary bypass surgery after coronary angioplasty: The National Heart, Lung, and Blood Institute's Percutaneous Transluminal Coronary Angioplasty Registry experience. Am J Cardiol 53(suppl):22C, 1984.

184. Golding LAR, Loop FD, Hollman JL, et al: Early results of emergency surgery after coronary angioplasty. Circulation 74(suppl III):III-26, 1984.

185. Killen DA, Hamaker WR, Reed WA: Coronary artery bypass following percutaneous transluminal coronary angioplasty. Ann Thorac Surg 40:133, 1985.

186. Reul GJ, Cooley DA, Hallman GL, et al: Coronary artery bypass of unsuccessful percutaneous transluminal coronary angioplasty. J Thorac Cardiovasc Surg 88:685, 1984.

187. Weintraub WS, Cohen CL, Curling PE, et al: Results of coronary surgery after failed elective coronary angioplasty in patients with prior coronary surgery. J Am Coll Cardiol 16:1341, 1990.

188. Connor AR, Vlietstra RE, Schaff HV, et al: Early and late results of coronary artery bypass after failed angioplasty. J Thorac Cardiovasc Surg 96:191, 1988.

189. Parsonnet V, Fisch D, Gielchinsky I, et al: Emergency operation after failed angioplasty. J Thorac Cardiovasc Surg 96:198, 1988.

190. Pepine CJ, Holmes DR, Block PC, et al: ACC expert consensus document: Coronary artery stents. J Am Coll Cardiol 28:782, 1996.

191. Murphy DA, Craver JM, Jones EL, et al: Surgical management of acute myocardial ischemia following percutaneous transluminal coronary angioplasty: Role of intra-aortic balloon pump. J Thorac Cardiovasc Surg 87:332, 1984.

192. Ishihara M, Sato M, Tateishi H, et al: Intra-aortic balloon pumping as the post angioplasty strategy in acute myocardial infarction. Am Heart J 122:385, 1991.

193. Suneja R, Hodgson JM: Use of intraaortic balloon counterpulsation for treatment of recurrent acute closure after coronary angioplasty. Am Heart J 125:530, 1993.

194. Kern MJ, Aguirre FV, Bach R, et al: Augmentation of coronary blood flow by intra-aortic balloon counterpulsation in patients after coronary angioplasty. Circulation 87:500, 1993.

195. Ohman EM, George BS, White CJ, et al: Use of aortic counterpulsation to improve sustained coronary artery patency during acute myocardial infarction: Results of a randomized trial. Circulation 90:78, 1994.

196. Ohman EM, Califf RM, George BS, et al: The use of intraaortic balloon pumping as an adjunct to reperfusion therapy in acute myocardial infarction. The Thrombolysis and Angioplasty in Myocardial Infarction (TAMI) study group. Am Heart J 121:895, 1991.

197. Ambrose JA: Thrombolysis as an adjunct to angioplasty. Am J Cardiol 72(suppl):34G, 1993.

198. Schieman G, Cohen BM, Cozina J, et al: Intracoronary urokinase for intracoronary thrombus accumulation complicating percutaneous transluminal coronary angioplasty in acute ischemic syndromes. Circulation 82:2052, 1990.

199. Vaitkus PT, Herrmann HC, Laskey WK: Management and immediate outcome of patients with intracoronary thrombus during percutaneous transluminal coronary angioplasty. Am Heart J 124:1, 1992.

200. Goudreau E, DiSciascio G, Vetrovec GW, et al: Intracoronary urokinase as an adjunctive to percutaneous transluminal coronary angioplasty in patients with complex native coronary narrowings or angioplasty induced complications. Am J Cardiol 69:57, 1992.

201. Gulba DC, Daniel WG, Simon R, et al: Role of thrombolysis and thrombin in patients with acute coronary occlusion during percutaneous transluminal coronary angioplasty. J Am Coll Cardiol 16:563, 1990.

202. Ambrose JA, Almeida OD, Sharma SK, et al: Adjunctive thrombolytic therapy during angioplasty for ischemic rest angina. Results of the TAUSA Trial. Circulation 90:69, 1994.

203. Vaitkus PT, Laskey WK: Efficacy of adjunctive thrombolytic therapy in percutaneous transluminal coronary angioplasty. J Am Coll Cardiol 24:1415, 1994.

204. Barry WL, Sarembock IJ: Antiplatelet and anticoagulant therapy in patients undergoing percutaneous transluminal coronary angioplasty. Cardiol Clin 12:517, 1994.

205. Schwartz L, Seidelin PH: Antithrombotic and thrombolytic therapy in patients undergoing coronary artery interventions: A review. Prog Cardiovasc Dis 38:67, 1995.

206. Bell WB, Kong DF: Anticoagulants, antithrombotics, and hemostatics. In Wolff ME (ed): Burger's Medicinal Chemistry and Drug Discovery, 5th ed, vol 4, p IV:179. New York: John Wiley, 1997.

207. The EPIC Investigators: Use of a monoclonal antibody directed against the platelet glycoprotein IIb/IIIa receptor in high-risk coronary angioplasty. N Engl J Med 330:956, 1994.

208. Bittl JA: Advances in coronary angioplasty. N Engl J Med 335:1290, 1996.

209. Muhlestein JB, Gomez MA, Karagounis LA, et al: "Rescue ReoPro": Acute utilization of abciximab for the dissolution of coronary thrombus developing as a complication of coronary angioplasty. Circulation 92(suppl I):I-607, 1995.

210. Tcheng JE, Lincoff AM, Sigmon KN, et al: Platelet glycoprotein IIb/IIIa inhibition with integrelin during percutaneous coronary intervention: The IMPACT II Trial. Circulation 92(suppl I):I-543, 1995.

211. Danchin N, Juillière Y, Kettani C, et al: Effect on early acute occlusion rate of adjunctive antithrombotic treatment with intravenously administered dipyridamole during percutaneous transluminal coronary angioplasty. Am Heart J 127:494, 1994.

212. van den Bos AA, Deckers JP, Heyndrickx GR, et al: Safety and efficacy of recombinant hirudin (CGP 39393) versus heparin in patients with stable angina undergoing coronary angioplasty. Circulation 88:2058, 1993.

213. Bittl JA, Strony J, Brinker JA, et al: Treatment with bivalirudin (Hirulog) as compared to heparin during coronary

angioplasty for unstable or postinfarction angina. N Engl J Med 333:764, 1995.

214. Hollman J, Gruentzig AR, Douglas JS, et al: Acute occlusion after percutaneous transluminal coronary angioplasty—A new approach. Circulation 68:725, 1983.

215. Jackman JD, Zidar JP, Tcheng JE, et al: Outcome following prolonged balloon inflations of over twenty minutes for initially unsuccessful percutaneous transluminal coronary angioplasty. Am J Cardiol 69:1471, 1992.

216. Little T, Majcher G, Doorey A, et al: Immediate and long-term results of the splinting for acute closure trial. Catheter Cardiovasc Diagn 38:341, 1996.

217. Ohman EM, Marquis JF, Ricci DR, et al: A randomized comparison of the effects of gradual prolonged versus standard primary balloon inflation on early and late outcome: Results of a multicenter clinical trial. Circulation 89:1118, 1994.

218. Ohman EM, Marquis JF, Ricci DR, et al: Effect of gradual prolonged inflation during angioplasty on in-hospital and long-term outcome: Results of a multicenter randomized trial. J Am Coll Cardiol 19(suppl):33A, 1992.

219. Ferguson TB, Hinohara T, Simpson J, et al: Catheter reperfusion to allow optimal coronary bypass grafting following failed transluminal coronary angioplasty. Ann Thorac Surg 42:399, 1986.

220. Sundram P, Harvey JR, Johnson RG, et al: Benefit of the perfusion catheter for emergency coronary artery grafting after failed PTCA. Am J Cardiol 63:282, 1989.

221. Hinohara T, Simpson JB, Phillips HR, et al: Transluminal intracoronary reperfusion catheter: A device to maintain coronary perfusion between failed coronary angioplasty and emergency coronary bypass surgery. J Am Coll Cardiol 11:977, 1988.

222. van Lierde JM, Glazier JJ, Stammen FJ, et al: Use of an autoperfusion catheter in the treatment of acute refractory vessel closure after coronary balloon angioplasty: Immediate and six-month follow-up results. Br Heart J 68:51, 1992.

223. Scott NA, Weintraub WS, Carlin SF, et al: Recent changes in the management and outcome of acute closure after percutaneous transluminal coronary angioplasty. Am J Cardiol 71:1159, 1993.

224. Leitschuh ML, Mills RM, Jacobs AK, et al: Outcome after major dissection during coronary angioplasty using the perfusion balloon catheter. Am J Cardiol 67:1056, 1991.

225. Stauffer JC, Eeckhout E, Vogt P, et al: Stand-by versus stent-by during percutaneous transluminal coronary angioplasty. Am Heart J 130:21, 1995.

226. Warner M, Chamy Y, Johnson D, et al: Directional coronary atherectomy for failed angioplasty due to occlusive coronary dissection. Catheter Cardiovasc Diagn 24:28, 1991.

227. Lee TC, Hartzler GO, Rutherford BD, et al: Removal of an occlusive coronary dissection flap by using an atherectomy catheter. Catheter Cardiovasc Diagn 20:185, 1990.

228. Vetter JW, Simpson JB, Gregory C, et al: Rescue directional coronary atherectomy for failed balloon angioplasty [Abstract]. J Am Coll Cardiol 17:384A, 1991.

229. Whitlow PL, Robertson GC, Selmon MR, et al: Use of directional coronary atherectomy for failed PTCA. Circulation 82(suppl III):III-1, 1990.

230. Harris WO, Berger PB, Holmes DR Jr, et al: "Rescue" directional coronary atherectomy after unsuccessful percutaneous transluminal coronary angioplasty. Mayo Clin Proc 69:717, 1994.

231. Serruys PW, Umans VAWM, Strauss PH, et al: Quantitative angioplasty after directional coronary atherectomy. Br Heart J 66:122, 1991.

232. Vetter J, Robertson G, Selmon M, et al: Perforation with directional coronary atherectomy. J Am Coll Cardiol 19(suppl A):76A, 1992.

233. van Suyien RJ, Serruys PW, Simpson JB, et al: Delayed rupture of right coronary artery after directional atherectomy for bailout. Am Heart J 121:914, 1991.

234. Kuntz RE, Piana R, Pomerantz RM, et al: Changing incidence and management of abrupt closure following coronary intervention in the new device era. Catheter Cardiovasc Diagn 27:189, 1992.

235. Lee BI, Becker GJ, Waller BF, et al: Thermal compression and molding of atherosclerotic vascular tissue with use of radiofrequency energy: Implications for radiofrequency balloon angioplasty. J Am Coll Cardiol 13:1167, 1989.

236. Reis GG, Pomerantz RM, Jenkins RD, et al: Laser balloon angioplasty: Clinical, angiographic and histologic results. J Am Coll Cardiol 18:193, 1991.

237. Spears JR, Reyes VP, Wynne J: Percutaneous coronary laser balloon angioplasty: Initial results of a multicenter experience. J Am Coll Cardiol 16:293, 1990.

238. Spears JF, Safian RD, Douglas JS, et al: Multicenter acute and chronic results of laser balloon angioplasty for refractory abrupt closure after PTCA. Circulation 84(suppl II):II-517, 1991.

239. Ferguson JJ, Dear WD, Leatherman LL, et al: A multi-center trial of laser balloon angioplasty for abrupt closure following PTCA. J Am Coll Cardiol 15(suppl):25A, 1990.

240. Yamashita K, Satake S, Ohira H, et al: Radiofrequency thermal balloon coronary angioplasty: A new device for successful percutaneous transluminal coronary angioplasty. J Am Coll Cardiol 23:335, 1994.

241. Lau KW, Sigwart U: Novel coronary interventional devices: An update. Am Heart J 123:497, 1992.

242. Lincoff AM, Topol EJ, Chapekis AT, et al: Intracoronary stenting compared with conventional therapy for abrupt vessel closure complicating coronary angioplasty: A matched-case control study. J Am Coll Cardiol 21:866, 1993.

243. Altmann DB, Racz M, Battleman DS, et al: Reduction in angioplasty complications after the introduction of coronary stents: Results from a consecutive series of 2242 patients. Am Heart J 132:503, 1996.

244. Lindsay J, Hong MK, Pinnow EE, et al: Effects of endoluminal coronary stents on the frequency of coronary artery bypass grafting after unsuccessful percutaneous transluminal coronary revascularization. Am J Cardiol 77:647, 1996.

245. Ray SG, Penn IM, Ricci DR, et al: Mechanism of benefit of stenting in failed PTCA: Final results from the Trial of Angioplasty and Stents in Canada (TASC II). J Am Coll Cardiol 25(suppl):156A, 1995.

246. de Muinck ED, den Heijer P, Dijk RB, et al: Autoperfusion balloon versus stent for acute or threatened closure during percutaneous transluminal coronary angioplasty. Am J Cardiol 74:1002, 1994.

247. Sigwart U, Urban PH, Golf S, et al: Emergency stenting for acute occlusion after balloon angioplasty. Circulation 78:1121, 1988.

248. Sigwart U, Puel J, Mirkovitch V, et al: Intravascular stents to prevent occlusion and restenosis after transluminal angioplasty. N Engl J Med 316:701, 1987.

249. Serruys PW, Strauss BH, Beatt KJ, et al: Angiographic follow-up after placement of a self-expanding coronary artery stent. N Engl J Med 324:13, 1991.

250. Sigwart U, Urban P, Sadeghi H, et al: Implantation of 100 coronary artery stents: Learning curve for incidence of acute early complications. J Am Coll Cardiol 13(suppl):107A, 1989.

251. Turi ZG, Campbell CA, Gottimukkala MV, et al: Preservation of distal coronary perfusion during prolonged balloon inflation with an autoperfusion angioplasty catheter. Circulation 75:1273, 1987.

252. Sutton JM, Ellis SG, Roubin GS, et al: Differences in clinical characteristics and outcome for acute versus elective coronary artery stent placement [Abstract]. Circulation 84(suppl II):II-301, 1991.

253. Sutton JM, Ellis SG, Roubin GS, et al: Major clinical events after coronary stenting: The multicenter registry of acute and elective Gianturco-Roubin stent placement. Circulation 89:1126, 1993.

254. Grinstead WC, Raizner AE, Churchill DA, et al: Intracoronary thrombosis prior to stenting: Impact on angiographic success and clinical outcome [Abstract]. J Am Coll Cardiol 21:30A, 1993.

255. Nath FC, Muller DW, Ellis SG, et al: Thrombosis of a flexible coil coronary stent: Frequency predictors in clinical outcome. J Am Coll Cardiol 21:622, 1993.

256. Hearn JA, King SB III, Douglas JS Jr, et al: Clinical and

angiographic outcomes after coronary artery stenting for acute or threatened closure after percutaneous transluminal coronary angioplasty: Initial results with a balloon-expandable, stainless steel design. Circulation 88:2086, 1993.

257. Leon MB, Fry ETA, O'Shaughnessy CD, et al: Preliminary multicenter experiences with the new GR-II stent for abrupt and threatened closure syndrome. Circulation 94(suppl I):I-207, 1996.

258. Palmaz JC, Sibbitt RR, Reuter SR, et al: Expandable intraluminal graft: Preliminary study. Radiology 156:73, 1985.

259. Palmaz JC, Garcia O, Kopp DT, et al: Balloon expandable intraarterial stents: Effects of antithrombotic medication on thrombus formation. In Zeitler E, Seyforth W (eds): Pros and Cons in PTA and Auxiliary Methods, p 170. Berlin: Springer-Verlag, 1989.

260. Schatz RA, Palmaz JC: Balloon expandable intravascular stents (BEIS) in human coronary arteries: Report of initial experience. Circulation 78(suppl II):II-408, 1988.

261. Schatz RA, Palmaz JC, Tio F, et al: Report of a new articulated balloon expandable intravascular stent (ABEIS), abstracted. Circulation 78(suppl II):II-449, 1988.

262. Schatz RA, Baim DS, Leon M, et al: Clinical experience with the Palmaz-Schatz coronary stent: Initial results of a multicenter study. Circulation 83:148, 1991.

263. Carrozza JP Jr, Kuntz RE, Levine MJ, et al: Angiographic and clinical outcome of intracoronary stenting: Immediate and long-term results from a large single-center experience. J Am Coll Cardiol 20:328, 1992.

264. Strumpf RK, Mehta SS, Ponder R, et al: Palmaz-Schatz stent implantation in stenosed saphenous vein grafts: Clinical and angiographic follow-up. Am Heart J 123:1329, 1992.

265. Serruys PW, de Jaegere P, Kiemeneij F, et al: A comparison of balloon-expandable stent implantation with balloon angioplasty in patients with coronary artery disease. N Engl J Med 331:489, 1994.

266. Macaya C, Serruys PW, Ruygrok P, et al: Continued benefit of coronary stenting versus balloon angioplasty: One-year clinical follow-up of BENESTENT trial. J Am Coll Cardiol 27:255, 1996.

267. Herrmann HC, Buchbinder M, Clemen MW, et al: Emergent use of balloon-expandable coronary artery stenting for failed percutaneous transluminal coronary angioplasty. Circulation 87:812, 1992.

268. de Jaegere PP, Serruys PW, Bertrand M, et al: Wiktor stent implantation in patients with restenosis following balloon angioplasty of a native coronary artery. Am Heart J 69:598, 1992.

269. Burger W, Krieken T, de Jaegere P, et al: Mid-term follow-up after Wiktor stent implantation for prevention of restenosis [Abstract]. J Am Coll Cardiol 21:30A, 1993.

270. Agrawal SK, Hearn JA, Liu MW, et al: Stent thrombosis and ischemic complications following coronary artery stenting. Circulation 86(suppl I):I-113, 1992.

271. Fischman DL, Leon MB, Baim DS: A randomized trial of stents and angioplasty in the treatment of coronary artery disease. N Engl J Med 331:496, 1994.

272. Haude M, Erbel R, Straub U, et al: Short and long term results after intracoronary stenting in human coronary arteries: Monocentre experience with the balloon-expandable Palmaz-Schatz stent. Br Heart J 66:337, 1991.

273. Fajadet J, Jenny D, Guagliumi G, et al: Does the indication for coronary stenting influence clinical results? J Am Coll Cardiol 19(suppl):198A, 1992.

274. Kimura T, Nosaka H, Yokoi H, et al: Emergency coronary stenting for abrupt closure and dissection after balloon angioplasty. J Am Coll Cardiol 19(suppl):198A, 1992.

275. Penn I, Brown R, MacDonald R, et al: Stent complications are dependent on the "stent environment." J Am Coll Cardiol 19(suppl):47A, 1992.

276. Kiemeneij F, Laarman G, Suwarganda J, et al: Emergency coronary stenting after failed coronary angioplasty: Immediate and mean term results with the Palmaz-Schatz stent. J Am Coll Cardiol 19(suppl):47A, 1992.

277. Fajadet J, Marco J, Cassagneau B, et al: Clinical and angiographic follow-up in patients receiving a Palmaz-Schatz stent for prevention or treatment of abrupt closure after coronary angioplasty. Eur Heart J 12(suppl):165, 1991.

278. Reifart N, Langer A, Hofmann M, et al: Warning against extensive use of a stent in dissection after PTCA. Eur Heart J 12(suppl):167, 1991.

279. Haude M, Erbel R, Issa H, et al: Subacute thrombotic complications after intracoronary implantation of Palmaz-Schatz stents. Am Heart J 126:15, 1993.

280. Eeckhout E, van Melle G, Stauffer JC, et al: Can early closure and restenosis after endoluminal stenting be predicted from clinical, procedural, and angiographic variables at the time of intervention? Br Heart J 74:592, 1995.

281. Mak KH, Belli G, Ellis SG, et al: Subacute stent thrombosis: Evolving issues and current concepts. J Am Coll Cardiol 27:494, 1996.

282. Herrmann HC, Malosky SA, Guidera SA, et al: Patient selection reduces thrombotic complications of emergent stenting for failed PTCA. Catheter Cardiovasc Diagn 34:286, 1995.

283. Agrawal SK, Ho DSW, Liu MW, et al: Predictors of thrombotic complications following placement of the flexible coil stent. Am J Cardiol 73:1216, 1994.

284. Scott NA, Robinson KA, Nunes GL, et al: Comparison of the thrombogenicity of stainless steel and tantalum coronary stents. Am Heart J 129:866, 1995.

285. Maiello L, Colombo A, Gianrossi R, et al: Coronary stenting for treatment of acute or threatened closure following dissection after coronary balloon angioplasty. Am Heart J 125:1570, 1993.

286. Chan CN, Tan AT, Koh TH, et al: Intracoronary stenting in the treatment of acute or threatened closure in angiographically small coronary arteries (<3.0 mm) complicating percutaneous transluminal coronary angioplasty. Am J Cardiol 75:23, 1995.

287. Tresukosol D, Schalij MJ, Savalle LH, et al: Micro stent, quantitative angiography, and procedural results. Catheter Cardiovasc Diagn 38:135, 1996.

288. Schwartz L, Bourassa MG, Lesperance J, et al: Aspirin and dipyridamole in the prevention of restenosis after percutaneous transluminal coronary angioplasty. N Engl J Med 318:1714, 1988.

289. Popma JJ, Satler LF, Pichard AD, et al: Vascular complications after balloon and new device angioplasty. Circulation 88:1569, 1993.

290. Metz D, Urban P, Camenzind E, et al: Improving results of bailout coronary stenting after failed balloon angioplasty. Catheter Cardiovasc Diagn 32:117, 1994.

291. Fail PS, Maniet AR, Banka VS: Subcutaneous heparin in postangioplasty management: Comparative trial with intravenous heparin. Am Heart J 126:1059, 1993.

292. Lablanche JM, Grolber G, Danchin N, et al: Full antiplatelet therapy without anticoagulation after coronary stenting. J Am Coll Cardiol 25(suppl):181A, 1995.

293. Van Belle E, McFadden EP, Lablanche JM, et al: Two-pronged antiplatelet therapy with aspirin and ticlopidine without systemic anticoagulation: An alternative therapeutic strategy after bailout stent implantation. Coron Artery Dis 6:341, 1995.

294. Morice MC, Zemour G, Benveniste E, et al: Intracoronary stenting without coumadin: One month results of a French multicenter study. Catheter Cardiovasc Diagn 35:1, 1995.

295. Schomig A, Neumann F, Kastrati A, et al: A randomized comparison of antiplatelet and anticoagulant therapy after the placement of coronary artery stents. N Engl J Med 334:1084, 1996.

296. Sankardas MA, Garrahy PJ, McEniery PT: Sequential implantation of dissimilar tandem stents for long dissections complicating percutaneous transluminal coronary angioplasty. Catheter Cardiovasc Diagn 34:155, 1995.

297. Eeckhout E, Stauffer JC, Vogt P, et al: Placement of multiple and different stent types for very long dissections during coronary angioplasty. Catheter Cardiovasc Diagn 39:302, 1996.

298. Scott NA, Candal FJ, Robinson KA, et al: Seeding of intracoronary stents with immortalized human microvascular endothelial cells. Am Heart J 129:860, 1995.

299. Tanguay JF, Zidar JP, Phillips HR 3rd, et al: Current status of biodegradable stents. Cardiol Clin 12:699, 1994.

300. Stefanadis C, Kallikazaros I, Vlachopoulos C, et al: A new adjustable temporary stent catheter for management of acute dissection during balloon angioplasty. Catheter Cardiovasc Diagn 37:89, 1996.

301. Collins GJ, Ramirez NM, Hinohara T, et al: The perfusion balloon catheter: A new method for safe prolonged coronary dilatation. J Am Coll Cardiol 9:106A, 1987.

302. Campbell CA, Rezkella S, Kloner RA, et al: The autoperfusion balloon angioplasty catheter limits myocardial ischemia and necrosis during prolonged balloon inflation. J Am Coll Cardiol 14:1045, 1989.

303. Zalewski A, Berry C, Kossman ZK, et al: Myocardial protection with autoperfusion during prolonged coronary artery occlusion. Am Heart J 119:41, 1990.

304. Christensen CW, Lassar TA, Daley LC, et al: Regional myocardial blood flow with a reperfusion catheter and an autoperfusion balloon catheter during total coronary occlusion. Am Heart J 119:242, 1990.

305. Quigley PJ, Hinohara T, Phillips HR, et al: Myocardial protection during coronary angioplasty with an autoperfusion balloon catheter in humans. Circulation 78:1128, 1988.

306. Smith JE, Quigley PJ, Tcheng JE, et al: Can prolonged perfusion balloon inflations salvage vessel patency after failed angioplasty? Circulation 80(suppl II):II-373, 1989.

307. Thomas CN, Weintraub WS, Shen Y, et al: "Bailout" coronary stenting in patients with a recent myocardial infarction. Am J Cardiol 77:653, 1996.

308. de Feyter PJ, De Scheerder IK, van den Brand M, et al: Emergency stenting for refractory acute coronary artery occlusion during coronary angioplasty. Am J Cardiol 66:1147, 1990.

309. Goy JJ, Sigwart U, Vogt P, et al: Long-term clinical and angiographic follow-up of patients treated with the self-expanding coronary stent for acute occlusion during balloon angioplasty of the right coronary artery. J Am Coll Cardiol 19:1593, 1992.

310. Maiello L, Colombo A, Almagor Y, et al: Results with a novel strategy of stenting of acute or threatened closure complicating coronary angioplasty. Circulation 88(suppl I):I-123, 1993.

311. Foley JB, Brown RIG, Penn IM: Thrombosis and restenosis after stenting in failed angioplasty: Comparison with elective stenting. Am Heart J 128:12, 1994.

312. Schomig A, Kastrati A, Mudra H, et al: Four-year experience with Palmaz-Schatz stenting in coronary angioplasty complicated by dissection with threatened or present vessel closure. Circulation 90:2716, 1994.

313. Goy JJ, Eeckhout E, Stauffer JC, et al: Emergency endoluminal stenting for abrupt vessel closure following coronary angioplasty: A randomized comparison of the Wiktor and Palmaz-Schatz stents. Catheter Cardiovasc Diagn 34:128, 1995.

314. Vrolix M, van der Krieken T, Piessens J: Wiktor stent for acute and threatened closure after coronary angioplasty: An update of the European Registry. Circulation 86(suppl):987A, 1992.

315. Garratt KN, Berger PB, MacIsaac A, et al: Urgent placement of Wiktor intracoronary stent: Results in first 125 patients. A report from the U.S. Wiktor stent investigators. Circulation 88(suppl I):I-123, 1993.

316. Vrolix M, Piessens J: Usefulness of the Wiktor stent for treatment of threatened or acute closure complicating coronary angioplasty. The European Wiktor Stent Study Group. Am J Cardiol 73:737, 1994.

317. Eeckhout E, Goy JJ, Vogt P, et al: Complications and follow-up after intracoronary stenting: Critical analysis of a 6-year single-center experience. Am Heart J 127:262, 1994.

318. Hamm CW, Beythien C, Sievert H, et al: Multicenter evaluation of the Strecker tantalum stent for acute coronary occlusion after angioplasty. Am Heart J 129:423, 1995.

319. Ozaki Y, Keane D, Ruygrok P, et al: Acute clinical and angiographic results with the new AVE Micro coronary stent in bailout management. Am J Cardiol 75:112, 1995.

320. Waigand J, Uhlich F, Gulba DC, et al: Intracoronary stenting with the Multi-link stent—Single center experience. Circulation 94(suppl I):I-88, 1996.

321. Haude M, Erbel R, Straub U, et al: Results of intracoronary stents for management of coronary dissection after balloon angioplasty. Am J Cardiol 67:691, 1991.

322. Hinohara T, Selmon MR, Robertson GC, et al: Directional atherectomy. New approaches for treatment of obstructive coronary and peripheral vascular disease. Circulation 81(suppl IV):79, 1990.

323. Flynn MS, Aguirre FV, Donohue TJ, et al: Conservative management of guidewire coronary artery perforation with pericardial effusion during angioplasty for acute inferior myocardial infarction. Catheter Cardiovasc Diagn 29:285, 1993.

324. Ajluni SC, Glazier S, Blankenship L, et al: Perforations after percutaneous coronary interventions: Clinical, angiographic, and therapeutic observations. Catheter Cardiovasc Diagn 32:206, 1994.

325. Ellis SG, Ajluni S, Arnold AZ: Increased coronary perforation in the new device era: Incidence, classification, management, and outcome. Circulation 90:2725, 1994.

326. Finch I, Krouse JR: Pericardial tamponade from iatrogenic coronary artery perforation treated with transcatheter embolization. J Vasc Interv Radiol 7:147, 1996.

327. Meng RL, Harlan JL: Left anterior descending coronary artery–right ventricle fistula complicating percutaneous transluminal coronary angioplasty. J Thorac Cardiovasc Surg 90:387, 1985.

328. Cherry S, Vandormael M: Rupture of a coronary artery and hemorrhage into the ventricular cavity during coronary angioplasty. Am Heart J 113:386, 1987.

329. Dorros G, Jain A, Kumar K: Management of coronary artery rupture: Covered stent or microcoil embolization. Catheter Cardiovasc Diagn 36:148, 1995.

330. Kimbiris D, Iskandrian AS, Goel I, et al: Transluminal coronary angioplasty complicated by coronary artery perforation. Catheter Cardiovasc Diagn 8:481, 1982.

331. Saffitz J, Rose T, Oaks J, et al: Coronary artery rupture during coronary angioplasty. Am J Cardiol 51:902, 1983.

332. Topol EJ: Promises and pitfalls of new devices for coronary artery disease. Circulation 83:689, 1991.

333. Cohen EA, Naqvi SZ, Fremes SE: Perforation of nontarget artery during directional coronary atherectomy. Catheter Cardiovasc Diagn 35:240, 1995.

334. Hinohara T, Simpson JB: Lessons from the CAVEAT: Will the BOAT answer the questions? Coron Artery Dis 7:282, 1996.

335. Garratt KN, Kaufmann UP, Edwards WD, et al: Safety of percutaneous coronary atherectomy with deep arterial resection. Am J Cardiol 64:538, 1989.

336. Phillips HR, Sketch MH Jr, Meany TB, et al: Coronary transluminal extraction-endarterectomy: A multicenter experience. Circulation 84(suppl II):II-82, 1991.

337. Ellis SG, Popma JJ, Buchbinder M, et al: Relation of clinical presentation, stenosis morphology, and operator technique to the procedural results of rotational atherectomy and rotational atherectomy-facilitated angioplasty. Circulation 89:882, 1994.

338. Cohen BM, Weber VJ, Reisman M, et al: Coronary perforation complicating rotational ablation: The U.S. multicenter experience. Catheter Cardiovasc Diagn Suppl 3:55, 1996.

339. Holmes DR, Bresnahan JF, Reeder CS, et al: Coronary perforation following excimer laser coronary angioplasty (ELCA). J Am Coll Cardiol 19(suppl A):76A, 1992.

340. Holmes DR, Reeder GS, Ghazzal ZMB, et al: Coronary perforation after excimer laser coronary angioplasty: The excimer laser coronary angioplasty registry experience. J Am Coll Cardiol 23:330, 1994.

341. Isner JM, Donaldson RF, Funai JT, et al: Factors contributing to perforations resulting from laser coronary angioplasty: Observations in an intact human postmortem preparation of intraoperative laser coronary angioplasty. Circulation 72(suppl II):II-191, 1985.

342. Ribeiro PA, Gallo R, Antonius J, et al: A new expandable intracoronary tantalum (Strecker) stent: Early experimental

results and follow up to twelve months. Am Heart J 125:501, 1993.

343. Shammas NW, Thondapu VR, Winniford MD, et al: Perforation of saphenous vein graft during coronary stenting: A case report. Catheter Cardiovasc Diagn 38:274, 1996.

344. Mendzelevski B, Sigwart U: Rupture of coronary artery and cardiac tamponade complicating Wallstent implantation. Catheter Cardiovasc Diagn 40:368, 1997.

345. Reimers B, von Birgelen C, van der Giessen WJ, et al: A word of caution on optimizing stent deployment in calcified lesions: Acute coronary rupture with cardiac tamponade. Am Heart J 131:192, 1996.

346. Alfonso F, Goicolea J, Hernandez R, et al: Arterial perforation during optimization of coronary stents using high-pressure balloon inflations. Am J Cardiol 78:1169, 1996.

347. Chae JK, Park SW, Kim YH, et al: Successful treatment of coronary artery perforation during angioplasty using autologous vein graft–coated stent. Eur Heart J 18:1030, 1997.

348. Meier B: Benign coronary perforation during percutaneous transluminal coronary angioplasty. Br Heart J 54:33, 1985.

349. Grollier G, Bories H, Commeau P, et al: Coronary artery perforation during coronary angioplasty. Clin Cardiol 9:27, 1986.

350. Tierstein PS, Hartzler GO: Nonoperative management of aortocoronary saphenous vein graft rupture during percutaneous transluminal coronary angioplasty. Am J Cardiol 60:377, 1987.

351. Parker JD, Ganz P, Selwyn AP, et al: Successful treatment of an excimer laser–associated coronary artery perforation with the Stack perfusion catheter. Catheter Cardiovasc Diagn 22:118, 1991.

352. Altman F, Yazdanfar S, Wertheimer J, et al: Cardiac tamponade following perforation of the left anterior descending coronary system during percutaneous transluminal coronary angioplasty: Successful treatment by pericardial drainage. Am Heart J 111:1196, 1986.

353. Robicsek F, Bersin RM, Kowalchuk G, et al: Surgical management of instrumentation-induced coronary artery dissection. J Card Surg 10:626, 1995.

354. Gonzalez-Santos JM, Vallejo JL, Pineda T, et al: Emergency surgery after coronary artery disruption complicating PTCA. Thorac Cardiovasc Surg 33:244, 1985.

355. Dralle JG, Turner C, Hsu J, et al: Coronary artery aneurysms after angioplasty and atherectomy. Ann Thorac Surg 59:1030, 1995.

356. Cohen AJ, Banks A, Cambier P, et al: Post-atherectomy coronary artery aneurysm. Ann Thorac Surg 54:1216, 1992.

357. Saito S, Arai H, Kim K, et al: Pseudoaneurysm of coronary artery following rupture of coronary artery during coronary angioplasty. Catheter Cardiovasc Diagn 26:304, 1992.

358. Thomas MR, Wainwright RJ: Use of an intracoronary stent to control intrapericardial bleeding during coronary artery rupture complicating coronary angioplasty. Catheter Cardiovasc Diagn 30:169, 1993.

359. Rath PC, Tripathy MP: Management of coronary artery dissection and perforation following coronary angioplasty by intracoronary stent. J Invasive Cardiol 9:197, 1997.

360. Heuser RR: Stents in jackets: The latest in endovascular haute couture. Catheter Cardiovasc Diagn 38:179, 1996.

361. Colombo A, Itoh A, di Mario C, et al: Successful closure of a coronary vessel rupture with a vein graft stent: Case report. Catheter Cardiovasc Diagn 38:172, 1996.

362. Colon PJ 3rd, Ramee SR, Mulingtapang R, et al: Percutaneous bailout therapy of a perforated vein graft using a stent–autologous vein patch. Catheter Cardiovasc Diagn 38:175, 1996.

363. Kaplan BM, Stewart RE, Sakwa MP, et al: Repair of a coronary pseudoaneurysm with percutaneous placement of a saphenous vein allograft attached to a biliary stent. Catheter Cardiovasc Diagn 37:208, 1996.

364. Wong SC, Kent KM, Mintz GS, et al: Percutaneous transcatheter repair of a coronary aneurysm using a composite autologous cephalic vein–coated Palmaz-Schatz biliary stent. Am J Cardiol 76:990, 1995.

# 29

# Left Main Coronary Interventions

*Ellen C. Keeley*    *Stephen G. Ellis*    *Cindy L. Grines*

Since its first clinical description by Herrick in 1912,[1] obstruction of the left main coronary artery (LMCA), or left main coronary disease (LMCD), has been shown to be of critical prognostic importance (Table 29–1).[2, 3] Obstructive disease of this short vessel before the bifurcation into the left anterior descending and circumflex arteries jeopardizes the blood supply to all but the inferior and posterior surfaces of the left ventricle. Thus, some 80% of the blood supply to the left ventricle is delivered through the LMCA. Critical narrowing of this vessel is potentially the most lethal form of coronary atherosclerosis.[4]

## ETIOLOGY

LMCD usually occurs concomitantly with disease of the other coronary arteries. Isolated LMCD is rare and is often associated with pathologic states of the aorta and left main ostium.[5] Stenosis of the ostium is a lesion of the aortic wall that can be separated anatomically from LMCD. Although both lesions are usually caused by atherosclerosis, they differ in their natural history. Atherosclerotic coronary ostial lesions have been reported in 0.1% to 3% of patients with coronary artery disease.[6, 7] Uncommon causes of left main ostial disease are mediastinal lymphoma, syphilitic aortitis, rheumatoid arthritis, Takayasu's arteritis, Kawasaki's disease, congenital malformations of the aorta, and homozygous familial hypercholesterolemia (Table 29–2).[8–13] The incidence of syphilitic aortitis has decreased significantly since the 1970s, leaving atherosclerosis as the most common cause. The high frequency of left main ostial lesions in autopsy series of victims of sudden death has led some researchers to conclude that these lesions are associated with a higher mortality.[6]

The association of mediastinal radiation and coronary artery disease has been well documented since the 1970s. Radiation aortitis involving the coronary ostium may occur 5 to 16 years after radiation therapy.[14–18] Higher survival rates after radiation therapy have led to an enlarging young population susceptible to early development of ischemic heart disease.

Disease of the aortic valve with extensive calcification has been reported to obstruct the left main ostium.[5] Left main ostial stenosis has also been reported after aortic valve replacement and coronary artery bypass surgery,[19–23] in which intimal proliferation is caused by coronary perfusion cannulas used for antegrade cardioplegia. This complication can be avoided with the use of retrograde delivery of cardioplegia for myocardial protection.

Caged-ball prosthetic aortic valves have been implicated in several cases of accelerated atherosclerosis.[5] This complication results from turbulent flow around the left main ostium. Thrombus extending from the valve, and the poppet itself, have also been reported to obstruct the ostium.[24] The onset of ischemic symptoms or refractory ventricular arrhythmias in the first 6 months after aortic valve replacement is highly suggestive of iatrogenic LMCA stenosis.

Damage to the LMCA can occur as a complication of coronary arteriography as well as percutaneous transluminal coronary angioplasty (PTCA).[25] Dissection and thrombosis of this vessel can occur during guide catheter positioning, guide wire manipulation, and balloon catheter advancement and inflation.[26–29] Retrograde extension of restenosis from an adjacent proximal coronary segment in the left anterior descending artery or left circumflex artery may impinge upon the distal LMCA.[30–36] Aneurysms of the LMCA that cause areas of stenosis are rare but

**TABLE 29–1.    NATURAL HISTORY OF NONSURGICAL TREATMENT OF LEFT MAIN CORONARY DISEASE**

|                        | BRUSCHKE ET AL (1973)[3] | LIM ET AL (1975)[2] |
| ---------------------- | ------------------------ | ------------------- |
| Number of patients     | 590                      | 141                 |
| Length of follow-up    | 7 years                  | 6 years             |
| 5-year mortality rate (%) | 34%                   | 51%                 |
| 1-vessel involvement   | 15%                      | 47%                 |
| 2-vessel involvement   | 38%                      | 41%                 |
| 3-vessel involvement   | 53%                      | 57%                 |

**TABLE 29-2.**  **NONATHEROSCLEROTIC CAUSES OF LEFT MAIN CORONARY DISEASE**

Idiopathic
Radiation aortitis
Syphilitic aortitis
Rheumatoid arthritis
Takayasu's arteritis
Aortic valve disease
Aortic valve replacement
Kawasaki's disease
Congenital malformations
Homozygous familial hypercholesterolemia
Injury after coronary intervention
Injury after cardiac surgery

can occur in patients with hypertensive heart disease, extensive atherosclerotic disease, and Kawasaki's disease.[37, 38]

## DIAGNOSIS

History, physical examination, and laboratory tests do not reliably identify patients with LMCD. Results of certain noninvasive tests, however, have been shown to support the diagnosis of LMCD.

During qualitative exercise thallium-201 scintigrams, patients with LMCD often experience hypotension. The electrocardiogram typically reveals a marked, early ischemic response to exercise. A "high-risk" scintigram has been defined as showing (1) 25% or greater homogeneous decrease in thallium-201 activity, (2) increased lung uptake, or (3) abnormal thallium-201 uptake or washout in multiple segments.[39–44] High-risk scintigrams are significantly more common in patients with LMCA stenoses than those with one-, two-, or three-vessel coronary artery disease.[45]

Studies have shown that biplane transesophageal echocardiography can detect significant LMCA stenoses of greater than 50% of luminal diameter with a positive predictive value of 100% and a negative predictive value of 98%.[46–50]

LMCD can also be detected from the fluoroscopic observation of calcification near the LMCA at the time of cardiac catheterization. Coronary artery calcification is a sensitive but nonspecific finding consistent with LMCD.[51]

Definitive diagnosis of LMCD requires coronary angiography. In 1989, The Society for Cardiac Angiography and Interventions reported data on a series of 222,553 patients who underwent coronary arteriography between July 1, 1984, and December 31, 1987.[52] Subsets of patients with higher procedural mortality rate included patients with greater than 50% stenosis of the LMCA 0.94% of patients, left ventricular (LV) ejection fraction less than 30%

(0.54%), New York Heart Association (NYHA) functional class III or IV heart failure (0.24%), age greater than 60 years (0.23%), aortic valvular disease (0.23%), and three-vessel coronary artery disease (0.13%).

Other factors may increase the risk of periprocedure complications associated with cardiac catheterization.[53–59] Patients experiencing angina in the 24 hours prior to catheterization are at higher risk of complications. The distance from the tip of the catheter to the lesion in the LMCA is also associated with complications (24% complication rate when the catheter tip is 6 mm or less from the lesion, and 3% when the catheter tip is more than 6 mm from the lesion).[56] Coronary spasm, intimal damage, or reduced flow caused by the catheter in the ostium may also raise the complication rate. In the setting of coexisting disease in other coronary arteries, progressive drops in perfusion pressure at successive stenoses lead to global ischemia.[51, 60]

Unsuspected LMCA stenosis may be discovered during cardiac catheterization performed for chest pain syndrome. Hermiller and associates[61] found that an intravascular ultrasound study detected plaque in 100% of angiographically abnormal LMCAs and in 89% of the arteries deemed normal on angiography.[61] Advancement and seating of the catheter should, therefore, avoid deep insertion into the left main ostium. We recommend a nonselective left coronary angiogram before cannulation to detect proximal disease. This maneuver is achieved by hand-injection of contrast agent into the aortic sinus, with the catheter positioned inferior to the ostium, and viewing of the result with the patient in an anteroposterior or shallow right anterior oblique position.[5] We also recommend close monitoring of the pressure waveform. Damping of pressure or pressure drops indicate impingement of the catheter against the arterial wall or obstruction of coronary blood flow as a result of ostial narrowing.[51]

LMCD rarely occurs as an isolated lesion. Arterial spasm should be suspected if an isolated lesion of the LMCA is found. Another indication of a significant left main ostial lesion is the absence of reflux of contrast agent into the sinus of Valsalva during coronary injection. The side holes in the Sones catheter, however, make both of these signs, pressure damping and lack of reflux, less reliable.[5] Artifactual ostial disease should be suspected if (1) the catheter tip is seated deeply in the ostium, (2) contrast agent is injected too slowly, (3) the catheter has only one end hole, or (4) the catheter tip is directed at the vessel wall.[6]

To allow for safe early ambulation after outpatient cardiac catheterization, small-caliber catheters are often used.[62–64] Occasionally, an ostial stenosis may be completely missed if it is not severe enough to prevent a small-caliber diagnostic catheter or a catheter with a tapered tip from crossing it.[65] For example, in a 4.0-mm LMCA, an ostial narrowing of 50% results in a 2.0-mm lumen. The artery's lumen could, therefore, accommodate a 5-French (1.65-mm) catheter without showing angiographic and hemodynamic evidence of ostial disease.

Boehrer and colleagues[53] examined the periprocedure mortality in patients with LMCD undergoing cardiac catheterization to compare it with periprocedure mortality in subjects with less coronary artery disease and to identify the variables associated with pericatheterization mortality in this patient cohort. Of 4009 patients undergoing elective coronary arteriography from 1978 to 1992, 176 had LMCD. Of the 10 deaths during or within 24 hours of catheterization, 5 occurred in these 176 subjects. The periprocedure mortality in patients with LMCD (2.8%) was more than 20 times that in patients without LMCD (0.13%). In comparison with the 171 patients with LMCD who survived, the 5 who died were older ($67 \pm 8$ vs. $58 \pm 12$ years), and had more severe LMCD ($92 \pm 10\%$ vs. $72 \pm 16\%$) and a lower cardiac index ($1.9 \pm 0.4$ vs. $2.6 \pm 0.7$ L/min/m²) ($p < 0.05$ for all three variables). These researchers concluded that patients with LMCD have a high pericatheterization mortality, especially those who are older and have severe LMCD.

Once a critical LMCA stenosis is identified, the major purpose of the angiogram is to identify vessels that can be targeted for coronary bypass. Each time the catheter engages the LMCA and the contrast jet disturbs the lesion, coronary spasm, dissection, or occlusion may cause irreversible hemodynamic instability. Contrast medium–induced hypotension and bradycardia, once serious dangers in patients with LMCD, have been virtually eliminated with the advent of low-osmolar or nonionic contrast media.[66] Whether the risks of a left ventriculogram are outweighed by its benefits is the subject of controversy.[5] Safe ventriculography can often be performed with the use of less than 40 mL of a low-osmolar contrast agent. Even minor catheter manipulations may cause irreversible hemodynamic instability by inducing a transient arrhythmia or vasovagal response. Left ventriculography should be performed only in patients with favorable risk-benefit ratio. Otherwise, noninvasive assessments of ventricular function and mitral regurgitation by means of transthoracic two-dimensional echocardiography, nuclear, or magnetic resonance techniques are appropriate.

## POSTCATHETERIZATION CARE

In the postcatheterization period, patients with significant LMCD remain at increased risk for hemodynamic instability, including hypotension during the subsequent 1 to 2 hours, which is caused by the negative inotropic and vasodilatory effects of the contrast medium and post–contrast injection diuresis.[67, 68] American College of Cardiology/American Heart Association (ACC/AHA) guidelines state that such patients must be admitted to a monitored unit.[69, 70] The timing of bypass surgery after cardiac catheterization is a clinical decision based on the severity of symptoms, clinical presentation, and severity of the identified lesion.

In patients with critical LMCA stenosis who are to undergo urgent bypass surgery, the femoral sheaths should be left in place. They serve as easy access for possible placement of intra-aortic balloon pumps and decrease the likelihood of vagally mediated hypotension secondary to groin compression at the time of sheath removal. Prophylactic and therapeutic applications of intra-aortic balloon counterpulsation have been shown to improve outcome for patients with serious LV dysfunction or impending myocardial infarction (MI) for whom cardiac surgery was planned.[71] Vascular plugs should be used with caution in patients with LMCD. Although their use obviates prolonged groin compression and may lessen the likelihood of vagally mediated hypotension, vascular plugs may limit future placement of intra-aortic balloon pumps.

## NATURAL HISTORY AND REVASCULARIZATION

Natural history studies based on coronary angiography indicate a high risk of death in the first 5 years after documentation of a lesion in the LMCA. Two observational studies from the Cleveland Clinic are of particular value in the description of the natural history of LMCD, because they include patients diagnosed at a time when less coronary artery surgery was performed. Bruschke and coworkers[3] found a survival rate of 37.4% at 7 years in patients with LMCD, similar to the 34% survival rate found in patients with three-vessel disease. Because many patients had two- or three-vessel disease in addition to LMCD, the impact of the left main artery lesion on mortality is difficult to assess. In the second study, the 6-year survival of patients with LMCA stenoses of greater than 50% was 46.1%,[2] indicating that prolonged survival is possible without surgery. Although prognosis is related to coexisting disease and extent of ventricular dysfunction, the prognosis in the individual patient remains highly unpredictable.

Total occlusion of the LMCA is rarely demonstrated with coronary angiography.[72] It was found, in the Coronary Artery Surgery Study (CASS), in

0.06% of the patients registered.[73] Conceivably, the low prevalence of patients with total LMCA occlusion is due to their high mortality. Although surgical management has not proved to be superior to medical treatment in patients with total occlusion, the favorable responses to surgery suggest that surgery is a reasonable therapeutic option for patients with this uncommon lesion.

## SURGICAL VERSUS MEDICAL TREATMENT

Since the first report by Cohen and associates[4] in 1972 on the surgical and medical treatment of patients with significant stenosis of the LMCA, relatively few published studies have directly compared surgical and medical therapies.[74–78] LMCD has traditionally been treated with coronary artery bypass surgery. Coronary bypass surgery has been shown to confer better survival than medical therapy in patients with significant LMCD.

The largest randomized trials assessing medical versus surgical therapy for LMCD are the CASS,[79] the European Coronary Surgical Study (ECSS),[80] and the Veterans Administration Cooperative Randomized Trial (VA-Coop)[81, 82] (Table 29–3). Among 1484 patients enrolled in the CASS Registry who had more than 50% stenosis of the LMCA, median survival was 13.3 years for the surgically treated group but only 6.6 years for the medically treated group. The 3-year survival was 69% for patients with LMCD treated medically. In patients treated surgically, the 1-year, 2-year, and 3-year survival rates were 95%, 92% and 91%, respectively. The survival benefit was confined mainly to patients who had greater than 60% stenosis, particularly in the presence of LV dysfunction.[79]

The ECSS demonstrated 1-year and 3-year survival rates of 95% and 82% percent, respectively, in patients treated medically, and of 92% and 91%, respectively, in patients treated surgically. However, these patients differed from those in the VA-Coop Study in that all were less than 65 years old and had preserved LV function.[80]

**TABLE 29–3. SURGICAL VERSUS MEDICAL TREATMENT FOR LEFT MAIN CORONARY DISEASE**

| STUDY | 3-YEAR SURVIVAL RATE (%) | |
| --- | --- | --- |
| | SURGICAL TREATMENT | MEDICAL TREATMENT |
| Coronary Artery Surgery Study[78, 79] | 91 | 69 |
| European Coronary Surgical Study[80] | 91 | 82 |
| Veterans Administration Cooperative Study[81, 82] | 82 | 60 |

The majority of the deaths in the medically treated patients in the VA-Coop Study occurred within the first year of diagnosis. The 1-year and 3-year survival rates for the medically treated patients were 67% and 60%, respectively, whereas those for surgically treated patients were 87% and 82%, respectively.[81, 82]

The Cleveland Clinic nonsurgical series of LMCD found a 51% 5-year mortality rate.[2] A history of congestive heart failure, depressed LV ejection fraction, and three-vessel disease adversely affected survival.

Other studies have shown that patients with LMCD can undergo coronary bypass surgery with a relatively low and acceptable risk. In addition, patients who undergo coronary artery bypass have improved survival time and greater relief of symptoms compared with similar subsets of patients who receive medical treatment.[83–85]

## PERCUTANEOUS REVASCULARIZATION

PTCA of the left main coronary artery remains a controversial issue. Gruentzig and associates[86, 87] dilated the LMCA in two of the first five patients to undergo the procedure. Owing to procedural difficulties and early cardiac death in one patient, these researchers subsequently concluded that significant LMCA stenosis was an absolute contraindication to PTCA. During the ensuing decade, LMCD remained the most solid contraindication to coronary angioplasty. The 1993 ACC/AHA Task Force Report on Guidelines for PTCA listed significant LMCA obstruction in the absence of a patent bypass graft to the coronary system as the single major contraindication to PTCA.[88]

Percutaneous revascularization of the LMCA has been sporadic and controversial.[89–92] PTCA in patients with LMCA stenoses has been divided into the following three groups: (1) angioplasty of an elective "protected" LMCA (defined as the existence of at least one patent bypass graft to the left anterior descending artery or left circumflex artery), (2) elective angioplasty of an "unprotected" artery, and (3) emergent procedures for an evolving acute MI.[89]

Studies have shown that elective PTCA of a "protected" LMCA is an effective alternative to a second coronary bypass procedure and can be performed safely with a high success rate (Table 29–4).[89–92] Angioplasty in "protected" LMCA may be treated as a general complex PTCA procedure if at least one major branch of the left coronary artery either has good collateral flow or a functional bypass graft. O'Keefe and associates[89] published a retrospective analysis of 127 LMCA dilations,[89] in which 66% (84 lesions) of the arteries were "protected" by one or

**TABLE 29–4.  RESULTS OF "PROTECTED" LEFT MAIN CORONARY ANGIOPLASTY**

| STUDY (YEAR) | NO. OF PATIENTS | MI | PTCA | CABG |
|---|---|---|---|---|
| Stertzer et al (1985)[90] | 8 | 25% | 75% | 38% |
| O'Keefe et al (1989)[89] | 84 | 6% | 15% | 10% |
| Eldar et al (1991)[91] | 8 | NR | 25% | 13% |
| Crowley et al (1994)[92] | 12 | 0% | 17% | 0% |

Header: RATE OF EVENTS DURING SUBSEQUENT FOLLOW-UP (MEAN, 3 YEARS, %)

CABG, coronary artery bypass grafting; MI, myocardial infarction; NR, not reported; PTCA, percutaneous transluminal coronary angioplasty.

more patent bypass grafts to the left coronary system. The rate of late mortality for patients with a "protected" left coronary system was 12.5%, compared with 56% for patients with "unprotected" systems ($p < 0.01$). Three-year survival in "protected" patients was 87%, compared with 40% patients with in "unprotected" systems.

Elective "unprotected" PTCA of the LMCA is technically feasible but carries a high procedural mortality rate and poor long-term survival. Rates of procedural mortality of up to 9% and 3-year mortality of 64% have been reported[89–92] (Table 29–5). Some studies have suggested that angioplasty of "unprotected" LMCA stenosis is a viable option in patients for whom the risk of surgery is prohibitive. Selection bias and the small number of patients studied weakens this conclusion, however. The poor prognosis of PTCA in the "unprotected" LMCA is, at least in part, related to the high incidence of restenosis in this setting. Restenosis is poorly tolerated in this population and can be life threatening because of the large amount of myocardium at risk. Early angiographic follow-up has therefore been recommended for early detection of restenosis in patients who undergo PTCA of "unprotected" vessels.

**TABLE 29–5.  RESULTS OF "UNPROTECTED" LEFT MAIN CORONARY ANGIOPLASTY**

| STUDY (YEAR) | NO. OF PATIENTS | MI | PTCA | CABG |
|---|---|---|---|---|
| Stertzer et al (1985)[90] | 11 | 0% | 55% | 45% |
| O'Keefe et al (1989)[89] | 33 | 8% | 23% | 23% |
| Eldar et al (1991)[91] | 8 | 0% | 25% | 13% |
| Crowley et al (1994)[92] | 3 | 100% | 100% | 0% |

Header: RATE OF EVENTS DURING SUBSEQUENT FOLLOW-UP (MEAN, 3 YEARS, %)

CABG, coronary artery bypass grafting; MI, myocardial infarction; PTCA, percutaneous transluminal coronary angioplasty.

Acute LMCA stenosis usually results in rapid hemodynamic deterioration. In certain circumstances, therefore, benefits of an immediate improvement in myocardial perfusion make LMCA PTCA a potentially life-saving procedure.[93, 94] The procedural mortality is high (40% to 50%), but most of the patients who undergo the procedure are unlikely to survive unless patency of the LMCA is promptly reestablished: Emergent LMCA PTCA may improve the outcome in patients with cardiogenic shock and may be used as a bridge to coronary artery bypass surgery. In exceptional circumstances, a clinically unstable patient may be considered for emergency PTCA of the LMCA if the risk of emergency bypass is unacceptable; for example, in a patient with hemodynamic or rhythmic instability despite full medical therapy and intra-aortic balloon counterpulsation or with concurrent disease that prohibits surgery.

Despite technologic advances in dilation catheter and guide-wire design, "unprotected" angioplasty of the left main coronary artery remains relatively contraindicated because of the risk of acute closure and cardiogenic shock and the inability to perform prolonged balloon inflations in such situations. During conventional balloon angioplasty, myocardial ischemia may be minimized by using either an autoperfusion balloon catheter (which maintains some left coronary artery blood flow) or short balloon inflation times.[95] If hemodynamic instability prohibits balloon dilation, percutaneous cardiopulmonary support or intra-aortic balloon counterpulsation may be necessary. Although these strategies may permit prolonged balloon inflations (>30 seconds), they have not been shown to reduce the incidence of intimal dissection or restenosis.

LMCD is often characterized by aorto-ostial involvement and bulky, eccentric stenoses. These lesion characteristics impose limitations on conventional balloon angioplasty. Balloon angioplasty of the LMCA (Fig. 29–1) has typically resulted in residual stenoses of 20% to 35%, leading to restenosis and the need for second revascularization procedures in 30% to 50% of patients.[89] The high content of elastic fibers in the proximal segment of the left main coronary artery has been proposed as a possible explanation for the frequency of elastic recoil and the high rate of restenosis after conventional balloon angioplasty at this site.

The availability of newer interventional techniques, such as directional coronary atherectomy (DCA),[96, 97] mechanical rotational atherectomy (MRA) (Fig. 29–2),[98, 99] excimer laser coronary angioplasty (ELCA),[100] and placement of intracoronary stents,[101–106] has rekindled interest in percutaneous treatment of left LMCA stenoses. These techniques have been used with varying degrees of success in

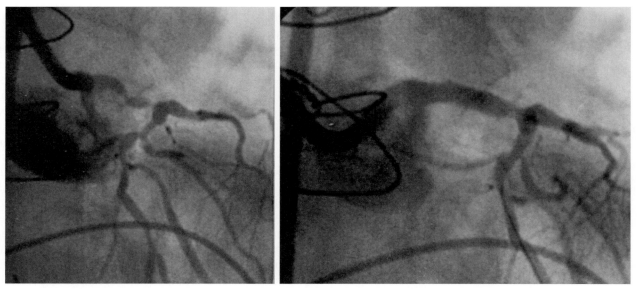

FIGURE 29–1. Before *(left panel)* and after *(right panel)* conventional balloon angioplasty of a "protected" left main coronary artery.

the treatment of LMCD. Their potential advantages include lower risks of dissection, abrupt closure, elastic recoil, and restenosis.

Despite the increasing availability of the new techniques, however, adjunctive angioplasty is commonly required to optimize lumen enlargement, manage technique-induced complications, or salvage procedural failures. This combination is referred to as *facilitated angioplasty*. Safian and colleagues[100] have shown that the success of facilitated angioplasty depends on the type of interventional device used and the morphology of the target lesion.

In 71 left main lesions in their study, facilitated angioplasty using rotational atherectomy was found to be superior to conventional PTCA in ulcerated, eccentric, and calcified lesions, in lesions involving a bend in the vessel, and lesions longer than 20 mm in length. Adjunctive angioplasty using extraction atherectomy or the excimer laser was no better than angioplasty alone. Facilitated angioplasty was not superior to conventional PTCA in treatment of chronic total occlusions or lesions with thrombus.

Lopez and associates[107] found a lesion-specific approach to be safe and effective in the treatment

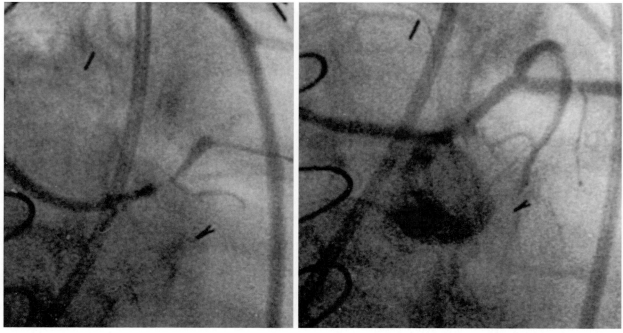

FIGURE 29–2. Before *(left panel)* and after *(right panel)* mechanical rotational atherectomy of a "protected" left main coronary artery.

**TABLE 29–6. RESULTS OF INTERVENTIONAL TECHNIQUES FOR TREATMENT OF LEFT MAIN CORONARY ARTERY STENOSIS**

| | STUDY (YEAR) | | | | | |
|---|---|---|---|---|---|---|
| | Macaya et al (1992)[104] | Laster et al (1994)[97] | Fajadet et al (1996)[105]* | Itoh et al (1996)[106]* | Lopez et al (1997)[107] | Ellis et al (1997)[108]* |
| No. of patients | 3 | 22 | 34 | 33 | 46 | 100 |
| Technique(s) | Stent | DCA | Stent | Stent | DCA, MRA, stent | DCA, stent, MRA, PTCA |
| Mean follow-up (months) | 4 | 24 | 13 | NR | 9 | 15 |
| Death rate | 33% | 0% | 3% | 9% | 2% | 11% |
| Rate of subsequent Q wave myocardial infarction | 0% | 0% | NR | 3% | 2% | 4.5% |
| Rate of second left main coronary intervention (%) | 0% | 9% | 12% | NR | 13% | NR |

*Abstract.

DCA, directional coronary atherectomy; MRA, mechanical rotational atherectomy; NR, not reported; PTCA, percutaneous transluminal coronary angioplasty.

of primarily "protected" LMCA stenoses[107] (Table 29–6). In 46 left main lesions (four "unprotected" and 42 "protected" LMCA lesions), procedural success was 100%, with no major in-hospital complications. The use of specific new device technology resulted in excellent immediate angiographic outcomes and a 1-year event-free survival rate of 71%. The use of coronary stents, either alone or after initial rotational atherectomy (pretreatment for heavily calcified lesions to facilitate optimal stent deployment), produced the best immediate angiographic results. The benefits of stenting were most pronounced for aorto-ostial lesions which are prone to elastic recoil. Figure 29–3 illustrates the results of intracoronary stent placement in a "protected" LMCA.

Laster and colleagues[97] analyzed the acute and long-term results of 24 DCA procedures in 22 patients with "protected" LMCA lesions (see Table 29–6). DCA was the initial choice in 13 of the 24 cases and was employed as an adjunctive procedure in 11 of 24 cases after suboptimal results of balloon angioplasty. Mean LMCA stenosis was reduced from 86% to 13% with DCA. Long-term follow-up showed a clinical restenosis rate of 16% and an event-free survival rate of 89%. Figure 29–4 illustrates the results of DCA of a "protected" LMCA.

The results of LMCA stent placement have been reported. Fajadet and coworkers[105] deployed coronary stents in 21 patients with "unprotected" LMCD and 13 patients with "protected" LMCD. Procedural success was 100%, and stent thrombosis occurred in 3% of cases. At 13 months, sudden death had occurred in 3% of patients, and second PTCA procedures were required for in-stent restenosis in 12%. Itoh and colleagues[106] reported a 94% success rate of LMCA stent placement for 33 "protected" LMCA lesions.[106] Emergency coronary bypass surgery was required in 3% of patients, and 9% died within 3 months of the procedure. Stent placement in an "unprotected" LMCA has been shown to be very effective as a salvage procedure in patients with acute occlusion or dissection. The procedure restores coronary flow, permitting the patient to un-

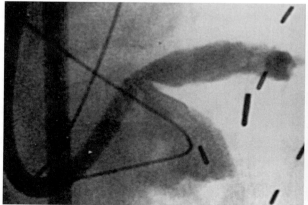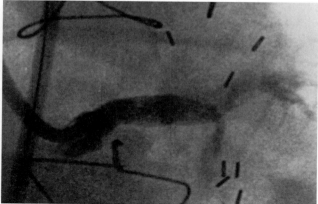

FIGURE 29–3. Before *(left panel)* and after *(right panel)* intracoronary stent placement in a "protected" left main coronary artery.

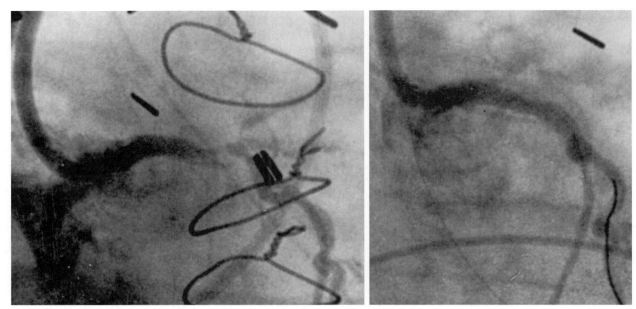

FIGURE 29–4. Before *(left panel)* and after *(right panel)* directional coronary atherectomy of a "protected" left main coronary artery.

dergo emergent revascularization surgery of the LMCA.[102] Macaya and associates[104] reported on three patients with "unprotected" ostial lesions of the LMCA in whom significant elastic recoil after balloon angioplasty was successfully managed with coronary stent placement.

Ellis and colleagues[108] described the results from a multicenter registry (Unprotected Left Main Trunk Intervention Multi-center Assessment [ULTIMA] Registry).[108] Of patients treated for acute MI, 88% were in cardiogenic shock, and the in-hospital survival rate was only 25%. The most powerful predictor of both in-hospital and late outcomes for the patients treated for indications other than acute MI was LV ejection fraction. For patients with LV ejection fractions less than 40%, the in-house mortality (cardiac and noncardiac) was 25%, and the 13-month survival was only 50%. For those patients with ejection fractions greater than 40%, however, the in-house mortality was only 1.8%, and the 13-month mortality was 16%. Half the patients were treated with prophylactic intra-aortic balloon counterpulsation, and 6% were treated with prophylactic cardiopulmonary support.

Although DCA and stent placement for patients who had stable angina or were candidates for cardiopulmonary bypass surgery led to fair in-hospital results, sudden death occurred within 6 months in 5% to 7%. In addition, 6-month follow-up in patients who had unstable angina or were not surgical candidates showed restenosis rates of 48% to 86%, all-cause death rates of 39% to 65%, and cardiac death, subsequent MI, and subsequent coronary bypass surgery rates of 49% to 70%. Ellis and colleagues[108] concluded that if the early postdischarge

events could be minimized, DCA or stent placement for LMCA lesions in patients with stable or new-onset angina and well-preserved LV function performed by highly experienced operators may be a reasonable approach. DCA has been shown in other studies to successfully debulk eccentric atherosclerotic plaque and limit elastic recoil, leading to larger final luminal diameters.[96, 97] Intracoronary stents have also been shown to limit elastic recoil, improve the final minimal luminal diameter, and, therefore, reduce the incidence of subsequent restenosis in this high-risk population.[104, 107] The researches in the ULTIMA Registry propose close angiographic follow-up at 6 to 8 weeks after LMCA interventions to identify patients with early, aggressive restenosis.[107] However, given the high rate of early postdischarge cardiac mortality after this procedure, coronary bypass surgery is still preferred to percutaneous revascularization of "unprotected" LMCA lesions in most patients. In terms of procedural difficulty and long-term outcome, LMCA stenting can be divided into treatment of ostial, body, and distal bifurcation stenting. Procedural difficulty increases and recurrent events increase in ostial, body, and bifurcation lesions, respectively.[109]

Cardiopulmonary bypass has been used as adjunctive therapy in patients undergoing coronary intervention for whom the procedure is considered high risk. The National Registry of Elective Supported Angioplasty was formed as a voluntary registry that gathered data from operators in the United States about patients who had undergone angioplasty with cardiopulmonary bypass *(supported angioplasty)*. Of the 458 patients whose data were submitted to the registry, 61 (13.3%) had LMCA

**TABLE 29-7.    LEFT MAIN CORONARY INTERVENTIONS—WILLIAM BEAUMONT HOSPITAL EXPERIENCE, 1990–1996**

| INTERVENTION | BASELINE | | AFTER INTERVENTION | | AFTER ADJUNCT PTCA | |
|---|---|---|---|---|---|---|
| | AVERAGE MLD | % STENOSIS | AVERAGE MLD | % STENOSIS | AVERAGE MLD | % STENOSIS |
| PTCA (n = 52) | 1.13 ± 0.41 | 67 ± 11 | 2.22 ± 0.91 | 36 ± 14 | — | — |
| ELCA (n = 28) | 0.79 ± 0.25 | 71 ± 7.8 | 2.81 ± 0.39 | 30 ± 8.0 | 2.79 ± 0.36 | 28 ± 7.9 |
| MRA (n = 34) | 0.97 ± 0.32 | 66 ± 10 | 1.55 ± 0.48 | 38 ± 13 | 1.88 ± 0.39 | 28 ± 12 |
| DCA (n = 13) | 1.16 ± 0.47 | 62 ± 13 | 2.94 ± 0.25 | 27 ± 4.0 | 3.02 ± 0.31 | 28 ± 5.0 |
| TEC (n = 5) | 1.11 ± 0.47 | 65 ± 11 | 2.78 ± 0.59 | 24 ± 11 | 2.82 ± 0.62 | 22 ± 11 |
| Stent (n = 9) | 0.94 ± 0.33 | 63 ± 12 | 2.79 ± 0.31 | 5.0 ± 7.0 | 2.99 ± 0.30 | 4.0 ± 6.0 |

DCA, directional coronary atherectomy; ELCA, excimer laser coronary angioplasty; MLD, minimal luminal diameter (in millimeters); MRA, mechanical rotational atherectomy; PTCA, percutaneous transluminal coronary angioplasty; TEC, transluminal extraction catheter atherectomy.

stenosis of greater than 60%.[110, 111] The mortality of "high-risk" patients undergoing angioplasty of the LMCA was significantly higher than that of "high-risk" patients undergoing angioplasty of another vessel who also had an LMCA stenosis less than 60%.

In the presence of significant LMCA disease, there was an increased risk of complications during and after angioplasty of vessels other than the LMCA. This risk was not limited to the procedure itself but extended over several days after a successful procedure. These results differ from those of most routine angioplasty procedures, for which 84% of postprocedural closures occur within 6 hours, and the acute closure rate after the first 24 hours is very low.[91, 92] Possible explanations for the differences include (1) promotion of elastic recoil by higher amounts of elastic tissue and (2) a possible rebound coagulant effect after the large doses of heparin. Additional risks factors for supported angioplasty are hypotension, excessive blood loss, and the need for surgical repair of the femoral artery. The addition of cardiopulmonary bypass does not significantly alter the outcome of patients undergoing interventions in the LMCA. Thus, even with percutaneous cardiopulmonary bypass, LMCA intervention should be considered only in patients whose disease would otherwise be deemed inoperable and who are willing to accept the risk involved.

Results of the analysis of all LMCA interventions performed at William Beaumont Hospital are presented in Table 29–7. Between 1990 and 1996, we performed conventional balloon angioplasty, MRA, DCA, ELCA, and coronary stent placement in 141 LMCA stenoses of at least 50% severity. The majority of the procedures were performed for unstable angina (89%) and were "protected" procedures (80%). DCA and coronary stent placement resulted in the largest average luminal diameters after adjunctive balloon angioplasty. There was an 11% incidence of in-hospital cardiac death, a 37% incidence of death within 6 months of the procedure,

a 22% incidence of procedure-related MI, a 13% incidence of need for urgent coronary bypass surgery, a 5% incidence of "bail-out" stent placement (stent placement as an alternative to emergency bypass surgery), and a 3% incidence of stroke.

## SUMMARY

Because there are no specific historical, physical, or laboratory features that identify patients with LMCD, disease of the LMCA should always be suspected in patients who undergo diagnostic cardiac catheterization. The stenosis is most commonly due to atherosclerosis and is generally associated with involvement of other major epicardial vessels. Disease limited to the left main ostium is rare and is likely due to conditions that affect the aorta.

Caution must be exercised in the performance of cardiac catheterization in patients with LMCD. Because of their tenuous condition, otherwise benign occurrences, such as a brief vasovagal response or an nonsustained atrial arrhythmia, can lead to rapid and irreversible hemodynamic collapse. Nonetheless, proper technique and careful hemodynamic monitoring limits the potential for complications.

Treatment of LMCD has historically been surgical. When the vessel is "protected," catheter-based interventions can be performed with acceptable early and late outcomes. In contrast, "unprotected" LMCA stenosis remains largely a surgical disease. Preliminary data suggest that treatment of "unprotected" LMCA stenoses is associated with significant morbidity and mortality and should be reserved for those patients who are deemed not to be surgical candidates and who are willing to accept the risks involved.

## REFERENCES

1. Herrick J: Clinical features of sudden obstruction of the coronary arteries. JAMA 59:2015, 1912.

2. Lim JS, Proudfit WL, Sones FM: Left main coronary arterial obstruction: Follow-up of 141 nonsurgical cases. Am J Cardiol 36:131, 1975.

3. Bruschke AV, Proudfit WL, Sones FM: Progress study of 590 consecutive nonsurgical cases of coronary disease followed 5–9 years: I. Arteriographic correlations. Circulation 47:1147, 1973.

4. Cohen MV, Cohn PF, Herman MV, et al: Diagnosis and prognosis of main left coronary artery obstruction. Circulation 45(suppl I):I-57, 1972.

5. Bergelson BA, Tommaso CL: Left main coronary artery disease: Assessment, diagnosis, and therapy. Am Heart J 129:350, 1995.

6. Salem BI, Terasawa M, Mathur VS, et al: Left main coronary artery ostial stenosis: Clinical markers, angiographic recognition and distinction from left main disease. Cathet Cardiovasc Diagn 5:125, 1979.

7. Barner HB, Reese J, Standeven J, et al: Left coronary ostial stenosis: Comparison with left main coronary artery stenosis. Ann Thorac Surg 47:293, 1989.

8. Josa M, Danielson GK, Weidman WH, et al: Congenital ostial membrane of left main coronary artery. J Thorac Cardiovasc Surg 81:338, 1981.

9. Chun PKC, Jones R, Robinowitz M, et al: Coronary ostial stenosis in Takayasu's arteritis. Chest 78:330, 1980.

10. Martin de Dios R, Pey J, Cazzanigam M: Coronary artery stenosis and subclavian steal in Takayasu's arteritis. Eur J Cardiol 12:229, 1981.

11. Frater FWM, Jordan A: Syphilitic coronary ostial stenosis. Ann Thorac Surg 6:463, 1968.

12. Riberio P, Shapiro L, Gonzalez A, et al: Cross sectional echocardiographic assessment of the aortic root and coronary ostial stenosis in familial hypercholesterolemia. Br Heart J 50:432, 1983.

13. Roberts W, Ferrans V, Levy R, et al: Cardiovascular pathology in hyperlipoproteinemia. Am J Cardiol 31:557, 1973.

14. Chinnasami BR, Schwartz RC, Pink SB, et al: Isolated left main coronary stenosis and mediastinal irradiation. Clin Cardiol 15:459, 1992.

15. Tommaso CL, Applefeld MM, Singleton RT: Isolated left main coronary artery stenosis and mediastinal radiotherapy as an etiologic factor. Am J Cardiol 61:1119, 1988.

16. Tenet W, Missri J, Hager D: Radiation-induced stenosis of the left main coronary artery. Cathet Cardiovasc Diagn 12:169, 1986.

17. Zeymer U, Hirschmann WD, Neuhaus KL: Left main coronary stenosis by a mediastinal lymphoma. Clin Invest 70:1024, 1992.

18. Radwaner BA, Geringer R, Goldman AM, et al: Left main coronary artery stenosis following mediastinal irradiation. Am J Med 82:1017, 1987.

19. Prachar H, Muhlbauer J, Pollak H, et al: Iatrogenic left main coronary artery stenosis following aortic valve replacement. Eur Heart J 9:1151, 1988.

20. Bashour TT, Hanna ES, Edgett J, et al: Iatrogenic left main coronary artery stenosis following PTCA or valve replacement. Clin Cardiol 8:114, 1985.

21. Winkelmann BR, Ihnken V, Beyersdorf F, et al: Left main coronary artery stenosis after aortic valve replacement: Genetic disposition for accelerated arteriosclerosis after injury of the intact human coronary artery. Coron Artery Dis 4:659, 1993.

22. Hazan E, Rioux C, Deqirot A, et al: Postperfusion stenosis of the common left coronary artery. J Thorac Cardiovasc Surg 69:703, 1975.

23. Trimble AS, Bigelow WG, Wigle ED, et al: Coronary ostial stenosis: A late complication of coronary perfusion in open heart surgery. J Thorac Cardiovasc Surg 57:792, 1969.

24. Jain A, Mazanek GJ, Armitage JM: Unstable angina secondary to left main coronary thrombus extending from prosthetic aortic valve. Cathet Cardiovasc Diagn 15:271, 1988.

25. Zelinger AB, Shulruff S, Pouget JM: Significant left main stenosis following asymptomatic dissection during coronary arteriography. Chest 83:568, 1983.

26. Keltai M, Bartek I, Biro V: Guidewire snap causing left main

27. Lotan C, Milgalter E, Gotsman M: Dissection of the left main coronary artery: A complication of PTCA to the left anterior descending artery. Clin Cardiol 11:120, 1988.

28. Harlan JL, Meng R: Thrombosis of the left main coronary artery following percutaneous transluminal coronary angioplasty. Ann Thorac Surg 43:220, 1987.

29. Slack JD, Pinkerton CA, VanTassel JW, et al: Left main coronary artery dissection during percutaneous transluminal coronary angioplasty. Cathet Cardiovasc Diagn 12:255, 1986.

30. Slack JD, Pinkerton CA: Subacute left main coronary stenosis: An unusual but serious complication of percutaneous transluminal coronary angioplasty. Angiology 36(2):130–136, 1985.

31. Haraphongse M, Rossall RE: Subacute left main coronary stenosis following percutaneous transluminal coronary angioplasty. Cathet Cardiovasc Diagn 13:410, 1987.

32. Waller BF, Pinkerton CA, Foster LN: Morphologic evidence of accelerated left main coronary artery stenosis: A late complication of percutaneous transluminal balloon angioplasty of the left anterior descending coronary artery. J Am Coll Cardiol 9:1019, 1987.

33. Vardhan IN, Aharonian VJ, Gordon S, et al: A rare complication of percutaneous transluminal coronary angioplasty—Left main disease. Am Heart J 121:902, 1991.

34. Hamad N, Pichard A, Oboler A, et al: Left main coronary artery stenosis as a late complication of percutaneous transluminal coronary angioplasty. Am J Cardiol 60:1183, 1987.

35. Wayne VS, Harper RW, Pitt A: Left main coronary artery stenosis after percutaneous transluminal coronary angioplasty. Am J Cardiol 61:459, 1988.

36. Kells CM, Miller RM, Henderson MA, et al: Left main coronary artery disease progression after percutaneous transluminal coronary angioplasty. Am J Cardiol 65:513, 1990.

37. Smith MD, Cowley MJ, Vetrovec GW: Aneurysms of the left main coronary artery: A report of three cases and a review of the literature. Cathet Cardiovasc Diagn 10:583, 1984.

38. Lenihan DJ, Zeman HS, Collins GJ: Left main coronary artery aneurysm in association with severe atherosclerosis: A case report and review of the literature. Cathet Cardiovasc Diagn 23:28, 1991.

39. Gill JB, Ruddy TD, Newell JB, et al: Prognostic importance of thallium uptake by the lungs during exercise in coronary artery disease. N Engl J Med 317:1485, 1987.

40. Gibbons RJ, Fyke FE, Clements IP, et al: Noninvasive identification of severe coronary artery disease using exercise radionuclide angiography. J Am Coll Cardiol 11:28, 1988.

41. Gibson RS, Watson DD, Craddock GB, et al: Prediction of cardiac events after uncomplicated myocardial infarction: A prospective study comparing predischarge exercise thallium-201 scintigraphy and coronary angiography. Circulation 68:321, 1983.

42. Giubbini R, Campini R, Milan E, et al: Evelution of technetium-99m-sestamibi lung uptake: Correlation with left ventricular function. J Nucl Med 36:58, 1995.

43. Machecourt J, Longere P, Fagret D, et al: Prognostic value of thallium-201 single-photon emission computed tomographic myocardial perfusion imaging according to extent of myocardial defect: Study in 1,926 patients with follow-up at 33 months. J Am Coll Cardiol 23:1096, 1994.

44. Abraham RD, Freedman SB, Dunn RF, et al: Prediction of multivessel coronary artery disease and prognosis early after acute myocardial infarction by exercise electrocardiography and thallium-201 myocardial perfusion scanning. Am J Cardiol 58:423, 1986.

45. Nygaard TW, Gibson RS, Ryan JM, et al: Prevalence of high risk thallium-201 scintigraphic findings in left main coronary artery stenosis: Comparison with patients with multiple- and single-vessel coronary artery disease. Am J Cardiol 53:462, 1984.

46. Tardif JC, Vannon MA, Taylor K, et al: Delineation of extended lengths of coronary arteries by multi-plane transesophageal echocardiography. J Am Coll Cardiol 24:909, 1994.

47. Memmola C, Iliceto S, Rizzon P: Detection of proximal stenosis of the left coronary artery by digital transesophageal echocardiography: Feasibility, sensitivity and specificity. J Am Soc Echocardiogr 6:149, 1993.

48. Yamagishi M, Yasu T, Ohara K, et al: Detection of coronary blood flow associated with left main coronary artery stenosis by transesophageal Doppler color flow echocardiography. J Am Coll Cardiol 17:87, 1991.

49. Heublein B, Kanemoto N, Steidl C, et al: Detection and quantification of left main coronary artery stenosis by two-dimensional echocardiography. Jpn Heart J 24:689, 1983.

50. Yoshida K, Yoshikawa J, Hozumi T, et al: Detection of left main coronary artery stenosis by transesophageal color Doppler and two-dimensional echocardiography. Circulation 81:1271, 1990.

51. DeMots H, Rosch J, McAnulty JH, et al: Left main coronary artery disease. Circulation 50:972, 1974.

52. Lozter EC, Johnson LW, Johnson S, et al: Coronary arteriography 1984–1987: A report of the Registry of the Society for Cardiac Angiography and Interventions. II. An analysis of 218 deaths related to coronary arteriography. Cathet Cardiovasc Diagn 17:11, 1989.

53. Boehrer JD, Lange RA, Willard JE et al: Markedly increased periprocedure mortality of cardiac catheterization in patients with severe narrowing of the left main coronary artery. Am J Cardiol 70:1388, 1992.

54. Kovac JD, de Bono DP: Cardiac catheter complications related to left main stem disease. Heart 76:76, 1996.

55. Ko JK, Nishimura RA, Holmes DR, et al: Predictors of early mortality in patients with angiographically documented left main coronary artery disease. Cathet Cardiovasc Diagn 24:84, 1991.

56. Gordon PR, Abrams C, Gash AK, et al: Pericatheterization risk factors in left main coronary artery stenosis. Am J Cardiol 59:1080, 1987.

57. DeMots H, Bonchek L, Rosch J, et al: Left main coronary artery disease: Risks of angiography, importance of coexisting disease of other coronary arteries and effect of revascularization. Am J Cardiol 36:136, 1975.

58. Kennedy JW: Complication associated with cardiac catheterization and angiography. Cathet Cardiovasc Diagn 8:13, 1982.

59. Laskey W, Boyle J, Johnson JW, and the Registry Committee of the Society for Cardiac Angiography and Interventions: Multivariable model for prediction of risk of significant complication during diagnostic cardiac catheterization. Cathet Cardiovasc Diagn 30:185, 1993.

60. Gould KL, Lipscomb K: Effects of coronary stenoses on coronary reserve and resistance. Am J Cardiol 34:48, 1974.

61. Hermiller JB, Buller CE, Tenaglia AN: Unrecognized left main coronary artery disease in patients undergoing interventional procedures. Am J Cardiol 71:173, 1993.

62. Skinner JS, Adams PC: Outpatient cardiac catheterization. Int J Cardiol 53:209, 1996.

63. Klinke WP, Kubac G, Talibi T, et al: Safety of outpatient cardiac catheterizations. Am J Cardiol 56:639, 1985.

64. Clark DA, Moscovich MD, Vetrovec GW, et al: Guidelines for the performance of outpatient catheterization and angiographic procedures. Cathet Cardiovasc Diagn 27:5, 1992.

65. Feld H, Fisher M, Shani J: Coronary angiography with 5 French catheters may miss an ostial left main stenosis. J Intervent Cardiol 6:131, 1993.

66. Barrett BJ, Parfrey PS, Vavasour HM, et al: A comparison of nonionic, low-osmolality radiocontrast agents with ionic, high-osmolality agents during cardiac catheterization. N Engl J Med 326:431, 1992.

67. Hwang MH, Piao ZE, Murdock DK, et al: Effects of contrast media on the conducting system of the heart during coronary angiography: A comparison of Renografin-76 to Hypaque-76. Invest Radiol 23:748, 1988.

68. Wolfson S, Grant D, Ross AM, et al: Risk of death related to coronary arteriography; Role of left coronary arterial lesions. Am J Cardiol 37:210, 1976.

69. Ross J, Brandenburg RO, Dinsmore RE, et al: Guidelines for coronary angiography. A report of the American College of Cardiology/American Heart Association Task Force on the Assessment of Diagnostic and Therapeutic Cardiovascular Procedures (Subcommittee on Coronary Angiography). J Am Coll Cardiol 10:935, 1987.

70. Pepine CJ, Allen HD, Bashore TM, et al: ACC/AHA guidelines for cardiac catheterization and cardiac catheterization laboratories. American College of Cardiology/American Heart Association Ad Hoc Task Force on Cardiac Catheterization. J Am Coll Cardiol 18:1149, 1991.

71. Tahan SR, Geha AS, Hammond GL, et al: Bypass surgery for left main coronary artery disease—Reduced perioperative myocardial infarction with preoperative intra-aortic balloon counterpulsation. Br Heart J 43:191, 1979.

72. Shahian DM, Butterly JR, Malacoff RF: Total obstruction of the left main coronary artery. Ann Thorac Surg 46:317, 1988.

73. Zimmern SH, Rogers WJ, Bream PR, et al: Total occlusion of the left main coronary artery: The Coronary Artery Surgery Study (CASS) experience. Am J Cardiol 49:2003, 1982.

74. Cohen MV, Gorlin R: Main left coronary artery disease: Clinical experience from 1964–1974. Circulation 52:275, 1975.

75. Oberman A, Harrell RR, Russell RO, et al: Surgical versus medical treatment in disease of the left main coronary artery. Lancet 2:591–594, 1976.

76. Mehta J, Hamby RI, Hoffman I, et al: Medical-surgical aspects of left main coronary artery disease. J Thoracic Cardiovasc Surg 71:137, 1976.

77. Coles JC, Goldbach MM, Ahmed SN, et al: Left main-stem coronary artery disease: Surgical versus medical management. Can J Surg 27:571, 1984.

78. Caracciolo EA, Davis KB, Sopko G, et al: Comparison of surgical and medical group survival in patients with left main coronary artery disease. Circulation 91:2325, 1995.

79. Chaitman BR, Fisher LD, Bourassa MG, et al: Effect of coronary bypass surgery on survival patterns in subsets of patients with left main coronary artery disease. Am J Cardiol 48:765, 1981.

80. European Coronary Surgery Study Group: Prospective randomized study of coronary artery bypass in stable angina pectoris. Lancet 2:491, 1980.

81. Takaro T, Peduzzi P, Detre KM, et al: Survival in subgroups of patients with left main coronary artery disease: Veterans Administration Cooperative Study of Surgery for Coronary Arterial Occlusive Disease. Circulation 66:14, 1982.

82. Detre K, Murphy ML, Hultgren H: Effect of coronary bypass surgery on longevity in high and low risk patients. Report from the V.A. Cooperative Coronary Surgery Study. Lancet 2:1243–1245, 1977.

83. Zajtchuk R, Albus R, Bowen TE, et al: Surgical treatment of left main and left main equivalent coronary artery disease. J Thorac Cardiovasc Surg 78:452, 1979.

84. Killen DA, Reed WA, Kinded L, et al: Surgical therapy for left main coronary artery disease. J Thorac Cardiovasc Surg 80:255, 1980.

85. McConahay DR, Killen DA, McCallister BD, et al: Coronary artery bypass surgery for left main coronary artery disease. Am J Cardiol 37:885, 1976.

86. Gruentzig AR: Transluminal dilatation of coronary artery stenosis. Lancet 1:263, 1978.

87. Gruentzig AR, Senning A, Siegenthaler WE: Nonoperative dilatation of coronary artery stenosis. N Engl J Med 301:61, 1979.

88. Ryan TJ, Bauman WB, Kennedy JW, et al: Guidelines for percutaneous transluminal coronary angioplasty. A report of the American College of Cardiology/American Heart Association Task Force on Assessment of Diagnostic and Therapeutic Cardiovascular Procedures (Subcommittee on Percutaneous Transluminal Coronary Angioplasty). J Am Coll Cardiol 22:2033, 1993.

89. O'Keefe JH, Hartzler GO, Rutherford BD, et al: Left main coronary angioplasty: Early and late results of 127 acute and elective procedures. Am J Cardiol 64:144, 1989.

90. Stertzer SH, Myler RK, Insel H: Percutaneous transluminal coronary angioplasty in left main stem coronary stenosis: A five-year appraisal. Int J Cardiol 9:149, 1985.

91. Eldar M, Schulhoff N, Herz I, et al: Results of percutaneous

transluminal angioplasty of the left main coronary artery. Am J Cardiol 68:255, 1991.

92. Crowley ST, Morrison DA: Percutaneous transluminal coronary angioplasty of the left main coronary artery in patients with rest angina. Cathet Cardiovasc Diagn 33:103, 1994.

93. Nakhjavan FK, Goldman AP, Hutt GH: Emergency percutaneous transluminal coronary angioplasty of left main stenosis. Am Heart J 114:643, 1987.

94. Groves PH, Ikram S, Hayward WJ: Emergency angioplasty of the left main coronary artery. Eur Heart J 10:1123, 1989.

95. Turi ZG, Rezkella S, Campbell CA, et al: Left main percutaneous transluminal coronary angioplasty with the autoperfusion catheter in an animal model. Cathet Cardiovasc Diagn 21:45, 1990.

96. Muller DW, Ellis SG, Topol EJ: Atherectomy of the left main coronary artery with percutaneous cardiopulmonary bypass support. Am J Cardiol 64:114, 1989.

97. Laster SB, Rutherford BD, McConahay DR, et al: Directional atherectomy of left main stenoses. Cathet Cardiovasc Diagn 33:317, 1994.

98. Rozenman Y, Lotan C, Weiss AT, et al: Emergency rotational ablation of a calcified left main coronary artery stenosis in a patient with ischemic induced cardiogenic shock. Cathet Cardiovasc Diagn 36:63, 1995.

99. Chaix AF, Barragan P, Silvestri M, et al: Rotablator and endoprosthesis in the left main trunk. Arch Mal Coeur Vaiss 88:95, 1995.

100. Safian RD, Freed M, Reddy V, et al: Do excimer laser angioplasty and rotational atherectomy facilitate balloon angioplasty? Implications for lesion-specific coronary intervention. J Am Coll Cardiol 27:552, 1996.

101. Lee S, Chan HW, Lam L, et al: Stand-alone stenting of the left main coronary artery and 16-month patency despite sepsis and complicated hospital course. Am Heart J 130:1289, 1995.

102. Sathe S, Sebastian M, Vohra J, et al: Bail-out stenting for left main coronary artery occlusion following diagnostic angiography. Cathet Cardiovasc Diagn 31:70, 1994.

103. Garcia-Robles JA, Garcia E, Rico M, et al: Emergency coronary stenting for acute occlusive dissection of the left main coronary artery. Cathet Cardiovasc Diagn 30:227, 1993.

104. Macaya C, Alfonso F, Iniguez A, et al: Stenting for elastic recoil during coronary angioplasty of the left main coronary artery. Am J Cardiol 70:105, 1992.

105. Fajadet J, Brunel P, Jordan C, et al: Stenting of unprotected left main coronary artery stenosis without Coumadin. J Am Coll Cardiol 27:277A, 1996.

106. Itoh A, Colombo A, Hall P, et al: Stenting in protected and unprotected left main coronary artery: Immediate and follow-up results. J Am Coll Cardiol 27:277A, 1996.

107. Lopez JJ, Ho KK, Stoler RC: Percutaneous treatment of protected and unprotected left main coronary stenoses with new devices: Immediate angiographic results and intermediate-term follow-up. J Am Coll Cardiol 29:345, 1997.

108. Ellis SG, Tamai H, Nobuyoshi M, et al: Contemporary percutaneous treatment of unprotected left main coronary stenoses. Initial results from a multicenter registry analysis 1994–1996. Circulation 96:3867–3872, 1997.

109. Lefevre T, Louvard Y, Morice MC, et al: Stenting of bifurcation lesions: Classification, treatments, and results. Catheter Cardiovasc Interv 49:274–283, 2000.

110. Tommaso CL, Vogel JH, Vogel RA: Coronary angioplasty in high-risk patients with left main coronary stenosis: Results from the National Registry of Elective Supported Angioplasty. Cathet Cardiovasc Diagn 25:169, 1992.

111. Vogel JH, Ruiz CE, Jahnke RB, et al: Percutaneous (nonsurgical) supported angioplasty in unprotected left main disease and severe left ventricular dysfunction. Clin Cardiol 12:297, 1989.

# 30

# Emergency Coronary Artery Bypass Grafting

*James M. Douglas, Jr.*     *Thomas F. Slaughter*     *Donald D. Glower*     *J. G. Reves*

Soon after the development and propagation of coronary artery bypass grafting (CABG) as a therapeutic option for coronary artery disease, reports appeared in the literature confirming the feasibility of performing this procedure in the emergent situation.[1–4] Over the ensuing years, many investigators have attempted to define the role of emergency CABG in the treatment of unstable angina, evolving myocardial infarction, and postinfarction angina. Although many questions remain unanswered, these studies have clearly shown that CABG can be performed successfully in the acutely ischemic patient.

The introduction of percutaneous transluminal coronary angioplasty by Gruntzig in 1977 produced a new population of patients who were candidates for iatrogenic cardiac emergencies.[5] The successful development of this technique relied on the ability to salvage unstable patients by the use of CABG. In this chapter, we examine the application of emergency CABG with specific emphasis on its use in the treatment of failed angioplasty. Emergency CABG is defined as that occurring in the setting of ongoing ischemia or infarction.

## INDICATIONS FOR EMERGENCY CORONARY ARTERY BYPASS GRAFTING

Percutaneous transluminal coronary angioplasty has spread rapidly since its inception. As experience has been gained, the safety of the technique has increased, despite the greater complexity of cases currently being approached. The overall immediate failure rate, requiring emergent bypass surgery is less than 5% in collected series.[6–18] The most common indication for emergency CABG has been acute vessel occlusion with or without intimal dissection. Other indications include vessel perforation and persistent ischemia with hemodynamic or electrical instability. Occasionally, a diagnosis of myocardial rupture, ischemic mitral regurgitation, or ventricular septal defect may be made at the time of attempted angioplasty. The decision for surgery and the timing of repair are then dependent on the hemodynamic status of the patient.

## PATIENT PREPARATION

The goals of emergency CABG are to relieve ischemia, minimize the extent of infarction, restore hemodynamic and electrical stability, and improve long-term mortality. Although the degree of myocardial salvage is dependent on numerous factors, including the territory at risk, the degree of collateral flow present, and the perfusion pressure, clearly one of the most important factors is the time between the development of ischemia and the provision of reperfusion. Minimizing the ischemic interval that precedes surgical revascularization requires an orchestrated effort by the cardiologist, surgeon, and anesthesiologist. Additionally, several methods may be employed to minimize progression of ischemia or to maintain flow through occluded vessels. The intra-aortic balloon pump may provide hemodynamic stability and augmentation of coronary blood flow. Also, placement of an intraluminal perfusion catheter across the area of occlusion may allow for continued blood flow while surgical preparations are made.[19]

After the decision is made to proceed with surgery, certain considerations become important. Despite the urgency of the situation, it is in the best interest of the patient that the cardiologist convey information on the patient's status before the patient is transported to the operating room. In addition to routine preoperative information regarding past medical history, current medications, and allergies, the anesthesiologist is interested in current hemodynamic support, episodes of dysrhythmia and effectiveness of any antiarrhythmic drugs administered, vascular access available, time of last oral intake, and complete history of administration of anticoagulants and thrombolytics. Review of the history, review of the coronary and other angiographic studies, and repeat physical examination by the surgeon are important first steps before any operation. It has not been unheard of for a patient to reach the operating room for emergency bypass surgery only to learn that he or she has had bilateral saphenous vein strippings. Although there are methods to circumvent this problem, clearly it is better for the surgeon to know of it in advance so that appropriate adjustments can be made.

## IMPLICATIONS OF THROMBOLYTIC THERAPY

### Mechanism of Action

Administration of thrombolytic therapy during the acute phase of myocardial infarction has become an increasingly widespread practice. Thrombolytic therapy rapidly achieves reperfusion of the occluded vessel in most patients; however, as many as 20% of vessels fail to reperfuse and require, in some cases, emergent CABG in a patient in a fibrinolytic state.[20] Each of the thrombolytic agents in current clinical use produces the conversion of plasminogen to the active serine protease plasmin. Degradation of fibrinogen is the most notable laboratory finding associated with thrombolytic therapy. Indeed, this is likely the most common cause of bleeding after thrombolytic therapy, but plasmin also exerts numerous other effects on the hemostatic system.[21] Fibrinogen fragments produced after exposure to plasmin inhibit fibrin polymerization essential to formation of the clot.[22] In addition, plasmin causes proteolysis of the cofactors V and VIII, which are necessary in the formation of thrombin.[21, 23] After exposure to plasmin in vitro, platelet function is impaired by interference with arachidonic acid production and proteolysis of the surface glycoproteins Ib and IIb/IIIa.[21]

### Incidence of Bleeding Complications

Thrombolytic therapy itself is a relatively infrequent cause of bleeding; however, in the setting of a major surgical procedure, exsanguination becomes a significant concern. Intracoronary streptokinase administered immediately before CABG is associated with increased postoperative bleeding, requiring greater exposure to blood products; however, thrombolytic therapy does not appear to contribute to perioperative mortality.[20, 24, 25] No correlation has been noted between the dose of thrombolytic agent and perioperative bleeding.[24] Kereiakes and coworkers[26] examined the incidence of postoperative bleeding for patients undergoing CABG within 6 hours of intravenous tissue plasminogen activator administration and failed angioplasty. Eight percent of the patients required surgical reexploration attributable

to a postoperative coagulopathy, and the patients exposed to thrombolytic therapy required an average of 5.6 units of packed red blood cells during the 24 hours after surgery. A retrospective study performed at Duke University correlated the incidence of bleeding associated with CABG surgery to the interval since the administration of intravenous streptokinase.[27] Patients receiving streptokinase within 12 hours of surgery experienced significantly greater postoperative hemorrhage than those whose surgery was delayed after thrombolytic therapy.

### Management of Bleeding Complications

Any approach to the management of hemorrhage after thrombolytic therapy and CABG must take into consideration the multitude of factors contributing to abnormal hemostasis following cardiopulmonary bypass.[28] Cryoprecipitate, with high concentrations of both fibrinogen and factor VIII, provides the best initial therapy for postoperative bleeding following thrombolytic therapy.[21] Although fresh frozen plasma could also be used to replete factors V and VIII, platelet defects following cardiopulmonary bypass and plasmin exposure would best be managed by the administration of platelet concentrates. Platelet concentrates contain intracellular factor V as well as factors V and VIII in the plasma diluent.[29] Aprotinin and the synthetic antifibrinolytics ε-aminocaproic acid and tranexamic acid may further limit postoperative hemorrhage after thrombolytic therapy. Although antifibrinolytic drugs have proved effective at decreasing blood loss associated with cardiac surgery under most circumstances, the efficacy of these drugs in the setting of thrombolytic therapy remains to be investigated.[30]

## CONDUCT OF THE OPERATION

### Anesthetic Induction

On arrival in the operating room, the patient is preoxygenated as surgical preparation begins. Premedication has usually been accomplished in the catheterization laboratory. Peripheral venous access in the form of at least one 14-gauge intravenous catheter and a radial arterial line are placed before anesthetic induction. If the patient arrives with arterial access in the form of a femoral sheath or an intra-aortic balloon pump, we transduce that line while performing the anesthetic induction. We believe that the beneficial effects of general anesthesia on myocardial ischemia outweigh the risks associated with less than optimal monitoring. After anesthetic induction, additional invasive monitoring may be inserted while final surgical preparation occurs. Pulmonary artery catheters with or without continuous mixed venous oximetry and transesophageal echocardiography are used more frequently in emergency CABG than in elective CABG.

If an intra-aortic balloon pump or an intraluminal perfusion catheter has been placed, this instrumentation is cleansed appropriately near the entry sites and draped out of the operative field. In the case of perfusion catheters, provisions are made to allow the operating room personnel access to this catheter so that it may be withdrawn before cross-clamping of the aorta.

## Choice of Conduit

The choice of conduit during emergency CABG requires some thought. Traditionally, most surgeons have employed saphenous vein bypass grafts without the use of the internal mammary artery in order to minimize operative time and to ensure ample perfusion. In addition, the increased risk of chest wall bleeding after thrombolytic agents has been a consideration. However, in recent years, we have used the internal mammary artery as often as possible, even in emergency situations, because of its proven increased long-term patency rates. Clinical studies have demonstrated a 10-year patency rate of 95% with internal mammary artery grafts, as opposed to approximately 50% with saphenous vein bypass grafts.[31, 32] As experience has been gained, the time required to harvest the internal mammary artery has not been excessive. Also, the presence of a perfusion catheter allows the luxury of harvesting the graft while perfusion of the coronary artery is maintained. Frequently the internal mammary artery has been taken down after the patient is placed on cardiopulmonary bypass. This is less cumbersome than might be expected, and harvesting of the graft has been somewhat easier with the lung deflated.

Regardless of the conduits chosen, complete revascularization has been the goal in our institution. Preferably, the acutely ischemic arterial bed is grafted first when the saphenous vein is the sole conduit source. However, when the internal mammary artery is used, this frequently is the last vessel to be anastomosed.

## ANESTHETIC CONSIDERATIONS

The occurrence of myocardial ischemia detected by electrocardiography, lactate production, and thallium perfusion scans is common during surgery for patients with ischemic heart disease.[33–35] The incidence of ischemia has been associated with tachycardia and hypotension, but frequently occurs in the absence of hemodynamic changes.[33–36]

General anesthesia favorably influences myocardial ischemia by altering the hemodynamic determinants of global myocardial oxygen supply and demand. Anesthetic drugs reduce oxygen demand by slowing heart rate, decreasing ventricular wall tension, and decreasing contractility. Oxygen supply is increased by supporting diastolic coronary perfusion pressure, lengthening diastolic time for perfusion, and decreasing intraventricular pressure.[37, 38] In addition, many anesthetics blunt the release of endogenous catecholamines in response to the stress of surgery.[39] This may improve myocardial tolerance to ischemia. It is conceivable that anesthetics that decrease intracellular calcium concentration may also render myocardial cells less vulnerable to ischemic injury. Most general anesthetic agents favorably affect the determinants of myocardial oxygen supply and demand.

Clinical investigations provide support for the protective effects of inhalation anesthetics. Moffitt and associates[40–42] conducted a series of investigations during CABG surgery to determine the effects of the inhalation anesthetics (halothane, enflurane, and isoflurane) on myocardial metabolism and hemodynamics in patients with significant coronary artery disease. Twelve patients were given halothane with either intravenous thiopental or intramuscular morphine. Mean arterial pressure declined 17% and 30%, respectively, as did myocardial oxygen consumption. Coronary sinus oxygen content increased.[40] In another investigation, 10 patients receiving β-blockers were anesthetized with enflurane in initial concentrations sufficient to decrease blood pressure by 30%. During stimulation, enflurane was titrated to maintain blood pressure slightly below awake levels. Coronary blood flow remained proportional to myocardial oxygen consumption, and no patients experienced myocardial lactate production.[41]

In clinical studies of myocardial metabolism involving both healthy subjects and patients with ischemic heart disease complicated by moderate heart failure, halothane did not affect coronary vascular resistance.[43] Myocardial oxygenation was adequately maintained in both groups without evidence of myocardial lactate production.

The administration of isoflurane to patients with ischemic heart disease continues to be a controversial topic. Reiz and colleagues[44] found that isoflurane reduced coronary vascular resistance in patients with ischemic heart disease, whether it was administered as the sole anesthetic agent or in combination with nitrous oxide. Although myocardial lactate extraction was significantly reduced in both groups, electrocardiographic evidence of ischemia occurred in 10 of 21 patients receiving isoflurane alone and in 7 of 13 patients receiving isoflurane in combination with nitrous oxide. In a group of 10 patients receiving β-blockers—all of whom were anesthetized with isoflurane—average coronary vascular resistance and myocardial lactate extraction were reduced; however, lactate production, indicating the presence of ischemia, was evident in 3 of the 10 patients.[42] In other circumstances, isoflurane has demonstrated a protective influence on ischemia. Tarnow and associates[45] found that isoflurane (0.5%) and nitrous oxide (50%) increased the threshold for the development of pacing-induced myocardial ischemia in patients with multivessel coronary artery disease.

Intravenous anesthetic agents have also been investigated for their effects on myocardial oxygen consumption and coronary blood flow. Fentanyl (109 μg/kg) was associated with a proportional reduction of both coronary blood flow (32%) and myocardial oxygen consumption (29%).[46] Only 1 of 10 patients exhibited myocardial lactate production. Skourtis and coworkers[47] found myocardial lactate production in only one of six coronary surgical patients given fentanyl as the primary anesthetic. When combined with droperidol and nitrous oxide in eight patients with coronary artery disease, fentanyl (15 μg/kg) produced similar declines in both myocardial blood flow and oxygen consumption without any evidence of lactate production or electrocardiographic signs of ischemia.[48]

Sufentanil may offer more intense blockade of the surgical stress response.[49] Administering sufentanil as the primary anesthetic in doses of 10, 20, or 30 μg/kg, Lappas and colleagues[50] found minimal changes in coronary blood flow or myocardial oxygen consumption. Myocardial lactate production occurred in only 2 of 20 patients with coronary artery disease.

The benzodiazepines produce minimal changes in coronary vascular resistance in patients with coronary artery disease. Cote and associates[51] demonstrated that diazepam (5 to 8 mg) reduced left ventricular diastolic pressure, which was accompanied by minimal decreases in coronary blood flow and myocardial oxygen consumption. No change in coronary vascular resistance or myocardial lactate production occurred in 12 patients. In a similar study, midazolam (0.2 mg/kg) produced moderate decreases in coronary blood flow (24%) and myocardial oxygen consumption (26%) without changing coronary vascular resistance.[52] There was no myocardial lactate production or electrocardiographic evidence of ischemia in any of eight patients.

Patschke and coworkers[53] have demonstrated that etomidate (0.3 mg/kg) decreases myocardial oxygen consumption in healthy patients. In addition, the safety of etomidate as an induction agent in patients after acute myocardial infarction has been demonstrated.[54] It is possible to plan a "fast-track" course for these patients, using relatively high doses of inhalation anesthesia and lower opioids.

Clinical investigations of the inhalation agents in patients with coronary artery disease support the use of halothane and enflurane with a low incidence of ischemic events. The association of isoflurane with myocardial ischemia in some patients would appear to be related to specific "steal-prone" anatomy, which manifests itself with decreasing coronary vascular resistance.[55–57] Our approach to the emergency situation is similar to the elective one[58] in terms of maintenance of anesthesia. For induction of anesthesia in emergency situations, bolus administration of midazolam or etomidate along with succinylcholine for relocation may be preferred.

## INTRAOPERATIVE MYOCARDIAL PROTECTION

The issue of optimal myocardial protection continues to be a very controversial, evolving subject.[59] It may be especially important in emergency CABG. Of the numerous published reports demonstrating good long-term results with low operative mortality after emergency bypass CABG, various methods of myocardial protection have been used. These have included intermittent cross-clamping, crystalloid cardioplegia, oxygenated crystalloid cardioplegia, blood cardioplegia, retrograde crystalloid, or blood cardioplegia, and even complete avoidance of cardiopulmonary bypass.[60] The best of these methods remains unclear; however, laboratory studies examining myocardial protection have steered many surgeons toward the more sophisticated techniques.

An increasing amount of attention has been paid to the concept of reperfusion injury.[59, 61–68] As a result of very elegant experimental studies, it would appear that both the manner of reperfusion and the composition of the perfusate are important in determining the ultimate degree of myocardial damage. The addition of substrates such as aspartate and glutamate to hyperkalemic blood, and its infusion during the initial phases of reperfusion, have been shown to improve myocardial recovery. Theoretically, this allows for the diversion of substrate toward cellular repair and maintenance of membrane integrity, rather than for mechanical work. Furthermore, oxygenated cardioplegia has been shown to delay the onset of ischemic contracture, to increase coronary flow and oxygen consumption during reperfusion, to improve systolic recovery, and to minimize diastolic stiffness in animal models. Because blood has a high oxygen affinity at low temperatures, crystalloid compositions have been favored by some. These findings support arrest of the heart with an oxgenated crystalloid solution. This is followed by controlled reperfusion of the empty beating heart at physiologic pressures with oxgenated blood containing nutrients and decremental doses of potassium.[69–72]

## SURGICAL RESULTS

The published results for surgical mortality in association with emergency CABG have been acceptable. In a retrospective study conducted at our institution, outcome of patients undergoing emergency CABG surgery for acute myocardial infarction (AMI) was compared with that of patients undergoing elective CABG.[73] Twenty-three patients undergoing emergent CABG surgery for AMI over an 18-month period were identified from a computer-generated database of all cardiac surgical patients at Duke University Medical Center. Criteria for inclusion in the study were documentation of the onset of persistent chest pain within 12 hours of induction of anesthesia and associated ST-segment elevation of at least 0.2 mV on two or more leads of a standard 12-lead electrocardiogram. Using the same computerized databank investigators individually matched for gender, operating surgeon, similar preoperative angiographic ejection fraction (within an average of 8%), and aortic cross-clamp time (within an average of 12 minutes) with 23 patients who underwent elective CABG over the same time period.

The 23 AMI patients were anesthetized 6 + 3.0 (range, 1.5 to 11.00) hours after the onset of chest pain. Fifteen AMI patients received streptokinase. In addition, angioplasty was attempted in seven patients before CABG. Before surgery, the AMI patients more frequently required inotropic support (4 versus 0; $p < 0.05$) and intra-aortic balloon counter pulsation (9 versus 0; $p < 0.005$). Ventricular dysrhythmias requiring intravenous lidocaine also occurred more frequently in the AMI group (13 versus 1; $p < 0.005$). Despite similar aortic cross-clamp and cardiopulmonary bypass times, inotropic and antiarrhythmic drugs were required more frequently in the AMI group both before and after cardiopulmonary bypass. No intraoperative deaths occurred; however, three AMI patients died after surgery. All patients receiving elective CABG survived to be discharged from the hospital.

In these patients undergoing CABG surgery by the same surgical and anesthetic teams, significantly increased risks were associated with emergent surgery after an AMI. Patients with AMI came to the operating room with inotropic and intra-aortic balloon pump support more often than elective patients. Importantly, the induction of general anesthe-

sia did not increase the incidence of this support. The interval from induction to cardiopulmonary bypass was free of new inotropic interventions in the AMI group. However, there was a much more frequent requirement for inotropic support at discontinuation of cardiopulmonary bypass in the AMI group. This suggests that myocardial ischemia before bypass leads to poor tolerance of hypothermic cardiac arrest with cardioplegia. The postoperative course for the AMI group is more complex, as indicated by the increased frequency of prolonged ventilation and time in the intensive care unit, although the incidence of individual complications was not statistically different from that in the elective group.

Overall postoperative death rates in large recent series have ranged from 2% to 12% after failed angioplasty.[6, 7, 16–18, 74] The incidence of postoperative myocardial infarction has ranged from 18% to 63%, with an average of approximately 40%.[6–13, 16–18] The complication rate has been approximately 19%.[18] In all series, there appears to be a higher incidence of myocardial infarction and other complications in patients with multivessel coronary artery disease.[18, 75] Furthermore, it is clear that the incidence of death and complications is higher than that seen in the elective surgical population. Although no controlled studies have been performed with matched patients who have received only medical therapy, it is apparent based on historical data that emergency bypass surgery provides a better outcome than medical therapy alone.

## CONCLUSION

The management of patients requiring emergent CABG surgery after failed percutaneous transluminal coronary angioplasty involves considerations not associated with elective surgical patients. Rapid assessment and transport of a hemodynamically unstable patient to a hastily prepared operating room, management of anesthetic induction in a nonfasting individual, establishment of invasive monitoring after systemic anticoagulation, and optimization of postoperative care after acute myocardial infarction complicate the perioperative care of these high-risk patients. Early preoperative notification of the surgical team will minimizes the time to myocardial revascularization. Appropriate availability of blood products, including platelets and cryoprecipitate, decrease bleeding complications in patients receiving thrombolytic agents. The institution of intra-aortic balloon pumping in the unstable, ischemic patient or the placement of intracoronary perfusion catheters can aid in the safe delivery of the patient to the operating room. In addition, laboratory and clinical evidence supports the hypothesis that general anesthesia provides a protective effect for the myocardium in the interval preceding surgical revascularization. Total revascularization is performed whenever possible, and the internal mammary artery is included in most cases. If these principles are used, good surgical results can be obtained. Further refinement of surgical techniques and myocardial preservation may produce further decreases in morbidity and mortality.

## REFERENCES

1. Favaloro RG, Effler DB, Cheanvechai C, et al: Acute coronary insufficiency (impending myocardial infarction and myocardial infarction): Surgical treatment by the saphenous vein graft technique. Am J Cardiol 28:598, 1971.
2. Cohn LH, Fogarty TJ, Daily PO, et al: Emergency coronary artery bypass. Surgery 70:821, 1971.
3. Hill JD, Kerth WJ, Kelly JJ, et al: Emergency aortocoronary bypass for impending or extending myocardial infarction. Circulation 43:I105, 1971.
4. Pifarre R, Spinazzola A, Nemickas R, et al: Emergency aortocoronary bypass for acute myocardial infarction. Arch Surg 103:525, 1971.
5. Gruntzig AR: Transluminal dilatation of coronary artery stenosis. Lancet 1:263, 1978.
6. Craver JM, Weintraub WS, Jares EL, et al.: Emergency coronary artery bypass surgery for failed percutaneous coronary angioplasty: A 10 year experience. Ann Thorac Surg 215:425, 1992.
7. Cowley MG, Dorros G, Kelsey SF, et al: Emergency coronary bypass surgery after coronary angioplasty: The National Heart, Lung, and Blood Institute's Percutaneous Transluminal Coronary Angioplasty Registry experience. Am J Cardiol 53:22, 1984.
8. Pelletier LC, Pardini A, Renkin J, et al: Myocardial revascularization after failure of percutaneous transluminal coronary angioplasty. J Thorac Cardiovasc Surg 90:265, 1985.
9. Killen DA, Hamaker WR, Reed WA: Coronary artery bypass following percutaneous transluminal coronary angioplasty. Ann Thorac Surg 40:133, 1985.
10. Golding LA, Loop FD, Hollman JL, et al: Early results of emergency surgery after coronary angioplasty. Circulation 74:26, 1986.
11. Page US, Okies JE, Colburn LQ, et al: Percutaneous transluminal coronary angioplasty: A growing surgical problem. J Thorac Cardiovasc Surg 92:847, 1986.
12. Lazar HL, Haan CK: Determinants of myocardial infarction following emergency coronary artery bypass for failed percutaneous coronary angioplasty. Ann Thorac Surg 44:646, 1987.
13. Parsonnet V, Fisch D, Gielchinsky I, et al: Emergency operation after failed angioplasty [see comments]. J Thorac Cardiovasc Surg 96:198, 1988. [Published erratum appears in J Thorac Cardiovasc Surg 97:503, 1989.]
14. Boylan MJ, Lytle BW, Taylor PC, et al: Have PTCA failures requiring emergent bypass operation changed? Ann Thorac Surg 59:283, 1995.
15. Caes FL, Van Nooten GJ: Use of internal mammary artery for emergency grafting after failed coronary angioplasty. Ann Thorac Surg 57:1295, 1994.
16. Connor AR, Vliestra RE, Schaff HV, et al: Early and late results of coronary artery bypass after failed angioplasty: Actuarial analysis of late cardiac events and comparison with initially successful angioplasty. J Thorac Cardiovasc Surg 96:191, 1988.
17. Naunheim KS, Fiore AC, Fagan DC, et al: Emergency coronary artery bypass grafting for failed angioplasty: Risk factors and outcome. Ann Thorac Surg 47:816, 1989.
18. Greene MA, Gray LAJ, Slater AD, et al: Emergency aortocoronary bypass after failed angioplasty. Ann Thorac Surg 51:194, 1991.
19. Ferguson TBJ, Hinohara T, Simpson J, et al: Catheter perfusion to allow optimal coronary bypass grafting following failed transluminal coronary angioplasty. Ann Thorac Surg 42:399, 1986.
20. Marder VJ, Sherry S: Thrombolytic therapy: Current status. N Engl J Med 318:1512, 1988.
21. Sane DC, Califf RM, Topol EJ, et al: Bleeding during thrombolytic therapy for acute myocardial infarction: Mechanisms and management. Ann Intern Med 111:1010, 1989.
22. Marder VJ, Shulman NR: High molecular weight derivatives of human fibrinogen produced by plasmin: II. Mechanisms of their anticoagulant activity. J Biol Chem 244:2120, 1969.
23. Omar MN, Mann KG: Inactivation of factor Va by plasmin. J Biol Chem 262:9750, 1987.
24. Kay P, Ahmad A, Floten S, et al: Emergency coronary artery bypass surgery after intracoronary thrombolysis for evolving myocardial infarction. Br Heart J 53:260, 1985.
25. Skinner JR, Phillips SJ, Zeff RH, et al: Immediate coronary bypass following failed streptokinase infusion in evolving myocardial infarction. J Thorac Cardiovasc Surg 87:567, 1984.
26. Kereiakes DJ, Topol EJ, George BS, et al: Emergency coronary artery bypass surgery preserves global and regional left ventricular function after intracoronary tissue plasminogen activator therapy for acute myocardial infarction. J Am Coll Cardiol 11:899, 1988.
27. Lee KF, Mandell J, Rankin JS, et al: Immediate versus delayed coronary grafting after streptokinase treatment. J Thorac Cardiovasc Surg 95:216, 1988.
28. Campbell FW: The contribution of platelet dysfunction to postbypass bleeding. J Cardiothorac Vasc Anesth 5:8, 1991.
29. Simon TL, Henderson R: Coagulation factor activity in platelet concentrates. Transfusion 19:186, 1979.
30. Hardy JF, Belisle S: Natural and synthetic antifibrinolytics in adult cardiac surgery: Efficacy, effectiveness and efficiency. Can J Anaesth 41:1104, 1994.
31. Ivert T, Huttunen K, Landou C, Bjork V: Angiographic studies of internal mammary artery grafts 11 years after coronary artery bypass grafting. J Thorac Cardiovasc Surg 96:1, 1988.
32. Acinopura AJ, Rose DM, Cunningham JN, et al: Internal mammary artery bypass: Effect on longevity and recurrent angina pectoris in 2900 patients. Eur J Cardiothorac Surg 3:321, 1989.
33. Slogoff S, Keats AS: Does perioperative myocardial ischemia lead to postoperative myocardial infarction? Anesthesiology 62:107, 1985.
34. Wilkinson PL, Hamilton WK, Moyers JR, et al: Halothane and morphine-nitrous oxide anesthesia in patients undergoing coronary artery bypass operation. J Thorac Cardiovac Surg 82:372, 1981.
35. Kleinman B, Henkin RE, Glisson SN, et al: Qualitative evaluation of coronary flow during anesthetic induction using thallium-201 perfusion scans. Anesthesiology 64:157, 1986.
36. Lieberman RW, Orkin FK, Jobes DR, et al: Hemodynamic predictors of myocardial ischemia during halothane anesthesia for coronary-artery revascularization. Anesthesiology 59:36, 1983.
37. Maroko PR, Kjekshus JK, Sobel BE, et al: Factors influencing infarct size following experimental coronary artery occlusions. Circulation 43:67, 1971.
38. Sonnenblick EH, Skelton CL: Myocardial energetics: Basic principles and clinical applications. N Engl J Med 285:668, 1971.
39. Roizen MF, Horrigan RW, Frazer BM: Anesthetic doses blocking adrenergic (stress) and cardiovascular responses to incision-Mac Bar. Anesthesiology 54:390, 1981.
40. Moffitt EA, Sethna DH, Bussell JA, et al: Myocardial metabolism and hemodynamic responses to halothane or morphine anesthesia for coronary artery surgery. Anesth Analg 61:979, 1982.
41. Moffitt EA, Imrie DD, Scovil JE, et al: Myocardial metabolism and haemodynamic responses with enflurane anesthesia for coronary artery surgery. Can Anaesth Soc J 31:604, 1984.
42. Moffitt EA, Barker RA, Glenn JJ, et al: Myocardial metabolism and hemodynamic responses with isoflurane anesthesia for coronary arterial surgery. Anesth Analg 65:53, 1986.
43. Reiz S, Balfors E, Gustavsson B, et al: Effects of halothane

on coronary haemodynamics and myocardial metabolism in patients with ischaemic heart disease and heart failure. Acta Anaesth Scand 26:133, 1982.

44. Reiz S, Balfors E, Sorensen MB, et al: Isoflurane: A powerful coronary vasodilator in patients with coronary artery disease. Anesthesiology 59:91, 1983.

45. Tarnow J, Markschies-Hornung A, Schulte-Sasse U: Isoflurane improves the tolerance to pacing-induced myocardial ischemia. Anesthesiology 64:147, 1986.

46. Moffitt EA, Scovil JE, Barker RA, et al: Myocardial metabolism and haemodynamic responses during high-dose fentanyl anaesthesia for coronary patients. Can Anaesth Soc J 31:611, 1984.

47. Skourtis CT, Nissen M, McGinnis LA, et al: The effect of high-dose fentanyl on cardiac metabolic balance and coronary circulation in patients undergoing coronary artery surgery [Abstract]. Anesthesiology 61:A6, 1984.

48. Reiz S, Balfors E, Haggmark S, et al: Myocardial oxygen consumption and coronary haemodynamics during fentanyl-droperidol-nitrous oxide anaesthesia in patients with ischemic heart disease. Acta Anaesth Scand 25:286, 1981.

49. deLange S, Boscoe M, Stanley T, et al: Comparison of sufentanil-$O_2$ and fentanyl-$O_2$ for coronary artery surgery. Anesthesiology 56:112, 1982.

50. Lappas DG, Palacios I, Athanasiadis C, et al: Sufentanil dosage and myocardial blood flow and metabolism in patients with coronary artery disease [Abstract]. Anesthesiology 63:A58, 1985.

51. Cote P, Gueret P, Bourassa M: Systemic and coronary hemodynamic effects of diazepam in patients with normal and diseased coronary arteries. Circulation 50:1210, 1974.

52. Marty J, Nitenberg A, Blanchet F, et al: Effects of midazolam on the coronary circulation in patients with coronary artery disease. Anesthesiology 64:206, 1986.

53. Patschke D, Brucker JB, Eberlein HJ, et al: Effects of althesin, etomidate, and fentanyl on haemodynamics and myocardial oxygen consumption in man. Can Anaesth Soc J 24:57, 1977.

54. Kates RA, Stack RS, Hill RF, et al: General anesthesia for patients undergoing percutaneous transluminal coronary angioplasty during acute myocardial infarction. Anesth Analg 65:815, 1986.

55. Buffington CW, Romson JL, Levine A, et al: Isoflurane induces coronary steal in a canine model of chronic coronary occlusion. Anesthesiology 66:280, 1987.

56. Priebe HJ, Foex P: Isoflurane causes regional myocardial dysfunction in dogs with critical coronary artery stenosis. Anesthesiology 66:293, 1987.

57. Sill JC, Bove AA, Nugent M, et al: Effects of isoflurane on coronary arteries and coronary arterioles in the intact dog. Anesthesiology 66:273, 1987.

58. Theil DR, Stanley TE III, White WD, et al: Midazolam and fentanyl continuous infusion anesthesia for cardiac surgery: A comparison of computer-assisted versus manual infusion systems. J Cardiothorac Vasc Anesth 7:300, 1993.

59. Beyersdast F: Protection of evolving myocardial infarction and failed PTCA. Ann Thorac Surg 60:833, 1995.

60. Laborde F, Abdelmeguid I, Piwnica A: Aortocoronary bypass without extracorporeal circulation: Why and when? Eur J Cardiothorac Surg 3:152, 1989.

61. Allen BS, Okamoto F, Buckberg G, et al: Immediate functional recovery after six hours of regional ischemia by careful control of conditions of reperfusion and composition of reperfusate. J Thorac Cardiovasc Surg 92:621, 1986.

62. Allen BS, Okamoto F, Buckberg GD, et al: Reperfusion conditions: Critical importance of total ventricular decompression during regional reperfusion. J Thorac Cardiovasc Surg 92:605, 1986.

63. Allen BS, Okamoto F, Buckberg GD, et al: Reperfusate composition: Benefits of marked hypocalcemia and diltiazem on regional recovery. J Thorac Cardiovasc Surg 92:564, 1986.

64. Allen BS, Buckberg GD, Schwaiger M, et al: Early recovery of regional wall motion in patients following surgical revascularization after eight hours of acute coronary occlusion. J Thorac Cardiovasc Surg 92:636, 1986.

65. Okamoto F, Allen BS, Buckberg GD, et al: Reperfusion conditions: Importance of ensuring gentle versus sudden reperfusion during relief of coronary occlusion. J Thorac Cardiovasc Surg 92:613, 1986.

66. Okamoto F, Allen BS, Buckberg GD, et al: Reperfusate composition: Interaction of marked hyperglycemia and marked hyperosmolarity in allowing immediate contractile recovery after four hours of regional ischemia. J Thorac Cardiovasc Surg 92:583, 1986.

67. Okamoto F, Allen BS, Buckberg GD, et al: Reperfusate composition: Supplemental role of intravenous and intracoronary coenzyme Q10 in avoiding reperfusion damage. J Thorac Cardiovasc Surg 92:573, 1986.

68. Vinten JJ, Buckberg GD, Okamoto F, et al: Metabolic and histochemical benefits of regional blood cardioplegic reperfusion without cardiopulmonary bypass. J Thorac Cardiovasc Surg 92:535, 1986.

69. Bodenhamer RM, DeBoer LWV, Geffin GA, et al: Enhanced myocardial protection during ischemic arrest. J Thorac Cardiovasc Surg 85:769, 1983.

70. Digerness SB, Vanini V, Wideman FE: In vitro comparison of availability from asanguinous and sanguinous cardioplegic media. Circulation 64:80, 1981.

71. Buckberg GD: Strategies and logic of cardioplegia delivery to prevent, avoid, and reverse ischemic and reperfusion damage. J Thorac Cardiovasc Surg 93:127, 1987.

72. Follette DM, Steed DL, Foslia RP, et al: Reduction of postischemic myocardial damage by maintaining arrest during initial reperfusion. Surg Forum 28:281, 1977.

73. Hill RF, Kates RA, Davis D, et al: Anesthetic implications for the management of patients with acute myocardial infarction: A matched cohort study of patients undergoing emergency myocardial revascularization. J Cardiothorac Anesth 2:23, 1988.

74. Bredlau CE, Roubin GS, Leimgruber PP, et al: In-hospital morbidity in patients undergoing elective coronary angioplasty. Circulation 72:1044, 1985.

75. Klepzig HJ, Kober G, Satter P, et al: Analysis of 100 emergency aortocoronary bypass operations after percutaneous transluminal coronary angioplasty: Which patients are at risk for large infarctions? Eur Heart J 12:946, 1991.

# 31

# Mechanical Rotational Atherectomy

*William W. O'Neill*

Since publication of the first edition of this textbook, the landscape for the practice of interventional cardiology has been radically altered. The safety of interventional procedures has been dramatically improved.[1] The need for emergency bypass has almost been eliminated by bail-out stents.[2] Dramatic advances have been made in pharmacologic adjunctive therapy.[3] Even the great implacable nemesis of percutaneous intervention, restenosis, has been partially tamed.[4, 5] Without a doubt, the greatest change to occur since the first edition has been the ever expanding role of intracoronary stents. At the time of publication of the first edition, no stents approved by the U.S. Food and Drug Administration existed in the United States, and no randomized clinical trials validated their use. Since then, stents have gained a dominant role in the field of interventional cardiology and are now used in 50% to 70% of cases in the United States and Europe. Multiple chapters of this text are thus devoted to this important topic.

In the current interventional landscape, atherectomy devices have taken a much lower profile. Atherectomy devices were developed to overcome the deficiencies of balloon angioplasty. These deficiencies included elastic recoil, occlusive dissection, nondilatable lesions, and restenosis. Some would argue that stents have largely corrected these deficiencies and there is no need for atherectomy devices. In Europe, in fact, atherectomy devices are rarely used.

With these thoughts in mind, one must seriously ask whether atherectomy devices truly have any relevance or whether they should merely be viewed as historical anecdotes? This chapter addresses this fundamental question. An argument is made for continued optimism about the current and future role of atherectomy, not as an alternative to stent implantation but as a valuable tool to further expand percutaneous revascularization. Small vessels, diffusely diseased vessels, calcified vessels, diseased side branches, ostial lesions, and in-stent restenosis

all remain as unsolved challenges for stent implantation. Mechanical rotational atherectomy has an important role in these areas. This chapter comprehensively reviews the current status of mechanical rotational atherectomy. The mechanics of the system are described, basic experiments and early clinical trials are reviewed, and randomized trials are highlighted. With this information, interventionalists should be able to integrate this tool into a cohesive algorithm for the care of an increasingly aged population and an increasingly complex practice of interventional cardiology.

## HISTORICAL NOTE

The Rotablator catheter (Boston Scientific, Natick, MA) was invented by David Auth, PhD, from Seattle. Dr. Auth's original biomedical inventions consisted of the biomedical uses for laser technology. He invented a commonly used system for laser cautery of gastric bleeding ulcers. Because of his physics background and experience with laser technology, he was approached in the early 1980s to develop a coronary laser ablation system. On a theoretical basis, he recognized the three major limitations of laser technology. First, the laser beam could not be directed, and bend points and tortuosity could not be treated safely. Second and most important, laser vaporization of plaque could cause acoustic and barotrauma that would cause major vessel dissection. Last, laser energy could not be very efficiently used to ablate calcium. As an alternative to laser, Auth postulated that mechanical microabrasion might be more effective. The first prototype catheter (Fig. 31–1) was used in cadaver coronaries at the University of Michigan in 1983. Apart from microembolization, the most important early question concerned the efficacy of the Rotablator in removing atheroma. Lai and coworkers[6] first demonstrated that the Rotablator could effectively ablate human coronary atheroma. They performed mechanical rotational atherectomy (MRA) on hu-

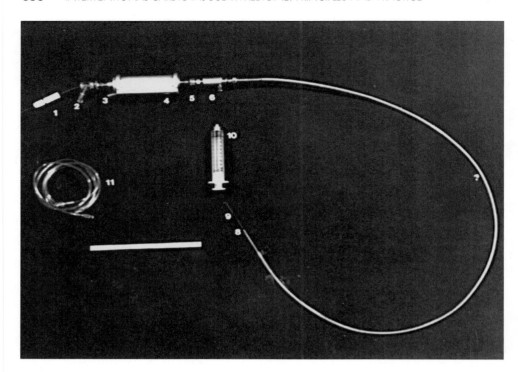

FIGURE 31–1. The original prototype of the Rotablator used in the original canine studies was 11-French and had a steel burr at its tip.

man cadaver atherosclerotic coronary arteries. These vessels were anastomosed end-to-side into canine femoral arteries. Angiography and trans-stenotic gradients were measured before and after atherectomy. MRA resulted in decreased trans-stenotic gradient from 15.7 ± 38 to 5.5 ± 2 mm Hg ($p$ <0.05). An improvement in angiographic lumen diameter occurred in 11 of 13 vessels.

The catheter was redesigned after this initial protocol, and a smaller, more usable system was developed. Soon thereafter, the system that was used from 1988 to 1997 was developed (Fig. 31–2). The basic mechanics of the front tip and the concept of microabrasion have not changed since the first prototype. Although the system is now smaller, sleeker, and more user friendly, microabrasion by high-

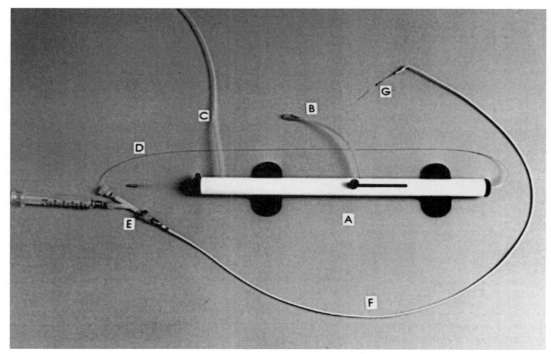

FIGURE 31–2. The second-generation device was well engineered and remained basically unchanged for the next 10 years. The original device did not have a tachometer for revolution-per-minute read-out.

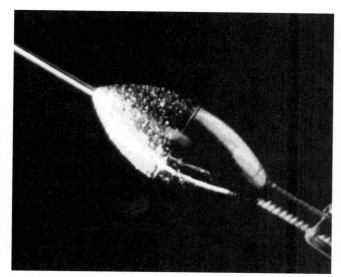

FIGURE 31–3. The unique feature of the Rotablator is its diamond-coated ovoid cutting burr. Diamond microparticles are coated only at the front ends so that cutting can only occur in a forward motion.

speed rotation of a diamond tip burr remains the hallmark of this device.

## MECHANICS OF THE ROTABLATOR CATHETER

### Catheter Tip

The catheter tip has an ovoid shape with diamond microparticles annealed to the forward tip of the burr (Fig. 31–3). Burr diameter sizes for coronary use range from 1.25 to 2.5 mm. The 1.25-mm burr can be placed thru a 6-French guiding catheter, the

1.5-mm and 1.75-mm burr through a 7-French guide, the 2.0-mm and 2.15-mm burrs through an 8-French guide, the 2.25-mm and 2.38-mm burrs through 9-French guide, and the 2.5-mm through a 10-French guiding catheter. Because modern guides are thin walled and change in configuration frequently, if doubt arises about the fit of a burr, the burr should be tested out of the body in the guide. Additionally, great care should be used in advancing the burr through large-lumen thin-walled guides. Kinking can occur at the secondary bends and at the catheter tip. This may prevent advancement of burrs that are appropriately sized. This phenomenon can be recognized immediately because the burr easily advances to the point of kinking. Gentle withdrawal or counter torquing of the guide can sometimes allow the burr to advance. Similarly, transient burr activation may allow orthogonal displacement of friction and allow burr advancement. The burr must *never* be activated for long times at the spot in the guiding catheter where resistance occurs, because guide transection or embolization of guide material could occur. The burr is attached to a helical torque cable that is now detachable (Fig. 31–4). The burr is activated through a gas-powered turbine with calibration via a tachometer. The turbine is activated by a foot pedal with two speed levels (60 to 80,000 rpm for low speed advancement and 120,000 to 200,000 rpm for high speed atheroablation). Low-speed activation can be used for catheter advancement in the guide and in the proximal vessel.

The catheter has diamond particles only on the forward section of the burr, and, for this reason, only forward cutting of the blood vessels can occur. Normal blood vessel wall is viscoelastic and is

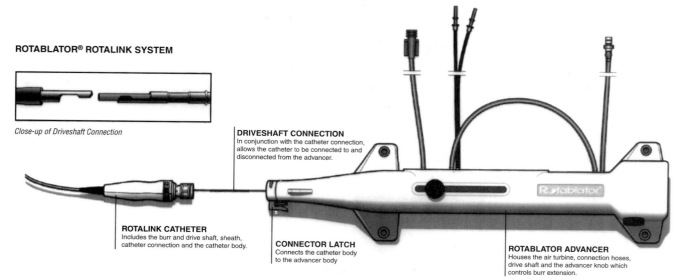

**ROTABLATOR® ROTALINK SYSTEM**

*Close-up of Driveshaft Connection*

**DRIVESHAFT CONNECTION**
In conjunction with the catheter connection, allows the catheter to be connected to and disconnected from the advancer.

**ROTALINK CATHETER**
Includes the burr and drive shaft, sheath, catheter connection and the catheter body.

**CONNECTOR LATCH**
Connects the catheter body to the advancer body

**ROTABLATOR ADVANCER**
Houses the air turbine, connection hoses, drive shaft and the advancer knob which controls burr extension.

FIGURE 31–4. The latest advance in Rotablator design allows for a detachable tip that allows up-sizing of burrs without change in the advancer. (Printed with permission of Boston Scientific Corporation.)

pushed aside, whereas the more rigid atheroma can be selectively ablated. The entire concept by which the Rotablator catheter works is demonstrated in Figure 31–5. The theory of selective ablation of atheroma is demonstrated. The rigid diamond particles selectively abrade rigid atherosclerotic plaque. The normal viscoelastic blood vessel is pushed or stretched aside, and no ablation occurs in this area. Because most coronary lesions are eccentric, this provides a great safety feature in that the more rigid atheroma is selectively ablated, whereas the normal blood vessel wall is pushed aside so that perforation does not occur.

Figure 31–6 demonstrates a schematic of the entire system. The Rotablator catheter is attached to an air-powered turbine. The catheter itself is a very flexible steel-wound shaft housed over a plastic sheath. The sheath allows the catheter to rotate without traumatizing the blood vessel wall. An advancer knob is present on the roof of the device. This permits selective advancement of the diamond burr. In addition, an infusion port is present that permits forceful infusion of saline through the sheath so that saline can provide lubrication between the plastic sheath and the drive shaft. Thus,

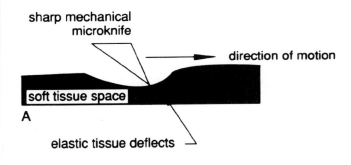

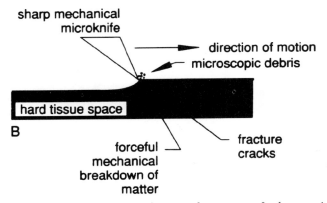

FIGURE 31–5. Theory of selective atherectomy of atheroma is demonstrated. *A*, Soft tissue is able to deflect out of the way. *B*, Hard tissue is unable to deflect out of the way, resulting in fracture and mechanical break-up.

in spite of the fact that the catheter rotates at ultra-high speed, heating of the shaft does not occur. Finally, the device is attached to a nitrogen tank so that compressed gas can operate the air turbine. The stainless steel guide wire is 300 cm long and allows exchange guide wire technique to be employed. Various stiffnesses of the guide wire tip have been manufactured.

## Guide Wire

The second critical and unique component of the Rotablator system is the guide wire. In order to allow high-speed rotation of the torque tube, a non-coated stainless steel guide wire is required. The Rotablator guide wires are all 0.009 inches in diameter with a 0.014 moldable tip. Tips of different flexibility now exist. More important, the body of the guide wire itself is now more malleable. This has allowed a major advance in technique. Previously, the clinically used guide wires were extremely rigid. As a result, pseudolesions could occur in tortuous vessels. More importantly, Reisman and Harms[7] demonstrated that rigid guide wires could inadvertently bias the burr activation so that selective atheroablation on the inner radius of vessel bend points could occur. If atheroma exists on the inner radius, this is beneficial. However, if the inner radius of bends were disease free, then severe dissection or even coronary perforation could occur. This selective ablation due to guide wire bias is not unique to rotational atherectomy and has been documented in laser angioplasty and transluminal extraction coronary atherectomy as well.[8] More mobile guide wires and more flexible catheter tips have been developed. These advances should greatly improve the trackability of the Rotablator system and should improve the safety of activation in bend points and tortuous vessel segments.

## MECHANISM OF ACTION

### Impact of Microparticle Embolization: Preclinical Trials

Unlike any other revascularization device, the Rotablator enlarges lumen area by pulverization and distal embolization of atheroma. Because no attempt is made to aspirate or retrieve atheroma, concern about the sequelae of downstream embolization existed from the start of development of this tool. It was hoped that micropulverization would create particles sufficiently small to pass harmlessly through the coronary capillary microcirculation. However, extensive testing was required before initiation of human clinical trials.

Ahn and associates[9] carefully analyzed micropar-

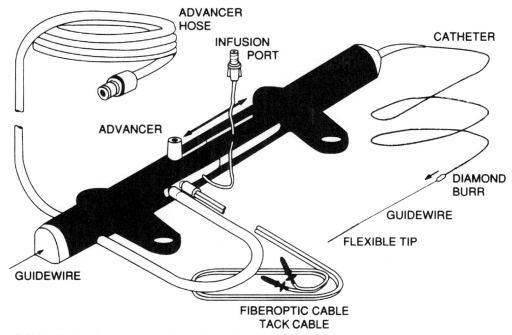

FIGURE 31–6. Schematic of entire Auth Rotablator system.

ticles from 68 atherosclerotic cadaver peripheral vessels treated with rotational atherectomy (Fig. 31–7). Coulter counter analysis revealed that most particles from vessels treated with a 2.5-mm burr were less than 10 μm in size. Vessels treated with the larger 4.5-mm burr had particle sizes that were less than 20 μm in size. When this effluent was injected into canine femoral arteries, no peripheral changes

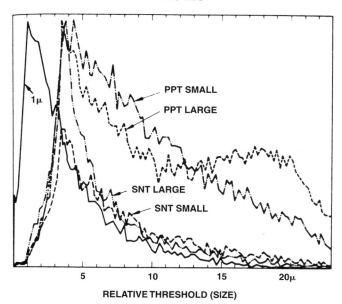

**DISTRIBUTION OF ATHERECTOMIZED PARTICLES**

FIGURE 31–7. Microparticle analysis of debris generated from atherosclerotic tissue.

were seen. Technetium-labeled atherectomy samples passed through the peripheral circulation and were taken up by the lungs, the liver, and the spleen in their reticuloendothelial system.

Friedman and colleagues[10] studied the effluent generated from human cadaver coronary atherectomy. Microparticle size was generally less than 0.1 mm, and the largest particles were less than 0.2 mm. Particles were injected into the canine coronary circulation. Coronary blood flow and coronary flow reserve of control and embolized myocardial territories were compared. A slight transient decline in regional wall motion occurred within 60 minutes. No change in resting coronary blood flow or decline in hyperemic reserve occurred. Histologic analysis of the myocardium demonstrated that only rare spotty areas of micronecrosis occurred. Zacca and coworkers[11] similarly embolized effluent collected from the clinical peripheral MRA cases and injected to embolize these into a porcine coronary model. The porcine model was chosen because of its exquisite sensitivity to ischemia and the known poor collateral circulation that exists in this model. No ischemic changes or arrhythmias were noted. Analysis of particles revealed that 87% of the particles were less than 50 μm and only 1.4% were 100 to 180 μm.

In contradistinction to these comforting initial observations, Prevosti and associates[12] noted deleterious effects of microparticle embolization. The Rotablator was used to atherectomize human atherosclerotic aorta. Effluent was analyzed and injected into a canine model. Although 87% of the particles were less than 12 μm and only 0.001%

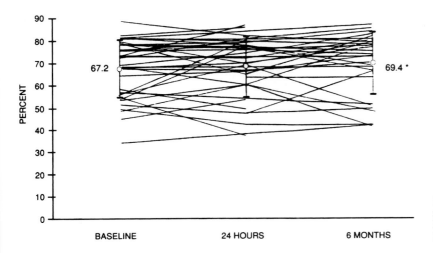

FIGURE 31–8. Ejection fraction changes with mechanical rotational atherectomy employing the Rotablator catheter. $*p$ = NS, not significant (ANOVA).

were greater than 40 μm, severe ischemic changes were noted. Overt heart failure was detected after large-volume effluent embolization.

## Impact of Microembolization: Clinical Trials

Although preclinical trials were encouraging, the ultimate impact of microparticle embolization could not be delineated without careful clinical observations. Concerned by the observations of Prevosti and associates[12] we specifically limited our first cases to short, complex lesions. The first 38 patients were treated and underwent right anterior oblique contrast ventriculography at baseline, 24 hours, and 6 months (Fig. 31–8). We found no decline in global function or regional wall motion. To further evaluate the impact of microembolization, we performed transesophageal echocardiography on 17 patients during rotational atherectomy. Pavlides and colleagues[13] reported these observations and determined that regional wall motion transiently deteriorated but returned to baseline immediately after atherectomy (Fig. 31–9).

In contradistinction to these observations, Teirstein and coworkers[14] reported severe regional dysfunction and a 19% incidence of creatine phosphokinase (CPK) elevation in a cohort of patients with long, diffuse coronary lesions. Williams and associates[15] performed serial echos on 10 patients treated with percutaneous transluminal coronary angioplasty (PTCA) alone and 22 patients treated with rotational atherectomy. The PTCA patients had normalization of regional wall motion within 2.6 minutes of treatment, whereas 153 minutes elapsed before the rotational atherectomy group experienced normalization. In only 1 of 22 patients (the only patient with non–Q wave myocardial infarction) did regional wall motion not return to normal within 30 hours of treatment. Disturbingly, severe regional

wall motion abnormalities often persisted without clinical or electrocardiographic findings.

More serious cases of embolization have been reported.[16–18] van de Rijn and colleagues[17] and Bowles and coworkers[16] also reported cases of fatal embolization. In both reports, intraluminal thrombus existed before atherectomy. Hetterick and McEniery[18] reported on a case of severe right ventricular infarction as a sequela of transient right ventricular side branch occlusion.

The availability of Doppler flow wire catheters has allowed determination of the impact of rotational atherectomy on distal coronary vascular reserve. Khoury and Kern,[19] Nunez and colleagues,[20] and Bowers and colleagues[21] performed serial flow reserve measurements after rotational atherectomy. Consistently, flow reserve, average peak velocity at base, and hyperemic peak velocities increase but do not normalize (Fig. 31–10). Flow reserves of 1.4

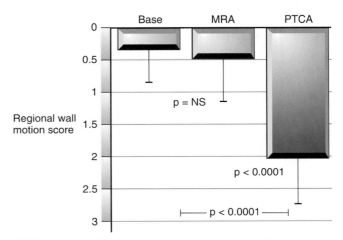

FIGURE 31–9. Wall-motion score of regions perfused by the target vessels during mechanical rotational atherectomy (MRA) and during subsequent adjunctive percutaneous transluminal coronary angioplasty (PTCA) in patients undergoing Rotablator atherectomy.

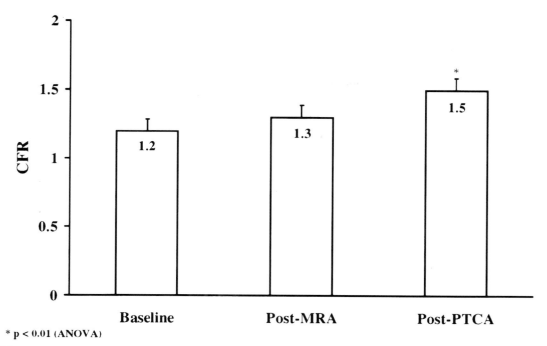

FIGURE 31–10. Coronary flow reserve at baseline, after mechanical rotational atherectomy, and after percutaneous transluminal coronary angioplasty is depicted.

to 1.6 have been reported. More recently, Bowers (personal communication) treated 10 patients with elective planned stents after rotational atherectomy and found further improvement in flow reserve up to 2.8. These findings suggest that flow reserve is improved but not normalized, in part because of distal particle embolization, but also in part because of partial residual stenosis that can be improved by adjunctive stent implantation.

Taken in context, the functional and pathologic studies suggest that a real but manageable risk exists from microparticle embolization. The basic studies demonstrated that rotational atherectomy does indeed cause micropulverization of human atherosclerotic tissue. Particle sizes generally smaller than red blood corpuscles are generated. Particle size appears to correlate with burr size, with larger burrs causing larger particles. In addition to particle size, volume of atheromatous effluent appears critical. Short segment occlusions, as in the experiments by Friedman and colleagues[10] and Zacca and colleagues,[11] appear to be well tolerated. Larger-volume effluent, as in the experiments by Prevosti and associates,[12] do have potential for serious transient or permanent myocardial damage. Thus, not only is particle size important but the size of the vascular bed is as well. Large vascular beds have a greater capacity to handle large volumes of effluent than smaller beds. To minimize the risk of adverse sequelae of microparticles, smaller burr sizes decrease particle size, and short-segment occlusions minimize the volume of tissue embolized. These studies suggest that dif-

fusely diseased vessels supplying small vascular beds have the potential risk of embolus-induced ischemia. Conversely, large vascular beds with short-segmented occlusions should easily handle the microparticle burden.

## MECHANISM OF LUMEN ENLARGEMENT

Experimental and pathologic studies have demonstrated that rotational atherectomy does in fact micropulverize atheroma and leave a clean smooth groove in vessels at the atherectomy site. Observations with quantitative angiography and intravascular ultrasound (IVUS) have greatly advanced our understanding of the mechanism of lumen enlargement in vivo. It is now understood that lumen enlargement after percutaneous revascularization is related to both changes in plaque mass and vessel stretch. Balloon angioplasty causes stretch of nondiseased vessel wall and a controlled medial dissection. Stent implantation causes mild plaque compression and primarily vessel stretch. Rotational atherectomy in combination with balloon angioplasty is a much more complicated process. Safian and coworkers[22] performed quantitative angiography in 211 lesions treated with rotational atherectomy. They found that in comparison with PTCA alone, vessel recoil was substantially diminished by rotational atherectomy. Recoil was 31% after PTCA and 22% after rotational atherectomy. These data suggest that less stretch and thus less recoil occurs after rotational atherectomy. These observations appear to corroborate our original observations that vessel size does not deteriorate at 24 hours.[23] Rodriguez and coworkers[24] demonstrated that up to 40% of patients have significant vessel recoil at angiography 24 hours after PTCA. This is presumably related to recoil of normal vessel wall that was stretched initially. If rotational atherectomy occurs primarily by plaque ablation, then early deterioration of lumen caliber should not occur.

IVUS has further defined the exact mechanism of lumen enlargement. Dussaillant and associates[25] performed IVUS and found that the ratio to final lumen/burr area was 1.01 ± 0.26. Thus, rotational atherectomy very efficiently enlarged the coronary lumen to the cross-sectional area of the burr by plaque ablation and not vessel stretch. One exception to this correlation between final lumen area to burr size is the furrowing effect that can occur as a result of guide wire bias. Stuver and Ling[26] reported that final lumen areas could be dramatically larger than the burr size when the burrs are activated in bend point lesions. Kovach and coworkers[27] found that lumen area increased from 1.8 to 3.9 $mm^2$. Plaque area decreased from 15.7 to 13.0 $mm^2$ after atherectomy. Thus, lumen enlargement was almost entirely related to plaque ablation. After adjunctive PTCA, lumen area increased to 5.2 $mm^2$. The further lumen enlargement was due to vessel stretch and plaque dissection. In this careful IVUS study, dissection was present in only 22% of cases after rotational atherectomy. After adjunctive PTCA, however, dissections were documented in 77% of cases. Quantitative angiography has been reported in numerous series and provides further insight into the efficacy of MRA. Zacca and associates[28] first reported that minimum lumen diameter (MLD) increased from 1.0 ± 0.4 mm to 1.9 ± 0.3 mm in the first 23 patients treated at their institution. Later, from the same group, Rodriguez and colleagues[29] found that the use of large burrs (2.5 or 2.5 mm) resulted in a MLD increase from 0.9 ± 0.3 to 2.1 ± 0.4 mm. Schieman and coworkers[30] analyzed quantitative arteriography in 52 lesions and also found an increase in lesion diameter from 0.92 ± 2.8 to 1.7 ± 0.35 mm after MRA. In this study, angiography was available at 24 hours. No decrease in lumen diameter occurred. Similarly, Harris and coworkers[31] reported that MLD increased from 1.0 ± 0.4 to 1.5 ± 0.4 and further increased to 2.1 ± 0.3 mm at 24 hours. These quantitative findings demonstrate that final MLD is approximately 80% of the final burr diameter employed. Importantly, arterial recoil does not occur, and thus, this potential mechanism of restenosis does not appear to apply for MRA. These findings further demonstrate that large vessels (> 3 mm in diameter) cannot be treated solely with

MRA. Even with the largest burr sizes used (2.5 mm), adjunctive balloon angioplasty is required to optimize lumen diameter in these large vessels.

These angiographic and ultrasound studies nicely corroborate the pathologic studies that demonstrated a smooth, nontraumatic lumen enlargement for most lesions that are treated. The mechanisms of initial lumen enlargement also assist us in understanding the mechanism of restenosis. In cases in which rotational atherectomy is employed as a stand-alone procedure, restenosis must be predominantly related to fibrointimal hyperplasia. After adjunctive PTCA, restenosis is complex. It can be due to vessel recoil, thrombus deposition at dissection sites, or fibrointimal hyperplasia. As the burr-to-artery ratio increases, more and more lumen enlargement is due to atheroablation and less and less to vessel stretch and plaque compression or dissection. In parallel, restenosis is increasingly due to fibrointimal hyperplasia. To summarize, the smaller the final burr-to-artery diameter ratio is, the more the vessel reacts in a manner similar to PTCA. Small burr-to-artery ratios (as in large vessels) require adjunctive stent implantation to maximize lumen dimension and decrease restenosis risk. Large burr-to-artery ratios will require adjunctive antimitotic therapy, perhaps pharmacologic therapy or perhaps radiation to minimize restenosis risk.

## PERIPROCEDURAL MANAGEMENT OF PATIENTS

Patients treated with the Rotablator catheter undergo pharmacologic therapy quite similar to that given to patients requiring balloon angioplasty. However, a few major differences exist in the care of these patients. Patients are all pretreated with aspirin therapy (325 mg/day orally) before the procedure. Patients routinely have been given oral calcium channel blockers. At catheterization, 10,000 units of heparin are employed. Activated clotting times (ACTs) are obtained in the laboratory to ensure that therapeutic anticoagulation is achieved and that ACTs greater than 300 seconds are present before initiation of therapy. Patients are given intravenous nitroglycerin sufficient to decrease systolic blood pressure by 10 mm Hg. The adjunctive use of glycoprotein receptor blockers is being explored, but at present, no randomized controlled data validate their routine use.

Once intracoronary nitroglycerin is given, the Rotablator catheter can be selectively advanced into the blood vessel to be treated. Prophylaxis for coronary artery spasm must occur. Our experience initially demonstrated that severe coronary spasm could occur if patients were not optimally premedicated. Once a catheter advances near the origin of the guiding catheter, some resistance of passage of the Rotablator around the bend points of the Judkins catheter often occurs. Very brief activation of the motor allows for advancement of the catheter. Once the catheter is advanced into the coronary artery, it is advanced near the atheroma. At this point, the Rotablator catheter is activated. Very gentle imperceptible initial motion of the catheter should originally occur. The Rotablator itself should be very gently advanced. The catheter is activated so that it rotates at 170,000 to 200,000 rpm. It is imperative that forceful pressure not be applied. If the speed of the catheter decreases to less than 130,000 rpm, it is very possible that the diamond particles will actually grab the blood vessel wall and cause dissection to occur. For this reason; the Rotablator is very gently advanced until the atheroma is ablated. Acoustical feedback is present from the rotation of the Rotablator. It is important that a decrease in rotation of less than 130,000 rpm not occur. Once the catheter is advanced across the atheroma, our practice is to gently advance the catheter back and forth across the lesion so that continuous-abrasion "sanding" of the blood vessel occurs. When the Rotablator catheter can be passed smoothly without friction and with no further resistance, it can be removed. The exchange guide wire technique is then employed, and the Rotablator catheter is removed completely from the coronary artery. Intracoronary nitroglycerin is again readministered, and coronary angiograms are performed. If the artery is incompletely treated, larger burr sizes can be employed. Again, for coronary arteries that are 3 mm or less in size, Rotablator burrs of 2 mm or less provide for partial-debulking atherectomy. Once the largest Rotablator available has been used, completion of the procedure can occur with adjunctive balloon angioplasty or stent implantation. Our practice is to attempt to achieve an optimal lumen expansion so that a residual stenosis of 10% or less occurs. Usually, this requires stent implantation.[32, 33] At the termination of the procedure, if the anatomic appearance of the blood vessel is smooth and stable lumen is present, no further heparin therapy is required. If dissections are present, then the patients can be heparinized overnight or adjunctive stent therapy can be employed. In our experience, delayed closure has not occurred out of the catheterization laboratory because of the extremely stable luminal appearance after the Rotablator therapy. Patients are maintained on intravenous nitroglycerin for 24 hours, and vascular sheaths are removed as indicated. Follow-up of patients is similar to that of other interventional patients.

## COMPLICATIONS

Complications can occur during Rotablator therapy and are important to anticipate and recognize. When the right coronary artery or a dominant circumflex artery is treated, invariably, transient bradycardia or transient asystole occurs. The actual mechanism by which this happens is unknown. It is postulated that either microparticle embolization or microcavitation of the blood itself causes transient ischemia to the conduction system and transient heart block. In any event, these phenomena are very self-limiting. However, when these types of patients are treated, temporary pacemakers must be employed and an adequate underlying rate must be present.

## Coronary No-Reflow

A major complication called coronary no-reflow can occur during Rotablator therapy. This is demonstrated in Figure 31–11. Coronary no-reflow is presumed to occur as the sequela of distal microparticle embolization. The reported incidence of this phenomenon is between 1% and 5%. No-reflow is recognized after the Rotablator therapy, when it is apparent that occlusive dissection is not present in the blood vessel, yet cessation of blood flow has occurred. The phenomenon can be easily treated with very large doses of intracoronary nitroglycerin. Nitroglycerin doses between 1 and 2 mg should be used. With this therapy and with supportive measures, that phenomenon resolves over 5 to 15 minutes. In addition, intracoronary verapamil (250 to 1000 $\mu$g) has been tried and may have some value in the treatment of coronary no-reflow. It is important to recognize this phenomenon and to distinguish it from occlusive dissection.

## Occlusive Dissection

Occlusive dissections may require prolonged balloon inflation with autoperfusion catheters. They may require intracoronary stents but constitute a mechanical problem that requires some mechanical correction. One method of differentiating no-reflow from occlusive dissection is by placement of an autoperfusion catheter. If flow can be reestablished only with the autoperfusion balloon, then it is likely that an occlusive dissection is present. On the other hand, if the autoperfusion catheter does not allow for reestablishment of flow, the diagnosis of coronary no-reflow is made. Usually, it is not difficult to tell whether no-reflow occurs. The anatomic appearance of the blood vessel itself appears to be quite stable without the presence of angiographic dissection and with no contrast opacification of the distal coronary bed. The reason why the differentiation is important is because no-reflow is a transient phenomenon that resolves over a 5- to 15-minute period. In our initial experience, one patient with this phenomenon occurring was referred for emergency bypass surgery. At emergency bypass, the artery was widely patent, and brisk antegrade flow had been

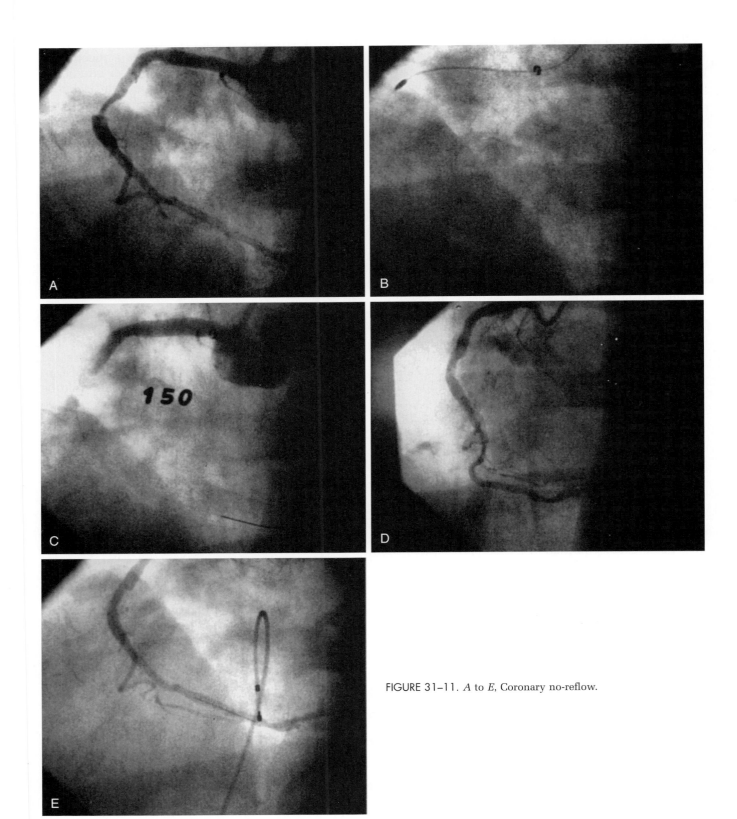

FIGURE 31–11. *A* to *E*, Coronary no-reflow.

reestablished. For this reason, it is important to understand that no-reflow is not a mechanical problem and does not need mechanical correction or emergency bypass.

## Coronary Perforation

The other potential catastrophic complication is that of coronary perforation. Presently, the risk of coronary perforation appears to be negligible. There have been no reported cases of coronary perforation occurring when guide wires are properly positioned. However, there is a theoretical risk of perforation. This would manifest itself by a dye stain present around a coronary artery. Temporary treatment with an autoperfusion catheter has corrected the problem, preventing tamponade from developing. However, tamponade can quickly develop if a coronary perforation occurs, and this may result in very rapid development to electromechanical dissociation. For this reason, whenever atherectomy is employed, a percutaneous pericardiocentesis tray should be immediately available.

## Microparticle Embolization

There was initial concern expressed about the myocardial effects of microparticle embolization. Initially, to assess the impact of MRA on systolic ventricular function, we performed serial paired ventriculograms before treatment and 24 hours later in the first 38 patients treated at our center. We found no deterioration of global or regional wall motion in these patients. In addition, Pavlides and colleagues[13] reported that MRA had no deleterious effect on regional myocardial function, as assessed by transesophageal echocardiography. Teirstein and coworkers[14] reported on a small subgroup of patients who experienced severe wall-motion abnormalities in treated vessels with very long lesions. Cheirif and associates[34] also compared echocardiographic wall-motion changes induced by MRA in 12 patients with those occurring in 19 patients treated with balloon angioplasty. A semiquantitative wall-motion score was used. Wall motion decreased by at least 2 grades in 58% of patients during balloon inflation and in only 8% of patients during MRA. Time-to-recovery function was $39 \pm 35$ seconds after balloon inflation and $18 \pm 5$ seconds after MRA. These studies suggest that MRA has little deleterious effect on myocardial function when short segments are treated.

In addition to transient loss of myocardial function, microembolization could also cause microinfarction with release of CPK. Teirstein and associates[14] found that 20% of patients in their series had CPK elevations. These were not associated with Q-wave myocardial infarction. Popma and coworkers[35] carefully analyzed a multicenter registry experience. They reported that an elevation of CPK of more than 1.5 times normal occurred in 8.5% of patients, and elevations of more than 5 times normal occurred in 2.9% of patients. CPK elevations were most likely in long lesions and in patients with abrupt closure and coronary spasm. These results suggest that mechanical occlusion as well as microparticle embolization was responsible for the CPK elevation in the multicenter registry. Basnight and colleagues[36] reported on the San Francisco Heart Institute experience in 149 patients. CPK elevation occurred in 13% of patients. Of importance is that CPK levels continue to increase after 24 hours of the procedure. The kinetics of CPK elevation in this study are similar to those of acute myocardial infarction without coronary reperfusion. The long-term prognostic impact of CPK elevation has not been determined.

## Abrupt Closure and Emergency Bypass

Apart from the adverse effect of particle embolization, the actual risk of coronary artery injury is now being defined. The American College of Cardiology/American Heart Association (ACC/AHA) lesion morphology type does appear to segregate risks. Although risk may be lower than with balloon angioplasty for complex (type C) lesions, increased complexity of lesion morphology increases risk. Whitlow[37] found a 15% incidence of major cardiac events for type C lesions, compared with zero and 7% for type A and $B_1$ lesions. Fajadet and colleagues[38] similarly found a 28% incidence of major cardiac events for type C lesions, compared (with zero) for $B_1$ and 5.9% for $B_2$ lesions. Whitlow[37] has most extensively analyzed risk factors for complications after MRA by use of the multicenter registry database. In addition to lesion type, lesion length and lesion eccentricity also increase the risk of complications. Mortality was twice as high in patients with lesions greater than 10 mm. Rates of emergency bypass were 2.6% and 1.1% for eccentric and concentric lesions, respectively. MacIsaac and coworkers[39] found that calcified, eccentric lesions had an increased rate of need for urgent bypass. Satler and Warth[40] analyzed high-risk factors for dissection in the multicenter registry. The overall rate of dissection was 13% in 1688 treated lesions. Eccentric lesions, lesions in tortuous vessels, and long lesions have increased predisposition to dissect. As in balloon angioplasty, coronary dissection was associated with poor outcome. Rates of abrupt closure were 14% and 4% for lesions with dissection versus those without dissection, respectively. Rates of emergency bypass were 9.5% and 1.5% and mortality was 2.2% and 0.7% for lesions with dissection and those without dissection, respectively. Leon and associates[41] found that lesion calcification does increase risk of dissection as well. Although the rates of emergency bypass and mortality were the same, dissection occurred in 10.5% of the 220 calcified lesions, compared with 5.1% of the noncalcified lesions. To date, intracoronary thrombus has been a contraindication to MRA, and no data are available concerning this historic risk factor for balloon angioplasty. When procedural risk after MRA is assessed, both risk of embolization and coronary artery injury must be calculated. Lesion length appears to increase risk of myocardial dysfunction, coronary dissection, and rate of emergency bypass and mortality. Lesion eccentricity increases the risk of dissection and the need for emergency bypass, and lesion calcification increases the risk of dissection. These findings suggest that optimum risk benefit exists for the use of MRA in sort-segment complex lesions that are anatomically unsuited for balloon angioplasty. Caution must be applied for the use in long arterial segments and for eccentric coronary lesions.

## CLINICAL TRIALS

### Multicenter Registry

A multicenter registry was organized to incorporate patients treated at facilities in Houston; San Diego; Palo Alto; Seattle; Royal Oak, Michigan; and Washington, D.C.[42] In this registry, 745 patients were enrolled, and 847 lesions were treated. A broad spectrum of lesion location and lesion types were treated (Table 31–1). Unfavorable lesion morphology, such as lesion tortuosity (26%) lesions longer than 10

mm (25%), and restenosis lesions (30%), were very common. Angiographic success (<50% residual stenosis) was achieved by MRA alone in 53% of cases. With adjunctive angioplasty, success rate was increased in 82%. MRA was unsuccessful in 13% of cases, but PTCA salvaged the procedure. Finally, in 5% of cases, both MRA and PTCA were unsuccessful. Employing an "intention to treat" criterion, the combination of MRA and PTCA resulted in a 95% success rate. The low sole therapy success of MRA in this trial is in part related to the small burr sizes available; only sizes of up to 2 mm were available for much of the study. In addition, many centers used the device strictly for debulking. A combination of MRA and angioplasty did provide an extremely high procedural success. Major complications occurred in 3.9% of patients. Death occurred in 0.8%. Q-wave myocardial infarction occured in 0.9% and emergency bypass in 2.1%. Nonocclusive dissection occurred in only 10.6% of cases.

Other clinical series have been published.[43–47] The first five trials are summarized in Table 31–2. We treated 104 patients in the initial U.S. experience, Bertrand treated 129 patients in the initial European experience, and Teirstein reported on 42 patients in an initial American experience. Reifart and colleagues[48] presented a randomized trial comparing MRA to PTCA and laser. An overview of these clinical series provides added insight into the efficacy of MRA.

These series have preponderantly male populations. Target arteries are well distributed throughout the coronary tree. Stand-alone device success was only achieved in 50% to 60% of cases. Again, this result may be related to burrs' being undersized for target arteries as well as frequent planned adjunctive PTCA being performed. In the Teirstein study, in which PTCA was not performed, a success rate of 76% was achieved; in our own series, adjunctive PTCA was performed in 70% of cases, and a final procedural success of 96% was achieved. Angiographic dissection occurred in 10% of cases. In these series, emergency bypass occurred in 2% of cases. Given the preponderance of anatomically high-risk (B and C) lesions, this appears to be a major safety advance of MRA. Q-wave and non-Q myocardial infarction incidence varies widely. In part, this related to intensity of scrutiny. Some inherent differences in myocardial infarction rate, no doubt, are presented related to lesion selection. Teirstein's series had the highest incidence of myocardial infarction and also treated very long lesions. Perforation appears to be an extremely rare complication of MRA.

### ERBAC Study

Great insight has been gleaned from the randomized study conducted at the Red Cross Hospital in Frank-

## TABLE 31–1.　MULTICENTER REGISTRY

| BASELINE CHARACTERISTICS OF TREATED LESIONS | N | % |
|---|---|---|
| Male | 576 | 77 |
| Female | 169 | 23 |
| Location (artery) | | |
|   Left anterior descending | 433 | 50 |
|   Right | 258 | 30 |
|   Circumflex | 166 | 19 |
|   Left main | 17 | 2 |
| Characteristics* (Yes/No) | | |
|   Bifurcated | 164/446 | 27 |
|   Calcified | 277/434 | 39 |
|   Eccentric | 430/275 | 61 |
|   Long (11–25 mm) | 196/585 | 25 |
|   Tortuous | 159/444 | 26 |
| Previous restenosis | 229/532 | 30 |

*Lesion morphology data requested in most recent 761 cases, reported as percentage responding yes or no to each characteristic. Lesions may have more than one characteristic or involvement: bifurcated, major or moderate-sized branch point; calcified, angiographically visible calcium; eccentric, >75% of lesion unilateral; long, >10 mm; tortuous, >30-degree angulation within diseased segment.

**TABLE 31–2.    ROTABLATOR CLINICAL TRIALS**

| | MULTICENTER | BEAUMONT HOSPITAL | FRANKURT | EUROPEAN | CALIFORNIA |
|---|---|---|---|---|---|
| N | 745 | 104 | 130 | 129 | 42 |
| Males, 576/745 (77) | | 81 (78%) | NR | 107 (83%) | 28 (66%) |
| Lesion location | | | | | |
|   LAD, N = 433 | (50) | 36 (35%) | | 63 (49%) | 48% |
|   RCA, N = 258 | (30) | 40 (39%) | | 47 (36%) | 33% |
|   LCX, N = 166 | (19) | 15 (15%) | | 19 (15%) | 12% |
|   LMCA, N = 17 | (02) | 07 (07%) | | | |
| MRA success | 53% | 50% | 66% | 57% | 76% |
| Overall success | 95% | 96% | 93% | 86% | 76% |
| Death | 0.8% | 1.0% | 0% | 0% | 2% |
| QMI | 0.9% | 4.0% | NR | 2.3% | 0% |
| ER CABG | 2.1% | 1.9% | 0.7% | 2% | 2% |
| Dissection | 10.0% | 11% | 11% | NR | NR |
| Non–Q wave | 4.2% | 2.9% | NR | 5.4% | 19% |
| Perforation | 0.7% | 0% | 0% | 0% | 2% |

ER CABG, emergency coronary artery bypass graft; LAD, left anterior descending artery; LCX, left circumflex artery; LMCA, left main coronary artery; RCA, right coronary artery; MRA, mechanical rotational ablation; MI, myocardial infarction; NR, not reported.

furt by Reifart and colleagues.[48] Patients with type B and C lesions were randomly assigned to PTCA, MRA, or excimer laser therapy. Overall procedural success was better for MRA than for balloon angioplasty (85% vs. 93%). Stenosis severity was less (33% vs. 26%) for MRA. Conversely, dissections were more common after MRA (11% vs. 5%). Rates of bypass were very low for all groups, as was mortality. Calcified lesions, long lesions, and eccentric lesions appear to have higher success rates with MRA than with balloon angioplasty. Rotablator therapy resulted in a higher initial procedural success (83% vs. 90.5%, $p = 0.025$) than PTCA. No difference in major adverse cardiac events occurred. At follow-up, target vessel revascularization rates were higher for rotational atherectomy (42% vs. 32%, $p = 0.013$), and angiographic restenosis occured at a higher level (57% vs. 47%, $p = 0.14$) for rotational atherectomy. Like other early randomized device trials, ERBAC had great influence on use of the Rotablator in Europe. This trial took place early in development of the Rotablator technique. Small, undersized burrs were used, burrs greater than 2.0 mm were not available at the time this trial was performed, and burr-to-artery ratios of less than 0.6 existed. Irrespective of these drawbacks, this study was the first to limit hope that rotational atherectomy would have a significant impact on restenosis.

## Lesion Selection for MRA

Controlled atheromatous ablation with a well-defined angiographic lumen was the initial goal of MRA. It was hoped that this would provide a predictable angiographic response and a low incidence of complications. Because balloon angioplasty is associated with such a low rate of immediate complications in simple lesions (short segment, concentric), it was unlikely that MRA would have a selective advantage in this setting. From the onset, MRA was selectively applied to anatomically high-risk lesions. Sufficient experience now exists to provide insight into specific lesions in which MRA may have superior efficacy.

We first examined our experience with MRA in ACC/AHA type C lesions.[49] We compared the success and complication rates of type C lesions treated with MRA with rates in a contemporaneous group of patients treated with balloon angioplasty (Table 31–3). We found that the success rate was higher, and a trend toward lower complications occurred in patients treated with MRA. Whitlow[50] also stratified lesions according to ACC/AHA lesion type. This study was performed based on the multicenter registry. Success rate was equally high (95%) in the two groups. In the registry, there was a higher frequency of major cardiac events for more complex lesions. No adverse events occurred in type A lesions, major adverse events occurred in 7% of $B_1$ lesions, in 8% of $B_2$ lesions, and in 15% of type C lesions. These two reports demonstrate that complex lesions have a

**TABLE 31–3.    RESULTS OF MECHANICAL ROTATIONAL ATHERECTOMY OF TYPE C LESIONS**

| OUTCOME | MRA (N = 27) | PTCA (N = 196) | p |
|---|---|---|---|
| Successful | 26 (96%) | 149 (76%) | <0.03 |
| Major cardiac event | 1 (3.7%) | 11 (5.6%) | NS |
|   Emergency CABG | 1 (3.7%) | 5 (2.6%) | NS |
|   Abrupt closure | 0 | 4 (2.0%) | NS |
|   Death | 0 | 2 (1.0%) | NS |

CABG, coronary artery bypass grafting; MRA, mechanical rotational atherectomy; NS, not significant; PTCA, percutaneous transluminal coronary angioplasty.

high success rate, perhaps superior to that of PTCA. These findings appear to be consistent with those of the Frankfurt prospective randomized trial.

## Lesion Length

Lesion length has long been considered a major risk of poor outcome of balloon angioplasty. The Rotablator has now been extensively tested in this setting. Teirstein and coworkers[14] first reported the use of MRA in this setting. Although a high technical success rate was achieved, 20% of patients experienced CPK elevations, and many patients had severe wall-motion abnormalities after therapy. In addition, restenosis rates of up to 75% occurred for extremely long lesions. Bertrand and colleagues[51] reviewed the initial 315-patient multicenter experience and found that lesion length was not associated with poor procedural outcome. As experience in the multicenter registry progressed, lesion length did start to become an adverse prognostic feature. Whitlow[50] reported that mortality was 1.9% for lesions greater than 10 mm, compared with 0.7% for lesions less than 10 mm. Popma and associates[35] reported that lesion length was independently correlated with CPK elevation in the multicenter experience. These reports provided a mixed picture concerning the use of MRA in long lesions. Technically, high procedural success appears possible. Dissection and abrupt closure appear to be very low for these lesions. Unfortunately, adverse events (especially CPK elevation) and procedural mortality appear to be increased. Long-term outcome may also be suboptimal because a substantial risk of restenosis is present. These findings suggest that judicious case selection is required in this setting. For some patients, no other revascularization modality is available. Diffusely diseased vessels may not be revascularized by any other method. If these patients have well-preserved ventricular function, the transient decrease of ventricular function occurring in this setting may be well tolerated. Patients with poor ventricular function may not tolerate even transient further impairment of function. Use of MRA may thus be reasonable in patients with well-preserved left ventricular function who have no other revascularization options. MRA should not be used in diffusely diseased vessels in patients with poor ventricular function.

## Vessel Calcification

Because of the mechanical property of microabrasion, heavily calcified vessels may be very effectively treated. Leon and associates[41] reviewed their experience with MRA of 190 patients with 220 calcified lesions. These investigators compared these calcified vessels to 275 lesions in 237 patients treated without fluoroscopic calcification. Success

rate was equally high (82% vs. 86%). Dissection occurred in 5% if no calcification was present, versus 10.5% if calcification was present. No difference in major complications existed. Mortality was 0.5%, urgent coronary bypass surgery was necessary in 1.1%, and Q-wave myocardial infarction occurred in 1.6%. MacIsaac and associates[39] analyzed the multicenter registry and also found a high (94%) success rate for calcified vessels. However, there was a 2.6% rate of CPK elevation for these lesions. These studies suggest that heavily calcified vessels may be safely and successfully treated by MRA. These findings are in marked disparity with the poor procedural outcome from calcified vessels treated with DVI or transluminal extraction coronary atherectomy. Also, excimer laser angioplasty has a less favorable outcome for heavily calcified vessels. Thus, MRA may become the tool of choice for these heavily calcified lesions.

## Ostial Lesions

Koller and coworkers,[52] Zimarino and colleagues,[53] and Popma and colleagues[54] have reported on the use of MRA in ostial lesions. The MRA catheter has several unique properties that aid in the removal of this lesion. Aorta ostial lesions are heavily calcified and invariably reocclude after balloon inflation, and the lesions are often eccentric. Lesions in the ostium of the left anterior descending artery and circumflex arteries may have extreme perpendicular take-off from the left main coronary artery. These features make them poorly suited for balloon angioplasty, directional atherectomy, and excimer laser. The Rotablator works very effectively in calcified plaque and can be activated on bend points of vessels. For these reasons, ostial lesions may be effectively treated. Koller and coworkers[52] reported on the use of MRA in 28 lesions. A success rate of 96% was achieved. Angiographic restenosis occurred in 40% of lesions. These findings suggest that the Rotablator is uniquely suited for this lesion.

## Undilatable Lesions

A final subgroup of lesions in which the Rotablator may have benefit are those that failed to dilate with balloon angioplasty.[55–58] Some lesions failed to expand with balloon inflation pressures of 20 atm or more. Other lesions are extremely elastic and have extensive recoil. Buchbinder (personal communication) employed MRA in 114 patients with undilatable lesions. Angiographic success (< 50% residual stenosis) was achieved in 93% of patients.

## OPTIMAL ROTATIONAL ATHERECTOMY

Since the publication of the first edition of this textbook, major advances in our understanding of the mechanism of lumen enlargement after rotational atherectomy have occurred. In addition, a great deal has been learned from improvements in operator technique.[59, 60] Stertzer and associates[60] have quantified improvements occurring at their institution. These investigators evaluated the impact of improved technique and on outcome for 710 patients treated from 1990 to 1994. Improvements in technique included initiation of verapamil/nitroglycerin flush solution, stepwise increase in burr size, very slow burr advancement, and strict control of rpm. This improvement resulted in the elimination of no-reflow and a decrease in coronary artery spasm.

We wish to determine optimal burr-to-artery ratios that would provide the least risk of restenosis. Kaplan and colleagues[61] reviewed the outcome of 311 patients (339 lesions) treated at William Beaumont Hospital between 1993 and 1994. Hospital outcome and 6-month follow-up were reported. It was apparent that to decrease restenosis risk, burr-to-artery ratios of 0.6 to 0.8 were required (Fig. 31–12). At these ranges, target vessel revascularization rates comparable to those in stent implantation occurred.

Controversy has existed concerning the philosophy of sizing of burrs and balloon inflation pressures of adjunctive balloon angioplasty. One school believed that to achieve optimal results, an aggressive burr-to-artery ratio was required to optimally ablate plaque. In addition, low balloon inflation pressures were required to achieve less deep tissue

injury and to limit restenosis risk. These issues were settled by two randomized trials. Safian and colleagues[62] have reported the Coronary Angioplasty and Rotablator Atherectomy Trial (CARAT) results. In this trial, 220 patients were randomly assigned to a strategy of a small burr-to-artery ratios (≤0.7) or a large burr-to-artery ratio (>0.7). Balloon sizing to a 1:1 ratio and balloon inflation pressures of 8 atm were employed. A second study, the Study to determine Rotablator and Transluminal Angioplasty Strategy (STRATAS), has also been completed, and Whitlow and colleagues[63] have presented initial and 6-month results. In this study, patients were randomly assigned to an aggressive strategy (burr-to-artery ratio ≥9.7) or usual care. Balloon inflation pressures of 3 atm or less were mandated.

The CARAT study could not demonstrate an advantage of larger burr-to-artery ratios. In fact, more dissections and more no-reflow occurred with aggressive burr sizing. The STRATAS study confirmed the increased periprocedural risk of an aggressive burr sizing strategy. In addition, neither the CARAT nor the STRATAS trial found an impact on 6-month target lesion revascularization for an aggressive burr sizing. In both studies, target vessel revascularization rates of greater than 25% occurred. In the CARAT study, final luminal stenosis was 27% and 23% for conservative and aggressive burr sizing, respectively. In the STRATAS study, final percentage of stenosis was 26% and 27% for routine and aggressive burr sizing, respectively. These studies have determined that for vessels greater than 2.5

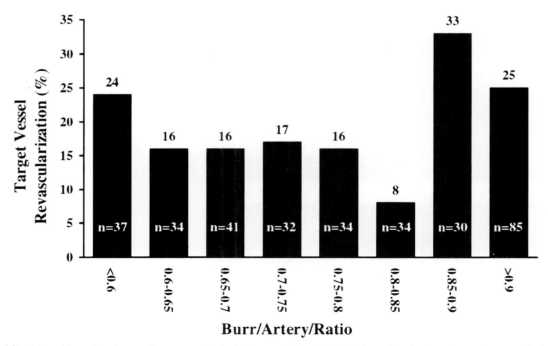

FIGURE 31–12. Optimal burr-to-artery ratios appear to be between 0.7 and 0.8. At these levels, target vessel revascularization (TVR) rates comparable to those achieved with stent implantation occur.

mm, it is unlikely that rotational atherectomy with or without angioplasty can achieve final target vessel revascularization rates comparable to those achieved with stent therapy. It is therefore unlikely that MRA will compete for lesions that are well suited for stent implantation.

## ROTABLATOR AND STENT THERAPY

In spite of the inability of MRA to replace stent implantation, a substantial role for this device still exists. A major role will exist in heavily calcified lesions: these lesions are difficult to cross with current stents. Even if a stent can be placed across heavily calcified lesions, optimal stent expansion is difficult; even with high balloon inflation pressures, stents may not fully deploy in heavily calcified vessels. The Rotablator has proved to be useful in aorto-ostial lesions. In these lesions, the pretreatment with MRA before stent implantation is beneficial, especially if heavy calcification is present. Furthermore, stent delivery and placement are often expedited because recoil is limited by MRA pretreatment. Bifurcation lesions remain a major obstacle to stent therapy. Our favorite approach is to sequentially treat the side branch, then the major vessel, with MRA and follow this with a kissing balloon technique. If a suboptimal result persists, then stenting of the major branch alone is sufficient. The initial pretreatment of the two branches markedly reduces plaque shift and decreases the risk of sidebranch occlusion.

Finally, a major new use for the Rotablator has been developed for the treatment of in-stent restenosis[64-68] (Fig. 31–13). Our own approach is to aggressively treat the restenotic tissue with large burrs and use IVUS to guide us in selecting the burr size. This technique has limited the need for retreatment with additional stents. Sharma and coworkers[69] have completed a randomized trial for in-stent restenosis and have found a significant decrease in the rate of in-stent re-restenosis after MRA. Whether these results are superior to radiation therapy or the cutting balloon is uncertain. At present, MRA and laser are the only two nonballoon devices commonly used to treat in-stent restenosis.

## CONCLUSION

At the present time, rotational atherectomy has found an important niche in the interventional armamentarium. Although the initial promise of the device to decrease restenosis has not been realized, important treatment applications still exist. Without a doubt, heavily calcified vessels will remain an important environment for rotational atherectomy. As limitations of stent therapy (small vessels, heavy calcium deposits, bifurcated lesions, long diffuse disease) become more apparent, we are convinced that rotational atherectomy will increase in use in these areas. At present, a great body of knowledge exists on how to perform a safe, effective, rotational atherectomy procedure. Information is increasing on how to combine rotational atherectomy with stent

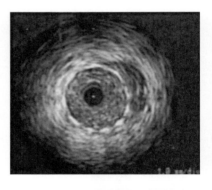
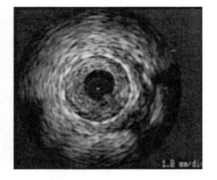
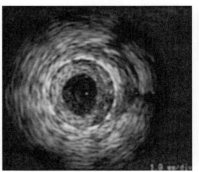
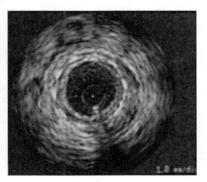

FIGURE 31–13. The diffuse process of in-stent restenosis is depicted in the *upper left panel*. Sequentially up-sized burrs were used with intravascular ultrasound images after a 1.5 burr (*upper right*), after a 2.15 burr (*lower left*), and finally after adjunctive percutaneous transluminal coronary angioplasty (*lower right*). (From Van Dahl J, et al: Am J Cardiol 1999; 83:862).

implantation. If an effective pharmacologic or radiation treatment for fibrointimal hyperplasia were developed, it is possible that rotational atherectomy would take on an even larger role in interventional practice. It behooves interventionalists to remain current on the indications for this device and on improvements in design because it is quite likely that rotational atherectomy will play an important role in interventional cardiology for the foreseeable future.

# REFERENCES

1. Sandborn EL: Reduction in angioplasty complications after the introduction of coronary stents: Results from a consecutive series of 2242 patients. Am Heart J 132:503–507, 1996.
2. Bergelson BA, Fishman RF, Tommaso CL: Abrupt vessel closure: Changing importance, management, and consequences. Am Heart J 134:362–381, 1997.
3. Topol EJ, Byzova TV, Plow EF: Platelet GPIIb–IIIa blockers. Lancet 353:227–231, 1999.
4. Serruys PW, DeJaegere P, Kiemeneij F, et al: A comparison of balloon-expandable-stent implantation with balloon angioplasty in patients with coronary artery disease. N Eng J Med 331:489–495, 1994.
5. Fischman DL, Leon MBM, Baim DS, et al: A randomized comparison of coronary stent placement and balloon angioplasty in the treatment of coronary artery disease. N Engl J Med 331:496–501, 1994.
6. Lai P, O'Neill WW, Auth D, et al: Non-surgical human coronary endarterectomy: Use of a mechanical rotary catheter [Abstract]. Circulation 72(suppl III):III-371, 1985.
7. Reisman M, Harms V: Guidewire bias: Potential source of complications with rotational atherectomy. Cathet Cardiovasc Diagn 3:64–68, 1996.
8. Safian RD, May MA, Lichtenberg A, et al: Detailed clinical and angiographic analysis of transluminal extraction coronary atherectomy for complex lesions in native coronary arteries. J Am Coll Cardiol 25:848–854, 1995.
9. Ahn SS, Auth D, Marcus DR, et al: Removal of focal atheromatous lesions by angioscopically guided high-speed rotary atherectomy: Preliminary experimental observations. J Vasc Surg 7:292, 1988.
10. Friedman HZ, Elliott MA, Gottlieb GJ, et al: Mechanical rotary atherectomy: The effects of microparticle embolization on myocardial blood flow and function. J Intervent Cardiol 2:77, 1989.
11. Zacca NM, Raizner AE, Noon GP, et al: Short term follow up of patients treated with a recently developed rotational atherectomy device and in vivo assessment of the particles generated [Abstract]. J Am Coll Cardiol 11:109A, 1988.
12. Prevosti LG, Cook JA, Unger EF, et al: Particulate debris from rotational atherectomy: Size distribution and physiologic effects [Abstract]. Circulation 78(suppl II):II-83, 1988.
13. Pavlides GS, Hauser AM, Grines CL: Clinical, hemodynamic, electrocardiographic and mechanical events during nonocclusive, coronary atherectomy and comparison with balloon angioplasty. Am J Cardiol 70:841–845, 1992.
14. Teirstein PS, Warth DC, Haq N: High speed rotational coronaryatherectomy for patients with diffuse coronary artery disease. J Am Coll Cardiol 18:1694–1701, 1991.
15. William MJA, Dow CJ, Newell JB, et al: Prevalence and timing of regional myocardial dysfunction after rotational coronary atherectomy. J Am Coll Cardiol 28:861, 1996.
16. Bowles M, Palko W, Beaver C, et al: Clinical and postmortem outcome of "no-reflow" phenomenon in a patient treated with rotational atherectomy. South Med J 89(8):820, 1996.
17. van de Rijn M, Regula DP Jr, Billingham M: Autopsy findings after coronary rotational atherectomy. Am J Cardiovasc Pathol 3:301–304, 1990.
18. Hetterich FS, McEniery PT: Right ventricular infarction following percutaneous coronary rotational atherectomy. Cathet Cardiovasc Diagn 34:321–324, 1995.
19. Khoury A, Kern MJ: Coronary physiology of percutaneous rotational atherectomy. Cathet Cardiovasc Diagn 3(suppl):15–22, 1996.
20. Nunez BD, Keelan ET, Higano ST, et al: Coronary hemodynamics before and after rotational atherectomy with adjunctive balloon angioplasty. Cathet Cardiovasc Diagn 3 (suppl): 40–49, 1996.
21. Bowers TR, Stewart RE, O'Neill WW, et al: Effect of Rotablator atherectomy and adjunctive balloon angioplasty on coronary blood flow. Circulation 95:1157–1164, 1997.
22. Safian RD, Freed M, Reddy V: Do excimer laser angioplasty and rotational atherectomy facilitate balloon angioplasty? Implications for lesion-specific coronary intervention. J Am Coll Cardiol 27:552, 1996.
23. O'Neill WW: Mechanical rotational atherectomy. Am J Cardiol 69:12F, 1992.
24. Rodriguez A, Santaera O, Larribeau M, et al: Early decrease in minimal luminal diameter after successful percutaneous transluminal coronary angioplasty predicts late restenosis. Am J Cardiol 71:1391–1395, 1993.
25. Dussaillant GR, Mintz GS, Pichard AD, et al: Effect of rotational atherectomy in noncalcified atherosclerotic plaque: A volumetric intravascular ultrasound study. J Am Coll Cardiol 28:856, 1996.
26. Stuver TP, Ling FS: The "furrowing effect": Guidewire-induced "directional" lesion ablation in rotational atherectomy of angulated coronary artery lesions. Cathet Cardiovasc Diagn 39:385–395, 1996.
27. Kovach J, Mintz G, Pichard A: Sequential intravascular ultrasound characterization of the mechanisms of rotational atherectomy and adjunct balloon angioplasty J Am Coll Cardiol 22:1024–1032, 1993.
28. Zacca NM, Kleiman NS, Rodriguez AR, et al: Rotational atherectomy: Rotational ablation of coronary artery lesions using single, large burrs. Cathet Cardiovasc Diagn 26:92, 1992.
29. Rodriguez AR, Zacca N, Heibig J, et al: Coronary rotary ablation using a single large burr and without balloon assistance [Abstract]. Circulation (suppl 82):III-310, 1990.
30. Schieman G, McDaniel M, Fenner J, et al: Quantitative angiographic assessment of percutaneous transluminal coronary rotational ablation [Abstract]. Circulation (suppl 82):III-493, 1990.
31. Harris SL, Staudacher RA, Heibig JP, et al: Rotational coronary ablation achieves lumen size comparable to balloon angioplasty without stretching the arterial wall [Abstract]. J Am Coll Cardiol 17:124A, 1991.
32. Hoffmann R, Mintz GS, Kent KM, et al: Comparative early and nine-month results of rotational atherectomy, stents, and the combination of both for calcified lesions in large coronary arteries. Am J Cardiol 81:552–557, 1998.
33. Moussa I, Di Mario C, Moses J, et al: Coronary stenting after rotational atherectomy in calcified and complex lesions: Angiographic and clinical follow-up results. Circulation 96:128–136, 1997.
34. Cheirif JB, Heibig J, Harris S, et al: Rotational ablation is associated with less myocardial ischemia than PTCA [Abstract]. Circulation 82(suppl III):III-493, 1990.
35. Popma J, Leon M, Buchbinder M, et al: Predictors and prognostic significance of CPK elevation after percutaneous transluminal rotational coronary atherectomy [Abstract]. J Am Coll Cardiol 19:77A, 1992.
36. Basnight M, Zipkin R, Stertzer S, et al: Myocardial injury following coronary rotational ablation: Mechanisms and incidence [Abstract]. J Am Coll Cardiol 19:334A, 1992.
37. Whitlow PL: Rotablator technique and complications. Cathet Cardiovasc Diagn 36:311–312, 1995.
38. Fajadet J, Doucet S, Caillard J, et al: Coronary rotational ablation in complex lesions: Clinical, angiographic and procedural predictors of success and complications [Abstract]. Circulation 86(suppl I):I-2034, 1992.
39. MacIsaac AI, Bass TA, Buchbinder M, et al: High speed rotational atherectomy: Outcome in calcified and non-

calcified coronary artery lesions. J Am Coll Cardiol 26:731–736, 1995.

40. Satler LF, Warth D: Dissections after high-speed rotational atherectomy: Frequency, predictive factors and clinical consequences [Abstract]. Circulation 86(suppl I):I-3124, 1992.

41. Leon M, Kent K, Pichard A, et al: Percutaneous transluminal coronary rotational angioplasty of calcified lesions [Abstract]. Circulation 84(suppl II):II-82, 1991.

42. Fajadet J, Doucet S, Caillard J, et al: Coronary rotational ablation in complex lesions: Clinical, angiographic and procedural predictors of success and complications [Abstract]. Circulation 86(suppl I):I-2034, 1992.

43. Levin TN, Carroll J, Feldman T: High-speed rotational atherectomy for chronic total coronary occlusions. Cathet Cardiovasc Diagn (suppl 3):34, 1996.

44. Brown DL, George CJ, Steenkiste AR, et al: High-speed rotational atherectomy of human coronary stenoses: Acute and one-year outcomes from the new approaches to coronary intervention (NACI) registry. Am J Cardiol 80(10A):60k, 1997.

45. Guérin Y, Spalding C, Desnos M, et al: Rotational atherectomy with adjunctive balloon angioplasty versus conventional percutaneous transluminal coronary angioplasty in type B2 lesions: Results of a randomized study. Am Heart J 131:879, 1996.

46. Hoffmann R, Mintz Gary S, Kent Kenneth M, et al: Comparative early and nine-month results of rotational atherectomy, stents, and the combination of both for calcified lesions in large coronary arteries. Am J Cardiol 81:552, 1998.

47. Hong MK, Mintz GS, Popma JJ, et al: Safety and efficacy of elective stent implantation following rotational atherectomy in large calcified coronary arteries. Cathet Cardiovasc Diagn 3(suppl 1):50, 1996.

48. Reifart N, Vandormael M, Krajcar M, et al: Randomized comparison of angioplasty of complex coronary lesions at a single center. Circulation 96:91, 1997.

49. O'Neill WW, Bates RE, Kirsch M, et al: Mechanical transluminal coronary endarterectomy: Initial clinical experience with the Auth mechanical rotary catheter [Abstract]. J Am Coll Cardiol 13:227A, 1989.

50. Whitlow PL: Is rotational atherectomy here to stay? Heart 78(suppl 2):35, 1997.

51. Bertrand ME, Fourrier JL, Dietz U, et al: European experience with percutaneous transluminal coronary rotational ablation: Immediate results [Abstract]. Circulation 82(suppl III):III-310, 1990.

52. Koller PT, Freed M, Grines CL, et al: Success, complications and restenosis following rotational transluminal extraction atherectomy of ostial stenosis. Cathet Cardiovasc Diagn 31:255, 1994.

53. Zimarino M, Corcos T, Favereau X, et al: Rotational coronary atherectomy with adjunctive balloon angioplasty for the treatment of ostial lesions. Cathet Cardiovasc Diagn 33:22, 1994.

54. Popma JJ, Brogan WC III, Pichard AD, et al: Rotational coronary atherectomy of ostial stenoses. Am J Cardiol 71:436, 1993.

55. Topol EJ: Rotablator to the rescue. Am J Cardiol 71:858, 1993.

56. Dietz U, Erbel R, Rupprecht H-J, et al: High-frequency rotational ablation following failed percutaneous transluminal coronary angioplasty. Cathet Cardiovasc Diagn 31:179, 1994.

57. Brown RIG, Penn IM: Coronary rotational ablation for unsuccessful angioplasty due to failure to cross the stenosis with a dilatation catheter. Cathet Cardiovasc Diagn 26:110, 1992.

58. Brogan WC III, Popma JJ, Pichard AD, et al: Rotational coronary atherectomy after unsuccessful coronary balloon angioplasty. Am J Cardiol 71:794, 1993.

59. Reisman M: Technique and strategy of rotational atherectomy. Cathet Cardiovasc Diagn 3(suppl):2, 1996.

60. Stertzer SH, Pomerantsev EV, Fitzgerald PJ, et al: Effects of technique modification on immediate results of high speed rotational atherectomy in 710 procedures on 656 patients. Cathet Cardiovasc Diagn 36:304, 1995.

61. Kaplan BM, Safian RD, Mojares JJ, et al: Optimal burr and adjunctive balloon sizing reduces the need for target artery revascularization after coronary mechanical rotational atherectomy. Am J Cardiol 78:1224, 1996.

62. Safian RD, Feldman T, Muller DWM, et al: Coronary Angioplasty and Rotablator Atherectomy Trial (CARAT): Immediate and late results of a prospective multicenter randomized trial. In press.

63. Whitlow PL, Cowley MJ, Kuntz RE, et al: Study to determine Rotablator and Transluminal Angioplasty Strategy (STRATAS). In press.

64. Lee S-G, Lee CW, Cheong S-S, et al: Immediate and long-term outcomes of rotational atherectomy versus balloon angioplasty alone for treatment of diffuse in-stent restenosis. Am J Cardiol 82:140, 1998.

65. Sharma SK, Duvvuri S, Dangas G, et al: Rotational atherectomy for in-stent restenosis: Acute and long-term results of the first 100 cases. J Am Coll Cardiol 32:1358, 1998.

66. Schiele F, Meneveau N, Vuillemenot A, et al: Treatment of in-stent restenosis with high speed rotational atherectomy and IVUS guidance in small <3.0 mm vessels. Cathet Cardiovasc Diagn 44:77, 1998.

67. Belli G, Whitlow PL: Should we spark interest in rotational atherectomy for in-stent restenosis? Cathet Cardiovasc Diagn 40:150–151, 1997.

68. Stone GW: Rotational atherectomy for treatment of in-stent restenosis: Role of intracoronary ultrasound guidance. Cathet Cardiovasc Diagn 3(suppl): 73, 1996.

69. Sharma SK, Kini A, Shalouh E, et al: Rotational atherectomy achieves a higher acute luminal gain vs. PTCA in the treatment of diffuse in-stent restenosis: Insight from the randomized ROSTER trial [Abstract]. J Am Coll Cardiol 49A:1098–1058, 1999.

# 32

# Coronary Transluminal Extraction Catheter Atherectomy

*Joseph A. Puma*    *Marino Labinaz*    *Michael H. Sketch, Jr.*

Percutaneous transluminal coronary angioplasty (PTCA) has enjoyed explosive acceptance and success since the 1980s and is now the leading form of coronary revascularization in the United States. Restenosis continues to be the cause of significant morbidity and the need for second intervention despite the success of intracoronary stents and intravenous glycoprotein IIb/IIIa platelet inhibitors.[1, 2]

The early pioneers of PTCA understood the intuitive and practical limitations of balloon expansion within the coronary artery to maintain long-term luminal enlargement in the presence of obstructive atherosclerotic plaque and thrombus. The initial concept of mechanical excision of atheromatous material from diseased arterial segments was introduced by John B. Simpson and termed *atherectomy*. Three types of percutaneous atherectomy devices are currently approved for use in humans in the United States: directional (Guidant Corp.; Temecula CA), rotational (Boston Scientific Corp.; Maple Grove MN), and extraction (InterVentional Technologies, Inc.; San Diego CA). Directional and rotational atherectomy procedures are discussed in detail in other chapters.

The transluminal extraction catheter (TEC) was developed by the manufacturer in conjunction with Richard S. Stack at Duke University Medical Center. The device was approved for use in the United States by the U.S. Food and Drug Administration (FDA) in May 1989 to treat obstructive peripheral arterial disease. The FDA subdivision on the circulatory system authorized the TEC for use in native coronary arteries and saphenous vein bypass grafts (SVBGs) in June 1992. The purposes of this chapter are to give an overview of the scientific data on the outcomes of use of the TEC device and to define its current role in the percutaneous treatment of coronary artery disease.

## THE DEVICE

The TEC is a percutaneous, over-the-wire, cutting and aspirating device. The tip of the catheter consists of two stainless steel blades and two adjacent windows arranged in a conical configuration attached to the distal end of a flexible, hollow torque tube (Fig. 32–1). The TEC device is guided over a 0.014-inch steerable floppy-tip guide wire, which is passed through the central lumen of the catheter and through the conical head. The tip of this guide wire is radiopaque and has a terminal 0.021-inch ball to prevent entrapment of the wire tip and advancement of the cutting blades beyond it. Once the catheter is positioned in the coronary artery, the guide wire can be fixed in position by being secured to the catheter drive unit. The 153-cm torque-tube is connected to the catheter drive unit, which is battery powered and hand held. The catheter drive unit houses the trigger, which, when compressed, simultaneously activates the cutting blades (750 rpm) and vacuum suction (Fig. 32–2). Attached to the drive unit are a remote battery power source and tubing that leads to a glass vacuum bottle for collection of excised material.

## ANIMAL STUDIES AND HUMAN PERIPHERAL EXPERIENCE

Development of TEC atherectomy was undertaken to overcome the limitations of balloon angioplasty, such as abrupt closure, restenosis, and an inability

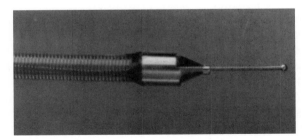

FIGURE 32–1. Close-up of the torque tube and cutter head of the TEC transluminal extraction catheter over the unique 0.014-inch TEC guide wire. (From Sketch MH Jr., Phillips HP, Lee MM, et al: Coronary transluminal extraction-endarterectomy. J Invas Cardiol 3:23, 1991.)

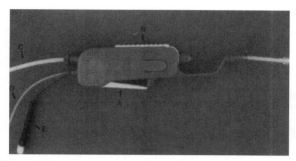

FIGURE 32–2. Drive unit for the TEC transluminal extraction catheter. *A,* trigger; *B,* advancement control level; *C,* rear extension tubing; *D,* suction tubing; *E,* power connector. (From Sketch MH Jr., Phillips HP, Lee MM, et al: Coronary transluminal extraction-endarterectomy. J Invas Cardiol 3:23, 1991.)

to adequately treat thrombus-laden lesions. Initial in vivo studies of the TEC device were carried out in normal canine arteries.[3] Histologic analysis of treated segments revealed focal intimal dissection with subintimal excision of less than 25% of the media. In diseased segments, excision was typically limited to the media, although there was occasional disruption of external elastic lamina.

In human peripheral arterial evaluation, examination of extracted material revealed a mixture of collagen, elastic tissue, moderate numbers of smooth muscle cells, and cholesterol crystals ranging in size from 0.1 to 2.8 mm in maximum dimensions.[4] Subsequent registry and multicenter trial analysis of the use of the TEC in human peripheral arterial disease, to treat 189 lesions in 129 patients, demonstrated a success rate greater than 90% and a restenosis rate of 20% to 25%, without any perforations or distal emboli.[5, 6]

## THE PROCEDURE

Coronary TEC atherectomy is performed via a percutaneous transfemoral approach. As with standard balloon sheaths, intravenous heparin is administered to achieve an activated clotting time of 300 to 350 seconds during the procedure. There are no randomized data regarding the use of glycoprotein receptor blockers during TEC atherectomy, but we recommend their use for high-risk procedures and strongly suggest that it be considered for all TEC procedures. If the patient receives these agents, the dose of heparin should be lowered to obtain an activated clotting time of 200 to 300 seconds.

A 10.5-French arterial sheath is required to permit insertion of a 10-French guide catheter, preferably with side holes. Size 10-French guide catheters can accommodate all cutter sizes, although smaller guide catheters may be used for smaller cutters (Table 32–1). Predominantly 9-French guides with 6.5-French cutters are used for vein graft interventions,

and predominantly 8-French guides with 5.5-French cutters are used in native coronary arteries. The guide catheter is advanced to the aortic root over a 0.063-inch J-tip guide wire to reduce trauma to the arterial wall. The guide tip is soft, atraumatic, and unlikely to cause ostial trauma.

After the lesion is localized with injection of contrast media, a 0.014-inch TEC guide wire is placed across the lesion. The wire should be placed as distal as possible to ensure that the cutter can be positioned on the more proximal, stiff portion of the wire to minimize lateral displacement. A more steerable conventional PTCA wire can be used to cross complex or tortuous vessels and then exchanged for the TEC wire with any transport catheter that can accommodate a 0.021-inch ball.

The TEC device should be assembled and the catheter drive unit tested on the operating table before each use. The vacuum system should be tested, and the entire system flushed with heparinized saline. A fresh vacuum bottle should be attached to the vacuum tubing. Once proper functioning has been confirmed, the catheter is carefully positioned over the guide wire so that the conical head is 3 to 4 mm proximal to the lesion. Activation of the cutter within the lesion must be avoided, because it may increase the risk of dissection and embolization. Intracoronary nitroglycerin (0.1 to 0.3 mg) is administered to prevent spasm prior to activation of the cutter. Lactated Ringer's solution is infused under pressure through the guide catheter during cutter operation to create a particulate slurry, facilitating aspiration of excised material.

Three to five passes across the lesion, of 10 to 15 seconds each, are made. Special care should be taken to ensure the presence of flow into the vacuum bottle. If there is no flow, cutting should be stopped immediately, and the function of the vacuum system should be reassessed. The cutter should not be activated within the guide catheter, nondiseased segments, or a bend or tortuous segment. If angiographic evaluation shows the result of TEC to

**TABLE 32–1.** **CUTTER AND VESSEL SIZE AND GUIDE CATHETER CORRELATES FOR THE TRANSLUMINAL EXTRACTION CATHETER**

| CUTTER SIZE (FRENCH) | CUTTER DIAMETER (mm) | MINIMAL VESSEL DIAMETER (mm) | MINIMAL GUIDE CATHETER INTERNAL DIAMETER (INCH) |
|---|---|---|---|
| 5.5 | 1.8 | 2.5 | 0.86 |
| 6.0 | 2.0 | 2.75 | 0.92 |
| 6.5 | 2.17 | 3.0 | 0.92 |
| 7.0 | 2.33 | 3.25 | .104 |
| 7.5 | 2.5 | 3.5 | .104 |

be suboptimal (greater than 25% luminal diameter narrowing), adjunctive balloon angioplasty or stenting is performed to optimize the result.

Optimal criteria for cutter size selection have not been determined. Several sizes, from 5.5- to 7.5-French (1.8- to 2.5-mm), are currently available (see Table 32–1). In general, a cutter diameter at least 1 mm smaller than the reference vessel diameter is preferred. Smaller cutters should be employed in tortuous vessels to prevent perforation. In thrombus-laden lesions, a larger cutter (i.e., 7.0- or 7.5-French) is initially selected to facilitate clot aspiration. In severely stenotic lesions, a smaller cutter is initially used, with progression to larger cutters as necessary to maximize resection of the lesion.

Thrombus removal is almost always accomplished by TEC atherectomy, although tissue removal is less reliable, and angiographic evidence of improvement may be associated with a "Dotter" effect.[7–9] Adjunctive intervention is therefore generally required.

Postprocedure care is the same as for standard percutaneous interventions. The sheath should be removed as soon as feasible to reduce vascular complications. Aspirin therapy is continued indefinitely.

## CLINICAL APPLICATION

The early published experience of TEC atherectomy was limited to patients enrolled in the Duke Multicenter Coronary Transluminal Extraction-endarterectomy Registry and the U.S. Transluminal Extraction-endarterectomy Catheter Registry, and to small studies of nonrandomized patients. We attempt to combine the results of available literature here, in hopes of developing a statistical rationale for use of the device.

Interesting observations from the early use of the TEC include a disproportionate use in SVBGs compared with native arteries (typically, up to 50% of TEC procedures are performed in SVBGs). One possible explanation is the assumption that the unique

excision and vacuum removal properties of the TEC would make it suitable for more complex lesions thought to be laden with thrombus or filled with debris. Furthermore, an operator inexperienced with a new device that is significantly more complicated to use than standard balloon PTCA might be less enthusiastic about using the TEC for less complex lesions and might tend to refrain from performing complex angioplasty.

## Native Coronary Arteries

There is limited experience with use of the TEC device in native coronary arteries (Table 32–2). The point estimate of success is 91%. Adjunctive PTCA is usually required. In the U.S. TEC Registry, the success rate did not appear to be affected by lesion location, and success was achieved in all patients with angiographic evidence of thrombus or total occlusion.[10, 11] The complication rate for TEC atherectomy is greater than that for standard PTCA.

## Saphenous Vein Bypass Grafts

Instrumentation of SVBGs is often an unrewarding experience because of complications associated with intraluminal thrombus and distal embolization. Older, more degenerated grafts are more prone to poor outcomes with PTCA than younger grafts. There has been extensive experience with TEC atherectomy and SVBGs (Table 32–3).[12–16] As in use of the TEC in native coronary arteries, success rates for use in SVBGs are acceptable, and adjunctive PTCA is typically required. The point estimate of success is 88%. In the U.S. TEC Registry, success rates were similar for all lesion sites, although longer lesions (>20 mm) were less likely to be successfully opened than shorter lesions (85% and 96%, respectively).[10] The complication rate is somewhat higher than that of PTCA of SVBGs, although this difference may be explained, at least in part, by a selection bias toward more complex cases for TEC atherectomy (as evidenced by 183 lesions with thrombus and 68 total occlusions in the U.S. TEC Registry).[10]

## TABLE 32–2. RESULTS OF TRANSLUMINAL EXTRACTION CATHETER ATHERECTOMY IN NATIVE CORONARY ARTERIES

| STUDY (YEAR) | NO. OF LESIONS | RATE OF ADJUNCTIVE PTCA (%) | RATE OF SUCCESS (%) | COMPLICATION RATES (%) | | | | |
|---|---|---|---|---|---|---|---|---|
| | | | | MI | DEATH | AC | DE | NO REFLOW |
| O'Neill et al (1992)[10] | 662 | 75 | 93 | 1.2 | 1.6 | | | |
| Safian et al (1995)[11] | 181 | 84 | 84 | 3.4 | 2.3 | 11 | 5 | — |
| Total | 843 | 76 | 914 | | | | | |
| 95% confidence interval | | .73–.79 | .89–.93 | | | | | |

AC, acute closure; DE, distal embolization; MI, myocardial infarction.

**TABLE 32–3. RESULTS OF TRANSLUMINAL EXTRACTION CATHETER ATHERECTOMY IN SAPHENOUS VEIN BYPASS GRAFTS**

| STUDY (YEAR) | NO. OF LESIONS | RATE OF ADJUNCTIVE PTCA (%) | RATE OF SUCCESS (%) | COMPLICATION RATES (%) | | | | |
|---|---|---|---|---|---|---|---|---|
| | | | | MI | DEATH | AC | DE | No REFLOW |
| Popma et al (1992)[15] | 29 | 86 | 82 | 3.7 | 10.3 | — | 17 | — |
| Safian et al (1994)[13] | 158 | 91 | 84 | 2 | 2 | 5 | 11.9 | 8.8 |
| Twidale et al (1994)[16] | 88 | 95 | 86 | 3.4 | 0 | 5 | 4.5 | — |
| Meany (1995)[24] | 650 | 74 | 89 | 0.7 | 3.2 | 2 | 2 | — |
| Misumi et al (1996)[20] | 103 | — | 90 | 3.9 | 0 | — | 13 | — |
| Bejarano et al (1997)[14] | 127 | 85 | 91 | 6.6 | — | — | 11.8 | — |
| Total | 1155 | 80 | 88 | | | | | |
| 95% confidence interval | | .78–.82 | .86–.90 | | | | | |

AC, acute closure; DE, distal embolization; MI, myocardial infarction.

## Restenosis

Restenosis remains a major limitation of coronary angioplasty. The use of intracoronary stents and intravenous abciximab has been demonstrated to reduce restenosis in randomized clinical trials. These agents have not been studied in patients undergoing TEC atherectomy, however, and therefore no conclusions can be drawn.

Published restenosis rates with TEC atherectomy for native coronary arteries and SVBGs are summarized in Tables 32–4 and 32–5, respectively. Restenosis is significant with the use of the TEC and may be considered prohibitive. Subgroup analysis from the Duke registry suggests that the likelihood of restenosis may be inversely related to the immediate gain at the time of the procedure.[17] In this registry, patients undergoing native artery TEC atherectomy alone had only an 18% restenosis rate if the final residual stenosis was less than 25%. Similar findings were observed in the patients undergoing TEC atherectomy of SVBGs. If this relationship is proven, it would suggest that TEC atherectomy alone may not be a good option, particularly in vein grafts, because of the limitations in the size of the TEC cutters now available. It would also suggest that adjunctive intervention (particularly with stents) may be a preferable planned approach to TEC atherectomy of both native coronary arteries and SVBGs.

## OTHER APPLICATIONS
### Acute Ischemic Syndromes

Acute ischemic syndromes are pathologically associated with the formation of intracoronary thrombus, causing varying degrees of lumen obstruction that can be correlated with the patient's clinical presentation, ranging from partial occlusion (unstable angina pectoris) to complete occlusion (acute myocardial infarction [MI]). Patients with acute ischemic syndromes who undergo percutaneous intervention have considerably worse outcomes when there is angiographic evidence of thrombus in the culprit lesion.[18] Furthermore, patients with visible thrombus have high-risk clinical profiles with lower left ventricular ejection fractions, more three-vessel and left main artery disease, and a higher incidence of prior MI and bypass surgery.

Theoretically, the design of the TEC device should offer an advantage in thrombus-laden lesions because of its unique ability to cut and suction intracoronary plaque and debris. Sketch and colleagues[19] found TEC atherectomy to be associated with lower rates of distal embolization in vein grafts with thrombus than was PTCA (5.6% and 31.8%, respectively; $p = 0.004$). This difference was not translated into better outcomes for the patients undergoing TEC atherectomy in this study, however; no difference was seen in the rates of procedural suc-

**TABLE 32–4. RESTENOSIS RATE AFTER TRANSLUMINAL EXTRACTION CATHETER ATHERECTOMY OF NATIVE CORONARY ARTERIES**

| STUDY (YEAR) | NO. OF LESIONS (NO. OF PATIENTS) | RATE OF ANGIOGRAPHIC FOLLOW-UP (%) | RATE OF RESTENOSIS (%) |
|---|---|---|---|
| Safian et al (1995)[11] | 181 (175) | 83 (143/172) | 61 |
| O'Neill et al (1992)[10] | 662 (609) | 73 | 51 |
| Total | 843 (784) | 75 | 53 |
| 95% confidence interval | | .72–.78 | .50–.53 |

**TABLE 32–5.** **RESTENOSIS RATE AFTER TRANSLUMINAL EXTRACTION CATHETER ATHERECTOMY OF SAPHENOUS VEIN BYPASS GRAFTS**

| STUDY (YEAR) | NO. OF LESIONS (NO. OF PATIENTS) | RATE OF ANGIOGRAPHIC FOLLOW-UP (%) | RATE OF RESTENOSIS (%) |
|---|---|---|---|
| Safian et al (1994)[13] | 158 (146) | 66 | 69 |
| O'Neill et al (1992)[10] | 650 (538) | 41 | 60 |
| Dooris et al (1995)[21] | 183 (175) | 74 | 69 |
| Total | 991 (859) | 49 | 64 |
| 95% confidence interval | | .46–.52 | .61–.67 |

cess or complications (death, MI, or emergent bypass surgery).[19] Patients who undergo TEC atherectomy of SVBGs with thrombus have higher rates of acute MI, need for vascular repair, abrupt closure, distal embolization, and no-reflow than patients undergoing the procedure in SVBGs without thrombus.[20, 21] There are no randomized studies comparing TEC atherectomy and PTCA in vein graft lesions with thrombus.

Kaplan and associates,[22] in a randomized, multicenter trial, compared TEC atherectomy with PTCA in native coronary arteries in patients with acute ischemic syndromes. A total of 251 patients were randomly assigned to undergo either procedure (116 to TEC atherectomy and 135 to PTCA), with angiographic evidence of thrombus noted in 52% of lesions. The primary composite end point of procedure-related angiographic or clinical complications was 4.3% in the TEC group and 8.1% in the PTCA group ($p = 0.22$). Subanalysis of the groups with unstable angina and postinfarction angina revealed a statistically significant reduction in postprocedure creatine phosphokinase (CPK) elevations in the TEC patients compared with the PTCA patients (7.1% versus 31.3%; $p < 0.05$). This study, therefore, demonstrated that the safety profile for TEC atherectomy is equivalent to that of PTCA in the treatment of patients with acute ischemic syndromes and may reduce the risk of postprocedure CPK elevations.

## Adjunctive Use

The utility of TEC atherectomy remains limited in its ability to independently produce adequate lumen enlargement. This limitation is particularly apparent in the treatment of vein grafts, which are typically larger than native coronary arteries. TEC atherectomy is therefore often coupled with adjunctive PTCA or stent placement. A study by Braden and colleagues[23] analyzed the effectiveness of a strategy of TEC atherectomy for debulking followed by Palmaz-Schatz stenting and PTCA for optimal luminal gain in 53 SVBGs in 49 consecutive patients. Despite an average vein graft age of 9.2 years, proce-

dural success was achieved in 98% of patients, with an improvement in minimal luminal diameter from 1.3 mm to 3.9 mm. Graft perforation and distal embolization occurred in 2 patients, 2 other patients had non–Q-wave MI, and 3 patients died in hospital, for an in-hospital event-free survival rate of 90%. At 13-month clinical follow-up, 5 patients required second revascularization procedures. There were four nonfatal MIs and five more deaths, for a total of 13 adverse events in 46 patients. A randomized trial comparing a TEC-stent procedure with a PTCA-stent procedure in vein graft lesions is presently enrolling patients.

## CONCLUSION

TEC atherectomy may have application in vein graft intervention or in thrombus-laden native vessel disease. The unique design of the TEC device makes it seem most practical for debulking lesions and removing thrombus. This attitude may explain, in part, the preponderance of data regarding the use of the TEC in vein grafts.[24] There remains a paucity of controlled randomized data to guide the use of TEC atherectomy, although it may be equally as effective as PTCA in treatment of native coronary arteries in patients with acute ischemic syndromes.

Although procedural success of TEC atherectomy in both native coronary arteries and SVBGs is similar to that of PTCA alone, adjunctive PTCA is often required, and both the restenosis rate and the complication rate are high (although these data may be partially explained by the use of the TEC to treat more complex lesions and in patients at increased risk of morbidity and mortality). Rigorous randomized analysis is needed to determine whether TEC atherectomy is valuable in improving patient outcome or merely remains in an ambiguous role, whose use by the interventional cardiologist should be questioned.

## REFERENCES

1. Serruys PW, deJaegere P, Kiemeneij F, et al: A comparison of balloon-expandable-stent implantation with balloon angio-

plasty in patients with coronary artery disease. N Engl J Med 331:489–501, 1994.

2. The EPIC Investigators: Use of a monoclonal antibody directed against the platelet glycoprotein IIb/IIIa receptor in high-risk coronary angioplasty. N Engl J Med 330:956–961, 1994.

3. Stack RS, Califf RM, Phillips HR, et al: Advances in cardiovascular technologies: Interventional cardiac catheterization at Duke Medical Center. Am J Cardiol (suppl) 62–1F, 1988.

4. Perez JA, Hinohara T, Quigley PJ, et al: In-vitro and in-vivo experimental results using a new wire-guided concentric atherectomy device. J Am Coll Cardiol 11:109A, 1988.

5. Sketch MH Jr, Newman GE, McCann RL, et al: Transluminal extraction-endarterectomy in peripheral vascular disease: Late clinical and angiographic follow-up. Circulation 80(suppl II):II-305, 1989.

6. Wholey MH, Jarmolowski CR: New reperfusion devices: The Kensey catheter, the atherolytic reperfusion wire device and the transluminal extraction catheter. Radiology 172:947–952, 1989.

7. Annex BH, Larkin TJ, O'Neill WW, et al: Evaluation of thrombus removal by transluminal extraction coronary atherectomy by percutaneous coronary angioplasty. Am J Cardiol 74:606–609, 1994.

8. Kaplan BM, Safian RS, Grines CL, et al: Usefulness of adjunctive angioscopy and extraction atherectomy before stent implantation in high risk narrowings in aorto-coronary artery saphenous vein grafts. Am J Cardiol 76:822–824, 1995.

9. Moses JW, Lieberman SM, Knopf WD, et al: Mechanism of transluminal extraction catheter (TEC) atherectomy in degenerative saphenous vein grafts (SVG): An angioscopic observational study. J Am Coll Cardiol 21:442A, 1993.

10. O'Neill WW, Kramer BL, Sketch MH Jr, et al, and the U.S. TEC Registry Investigators: Mechanical extraction atherectomy: Report of the U.S. Transluminal Extraction Catheter Investigation. Circulation 86(suppl I):I-779, 1992.

11. Safian RD, May MA, Lichtenberg A, et al: Detailed clinical and angiographic analysis of transluminal extraction coronary atherectomy for complex lesions in native coronary arteries. J Am Coll Cardiol 25: 848–854, 1995.

12. Platko WP, Hollman J, Whitlow PL, et al: Percutaneous transluminal angioplasty of saphenous vein graft stenoses: Long-term follow-up. J Am Coll Cardiol 14:1545–1650, 1989.

13. Safian RD, Grines CL, May MA, et al: Clinical and angiographic results of transluminal extraction coronary atherectomy in saphenous vein bypass grafts. Circulation 89:302–312, 1994.

14. Bejarano J, Margolis J, Kramer B: Extraction atherectomy for recently occluded saphenous vein grafts: A retrospective study. J Invasive Cardiol 9:263–269, 1997.

15. Popma JJ, O'Neill WW, Kramer BL, et al: A quantitative analysis of late angiographic outcome after transluminal extraction-endarterectomy (TEC) abstracted. Circulation 86(suppl I):I-457, 1992.

16. Twidale N, Barth CW III, Kipperman RM, et al: Acute results and long term outcome of transluminal catheter atherectomy for saphenous vein graft stenoses. Cath Cardiovasc Diagn 31:191–197, 1994.

17. Sketch MH, O'Neill WW, Galichia JP, et al: The Duke multicenter coronary transluminal extraction-endarterectomy registry: Acute and chronic results [Abstract]. Circulation (Suppl) J Am Coll Cardiol 17:31A, 1991.

18. Freed M, Grines C, Safian R: The New Manual of Interventional Cardiology, p 16. Birmingham, MI: Physicians' Press, 1996.

19. Sketch MH Jr, Davidson CH, Yah W, et al: Predictors of acute and long-term outcome with transluminal extraction atherectomy: The New Approaches to Coronary Intervention (NACI) registry. Am J Cardiol 80:68K–77K, 1997.

20. Misumi K, Matthews RV, Sun G-W, et al: Reduced distal embolization with transluminal extraction atherectomy compared to balloon angioplasty for saphenous vein graft disease. Cathet Cardiovasc Diagn 39:246–251, 1996.

21. Dooris M, Hoffmann M, Glazier S, et al: Comparative results of transluminal extraction coronary atherectomy in saphenous vein graft lesions with and without thrombus. J Am Coll Cardiol 25:1700–1705, 1995.

22. Kaplan BM, Gregory M, Schreiber TL, et al: Transluminal extraction atherectomy versus balloon angioplasty in acute ischemic syndromes: An interim analysis of the TOPIT trial [Abstract 1846A]. Circulation 94(suppl I):I-317, 1996.

23. Braden GA, Xenopoulos NP, Young T, et al: Transluminal extraction catheter atherectomy followed by immediate stenting in treatment of saphenous vein grafts. J Am Coll Cardiol 30:657–663, 1997.

24. Meany TB, Leon MB, Kramer BL, et al: Transluminal Extraction Catheter for the Treatment of Diseased Saphenous Vein Grafts: A Multicenter Experience. Catheter Cardiovasc Diagn 341:112–120, 1995.

# 33

# Direct Laser Ablation

*James E. Tcheng*

Because of the safety, efficacy, and ease of performance of coronary intervention, percutaneous revascularization has become the preferred strategy for the management of the patient with atherosclerotic coronary artery disease. A remarkable evolution in the technology of coronary intervention now permits more than half of patients to be treated with this modality. Among the new technologies, direct laser ablation was initially hailed as one of the major solutions that would address the limitations of conventional balloon angioplasty. Not well understood were the complexity and enormity of the task of bringing this technology into the mainstream of cardiology. Although the laser has not lived up to the high early expectations, it nonetheless continues to play a specialized role in tackling problems not easily addressed with other interventional modalities.

The purpose of this chapter is to examine the current state of the art of direct laser ablation in the treatment of the patient with cardiovascular disease. It contains sections on the fundamentals of laser ablation, clinical data, technical caveats, and promising applications of laser technology. Also incorporated is a brief discussion of the costs of implementation and use of laser ablation. The concluding remarks include an overview of current trends and future directions to put into perspective the potential applicability of this technology.

## LASER FUNDAMENTALS

The term *laser* is actually an acronym for the descriptive phrase *l*ight *a*mplification by the *s*timulated *e*mission of *r*adiation. The theoretical existence of laser light was first proposed by Albert Einstein[1] in the early 1900s. It was not until the late 1950s, however, that the first visible-light laser was actually constructed. Credit for this accomplishment is given to T. H. Maiman[2] of Hughes Aircraft, who used a ruby crystal in the first laser device.

Several properties distinguish laser energy as a unique form of electromagnetic radiation (Table 33–1). First, laser radiation is monochromatic; for any given laser, energy is usually produced at a single, specific wavelength. This fundamental wavelength is determined by the physical properties of the *active medium*, the substrate in the laser that is excited to produce laser energy. Second, the radiation emitted by the laser exists as a beam of photons that have both spatial and temporal *coherence*; that is, the photons in the laser beam are collimated and in synchrony in both space and time. Coherence results in the third important attribute of laser radiation, constancy in the energy density of the laser beam regardless of distance from the laser energy source. Indeed, if it were not for the scattering of light that occurs as photons strike gas molecules and particulate matter suspended in the atmosphere, a laser beam could exist into infinity.

## Physical Properties of a Laser

Five characteristics describe the physical properties of a given laser. They are (1) the active medium, (2) wavelength, (3) energy density, (4) operational mode (pulsed versus continuous), and (5) for pulsed lasers, the pulse duration. It is important to understand that there is no such thing as a "generic" laser; the properties of the light emitted by a laser are intrinsic to the specific laser and differ from one laser to another.

The active medium can be any substrate that, when excited, results in the emission of laser light. This active medium may exist in any physical state, such as solid crystals (ruby, neodymium:yttrium-aluminum-garnet [Nd:YAG], erbium, holmium, thulium), liquid (tunable dye), and gas (argon, $CO_2$, excimer). Depending on both the laser medium and the excitation and mechanical properties of the laser system, activation of a laser results in laser radiation that may be emitted continuously or as a series of pulses. The pulse duration of pulsed lasers typically is on the order of nanoseconds to microseconds separated by relatively long energy-free periods. The amount of energy emitted depends on the efficiency and size of the laser; for continuous-wave lasers, energy output is typically measured in watts, whereas for pulsed lasers, the output is usually in millijoules per square millimeter ($mJ/mm^2$).

**TABLE 33-1.  UNIQUE PROPERTIES OF LASER ENERGY**

| | |
|---|---|
| Monochromatic radiation | Photons are of same wavelength |
| Temporal and spatial coherence | Photons are in phase through time and space |
| Beam collimation | Photons are emitted as a single nondivergent beam (except for laser generator imperfections) |
| Uniform energy density | Energy remains constant with distance (except for transmission losses) |

## Physical Effects of Laser Energy

The physical effects of laser energy on tissue (or for that matter, any substance) are determined by (1) radiation wavelength, (2) duration of exposure, (3) energy density, and (4) intrinsic properties of the target substrate.[3-6] With regard to laser-tissue interactions, three mechanisms for ablation resulting in tissue removal have been described; they are thermal ablation, photoacoustic ablation, and photodecomposition.[7, 8] The first, ablation of tissue by thermal mechanisms, is typical of continuous-wave and infrared lasers. *Tissue ablation* is produced by a sequence of events that start with absorption of laser energy by water, rapid conversion of water into steam, and expansion of steam, leading to tissue fragmentation, disruption, and tissue ejection. *Photoacoustic ablation* occurs when tissue is exposed to brief pulses of extremely high intensity laser energy. In this situation, the incident energy creates a local photoplasma, resulting in an intense shock wave, tissue disruption, fragmentation, and consequent tissue removal.

Because of the disruptive nature of these first two mechanisms, current laser systems minimize these types of laser-tissue interactions. Instead, today's systems rely upon a third mechanism, *photochemical ablation* (or photodecomposition), wherein exposure leads directly to the breaking of molecular bonds. Bond breaking in organic compounds can occur when the energy per photon exceeds approximately 3.5 electron volts; photons with a wavelength of approximately 310 nm and shorter (including the excimer laser) possess this level of energy. The sequence of events resulting in removal of tissue by photochemical ablation is as follows[9]:

1. Strong local absorption of the ionizing laser radiation (primarily by organic substrates).
2. Electronic excitation.
3. Direct molecular bond breaking with conversion of solids into the gas phase.

Lasers that use this mechanism to achieve tissue removal (e.g., the excimer lasers) can effect precise, scalpel-like excision and ablation, as opposed to the longer-wavelength lasers (including the argon, Nd:YAG, and holmium lasers), which must rely on thermal ablation to remove tissue.

## EARLY SYSTEMS

The theoretical basis for using laser energy to treat obstructive cardiovascular disease is straightforward; application of laser energy to remove atherosclerotic tissue might result in improved procedural outcomes or lowered rates of restenosis, or both.[10] The first reports of ablation of human atheroma (in autopsy specimens) with a laser are attributed to the 1963 report of McGuff and coworkers.[11] However, the first investigations of laser ablation in patients did not begin until around 1980, when the concomitant introduction of percutaneous balloon angioplasty, flexible fiberoptics, and commercially available laser sources made it feasible to deliver laser energy directly to atheroma in situ.[3, 12-16]

Development of clinically useful laser systems has proved to be a difficult technologic challenge. The first systems coupled commercially available laser generators to simplistic fiberoptic catheters to deliver thermal energy to the target tissue. Clinical experience with these early systems, however, was uniformly dismal, with unacceptably high rates of spasm, thrombosis, coronary perforation, myocardial infarction, restenosis, and other clinical complications. These first devices are now but a footnote in the annals of interventional cardiology, having been universally abandoned.[17-24]

## DIRECT ABLATION SYSTEMS

In response to the limitations observed with continuous-wave systems, investigators began evaluating the effects of altering wavelength, output mode (pulsed versus continuous-wave operation), pulse duration, and energy exposure, searching for that ideal combination of parameters that would result in precise, controlled tissue removal, reasonable cutting efficiency, and minimal thermal injury to adjacent tissue.[4, 5, 25] By using pulsed lasers with pulse durations shorter than the thermal relaxation time (the time required for diffusion of thermal energy to the surrounding tissue) and with instantaneous peak power densities exceeding ablation thresholds, several laboratories demonstrated that true tissue ablation without adjacent tissue damage could be achieved. Other theoretical considerations suggested that the ideal radiation spectrum for the ablation of cardiovascular plaque would be limited to those wavelengths for which there was intense energy absorption by the target tissue.[26] Finally, a practical consideration, delivery of energy light via quartz silica of optical fibers, dictated that the laser wavelength had to be no shorter than approximately 300 nm.

Of the lasers meeting the preceding qualifications, pulsed excimer lasers were observed to ablate tissue not only without local thermal injury but also with nearly microsurgical precision.[27] On the basis of these experimental observations, several companies have now tested and marketed 308-nm XeCl (xenon-chloride) excimer lasers for clinical use in cardiovascular disease.

The consensus today is that the goal of laser ablation is the precise removal of obstructive atherosclerotic material by direct ablation. Intrinsic to this "microsurgical" approach is minimizing the potential for detrimental local or distant effects. As discussed previously, the only laser wavelength fulfilling the myriad of theoretical requirements with respect to direct ablation is the 308-nm XeCl excimer laser. *Excimer* is an acronym for *exci*ted di*mer*. In the excimer laser, the active medium consists of a mixture of dilute hydrogen chloride gas contained in a laser chamber containing mostly inert noble gases. The laser wavelength (308 nm) is determined by the xenon-chloride laser medium. *Excimer* specifically refers to the metastable dimeric molecule of xenon and chloride formed during the excitation phase of laser light production. Two systems, the LAIS Dymer 200+ and the Spectranetics CVX-300 system (both available from Spectranetics; Colorado Springs CO) remain in clinical use today.

## LASER ANGIOPLASTY TECHNIQUE

The procedure of excimer laser angioplasty uses techniques familiar to the interventional cardiologist, with the main difference being substitution of a laser catheter for the primary treatment device (Table 33–2). Patients should be pretreated with aspirin. After vascular access is established, heparin anticoagulation is given to achieve an activated clotting time of approximately 300 seconds. Because of a small risk of perforation, glycoprotein receptor blockers should be avoided. Standard guide catheters are used to access the coronary circulation; laser catheters larger than 1.7 mm require a large-lumen 8-French guide, whereas smaller-diameter laser catheters are compatible with standard 8-French (and large-lumen 7-French) guide catheters (Table 33–3). Use of side-hole guide catheters should be avoided unless critical catheter-induced damping of arterial pressure occurs.

After angiographic roadmap images are obtained, the lesion is crossed with a stiff 0.014-inch coronary guide wire. The laser catheter is brought into the coronary circulation over the coronary guide wire

## TABLE 33–2. TECHNIQUE OF EXCIMER LASER CORONARY ANGIOPLASTY

### Preparing the Patient

Perform typical preangioplasty patient management (including aspirin).
Obtain consent for laser procedure.

### Procedure Preparation

1. Establish vascular access.
2. Administer heparin to achieve an activated clotting time of 300 sec.
3. Avoid use of glycoprotein IIb/IIIa inhibitor before ablation.
4. Advance guide catheter:
   a. 7-French for 1.4-mm or 1.7-mm laser catheter; 8-French for 2.0-mm laser catheter.
5. Cross lesion with 0.014-inch coronary guide wire
   a. Stiffer guide wire recommended.
6. Advance laser catheter to lesion
   a. Position laser catheter with contrast as needed.

### Ablation/Saline Flush Cycle

1. Flush manifold and guide catheter clear of blood and contrast agent.
   a. Replace control syringe with a fresh 20-cc syringe for saline flush.
2. Immediately before ablation, inject 5–10 mL saline bolus as rapidly as possible.
3. Activate the laser, continuing the saline infusion at a rate of 2–3 mL/sec.
4. Advance the laser catheter at a rate of 0.5 to 1 mm/sec (until laser terminates); repeat cycle until lesion is traversed.

### Adjunctive Intervention

1. Adjunctive balloon angioplasty, stent implantation as needed.
2. Administer glycoprotein IIb/IIIa when needed after ablation completed.

### After the Procedure

Depends on final angiographically demonstrated results (no special considerations).

and advanced until the distal tip of the catheter is in contact with the target lesion. Once it is in place, saline is injected to clear blood and contrast agent from the guide catheter. Immediately before activation of the laser, saline is aggressively flushed; the laser system is then activated, delivering energy through the fiberoptic catheter to the lesion. As tissue is ablated, the catheter is slowly advanced at a rate of 0.5 to 1 mm/sec, with use of minimal antegrade pressure. The saline infusion technique is used whenever laser ablation is performed, to reduce the potential for vessel dissection.[28–30]

To lower the risk of mechanical trauma to the lesion, care must be used to avoid rapid advancement of the laser system during active ablation. The lesion should then be assessed angiographically after passage of the laser catheter. A single-pass technique is usually employed, but depending on the alignment of the laser catheter relative to the residual stenosis and normal vessel wall, the catheter may be passed again to enlarge the result. The laser catheter is then totally withdrawn, and the postprocedure result is documented angiographi-

**TABLE 33–3.  SPECTRANETICS LASER CATHETER SIZES AND COMPATIBILITY**

| CATHETER TIP DIAMETER (mm) AND STYLE | TIP DIAMETER (INCH) | GUIDE WIRE(S) (INCH) | RECOMMENDED GUIDE CATHETER SIZE (FRENCH) | MINIMUM VESSEL DIAMETER (mm) |
|---|---|---|---|---|
| 1.4, concentric | 0.056 | 0.014 | 7 | 2.0 |
| 1.7, concentric | 0.064 | 0.014–0.018 | 7 | 2.5 |
| 2.0, concentric | 0.077 | 0.014–0.018 | 8 | 3.0 |
| 1.7, eccentric | 0.065 | 0.014 | 7 | 2.5 |
| 2.0, eccentric | 0.078 | 0.014 | 8 | 3.0 |

cally. Additional adjunctive balloon angioplasty, stent implantation, or both should be performed to optimize the luminal result. Decisions about post-procedure management depend on the final result without special consideration for the application of laser energy during the procedure.

Formal training and certification are required before one can perform excimer laser angioplasty. The skill requirements set forth by the American Heart Association/American College of Cardiology (AHA/ACC) Task Force on Assessment of Diagnostic and Therapeutic Cardiovascular Procedures (Committee on Percutaneous Transluminal Coronary Angioplasty) should be considered minimal for the performance of laser angioplasty.[31] Ideally, the operator should have performed at least 250 coronary interventional procedures and should be competent in the treatment of complex coronary disease and the management of the complications of angioplasty. Specific aspects addressed in training courses include patient and case selection, laser physics, laser safety, and system troubleshooting, in addition to the technique of laser angioplasty. Fortunately, the procedure itself is straightforward, and in general, few additional technical skills must be mastered.

## CLINICAL REGISTRY RESULTS

The first successful human excimer laser coronary angioplasty procedure was performed at Cedars-Sinai Medical Center in Los Angeles in 1988. Since then, large clinical experiences involving tens of thousands of patients have accrued. The majority of reports detail the registry experiences with the LAIS Dymer 200+ and the Spectranetics CVX-300 systems. These registry reports reflect the design, performance, and results of the early trials conducted to gain approval for sale of the systems from the U.S. Food and Drug Administration (FDA).

Clinical experience with the first 3000 patients treated with the LAIS Dymer 200+ system was reported by Litvack and colleagues[32] in 1994. In this report, results of patients treated between July 1988 and March 1992 at 33 centers were analyzed. Entry criteria were liberal, symptomatic coronary artery

disease with objective evidence of ischemia being the only specific entry requirement. In the study, 10% of lesions were total occlusions, with the complexity of lesions treated growing toward the end of the study. Clinical success was achieved in 90% of patients; complication rates are listed in Table 33–4. The angiographic restenosis rate (50% rate of angiographic follow-up) was 58%.

Similarly, Bittl and coworkers[33, 34] have reported the results of treatment of the first 2041 patients treated with the Spectranetics CVX-300 system. In this registry of patients, treated between May 1989 and October 1993, results strikingly similar to those obtained with the LAIS were noted. Almost 14% of lesions treated were total occlusions. Clinical success was achieved in 89% of cases. Complication rates, listed in Table 33–4, were similar to those reported for the LAIS system, and angiographic restenosis rates approached 50%.

On the basis of these studies, the FDA granted approval in February 1992 to Advanced Interventional Systems, original developer of this product, for the use of the Dymer 200+ system in the treatment of lesions longer than 20 mm. One year later,

**TABLE 33–4.  MAJOR COMPLICATIONS REPORTED IN THE TWO UNITED STATES EXCIMER LASER ANGIOPLASTY REGISTRIES**

|  | SPECTRANETICS* LASER REGISTRY | LAIS† REGISTRY |
|---|---|---|
| No. of patients | 2041 | 3000 |
| No. of lesions | 2324 | 3592 |
| Age (years; mean ± SD) | 63 ± 11 | 62 ± 11 |
| Male patients (%) | 72 | 75 |
| Clinical complications (% of patients) |  |  |
| Q-wave myocardial infarction | 1.1 | 2.1 |
| Coronary bypass surgery | 3.8 | 3.8 |
| Death | 1.0 | 0.5 |
| Procedural complications (% of lesions) |  |  |
| Major dissection | 16.6 | 13.0 |
| Perforation | 2.1 | 1.0 |

*Data from reference 33.
†Data from reference 32.

in February 1993, the FDA granted a similar approval to Spectranetics for use of the CVX-300 system to treat long lesions (longer than 20 mm), moderately calcified lesions, total occlusions, saphenous vein graft lesions, ostial lesions, and lesions not dilatable with balloon angioplasty. A subsequent merger between the two companies resulted in the corporate entity Spectranetics, which currently markets the excimer laser.

What was learned from the "learning curve" registries of excimer laser angioplasty? It is well recognized that the primary limitation of nonrandomized registry studies is the inability to apply formal statistical methodologies to quantitate differences among treatment approaches. Even with this limitation, however, several important messages emerged from the early work. As the studies progressed, significant differences in patient and lesion characteristics developed, the complexity of lesions increasing with time.[34, 35] Despite these trends, procedural and clinical success rates were at least maintained if not actually improved.

It is now clear, however, that excimer laser angioplasty adds little if anything to the treatment of straightforward, ACC/AHA type A lesions. In other words, the lower success rates of conventional balloon angioplasty associated with greater lesion complexity were not observed in the patients selected for inclusion in the excimer laser registries. These observations have led directly to the current patient and lesion selection algorithms, which reserve the use of the excimer laser to situations in which other, more conventional technologies are less likely to succeed.

A second major issue identified in the registries was the vexing problem of laser-induced dissection. Although numerically, the overall rates of dissection were similar to those reported in contemporary balloon angioplasty registries, laser-related dissections were both unpredictable and, in some cases, qualitatively far worse than expected.[36] This problem became the Achilles' heel of excimer laser angioplasty and led to disaffection for the technique in many interventional cardiologists.

Fortunately, this problem now appears to be largely resolved. Work by van Leeuwen and colleagues[37, 38] clearly documents that excimer laser energy is avidly absorbed by both blood and contrast agent and that the interaction between tissue and excimer laser light in the presence of blood or contrast agent is explosive. This finding led to the development of the saline "flush and bathe" technique for replacing blood and contrast with crystalloid during laser ablation, an approach that has reduced the incidence of dissection and improved clinical outcomes.[28, 29]

## RANDOMIZED TRIALS

Two randomized trials of excimer laser angioplasty have been conducted. The Amsterdam-Rotterdam trial (AMRO) compared excimer laser coronary angioplasty with conventional balloon angioplasty in 308 patients with lesions longer than 10 mm.[39] In the AMRO trial, total occlusion was the target lesion in 33% of patients. Analysis performed by an independent angiographic core laboratory demonstrated that procedural success was achieved in 80% of the excimer laser angioplasty group and in 79% of the balloon angioplasty group. Likewise, rates of adverse clinical events (death, myocardial infarction, bypass surgery, and second angioplasty) were essentially the same up to 6 months after the procedure.

In a second trial, the Excimer Laser, Rotational Atherectomy, and Balloon Angioplasty Comparison (ERBAC) study, 620 patients with ACC/AHA type B or C lesions were randomly assigned to undergo excimer laser angioplasty, rotational atherectomy, or conventional balloon angioplasty.[40] A high proportion (almost 40%) of patients had calcified lesions, but patients with total occlusions, aorto-ostial lesions, and vein graft disease were specifically excluded. Procedural success was achieved in 84% of patients with balloon angioplasty, in 88% with the excimer laser, and in 93% with rotational atherectomy. At 6-month follow-up, the cumulative incidence of adverse clinical events (death, myocardial infarction, bypass surgery, or second intervention) was greatest with rotational atherectomy (53%); incidences of 49% and 45% were observed with excimer laser angioplasty and balloon angioplasty, respectively.

What conclusions can be drawn from these trials? First, results of these studies remain largely consistent with the early registry evaluations. In lesions amenable to balloon angioplasty, no particular advantage (with regard to immediate or long-term outcome) is achieved with adjunctive excimer laser ablation. Second, selection bias in randomized studies reduced the potential for a salutary finding; entry criteria for the AMRO and ERBAC studies specifically excluded lesion morphologies that today represent the bulk of the target lesions to which excimer laser angioplasty is applied. Third, trials conducted early in the development of a device may not provide the best insight into the clinical utility of the device; as a case in point, neither the AMRO trial nor the ERBAC study incorporated saline infusion into the protocol for laser procedures. Indefinite delays in conducting randomized trials are arguably just as bad as premature studies; further trials to clearly delineate the maximal utility of excimer laser angioplasty are indeed currently under way. Notably, the LARS trial of excimer laser ablation compared to balloon angioplasty to treat in-stent restenosis should be completed in 2001.

## ECONOMICS

Compared with other percutaneous revascularization technologies, laser angioplasty is expensive because of capital equipment costs. The initial outlay for an excimer laser generator is approximately $250,000. Annual maintenance costs must also be considered. These high capital costs are unique among interventional devices, because most other devices require only a minimal infrastructure investment. Even the expendable supplies are not inexpensive; the technology and materials required to produce a laser catheter dictate a minimum retail cost approaching $1000 per device. However, most excimer laser procedures are completed with the use of only 1 catheter; thus (particularly in comparison with rotational atherectomy, in which use of multiple burs is the norm), the cost of expendables remains controlled.

To warrant the use of a technique such as excimer laser angioplasty, an additional benefit therefore must accrue to justify the added expense. The primary additional benefit of excimer laser angioplasty appears to be the ability to treat patients who otherwise would be relegated to medical therapy or would require bypass surgery. In the former situation, laser treatment may render a patient asymptomatic who, with only medical management, would have required antianginal medications into perpetuity and who might have continued to have angina even with treatment. For the patient facing coronary bypass surgery, an interventional approach would offer the promise of a shorter hospital stay, more rapid return to productivity, and fewer side effects, all at an initial cost significantly lower than that of a bypass operation.

Excimer laser angioplasty offers an additional benefit to the patient who has undergone bypass surgery and returns with graft disease. With better procedural outcomes and a 30% to 40% incidence of restenosis, excimer laser angioplasty treatment might obviate a second bypass procedure, with its attendant risks and costs. Thus, a calculation of the true cost of excimer laser angioplasty not only must take into account the direct, billable charges but also consider the direct and indirect costs to the patient and the health care system. Only then can one justify the additional expense of the laser; in terms of procedures avoided and lives improved, the benefits of excimer laser angioplasty may indeed be great.

## INTEGRATION: PRACTICAL REALITIES

Recommendations for the practice of excimer laser angioplasty today are derived via a compilation and integration of information gleaned from clinical trials coupled with practical experience, factoring in patient safety and economic constraints. Excimer laser angioplasty is not for everyone; it is best performed by experienced operators with high-volume practices at large centers performing a minimum of 300 to 400 procedures per year. No specific clinical factors mitigate against the use of the excimer laser; in fact, because ischemia time is generally very limited, this intervention is actually one of the better choices for the patient with a low left ventricular ejection fraction.

The primary determinants of suitability for excimer laser angioplasty are anatomic and morphologic. Patients excluded from consideration are those with a large thrombus burden or excessive vessel tortuosity proximal to the target lesion. The two general rules that seem to work the best for choosing ideal candidates are as follows. First, if treatment with a different technology provides ideal results, one should choose the alternative; excimer laser ablation works best in situations in which other technologies would have suboptimal results. Second, the tighter the lesion, the better for laser angioplasty; because the laser ablates only the tissue in direct contact with the end of the fiber, maximal ablation is achieved when the plaque mass fills the vessel lumen.

Examples of the use of excimer laser angioplasty in the treatment of several lesion types are shown in the illustrations. Figure 33–1 shows excimer laser ablation of a chronic total occlusion, and Figure 33–2, treatment of an aorto-ostial lesion in a native right coronary artery. A summary of the lesion types, in relative order of preference, for treatment in a typical excimer laser angioplasty practice, is shown in Table 33–5.

A specific morphology that has emerged as an ideal lesion target is in-stent restenosis; compared

**TABLE 33–5. PRACTICAL APPLICATIONS OF THE EXCIMER LASER**

Coronary artery disease
   In-stent restenosis
   Total occlusions
   Aorto-ostial lesions
   Vein graft disease
   Diffuse, extensive (99%) lesions
   Lesions failing to dilate (after being crossed with a guide wire)
Extraction of pacemaker leads
Peripheral vascular disease
   Superficial femoral artery disease
   Small vessel runoff disease

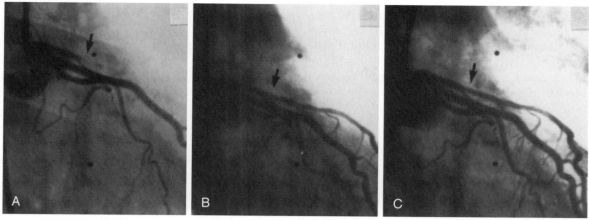

FIGURE 33–1. Treatment of a chronic total occlusion with excimer laser angioplasty. The estimated age of this lesion was 6 months; the patient continued to have Canadian Cardiovascular Society class III angina despite maximal medical therapy. *A,* The lesion *(arrow)* was crossed with a coronary guide wire and treated with a 1.7-mm excimer laser catheter. *B,* A 30% residual stenosis remained *(arrow)* after laser ablation. *C,* Balloon angioplasty reduced the lesion to a 10% final stenosis *(arrow).* The patient was asymptomatic at 1-year follow-up.

with other modalities (directional atherectomy, rotational atherectomy, and balloon angioplasty), the anecdotal experience is that excimer laser angioplasty is more straightforward, takes less time, and reliably produces excellent angiographically confirmed results. Whether these observational results will translate into demonstrable clinical efficacy in randomized comparisons remains to be seen.

## NEW PROGRAMS AND FUTURE DIRECTIONS

Several development programs have led to a resurgence of interest in the excimer laser. At Spectranetics, the five most active development programs for the laser are homogeneous light distribution, the total occlusion guide wire, removal of pacemaker leads, clinical trials of excimer laser ablation of in-stent restenosis, and peripheral vascular applications. The homogeneous light distribution program, under the direction of Patrick Serruys, is an engineering effort directed at improving the uniformity and efficiency of laser ablation while simultaneously lowering the potential for injury to adjacent tissue.[41] It is expected that this research will result in significant technical improvements.

The investigational Prima total occlusion guide wire consists of a hypotube through which 12 45-micron fibers deliver 308-nm laser radiation to the target tissue (see Chapter 25). In clinical trials, this device has succeeded in more than half of totally occluded coronary arteries in which prolonged attempts with conventional guide wires have failed to cross the occlusion.[42] In 1997, as the culmination of a development program led by Dr. Charles Byrd,[43] the FDA granted approval of a sheath for the excimer laser that would enable extraction of pacemaker leads. Intensive investigation of excimer laser ablation of in-stent restenosis already has documented

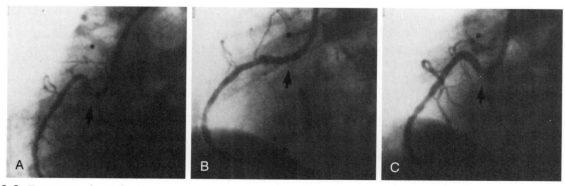

FIGURE 33–2. Treatment of a right coronary ostial stenosis with excimer laser angioplasty. The patient presented with Canadian Cardiovascular Society class II to III angina poorly controlled by medical therapy. *A,* Diagnostic catheterization demonstrated one vessel disease consisting of a 90% stenosis of the right coronary ostium *(arrow).* *B,* A 30% residual stenosis remained *(arrow)* after excimer laser ablation. *C,* Adjunctive balloon angioplasty resulted in a final residual stenosis of 20% *(arrow).* The patient was asymptomatic at 1-year follow-up.

the ability to achieve excellent luminal results; randomized trials are currently under way to assess overall clinical efficacy.[44–50] Finally, peripheral vascular disease, in particular, chronic occlusion of the superficial femoral artery, is being approached with a novel technique developed by Professor Giancarlo Biamino in Germany.

## CONCLUSION

Today, the practice of laser angioplasty is directed at the debulking of plaque mass in preparation for further definitive treatment. As such, it is relegated to a fairly small niche in the compendium of interventional practice. What will lead to more widespread (and appropriate) use of this technique? The potential for catheter improvement and refinement remains great; compared with other interventional technologies introduced in the latter half of the 1980s and the early 1990s, laser angioplasty emerged as the least mature and even now is at a relatively early stage in evolutionary development. Fortunately, the laser generators incorporate relatively mature engineering technology, so that only minor changes should be necessary to adapt the systems to accommodate changes in catheter design and construction. Another long-sought goal is feedback control to prevent perforation. As the technology evolves, appropriate randomized clinical trials will be needed to quantitatively ascertain clinical value. Only when the excimer laser technology truly matures will the full potential of direct ablative treatment in cardiovascular disease be realized.

## REFERENCES

1. Einstein A: Quantentheorie der Strahlung. Physiol Z 18:121, 1917.
2. Maiman TH: Stimulated optical radiation in ruby. Nature 187:493, 1960.
3. Abela GS, Normann SJ, Cohen DM, et al: Effects of carbon dioxide, Nd-YAG, and argon laser radiation on coronary atheromatous plaques. Am J Cardiol 50:1199, 1982.
4. Deckelbaum LI, Isner JM, Donaldson RF, et al: Reduction of laser-induced pathologic tissue injury using pulsed energy delivery. Am J Cardiol 56:662, 1985.
5. Grundfest WS, Litvack F, Forrester JS, et al: Laser ablation of human atherosclerotic plaque without adjacent tissue injury. J Am Coll Cardiol 5:929, 1985.
6. van Leeuwen TG, Borst C: Fundamental laser-tissue interactions. Semin Intervent Cardiol 1:121, 1996.
7. Livesay JJ, Hogan PJ, McAllister HA: The development of laser angioplasty. Herz 10:343, 1985.
8. Grundfest WS, Segalowitz J, Laudenslager J: The physical and biological basis for laser angioplasty. In Litvack F (ed): Coronary Laser Angioplasty, p 1 (Series in Interventional Cardiology). Boston: Blackwell Scientific, 1992.
9. Srinvasan R: Ablation of polymers and biological tissues by ultraviolet laser. Science 234:559, 1986.
10. Waller BF: "Crackers, breakers, stretchers, drillers, scrapers, shavers, burners, welders and melters"—the future treatment of atherosclerotic coronary artery disease? A clinical-morphologic assessment. J Am Coll Cardiol 13:969, 1989.
11. McGuff PE, Bushness D, Saroff HS, et al: Studies of the surgical applications of laser (light amplification by stimulated emission of radiation). Surg Forum 14:143, 1963.
12. Macruz R, Martins JRM, Tupinamba A, et al: Therapeutic possibilities of laser beams in atheromas. Arq Bras Cradiol 34:9, 1980.
13. Choy DSJ, Stertzer SH, Rotterdam HZ, et al: Laser coronary angioplasty: Experience with 9 cadaver hearts. Am J Cardiol 50:1209, 1982.
14. Lee G, Ikeda R, Herman I, et al: The qualitative effects of laser irradiation on human arteriosclerotic disease. Am Heart J 105:885, 1983.
15. Abela GS, Normann SJ, Cohen DM, et al: Laser recanalization of occluded atherosclerotic arteries in vivo and in vitro. Circulation 71:403, 1985.
16. Livesay JJ, Johansen WE, Sutter LV, et al: Can laser endarterectomy extend the limits of coronary revascularization? Lasers Surg Med 3:173, 1983.
17. Sanborn TA, Faxon DP, Kellett MA, et al: Percutaneous coronary laser thermal angioplasty. J Am Coll Cardiol 8:1437, 1986.
18. Linnemeier TJ, Cumberland DC: Percutaneous laser coronary angioplasty without balloon angioplasty. Lancet 1:154, 1989.
19. Leon MB, Lu DY, Prevosti LG, et al: Human arterial surface fluorescence: Atherosclerotic plaque identification and effects of laser atheroma ablation. J Am Coll Cardiol 12:94, 1988.
20. Spears JR, Reyes VP, Wynne J, et al: Percutaneous coronary laser balloon angioplasty: Initial results of a multicenter experience. J Am Coll Cardiol 16:293, 1990.
21. Geschwind H, Fabre M, Chaitman BR, et al: Histopathology after Nd:YAG laser percutaneous transluminal coronary angioplasty of peripheral arteries. J Am Coll Cardiol 8:1089, 1986.
22. Forrester JS, Litvack F, Grundfest W: Vaporization of atheroma in man: The role of lasers in the era of balloon angioplasty. Int J Cardiol 20:1, 1988.
23. Knopf W, Parr K, Moses J, et al: Holmium laser angioplasty in coronary arteries. J Am Coll Cardiol 19:352A, 1992.
24. Sanborn TA: Laser angioplasty: Historical perspective. Semin Intervent Cardiol 1:117, 1996.
25. Isner JM, Donaldson RF, Deckelbaum LI: The excimer laser: Gross, light microscopic and ultrastructural analysis of potential advantages for use in laser therapy of cardiovascular disease. J Am Coll Cardiol 6:1102, 1985.
26. Wolbarsht ML: Laser surgery: $CO_2$ or HF. IEEE J Quantum Electron QE 20:1427, 1984.
27. Grundfest WS, Litvack F, Goldenberg T, et al: Pulsed ultraviolet lasers and the potential for safe laser angioplasty. Am J Surg 150:220, 1985.
28. Tcheng JE, Wells LD, Phillips HR, et al: Development and evaluation of a new technique for reducing pressure pulse generation during 308-nm excimer laser coronary angioplasty. Cathet Cardiovasc Diagn 34:15, 1995.
29. Deckelbaum LI, Natarajan MK, Bittl JA, et al, for the Percutaneous Excimer Laser Coronary Angioplasty (PELCA) Investigators: Effect of intracoronary saline infusion on dissection during excimer laser coronary angioplasty: A randomized trial. J Am Coll Cardiol 26:1264, 1995.
30. Pizzulli L, Jung W, Pfeiffer D, et al: Angiographic results and elastic recoil following coronary excimer laser angioplasty with saline perfusion. J Intervent Cardiol 9:9, 1996.
31. Ryan TJ, Bauman WB, Kennedy JW, et al: Guidelines for percutaneous transluminal coronary angioplasty: A report of the American Heart Association/American College of Cardiology Task Force on Assessment of Diagnostic and Therapeutic Cardiovascular Procedures (Committee on Percutaneous Transluminal Coronary Angioplasty). Circulation 88:2987, 1993.
32. Litvack F, Eigler N, Margolis J, et al: Percutaneous excimer laser coronary angioplasty: Results in the first consecutive 3,000 patients. The ELCA Investigators. J Am Coll Cardiol 23:323, 1994.
33. Bittl JA, Sanborn TA, Tcheng JE, et al: Clinical success, complications and restenosis rates with excimer laser coro-

nary angioplasty. The Percutaneous Excimer Laser Coronary Angioplasty Registry. Am J Cardiol 70:1533, 1992.

34. Bittl JA, Brinker JA, Sanborn TA, et al, on behalf of the participating investigators of the Percutaneous Excimer Laser Angioplasty Registry: The changing profile of patient selection, procedural techniques, and outcomes in excimer laser coronary angioplasty. J Interv Cardiol 8:653, 1995.

35. Cook SL, Eigler NL, Shefer A, et al: Percutaneous excimer laser coronary angioplasty of lesions not ideal for balloon angioplasty. Circulation 84:632, 1991.

36. Isner JM, Pickering JG, Mosseri M: Laser-induced dissections: Pathogenesis and implications for therapy. J Am Coll Cardiol 19:1619, 1992.

37. van Leeuwen TG, van Erven L, Meertens JH, et al: Origin of arterial wall dissections induced by pulsed excimer and mid-infrared laser ablation in the pig. J Am Coll Cardiol 19:1610, 1992.

38. van Leeuwen TG, Meertens JH, Velema E, et al: Intraluminal vapor bubble induced by excimer laser causes microsecond arterial dilatation and invagination leading to extensive wall damage in the rabbit. Circulation 87:1258, 1993.

39. Appelman YEA, Piek JJ, Strikwerda S, et al: Randomised trial of excimer laser versus balloon angioplasty for treatment of obstructive coronary artery disease. Lancet 347:79, 1996.

40. Reifart N, Vandormael M, Krajcar M, et al: Randomized comparison of angioplasty of complex coronary lesions as a single center. Excimer Laser, Rotational Atherectomy, and Balloon Angioplasty Comparison (ERBAC) study. Circulation 96:91, 1997.

41. Gijsbers GHM, Hamburger JN, Serruys PW: Homogenous light distribution to reduce vessel trauma during excimer laser angioplasty. Semin Intervent Cardiol 1:143, 1996.

42. Hamburger JN, Gijsbers GHM, Ozaki Y, et al: Recanalization of chronic total coronary occlusions using a laser guide wire: A pilot study. J Am Coll Cardiol 30:649, 1997.

43. Byrd CL: Extracting chronically implanted pacemaker leads using the Spectranetics excimer laser: Initial clinical experience. Pac Clin Electrophys 19:567, 1996.

44. Mehran R, Mintz GS, Popma JJ, et al: Excimer laser angioplasty in the treatment of in-stent restenosis: An intravascular ultrasound study [Abstract]. J Am Coll Cardiol 27:362A, 1996.

45. Giri S, Ito S, Lansky AJ, et al: Clinical and angiographic outcome in the Laser Angioplasty for Restenotic Stents (LARS) multicenter registry. Catheter Cardiovasc Interv 52:24–34, 2001.

46. Hamburger JN, Foley DP, de Feyter PJ, et al: Six-month outcome after excimer laser coronary angioplasty for diffuse in-stent restenosis in native coronary arteries. Am J Cardiol 86:390–394, 2000.

47. Koster R, Kahler J, Terres W, et al: Six-month clinical and angiographic outcome after successful excimer laser angioplasty for in-stent restenosis. J Am Coll Cardiol 36:69–74, 2000.

48. Mehran R, Dangas G, Mintz GS, et al: Treatment of in-stent restenosis with excimer laser coronary angioplasty versus rotational atherectomy: Comparative mechanisms and results. Circulation 101:2484–2489, 2000.

49. Koster R, Hamm CW, Seabra-Gomes R, et al: Laser angioplasty of restenosed coronary stents: Results of a multicenter surveillance trial. The Laser Angioplasty of Restenosed Stents (LARS) investigators. J Am Coll Cardiol 34:25–32, 1999.

50. Koster R, Hamm CW, Terres W, et al: Treatment of in-stent coronary restenosis by excimer laser angioplasty. Am J Cardiol 80:1424–1428, 1997.

# 34

# Perfusion Balloon Catheter

*Wayne B. Batchelor*     *Joseph B. Muhlestein*     *Michael H. Sketch, Jr.*

The therapeutic approach to coronary artery disease was revolutionized by the introduction of percutaneous transluminal coronary angioplasty (PTCA) by Gruentzig and coworkers in 1979.[1] More than 400,000 PTCA procedures are performed annually in the United States, and percutaneous interventions have replaced coronary artery bypass graft (CABG) surgery as the most common method of coronary revascularization. Since 1980, increasing operator experience, advances in angioplasty technique and catheter design, intracoronary stent implantation, and adjunctive antiplatelet therapy have allowed percutaneous revascularization to achieve its current high degree of success and safety. The development of perfusion balloon angioplasty technique constitutes one of several important developments contributing to this evolution.

The major mechanism by which balloon angioplasty appears to increase intravascular lumen diameter involves atherosclerotic plaque breaking, cracking, fracturing, or splitting.[2] Although successful angioplasty may necessitate this disruptive process, the biologic response (thrombosis, dissection, or both) to this injury may lead to acute occlusion in 2% to 12% of patients.[3] This and other sequelae of PTCA-related vessel injury, including elastic recoil, neointimal hyperplasia, and extracellular matrix elaboration, contribute to the 30% to 45% incidence of restenosis observed after balloon PTCA.[4, 5] Furthermore, the maximal duration of balloon inflation during conventional PTCA is usually short (30 to 120 seconds), limited by patient intolerance to chest pain and hemodynamic or electrical instability. These shortcomings of conventional PTCA have served as the impetus behind the development of new interventional techniques such as perfusion balloon angioplasty.

Numerous pharmacologic and mechanical techniques have been aimed at facilitating longer balloon catheter inflation durations. These techniques have included pretreatment with β blockers, calcium channel blockers, or nitrates; attempts at alternative perfusion using fluorocarbons; retrograde perfusion via the coronary sinus; and perfusion pump systems.[6] The majority of these techniques have resulted in only modest increases in balloon inflation duration and have occasionally been associated with significant ventricular arrhythmias. A subsequent solution was the development of a perfusion balloon catheter (PBC), which would allow continuous myocardial perfusion through a central lumen in the inflated balloon, thus maintaining distal coronary blood flow and allowing more gradual and prolonged balloon catheter inflation. Prolonged and gradual expansion of the balloon is believed to result in less trauma to the vessel wall, thus lessening the risk of a large dissection and acute occlusion. In addition, it has been postulated that prolonged balloon dilatation, through plaque desiccation and compression of the vasa vasorum, may lead to a reduction in nutrient flow to the media, thereby potentially mitigating the proliferation of smooth muscle cells that leads to restenosis.

Since the development of PBCs, studies both in animals and in humans have demonstrated beneficial effects of prolonged perfusion balloon dilatations with regard to elastic recoil, intimal dissection, and acute ischemic complications.[7–9] Although results of initial investigation suggested a beneficial effect on restenosis,[10] subsequent randomized and nonrandomized studies failed to confirm this.[11] With the rapid evolution of interventional techniques that improve acute and long-term PTCA results, such as intracoronary stent implantation[12, 13] and adjunctive glycoprotein (GP) IIb/IIIa antiplatelet therapy,[14] the role of the PBC is currently being redefined.

## DEVELOPMENTAL STUDIES

The desire to approach PTCA with more prolonged dilatations has existed since the early developmental stages of the procedure. Realizing the risk of prolonged coronary ischemia, Andreas Gruentzig made the first attempt at preservation of autologous blood flow during angioplasty.[1] He designed an active perfusion system in which femoral arterial blood was infused (60 to 100 mL/minute) through a dilating catheter into the coronary artery during 3-

minute periods of coronary angioplasty, resulting in a reduction in the frequency and amount of ST segment elevation. Another antegrade active external infusion pump system was described by Lehmann and coworkers[15]; however, there was concern about the possible induction of erythrocyte hemolysis at higher flow rates. Other systems have used oxygen-containing perfluorocarbons,[16] artificial hemoglobin,[17] or coronary sinus retroperfusion[18] as methods of myocardial perfusion. In view of the complexity, cost, and limited myocardial protection afforded by these active perfusion techniques, a simpler method of providing adequate blood flow to the distal coronary artery bed was desirable.

In 1984, the Interventional Cardiovascular Program at Duke University Medical Center, in conjunction with John Simpson and Advanced Cardiovascular Systems, Inc. (Santa Clara CA), developed a simple coronary reperfusion catheter that could be placed across an area of occlusion, after failed PTCA, to maintain myocardial perfusion while patients were transferred to the operating room.[19, 20] The distal 10 cm of the device contained 30 holes that allowed blood to enter proximal and exit distal to the occlusion by passive perfusion. This and other similar devices[21] simplified the process of providing distal hemoperfusion by eliminating the need for external pump systems. This concept of passive reperfusion led to the development of passive autoperfusion balloon angioplasty systems designed to reduce myocardial ischemia during prolonged balloon inflation by maintaining myocardial perfusion through side holes in the catheter shaft, proximal and distal to the balloon. Initially, autoperfusion catheter systems were independently developed by United States Catheter, Inc. (USCI) (USCI-Bard, Inc.; Billerica MA), Schneider, Inc. (Minneapolis MN) and Advanced Cardiovascular Systems, Inc. (ACS; Santa Clara CA), and were used to document the safety and efficacy of prolonged balloon inflation in

animal models and patients.[22, 23] Flow rates through these catheters, determined by means of a standardized in vitro system (generally 38% glycerol, perfusion pressure of 80 mm Hg, inflation pressure of 60 psi), ranged from 40 to 60 mL/minute. It has subsequently been demonstrated that flow rates are very sensitive to perfusion pressure and hematocrit, which highlights the potential unpredictability of true flow rates in the in vivo setting[24] (Fig. 34–1).

Studies in animals and humans have been designed to determine the capability of the autoperfusion catheter to provide antegrade perfusion adequate for preventing myocardial ischemia during coronary balloon angioplasty. Various methods to assess myocardial ischemia included quantification of symptoms and electrocardiographic, hemodynamic, and left ventricular wall motion parameters. Also, experiments were designed to address concerns regarding side branch occlusion and potential hemolysis as a result of the mechanical trauma to erythrocytes passing through the catheter. The insight gained from this work proved unequivocally the efficacy and safety of PBCs, by which an important role for such catheters in a variety of clinical situations was rapidly established.

Initial animal studies were designed to demonstrate the effectiveness of autoperfusion, in comparison with standard angioplasty, in attenuating myocardial ischemia during prolonged coronary inflation. In canine studies performed by Turi and coworkers,[25, 26] a standard balloon inflation for 3 minutes in the left anterior descending, left circumflex, or left main coronary artery resulted in marked ischemia, as indicated by ST segment elevation, and in marked reduction in regional myocardial blood flow, as demonstrated by radioactive microsphere techniques. In contrast, balloon inflation with the perfusion catheter for 3 minutes resulted in no ST segment changes and in preservation of near-baseline regional myocardial blood flow in every in-

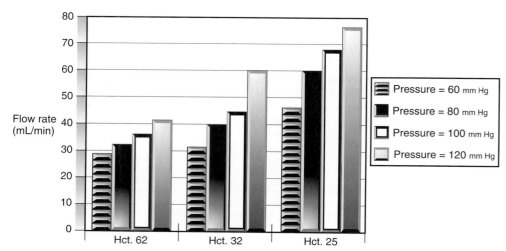

FIGURE 34–1. The blood flow rates obtained in vitro through a perfusion balloon catheter (Rx-60, ACS) under varying continuous pressures (40 to 120 mm Hg) and varying hematocrit levels (25% to 62%) at 37°C. Blood flow rates can be seen to vary drastically with both pressure and hematocrit. (Adapted from de Muinck ED, Angelini P, Dougherty K, et al: In vitro evaluation of blood flow through autoperfusion catheters. Catheter Cardiovasc Diagn 30:58–62, 1993.)

stance. In a similar study performed by Collins and coworkers, canines were found to tolerate autoperfusion balloon inflations up to a mean of 37 minutes without any evidence of ST-segment elevation, ventricular arrhythmias, or left ventricular wall motion abnormalities.[27, 28] White and associates also found the same protective effect during 30 minutes of autoperfusion angioplasty in a miniature swine model.[29] To determine the safe upper limit to the duration of autoperfusion angioplasty, canine studies with the use of radiolabeled microspheres revealed a myocardial protective effect persisting for up to 90 minutes of inflation in the left anterior descending and circumflex coronary arteries.[30, 31] However, when autoperfusion balloon inflation times were extended significantly longer, up to 6 hours, some degree of inadequate coronary perfusion was detected, as evidenced by the presence of necrosis of 25% of the area of myocardium at risk. This nonetheless compared favorably with results of standard balloon inflations, in which myocardial necrosis of 84% of the area at risk was noted.[32]

After establishing the safety of prolonged balloon inflations in animals, studies in humans were begun to confirm these findings.[33] Quigley and coworkers[34] compared autoperfusion angioplasty with standard angioplasty in 11 patients undergoing routine PTCA. In order to exclude the role of "fading ischemia" in which subsequent occlusions are better tolerated, possibly because of the recruitment of collateral vessels, each lesion was dilated three times: the first and third times with standard catheters and the second time with autoperfusion. Standard balloon inflations were continued until the development of severe chest pain (7 on a scale of 0 to 10), ST segment elevation of more than 4 mm, widened QRS interval, arrhythmias, or hypotension. During dilatation with the PBC, inflation was maintained either until the development of any of the indications of ischemia just mentioned or for a period of at least 10 minutes. Inflation duration during autoperfusion angioplasty (513 seconds) was significantly longer ($p < 0.001$) than for the first (107 seconds) and third (139 seconds) standard dilatations. In addition, there were significant reductions, although not complete elimination, in the degree of ST segment changes and chest pain scores during autoperfusion angioplasty in comparison to standard angioplasty (Table 34–1). This demonstrated that in humans, the PBC significantly reduces ischemic signs and symptoms during coronary angioplasty, thus allowing for prolonged periods of balloon inflation.

Autoperfusion angioplasty has also been shown to have a protective effect on left ventricular function. In a report by Simonton and associates,[35] echocardiographic assessment of regional myocardial function was performed during standard balloon coronary angioplasty followed by autoperfusion balloon angioplasty of stenosis of the proximal left anterior descending artery. Although septal and apical akinesis occurred within 60 seconds of standard balloon inflation, regional function remained well preserved for 15 minutes with autoperfusion angioplasty. Muhlestein and coworkers[36] assessed quantitative left ventriculography, including left ventricular ejection fraction and regional wall motion analysis, before and immediately after balloon inflation in a subgroup of 15 patients from a series of 50 consecutive patients undergoing 15-minute prolonged autoperfusion angioplasty. No statistically significant change in overall left ventricular function was noted, which indicates that perfusion balloon angioplasty provided adequate perfusion to prevent ischemic systolic ventricular dysfunction.

The procedural safety of prolonged autoperfusion coronary angioplasty was examined in a study involving 62 consecutive patients undergoing elective PTCA with autoperfusion balloon dilatation for an average of 14 minutes.[37] Mean chest pain score (range, 0 to 10) was 4. Electrocardiographic or biochemical evidence of myocardial infarction was not observed in any patient despite the presence of nonmajor (<2.5 mm diameter) side branches close enough to the target lesion to be transiently occluded by the inflated balloon in 60% of patients.

**TABLE 34–1. COMPARISON OF ELECTROCARDIOGRAPHIC AND CLINICAL DATA DURING STANDARD AND AUTOPERFUSION ANGIOPLASTY**

| PROCEDURE | ST ELEVATION (mm) | ST DEPRESSION (mm) | CHEST PAIN SCORE (0–10) | HEART RATE (BEATS/MINUTE) | MEAN AORTIC PRESSURE (mm Hg) |
|---|---|---|---|---|---|
| SR1 | 2.4 ± 1.7* | 2.2 ± 1.3* | 6.1 ± 2.1* | 70 ± 17 | 90 ± 10 |
| PBC | 0.3 ± 0.5† | 0.6 ± 0.8† | 3.2 ± 3.5† | 71 ± 14 | 91 ± 18 |
| SR2 | 1.9 ± 1.3 | 1.6 ± 1.3 | 5.2 ± 3.1 | 76 ± 13 (NS) | 95 ± 14 (NS) |

Values are expressed as mean ± standard deviation.
SR1, standard dilatation before PBC; PBC, perfusion balloon catheter (autoperfusion angioplasty); SR2, standard dilatation after PBC.
*$p < 0.05$ (PBC vs. SR1); †$p < 0.05$ (PBC vs. SR2); NS, not significant (SR1 vs. PBC or SR2).
Adapted from Quigley PH, Hinohara T, Phillips HR, et al: Myocardial protection during coronary angioplasty with an autoperfusion balloon catheter in humans. Circulation 78:1128–1134, 1988.

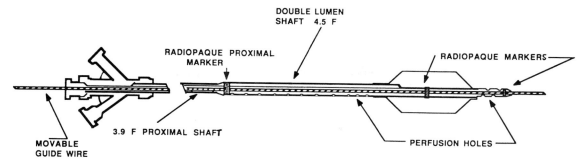

FIGURE 34–2. Design of the Stack Perfusion Balloon Catheter. (From Muhlestein JB, Quigley PJ, Ohman EM, et al: A prospective analysis of possible myocardial damage or hemolysis occurring as a result of prolonged autoperfusion angioplasty in humans. J Am Coll Cardiol 20:594–598, 1992.)

The presence of side branches did not result in creatine phosphokinase elevation; however, it did correlate with the degree of chest pain experienced by the patients. All patients with involvement of large side branches had a chest pain score of 6 or higher, as did 36% of patients with medium-sized or small side branches. Only 20% of patients with no side branches experienced chest pain. Although concern had been raised about the possibility of clinically detectable hemolysis occurring as a result of the passage of blood through the central lumen of the autoperfusion catheter, no hemolysis was evident on the basis of levels of serum and plasma markers of hemolysis. After these early studies documenting the safety of prolonged dilatation with the autoperfusion catheter, the first device to be approved for general use by the U.S. Food and Drug Administration was the ACS Stack Perfusion Catheter. Soon thereafter, the use of autoperfusion catheters in the clinical practice of interventional cardiology became widespread, and a variety of other designs have become available.

## CATHETER DESIGN AND PROCEDURE TECHNIQUE

### Catheter Design

The basic design feature of the autoperfusion catheter is the presence of proximal and distal side holes through which blood enters and exits a noncollapsing central lumen (Fig. 34–2). The amount of blood flow distal to the catheter depends on the diameter and length of the central lumen, the mean arterial pressure, and blood viscosity. In view of these constraints, the challenge of designing autoperfusion balloon catheters has been to make a catheter with an adequately low profile to be used in the majority of lesions in the coronary tree, while maintaining adequate flow to minimize myocardial ischemia.

The original ACS Stack Perfusion Catheter consisted of a 4.5-French polyethylene, double-lumen, PTCA catheter with 10 side holes in the shaft proximal to the 1.8-cm balloon and 4 side holes distally (see Fig. 34–2). This catheter had an in vitro flow rate of 60 mL/min during autoperfusion with 38% glycerol at a mean pressure of 80 mm Hg. Newer generation ACS catheters have since been designed with similar flow rates ranging from 40 to 60 mL/minute, but with shorter tips, lower and more flexible profiles, and the ability to inflate to higher pressures (up to 14 atm) without compromising flow rates. These catheters are designed to be used with standard 0.014-inch angioplasty guide wires, although the ACS Rx Perfusion and ACS Rx Flowtrack may be used with a 0.018-inch guide wire. Currently available sizes range from 2.0 to 4.0 mm in diameter and 10 to 40 mm in length. The ACS OTW Lifestream has replaced the Stack perfusion balloons as this company's standard over the wire perfusion balloon. In addition, ACS perfusion balloons with short guide wire lumens and a monorail design (Rx) have been introduced (ACS Rx Lifestream, ACS Rx Flowtrack, ACS Rx Perfusion). Such monorail systems allow for more rapid replacement of the catheter and simplified single-operator usage.

Two new over-the-wire perfusion catheters, the WAVE and the SURPASS, have been designed recently by SCIMED Life Systems (SCIMED; Maple Grove MN). These perfusion catheters have a patented Superfusion design that allows for the guide wire position to be maintained in situ without wire pullback while not compromising coronary perfusion (Fig. 34–3). Both SCIMED perfusion catheters afford respectable flow rates with the wire in situ (~45 mL/minute); however, the SURPASS has a

FIGURE 34–3. Diagram of Superfusion balloon catheters.

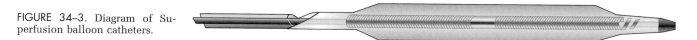

higher rated burst pressure (12 vs. 8 atm) and smaller distal tip (lesion entry profile), modifications that are thought to improve catheter performance. Comparisons of the specifications of currently U.S. Food and Drug Administration–approved PBCs are shown in Table 34–2. The design modifications in the new ACS and SCIMED prototypes have enhanced catheter performance, particularly in more distal lesions and tortuous vessels, making possible the use of a PBC as the primary dilatation catheter in a majority of lesions as well as for high-pressure stent deployment.

## Technique for Autoperfusion Angioplasty

At our institution, patients are pretreated with aspirin, 325 mg, and, if coronary stent implantation is anticipated, clopidogrel, 300-mg loading dose, followed by 75 mg orally every day, ideally 24 hours before PTCA. Concomitant medical therapy with a GPIIb/IIIa platelet receptor inhibitor, β blockers, calcium channel blockers, and nitrates is administered at the discretion of the individual physician. Angioplasty is performed generally via the femoral approach with 8-French or large-lumen 7-French guide catheters. Heparin is administered at the beginning of each procedure after vascular access is established, and additional heparin is administered as necessary during the procedure to maintain an activated clotting time (ACT) of more than 300 seconds. Lower heparin dosing (50-mg/kg bolus and additional heparin to keep ACT at >200) is recommended if adjunctive GPIIb/IIIa receptor inhibitor is administered. Intracoronary nitroglycerin (0.1 to 0.3 μg) may be given before cinearteriography, which is performed in two orthogonal views.

An autoperfusion balloon catheter suitably sized to produce an approximate balloon-to-artery ratio of 1.1:1 is then prepared with standard aspiration techniques and advanced across the lesion over a 0.014- or 0.018-inch guide wire. If a coaxial version of the catheter is used, it is advisable to use a wire of exchangeable length that allows retraction of the balloon catheter out of the guide catheter far enough to provide easy opacification of the vessel after the dilatation. If the target lesion is considered too severely narrowed to allow easy primary passage of the autoperfusion catheter, an initial dilatation may be performed with a standard 2.0-mm angioplasty catheter for a period of 60 seconds. However, this is very rarely required if the newer high-performance catheter, low profile designs are used.

The usual protocol for autoperfusion dilatation consists of gradual balloon expansion at a rate of 1 atm every 30 seconds to a nominal pressure of 6 atm,[7, 8] with a target inflation period of 10 to 20 minutes. If necessary to obtain adequate expansion, the balloon inflation pressure may be increased to 8 to 14 atm. Newer designs such as the ACS Lifestream and SCIMED SURPASS catheters have allowed for balloon inflation to high pressures (up to 14 atm) without compromising flow rates. With ACS perfusion balloons, once the balloon is inflated, the guide wire is pulled back proximal to the side holes, and the distal perfusion is documented by a small injection of contrast material with the balloon inflated. If an Rx design is used, extreme care must be made not to pull the wire back so far that it exits the catheter. The guide catheter is then withdrawn slightly from the coronary ostium (0.5 to 1.0 cm) to facilitate entry of blood into the proximal side holes. In some instances, because of distal disease or tortuosity of the vessel, it may be desirable to leave the guide wire across the lesion during the entire prolonged inflation. In these cases, if a 0.014-inch guide wire is used in a version of the autoperfusion catheter that will accept a 0.018-inch guide wire, adequate distal perfusion can often be obtained with the guide wire left in place.

In the use of ACS perfusion balloons, to prevent possible formation of fibrin or thrombus on the distal perfusion tip of the catheter during prolonged inflations, a heparin solution (500 U/mL of normal

## TABLE 34–2. PERFUSION BALLOON SPECIFICATIONS

| PERFUSION BALLOON CATHETER | BALLOON LENGTHS (mm) | CROSSING PROFILE (INCHES)* | RATED BURST PRESSURE (atm)† | FLOW RATE (mL/MINUTE)‡ |
|---|---|---|---|---|
| ACS OTW Lifestream | 20, 30 | 0.041 | 12 | 40 |
| ACS Rx Lifestream | 10, 20, 30 | 0.041 | 12 | 40 |
| ACS Rx Flowtrack | 20 | 0.048 | 8 | 40 |
| ACS Rx Flowtrack Long | 30, 40 | 0.050 | 8 | 40 |
| ACS Rx Perfusion | 20, 30 | 0.053 | 8 | 60 |
| SCIMED WAVE | 20 | 0.055 | 8 | 44 |
| SCIMED SURPASS | 20 | 0.048 | 12 | 45 |

*For 2.0 × 20 mm balloon size.
†For a 2.5-mm balloon.
‡Flow rates for ACS catheters are with wire pulled back. Flow rate for SURPASS is with wire in situ.

saline) can be administered through the central lumen of the balloon catheter in 2-mL (1000-U) boluses every 3 minutes. If an Rx design of the catheter is used, the heparin is administered through the engaged guide catheter. In cases of very prolonged (>30 minutes) or repeated inflations, the total dose of heparin administered to the patient may lead to an elevation of the ACT above 400 seconds. If this is the case, it is recommended that the dose of heparin administration be reduced to 500 U and that the interval between administrations be prolonged to 5 to 8 minutes.

Inflation is terminated, either at the end of the target period or when intolerable symptoms of angina or electrocardiographic or hemodynamic signs of severe ischemia develop. After dilatation is completed, the guide catheter is reseated, and the guide wire is reinserted across the lesion. During reinsertion of the guide wire, care must be taken not to pass the wire out the side holes. Once deflated, the balloon is withdrawn into the guide, and arteriography is repeated. If the initial inflation is not successful (stenosis persists; thrombosis, filling defect, large dissection, or other complications develop), the balloon is repassed across the lesion, and further dilatations, at higher inflation pressures or for longer durations, are performed. In instances of adequate reduction of lesion stenosis but a persistent obstructive dissection, a prolonged low-pressure (3- to 4-atm) inflation with a half-size larger autoperfusion balloon is often successful in creating a persistent adequate vessel lumen. If successful PTCA cannot be performed because of persistent occlusive dissection and emergency CABG is contemplated, the deflated autoperfusion catheter may be left in place across the lesion to provide adequate distal perfusion until preparations for surgery are made.

## POTENTIAL APPLICATIONS

There are five potential applications for the use of the perfusion balloon catheter in coronary arteries: routine balloon PTCA, intracoronary stent implantation, high-risk PTCA, salvaging of failed PTCA, and maintaining perfusion before emergency bypass surgery (Table 34–3).

### Routine PTCA

To assess the efficacy of the PBC as a primary device for PTCA, the acute and long-term outcomes of 140 consecutive patients undergoing elective coronary angioplasty was evaluated by Tenaglia and colleagues.[38] Perfusion balloon angioplasty was successful (stenosis affecting ≤50% of the luminal diameter) in 138 patients (98.6%). This compares favorably with lesion success rates of 88% to 96%

**TABLE 34–3. POTENTIAL APPLICATIONS FOR THE PERFUSION BALLOON CATHETER**

Primary angioplasty strategy in complex lesions (i.e., irregular, ulcerated, or eccentric, or thrombus)
Intracoronary stent implantation
Treatment of target lesion in vessels supplying greater than 50% of the myocardium
Treatment for LVEF less than 30%
Salvaging failed PTCA
Maintaining perfusion before emergency bypass surgery

reported in larger series of standard angioplasty.[39–41] Abrupt closure occurred in 3% of lesions in this study, in comparison with a 2% to 12% rate reported with standard angioplasty.[3] The angiographic restenosis rate in this series of patients with an 87% angiographic follow-up rate was 42%. This rate is comparable with a restenosis rate of 43% in a consecutive series of 2191 patients with an 84% angiographic follow-up rate.[5] Although these results reflected favorably on the use of the PBC as a first-choice catheter for routine PTCA, the major limitation of this study was the absence of a direct comparison with standard balloon angioplasty.

### The Randomized PBC Trial

To further evaluate the advantages of prolonged inflations over standard inflation duration, a randomized multicenter clinical trial was initiated to test the hypothesis that a strategy of a primary gradual, prolonged 15-minute balloon inflation, in comparison with repeated short 1-minute inflations with the PBC, would result in a higher primary procedural success rate, lower rates of in-hospital complications, and a lower restenosis rate.[11] The clinical inclusion criteria included undergoing elective angioplasty for either stable or unstable angina. Patients who had had an acute myocardial infarction within 24 hours before angioplasty or who were unable to return for 6-month follow-up angiography were excluded. The angiographic exclusion criteria were those that predominantly would limit prolonged inflation durations with the perfusion balloon catheter, including major side branch (≥2 mm) at lesion site, target vessel less than 2 mm in diameter, stenosis affecting 50% of the luminal diameter proximal to the target lesion, tandem lesions, ostial lesions, severely angulated lesions, and lesions in bypass grafts.

The design of this study (Fig. 34–4) involved patients' being randomly assigned to undergo two different primary inflation strategies (standard vs. prolonged). The standard inflation strategy consisted of a dilatation up to 6 atm over 20 seconds for a total inflation duration of 60 seconds. This dilatation

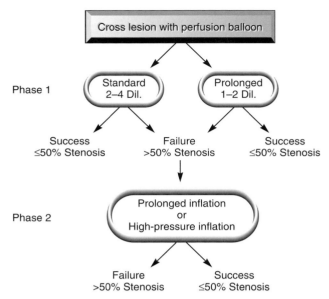

FIGURE 34–4. Design of the randomized Perfusion Balloon Catheter Trial outlining the two phases. The randomization strategy applied to dilatations (Dil.) only during phase I of the procedure. After phase I, further dilatations in phase II were performed at the discretion of the angioplasty operator. (From Ohman EM, Marquis JF, Ricci DR, et al: A randomized comparison of the effects of gradual prolonged versus standard primary balloon inflation on early and late outcome. Results of a multicenter clinical trial. Perfusion Balloon Catheter Study Group. Circulation 89:1119, 1994.)

could be repeated up to a total of four times in phase I of the study. The prolonged inflation strategy consisted of a gradual increase in balloon pressure of 1 atm every 30 seconds to a maximum of 6 atm. The inflation duration in this strategy was 15 minutes, and two dilatations were allowed in phase I. If the lesion was not successfully dilated to the point at which stenosis affected 50% or less of the luminal diameter after completion of phase I in this inflation strategy, the strategy was deemed unsuccessful, and the patient went into phase II, in which further dilatations were performed. In phase II, the physician was at liberty to treat the residual stenosis with up to a 30-minute inflation or with higher inflation pressures.

A total of 547 patients were enrolled in this study at 11 clinical sites in both the United States and Canada. Of these patients, 69 required predilatation with a 2.0-mm balloon catheter and were randomly assigned separately. Of the remaining 478 patients with primary perfusion balloon catheter inflations, 236 were randomly assigned to undergo the standard strategy and 242 to undergo the prolonged strategy. The baseline patient characteristics were similar. The majority of target lesions were in either the left anterior descending artery or the right coronary artery, and these lesions were similarly distributed between American College of Cardiology/ American Heart Association (ACC/AHA) Classification types A and B, with a few type C.

This study revealed a significantly higher angiographic success rate at the end of phase I with the prolonged inflation strategy (95%) than with the standard inflation strategy (89%). In addition, there was a significantly lower incidence of major dissections at the end of phase I with the prolonged inflation strategy (3%) than with the standard inflation strategy (9%). There was no significant difference in the incidence of restenosis between the two strategies. In view of these results, prolonged inflation with the perfusion balloon catheter may be a better primary angioplasty strategy than is short inflation. The efficacy and safety of using the newer, low profile designs as the initial balloon in PTCA have also been confirmed.[42] Waksman and associates retrospectively assessed the performance of the ACS RX Flowtrack at their institution in 61 patients with predominantly type A and B lesions. PTCA was successful in all but one patient (98.4%), and complication rates were low; the complications included only one (1.6%) in-hospital reocclusion and six mild intimal tears (9.8%), and there were no deaths or CABG. The complication rates were noted to be similar to those of historical controls.

There are, however, some limitations in applying a universal strategy of perfusion balloon PTCA as a primary strategy in all patients. First, perfusion balloons are more costly than standard PTCA balloons. In addition, the presence of side branches, distal lesions, severe angulation, or tortuosity may preclude the use of a perfusion balloon. In the Randomized PBC Trial, during a 1-year screening log of 1687 patients, only 10% were eligible for enrollment. As a result of these limitations of PBC angioplasty for routine use, Eltchaninoff and colleagues investigated a strategy of using several balloon inflations of 3 to 5 minutes each with a standard PTCA balloon to achieve a cumulative occlusion time comparable with that of perfusion balloon PTCA (≥12 minutes).[43] This prolonged cumulative dilatation strategy was compared with standard PTCA (3 to 5 inflations of ≤1 minute each) in a randomized, prospective manner in 310 lesions with repeat catheterization performed in 4 to 6 months. The success rate was higher with the prolonged dilatation strategy than with standard dilatation (92% vs. 80%; $p < 0.002$), and dissections were less frequent (14% vs. 30%; $p < 0.0009$). There was no difference in restenosis rates. These results suggest that the acute benefits of prolonged inflations may in fact be achieved by using less expensive standard balloons.

## Intracoronary Stent Implantation

With the development of perfusion balloons that may be inflated under high pressure without compromising coronary flow, a strategy of single–perfusion balloon catheter use for stent deployment has been investigated. The safety and feasibility of dilatation before stent implantation and high-pressure dilatation afterward with the same perfusion balloon has been prospectively investigated by Waksman and associates.[44] All 77 lesions in consecutive patients undergoing stent implantation at a single center were successfully dilated before implantation, and 76 lesions (98.7%) successfully dilated after implantation (16.2 ± 0.8 atm) with the same PBC (ACS Rx Lifestream). The balloon burst rate was 6.5%, and the average number of PBCs used per stent was 1.1. There were no major complications or incidents of stent thrombosis. This confirms that the use of a single PBC is safe and feasible and may reduce the number of balloons used per procedure, in comparison to a strategy in which separate balloons are used for dilatation before and after stent implantation. However, because no comparison directly with standard high-pressure balloon catheters was performed, it is unclear that the use of the PBC balloon for intracoronary stent implantation in this manner is either more efficacious or less costly.

## High-Risk PTCA

The indications for coronary angioplasty have expanded to include more patients at high risk for complications. These expanded indications include severe or unstable coronary disease with one or more technically approachable lesions in the setting of either a target lesion in a vessel supplying more than 50% of the myocardium or a left ventricular ejection fraction of less than 30%. In addition to the patient's intolerance to chest pain, an unsuccessful result in these settings could result in either electrical or hemodynamic instability. The use of the perfusion balloon catheter in these high-risk lesions provides not only a means of protecting against coronary ischemia but also a potential method for improving angiographic outcome.[45–49] In a substudy of

the PBC Trial, angiographic outcome in complex coronary stenoses (ACC/AHA type $B_2$; irregular; ulcerated; thrombus; eccentric) treated with the perfusion balloon catheter was evaluated.[49] The angiographic success rate in type $B_2$ lesions ($N = 129$) was 91% for standard dilatations (up to four dilatations for 1 minute each) and 97% for prolonged dilatations (up to two dilatations for 15 minutes each). In irregular, ulcerated, or thrombus-laden lesions ($N = 114$) the angiographic success rates were 88% for standard dilatations and 98% for prolonged dilatations. Eccentric lesions ($N = 290$) had a similar trend toward improved angiographic outcome with prolonged dilatations (97%) in comparison with standard dilatations (92%).

## Salvaging Failed PTCA

The major significant limitations of PTCA are coronary dissection and abrupt closure. These events occur in 2% to 12% of patients and can lead to such major complications as death, myocardial infarction, and the need for emergency CABG. Clinical experience supports the benefit of prolonged balloon inflations with a PBC in obtaining successful revascularization and avoiding surgery in patients who underwent initially unsuccessful PTCA (Table 34–4; Fig. 34–5).[50–56] The angiographic success rate with the PBC in these series ranged from 57% to 86%; the mean inflation duration ranged from 10 to 29 minutes. The incidence of emergency CABG for initial unsuccessful PTCA was reduced to 8% to 36% in these series of patients treated with the PBC. Leitschuh and coworkers reported the outcome of prolonged inflations with PBCs in 36 patients with major dissection and compared the results with those of historical control subjects with similar dissections before the availability of perfusion balloons.[54] The angiographic success rate was 84% among the patients treated with perfusion balloons and 62% among those who received conventional treatment; the patients treated with perfusion balloons also had a significantly lower rate of major

**TABLE 34–4.  STUDIES OF SALVAGE OF FAILED PTCA WITH THE PERFUSION BALLOON CATHETER**

| AUTHORS (YEAR) | NO. OF PATIENTS | INFLATION DURATION (MINUTES) | SUCCESS (%) | EMERGENCY CABG (%) |
|---|---|---|---|---|
| Smith et al. (1989)[50] | 28 | 21 | 57 | 36 |
| DeMuinck et al. (1991)[52] | 33 | 25* | 67 | 33 |
| Haerer et al. (1991)[53] | 22 | 10 | 86 | 14 |
| Leitschuh et al. (1991)[54] | 36 | 18 | 84 | 11 |
| Van Lierde et al. (1991)[55] | 24 | 29 | 63 | 29 |
| Jackman et al. (1992)[51] | 40 | 21 | 80 | 8 |

CABG, coronary artery bypass grafting; PTCA, percutaneous transluminal coronary angioplasty.
*Inflation duration reported as median, in contrast to all other studies which were reported as mean.

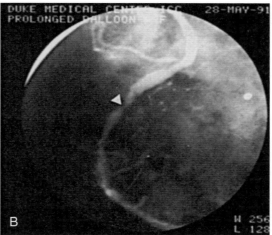

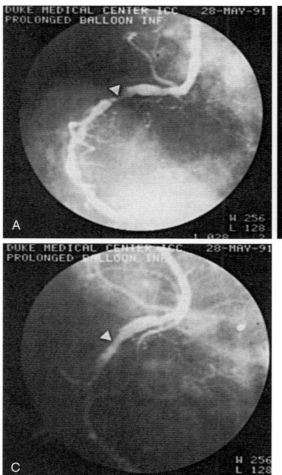

FIGURE 34–5. Angiogram *(A)* demonstrating a subtotal proximal right coronary artery stenosis *(arrow)* in a left anterior oblique projection before standard balloon angioplasty. *(B)* Persistent subtotal occlusion *(arrow)* despite multiple standard balloon dilatations. *(C)* Final result *(arrow)* following 15-minute inflation with the perfusion balloon catheter.

complications. The majority of patients in this study received several short inflations without more extended inflations before the perfusion balloon inflation. In follow-up to this study, Jackman and coworkers evaluated the efficacy of prolonged balloon inflations of more than 20 minutes' duration in patients with unsuccessful angioplasty despite both conventional and more extended inflations.[51] The population reported in this study represented patients in whom disease remained refractory to aggressive angioplasty efforts, as evidenced by the fact that before the prolonged inflation, 80% had a total inflation duration of more than 10 minutes. Prolonged inflations longer than 20 minutes resulted in a significant improvement in the degree of stenosis and an 80% angiographic success rate.

In a series of 14 patients, a PBC was inflated for more than 12 hours (range, 12 to 19 hours).[57] The result of this prolonged inflation duration was that all but one vessel remained widely patent without evidence of dissection or thrombosis. In fact, if large side branches are avoided and catheters are infused with heparinized saline, balloon inflation durations of 5 to 24 hours are possible, albeit with some atten-

dant risk of elevation of creatine kinase with muscle and brain subunits (CK-MB).[58, 59] In a consecutive series of abrupt vessel closures at the Cleveland Clinic, Lincoff and coworkers showed that prolonged balloon inflations were independently correlated with a successful outcome.[60] Therefore, there is abundant evidence that prolonged PBC inflations provide an effective "bail-out" option for abrupt vessel closure that complicates standard balloon angioplasty. The exact mechanism of arterial repair or salvage with the use of PBCs is unknown but believed to be related to a reduction in elastic recoil and the "sealing" of intimal flaps.

Despite these earlier trials demonstrating the efficacy of PBC dilatations for abrupt closure, the advent of intracoronary stent implantation has drastically revolutionized the approach to abrupt closure. Most cases of abrupt closure are caused by vessel dissection; a minority result from acute vessel thrombosis (an exception to this is with directional coronary atherectomy, in which thrombosis may account for >50% of abrupt closures). It has become clear that the mechanical radial forces of an intracoronary stent are highly efficacious in sealing dissections in vessels 3 mm or more in diameter. Several trials have compared prolonged PBC inflations with stent implantation for abrupt vessel closure and have demonstrated the superiority of stent implantation.[61–64] In comparison with the PBC, stent implantation results in more favorable acute angiographic results, a larger minimal luminal diameter, improved restoration of Thrombosis In Myocardial Infarction (TIMI) grade 3 flow, and a reduced need for CABG. Furthermore, the rates of stent thrombosis and bleeding, the early major limitations of stent implantation, have been reduced with antiplatelet therapy without warfarin (Coumadin).[65, 66] Therefore, intracoronary stent implantation is the current therapy of choice for abrupt vessel closure, particularly in vessels 3.0 mm in diameter; the PBC is an optional strategy when intracoronary stent implantation is not feasible (i.e., because of vessel tortuosity, calcification, or small vessel diameter).

## Maintaining Perfusion Before Emergency Bypass Surgery

Emergency CABG continues to be needed in 1% to 3% of attempted PTCA procedures, despite progressive improvements in technique and operator experience. Even with in-hospital surgical standby, emergency CABG for abrupt closure is associated with a 3% to 6% rate of mortality and up to a 50% frequency of perioperative myocardial infarction.[67, 68] To improve outcome by minimizing the duration of ischemia before CABG, both the reperfusion catheter and the PBC have been used. The reperfusion, or "bail-out," catheter is a 4.3-French tapered-tip catheter with 30 holes arranged in a spiral pattern over its distal 10 cm. This catheter can provide up to 80 mL/minute of passive blood flow across the coronary stenosis. Use of this catheter has been documented to be a safe and effective method of reestablishing and maintaining coronary blood flow before bypass surgery after failed coronary angioplasty in the majority of patients.[20, 69–72] In a retrospective series of 31 patients in whom abrupt closure developed after coronary angioplasty, the reperfusion catheter was successfully placed in 11 (61%) of 18 attempts.[72] The rate of Q-wave infarction was 9% among patients managed with the reperfusion catheter, in contrast to 75% among patients who underwent intra-aortic balloon counterpulsation or no mechanical intervention. Reperfusion catheter use was also associated with more consistent resolution of ST segment elevation and greater use of internal mammary artery grafts than was intra-aortic balloon counterpulsation alone. Like the reperfusion catheter, the perfusion balloon catheter has also been used to mechanically maintain myocardial perfusion in patients en route to surgery.[73] Coronary perfusion may be maximized by disengaging the coronary ostium and removing the guide wire. Maintenance of coronary blood flow may then allow the surgeon time to perform a more optimal revascularization procedure with the use of the internal mammary artery graft.

## LIMITATIONS OF THE DEVICE

Despite the many advantages offered by autoperfusion angioplasty, not all lesions are suitable for prolonged inflations with current PBC designs (Table 34–5). In lesions close to major side branches, balloon inflation may occlude these vessels and produce ischemia, thus preventing prolonged dilatations. In addition, some patients, even in the absence of involved side branches, cannot tolerate prolonged inflations. This may result either from inadequate distal perfusion despite the use of the autoperfusion catheter[74] or from discomfort not related to coronary ischemia at all but rather associated with the stretching of the vessel wall itself.[75] Because perfusion of the distal coronary bed is dependent on driving pressure, the usefulness of the autoperfusion catheter is reduced when systemic blood pressure is low.

The relatively higher profile of autoperfusion balloon catheters may make it difficult to cross tight, rigid lesions, and preprocedure dilatation with a smaller standard balloon catheter may be required. However, with the use of newer low-profile devices, the number of lesions that necessitate preprocedure dilatation has decreased to a small minority. Angulated lesions, tandem lesions, or vessels with tortuous bends, which previously posed a problem for PBC use, are also much more readily crossed with newer flexible, shorter tipped designs. When the guide wire is retracted proximal to the side holes to allow adequate distal perfusion during balloon inflation, guide wire reinsertion may be unsuccessful, and distal access may consequently be lost after balloon deflation. The risk of trauma to the vessel by the catheter tip, and maintenance of guide wire

## TABLE 34–5. LIMITATIONS OF PERFUSION BALLOON ANGIOPLASTY

Anatomic limitations*
  Tandem lesions
  Major sidebranch
  Sharp angulation
High profile, increased stiffness*
Tip positioning
Loss of guide wire access
Possible activation of stretch receptors
Decreased autoperfusion at low blood pressures

*Less of a problem with new perfusion balloon catheter designs.

position, can be reduced by leaving the guide wire across the lesion for the entire inflation duration.

## CONCLUSION

Development of perfusion balloon technology has been a major contribution to the practice of interventional cardiology. As a result of the use of the PBC, the number of patients able to undergo safe and successful procedures (despite high-risk characteristics or failed conventional PTCA) has been expanded. With advances in catheter design, perfusion balloon performance has improved substantially since the original prototypes. Prolonged inflation with the PBC catheter may be a better primary angioplasty strategy than is short inflation. Although the PBC also has proven clinical value in salvaging for failed angioplasty and acting as a bridge to emergency bypass surgery, intracoronary stent implantation in vessels 3.0 mm in diameter appears to be more effective in treating the major dissections often seen associated with threatened or abrupt closure. The new thermal balloon catheter, which combines radiofrequency thermal capability and perfusion balloon technology, may also be used to repair intimal dissections.[76] However, the safety and efficacy of this new development awaits further clinical investigation. Despite the significant advances in PBC design and technology, its future role is subject to change with the rapid evolution of other highly effective modalities such as intracoronary stent implantation and adjunctive therapies such as GPIIb/IIIa inhibition.

## REFERENCES

1. Gruentzig AR, Senning A, Siegenthaler WE: Nonoperative dilatation of coronary-artery stenosis: Percutaneous transluminal coronary angioplasty. N Engl J Med 301:61–68, 1979.
2. Waller BF: "Crackers, breakers, stretchers, drillers, scrapers, shavers, burners, welders and melters"—the future treatment of atherosclerotic coronary artery disease? A clinical-morphologic assessment. J Am Coll Cardiol 13:969–987, 1989.
3. Simpfendorfer C, Belardi J, Bellamy G, et al: Frequency, management and follow-up of patients with acute coronary occlusion after percutaneous transluminal angioplasty. Am J Cardiol 59:267–269, 1987.
4. Blackshear JL, O'Callaghan WG, Califf RM: Medical approaches to prevention of restenosis after coronary angioplasty. J Am Coll Cardiol 9:834–848, 1987.
5. Tcheng JE, Fortin DF, Frid DJ, et al: Conditional probabilities of restenosis following coronary angioplasty. Circulation 82(suppl III):III-1, 1990.
6. Lasala JM, Cleman NW. Myocardial protection during percutaneous transluminal coronary angioplasty. Cardiology Clinics 6:329–343, 1988.
7. Remetz MS, Cabin HS, McConnel S, et al: Gradual balloon inflation protocol reduces arterial damage following percutaneous transluminal angioplasty [Abstract]. J Am Coll Cardiol 11(suppl A):131A, 1988.
8. Berland J, Farcot JC, Stix G, et al: Gradual, low-pressure and sustained inflations with the physiologic anteroperfusion system improve the immediate results of LAD angioplasty [Abstract]. J Am Coll Cardiol 19:350A, 1992.
9. Quigley PH, Hinohara T, Phillips HR, et al: Myocardial protection during coronary angioplasty with an autoperfusion balloon catheter in humans. Circulation 78:1128–1134, 1988.
10. Quigley PH, Kereiakes DJ, Hinohara T, et al: Efficacy of gradual, prolonged balloon inflation during coronary angioplasty in humans using a perfusion catheter [Abstract]. J Am Coll Cardiol 11(suppl II):II-449, 1988.
11. Ohman EM, Marquis JF, Ricci DR, et al: Effect of gradual prolonged balloon inflation during angioplasty on in-hospital and long term outcome: Results of a multicenter randomized trial [Abstract]. J Am Coll Cardiol 19:33A, 1992.
12. Fischmann DL, Leon MB, Baim DS, et al: A randomized comparison of balloon expandable stent implantation with balloon angioplasty in the treatment of coronary artery disease. N Engl J Med 331:496–501, 1994.
13. Serruys PW, De Jaegere P, Kiemeneij F, et al: A comparison of balloon expandable stent implantation with balloon angioplasty in patients with coronary artery disease. N Engl J Med 331:489–495, 1994.
14. The Epic Investigators: Use of a monoclonal antibody directed against the platelet glycoprotein IIb/IIIa receptor in high-risk coronary angioplasty. N Engl J Med 330:956–961, 1994.
15. Lehmann KG, Atwood JE, Snyder EL, et al: Autologous blood perfusion for myocardial protection during coronary angioplasty: A feasibility study. Circulation 76:312–323, 1987.
16. Kent KM, Clemann M, Cowley M, et al: Reduction of ischemia during percutaneous transluminal coronary angioplasty (PTCA) with oxygenated fluosol [Abstract]. Circulation 76(suppl IV):IV-27, 1987.
17. Rossen JD, Snyder SR, Marcus ML, et al: Coronary perfusion with modified hemoglobin prevents myocardial dysfunction during coronary occlusion. Circulation 76(suppl IV):IV-27, 1987.
18. Chang B, Drury JK, Meerbaum S, et al: Enhanced myocardial washout and retrograde blood delivery with synchronized retroperfusion during acute myocardial ischemia. J Am Coll Cardiol 9:1091–1098, 1987.
19. Hinohara T, Simpson JB, Phillips HR, et al: Transluminal catheter reperfusion: A new technique to reestablish blood flow after coronary occlusion during percutaneous transluminal coronary angioplasty. Am J Cardiol 57:684–686, 1986.
20. Hinohara T, Simpson JB, Phillips HR, et al: Transluminal intracoronary reperfusion catheter: A device to maintain coronary perfusion between failed coronary angioplasty and emergency coronary bypass surgery. J Am Coll Cardiol 11:977–982, 1988.
21. Moreyra AE, Macris A, Kostis JB, et al: Coronary Perfusion Catheter: Its effectiveness in an experimental model of acute coronary occlusion. Am Heart J 120:1031–1038, 1990.
22. Erbel R, Clas W, Busch U, et al: New balloon catheter for prolonged percutaneous transluminal coronary angioplasty and bypass flow in occluded vessels. Catheter Cardiovasc Diagn 12:116–123, 1986.
23. Turi ZG, Campbell CA, Gottimukkala MV, et al: Preservation of distal coronary perfusion during prolonged balloon inflation with an autoperfusion angioplasty catheter. Circulation 75:1273–1280, 1987.
24. de Muinck ED, Angelini P, Dougherty K, et al: In vitro evaluation of blood flow through autoperfusion catheters. Catheter Cardiovasc Diagn 30:58–62, 1993.
25. Turi ZG, Campbell CA, Gottimukkala MV, et al: Preservation of distal coronary perfusion during prolonged balloon inflation with an autoperfusion angioplasty catheter. Circulation 75:1273–1280, 1987.
26. Turi ZG, Rezkella S, Campbell CA, et al: Left main percutaneous transluminal coronary angioplasty with the autoperfusion catheter in an animal model. Catheter Cardiovasc Diagn 21:45–50, 1990.
27. Stack RS, Quigley PJ, Collins G, et al: Perfusion balloon catheter. Am J Cardiol 61:77G–80G, 1988.
28. Collins GJ, Ramirez NM, Hinohara T, et al: The perfusion balloon catheter: A new method for safe prolonged coronary dilatation. J Am Coll Cardiol 9:106A, 1987.
29. White CJ, Ramee SR, Banks AK, et al: New passive perfusion PTCA catheter. Catheter Cardiovasc Diagn 19:264–268, 1990.

30. Campbell CA, Rezkalla S, Kloner RA, et al: The autoperfusion balloon angioplasty catheter limits myocardial ischemia and necrosis during prolonged balloon inflation. J Am Coll Cardiol 14:1045–1050, 1989.

31. Christensen CW, Lassar TA, Daley LC, et al: Regional myocardial blood flow with a reperfusion catheter and an autoperfusion balloon catheter during total coronary occlusion. Am Heart J 119:242–248, 1990.

32. Zalewski A, Berry C, Kosman AK, et al: Myocardial protection with autoperfusion during prolonged coronary artery occlusion. Am Heart J 119:41–46, 1990.

33. Turi ZG, Rezkalla S, Campbell CA, et al: Amelioration of ischemia during angioplasty of the left anterior descending coronary artery with an autoperfusion catheter. Am J Cardiol 62:513–517, 1988.

34. Quigley PH, Hinohara T, Phillips HR, et al: Myocardial protection during coronary angioplasty with an autoperfusion balloon catheter in humans. Circulation 78:1128–1134, 1988.

35. Simonton CA, Kowalchuk GJ, Austin W: Preservation of regional myocardial function during coronary angioplasty with an autoperfusion balloon catheter: A case report. Catheter Cardiovasc Diagn 22:28–34, 1991.

36. Muhlestein JB, Quigley PJ, Phillips HR, et al: Does myocardial damage or hemolysis occur during prolonged perfusion balloon anigoplasty? [Abstract]. J Am Coll Cardiol 15:250A, 1990.

37. Muhlestein JB, Quigley PJ, Ohman EM, et al: A prospective analysis of possible myocardial damage or hemolysis occurring as a result of prolonged autoperfusion angioplasty in humans. J Am Coll Cardiol 20:594–598, 1992.

38. Tenaglia AN, Quigley PJ, Kereiakes DJ, et al: Coronary angioplasty performed with gradual and prolonged inflation using a perfusion balloon catheter: Procedural success and restenosis rate. Am Heart J 124:585–589, 1992.

39. Ellis, SG, Roubin GS, King SB III, et al: Angiographic and clinical predictors of acute closure after native vessel coronary angioplasty. Circulation 77:372–379, 1988.

40. Detre K, Holubkov R, Kelsey S, et al: Percutaneous transluminal coronary angioplasty in 1985–86 and 1977–81. The National Heart, Lung, and Blood Institute registry. N Engl J Med 318:265–270, 1988.

41. Savage MP, Goldberg S, Hirshfeld JW, et al: Clinical and angiographic determinants of primary coronary angioplasty success. J Am Coll Cardiol 17:22–28, 1991.

42. Waksman R, Ghazzal ZMB, Scott NA, et al: Efficacy and safety of using perfusion dilatation catheter as initial balloon in coronary angioplasty. Catheter Cardiovasc Diag 32:319–322, 1994.

43. Eltchaninoff H, Cribier A, Koning R, et al: Effects of prolonged sequential balloon inflations on results of coronary angioplasty. Am J Cardiol 77:1062–1066, 1996.

44. Waksman R, Shafer CD, Seung KB, et al: Intracoronary stent implantation using a single high pressure perfusion balloon catheter. Catheter Cardiovasc Diagn 40:140–143, 1997.

45. Tommaso CL: Management of high-risk coronary angioplasty. Am J Cardiol 64(suppl E):33E–37E, 1989.

46. Saenz CB, Schwartz KM, Slysh SJ, et al: Experience with the use of coronary autoperfusion catheter during complicated angioplasty. Catheter Cardiovasc Diagn 20:276–278, 1990.

47. Lincoff AM, Popma JJ, Ellis SG, et al: Percutaneous support devices for high risk or complicated coronary angioplasty. J Am Coll Cardiol 17:770–780, 1991.

48. Turi ZG, Rezkalla S, Campbell CA, et al: Amelioration of ischemia during angioplasty of the left anterior descending coronary artery with an autoperfusion catheter. Am J Cardiol 62:513–517, 1988.

49. Kereiakes DJ, Knudtson MJ, Ohman EM, et al: Prolonged dilatation improves initial results during PTCA of complex coronary stenoses: Results from a randomized trial [Abstract]. J Am Coll Cardiol 21:290A, 1993.

50. Smith JE, Quigley PJ, Tcheng JE, et al: Can prolonged perfusion balloon inflations salvage vessel patency after failed angioplasty? Circulation 80(suppl II):II-373, 1989.

51. Jackman JD, Zidar JP, Tcheng JE, et al: Outcome after prolonged balloon inflations of >20 minutes for initially unsuc-

52. De Muinck E, Van Dijk R, Den Heijer P, et al: Prolonged autoperfusion balloon inflation for acute failure of conventional coronary angioplasty: A prospective study with retrospective controls. Eur Heart J 12:155, 1991.

53. Haerer W, Schmidt A, Eggeling T, et al: The impact of an autoperfusion device on the outcome of patients with PTCA complications. Eur Heart J 12(abstract suppl):154, 1991.

54. Leitschuh ML, Mills RM, Jacobs AK, et al: Outcome after major dissection during coronary angioplasty using the perfusion balloon catheter. Am J Cardiol 67:1056–1060, 1991.

55. Van Lierde J, Vrolix M, Sionis D, et al: Efficacy of Stack autoperfusion catheter in acute complications of balloon angioplasty: Short and intermediate-term results. Eur Heart J 12(abstract suppl):154, 1991.

56. Saenz CB, Schwartz KM, Slysh SJ, et al: Experience with the use of coronary autoperfusion catheter during complicated angioplasty. Catheter Cardiovasc Diagn 20:276–278, 1990.

57. Tjonjoegin RM, Bal ET, Ernst S, et al: Can coronary perfusion balloon inflations of more than 12 hours serve as a bail-out system for recurrent coronary artery occlusion during PTCA? Circulation 86(suppl I):I-248, 1992.

58. Brenner AS, Browne KF: Five-hour balloon inflation to resolve recurrent reocclusion during coronary angioplasty. Catheter Cardiovasc Diagn 22:107–111, 1991.

59. Tjonjoegin RM, Bal ET, Ernst S, et al: Can coronary perfusion balloon inflations of more than 12 hours serve as a bail-out system for recurrent coronary artery occlusion during PTCA? Circulation 86:I-248, 1992.

60. Lincoff AM, Popma JJ, Ellis SG, et al: Abrupt vessel closure complicating coronary angioplasty: Clinical, angiographic and therapeutic profile. J Am Coll Cardiol 19:926–935, 1992.

61. Ricci HR, Ray S, Buller CE, et al: Six month followup of patients randomized to prolonged inflation or stent for abrupt occlusion during PTCA-Clinical and angiographic data: TASC II. Circulation 92(suppl I):I-475, 1995.

62. Lincoff M, Topol E, Chapekis A, et al: Intracoronary stenting compared with conventional therapy for abrupt vessel closure complicating coronary angioplasty: A matched case-control study. J Am Coll Cardiol 21:866–875, 1993.

63. de Muinck E, den Heijer P, van Dijk R: Autoperfusion balloon versus stent for acute or threatened closure during percutaneous transluminal coronary angioplasty. Am J Cardiol 74:1002–1005, 1994.

64. Barberis P, Marsico F, De Servi S, et al: Treatment of failed PTCA with perfusion balloon versus intracoronary stent: A short-term follow-up [Abstract]. J Am Coll Cardiol (Special Issue), p 136A, February 1994.

65. Schomig A, Neumann F, Kastrati A, et al: A randomized comparison of antiplatelet and anticoagulant therapy after the placement of coronary artery stents. N Engl J Med 334:1084–1089, 1996.

66. Columbo A, Hall P, Nakamura S, et al: Intracoronary stenting without anticoagulation accomplished with intravascular ultrasound guidance. Circulation 91:1676–1688, 1995.

67. Bredlau CE, Roubin GS, Leimgruber PP, et al: In-hospital morbidity and mortality in patients undergoing elective coronary angioplasty. Circulation 72:1044–1052, 1965.

68. Cowley MJ, Dorros G, Kelsey SH, et al: Emergency coronary bypass surgery after coronary angioplasty: The National Heart, Lung and Blood Institute's percutaneous transluminal coronary angioplasty registry experience. Am J Cardiol 53(suppl C):22C–26C, 1984.

69. Kereiakes DJ, Abbottsmith CW, Callard GM, et al: Emergent internal mammary artery grafting following failed percutaneous transluminal coronary angioplasty: Use of transluminal catheter reperfusion. Am Heart J 113:1018–1020, 1987.

70. Tebbe V, Ruschewski W, Korb H, et al: Autoperfusion catheter after failed percutaneous transluminal coronary angioplasty. Z Kardiol 78:63–67, 1989.

71. Ciampricotti R, Dekkers P, El Gamal M, et al: Catheter reperfusion for failed emergency coronary angioplasty without subsequent bypass surgery. Catheter Cardiovasc Diagn 18:159–164, 1989.

72. Sundram P, Harvey JR, Johnson RG, et al: Benefit of the

perfusion catheter for emergency coronary artery grafting after failed percutaneous transluminal coronary angioplasty. Am J Cardiol 63:282–285, 1989.

73. Kereiakes DJ, Topol EJ, George BS, et al: Emergency coronary artery bypass surgery preserves global and regional left ventricular function after intravenous tissue plasminogen activator therapy for acute myocardial infarction. J Am Coll Cardiol 11:899–907, 1988.

74. Coghlan J, Flitter W, Paul V, et al: Myocardial protection with the ACS Rx Perfusion Balloon Catheter. Ischemic or Non-ischemic? [Abstract]. J Am Coll Cardiol 19:293A, 1992.

75. Katz LN: Mechanism of pain production in angina pectoris. Am Heart J 10:322–327, 1935.

76. Buller CE, Culp SC, Sketch MH Jr, et al: Thermal/perfusion balloon coronary angioplasty: In vivo evaluation. Am Heart J 125:226–233, 1993.

# 35

# Percutaneous Balloon Valvuloplasty

*Larry S. Dean*

After the introduction of percutaneous transluminal coronary angioplasty by Andreas Gruentzig[1] in 1977, investigators broadened the use of percutaneous techniques for the correction of other cardiac abnormalities. This chapter discusses the percutaneous approach to valvular stenosis involving the aortic, mitral, pulmonic, and tricuspid valves. Many hemodynamic, clinical, and follow-up data for these procedures have been generated since 1985. This chapter also discusses the mechanisms, techniques, outcomes, and recommendations for percutaneous balloon valvuloplasty procedures.

## PATHOPHYSIOLOGY AND NATURAL HISTORY

### Mitral Stenosis

Most cases of mitral stenosis are products of prior rheumatic fever and subsequent damage to the valve that develops in the 10 to 30 years following the initial episode. The mitral apparatus is variably involved with the process, but there is almost always commissural fusion as well as thickening and calcification of the valve leaflets. Also, the chordae tendineae are usually involved and are shortened as well as thickened. The process leads to the development of progressive damage to the valvular apparatus and subsequent stenosis with associated variable degrees of regurgitation (Fig. 35–1).

During the latent period, clinical symptoms develop because of progressive damage to the valve and its supporting apparatus. Symptoms such as progressive dyspnea on exertion, paroxysmal nocturnal dyspnea, and hemoptysis as well as atrial fibrillation are insidious and, once developed, portend a poor prognosis. The propensity for development of left atrial thrombi is important in the assessment of patients with mitral stenosis.

### Aortic Stenosis

Unlike mitral stenosis, aortic stenosis can occur from a number of different causes, mostly depending on the age of the patient. In adolescents, aortic stenosis is congenital, and etiologies include unicuspid and bicuspid aortic valves. In the fifth and sixth decades of life, the most likely etiology is a congenitally bicuspid aortic valve that has undergone progressive fibrosis and calcification from continuous damage by abnormal flow over time (Fig. 35–2). The development of rheumatic aortic stenosis also occurs in this age group. Isolated aortic stenosis from a rheumatic cause is uncommon. The pathol-

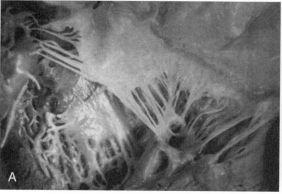
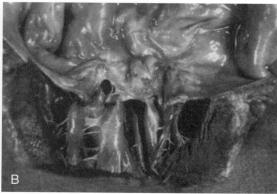

FIGURE 35–1. *A*, Normal mitral valve. Note the thin leaflets and featherlike chordae tendineae. *B*, Effect of the rheumatic process on the mitral valve, showing severe thickening of the mitral valve leaflets and subvalvular apparatus.

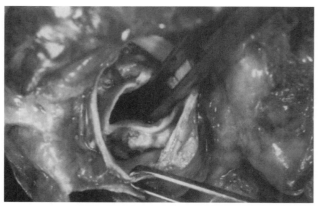

FIGURE 35–2. Pathologic specimen showing the typical features of bicuspid aortic valve with heavy nodular calcification of the valve leaflets. The calcific nodule at the 11 o'clock position in the picture is fractured from an aortic balloon valvuloplasty performed 4 weeks prior to autopsy. The patient died of clinically undetected diffuse myocarditis.

ogy of rheumatic aortic stenosis is similar to that seen in rheumatic mitral stenosis, in that the commissures of the valve leaflets are fused and thickened (Fig. 35–3). In the seventh and eighth decades of life, the most common etiology is senile degeneration and calcification of a tricuspid valve.

The natural history of aortic stenosis is similar, whatever the etiology. Patients typically experience dyspnea on exertion, angina, and syncope. Once congestive heart failure has developed, the prognosis is poor, with an average survival of 1 to 2 years. Angina and syncope confer an intermediate prognosis.

## Pulmonic Stenosis

Stenosis of the pulmonic valve is one of the more common isolated congenital valvular abnormalities found in the adult population. The pathology involves a congenital abnormality in which doming of the valve leaflets occurs as a result of fusion of the pulmonic valve commissures (Fig. 35–4). Less common is a dysplastic pulmonic valve. Acquired causes of pulmonic stenosis include rheumatic involvement (which is not isolated) and the involvement seen with carcinoid heart disease. Carcinoid heart disease produces a unique pathologic picture that consists of thickening and the development of plaquelike material involving the valve leaflets. Unlike the rheumatic process, carcinoid involvement does not produce commissural fusion.

Patients with significant pulmonic valve stenosis typically present with signs and symptoms of right heart failure, including fatigue, dyspnea, ascites, and peripheral edema. Severe pulmonic stenosis subsequently leads to profound right heart failure with progressive and severe tricuspid regurgitation and death.

## Tricuspid Stenosis

The most common cause of tricuspid stenosis by far is rheumatic heart disease. Such stenosis is rarely isolated and is typically associated with rheumatic involvement of the mitral valve. There are a number of rare causes of tricuspid stenosis. The only one potentially amenable to percutaneous balloon valvuloplasty is that seen with carcinoid heart disease. Unfortunately, most patients with carcinoid heart disease present with significant tricuspid regurgitation rather than isolated severe tricuspid stenosis, although the latter presentation has been reported. Patients with significant tricuspid stenosis present with fatigue and signs of right heart failure that are out of proportion to the symptom of dyspnea. Once symptoms of right heart failure become manifest, the mean pressure gradient across the valve is usually 5 mm Hg or more, and the valve area is 2 cm² or less. Intervention should be seriously considered.

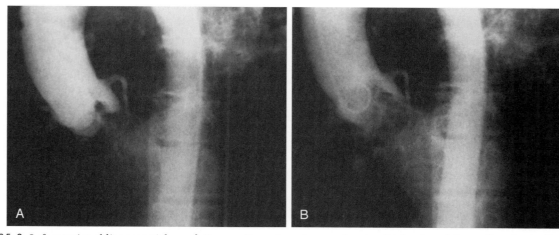

FIGURE 35–3. Left anterior oblique cranial angulation, aortic root angiogram showing thickening of the aortic valve leaflets, especially of the left coronary cusp, during diastole *(A)* and restricted motion with doming during systole *(B)*.

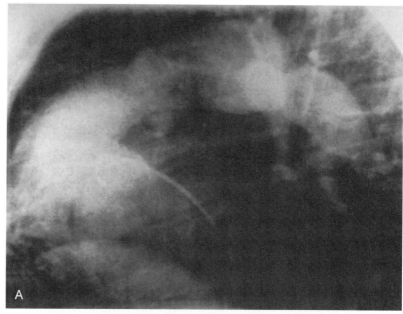

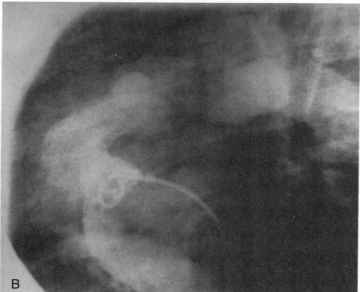

FIGURE 35–4. Left lateral cineangiogram. *A*, Diastolic frame from a patient with pulmonic stenosis. *B*, Typical systolic doming and restricted opening of pulmonic valve. Note the markedly enlarged left pulmonary artery, which is a typical finding of pulmonic stenosis.

## MITRAL VALVULOPLASTY

Although surgical commissurotomy is one of the oldest cardiac surgical procedures performed, the first report on a percutaneous approach to mitral stenosis, by Inoue and colleagues,[2] did not appear until 1984. Since then, numerous other reports have appeared in the literature documenting various techniques and noting both clinical and hemodynamic improvement after percutaneous mitral valvuloplasty in numerous institutions throughout the world.[3–5]

## Mechanism of Action

Both in vivo and in vitro experiments have shown that the primary mode of action in percutaneous

mitral balloon valvuloplasty involves the splitting of the anterolateral commissure, the posterior medial commissure, or both, of the mitral valve by means of balloon inflation.[6, 7] There may also be some component of mitral annular stretching as well as fracture of thickened calcific deposits in the valve.[8] In addition, in patients who have significant subvalvular disease, some modification of the subvalvular apparatus may improve the overall size of the orifice.

## Technique

The initial technique described by Inoue and colleagues[2] involved the placement of a single balloon through a transseptal approach across the mitral

FIGURE 35–5. The 60-cm Mullins sheath, dilator, and Brocken-brough needle in their normal positions. Note that when the needle is fully extended, it protrudes slightly from the tip of the dilator. Prior to use, it is important to confirm that the needle will traverse the opening of the dilator.

valve orifice. Modifications of this initial technique have involved the use of a transseptal approach and either single or multiple balloons. An arterial approach has been described by Babic and associates.[9]

Most institutions initially used the double-balloon technique described by Al Zaibag and others.[4, 10] The transseptal approach is from the right femoral vein, and the Brockenbrough transseptal needle is placed in a Mullins sheath (Fig. 35–5). Over a 0.032-inch guide wire placed in the superior vena cava, the Mullins sheath and Brockenbrough needle are advanced into the superior vena cava and then slowly withdrawn, with the tip oriented in a 4 to 6 o'clock position. In patients with significant mitral stenosis, there is distortion of the usual anatomy, which usually requires that the needle and sheath be pointed more posteriorly (closer to 6 o'clock) for the fossa to be entered and a successful transseptal puncture obtained (Fig. 35–6). As the needle and sheath are withdrawn, there are three pronounced movements of the sheath-needle combination toward the spine in the anteroposterior (AP) projection. The first reflection or movement is due to the passage of the sheath-needle across the reflection of the superior vena cava with the right atrium. The second is due to movement along the reflection of the aorta and the right atrium,

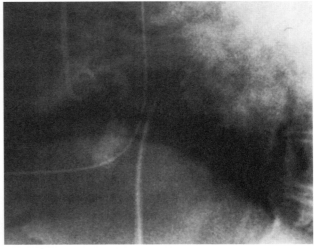

FIGURE 35–7. Lateral cineframe in the same patient as shown in Figure 35–6. Note the posterior orientation of the needle in the lateral projection. Also note the heavily calcified mitral annulus in this patient. A pigtail catheter has been placed at the level of the aortic valve to confirm its anterior location.

and the third is due to engagement of the fossa ovalis, upon which one notes that atrial pulsations are felt in the sheath. In addition, the sheath-needle combination often is restrained, and its superior movement is met with some resistance. We always confirm the proper location of the sheath-needle combination by means of lateral fluoroscopy, with a pigtail catheter placed in the area of the aortic valve to mark the anterior location of the aorta and decrease the likelihood of inadvertent puncture of the aorta by a too-anterior approach. Likewise, the use of the lateral or left anterior oblique (LAO) projection prior to puncture shows the correct posterior orientation of the sheath-needle combination (Fig. 35–7).

Once the location of the sheath-needle combination has been confirmed in the fossa ovalis, we gingerly advance the sheath without advancing the needle, on the chance that the patient has a patent fossa. A probe-patent foramen ovale has been reported in approximately 10% of patients.[11] If the sheath does not advance, we slowly advance the needle through the sheath, monitoring the pressure at the tip of the needle during the entire procedure. Usually, when the intra-atrial septum has been punctured, a left atrial pressure waveform is obtained. If not, aspiration through the needle generally reveals arterialized blood, which can be confirmed by oxygen saturation determination in the catheterization suite.

When a successful left atrial puncture has been documented, the sheath-needle combination is slowly advanced until the tip of the dilator is in the left atrium. The needle is then withdrawn, and the sheath is further advanced. We reconfirm hemodynamics using left atrial/left ventricular simultane-

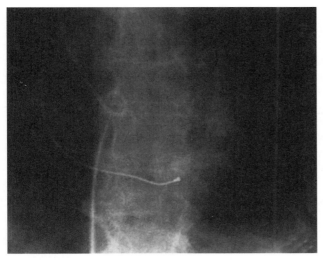

FIGURE 35–6. Anteroposterior cineframe following successful transseptal puncture of the fossa ovalis.

ous pressures to measure the severity of mitral stenosis.

Next, we place at least one or two 300-cm, Amplatz-type, 0.038-inch guide wires in the descending aorta, using a flotation balloon inserted through the Mullins transseptal sheath into the left ventricle and, in some instances, across the aortic valve and into the descending aorta. Then a wire is inserted in either the left ventricular apex or the aorta, depending on the site of the previously placed flotation balloon catheter. We next perform an atrial septostomy using a 5- or 8-mm dilating balloon placed over the wire. The balloon is withdrawn and the groin access site is dilated, allowing easier passage of the balloon dilation catheters. A second wire can then be placed either in the left ventricle or, in many instances, into the aorta. If an aortic location is desired for the wire, the Mullins sheath and flotation balloon are removed, and a specially designed double-lumen catheter is negotiated into the ascending aorta.

A second wire is then placed through the dual lumen, leaving two wires traversing the left ventricular apex and descending aorta (Fig. 35–8). It is

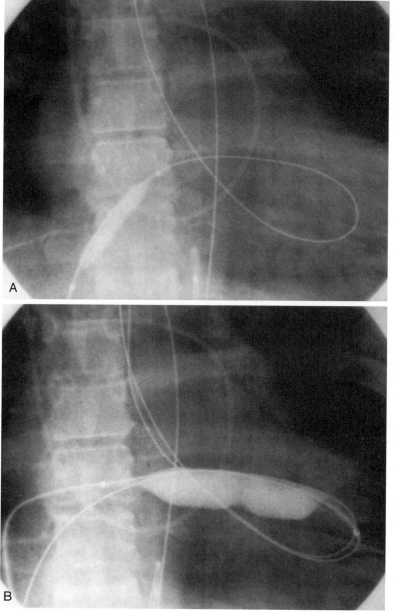

FIGURE 35–8. *A*, Anteroposterior cineangiogram of the correct placement of the wire, which has passed through the intra-atrial septum to the left ventricular apex and out the outflow tract, and terminally placed in the descending aorta. Note full inflation of an 8-mm balloon, which produces the desired atrial septostomy. *B*, Two wires placed across the intra-atrial septum through to the left ventricular apex, out the left ventricular outflow tract, and into the descending aorta. A single balloon has been inflated across the mitral annulus. Note the constriction present at the level of the mitral valve.

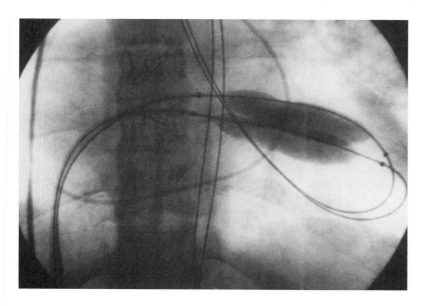

FIGURE 35–9. Right anterior oblique projection showing two balloons completely inflated in the mitral annulus. Note indentations in the balloons in this early cineframe. Subsequent inflation produced completed resolution, indicating complete dilation of the mitral valve.

critical that the loop in the two wires crosses the mitral valve and extends to the apex and out the left ventricular outflow track. If the loop is lost during the placement of the wires or during the procedure, one must begin again, maintaining the loop in the appropriate orientation. If dilation is attempted without an adequate loop, the result of the procedure will be suboptimal, and damage to the mitral apparatus can occur. After the balloons are properly placed, they are inflated, typically for approximately 10 to 15 seconds. The valve has been dilated when the typical "waist" in the balloon has resolved, indicating splitting of the commissures. This resolution often occurs after one or two inflations. We do not continue inflations once the waist has resolved (Fig. 35–9).

Now that the Inoue balloon (Toray Medical Co., Ltd.; Tokyo, Japan) has become available in the United States, most centers have been using this device exclusively. The approach is similar to that in the double-balloon technique, in that it requires transseptal catheterization. However, after the catheterization, a special pigtail-configured 0.025-inch guide wire is placed in the left atrium (Fig. 35–10), and a 14-French dilator is passed through the right femoral puncture site and across the atrial septum, dilating both areas. The dilator is then withdrawn, and the prepared Inoue balloon is placed across the intra-atrial septum and above the mitral annulus. We commonly use 1 or 2 mL of contrast agent in the balloon to visualize it better as well as to allow its passage across the valve without entrapment in the subvalvular apparatus. A specially designed J-wire supplied with the balloon is placed in the catheter, rotated in a counterclockwise fashion, and withdrawn slightly from the catheter. This maneuver produces anterior and forward displacement of the balloon. With proper balloon position, the valve is usually easy to cross with use of this device.

The balloon is then inflated. Owing to its unique design, the distal portion inflates first, and the catheter is slightly withdrawn, locking the balloon into the mitral annulus; complete balloon inflation is then undertaken, which results in an hourglass type of configuration and splitting of the commissures (Fig. 35–11). The balloon is usually inflated more than once, echocardiographic guidance being used to assess the extent of mitral regurgitation after each inflation. The procedure is stopped once either an increase in mitral regurgitation occurs or hemodynamic success has been obtained.

Determination of correct balloon size has not undergone rigorous scientific evaluation. Palacios and colleagues[5] have reported that balloon size can be estimated by the formula shown in Table 35–1. We usually use two 18-mm balloons for a smaller patient, one 18-mm and one 20-mm balloon for a mod-

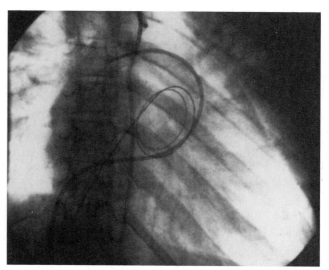

FIGURE 35–10. Anteroposterior cineframe showing the correct orientation of the pigtail-shaped 0.025-inch guide wire required for correct placement of the Inoue balloon in the left atrium.

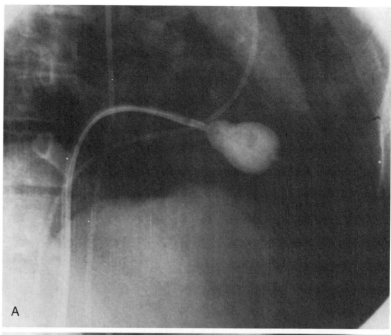

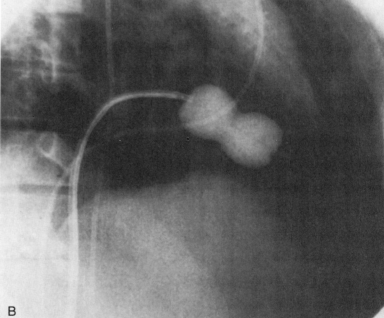

FIGURE 35–11. Cineframe showing a 26-mm Inoue balloon across the inflow tract of the left ventricle. *A,* Configuration of the distal balloon. *B,* Hourglass configuration when the balloon is fully inflated. This allows the balloon to be "locked" in the mitral annulus, producing the desired splitting of the fused mitral commissures.

## TABLE 35–1.    EFFECTIVE BALLOON DILATING AREA (cm²)*

| FIRST BALLOON SIZE (mm) | SECOND BALLOON SIZE (mm) | | | |
|---|---|---|---|---|
| | 0 | 15 | 18 | 20 |
| 15 | 1.77 | 4.02 | 4.89 | 5.55 |
| 18 | 2.54 | 4.89 | 5.78 | 6.46 |
| 20 | 3.14 | 5.55 | 6.46 | 7.14 |
| 23 | 4.15 | 6.57 | 7.55 | 8.27 |
| 25 | 4.91 | 7.46 | 8.41 | 9.11 |

*Diagrammatic representation of the effective balloon dilating area (EBDA) for any two-balloon combinations in which EBDA = $h[L_1 + L_2/2] + \pi[(r_1^2 + r_2^2)/2]$, where $L_1$ and $L_2$ = diameters of the balloons, $r_1$ and $r_2$ = radii of the balloons, and h = height of the trapezoid formed by the diameters of the balloons. An EBDA/BSA (body surface area) ratio of 3.1 to 4.0 cm²/m² is considered optimal.

Modified from Roth RB, Block PC, Palacios IF: Predictors of increased mitral regurgitation after percutaneous mitral balloon valvulotomy. Cathet Cardiovasc Diagn 20:17, 1990.

**TABLE 35-2.** **GUIDELINES FOR DETERMINING INOUE BALLOON SIZE ACCORDING TO PATIENT CHARACTERISTICS**

| INOUE BALLOON | | PATIENT CHARACTERISTIC | | |
|---|---|---|---|---|
| CATALOG NO. | DIAMETER RANGE (mm) | WEIGHT (kg) | BODY SURFACE AREA (m²) | HEIGHT (cm) |
| PTMC-30 | 26–30 | >70 | >1.9 | >180 |
| PTMC-28 | 24–28 | 45–70 | 1.6–1.9 | 160–180 |
| PTMC-26 | 22–26 | ≤45 | ≤1.6 | <160 |

Adapted from Inoue Balloon Catheter, Package Insert. Toray Medical Co., Ltd., Tokyo, Japan.

erate-sized patient, and two 20-mm balloons for a larger patient. Various formulas have been proposed for calculating the size of an Inoue balloon (Table 35-2). We currently use the formula of patient height (in centimeters) divided by 10 with the addition of 10; this is an empiric formula for the calculation of balloon size that is simple to remember. We undersize the balloon during the initial inflation by approximately 4.0 mm and then increase the balloon size by 1.0 mm with each subsequent inflation until we have reached the maximum diameter or we have obtained either hemodynamic success or an increase in mitral regurgitation. Experience shows that it is important not to oversize the Inoue balloon, because damage to the subvalvular apparatus and valve can result in the development of significant mitral regurgitation. This balloon produces acceptable hemodynamic results when properly used and is easier to use as well as safer than the double-balloon technique.

Interventional cardiologists relied almost completely on the echocardiographic mitral valve mor-phology scoring system originally reported by the group at the Massachusetts General Hospital[12] to determine which cases are appropriate for the procedure (Table 35-3). Although this scoring system is not perfect with respect to identifying patients who will have good initial and long-term results, some data suggest that it does have predictive value. Patients with an echocardiographic mitral valve score less than 8, the results are excellent; in patients with a score between 8 and 10, the results are intermediate; and in patients with a score of 12 or greater, our results, as well as those reported by others, have been less than optimal, with higher complication rates.[5]

Interventional cardiologists have usually not performed valvuloplasty in patients who have high echocardiographic mitral valve scores unless they have other comorbid diseases that prohibit operative replacement of the valve. We believe that valvuloplasty is best suited for patients who would be considered good candidates for surgical commissurotomy, either open or closed. All candidates for

**TABLE 35-3.** **GRADING OF CHARACTERISTICS OF MITRAL VALVE MORPHOLOGY FROM ECHOCARDIOGRAPHIC EXAMINATION***

| GRADE | CHARACTERISTIC | | | |
|---|---|---|---|---|
| | LEAFLET MOBILITY | VALVULAR THICKENING | SUBVALVULAR THICKENING | VALVULAR CALCIFICATION |
| 1 | Highly mobile valve with restriction of only the leaflet tips | Leaflets near normal (4–5 mm) | Minimal thickening of chordal structures just below the valve | A single area of increased echo brightness |
| 2 | Midportion and base of leaflets have reduced mobility | Midleaflet thickening, marked thickening of the margins | Thickening of chordae tendineae cordis extending up to one third of chordal length | Scattered areas of brightness confined to leaflet margins |
| 3 | Valve leaflets move forward in diastole mainly at the base | Thickness extends through the entire leaflets (5–8 mm) | Thickening extending to the distal third of the chordae | Brightness extending into the midportion of leaflets |
| 4 | No or minimal forward movement of the leaflets in diastole | Marked thickening of all leaflet tissue (>8–10 mm) | Extensive thickening and shortening of all chordae extending down to the papillary muscle | Extensive brightness through most of the leaflet tissue |

*Echocardiographic scores are derived from the analysis of leaflet mobility, valvular and subvalvular thickening, and valvular calcification, and graded from 1 to 4 according to the above criteria; the total score is the sum of scores for these echocardiographic features (maximum 16).
Adapted from Wallace AG: Pathophysiology of cardiovascular disease. In Smith LH Jr, Thiur SO (eds): The Biological Principles of Disease, p 1200. Philadelphia: WB Saunders, 1981.

mitral valvuloplasty should undergo transesophageal echocardiography before the procedure to exclude left atrial thrombus. A history of cerebrovascular accident or peripheral embolization is not a contraindication to mitral valvuloplasty, provided that the patient has received anticoagulation therapy for 2 to 3 months and the transesophageal echocardiogram is negative for left atrial thrombus.

## Results and Complications

Since first described by Inoue and colleagues,[2] mitral balloon valvuloplasty has steadily grown in use both in the United States and throughout the world. The immediate hemodynamic results have been published by numerous investigators: In general, the mean transvalvular mitral valve pressure gradients are reduced from approximately 15 mm Hg before the procedure to 5 or 6 mm Hg after it.[13–15] Also, the valve area before the procedure has been in the 1 cm² range, improving to approximately 2 cm² after successful dilation. We consider successful a procedure that yields a final mitral valve area of 1.5 cm² or more, with mild mitral regurgitation. Generally, the cardiac output either remains unchanged or increases slightly. Pulmonary capillary wedge pressure typically decreases after the procedure. However, we have seen certain patient subgroups, typically those with more severe pulmonary hypertension or more prolonged symptoms, in which the pulmonary capillary wedge pressure does not fall immediately but may decrease in the first few minutes to hours after the procedure. In general only the left atrial pressure, not the pulmonary capillary wedge pressure, is monitored after the procedure. Pulmonary artery and right heart pressures may not decrease immediately but may do so subsequently.

In short-term follow-up, patients who have a successful procedure (i.e., a mitral valve area ≥1.5 cm² after dilation) typically do well.[15–18] The patient's New York Heart Association (NYHA) function classification usually improves by two grades or more, and exercise treadmill time has been shown to be improved.[19]

Long-term follow-up data for 10 or more years are not currently available for large numbers of patients. Reports with a mean follow-up of 3 to 4 years have been published, however.[20, 21] In one study of 146 patients with a mean follow-up of 36 months, echocardiographic mitral valve score of 8 or less, left ventricular end-diastolic pressure (LVEDP) of 10 mm or less, and NYHA functional class II or III were factors that predicted improved event-free survival. Survival was 96% at 1 year, 89% at 3 years, and 84% at 5 years.[20]

National Heart, Lung, and Blood Institute (NHLBI)

Balloon Valvuloplasty Registry participants reported the 4-year follow-up for patients undergoing percutaneous balloon mitral commissurotomy.[21] The maximum follow-up in this study was 5.2 years, with a mean of 4 years. Eighty percent of the patients were alive and without the need for mitral surgery or second balloon mitral commissurotomy at 1 year. Actuarial survival was 93% at 1 year, 90% at 2 years, 87% at 3 years, and 84% at 4 years. The event-free survival was 80% at 1 year, 71% at 2 years, 56% at 3 years, and 60% at 4 years. The univariable predictors of mortality at 4 years were age greater than 70 years, NYHA functional class IV, and baseline echocardiographic mitral valve score greater than 12. Multivariable predictors of mortality were NYHA functional class IV, higher echocardiographic mitral valve score and higher postprocedure LVEDP and pulmonary artery systolic pressure. Figure 35–12 shows the Kaplan-Meier estimate of survival, and Figure 35–13 shows the actuarial estimates of survival based on echocardiographic mitral valve scores.

It seems that the 5- to 10-year follow-up results should be similar to those for patients who have undergone closed surgical commissurotomy, which this procedure most closely mimics.[22, 23] The similarity depends, to some degree, on the underlying severity of the valve disease prior to the procedure. Complications that have been reported with mitral valvuloplasty include death, cardiac perforation either from the transseptal catheterization or from guide wires, worsening mitral regurgitation, left-to-right shunting, and cerebrovascular accidents.[24, 25]

The NHLBI registry of valvuloplasty contains data from 738 patients who underwent mitral valvuloplasty at 23 centers throughout North America.[24] Complications reported in this registry include

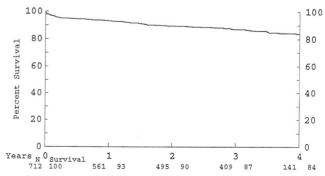

FIGURE 35–12. Overall survival: censored at mitral valve surgery or second balloon mitral commissurotomy in patients undergoing percutaneous balloon mitral commissurotomy. (From Dean LS, Mickel M, Bonan R, et al: Four year follow-up of patients undergoing percutaneous balloon mitral commissurotomy. A report from the National Heart, Lung, and Blood Institute Balloon Valvuloplasty Registry. J Am Coll Cardiol 28:1452, 1996. Reprinted with permission from the American College of Cardiology.)

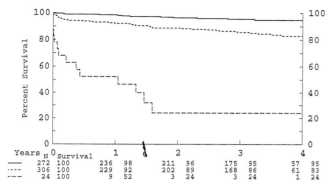

| Years | N | 0 Survival | | 1 | | 2 | | 3 | | 4 | |
|-------|---|-----------|---|---|---|---|---|---|---|---|---|
| —— | 272 | 100 | | 236 | 98 | 211 | 96 | 175 | 95 | 57 | 95 |
| ---- | 306 | 100 | | 229 | 92 | 202 | 89 | 168 | 86 | 61 | 83 |
| --- | 24 | 100 | | 9 | 52 | 3 | 24 | 3 | 24 | 1 | 24 |

FIGURE 35–13. Patient survival after balloon mitral commissurotomy by baseline echocardiographic mitral valve score: 8 *(solid line)*, 8 to 12 *(short dashed line)*, and 12 *(long dashed line)*. p<0.0001 (log rank statistic, 133.675). (From Dean LS, Mickel M, Bonan R, et al: Four year follow-up of patients undergoing percutaneous balloon mitral commissurotomy. A report from the National Heart, Lung, and Blood Institute Balloon Valvuloplasty Registry. J Am Coll Cardiol 28:1452, 1996. Reprinted with permission from the American College of Cardiology.)

death in the cardiac catheterization laboratory in 1% of patients, cerebrovascular accident in 2%, embolic event in 2%, development of cardiac perforation in 4% and cardiac tamponade in 4%, each, and the need for emergency cardiac surgery in 4% (Table 35–4). It should be noted that the death rate at 30 days was significantly better in the second year of enrollment in the registry than in the first year, as were rates for the need for pericardiocentesis, the development of tamponade, mitral regurgitation, and cardiac perforation, and the need for transfusion. It was also noted in this registry that complications were more frequently seen in those centers with the least experience in the technique. This observation was true for almost all complications,

either minor or major, occurring in the hospital. By and large, one can safely state that the patients in the NHLBI registry who died early after the procedure were either elderly or quite ill prior to it.

Patients with prior surgical or percutaneous commissurotomy can undergo percutaneous mitral balloon valvuloplasty, although the immediate and long-term results do not appear to be as good as in patients who have never undergone surgical commissurotomy. However, patients with previous procedures who have continued good valve morphology on echocardiography, that is, an echocardiographic mitral valve score less than or equal to 8, do as well as those who have not had surgical commissurotomy previously.[26]

The presence of severe tricuspid regurgitation prior to mitral balloon valvuloplasty has also been shown to be associated with poor long-term outcome.[27] The group at the Massachusetts General Hospital identified tricuspid regurgitation as an independent predictor of late outcome in their patient cohort. The estimated 4-year event-free survival in patients with severe tricuspid regurgitation was noted to be lower than in those without it (35% and 68%, respectively). Overall survival at 4 years was likewise affected by the presence of severe tricuspid regurgitation, being 94% in patients with mild tricuspid regurgitation and 69% in those with severe regurgitation. Severity of tricuspid regurgitation on echocardiography should therefore be critically assessed and should be a factor in determining which patients are candidates for the procedure. In patients with severe tricuspid regurgitation who do not have contraindications to the surgical procedure, mitral commissurotomy or mitral valve replacement with tricuspid annuloplasty may be the best procedure.

## Recommendations

Although the follow-up period for balloon mitral valvuloplasty reported in the literature is not as long as that documented for closed and open commissurotomy procedures, it appears that this technique has the same ability to improve mitral valve area (in patients for whom the procedure is suitably chosen) as the surgical procedure. Patient selection is critical if one is to produce excellent short-term and long-term results. Patients with echocardiographic mitral valve scores are good candidates. Because fewer complications seem to occur in those centers with the most experience and because, at least in the United States, mitral stenosis is not particularly common, it seems reasonable to suggest that either those centers or experienced physicians should perform the procedure.

Advantages of percutaneous mitral balloon valvu-

**TABLE 35–4.** **SERIOUS COMPLICATIONS BEGINNING IN THE CATHETERIZATION LABORATORY IN 738 PATIENTS UNDERGOING MITRAL VALVULOPLASTY**

| | NO. | % |
|---|-----|---|
| Emergency cardiac surgery | 29 | 4 |
| Cardiac perforation | 27 | 4 |
| Cardiac tamponade | 27 | 4 |
| Acute mitral regurgitation | 24 | 3 |
| Cerebrovascular accident | 16 | 2 |
| Embolic event | 16 | 2 |
| Pulmonary edema | 14 | 2 |
| Cardiogenic shock | 8 | 1 |
| Death | 8 | 1 |
| Myocardial infarction | 4 | 0.5 |
| Pulmonary embolus | 1 | 0.1 |

Adapted from Complications and mortality of percutaneous balloon commissurotomy: A report from the NHLBI Valvuloplasty Registry. Circulation 85:2014, 1992. By permission of the American Heart Association.

loplasty include a shorter hospital stay and less recovery time compared with the surgical approach. However, as noted previously, long-term follow-up data are needed to allow comparison of the surgical and nonsurgical approaches; also, patient selection for the balloon procedure is paramount, because such excellent results have been obtained with the surgical approach. Randomized studies comparing the results of mitral balloon valvuloplasty with surgical commissurotomy, both open and closed, have shown comparable results in both short-term and long-term follow-up.[28, 29] Patients with mitral valve heterografts should not undergo balloon valvuloplasty because of possible valve leaflet fractures and the potential for their embolization into the systemic circulation.

## AORTIC VALVULOPLASTY

Percutaneous aortic balloon valvuloplasty was first described by Lababidi and associates[30] in 1984, for the treatment of congenital aortic stenosis in children. In 1986, Cribier and colleagues[31] described the use of this procedure in adult patients with aortic stenosis. Although there was initially great enthusiasm for this use of this procedure in adults, further long-term follow-up has shown that such patients generally do not do well because of restenosis of the valve and sudden cardiac death. The procedure may play a limited role in certain subsets of patients.

### Mechanisms of Action

As previously described, the primary causes of aortic stenosis in the adult population are (1) a congenitally bicuspid aortic valve with fibrosis and calcification and (2) in the elderly, senile degeneration of a tricuspid valve. Pediatric patients with aortic stenosis have a congenitally malformed valve, often resulting from either unicuspid or severe bicuspid abnormalities. The mechanism of action of percutaneous aortic balloon valvuloplasty in pediatric patients appears to be tearing of the fused commissures or actual splitting of one or more valve leaflets. In the adult population, its primary mode of action appears to be the splitting of calcific nodules on the valve, which improves leaflet mobility. There may be, in addition, some dilation of the aortic annulus. In patients who have rheumatic aortic stenosis, the primary mechanism appears to be splitting of the fused valve commissures as seen with mitral valvuloplasty.

The procedure does not result in a significant increase in calculated valve area. Because of the curvilinear nature of aortic valve flow, however, with a change in the transvalvular aortic pressure gradient (Fig. 35–14), minor changes in the gradient

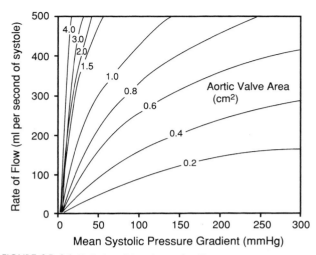

FIGURE 35–14. Relationship of systolic flow to aortic valve area. As seen, the curves are not linear; therefore, small changes in the aortic valve area produce substantial improvements in systolic flow. This relationship is at least partially responsible for the clinical improvement seen in patients undergoing aortic valve valvuloplasty. (From Wallace AG: Pathophysiology of cardiovascular disease. *In* Smith LH Jr, Thiur SO [eds]: The Biological Principles of Disease, p 1200. Philadelphia: WB Saunders, 1981.)

produce substantial improvements in flow across the aortic valve. Therefore, the small changes in pressure gradient with greater increase in transvalvular flow produced by this technique appear to be responsible for the clinical improvement seen.

## Technique

The procedure is typically performed from the right or left femoral artery using balloons in the 18- to 23-mm range. A standard left heart catheterization is performed, and the aortic valve is usually crossed with the use of a 0.038-inch straight wire and an AL1 Amplatz-type diagnostic catheter. Once the valve has been crossed, a double-lumen pigtail catheter (Cordis) is used to measure simultaneous pressure gradients across the aortic valve for calculation of the valve area. Next, the catheter is removed with a long, 300-cm Amplatz 0.038-inch wire, and an 18- to 23-mm balloon is placed across the aortic valve. The balloon is usually inflated more than once or until any "waist" in the valve has resolved. The balloon is then removed, and hemodynamic measurements are repeated. Typically, a 14-French hemostatic sheath (Cook, Daig) is used for vascular access. This sheath allows the passage of a low-profile balloon, up to a 23-mm (Boston Scientific), without difficulty. However, a 23-mm balloon cannot generally be removed through the sheath. The sheath and balloon must be removed in combination (as with removal of an intra-aortic balloon).

Balloon sizing has not undergone significant scientific evaluation, but it appears that in an adult patient of moderate size, a 20-mm balloon is a reasonable first choice. If this balloon inflates completely without a waist, or if there is a significant pressure gradient after its use, a 23-mm balloon may be used. Occasionally, a 25-mm balloon may be used if the aortic annulus will so permit. Several studies have shown that oversizing of the balloon can lead to vascular complications, including the development of severe aortic regurgitation, rupture of the aortic annulus, and death.[32–34] Helgason and associates[35] suggested that the balloon size should not exceed 120% of the aortic annulus size as estimated on echocardiography.[35]

It is possible to use a double-balloon technique with an approach from both femoral arteries or from one femoral artery and the brachial artery.[36] There is no conclusive evidence that patients have a lower restenosis rate or do better in follow-up with the double-balloon approach than with the single-balloon approach. There may possibly be more hemodynamic stability with a double-balloon approach, but this feature is rarely of significant clinical importance.

An antegrade approach for aortic balloon valvuloplasty has also been described.[37] The primary indication for this approach is severe peripheral arterial disease when retrograde access is not possible. It is performed via a transseptal catheterization with placement of the aortic balloon into the left ventricular outflow track and across the aortic valve with the use of a previously placed stiff (Amplatz) wire inserted as for mitral valvuloplasty. It is important to make sure that the loop into the outflow track is not too "tight," because the mitral valve apparatus can be damaged either with passage of the balloon or with inflation. Severe mitral regurgitation has been described with this technique.[38]

## Results and Complications

As noted, reports of the initial results of aortic balloon valvuloplasty in adults were met with great enthusiasm. It is clear from the data of multiple centers and investigators that the procedure results in improved hemodynamics and clinical status in the majority of patients.[39–41] As reported by the NHLBI Aortic Balloon Valvuloplasty Registry investigators,[41] the average aortic valve area increased from 0.5 to 0.8 cm² after the procedure. The increase was accompanied by a change in the mean aortic pressure gradient from 55 to 29 mm Hg. There was likewise a small increase in cardiac output and aortic pressure and small declines in the LVEDP.

Complications were not insignificant, however. At least one complication occurred in 25% of patients within the first 24 hours. Additionally, 31% experienced a significant complication before hospital discharge. The most common complications before discharge were the need for transfusion (23%), vascular surgery (7%), cerebrovascular accident (3%), systemic embolization (2%), and myocardial infarction (2%). The mortality rate was 3%, mostly from cardiovascular causes. Logistic regression analysis revealed that death was related to multisystem failure and poor left ventricular systolic function before the procedure. In the patients who survived to 30 days, there was symptomatic improvement; at least 75% experienced improvement by at least one NYHA functional class.

Additional long-term studies have shown a poor outcome, with a restenosis rate at 6 to 12 months approaching 50% to 100%.[42, 43] However, a small group of patients has shown greater long-term symptomatic improvement; some of them manifest evidence of restenosis but remain relatively asymptomatic at follow-up.[44] To date, it has not been possible to determine which patients are likely to have a long-term improvement in symptoms.

Other complications that have been noted are the development of worsened aortic regurgitation and high-degree atrioventricular block.[32, 34, 41] Perforation of the left ventricle has also been reported.[41, 45]

## Recommendations

Although aortic balloon valvuloplasty does result in both hemodynamic and symptomatic improvement, it does not have a good long-term efficacy in most patients. However, the natural history of untreated aortic stenosis in a similar patient population has shown that untreated patients uniformly do very poorly.[46] Therefore, as a purely palliative technique, this procedure appears to have some merit with what appears to be acceptable morbidity and mortality in this aged patient population. It would seem reasonable to perform the procedure to improve symptoms in patients who have intractable symptoms of heart failure despite medications or who cannot be discharged from the hospital because of difficulty with weaning from catecholamines and other supportive measures.

It has also been suggested that this procedure may have some benefit in patients with aortic stenosis, low cardiac output, and low transvalvular pressure gradient. Such patients often represent a difficult clinical decision because it is not clear, on presentation, whether they have a primary cardiomyopathy or poor left ventricular systolic function due to severe aortic stenosis. A small subset show improvement in left ventricular systolic function after aortic balloon valvuloplasty and therefore may become surgical candidates for aortic valve replacement. Experience shows that patients with low-output, low-gradient aortic stenosis generally do not improve after aortic balloon valvuloplasty. The subset of patients that appears to improve comprises those who have low cardiac output but maintained transvalvular gradients.[47] Such a patient would probably benefit from surgical intervention if systolic function improves after valvuloplasty.

Percutaneous aortic balloon valvuloplasty may serve to stabilize the hemodynamically unstable patient prior to operative intervention, thereby lowering the perioperative risk of aortic valve replacement or noncardiovascular surgical procedures.[48] The procedure is not indicated for patients with heterografts, and its use will remain limited in the future.

## PULMONIC VALVULOPLASTY

As previously discussed, pulmonic stenosis is one of the most common isolated congenital heart lesions found in the adult population. Percutaneous valvuloplasty of the pulmonic valve was first described by Semb and coworkers[49] in 1979. Most of the published literature on the procedure has dealt with its use in children and adolescents. Some data from its performance in adults suggest that the procedure may be efficacious in this age group as well.

### Mechanism of Action

The mechanism of action of balloon pulmonic valvuloplasty depends on the disease and its cause—splitting of fused commissures if the condition is rheumatic or, in some cases, congenital, or actual tearing of a portion of the valve. Although this tearing may result in some pulmonic valve insufficiency, most patients with pulmonic stenosis have normal pulmonary artery pressures, and the degree of regurgitation is small and usually well tolerated.

There are reports of infundibular narrowing after pulmonic valvuloplasty.[50] A small percentage of all patients undergoing the procedure experience significant outflow track obstruction, which may cause acute hemodynamic compromise. This complication appears to be more common in the pediatric age group. Typically, pretreatment of all patients undergoing this procedure with fluid loading, making sure that they are well hydrated, is indicated. Also used are either β blockers or calcium channel blockers (verapamil) in an attempt to decrease myocardial contractility. The infundibular hypertrophy seen in patients with pulmonic stenosis undergoing valvuloplasty has also been reported to regress within a few weeks after the procedure in the majority of cases.[51]

### Technique

Generally, a right or left femoral vein approach is used for pulmonic valvuloplasty. A pulmonary artery flotation balloon catheter that allows a 0.038-inch guide wire to be placed in the distal right or left pulmonary artery is used initially. A stiff guide wire is usually placed in the left pulmonary artery, allowing a more direct approach to the pulmonic valve (Fig. 35–15). Prior to placement of the balloon and wire, a right anterior oblique and lateral right ventricular angiograms are obtained to outline the area of interest and also to enable calculation of the approximate balloon size to use. In adult patients, generally a 23-mm balloon is used initially, but it is possible to oversize the valve by 20% to 30% with regard to the annulus diameter as determined from echocardiography or ventriculography.[52] However, care must be taken in the adult patient, whose pulmonary vasculature is not as elastic as that of children. After balloon inflation and resolution of the balloon "waist," hemodynamic measurements are repeated. A repeat right ventricular angiogram is usually not obtained after the procedure.

It is also possible to perform the procedure using two balloons. This approach is especially useful in patients who have a large pulmonary annulus. It may be that patients tolerate the two-balloon approach better from a hemodynamic standpoint because the use of two balloons allows flow through the outflow track and into the pulmonary artery during balloon inflation.

The surgical literature suggests that pulmonic balloon valvuloplasty should be performed in patients who have at least a 50-mm peak pressure gradient across the valve at the time of catheterization.[53] This feature is typically found in patients who have significant pulmonic stenosis with signs of right ventricular dysfunction. Other researchers have recommended a more aggressive approach with percutaneous pulmonic valvuloplasty, because it has a lower morbidity than that associated with the surgical procedure. Clearly, one wishes to intervene prior to the development of significant tricuspid incompetence and right ventricular failure.

### Results and Complications

NHLBI Balloon Valvuloplasty Registry participants have reported on 37 adult patients undergoing pulmonic valvuloplasty.[54] The mean age of the patients was 38 years, and the majority were female. The procedure was completed in 97% of patients, and a double-balloon technique was used in 44%. The peak transvalvular pressure gradient fell from 46 to 18 mm Hg, and there were no significant procedural complications. At 5 weeks of follow-up, 75% of patients remained improved. Hospital mortality was 3%.

Longer-term follow-up has generally indicated a favorable intermediate-term prognosis in the first 5

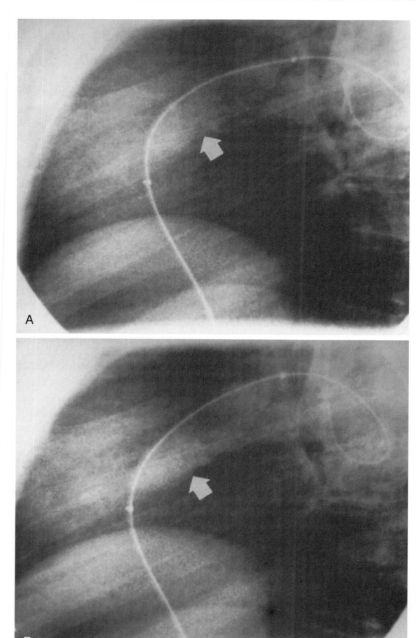

FIGURE 35–15. Cineframe of a 23-mm balloon inflated in a stenotic pulmonic valve. *A*, Note the indentation *(arrow)* in the balloon at the level of the pulmonic valve. *B*, Subsequent resolving with additional inflation *(arrow)*. Also note the placement of the 0.038-inch exchange wire into the left pulmonary artery.

to 7 years after pulmonic balloon valvuloplasty. Kasab and associates[55] have reported on 21 consecutive patients undergoing pulmonic valvuloplasty with a mean follow-up of 17 months. All patients had good continued symptomatic and hemodynamic improvement. Kaul and colleagues[56] have reported on 40 adult patients undergoing pulmonary valvuloplasty with a mean follow-up of 24.5 months. Follow-up status was generally favorable, and the researchers noted that in 8 patients with a residual pressure gradient following valvuloplasty, the gradient tended to decrease over time.

Complications have been minimal but include the development of significant pulmonic insufficiency, which is usually well tolerated, perforation of a cardiac chamber, including the pulmonary artery or pulmonic annulus, and the high-degree atrioventricular block.

## TRICUSPID VALVULOPLASTY

There are few data on the use of percutaneous balloon techniques in the treatment of tricuspid stenosis. NHLBI Balloon Valvuloplasty Registry participants have reported on seven patients undergoing the procedure.[54] The majority were female, and the procedure was successful in all patients. In four of the patients, the procedure was performed in porcine heterografts. In six patients, the procedure was performed with a two-balloon technique. The valve area increased from 0.9 to 1.6 cm², and no serious procedural complications were noted. Long-term follow-up has not been reported on these patients.

There are isolated reports of the use of this technique in the treatment of tricuspid stenosis due to carcinoid heart disease.[57, 58] In general, the procedure has shown success; however, it must be remembered that carcinoid heart disease of the tricuspid valve is different from rheumatic heart disease. Patients with carcinoid heart disease typically have thickened valves with plaquelike deposits. Therefore, their response to the technique may be somewhat variable. Unfortunately, most patients with carcinoid involvement of the tricuspid valve present with significant tricuspid incompetence, which cannot be handled with balloon techniques.

## CONCLUSIONS

The greater use of percutaneous balloon valvuloplasty techniques for treatment of stenotic cardiac valves appears to have been generally successful, mostly in patients with mitral stenosis or pulmonic stenosis. The use of balloon valvuloplasty in the treatment of aortic stenosis remains somewhat controversial and, at present, can be recommended only for palliation. Use of the procedure in the tricuspid valve remains promising, but there still are few data in this regard.

## REFERENCES

1. Gruentzig A: Transluminal dilatation of coronary artery stenosis. Lancet 1:263, 1978.
2. Inoue K, Owaki T, Nakamura T, et al: Clinical application of transvenous mitral commissurotomy by a new balloon catheter. J Thorac Cardiovasc Surg 87:394, 1984.
3. Lock JE, Khalilullah M, Shrivastava S, et al: Percutaneous catheter commissurotomy in rheumatic mitral stenosis. N Engl J Med 313:1515, 1985.
4. Al Zaibag M, Al Kasab S, Ribeiro PA, et al: Percutaneous double-balloon mitral valvotomy for rheumatic mitral-valve stenosis. Lancet 1:757, 1986.
5. Palacios IF, Block PC, Wilkins GT, et al: Follow-up of patients undergoing percutaneous mitral balloon valvotomy. Circulation 79:573, 1989.
6. Reid CL, McKay CR, Chandraratna PAN, et al: Mechanisms of increase in mitral valve area and influence of anatomical features in double-balloon, catheter balloon valvuloplasty in adults with rheumatic mitral stenosis: A Doppler and two-dimensional echocardiographic study. Circulation 79:628, 1987.
7. Kaplan JD, Isner JM, Karas RH, et al: In vitro analysis of mechanisms of balloon valvuloplasty of stenotic mitral valves. Am J Cardiol 59:318, 1987.
8. McKay RG, Lock JE, Safian RD, et al: Balloon dilatation of mitral stenosis in adult patients: Postmortem and percutaneous mitral valvuloplasty studies. J Am Coll Cardiol 9:723, 1987.
9. Babic UU, Pejcic P, Djurisic Z, et al: Percutaneous transarterial balloon valvuloplasty for mitral valve stenosis. Am J Cardiol 57:1101, 1986.
10. McKay CR, Kawanishi DT, Rahimtoola SH: Catheter balloon valvuloplasty of the mitral valve in adults using a double-balloon technique. JAMA 257:1753, 1987.
11. Bain DS, Grossman W: Percutaneous approach and transseptal catheterization: Transseptal left heart catheterization. *In* Grossman W (ed): Cardiac Catheterization and Angiography, 3rd ed, p 71. Philadelphia: Lea & Febiger, 1986.
12. Abascal VM, Wilkins GT, Choong CY, et al: Mitral regurgitation after percutaneous balloon mitral valvuloplasty in adults: Evaluation by pulsed Doppler echocardiography. J Am Coll Cardiol 11:257, 1988.
13. Ruiz CE, Allen JW, Lau FYK: Percutaneous double balloon valvotomy for severe rheumatic mitral stenosis. Am J Cardiol 65:473, 1990.
14. Babic UU, Prejcic P, Djurisic Z, et al: Percutaneous transarterial balloon mitral valvuloplasty: 30 months experience. Herz 13:91, 1988.
15. Multicenter experience with balloon mitral commissurotomy: The NHLBI Balloon Valvuloplasty Registry report on immediate and 30-day follow-up results. Circulation 85:448, 1992.
16. Dean LS, Baxley WA, Anderson JC, et al: Mitral valvuloplasty: Immediate and long-term follow-up. Clin Res 37:2A, 1989.
17. Tuzcu EM, Block PC, Griffin BP, et al: Clinical investigation: Immediate and long-term outcome of percutaneous mitral valvotomy in patients 65 years and older. Circulation 85:963, 1992.
18. Babic UU, Grujicic S, Popovic Z, et al: Percutaneous transarterial balloon dilatation of the mitral valve: Five year experience. Br Heart J 67:185, 1992.
19. McKay CR, Kawanishi DT, Kotlewski A, et al: Improvement in exercise capacity and exercise hemodynamics 3 months after double-balloon catheter balloon valvuloplasty treatment of patients with symptomatic mitral stenosis. Circulation 77:1013, 1988.
20. Cohen DJ, Kuntz RE, Gordon SPF, et al: Predictors of long-term outcome after percutaneous balloon mitral valvuloplasty. N Engl J Med 327:1329, 1992.
21. Dean LS, Mickel M, Bonan R, et al: Four year follow-up of patients undergoing percutaneous balloon mitral commissurotomy. A report from the National Heart, Lung and Blood Institute Balloon Valvuloplasty Registry. J Am Coll Cardiol 28:1452, 1996.
22. Rutledge R, McIntosh CL, Morrow AG, et al: Mitral valve replacement after closed mitral commissurotomy. Circulation 66(suppl I):I-162, 1982.
23. Hickey MSJ, Blackstone EH, Kirklin JW, et al: Outcome probabilities and life history after surgical mitral commissurotomy: Implications for balloon commissurotomy. J Am Coll Cardiol 17:29, 1991.
24. Complications and mortality of percutaneous balloon commissurotomy: A report from the NHLBI Valvuloplasty Registry. Circulation 85:2014, 1992.
25. Feldman T, Carroll JD, Isner JM, et al: Effect of valve deformity on results and mitral regurgitation after Inoue balloon commissurotomy. Circulation 85:180, 1992.
26. Jang IK, Block PC, Newell JB, et al: Percutaneous mitral balloon valvotomy for recurrent mitral stenosis after surgical commissurotomy. Am J Cardiol 75:601, 1995.
27. Sagie A, Schwammenthal E, Newell JB, et al: Significant tricuspid regurgitation is a marker for adverse outcome in patients undergoing percutaneous balloon mitral valvuloplasty. J Am Coll Cardiol 24:696, 1994.
28. Turi ZG, Reyes VP, Raju BS, et al: Clinical investigation: Percutaneous balloon versus surgical closed commissurotomy for mitral stenosis: A prospective, randomized trial. Circulation 83:1179, 1991.
29. Reyes VP, Rajub S, Wynne J, et al: Percutaneous balloon valvuloplasty compared with open surgical commissurotomy for mitral stenosis. N Engl J Med 331:961, 1994.
30. Lababidi Z, Wu J-R, Walls JT: Percutaneous balloon aortic valvuloplasty: Results in 23 patients. Am J Cardiol 53:194, 1984.

31. Cribier A, Savin T, Saoudi N, et al: Percutaneous transluminal valvuloplasty of acquired aortic stenosis in elderly patients: An alternative to valve replacement? Lancet 1:63, 1986.

32. Treasure CB, Schoen FJ, Treseler PA, et al: Leaflet entrapment causing acute severe aortic insufficiency during balloon aortic valvuloplasty. Clin Cardiol 12:405, 1989.

33. Lembo NJ, King SB, Roubin GS, et al: Fatal aortic rupture during percutaneous balloon valvuloplasty for valvular aortic stenosis. Am J Cardiol 60:733, 1987.

34. Dean LS, Chandler JW, Saenz CB, et al: Severe aortic regurgitation complicating percutaneous aortic valve valvuloplasty. Cathet Cardiovasc Diagn 16:130, 1989.

35. Helgason H, Keane JF, Fellows KE, et al: Balloon dilation of the aortic valve: Studies in normal lambs and in children with aortic stenosis. J Am Coll Cardiol 9:816, 1987.

36. Lewin RF, Dorros G, King JF, et al: Percutaneous transluminal aortic valvuloplasty: Acute outcome and follow-up of 125 patients. J Am Coll Cardiol 14:1210, 1989.

37. Block PC, Palacios IF: Comparison of hemodynamic results of anterograde versus retrograde percutaneous balloon aortic valvuloplasty. Am J Cardiol 60:659, 1987.

38. Farb A, Galloway JR, Davis RC, et al: Mitral valve lacerations and papillary muscle rupture secondary to percutaneous balloon aortic valvuloplasty. Am J Cardiol 69:829, 1992.

39. Sherman W, Hershman R, Lazzam C, et al: Balloon valvuloplasty in adult aortic stenosis: Determinants of clinical outcome. Ann Intern Med 110:421, 1989.

40. Safian RD, Berman AD, Diver DJ, et al: Balloon aortic valvuloplasty in 170 consecutive patients. N Engl J Med 319:125, 1988.

41. NHLBI Balloon Valvuloplasty Registry Participants: Percutaneous Balloon Aortic Valvuloplasty: Acute and 30-day follow-up results in 674 patients from the NHLBI Balloon Valvuloplasty Registry. Circulation 84:2383, 1991.

42. Block PC, Palcios IF: Clinical and hemodynamic follow-up after percutaneous aortic valvuloplasty in the elderly. Am J Cardiol 62:760, 1988.

43. Kennedy JW, Otto CM, Mickel M, et al: Longterm outcome following balloon aortic valvuloplasty (BAV). Eur Heart J 13:409, 1992.

44. O'Neill WW, Bashore TM, Davidson CJ: Seminar on balloon aortic valvuloplasty: V Follow-up recatheterization after balloon aortic valvuloplasty. J Am Coll Cardiol 17:1188, 1991.

45. Isner JM: Acute catastrophic complications of balloon aortic valvuloplasty. J Am Coll Cardiol 17:1436, 1991.

46. O'Keefe JH Jr, Vlietstra RE, Bailey KR, et al: Natural history of candidates for balloon aortic valvuloplasty. Mayo Clin Proc 62:986, 1987.

47. Nishimura RA, Holmes DR Jr, Michela MA: Follow-up of patients with low output, low gradient hemodynamics after percutaneous balloon aortic valvuloplasty: The Mansfield Scientific Aortic Valvuloplasty Registry. J Am Coll Cardiol 17:828, 1991.

48. Hayes SN, Holmes DR Jr, Nishimura RA, et al: Palliative percutaneous aortic balloon valvuloplasty before non-cardiac operations and invasive diagnostic procedures. Mayo Clin Proc 64:753, 1989.

49. Semb BKH, Tjonneland S, Stake G, et al: "Balloon valvulotomy" of congenital pulmonary valve stenosis with tricuspid valve insufficiency. Cardiovasc Radiol 2:239, 1979.

50. Ben-Shachar G, Cohen MH, Sivakoff MC, et al: Development of infundibular obstruction after percutaneous pulmonary balloon valvuloplasty. J Am Coll Cardiol 5:754, 1985.

51. Fontes VF, Esteves CA, Euardo J, et al: Regression of infundibular hypertrophy after pulmonary valvuloplasty for pulmonic stenosis. Am J Cardiol 62:977, 1988.

52. Radtke W, Keane JF, Fellows KE, et al: Percutaneous balloon valvotomy of congenital pulmonary stenosis using oversized balloons. J Am Coll Cardiol 8:909, 1986.

53. Hayes CJ, Gersony WM, Driscall DJ, et al: Second natural history study of congenital heart defects. Results of treatment of patients with pulmonary valvular stenosis. Circulation 87(suppl I):I-28, 1993.

54. Feit F, Davis K, Kennedy JW: Percutaneous balloon pulmonic and tricuspid valvuloplasty in adults. Circulation 82(suppl III):III-78, 1992.

55. Kasab SA, Ribeiro PA, Zaibag MA, et al: Percutaneous double balloon pulmonary valvotomy in adults: One- to two-year follow-up. Am J Cardiol 62:822, 1988.

56. Kaul UA, Singh B, Tyagi S, et al: Long term results after balloon pulmonary valvuloplasty in adults. Am Heart J 126:1152, 1993.

57. Cheng TO: Nonsurgical treatment of carcinoid heart disease. Ann Thorac Surg 51:1046, 1991.

58. Dalvi B, Mullins P, Hall J, et al: Balloon dilatation of tricuspid stenosis caused by carcinoid heart disease. Br Heart J 65:113, 1991.

59. Roth RB, Block PC, Palacios IF: Predictors of increased mitral regurgitation after percutaneous mitral balloon valvotomy. Cathet Cardiovasc Diagn 20:17, 1990.

60. Inoue-Balloon Catheter, Package Insert. Toray Medical Co., Ltd, Tokyo, Japan.

61. Wallace AG: Pathophysiology of cardiovascular disease. In Smith LH Jr, Thiur SO (eds): Pathophysiology: The Biological Principles of Disease, p 1200. Philadelphia: WB Saunders, 1981.

# Practice and Approaches to Coronary Stenting

# Selection of Coronary Stents for Particular Anatomy

*Antonio Colombo    Issam Moussa    Yoshio Kobayashi    Giovanni Martini*

The implantation of coronary stents is an integral part of most interventional procedures of percutaneous revascularization since the data of the Belgian-Netherlands Stent (BENESTENT) study[1] and Stent Restenosis Study (STRESS)[2] became available and since the elimination of anticoagulant therapy after stent implantation.[3-5]

The growth in stent implantation[6] stimulated the introduction in the market of a number of different stents. Table 36–1 illustrates the characteristics of most of the stents available in Europe in early 1997. The rapid increase in the number of designs available is such that any list rapidly becomes outdated. This table shows that some stent designs are quite similar to others, but it is also clear that some designs are very different from others.

The reasons why different designs have been proposed are multiple. Besides the need to overcome a specific patent, there are conceptual grounds that stimulated inventors to introduce a new design. The need to increase the flexibility in order to allow better and safe deliverability of the stent is one of the most important reasons to improve a stent design. Manufacturers try to achieve this goal without compromising radial support and lesion coverage. Another element, not specifically part of the design but very specific to the stent, is its radiologic visibility.

Many of these characteristics were not introduced with the idea to make a stent more suitable for a specific lesion. Every stent manufacturer is likely to assume that its stent will be employed in the largest number of lesions as possible.

This chapter focuses on the specific features of a stent design that make a specific stent more suitable or less suitable for a particular type of lesion or anatomy. We also review our experience and the results obtained at Columbus Hospital since 1992 in which different types of stents have been used.

## TYPES OF STENTS

Stents can be classified according to their type of delivery system (self-expanding, balloon expand-

able), their composition (stainless steel, cobalt-based alloy, tantalum, nitinol, biodegradable, polymeric), and their design (mesh structure, slotted tube, coil). According to the manufacturers, all stents are suitable for implantation in native coronary arteries of appropriate size, and the indications for the Palmaz-Schatz stent have been expanded to lesions located in vein grafts. No stent is specifically designed to be implanted in a particular lesion, and the absolute or relative contraindications to the use of stents apply to stents in general and not to a specific stent.

Described as follows is our view of selective use of different stents in different lesions.

## Proximal Lesions Not Located at a Bend (>45 Degrees) Without Significant Tortuosity in the Proximal Segment and Without a Significant Angle at the End of the Lesion to Create a Hinge Point

The ideal stents for these types of lesions are the ones with slotted tubular design. The lesion coverage, the recoil, and the risk of plaque prolapse are reduced with this type of design. These features are important for offering the largest possible final diameter. Currently, the achievement of a large final diameter remains the most solid approach to limiting late restenosis.[3]

These types of lesions were the ones included in the initial evaluation of the Palmaz-Schatz stent. Three large studies employed this stent in lesions that are similar to the ones referred to in this paragraph.[1, 2, 7] The first study was a multicenter clinical trial with the Palmaz-Schatz stent[7] that extended from December 1987 to September 1989. In this study, 226 patients underwent stent implantation of native coronary arteries with a rigid prototype and subsequently with the Palmaz-Schatz stent in the United States. The other two studies were the BENESTENT[1] and the STRESS[1] study. The common

# TABLE 36–1. STENT ENGINEERING DATA

| BRAND | MANUFACTURER | STRUCTURE | MATERIAL | STRUT (WIRE) THICKNESS, MM | METAL ARTERY (%) | RECOIL | FORE-SHORT-ENING | RADIO-PACITY | MARKERS | LENGTH (MM) | DIAMETERS (MM) |
|---|---|---|---|---|---|---|---|---|---|---|---|
| ACS MultiLink | ACS | Etched tube | Stainless steel | 0.06 | 7–15 | <5% | 3% | Low | No | 15 | 3.0; 3.25; 3.5 |
| ACT One | PAS | Slotted tube | Nitinol | 0.177 | 36 | 3–6% | 11% | Moderate | No | 7; 15 | 3.0–6.0 |
| AngioStent | Angiodynamics | Single wire, long spine | Platinum, iridium | 0.127 | 10–1 | 7% | 12% | High | No | 15; 25; 35 | 3.0–6.0 |
| AVE Micro II | AVE | Wire crown | Stainless steel | 0.15–0.20 | 8,5 | 8% | Minimal | Moderate | No | 6; 12; 18; 30; 39 | 2.5–3.5–4.0 |
| AVE Gfx | AVE | Eliptorectangular | Stainless steel | 0.127 | 21 | 4% | Minimal | Moderate | No | 8; 12; 18; 24; 30; 40 | 3.0–3.5–4.0 |
| Bard-XT | Bard | Modular zigzag | Stainless steel | 0.15 | 13–20 | Minimal | None | Moderate | Yes | 6; 11; 15; 19; 24; 30; 37 | 2.5–4.0 |
| BeStent | Medtronic | Slotted tube | Stainless steel | 0.075 | 12–18 | Minimal | None | Low | Yes | 15; 25; 35 | 3.0–5.5 |
| DiVisio | Biocompatibles | Interlocking arrowhead | Stainless steel | 0.075 | 14 | 2% | <2% | Low | | 8; 15; 28; 40 | 2.5–3.5,3.0–8.0* |
| Cook Gianturco-Roubin II | Cook | Coil spine | Stainless steel | 0.076 | 15–20 | 9–11% | None | Low | Yes | 20; 40 | 2.5–3.0–3.5–4.0 |
| Cordis | Cordis JJ | Single sinusoidal helical coil | Tantalum | 0.127 | 15 | <10% | 10% | High | No | 15 | 3.0–3.5–4.0 |
| Cross-Flex | Cordis JJ | Single wire | Stainless steel | 0.15 | 15 | Minimal | 5% | Low | No | 15 | 3.0–3.5–4.0 |
| Cross-Flex II | Cordis JJ | Single sinusoidal, helical coil welded | Stainless steel wire | 0.15 | 15-18-21 | <5% | <10% | Good | 2 | 15; 25; 35 | 3.0; 3.5; 4 |
| Crown | Cordis JJ | Slotted tube | Stainless steel | 0.069 | 17–20 | 2% | 5% | Low | No | 15; 22; 30 | 3.0–3.5–4.0 |
| Freedom | Global Therapeutics | Single wire fishbone | Stainless steel | 0.178 | 11–15 | 5–9% | Minimal | Low | No | 12; 16; 20; 24; 30; 40 | 2.5–4.5 |
| NIR seven-cell | Medinol | Multicell design | Stainless steel | 0.06–0.10 | 14–19 | 2% | Minimal | Low | No | 9; 16; 25; 32 | 2.0–3.5 |
| NIR nine-cell | Medinol | Multicell design | Stainless steel | 0.064; 0.1 spiral | 20 | 2% | Minimal | Low | No | 9; 16; 25; 32 | 3.0–5.0 |
| Palmaz-Schatz | Cordis JJ | Slotted tube | Stainless steel | | | 5% | Minimal | Low | No | 8; 9; 14; 18 | 3.0–5.0 |
| Pura | Devon JJ | Slotted tube | Stainless steel | 0.10 | 24 | <1.9% | 3.14% | Low | No | 7; 15 | 3.0–5.0 |
| Pura Vario | Devon JJ | Slotted tube | Stainless steel | 0.13 | 17–21 | <2.5% | 3.14% | Low | No | 10; 16; 22; 28; 34; 40 | 3.0–5.0 |
| IRIS | Uni-Cath | Slotted tube | Stainless steel | NA | 14 | NA | <10% | Low | No | 17; 27; 37 | 3.5–4.0 |
| Wiktor | Medtronic | Single wire | Tantalum | 0.13 | 8 | 9% | 4% | High | No | 16 | 3.0–3.5–4,0–4.5 |
| Wallstent | Schneider | Multiple wire braid | Elgiloy† | 0.10 | 20 | NA | 30% | Moderate | No | 15–45 | 4.0–6.0 |
| TENSUM | Biotronic | Slotted tube | Tantalum | 0.20 | 13 | NA | NA | Good | No | 14 | 3.0–4.0 |

NA, not available.

*Five element structure for 2.5–3.5 mm and six element structure for 3.0–8.0 mm.

†Cobalt-based alloy

denominator of these studies is the implantation of this stent in relatively straight lesions, located in the proximal segment of the vessel and usually shorter than 10 mm. One important element of these early studies is the lesion selection.

The characteristics of the Palmaz-Schatz stent are such that implantation of this stent in complex anatomy is quite difficult. This statement is particularly true in view of the time period in which those studies were performed, when no high support guide wires were available. In the BENESTENT study,[1] 50% of the lesions treated with stents were concentric, and only 11% showed some calcifications; in the STRESS study,[2] only 13% of the lesions with stents showed an angle over 45 degrees at the lesion site. This particular selection resulted from the difficulties in deploying this stent in complex anatomy. All these features show that the stent itself contributed to a "favorable" lesion selection.

The introduction of the spiral articulated stent has improved the lesion coverage at the articulation site without significantly affecting the neointima formation, which appears to reach its maximal thickness at the center of the lesion.[8] The ability to deliver the new spiral articulated Palmaz-Schatz stent (PS 154) appears slightly inferior to that of the one with the bridge articulation (PS 153).

For the lesions treated in these studies, we think the Palmaz-Schatz stent, its updated versions (spiral articulated PS154 and the Crown stent), or other types of slotted tubular stents (e.g., the NIR, ACS MultiLink, BeStent, Pura Vario) are most probably the most suitable.

Among the new stents with designs relatively similar to that of the Palmaz-Schatz stent, the Pura Vario A series (Davon Medical, Hamburg, Germany) should be mentioned in particular. This stent has a few positive features in addition to the ones of the classic Palmaz-Schatz: rounded edges at the free ends of each strut, absence of transversal bridge connection between the struts (to decrease the crimped profile), absence of the longitudinal bridge, and availability in two designs and thicknesses for vessels larger and smaller than 3.5 mm in diameter.

What needs to be kept in mind in that the Palmaz-Schatz stent still holds a unique track record that can be challenged only with comparable data rather than with theoretical assumptions.

We have analyzed in our database 1059 lesions (in 890 patients) treated with the Palmaz-Schatz stent. The summary findings are reported in Tables 36–2 and 36–3. It is evident from these data that the reference vessel size for these lesions is relatively large—3.10 ± 0.53 mm—and therefore, in the interpretation of these results, it must be remembered that the deliverability of this stent performs a favorable lesion selection. The overall trend is what will

**TABLE 36–2.    GLOBAL PALMAZ-SCHATZ EXPERIENCE**

| | |
|---|---|
| No. patients | 890 |
| No. lesions | 1059 |
| No. stents/lesion | 1.4 |
| Rate of procedural success | 98% |
| Thrombosis | 1.8 |
| No. vessels with ref ≥3 mm | 615 (59%) |
| No. vessels with ref <3 mm | 423 (41%) |
| Average ref vessel size | 3.10 ± 0.53 |
| Average size of large vessels | 3.46 ± 0.42 |
| Average size of small vessels | 2.66 ± 0.27 |

Ref = reference.

be seen with the other stents: high delivery success (the operator knows where the delivery will not be successful and avoids attempts to deliver in such vessels), thrombosis rate slightly over 1%, and restenosis rates that depend on reference vessel size and lesion length.

One element to be considered when a slotted tubular stent is used is the relation of the extremities of the stent with the non–stent-implanted vessel. If there is a significant angulation between one extremity of the stent and the proximal or distal vessel (it is more common with the distal vessel) or if this angulation is created by the rigid stent, the resulting hinge may alter the lumen size, the flow dynamics, or both and have a negative impact on stent restenosis.[9] Figure 36–1 demonstrates this hinge effect caused by an NIR stent, which becomes rigid upon deployment. This particular lesion restenosed 4 months later at the distal extremity of the stent (Fig. 36–2). The operator should be aware of these situations and select a different type of stent.

## Lesions Situated on a Curve (>45 Degrees) or Immediately Followed by a Curve

No specific study has examined this issue. In view of the straightening effect caused by a slotted tubu-

**TABLE 36–3.    FOLLOW-UP RESULTS OF THE GLOBAL PALMAZ-SCHATZ EXPERIENCE**

| | |
|---|---|
| No. lesions eligible for FU | 1032 |
| No. lesions assessed in FU | 619 (61%) |
| Global restenosis rate | 19 (CI, 16%–22%) |
| Ref ≥3 mm, lesion length <10 mm | 280 (RR, 13%; CI, 9%–17%) |
| Ref ≥3 mm, lesion length >10 mm | 93 (RR, 24%; CI, 15%–33%) |
| Ref <3 mm, lesion length <10 mm | 171 (RR, 23%; CI, 17%–30%) |
| Ref <3 mm, lesion length <10 mm | 72 (RR, 30%; CI, 19%–41%) |

CI, confidence interval; FU, follow-up; Ref, reference; RR, relative risk.

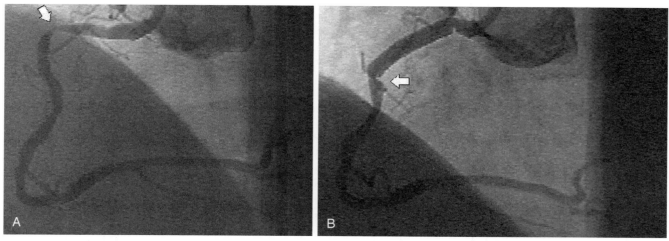

FIGURE 36–1. *A*, Baseline angiogram of a lesion *(arrow)* in the proximal right coronary artery. *B*, After implantation of a nine-cell, 16-mm-long NIR stent. The hinge site at the end of the stent is clear *(arrow)*.

lar stent and the possible consequences on restenosis, the operator should consider using a stent that conforms better to the original anatomy.

The choices are among the classic coil stents as the Gianturco-Roubin II stent, the Wiktor-*i* stent (similar to the original Wiktor stent but with tighter waves), the Cross-Flex stent, and the Cross-Flex II stent (similar to the original Cross-Flex but with welding among the coils). Another alternative is the AVE Micro II stent; concerns regarding this stent are related to the wire thickness (0.20 mm) and to the gaps, which may result in curved segments after attempts to optimize the lumen diameter. The new and improved Gfx stent (oval wire thickness, 0.012 mm; crown length, 2 mm) is probably free from these limitations and may be considered another good alternative.

The ACS MultiLink stent, despite being a slotted

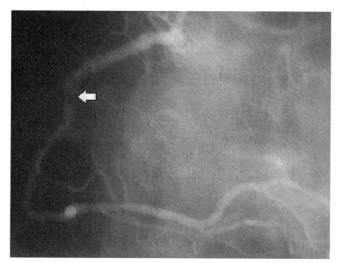

FIGURE 36–2. Follow-up angiogram of the lesion in Figure 36–1, 4 months later, showing restenosis at the hinge site *(arrow)*. LAD, left anterior descending artery.

tubular stent, has unique flexibility that could make this stent suitable for a lesions on a bend. Another alternative, the Wallstent, is also a flexible stent.

Our initial evaluation of the Cross-Flex stent and its latest version, Cross-Flex II, has been positive in terms of final lumen achieved and conformability to the anatomy. No long-term follow-up data are available. The thickness of the stainless steel wire (0.15 mm) could be a concern in vessels 3 mm in diameter or smaller.

We do not know the results of any large randomized study comparing different coil stents. In our database, we found 163 lesions located at a bend of more than 45 degrees in which stents were implanted. The overall restenosis rate (64% of patients underwent angiographic follow-up) was 33%. The Palmaz-Schatz stent was associated with a 21% restenosis rate; there was no trend to suggest that other specific stents yielded a better restenosis rate.

## Ostial Lesions

Ostial lesions are classified as either aorto-ostial or coronary ostial.

For aorto-ostial lesions, the slotted tubular design, preferably with strong radial support and radiologic visibility, is the most appropriate one.[10] For vessels 4 mm in diameter or larger, the Palmaz biliary stent seems very suitable because it has good radial support at this size and good radiologic visibility. For aorto-ostial lesions located in vessels smaller than 4.0 mm, we favor the spiral articulated Palmaz-Schatz stent, which, with a strut thickness of 0.1 mm (0.064 mm for the model with the bridge articulation), has good radial support and fair radiopacity. It is conceivable that the NIR stent with its radiopaque version (NIR Royal) is also useful for this application.

For lesions that are located at a coronary ostium

and are not aorto-ostial, the decision is quite open among the different slotted tubular designs; the presence of a proximal marker or the radiopacity of the stent are favorable features.

## Bifurcational Lesions

The most important element in stent implantation in a bifurcational lesion is to decide whether (1) both branches of the bifurcation need to receive stents or (2) only the major one needs a stent while the other branch is dilated through the deployed stent. In implanting stents in bifurcational lesions, the operator should be aware that no report, registry, or selected case series has ever shown that implanting stents in both branches of the bifurcation has a positive impact on restenosis (Table 36–4). In our opinion, the possible exception to this statement is a situation where both branches are quite large (3.5 mm or more) and the operator has been able to effectively debulk the lesions.

The goal is to try not to implant stents in both branches. Placement of the stent in the large branch and dilating into the small one is a very practical solution. When this approach is not appropriate, both branches do require stent implantation.

There are situations in which, for whatever reasons (the most common one being the size of the branch in association with a poor result after angioplasty), the operator decides to deploy stents in both branches. The approaches we consider more friendly and successful are the V approach, the T approach, and the Y approach. At the present time we favor the use of various slotted tubular stents or the Gfx stent for all these approaches; we also consider the Gianturco-Roubin II and Cross-Flex II stents for the T and Y approaches.

The V approach is performed with the intent to create a new carina slightly proximal to the actual bifurcation. The stents should be advanced separately, should be at the site of the lesion at the time of deployment, should initially be inflated separately (to prevent one stent from slipping forward), and should finally be inflated again simultaneously. Intravascular ultrasound guidance is important in this situation to check that both stents are well expanded at their proximal ends (Figs. 36–3, 36–4). We performed several implantations with this technique, and the creation of a proximal carina did not lead to stent thrombosis.

The T approach is performed by advancing the first stent into the branch (the vertical segment of the T) and advancing the other stent into the major vessel (the horizontal segment of the T); the first stent is then pulled back exactly to the ostium, even with minimal protrusion into the main vessel, and then deployed. The fact that the stent into the main vessel is already in place (but not deployed) allows the operator to deploy the first stent, even protruding slightly into the main vessel. The wire and the

## TABLE 36–4. RESULTS OF BIFURCATIONAL STENT IMPLANTATION WITH STENTS IN BOTH BRANCHES

| No. patients | 32 |
| No. stents/lesion | $1.2 \pm 0.8$ |
| Lesion success rate | 95% |
| Balloon-vessel ratio | $1.2 \pm 0.2$ |
| Final balloon size (mm) | $3.3 \pm 0.4$ |
| Final pressure (mm Hg) | $15.0 \pm 3.3$ |
| Angiographic follow-up | 67% |
| Restenosis rate | 29% |

| ANGIOGRAPHIC DATA | PREIMPLANTATION | FINAL | FOLLOW-UP |
|---|---|---|---|
| Reference diameter (mm) | $2.8 \pm 0.5$ | — | — |
| Minimal luminal diameter (mm) | $1.1 \pm 0.7$ | $2.8 \pm 0.7$ | $1.6 \pm 0.8$ |
| % stenosis* | $61.3 \pm 24.2$ | $5.1 \pm 18.3$ | $43.5 \pm 25.4$ |
| Lesion length (mm) | $8.2 \pm 6.2$ | — | — |

| FOLLOW-UP RESULTS | % | ANGIOGRAPHIC FOLLOW-UP (%) | RESTENOSIS RATE (%) |
|---|---|---|---|
| Palmaz-Schatz stent only | 31 | 47 | 38 |
| Combination | 4 | 33 | 0 |
| Cook stent | 16 | 78 | 43 |
| Wiktor stent | 2 | 100 | 100 |
| Micro stent | 22 | 85 | 36 |
| Cordis stent | 2 | 100 | 0 |
| NIR stent | 19 | 80 | 18 |
| ACS stent | 2 | 0 | — |
| Pura Vario stent | 2 | 0 | — |

*Percentage of luminal diameter affected by stenosis.

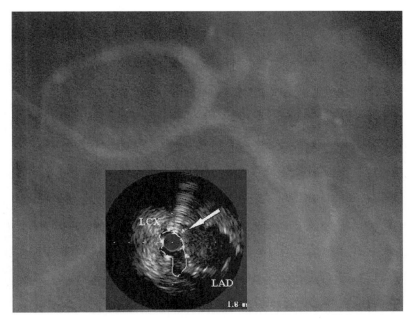

FIGURE 36–3. Angiogram showing a bifurcational lesion involving the origin of the left anterior descending artery (LAD) and of the circumflex artery after deployment of two MultiLink stents with the V "kissing" approach. Despite a good angiographic result after kissing inflation, intravascular ultrasound interrogation shows that the stent at the origin of the circumflex artery is partially compressed *(arrow)*.

balloon are then removed from the side vessel, and the other stent is deployed into the major vessel. If necessary, the stent into the side branch will have to be recrossed (usually with a fixed wire system) to perform a kissing inflation (Figs. 36–5, 36–6).

The Y approach is performed in the same manner as the V approach except that a third stent is sandwiched between two balloons, which are then advanced on the two wires left in place. This third stent is attached to the V stents, and the two balloons are inflated, partially protruding into the two arms of the V (which has now become a Y) to allow spreading of the distal part of the proximal stents toward the two branches with the V stents. This approach, which was quite demanding with the original Palmaz-Schatz stent, can now be performed

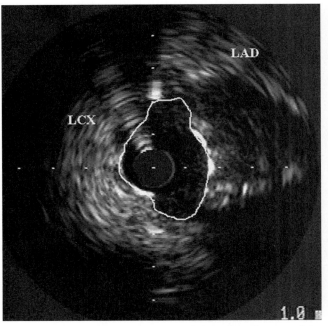

FIGURE 36–4. Intravascular ultrasound (IVUS) evaluation of the lesion in Figure 36–3, after a higher pressure "kissing" inflation. There is now a better expansion of the stent at the ostium of the left circumflex artery (LCX). IVUS evaluation of the left anterior descending artery (LAD) confirmed persistent good expansion of this second stent.

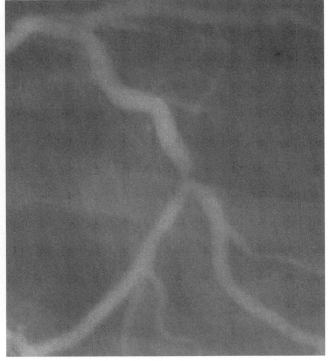

FIGURE 36–5. Baseline angiogram of a stenosis involving the bifurcation of the circumflex artery and of the obtuse marginal branch.

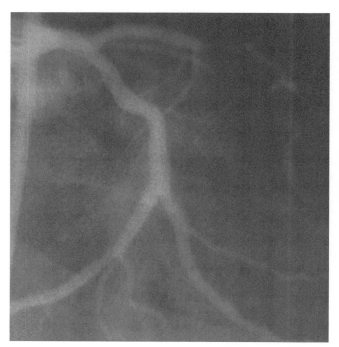

FIGURE 36–6. Result after directional atherectomy and deployment of two NIR stents with the T approach.

more easily with new-generation, low-profile, slotted tubular stents. The seven-cell NIR stent (when the proximal vessel is 3.5 mm or less in diameter) is particularly suited to be mounted on the two balloons because of its low profile.

The availability, at least in Europe, of a number of low-profile stents increased the success of these approaches. With appropriate case selection, success (stent delivery, angiographic patency, no Q-wave myocardial infarction, no need for emergency CABG, no death) can now be expected in 95% of the lesions in which stent implantation is attempted.

In kissing stent implantation with slotted tubular stents, one important problem that should always be kept in mind is the risk of balloon rupture, caused by puncturing of the balloon by the strut extremities of the stent positioned in the side branch or vice versa. We noticed that this risk decreased, but did not disappear, with the new generation of slotted tubular stents. This type of complication can sometimes be difficult to solve, especially if stent optimization in both branches is one goal to be achieved. The availability of strong balloons can help, but sometimes, because of their high profile, they cannot be advanced in the deployed stent, which may need further dilatation. For these reasons, the best approach is to avoid situations in which this complication can occur. Stent selection is therefore an important element.

In view of all these elements at present time, we think that the most appropriate stent for a kissing bifurcational lesion is probably the new AVE Gfx stent. This stent is free of sharp edges, it has good radial support, it has lesion coverage quite similar to that of a slotted tubular stent, it is moderately visible radiologically (an important element in dealing with bifurcational lesions), and it is reasonably amenable to being recrossed even by another stent. This last issue is also important because it is always possible that after the deployment of both kissing stents, a dissection appears distally to one of the two stents, creating the need to implant another stent distally to a deployed stent in the bifurcation. These considerations do not mean that bifurcational stent implantation will not be successful with other stent types (as a matter of fact, most of our bifurcation have been successfully performed with other stents besides the Gfx); rather, there are some theoretical advantages of some new stent designs and their possible impact in facilitating stent implantation of this still complex lesion subset. Experience will confirm whether these considerations will lead to higher success and better efficiency.

Another important stent for treating bifurcations is the Mini Crown on a low-profile delivery system. The availability of this stent with a very thin sheath allows safe stent implantation in a branch through the struts of a deployed stent. This modality gives to the operator the option to place a stent into the branch if angioplasty has not been successful. This protected stent can also be placed distally to a bifurcation treated with kissing stents in case a dissection develops distally to one deployed stent.

In Milan, we treated bifurcations with kissing stent implantation (excluding left main artery bifurcations) in 32 patients. We used the Palmaz-Schatz stent in 38% of the lesions, the AVE MicroStent in 22%, and the NIR and Gianturco-Roubin stents in the remaining 40%. The overall restenosis rate was 29%; no stent performed particularly better than another one.

The approach of using a stent in one branch and dilating the other branch through the struts is more simple, is less expensive, and yields results comparable with those of using two or more stents (Table 36–5).

An interesting new approach in treating bifurcational lesions is the use of debulking with rotational atherectomy or directional atherectomy (when possible) before stent implantation. Preliminary follow-up results so far are encouraging. It will be determined whether the reduction in restenosis is sufficient to justify the complexity and the cost of the procedure.

## Lesions Located at the Left Main Stem

Percutaneous treatment of left main lesions is currently performed on a protected left main artery or

**TABLE 36–5.  RESULTS OF BIFURCATIONAL STENT IMPLANTATION WITH STENTS IN ONE BRANCH**

| | | | |
|---|---|---|---|
| No. patients | 78 | | |
| No. stents/lesion | 1.2 ± 0.5 | | |
| Lesion success rate | 99% | | |
| Balloon-vessel ratio | 1.2 ± 0.2 | | |
| Final balloon size (mm) | 3.4 ± 0.4 | | |
| Final pressure (mm Hg) | 16.2 ± 3.8 | | |
| Angiographic follow-up | 59% | | |
| Restenosis rate | 34% | | |
| ANGIOGRAPHIC DATA | PREIMPLANTATION | FINAL | FOLLOW-UP |
| Reference diameter (mm) | 2.9 ± 0.4 | — | — |
| Minimal luminal diameter (mm) | 0.9 ± 0.5 | 2.9 ± 0.6 | 1.8 ± 0.9 |
| % stenosis* | 68.9 ± 17.7 | 6.5 ± 10.8 | 38.1 ± 27.2 |
| Lesion length (mm) | 10.3 ± 6.0 | — | — |
| FOLLOW-UP RESULTS | % | ANGIOGRAPHIC FOLLOW-UP (%) | RESTENOSIS RATE (%) |
| Palmaz-Schatz stent only | 27 | 67 | 21 |
| Combination | 5 | 67 | 0 |
| Cook stent | 15 | 75 | 33 |
| Wiktor stent | 2 | 50 | 100 |
| Micro stent | 12 | 60 | 67 |
| Cordis stent | 2 | 50 | 0 |
| NIR stent | 20 | 44 | 29 |
| ACS stent | 6 | 0 | — |
| Crown stent | 6 | 80 | 50 |
| BeStent | 4 | 100 | 33 |
| Cross-Flex II stent | 1 | 0 | — |

*Percentage of luminal diameter affected by stenosis.

on selected patients without protected circulation. The clinical indications for treating these lesions with stent implantation are not discussed here; we discuss only the technical aspects involved in stent selection.

Treatment of left main lesions frequently involves treatment of both an aorto-ostial lesion and a bifurcational lesion. The stent selected is almost always a slotted tubular one or an AVE MicroStent. The size of the left main artery is quite favorable to stent implantation in terms of restenosis rate. The major problem is that in an unprotected left main artery, stent restenosis may manifest either with sudden death or with unstable angina rapidly followed by death. For this reason, when stent implantation in an unprotected left main artery is clinically indicated, we invariably debulk the lesion before the procedure to minimize the risk of restenosis.

The results of our experience involving stent implantation of protected and unprotected left main arteries are summarized in Table 36–6.

## Calcified Lesions

Despite the widespread notion that calcium affects stent expansion,[11] there are only few reports specifically dealing with this issue.[12–14] The general view is that stent expansion in a calcified lesion will yield a smaller final lumen than will expansion in a noncalcified lesion. Adequate final expansion is usually achieved by stretching the softer part of the wall. If an adequate final lumen is achieved, this approach does not seem to affect restenosis.[15] In order to obtain a good final lumen size, it is important to have a stent with minimal recoil and good radial strength. Therefore, a slotted tubular stent should be used in calcified lesions.

The best slotted tubular models are the Palmaz-Schatz stent with the spiral articulation, the NIR stent, and other variations of the two (Pura Vario, Sito). The best nonslotted tubular models are the AVE MicroStent II, the AVE Gfx, and the Cross-Flex. If the operator successfully debulks the lesion, the ACS MultiLink stent could also be used.

Our experience in implanting stents into lesions with angiographic calcifications is summarized in Table 36–7. It must be kept in mind that most of the complex and longer lesions were treated with the new stents. This type of lesion selection affects the results.

## Chronic Total Occlusions

Stent implantation for chronic total occlusions has to deal with two problems: (1) The amount of plaque mass in these types of lesions is large, and (2) it is not rare that the passage through the occluded segment occurs by creating a false lumen with reentry.

## TABLE 36–6. RESULTS OF LEFT MAIN ARTERY STENT IMPLANTATION

| | | | |
|---|---|---|---|
| No. patients | 48 | | |
| Lesion success rate | 88% | | |
| Balloon-vessel ratio | 1.1 ± 0.2 | | |
| Final balloon size (mm) | 3.9 ± 0.6 | | |
| Final pressure (mm Hg) | 15.6 ± 4.1 | | |
| Angiographic follow-up | 76% | | |
| Restenosis rate | 16% | | |

| ANGIOGRAPHIC DATA | | PREIMPLANTATION | FINAL | FOLLOW-UP |
|---|---|---|---|---|
| Reference diameter (mm) | | 3.8 ± 0.8 | — | — |
| Minimal luminal diameter (mm) | | 1.5 ± 0.8 | 3.6 ± 0.9 | 2.6 ± 0.9 |
| % stenosis* | | 65.4 ± 19.1 | 6.1 ± 16.8 | 36.3 ± 32.4 |
| Lesion length (mm) | | 6.3 ± 3.4 | — | — |

| FOLLOW-UP RESULTS | % | ANGIOGRAPHIC FOLLOW-UP (%) | RESTENOSIS RATE (%) |
|---|---|---|---|
| Palmaz-Schatz stent only | 82 | 79 | 15 |
| Combination | 4 | 100 | 0 |
| Micro stent | 4 | 100 | 50 |
| NIR stent | 6 | 67 | 0 |
| ACS stent | 4 | 0 | — |

*Percentage of luminal diameter affected by stenosis.

These two elements mandate the insertion of a stent with good lesion coverage and radial support. The Palmaz-Schatz stent was the one used in the Stenting In Chronic Coronary Occlusion (SICCO) study,[16] which reported significant benefit of stent implantation (32% restenosis) in comparison with PTCA (74% restenosis) after recanalization of chronic total occlusions.

In addition to various slotted tubular stents, the Wallstent should be considered for dealing with a large vessel, especially the right coronary artery.[17, 18]

Our results and experience with stent implanta-

## TABLE 36–7. RESULTS OF STENT IMPLANTATION CALCIFIED LESIONS

| | | | |
|---|---|---|---|
| No. patients | 254 | | |
| No. stents | 1.5 ± 1.1 | | |
| Lesion success rate | 95% | | |
| Balloon-vessel ratio | 1.2 ± 0.2 | | |
| Final balloon size (mm) | 3.6 ± 0.5 | | |
| Final pressure (mm Hg) | 16.0 ± 3.3 | | |
| Use of Rotablator | 33% | | |
| Angiographic follow-up | 76% | | |
| Restenosis rate | 26% | | |

| ANGIOGRAPHIC DATA | | PREIMPLANTATION | FINAL | FOLLOW-UP |
|---|---|---|---|---|
| Reference diameter (mm) | | 3.1 ± 0.5 | — | — |
| Minimal luminal diameter (mm) | | 0.9 ± 0.6 | 3.1 ± 0.6 | 2.0 ± 1.0 |
| % stenosis* | | 71.1 ± 17.0 | 1.8 ± 15.4 | 34.8 ± 28.7 |
| Lesion length (mm) | | 11.3 ± 7.3 | — | — |

| FOLLOW-UP DATA | % | ANGIOGRAPHIC FOLLOW-UP (%) | RESTENOSIS RATE (%) |
|---|---|---|---|
| Palmaz-Schatz stent | 48 | 80 | 16 |
| Combination | 9 | 79 | 37 |
| Cook stent | 8 | 84 | 43 |
| Wiktor stent | 1 | 75 | 0 |
| Micro stent | 8 | 61 | 50 |
| Cordis stent | 1 | 33 | 0 |
| Wallstent | 2 | 71 | 40 |
| AngioStent | 1 | 100 | 0 |
| NIR stent | 12 | 67 | 38 |
| ACS stent | 1 | 0 | — |
| Crown stent | 4 | 75 | 33 |
| BeStent | 5 | 73 | 27 |

*Percentage of luminal diameter affected by stenosis.

tion in chronic total occlusions are summarized in Table 36–8.

## Vessels Smaller than 3.0 Millimeters in Diameter

Stent implantation in small vessels is accompanied by a number of problems. First, no stents were specifically made to be expanded in small vessels with the capacity to gain optimal radial support at diameters between 2.5 and 3.0 mm. Only recently have stents such as the Mini Crown, the five-cell NIR, the small-vessel BeStent, and the small-vessel Pura Vario A, which are designed to fit vessels below 3 mm, been available. There are no follow-up data regarding these new stents; the initial findings are of good flexibility and capacity to reach quite distal lesions. For these reasons, we cannot make any specific recommendation.

Our experience with the stents that have been available so far indicates that the initial and follow-up results are quite good for lesions that are short (one 15-mm stent or smaller). We treated 782 lesions located in vessels smaller than 3 mm in 576 patients. Two important findings stand out: the thrombosis rate with optimal deployment and only antiplatelet therapy was 1.5% (not statistically different from the thrombosis rate in larger vessels), and the restenosis rate was significantly higher (32%) than that in larger vessels but not particularly high in focal lesions treated. The four stents that we used most frequently in small vessels were the Palmaz-Schatz, the Gianturco-Roubin I and II stents, and the NIR stent (initially the nine-cell and then the seven-cell versions). The NIR stent and the Gianturco-Roubin II stents have been used more frequently in distal locations and in vessels with a slightly smaller reference diameter. These are the most probable reasons why the restenosis rate has been higher with these two stents than with the Palmaz-Schatz stent.

One particular feature of our experience of implanting stents in vessels with angiographic diameter less than 3 mm is that the balloon-artery ratio for the final stent dilatation is significantly higher than the ratio employed in larger vessels (1.29 for small vessels vs. 1.09 for larger vessels; $p < 0.0001$). The explanation for this choice is that we use the information obtained by intravascular ultrasound study in order to maximize the lumen gain, particu-

## TABLE 36–8. RESULTS OF STENT IMPLANTATION IN CHRONIC TOTAL OCCLUSIONS

| | |
|---|---|
| No. patients | 280 |
| No. lesions | 294 |
| No. stents | $1.9 \pm 1.3$ |
| Lesion success rate | 94% |
| Balloon-vessel ratio | $1.2 \pm 0.2$ |
| Final balloon size (mm) | $3.6 \pm 0.5$ |
| Final pressure (mm Hg) | $14,9 \pm 4,1$ |
| Angiographic follow-up | 77% |
| Restenosis rate | 30% |
| Location of chronic total occlusions | |
|     LAD | 45% |
|     Diagonal | 2% |
|     RCA | 32% |
|     Cx | 14% |
|     OM | 5% |
|     SVG | 2% |

| ANGIOGRAPHIC DATA | PREIMPLANTATION | FINAL | FOLLOW-UP |
|---|---|---|---|
| Reference diameter (mm) | $3.1 \pm 0.2$ | — | — |
| Minimal luminal diameter (mm) | 0 | $3.0 \pm 0.6$ | $1.8 \pm 1.0$ |
| % stenosis* | 100 | $3.2 \pm 13.8$ | $40.7 \pm 34.6$ |
| Lesion length (mm) | | | |

| FOLLOW-UP RESULTS | % | ANGIOGRAPHIC FOLLOW-UP (%) | RESTENOSIS RATE (%) |
|---|---|---|---|
| Palmaz-Schatz stent only | 39 | 73 | 26 |
| Combination | 12 | 66 | 21 |
| Cook stent | 14 | 56 | 56 |
| MicroStent | 10 | — | — |
| NIR stent | 10 | 25 | 30 |
| Wallstent | 7 | 81 | 44 |
| Wiktor stent | 4 | 92 | 27 |
| BeStent | 4 | 91 | 40 |

Cx, circumflex artery; LAD, left anterior descending artery; RCA, right coronary artery; SVG, saphenous vein graft.
*Percentage of luminal diameter affected by stenosis.

# Stenting Small Vessels

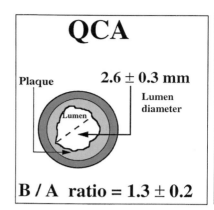

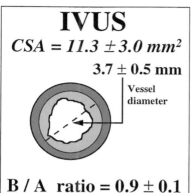

FIGURE 36–7. Evaluation of balloon-artery (B/A) ratio by quantitative coronary angiography (QCA) compared with the evaluation by intravascular ultrasound (IVUS). The presence of diffuse disease and of vascular remodeling explains the differences.

larly in small vessels. The amount of plaque (which decreases the angiographic lumen size) and the arterial remodeling (which enlarges the vessel size as measured, by intravascular ultrasound study) explain the differences between angiographic balloon sizing in comparison with sizing by intravascular ultrasound study (Fig. 36–7). At follow-up, the higher restenosis rate seen in small vessels was associated with a loss index that was significantly higher than that obtained in large vessels (0.55 vs. 0.47; $p = 0.0074$). We can only speculate on the possible causes for this higher loss index. Possible explanations include wall trauma resulting from aggressive dilatation, the use of stents not perfectly suited to be implanted in vessels smaller than 3 mm (higher recoil, more metal in relation to the vessel surface area), or a combination of the two. Independently from the explanation of these findings, the goal is to produce the largest possible lumen inside the stent.

Table 36–9 summarizes the evaluation of the most significant factors predictive of restenosis in large and small vessels. The size of final cross-sectional area inside the stent-implanted segment is the vari-

able with the strongest negative predictive value for restenosis. This association seems to be even stronger for small vessels.

## Saphenous Vein Grafts

Implanting stents in lesions located in a saphenous vein graft usually involves dealing with a long lesion located on a large vessels. This is why we consider the Wallstent the most suitable device for lesions in these locations, despite unsatisfactory early results: a reported 7.6% rate of mortality and a 24% rate of complete occlusion reported in 1991.[19, 20] Results subsequently improved, with a decrease in the incidence of stent occlusion (3.4%), but there remained a high incidence of hemorrhagic complications (17%).[21] During the following years, results improved mainly because of increased experience.[22] The introduction of the Palmaz-Schatz stent in the United States allowed a significant increase in the numbers of patients treated with sustained improvement in the results: a procedural success rate exceeding 97% and a thrombosis rate of

**TABLE 36–9.    MULTIVARIATE ANALYSIS FOR RESTENOSIS OF LARGE AND SMALL VESSELS EVALUATED BY IVUS STUDY**

| VARIABLE | ODDS RATIO | CONFIDENCE INTERVAL | $p$ |
|---|---|---|---|
| **Total Cohort: 1673 Lesions*** | | | |
| Final stent IVUS CSA | 1.202 | 1.09–1.33 | 0.0005 |
| Angiographic reference diameter | 1.866 | 1.16–3.00 | 0.0103 |
| Lesion length | 1.043 | 1.02–1.07 | 0.0006 |
| **Small Vessel Cohort: 782 Lesions†** | | | |
| Final stent CSA | 1.263 | 1.09–1.46 | 0.0014 |

CSA, cross-section area; IVUS, intravascular ultrasound.
*These are the only three variables that remained significant with the stepwise logistic regression.
†Only this variable remained significant.

0.6% to 1.4%.[23, 24] In addition to the Palmaz-Schatz stent, the Palmaz biliary stent is frequently employed in large grafts and in the aorto-ostial location (because of its good visibility).[25]

Stent implantation can currently be considered the necessary final step of any intervention performed in vein grafts. Early reports referred to a high incidence of adverse events or graft occlusion; the subsequent elimination of anticoagulant therapy contributed to the decrease in these procedural complications.

One persisting problem with stent implantation in vein grafts is that future adverse events may result from progression of other lesions that were not considered critical at the time of initial stent implantation on the target lesion.[26] This issue will be evaluated by prospective studies comparing a strategy of focal stent implantation on the critical lesions with a strategy aimed also to implant stents in lesions not angiographically critical.

For all these reasons, vein graft stent implantation must be performed with a stent with optimal lesion coverage and available in different lengths (vein grafts require longer stents). The Wallstent best satisfies these requirements. For more focal lesions, the Palmaz-Schatz stent, the Crown stent (its more current version), and the nine-cell NIR stent are good choices.

The other issue quite unique to vein graft is the risk of distal embolization. It has been our experience that no particular stent currently available is more likely than another to limit this complications. In this regard, other options such as infusion of ReoPro, transluminal extraction catheter (TEC) atherectomy,[27] or both performed before stent implantation may be more effective.

## Acute Closure and Threatened Closure

Closure is the typical situation in which stents were originally applied.[28, 29] The stents used most extensively are the Gianturco-Roubin I stent[30, 31] and the Palmaz-Schatz stent.[32] Higher rates of success, even in complex anatomy and long dissections, have been reported with the Gianturco-Roubin II stent[33] and with the AVE II MicroStent.[34]

We think that the ideal stent for treating a dissection with impending closure should be available premounted (possibly on a high-pressure balloon), should be easy to deliver even in complex anatomy, should have a reasonable lesion coverage capacity, and should be available in different lengths. The new Gianturco-Roubin II stent, the AVE II MicroStent, the AVE Gfx stent, and the Cross-Flex II stent satisfy these requirements better than do other stents.

Treatment of dissections may include placing a short stent distally to an already deployed stent, usually to treat a residual distal dissection not evident at the time of the first stent implantation. The AVE MicroStent II stent, the new Gfx stent, and the Mini Crown stent on a low-profile delivery system are the most appropriate choices for this situation. The possibility of completely sealing a dissection, especially in the setting of impending closure, remains one important predictor of stent occlusion even with the use of high-pressure dilatation after stent implantation and with administration of aspirin and ticlopidine.[35] Therefore, the stent with the best predictable delivery is likely to be the preferred one. It will also be the one with the lowest incidence of stent thrombosis if it provides good dissection coverage (no prolapse) and has been implanted correctly.

## Special Situations

There are instances in which the operator needs to modify the tools available in order to provide a new device capable of satisfying a need. Three of these conditions are the treatment of severe focal aneurysmatic dilatation of the coronary arteries, the treatment of more diffuse aneurysmatic disease of vein grafts, and, occasionally, the treatment of coronary perforations. The use of an autologous vein graft–coated stent is an interesting solution pioneered by Stefanadis and associates.[36, 37] The Palmaz-Schatz stent, the NIR stent, and other slotted tubular stents are good platforms on which the autologous vein is mounted.

Another use for this solution is the treatment of restenotic saphenous vein graft ostial lesions. Because of the high incidence of a second restenosis in this type of aorto-ostial lesions, the vein-covered stent should be considered among the options.

## CONCLUSIONS

Among all the theoretical and practical considerations and reasons we gave for selecting a particular stent to treat a specific lesion, the experience and confidence of the operator should top of the list.

Table 36–10 is a "consumer's guide" summarizing what we believe are the typical features of that make certain stents more suitable than others for a specific indication. No rationale for choosing is yet supported by randomized trials. Nonetheless, a large number of observational studies support the views expressed in this chapter.

Except for bail-out stent implantation, stents are implanted with the intent to prevent restenosis. Therefore, the operator should strive to reach this goal in the frame of patient's safety. Optimal stent

## TABLE 36–10. SUMMARY OF STENTS FOR SPECIFIC LESIONS

| STENT | DISCRETE | LONG | CALCIFIED | OSTIAL | BIFURCATIONS | AT SIDE BRANCH | AT BEND | DISSECTIONS | TORTUOSITY | SVG |
|---|---|---|---|---|---|---|---|---|---|---|
| Palmaz-Schatz | ++ | − | + | ++ | + | − | − | − | − | + |
| Crown | ++ | ++ | ++ | ++ | + | − | − | − | − | ++ |
| NIR | ++ | ++ | ++ | ++ | + | ++* | + | +* | +* | ++ |
| BeStent | ++ | ++ | + | ++ | − | + | − | + | | ++ |
| ACT 1 | ++ | − | | | | | | | | |
| Gianturco-Roubin (GR) stent | | | | | | | | | | |
|   GR I | − | − | − | − | − | + | + | ++ | − | − |
|   GR II | − | + | − | − | + | +++ | ++ | +++ | +++ | − |
| Wiktor | + | − | − | − | − | +++ | ++ | + | ++ | − |
| Flex Stent | + | − | − | − | + | + | ++ | − | ++ | − |
| AngioStent | + | − | − | − | − | + | ++ | − | ++ | − |
| Freedom | | − | − | − | − | + | | − | | − |
| MultiLink | +++ | − | + | + | + | ++ | + | + | + | − |
| AVE | ++ | ++ | ++ | ++ | ++ | +++ | − | +++ | +++ | − |
| Wallstent | − | + | − | − | − | − | − | − | − | +++ |

SVG, saphenous vein graft.

−, Not recommended; +, good; ++, very good; +++, excellent.

*For the seven-cell design.

selection in order to achieve an optimal result (minimal luminal diameter) most important.

## REFERENCES

1. Serruys PW, de Jaegere P, et al: A comparison of balloon-expandable-stent implantation with balloon angioplasty in patients with coronary artery disease. N Engl J Med 331:489, 1994.
2. Fischman DL, Leon MB, Baim DS, et al: A randomized comparison of coronary-stent placement and balloon angioplasty in the treatment of coronary artery disease. N Engl J Med 331:496, 1994.
3. Colombo A, Hall P, Nakamura S, et al: Intracoronary stenting without anticoagulation accomplished with intravascular ultrasound. Circulation 91:1676, 1995.
4. Schömig A, Neumann FJ, Kastrati A, et al: A randomized comparison of antiplatelet and anticoagulation therapy after the placement of coronary-artery stents. N Engl J Med 334:1084, 1996.
5. Karrillon GJ, Morice MC, Benveniste E, et al: Intracoronary stent implantation without ultrasound guidance and with replacement of conventional anticoagulation by antiplatelet therapy: 30-day clinical outcome of the French Multicenter Registry. Circulation 94:1519, 1996.
6. Meyer BJ, Meyer B, Bonzel T, et al: Interventional cardiology in Europe 1994. Eur Heart J 17:1318, 1996.
7. Schatz RA, Baim DS, Leon M, et al: Clinical experience with the Palmaz-Schatz coronary stent. Initial results of a multicenter study. Circulation 83:148, 1991.
8. Werner F, Regar E, Klauss V et al: Does a different stent design lead to a different pattern of neointimal proliferation? Eur Heart J 17:373, 1996.
9. Phillips PS, Alfonso F, Segovia J, et al: Effects of Palmaz-Schatz stents on angled coronary arteries. Am J Cardiol 79:191, 1997.
10. Zampieri P, Colombo A, Almagor Y, et al: Results of coronary stenting of ostial lesions. Am J Cardiol 73:901, 1994.
11. Hodgson JMcB: Oh no, even stenting is affected by calcium! Catheter Cardiovasc Diagn 38:236, 1996.
12. Albrecht D, Kaspers S, Fussl R, et al: Coronary plaque morphology affects stents deployment: Assessment by intracoronary ultrasound. Catheter Cardiovasc Diagn 38:229, 1996.
13. Goldberg SL, Hall P, Almagor Y, et al: Intravascular ultrasound guided rotational atherectomy of fibro-calcific plaque prior to intracoronary deployment of Palmaz-Schatz stents. J Am Coll Cardiol 775–4:290A, 1994.
14. Moussa i, Di Mario C, Blengino S, et al: Coronary stenting after rotational atherectomy in calcified and complex lesions: Angiographic and clinical follow-up results. Eur Heart J 17:2456, 1996.
15. Nakamura S, Hall P, Blengino S, et al: Does focal overstretch increase restenosis? Ultrasound evaluation after Palmaz-Schatz coronary stent deployment. Circulation 23:I-114, 1994.
16. Sirnes PA, Golf S, Myreng Y, et al: Stenting In Chronic Coronary Occlusion (SICCO): A randomized, controlled trial of adding stent implantation after successful angioplasty. J Am Coll Cardiol 28:1444, 1996.
17. Ozaki Y, Violaris AG, Hamburger J et al: Short- and long-term clinical and quantitative angiographic results with the new, less shortening Wallstent for vessel reconstruction in chronic total occlusion: A quantitative angiographic study. J Am Coll Cardiol 28:354, 1996.
18. Ozaki Y, Keane D, Ruygrok P, et al: Six-month clinical and angiographic outcome of the new, less shortening Wallstent in native coronary arteries. Circulation 93:2114, 1996.
19. Serruys PW, Strauss BH, Beatt KJ, et al: Angiographic follow-up after placement of a self-expanding coronary-artery stent. N Engl J Med 3:13, 1991.
20. de Scheerder JK, Strauss BH, de Feyter PJ, et al: Stenting of venous bypass grafts: A new treatment modality for patients who are poor candidates for reintervention. Am Heart J 123:1046, 1992.
21. Buis KB, Reifart N, Plokker TH, et al: Clinical and angiographic outcome following implantation of the new less shortening Wallstent in aortocoronary vein grafts: Introduction of a second generation stent in the clinical arena. J Intervent Cardiol 7:557, 1994.
22. de Jaegere PP, van Domburg RT, de Feyter PJ, et al: Long-term clinical outcome after stent implantation in saphenous vein grafts. J Am Coll Cardiol 28:89, 1996.
23. Wong SC, Baim DS, Schatz RA, et al: Immediate results and late outcomes after stent implantaion in saphenous vein graft lesions: The multicenter U.S. Palmaz-Schatz stent experience. J Am Coll Cardiol 26:704, 1995.
24. Piana RN, Moscucci M, Cohen DJ, et al: Palmaz-Schatz stenting for treatment of focal vein graft stenosis: Immediate results and long-term outcome. J Am Coll Cardiol 23:1296, 1994.
25. Wong SC, Popma JJ, Pichard AD, et al: Comparison of clinical and angiographic outcomes after saphenous vein graft angioplasty using coronary versus "biliary" tubular sotted stents. Circulation 91:339, 1995.
26. Hartmann JR, McKeever LS, O'Neill WW, et al: Recanalization of chronically occluded aortocoronary saphenous vein bypass grafts with long-term, low dose direct infusion of

urokinase (ROBUST): A serial trial. J Am Coll Cardiol 27:60, 1996.

27. Misumi K, Matthews RV, Sun GW, et al: Reduced distal embolization with transluminal extraction atherectomy compared to balloon angioplasty for saphenous vein graft disease. Catheter Cardiovasc Diagn 39:246, 1996.

28. Roubin G, Cannon A, Agrawal S, et al: Intracoronary stenting for acute and threatened closure complicating percutaneous transluminal coronary angioplasty. Circulation 85:916, 1992.

29. Hermann H, Buchbinder M, Cleman M, et al: Emergent use of balloon-expandable coronary artery stenting for failed percutaneous coronary angioplasty. Circulation 86:812, 1992.

30. George B, Woorhees W, Roubin G, et al: Multicenter investigation of coronary stenting to treat acute or treated closure after percutaneous transluminal coronary angioplasty: Clinical and angiographic outcomes. J Am Coll Cardiol 22:135, 1993.

31. Suttonh J, Ellis S, Roubin G, et al: Major clinical events after coronary stenting. The multicenter registry of acute and elective Gianturco-Roubin stent placement. Circulation 89:1126, 1994.

32. Schömig A, Kastrati A, Mudra H, et al: Four-year experience with Palmaz-Schatz stenting in coronary angioplasty complicated by dissection with threatened or present vessel closure. Circulation 90:2716, 1994.

33. Leon MB, Fry ETA, O'Shaughnessy CD, et al: Preliminary multicenter experiences with the new GR-II stent for abrupt and threatened closure syndrome. Circulation 94(suppl I):I-207, 1996

34. Ozaky Y, Keane D, Ruygrok P, et al: Acute clinical and angiographic results with the new AVE Micro coronary stent in bailout management. Am J Cardiol 76:112, 1995.

35. Moussa I, Di Mario C, Reimer B, et al: Subacute stent thrombosis in the era of intravascular ultrasound-guided coronary stenting without anticoagulation: Frequency, predictors and clinical outcome. J Am Coll Cardiol 29:6, 1997.

36. Stefanadis C, Toutouzas KP: Percutaneous implantation of autologous vein graft stent for treatment of coronary artery disease [Letter]. Lancet 345:1509, 1995.

37. Stefanadis C, Toutouzas K, Vlachopoulos C, et al: Autologous vein graft–coated stent for treatment of coronary artery disease. Catheter Cardiovasc Diagn 38:159, 1996.

# 37

# Optimal Technique for Stent Deployment

*Guido Belli     Stephen G. Ellis*

Improved understanding and evolution of implantation techniques and adjunctive pharmacotherapy have fueled the exponential rise in intracoronary stent placement that is revolutionizing the field of interventional cardiology. This chapter reviews some of the technical aspects of optimal stent deployment, such as use of angiography or intravascular ultrasound study, preprocedure dilatation of the lesion, stent sizing, postprocedure high-pressure balloon dilatation, and the most effective adjunctive therapy for preventing stent thrombosis.

## BACKGROUND

Intracoronary stents have been developed to improve results of balloon angioplasty (percutaneous transluminal coronary angioplasty [PTCA]) and overcome the major limitations of abrupt vessel closure[1] and restenosis.[2] Initial experimental animal data suggested relatively low thrombogenicity of metallic stents.[3–6] Nevertheless, the risk of death and acute myocardial infarction associated with stent thrombosis[7] was a major deterrent to clinical development. The early European experience with the Wallstent was complicated by a 24% overall rate of stent thrombosis. The highest incidence (39%) was observed in the first patients, who were treated with heparin and thrombolysis during the procedure but with only aspirin and dipyridamole afterwards. A more aggressive anticoagulation strategy, with prolonged heparin infusion and oral vitamin K antagonist therapy, empirically ensued.[8] In the first multicenter clinical trial with the Palmaz-Schatz stent, subacute thrombosis occurred in 18% of the first 39 patients who did not receive oral anticoagulation. Of note is that 4 of these 7 patients were also not taking aspirin. Treatment with heparin and dextran during the procedure, followed by aspirin, dipyridamole, and warfarin for 1 to 3 months in the next 174 patients resulted in a decrease in the rate of thrombotic events to 1.8%.[9]

The implantation technique usually consisted of mounting the stents on regular, compliant angioplasty balloons that were inflated at nominal pressures of 6 to 10 atm. Angiographically documented residual stenosis affecting close to 0% of the luminal diameter (or even overdilatation to −10%) of the normal reference vessel diameter was considered optimal.[9] However, residual stenoses affecting 10% to 20% of the luminal diameter according to visual estimate (or about 20% by quantitative coronary angiography[10, 11]), which already represented a marked improvement over results of balloon angioplasty, were generally accepted as satisfactory. In retrospect, it is quite likely that technical factors, patient and lesion selection, and lack of operator experience (learning curve) were factors in the unfavorable outcomes in these early trials. Nonetheless, subsequent studies adopted a very aggressive anticoagulation regimen with heparin and dextran during the procedure, followed by warfarin in addition to aspirin and dipyridamole.[10–20] A markedly increased risk of vascular and bleeding complications (range, 4% to 20%) prevented more extensive use of stents.

## INTRAVASCULAR ULTRASOUND STUDIES

The development of intravascular ultrasound (IVUS) technology for direct visualization of endoluminal structures has had a formidable influence on stent deployment techniques. Miniaturization of ultrasound probes allowed safe interrogation of stented segments, which suggested a role for IVUS in assessing results.[20–24] The Milan group comprised the first investigators to clearly demonstrate the limitation of angiographic evaluation of "adequate" stent placement. In 62 patients with satisfactory angiographic results (residual stenosis affecting mean of 9% ± 13% of the luminal diameter), IVUS study showed suboptimal deployment in up to 80% of cases, with incomplete apposition of the struts or global underexpansion of the stent. The use of larger balloons, or higher inflation pressures with noncompliant balloons, was required for adequate stent enlargement; IVUS guidance led to improved results in 87% of patients.[25, 26] Other groups substantiated these findings. Kiemeneij and coworkers showed that the standard delivery balloon of the Palmaz-Schatz stent at nominal pressure led to complete and symmetric apposition of the struts in only 28% of patients.[27] A study by Mudra and colleagues with a combined ultrasound and angioplasty balloon catheter revealed a smaller in-stent minimal luminal diameter than assessed angiographically (2.1 vs. 2.6 mm; $p < 0.0001$) and poor correlation between the two measurements ($r = .27$) after traditional deployment techniques. The correlation improved ($r = .60$) after an average of three additional balloon inflations were performed (at higher pressure, with larger balloons, or both) to optimize stent deployment.[28]

The impact of these studies has been twofold. They have led to an evolution and refinement in stent implantation techniques, which emphasizes the importance of optimal stent expansion obtained with accurate balloon sizing and high-pressure postprocedure dilatation, as discussed in more detail in the subsequent paragraphs. Of more importance is that they suggested that inadequate stent deployment, as opposed to the intrinsic thrombogenicity of the device itself or the level of anticoagulation achieved, has a primary role in increasing the risk of subsequent thrombosis.[29] Colombo and associates reported on a consecutive series of 321 patients who, after "optimal" stent deployment with IVUS guidance and high-pressure balloon postprocedure dilatation, were treated with antiplatelet therapy alone (aspirin and ticlopidine in 252 patients and aspirin alone in 69 patients). Criteria of adequate stent expansion evolved during the course of the study. They included complete and symmetric strut apposition to the vessel wall and avoidance of any

potential impediment to blood flow, with treatment of the full extent of the lesion or any residual dissection. With on-line quantitative assessment by IVUS study, an intrastent luminal cross-sectional area equal to or greater than the distal reference segment area was pursued. Any adjacent segment without a stent and with stenosis affecting more than 60% of the area was also treated with more stents or balloon angioplasty. In a population relatively nonselected for clinical and angiographic characteristics, stent thrombosis occurred in only 0.9% of patients in the first 2 months. Adverse cardiac events at 6 months were limited to death in 1.9%, myocardial infarction in 5.7%, the need for bypass surgery in 6.4%, and the need for repeat angioplasty in 13.1% of patients. Only one patient had a peripheral vascular complication.[30]

## Unresolved Issues: Need for Routine Intravascular Ultrasound Study

With increasing operator experience and better patient and lesion selection, simple empirical high-pressure postprocedure dilatation with combined antiplatelet therapy alone has also been associated with remarkably low rates of stent thrombosis, as illustrated in Table 37–1. Therefore, at present the need for routine IVUS study after stent implantation remains undefined. Several studies have reported that IVUS interrogation can still lead to further interventions in 24% to 53% of patients even after systematic high-pressure postprocedure dilatation. Depending on variable criteria of "optimal" stent deployment, more dilatations, with larger balloons or higher inflation pressures, or additional stents can improve lumen morphology.[31–36] Independent core laboratory analysis in the Optimal Stent Im-

**TABLE 37–1. LARGE SERIES OF CORONARY STENT IMPLANTATION WITHOUT WARFARIN OR INTRAVASCULAR ULTRASOUND: SHORT-TERM (30-DAY) RESULTS**

| AUTHOR | YEAR | N | STENT TYPE | STENT THROMBOSIS (%) | DEATH (%) | MYOCARDIAL INFARCTION (%) | NON–Q-WAVE MYOCARDIAL INFARCTION (%) | CABG (%) |
|---|---|---|---|---|---|---|---|---|
| Barragan et al[121] | 1994 | 387 | Mixed | 3.0 | 1.3 | 1.3 | NR | 0 |
| Lablanche et al[160] (TASTE) | 1995 | 334 | Mixed | 2.1 | 1.2 | 2.1 | NR | 0 |
| Karrillon et al[87] | 1996 | 2900 | Mixed | 1.8 | 0.5 | 0.6 | NR | 0.3 |
| Sainsous et al[141] | 1996 | 1336 | Mixed | 1.3 | 1.1 | 0.4 | NR | NR |
| Goodhart et al[161] | 1996 | 330 | Mixed | 1.2 | 0.3 | | 1.2 | 0 |
| Lawrence et al[162] | 1996 | 322 | Mixed | 0.3 | 0 | 0 | 3 | 0 |
| Morice et al[163] (MUST) | 1996 | 260 | Palmaz-Schatz | 1.2 | 0 | 1.9 | NR | 0.4 |
| Goods et al[164] | 1996 | 216 | Gianturco-Roubin | 0.9 | 0.5 | 0 | 3.7 | 0.9 |
| Sankardas et al[165] | 1996 | 168 | Mixed | 1.2 | 0 | 0 | 1.2 | 0 |
| Goods et al[166] | 1996 | 137 | Palmaz-Schatz | 0 | 0 | 0 | 2.2 | 0 |
| Pooled | | 6390 | | 1.6 | | | | |

CABG, coronary artery bypass grafting; MUST, Multicenter Stent Ticlopidine study; TASTE, Ticlopidine Aspirin Evaluation study.

plantation (OSTI) trial showed that although progressive expansion of the Palmaz-Schatz stent occurs as implantation pressure is increased from 12 to 18 atm, commonly used IVUS criteria for optimal expansion are not met in 25% to 40% of cases even after a final inflation pressure of 18 atm (Table 37–2).[37] In the Multicenter Ultrasound Intracoronary Stent (MUSIC) registry, 83% of 160 consecutive patients were treated with aspirin alone after IVUS study demonstrated optimal stent expansion. In this small cohort, short-term complications were limited to subacute thrombosis in only 0.6% of patients, emergency coronary artery bypass grafting (CABG) in 0.6%, and Q-wave myocardial infarction in 0.6%.[38] In the Anti-Platelet Treatment After Intravascular Ultrasound Guided Optimal Stent Expansion (APLAUSE) trial, a thrombosis rate of less than 1% and a rate of target vessel revascularization at 1 year of less than 20%, in either native vessels or saphenous vein grafts, were obtained in 222 consecutive patients with full stent strut apposition and cross-section area of 80% or more of the reference lumen area according to IVUS study.[39]

The benefit and cost effectiveness of routine IVUS study, together with the clinical relevance of specific parameters of adequate placement, are being tested by several ongoing randomized studies. In the Can Routine Ultrasound Impact Stent Expansion (CRUISE) study, outcomes at 9 and 12 months after IVUS-guided or IVUS-documentary (with the operator unaware of results) stent implantation will be analyzed. A preliminary report on 108 patients confirmed the larger final minimal luminal diameter obtained with IVUS guidance.[40] The Angiography Versus Ultrasound-Directed stent placement (AVID) trial will also compare 6-month clinical outcome after IVUS- or angiography-guided stent placement. No difference in the incidence of subacute stent thrombosis (1.8% vs. 1.9% after angiography or IVUS guidance, respectively) was found in a preliminary 30-day analysis of 218 patients.[41] Interim results from the third Stent Restenosis Study (STRESS-III) show no difference in acute complications or target lesion revascularization between IVUS-guided and non–IVUS-guided stent implantation in the first 160 patients. However, this was not a randomized comparison; use of IVUS was optional.[42] IVUS may also be of value in assessment of difficult lesions or equivocal angiographic results after stent implantation[43] and in accelerating the learning curve and refining the stent implantation technique of new operators.[44] On the basis of our own experience and preliminary data, tentative recommendations on when use of IVUS, after stent implantation with current techniques, may be most beneficial can be summarized as follows: (1) when angiographic results are suboptimal, to help define causative factors such as inadequate stent apposition, edge trauma, small dissection flaps, or heavy residual plaque burden, which require further specific treatment and are often seen angiographically as residual stenosis or ill-defined localized "haziness"[45]; (2) in situations with higher risk of partial stent underexpansion, such as with multiple overlapping stents, or in angulated, heavily calcified or bifurcating stenoses; (3) after bail-out stent implantation for large dissections, which are at highest risk of subsequent stent thrombosis; (4) after stent implantation in the ostium or most proximal portion of major vessels (left anterior descending artery, right circumflex coronary artery), when absolute certainty about exact location and adequate expansion of the stent is vital because of the very large territory of myocardium at risk; (5) to assess complications, such as to help localize radiolucent stents in the coronary circulation after inadvertent detachment from the delivery balloon; and (6) when initiating a new program or implanting stents with new designs, as a learning tool.

## STENT IMPLANTATION TECHNIQUE

Successful coronary stent implantation is associated with better immediate angiographic results than is angioplasty.[10, 11] However, this procedure is generally more technically demanding than simple balloon dilatation. Careful advance planning is required and should incorporate both (1) correct indications, based on available evidence of clinical benefit and cost effectiveness,[46] and (2) the likeli-

**TABLE 37–2. RELATIONSHIP BETWEEN STENT IMPLANTATION PRESSURE AND OPTIMAL EXPANSION IN THE OPTIMAL STENT IMPLANTATION (OSTI) TRIAL**

| IVUS MEASURE | 12 atm | 15 atm | 18 atm |
|---|---|---|---|
| Mean MLD (mm) | 2.72 | 2.91 | 3.04 |
| Mean diameter stenosis (%) | 6.2 | −0.3 | −4.7 |
| % Patients meeting predefined IVUS criteria | | | |
| LA ≥ 70% balloon area | 55% | 79% | 85% |
| LA ≥ 90% reference area | 28% | 44% | 60% |
| LA ≥ 100 minimal reference area | 35% | 50% | 60% |
| LA ≥ 9 mm² | 21% | 37% | 41% |

Note: Although progressive stent expansion is obtained with increased implantation pressures, commonly used IVUS criteria for optimal expansion are still not met after postinflation pressures of 18 atm in a substantial proportion of patients.

IVUS, intravascular ultrasound; LA, luminal area; MLD, minimal luminal diameter.

Modified from Stone GW, Linnemeier TJ, Saint Goar FG, et al: Refining the relationship between implantation pressure and optimal expansion—Core lab analysis from the OSTI trial [Abstract]. Circulation 94:I-259, 1996.

hood of successful delivery to the intended site. New and specific potential complications, such as stent embolization, obligatory deployment of a permanent implant at a site where it is unwanted, or iatrogenic stent-edge dissection leading to unplanned placement of multiple stents, should be taken into account. More guiding catheter and guide wire support is required than for most angioplasty balloons, for satisfactory ability of the bulkier and more rigid stents currently available to be pushed and tracked. To achieve better support, the use of stiffer guide wires, or excessively distal wire positioning, can lead to an increased risk of coronary perforation. Precise angiographic assessment and use of multiple projections are necessary for stent sizing and positioning and for evaluating lesion accessibility. Specifically, a correct evaluation of vessel tortuosity, the presence of proximal or distal disease (preventing stent advancement or compromising distal flow), lesion length, angulation, and degree of calcification or presence of thrombus, is necessary to avoid unsuccessful or suboptimal deployment, with risk of subsequent stent thrombosis. The presence, size, and exact location of side branches should be noted: slight modification of stent location may be necessary to prevent "jailing" and acute side branch closure. Side branch location can also be used as a reference for placing radiolucent stents. Figure 37–1 summarizes some general technical aspects of optimal stent implantation technique.

## PREPROCEDURE DILATATION OF LESIONS

Currently available stents, whether premounted and covered by a sheath delivery system or hand-crimped on a balloon, are more rigid and have a larger profile than most angioplasty balloons. One of the most important technical aspects of stent implantation is the correct evaluation of the degree of preprocedure dilatation necessary for accessibility of severely stenotic lesions. Two different preprocedure dilatation strategies are described.

### Primary Stent Implantation with Limited Balloon Preprocedure Dilatation

The Belgium Netherlands Stent (BENESTENT-1) study and the STRESS-I demonstrated lower restenosis rates after primary stent implantation than after balloon angioplasty, in large native vessels with focal, de novo lesions.[10, 11] Because commitment to place a stent preceded balloon preprocedure dilatation, the objective was only to be able to negotiate the device itself across the stenosis. The intentional use of preprocedure dilatation balloons well undersized in relation to the vessel diameter (0.5:0.7

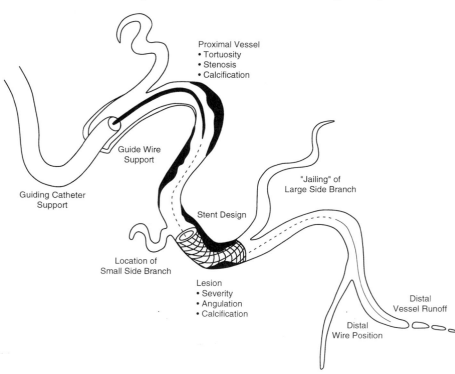

Schematic Diagram of Factors Related to Correct Stenting Technique

FIGURE 37–1. General aspects of optimal stent implantation technique.

balloon-artery ratio) and of low inflation pressures was aimed at limiting local vessel trauma and the risk of dissection. Advocates of only limited balloon preprocedure dilatation in routine primary stent implantation in suitable lesions argue that this is the only proven strategy for clinical benefit and decreased restenosis rates after stent implantation.[47]

Furthermore, evidence from animal studies, discussed in more detail later, suggest that the degree of in-stent and peristent reactive neointimal hyperplasia may be directly related to deep vessel injury.[48, 49] Another study in the rabbit model also showed that even minimizing *superficial* endothelial injury, by limiting or avoiding balloon preprocedure dilatation, may be important for limiting restenosis.[50] Some of the "second-generation" stents may be suitable for direct implantation without preprocedure dilatation in up to 62% of selected patients.[51] Conversely, stents with less radial strength, such as most currently available coiled stents, may become deformed if implanted without adequate preprocedure treatment of fibrotic or calcific lesions.

Limited balloon dilatation before the procedure, aimed at minimizing deep and superficial vessel trauma, appears to be the most rational strategy whenever the operator is primarily committed to deploy a stent, as indicated by lesion or vessel characteristics.

## PTCA with Provisional or "Ad Hoc" Stent Implantation

A conceptually different approach consists of an initial attempt to obtain the best angiographic outcome with angioplasty alone and reserving stent implantation only for suboptimal results, usually caused by significant vessel recoil or residual dissection. The rationale for limiting the use of stents to lesion or patient subsets at highest risk of restenosis after angioplasty is to maximize cost effectiveness and relative clinical benefit. With an unrestricted stent implantation strategy, a large proportion of patients with a high likelihood of good clinical outcome with angioplasty alone would nonetheless receive a stent; thus stents would be used unnecessarily in approximately 50% of cases.[46] In the BENESTENT-1 trial, 35% of patients in the angioplasty cohort had achieved an optimal, or "stent-like" result (defined as residual stenosis affecting ≤30% of the luminal diameter, according to quantitative coronary angiography). Their outcomes were compared with those of the 213 stent recipients with similar angiographic results and those of the whole cohort that received stents ($N = 259$). At 7-month follow-up, the restenosis rates were 16% after "stent-like" angioplasty, 18% after optimal stent implantation, and 22% in the whole cohort ($p$

= NS).[52] Different results, however, were found in a smaller retrospective study of 89 patients after optimal PTCA (residual stenosis affecting ≤20% of the luminal diameter) or stent implantation of saphenous vein grafts: at 1 year, major adverse cardiac events (death, myocardial infarction, or need for reintervention) had occurred in 12% after elective stent implantation, in comparison with 46% after angioplasty.[53]

Maximal relative advantage from stent implantation may be obtained after suboptimal results with balloon dilatation alone. With repeat angiography after 24 hours, Rodriguez and associates demonstrated that, in comparison with continued observation alone, stent implantation of lesions with significant recoil after PTCA results in a very marked decrease in restenosis (21% vs. 76%) and need for repeat revascularization (21% vs. 73%).[54] In the same cohort, more than 80% of treated stenoses with subsequent significant diameter loss, as a result of recoil or residual dissection, could be identified within 1 hour of the index procedure.[55] Thus, a selective strategy clearly may not reduce risk of restenosis in some patients.[46] The availability of stents as a backup, however, by limiting the risks of coronary dissection or abrupt vessel closure, may allow operators to perform more aggressive balloon angioplasty, as suggested by the significant increase in mean balloon-artery ratio over time (from 1.03 to 1.10; $p = 0.03$) observed in two large-scale clinical trials that were conducted only 3 years apart but spanned the widespread implementation of stent implantation (unpublished data from the Evaluation of 7E3 for the Prevention of Ischemic Complications (EPIC) and Evaluation of PTCA to Improve Long-term Outcome by c7E3 GP IIb/IIIa receptor blockade (EPILOG) trials; data on file).

## Lesion Debulking

The availability of atherectomy devices capable of removing plaque or calcific material has led to intense clinical research on the possibility of combining these technologies with stents. The goals of lesion debulking before stent implantation are to achieve the best possible immediate luminal gain (the most important predictor of restenosis[10, 11, 56–58]), to gain access to calcified lesions not amenable to adequate balloon preprocedure dilatation, and to decrease plaque burden, which recent ultrasound studies after angioplasty have proved to be another very important determinant of restenosis.[59] The potential drawback, however, is that a higher degree of lumen renarrowing may be paradoxically induced because of deeper tissue injury, antagonizing the benefit of stent implantation.[60]

Data for directional atherectomy are mixed. Deep wall resection after atherectomy alone was not associated with worse procedural or long-term outcome in the first and second Coronary Angioplasty Versus Excisional Atherectomy Trials (CAVEAT-I and CAVEAT-II), although a trend was found for higher restenosis rates in saphenous vein grafts (40% intimal resection vs. 57% subintima resection; $p = 0.14$).[61] In a case-control study of 117 pairs of patients matched for baseline lesion and clinical characteristics, stent implantation resulted in larger immediate gain than did atherectomy and in a similar late rate of loss, with larger lumen at late follow-up (1.96 vs. 1.66 mm; $p < 0.0001$). Of interest is that in a subgroup of 75 pairs with identical rates of immediate luminal gain after either procedure, subsequent lumen loss was more pronounced after atherectomy than after stent implantation, with more repeat target-vessel revascularization at follow-up (Fig. 37–2).[62] This study and other observations[63, 64] suggest a device-specific effect on restenosis. Although lower restenosis rates after stent implantation may predominantly derive from lack of significant vessel recoil[65–69] or from "negative" arterial remodeling with shrinkage of the external elastic lamina,[70–72] an independent effect of reduced trauma to the vessel wall cannot be excluded.[73]

Rotational atherectomy may be valuable in pre-

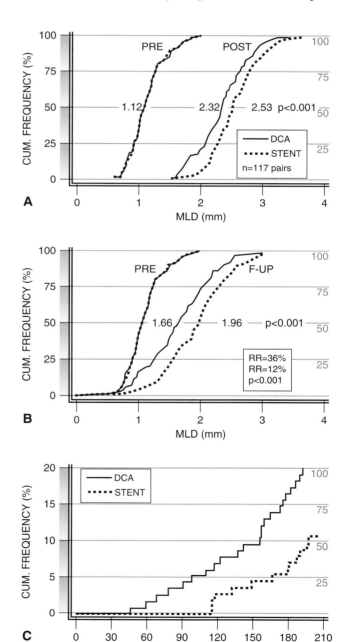

FIGURE 37–2. Cumulative (CUM) frequency curves for immediate *(A)* and follow-up (F-UP) *(B)* effects on minimal lumen diameter (MLD) and cumulative frequency of target lesion revascularization *(C)* for directional coronary atherectomy (DCA) and stent implantation in 117 patients matched for lesion location and severity (see text for details). In lesions with similar severity, stenting was associated with larger immediate *(A)* and follow-up *(B)* luminal diameter and reduced requirement for target vessel revascularization with either repeat percutaneous transluminal coronary angioplasty (PTCA) or coronary artery bypass grafting (CABG) *(C; $p = 0.05$ between curves)* when indirectly compared with DCA. PRE, before DCA or stent implantation; POST, after DCA or stent implantation; RR, relative ratio. (From Umans VA, Melkert R, Foley DP, et al: Clinical and angiographic comparison of matched patients with successful directional coronary atherectomy or stent implantation for primary coronary artery lesions. J Am Coll Cardiol 28:637–644, 1996.)

procedure treatment of severely calcified lesions.[74-76] "Hard," densely fibrotic plaque or lesion calcification, as more accurately assessed by IVUS,[77] is associated with a higher risk of limited stent expansion[78, 79] and may not be detected by angiography alone.[79] Yokoi and coworkers retrospectively compared clinical outcomes after stent implantation in 200 calcified and 804 noncalcific lesions. Severe calcification was associated with worse clinical success rates (83% vs. 97%, in severely calcified or noncalcified lesions, respectively; $p = 0.0001$) and lower rates of event-free survival at 6 months (82% vs. 92%; $p = 0.02$), with a trend toward an increase in restenosis rates (33% vs. 23%).[80] In a nonrandomized comparison of calcified lesions matched for vessel area and total amount of calcium after rotablation followed by PTCA, directional atherectomy, or stent implantation, final lumen areas as measured by IVUS were $5 \pm 1$ mm², $6.5 \pm 2$ mm², and $7.1 \pm 2$ mm² ($p < 0.0001$) and final diameter sizes affected by stenosis were 24% $\pm$ 13%, 16% $\pm$ 13%, and 12% $\pm$ 12% ($p < 0.0001$), respectively.[81] Adjunctive stent implantation can lead to marked improvement in immediate angiographic results after suboptimal rotational atherectomy of calcified stenoses.[82] However, the risk of slow flow (secondary to excessive distal microembolization) after rotational atherectomy should also be considered, because it may increase the risk of acute periprocedural complications (namely, non–Q-wave myocardial infarction) and theoretically predispose to subacute stent thrombosis.

Results of clinical trials directly comparing combined atherectomy procedure, followed by stent implantation, with stent implantation alone are not available at the time of this writing.

## Stent and Balloon Sizing

The large randomized clinical trials with balloon angioplasty showed that decreased restenosis rates after stent implantation resulted from a larger immediate gain in luminal diameter.[10, 11] The rate of critical restenosis over time is decreased because the wider lumen, with lack of significant chronic recoil, can accommodate even a proportionately higher degree of intimal hyperplasia within the stent itself. However, simple application of the popular "bigger is better" principle[56] of balloon angioplasty to stent implantation may not be warranted. Because of unique mechanical and scaffolding properties, a higher degree of stretching of the vessel wall can indeed be achieved more safely with stents than with angioplasty. Excessive balloon sizing, however, especially in conjunction with high-pressure dilatations, may nonetheless be associated with severe acute complications and possibly also worse long-

term outcome. In the landmark study of Colombo and associates, the initial empirical attempt to use oversized balloons (mean balloon-artery ratio of 1.2) for full stent expansion was associated with a 1.2% risk of vessel rupture and a 5.7% incidence of major intraprocedural complications (death, myocardial infarction, or need for emergency CABG). More appropriately sized noncompliant balloons (1.05 ratio), even when inflated at high pressures of more than 14 atm, resulted in a significant reduction in intraprocedural complications to 1% ($p = 0.04$), no coronary perforations, and still adequate stent expansion when assessed by IVUS.[30] In another study of 435 patients, angiographic features associated with increased risk of coronary perforation (occurring in 2.3% of patients) also included excessively oversized stents (stent-artery ratio of 1.4) and small vessel diameter (mean, 2.6 mm).[83] Therefore, it appears that extremely accurate sizing of stents, post-inflation balloons, or both and a conservative balloon-artery ratio in the range of 1:1 to 1.1:1, is necessary to minimize acute complications. This is especially true if the length of the balloon used for postprocedure dilatation exceeds that of the stent itself, leading to partially "unprotected" complete expansion of one or both of the balloon shoulders outside the stent.

Preliminary evidence from animal studies suggest the hypothesis that minimizing vessel overstretch and injury may be the most effective strategy for preventing excessive neointimal growth and in-stent restenosis. In the porcine restenosis model, the degree of neointimal proliferation is proportional to the depth of injury into the vessel wall by the stent struts.[48] Another study in rabbits suggested that geometric configuration of the stent, which affects vascular injury by altering radial force, may be more important than postprocedure luminal diameter in determining thrombosis and neointimal hyperplasia.[49] Some indicative clinical data, albeit extremely limited and controversial, also exist. Post-hoc analysis of the BENESTENT-I) results suggested that using the smallest balloon diameter to provide full stent expansion may be associated with decreased rates of restenosis.[84] In another small, retrospective, observational study, a quadratic relationship was found between postprocedure luminal stenosis after stent implantation and restenosis, increasing from 24% after optimal deployment (±10% residual stenosis) to 80% after excessive overexpansion (< −10% residual stenosis).[85]

In view of the paucity of available studies and the complex interplay of clinical scenarios, operator's experience or preferences, morphologic variations, stent designs, and interventional equipment, it is difficult to derive guidelines on stent sizing. At present, however, it appears that a strategy aimed at optimal rather than than maximal and a stent-vessel ratio close to 1:1 may be preferable. The use of slightly oversized high-pressure balloons (balloon-vessel ratio ~1.1) is usually necessary to overcome a small degree of acute vessel and stent recoil and balloon subexpansion occurring in vivo in most lesions.[86]

## High-Pressure Postprocedure Dilatation

Several factors affect the degree of inflation pressure necessary for adequate stent deployment. The stent metallic composition and, of more importance, its design, length, and deployment system (balloon- or self-expandable) affect the degree of radial strength required for full stent expansion. Data acquired on tubular slotted or MultiLink stents, with highest radial compressive strength, should not be directly extrapolated to stents with different designs. Use of excessively high postprocedure dilatation pressure or oversized balloons can lead to deformation or extramural strut protrusion of coiled stents. Lesion characteristics—of most importance, the degree of calcification,[78, 79] but also, more in general, vessel wall elasticity and luminal size, geometry, tapering, and degree of lesion angulation—will all affect resistance to balloon dilatation. For example, adequate stent deployment in a large, straight segment of an old saphenous graft may not require the same degree of expansion pressure used in a tortuous, calcified segment of a circumflex coronary artery. Finally,

required balloon size or inflation pressure may vary according to specific IVUS or angiographic criteria of "adequate" stent deployment (see previous paragraphs and Table 37–2).

Most available data on adequate inflation pressure required for full stent expansion is derived from studies of the tubular slotted Palmaz-Schatz stent. Colombo and associates defined inflation pressures above nominal but less than 14 atm as "moderate," and any pressure more than 14 atm as "high,"[30] but other researchers consider postprocedure dilatation pressures more than 10 atm as high.[87] As assessed by IVUS, use of noncompliant balloons, able to withstand high-pressures with low risk of rupture, consistently leads to adequate stent expansion in a higher percentage of patients than does use of oversized but compliant balloons.[30] Stone and colleagues showed that full deployment of a Palmaz-Schatz stent, to achieve 70% of the balloon cross-sectional area, requires at least 18 atm of pressure, with further increases in either balloon size or postprocedure dilatation pressure (>18 atm) still necessary in 29% of patients to optimize lumen morphology.[88] Published preliminary data suggest the need for postprocedure inflation up to 16 atm for the ACS MultiLink stent[89] and of at least 13 atm for the Medtronic-Wiktor stent.[90] In the future, charts and tables may be needed for each balloon and stent, similar to the currently used burst and compliance charts of angioplasty balloons, rating the in vitro performance in terms of stent expansion. Table 37–3 illustrates the current coronary artery stent designs

**TABLE 37–3.    CURRENT STENT DESIGNS THAT ARE FOOD AND DRUG ADMINISTRATION APPROVED OR ARE UNDERGOING TESTING**

| STENT | STRUCTURE | DELIVERY/ EXPANSION METHOD | MATERIALS |
|---|---|---|---|
| ACS MultiLink | Rings joined by linked, etched tube | Balloon | 316L SS |
| ACT One | Slotted tube | Balloon | Nitinol |
| AngioDynamics/AngioStent | Single wire, simple coil | Balloon | Platinum/iridium |
| Angiomed—USCI | Multiple-wire braid | Self | Nitinol |
| AVE Microstent | Wire zigzags; welded/unwelded in series | Balloon | 316L SS |
| BeStent (Medtronic) | Slotted tube | Balloon | 316L SS |
| Duke Biodegradable Stent | NA | NA | NA |
| Cook Gianturco-Roubin Flex Stent* | Flexible coil stent | Balloon | 316L SS |
| Cordis | Single sinusoidal helical coil | Balloon | Tantalum |
| Global Therapeutics Freedom Stent | Wire mesh | Balloon | 316L SS |
| INSTENT CardioCoil | Single wire, simple coil | Self | Nitinol |
| Isostent (Fischell) | Johnson & Johnson stent dosed with radioactivity | Balloon | Coated with radioactive isotope |
| Johnson & Johnson Palmaz-Schatz* | Slotted tube | Balloon | 316L SS |
| Mayo Stent | Fibrin-waffled metallic stent | Balloon | Tantalum |
| Medivent-Schneider Wallstent | Multiple-wire braid | Self | Eligiloy (cobalt-based alloy) |
| Medtronic Wiktor | Single-wire sinusoidal helix | Balloon | Tantalum |
| NIR Stent (SCIMED/Medinol) | Slotted tube | Balloon | 316L SS |
| SCIMED | Slotted tube | Balloon | Nitinol |

*Food and Drug Administration approved.
NA, not available at this time; SS, stainless steel.
Modified from Pepine CJ, Holmes DR, Block PC, et al: ACC Expert Consensus Document. Coronary artery stents. J Am Coll Cardiol 28:782–794, 1996.

that are approved by the U.S. Food and Drug Administration (FDA) or are undergoing testing. As a general guideline, Table 37–4 shows when high-pressure inflations were used in published series with second-generation stent designs, reflecting current clinical practice by most experienced operators.

The use of high pressure entails a much higher risk of balloon rupture. In our initial experience, balloon rupture occurred in 13% of the first 228 patients treated with high-pressure postprocedure dilatation. Major acute complications in 2 patients (7%) were severe diffuse spasm of the left anterior descending artery with asystole, resolved after cardiopulmonary resuscitation and pressor use, and a large dissection with probable perforation of the right coronary artery, treated with multiple stents (unpublished data, Cleveland Clinic Interventional registry). Pinpoint balloon rupture leading to coronary perforation and tamponade has also been reported.[91] In addition, there appears to be an increased risk of peristent dissection, often unrecognized on angiography but detected with IVUS.[45] A generally accepted misconception among interventional cardiologists is that "high pressure" is a direct cause of coronary dissection. In theory, it is obviously not the absolute inflation pressure per se that causes the damage, inasmuch as this is transmitted only to the balloon, but the fact that the actual nominal (or slightly higher) size of the balloon itself is reached within the vessel. As already discussed, accurate and conservative sizing of postprocedure inflation balloons should limit this complication.

## DIFFICULT LESIONS

### Aorto-ostial Stenoses

Encouraging immediate angiographic results with low restenosis rates, in comparison to historic angioplasty controls, have been reported after stent implantation of aorto-ostial lesions in either native vessels or saphenous vein grafts.[92–96] Special attention must be directed to the choice of the guiding catheter, and extreme precision is required in device placement. With true ostial stenoses, initial positioning of the stent within 2 to 3 mm of the aortic origin, with the most proximal end 1 or 2 mm in the aorta, is usually necessary to cover the lesion adequately and accounts for partial stent shrinkage upon expansion. The shape, position in relation to the ostium, and maneuverability of the guiding catheter tip determine the ability to deploy the stent while avoiding impingement against the free proximal edge with risk of stent deformation, which most often occurs when the deflated balloon is retrieved proximally or inside the guide. After stent expan-

sion, an attempt should be made to "flare" or "trumpet" the proximal portion of the stent itself against the aortic wall.[92, 94, 95] This can be achieved with high-pressure inflations with the balloon partially freed in the aorta and directed as necessary with the guiding catheter (Fig. 37–3).

## Bifurcation Stenoses

Treatment of bifurcation stenoses remains problematic with current interventional techniques. Higher complication rates and worse long-term outcome with PTCA or atherectomy[97–100] are thought to result from a greater tendency for vessel recoil and heavier atherosclerotic burden, with plaque "shifting" among involved subdivisions and preventing optimal angiographic results. Scaffolding of plaque is a potential theoretical advantage of stent implantation for bifurcations. Preliminary results indicate that it is possible to obtain gratifying immediate angiographic results, albeit at the price of significant technical difficulties and complications. Incorrect stent placement may prevent treatment of the full extent of the lesion or lead to acute side branch closure with difficulties in renegotiating the vessel through the stent struts ("stent-jail"). Figures 37–4 to 37–6 illustrate some of the different stent implantation techniques described in the literature in a very limited number of cases. When significant discrepancy in size between subdivisions exists, a simple approach consists of stent implantation in the main vessel and then performing simple balloon dilatation of the side branch (see Fig. 37–4A). This requires rewiring of the side branch through the stent, which can easily be accomplished only with coiled stents and possibly with some of the second-generation stents. Access through tubular slotted stent struts is usually much more difficult. Use of very low-profile balloons or fixed-wire systems, limited to diameters of 2.5–2.75 mm or less, is usually necessary, with attempts to maintain as much of the balloon length as possible inside the stent itself in order to prevent trapping upon deflation with inability to retrieve the balloon. Another possibility is to initially perform rotational atherectomy of the smaller subdivision and then deploy a stent in the main branch. In true bifurcation lesions, with vessels of equal diameter, more difficult approaches have included T stent implantation, with placement of the first stent at the ostium of the side branch, followed by a second stent in the main vessel, overriding the origin of the first[101] (see Fig. 37–4B); "kissing" or "touching" stents in both distal branches, with a third stent proximally, before the bifurcation and a small gap in-between[102] (see Fig. 37–4C); and "kissing" stents with a double-barrel lumen in the main vessel (with proximal stent metal-on-metal de-

**TABLE 37–4.   DEPLOYMENT TECHNIQUE WITH "SECOND GENERATION" STENTS**

| AUTHOR (REFERENCE) | N | NO. STENTS | STENT TYPE | B/A RATIO | HPP | ATMOSPHERES | ASA | TICLOPIDINE | WARFARIN | STENT THROMBOSIS (%) |
|---|---|---|---|---|---|---|---|---|---|---|
| Priestly et al[167] | 10 | 10 | ACS MultiLink | 1–1.1 | – | NR | + | – | + | 0 |
| Wong et al[168] | 40 | 56 | ACS MultiLink | 1–1.1 | + | 16–20 | + | + | + | 0 |
| Hermiller et al[169] | 50 | 55 | ACS MultiLink | NR | + | 16 | + | – | + | 0 |
| Waigand et al[170] | 133 | 219 | ACS MultiLink | NR | 42% | >12 | + | + | – | 1.5 |
| Chevalier et al[51] | 160 | 180 | ACS MultiLink | NR | + | 12 | + | + | – | 0 |
| Thomas et al[110] | 110 | 129 | LSWall | * | – | – | NR | NR | NR | 5 |
| Ozaki et al[119] | 35 | 44 | LSWall | + | + | 14 | + | – | + | 2.9 |
| Ozaki et al[118] | 20 | 25 | LSWall | + | + | 14 | + | – | + | 5 |
| Tresukosol et al[171] | 85 | 127 | AVE Microstent | NR | + | 12 | + | – | ± | 6 |
| Rau et al[172] | 384 | 66 | AVE Microstent | NR | + | NR | + | + | – | 0.8 |
| Schiele et al[173] | 109 | 127 | AVE Microstent | 1.1 | + | 12 | + | + | – | 1.8 |
| Chevalier et al[174] | 100 | 110 | Freedom | ~1 | + | 11 | + | + | – | 1 |
| Chevalier et al[175] | 1000 | 1185 | Freedom | ~1 | + | 11 | + | + | – | 2 |
| De Scheerder et al[176] | 169 | 233 | Freedom | 1.1 | + | 14–16 | + | + | – | 0.6 |
| Fajadet et al[177] | 85 | 88 | NIR | NR | + | NR | + | + | – | 0 |
| Almagor et al[178] | 214 | 300 | NIR | NR | + | 12–16 | + | ± | – | 0 |
| Beyar et al[179] | 45 | 69 | BeStent | NR | + | NR | + | ± | – | 2.2 |
| Leon et al[180] | 83 | 83 | Cook Gianturco-Roubin II stent | NR | + | NR | + | ± | ± | 2.4 |

ASA, acetylsalicylic acid; B/A, balloon-artery; LSWall, less-shortening Wallstent; NR, not reported.
*Nominal stent diameter 0.75 to 1.5 mm larger than reference segment diameter.
†Nominal stent diameter 1.4 to 1.8 mm larger than reference segment diameter.

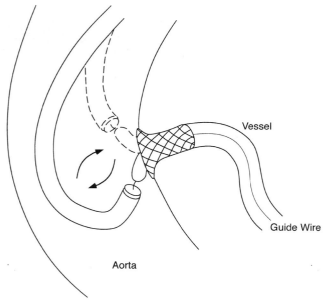

FIGURE 37–3. Stent implantation for ostial stenoses. After stent expansion, an attempt is made to "flare" or "trumpet" the proximal end of the stent against the aortic wall by leaving the proximal end of the balloon in the aorta and maneuvering the guiding catheter-balloon unit as a whole (see text for details).

formity) and their distal segments in the daughter vessels[103] (see Fig. 37–4D). The inverted Y technique of Colombo consists of initially deploying two guide wires and stents in the nonmajor vessels, followed by manual crimping of a single larger stent over two balloons, with the whole apparatus advanced as a unit to the proximal segment of the major vessel (over both wires; see Fig. 37–4E). Placement of the third stent is exceedingly difficult and not possible in probably 50% of attempted cases,[104, 105] but in the future, preformed bifurcation stents may follow a similar principle for delivery. With newer stent designs, allowing easier access to side branches, slight variations of these techniques may be used. In the so-called monoclonal antibody approach of the Thoraxcenter in Rotterdam, The Netherlands, after insertion of two guide wires, the first stent is deployed across the side branch, "jailing" the guide wire of the daughter branch against the vessel wall. A second wire is passed into the same branch through the stent struts, guided by the first guide wire (usually 0.010 mm in diameter), which is then retracted. The struts are adequately opened with balloon inflations, to allow passage of the second stent, which is positioned at the ostium of the daughter branch[104] (Fig. 37–5). The "Culotte" technique has been described by the French group of Chevalier and Glatt using two Freedom stents, with interlocking of the metal struts in the proximal portion of the vessel[104] (Fig. 37–6). At present, there are no available data on the relative merits and long-term outcome of

different strategies for stent implantation for bifurcation stenoses. Apart from the risks of stent misplacement, trapping of uncovered stents, and metal-on-metal deformity, there is suspicion of significant increased restenosis rates with most current techniques.

## Long, Diffuse Lesions

Stent implantation of long, diffusely diseased segments can lead to immediate angiographic results usually not achievable with balloon angioplasty alone.[106–112] Determining the relative merit of this

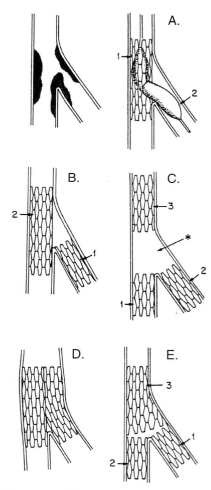

FIGURE 37–4. Stent implantation for side branches and bifurcation lesions. *A*, Stent implantation across the main branch, followed by balloon dilatation of the side branch through stent struts. *B*, T stent implantation with initial placement of the first stent at the side branch ostium, followed by placement of the second stent across the main branch. *C*, "Kissing" or "touching" stents in both distal branches, with a third stent placed proximally and a variable gap in between. *D*, "Kissing" or "trousers" stents with a double-barrel lumen and stent-on-stent deformity proximally. *E*, inverted Y stent implantation, with two distal stents and the third proximal stent mounted on two balloons. (Adapted and reprinted from Baim DS: Is bifurcation stenting the answer? Catheter Cardiovasc Diagn 37:314–316, 1996.)

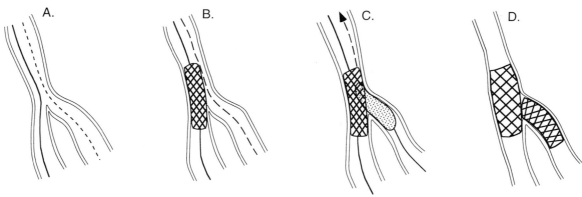

FIGURE 37–5. "Monoclonal antibody" approach of the Thoraxcenter, Rotterdam, The Netherlands, for bifurcation lesions. This technique may be possible with the use of second-generation stents, which allow easier access to side branches. A smaller (0.010-mm) guide wire is inserted in the smaller subdivision, whereas a regular wire is advanced into the main vessel (A). The first stent is initially deployed, but *not* postprocedurally dilated, in the main vessel and across the subdivision, "jailing" the smaller guide wire against the vessel wall (B). A second wire is then passed into the same side branch and through the stent struts, guided by the first 0.010-mm wire, which is then retracted. The struts are opened to allow passage of the second stent (C), positioned at the ostium of the side branch. This is followed by postdilatation of both stents (D) (see text for details). (From Foley DP, Serruys PW: Bifurcation lesion stenting. Thoraxcentre J 8/4:32–36, 1996.)

strategy in terms of cost effectiveness and long-term outcome, however, requires results from comparative clinical trials.

General technical considerations in approaching this type of lesion include the accurate estimate of the number of stents or stent length necessary to form an adequate scaffold for a diffusely stenotic vessel or a long dissection, the size of the vessel, and especially the degree of tapering, which for long lesions may determine a significant mismatch between the proximal and distal segments and the number and size of side branches that may be "jailed." Multiple short stents or second-generation long stents can be deployed. Without the use of high-pressure postprocedure dilatation, the number of deployed stents, and possibly also the degree of metal overlap, has been associated with significantly higher restenosis rates.[113, 114] With current tech-

niques, multiple stents may portend a more favorable prognosis.[111, 115, 116] Nevertheless, the use of a single, longer stent seems intuitively preferable for ease of deployment and to avoid excessive metal overlap. The new self-expanding, less-shortening Wallstent may be suitable for covering long lesions,[110, 117] such as in recanalized total coronary occlusions[118] or after acute or threatened vessel closure.[119] The use of oversized stents, with nominal diameters of 1.4 mm larger than the vessel diameter, and of postprocedure dilatation pressures of 14 atm or more was achieved safely with this particular stent design, accommodating a higher degree of intimal hyperplasia. The fine wire-mesh design, however, prevents adequate accessibility to side branches.[118, 119] Although the presence of residual uncovered dissections may entail a higher risk of subacute stent occlusion,[7] use of more stents, and

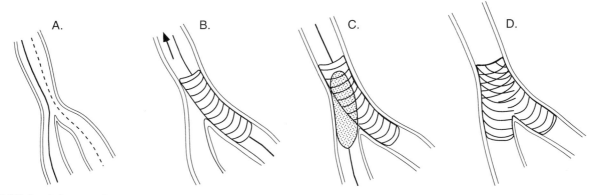

FIGURE 37–6. "Culotte" technique for bifurcation lesions, using two Freedom stents (Global Therapeutics, Inc.; Broomfield CO). After preprocedural dilatation (A), the first stent is placed in the smaller subdivision but with its proximal portion extending in the main vessel (B). The stent is rewired, with balloon dilatation to stretch the struts extending across the main lumen (C), followed by deployment of a second stent in the main vessel, with its proximal portion overlapping and interlocking with the proximal portion of the first stent (D) (see text for details). This technique may be possible with new stent designs or coiled stents, to prevent excessive metal-on-metal deformity in the proximal segment of the bifurcation. (From Foley DP, Serruys PW: Bifurcation lesion stenting. Thoraxcentre J 8/4:32–36, 1996.)

particularly the use of a combination of different stent designs, is also associated with subsequent increased risk of thrombosis, even after IVUS-optimized deployment and high-pressure postprocedure dilatation.[120] Several new stents with lengths of 20 mm or more are undergoing clinical evaluation, and in the near future their role will be better defined.

## ADJUNCTIVE PHARMACOTHERAPY

### Antiplatelet Versus Anticoagulant Therapy

Evolution of antithrombotic strategies has paralleled the improvement in technical aspects of stent implantation. With current deployment techniques and antiplatelet therapy alone, stent thrombosis rates of considerably less than 2% can be achieved (see Table 37–1) without risk of excessive bleeding. The addition of ticlopidine to a regimen of aspirin was initially based on the empirical experience of several groups in France, comprising several thousands of patients treated with this regimen after PTCA or stent implantation.[121–124] Ticlopidine interferes with platelet function through a different mechanism than does aspirin,[125] involving adenosine diphosphate (ADP)–mediated inhibition of fibrinogen binding[126]; combination therapy results in a synergistic antiplatelet effect.[127–130] The most feared side effect of ticlopidine is bone marrow suppression with risk of neutropenia, which occurs in 1% to 2% of patients, is usually reversible upon discontinuation of the drug, and probably requires at least 2 to 3 weeks of therapy to occur.[131, 132] The superior efficacy over anticoagulant therapy of a combined aspirin plus ticlopidine regimen after stent implantation was demonstrated in 517 patients in the Intracoronary Stenting and Antithrombotic Regimen (ISAR) trial. More than 40% of patients in both groups had unstable angina at the time of enrollment. The combined primary clinical end point of death, myocardial infarction, and need for bypass surgery or repeat PTCA occurred in 6.2% of patients after treatment with phenprocoumon (an oral vitamin K antagonist), but in only 1.6% after ticlopidine plus aspirin therapy (relative risk, 0.25; 95% confidence interval, 0.06 to 0.77). Antiplatelet therapy resulted in significant decreases in stent thrombosis (from 5.4% to 0.8%; $p = 0.004$), hemorrhagic complications (from 6.5% to 0%; $p < 0.001$), and peripheral vascular events (from 6.2% to 0.8%; $p = 0.001$) (Fig. 37–7).[133] In the subgroup of 123 patients with acute myocardial infarction within 48 hours of the index procedure, markedly lower rates of 30-day clinical events (3.3% vs. 21%; $p = 0.005$) and stent occlusion (0% vs. 9.7%; $p = 0.03$) were found after combined antiplatelet therapy than after anticoagulation, respectively, with lower 6-month

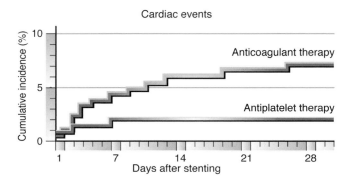

Cardiac events

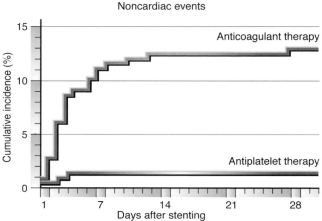

Noncardiac events

FIGURE 37–7. Incidence of the primary composite cardiac end point (consisting of death, Q-wave myocardial infarction, bypass surgery, or repeat PTCA) and noncardiac end point (noncardiac death, cerebrovascular accident, severe hemorrhagic or peripheral vascular complications) in the Intracoronary Stenting and Antithrombotic Regimen (ISAR) trial, in which patients were randomly assigned, after intracoronary stent implantation, to receive either antiplatelet therapy with a combination of aspirin and ticlopidine or oral anticoagulant therapy with phenprocoumon. (From Schomig A, Neumann F-J, Kastrati A, et al: A randomized comparison of antiplatelet and anticoagulant therapy after the placement of coronary artery stents. N Engl J Med 334:1084–1089, 1996.)

rates of reinfarction (0% vs. 9.7%; $p < 0.01$) and stent occlusion (1.6% vs. 14.5%; $p = 0.02$) but comparable restenosis rates (26.5% vs. 26.9%; $p = 0.87$).[134] A corollary of this study showed prevention of enhanced platelet activation after stent implantation by combined aspirin plus ticlopidine but not with oral anticoagulation.[135] In the Full Anticoagulation versus Ticlopidine plus Aspirin after Stent Implantation (FANTASTIC) trial of 476 patients, the rate of occurrence of the primary end point of death, myocardial infarction, or bypass surgery decreased from 4.3% after the combination of aspirin and warfarin to 0.8% ($p = 0.03$) after combination therapy with ticlopidine and aspirin.[136]

### Aspirin Versus Combined Antiplatelet Therapy (Aspirin and Ticlopidine)

Several studies have addressed the question of the relative additive clinical benefit of ticlopidine with aspirin. A small, open-label, randomized trial of 226 patients found a rate of stent thrombosis of 2.9% with aspirin alone and 0.8% with combined aspirin plus ticlopidine therapy ($p = 0.2$) but was prematurely terminated because of three unexpected deaths among the patients taking only aspirin.[137] In a retrospective and nonrandomized comparison, significant increases in risks of stent thrombosis (6.5% vs. 0.9%; $p = 0.02$), death (4.4% vs. 0.3%; $p = 0.04$), and Q-wave infarction (6.5% vs. 0%; $p = 0.002$) was found after aspirin alone than after combined aspirin plus ticlopidine therapy, respectively.[138] With adjunctive routine use of IVUS as in the MUSIC registry, however, subacute thrombosis occurred in only 1 (0.7%) of 133 selected patients with optimal stent results and treated only with aspirin.[38] Three antithrombotic strategies after stent implantation—aspirin alone, combined aspirin and warfarin, or combined aspirin and ticlopidine—were tested in 1652 patients in the multicenter, randomized Stent Anticoagulation Regimen Study (STARS) trial. The primary composite end point, consisting of death, Q-wave myocardial infarction, need for bypass surgery, or stent thrombosis at 30 days, occurred in 3.6%, 2.4%, and 0.6% of patients (with stent thrombosis in 2.9%, 2.4%, and 0.6%) after aspirin, aspirin plus warfarin, or aspirin plus ticlopidine, respectively ($p < 0.05$ for both composite and thrombosis end points) (Fig. 37–8).[139] Overall, these studies indicate additive benefits of combined antiplatelet therapy over aspirin alone.

Ticlopidine is usually started during or immediately after the procedure, with the first dose of 250 to 500 mg followed by 250 mg twice a day, and is continued for about 3 to 4 weeks, which is considered an average time for stent re-endothelialization and the period of highest risk of subacute stent thrombosis.[7] Clinical testing of different strategies,

limiting the duration of therapy with ticlopidine to avoid side effects,[131, 140] or starting the drug at least 48 to 72 hours before the procedure to attain a full antiplatelet effect,[129, 141] is under way; preliminary results have been encouraging. In a multicenter French registry, an overall rate of stent thrombosis of 1.7% was reported in a consecutive series of 1336 patients after preprocedure treatment with ticlopidine alone and intraprocedural heparin. Adequate stent deployment was achieved without use of IVUS or postprocedure high-pressure balloon dilatation.[141]

## New Antiplatelet Agents

Clinical efficacy of antiplatelet therapy has led to rediscovery of the central role of platelets in stent thrombosis and renewed interest in the potential additive benefit of more potent agents, such as the glycoprotein (GP) IIb/IIIa inhibitors.[142] Greater surface expression of the GPIIb/IIIa receptor (activated fibrinogen receptor),[143] a marker of platelet activation, is present after stent implantation than after angioplasty and can be prevented by combined ticlopidine plus aspirin therapy but not by vitamin K antagonists.[135] In 140 consecutive patients, Neumann and associates demonstrated a strong association between higher surface expression of GPIIb/IIIa platelet receptor and increased risk of stent thrombosis, independent of other angiographic or coagulation parameters.[144]

Patients pretreated with GPIIb/IIIa blockers in the Integrilin to Minimize Platelet Aggregation and Prevent Coronary Thrombosis (IMPACT) II trial exhibited a reduction in the incidence of periprocedural myocardial infarction from 32% to 16% ($p = 0.01$) when bail-out stent implantation became necessary during the procedure.[145] In a subgroup of 325 patients with bail-out stent implantation in the

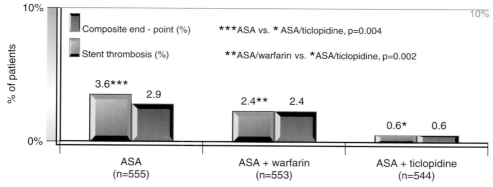

FIGURE 37–8. Incidence of the primary composite end point, consisting of death, Q-wave myocardial infarction, bypass surgery, or stent thrombosis at 30 days, and of stent thrombosis alone in the randomized Stent Anticoagulation Regimen Study (STARS), in which patients were treated with aspirin (ASA) alone, aspirin and warfarin, or aspirin and ticlopidine. Data are expressed as percentages of patients. There was a statistically significant decrease in the incidence of the combined primary end point in the group treated with the combination aspirin and ticlopidine in comparison with aspirin alone ($p = 0.004$) and aspirin and warfarin therapy ($p = 0.02$). (From Leon MB, Baim DS, Gordon P, et al: Clinical and angiographic results from the Stent Anticoagulation Regimen Study (STARS) [Abstract]. Circulation 94:I-685, 1996.)

**TABLE 37–5. RETROSPECTIVE, NONRANDOMIZED COMPARISON OF SHORT-TERM CLINICAL OUTCOME IN PATIENTS AFTER BAIL-OUT STENT IMPLANTATION WITH AND WITHOUT ABCIXIMAB AT THE CLEVELAND CLINIC FOUNDATION**

| DEMOGRAPHICS | NO ABCIXIMAB | PRESTENT IMPLANTATION ABCIXIMAB | BAIL-OUT ABCIXIMAB |
|---|---|---|---|
| N | 368 | 149 | 30 |
| Age (years) | 63 ± 12 | 62 ± 11 | 63 ± 10 |
| Rest angina (%) | 42 | 46 | 36 |
| MI <2 weeks (%) | 14 | 26 | 30 |
| Type C lesion (%) | 24 | 36 | 30 |
| LVEF (%) | 57 ± 11 | 53 ± 12 | 54 ± 14 |
| Death (%) | 1.6 | 2.8* | 10 |
| Q-wave MI (%) | 0.6 | 0.7† | 6.7 |
| Non–Q-wave MI (%) | 13 | 10‡ | 20 |
| CABG (%) | 1.4 | 1.4 | 3.3 |
| MACE (%) | 15.3 | 13.2 | 30 |
| Transfusion (%) | 8 | 13 | 13 |

CABG, coronary artery bypass graft surgery; LVEF, left ventricular ejection fraction; MACE, major adverse cardiac events, comprising death, MI, CABG, or emergency revascularization; MI, myocardial infarction.
*$p = 0.11$.
†$p = 0.04$.
‡$p = 0.04$.
Unpublished data from the Cleveland Clinic Interventional registry.

EPILOG study, the incidence of the combined clinical end point of death, myocardial infarction, and need for urgent revascularization decreased from 22.6% to 9.3% ($p = 0.004$) in the placebo-treated group (heparin only) and the c7E3-treated group, respectively (unpublished data, on file).

In practice, because the requirement for bail-out stent implantation cannot be anticipated, data on the use of GPIIb/IIIa inhibitors on "ad hoc" basis, after the complication has occurred, are needed to elucidate their role (Table 37–5).

However, it seems reasonable to extrapolate from the available evidence that patient subsets at highest risk for thrombosis may derive additive clinical benefit of GPIIb/IIIa inhibition after stent implantation. Potential indications may include unstable coronary syndromes such as severe unstable angina or acute myocardial infarction, thrombus-laden lesions, and old degenerated saphenous vein grafts.

The ongoing EPILOG-Stent study will help better define the role of c7E3 (abciximab, or ReoPro) after stent implantation. The Evaluation of ReoPro And Stenting to Eliminate Restenosis (ERASER) study will analyze the effects of GPIIb/IIIa inhibition on in-stent restenosis with IVUS.

## Low Molecular Weight Heparin

Low molecular weight heparin (LMWH) was initially used as adjunctive therapy after stent implan-

tation as an alternative to warfarin, to decrease the incidence of bleeding complications.[121, 122, 146] In phase I of the French Multicenter registry study, subacute stent occlusion in 10.4% of the first 237 patients treated with LMWH instead of warfarin (Coumadin) led to replacement with a combination of aspirin and ticlopidine.[87] No subacute stent thrombosis was found in a consecutive series of 539 patients treated with LMWH in addition to aspirin and ticlopidine, without increased bleeding complications.[147] In view of the need for daily subcutaneous injections with patient discomfort, however, the routine use of LMWH after stent implantation cannot be advocated until further supporting evidence of additive clinical benefit to standard combined antiplatelet therapy is available. Ongoing research will explore the potential benefit in terms of antiproliferative action for restenosis prevention, possibly after local delivery,[148] and as additive anticoagulation therapy in patients at high prothrombotic risk.[147, 149, 150]

## NEW TECHNOLOGIES

Besides ongoing evolution of new designs, to find the most effective combination of scaffolding properties, radial strength, and flexibility (see Tables 37–3 and 37–4), several lines of research are aimed at further decreasing stent thrombogenicity and the elicited neointimal proliferative response. Very promising results for preventing restenosis have been obtained in different animal models with radioactive stents[151–155] or with local radiation therapy to the treated vessel,[156] which is already in early clinical development.[157] Although it is quite premature to draw conclusions on the clinical applicability, the interventional cardiologist may soon be faced with a need for specialized training and expertise on appropriate handling of radioactive sources (stents, delivery catheters, or both) and more technically demanding procedures for accurate placement and dosing of the delivered radiation.[158]

Conversely, the use of heparin-coated stents[159] may in the near future provide the operator with a "safety net" after suboptimal deployment or in high-risk situations.

## CONCLUSION

Intracoronary stent implantation represents the most important development since movable guide wires in the brief history of interventional cardiology. Concomitant progress in indications, deployment techniques, and adjunctive pharmacotherapy have spurred the current widespread use of stents in daily practice. As reviewed in this chapter, great progress has been made in understanding some technical aspects unique to this procedure, with refinement of implantation strategies. Optimal stent implantation should begin from advanced planning on correct indications and feasibility, with the recognition that the procedure will generally be more technically demanding than simple balloon dilatation, with unique potential complications, and that the often impressive immediate angiographic results may not always translate to equivalent overall long-term clinical benefit. The risk of stent thrombosis has indeed been greatly limited with combined antiplatelet therapy alone, but only in the setting of adequate stent expansion and absence of an excessively prothrombotic milieu. IVUS may still be of benefit after stent implantation, either as a learning tool or for assessing suboptimal results. The field is in rapid and exponential evolution, and ongoing studies will address several unanswered questions in the near future.

# REFERENCES

1. Lincoff AM, Popma JJ, Ellis SG, et al: Abrupt vessel closure complicating coronary angioplasty: Clinical, angiographic and therapeutic profile. J Am Coll Cardiol 19:926–938, 1992.
2. Moliterno DJ: Restenosis following percutaneous coronary intervention. In Topol EJ (ed): Textbook of Interventional Cardiology, vol update 17. Philadelphia: WB Saunders, 1995, pp 257–272.
3. Palmaz JC, Sibbitt RR, Reuter SR, et al: Expandable intraluminal graft: A preliminary study. Radiology 156:73–77, 1985.
4. Palmaz JC, Garcia OJ, Copp DT, et al: Balloon-expandable intra-arterial stents: Effect of anticoagulation on thrombus formation. Circulation 76(suppl IV):IV-45A, 1987.
5. Schatz RA, Palmaz C, Tio FO, et al: Balloon-expandable intracoronary stents in the adult dog. Circulation 76:450–457, 1987.
6. Cragg A, Lund G, Rysavy J, et al: Non-surgical placement of arterial endoprosthesis: A new technique using nitinol wire. Radiology 147:261–263, 1993.
7. Mak KH, Belli G, Ellis SG, et al: Subacute stent thrombosis: Evolving issues and current concepts. J Am Coll Cardiol 27:494–503, 1996.
8. Serruys PW, Strauss BH, Beatt KJ, et al: Angiographic follow-up after placement of a self-expanding coronary artery stent. N Engl J Med 324:13–17, 1991.
9. Schatz RA, Baim DS, Leon M, et al: Clinical experience with the Palmaz-Shatz coronary stent: Initial results of a multicenter study. Circulation 83:148–161, 1991.
10. Serruys PW, DeJaegere P, Kiemeneij F, et al: A comparison of balloon-expandable stent implantation with balloon angioplasty in patients with coronary artery disease. N Engl J Med 331:489–495, 1994.
11. Fischman DL, Leon MB, Baim DS, et al: A randomized comparison of coronary stent placement and balloon angioplasty in the treatment of coronary artery disease. N Engl J Med 331:496–501, 1994.
12. Sutton JM, Ellis SG, Roubin GS, et al: Major clinical events after coronary stenting. The multicenter registry of acute and elective Gianturco-Roubin stent placement. Circulation 89:1126–1137, 1994.
13. Wong SC, Baim DS, Schatz RA, et al: Immediate results and late outcomes after stent implantation in saphenous graft lesions: the multicenter U.S. Palmaz-Schatz stent experience. J Am Coll Cardiol 26:704–712, 1995.
14. Roubin GS, Cannon AD, Agrawal SK, et al: Intracoronary stenting for acute and threatened closure complicating percutaneous transluminal coronary angioplasty. Circulation 85:916–927, 1992.
15. Carrozza JP, Kuntz RE, Levine MJ, et al: Angiographic and clinical outcome of intracoronary stenting: Immediate and long-term results from a large single-center experience. J Am Coll Cardiol 20:328–337, 1992.
16. Piana RN, Moscucci M, Cohen DJ, et al: Palmaz-Schatz stenting for treatment of focal vein graft stenosis: Immediate results and long-term outcome. J Am Coll Cardiol 23:1296–1304, 1994.
17. Fenton SH, Fischman DL, Savage MP, et al: Long-term angiographic and clinical outcome after implantation of balloon-expandable stents in aortocoronary saphenous vein grafts. Am J Cardiol 74:1187–1191, 1994.
18. Dorros G, Bates MC, Iyer S, et al: The use of Gianturco-Roubin flexible metallic coronary stents in old saphenous vein grafts: In hospital outcome and 7 day angiographic patency. Eur Heart J 15:1456–1462, 1994.
19. Eeckhout E, Goy JJ, Vogt P, et al: Complications and follow-up after intracoronary stenting: Critical analysis of a 6-year single-center experience. Am Heart J 127:262–272, 1994.
20. Strumpf RK, Mehta SS, Ponder R, et al: Palmaz-Schatz stent implantation in stenosed saphenous vein grafts: Clinical and angiographic follow-up. Am Heart J 123:1329–1336, 1992.
21. Yock PG, Fitzgerald PJ, Linker DT, et al: Intravascular ultrasound guidance for catheter-based coronary interventions. J Am Coll Cardiol 17:39B–45B, 1991.
22. Slepian MJ: Application of intraluminal ultrasound imaging to vascular stenting. Int J Cardiac Imaging 6:285–311, 1991.
23. Keren G, Douek P, Oblon C, et al: Atherosclerotic saphenous vein grafts treated with different interventional procedures assessed by intravascular ultrasound. Am Heart J 124:198–206, 1992.
24. Tenaglia AN, Kisslo K, Kelly S, et al: Ultrasound guide wire–directed stent deployment. Am Heart J 125:1213–1216, 1993.
25. Nakamura S, Colombo A, Gaglione A, et al: Intracoronary ultrasound observations during stent implantation. Circulation 89:2026–2034, 1994.
26. Goldberg SL, Colombo A, Nakamura S, et al: Benefit of intracoronary ultrasound in the deployment of Palmaz-Shatz stents. J Am Coll Cardiol 24:996–1003, 1994.
27. Kiemeneij F, Laarman G, Slagboom T: Mode of deployment of coronary Palmaz-Schatz stents after implantation with the stent delivery system: An intravascular ultrasound study. Am Heart J 129:638–644, 1995.
28. Mudra H, Klauss V, Blasini R, et al: Ultrasound guidance of Palmaz-Schatz intracoronary stenting with a combined intravascular ultrasound balloon catheter. Circulation 90:1252–1261, 1994.
29. Serruys PW, Di Mario C: Who was thrombogenic: The stent or the doctor? Circulation 91:1891–1893, 1995.
30. Colombo A, Hall P, Nakamura S, et al: Intracoronary stenting without anticoagulation accomplished with intravascular ultrasound guidance. Circulation 91:1676–1688, 1995.
31. Belli G, Whitlow PL, Gross L, et al: Intracoronary stenting without oral anticoagulation: The Cleveland Clinic Registry [Abstract]. Circulation 92:I-796, 1995.
32. Allen KM, Undemir C, Shaknovich A, et al: Is there a need for intravascular ultrasound after high-pressure dilatations of Palmaz-Schatz stents? [Abstract]. J Am Coll Cardiol 27:138A, 1996.
33. Nunez BD, Holmes DR, Lerman A, et al: Detailed intravascular ultrasound analysis after routine high-pressure assisted intracoronary stent implantation [Abstract]. J Am Coll Cardiol 27:199A, 1996.
34. Werner GS, Diedrich J, Ferrari M, et al: Can additional ultrasound improve the luminal area gain after high-pressure stent deployment? [Abstract]. J Am Coll Cardiol 27:225A, 1996.
35. Goldberg SL, Hall P, Nakamura S, et al: Is there a benefit from intravascular ultrasound when high-pressure stent

expansion is routinely performed prior to ultrasound imaging? [Abstract]. J Am Coll Cardiol 27:306A, 1996.

36. Vardi GM, Fishman RF, Meyers SN, et al: Benefit of intracoronary ultrasound after angiographically optimal Palmaz-Schatz stent deployment. Circulation 94:I-262, 1996.

37. Stone GW, Linnemeier TJ, Saint Goar FG, et al: Refining the relationship between implantation pressure and optimal expansion—Core lab analysis from the OSTI trial [Abstract]. Circulation 94:I-259, 1996.

38. de Jaegere P, Mudra H, Almagor Y, et al, for the MUSIC study Investigators: In-hospital and 1-month clinical results of an international study testing the concept of IVUS guided optimized stent expansion alleviating the need of systemic anticoagulation [Abstract]. J Am Coll Cardiol 27:137A, 1996.

39. Hong MK, Wong SC, Pichard AD, et al: Long-term results of patients enrolled in the Anti-Platelet After Intravascular Ultrasound Guided Optimal Stent Expansion (APLAUSE) trial [Abstract]. Circulation 94:I-686, 1996.

40. Metz JA, Fitzgerald PJ, Oshima A, et al: Impact of intravascular ultrasound guidance on stenting in the CRUISE substudy [Abstract]. Circulation 94:I-199, 1996.

41. Russo RJ, Teirstein PS, for the AVID Investigators: Angiography versus intravascular ultrasound-directed stent placement [Abstract]. Circulation 94:I-263, 1996.

42. Strain JE, Rehman DE, Fischman D, et al, for the STRESS-III Investigators: STRESS-III: Preliminary acute results of IVUS vs. non-IVUS stenting [Abstract]. Circulation 94:I-200, 1996.

43. Werner F, Regar E, Klauss V, et al: What is the benefit of intravascular ultrasound guidance after angiographically optimized high-pressuure stenting? [Abstract]. Eur Heart J 17(Abstract suppl):187, 1996.

44. Tobis JM, Colombo A: Do you need IVUS guidance for coronary stent deployment? [Editorial]. Catheter Cardiovasc Diagn 37:360–361, 1996.

45. Ziada KM, Tuzcu EM, DeFranco AC, et al: Angiographic "haziness" following stent deployment: Differential diagnosis using intravascular ultrasound [Abstract]. J Am Coll Cardiol 27:224A, 1996.

46. Pepine CJ, Holmes DR, Block PC, et al: ACC Expert Consensus Document. Coronary artery stents. J Am Coll Cardiol 28:782–794, 1996.

47. Fishman dL, Savage MP, Goldberg S: Coronary stent placement compared with balloon angioplasty [Letter]. N Engl J Med 332:536–538, 1995.

48. Schwartz RS, Huber KC, Murphy JG, et al: Restenosis and the proportional neointimal response to coronary artery injury: Results in a porcine model. J Am Coll Cardiol 19:267–274, 1992.

49. Rogers C, Edelmann ER: Endovascular stent design dicates experimental restenosis and thrombosis. Circulation 91:2995–3001, 1995.

50. Rogers C, Parikh S, Seifert P, et al: Endogenous cell seeding. Remnant endothelium after stenting enhances vascular repair. Circulation 94:2909–2914, 1996.

51. Chevalier B, Royer T, Glatt B, et al: Early clinical experience with the MultiLink coronary stent [Abstract]. Circulation 94:I-206, 1996.

52. Serruys PW, Azar AJ, Sigwart U, et al, on behalf of the BENESTENT Group: Long-term follow-up of "stent-like" (<30% diameter stenosis post) angioplasty: A case for provisional stenting [Abstract]. J Am Coll Cardiol 27:15A, 1996.

53. Abhyankar A, Bernstein L, Harris PJ, et al: Reintervention and clinical events after saphenous vein angioplasty—A comparison of optimal PTCA versus stenting [Abstract]. Circulation 94:I-686, 1996.

54. Rodriguez AE, Santaera O, Larribau M, et al: Coronary stenting decreases restenosis in lesions with early loss in luminal diameter 24 hours after successful PTCA. Circulation 91:1397–1402, 1995.

55. Rodriguez AE, Palacios IF, Fernandez MA, et al: Time course and mechanism of early luminal diameter loss after percutaneous transluminal coronary angioplasty. Am J Cardiol 76:1131–1134, 1995.

56. Kuntz RE, Gibson CM, Nobuyoshi M, et al: Generalized

model of restenosis after conventional balloon angioplasty, stenting and directional atherectomy. J Am Coll Cardiol 21:15–25, 1993.

57. Umans V, Hermans W, Foley D, et al: Restenosis after directional coronary atherectomy and balloon angioplasty: Comparative analysis based on matched lesions. J Am Coll Cardiol 21:1382–1390, 1993.

58. Umans V, Robert A, Foley D, et al: Clinical, histologic and quantitative angiographic predictors of restenosis after directional coronary atherectomy: A multivariate analysis of the renarrowing process and late outcome. J Am Coll Cardiol 23:49–58, 1994.

59. Mintz GS, Popma JJ, Pichard AD, et al: Intravascular ultrasound predictors of restenosis after percutaneous transcatheter coronary revascularization. J Am Coll Cardiol 27:1678–1687, 1996.

60. Mehran R, Mintz G, Pichard AD, et al: Impact of vessel wall injury on in-stent restenosis: A serial quantitative angiographic and intravascular ultrasound study [Abstract]. Circulation 94:I-262, 1996.

61. Holmes DR, Garratt KN, Isner JM, et al, for the CAVEAT-I and II Investigators: Effect of subintimal resection on initial outcome and restenosis for native coronary lesions and saphenous vein graft disease treated by directional coronary atherectomy. J Am Coll Cardiol 28:645–651, 1996.

62. Umans VA, Melkert R, Foley DP, et al: Clinical and angiographic comparison of matched patients with successful directional coronary atherectomy or stent implantation for primary coronary artery lesions. J Am Coll Cardiol 28:637–644, 1996.

63. Umans VAWM, Keane D, Foley D, et al: Optimal use of directional coronary atherectomy is required to ensure long-term angiographic benefit: A study with matched procedural outcome after atherectomy and angioplasty. J Am Coll Cardiol 24:1652–1659, 1994.

64. Lehmann KG, Melkert R, Serruys PW: Contributions of frequency distribution analysis to the understanding of coronary restenosis. A reappraisal of the Gaussian curve. Circulation 93:1123–1132, 1996.

65. Gordon PC, Gibson MC, Cohen DJ, et al: Mechanisms of restenosis and redilation with coronary stents. Quantitative angiographic assessment. J Am Coll Cardiol 21:1166–1174, 1993.

66. Haude M, Erbel R, Issa H, et al: Quantitative analysis of elastic recoil after balloon angioplasty and after intracoronary implantation of balloon-expandable Palmaz-Schatz stents. J Am Coll Cardiol 21:26–34, 1993.

67. de Jaegere P, Serruys PW, van Es G-A, et al: Recoil following Wiktor stent implantation for restenotic lesions of coronary arteries. Catheter Cardiovasc Diagn 32:147–156, 1994.

68. Dussaillant GR, Mintz GS, Pichard AD, et al: Small stent size and intimal hyperplasia contribute to restenosis: A volumetric intravascular ultrasound analysis. J Am Coll Cardiol 26:720–724, 1995.

69. Hoffman R, Mintz GS, Dussaillant GR, et al: Patterns and mechanism of in-stent restenosis. A serial intravascular ultrasound study. Circulation 94:1247–1254, 1996.

70. Mintz GS, Popma JJ, Pichard AD, et al: Arterial remodeling after coronary angioplasty. A serial intravascular ultrasound study. Circulation 94:35–43, 1996.

71. Isner JM: Vascular remodeling. Honey, I think I shrunk the artery [Editorial]. Circulation 89:2937–2941, 1994.

72. Post MJ, Borst C, Kuntz RE: The relative importance of arterial remodeling with intimal hyperplasia in lumen renarrowing after balloon angioplasty. A study in the normal rabbit and the hypercholesterolemic Yucatan micropig. Circulation 89:2816–2821, 1994.

73. Baptista J, Umans V, Di Mario C, et al: Mechanisms of luminal enlargment and quantification of vessel wall trauma following balloon coronary angioplasty and directional coronary atherectomy. A study using intracoronary ultrasound, angioscopy and angiography. Eur Heart J 16:1603–1612, 1995.

74. Ellis S, Popma J, Buchbinder M, et al: Relation of clinical presentation, stenosis morphology, and operator technique to the procedural results of rotational atherectomy and rota-

tional atherectomy-facilitated angioplasty. Circulation 89:882–892, 1994.

75. MacIsaac AI, Bass TA, Buchbinder M, et al: High speed rotational atherectomy: Outcome in calcified and non-calcified coronary artery lesions. J Am Coll Cardiol 26:731–736, 1995.

76. Safian RD, Freed M, Reddy V, et al: Do excimer laser and rotational atherectomy facilitate balloon angioplasty? Implications for lesion-specific coronary intervention. J Am Coll Cardiol 27:552–559, 1996.

77. Mintz GS, Popma JJ, Pichard AD, et al: Patterns of calcification in coronary artery disease. A statistical analysis of intravascular ultrasound and coronary angiography in 1155 lesions. Circulation 91:1959–1965, 1995.

78. Albrecht D, Kaspers S, Fussl R, et al: Coronary plaque morphology affects stent deployment: Assessment by intracoronary ultrasound. Catheter Cardiovasc Diagn 38:229–235, 1996;

79. Komiyama M, Stone GW, Alderman EL, et al: Relative stent expansion is dependent upon target segment calcification: An intravascular ultrasound assessment [Abstract]. Circulation 94:I-262, 1996.

80. Yokoi H, Nobuyoshi M, Nosaka H, et al: Palmaz-Schatz stent implantation in calcified lesions: Immediate and follow-up results [Abstract]. Circulation 94:I-453, 1996.

81. Dussaillant GR, Mintz GS, Pichard AD, et al: The optimal strategy for treating calcified lesions in large vessels: Comparison of intravascular ultrasound results of rotational atherectomy with adjunctive PTCA, DCA or stents [Abstract]. J Am Coll Cardiol 27:153A, 1996.

82. Guarneri EM, Norman SL, Stevens M, et al: Rotational atherectomy prior to stent implantation [Abstract]. J Am Coll Cardiol 27:252A, 1996.

83. Benzuly KH, Glazier S, Grines CL, et al: Coronary perforation: An unreported complication after intracoronary stent implantation [Abstract]. J Am Coll Cardiol 27:252A, 1996.

84. Buszman P, Stables R, Sigwart U, et al, on behalf of the BENESTENT Study Group: Endothelial hyperplasia and restenosis depend on the technique of coronary stent implantation [Abstract]. J Am Coll Cardiol 27:226A, 1996.

85. MacIsaac AI, Elliott JM, Ellis SG, et al: Predictors of restenosis in Palmaz-Schatz biliary stents used for coronary stenosis: Is overdilation important? [Abstract]. Circulation 90:I-611, 1994.

86. Bermejo J, Botas J, Garcia EJ, et al: Mechanisms of residual lumen stenosis after high-pressure stent implantation: A QCA and IVUS study [Abstract]. Circulation 94:I-199, 1996.

87. Karrillon GJ, Morice MC, Benveniste E, et al: Intracoronary stent implantation without ultrasound guidance and with replacement of conventional anticoagulation by antiplatelet therapy. 30-day clinical outcome of the French multicenter registry. Circulation 94:1519–1527, 1996.

88. Stone GW, Linnemeier T, St. Goar F, et al: What is optimal pressure for stent implantation (how high is high)? [Abstract]. J Am Coll Cardiol 27:225A, 1996.

89. Carrozza JP, Yock PG, Linnemeier TJ, et al: Serial expansion of the ACS MultiLink stent after 8, 12, and 16 atmospheres: A QCA and IVUS pilot study [Abstract]. Circulation 94:I-88, 1996.

90. Yang P, Hassan A, Heyer G, et al: High-pressure post-dilatation of the Medtronic-Wiktor stent: Iintravascular ultrasound and quantitative angiographic data from the Austrian multicenter trial. Circulation 94:I-207, 1996.

91. Alfonso F, Goicolea J, Hernandez R, et al: Arterial perforation during optimization of coronary stents using high-pressure balloon inflations. Am J Cardiol 78:1169–1172, 1996.

92. Zampieri P, Colombo A, Almagor Y, et al: Results of coronary stenting of ostial lesions. Am J Cardiol 73:901–903, 1993.

93. Nordrehaug JE, Priestley K, Chronos N, et al: Implantation of half Palmaz-Schatz stents in short aorto-ostial lesions of saphenous vein grafts. Catheter Cardiovasc Diagn 29:141–143, 1993.

94. Rechavia E, Litvack F, Macko G, et al: Stent implantation of saphenous vein graft aorto-ostial lesions in patients with unstable ischemic syndromes: Immediate angiographic re-

sults and long-term clinical outcome. J Am Coll Cardiol 25:866–870, 1995.

95. Rocha-Singh K, Morris N, Wong SC, et al: Coronary stenting for treatment of ostial stenoses of native coronary arteries or aortocoronary saphenous venous grafts. Am J Cardiol 75:26–29, 1995.

96. Wong SC, Popma JJ, Pichard AD, et al: Comparison of clinical and angiographic outcomes after saphenous vein graft angioplasty using coronary versus "biliary" tubular slotted stents. Circulation 91:339–350, 1995.

97. Myler RK, McConahay DR, Stertzer SH, et al: Coronary bifurcation stenoses: The kissing balloon probe technique via a single guiding catheter. Catheter Cardiovasc Diagn 16:267–278, 1989.

98. Renkin J, Wijns W, Hanet C, et al: Angioplasty of coronary bifurcation stenoses: Immediate and long-term results of the protecting branch technique. Catheter Cardiovasc Diagn 22:167–173, 1991.

99. Weinstein JS, Baim DS, Sipperly ME, et al: Salvage of branch vessels during bifurcation lesion angioplasty: Acute and long-term follow-up. Catheter Cardiovasc Diagn 22:1–6, 1991.

100. Lewis B, Leya FS, Johnson SA, et al: Acute procedural results in the treatment of 30 coronary artery bifurcation lesions with a double-wire atherectomy technique for side-branch protection. Am Heart J 127:1600–1607, 1994.

101. Carrie D, Karouny E, Chouairi S, et al: "T"-shaped stent placement: A technique for the treatment of dissected bifurcation lesions. Catheter Cardiovasc Diagn 37:311–313, 1996.

102. Teirstein PS: Kissing Palmaz-Schatz stents for coronary bifurcation stenoses. Catheter Cardiovasc Diagn 37:307–310, 1996.

103. Colombo A, Gaglione A, Nakamura S, et al: "Kissing" stents for bifurcational coronary lesions. Catheter Cardiovasc Diagn 30:327–330, 1993.

104. Foley DP, Serruys PW: Bifurcation lesion stenting. Thoraxcentre J 8/4:32–36, 1996.

105. Baim DS: Is bifurcation stenting the answer? Catheter Cardiovasc Diagn 37:314–316, 1996.

106. Cannon AD, Roubin GS, Hearn JA, et al: Acute angiographic and clinical results of long balloon percutaneous transluminal coronary angioplasty and adjuvant stenting for long narrowings. Am J Cardiol 73:635–641, 1994.

107. Shaknovich A, Moses JW, Undemir C, et al: Procedural and short-term clinical outcomes of multiple Palmaz-Schatz stents in very long lesions/dissections [Abstract]. Circulation 92:I-535, 1995.

108. Reimers B, Di Mario C, Nierop P, et al: Long-term restenosis after multiple stent implantation. A quantitative angiographic study [Abstract]. Circulation 92:I-327, 1995.

109. Akira I, Hall P, Maiello L, et al: Coronary stenting of long lesions (greater than 20 mm)—A matched comparison of different stents [Abstract]. Circulation 92:I-688, 1995.

110. Thomas MR, Wainwright RJ, Robinson NM, et al: Treatment of diffuse coronary and graft disease using the less-shortening Wallstent [Abstract]. Circulation 94:I-87, 1996.

111. Liu MW, Luo JF, Dean LS, et al: Coronary vessel reconstruction with multiple stents—A follow-up study [Abstract]. Circulation 94:I-258, 1996.

112. Kelly PA, Kurbaan AS, Sigwart U: Total endovascular reconstruction of occluded saphenous vein grafts using coronary or peripheral Wallstents [Abstract]. Circulation 94:I-258, 1996.

113. Ellis SG, Savage M, Fischman D, et al: Restenosis after placement of Palmaz-Schatz stents in native coronary arteries. Initial results of a multicenter experience. Circulation 86:1836–1844, 1992.

114. Strauss BH, Serruys PW, De Scheerder IK, et al: Relative risk analysis of angiographic predictors of restenosis within the coronary wallstent. Circulation 84:1636–1643, 1991.

115. Savage M, Fernandes L, Fischman D, et al: Radical endoluminal reconstruction of diffusely diseased coronary arteries using multiple stents [Abstract]. Circulation 94:I-258, 1996.

116. Eccleston DS, Belli G, Penn IM, et al: Are multiple stents

associated with multiplicative risk in the optimal stent era? [Abstract]. Circulation 94:I-454, 1996.

117. Fajadet J, Mehta S, Loubeyre C, et al: Lesion-specific coronary stenting [Abstract]. Circulation 94:I-332, 1996.

118. Ozaki Y, Violaris AG, Hamburger J, et al: Short- and long-term clinical and quantitative angiographic results with the new, less shortening Wallstent for vessel reconstruction in chronic total occlusion: A quantitative angiographic study. J Am Coll Cardiol 28:354–360, 1996.

119. Ozaki Y, Keane D, Ruygrok P, et al: Six-month clinical and angiographic outcome of the new, less-shortening Wallstent in native coronary arteries. Circulation 93:2114–2120, 1996.

120. Moussa I, Di Mario C, Reimers B, et al: Subacute stent thrombosis in the era of intravascular ultrasound-guided coronary stenting without anticoagulation: Frequency, predictors and clinical outcome. J Am Coll Cardiol 29:6–12, 1997.

121. Barragan P, Sainsous J, Silvestri M, et al: Etude pilote de l'efficacité de la ticlopidine dans la permeabilité precoce des endoprotheses coronaires. Arch Mal Coeur Vaiss 87:1431–1437, 1994.

122. Barragan P, Sainsous J, Silvestri M, et al: Ticlodipine and subcutaneous heparin as an alternative regimen following coronary stenting. Catheter Cardiovasc Diagn 32:133–138, 1994.

123. Morice M-C, Zermour G, Beneviste E, et al: Intracoronary stenting without Coumadin: One month results of a French multicenter study. Catheter Cardiovasc Diagn 35:1–7, 1995.

124. Lablanche J-M, Grollier G, Danchin N, et al: Full antiplatelet therapy without anticoagulation after coronary stenting [Abstract]. J Am Coll Cardiol 25:181A, 1995.

125. Mc Tavish D, Faulds D, Goa KL: Ticlopidine: An updated review of its pharmacology and therapeutic use in platelet dependent disorders. Drugs 40:238–259, 1990.

126. Cattaneo M, Akkawat B, Lecchi A, et al: Ticlopidine selectively inhibits human platelet response to adenosine diphosphate. Thromb Haemost 66:694–699, 1991.

127. Uchiyama S, Sone R, Nagayama T, et al: Combination therapy with low-dose aspirin and ticlopidine in cerebral ischemia. Stroke 20:1643–1647, 1989.

128. De Caterina R, Sicari R, Bernini W, et al: Benefit/risk profile of combined antiplatelet therapy with ticlopidine and aspirin. Thromb Haemost 65:504–510, 1991.

129. Gregorini L, Marco J, Fajadet J, et al: Ticlopidine and aspirin pretreatment reduces coagulation and platelet activation during coronary dilation procedures. J Am Coll Cardiol 29:13–20, 1997.

130. Darius H, Veit K, Rupprecht HJ, et al: Synergistic inhibition of platelet aggregation by ticlopidine plus aspirin following intracoronary stent placement [Abstract]. Circulation 94:I-257, 1996.

131. Berger PB, Melby SJ, Grill DE, et al: How long should ticlopidine be administered to intracoronary stent patients not treated with Coumadin? [Abstract]. Circulation 94:I-256, 1996.

132. Hass WK, Easton JD, Adams JP, et al: A randomized trial comparing ticlopidine hydrochloride with aspirin for the prevention of stroke in high-risk patients. N Engl J Med 321:501–507, 1989.

133. Schomig A, Neumann F-J, Kastrati A, et al: A randomized comparison of antiplatelet and anticoagulant therapy after the placement of coronary-artery stents. N Engl J Med 334:1084–1089, 1996.

134. Schomig A, Neumann F-J, Walter H, et al: Coronary stent placement in patients with acute myocardial infarction: Comparison of clinical and angiographic outcome after randomization to antiplatelet or anticoagulant therapy. J Am Coll Cardiol 29:28–34, 1997.

135. Gawaz M, Neumann FJ, Ott I, et al: Platelet activation and coronary stent implantation. Effect of antithrombotic therapy. Circulation 94:279–285, 1996.

136. Bertrand M, Legrand V, Boland J, et al: Full anticoagulation versus ticlopidine plus aspirin after stent implantation: A randomized multicenter European study, the FANTASTIC trial [Abstract]. Circulation 94:I-685, 1996.

137. Hall P, Nakamura S, Maiello L, et al: A randomized comparison of combined ticlopidine and aspirin therapy versus aspirin therapy alone after successful intravascular ultrasound-guided stent implantation. Circulation 93:215–222, 1996.

138. Goods CM, Al-Shaibi KF, Liu MW, et al: Comparison of aspirin alone versus aspirin plus ticlopidine after coronary artery stenting. Am J Cardiol 78:1042–1044, 1996.

139. Leon MB, Baim DS, Gordon P, et al: Clinical and angiographic results from the Stent Anticoagulation Regimen Study (STARS) [Abstract]. Circulation 94:I-685, 1996.

140. Kataoka K, Sato Y, Ito S, et al: Palmaz-Schatz stenting with 10 days ticlopidine treatment [Abstract]. Circulation 94:I-684, 1996.

141. Sainsous J, Silvestri M, Baaayet G, et al: Coronary artery stenting without anticoagulation, intravascular ultrasound or high pressure balloon: Immediate results and one month follow-up [Abstract]. Circulation 94:I-262, 1996.

142. Lefkovits J, Plow EF, Topol EJ: Platelet glycoprotein IIb/IIIa receptors in cardiovascular medicine. N Engl J Med 332:1553–1559, 1995.

143. Gawaz M, Neumann F-J, Ott I, et al: Changes in membrane glycoproteins of circulating platelets after coronary stent implantation. Heart 76:166–172, 1996.

144. Neumann FJ, Gawaz M, Ott I, et al: Prospective evaluation of hemostatic predictors of subacute stent thrombosis after coronary Palmaz-Schatz stenting. J Am Coll Cardiol 27:15–21, 1996.

145. Zidar JP, Kruse KR, Thel MC, et al: Integrilin for emergency coronary artery stenting [Abstract]. J Am Coll Cardiol 27:138A, 1996.

146. Fernandes-Aviles F, Alonso JJ, Duran JM, et al: Subacute occlusion, bleeding complications, hospital stay and restenosis after Palmaz-Schatz coronary stenting under a new antithrombotic regimen. J Am Coll Cardiol 27:22–29, 1996.

147. Pan M, Suarez de Lezo J, Velasco F, et al: Reduction of thrombotic and hemorrhagic complications after stent implantation. Am Heart J 132:119–126, 1996.

148. Kiesz SR, Martin JL, Buszman P, et al: Intramural low molecular weight heparin delivery at the time of predilation permits safe intracoronary stent deployment with reduced systemic anticoagulation and early ambulation [Abstract]. Circulation 94:I-325, 1996.

149. Monassier JP, Elias J, Meyer P, et al: STENTIM I: The French registry of stenting at acute myocardial infarction [Abstract]. J Am Coll Cardiol 27:68A, 1996.

150. Goods CM, Liu MW, Jain SP, et al: Low molecular weight heparin versus standard heparin in patients at high risk for stent thrombosis: Clinical outcomes [Abstract]. Circulation 94:I-684, 1996.

151. Fischell tA, Kharma BK, Fischell DR, et al: Low-dose, β-particle emission from "stent" wire results in complete, localized inhibition of smooth muscle cell proliferation. Circulation 90:2956–2963, 1994.

152. Hehrlein C, Gollan C, Donges K, et al: Low-dose radioactive endovascular stents prevent smooth muscle cell proliferation and neointimal hyperplasia in rabbits. Circulation 92:1570–1575, 1995.

153. Laird JR, Carter AJ, Kufs WM, et al: Inhibition of neointimal proliferation with low-dose irradiation from a β-particle–emitting stent. Circulation 93:529–536, 1996.

154. Hehrlein C, Stintz M, Kinscherf R, et al: Pure β-particle–emitting stents inhibit neointima formation in rabbits. Circulation 93:641–645, 1996.

155. Carter AJ, Laird JR, Bailey LR, et al: Effects of endovascular radiation from a β-particle–emitting stent in a porcine coronary restenosis model. A dose-response study. Circulation 94:2364–2368, 1996.

156. Waksman R, Robinson KA, Crocker IR, et al: Intracoronary radiation before stent implantation inhibits neointima formation in stented porcine coronary arteries. Circulation 92:1383–1386, 1995.

157. Teirstein PS, Massullo V, Jani S, et al: Radiation therapy following coronary stenting—6-month follow-up of a randomized clinical trial [Abstract]. Circulation 94:I-210, 1996.

158. Van der Giessen WJ, Serruys PW: β-particle emitting stents

radiate enthusiasm in the search for effective prevention of restenosis [Editorial]. Circulation 94:2358–2360, 1996.

159. Serruys PW, Emaneulsson H, van der Giessen W, et al: Heparin-coated Palmaz-Schatz stents in human coronary arteries. Early outcome of the BENESTENT-II Pilot Study. Circulation 93:412–422, 1996.

160. Lablanche JM, Grollier G, Bonnet JL, et al: Ticlopidine Aspirin Stent Evaluation (TASTE); a French multicenter study [Abstract]. Circulation 92:I-476, 1995.

161. Goodhart DM, Traboulsi M, Anderson TJ, et al: Intracoronary stenting guided by mangiography alone: A safe approach [Abstract]. Circulation 94:I-453, 1996.

162. Lawrence ME, Burtt DM, Shaftel PA, et al: Intracoronary stent placement without Coumadin or intravascular ultrasound. J Invas Cardiol 8:428–432, 1996.

163. Morice MC, Valeix B, Marco J, et al: Preliminary results of the MUST trial. Major clinical events during the first month [Abstract]. J Am Coll Cardiol 27:137A, 1996.

164. Goods CM, Al-Shaibi KF, Yadav SS, et al: Utilization of the coronary balloon-expandable coil stent without anticoagulation or intravascular ultrasound. Circulation 93:1803–1808, 1996.

165. Sankardas MA, McEniery PT, Aroney CN, et al: Elective implantation of intracoronary stents without intravascular ultrasound guidance or subsequent warfarin. Catheter Cardiovasc Diagn 37:355–359, 1996.

166. Goods CM, Mathur A, Liu MW, et al: Intracoronary stenting using slotted tubular stents without intravascular ultrasound and anticoagulation. Catheter Cardiovasc Diagn 39:341–345, 1996.

167. Priestley KA, Clague JR, Buller NP, et al: First clinical experience with a new flexible low profile metallic stent and delivery system. Eur Heart J 17:438–444, 1996.

168. Wong P, Wong C-M, Cheng C-H, et al: Early clinical experience with the Multi-Link coronary stent. Catheter Cardiovasc Diagn 39:413–419, 1996.

169. Hermiller JB, Baim DS, Linnemeier TJ, et al: Clinical results with the ACS Multi-Link stent in the US pilot phase [Abstract]. Circulation 94:I-88, 1996.

170. Waigand J, Uhlich F, Gulba D, et al: Intracoronary stenting with the Multi-Link—Single center experience [Abstract]. Circulation 94:I-88, 1996.

171. Tresukosol D, Schalij MJ, Savalle LH, et al: Micro Stent, quantitative coronary angiography and procedural results. Catheter Cardiovasc Diagn 38:135–143, 1996.

172. Rau T, Mathey DG, Miesch M, et al: The A.V.E. Micro stent to treat difficult to reach coronary artery stenoses [Abstract]. Circulation 94:I-87, 1996.

173. Schiele FJ, Meneveau NF, Vuillemenot AR, et al: A single center prospective experience with two generations of coronary AVE micro-stent: Acute clinical and angiographic results. Circulation 94:I-88, 1996.

174. Chevalier B, De Scheerder I, Simon R, et al: Long bare stent registry [Abstract]. Circulation 94:I-207, 1996.

175. Chevalier B, Montserrat P, Haguet R, et al: French Freedom stent registry: Short term results [Abstract]. Circulation 94:I-207, 1996.

176. De Scheerder IK, Wang K, Kerdsinchai P, et al: Clinical and angiographic experience with coronary stenting using Freedom stent. J Invas Cardiol 8:418–427, 1996.

177. Fajadet J, Mehta S, Loubeyre C, et al: Encouraging initial experience with the NIR stent [Abstract]. Circulation 94:I-88, 1996.

178. Almagor Y, Kiemeneij F, Serruys PW, et al: Preliminary results from the multicenter NIR stent registry. Circulation 94:I-207, 1996.

179. Beyar R, Saalman A, Hamburger J, et al: Initial report of a multi-center pilot phase evaluation of serpentine design balloon expandable stent (BeStent) [Abstract]. Circulation 94:I-206, 1996.

180. Leon MB, Fry ETA, O'Shaughnessy CD, et al: Preliminary multicenter experience with the new GR-II stent for abrupt and threatened vessel closure [Abstract]. Circulation 94:I-207, 1996.

# 38

# Stent Complications

*Darius Aliabadi    Robert D. Safian*

The Wallstent was the first stent implanted in a human coronary artery in 1985. Since then, improvements in stent design, deployment techniques, anticoagulation regimens, and operator experience have contributed to a lower incidence of complications with contemporary stenting compared with earlier experience. Nevertheless, although intracoronary stenting has decreased the incidence of some complications associated with percutaneous intervention, it is associated with other complications, some unique to stenting. In general, stent complications can be divided into two broad categories: angiographic complications (stent thrombosis, side branch occlusion, perforation, marginal dissection, stent embolization, stent migration, and stent misplacement) and clinical complications (death, myocardial infarction, coronary artery bypass surgery, bleeding, vascular injury, and infection).

## ANGIOGRAPHIC COMPLICATIONS

### Stent Thrombosis

#### Incidence and Timing

Acute stent thrombosis (Tables 38–1 to 38–5) is usually a dramatic event that occurs within minutes to hours of stent implantation, often before the patient leaves the catheterization laboratory (Fig. 38–1). Acute stent thrombosis is rare (<1% of cases) and is usually due to readily identifiable mechanical and anatomic problems, such as unstented dissection proximal or distal to the stent (marginal dissections), incomplete stent expansion, or inadequate stent apposition. Thus, many cases of acute stent thrombosis are due to operator failure or to anatomic constraints (e.g., small vessel caliber) that preclude placement of additional stents. Because patients with acute stent thrombosis are usually in-hospital, they are quickly diagnosed and often successfully treated. In selected cases of acute stent thrombosis, intravascular ultrasound may help identify the adequacy of stent expansion and guide management. In contrast, subacute stent thrombosis is a more insidious event that occurs within 3 to 5 days of implantation, typically after the patient has been discharged, and accounts for more than 95% of stent thromboses. The incidence of subacute stent thrombosis is zero to 5% between 3 and 5 days, less than 1% between 5 and 8 days, and exceedingly rare beyond 2 weeks after stent implantation.[4, 107] Because many patients with subacute stent thrombosis have been discharged, rapid revascularization is often not possible and ischemic complications are more likely.

### Clinical Presentation

Patients with stent thrombosis typically present with chest pain and electrocardiographic evidence

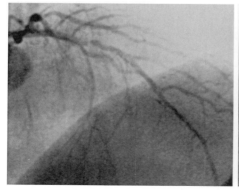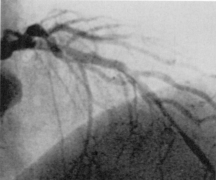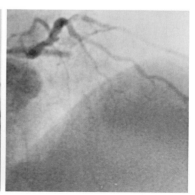

FIGURE 38–1. Acute stent thrombosis. A 90% mid–left anterior descending artery stenosis (*left panel*) was successfully treated with a 3.0 Palmaz-Schatz stent (*middle panel*). The patient underwent urgent repeat catheterization within 1 hour of stent implantation because of chest pain and ST-segment elevation, revealing an acute stent thrombosis site (*right panel*). He was subsequently successfully treated with ReoPro and repeat in-stent high-pressure balloon inflations.

## TABLE 38–1. COMPLICATIONS FOLLOWING BAIL-OUT STENTING

| SERIES (STUDY PERIOD) [YEAR PUBLISHED] | STENT | N | SAT (%) | D/MI/CABG (%) | ARS (%) | VSR/XF (%) | REGIMEN |
|---|---|---|---|---|---|---|---|
| Goy et al[1] (1991–1993) | PSS | 32 | 13 | 8/6.3/0 | 27 | — | APUC |
| Urban et al[2] (1992–1994) | PSS | 52 | 4 | 0/10/4 | — | 6/4 | AC |
| Metz et al[3] (1988–1993) | PSS | 88 | 9 | 3/26/8 | — | —/17 | AC |
| Schomig et al[4] (1989–1993) | PSS | 339 | 6.9 | 1.3/4.0/9 | 29.6 | 5.6/9 | AC |
| Maiello et al[5] (1990–1992) | PSS | 32 | 6 | 6/6/6 | 54 | — | ADPC |
| Kiemeneij et al[6] (1990–1991) | PSS | 52 | 23 | 3/—/15 | 29 | 4/4 | ADPC |
| Reifart et al[7] (1992) | PSS | 25 | 12 | 6/3/5 | — | — | ADPC |
| Haude et al[8] [1991] | PSS | 15 | 6.7 | 0/0/6.7 | 21 | —/9.5 | AC |
| Alfonso et al[9] (1990–1993) | PSS | 42 | 5 | 0/5/2.5 | 16 | 2.7/5.4 | ADPC |
| Foley et al[10] (1990–1992) | PSS | 60 | 16.7 | 0/21.6/7 | 50 | 0/— | ADPC |
| Hermann et al[11] (1992) | PSS | 56 | 16 | 0/5.3/3.6 | 23 | 3.5/16 | — |
| Chan et al[12] (1991–1994) | GRS | 42 | 4.8 | 0/4.8/7.1 | 66 | —/— | ADC |
| Sutton et al[13] (1989–1991) | GRS | 415 | — | 3/5/12 | — | —/— | ADPC |
| Agrawal et al[14] (1989–1992) | GRS | 240 | 7 | 3/18/— | — | — | ADPC |
| Hearn et al[15] (1987–1990) | GRS | 116 | 8.6 | 4/4/28 | 53 | 7/— | ADPC |
| George et al[16] (1988–1991) | GRS | 518 | 8.7 | 2.2/5.5/4.3 | 39 | —/16.8 | ADPC |
| Roubin et al[17] (1989–1991) | GRS | 115 | 7.6 | 1.7/16/4.2 | 41 | 4.2/10.2 | ADPC |
| Goy et al[1] (1995) | Wik | 33 | 18 | 9/8/3 | 38 | — | APUC |
| Vrolix et al[18] (1990–1992) | Wik | 180 | 13.3 | 3.3/12/16.5 | 27 | 3.9/3.9 | ADPC |
| Garratt et al[19] (1994) | Wik | 308 | 3 | 3.7/2.7/8.7 | — | — | AC |
| Reifart et al[20] (1990–1991) | Wik | 48 | 21 | 10/2/6 | — | — | — |
| Reifart et al[7] (1992) | Strk | 25 | 16 | 8/16/16 | — | — | ADPC |
| Ozaki et al[21] (1995) | AVE | 20 | 0 | 0/10/5 | — | — | ADPC |
| Goy et al[22] (1986–1989) | Wall | 17 | 5.8 | 0/5.8/0 | 25 | — | APCUS |
| Sigwart et al[23] (1986–1988) | Wall | 11 | 9 | 9/9/0 | — | 20/10 | AUCP |
| de Feyter et al[24] (1989–1990) | Wall | 15 | 20 | 6.6/13.3/— | — | — | AUPC |

AVE, AVE micro stent; PSS, Palmaz-Schatz stent; GRS, Gianturco-Roubin stent; Wik, Wiktor stent; SAT, stent thrombosis; Strk, Strecker stent; Wall, Wallstent; D, death; MI, myocardial infarction; CABG, coronary artery bypass surgery; ARS, angiographic restenosis; VSR, vascular injury requiring surgical repair; XF, bleeding requiring transfusion; A, aspirin; D, dextran; U, urokinase; P, Persantine; C, Coumadin; S, sulfinpyrazone; —, not reported.

**TABLE 38–2.    COMPLICATIONS AFTER ELECTIVE STENTING IN NATIVE VESSELS**

| SERIES (STUDY PERIOD) [YEAR PUBLISHED] | STENT | N | SAT (%) | D/MI/CABG (%) | ARS (%) | VSR/XF (%) | REGIMEN |
|---|---|---|---|---|---|---|---|
| STRESS[25] (1994) | PSS | 205 | 3.4 | 0/4.4/2.0 | 31.6 | 3.9/4.9 | ADPC |
| Benestent[26] (1994) | PSS | 259 | 3.5 | 0/3.9/3.1 | 22 | 13.5* | ADPC |
| Levine et al[27] (1988–1989) | PSS | 37 | 3 | 0/—/0 | 28 | — | ADPC |
| Schatz et al[28] (1987–1989) | PSS | 226 | 3.7 | 0.9/2.8/0.9 | — | 5.7* | ADPC |
| Colombo et al[29] (1994) | PSS | 97 | 2 | 1/1/1 | 19 | — | — |
| Savage et al[30] (1987–1990) | PSS | 217 | 4.7 | 0.7/3.7/8 | 39 | 10* | ADPC |
| Carrozza et al[31] (1988–1991) | PSS | 220 | 0.4 | 0/0/0.4 | 25 | 11/5 | ADPC |
| Strauss et al[32] (1986–1990) | Wall | 107 | 19 | 6.6/—/— | 18 | — | ADUPCS |
| Serruys et al[33] [1991] | Wall | 105 | 24 | 7.6/—/— | 14 | — | AUPC |
| Sigwart et al[34] (1986–1988) | Wall | 44 | 4.4 | 6.8/—/4.5 | — | — | ACPS |
| Eeckhout et al[35] (1985–1991) | Wall | 59 | 12 | 2/5/3 | 17 | — | — |
| de Jaeger et al[36] (1990–1992) | Wik | 109 | 11.9 | 0.9/—/4.6 | 30 | — | — |

PSS, Palmaz-Schatz stent; Wik, Wiktor stent; SAT, stent thrombosis; Wall, Wallstent; D, death; MI, myocardial infarction; CABG, coronary artery bypass surgery; ARS, angiographic restenosis; VSR, vascular injury requiring surgical repair; XF, bleeding requiring transfusion; A, aspirin; D, dextran; U, urokinase; P, Persantine; C, Coumadin; S, sulfinpyrazone; —, not reported.
*Composite of both vascular complications requiring surgery and bleeding complications requiring transfusion.

**TABLE 38–3.    COMPLICATIONS AFTER STENTING IN ACUTE MYOCARDIAL INFARCTION**

| SERIES (STUDY PERIOD) [YEAR PUBLISHED] | STENT | N | SAT (%) | D/MI/CABG (%) | ARS (%) | VSR/XF (%) | REGIMEN |
|---|---|---|---|---|---|---|---|
| Neumann et al[37] [1995] | PSS | 74 | 9.6 | 0/—/— | — | — | AT (100%) C (44%) |
| Monassier et al[38] (1994–1995) | PSS, GRS, AVE, Wik | 340 | 2 | 3/—/1 | — | —/2.0 | ATL |
| Verna et al[39] (1994–1995) | — | 51 | 7.1 | 0/—/3.5 | — | — | AT |
| Levy et al[40] (1992–1995) | — | 54 | 1.8 | 5.5/—/0 | — | 0/— | ATL |
| Benzuly et al[41] (1993–1995) | GRS, PSS, biliary | 31 | 2.8 | 6.9/—/10.3 | — | —/34 | ATC |
| Romero et al[42] [1995] | PSS | 51 | 0 | 0/4/0 | 34 | —/— | AC (21) ATL (30) |
| Rodriquez et al[43] (1993–1995) | GRS, PSS, Wik | 30 | 3 | 3/—/— | — | 0/10 | ADPC (23) AT (7) |
| Steinhubl et al[44] [1996] | — | 44 | 5 | 7/—/5 | — | — | AU(27) R(19) T (1) |
| Stone et al[45] [1996] | PSS | 109 | 0 | 0/0/1.1 | — | — | AT |
| Lefevre et al[46] [1996] | PSS, AVE | 85 | 1.2 | 8/2.4/1.2 | — | — | ATH |

AVE, AVE micro stent; biliary, biliary stent; PSS, Palmaz-Schatz stent; GRS, Gianturco-Roubin stent; Wik, Wiktor stent; SAT, stent thrombosis; D, death; MI, myocardial infarction; CABG, coronary artery bypass surgery; ARS, angiographic restenosis; VSR, vascular injury requiring surgical repair; XF, bleeding requiring transfusion; A, aspirin; D, dextran; U, urokinase; P, Persantine; C, Coumadin; S, sulfinpyrazone; —, not reported; L, low molecular weight heparin; H, subcutaneous heparin; T, ticlopidine.

**TABLE 38–4.     COMPLICATIONS AFTER STENTING IN SAPHENOUS VEIN GRAFTS**

| SERIES (STUDY PERIOD) | STENT | N | SAT (%) | D/MI/CABG (%) | ARS (%) | VSR/XF (%) | REGIMEN |
|---|---|---|---|---|---|---|---|
| Wong et al[47] (1990–1992) | PSS | 624 | 1.4 | 1.7/0.3/0.9 | 30 | 8.0/6.3 | ADPC |
| Rechavia et al[48] (1992–1994) | PSS, Biliary | 29 | 0 | 0/0/0 | — | 3.4/6.8 | APC |
| Wong et al[47] (1990–1993) | PSS, Biliary | 205 | 1.7 | 1.3/0.9/0.4 | — | 15.9/25 | ADPC |
| Piana et al[49] (1988–1993) | PSS, Biliary | 200 | 0.6 | 0.6/0/0 | 17 | 8.5/14 | ADPC |
| Fenton et al[50] (1990–1991) | PSS | 209 | 0.5 | 0.4/0/0 | 34 | 17.2/12 | ADC |
| Leon et al[51] (1993) | PSS | 589 | 1.4 | 1.7/0.3/0.9 | 30 | 7.5/15.5 | ADC |
| Pomerantz et al[52] (1988–1991) | PSS | 84 | 0 | 0/0/0 | 25 | 5 | ADPC |
| Eeckhout et al[53] (1986–1993) | Wall, Wik | 58 | — | 2/0/2 | 25 | 14 | APC |
| Keane et al[54] (1991–1993) | New, Wall | 29 | 3.4 | 0/0/0 | 32 | 3.4/6.8 | ADPC |
| Strauss et al[32] (1986–1990) | Wall | 145 | 8 | — | 39 | — | ADUPCS |
| de Scheerder et al[55] (1988–1990) | New, Wall | 69 | 10 | 1.4/4.3/2.8 | 47 | 33 | AUDPC |
| Urban et al[56] (1986–1988) | Wall | 14 | 0 | 0/0/0 | 20 | 7.7/7.7 | AUPC |
| Fortuna et al[57] (1993) | Wik | 101 | 2 | 1/3/1 | — | — | — |
| Bilodeau et al[58] (1988–1991) | GRS | 37 | — | 0/2.5/0 | 35 | 2.7/21 | — |

Biliary, biliary stent; PSS, Palmaz-Schatz stent; GRS, Gianturco-Roubin stent; Wik, Wiktor stent; SAT, stent thrombosis; Wall, Wallstent; D, death; MI, myocardial infarction; CABG, coronary artery bypass surgery; ARS, angiographic restenosis; VSR, vascular injury requiring surgical repair; XF, bleeding requiring transfusion; A, aspirin; D, dextran; U, urokinase; P, Persantine; C, Coumadin; S, sulfinpyrazone; —, not reported.

of acute myocardial infarction; chest pain without electrocardiographic changes is rarely related to stent thrombosis. However, in vessels that were chronically occluded or well collateralized before stenting, stent thrombosis may be clinically silent or may manifest only as mild chest pain resulting from recruitment of collaterals.

### Predictors

The development of stent thrombosis depends on many factors, including angiographic factors, clinical factors, lesion and vessel factors, stent factors, and technical factors.

**ANGIOGRAPHIC FACTORS.** Early data obtained before the routine use of high-pressure adjunctive percutaneous transluminal coronary angioplasty (PTCA) suggested that the strongest angiographic predictors of stent thrombosis were unstented distal disease or dissection (odds ratio, 10.6), stent diameter less than 3.0 mm (odds ratio, 14.7), residual filling defect inside the stent (odds ratio, 14.7), and multiple stents (odds ratio, 3.7).[14] Other predictors included smaller reference target diameter, stent placement in the left anterior descending artery, high platelet count, presence of thrombus after predilatation, and

postprocedure bleeding complications.[107] In a series in which stenting was accomplished with ultrasound guidance and reduced anticoagulation, predictors of stent thrombosis included low ejection fraction, use of different stent designs, postprocedure dissection, and slow flow.[108]

**CLINICAL FACTORS.** The clinical indication for stent implantation may be an important determinant of subsequent stent thrombosis. In abrupt closure, vessel wall injury results in exposure of collagen and tissue factor and activation of platelets and coagulation factors, thus creating an environment suitable for stent thrombosis. In fact, earlier studies of stents used for abrupt closure reported subacute stent thrombosis in up to 23% of patients using warfarin (Coumadin)–based anticoagulation strategies and older deployment techniques; the incidence of stent thrombosis is much lower for elective planned stent implantation (see Tables 38–1 and 38–2). In one study,[10] the risk of subacute stent thrombosis was eight times higher after "bail-out stenting" than after elective stenting. In the Stent Restenosis Study, the incidence of subacute stent thrombosis was 21.4% for PTCA patients requiring bail-out stenting, which was six times higher than for planned stenting.

Unstable angina and acute myocardial infarction

**TABLE 38–5.    COMPLICATIONS AFTER STENTING OTHER LESION SUBTYPES**

| SERIES (STUDY PERIOD) [YEAR PUBLISHED] | STENT | N | SAT (%) | D/MI/CABG (%) | ARS (%) | VSR/XF (%) | REGIMEN |
|---|---|---|---|---|---|---|---|
| Colombo et al[59] [1996] | PSS, GRS, Wik | 35 Ostial | — | — | 23 | — | — |
| Rocha-Singh et al[60] (1989–1992) | PSS | 41 Ostial | 4.9 | 4.9/2.5/0 | 28 | —/2.5 | ADPC |
| Medina et al[61] [1994] | PSS | 30 CTO | 9 | 0/0/0 | 15 | 9/9 | ADPC |
| Hsu et al[62] [1995] | PSS, Wik | 36 CTO | 5 | — | 20 | — | — |
| Ooka et al[63] (1992–1994) | PSS, GRS | 33 CTO | 5 | — | 24 | — | — |
| Ooka et al[64] [1995] | PSS, GRS | 47 CTO | 10 | — | 44 | — | — |
| Goldberg et al[65] (1989–1993) | PSS | 60 CTO | 5 | 0/2/0 | 20 | — | ADPC |
| Maiello et al[66] [1995] | PSS, GRS, Wik | 89 Diffuse | 1.2 | 0/3/3 | 35 | — | AT |
| Reimers et al[67] [1995] | PSS, GRS, Wall, AVE | 48 Diffuse | 4 | — | 25 | — | AHC |
| Shaknovich et al[68] [1995] | PSS | 54 Diffuse | 3.7 | 2/0/2 | — | 3.7/— | AHC |
| Mintz et al[69] [1995] | PSS, MRA | 88 Calcified | 0 | 0/0/0 | — | — | — |
| Teirstein et al[70] (1994–1995) | PSS | 145 <3 mm | 0 | 0/3.4/0 | — | — | A or T: 56% ATC: 44% |
| Hall et al[71] [1995] | GRS | 68 <3 mm | 3 | 1.5/—/— | 31 | —/0 | AT |
| Colombo et al[72] [1995] | AVE | 16 <3 mm | 0 | — | — | — | AT |

AVE, AVE micro stent; PSS, Palmaz-Schatz stent; GRS, Gianturco-Roubin stent; Wik, Wiktor stent; Wall, Wallstent; CTO, chronic total occlusion; SAT, stent thrombosis; D, death; MI, myocardial infarction; CABG, coronary artery bypass surgery; ARS, angiographic restenosis; VSR, vascular injury requiring surgical repair; XF, bleeding requiring transfusion; A, aspirin; D, dextran; H, subcutaneous heparin; P, Persantine; C, Coumadin; —, not reported; MRA, mechanical rotational atherectomy; T, ticlopidine.

are associated with plaque rupture, intracoronary thrombus, and increased thrombogenic potential, all of which theoretically predispose to stent thrombosis. Although early data suggested that stenting in unstable ischemic syndromes was associated with an increased risk of stent thrombosis,[33, 109, 110] more contemporary data suggest that stent thrombosis is not influenced by the presence of an unstable ischemic syndrome.[111, 112] However, comparisons of these studies are confounded by differences in deployment technique, anticoagulation strategy, and patient selection; available data suggest that it is reasonable and safe to deploy stents in patients with unstable angina.

In bail-out stenting after failed PTCA for acute myocardial infarction, small observational studies reported stent thrombosis in up to 30% of patients,[113–117] suggesting that intraluminal thrombus was an absolute contraindication to stenting. Other studies suggested that favorable outcomes can be achieved when optimal stent techniques and reduced anticoagulation are employed in the setting of planned or bail-out stenting after acute myocardial infarction (see Table 38–3). In one report, major in-hospital complications after bail-out stenting for acute myocardial infarction were similar to those

for bail-out stenting without acute myocardial infarction.[41] In aggregate, these data suggest that stenting in carefully selected patients with acute myocardial infarction is feasible. The safety and efficacy of primary stenting for acute myocardial infarction are currently being studied in the Stent Primary Angioplasty in Myocardial Infarction trial, a multicenter randomized trial comparing the heparin-coated Palmaz-Schatz stent with PTCA.

**LESION- AND VESSEL-RELATED FACTORS.** During the early stent experience, a key observation was the inverse relationship between vessel caliber and stent thrombosis,[16, 17] with rates of stent thrombosis as high as 25% for vessels less than 3.0 mm. With older deployment techniques and anticoagulation strategies, vessel diameter of less than 3.0 mm was shown to be one of the strongest independent predictors of stent thrombosis,[14] possibly because of lower blood flow and increased metal density in smaller vessels.[110, 118] Thus, some operators in the United States do not implant stents in vessels of less than 3.0 mm. However, using optimal deployment techniques and reduced anticoagulation regimens, some studies reported subacute thrombosis rates of zero to 3% for vessels of less than 3.0 mm (see Table

38–5), suggesting that the role of stenting in small vessels needs further investigation. Although older studies of long lesions, chronic total occlusions, and ostial lesions reported an increased incidence of stent thrombosis, subsequent studies using optimal stent techniques reported a lower incidence of stent thrombosis (see Table 38–5).

Several studies suggest that subacute stent thrombosis is less common in saphenous vein grafts than in native vessels.[32, 119] The European Wallstent experience suggested that the risk of stent thrombosis in saphenous vein grafts was three times lower than for native vessels (see Table 38–4). For focal lesions in nondegenerated saphenous vein grafts, stent thrombosis was reported in zero to 1.7% of patients after implantation of Palmaz-Schatz coronary or biliary stents. In degenerated vein grafts, a thrombus-debulking strategy with transluminal extraction coronary atherectomy or AngioJet before stenting is reasonable but of unproven value in preventing stent thrombosis. Impaired runoff in any vessel probably predisposes to stent thrombosis.

**STENT FACTORS.** The impact of stent design, stent material, stent length, and number of implanted stents on stent thrombosis is unknown. Available data are clouded by the fact that long stents and multiple stents are often used to treat long dissections and diffuse disease, anatomic settings that may predispose to stent thrombosis. Although some data[14] suggest that use of multiple stents is an independent risk factor for stent thrombosis, other data do not.[10, 16, 110] With the data taken in aggregate, the risk of thrombosis with multiple stents is probably not increased with optimal deployment techniques.

There are currently more than 40 different stents in use worldwide. These stents differ with respect to metal surface area, strut diameter, material, and fundamental design (slotted tube, coil, and crossing wires). Theoretically, such differences could influence thrombosis rates. For example, in early stent designs the larger strut diameter of the Gianturco-Roubin stent (125 μm) in comparison with the Palmaz-Schatz stent (70 μm) may partly explain the longer time course to neointimal coverage[120]; however, clinical studies do not suggest a greater risk of stent thrombosis. The 21% incidence of stent thrombosis after implantation of the Strecker stent for abrupt closure was initially attributed to its unique design (wire crossings), but randomized data failed to show a difference in stent thrombosis rates between the Strecker and the Palmaz-Schatz stents for bail-out indications.[7]

Stent materials include stainless steel (Palmaz-Schatz, Gianturco-Roubin, Microstent, Multilink, Wallstent), tantalum (Wiktor and Strecker stents), and nitinol (Radius stent), but the clinical impact of stent material on stent thrombosis is unknown. Extensive in vitro and in vivo animal models have failed to show superiority of tantalum over stainless steel for reducing thrombogenicity.[121] Some series suggest that with optimal deployment techniques and reduced anticoagulation, thrombosis rates are remarkably low (zero to 3.6%), irrespective of stent material (Table 38–6). However, several multicenter randomized trials are underway to compare the early and late results of different stent designs.

A promising method to reduce thrombosis is the use of polymers to bond pharmacologic agents such as heparin to metallic stents. This technology offers the potential opportunity for improving current stent designs by altering the surface properties of the stent. Experimental studies with heparin-bonded stents reported less thrombosis.[122, 123] Preliminary human experience is also promising; during the pilot phase of the Benestent-II trial, in which the heparin-coated Palmaz-Schatz stent was implanted in 202 patients, there were no stent thromboses.[124] In summary, with optimal stent technique and reduced anticoagulation, stent material and stent design probably do not significantly affect thrombosis.

**TECHNICAL FACTORS.** During the early stent era, stent thrombosis was attributed to inadequate antiplatelet and anticoagulation therapy; intense anticoagulation regimens (aspirin, heparin, dextran, dipyridamole [Persantine], and warfarin with or without urokinase) were often recommended. Despite these intense anticoagulation regimens, relatively high thrombosis rates were reported (see Tables 38–1 and 38–2). It now appears that implantation technique plays the most important role in subsequent thrombosis rates. Based on the studies by Colombo and colleagues[79] and Goldberg and colleagues,[125] stent thrombosis is now viewed as a mechanical problem that can be prevented by "optimal stenting." Optimal stenting involves the use of high-pressure (>15 atm) adjunctive PTCA to ensure complete stent expansion, symmetry, and apposition of the stent to the vessel wall, as well as complete coverage of the lesion or dissection. With this technique, the incidence of subacute thrombosis has been reduced to less than 3% (see Table 38–6), despite the elimination of aggressive anticoagulation. The superiority of antiplatelet therapy (aspirin and ticlopidine [Ticlid]) over anticoagulation therapy (aspirin and warfarin) in reducing cardiac events was demonstrated in two prospective randomized trials. In STARS, the incidence of clinical subacute closure within 30 days (death, emergency coronary artery bypass grafting, Q-wave myocardial infarction, and subacute stent thrombosis with repeat revascularization) was 0.6% in the antiplatelet arm and 2.4%

| SERIES (STUDY PERIOD) [YEAR PUBLISHED] | STENT | N | SAT (%) | D/MI/CABG (%) | ASR (%) | VSR/XF (%) | REGIMEN |
|---|---|---|---|---|---|---|---|
| Morice et al[73] (1995) | PSS | 260 | 1.2 | 0/1.9/0.4 | — | — | ATL |
| Hall et al[74] [1995] | PSS | 411 | 1.0 | 0.3/1.0/0.5 | — | — | A or T |
| Wong et al[75] [1995] | PSS | 33 | 0 | 0/0/0 | — | 1/1 | AT |
| Buszman et al[76] [1995] | PSS | 100 | 1 | 1/—/— | — | 1/1 | AL |
| Fajadet et al[77] [1995] | PSS | 119 | 0 | 1/1/9 | — | Radial site | AL |
| Blasini et al[78] [1995] | PSS | 60 | 0 | 0 | — | 1.6* | AT |
| Colombo et al[79] (1993–1994) | PSS | 359 | 0.9 | 1.1/3.9/3.9 | — | 0.3/1 | A or T |
| Mehan et al[80] [1995] | PSS | 8 | 0 | 0/0/0 | — | 0/0 | A |
| Russo et al[81] (1994–1995) | PSS | 105 | 0 | — | 13* | — | AT |
| Haase et al[82] (1994–1995) | PSS | 46 | 0 | 0/0/0 | — | 0/0 | AT |
| Saito et al[83] (1994–1995) | PSS | 32 | 0 | — | 18 | — | AT |
| Jordan et al[84] (1993–1994) | PSS | 132 | 0 | — | — | — | ATL |
| Wong et al[85] [1994] | PSS | 28 | 0 | 0/0/0 | — | 0/0 | AT |
| Goods et al[86] (1994–1995) | GRS | 296 | 0.7 | —/1.9/0.4 | — | — | AT |
| Marco et al[87] [1996] | GRS | 18 | 0 | 0/0/0 | — | — | — |
| Colombo et al[88] [1995] | GRS | 60 | 0 | 1/—/4.0 | 32 | 0/0 | AT |
| Reifart et al[89] [1995] | GRS | 98 | — | 1/0/1 | — | —/1 | AT |
| Goods et al[90] (1994–1995) | GRS | 152 | 0.7 | 0/0/0.7 | — | 2/1.3 | AT |
| Carvalho et al[91] (1993–1994) | GRS | 87 | 1.1 | 0/1.1/0 | — | 2.3* | ATL |
| Hall et al[92] [1994] | GRS | 44 | 0 | —/—/— | — | — | AT |
| Elias et al[93] (1993–1995) | Wik | 240 | 3.6 | 1.2/—/1.2 | 13–20 | — | ATL |
| Elias et al[93] (1993–1995) | Wik | 182 | 1.0 | 1/—/0 | 18 | — | AT |
| Elias et al[94] (1993–1994) | Wik | 79 | 1.3 | 0/1.3/0 | — | 1.3/1.3 | ATL |
| Colombo et al[95] [1995] | Wik | 68 | 1.7 | 1.7/—/3.4 | 23 | 1.5/1.5 | — |
| Colombo et al[96] [1994] | Wik | 50 | 2.2 | —/—/— | — | — | AT |
| Morice[97] [1995] | All | 1250 | 1.7 | 0.7/0.6/0.4 | — | — | ATL |
| Morice et al[98] (1993–1994) | PSS, Wik, GRS | 397 | 1.5 | 1.0/0.3/1.0 | — | 3.8* | ATL |
| Morice et al[99] (1992–1993) | PSS, GRS, Wik | 246 | 1.2 | 0.4/0/0.8 | — | 2/1.6 | ATL |
| Morice et al[100] (1994–1995) | PSS, GRS, Wik | 1156 | 1.6 | 0.3/2.7/0.3 | — | 0.6* | AT |
| Lablanche et al[101] [1995] | PSS, GRS, Wik | 98 | 0 | 2.0/4.0/3.0 | — | 0.6/1.2 | ATD |
| Barragan et al[102] [1994] | GRS, PSS | 208 | 0.5 | 1.0/1.0/0.5 | — | 0.5/0.5 | AT |
| Barragan et al[103] (1990–1993) | Strk, PSS | 238 | 3.8 | 2/2.9/— | — | 3.8/0.8 | ATH |
| Aubry et al[104] (1992–1994) | PSS, GRS, Wik | 643 | 2.5 | 3.7/3.7/1.3 | — | — | ATL |
| Blengino et al[105] [1994] | PSS, GRS, Wik | 74 | 0 | —/—/— | — | — | A or AT |
| Lefevre et al[106] (1991–1995) | All | 245 | 2.0 | 3/1.6/0 | — | 1.2/— | ATL |

PSS, Palmaz-Schatz stent; GRS, Gianturco-Roubin stent; Wik, Wiktor stent; Strk, Strecker stent; SAT, stent thrombosis; D, death; MI, myocardial infarction; CABG, coronary artery bypass surgery; ARS, angiographic restenosis; VSR, vascular injury requiring surgical repair; XF, bleeding requiring transfusion; A, aspirin; D, dextran; H, subcutaneous heparin; L, low molecular weight heparin; T, ticlopidine; —, not reported.

in the anticoagulation arm. Similarly, in ISAR, the incidence of "clinical" stent thrombosis was 1.6% in the antiplatelet arm and 6.2% in the anticoagulation arm.[126]

**INTRAVASCULAR ULTRASOUND FACTORS.** Intravascular ultrasound has been invaluable in documenting optimal stent placement; whether intravascular ultrasound will affect stent thrombosis is unclear. Preliminary data from the POST registry suggest that intravascular ultrasound findings associated with stent thrombosis include stent malapposition, stent underexpansion, plaque protrusion, thrombus, and marginal dissections.[127] Whether intravascular ultrasound–guided stent placement will improve clinical outcomes is also unclear. Preliminary findings from the Angiography Versus Intravascular Ultrasound-Directed Stent Placement Study, a randomized multicenter study, suggest that intravascular ultrasound–directed stent implantation improves acute stent dimensions but does not influence 30-day clinical event rates, including in-hospital stent thrombosis, myocardial infarction, coronary artery bypass grafting, and death.[128]

### Treatment

All patients with suspected stent thrombosis should undergo immediate angiography and revascularization. Mechanical causes of stent thrombosis must be specially sought and corrected, including uncovered dissection, inadequate stent expansion/apposition, improper sizing, and intimal flaps protruding through the stent struts. Intravascular ultrasound may be helpful in selected cases to identify the mechanical problem. When recrossing a recently deployed stent, a large J-tip should be placed on a flexible wire to minimize the chance of crossing between a stent strut (or coil) and the vessel wall. If such a wire position is inadvertently achieved, excessive resistance results when attempts are made to pass a balloon. Subsequent balloon inflations can separate the stent from the vessel wall and can lead to stent compression or possible embolization. In most cases of stent thrombosis, repeat PTCA within the stented segment (>15 atm) restores flow. If uncovered distal dissection or protruding intimal flaps are suspected, then placement of multiple overlapping stents is recommended. For resistant thrombus, potential adjunctive strategies include the use of thrombolytic agents (urokinase, 250,000- to 500,000-U bolus over 2 to 5 minutes followed by an infusion of 100,000 to 200,000 U/hour for 8 to 24 hours), ReoPro (using the EPILOG guidelines), or the Angio-Jet. After successful revascularization, if a clear mechanical problem has been identified and reversed, patients should be treated with aspirin and ticlopidine. If the cause of stent thrombosis has not been

identified and corrected, the ideal medical regimen is unknown. Commonly employed regimens include prolonged intravenous heparin, warfarin (international normalized ratio, 2.5 to 3.5), ticlopidine (250 mg twice daily), and soluble aspirin (325 mg daily). The role of glycoprotein IIb/IIIa inhibitors remains to be determined. However, if the angiographic result is suboptimal, intense anticoagulation therapy can increase the risk of bleeding and vascular complications without necessarily reducing stent thrombosis; coronary artery bypass grafting should be considered. The reported success rate of treating patients with subacute thrombosis after placement of the Gianturco-Roubin stent with PTCA or thrombolytic therapy is up to 58%.[119] The use of low molecular weight heparin as an adjunct after "suboptimal" stenting is under evaluation in the ATLAST trial, and the role of ReoPro during stenting is being studied in the EPILOG-Stent trial.

## Side Branch Occlusion

Side branch occlusion is a known complication of percutaneous intervention[129–135] and occurs in 1% to 17% of cases.[132–135] A detailed review of 358 stented lesions from our institution revealed side branch occlusion in 19%; 67% occurred after high-pressure adjunctive PTCA.[136] Side branch ostial disease (Fig. 38–2) was a strong predictor of side branch occlusions (odds ratio, 40). Despite the high incidence of side branch occlusion, in-hospital and long-term adverse ischemic complications are unusual. However, although the occlusion of small side branches is generally well tolerated,[129] occlusion of large side branches may result in significant adverse clinical events.[131] PTCA of the side branch through the stent can be readily accomplished with most stents.[137] Early angiographic follow-up suggests that antegrade flow may spontaneously return to normal in previously occluded side branches.[132] Furthermore, stenting can often result in reappearance of side branches that are initially occluded after balloon dilatation.[135] Angiographic follow-up of "jailed" (but not occluded) side branches reveals a low incidence of late side branch occlusion.[133, 134] Strategies to prevent side branch occlusion, particularly if the side branch has ostial disease, include the use of kissing stents or T-stents and pretreatment of the side branch ostium with PTCA or atherectomy, before stenting of the parent vessel.[138–141]

## Perforation

The reported incidence of coronary perforations is 0.1% to 0.6% after PTCA and up to 3% after laser and atherectomy.[142–144] Perforation following stent deployment is rare and typically occurs as a consequence of high-pressure adjunctive PTCA (Fig. 38–

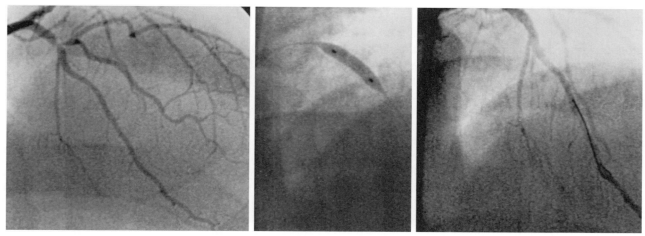

FIGURE 38–2. Side branch occlusion after stent placement. A complex bifurcation lesion involving the left anterior descending artery and the diagonal branch (*left panel*). After high-pressure poststent inflations (*middle panel*), occlusion of the diagonal side branch is noted (*right panel*). Retrieval of the side branch could not be accomplished.

3).[145] The reported incidence of coronary perforations after stent placement is 0.2% to 2.3%.[145–149] Angiographic features associated with perforation include use of an oversized stent (stent/artery ratio >1.3), high-pressure balloon inflations distal to the stent, stenting vessels with significant distal tapering, and need to recross a severe dissection with a guide wire.[148] Initial management strategies include prolonged balloon inflations and reversal of anticoagulation with protamine. If this strategy fails, stenting the perforated area with a vein-patch stent or bare stent[149] has been reported with success; however, a low threshold for surgery is appropriate.

## Marginal Dissection

The use of high pressures to dilate stents after implantation has lowered the incidence of stent throm-

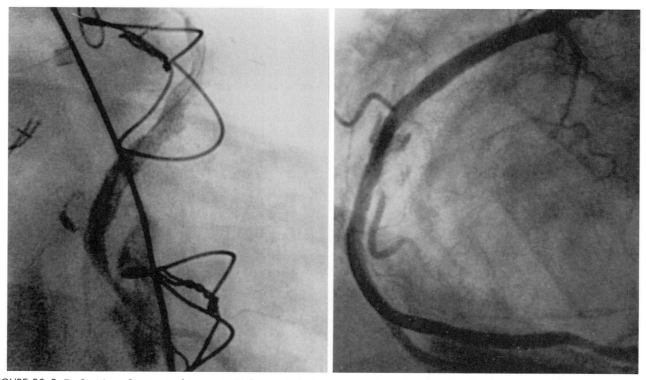

FIGURE 38–3. Perforation after stent placement. *Right panel*, A large, noncontained perforation develops in a saphenous vein graft to the obtuse marginal after transluminal extraction coronary atherectomy and high-pressure adjunctive percutaneous transluminal coronary angioplasty (PTCA) with an oversized balloon, requiring emergent open heart surgery. *Left panel*, A small, contained perforation is noted at the stent site in the mid–right coronary artery after poststent high-pressure PTCA. The patient was successfully treated with prolonged low-pressure balloon inflations and reversal of anticoagulation.

bosis and bleeding and vascular complications caused by elimination of aggressive anticoagulation protocols. However, high-pressure adjunctive PTCA can lead to marginal dissections as a result of balloon rupture[150, 151] or barotrauma beyond the stent margin. Marginal dissections can be avoided by employing high-resolution fluoroscopic equipment to ensure identification of the ends of the stent, noncompliant high-pressure balloons to avoid overdilating the stent and adjacent segments, and short (9- to 15-mm) double-marker balloons to accurately position the balloon inside the stent. When dilating with a balloon that is longer than the stent, the excess balloon length should be placed at the proximal end of the stent to minimize the likelihood of distal dissection and the subsequent need to deploy another stent distal to the first stent. This technique also reduces the chance of balloon entrapment within the distal stent margins if balloon rupture occurs.[150]

## Stent Migration

Stent migration after deployment is unusual after intracoronary stenting. Stent migration may be more common with self-expanding and thermal memory stents than with balloon-expandable stents, and with coil designs rather than with tubular slotted stents. Migration of the original coronary Microstent was reported with the 12- and 16-mm stents,[21, 152] but this has been corrected by further design modifications. The round, thick (0.008-inch), and longitudinal orientation of the struts of the older Microstents may have prevented complete embedding of the struts into the vessel wall and allowed sliding of the stent along the long axis when balloon catheters were removed or advanced.[152] These problems have been completely corrected.

## Stent Embolization

Stent embolization is rare (<0.5%) but may occur more frequently with manually crimped uncovered stents, such as the Palmaz biliary stent. Other risk factors for stent embolization include proximal vessel tortuosity and inability to cross the lesion.[153] The most common management strategy is to deploy the stent at the site of embolization. Successful retrieval of embolized stents with snare devices or balloons has been reported[154–157] but can be technically challenging (especially if the stent is partially expanded). Computed tomographic scanning may localize the embolization site and reveal coaxial alignment relative to the artery if fluoroscopy fails to localize the stent; coaxial alignment of an undeployed stent may predict a begin course.[153] Radiolucent nonferromagnetic metallic stents can be successfully localized by use of magnetic resonance imaging.[158] Measures to avoid stent embolization include alignment of coaxial guide, use of extra-support wires, and careful stent selection for the specific anatomy. For ostial lesions, it is important to fully expand the ostium with PTCA, rotational atherectomy, or directional atherectomy before stent placement, to minimize the chance of embolization.

## Stent Misplacement

Many factors may contribute to stent misplacement, including inadequate predilatation, excessive vessel tortuosity, and heavy calcification, particularly if unsheathed stents are used. Some self-expanding stents, such as the Wallstent, may be associated with inadvertent misplacement because of stent shortening. For the self-expanding Radius stent, it is important to ensure that the "tension" has been removed from the stent delivery system before deployment, to avoid misplacement.

## CLINICAL COMPLICATIONS

## Ischemic Complications

Most ischemic complications after stenting are associated with stent thrombosis, which is associated with significant morbidity and mortality (death, 7% to 19%; myocardial infarction, 57% to 85%; emergency coronary artery bypass grafting, 30% to 44%).[159] Ischemic complications are more common when stents are placed for abrupt closure; these include myocardial infarction in 2% to 26%, emergency coronary artery bypass grafting in zero to 16%, and death in zero to 10% (see Table 38–2). Independent predictors of ischemic complications include delayed use of stents for abrupt closure, side branch occlusion, need for multiple stents, and incomplete coverage of dissection.[159] In contrast, the overall incidence of ischemic complications for elective stent placement is lower than for the bailout stenting (see Tables 38–1 to 38–3).

## Infection

Endovascular infection attributable to stents is exceedingly rare; only one reported perivascular abscess is directly attributable to Palmaz-Schatz stent implantation in a right coronary artery.[160] Although no data suggest a routine need for antibiotics in patients receiving stents, stent implantation should be deferred in patients who are suspected of having bacteremia. It is reasonable to use antibiotic prophylaxis in patients who undergo procedures associated with bacteremia (dental work, endoscopy, colonoscopy) within 3 months of stent placement.

## Bleeding and Vascular Injury

The use of prolonged heparin infusion and oral warfarin after stent implantation is associated with serious vascular complications, requiring surgical repair in 2% to 20% of cases and blood transfusion in 4% to 10% (see Tables 38–1 to 38–5). With antiplatelet therapy alone, the incidence of major vascular complications is 0.5% to 3%, and blood transfusion is required in 0.5% to 1.5% of cases. In the ISAR trial, hemorrhagic complications occurred only in the anticoagulation group (6.5%), and there was an 87% reduction in the risk of peripheral vascular complications in the antiplatelet group. Risk factors for bleeding and vascular complications are age greater than 70 years, female gender, use of warfarin, multiple procedures during the same hospitalization, and low platelet count.[161–163] The puncture site is the most common site of vascular bleeding, although retroperitoneal bleeding may occur less commonly. If prolonged intravenous heparin therapy is clinically indicated, vascular sheaths should be removed early after the procedure (with resumption of heparin several hours after achieving homeostasis), rather than continuing heparin overnight. With this strategy, a twofold to threefold reduction in bleeding and vascular injury has been demonstrated.[164] Use of the radial or brachial artery as an access site for stent implantation has been shown to be safe and feasible, with fewer vascular complications than the femoral approach.[165–168] The use of collagen implants and other vascular closure devices may further reduce vascular complications.[169–172]

## CONCLUSION

The use of optimal stenting techniques, combined with antiplatelet therapy, has reduced the incidence of both angiographic and clinical complications associated with stent placement. Whether improvements in stent design will further decrease stent complications remains to be seen in randomized trials.

## REFERENCES

1. Goy JJ, Eeckhout E, Stauffer JC, et al: Emergency endoluminal stenting for abrupt vessel closure following coronary angioplasty: A randomized comparison of the Wiktor and Palmaz-Schatz stents. Cathet Cardiovasc Diagn 34:128, 1995.
2. Urban P, Chatelain P, Brzostek T, et al: Bailout coronary stenting with 6F guiding catheters for failed balloon angioplasty. Am Heart J 129:1078, 1995.
3. Metz D, Urban P, Camenzind E, et al: Improving results of bailout coronary stenting after failed balloon angioplasty. Cathet Cardiovasc Diagn 32:117, 1994.
4. Schomig A, Kastrati A, Mudra H, et al: Four-year experience with Palmaz-Schatz stenting in coronary angioplasty complicated by dissection with threatened or present vessel closure. Circulation 90:2716, 1994.
5. Maiello L, Colombo A, Gianrossi R, et al: Coronary stenting for treatment of acute or threatened closure following dissection after coronary balloon angioplasty. Am Heart J 125:1570, 1993.
6. Kiemeneij F, Laarman G, van der Wieken R, et al: Emergency coronary stenting with the Palmaz-Schatz stent for failed transluminal coronary angioplasty: Results of a learning phase. Am Heart J 126:23, 1993.
7. Reifart N, Haase J, Massa TH, et al: Randomized trial comparing two devices: The Palmaz-Schatz stent and the Strecker stent in bail-out situations. J Intervent Cardiol 7:539, 1994.
8. Haude M, Erbel R, Straub U, et al: Results of intracoronary stents for management of coronary dissection after balloon angioplasty. Am J Cardiol 67:691, 1991.
9. Alfonso F, Hernandez R, Coicolea J, et al: Coronary stenting for acute coronary dissection after coronary angioplasty: Implications of residual dissection. J Am Coll Cardiol 24:989, 1994.
10. Foley JB, Brown RIG, Penn IM: Thrombosis and restenosis after stenting in failed angioplasty: Comparison with elective stenting. Am Heart J 128:12, 1994.
11. Hermann H, Buchbinder M, Cleman M, et al: Emergent use of balloon-expandable coronary artery stenting for failed percutaneous coronary angioplasty. Circulation 86:812, 1992.
12. Chan C, Tan A, Koh T, et al: Intracoronary stenting in the treatment of acute or threatened closure in angiographically small coronary arteries (<3.0 mm) complicating percutaneous transluminal coronary angioplasty. Am J Cardiol 75:23, 1995.
13. Sutton J, Ellis S, Roubin G, et al: Major clinical events after coronary stenting: The multicenter registry of acute and elective Gianturco-Roubin stent placement. Circulation 89:1126, 1994.
14. Agrawal S, Ho D, Liu M, et al: Predictors of thrombotic complications after placement of the flexible coil stent. Am J Cardiol 73:1216, 1994.
15. Hearn JA, King SB III, Douglas JS, et al: Clinical and angiographic outcomes after intracoronary artery stenting for acute or threatened closure after percutaneous transluminal coronary angioplasty: Initial results with a balloon-expandable, stainless steel design. Circulation 88:2086, 1993.
16. George B, Voorhees W, Roubin G, et al: Multicenter investigation of coronary stenting to treat acute or threatened closure after percutaneous transluminal coronary angioplasty: Clinical and angiographic outcomes. J Am Coll Cardiol 22:135, 1993.
17. Roubin G, Cannon A, Agrawal S, et al: Intracoronary stenting for acute and threatened closure complicating percutaneous transluminal coronary angioplasty. Circulation 85:916, 1992.
18. Vrolix MC, Rutsch W, Piessens J, et al: Bail-out stenting with Medtronic Wiktor: Results from the European stent study group. J Intervent Cardiol 7:549, 1994.
19. Garratt K, White C, Buchbinder M, et al: Wiktor stent placement for unsuccessful coronary angioplasty. Circulation 90:I-279, 1994.
20. Reifart N, Langer A, Stroger H, et al: Strecker stent as a bailout device following percutaneous transluminal coronary angioplasty. J Intervent Cardiol 5:79, 1992.
21. Ozaki Y, Keane D, Ruygrok P, et al: Acute clinical and angiographic results with the new AVE micro coronary stent in bailout management. Am J Cardiol 76:112, 1995.
22. Goy JJ, Sigwart U, Vogt P, et al: Long-term clinical and angiographic follow-up of patients treated with the self-expanding coronary stent for acute occlusion during balloon angioplasty of the right coronary artery. J Am Coll Cardiol 19:1593, 1992.
23. Sigwart U, Urban P, Golf S, et al: Emergency stenting for acute occlusion after coronary balloon angioplasty. Circulation 78:1121, 1988.
24. de Feyter PJ, De Scheerder IK, van den Brand M, et al: Emergency stenting for refractory acute coronary artery oc-

clusion during balloon angioplasty. Am J Cardiol 66:1147, 1990.

25. Fischman DL, Leon MB, Baim DS, et al: A randomized comparison of coronary stent placement and balloon angioplasty in the treatment of coronary artery disease. N Engl J Med 331:496, 1994.

26. Serruys P, de Jaegere P, Kiemeneij F, et al: A comparison of balloon expandable stent implantation with balloon angioplasty in patients with coronary artery disease. N Engl J Med 331:489, 1994.

27. Levine M, Leonard B, Burke J, et al: Clinical and angiographic results of balloon-expandable intracoronary stents in right coronary artery stenoses. J Am Coll Cardiol 16:332, 1990.

28. Schatz RA, Baim DS, Leon MB, et al: Clinical experience with the Palmaz-Schatz coronary stent: Initial results of a multicenter study. Circulation 83:148, 1991.

29. Colombo A, Almagor Y, Maiello L, et al: Results of coronary stenting for restenosis. J Am Coll Cardiol 25:118A, 1994.

30. Savage M, Fischman D, Schatz R, et al: Long-term angiographic and clinical outcome after implantation of a balloon-expandable stent in the native coronary circulation. J Am Coll Cardiol 24:1207, 1994.

31. Carrozza J, Kuntz R, Levine M, et al: Angiographic and clinical outcome of intracoronary stenting: Immediate and long-term results from a large single-center experience. J Am Coll Cardiol 20:328, 1992.

32. Strauss B, Serruys P, Bertrand M, et al: Quantitative angiographic follow-up of the coronary Wallstent in native vessels and bypass grafts (European experience—March 1986 to March 1990). Am J Cardiol 69:475, 1992.

33. Serruys PW, Strauss BH, Beatt KJ, et al: Angiographic follow-up after placement of a self-expanding coronary-artery stent. N Engl J Med 324:13, 1991.

34. Sigwart U, Kaufman U, Goy JJ, et al: Prevention of coronary restenosis by stenting. Eur Heart J 9:31, 1988.

35. Eeckhout E, Stauffer JC, Vogt P, et al: A comparison of intracoronary stenting with conventional balloon angioplasty for the treatment of new onset stenoses of the right coronary artery. J Am Coll Cardiol 25:196A, 1995.

36. de Jaeger P, Serruys P, Bertrand M, et al: Angiographic predictors of recurrence of restenosis after Wiktor stent implantation in native coronary arteries. Am J Cardiol 72:165, 1993.

37. Neumann FJ, Walter H, Schmitt C, et al: Coronary stenting as an adjunct to direct balloon angioplasty in acute myocardial infarction. Circulation 92:I-609, 1995.

38. Monassier JP, Elias J, Meyer P, et al: STENTIMI I: The French Registry of Stenting at Acute Infarction. J Am Coll Cardiol 27:68A, 1996.

39. Verna E, Castiglioni B, Onofri M, et al: Intracoronary stenting of the infarct-related artery without anticoagulation in acute myocardial infarction. Eur Heart J 16:12, 1995.

40. Levy G, deBoisgelin, Volpiliere R, et al: Intracoronary stenting in direct infarct angioplasty: Is it dangerous? Circulation 92:I-139, 1995.

41. Benzuly KH, Goldstein JA, Almany SL, et al: Feasibility of stenting in acute myocardial infarction. Circulation 92:I-616, 1995.

42. Romero M, Medina A, Suarez J, et al: Elective Palmaz-Schatz stent implantation in acute coronary syndromes induced by thrombus-containing lesions. Eur Heart J 16:179, 1995.

43. Rodriquez A, Fernanadez M, Santaera D, et al: Coronary stenting in patients undergoing PTCA during acute myocardial infarction. Am J Cardiol 77:685, 1996.

44. Steinhubl S, Moliterno D, Teirstein P, et al: Stenting for acute myocardial infarction: The early United States Multicenter Experience. J Am Coll Cardiol 27:279A, 1996.

45. Stone G, Morice M, Brodie B, et al: Primary stenting in acute MI: Interim report from the PAMI-3 Pilot study. European Congress of Cardiology, August 1996.

46. Lefevre T, Morice M-C, Karrillon G, et al: Coronary stenting during acute myocardial infarction: Results from the Stent Without Coumadin French Registry. J Am Coll Cardiol 27:69A, 1996.

47. Wong SC, Popma J, Pichard A, et al: Comparison of clinical and angiographic outcomes after saphenous vein graft angioplasty using coronary versus "biliary" tubular slotted stents. Circulation 91:339, 1995.

48. Rechavia E, Litvack F, Macko G, et al: Stent implantation of saphenous vein graft aorto-ostial lesions in patients with unstable ischemic syndromes: Immediate angiographic results and long-term clinical outcome. J Am Coll Cardiol 25:866, 1995.

49. Piana R, Moscucci M, Cohen D, et al: Palmaz-Schatz stenting for treatment of focal vein graft stenosis: Immediate results and long-term outcome. J Am Coll Cardiol 23:1296, 1994.

50. Fenton S, Fischman D, Savage M, et al: Long-term angiographic and clinical outcome after implantation of balloon-expandable stents in aortocoronary saphenous vein grafts. Am J Cardiol 74:1187, 1994.

51. Leon MB, Wong SC, Pichard A: Balloon expandable stent implantation in saphenous vein grafts. In Hermann HC, Hisrschfeld JW (eds): Clinical Use of the Palmaz-Schatz Intracoronary Stent, pp 111–121. Futura, 1993.

52. Pomerantz R, Kuntz R, Carrozza J, et al: Acute and long-term outcome of narrowed saphenous venous grafts treated by endoluminal stenting and directional atherectomy. Am J Cardiol 70:161, 1992.

53. Eeckhout E, Goy J, Stauffer J, et al: Endoluminal stenting of narrowed saphenous vein grafts: Long-term clinical and angiographic follow-up. Cathet Cardiovasc Diagn 32:139, 1994.

54. Keane D, Buis B, Reifart N, et al: Clinical and angiographic outcome following implantation of the new less shortening Wallstent in aortocoronary vein grafts: Introduction of a second generation stent in the clinical arena. J Intervent Cardiol 7:557, 1994.

55. de Scheerder I, Strauss B, de Feyter P, et al: Stenting of venous bypass grafts: A new treatment modality for patients who are poor candidates for reintervention. Am Heart J 123:1046, 1992.

56. Urban P, Sigwart U, Golf S, et al: Intravascular stenting for stenosis of aortocoronary venous bypass grafts. J Am Coll Cardiol 13:1085, 1989.

57. Fortuna R, Heuser R, Garratt K, et al: Intracoronary stent: Experience in the first 101 vein graft patients. J Am Coll Cardiol 26:I-308, 1993.

58. Bilodeau L, Iyer S, Cannon A, et al: Flexible coil stent (Cook, Inc.) in saphenous vein grafts: Clinical and angiographic follow-up. J Am Coll Cardiol 19:264A, 1992.

59. Colombo A, Itoh A, Maiello L, et al: Coronary stent implantation in aorto-ostial lesions: Immediate and follow-up results. J Am Coll Cardiol 27:253A, 1996.

60. Rocha-Singh K, Morris N, Wong C, et al: Coronary stenting for treatment of ostial stenoses of native coronary arteries or aortocoronary saphenous venous grafts. Am J Cardiol 75:26, 1995.

61. Medina A, Melian F, deLezo J, et al: Effectiveness of coronary stenting for the treatment of chronic total occlusion in angina pectoris. Am J Cardiol 73:1222, 1994.

62. Hsu Y-S, Tamai H, Ueda K, et al: Clinical efficacy of coronary stenting in chronic total occlusions. Circulation 90:I-613, 1994.

63. Ooka M, Suzuki T, Kosokawa H, et al: Stenting vs. nonstenting after revascularization of chronic total occlusion. Circulation 90:I-613, 1994.

64. Ooka M, Suzuki T, Yokoya K, et al: Stenting after revascularization of chronic total occlusion. Circulation 92:I-94, 1995.

65. Goldberg SL, Colombo A, Maiello L, et al: Intracoronary stent insertion after balloon angioplasty of chronic total occlusion. J Am Coll Cardiol 26:713, 1995.

66. Maiello L, Luigi S, Hall P, et al: Results of stent implantation for diffuse coronary disease assisted by ultravascular ultrasound. J Am Coll Cardiol 25:156A, 1995.

67. Reimers B, Di Mario C, Nierop P, et al: Long-term restenosis after multiple stent implantation: A quantitative angiographic study. Circulation 92:I-327, 1995.

68. Shaknovich A, Moses J, Undemir C, et al: Procedural and

short-term clinical outcomes of multiple Palmaz-Schatz stents (PSS) in very long lesions/dissections. Circulation 92:I-535, 1995.

69. Mintz G, Dussaillant G, Wong SC, et al: Rotational atherectomy followed by adjunct stents: The preferred therapy for calcified lesions in large vessels? Circulation 92:I-329, 1995.

70. Teirstein P, Schatz R, Russo R, et al: Coronary stenting of small diameter vessels: Is it safe? Circulation 92:I-281, 1995.

71. Hall P, Colombo A, Itoh A, et al: Gianturco-Roubin stent implantation in small vessels without anticoagulation. Circulation 92:I-795, 1995.

72. Colombo A, Maiello L, Nakamura S, et al: Preliminary experience of coronary stenting with the MicroStent. J Am Coll Cardiol 25:239A, 1995.

73. Morice MC, Valelx B, Marco J, et al: Preliminary results of the MUST trial, major clinical events during the first month. J Am Coll Cardiol 27:137A, 1996.

74. Hall P, Nakamura S, Maiello L, et al: Clinical and angiographic outcome after Palmaz-Schatz stent implantation guided by intravascular ultrasound. J Invasive Cardiol 7:12A, 1995.

75. Wong C, Popma J, Chuang Y, et al: Economic impact of reduced anticoagulation after saphenous vein graft stent placement. J Am Coll Cardiol 25:80A, 1995.

76. Buszman P, Clague J, Gibbs S, et al: Improved post stent management: High gain at low risk. J Am Coll Cardiol 25:182A, 1995.

77. Fajadet J, Jordon C, Carvalho H, et al: Percutaneous transradial coronary stenting without Coumadin can reduce vascular access complications and hospital stay. J Am Coll Cardiol 25:182A, 1995.

78. Blasini R, Mudra H, Schuhlen H, et al: Intravascular ultrasound guided optimized emergency coronary Palmaz-Schatz stent placement without post procedural systemic anticoagulation. J Am Coll Cardiol 25:197A, 1995.

79. Colombo A, Hall P, Nakamura S, et al: Intracoronary stenting without anticoagulation accomplished with intravascular ultrasound guidance. Circulation 91:1676, 1995.

80. Mehan V, Saizmann C, Kaufmann U, et al: Coronary stenting without anticoagulation. Cathet Cardiovasc Diagn 34:137, 1995.

81. Russo R, Schatz R, Morris N, et al: Ultrasound-guided coronary stent placement without warfarin anticoagulation: Six-month clinical follow-up. Circulation 92:I-543, 1995.

82. Haase H, Reifart N, Baier T, et al: Bail-out stenting (Palmaz-Schatz) without anticoagulation. Circulation 92:I-795, 1995.

83. Saito S, Kim K, Hosokawa G, et al: Primary Palmaz-Schatz implantation without Coumadin in acute myocardial infarction. Circulation 92:I-796, 1995.

84. Jordan C, Carvalho H, Fajadet J, et al: Reduction of acute thrombosis rate after coronary stenting using a new anticoagulant protocol. Circulation 90:I-125, 1994.

85. Wong SC, Popma J, Mintz G, et al: Preliminary results from the Reduced Anticoagulation in Saphenous Vein Graft Stent (RAVES) Trial. Circulation 90:I-125, 1994.

86. Goods CM, Al-Shaibi KF, Dean LS, et al: Is ticlopidine a necessary component of antiplatelet regimens following coronary artery stenting? J Am Coll Cardiol 27:137A, 1995.

87. Marco J, Fajadet J, Brunel P, et al: First use of the second-generation Gianturco-Roubin stent without Coumadin. Am J Cardiol, in press.

88. Colombo A, Nakamura S, Hall P, et al: A prospective study of Gianturco-Roubin coronary stent implantation without anticoagulation. J Am Coll Cardiol 25:50A, 1995.

89. Reifart N, Haase J, Vandormael M, et al: Gianturco-Roubin Stent Acute Closure Evaluation (GRACE): Thirty-day outcomes compared to drug regimen. Circulation 92:I-409, 1995.

90. Goods C, Al-Shaibi K, Iyer S, et al: Flexible coil coronary stenting without anticoagulation or intravascular ultrasound: A prospective observational study. Circulation 92:I-795, 1995.

91. Carvalho H, Fajadet J, Jordan C, et al: A lower rate of complications after Gianturco-Roubin coronary stenting using a new antiplatelet and anticoagulant protocol. Circulation 90:I-125, 1994.

92. Hall P, Colombo A, Nakamura S, et al: A prospective study of Gianturco-Roubin coronary stent implantation without subsequent anticoagulation. Circulation 90:I-124, 1994.

93. Elias J, Monassiers JP, Carrie D, et al: Final results of phases II, III, IV and V of Medtronic Wiktor stent implantation without Coumadin. J Am Coll Cardiol 27:15A, 1996.

94. Elias J, Monassiers JP, Puel J, et al: Medtronic Wiktor stent implantation without Coumadin: Hospital outcome. Circulation 90:I-124, 1994.

95. Colombo A, Nakamura S, Hall P, et al: A prospective study of Wiktor coronary stent implantation without anticoagulation. J Am Coll Cardiol 25:239A, 1995.

96. Colombo A, Nakamura S, Hall P, et al: A prospective study of Wiktor coronary stent implantation treated only with antiplatelet therapy. Circulation 90:I-124, 1994.

97. Morice M-C: Advances in post stenting medication protocol. J Invasive Cardiol 7:32A–35A, 1995.

98. Morice M-C, Bourdonnec C, Lefevre T, et al: Coronary stenting without Coumadin: Phase III. Circulation 90:I-125, 1994.

99. Morice M, Zemour G, Benveniste E, et al: Intracoronary stenting without Coumadin: One month results of a French multicenter study. Cathet Cardiovasc Diagn 35:1, 1995.

100. Morice M, Breton C, Bunouf P, et al: Coronary stenting without anticoagulant, without intravascular ultrasound: Results of the French Registry. Circulation 92:I-796, 1995.

101. Lablanche J-M, Grollier G, Danchin N, et al: Full antiplatelet therapy without anticoagulation after coronary stenting. J Am Coll Cardiol 25:181A, 1995.

102. Barragan P, Silvestri M, Sainsous I, et al: Prevention of subacute occlusion after coronary stenting with ticlopidine regimen without intravascular ultrasound guided stenting. J Am Coll Cardiol 25:182A, 1995.

103. Barragan P, Sainsous J, Silvestri M, et al: Ticlopidine and subcutaneous heparin as an alternative regimen following coronary stenting. Cathet Cardiovasc Diagn 32:133, 1994.

104. Aubry P, Royer T, Spaulding C, et al: Coronary stenting without Coumadin: Phase II and III, the bail-out group. Circulation 90:I-124, 1994.

105. Blengino S, Maiello L, Hall P, et al: Randomized trial of coronary stent implantation without anticoagulation: Aspirin vs. ticlopidine. Circulation 90:I-124, 1994.

106. Lefevre T, Morice M, Larunie B, et al: Coronary stenting in elderly patients: Results from the Stent Without Coumadin French Registry. J Am Coll Cardiol 27:252A, 1996.

107. Shaknovich A, Rocha-Singh K, Teirstein PS, et al: Subacute stent thrombosis in native coronary arteries: Time course, acute management and outcome. US multicenter experience. 65th Annual Scientific Sessions of the American Heart Association, November 1992.

108. Moussa I, Di Mario C, Reimers B, et al: Subacute stent thrombosis in the era of intravascular ultrasound-guided coronary stenting without anticoagulation: Frequency, predictors and clinical outcome. J Am Coll Cardiol 29:6, 1997.

109. Malosky SA, Hirshfeld JWJ, Hermann HC: Comparison of results of intracoronary stenting in patients with unstable vs stable angina. Cathet Cardiovasc Diagn 31:95, 1994.

110. Nath CF, Muller DWM, Ellis SG, et al: Thrombosis of a flexible coil coronary stent: Frequency, predictors and clinical outcome. J Am Coll Cardiol 21:622, 1993.

111. Robinson NMK, Thomas MR, Wainright RJ, et al: Unstable angina is not a contraindication to intracoronary stent insertion. J Invasive Cardiol 7:6A, 1995.

112. Guameri EM, Schatz RA, Sklar MA, et al: Acute coronary syndromes: Is it safe to stent? Circulation 92:I-616, 1995.

113. Walton AS, Oesterle SN, Yeung AC: Coronary artery stenting for acute closure complicating primary angioplasty for acute myocardial infarction. Cathet Cardiovasc Diagn 34:142, 1995.

114. Ahmad T, Webb JG, Carere RR, et al: Coronary stenting for acute myocardial infarction. Am J Cardiol 76:77, 1995.

115. Wong PH, Wong CM: Intracoronary stenting in acute myocardial infarction. Cathet Cardiovasc Diagn 33:39, 1994.

116. Iyer S, Bilodeau L, Cannon A, et al: Stenting the infarct related artery within 15 days of the acute event: Immediate and long term outcome using the flexible metallic coil stent. J Am Coll Cardiol 21:291A, 1993.

117. Capers Q, Thomas C, Weintraub W, et al: Emergent stent placement: Worse out come in the patients with a recent myocardial infarction. J Am Coll Cardiol 23:71A, 1994.

118. Metz D, Urban P, Hoang V, et al: Predicting the risk of ischemic complications after bail-out stenting for failed angioplasty. J Am Coll Cardiol 23:72A, 1994.

119. Shaknovich A: Complications of coronary stenting. Coron Artery Dis 5:583, 1994.

120. Hosokawa H, Tani T: Time course of neointimal stent coverage by coronary angioscopy: Palmaz-Schatz vs Gianturco-Roubin stents. Circulation 92:I-27, 1995.

121. Nunes GL, Hanson SR, Rowland SM, et al: A comparison of the thrombogenicity of stainless and tantalum coronary stents. Circulation 84:I-332, 1992.

122. Bailey SR, Page S, Lunn A, et al: Heparin coating of endovascular stents decreases subacute thrombosis in a rabbit model. Circulation 86:I-186, 1992.

123. van der Giessen WJ, Hardhammar PA, van Beusexon MM, et al: Prevention of (sub)acute thrombosis using heparin-coated stents. Circulation 90:I-650, 1994.

124. Serruys PW, Emanuelsson H, van der Giessen W, et al: Heparin-coated Palmaz-Schatz stents in human coronary arteries: Early outcome of the Benestent-II Pilot Study. Circulation 93:412, 1996.

125. Goldberg SL, Colombo A, Nakamura S, et al: Benefits of intracoronary ultrasound in the deployment of Palmaz-Schatz stents. J Am Coll Cardiol 24:996, 1994.

126. Schomig A, Neumann FJ, Kastrati A, et al: A randomized comparison of antiplatelet and anticoagulant therapy after the placement of coronary-artery stents. N Engl J Med 334:1085, 1996.

127. Uren NG, Schwarzacher SP, Meta JA, et al: Intravascular ultrasound prediction of stent thrombosis: Insights from the POST registry. J Am Coll Cardiol, p 60A, 1997.

128. Russo RJ, Nicosia A, Teirstein PS: Angiography versus intravascular ultrasound-directed stent placement. J Am Coll Cardiol 29:60A, 1997.

129. Meier B, Gruentzig AR, King SB III, et al: Risk of side branch occlusion during coronary angioplasty. Am J Cardiol 53:10, 1984.

130. Vetrovec GW, Cowely MJ, Wolfgang TC, et al: Effects of percutaneous transluminal coronary angioplasty on lesion-associated branches. Am Heart J 109:921, 1985.

131. Arora RR, Raymond RE, Dimas AP, et al: Side branch occlusion during coronary angioplasty: Incidence, angiographic characteristics and outcome. Cathet Cardiovasc Diagn 18:210, 1989.

132. Iniguez A, Macaya C, Alfonso F, et al: Early angiographic changes of side branches arising from a Palmaz-Schatz stented coronary segment: Results and clinical implications. J Am Coll Cardiol 23:911, 1994.

133. Fischman DL, Savage MP, Leon MB, et al: Fate of lesion-related side branches after coronary artery stenting. J Am Coll Cardiol 22:1641, 1993.

134. Pan M, Medina A, et al: Follow-up patency of side branches covered by intracoronary Palmaz-Schatz stent. Am Heart J 129:436, 1995.

135. Mazur M, Grinstead C, Hakim AH, et al: Fate of side branches after intracoronary implantation of the Gianturco-Roubin Flex-Stent for acute or threatened closure after percutaneous transluminal coronary angioplasty. Am J Cardiol 74:1207, 1994.

136. Aliabadi D, Safian RD, Tilli FV, et al: Side branch occlusion following high pressure coronary stenting: Incidence and angiographic predictors. J Am Coll Cardiol 29:274A, 1997.

137. Caputo RP, Chafizadeh ER, Stoler RC, et al: Stent jail: A minimum-security prison. Am J Cardiol 77:1226, 1996.

138. Colombo A, Gaglione A, Nakamura S, et al: Kissing stents for bifurcational coronary lesions. Cathet Cardiovasc Diagn 30:327, 1993.

139. Nakamura S, Hall P, Maiello L, et al: Techniques for Palmaz-Schatz stent deployment in lesions with a large side branch. Cathet Cardiovasc Diagn 34:353, 1995.

140. Carrie D, Karouny E, Chouairi S, et al: "T"-shaped stent placement: A technique for treatment of dissected bifurcation lesions. Cathet Cardiovasc Diagn 37:311, 1996.

141. Teirstein PS: Kissing Palmaz-Schatz stents for coronary bifurcation stenoses. Cathet Cardiovasc Diagn 37:307, 1996.

142. Ajluni SC, Glazier S, Blankenship L, et al: Perforations after percutaneous coronary interventions: Clinical, angiographic, and therapeutic observations. Cathet Cardiovasc Diagn 32:206, 1994.

143. Ellis SG, Ajluni S, Arnold AZ, et al: Increased coronary perforation in the new device era: Incidence, classification, management and outcome. Circulation 90:2725, 1994.

144. Freed M, Grines CL, Safian RD: Coronary artery perforation. In Freed M, Grines CL, Safian RD (eds): The New Manual of Interventional Cardiology, pp 405–411. Birmingham, MI: Physicians Press, 1996.

145. Hall P, Nakamura S, Maiello L, et al: Factors associated with procedural complications during high pressure optimized Palmaz-Schatz intracoronary stent implantation. Circulation 90:I-612, 1994.

146. Fukutomi T, Suzuki T, Hosokawa H, et al: Incidence and management of coronary perforation in different coronary interventions. J Am Coll Cardiol 29:277A, 1997.

147. Flood RD, Popma JJ, Chuang YC, et al: Incidence, angiographic predictors, and clinical significance of coronary perforation occurring after new device angioplasty. J Am Coll Cardiol 23:301A, 1994.

148. Benzuly KH, Glazier S, Grines CL, et al: Coronary perforation: An unreported complication after stent implantation. J Am Coll Cardiol 127:252A, 1996.

149. Shammas NW, Thondapu VR, Winniford MD, et al: Perforation of saphenous vein graft during coronary stenting: A case report. Cath Cardiovasc Diagn 38:274, 1996.

150. Esente P, Giambartolemei A, Reger MJ, et al: Extensive coronary dissection caused by balloon rupture at high pressure during stent deployment. Cathet Cardiovasc Diagn 38:263, 1996.

151. Dittel M, Prachar H, Mlczoch J: Dissection of the left main coronary artery induced by balloon rupture during stent implantation: A case report. Z Kardiol 83:161, 1994.

152. Wong P, Wing-hung L, Chi-mong W: Migration of the AVE Micro stent. Cathet Cardiovasc Diagn 38:267, 1996.

153. Lebowitz NE, Bergman G, Flyer JL, et al: Coronary stent embolization: Incidence, clinical outcome, and localization. Cathet Cardiovasc Diagn 41:109, 1997.

154. Eeckhout E, Stauffer JC, Goy JJ: Retrieval of a migrated coronary stent by means of an alligator forceps catheter. Cathet Cardiovasc Diagn 30:166, 1993.

155. Foster-Smith KW, Garrat KN, Higano ST, et al: Retrieval techniques for managing flexible intracoronary stent misplacement. Cathet Cardiovasc Diagn 30:63, 1993.

156. Cishek MB, Laslett L, Gershony G: Balloon catheter retrieval of dislodged coronary artery stents: A novel technique. Cathet Cardiovasc Diagn 34:350, 1995.

157. Rozenman Y, Burstein M, Hasin Y, et al: Retrieval of occluding unexpanded Palmaz-Schatz stent from a saphenous aorto-coronary vein graft. Cathet Cardiovasc Diagn 34:159, 1995.

158. Mohiaddin RH, Roberts RH, Underwood R, et al: Localization of a misplaced coronary artery stent by magnetic resonance imaging. Clin Cardiol 18:175, 1995.

159. Freed M, Grines C, Safian RD: Bifurcation stenosis. In Freed M, Grines CL, Safian RD (eds): The New Manual of Interventional Cardiology, pp 233–243. Birmingham, MI: Physicians Press, 1996.

160. Gunther HU, Strupp G, Volmar J, et al: Coronary stent implantation: Infection and abscess with fatal outcome. Z Kardiol 82:521, 1993.

161. Dean L, Voorhees W, Sutor C, et al: Female gender: A risk factor for complications following intracoronary stenting? A Cook multicenter registry report. Circulation 90:I-620, 1994.

162. Mansour K, Moscucci M, Kent C, et al: Vascular complications following directional coronary atherectomy or Palmaz-Schatz stenting. J Am Coll Cardiol 23:136A, 1994.

163. Moscucci M, Mansour KA, Kent KC, et al: Peripheral vascu-

lar complications of directional coronary atherectomy and stenting: Predictors, management, and outcome. Am J Cardiol 74:448, 1994.

164. Moscucci M, Mansour K, Kuntz R, et al: Vascular complications of Palmaz-Schatz stenting: Predictors, management and outcome. J Am Coll Cardiol 23:134A, 1994.

165. Resar JR, Wolff MR, Blumanthal RS, et al: Brachial approach for intracoronary stent implantation: A feasibility study. Am Heart J 126:300, 1993.

166. Kiemeneij F, Hofland J, Laarman GJ, et al: Cost comparison between two modes of Palmaz-Schatz coronary stent implantation: Transradial bare stent technique vs. transfemoral sheath-protected stent technique. Cathet Cardiovasc Diagn 35:301, 1995.

167. Kiemeneij F, Laarman GJ: Transradial artery Palmaz-Schatz coronary stent implantation: Results of a single-center feasibility study. Am Heart J 130:14, 1995.

168. Heuser RR, Mehta SS, Strumpf RK, et al: Intracoronary stent implantation via the brachial approach: A technique to reduce vascular bleeding complications. Cathet Cardiovasc Diagn 25:300, 1992.

169. Bartorelli A, Sganzerla P, Fabbiocchi F, et al: Prompt and safe femoral hemostasis with a collagen device after intracoronary implantation of Palmaz-Schatz stents. Am Heart J 130:26, 1995.

170. Radvan J, Calver AL, Dawkins KD, et al: Early experience with the Prostar percutaneous vascular closure device in patients following coronary intervention. Circulation 92:I-410, 1995.

171. Ribeiro E, Silva L, Vetter JW, et al: Single center multiple operator experience with a percutaneous vascular surgery device: A new method to close vascular access sites. Circulation 92:I-410, 1995.

172. Hinohara T, Vetter JW, Ribeiro E, et al: New percutaneous procedure to achieve immediate hemostasis following sheath removal. Circulation 92:I-410, 1995.

# 39

# The Gianturco–Roubin II Stent

*Alexandra J. Lansky     Martin B. Leon*

The first-generation Gianturco-Roubin FlexStent was initially evaluated in clinical trials in 1987. In 1993, U.S. Food and Drug Administration approval was granted on the basis of 30-day clinical outcome data demonstrating safety and effectiveness for the treatment of abrupt and threatened closure. The second-generation Gianturco-Roubin (GR-II) stent is an improved design that includes a sheathless, balloon-expandable flexible coiled stent composed of a polymer coated, single, 0.006-inch 316L stainless steel wire, coiled into interdigitating loops in a "clamshell" design (Fig. 39–1). The coil is linked by a longitudinal spine to prevent axial stent shortening or deformation, and radiopaque gold markers at the proximal and distal ends of the stent allow easy visualization of the stent margins. The GR-II stent is available in two standard stent lengths (20 and 40 mm), allowing single-stent use for longer lesions. This advanced version of the GR-II stent was approved by the U.S. Food and Drug Administration for abrupt or threatened closure syndrome in May 1997.

The performance and outcomes of the GR-II stent have been evaluated extensively in a large, multicenter, randomized clinical trial comparing the elective use of the GR-II stent with the Palmaz-Schatz (PS) stent in patients with complex native coronary stenoses. Several independent registries have also been performed to assess the clinical outcome of the GR-II for the treatment of abrupt and threatened closure and the elective stenting of restenotic lesions, small vessels (2.0 to 3.0 mm), and saphenous vein grafts (Table 39–1).

## THE GR-II FOR ACUTE AND THREATENED CLOSURE

The GR-II stent was approved by the U.S. Food and Drug Administration for the treatment of acute and threatened closure on May 12, 1997, on the basis of the results of a registry of 606 consecutive patients undergoing GR-II stenting for failed angioplasty in both native coronaries and saphenous vein grafts.[1-3] Patients qualified for study entry if at least two of the following criteria were met: chest pain, ischemic electrocardiographic changes, residual stenosis greater than 50%, or any dissection greater than 8.0 mm in length or associated with reduced or no flow. The indication for GR-II stent placement was acute closure in 10% and threatened closure in 90% of cases. Despite the high complexity of lesions treated (81% B2/C lesions), which were composed mostly of long lesions (18 ± 12 mm) with moderate-to-severe tortuosity in 41% and calcification in 35%, successful stent deployment was achieved in 96.4% of cases, with an average of 1.6 stents deployed per lesion. The reference vessel size averaged 2.84 ± 0.50 mm; final Thrombosis In Myocardial Infarction grade 3 (TIMI-3) flow was achieved in 99% of cases, and final stent diameter stenosis was 18 ± 10%. In this high-risk patient population, the 30-day stent thrombosis rate was 4% (2.2% occurred within 24 hours and 1.8% occurred 24 hours to 30 days after deployment) despite the use of the standard anticoagulation regimen of aspirin, 325 mg daily, and ticlopidine, 250 mg twice daily for a month. Clinical results after 1 and 9 months (Table

**TABLE 39–1.     SELECTION CRITERIA FOR THE GIANTURCO–ROUBIN II CLINICAL TRIALS**

|  | AC/TC REGISTRY | SMALL VESSEL REGISTRY | RESTENOTIC REGISTRY | SVG REGISTRY | RANDOMIZED TRIAL |
|---|---|---|---|---|---|
| Number of patients | 606 | 262 | 306 | 106 | 755 |
| Vessel location | Native and SVG | Native | Native | SVG | Native |
| Lesion selection | De novo and restenotic | De novo | Restenotic | De novo and restenotic | De novo |
| Lesion lengths | Not defined | <30 mm | <30 mm | <30 mm | <30 mm |
| Vessel size | 2.0–4.0 mm | 2.0–3.0 mm | 3.0–3.9 mm | 2.5–3.9 mm | 3.0–4.0 mm |

AC/TC, acute and threatened closure; SVG, saphenous vein graft.

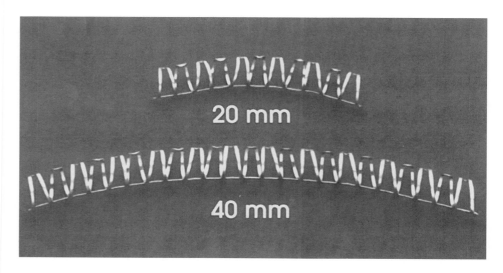

FIGURE 39–1. The 20-mm and 40-mm Gianturco-Roubin II stent with flat wire coil design and longitudinal spine.

39–2) were favorable compared to those of the first-generation FlexStent, with significant improvements in 30-day mortality (2.0% for GR-II vs. 4.8% for FlexStent, $p = 0.05$), Q-wave myocardial infarction (0.8% GR-II vs. 3.1% FlexStent, $p < 0.05$), and coronary artery bypass grafting (2.0% GR-II vs. 8.9% FlexStent, $p < 0.001$).[3] The overall 30-day major adverse cardiac event rate of 6.1% with the GR-II is favorable compared with currently accepted objective performance criteria for 30-day major adverse cardiac event rates of 10% and, compared with other currently approved second- and third-generation stents (Multilinks, ACS, Santa Clara, CA; NIR, Boston Scientific, Maple Grove, MN; AVE-GFX, Santa Rosa, CA). In the 105 patients assigned to angiographic follow-up, the mean follow-up stent diameter stenosis was 48.5% ± 22.8%. The overall 9-month target lesion revascularization in the 606-patient cohort was 12.2%. Among the clinical and angiographic characteristics tested, the independent predictors of target lesion revascularization in this registry included the number of stents implanted ($p = 0.015$), vessel taper ($p < 0.001$), and proximal tortuosity ($p = 0.015$).[4] The GR-II stent can be successfully delivered in most patients with acute or

threatened closure and is associated with reduced 30-day major adverse cardiac event rates compared with the first-generation FlexStent and with favorable 9-month clinical outcomes.

## THE GR-II FOR ELECTIVE STENTING OF DE NOVO LESIONS

The prospective multicenter randomized clinical trial of 755 patients conducted at 31 U.S. clinical sites (Appendix A) was designed to compare the long-term performance of elective stenting with the GR-II stent with that of the standard PS stent.[5, 6] Patients were randomly assigned to elective stent placement using the GR-II stent (N = 380) or the PS stent (N = 375), if they had objective evidence of myocardial ischemia, had a de novo native coronary lesion in a vessel between 3.0 to 4.0 mm in diameter by visual estimate, and required one or two 20-mm or a single 40-mm GR-II or one or two 15-mm PS stents. Lesions up to 30 mm in length were included. Patients were excluded if there was evidence of a recent (<7 days) myocardial infarction, angiographic thrombus, left ventricular ejection fraction less than 35%, unprotected left main disease, or unplanned stent use, such as the occurrence of a significant dissection or reduced (TIMI ≤2) flow after conventional percutaneous transluminal coronary angioplasty (PTCA).

Patients were premedicated with aspirin, 325 mg daily, and ticlopidine, 250 mg twice daily, for 48 hours before the procedure. Bolus intravenous heparin was administered to maintain the activated clotting time between 250 and 350 seconds. After the stent procedure, all patients received 325 mg of aspirin indefinitely and 250 mg of ticlopidine twice daily for 4 weeks. In patients assigned to receive the GR-II stent, the protocol recommended that a slightly oversized GR-II stent (0.1 to 0.5 mm larger

**TABLE 39–2.** **CLINICAL OUTCOMES OF THE ACUTE AND THREATENED CLOSURE REGISTRY**

|  | 30 DAYS (N = 606) | 9 MONTHS (N = 606) |
| --- | --- | --- |
| Death, % | 2.0 | 4.3 |
| Q-MI, % | 0.8 | 0.8 |
| PTCA, % | 2.1 | 8.4 |
| CABG, % | 2.0 | 3.8 |
| MACE (Death, Q-MI, TLR), % | 6.1 | 16.2 |

CABG, coronary artery bypass grafting; MACE, major adverse cardiac events; Q-MI, Q-wave myocardial infarction; PTCA, percutaneous transluminal coronary angioplasty; TLR, target lesion revascularization.

**TABLE 39–3.  BASELINE CLINICAL AND ANGIOGRAPHIC CHARACTERISTICS OF THE GIANTURCO–ROUBIN II (GR-II) RANDOMIZED TRIAL\***

|  | GR-II STENT (N = 380) N (%) | PS STENT (N = 375) N (%) | p VALUE |
|---|---|---|---|
| Age, years | 61 ± 11 | 61 ± 11 | 0.793 |
| Male gender | 261 (68.7) | 268 (71.5) | 0.450 |
| Hypercholesterolemia | 184 (48.4) | 166 (44.3) | 0.325 |
| Diabetes mellitus | 88 (23.2) | 84 (22.4) | 0.872 |
| Hypertension | 221 (58.2) | 225 (60.0) | 0.659 |
| LVEF, % | 55.7 ± 9.9 | 54.8 ± 10.4 | 0.214 |
| Multivessel disease | 175 (46.1) | 204 (54.4) | 0.070 |
| Vessel location |  |  | NS |
|   RCA | 145 (38.2) | 151 (40.3) |  |
|   LAD | 165 (43.4) | 149 (39.7) |  |
|   LCx | 70 (18.4) | 75 (20) |  |
| Ostial location | 8 (2.1) | 16 (4.3) | 0.237 |
| Eccentricity | 152 (40.0) | 141 (37.6) | 0.793 |
| Length, mm | 14.3 ± 8.4 | 14.0 ± 8.4 | 0.595 |
| Thrombus | 13 (3.4) | 9 (2.4) | 0.706 |
| Bend > 45 degrees | 43 (11.3) | 38 (10.1) | 0.850 |
| Total occlusion | 9 (2.4) | 15 (4.0) | 0.383 |
| Calcification | 71 (18.7) | 64 (17.1) | 0.845 |

LAD, left anterior descending artery; LCx, left circumflex coronary artery; LVEF, left ventricular ejection fraction; NS, not significant; PS, Palmaz-Schatz; RCA, right coronary artery.

\*A single culprit lesion is reported for each patient.

than the reference) be selected to achieve a 1.1 to 1.2/1.0 stent to reference artery ratio. Only GR-II stents between 3.0 and 4.0 mm in diameter were available for this study. The GR-II stent was deployed at 6 to 8 atmospheres by use of the stent delivery balloon; subsequent high-pressure (14 to 16 atmospheres) inflations were performed by use of a semicompliant or noncompliant balloon. Clinical follow-up was obtained at 30 days and 9 and 12 months. All adverse clinical events were adjudicated by an independent clinical events committee, and follow-up cineangiograms were obtained in the first 300 consecutive patients at approximately 9 months.

The prespecified primary end point of the trial was the 12-month target lesion revascularization-free survival. Secondary end points included procedure success, defined as the attainment of less than 50% diameter stenosis in the absence of death or emergent bypass surgery, stent thrombosis, and major adverse cardiac events, including death, myocardial infarction, and target lesion revascularization at

30 days and at 9 and 12 months. The secondary angiographic end point was the restenosis frequency defined as a greater than 50% follow-up diameter stenosis within the stent.

The study was powered to establish equivalence of the GR-II and the PS stents based on an estimated 12-month target lesion revascularization-free survival rate of 85% for the PS stent and a delta of less than 8% for the GR-II arm defining equivalence.[7, 7a] Three hundred forty-one patients (682 total patients) would be required per arm to achieve a statistical power of 90% with a type I (alpha) error of 0.05. Assuming a 10% dropout rate attributable to patient loss to clinical follow-up, 750 patients were required for this study.

Patient outcomes were analyzed by use of an "intention-to-treat" analysis (Tables 39–3 to 39–6). Multivariable logistic analyses were performed to identify clinical and angiographic predictors of (1) 30-day stent thrombosis, (2) 12-month target lesion revascularization (TLR), and (3) angiographic restenosis. (Tables 39–7 to 39–9). Variables included in

**TABLE 39–4.  PROCEDURE RESULTS OF THE GIANTURCO–ROUBIN II (GR-II) RANDOMIZED TRIAL**

| MORPHOLOGY | GR-II STENT N = 376 | PS STENT N = 369 | p VALUE |
|---|---|---|---|
| Maximum inflation pressure, atm | 16.0 ± 2.9 | 17.0 ± 3.3 | <0.01 |
| Number of stents | 1.27 ± 0.57 | 1.47 ± 0.72 | <0.001 |
| Total length of implanted stent, mm | 29.3 ± 15.1 | 22.0 ± 10.9 | <0.001 |
| Stent length/lesion length ratio | 2.5 ± 1.7 | 1.9 ± 1.2 | <0.001 |
| Stent/lesion length, mm | 14.8 ± 13.4 | 7.8 ± 8.5 | <0.001 |

PS, Palmaz-Schatz.

**TABLE 39–5. QUANTITATIVE ANGIOGRAPHIC RESULTS OF THE GIANTURCO–ROUBIN II (GR-II) RANDOMIZED TRIAL***

|  | GR-II STENT N = 368 | PS STENT N = 361 | p VALUE |
|---|---|---|---|
| Reference, mm |  |  |  |
| Baseline | 3.08 ± 0.49 | 3.08 ± 0.54 | 0.867 |
| Final | 3.15 ± 0.48 | 3.17 ± 0.53 | 0.676 |
| Follow-up | 2.97 ± 0.47 | 3.00 ± 0.50 | 0.732 |
| MLD, mm |  |  |  |
| Baseline | 1.08 ± 0.43 | 1.06 ± 0.45 | 0.607 |
| Final in-stent | 2.64 ± 0.41 | 2.83 ± 0.43 | <0.001 |
| Follow-up in-stent | 1.48 ± 0.73 | 1.90 ± 0.74 | <0.001 |
| Percent stenosis |  |  |  |
| Baseline | 64.7 ± 12.9 | 65.2 ± 13.9 | 0.636 |
| Final in-stent | 15.6 ± 10.7 | 9.8 ± 10.5 | <0.001 |
| Follow-up in-stent | 50.6 ± 22.3 | 36.4 ± 22.6 | <0.001 |
| Stent lumen changes |  |  |  |
| Acute gain, mm | 1.57 ± 0.52 | 1.76 ± 0.54 | <0.001 |
| Late loss, mm | 1.21 ± 0.69 | 0.92 ± 0.72 | 0.003 |
| Loss index | 0.76 | 0.57 | 0.007 |
| Restenosis rate, % | 47.3 | 20.6 | <0.001 |

*MLD, minimum lumen diameter; PS, Palmaz-Schatz. A single culprit lesion is reported for each patient. Follow-up was obtained in 110 patients for GR-II stents and in 107 patients for PS stents.

**TABLE 39–6. CLINICAL OUTCOME IN THE GIANTURCO–ROUBIN II (GR-II) RANDOMIZED CLINICAL TRIAL**

|  | GR-II STENT (N = 380) N (%) | PS STENT (N = 375) N (%) | p VALUE |
|---|---|---|---|
| In-hospital events |  |  |  |
| MACE (Death, Q-MI, TLR) | 12 (3.2) | 3 (0.8) | 0.039 |
| Death | 1 (0.3) | 2 (0.5) | 0.622 |
| Q-MI | 5 (1.3) | 2 (0.5) | 0.451 |
| TLR (PTCA or CABG) | 10 (2.6) | 0 (0.0) | 0.002 |
| Re-PTCA | 8 (2.1) | 0 (0.0) | 0.008 |
| CABG | 4 (1.1) | 0 (0.0) | 0.124 |
| 30-day cumulative events |  |  |  |
| MACE (Death, Q-MI, TLR) | 16 (4.2) | 5 (1.3) | 0.029 |
| Death | 1 (0.3) | 2 (0.5) | 0.622 |
| Q-MI | 5 (1.3) | 2 (0.5) | 0.451 |
| TLR (PTCA or CABG) | 15 (3.9) | 2 (0.5) | 0.004 |
| Re-PTCA | 10 (2.6) | 1 (0.3) | 0.016 |
| CABG | 7 (1.9) | 1 (0.3) | 0.079 |
| Stent thrombosis | 15 (3.9) | 1 (0.3) | 0.001 |
| 12-month follow-up |  |  |  |
| MACE (Death Q-MI, TLR) | 110 (28.9) | 65 (17.3) | <0.001 |
| Death | 10 (2.6) | 10 (2.7) | 0.976 |
| Q-wave MI | 5 (1.3) | 3 (0.8) | 0.725 |
| Non–Q-wave MI | 50 (13.2) | 41 (10.9) | 0.408 |
| TLR (PTCA or CABG) | 101 (26.6) | 56 (14.9) | <0.001 |
| CABG | 19 (5.0) | 16 (4.3) | 0.760 |
| PTCA | 84 (22.1) | 40 (10.7) | <0.001 |

CABG, coronary artery bypass grafting; MACE, major adverse cardiac events; Q-MI, Q-wave myocardial infarction; PTCA, percutaneous transluminal coronary angioplasty; TLR, target lesion revascularization.

**TABLE 39–7.    PREDICTORS OF 30-DAY STENT THROMBOSIS IN THE GIANTURCO–ROUBIN II (GR-II) RANDOMIZED TRIAL**

|  | UNIVARIATE OR | p VALUE | MULTIVARIATE OR (95% CI) | p VALUE |
|---|---|---|---|---|
| Stent/artery ratio | 16.96 | <0.0001 | 0.0006 (0.136, 0.000) | 0.001 |
| GR-II stent use | 6.750 | 0.009 | 13.560 (116.064, 1.584) | 0.017 |
| Diabetes mellitus | 4.573 | 0.032 | 3.129 (9.654, 1.014) | 0.047 |
| Total implanted stent length, mm | 3.261 | 0.071 | | |
| Incorrect sizing* | 8.217 | 0.042 | | |

CI, confidence interval; OR, odds ratio. Factors included in the univariate model include reference vessel size, left anterior descending artery location, lesion length, final minimal lumen diameter, stent/lesion length ratio, total length of implanted stent, stent/artery ratio, GR-II stent use, diabetes mellitus, and optimal stent sizing.

*Optimal sizing is defined as the selection of GR-II stent 0.1–0.5 mm larger than the reference diameter by Angiographic Core Laboratory assesment.

**TABLE 39–8.    MULTIVARIATE PREDICTORS OF 9-MONTH TARGET LESION REVASCULARIZATION IN THE GIANTURCO–ROUBIN II (GR-II) RANDOMIZED TRIAL**

|  | UNIVARIATE OR | p VALUE | MULTIVARIATE OR DDS RATIO | p VALUE |
|---|---|---|---|---|
| Final MLD, mm | 16.039 | <0.0001 | 2.494 | <0.001 |
| Diabetes mellitus | 11.932 | 0.001 | 2.137 | <0.001 |
| GR-II stent use | 10.538 | 0.001 | 1.779 | 0.004 |
| Reference vessel size, mm | 5.131 | 0.024 | | |
| Lesion length, mm | 4.324 | 0.038 | | |
| LAD location | 4.573 | 0.102 | | |

LAD, left anterior descending artery; MLD, minimum lumen diameter; OR, odds ratio.

Factors included in the univariate model include reference vessel size, LAD location, lesion length, final minimal lumen diameter, stent/lesion length ratio, total length of implanted stent, stent/artery ratio, GR-II stent use, diabetes mellitus, optimal stent sizing, final dissection ≥B.

*Optimal sizing is defined as the selection of a GR-II stent 0.1–0.5 mm larger than the reference diameter by Angiographic Core Laboratory assessment.

**TABLE 39–9.    MULTIVARIATE PREDICTORS OF 6-MONTH ANGIOGRAPHIC RESTENOSIS IN THE GIANTURCO–ROUBIN II (GR-II) RANDOMIZED TRIAL**

|  | UNIVARIATE OR | p VALUE | MULTIVARIATE OR (95% CI) | p VALUE |
|---|---|---|---|---|
| GR-II stent use | 9.858 | 0.002 | 3.244 (6.241, 1.686) | <0.001 |
| Diabetes mellitus | 5.130 | 0.024 | 2.461 (5.052, 1.199) | 0.014 |
| Lesion length, mm | 10.046 | 0.002 | 1.060 (1.102, 1.020) | 0.003 |
| Pre MLD, mm | 2.621 | 0.002 | 3.356 (0.710, 0.126) | 0.006 |
| Final MLD, mm | 3.692 | 0.055 | | |
| Total implanted stent length, mm | 10.432 | 0.001 | | |
| Stent/lesion length, mm | 4.795 | 0.029 | | |

CI, confidence interval; LAD, left anterior descending coronary artery; MLD, minimum lumen diameter; OR, odds ratio. Factors included in the univariate model include reference vessel size, LAD location, lesion length, final minimal lumen diameter, stent/lesion length ratio, total length of implanted stent, stent/artery ratio, GR-II stent use, diabetes mellitus, optimal stent sizing.

*Optimal sizing is defined as the selection of a GR-II stent 0.1–0.5 mm larger than the reference diameter by Angiographic Core Laboratory assessment.

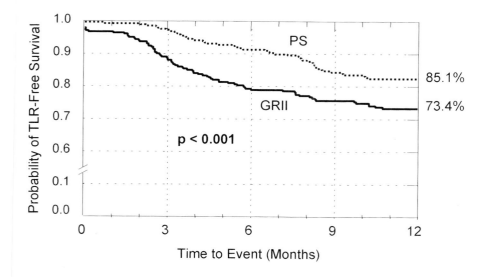

FIGURE 39–2. Target lesion revascularization (TLR)–free survival. Kaplan-Meier estimate of overall survival free of TLR. Freedom from TLR at 12 months was 73.4% for Gianturco-Roubin II (GR-II) vs. 85.1% for Palmaz-Schatz (PS) *(p < 0.001).*

the model were reference vessel size, left anterior descending artery location, lesion length, final minimal lumen diameter, stent/lesion length ratio, total length of implanted stent, stent/artery ratio, GR-II stent use, diabetes mellitus, and "incorrect" GR-II stent sizing (undersized and oversized). Binary stepwise multivariate logistic regression analysis utilized *p* values of 0.10 for entry and 0.20 for removal. A two-tailed *p* value of less than 0.05 was considered significant.

Patients treated with the GR-II stent had more early complications (stent thrombosis and 30-day composite events) and higher late angiographic and clinical restenosis rates than those given the PS stent (Fig. 39–2; see also Tables 39–4 and 39–5). Independent predictors of 9-month TLR-free survival (the primary end point of this randomized trial) were a smaller final minimum lumen diameter, diabetes mellitus, and implantation of a GR-II stent (see Table 39–8).

The likely explanation for increased early compli-

cations associated with the GR-II stent in this clinical trial was the reduced stent/artery ratio resulting from (1) increased acute recoil of this coiled stent design and (2) implantation of undersized stents—an operator-dependent variable (Table 39–10; see also Table 39–6). Other studies have demonstrated that small stent size and incompletely expanded stents are important predictors of subacute stent thrombosis.[8]

There are many potential reasons for the disappointing late outcomes of the GR-II stent when compared with the PS stent. First, late patient outcomes (both angiographic restenosis and TLR) are strongly influenced by the acute angiographic results after any coronary intervention.[9] In the current study, the final angiographic diameter stenoses were considerably higher in patients treated with GR-II stents (15.6% vs. 9.8% for PS, *p* <0.001) (Fig. 39–3). The design of the GR-II stent is different from most other tubular-slotted and multicellular stents; there is more acute stent recoil and more open space be-

**TABLE 39–10.   IMPACT OF GIANTURCO–ROUBIN II (GR-II) STENT SIZING ON 30-DAY AND 1-YEAR CLINICAL OUTCOMES IN THE GR-II RANDOMIZED TRIAL**

|  | CORRECT | OVERSIZED | UNDERSIZED | INCORRECTLY SIZED | PS STENT |
|---|---|---|---|---|---|
| N | 149 | 140 | 73 | 213 | 213 |
| **30-day events, %** | | | | | |
| MACE | 2.0 | 3.6 | 8.2* | 5.2 | 1.1 |
| SAT | 0.7 | 2.5 | 11‡ | 5.6* | 0.3 |
| MI | 0 | 0.7 | 5.5† | 2.3 | 0.3 |
| Death | 0 | 0 | 0 | 0 | 0.6 |
| TLR | 2.0 | 3.6 | 6.8 | 4.7 | 0.6 |
| **1-year events, %** | | | | | |
| MACE | 25.5 | 30.5 | 31.5 | 30.5 | 16.4† |
| Death | 1.3 | 2.1 | 4.1 | 2.8 | 2.0 |
| MI | 0 | 0.7 | 5.5† | 2.3 | 0.6 |
| TLR | 24.2 | 27.9 | 26.0 | 27.2 | 14.4† |

*p < 0.05; †p < 0.1; ‡p < 0.001.
MACE, major adverse cardiac event; MI, myocardial infarction; PS, Palmaz-Schatz; SAT, subacute thrombosis; TLR, target lesion revascularization.

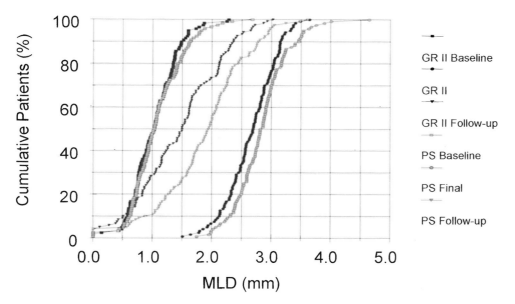

FIGURE 39–3. Cumulative distribution curves for the minimal lumen diameter (MLD) at baseline, final procedure, and 9-month follow-up in patients randomly assigned to the Gianturco-Roubin II (GR-II) and the Palmaz-Schatz (PS) stents. The MLD baselines are similar in both groups; however, the final procedure MLDs ($2.64 \pm 0.41$ for GR-II vs. $2.83 \pm 0.43$ for PS, $p < 0.001$) and the follow-up MLDs ($50.6 \pm 22.3$ for GR-II vs. $36.4 \pm 22.6$ for PS, $p < 0.001$) were significantly smaller for GR-II–treated patients.

tween stent struts, allowing increased tissue prolapse. Thus, implanting GR-II stents using a technique similar to that used for PS stents resulted in higher final diameter stenoses and worsened overall late outcomes in the GR-II stent patients. The problem was compounded by systematic operator undersizing of the GR-II stents in this study (this occurred in 20% of cases when vessel size was assessed quantitatively and an even greater number according to investigator estimates of reference vessel size) (Table 39–11). Previous studies have emphasized the importance of avoiding undersizing with coiled stents.[10] Second, the stent lengths available for this study inadvertently resulted in a much higher total stent length and stent/lesion length ratio

for the GR-II stent (29.3 mm vs. 22.0 mm for PS, $p <0.001$ and 2.5 versus 1.5 for PS, $p <0.001$, respectively) (see Table 39–6). In this trial and others,[11] stent length has been an important predictor of late angiographic and clinical restenosis (Fig. 39–4). Third, as with any new device, operator technique is critical for achieving optimal results.[12] There was a marked site-to-site variability in long-term patient outcomes in the GR-II group (Fig. 39–5), a finding not seen in the PS stent group. It is possible that a different stent implantation technique (i.e., a larger balloon/artery ratio to offset the acute recoil and tissue prolapse, resulting in lower final procedural diameter stenoses) would have produced better results in the GR-II arm of the current study.

**TABLE 39–11.    EFFECT OF VESSEL SIZE AND STENT SIZING ON 30-DAY AND 1-YEAR CLINICAL OUTCOMES IN THE GIANTURCO–ROUBIN II RANDOMIZED TRIAL**

| | CORRECT | | OVERSIZED | | UNDERSIZED | | PS STENT | |
|---|---|---|---|---|---|---|---|---|
| | <3.0 mm | >3.0 mm | <3.0 mm | >3.0 mm | <3.0 mm | >3.0 mm | <3.0 mm | >3.0 mm |
| N | 48 | 73 | 111 | 45 | 13 | 72 | 167 | 185 |
| **30-day events** | | | | | | | | |
| SAT | 0 | 0 | 4 (3.6) | 0 | 1 (7.7) | 4 (5.6) | 1 (0.6) | 0 |
| Death | 0 | 0 | 0 | 0 | 0 | 0 | 2 (1.2) | 0 |
| MI | 0 | 0 | 1 (0.9) | 0 | 0 | 4 (5.6) | 1 (0.6) | 0 |
| CABG | 1 (2.1) | 1 | 2 (1.8) | 0 | 0 | 2 (2.8) | 0 | 1 (0.5) |
| PTCA | 0 | 0 | 4 (3.6) | 1 (2.2) | 0 | 4 (5.6) | 1 (0.6) | 0 |
| TLR | 1 (2.1) | 1 (1.4) | 4 (3.6) | 1 (2.2) | 0 | 6 (8.3) | 1 (0.6) | 1 (0.5) |
| MACE | 1 (2.1) | 1 (1.4) | 4 (3.6) | 1 (2.2) | 0 | 7 (9.7) | 3 (1.8) | 1 (0.5) |
| **1-year events** | | | | | | | | |
| Death | 0 | 2 (2.7) | 1 (0.9) | 2 (4.4) | 0 | 3 (4.2) | 4 (2.4) | 3 (1.6) |
| MI | 0 | 0 | 1 (0.9) | 0 | 0 | 4 (5.6) | 2 (1.2) | 0 |
| CABG | 3 (6.3) | 3 (4.1) | 2 (1.8) | 0 | 1 (7.7) | 3 (4.2) | 8 (4.7) | 6 (3.2) |
| PTCA | 12 (25) | 10 (13.7) | 4 (3.6) | 8 (17.8) | 4 (31) | 14 (19.4) | 20 (12) | 17 (9.2) |
| TLR | 15 (31.3) | 13 (17.8) | 36 (32.4) | 8 (17.8) | 5 (38.5) | 17 (23.6) | 28 (16.6) | 23 (12.4) |
| MACE | 15 (31.3) | 15 (20.5) | 37 (33.3) | 10 (22.2) | 5 (38.5) | 21 (29.2) | 32 (19.0) | 26 (14.1) |

CABG, coronary artery bypass grafting; MACE, major adverse cardiac event; MI, myocardial infarction; PS, Palmaz-Schatz; PTCA, percutaneous transluminal coronary angioplasty; SAT, subacute thrombosis; TLR, target lesion revascularization.

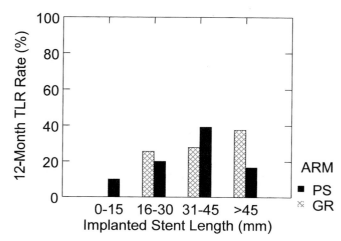

FIGURE 39–4. Frequency of 12-month target lesion revascularization (TLR) with increasing implanted stent length with the Gianturco-Roubin II (GR-II) and the Palmaz-Schatz (PS) stents.

## PATTERNS OF STENT HYPERPLASIA WITH THE GR-II STENT

The impact of stent design (coiled versus tubular slotted) on the pattern of stent hyperplasia and restenosis was assessed quantitatively in all patients assigned to the angiographic follow-up subset in the randomized clinical trial.[13] Hyperplasia associated with the GR-II stent was diffuse (mean length, 25 mm) and almost always more than 20 mm in length (Fig. 39–6). The diameter stenosis tended to be higher at all locations within the stent with the GR-II stent compared with the PS stent (Fig. 39–7). Similar to the articulated PS stent, the maximum stenosis tended to occur in the middle of the stent

with the GR-II, and stent margin hyperplasia and restenosis (<8%) were equally uncommon (Fig. 39–8). The mechanism of increased late lumen renarrowing in patients treated with GR-II stents remains speculative. Serial intravascular ultrasound studies have shown that late stent recoil is minimal with tubular slotted stents and that intimal hyperplasia is the dominant contributor to late lumen renarrowing in patients with PS stents.[14] Because late lumen loss and loss index were higher in the patients treated with the GR-II stent, it is clear that there was either late mechanical recoil of the GR-II coiled stent or increased intimal hyperplasia (or late tissue prolapse), or a combination of both.

## THE GR-II IN ELECTIVE STENTING OF SMALL VESSELS AND RESTENOTIC LESIONS

Small vessel (<3.0-mm) interventions are associated with high rates of restenosis and 30-day closure, and the definitive clinical benefit of small vessel stenting over balloon angioplasty has yet to be demonstrated. The performance of elective GR-II stenting in small vessels (2.1 to 3.0 mm in diameter) was evaluated in a 262-patient small vessel registry performed at 25 U.S. centers between January and September 1996.[15] Patients were mostly men (64%), with a mean age of 62 years; 30% had diabetes, 62% had hypertension, 66% had multivessel coronary disease, and 38% had had a prior myocardial infarction. Treated lesions included the left anterior descending (42%), left circumflex (31%), and right coronary (25%). Lesions were complex, with Ameri-

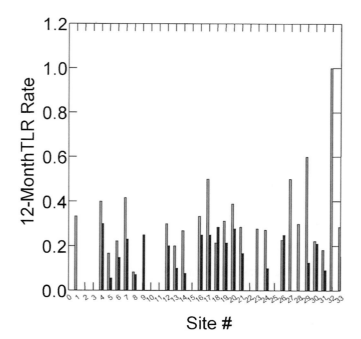

FIGURE 39–5. Site-to-site variation in 12-month target lesion revascularization (TLR). Site-to-site variation in TLR was greatest for the Gianturco-Roubin II (GR-II) group. PS, Palmaz-Schatz.

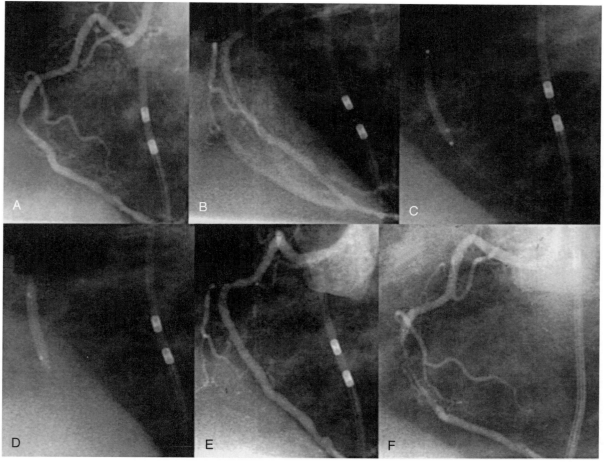

FIGURE 39–6. Focal mid–right coronary lesion *(A)* with a long, type D dissection after predilation *(B)*, Gianturco-Roubin II stent deployment for threatened closure indication *(C)* and then again after dilation *(D)*, with excellent final angiographic results *(E)*. Diffuse in-stent restenosis was present at follow-up *(F)*.

## Mean In-Stent and Stent Margin Diameter Stenosis

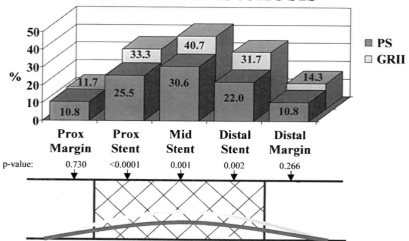

FIGURE 39–7. Comparison of the mean diameter stenosis between the Gianturco-Roubin II (GR-II) stent and the Palmaz-Schatz (PS) stent at five locations, including the proximal, mid, and distal stent and the proximal and distal stent margin.

# Frequency of In-Stent and Stent Margin Binary Restenosis

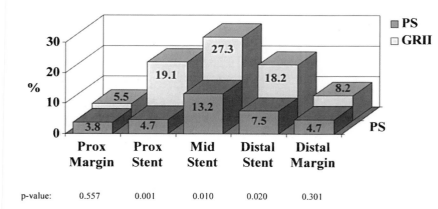

FIGURE 39–8. Comparison of the binary restenosis rates between the Gianturco-Roubin II (GR-II) stent and the Palmaz-Schatz (PS) stent at five locations, including the proximal, mid, and distal stent and the proximal and distal stent margin.

| p-value: | 0.557 | 0.001 | 0.010 | 0.020 | 0.301 |

can College of Cardiology/American Heart Association (ACC/AHA) grade B2/C in 62%, lesion length was 14.9 ± 11.4 mm, and the reference vessel size was 2.45 ± 0.45 mm. The 20-mm GR-II was used in 85% of cases, with 83% being either 2.5-mm or 3.0-mm stents. The GR-II was successfully deployed in 98.5% of cases, with 1.4 stents deployed per lesion. By quantitative angiography, the final stent diameter stenosis was 22.5 ± 14.8% with 20% acute recoil. Target lesion revascularization was 27.7% (Table 39–12). By multivariate analysis, the predictors of TLR included diabetes (odds ratio [OR] 3.06, 95% confidence interval [CI][1.59–5.90], $p = 0.001$), number of stents implanted (OR 1.60; 95% CI[1.0–2.55], $p = 0.049$), and left anterior descending artery location (OR 3.08; 95% CI[1.42–6.67], $p = 0.004$). Use of the GR-II stent for small vessels is associated with excellent procedural success, a 30-day stent thrombosis rate that is high but comparable to those observed in other small vessel studies, and follow-up clinical and angiographic results similar to historical rates with balloon angioplasty alone.[16] A comparative study of balloon angioplasty and stenting in this patient population is probably warranted to better define a comparative advantage of GR-II stenting over balloon angioplasty in this high-risk population.

The use of the tubular slotted PS stent results in a lower restenosis rate than that of balloon angioplasty in patients with restenotic lesions.[17] The GR-II was also evaluated for the elective treatment of restenotic lesions in a 306-patient registry. Men made up 70% of the population studied, and the mean age was 60 years; 24% were diabetic, 64% had hypertension, 52% had hypercholesterolemia, and 53% had had a prior myocardial infarction. The vessel distribution included 36% left anterior descending artery, 26% left circumflex coronary artery, and 37% right coronary artery. Lesions were complex (ACC/AHA grade B2/C in 62% of cases)

## TABLE 39–12.    CLINICAL OUTCOMES OF THE GIANTURCO-ROUBIN II (GR-II) REGISTRIES

|  | SMALL VESSEL | RESTENOTIC | SVG | AC/TC | GR-II RCT | PS RCT |
|---|---|---|---|---|---|---|
| N | 262 | 306 | 106 | 606 | 380 | 375 |
| **30-day events, %** | | | | | | |
| MACE | 4.8 | 2.9 | 4.7 | 6.1 | 4.2 | 1.3 |
| SAT | 4.0 | 2.0 | 1.9 | 4.0 | 3.9 | 0.3 |
| MI | 1.2 | 0.0 | 0.9 | 0.8 | 1.3 | 0.5 |
| Death | 1.6 | 0.0 | 2.8 | 2.0 | 0.3 | 0.5 |
| TLR | 3.2 | 3.0 | 1.9 | 4.1 | 3.9 | 0.5 |
| **1-year events, %** | | | | | | |
| MACE | 32.0 | 34.6 | 31.1 | 16.2 | 28.9 | 17.3 |
| Death | 4.3 | 2.0 | 5.7 | 4.3 | 2.6 | 2.7 |
| MI | 2.2 | 0.0 | 3.8 | 0.8 | 1.3 | 0.8 |
| TLR | 27.7 | 34.0 | 22.6 | 12.2 | 26.6 | 14.9 |

AC/TC, acute and threatened closure; MACE, major adverse cardiac event; MI, myocardial infarction; PS, Palmaz-Schatz; RCT, randomized clinical trial; SAT, subacute thrombosis; SVG, saphenous vein graft; TLR, target lesion revascularization.

and diffuse (lesion length $15.8 \pm 9.7$ mm). By quantitative angiography, the reference vessel size was 2.72 mm, and the final stent diameter stenosis was $15.4 \pm 11.6\%$ associated with 18% acute recoil. Overall, the 30-day clinical outcomes were comparable to those of other registries; however, at 9 months, the target lesion revascularization (34.0%) and major adverse cardiac event rates (34.6%) were higher than previously observed with this device (see Table 39–12).

## THE GR-II IN ELECTIVE STENTING OF SAPHENOUS VEIN GRAFTS

The treatment of older saphenous vein grafts can be problematic because of high periprocedural complications and restenosis rates after balloon angioplasty. Based on the results of the randomized Saphenous Vein de Novo (SAVED) trial, use of the PS tubular slotted stent has become the preferred alternative because of its higher procedure success rate (92% with PS vs. 69% with PTCA, $p = 0.001$) and lower major adverse cardiac events rates (25.9% with PS vs. 39.3% with PTCA, $p = 0.04$), despite similar restenosis rates.[18] The performance of elective GR-II stenting of saphenous vein grafts was evaluated in a 106-patient registry. Patients were mostly men (76%), with a mean age of 66 years; 33% had diabetes, 66% had hypertension, and 50% had had a prior myocardial infarction. Lesions were complex, with ACC/AHA grade B2/C in 74%, lesion length was $15.6 \pm 11.5$ mm, and reference vessel size was $3.17 \pm 0.70$ mm. On average, 1.36 stents were deployed per lesion. By quantitative angiography, the final stent diameter stenosis was $12.9 \pm 13.7\%$ with 14.5% acute recoil. Target lesion revascularization was 22.6%, and major adverse cardiac events occurred in 31% (see Table 39–12). Results with the GR-II stent are comparable to those observed in other registries using the PS stent in saphenous vein grafts, with major adverse cardiac rates of 25% to 30%.[19, 20]

## THE GR-II STENT IN ACUTE MYOCARDIAL INFARCTION

The benefits of primary stenting with the GR-II stent over primary angioplasty in patients presenting with acute myocardial infarction have been evaluated in the GR-II Stent in Acute Myocardial Infarction (GRAMI) Trial.[21] The study included 104 patients presenting within 24 hours of symptom onset who were randomly assigned to primary GR-II stenting (N = 52) or primary PTCA (N = 52). Baseline demographics were well matched between the groups. Procedural success was similar (98% with

stenting and 94% with PTCA, $p = $ NS) with a 25% crossover rate and bail-out stenting in the PTCA arm. Primary stenting with the GR-II stent resulted in a reduction of in-hospital major adverse cardiac events (19.2% with PTCA vs. 3.8% with GR-II, $p = 0.03$) and a higher incidence of TIMI 3 flow at 7 days (98% with GR-II vs. 83.3% with PTCA, $p = 0.028$). The 1-year event-free survival was significantly higher with the GR-II stent (82.7% vs. 65.4%, $p = 0.002$) than with primary PTCA; however, target lesion revascularization was not significantly different in the two groups (9.6% GR-II vs. 13.4% PTCA, $p = $ NS). Based on this small randomized clinical trial, primary stenting with the GR-II stent resulted in superior in-hospital and 1-year clinical events compared with primary angioplasty with conventional PTCA alone.

The Florence Randomized Elective Stenting in Acute Coronary Occlusion (FRESCO) Trial[22] was a randomized trial comparing primary stenting using the GR-II stent (N = 75) with primary PTCA (N = 75) in patients with acute myocardial infarction presenting within 6 hours of symptom onset. At 6-month follow-up, major adverse cardiac events (death, myocardial infarction, target vessel revascularization) were significantly reduced with the GR-II stent (9% vs. 28%, $p = 0.003$), and the GR-II stent was associated with a lower restenosis rate (17% GR-II vs. 43% PTCA, $p = 0.001$). The results of these two randomized clinical trials would suggest that in the setting of acute myocardial infarction, primary stenting with the GR-II improves clinical and angiographic outcomes over those of primary PTCA alone. A larger randomized clinical trial is warranted to confirm these results.

## IMPORTANCE OF CORRECT GR-II STENT SELECTION

As with any new device, operator technique is critical in achieving optimal results.[12] In the randomized clinical trial, correct sizing of the GR-II, as defined in the protocol, was achieved in only 41.2% of GR-II stented lesions when reference size was assessed by angiographic core analysis, and even fewer (35.5%) when investigator estimates of reference vessel diameter were used. Twenty percent of selected GR-II stents were undersized relative to the reference vessel diameter, likely contributing to the smaller stent/artery ratio ($p < 0.001$) and the higher final stent percent stenosis. Patients receiving an undersized stent had significantly more 30-day stent thrombosis (11.0% vs. 0.7% correct sizing, $p < 0.001$), Q-wave myocardial infarctions (5.5% vs. 0% correct sizing, $p < 0.01$), and major adverse cardiac events (8.2% vs. 2.0% correct sizing, $p < 0.05$)

(see Table 39–10). In vessels less than 3 mm, 65% of selected GR-II stents were oversized, and in vessels greater than 3 mm, 38% were undersized.[8] Compared with correct sizing, undersizing of the GR-II stent in patients with vessels greater than 3 mm resulted in the highest 30-day stent thrombosis, Q-wave myocardial infarction, and TLR rates. Oversizing of the GR-II stent (selection of a GR-II stent greater than 0.5 mm the reference vessel dimension) in small vessels (<3.0 mm) was also associated with a higher rate of stent thrombosis (see Table 39–11). Stent sizing was an important univariate determinant of stent thrombosis and angiographic restenosis in the randomized clinical trial (see Tables 39–7 and 39–8). This underscores the importance of correctly sizing the stent, as has been emphasized previously,[10] with slight oversizing of the stent by 0.1 to 0.5 mm in relation to the reference vessel diameter to achieve an optimal stent/artery ratio and to compensate for the acute recoil and tissue prolapse. Although this study had a smaller patient subset, patients with optimal GR-II stent sizing had a 12-month TLR that was similar to that of the PS stent.

The pronounced intersite variability in TLR observed in the randomized clinical trial (see Fig. 39–4) likely resulted from inconsistencies in operator technique and infrequent optimal GR-II size selection. Because greater variability was noted in the GR-II–treated patients, a "roll-in" learning phase may have reduced some of the observed differences. This should serve as an important lesson for future randomized clinical trials. Appropriate interdevice comparisons require that operator technique factors relating to new devices are completely understood and consistently applied by investigators before they launch definitive randomized controlled clinical trials.

## OPTIMAL GR-II STENT SELECTION AND DEPLOYMENT TECHNIQUES

Overexpansion of the GR-II stent beyond its intended range can result in separation of the stent arms, with subsequent tissue prolapse and suboptimal results.[23] For optimal stent selection, the proximal reference vessel diameter should be accurately assessed after predilation and vasodilation with intracoronary nitroglycerin. The selected stent should be larger than the reference vessel by no more than 0.5 mm. Long, tapering vessels are best treated with two correctly sized GR-II stents rather than with a single longer stent. Deployment of the GR-II is achieved slowly at low pressure (4 to 6 atmospheres) for 60 seconds. The balloon is then deflated and withdrawn 1 to 2 mm proximally so that the distal balloon marker is just inside the distal stent

marker. Inflation to 6 to 8 atmospheres in this position avoids overexpansion of the moderately compliant delivery balloon in the distal reference vessel segment. A final high-pressure (up to 16 atmospheres) postdilation is recommended with a noncompliant balloon that is slightly oversized to achieve a 1.15 to 1.0 balloon/artery ratio. This strategy overcomes the inherently higher stent recoil associated with the GR-II stent. These techniques used at some single centers participating in the randomized clinical trial achieved early and late clinical outcomes comparable to those of control patients. The widespread applicability of these techniques remains to be evaluated.

## CONCLUSIONS

The GR-II stent can be used safely and effectively in the treatment of acute and threatened closure after conventional balloon angioplasty. The elective use of the GR-II stent in complex de novo native coronary lesions is associated with higher stent thrombosis, angiographic restenosis, and late TLR rates than those of current alternative second- and third-generation stents. Similar rates of stent thrombosis and late restenosis are associated with the elective use of the GR-II for stenting of restenotic lesions, small vessels, and saphenous vein grafts. The benefit of the GR-II in such complex lesion subsets would require comparative evaluation with current standard therapies. Early and late outcomes with the GR-II stent are exquisitely sentitive to precise GR-II stent size selection. Specifically, slight oversizing of the stent is essential in reducing both early and late clinical events when the GR-II stent is used for the treatment of acute and threatened closure after conventional balloon angioplasty. Excellent early and late results have been achieved by single centers using a consistent deployment technique, after an initial learning curve. The GR-II multicenter randomized clinical trial and registries cannot confirm the generalizability of these single-center results, because of inconsistencies in deployment techniques that lead to wide site-to-site variations in clinical outcomes with the GR-II stent. The results of the GR-II trials underscore the necessity of defining (and controlling) optimal device performance techniques before the widespread use of this device in definitive randomized clinical trials.

### ACKNOWLEDGMENTS

The following investigators were participants in the clinical trial: R.R. Heuser, Arizona Heart Institute and Foundation, Phoenix, AZ; P.B. Moore, Montgomery Cardiovascular, Montgomery, AL; J.P. Carrozza Jr, Beth Israel Hospital, Boston, MA; J.A. Bittl, Brigham and Women's Hospital, Boston, MA; D.J. Kereiakes, Lindner Center for Cardiovascular Research, Cincinnati, OH; S.G. Ellis,

The Cleveland Clinical Foundation, Cleveland OH; J.P. Zidar, Duke North Hospital, Durham, NC; C.D. O'Shaughnessy, North Ohio Heart Center, Elyria, OH; L.A. Iannone, Iowa Heart Center, Des Moines, IA; J.A. Brinker, Johns Hopkins Hospital, Baltimore, MD; J.W. Moses, Lenox Hill Hospital, New York, NY; C.E. Ruiz, Loma Linda Hospital, Los Angeles, CA; D.R. Holmes, Mayo Clinic Foundation, Rochester, MN; A.E. Raizner, The Methodist Hospital, Houston, TX; D.A. Cox, Mid-Carolina Cardiology, Charlotte, NC; S.J. Yakubov, BS George, Midwest Cardiology Research Foundation, Columbus, OH; K. Rocha-Singh, Prairie Cardiovascular Consultants, Ltd., Springfield, IL; D.O. Williams, Rhode Island Hospital, Providence, RI; M.A. Thompson, Rochester General Hospital, Rochester, NY; E.W. Rogers, Sacred Heart Hospital, Pensacola, FL; W.D. Knoff, St. Joseph Hospital, Atlanta, GA; G. Dorros, St. Luke's Hospital, Milwaukee, WI; E.T.A. Fry, J.B. Hermiller, St. Vincent Hospital, Indianapolis, IN; C.A. Simonton, Sanger Clinic, PA, Charlotte, NC; D. Warth, Summit Cardiology, Seattle, WA; C.J. Cooper, Medical College of Ohio at Toledo, Toledo, OH; L.S. Dean, GS Roubin, University of Alabama at Birmingham, Birmingham, AL; R.E. Bowerman, University Hospital, Tampa FL; I.M. Penn, Vancouver Hospital and Health Science Center, Vancouver, BC; M.B. Leon, Washington Hospital Center, Washington DC; R.D. Safian, William Beaumont Hospital, Royal Oak, MI.

# REFERENCES

1. O'Shaughnessy CD: The new Gianturco-Roubin coronary stent is an improved therapy for abrupt and threatened closure syndrome. J Am Coll Cardiol 29:416A, 1997.
2. Garratt K, O'Shaughnessy CD, Leon MB: Improved early outcomes after coronary stent placement for abrupt and threatened closure: Results from a multicenter trial using second generation stents. Eur Heart J 18:388, 1997.
3. George BS: Early and late outcome following treatment of acute and threatened closure with the GR II coronary stent. Am J Cardiol 80:7A, 1997.
4. Fry ET: Effect of lesion characteristics and number of stents on 6 month outcome following treatment of acute and threatened closure with the GRII coronary stent. Am J Cardiol 80:7A, 1997.
5. Leon MB: A multicenter randomized trial comparing the second generation Gianturco-Roubin (GRII) and the Palmaz-Schatz coronary stents. J Am Coll Cardiol 29:170A, 1997.
6. Lansky AJ, Popma JJ, Hanzel GS, et al: Predictors of late clinical outcome after Gianturco Roubin II stent use: Final results of the GRII randomized clinical trial. Circulation 98:I-662, 1998.
7. Blackwelder WC: "Proving the null hypothesis" in clinical trials. Controll Clin Trials 3:345–353, 1982.
7a. Blackwelder WC, Chang MA: Sample size graphs for "proving the null hypothesis." Control Clin Trials 5(2):97–105, 1984.
8. Lansky AJ, Curran MI, Hanzel GS, et al: The impact of stent size selection on clinical outcome after use of the Gianturco-Roubin II stent: Results from the randomized clinical trial. Circulation 98:I-160, 1998.
9. Kuntz RE, Safian RD, Carrozza JP, et al: The importance of acute luminal diameter in determining restenosis after coronary atherectomy or stenting. Circulation 86:1827–1835, 1992.
10. Sutton JM, Ellis SG, Roubin GS, et al: Major clinical events after coronary stenting: The multicenter registry of acute and elective Gianturco-Roubin stent placement. Circulation 89:1126–1137, 1994.
11. Mehran R, Hong MK, Lansky AJ, et al: Vessel size and lesion length influence late clinical outcomes after native coronary artery stenting. Circulation 96(8):I-274, 1997.
12. Schatz R, Baim DS, Leon MB, et al: Clinical experience with the Palmaz-Schatz coronary stent: Initial results of a multicenter study. Circulation 83:148–161, 1991.
13. Hanzel G, Lansky AJ, Popma JJ, et al: Patterns of in-stent hyperplasia in the Gianturco-Roubin II compared to the Palmaz-Schatz stents: Results from the GR II randomized clinical trial. J Am Coll Cardiol 33:61A, 1999.
14. Hoffmann R, Mintz GS, Popma JJ, et al: Chronic arterial responses to stent implantation: A serial intravascular ultrasound analysis of Palmaz-Schatz stents in native coronary arteries. J Am Coll Cardiol 28(5):1134–1139, 1996.
15. Zidar JP, O'Shaughnessy CD, Dean LS, et al: Elective GRII stenting in small vessels: Multicenter results. J Am Coll Cardiol 31:274A, 1998.
16. Savage MP, Fischman DL, Rake R: Efficacy of coronary stenting versus balloon angioplasty in small coronary arteries: Stent Restenosis Study (STRESS) investigators. J Am Coll Cardiol 31:307–311, 1998.
17. Erbel R, Haude M, Hopp HW: Restenosis Stent (REST) study: Randomized trial comparing stenting and balloon angioplasty for treatment of restenosis after balloon angioplasty. J Am Coll Cardiol 27(suppl A):139A, 1996.
18. Savage MO, Douglas JS, Fischman DL: A randomized trial of coronary stenting and balloon angioplasty in the treatment of aortocoronary saphenous vein bypass graft disease. N Engl J Med 337:740–747, 1997.
19. Fenton SH, Fishman DL, Savage MP: Long-term angiographic and clinical outcome after implantation of balloon-expandable stents in aorto-coronary saphenous vein grafts. Am J Cardiol 74:1187–1191, 1994.
20. Wong SC, Baim DS, Schatz RA: Immediate results and late outcomes after stent implantation in saphenous vein graft lesions: The multicenter U.S. Palmaz-Schatz stent experience. J Am Coll Cardiol 26:704–712, 1995.
21. Rodrigez AE, Bernardi VH, Santaera OA, et al: Coronary stents improve outcome in acute myocardial infarction: Immediate and long term results of the GRAMI trial. J Am Coll Cardiol 31:64A, 1998.
22. Antoniucci D, Santoro GM, Bolognese L, et al: A clinical trial comparing primary stenting of the infarct-related artery with optimal primary angioplasty for acute myocardial infarction: Results from the Florence Randomized Elective stenting in acute coronary occlusions (FRESCO) trial. J Am Coll Cardiol 31:1234–1239, 1998.
23. Farhat NZ: GR II coronary stent deployment strategy for excellent late clinical outcome: A single center experience. Am J Cardiol 80:7A, 1997.

# In-Stent Restenosis: Mechanisms, Definitions, and Treatment

Gary S. Mintz     Rainer Hoffmann     Roxana Mehran
Mun K. Hong     Ron Waksman     Augusto D. Pichard
Kenneth M. Kent     Lowell F. Satler     Martin B. Leon

Stent implantation reduces periprocedural complications and restenosis rates in comparison with balloon and other new-device angioplasty.[1-3] Intravascular ultrasonography (IVUS) and quantitative coronary angiographic (QCA) studies have explained the latter observation. In *nonstented* lesions, late lumen loss is a combination of negative arterial remodeling and neointimal hyperplasia.[4, 5] Stents reduce restenosis by (1) achieving a larger final lumen,[6, 7] (2) eliminating acute recoil,[8] and (3) abolishing negative arterial remodeling[9, 10]; this offsets a stent-related increase in neointimal proliferation, which is the dominant mechanism of in-stent restenosis.[6]

The use of high-pressure balloon inflations and antithrombotic pharmacologic regimens have nearly abolished subacute thrombosis and anticoagulation-related bleeding complications. This has led to the acceptance of coronary stents as primary therapy, and in-stent restenosis has developed into a significant clinical problem. In part because of the rapid explosion in stent use, detailed information on in-stent restenosis has been lagging. The current review focuses on the mechanisms, demographics, predictors, and treatment of in-stent restenosis.

## MECHANISMS OF IN-STENT RESTENOSIS

In the porcine coronary artery model, Schwartz and colleagues showed that neointimal thickness correlated with (1) the severity of vessel injury as determined by depth of stent wire penetration and (2) degree of injury at adjacent stent wire sites.[11] Although stent design influenced the degree of vascular injury and the resulting neointimal hyperplasia,[12] the presence of normal media attenuated this response in eccentric lesions.[13] In this model there was late regression of the neointimal tissue.[14] There is also an inflammatory component to this development, occurring on both the luminal and the abluminal sides of the stent wires.[15-17]

Serial IVUS studies in humans showed that Palmaz-Schatz stents exhibit almost no chronic recoil and that in-stent restenosis was almost entirely neointimal hyperplasia. Lumen loss correlated strongly with the increase in neointimal tissue, regardless of whether planar or volumetric analysis was used.[9] There was no predilection for tissue accumulation within any one segment of the stent except perhaps in the middle (i.e., the location of the central articulation); however, this was significant only when normalized for the final lumen area, which was smallest at the central articulation. The findings of a smaller final lumen at the site of the central articulation and the increased neointimal hyperplasia in the middle of the stent explained the previous report of exaggerated restenosis at the central articulation of this stent.[18] Neointimal thickness was independent of stent size.[19] Palmaz-Schatz stents had an impact on adjacent reference segments.[9] Beginning at the stent-vessel margin and continuing proximally and distally for 5 to 10 mm, there appeared to be progressively more negative remodeling and progressively less neointimal hyperplasia. Stent implantation also led to an increase in peristent (or abluminal) plaque mass and attendant positive arterial remodeling,[20] which was perhaps similar to the animal model findings of a diffuse peristent inflammatory response.[15-17]

Some of these findings have been confirmed.[10] Of note, an increase in neointimal tissue in the middle of Palmaz-Schatz stents was found even in stent designs lacking a central articulation (i.e., Palmaz-Schatz stent with a spiral articulation). Although this study was not able to confirm the impact of stent implantation on adjacent reference segments (i.e., negative remodeling), it investigated only reference segments 1 to 3 mm from the edge of the stent (where stents may still have an anti-remodeling effect).

Finally, histologic analysis of retrieved specimens after the directional coronary atherectomy (DCA) treatment of in-stent restenosis has been reported. Findings included (1) intimal hyperplasia in 80% of the specimens, with 75% of the cells having morphologic features of a contractile phenotype; (2) no evidence of ongoing proliferation by proliferating cell nuclear antigen (PCNA) studies; and (3) a trend toward reduced cellularity over time.[21] This last finding is consistent with animal models that have shown late tissue regression.[14]

## PREVALENCE OF IN-STENT RESTENOSIS

It is difficult to assign an accurate frequency to the occurrence of in-stent restenosis without a detailed understanding of (1) definitions, (2) methodology, (3) patient and lesion subsets, and (4) stent designs and implantation techniques.

### Definitions of In-Stent Restenosis

Should the definition of angiographic in-stent restenosis be limited to just the axial length of the stent? The different restenosis rates in the Stent Restenosis Study (STRESS) and Belgium-Netherlands Stent (BENESTENT-I) study (early studies with similar inclusion criteria) have been explained by differences in QCA methodology: different analysis systems and intrastent versus intralesion analysis. Both intrastent and intralesion analyses were performed on the cineangiograms from the Scripps Coronary Radiation to Inhibit Proliferation Post Stenting (SCRIPPS) study. There was an almost twofold increase in angiographic restenosis according to intralesional analysis (to include reference segments 5 mm from the edges of the stents): 54% versus 36% in the lesions randomly assigned to placebo and 17% versus 8% in the lesions treated with catheter-based gamma iridium-192 irradiation.[22]

The preferred use of intralesional analysis is supported by IVUS and QCA studies showing an impact of stents on adjacent reference segments[23, 24] and by a report of a consecutive series of 282 in-stent restenosis lesions.[25] In the latter analysis, the restenotic process extended beyond the stent in 30% of cases and might have been missed by intrastent analysis.

Should angiographic or clinical restenosis rates be used? The commonly accepted QCA definition of restenosis is a 50% or greater diameter stenosis (DS) at follow-up. Because in-stent restenosis appears to plateau after 6 months,[26, 27] follow-up angiography normally is performed at 6 months. However, clinical definitions of restenosis are more vague; terms that are used include clinical restenosis, target lesion revascularization (TLR), target vessel failure, target vessel revascularization, and multiple adverse

clinical events (MACE). Although some authors use these terms interchangeably, others (and some multicenter studies) make subtle distinctions. Regardless, (1) clinical and angiographic restenosis rates parallel each other, (2) clinical rates are lower than angiographic rates, (3) clinical events lag behind angiographic events, (4) larger sample sizes are needed to show a statistical difference in clinical (vs. angiographic) restenosis, and (5) angiographic in-stent restenosis drives potentially unnecessary (and therefore overreported) TLR.[28, 29] The importance of avoiding unnecessary revascularization is magnified by serial QCA studies showing an increase in minimal lumen diameter (MLD) beginning 6 months after stent implantation and continuing for 3 years[30, 31] as well as by the paucity of late (>4 year) stent-related clinical events.[32] This is consistent with histologic data.[14, 20]

### Prevalence of In-Stent Restenosis

It is difficult to extrapolate the results of randomized clinical trials (typically restricted to favorable lesion subsets) to real-world experiences that include a wide range of lesions, indications, and stent types. For example, the angiographic restenosis rate after Palmaz-Schatz stent implantation was 32% in STRESS,[1] 22% in BENESTENT-I,[2] and 17% in BENESTENT-II[28]; the clinical restenosis rate in the Stent Antithrombotic Regimen Study (STARS) was approximately 9%, depending on the definition used.[33] In contrast, in unselected (or "real-world") patients (in whom study factors include restenotic lesions, smaller vessels, multiple stents, and so forth), the restenosis rates may be twofold or more higher.[34–36]

We have found similar extremes. In 137 of our patients enrolled in the IVUS-guided arm of the Can Routine Ultrasound Impact Stent Expansion (CRUISE) substudy of STARS—one or two native vessel lesions per patient, each lesion treated with one or two stents, 3.0- to 5.0-mm vessels, with a visual final angiographic DS of =10% and no perilesion dissections—the TLR rate was less than 5%. On the other hand, in long lesions (>15 mm in length) in small vessels (<2.75 mm in size) treated with multiple stents even with IVUS guidance, the TLR rate was as high as 58%.[37]

### Risk Factors and Predictors of In-Stent Restenosis

In a consecutive series of patients with native vessel lesions treated with stents at the Washington Hospital Center, Washington, D.C., the predictors of TLR included (1) diabetes, (2) unstable angina, (3) restenotic lesions, (4) reference vessel diameter, and (5) final MLD and DS.[35] An analysis from STARS showed similar predictors of TLR with the exception of unstable angina and restenotic lesions.[33, 38] In a series of 1753 lesions in 1349 patients, Kastrati and associates reported that diabetes, multiple stent use, and a smaller QCA final MLD predicted clinical restenosis.[39] (In this series, in which angiographic follow-up was available in 80% of cases, additional predictors of *angiographic* restenosis included previous percutaneous transluminal coronary angioplasty [PTCA], chronic total occlusions, and left anterior descending artery [LAD] lesion location.)

The importance of the final stent dimensions as a predictor of in-stent restenosis is supported by both angiographic and IVUS studies.[40–44] Because neointimal thickness is independent of stent size,[19] there is greater encroachment of the neointima on lumen dimensions in smaller stents than in larger stents. Finally, patients with the DD genotype of the angiotensin converting enzyme gene also appear to be at increased risk of in-stent restenosis.[45]

Three controversies exist with regard to predictors of in-stent restenosis: diabetes, restenosis in the same or companion lesions, and multiple stent use. (1) With regard to diabetes, most but not all studies have reported diabetes as a risk factor for in-stent restenosis.[33, 39, 46–51] Serial IVUS studies have shown that neointimal hyperplasia is exaggerated in diabetic patients.[52, 53] Whether insulin treatment or the level of glucose intolerance contributes to restenosis is not known, although one analysis suggested that insulin-treated diabetics are at increased risk.[54] (2) With regard to restenosis in the same or companion lesions, a report by Gibson of lesions treated with multiple devices (stents, balloons, or DCA) showed no interlesion dependence of restenosis in the same patient.[55] This is in contradistinction to a more recent report showing that stented lesions may not behave independently with regard to in-stent restenosis.[56] The impact of restenosis after a non–stent implantation procedure on subsequent in-stent restenosis may be related to the interval between the original angioplasty and the stent procedure.[57] (3) With regard to multiple stent use, some studies have indicated increased restenosis rates after multiple stent use[39, 58, 59] or stenting of long lesions.[60, 61] Others have not.[62] This issue becomes even more confusing as stents of various lengths become more available. There may also be an important *interaction* of lesion length and vessel size.[37, 63] The highest restenosis rates may be in long lesions in small vessels treated with multiple stents; conversely, lesion length and multiple stent use may not be important in large vessels.

Thus, patient-related variables (i.e., diabetes) and lesion-related variables (i.e., final lumen dimensions and vessel size) have a major impact on restenosis.

In the real world, only a minority of lesions fit the STARS inclusion criteria and are at low risk for in-stent restenosis.

## Impact of Stent Designs

The impact of new stent designs is under intense investigation, partly because of economic implications. Randomized clinical trials comparing balloon-expandable stents have shown approximately equivalent or occasionally superior restenosis rates in comparison with the Palmaz-Schatz stent,[64–67] with only one notable exception: the Gianturco-Roubin II stent.[68] The impact of self-expanding stents on restenosis is currently not known.[69] However, self-expanding stents appear to increase their dimensions over time and to have the same average neointimal thickness as do tubular-slotted stents.[70]

## THE HIGH-PRESSURE ADJUNCT PTCA CONTROVERSY

The abolition of subacute thrombosis has been attributed, in part, to use of high-pressure adjunct PTCA, which improves stent expansion and stent-vessel wall apposition. Final stent dimensions are an important predictor of in-stent restenosis, and progressively higher adjunct PTCA inflation pressures lead to progressively larger final stent dimensions.[71, 72] Nevertheless, several authors have suggested that there may be a down side to high-pressure adjunct PTCA.[73–81] This down side has been based primarily on (1) animal data showing that deep wall stent strut penetration elicits an aggressive proliferative response, (2) human clinical trials (i.e., the Saphenous Vein De Novo [SAVED] trial, a trial of stenting vs. PTCA in saphenous vein grafts, and the Stent Restenosis Study III) as well as experience from our own institution that suggests that high-pressure adjunct PTCA may be associated with more late lumen loss, and (3) empirical observations that new stent designs do not require the same high-pressure adjunct PTCA for optimal implantation.

In these studies, it has been difficult to separate the procedural variables (i.e., balloon/artery sizes and inflation pressures) from the lesion characteristics (i.e., larger balloon/artery ratios and higher inflation pressures are usually needed in smaller vessels). Some authors have suggested that these procedural variables have an impact only if optimal stent dimensions are not achieved; thus, again, the need for aggressive implantation techniques is tied to the underlying lesion.[74] The definition of high-pressure adjunct PTCA varies considerably among these studies. Finally, an analysis from STARS did not detect any deleterious impact of high-pressure inflations,[82] but this was in a subset of low-complexity lesions. In all probability, the high-pressure adjunct PTCA controversy will be settled only by a prospective randomized trial. Such a trial is currently under way; of note, in this trial high-pressure adjunct PTCA had no impact on 30-day events, including subacute thrombosis.[83]

## PREVENTION OF IN-STENT RESTENOSIS

With the exception of avoiding stent implantation in ultra–high-risk subsets (i.e., multiple stents to treat long lesions in small vessels in diabetic patients), the only currently available approach to reduce in-stent restenosis is to optimize the acute procedural result. This includes the use of atheroablation before stent implantation. Rotational atherectomy (RA) in heavily calcified lesions[84] and DCA in lesions with a larger plaque burden[85] may improve long-term outcome, at least in part by maximizing acute lumen dimensions. (This last is supported by one IVUS study indicating that preintervention plaque burden is an independent predictor of in-stent restenosis.[41]) Finally, results from the CRUISE substudy of STARS suggest that stent optimization is best accomplished with IVUS guidance and that larger IVUS-guided stent dimensions translate into reduced clinical restenosis rates.[86] This supports IVUS stent dimensions as important predictors of in-stent restenosis.[40–44]

## Pharmacologic Prevention of In-Stent Restenosis

Because in-stent restenosis is almost exclusively neointimal hyperplasia, in-stent restenosis is the ideal model for studying strategies to inhibit this process. Pharmacologic approaches that were unsuccessful in preventing restenosis in nonstented lesions (a combination of negative remodeling and intimal hyperplasia) may be efficacious in reducing in-stent restenosis (pure intimal hyperplasia). In general, drugs with positive results in animal studies have been novel drugs that are not clinically available and not approved by the U.S. Food and Drug Administration (FDA). These drugs have been administered systemically, locally at the time of stent implantation, and locally via prolonged elution from stents or biocompatible coatings.

When given systemically either from a subcutaneous minipump or from an intramuscular depot of slow-release formulation, the somatostatin analogue Angiopeptin reduced neointimal hyperplasia in a porcine coronary overstretch in-stent restenosis model.[87–89] Other promising systemic approaches include avb3 integrin[90] or leukocyte integrin Mac-1 blockade[91] in animals and cilostazol,[92, 93] tranilast,[94]

and estrogen replacement therapy in postmenopausal women.[95] Although promising in single center series,[96] antithrombotic regimens as well as systemic glycoprotein IIb/IIIa inhibitors have not proved efficacious in randomized clinical trials.[97, 98]

More recently, novel drugs delivered via local drug delivery catheters have been shown to reduce in-stent neointimal hyperplasia in animal models. These "drugs" include (1) vascular endothelial growth factor (VEGF), which accelerates reendothelialization,[99] and (2) chimeric ribozymes to DCD-2 kinase and PCNA genes, which interfere with gene expression.[100] The data on local delivery of low molecular weight heparin are inconclusive. One clinical study using the iontophoresis catheter as a delivery vehicle yielded negative results[101]; conversely, other studies have been promising.[102, 103] In addition, drugs such as c-*myc* antisense, which reduces neointimal hyperplasia in nonstent animal models of restenosis and in human smooth muscle cells studied ex vivo, are being introduced into clinical trials to reduce in-stent restenosis.[104, 105]

Various classes of drugs have been impregnated into either coatings of metallic stents or biodegradable polymeric stents. Positive results have been obtained with nitric oxide donors,[106] hirudin/prostacyclin analogues,[107, 108] tyrosine kinase inhibitors,[109] and paclitaxel.[110–112] Local delivery of glycoprotein IIb/IIIa inhibitors and heparin did not reduce in-stent neointima in animal models, although clinical studies are ongoing.[113, 114]

## Vascular Brachytherapy

Preclinical work in the porcine model of restenosis demonstrated that low doses (15 to 25 Gy) of radiation delivered intraluminally inhibit neointima formation after balloon overstretch injury with and without subsequent stent implantation.[115–118] In theory, both beta and gamma emitters can be used to prevent in-stent restenosis if the radiation is given before stent placement. Once the stent is implanted, however, dosimetry of beta radiation must be adjusted for the attenuation and shielding of the metallic stent struts.[119, 120]

User-friendly beta-emitting stents have been promising in preclinical studies.[121, 122] However, to date, results in patients have been equivocal.[123]

Seventeen patients were enrolled in the SCRIPPS trial during their initial stent implantation procedure.[124] Unlike patients with in-stent restenosis, this group showed no benefit from gamma irradiation.

## MECHANICAL PROBLEMS WITH STENT IMPLANTATION LEADING TO ADVERSE EVENTS AND RESTENOSIS: "PSEUDO–" IN-STENT RESTENOSIS

Mechanical problems with stent implantation occur despite routine high-pressure adjunct PTCA, and they can cause restenosis. IVUS can identify these problems and direct appropriate "reparative" measures. Mechanical problems include (1) missing the lesion, (2) stent underexpansion, (3) stent "crush," and (4) the stent's being stripped off the balloon during the implantation procedure. Because most stents are radiolucent, some lesions, especially aorto-ostial lesions, can be missed. Incomplete stent expansion during implantation can be missed angiographically because stents are porous and contrast can flow through and around them. If the guide wire is accidentally removed and, in recrossing the freshly placed (and presumably not fully implanted) stent, it courses adjacent to the stent and enters the stent through one of the diamonds, subsequent adjunct PTCA can crush part of the stent against the vessel wall. These mechanical problems constitute a minority of cases of in-stent restenosis. However, mechanical problems detected at follow-up were most likely present at implantation. Thus, the treatment of in-stent restenosis must begin by excluding these mechanical problems or, if they are present, by correcting them.

## TREATMENT OF IN-STENT RESTENOSIS

Three primary approaches have been used to treat in-stent restenosis: (1) PTCA, (2) atheroablation (using excimer laser coronary angioplasty [ELCA], RA, or DCA), and (3) additional stent implantation. In general, recurrence rates are high.

### PTCA of In-Stent Restenosis

Using QCA, Gordon concluded that lumen enlargement was entirely due to neointimal tissue compression or extrusion out of the stent.[125] Conversely, IVUS studies before and after PTCA showed that tissue extrusion and additional stent expansion (even in stents previously implanted using high-pressure adjunctive PTCA) contributed equally to lumen improvement.[126] In that study, (1) PTCA recovered only 85% of the minimum lumen area of the original stent implantation procedure, (2) post-PTCA there was significant residual neointimal tissue within the stent (averaging 32% of the stent area), and (3) the residual stenosis by QCA was relatively high (DS of 18%). These IVUS findings were confirmed by two other reports.[127, 128] Recurrence after PTCA ranged from 37% to 50% (angiographic restenosis) and from 14% to 30% (clinical restenosis).[129–133]

### Ablation of In-Stent Restenosis

Recently, atheroablative techniques have been used in an attempt to improve on these results. Both ELCA and RA increase lumen dimensions through ablation of neointimal tissue. Adjunct PTCA is needed after both ELCA and RA to optimize final lumen dimensions, and the mechanism of lumen enlargement during adjunct PTCA is similar to primary PTCA, a combination of additional stent expansion and neointimal tissue extrusion.[134, 135] Although tissue ablation with both ELCA and RA is modest, it appears to be slightly greater with RA, partly related to the larger burr sizes available and partly to greater ablation efficiency.[136] Like primary PTCA of in-stent restenosis, neither ELCA + PTCA nor RA + PTCA recover the lumen dimensions achieved during the initial stent implantation procedure.[134, 135] Compared to lesions treated with PTCA alone, lesions treated with ELCA + PTCA had (1) greater acute lumen gain, (2) more IH ablation/extrusion, and (3) larger final lumens.[134] However, one study reported a 52% angiographic restenosis rate after ELCA.[137] Clinical recurrence after RA has ranged from 28% to 50%, with one series reporting a 67% recurrence after stand-alone RA versus 42% after RA + PTCA.[138–140] There has been little quantitative data following the use of DCA to treat in-stent restenosis; however, it has been our observation that of the ablative devices, DCA removes the most tissue, causes the least additional stent expansion, and results in the largest lumens. MACE after DCA is said to be low (10.5%)[141]; however, this must be contrasted with cases of stent disruption during this procedure.[142, 143]

## Additional Stent Implantation

Preliminary observations indicate that additional stent implantation achieves the best acute results by recovering all of the lumen area of the original stenting procedure primarily via neointimal tissue extrusion out of the stent.[144] Angiographic recurrence after additional stent implantation has ranged from 30–35% while clinical recurrence has ranged from 17% to 40%.[144–148]

## Instant In-Stent Restenosis

Two IVUS observations may, in part, explain high recurrent rates: (1) treatment of in-stent restenosis with PTCA, excimer laser coronary angioplasty (ELCA) plus PTCA, or RA plus PTCA does not recover the lumen dimensions of the initial stent implantation procedure, and (2) there is early tissue reintrusion into the stent, analogous to recoil after PTCA of nonstented lesions. In a study of 32 lesions, an average of 42 ± 8 minutes after PTCA, ELCA plus PTCA, or RA plus PTCA, the delayed (42 ± 8 minutes) IVUS minimal lumen CSA decreased by 23%; and in 9 lesions (28%), there was a 2.0-mm² or greater decrease in minimum lumen CSA.[149] The mechanism of this early lumen loss appears to be neointimal tissue reintrusion back into the stent, rather than stent recoil. The correlation between early lumen loss and markers of in-stent restenosis severity indicates that this phenomenon may be more important in lesions with more diffuse in-stent restenosis and a larger neointimal tissue burden. Ablation with ELCA and RA does not reduce tissue reintrusion. Although additional stent implantation appears to prevent this process (as well as to recover all of the lumen dimensions of the original stent implantation procedure), long-term results after additional stent implantation appear to be disappointing (and probably not different from those of PTCA, ELCA plus PTCA, or RA plus PTCA).

## High-Risk Lesion Subsets

There are a number of problems with these studies, especially those comparing different treatment strategies: (1) Definitions of recurrence vary and include angiographic recurrence (often with incomplete follow-up), TLR, and MACE. (2) Most have small numbers or are registries with uncontrolled reporting rates. (3) There are few randomized trials, and even matched comparisons are unusual. In a matched comparison of lesions treated with ELCA plus PTCA versus PTCA alone, one study showed a trend toward less frequent need for TLR in the ELCA plus PTCA group (21%) than in the PTCA alone group (38%, $p = 0.0823$).[134] In a series of diffuse in-stent restenosis, a benefit was seen in "debulking" plus PTCA strategy versus PTCA alone.[150] (4) Different patterns of in-stent restenosis may be intentionally treated with different techniques. For example, at the Washington Hospital Center, 82% of lesions treated with additional stent implantation were at the margin or central articulation. (5) Of most importance, not all in-stent restenosis lesions carry a similar risk of recurrence. For example, it is important to differentiate between focal and diffuse in-stent restenosis and between the first episode of in-stent restenosis and recurrent in-stent restenosis. Yokoi and associates found an overall recurrence rate of 37% but a recurrence rate of 85% in diffuse in-stent restenosis.[130] The increased risk of recurrence in diffuse in-stent restenosis has been substantiated.[25, 133] For example, the TLR rate was 19% for focal in-stent restenosis (≤10 mm in length, occurring in 42%), 35% for diffuse intrastent restenosis (>10 mm in length and confined to the stent, in 22%), 50% for diffuse proliferative in-stent restenosis (>10 mm in length and extending into adjacent reference segments, in 30%), and 83% for total occlusions (occurring in 6%).[25] In this series, recurrence was also higher in the setting of previous in-stent restenosis (odds ratio, 11.9).[25] Similarly, in the placebo group of the SCRIPPS trial, the recurrence rate in lesions with previous in-stent restenosis was 70%. Conversely, the recurrence rate after PTCA of the first episode of in-stent restenosis is reported to be much lower.[132, 133]

## Vascular Brachytherapy

Vascular brachytherapy has emerged as the most promising way to treat in-stent restenosis, particularly the high-risk subsets of diffuse or recurrent in-stent restenosis. However, it is not known whether the target is the adventitia or the neointima. The first clinical use of endovascular gamma radiation was performed in peripheral arteries. Patients with restenosis of superficial femoral arterial stents were treated by atherectomy and PTA, followed by endovascular radiation ($^{192}$Ir at a prescribed dose of 12 Gy targeted to the vessel wall); at 5 years, the restenosis rate was less than 20%, and none of the patients developed adverse effects related to radiation.[151] In a prospective, placebo-controlled, double-blind, randomized study of catheter-based $^{192}$Ir gamma radiation (SCRIPPS trial), the treatment group had (1) a 17% restenosis rate (in comparison with 54% of the controls), (2) a 66% reduction in subsequent neointimal hyperplasia, and (3) a reduction in the need for late revascularization.[124] Several randomized trials have been initiated to prove the efficacy and safety of gamma intracoronary radiation for this application. Among these are the Washington Radiation for In-stent Restenosis Trial (WRIST),[152] Gamma-1, and ARTISTIC. SCRIPPS and Gamma-1 prescribe a dose to the adventitia on the basis of IVUS vessel dimensions; WRIST and ARTISTIC use a fixed dose prescription. Other trials were launched during 1998.

## CONCLUSIONS

The mechanism of in-stent restenosis is neointimal tissue proliferation, not chronic stent recoil. Although high-risk patient and lesion subsets can be identified, the only currently available approach to reduce in-stent restenosis is to optimize the acute result. Although in-stent restenosis may be related to mechanical problems or suboptimal results at the time of stent implantation (or at the time of treatment of in-stent restenosis), there appears to be a biologic subset of lesions and patients in whom in-stent restenosis is chronic and recurrent. Alternative therapies—such as brachytherapy or drugs for the prevention and/or treatment of in-stent restenosis, especially in high-risk lesion and patient subsets—may be important in the future.

# REFERENCES

1. Fischman DL, Leon MB, Baim DS, et al: A randomized comparison of coronary stent placement and balloon angioplasty in the treatment of coronary artery disease. N Engl J Med 331:496–501, 1994.
2. Serruys P, De Jaegere P, Kiemeneij F, et al: A comparison of balloon-expandable–stent implantation with balloon angioplasty in patients with coronary artery disease. N Engl J Med 331:490–495, 1994.
3. Versaci F, Gaspardone A, Tomai F, et al: A comparison of coronary-artery stenting with angioplasty for isolated stenosis of the proximal left anterior descending coronary artery. N Engl J Med 336:817–822, 1997.
4. Mintz GS, Popma JJ, Pichard AD, et al: Arterial remodeling after coronary angioplasty. A serial intrascular ultrasound study. Circulation 94:35–43, 1996.
5. Kimura T, Kaburagi S, Tamura T, et al: Remodeling responses of human coronary arteries undergoing coronary angioplasty and atherectomy. Circulation 96:475–483, 1997.
6. Mintz GS, Popma JJ, Hong MK, et al: Intravascular ultrasound to discern device-specific effects and mechanisms of restenosis. Am J Cardiol 78:18–22, 1996.
7. Umans VA, Melkert R, Foley DP, et al: Clinical and angiographic comparison of matched pateints with successful directional coronary atherectomy or stent implantation for primary coronary lesions. J Am Coll Cardiol 28:637–644, 1996.
8. Haude M, Erbel R, Issa H, et al: Quantitative analysis of elastic recoil after balloon angioplasty and after intracoronary implantation of balloon-expandable Palmaz-Schatz stents. J Am Coll Cardiol 21:26–34, 1993.
9. Hoffmann R, Mintz GS, Dussaillant GR, et al: Patterns and mechanisms of in-stent restenosis: A serial intravascular ultrasound study. Circulation 94:1247–1254, 1996.
10. Mudra H, Regar E, Klauss V, et al: Serial follow-up after optimized ultrasound-guided deployment of Palmaz-Schatz stents. In-stent neointimal proliferation without significant reference segment response. Circulation 95:363–370, 1997.
11. Schwartz RS, Huber KC, Murphy JG, et al: Restenosis and the proportional neointimal response to coronary artery injury: Results in a porcine model. J Am Coll Cardiol 19:267–274, 1992.
12. Rogers C, Edelman ER: Endovascular stent design dictates experimental restenosis and thrombosis. Circulation 91:2995–3001, 1995.
13. Carter AJ, Laird JR, Kufs WM, et al: Coronary stenting with a novel stainless steel balloon-expandable stent: Determinants of neointimal formation and changes in arterial geometry after placement in an atherosclerotic model. J Am Coll Cardiol 27:1270–1277, 1996.
14. Hong MK, Virmani R, Kornowski R, et al: Histologic responses during in-stent neointimal regression in a porcine coronary model. J Am Coll Cardiol 31:365A, 1998.
15. Karas SP, Gravanis MB, Santoian EC, et al: Coronary intimal proliferation after balloon injury and stenting in swine: An animal model of restenosis. J Am Coll Cardiol 20:467–474, 1992.
16. Kornowski R, Hong MK, Tio FO, et al: In-stent restenosis: Contributions of inflammatory responses and arterial injury to neointimal hyperplasia. J Am Coll Cardiol 31:224–230, 1998.
17. Inoue K, Nakamura N, Nagamatsu T, et al: Comparison of serial changes in coronary arteries after Palmaz-Schatz stent implantation and balloon angioplasty: A histopathological and immunohistochemical study. J Am Coll Cardiol 31:140A, 1998.
18. Ikari Y, Hara K, Tamura T, et al: Luminal loss and site of restenosis after Palmaz-Schatz coronary stent implantation. Am J Cardiol 76:117–120, 1995.
19. Hoffmann R, Mintz GS, Mehran R, et al: Intimal hyperplasia thickness is independent of stent size: A serial intravascular ultrasound study. J Am Coll Cardiol 31:366A, 1998.
20. Hoffmann R, Mintz GS, Popma JJ, et al: Chronic arterial responses to stent implantation: A serial intravascular ultrasound analysis of Palmaz-Schatz stents in native coronary arteries. J Am Coll Cardiol 28:1134–1139, 1996.
21. Strauss BH, Umans VA, van Suylen R-J, et al: Directional atherectomy for treatment of restenosis within coronary stents: Clinical, angiographic and histologic results. J Am Coll Cardiol 20:1465–1473, 1992.
22. Lansky AJ, Popma JJ, Mintz GS, et al: Stent margin restenosis after coronary intervention. A quantitative analysis of segmental lumen changes in the Scripps Radiation in Restenostic Lesion Study. J Am Coll Cardiol 29:77A, 1997.
23. Foley JB: Alterations in reference vessel diameter following intracoronary stent implantation: Important consequences for restenosis based on percent diameter stenosis. Catheter Cardiovasc Diagn 35:103–109, 1995.
24. Hoffmann R, Mintz GS, Popma JJ, et al: Overestimation of acute lumen gain and late lumen loss by quantitative coronary angiography (compared to intravascular ultrasound) in stented lesions. Am J Cardiol 80:1277–1281, 1997.
25. Mehran R, Abizaid AS, Mintz GS, et al: Patterns of in-stent restenosis: Classification and impact on subsequent target lesion revascularization. J Am Coll Cardiol 31:141A, 1998.
26. Kimura T, Nosaka H, Yokoi H, et al: Serial angiographic follow-up after Palmaz-Schatz stent implantation: Comparison with conventional balloon angioplasty. J Am Coll Cardiol 21:1557–1563, 1993.
27. Kastrati A, Schomig A, Dietz R, et al: Time course of restenosis during the first year after emergency coronary stenting. Circulation 87:1498–1505, 1993.
28. Serruys PW, Sousa E, Belardi J, et al: BENESTENT-II Trial: Subgroup analysis of patients assigned either to angiographic and clinical follow-up or clinical follow-up alone. Circulation 96:I-653, 1997.
29. Cutlip DE, Ho KKL, Kuntz RE, et al: Influence of routine angiographic follow-up on clinical restenosis outcome in the ASCENT Trial. J Am Coll Cardiol 31:139A, 1998.
30. Kimura T, Yokoi H, Nakagawa Y, et al: Three-year follow-up after implantation of metallic coronary-artery stents. N Engl J Med 334:561–566, 1996.
31. Nibler N, Kastrati A, Elezi S, et al: Angiographic and clinical follow-up of patients with asymptomatic restenosis after coronary stent implantation. J Am Coll Cardiol 31:65A, 1998.
32. Laham RJ, Carrozza JP, Berger C, et al: Long-term (4- to 6-year) outcome of Palmaz-Schatz stenting: Paucity of late clinical stent-related problems. J Am Coll Cardiol 28:820–826, 1996.
33. Kuntz RE, Baim DS, Popma JJ, et al: Late clinical results of the stent anticoagulation regimen study. Circulation 96:I-594, 1997.
34. Pizzulli LA, Zirbes M, Hagendorff A, et al: Indications, complications, and long-term follow-up of coronary stenting in an unselected patient population. Circulation 96:I-655, 1997.
35. Mehran R, Abizaid A, Hoffmann R, et al: Clinical and angiographic predictors of target lesion revascularization after stent placement in native coronary arteries. Circulation 96:I-472, 1997.
36. Danchin N, Lablanche JM, Grollier G, et al: Intracoronary stenting in patients with unstable angina. Results from the TASTE registry. Circulation 94:I-686, 1996.
37. Mehran R, Hong MK, Lansky AJ, et al: Vessel size and lesion length influence late clinical outcomes after native coronary stent placement. Circulation 96:I-274, 1997.
38. Kuntz RE, Ho KK, Senerchia C, et al: Prior restenosis does not increase the risk of restenosis following coronary stenting: An analysis from the Stent Anticoagulation Regimen Study (STARS) Trial. Circulation 96:I-2634, 1997.
39. Kastrati A, Schoemig A, Elezi S, et al: Predictive factors of restenosis after coronary stent placement. J Am Coll Cardiol 30:1428–1436, 1997.
40. Kuntz RE, Safian RD, Carrozza JP, et al: The importance of acute luminal diameter in determining restenosis after coronary atherectomy or stenting. Circulation 86:1827–1835, 1992.
41. Hoffmann R, Mintz GS, Mehran R, et al: Intravascular ultrasound predictors of angiographic restenosis in lesions

treated with Palmaz-Schatz stents. J Am Coll Cardiol 31:43–49, 1997.

42. Moussa I, DiMario C, Moses J, et al: The predictive value of different intravascular ultrasound criteria for restenosis after coronary stenting. J Am Coll Cardiol 29:60A, 1997.

43. Ziada KM, Kim MH, Potts W, et al: Predictors of target vessel revascularization following coronary stent deployment. J Am Coll Cardiol 29:239A, 1997.

44. Hayase M, Oshima A, Cleman MW, et al: Relation between target vessel revascularization and minimum stent area by intravascular ultrasound (CRUISE Trial). J Am Coll Cardiol 31:386A, 1998.

45. Ribichini F, Steffenino G, Dellavalle A, et al: Plasma activity and insertion/deletion polymorphism of angiotensin I–converting enzyme. A major risk factor and marker of risk for coronary stent restenosis. Circulation 97:147–154, 1998.

46. Aronson D, Bloomgarden Z, Rayfield EJ: Potential mechanisms promoting restenosis in diabetic patients. J Am Coll Cardiol 27:528–535, 1996.

47. Carrozza JP, Kuntz RE, Fishman RF, et al: Restenosis after arterial injury caused by coronary stenting in patients with diabetes mellitus. Ann Intern Med 118:344–349, 1993.

48. Gaxiola E, Vliestra RE, Brenner AS, et al: Diabetes and multiple stents independently double the risk of short-term revascularization I. Circulation 96:I-649, 1997.

49. Van Belle E, Bauters C, Hubert E, et al: Restenosis rates in diabetic patients. A comparison of coronary stenting and balloon angioplasty in native coronary vessels. Circulation 96:1454–1460, 1997.

50. Alonso J, Duran JM, Ramos B, et al: Initial and long term evolution of diabetic patients treated with stenting. J Am Coll Cardiol 31:415A, 1998.

51. Blankenbaker R, Ghazzal Z, Weintraub WS, et al: Clinical outcome of diabetic patients after Palmaz-Schatz stent implantation. J Am Coll Cardiol 31:415A, 1998.

52. Kornowski R, Mintz GS, Kent KM, et al: Increased restenosis in diabetes mellitus after coronary interventions is due to exaggerated intimal hyperplasia: A serial intravascular ultrasound study. Circulation 95:1366–1369, 1997.

53. Takagi T, Yoshida K, Akasaka T, et al: Increased intimal hyperplasia in patients with impaired glucose tolerance after coronary stent implantation: A serial intravascular ultrasound study. J Am Coll Cardiol 31:318A, 1998.

54. Abizaid A, Mintz GS, Oljaca B, et al: Predictors of target vessel revascularization in diabetic patients treated with Palmaz-Schatz stents. J Am Coll Cardiol 31:454A, 1998.

55. Gibson CM, Kuntz RE, Nobuyoshi M, et al: Lesion-to-lesion independence of restenosis following treatment by conventional angioplasty, stenting or directional atherectomy: Validation of lesion-based restenosis analysis. Circulation 87:1123–1129, 1993.

56. Kastrati A, Elezi S, Schuhlen H, et al: Intrapatient dependence of restenosis between lesions treated with intracoronary stenting. J Am Coll Cardiol 31:140A, 1998.

57. Savage MP, Fischman DL, Rake R, et al: Interprocedural interval as a predictor of stent restenosis after previous coronary angioplasty. Am J Cardiol 78:683–684, 1996.

58. Moussa I, Di Mario C, Moses J, et al: Single versus multiple Palmaz-Schatz stent implantation: Immediate and follow-up results. J Am Coll Cardiol 29:276A, 1997.

59. Aliabadi D, Bowers TR, Tilli FV, et al: Multiple stents increases target vessel revascularization rates. J Am Coll Cardiol 29:276A, 1997.

60. Joseph T, Fajadet J, Cassagneau B, et al: Clinical outcome of patients undergoing coronary stenting for extended lesions =30mm? J Am Coll Cardiol 31:273A, 1998.

61. Kobayashi Y, DeGregorio J, Reimers B, et al: The length of the stented segment is an independent predictor of restenosis. J Am Coll Cardiol 31:366A, 1998.

62. Haude M, Caspari G, Baumgart D, et al: Risk factor analysis for the development of restenosis after intracoronary stent implantation with adjunct high pressure stent dilatation. J Am Coll Cardiol 31:139A, 1998.

63. Kornowski R, Mehran R, Hong MK, et al: Procedural results and late clinical outcomes after placement of three or more stents in single coronary lesions. Circulation 97:1355–1361, 1998.

64. Baim DS, Cutlip DE, Midei M, et al: Acute 30-day and late clinical events in the randomized parallel-group comparison of the ACS MULTI-LINK coronary stent system and the Palmaz-Schatz. Circulation 96:I-593, 1997.

65. Heuser R, Kuntz R, Lansky A, et al: Six-month clinical and angiographic results of the SMART Trial. J Am Coll Cardiol 31:64A, 1998.

66. Hausleiter J, Dirschinger J, Schuhlen H, et al: A multicenter randomized trial comparing five different designs of slotted-tube stents. J Am Coll Cardiol 31:80A, 1998.

67. Lansky AJ, Popma JJ, Mehran R, et al: Late quantitative angiographic results after NIR stent use: Results from the NIRVANA randomized trial and registries. J Am Coll Cardiol 31:30A, 1998.

68. Leon MB, Popma JJ, O'Shaughnessy C, et al: Quantitative angiographic outcomes after Gianturco-Roubin II stent implantation in complex lesion subsets. Circulation 96:I-653, 1997.

69. Han RO, Schwartz RS, Mann JT, et al: Comparative efficacy of self expanding and balloon expandable stents for the reduction of restenosis. J Am Coll Cardiol 31:314A, 1998.

70. Kobayashi Y, Teirstein PS, Bailer SR, et al: Self-expandable stent versus-balloon expansable stent: A serial volumetric analysis by intravascular ultrasound. J Am Coll Cardiol 31:396A, 1998.

71. Stone GW, St. Goar F, Fitzgerald P, et al: The Optimal Stent Implantation Trial—Final core lab angiographic and ultrasound analysis. J Am Coll Cardiol 29:369A, 1997.

72. Abizaid A, Lefevre T, Lansky AJ, et al: Is the response to high pressure adjunct PTCA stent design specific? A sequential intravascular ultrasound study. J Am Coll Cardiol 31:493A, 1998.

73. Yokoi H, Nosaka H, Kimura T, et al: Influence of high-pressure stent dilatation on late angiographic and clinical outcome of Palmaz-Schatz stent implantation. J Am Coll Cardiol 29:312A, 1997.

74. Akiyama T, Di Mario C, Reimers B, et al: Does high-pressure stent expansion induce more restenosis? J Am Coll Cardiol 29:368A, 1997.

75. Goldberg SL, Colombo A, Di Mario C, et al: Does the use of aggressive stent implantation lead to more late loss and restenosis? J Am Coll Cardiol 29:368A, 1997.

76. Savage MP, Fischman DL, Douglas JS Jr, et al: The dark side of high pressure stent deployment. J Am Coll Cardiol 29:368A, 1997.

77. Hausleiter J, Schuhlen H, Elezi S, et al: Impact of high inflation pressures on six-month angiographic follow-up after coronary stent placement. J Am Coll Cardiol 29:369A, 1997.

78. Fernandez-Aviles F, Alonso JJ, Duran JM, et al: High pressure increases late loss after coronary stenting. J Am Coll Cardiol 29:369A, 1997.

79. Hoffmann R, Mintz GS, Mehran R, et al: Late tissue proliferation both within and surrounding Palmaz-Schatz stents is associated with procedural vessel wall injury. J Am Coll Cardiol 29:397A, 1997.

80. Fernandez-Aviles F, Alonso JJ, Duran JM, et al: High pressure impairs restenotic process after coronary stenting. Circulation 96:I-477, 1997.

81. Schofer J, Rau T, Golestani R, et al: Procedural vessel wall injury is not associated with late tissue proliferation within stents. Circulation 1997:I-402, 1997.

82. Mehran R, Popma JJ, Baim DS, et al: Routine high pressure post-stent dilatation did not influence clinical restenosis in STARS. J Am Coll Cardiol 31:80A, 1998.

83. Dirschinger J, Hausleiter J, Schuehlen H, et al: High versus normal balloon pressure dilatation for coronary stent placement: 6 month clinical and angiographic results from a randomized multicenter trial. J Am Coll Cardiol 31:17A, 1998.

84. Hoffmann R, Mintz GS, Kent KM, et al: Comparative early and nine-month results of rotational atherectomy, stents, and the combination of both for calcified lesions in large coronary arteries. Am J Cardiol 81:552–557, 1998.

85. Moussa I, Moses JW, Strain JE, et al: Angiographic and clinical outcome of patients undergoing "Stenting after Optimal Lesion Debulking": The SOLD Trial. Circulation 96:I-81, 1997.

86. Fitzgerald PJ, Hayase M, Mintz GS, et al: CRUISE: Can routine intravascular ultrasound influence stent expansion? Analysis of outcomes. J Am Coll Cardiol 31:396A, 1998.

87. Hong MK, Bhatti T, Matthews BJ, et al: The effect of porous infusion balloon delivered angiopeptin on myointimal hyperplasia following balloon injury in the rabbit. Circulation 88:638–648, 1993.

88. Hong MK, Kent KM, Mehran R, et al: Continuous subcutaneous angiopeptin treatment significantly reduces neointimal hyperplasia in a porcine coronary in-stent restenosis model. Circulation 95:449–454, 1997.

89. Hong MK, Kent KM, Tio FO, et al: Single-dose intramuscular administration of sustained-release angiopeptin reduces neointimal hyperplasia in a porcine coronary in-stent restenosis model. Coronary Artery Disease 8:101–104, 1997.

90. Srivatsa SS, Reilly TM, Holmes DR Jr, et al: Selective alpha v beta 3 integrin blockade limits neointimal hyperplasia and lumen stenosis in the stented porcine coronary artery injury model. Circulation 94:I-41, 1996.

91. Rogers C, Edelman ER, Simon DI: Blockade of the leukocyte integrin Mac-1 reduces experimental restenosis. Circulation 96:I-667, 1997.

92. Hara K, Yamasaki M, Kohzuma K, et al: Cilostazol reduces late lumen loss after the Palmaz-Schatz stent implantation. Circulation 94:I-91, 1996.

93. Nakamura T, Tsuchikane E, Sumitsuji S, et al: Impact of cilostazol on neointimal proliferation following Palmaz-Schatz stent implantation: A prospective randomized trial. J Am Coll Cardiol 31:404A, 1998.

94. Hsu Y, Tamai H, Ueda K, et al: Efficacy of tranilast on restenosis after coronary stenting. Circulation 94:I-620, 1996.

95. Singh D, Liu MW, Mather A, et al: Estrogen replacement therapy reduces repeat revascularization in post menopausal women after intracoronary stenting: A long term follow up. J Am Coll Cardiol 29:454A, 1997.

96. Sharma SK, Kini A, Dangas G, et al: Stenting with abciximab (ReoPro) decreases target lesion revascularization. J Am Coll Cardiol 31:237A, 1998.

97. Kastrati A, Schuhlen H, Hausleiter H, et al: Restenosis after coronary stent placement and randomization to a 4-week combined antiplatelet or anticoagulant therapy: Six-month angiographic follow-up of the Intracoronary Stenting and Antithrombotic Regimen (ISAR) Trial. Circulation 96:462–467, 1997.

98. Ellis SG, Serruys PW, Popma JJ, et al: Can abciximab prevent neointimal proliferation in Palmaz-Schatz stents? The final ERASER results. Circulation 96:I-86, 1997.

99. van Belle E, Maillard L, Tio FO, et al: Accelerated endothelialization by local delivery of recombinant human VEGF reduces in-stent intimal formation. J Am Coll Cardiol 29:77A, 1997.

100. Frimerman A, Eigler N, Makkar RR, et al: Chimeric DNA-RNA hammerhead ribozymes to CDC-2 kinase and PCNA reduce stent induced stenosis in a porcine coronary model. Circulation 96:I-87, 1997.

101. Gregoire J, Jeong MH, Camrud AR, et al: Does local iontophoretic low molecular weight heparin delivery reduce neointimal formation after stenting? J Am Coll Cardiol 29:238A, 1997.

102. Pavlides GS, Barath P, Manginas A, et al: Intramural delivery of low molecular weight heparin by direct injection within the arterial wall with a novel infiltrator catheter. Acute results and follow up in patients undergoing PTCA or stenting. Circulation 94:I-615, 1996.

103. Deutsch E, Kiesz S, Martin JL, et al: Favorable impact of intramural low molecular weight heparin delivered at the time of coronary stent deployment on late loss in de novo lesions. Circulation 96:I-710, 1997.

104. Bennett MR, Anglin S, McEwan JR, et al: Inhibition of vascular smooth muscle cell proliferation in vitro and in vivo by c-myc antisense oligodeoxynucleotides. J Clin Invest 93:820–828, 1994.

105. Shi Y, Hutchinson HG, Hail DJ, et al: Downregulation of c-myc expression by antisense oligonucleotides inhibits proliferation of human smooth muscle cells. Circulation 88:1190–1195, 1993.

106. Folts JD, Maalej N, Keaney JF Jr, et al: Palmaz-Schatz stents coated with a NO donor reduces reocclusion when placed in pig carotid arteries for 28 days. J Am Coll Cardiol 27:86A, 1996.

107. Prietzel K, Pasquantonio JD, Fliedner TU, et al: Inhibition of neointimal proliferation with a novel, hirudin/prostacyclin analog eluting stent coating in an animal overstretch model. Circulation 94:I-260, 1996.

108. Alt E, Beilharz C, Preter D, et al: Biodegradable stent coating with polylactic acid, hirudin and prostacyclin reduces restenosis. J Am Coll Cardiol 29:238A, 1997.

109. Yamawaki T, Shimokawa H, Kozai T, et al: Intraluminal delivery of tyrosine kinase inhibitor with biodegradable stent suppresses the restenotic changes of the coronary artery in pigs. Circulation 96:I-608, 1997.

110. Heldman AW, Cheng L, Heller P, et al: Paclitaxel applied directly to stents inhibits neointimal growth without thrombotic complications in a porcine coronary artery model of restenosis. Circulation 96:I-288, 1997.

111. Kornowski R, Hong MK, Ragheb AO, et al: Slow-release Taxol coated GR-II stents reduce neointima formation in a porcine coronary in-stent restenosis model. Circulation 96:I-341, 1997.

112. Farb A, Heller PF, Carter AJ, et al: Paclitaxel polymer-coated stents reduce neointima. Circulation 96:I-608, 1997.

113. Aggarwal RK, Martin WA, Azrin MA, et al: Effects of platelet GPIIb/IIIa antibody and antibody-urokinase conjugate adsorbed to stents on platelet deposition and neointima formation. Circulation 94:I-258, 1996.

114. Rogers C, Kjelsberg MA, Seifert P, et al: Heparin-coated stents eliminate mural thrombus deposition for days without affecting restenosis. Circulation 96:I-710, 1997.

115. Wiedermann JG, Marboe C, Schwartz A, et al: Intracoronary irradiation reduces restenosis after balloon angioplasty in a porcine model. J Am Coll Cardiol 23:1491–1498, 1994.

116. Waksman R, Robinson KA, Crocker IR, et al: Endovascular low dose irradiation inhibits neointima formation after coronary artery balloon injury in swine: A possible role for radiation therapy in restenosis prevention. Circulation 91:1533–1539, 1995.

117. Waksman R, Robinson K, Crocker I, et al: Intracoronary radiation prior to stent implantation inhibits neointima formation in stented porcine coronary arteries. Circulation 92:1383–1386, 1995.

118. Waksman R, Robinson K, Crocker I, et al: Intracoronary low dose irradiation inhibits neointima formation after coronary artery balloon injury in the swine restenosis model. Circulation 92:3025–3031, 1995.

119. Waksman R: Intracoronary radiation adjunct therapy to stenting. J Int Cardiol 10:2133–2136, 1997.

120. Weinberger J: Irradiation and stenting. Semin Intervent Cardiol 2:103–108, 1997.

121. Fischell TA, Carter AJ, Laird JR Jr: The beta-particle-emitting radioisotope stent (Isostent): Animal studies and planned clinical trials. Am J Cardiol 78:45–50, 1996.

122. Alt E, Herrmann RA, Rybnikar A, et al: Reduction of neointimal proliferation after implantation of a beta particle emitting gold Au-198 coated stent. J Am Coll Cardiol 31:350A, 1998.

123. Moses JW, Ellis SG, Bailer SR, et al: Short-term (1 month) results of the dose response IRIS feasibility study of a beta-particle emitting radioisotope stent. J Am Coll Cardiol 31:350A, 1998.

124. Teirstein PS, Massullo V, Jani S, et al: A double-blinded randomized trial of catheter-based radiotherapy to inhibit restenosis following coronary stenting. N Engl J Med 336:1697–1703, 1997.

125. Gordon PC, Gibson M, Cohen DC, et al: Mechanisms of restenosis and redilation within coronary stents—Quan-

titative angiographic assessment. J Am Coll Cardiol 21:1166–1174, 1993.

126. Mehran R, Mintz GS, Popma JJ, et al: Mechanisms and results of balloon angioplasty for the treatment of in-stent restenosis. Am J Cardiol 78:618–622, 1996.

127. Schiele F, Meneveau N, Vuillemenot A, et al: Assessment of balloon angioplasty in intrastent restenosis with intracoronary ultrasound. J Am Coll Cardiol 31:495A, 1998.

128. Gorge G, Konorza E, Voegle E, et al: Incomplete restoration of luminal dimensions after PTCA in restenotic stented segments: An intravascular ultrasound analysis. J Am Coll Cardiol 29:311A, 1997.

129. Baim DS, Levine MJ, Leon MB, et al: Management of restenosis within the Palmaz-Schatz coronary stent (the U.S. multicenter experience). Am J Cardiol 71:364–366, 1993.

130. Yokoi H, Kimura T, Nakagawa Y, et al: Long-term clinical and quantitative angiographic follow-up after the Palmaz-Schatz stent restenosis. J Am Coll Cardiol 27:224A, 1996.

131. Tan H-C, Sketch MH Jr, Tan ME, et al: Is there an optimal treatment for stent restenosis? Circulation 94:I-91, 1996.

132. Reimers B, Moussa I, Akiyama T, et al: Long-term clinical follow-up after successful percutaneous intervention for stent restenosis. J Am Coll Cardiol 30:186–192, 1997.

133. Bauters C, Banos J-L, Van Belle E, et al: Six-month angiographic outcome after successful repeat percutaneous intervention for in-stent restenosis. Circulation 97:318–321, 1998.

134. Mehran R, Mintz GS, Satler LF, et al: Treatment of in-stent restenosis with excimer laser coronary angioplasty. Mechanisms and results compared to PTCA alone. Circulation 96:2183–2189, 1997.

135. Mehran R, Mintz GS, Popma JJ, et al: Mechanisms of lumen enlargement during atheroablation of in-stent restenosis: A volumetric ultrasound analysis. J Am Coll Cardiol 29:497A, 1997.

136. Mehran R, Mintz GS, Abizaid A, et al: Mechanistic comparison of rotational atherectomy and excimer laser angioplasty in the treatment of in-stent restenosis: A volumetric intravascular ultrasound study. J Am Coll Cardiol 31:103A, 1998.

137. Koster R, Hamm CW, Reimers J, et al: Long term results of laser angioplasty for in-stent restenosis. J Am Coll Cardiol 31:141A, 1998.

138. Mehran R, Abizaid A, Abizaid A, et al: Rotational atherectomy for the treatment of in-stent restenosis: Long term outcome compared to balloon angioplasty alone. Am J Cardiol 80:23S, 1997.

139. Goldberg SL, Shawl F, Buchbinder M, et al: Rotational atherectomy for in-stent restenosis: The BARASTER registry. Circulation 96:I-80, 1997.

140. Sharma S, Duvvuri S, Kini A, et al: Rotational atherectomy for in-stent restenosis: Acute and long term results of first 100 cases. Circulation 96:I-88, 1997.

141. Pathan A, Butte A, Harrell L, et al: Directional coronary atherectomy is superior to PTCA for the treatment of Palmaz-Schatz stent restenosis. J Am Coll Cardiol 29:68A, 1997.

142. Meyer T, Schmidt T, Buchwald A, et al: Stent wire cutting during coronary directional atherectomy. Clin Cardiol 16:450–452, 1993.

143. Bowerman RS, Pinkerton CA, Kirk B, et al: Disruption of a coronary stent during atherectomy for restenosis. Catheter Cardiovasc Diagn 24:248–251, 1991.

144. Mehran R, Abizaid AS, Mintz GS, et al: Mechanisms and results after additional stent implantation to treat focal in-stent restenosis. J Am Coll Cardiol 31:455A, 1998.

145. Russo RJ, Massullo V, Jani SK, et al: Restenting vs PTCA for in-stent restenosis with or without intracoronary radiation therapy: An analysis of the SCRIPPS Trial. Circulation 96:I-219, 1997.

146. Elezi S, Kastrati A, Schuhlen H, et al: Stenting for restenosis of stented lesions: Acute and 6 month clinical and angiographic follow-up. Circulation 96:I-88, 1997.

147. Lefevre T, Louvard Y, Morice MC, et al: In-stent restenosis: Should we stent the stent? A single center prospective study. Circulation 96:I-88, 1997.

148. Goldberg SL, Loussararian AH, Di Mario C, et al: Stenting for in-stent restenosis. Circulation 96:I-88, 1997.

149. Shiran A, Waksman R, Abizaid A, et al: In recurrent in-stent restenosis INSTANT restenosis: An intravascular ultrasound study. Circulation 96:I-87, 1997.

150. Dauerman HL, Baim DS, Sparano AM, et al: Balloon angioplasty versus debulking for treatment of diffuse in-stent restenosis. J Am Coll Cardiol 31:455A, 1998.

151. Schoppel B, Liermann D, Pohlit, LJ, et al: 192-Ir endovascular brachytherapy for avoidance of intimal hyperplasia after percutaneous transluminal angioplasty and stent implantation in peripheral vessels: Years of experience. Int J Radiat Oncol Biol Phys 36:835–840, 1996.

152. Waksman R, White RL, Chan RC, et al: Localized intracoronary radiation therapy for patients with in-stent restenosis: Preliminary results from a randomized clinical study. Circulation 96:I-219, 1997.

# 41

# The Palmaz-Schatz Stent

*John P. Sweeney*    *Richard A. Schatz*

Since Gruentzig's[1] first description in 1978, percutaneous coronary angioplasty (PTCA) has become a widely accepted and generally safe treatment modality for selected patients with coronary artery disease. Despite improvements in initial success rates as a result of improved operator experience and refinements in equipment technology, the technique has been limited by procedural ischemic complications and an undesirable incidence of restenosis.

Restenosis remains the Achilles heel of conventional PTCA, occurring in 25% to 57% of cases within the first 6 months after the procedure.[2–4] Lesion sites such as saphenous vein grafts (SVG),[5–7] coronary ostial,[8] and left anterior descending artery,[9, 10] as well as certain patient subsets, such as diabetics,[11, 12] are associated with higher rates of restenosis. The pathogenesis appears to be multifactorial, refractory to pharmacologic manipulation, and unaffected by the use of newer devices such as directional coronary atherectomy, rotational atherectomy, and laser angioplasty.[13, 14] Ischemic complications secondary to abrupt closure still occur in 3% to 8% of cases,[15–17] often necessitating emergency bypass surgery. Most concerning is the associated reduction in survival in patients with this complication.[18, 19]

The common feature of these two limitations of conventional PTCA is luminal obstruction. In the case of restenosis, medial hyperplasia and arterial remodeling limit the late minimal luminal diameter.[20] In the case of abrupt closure, any combination of intimal flaps, spasm, or thrombus compromises the lumen.[21]

The limitations of balloon angioplasty as well as the failure of new devices and pharmacologic interventions to reduce the risk of restenosis provided the stimulus for the development of alternatives. Given that luminal obstruction appeared to be the cause of both the short-term and the long-term limitations of conventional PTCA, a mechanical solution to the problem was sought. It was in this context that the Palmaz-Schatz stent (Cordis Corporation, Miami Lakes, FL) was developed to provide a more effective interventional strategy than that provided by conventional PTCA.

## HISTORICAL PERSPECTIVE

The currently available Palmaz-Schatz stent delivery system was developed as a result of an accumulation of clinical experience that was critically evaluated, prompting several improvements and changes. The following is an overview of this evolution.

In 1987, Schatz and colleagues[22] reported on the implantation of coronary stents in dogs. In December 1987, clinical trials in humans began.[23, 24] The design was identical to those of stents originally implanted by Palmaz in rabbit aortas and consisted of a single tube of surgical grade, 316 L stainless steel, 15 mm in length, 1.6 mm in diameter, and with a wall thickness of 0.003 inches (0.08 mm). The design of the stent was based on the principle of plastic deformation whereby a metal will not change its shape after being stretched beyond a certain limit. The walls of the stent are etched into multiple rows of staggered rectangles that become diamond-shaped on balloon inflation and allow maximum expansion up to 5 to 6 mm (4:1 expansion ratio). The stent was retrogradely slipped over a delivery balloon and manually crimped down. Via an 8- or 9-French guiding catheter on a 0.014-inch wire, the stent was deployed at 6 to 8 atmospheres (atm). Because of difficulty in passing the rigid stent through the bends of the guiding catheter, the guide wire and the catheter had to be removed after the predilatation and replaced with a preloaded assembly. The lesion was then recrossed and the stent advanced to the lesion.

The delivery strategy was considerably simplified after a modification of the stent design by Schatz included a 1-mm articulation between two 7-mm-long rigid segments. This articulated flexible stent could be easily passed through an 8- or 9-French guiding catheter over a 0.014-inch guide wire, eliminating the necessity to recross the lesion with a guide wire.

Although the articulated design solved the problem of delivery to the proximal part of the vessel, the problem of advancing the balloon/stent assembly down tortuous and sometimes disrupted vessels

**793**

remained. In a small percentage of patients, stent snagging on diseased or dissected proximal segments resulted in failure of stent delivery and isolated cases of stent embolization. These problems were solved with the incorporation of a 5- or 6-French delivery sheath into the delivery system. Before the device was introduced into the patient, the balloon stent assembly was inserted into the delivery sheath with the tip of the balloon extending past the tip of the sheath. This prevented stent-wall contact during passage and created a gradual transition from the 3-French tip of the balloon to the tip of the sheath. Secondary to stiffness, the 6-French sheath was abandoned in favor of the 5-French sheath. With the 5-French stent delivery system, stent delivery success rates rose to 99% and embolization was effectively eliminated.

The current commercially available stent delivery system (Johnson & Johnson Interventional Systems, Warren, NJ) arrives as a preassembled unit with an articulated two-segment stent crimped on a specified diameter balloon between two radiopaque markers and preloaded into a transparent delivery sheath that has a radiopaque marker, which allows the operator to determine the position of the sheath with respect to the stent (Fig. 41–1).

## PROCEDURE

### Patient Selection

Candidates for intracoronary stent implantation include most of the patients eligible for percutaneous coronary revascularization based on clinical and angiographic criteria. The ideal candidate is a patient with symptoms of angina pectoris despite medical treatment and without contraindications for antiplatelet therapy or a history of aspirin allergy. Angiographically, the patient should have a discrete (<15 mm in length) de novo stenosis in a coronary artery or an SVG of at least 3 mm in diameter.

As experience and expertise with stenting accumulated, it became apparent that other types of lesions could be approached with excellent results using the Palmaz-Schatz stent, including ostial lesions, suboptimal results after conventional PTCA (including dissections), chronic occlusions, bifurcation lesions, long lesions (>15 mm), small vessels (2.5 to 3.0 mm), and acute myocardial infarction. Clinical results with these lesions are discussed later in this chapter.

### Vessel Selection

As noted earlier, many lesions can be treated with stenting, with excellent angiographic results. However, the operator needs to be mindful of features of the lesion that might make the procedure considerably more difficult or impossible.

Vessels in which stenting is being contemplated should be carefully evaluated for two potentially problematic characteristics: (1) proximal tortuosity or rigidity (secondary to heavy calcification) and (2) other areas of obstructive disease in the same vessel.

Proximal vessel tortuosity or rigidity may be significant enough to prevent passage of the stent delivery system to the lesion of interest. This is most effectively addressed with a well-seated guiding catheter in a power position coupled with a stiff guide wire to minimize the severity of the tortuosity.

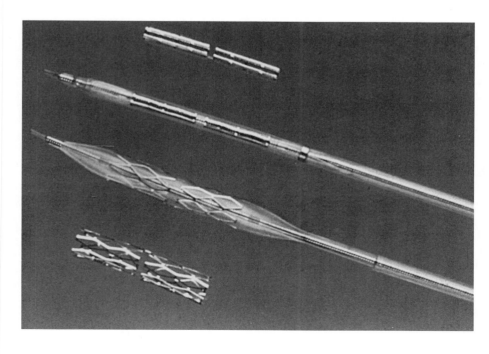

FIGURE 41–1. The Palmaz-Schatz coronary stent.

The presence of other areas of obstruction in the vessel to be treated must also be considered. Stenting of a segment that involves the origin of a significant branch can trap that branch in "stent jail." If the side branch does not have an obstructive lesion at its origin, it usually remains open at follow-up. If the side branch has a lesion at its ostium, the operator needs to be prepared to either treat the branch prophylactically with a stent (T-stenting procedure) or salvage the branch using conventional PTCA through the stent struts of the stent in the parent vessel. Another aspect of the problem with concomitant obstructive disease is the presence of distal disease that might obstruct distal runoff. This should be carefully evaluated and considered before a stent is implanted.

## Patient Preparation

Current experience dictates that the patient take 325 mg of noncoated Bayer aspirin once daily and 250 mg of ticlopidine once in the morning and once at night 24 hours before the procedure. On the day of stent implantation, aspirin is again given, as is the morning dose of ticlopidine.

## Procedural Anticoagulation

After access to the femoral artery is obtained, heparin is administered to maintain the activated clotting time at 200 to 300 seconds. After uncomplicated stent implantation, heparin is discontinued, and the activated clotting time measured every hour until it is less than 150 seconds, at which time the sheath is removed. Should heparin need to be restarted, a 2000- to 2500-unit bolus followed by a continuous infusion is administered 6 hours after sheath removal. Bed rest for 8 to 10 hours after sheath removal is strictly enforced.

## Guide Catheter Selection

Adequate internal luminal diameter is no longer a significant problem in choosing a guide catheter. The minimum internal diameter required is 0.082 inches, although a 0.086-inch internal diameter guide provides easier passage and better opacification of the vessel when the stent is being precisely placed.

The importance of choosing a guiding catheter that provides adequate support has seen a resurgence with the introduction of the relatively bulky Palmaz-Schatz system. This pivotal decision should be thoughtfully made because it becomes crucial in the setting of proximal tortuosity, a switchback right coronary artery, an angulated left circumflex, or a shepherd's crook right coronary artery. A simple maneuver known as the "push test" can be used to

anticipate how well the guide will transmit proximal force.

Under fluoroscopic guidance, forward advancement of the guide catheter should demonstrate a tendency to further intubate the coronary artery rather than prolapse to the aortic root. This has proved to be helpful in predicting the success or failure of the guiding catheter to provide adequate support. Failure to pass this test should result in rejection of the catheter.

## Stent Sizing

The long-term success of stenting is derived from achieving a large postprocedural lumen secondary to the stent's ability to minimize recoil and to allow full expansion of the lesion with minimal dissection. Oversizing of the stent can result in coronary rupture and marginal dissections. Thus, appropriate sizing directly affects short- and long-term outcomes. The stent delivery system should be chosen so that the stented region is slightly larger than the reference vessel in a ratio of approximately 1.1:1.0. This should produce the angiographic appearance of a slight "step-up" at the proximal edge and a "step-down" at the distal edge of the stent. The stents are uniform in size, with the deployment balloons sized according to the package labeling. This allows tremendous flexibility in sizing by simply changing the size of the postdilatation balloon.

## Technique of Implantation

After thoroughly reviewing the vessel morphology, selecting a catheter, and confirming prior ingestion of aspirin and ticlopidine as well as an activated clotting time of 200-300 seconds, the operator may now proceed.

Mapping views are obtained in several projections. Anatomic landmarks are carefully sought to aid positioning and include vessel calcification, bends, and side branches. In addition, other landmarks, including surgical clips and sternotomy wires, can be quite helpful in positioning the stent. The lesion is than crossed with a supportive 0.014-inch exchange length guide wire.

The lesion is then predilated with an appropriately sized balloon. Some operators prefer to slightly underdilate the lesion, and others prefer to use a noncompliant balloon that they anticipate will be used to postdilate the stent. Predilation facilitates passage of the stent delivery system (SDS). The goal of predilation is not to achieve a perfect angioplasty result, because this might eliminate angiographic features of the lesion that will ultimately serve as landmarks for stent deployment.

At this point, the lesion has been prepared for stent delivery. The stent arrives from the factory crimped down on a relatively noncompliant 20-mm balloon with two radiodense markers 17 mm apart. Proximally, there is a Y-adaptor with a side port for balloon inflation and a central port for wire passage. The catheter arrives with a 4.9-French delivery sheath, which has a single distal radiodense marker, and a Y-adaptor proximally, which serves as a flush port. The SDS is provided with a clamshell device proximally, which should be removed after the SDS is removed from its packaging. The central lumen and side port are flushed and the balloon port capped.

Attention is then directed toward the relationship of the components of the catheter. First, the position of the stent with respect to the two radiopaque markers should be noted. The location of the radiodense sheath marker with respect to the other markers is noted. The catheter is then advanced so that the distal balloon and 1 mm of stent remain exposed. This achieves the best transition from wire to balloon to stent to sheath in order to minimize snagging.

The SDS should then be advanced to the lesion and carefully positioned by use of predefined landmarks and the radiodense markers of the SDS. The sheath is then withdrawn by loosening the Tuohy-Borst valve of the delivery sheath and retracting the sheath to the hub of the Y-adaptor. Final adjustments can be made with the stent exposed; however, large movements risk stent migration and embolization. The balloon is then prepared with a single negative aspiration, and additional adjustments are made. The balloon is inflated to 8 atm for the 3.0-mm device, 7 atm for the 3.5-mm device, and 6 atm for the 4.0-mm device. Angiography is performed after stent deployment.

Stent implantation is then optimized by use of a properly sized noncompliant balloon to embed the stent struts into the vessel wall. A final inflation at 16 to 20 atm is recommended. A step-up proximally and step-down distally should be achieved at the conclusion of the procedure.

## Antithrombotic Regimen and Postprocedural Intravascular Ultrasound

The initial U.S. Food and Drug Administration (FDA)-approved anticoagulant regimen included periprocedural aspirin, dipyridamole, dextran, and heparin, followed by aspirin long-term, dipyridamole for 3 months, and warfarin (Coumadin) for 1 month after the procedure. This vigorous regimen was associated with a significant bleeding and vascular complication rate that threatened to impede the broad application of the technology.

Initial experience using intravascular ultrasound (IVUS) revealed that greater than 80% of stents may

be insufficiently dilated, despite apparent angiographic success.[25, 26] Colombo and associates[27] hypothesized that stent thrombosis may be caused in part by incomplete dilation and that anticoagulants may not be necessary when adequate expansion is achieved using IVUS. IVUS and adjunctive high-pressure balloon inflations were used to optimize deployment; 96% of patients were treated successfully and received only aspirin and ticlopidine after the procedure. Despite the absence of anticoagulants, the acute thrombosis rate was 0.6% and the subacute thrombosis rate was 0.3% at 2 weeks. At 6 months, the documented stent occlusion rate was 1.6%. This result lead the authors to conclude that if IVUS is used to confirm adequate expansion, anticoagulant therapy can be safely omitted.

The prospective, multicenter Angiography Versus Intravascular ultrasound-Directed (AVID) stent placement trial randomly assigned patients to IVUS-guided stent placement versus angiographically guided stent implantation. Interim results from 270 patients have been reported.[28] In the IVUS group, 33% of patients required additional therapy to fulfill IVUS criteria of optimal deployment. For those who underwent further therapy based on the IVUS, an increase in luminal diameter of 0.59 mm and a 32% increase in cross-sectional area (CSA) was noted. No patient experienced a complication as a result of IVUS-guided therapy. Patients were discharged receiving aspirin and ticlopidine only. At 30 days, 1.8% of angiography-guided patients and 1.9% of IVUS-guided patients experienced in-hospital stent thrombosis. The incidence of death, myocardial infarction (MI), or coronary artery bypass graft (CABG) was similar in both groups. The major clinical end point of target lesion revascularization or in-stent restenosis at 6 and 12 months is pending.

A randomized trial to compare antiplatelet therapy versus aspirin and an anticoagulant was undertaken to more definitively answer the question of anticoagulation after stent implantation. In the Intracoronary Stenting and Antithrombotic Regimen (ISAR) trial, 257 patients were randomly assigned to receive antiplatelet therapy (aspirin and ticlopidine), and 260 patients were randomly assigned to receive anticoagulant therapy (intravenous heparin, phenprocoumon, and aspirin).[29] The primary cardiac end point was a composite of death, MI, CABG, or repeat PTCA. The primary noncardiac end point was death from noncardiac causes, cerebrovascular accident, and severe hemorrhagic and peripheral vascular events. Of note, IVUS was not routinely used. The primary cardiac end point was reached by 1.6% of the patients assigned to antiplatelet therapy and 6.2% of the patients assigned to anticoagulants. Occlusion of the stented vessel occurred in 0.8% of the antiplatelet therapy group and in 5.4%

of the anticoagulant group. A primary noncardiac end point was reached by 1.2% of the antiplatelet group and 12.3% of the anticoagulant group. Hemorrhagic complications occurred only in the anticoagulant group (6.5%). The authors concluded that in comparison with anticoagulant therapy, antiplatelet therapy reduces the incidence of cardiac and noncardiac events as well as hemorrhagic complications.

Another trial comparing various postprocedural pharmacologic regimens has been reported. In the Stent Anticoagulation Regimen Study (STARS), three postprocedural regimens (aspirin, aspirin and ticlopidine, and aspirin and warfarin) in 1652 patients after optimal Palmaz-Schatz stent placement (<10% residual stenosis) were compared.[30] The primary end point was a 30-day composite of death, CABG, Q-wave MI, and subacute closure. The primary end point was reached by 3.6% of the aspirin group, 2.4% of the aspirin and warfarin group, and 0.6% of the aspirin and ticlopidine group (Fig. 41–2). The difference in reaching the primary endpoint in the aspirin and ticlopidine group was statistically significant when compared with the two other groups. The benefit of aspirin and ticlopidine was largely due to a reduction in Q-wave MI and subacute closure. A trend toward more frequent bleeding and vascular complications was noted in the aspirin and warfarin group.

From these data, it appears that the optimal regimen after stent implantation is aspirin (325 mg)

permanently and ticlopidine (250 mg) twice a day for 2 to 4 weeks. The role of IVUS remains controversial; however, if optimal stent deployment is achieved with adjunctive high-pressure balloon inflations, it appears to be safe to treat the patient with antiplatelet agents only, without the use of IVUS.

## CLINICAL RESULTS

In 1994, the Palmaz-Schatz stent was approved by the FDA for patients eligible for balloon angioplasty with symptomatic ischemia due to a discrete (length <15 mm), de novo (nonrestenotic) native coronary artery lesion with a reference vessel diameter in the range of 3 to 4 mm in order to produce a larger lumen diameter, maintain arterial patency, and reduce the incidence of restenosis at 6 months compared with balloon angioplasty. In practice, the use of Palmaz-Schatz stents has been expanded to a variety of non–FDA-approved indications. The following is a discussion of the various FDA- and non–FDA-approved indications.

### Elective Use in Native Coronary Arteries
#### STRESS Trial

The purpose of the STent REStenosis Study (STRESS) was to compare angiographic restenosis and outcome with coronary stenting versus balloon angioplasty.[31] The study population consisted of patients with symptoms of ischemic heart disease and de novo lesions of the native coronary circulation deemed suitable for stenting or PTCA. Angiographic inclusion criteria were a target stenosis of 70% or greater and lesion length of less than 15 mm with a reference diameter of 3.0 or greater. At 20 centers (14 United States and six international), 410 patients were randomly assigned to either stent placement (207 patients) or balloon angioplasty (203 patients). The patients underwent angiography at baseline, immediately after the procedure, and at 6 months. Quantitative coronary angiography was performed at a core laboratory.

The patients who underwent stenting had a higher procedural success rate than those who underwent balloon angioplasty (96.1% vs. 89.6%, $p = 0.011$), a larger increase in lumen diameter after the procedure (1.72 ± 0.46 mm vs. 1.23 ± 0.48 mm, $p <0.001$), and a larger luminal diameter immediately after the procedure (2.49 ± 0.43 mm vs. 1.99 ± 0.47, $p <0.001$). At 6 months, patients who underwent stenting continued to have a larger luminal diameter (1.74 ± 0.60 mm vs. 1.56 ± 0.65 mm, $p = 0.007$) and a lower rate of restenosis (31.6% vs. 42.1%) than those treated with balloon angioplasty

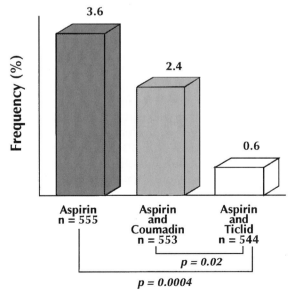

## STARS - Primary Endpoints

FIGURE 41–2. STARS: Incidence of primary end points (death, coronary artery bypass grafting, Q-wave myocardial infarction, and subacute closure). The difference between the aspirin and ticlopidine (ticlid) group and the other two treatment groups was statistically significant.

## STRESS
## p = 0.046

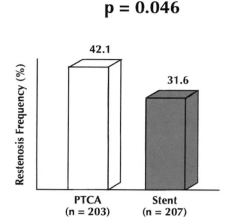

## BENESTENT
## p = 0.02

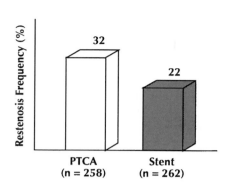

FIGURE 41–3. The incidence of restenosis at 6 months was significantly reduced in patients treated with stents compared with patients treated with balloon angioplasty in both the STRESS and the BENESTENT trials.

(Fig. 41–3). There were no coronary events (death, MI, CABG, vessel closure, or repeat PTCA) in 80.5% of the patients in the stent group or in 76.2% in the angioplasty group ($p = 0.16$). Revascularization of the original target lesion because of recurrent myocardial ischemia was performed less frequently in the stent group than in the PTCA group (10.2% vs. 15.4%, $p = 0.06$). The authors concluded that in selected patients, placement of an intracoronary stent affords patients an improved procedural success rate, a lower rate of angiographic restenosis, a similar rate of clinical events at 6 months, and a reduction in the need for revascularization of the original lesion.

### BENESTENT Trial

The BENESTENT study was also a multicenter trial comparing stent implantation and balloon angioplasty in patients with stable angina and de novo lesions in native coronary arteries.[32] A total of 520 patients were randomly assigned to receive either a Palmaz-Schatz stent (262 patients) or standard balloon angioplasty (258 patients). The primary clinical end points were death, MI, cerebrovascular accident, CABG, or a second intervention either at the time of the procedure or during the subsequent 7 months. The primary angiographic end point was the minimal luminal diameter at follow-up, as determined by quantitative coronary angiography.

A primary clinical end point was reached by 76 of the 257 patients assigned to balloon angioplasty (30%), compared with 52 of the 259 patients assigned to stent implantation (20%). The difference in clinical event rates was explained mainly by a reduced need for a second angioplasty in the stent group compared with the PTCA group (23.3% vs. 13.5%, $p = 0.005$).

The mean MLDs immediately after the procedure were 2.48 ± 0.39 mm in the stent group and 2.05

± 0.33 mm in the angiographic group. At follow-up, the diameters were 1.82 ± 0.64 mm in the stent group and 1.73 ± 0.55 mm in the PTCA group ($p = 0.09$), which corresponds to rates of restenosis (diameter stenosis ⩾50%) of 22% vs. 32% ($p = 0.02$) (see Fig. 41–3). Peripheral vascular complications requiring surgery or blood transfusion were more common after stenting than balloon angioplasty (13.5% vs. 3.19%, $p < 0.001$). The authors concluded that over 7 months of follow-up, both clinical and angiographic results were better in stent patients.

### Saphenous Vein Grafts

Balloon angioplasty of aortocoronary SVG lesions is associated with high restenosis and clinical event rates. Advantages of SVG stent placement over PTCA and other devices include its ability to scaffold the friable SVG surface, potentially reducing the risk of distal embolization and its ability to achieve a large postprocedure MLD, which might reduce the risk of restenosis. The role of the Palmaz-Schatz stent in treating these lesions was defined by several early observational studies, which noted restenosis rates and complication rates that compared quite favorably with PTCA. In a multicenter study of 198 patients, Fenton and colleagues[33] reported that elective stent placement was associated with a high initial success rate (98.5%) and a 34% angiographic restenosis rate at 6 months. The 6-month event-free (death, MI, CABG, and repeat PTCA) survival was 70%. Piana and associates[34] reported on stent placement in 200 SVG lesions treated with either coronary (146) or biliary (54) Palmaz-Schatz stents. Stent placement was successful in 98.5% of lesions with one acute stent thrombosis and no subacute stent thrombosis. One in-hospital death and no emergency bypass surgeries or Q-wave MIs occurred. Angiographic restenosis at

3 to 6 months was 17%. Wong and coworkers[35] reported on the Multicenter U.S. Palmaz-Schatz Stent Experience in 589 patients. Stent delivery was successful in 98.8% of procedures. Major in-hospital complications occurred in 2.9% of patients, stent thrombosis occurred in 1.4%, and major vascular or bleeding complications occurred in 14.3%. The 6-month angiographic restenosis rate was 29.7%.

The biliary stent design, with its greater radial compressive strength, enhanced visibility, larger diameter, and variable length, emerged as a potentially useful alternative to treat SVGs. Wong and associates[36] reported on 305 SVG lesions in 231 patients treated with biliary (123) and Palmaz-Schatz coronary (108) stents. Both biliary and coronary treated patients had similarly favorable short-term and long-term outcomes. The operator should be cautioned because this stent is not approved for coronary use, and the results are highly operator dependent.

As a result of these promising preliminary reports, a multicenter, randomized, controlled trial comparing stenting with PTCA was undertaken. In the Saphenous Vein Graft De Novo (SAVED) study, patients were eligible if they had angina pectoris or evidence of myocardial ischemia, new lesions of bypass grafts, SVG measuring 3.0 to 5.0 mm in diameter, and an ejection fraction of $\geq$25%.[37] Patients were excluded if they had an MI within 7 days, contraindications to full anticoagulation, evidence of thrombus, or a lesion that would require more than two stents. The average age of patients was 66 years, and the mean graft age 10 years. The postprocedure MLD was 2.81 mm in the stent group and 2.16 mm in the PTCA group ($p$ <0.001). Technical success (<50% residual stenosis) was achieved in 95% of the stent group, as opposed to 75% in the PTCA group ($p$ <0.0001). Clinical success (technical success without an in-hospital major cardiac event) was 92% in the stent group and 69% in the PTCA group ($p$ <0.0001). There was no significant difference in rates of Q-wave MI, death, or need for CABG. At 6 months, the late loss in the stent group was greater than in the PTCA group, but the net gain was significantly greater. The restenosis rates were not significantly different.

The major cardiac event (death, MI, CABG, repeat PTCA) rate at 6 months was 38% for the PTCA group versus 26% for the stent group ($p$ = 0.05). The authors concluded that in comparison with balloon angioplasty, elective stent placement in new lesions of SVGs results in a superior initial angiographic result, higher procedural success rates, and a reduction in the composite clinical end point of death, MI, CABG, or target lesion revascularization at 6 months.

## Unstable Angina

The safety of coronary stent implantation in the setting of coronary syndromes was initially questioned because of concerns that the risk of stent thrombosis might be enhanced. Guarneri and colleagues[38] reported on 92 patients who had unstable angina or acute MI treated with intracoronary stents. Procedural success was achieved in 94% of patients. In-hospital complications included new Q-wave MI in 3%, bypass surgery in 0%, death in 3%, and vascular complications in 5%. At 30 days' follow-up, no patient sustained stent thrombosis. In an observational study, Malosky and associates[39] compared stenting in patients with stable and unstable angina. There was no significant difference in 30-day complication rates in the two groups. At 6 months' follow-up, there was no difference in the rates of restenosis, angina class, or overall clinical success.

Thus, it appears that patients with unstable angina who receive intracoronary stents have complication, restenosis, and initial success rates similar to those of patients with stable angina. This differs from PTCA in these two patient populations and may be the result of the stents' ability to seal potentially thrombogenic dissections in an activated plaque.

## Emergency Use for Failed PTCA

Abrupt closure after PTCA occurs in as many as 11% of procedures and is associated with a high incidence of morbidity and mortality.[15–19] The stent's mechanism of action makes it very effective in salvaging certain PTCA failures by stabilizing dissections as well as by opposing elastic recoil and vessel spasm.

Herrmann and coworkers[40] described 56 patients who underwent emergency stent implantation: 23 patients with a suboptimal result, 15 with an impending closure, and 18 with a frank occlusion. Stents were successfully deployed in 55 of 56 (98%) patients, with 52 of 56 (93%) being free from death, CABG, or MI. Subacute thrombosis occurred in 16% of patients and major complications in 29% at 1 month, raising early concerns about this approach. Metz and associates[41] reviewed their experience with bailout stenting over time. Over the course of 7 years, the use of stents for bailout increased, although the success remained unchanged. There was a decreasing trend for stent thrombosis (14% vs. 5%), in-hospital death (5% vs. 2%), non–Q-wave MI (29% vs. 7%), and bleeding complications (27% vs. 7%) between group I (patients treated from 1988 to 1991) and group II (patients treated from 1991 to 1993). The main finding was a trend toward improved results that the authors attributed to the "learning curve" with stenting, earlier consideration of stent placement, and improved technique. Schömig and coworkers[42] reported on their 4-year experience with Palmaz-Schatz stenting for dissection with threatened or present closure. The procedure was successful in 96.5% of patients. At 4 weeks, there was a 1.3% cardiac mortality rate, a 4.0% nonfatal MI rate, a 1% CABG rate, and a 6.3% early repeat PTCA rate. Subacute closure was encountered in 6.3% of patients. At 6 months, the rate of restenosis was 29.6%, and at 2 years, 95.4% survived.

Thus, it appears that patients with threatened or frank closure after PTCA can be treated with bailout stenting with acceptable initial complication rates and excellent long-term outcome.

### Restenotic Lesions

The most common approach to the treatment of the restenotic lesion after PTCA has been repeat balloon dilatation and is associated with a restenosis rate of 25% to 40%.[43–45] Although stenting has been demonstrated to reduce restenosis in de novo lesions, data regarding its use in treating restenotic lesions are scarce.

Colombo and colleagues[46] analyzed the immediate and long-term angiographic outcome and clinical results of stent implantation for restenosis in 128 consecutive patients. Stent implantation was successful in 126 (98%), with a 1.8% ± 12 diameter stenosis at the conclusion. Four patients (3.1%) had complications, including one death. Angiographic restenosis occurred in 25% of patients. Late events (death, CABG, MI, emergency PTCA, or vascular complications) occurred in 19% of patients. Thus, it appears that stenting selected patients who have restenosis meets with a favorable outcome that is comparable to that of stenting of de novo lesions.

### Ostial Lesions

Coronary angioplasty of ostial lesions is fraught with technical difficulties and is hampered by a high restenosis rate.[8, 47] This high restenosis rate can be explained by involvement of the aortic wall in the lesion, resulting in a prominent component of elastic recoil. Stent deployment provides a scaffolding to prevent recoil and allows the operator to safely employ large balloons to achieve maximal luminal gain. Zampieri and coworkers[48] reported results on 13 patients with ostial stenoses, revealing a 100% angiographic success rate, no major complications, and a 16% restenosis rate. An observational study by Rocha-Singh and colleagues[49] of 41 patients with ostial native and SVG lesions revealed excellent initial success rates; however, 7.3% of patients had a major complication, and 5% died in hospital. In another observational study, Colombo and associates[50] described their experience with 35 ostial lesions. Angiographic success was achieved in 100% of patients, and the restenosis rate was 23% at follow-up.

Thus, it appears that ostial stenting is safe and feasible, with restenosis rates that compare favorably with historical controls. Because of a higher likelihood of restriction due to calcium at the aorto-ostial junction, adjunctive debulking with rotational atherectomy before stenting is an appealing strategy but has yet to be subjected to clinical trials. It is our philosophy to debulk ostial right coronary lesions before stenting in order to ensure the maximal stent expansion.

### Chronic Occlusion

Recanalization of chronic coronary occlusions has been reported to have a primary success rate of 54% to 81%, a restenosis rate of 44% to 77%, and a reocclusion rate of 14% to 40%.[51] Several nonrandomized studies have suggested that stenting of chronic occlusions may reduce restenosis rates after PTCA.[52–56]

Sirnes and associates[51] reported the results of the Stenting in Chronic Coronary Occlusion (SICCO) trial, which investigated whether stenting improves long-term results after recanalization of chronic coronary occlusions. One hundred nineteen patients with a satisfactory result after PTCA were randomly assigned to a control group or a group in which stenting was performed, followed by full anticoagulation. Angiography was performed at baseline, after stenting, and at 6 months. Subacute occlusion occurred in four patients in the stent group and in three patients in the PTCA group. At follow-up, 57% of the stent patients were free of angina, compared with 24% of the PTCA patients. Restenosis (>50% diameter stenosis) was noted in 32% of the patients with stents and in 74% of the patients with PTCA only ($p < 0.001$). Reocclusion occurred in 12% of the stent group and in 26% of the PTCA-only group ($p = 0.058$). It appears that stent implantation improved long-term clinical and angiographic outcome in chronic occlusions.

### Bifurcation Lesions

Previous studies have shown that more than half of the patients who underwent balloon angioplasty had side branches that were in jeopardy of occlusion.[56, 57] Of these, 5% were occluded after the PTCA. Side branches originating from a severely diseased segment had a 14% incidence of occlusion, whereas branches not directly involved (but within the segment covered by the balloon) had a 1% incidence of occlusion.[56, 57] Disease of the ostium of the branch appears to be a major risk factor for occlusion or further compromise. The impact of stenting on this phenomenon is of great concern to the interventionalist who treats similar patients with stents.

Fischman and associates[57] reported on 66 branches spanned by 57 stents. Twenty-seven (41%) of the branches had a greater than 50% ostial stenosis. Six side branches became occluded after PTCA and remained occluded after stent placement. Of the 60 branches patent after PTCA, 95% remained patent after stenting. All three that became occluded after stenting had a 50% or greater ostial stenosis at baseline. All 60 side branches, including those initially occluded after stenting, were patent at 6 months.

Iniguez and colleagues[58] reviewed their experience with 79 side branches crossed with intracoronary stents. Of the branches that were 1 mm or greater in diameter, 2/34 (6%) had flow impairment after stenting. Three patients experienced transient angina, but no patient had an acute MI.

Despite this relatively benign outcome, operators remain concerned when faced with a bifurcation if stenting is planned. This seems more reasonable if the branch is large and serves a substantial amount of myocardium, and particularly if the ostium of the branch is diseased. Several approaches to these lesions, including kissing stents (implantation of a stent into each vessel of a bifurcation with proximal overlap in the parent vessel), T-stenting (placement of a stent in the ostium of the branch and another stent across that branch in the parent vessel), stenting of the branch vessel through the struts of the stent in the parent vessel, and simple balloon dilatation of the struts of the stent in the parent vessel.[59, 60] Initial experience with these techniques has been somewhat disappointing, with reports of significant technical complexity and relatively high procedural event rates.[61] Long-term follow-up of lesions treated in this fashion has yet to be reported. In the United States, where sheathless systems are unavailable, strategic placement of a "stent through a stent" is problematic.

### Acute MI

Although superior to intravenous thrombolysis, primary PTCA has some limitations both in-hospital and in the first 6 months after the procedure. The incidence of recurrent ischemia of 10% to 15% necessitates repeat catheterization, which prolongs hospital stay and increases costs. At 6 months, the rate of restenosis is 30% to 50% and the reocclusion rate is 9% to 13%.[62–65] Angiographic predictors of recurrent ischemia in the PAMI II trial included a greater than 30% residual stenosis and the presence of dissection.[62, 63] Stents that achieve large lumens

and seal dissections seem to be a logical answer; however, they have been avoided because of the perceived increased risk of thrombosis. Despite these concerns, several investigators reported that intracoronary stenting is feasible.[66–69]

Schömig and associates[70] reported on the outcome of 123 patients treated with stents in the setting of acute MI from the ISAR trial. Patients were randomly assigned to aspirin and ticlopidine versus anticoagulant therapy. The 30-day event rate in patients treated with antiplatelet therapies was significantly lower (3.3% vs. 21.0%, $p = 0.005$), as was the stent vessel occlusion rate (0% vs. 9.7%, $p = 0.03$). At 6 months, survival free of recurrent MI was higher (100% vs. 90.3%, $p = 0.03$) and the rate of stent vessel occlusion lower (1.6% vs. 14.5%, $p = 0.02$) in the antiplatelet therapy group. Both groups had comparable restenosis rates (26.5% vs. 26.9%, $p = 0.87$). It appears from this study that stenting results compare quite favorably with historical PTCA results.

As a result of these promising studies, the PAMI investigators have undertaken the task of evaluating PTCA versus stent placement for acute MI. In the Multicenter PAMI Stent Pilot Study, 125 patients deemed eligible for stenting after PTCA (vessel >2.75 mm, two stents or less to treat lesion, no residual thrombus, no major side branches jeopardized, and feasible stent delivery) received stents.[62] Stents were deployed in 99% of patients; no in-hospital deaths occurred, and the recurrent ischemia rate was 2.1%. Currently, a multicenter, randomized trial evaluating PTCA versus stenting with the heparin-coated Palmaz-Schatz stent has been completed (see Chapter 12).

### Long Lesions

Early concerns that multiple stents might increase the risk of subacute thrombosis excluded long lesions from stent implantation. However, several studies have reported a much more favorable outcome than was originally predicted. Maiello and associates[71] described the experience with 108 lesions in 89 patients with diffuse disease (lesions >20 mm in length). IVUS was used to optimize stent deployment. Procedural complications included three MIs (3%), three emergency bypass surgeries (3%), and one elective bypass (1%). Follow-up angiography on 71% revealed a restenosis rate of 35%. Itoh and colleagues[72] reported their experience in treating long lesions. The Palmaz-Schatz stent achieved the greatest postprocedural MLD, compared with the Gianturco-Roubin and Wiktor stents; however, the restenosis rate of 40% proved disappointing.

Shaknovich and coworkers[73] reported their experience with multiple stents in very long lesions and dissections. The Palmaz-Schatz stent was implanted in native coronary arteries in 49 patients and in SVGs in five patients. Mean lesion length was 50 mm, with 31% of lesions being greater than 50 mm. Stents were placed electively in 19 patients and for bailout in 35 patients. The mean number of stents was four, and 13 patients received more than 5 stents per vessel. Procedural success was 98%. There were no MIs. Emergency CABG was required in one patient and elective CABG in three of 54 (3.7%) patients. Long lesions can be treated with stents with acceptable short-term results; however, restenosis rates appear to be considerably higher than with single stent placement.

### Small Vessels

Many operators have been reluctant to treat small vessels because of concern about the risk of stent thrombosis. However, subgroup analysis from the STRESS trial suggested that the impact of stenting versus PTCA was greater in vessels that were less than 3 mm compared with vessels that were greater than 3 mm. Although absolute restenosis rates were higher in vessels less than 3 mm (52% with PTCA vs. 36% with stents) compared with vessels greater than 3 mm (29% with PTCA vs. 26% with stents), the absolute reduction in restenosis was greater.[74] Teirstein and colleagues[75] showed that stenting of these small vessels can be performed safely. Palmaz-Schatz stents were placed in 145 patients with a reference vessel that was less than 3.0 mm by quantitative coronary angiography. Deployment was optimized with IVUS and high-pressure balloon inflations. Patients were discharged receiving aspirin and ticlopidine (56%) or aspirin, ticlopidine, and warfarin (44%). The procedural success (<50% diameter stenosis without Q-wave MI, CABG, or death) was achieved in 96% of patients. Thirty-day follow-up revealed a Q-wave MI in 3.4% of patients, bypass in 0%, and death in 0%. No stent thromboses were documented. These studies suggest that stenting of these vessels is feasible; however, additional studies are needed in order to reach any further conclusions.

### Left Main Coronary Stenosis

PTCA of the unprotected left main coronary artery (LMCA) is technically feasible; however, the procedure carries a high procedural mortality.[76] The role of stenting to treat LMCA disease has been addressed (see Chapter 29). Fajadet and coworkers[77] treated 26 patients who had unprotected LMCA with intracoronary stents. Thirteen patients received Palmaz-Schatz stents, 11 patients received Gianturco-Roubin stents, and two received AVE

stents. No acute or subacute thromboses occurred. No major cardiac events (repeat PTCA, CABG, MI, or death) occurred during the hospitalization. At a mean follow-up of 7 months, repeat PTCA was performed in five patients, and sudden death occurred in one patient. Two patients had class II angina, and 23 had no symptoms. Itoh and associates[78] reviewed their experience with unprotected LMCA stenting in 33 patients. Angiographic success was achieved in 94%, with 1 patient requiring emergent surgery (3%). There were three deaths (9%) within 3 months of the procedure: two preceded by unstable angina and subsequent closure and one of uncertain etiology.

Despite these results, the unprotected LMCA stenosis remains an indication for CABG. For selected patients who are not acceptable CABG candidates, LMCA stenting appears feasible and can be considered as an alternative to medical therapy alone.

## In-Stent Restenosis

Although stent placement has been shown to reduce restenosis rates compared with balloon angioplasty, in-stent restenosis still occurs in 20% to 30% of patients.[31, 32] Experience with the heparin-coated stent using optimal implantation technique revealed a restenosis rate of 17%.[79] With more and more patients receiving stents to treat coronary artery disease, the problem of in-stent restenosis has emerged as a growing and significant problem. The predictors remain poorly defined; however, placement of multiple stents and placement of stents in small vessels appear to be associated with higher restenosis rates.[71–74] The time course of in-stent restenosis appears to be similar to that reported for conventional PTCA.[80, 81] Reductions in coronary luminal dimensions appear to be largely confined to the first 6 months.[80, 81] However, late improvement in luminal diameter appears to occur between 6 months and 3 years. Kimura and colleagues[81] evaluated angiograms of patients treated with stents at 6 months, 1 year, and 3 years. At 6 months, the MLD decreased from $2.54 \pm 0.44$ mm to $1.87 \pm 0.56$ mm, but no further decrease had occurred at 1 year. A significant improvement in luminal diameter was observed at 3 years (Fig. 41–4). Fibrotic maturation of the intimal hyperplasia that initially compromises the luminal diameter has been postulated as the mechanism of this late improvement in luminal dimensions.

The mechanism of in-stent restenosis has been elucidated by serial IVUS studies.[20, 82] Late lumen loss correlated solely with neointimal tissue proliferation.[82] Stents appear to produce an exaggerated neointimal hyperplastic response compared with other interventions; however, because postintervention MLD is greater and because stents eliminate

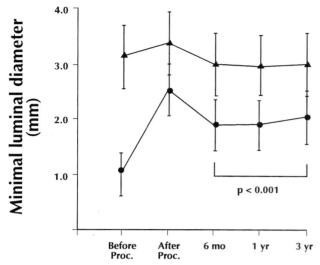

FIGURE 41-4. Serial changes in the minimal luminal diameter *(black circles)* as compared with the reference diameter *(black triangles)*. A significant improvement was noted in minimal luminal diameter from 6 months to 3 years after stent implantation ($p < 0.001$).

negative arterial remodeling (resulting in a reduction in vessel cross-sectional area), the vessel can accommodate a greater degree of tissue growth.[20]

The treatment of in-stent restenosis has been largely confined to repeat balloon dilatation. Procedural success rates of greater than 95% can be achieved with very low complication rates.[83] The mechanism of the approach appears to be a combination of tissue extrusion out of the stent as well as additional stent expansion.[84, 85] Despite improving lumen dimensions after PTCA, the procedure fails to achieve the same result as the original stent procedure because of significant residual neointimal tissue mass within the stent at the conclusion of the procedure.

Restenosis rates after balloon dilatation for in-stent restenosis are relatively high. Baim and coworkers[83] reported on the U.S. multicenter experience in which 54% of patients met angiographic criteria for restenosis. Yokoi and associates[86] demonstrated that restenosis rates after balloon dilatation for in-stent restenosis were dependent on the angiographic appearance of the in-stent restenosis before treatment. These groups of patients were defined: (1) those with diffuse (>10 mm) in-stent restenosis; (2) those with focal border stenosis; and (3) those with focal in-stent restenosis. Those with diffuse in-stent restenosis had the highest rate of restenosis (85%), and those with focal in-stent restenosis had the lowest rate of restenosis (12%) after PTCA.

Although PTCA may be adequate for focal in-stent restenosis, the results for diffuse in-stent restenosis appear to be inadequate. The role of devices such as the Rotablator, excimer laser, and directional coronary atherectomy that ablate tissue, thus debulking

the stent and reducing the amount of residual neointimal tissue, is being actively investigated.

Interest in directional coronary atherectomy has been limited by reports of stent strut excision and deep wall injury.[87] In addition, one report noted high restenosis rates with this technique.[88] The use of excimer laser to reduce tissue burden has also been disappointing, with one study demonstrating a residual stenosis of 28% after laser and adjunctive PTCA.[89] The feasibility of rotational atherectomy was reported by Bottner and colleagues[90]; however, long-term follow-up is not yet available.

The role of intracoronary irradiation to reduce the proliferative response to implanting stents was the focus of the SCRIPPS trial.[91] Teirstein and coworkers[91] reported on the initial results from 55 patients with in-stent restenosis or restenosis in an artery that was a candidate for stenting; the patients were randomly assigned to receive radiation (with a[192]Ir gamma source) or placebo after optimal intervention (additional stents were implanted if necessary). At 6 months, the incidence of angiographic restenosis in patients with stent and border restenosis was 53.6% in the untreated group and 16.7% in the treated group. In patients with restenosis within the stent only, the rate of restenosis was 35.2% in the untreated group and 8.3% in the treated group (Fig. 41-5). By 12 months, the rates of death, MI, and target lesion revascularization were 15.4% in the treatment group and 48.3% in the untreated group. When IVUS was used, this reduction in restenosis was attributed to a reduction in the neointimal proliferative response. Other radiation sources (beta emitting) and radioactive stents intended to reduce the proliferative response are under active investigation. Although radioactive stents have not been effective, $\beta$ radiation employing the Novoste system (Atlanta GA) has decreased in-stent restenosis. FDA approval has been obtained for this catheter to treat in-stent restenosis. This approach appears to be promising; however, larger numbers of patients need to be treated before the technique can be broadly applied.

## LONG-TERM CLINICAL OUTCOME

The long-term clinical outcome for patients treated with Palmaz-Schatz stents appears to be favorable. Savage and associates[92] reported on 300 patients treated with Palmaz-Schatz stents for stenoses in native coronary arteries. Clinical events after 1 year included death in 0.7%, MI in 3.7%, CABG in 8%, and repeat PTCA in 13%. Freedom from an adverse event occurred in 80%.

Macaya and associates[93] reported on 516 patients from the BENESTENT I trial. At 1 year, there was no significant difference in death, stroke, MI, or CABG between the stent and the PTCA group. However, the need for repeat PTCA was significantly

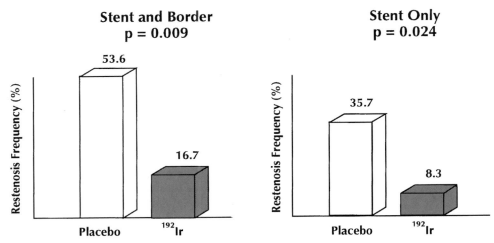

FIGURE 41–5. SCRIPPS Trial: Incidence of restenosis. *Left panel*, Patients with restenosis involving the stented region as well as the bordering vessel. *Right Panel*, Patients with restenosis involving only the stented region. Patients in both groups who received [192]Ir (a gamma source of radiation) had a statistically significant reduction in the rate of restenosis.

lower in the stent group (10%) than in the PTCA group (21%).

Laham and colleagues[94] described the 4- to 6-year outcome of 175 patients treated with Palmaz-Schatz stents. The survival rate at 5 years was 86.7%. The rate of repeat revascularization to the treatment site was 14.4% at 1 year, 17.7% at 3 years, and 19.8% at 5 years. At 5 years, the rate of target site revascularization was 21.9% for SVGs and 19.2% for native coronaries. The issue of late restenosis was addressed by Kimura and coworkers,[81] who demonstrated late improvement in luminal diameter from month 6 to the third year; this result was attributed to fibrotic maturation of the neointimal response (see section on restenosis).

The long-term follow-up of stenting reveals stability of the treated lesion from 1 year onward, with rare exception. Evidence of late luminal improvement has dispelled initial concerns about late restenosis in stented segments.

## STENT THROMBOSIS

The most feared complication related to stent implantation is early stent thrombosis. With refinements in implantation technique and changes in the postprocedural pharmacologic regimen, the risk has been reduced compared with the rate of 3.5% reported in the initial randomized trials.[31, 32] Stent occlusion rarely occurs in the laboratory; it usually occurs between days 3 and 14 but can occur up to 4 weeks after the procedure.[95, 96] Haude and colleagues[96] identified several variables that could be risk factors for stent thrombosis, including use for bailout, treatment of long lesions with multiple stents, symptomatic dissection after angioplasty, incomplete repair of dissection after stenting, and distal vessel irregularities. Others have identified small

target vessels, low ejection fraction, and recent MI as risk factors.[95, 97] Any mechanical factor that obstructs inflow or outflow or creates undue shear force can encourage stent thrombosis, likely through platelet activation.

The outcome of stent thrombosis is poor, despite early intervention. Haude and coworkers[96] reported on 10 patients with stent thrombosis. One patient underwent emergency bypass, and nine patients were treated with catheter-based procedures. Although eight of nine underwent recanalization within 2 hours of symptom onset, seven experienced MIs, two Q-wave and five non–Q-wave. Hasdai and coworkers[95] reported on 29 patients with stent thrombosis. Twenty-six patients (90%) had an acute MI (including 20 of 23 patients treated with catheter-based therapy), 10 were referred for emergent or urgent bypass surgery, and 5 died.

Because the consequences are severe and it appears that catheter-based interventions are limited, prevention appears to be the most prudent objective. The operator needs to pay careful attention to procedural details, including a careful inspection for residual filling defects, marginal dissections, or a suboptimal postprocedural lumen to direct further therapy. The role of IVUS remains controversial (see section on postprocedural IVUS). Technical improvements in the implantation procedure (e.g., adjunctive high-pressure balloon angioplasty), along with significant postprocedural pharmacologic regimens to include only aspirin and ticlopidine, have lead to a 0.8% stent thrombosis rate, as reported in the ISAR trial (see section on anticoagulation).[29] The additive role of IIb/IIIa platelet receptor blockage (e.g., 7E3) has not been addressed clinically; however, experimental work in an ex vivo model described a dose-dependent inhibition of stent thrombosis.[98]

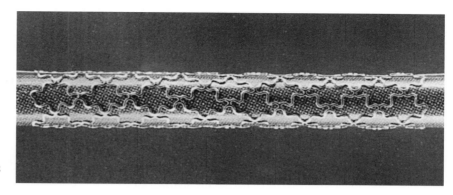

FIGURE 41–6. The Crown Palmaz-Schatz coronary stent.

The initial management of stent thrombosis should include immediate PTCA. Intravenous lytics should be avoided in favor of intracoronary lytics for residual thrombus. Hasdai and colleagues[95] reported limited success with this approach, attributing this poor outcome to the platelet-rich thrombus that appears to be present in most stent thromboses. Additional stents should be used if a mechanical cause (e.g., untreated dissections, proximal or distal disease) can be identified. The use of 7E3 (Repro, Eli Lily, IN) has been studied clinically in the CAD-ILLAC trial (see Chapter 12).

## NEW DEVELOPMENTS

As experience was gathered by operators implanting stents, several limitations of the Palmaz-Schatz SDS were noted. As a result of these limitations, several changes have emerged to address some of these problems.

Because stent thrombosis was a significant problem that had severe consequences in the early clinical experience, a novel approach to covalently binding heparin to the Palmaz-Schatz stent was developed in hopes of reducing this end point. Early animal studies indicated improved thromboresistance of the heparin-coated stent,[99] and thus clinical trials were undertaken. The BENESTENT II trial, which randomly assigned 827 patients to PTCA versus heparin-coated stent placement, has been reported.[79] Patients were treated with adjunctive high-pressure PTCA and discharged receiving aspirin and ticlopidine. The stent thrombosis rate was 0.2%. At 6 months, restenosis occurred in 17% of the stent patients and in 31% of the PTCA patients.

Despite the articulation at the midpoint of the Palmaz-Schatz stent, the device still suffers to some extent from longitudinal rigidity. The new Crown Palmaz-Schatz stent retains all the basic features of the Palmaz design but has greatly increased longitudinal flexibility without designated articulation points[100] (Fig. 41–6). Longitudinal flexibility is pro-

vided by cutting the slots in the stent in a sinusoidal fashion rather than as straight parallel slots. The stent will be available in 15-, 20-, and 31-mm lengths and will be provided on a high-pressure, power-grip balloon. Also, a smaller version of this design will be available worldwide that will be dedicated to vessels between 2.0 and 3.0 mm.

These new developments hope to improve the deliverability and clinical outcome of stents in the coming years.

## CONCLUSION

Restenosis has been the "holy grail" of contemporary interventional cardiology and has prompted the development of several new devices and pharmacologic agents directed at reducing this end point. Thus far, only the Palmaz-Schatz stent has proved effective in reducing the rate of restenosis.

As operators have gained experience with the device, the spectrum of lesions that can be treated has been continuously expanded. In addition, changes in the postprocedural pharmacologic regimen have substantially reduced complication rates. These changes have allowed broad application of the technology.

The future holds great promise for intracoronary stenting with the introduction of more flexible stents, stents of variable lengths, and heparin-coated stents. Ideally, the operator will be able to truly customize the procedure for each patient using an array of stents that will be on every interventional laboratory shelf.

## REFERENCES

1. Gruentzig AR: Transluminal dilatation of coronary artery stenosis [Letter]. Lancet 1:263, 1978.
2. Holmes DR, Vliestra RE, Smith HC, et al: Restenosis after percutaneous transluminal coronary angioplasty (PTCA): A report from the Coronary Angioplasty Registry of the National Heart, Lung, and Blood Institute. Am J Cardiol 53:77C–81C, 1984.
3. Nobuyoshi M, Kimura T, Nosaka H, et al: Restenosis after

successful percutaneous transluminal coronary angioplasty: Serial angiographic follow-up of 229 patients. J Am Coll Cardiol 12:616, 1988.

4. Serruys PW, Luijten HE, Beatt KJ, et al: Incidence of restenosis after successful coronary angioplasty: A time-related phenomenon. Circulation 77:361–371, 1988.

5. Cote G, Myler RK, Stertzer SH, et al: Percutaneous transluminal angioplasty of stenotic coronary artery bypass grafts: 5 years' experience. J Am Coll Cardiol 9:8–17, 1987.

6. Douglas JS, King SB, Roubin GS, et al: Percutaneous angioplasty of venous aortocoronary graft stenoses: Late angiographic and clinical outcome. Circulation 74(suppl II):II-281, 1986.

7. Webb JG, Myler RK, Shaw RE, et al: Coronary angioplasty after coronary bypass surgery: Initial results and late outcome in 422 patients. J Am Coll Cardiol 16:812–820, 1990.

8. Topol EJ, Ellis EG, Fishman J, et al: Multicenter study of percutaneous transluminal angioplasty for right coronary artery ostial stenosis. J Am Coll Cardiol 9:1214–1218, 1987.

9. Leimgruber PP, Roubin GS, Hollman J, et al: Restenosis after successful coronary angioplasty in patients with single-vessel disease. Circulation 73:710–717, 1986.

10. Vandormael MG, Deligonul U, Kern MJ, et al: Multilesion coronary angioplasty: Clinical and angiographic follow-up. J Am Coll Cardiol 10:246–252, 1987.

11. Myler RK, Topol EJ, Shaw RE, et al: Multiple vessel coronary angioplasty: Classification, results, and patterns of restenosis in 494 consecutive patients. Cathet Cardiovasc Diagn 13:1–15, 1987.

12. Fleck E, Regitz V, Lehnert A, et al: Restenosis after balloon dilatation of coronary stenosis: Multivariant analysis of potential risk factors. Eur Heart J 9:15–18, 1988.

13. Topol EJ, Leya F, Pinkerton CA, et al, the CAVEAT Study Group: A comparison of directional atherectomy with coronary angioplasty in patients with coronary artery disease. N Engl J Med 329:221–227, 1993.

14. Vandormael M, Reifart N, Preusler W, et al: Six months follow-up results following excimer laser angioplasty, rotational atherectomy and balloon angioplasty for complex lesions: ERBAC Study [abstract]. Circulation 90(suppl I):I-213, 1994.

15. Detre KH, Holmes DR, Holubkov R, et al: Incidence and consequences of periprocedural occlusion: The 1985–1986 NHLBI Percutaneous Transluminal Coronary Angioplasty Registry. Circulation 82: 739–750, 1990.

16. Kuntz RE, Piana R, Pomerantz RM, et al: Changing incidence and management of abrupt closure following coronary intervention in the new device era. Cathet Cardiovasc Diagn 27:183–190, 1992.

17. Gaul G, Hollman J, Simpfendorfer C, et al: Acute occlusion in multiple lesion coronary angioplasty: Frequency and management. J Am Coll Cardiol 13:283–289, 1989.

18. Dorros G, Crowley MJ, Janke L, et al: In-hospital mortality rate in the National Heart, Lung, and Blood Institute Percutaneous Transluminal Coronary Angioplasty Registry. Am J Cardiol 53:17C–21C, 1984.

19. Lincoff AM, Popma JJ, Ellis SG, et al: Abrupt vessel closure complicating coronary angioplasty: Clinical, angiographic therapeutic profile. J Am Coll Cardiol 19:926–935, 1992.

20. Mintz GS, Popma JJ, Hong MK, et al: Intravascular ultrasound to discern device-specific effects and mechanisms of restenosis. Am J Cardiol 78(suppl 3A):18–22, 1996.

21. de Feyter PJ, van den Brand M, Jaarman G, et al: Acute coronary artery occlusion during and after percutaneous transluminal coronary angioplasty. Frequency, prediction, clinical course, management, and follow-up. Circulation 83:927–936, 1991.

22. Schatz RA, Palmaz JC, Tio FO, et al: Balloon-expandable intracoronary stents in the adult dog. Circulation 76:450–457, 1987.

23. Schatz RA, Palmaz JC, Tio FC, et al: Report of a new articulated balloon-expandable intravascular stent (ABEIS). Circulation 78(suppl 3):1789, 1988.

24. Levine MJ, Leonard BM, Burke JA, et al: Clinical and angiographic results of balloon-expandable intracoronary stents

25. in right coronary artery stenoses. J Am Coll Cardiol 16:332–339, 1990.

25. Goldberg SL, Columbo A, Nakamura S, et al: Benefit of intracoronary ultrasound in the deployment of Palmaz-Schatz stents. J Am Coll Cardiol 24:996–1003, 1994.

26. Nakamura S, Colombo A, Gaglione A, et al: Intracoronary ultrasound observations during stent implantation. Circulation 89:2026–2034, 1994.

27. Colombo A, Hall P, Nakamura S, et al: Intracoronary stenting without anticoagulation accomplished with intravascular ultrasound guidance. Circulation 91:1676–1688, 1995.

28. Russo RJ, Teirstein PS, for the AVID Investigators. Angiography versus intravascular ultrasound-directed stent placement [Abstract]. Circulation 94(suppl I):I-263, 1996.

29. Schömig A, Neumann FJ, Kastrati A, et al: A randomized comparison of antiplatelet and anticoagulation therapy after coronary stent placement. N Engl J Med 334:1084–1089, 1996.

30. Leon MB, Baim DS, Gordon P, et al: Clinical and angiographic results from the stent anticoagulation regimen study (STARS) [Abstract]. Circulation 94 (suppl I):I-7685, 1996.

31. Fischman DL, Leon MB, Baim DS, et al: A randomized comparison of coronary-stent placement and balloon angioplasty in the treatment of coronary artery disease. N Engl J Med 331:496–501, 1994.

32. Serruys PW, de Jaegere P, Kiemeneij F, et al, for the Benestent Study Group. A comparison of balloon-expandable stent implantation with balloon angioplasty in patients with coronary artery disease. N Engl J Med 331:489–495, 1994.

33. Fenton SH, Fischman DL, Savage MP, et al: Long-term angiographic and clinical outcome after implantation of balloon-expandable stents in aortocoronary saphenous vein grafts. Am J Cardiol 74:1187–1191, 1994.

34. Piana RN, Moscucci M, Cohen DJ, et al: Palmaz-Schatz stenting for treatment of focal vein graft stenosis: Immediate results and long-term outcome. J Am Coll Cardiol 23:1296–1304, 1994.

35. Wong SC, Baim DS, Schatz RA, et al: Immediate results and late outcomes after stent implantation in saphenous vein graft lesions: The multicenter U.S. Palmaz-Schatz stent experience. J Am Coll Cardiol 26:704–712, 1995.

36. Wong SC, Popma JJ, Pichard AD, et al: A comparison of clinical and angiographic outcomes after saphenous vein graft angioplasty using coronary versus "biliary" tabular-slotted stents. Circulation 91:339–350, 1995.

37. Douglas JS, Savage MP, Bailey ST, et al: Randomized trial of coronary stent and balloon angioplasty in the treatment of saphenous vein graft stenosis [Abstract]. J Am Coll Cardiol 27(suppl A):178A, 1996.

38. Guarneri EM, Schatz RA, Sklar SL, et al: Acute coronary syndromes: Is it safe to stent? [Abstract]. Circulation 92(suppl 1):I-616, 1995.

39. Malosky SA, Hirshfeld JW, Herrmann HC: Comparison of results of intracoronary stenting in patients with unstable vs. stable angina. Cathet Cardiovasc Diagn 31:95–101, 1994.

40. Herrmann HC, Buchbinder M, Clemen MW, et al: Emergent use of balloon-expandable coronary artery stenting for failed percutaneous transluminal coronary angioplasty. Circulation 86:812–819, 1992.

41. Metz D, Urban P, Carmenzind E, et al: Improving results of bailout coronary stenting after failed balloon angioplasty. Cathet Cardiovasc Diagn 32:117–124, 1994.

42. Schömig A, Kastrati A, Mudra H, et al: Four-year experience with Palmaz-Schatz stenting in coronary angioplasty complicated by dissection with threatened or present vessel closure. Circulation 90:2716–2724, 1994.

43. Califf RM, Fortin DF, Frid DJ, et al: Restenosis after coronary angioplasty: An overview. J Am Coll Cardiol 66:3–6, 1991.

44. Dimas AP, Grigera F, Arora R, et al: Repeat coronary angioplasty as treatment of restenosis. J Am Coll Cardiol 19:1310–1314, 1992.

45. Serruys PW, Foley DP, Kirkeeide RL, et al: Restenosis revised: Insights provided by quantitative coronary angiography. Am Heart J 126:1243–1267, 1993.

46. Colombo A, Ferraro M, Itoh A, et al: Results of coronary stenting for restenosis. J Am Coll Cardiol 28:830–836, 1996.

47. Mathias DW, Mooney JF, Lange HW, et al: Frequency of success and complications of coronary angioplasty of a stenosis at the ostium of a branch vessel. Am J Cardiol 67:491–495, 1991.

48. Zampieri P, Colombo A, Almagor Y, et al: Results of coronary stenting of ostial lesions. Am J Cardiol 73:901–903, 1994.

49. Rocha-Singh KJ, Morris N, Wong CS, et al: Coronary stenting for treatment of ostial stenoses of native coronary arteries or aortocoronary saphenous venous grafts. Am J Cardiol 75:26–29, 1995.

50. Colombo A, Itoh A, Maiello L, et al: Coronary stent implantation in aorto-ostial lesions: Immediate and follow-up results [Abstract]. J Am Coll Cardiol 27(suppl A):253A, 1996.

51. Sirnes PA, Golf S, Myreng Y, et al: Stenting in chronic coronary occlusion (SICCO): A randomized, controlled trial of adding stent implantation after successful angioplasty. J Am Coll Cardiol 28:1444–1451, 1996.

52. Maiello L, Colombo A, Almagor Y, et al: Coronary stenting with a balloon-expandable stent after the recanalization of chronic total occlusions. Cathet Cardiovasc Diagn 25:293–296, 1992.

53. Medina A, Melián F, de Lezo SJ, et al: Effectiveness of coronary stenting for the treatment of chronic total occlusion in angina pectoris. Am J Cardiol 73:1222–1224, 1994.

54. Goldberg SL, Colombo A, Maiello L, et al: Intracoronary stent insertion after balloon angioplasty of chronic total occlusions. J Am Coll Cardiol 26:713–719, 1995.

55. Sheiban J, Marini A, Tonni S, et al: The use of coronary stents for the recanalization of chronic total occlusion reduces the restenosis rate [Abstract]. Eur Heart J 16:287, 1995.

56. Meier B, Gruentzig AR, King SB III, et al: Risk of side branch occlusion during coronary angioplasty. Am J Cardiol 53:10–14, 1984.

57. Fischman DL, Savage MP, Leon MB, et al: Fate of lesion-related side branches after coronary artery stenting. J Am Coll Cardiol 22:1641–1646, 1993.

58. Iniguez A, Macaya C, Alfonzo F, et al: Early angiographic changes of side branches arising from a Palmaz-Schatz stented coronary segment: Results and clinical implications. J Am Coll Cardiol 23:911–915, 1994.

59. Colombo A, Gaglione A, Nakamura S, et al: "Kissing" stents for bifurcational coronary lesion. Cathet Cardiovasc Diagn 30:327–330, 1993.

60. Nakamura S, Hall P, Maiello L, et al: Techniques for Palmaz-Schatz stent deployment in lesions with a large side branch. Cathet Cardiovasc Diagn 34:353–361, 1995.

61. Colombo A, Maiello L, Itoh A, et al: Coronary stenting of bifurcation lesions: Immediate and follow-up results [Abstract]. J Am Coll Cardiol 27(suppl A):277A, 1996.

62. Grines CL: Aggressive intervention for myocardial infarction: Angioplasty, stents, and intraaortic balloon pumping. Am J Cardiol 78(suppl 3A):29–34, 1996.

63. Stone GW, Grines CL, Browne KF, et al: Predictors of in-hospital and 6-month outcome after acute myocardial infarction in the reperfusion era: The Primary Angioplasty in Myocardial Infarction (PAMI) trial. J Am Coll Cardiol 25:370–377, 1995.

64. Brodie BR, Grines CL, Ivanhoe R, et al: Six-month clinical and angiographic follow-up after direct angioplasty for acute myocardial infarction. Circulation 90:156–162, 1994.

65. Grines C, Brodie B, Griffin J, et al: Which primary PTCA patients may benefit from new technologies? [Abstract]. Circulation 92(suppl I):I146, 1995.

66. Wong PHC, Wong CM: Intracoronary stenting in acute myocardial infarction. Cathet Cardiovasc Diagn 33:39–45, 1994.

67. Ahmad T, Webb JG, Carere RR, et al: Coronary stenting for acute myocardial infarction. Am J Cardiol 76:77–80, 1995.

68. Neumann F-J, Walker H, Richard G, et al: Coronary Palmaz-Schatz stent implantation in acute myocardial infarction. Heart 75:121–126, 1996.

69. Garcia-Cantu E, Spaulding C, Corcos T, et al: Stent implantation in acute myocardial infarction. Am J Cardiol 77:451–454, 1996.

70. Schömig A, Neumann F-J, Walker H, et al: Coronary stent placement: Comparison of clinical and angiographic outcome after randomization to antiplatelet or anticoagulant therapy. J Am Coll Cardiol 29:28–34, 1997.

71. Maiello L, Hall P, Nakamura S, et al: Results of stent implantation for diffuse coronary disease assisted by intravascular ultrasound. [Abstract]. J Am Coll Cardiol 25(suppl A):156A, 1995.

72. Itoh A, Hall P, Maiello L, et al: Coronary stenting of long lesions (greater than 20 mm): A matched comparison of different stents [Abstract]. Circulation 92 (suppl I):1-688, 1995.

73. Shaknovich A, Moses J, Undemin C, et al: Procedural and short-term clinical outcomes of multiple Palmaz-Schatz stents (PSSs) in very long lesions/dissections [Abstract]. Circulation 92(suppl I):1-535, 1995.

74. Wong C, Hirshfeld J, Teirstein P, et al: Differential impact of stent versus PTCA on restenosis in large ($\geq 3$ mm) and small ($<3$ mm) vessels in the STent REStenosis Study [Abstract]. J Am Coll Cardiol 25(suppl A):375A, 1995.

75. Teirstein PS, Schatz RA, Russo RJ, et al: Coronary stenting of small diameter vessels: Is it safe? Circulation 92:1–281, 1995.

76. O'Keefe JH, Hartzler GO, Rutherford BD, et al: Left main coronary angioplasty: Early and late results of 127 acute and elective procedures. Am J Cardiol 64:144–147, 1989.

77. Fajadet J, Brunel P, Jordan C, et al: Stenting of unprotected left main coronary artery stenosis without Coumadin [Abstract]. J Am Coll Cardiol 27:277A, 1996.

78. Itoh A, Colombo A, Hall P, et al: Stenting in protected and unprotected left main coronary artery: Immediate and follow-up results [Abstract]. J Am Coll Cardiol 27:277A, 1996.

79. Legrand V, Serruys PW, Emanuelsson H, et al: BENESTENT II Trial–Final results: I. A 15-day follow-up [Abstract]. J Am Coll Cardiol 29(suppl A):170A, 1997.

80. Kastrati A, Schömig A, Dietz R, et al: Time course of restenosis during the year after emergency coronary stenting. Circulation 87:1498–1505, 1993.

81. Kimura Y, Yokoi H, Nakugawa Y, et al: Three-year follow-up after implantation of metallic coronary-artery stents. N Engl J Med 334:561–566, 1996.

82. Hoffmann R, Mintz GS, Dussaillant GR, et al: Patterns and mechanisms of in-stent restenosis. Circulation 94:1247–1254, 1996.

83. Baim DS, Levine MJ, Leon MB, et al: Management of restenosis within the Palmaz-Schatz coronary stent (The U.S. multicenter experience). Am J Cardiol 71:364–366, 1993.

84. Gordon PC, Gibson CM, Cohen DJ, et al: Mechanisms of restenosis and redilatation within coronary stents: Quantitative angiographic assessment. J Am Coll Cardiol 21:1166–1174, 1993.

85. Mehran R, Mintz GS, Popma JJ, et al: Mechanisms and results of balloon angioplasty for the treatment of in-stent restenosis. Am J Cardiol 78:618–622, 1996.

86. Yokoi H, Kimura T, Nakagawa Y, et al: Long-term clinical and quantitative angiographic follow-up after the Palmaz-Schatz stent restenosis [Abstract]. J Am Coll Cardiol 27 (suppl A):224A, 1996.

87. Bowerman RE, Pinkerton CA, Kirk B, et al: Disruption of a coronary stent during atherectomy for restenosis. Cathet Cardiovasc Diagn 24:248–251, 1991.

88. Strauss BH, Umans VA, van Suylen RJ, et al: Directional atherectomy for treatment of restenosis within coronary stents: Clinical, angiographic and histologic results. J Am Coll Cardiol 20: 1465–1473, 1992.

89. Koster R, Hamm C, Koschyk DH, et al: Laser angioplasty of restenotic and occluded stents [Abstract]. Eur Heart J 17:308, 1996.

90. Bottner RK, Hardigan KR: High-speed rotational ablation for in-stent restenosis. Cathet Cardiovasc Diagn 40:144–149, 1997.

91. Teirstein PS, Massullo V, Jani S, et al: Radiation therapy following coronary stenting: 6-month follow-up of a randomized clinical trial. Circulation 94(suppl 1):1–210, 1996.

92. Savage RA, Fischman DL, Schatz RA, et al: Long-term angi-

ographic and clinical outcome after implantation of a balloon-expandable stent in the native coronary. Circulation 24:1207–1212, 1994.

93. Macaya C, Serruys PW, Ruygrok P, et al: Continued benefit of coronary stenting versus balloon angioplasty: One year clinical follow-up of Benestent trial. J Am Coll Cardiol 27:255–261, 1996.

94. Laham RJ, Carroza JP, Berger C, et al: Long-term (4- to 6-year) outcome of Palmaz-Schatz stenting: Paucity of late clinical stent-related problems. J Am Coll Cardiol 28:820–826, 1996.

95. Hasdai D, Garratt KN, Holmes DR, et al: Coronary angioplasty and intracoronary thrombolysis are of limited efficacy in resolving early intracoronary stent thrombosis. J Am Coll Cardiol 28:361–367, 1996.

96. Haude M, Erbel R, Issa H, et al: Subacute thrombotic complications after intracoronary implantation of Palmaz-Schatz stents. Am Heart J 126:15–22, 1993.

97. Moussa J, Di Mario C, DiFrancesco L, et al: Subacute stent thrombosis and the anticoagulation controversy: Changes in drug therapy, operator technique and the impact of intravascular ultrasound. Am J Cardiol 78(suppl 3A): 13–17, 1996.

98. Makkar RR, Litvack F, Eigler N, et al: Effects of GP IIb/IIIa receptor monoclonal antibody (7E3), heparin and aspirin in an *ex vivo* canine arteriovenous shunt model of stent thrombosis. Circulation 95:1015–1021, 1997.

99. Stratienko AA, Zhu D, Lambert CR, et al: Improved thrombo-resistance of heparin coated Palmaz-Schatz coronary stents in an animal model [Abstract]. Circulation 88(suppl I):1-596, 1993.

100. Schatz RA, Firth BG.: The Palmaz-Schatz coronary stent: New developments. *In* Serruys PW (ed): Handbook of Coronary Stents, pp 21–32, London: Martin Dunitz, 1997.

# 42

# The ACS MultiLink Stent

*James P. Zidar    James J. Crowley*

The efficacy of coronary artery stents were originally reported in two landmark studies that have demonstrated an advantage to stenting over conventional angioplasty.[1, 2] The incidence of major complications, such as acute thrombosis and hemorrhagic complications, has fallen significantly with the use of antiplatelet regimens, such as aspirin, glycoprotein IIb/IIIa agents, and ticlopidine, and the recognition of the importance of optimal stent deployment using intracoronary ultrasound.[3, 4] High-pressure intrastent dilatation is now possible because of the development of balloon catheters capable of withstanding high pressures. Despite these advances, restenosis continues to be a major limitation of stent usage.

In-stent restenosis is affected by many factors, and the mechanisms may differ from those of restenosis after balloon angioplasty. First, the struts of the expanding stent impose focal deep vascular trauma in comparison to the less-controlled stretching and fracturing of the vessel wall caused by balloon inflation alone.[5] Second, extensive early thrombus generated within days of stenting may provide a nidus for scaffolding and subsequent cell proliferation and neointimal hyperplasia.[6] Third, permanent rather than transient strain is applied to the vessel wall, producing lasting changes to the vessel geometry. Fourth, foreign material remains in the injured artery. The effect of each of these factors on neointimal hyperplasia may be minimized through the development of newer stent designs.[7]

It is apparent from animal studies that differences in stent design may provoke different responses in terms of neointimal proliferation. When animals are implanted with stents of identical material, weight, and surface area but of different configurations, a twofold difference in intimal growth may be observed.[6] Primary stenting without arterial predilation limits the extent of endothelial ablation and may reduce intimal hyperplasia still further.[8] Pasquantonio and coworkers[9] compared Palmaz-Schatz stent deployment characteristics with those of a novel stent design in 48 swine arteries. There were no differences in metallic surface area, deployment balloon characteristics, postprocedural angiographic luminal diameters, or balloon-to-vessel ratios. After 30 days, the novel stent showed significantly less neointimal thickness, and less lumen area loss by intravascular ultrasound, suggesting that vascular wall injury, depending on the stent design, is one of the factors responsible for restenosis. Hoffmann and colleagues[10, 11] used intravascular ultrasound to examine the fate of Palmaz-Schatz stents in 115 native coronary artery or saphenous vein bypass graft lesions over a mean follow-up period of 5.4 months. The accumulation of tissue within the stent proved to be the main contributor to lumen loss. The pattern of this loss was not uniform along the length of the stent but increased significantly where the two halves of the stent were joined by a bridging articulation. When two stents were placed in sequence without overlap (but also without articulation), no corresponding increase in tissue accumulation was found. Therefore, there is good reason to expect that further changes in stent design may have an even greater impact on in-stent restenosis in humans, just as they do in experimental animals.

Although early studies showed the Palmaz-Schatz stent provided better long-term results than angioplasty alone, this stent had many technical problems. It contained an articulation point in its midsegment that appeared to be the site most commonly associated with stent restenosis. It was relatively inflexible along its long axis, which made it difficult to deploy in tortuous vessels. Because only one length (15 mm) was available, multiple stents were required for long lesions.

## THE MULTILINK STENT

The ACS MultiLink stent is a highly flexible balloon expandable stent made of stainless steel. It is composed of individual corrugated rings, interconnected by numerous bridges. The metallic surface area is less than 15% in its expanded state. It is made in different lengths and has negligible shortening (6%) with expansion. The MultiLink design incorporates more metal at the sites where more stress is applied to the stent because of the continuing pressure fluctuations during the cardiac cycle. Computer-aided technique and finite element analysis have been used extensively throughout its development. The low strut thickness (approximately 50 μm, compared with 76 μm for the original Palmaz-Schatz stent) allows for good structural support, yet easy, safe delivery.

The stent is available as an over-the-wire system mounted on a balloon within a protective sheath (Fig. 42–1) or as a rapid-exchange system that does not have a protective sheath (Fig. 42–2). The nonexpanded profile is 4.1 French with the sleeve retracted or 5.2 French with the sleeve. For the rapid-exchange system, the nonexpanded profile is 4.0 French. Radiopaque markers are positioned on the balloon proximal and distal to the stent to improve the accuracy of stent deployment. The stent is deployed at 6 to 7 atm by use of the over-the-wire system and at 9 atm with the rapid-exchange system. There is also a high-pressure balloon rapid-exchange version (ACS Multilink HP system), which allows deployment at 10 to 11 atm. The sleeveless rapid-exchange versions are compatible with 6-French guiding catheters and may be suitable for branch artery access.

The stent is factory crimped onto specially folded balloons (propellor folded), which are covered by a protective elastic membrane. The balloons are prepared to provide expanded stent diameters of 3.0, 3.5, 3.75, or 4.0 mm (rapid exchange system only). The balloons are designed to provide many functions: even distribution of the inflation force for concentric stent expansion and optimal strut apposition to the arterial wall (the stent appears to be symmetrically deployed by intravascular ultrasound), rapid deflation times after stent deployment with a smooth balloon refolding, and reliable crimping of the stent on the balloon to guard against slipping and loss during deployment.

## ANIMAL STUDIES

Animal studies have suggested that the MultiLink stent may be delivered accurately and safely with a low acute thrombosis rate. Rogers and associates[12] deployed the device in the iliac artery of 17 rabbits after endothelial denudation. The thrombosis rate at 14 days was 15%, compared with 42% for a slotted tube design of identical material, mass, and surface area. This is also lower than that of earlier clinical trials.[12] The incidence of intimal hyperplasia was also lower. Sigwart and coworkers[13] implanted the device in 26 canine arteries and had no delivery failures. Angiographic follow-up revealed TIMI grade 3 angiographic patency at 3 days (N = 5), 2 weeks (N = 5), 1 month (N = 5), 6 months (N = 10), and 1 year (N = 1). There were no deaths and no acute thrombotic events. Carter and associates[14] deployed 20 MultiLink stents in 19 miniature swine with experimentally induced coronary atherosclerosis. Nineteen of the 20 stents were successfully deployed. There was minimal recoil after stent deployment. Angiographic and histologic follow-up at 72 hours (N = 7), 14 days (N = 4), and 56 days (N = 8) demonstrated that all stents were patent without evidence of migration, intraluminal filling defects, or side-branch occlusion. At 56 days, there was minimal in-stent neointimal proliferation, and mean in-stent lumen size remained significantly larger than in nonstented vessel segments.

## CLINICAL STUDIES

The first clinical experience with the MultiLink stent in humans was reported in 1993 by Priestley and coworkers.[16] Ten patients received the stent for suboptimal results with a visible coronary dissection after balloon angioplasty and were considered to be at high risk for abrupt closure. Stent deployment was successful in all patients. The stent delivery system readily negotiated tortuous vessels and was successfully deployed, even through bends in vessels. There was no failure of the stent delivery system. It was possible also to retract the whole delivery system so that the lesion could be dilated further with a balloon. The stent was then successfully deployed. There were no instances of balloon rupture. One patient required angioplasty at 6 weeks

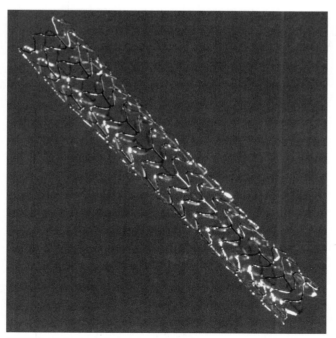

FIGURE 42–1. Over-the-wire system mounted on a balloon within a protective sheath.

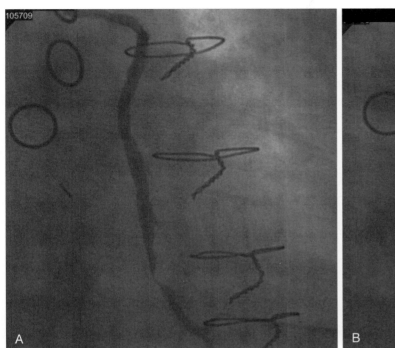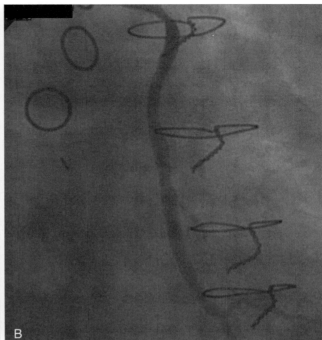

FIGURE 42–2. Rapid exchange system without a protective sheath.

for angina caused by in-stent restenosis. These results are encouraging, considering that these stents were implanted in patients at high risk for abrupt closure and in the era before the routine use of modern antiplatelet regimens and high-pressure balloon inflations.

A small number of single-center experiences with the MultiLink stent have been reported. Chevalier and colleagues[17] retrospectively assessed the results from 160 patients (168 arteries and 180 stents). The stent was delivered to the target by use of the over-the-wire system in 160 cases and a rapid-exchange 6-French compatible balloon in 20 cases. Clinical indications were predominantly unstable angina (48%) and recent myocardial infarction (22%). Stent indications were de novo lesions in 83% and a suboptimal angioplasty result in the remaining patients. In 62%, stent implantation was performed without prior balloon angioplasty. In this subgroup, the failure-to-cross rate was 9%, and implantation was successful after balloon inflation in all failure cases. Overall stent deployment was successful in 98.2%. The stent was successfully implanted after another stent failure in 5% of cases and distally to another stent in 5%. One patient had an acute myocardial infarction and died. There was no acute or subacute stent thrombosis or major local event in any patient.

Hermiller and associates[18] reported results from 50 patients with focal de novo lesions. After predilatation, a 3.5-mm MultiLink stent was deployed and postdilated to a mean of $16.2 \pm 2.3$ atm. The anticoagulation regime consisted of aspirin and warfarin. Stent placement was successful in all patients. There were no in-hospital major events. At 30-day follow-up, there were no acute stent thromboses, myocardial infarctions, or repeat revascularization procedures. Calver and coworkers[19] prospectively studied 98 patients who received 134 stents. Patients were pretreated with aspirin, 300 mg; given procedural heparin; and posttreated with aspirin alone. Clinical indications were elective in 78%, for a suboptimal result after angioplasty in 20%, and for abrupt or threatened vessel closure (bailout indication) in 2%. One patient had a subendocardial myocardial infarction. There were no other in-hospital cardiac complications. At mean follow-up at 74 days, no major cardiac events had occurred.

Five multicenter studies of the MultiLink stent are currently underway. The West European Stent Trial (WEST I) was a European multicenter feasibility and safety registry of the MultiLink stent. Stents were deployed in native lesions of 102 patients with stable angina. Patients were anticoagulated with warfarin and dextran and also received antiplatelet therapy with aspirin and dipyridamole. The 6-month follow-up is now complete and showed a target lesion revascularization of 12%, a target vessel revascularization of 5%, and a 6-month major adverse cardiac event rate (death, myocardial infarction, or target lesion revascularization) of 17.6%. These data compare favorably with the outcome of other stents analyzed prospectively in the era of full anticoagulation, such as the BENESTENT I trial.[1]

The WEST II study is a registry of stenting of native lesions using antiplatelet therapy alone with intravascular ultrasound. One hundred seventy patients have been enrolled.

The ASCENT study is a prospective randomized study comparing the long-term clinical outcomes of the MultiLink stent with those of the Palmaz-Schatz stent for the treatment of de novo lesions of native vessels. One thousand patients were enrolled. Clinical follow-up will continue for 9 months, and 500 patients will undergo repeat coronary angiography to determine angiographic restenosis. A registry of 200 additional patients with prior restenosis were also enrolled to determine the efficacy of MultiLink stent implantation in this group of patients.

The U.S. intravascular study will include at least 60 patients and up to 100 de novo or restenotic lesions. Serial ultrasound will be performed after mandatory postdilatation with a noncompliant balloon at 12 atm and 16 atm to help determine the optimal procedural technique for attaining adequate stent expansion and vessel apposition. Preliminary results indicate that dilatation to 16 atm produces progressive increases in mean cross-sectional area and that this high-pressure dilatation may be indicated to achieve adequate stent apposition with the vessel wall.

A Japanese registry has enrolled 112 patients with lesions of native vessels. Stents were implanted for multiple indications. The 6-month in-stent restenosis rate was 13.9%

## CONCLUSION

The MultiLink stent is a promising new stent that has been specifically designed to address the shortcomings identified during the widespread use of first-generation stents. Advantages include the flexibility and low profile of the sheathed stent and delivery system. The stent appears to provide good structural support along the vessel, combined with a very low metallic burden because of the small diameter of the corrugated struts. The system is designed to reduce shortening during expansion and to provide easy side-branch access. The stent expands evenly because of its innovative delivery balloon wrapping. A possible limitation is its radiolucency, which makes the positioning of noncompliant balloons more difficult when postdelivery high-pressure inflations are required. Preliminary clinical data indicate that this stent may have a broader range of indications than those currently available

and that it has an acceptable acute and 6-month complication rate.

## REFERENCES

1. Serruys PW, de Jaegere P, Kiemeneij F, et al: A comparison of balloon-expandable-stent implantation with balloon angioplasty in patients with coronary artery disease. Benestent Study Group. N Engl J Med 331:489–495, 1994.
2. Fischman DL, Leon MB, Baim DS, et al: A randomized comparison of coronary-stent placement and balloon angioplasty in the treatment of coronary artery disease. Stent Restenosis Study Investigators. N Engl J Med 331:496–501, 1994.
3. Schomig A, Neumann FJ, Kastrati A, et al: A randomized comparison of antiplatelet and anticoagulant therapy after the placement of coronary-artery stents. N Engl J Med 334:1084–1089, 1996.
4. Colombo A, Hall P, Nakamura S, et al: Intracoronary stenting without anticoagulation accomplished with intravascular ultrasound guidance. Circulation 91:1676–1688, 1995.
5. Schwartz RS, Huber KC, Murphy JG, et al: Restenosis and the proportional neointimal response to coronary artery injury: Results in a porcine model [see comments]. J Am Coll Cardiol 19:267–274, 1992.
6. Rogers C, Edelman ER: Endovascular stent design dictates experimental restenosis and thrombosis. Circulation 91:2995–3001, 1995.
7. Murphy JG, Schwartz RS, Edwards WD, et al: Percutaneous polymeric stents in porcine coronary arteries. Circulation 86:1596–1604, 1992.
8. van Beusekom HM, van der Giessen WJ, van Suylen R, et al: Histology after stenting of human saphenous vein bypass grafts: Observations from surgically excised grafts 3 to 320 days after stent implantation. J Am Coll Cardiol 21:45–54, 1993.
9. Pasquantonio EAJ, Fliedner T, Janczewski M, et al: Effect of endovascular stent design on experimental restenosis. J Am Coll Cardiol 29(suppl A):242A, 1997.
10. Hoffmann R, Mintz GS, Dussaillant GR, et al: Patterns and mechanisms of in-stent restenosis: A serial intravascular ultrasound study. Circulation 94:1247–1254, 1996.
11. Hoffmann R, Mintz GS, Popma JJ, et al: Chronic arterial responses to stent implantation: A serial intravascular ultrasound analysis of Palmaz-Schatz stents in native coronary arteries. J Am Coll Cardiol 28:1134–1139, 1996.
12. Rogers C, Karnovsky MJ, Edelman ER: Inhibition of experimental neointimal hyperplasia and thrombosis depends on the type of vascular injury and the site of drug administration. Circulation 88:1215–1221, 1993.
13. Sigwart U, Haber RH, G.J K, et al: A new balloon-expandable coronary stent. Eur Heart J 14(suppl):349, 1993.
14. Carter AJ, Laird JR, Kufs WM, et al: Coronary stenting with a novel stainless steel balloon-expandable stent: Determinants of neointimal formation and changes in arterial geometry after placement in an atherosclerotic model. J Am Coll Cardiol 27:1270–1277, 1996.
15. Poermer T, Voelker W, Teubner J, et al: Effect of high pressure balloon dilation upon the deployment of different coronary stents: An in vitro study using direct magnification radiography. J Am Coll Cardiol 29:274A, 1997.
16. Priestley KA, Clague JR, Buller NP, et al: First clinical experience with a new flexible low profile metallic stent and delivery system. Eur Heart J 17:438–444, 1996.
17. Chevalier B, Royer T, Glatt B, et al: Early experience with a multilink coronary stent.
18. Hermiller JB, Baim DS, Linnemeier TJ, et al.
19. Calver AL, Dawkins KD, Haywood GA, et al: Multilink stenting, a minimalist approach using aspirin alone: no ticlopidine, no Coumadin, no IVUS and no QCA. J Am Coll Cardiol 29:95A, 1997.

# 43

# The Wallstent

*U. Sigwart*

Stents provide a "scaffolding" to support the vessel wall, tack down intimal flaps, smooth the luminal surface, thereby improving blood flow and preventing vessel wall recoil. In 1986, the self-expanding mesh stent was the first of these devices deployed in a coronary vessel.[1] Over the following years, we have examined the role of the self-expanding mesh stent under circumstances of abrupt closure,[2] restenosis of native coronary vessels,[3] and restenosis of bypass graft vessels.[4] The self-expanding mesh stent has also been studied by others around the world. This chapter describes the use of the self-expanding mesh stent and its potential advantages.

## HISTORY

Following Senning's suggestions, Maass and coworkers[5] in Zürich described the experimental use of several different self-expanding stents that could be elongated by torsion onto an ad hoc introducing device and then released into the vascular lumen, where they expanded as a result of their elastic properties. One hundred eighty stents were implanted into the peripheral arteries or veins of 75 dogs. Tilting (11%), migration (5%), or thrombosis (10%) of the prosthesis remained a problem with the early stent design, but marked improvement was noted when the "double helix" stent was used because this proved more stable (tilting in 6%, no migration), and no occlusive thrombus formation was observed. However, the design required a bulky introducing system and was unsuitable for small arteries. All stents were made of surgical stainless steel (Mediloy, Medinvent SA, Switzerland), as either wire (0.3- to 0.5-mm diameter) or metal bands (0.08 to 0.30 mm thick and 1.5 mm wide). Positioning of such prostheses could be achieved without inducing pressure necrosis, and endothelial covering in previously normal arteries was complete within 6 weeks. A combination of intimal cell proliferation and microthrombi was observed more frequently in veins than in arteries.

Wright and coworkers[6] and Charnsangavej and associates[7] described a spring-loaded stainless steel stent with a zig-zag pattern that was implanted into large vessels, but stent migration was observed in some cases, and prosthesis stability appeared to be suboptimal. The stent's design also restricted its use to the covering of short vascular segments.

Several of the initial problems of self-expanding stents were solved when the coil concept was further developed and led to the use of a mesh design with several interwoven strands (see Figs. 43–1, 43–3, and 43–4). This device, later termed the *Sigwart*-Wallstent (Medinvent, Lausanne, Switzerland), was the first stent to be used for clinical purposes, and a large part of the early experience with clinical coronary stenting was obtained with it.

## TECHNICAL FEATURES

The stent now consists of 16 to 20 strands of 0.06- to 0.09-mm diameter, arranged into a self-expanding mesh design (Fig. 43–1). The material is a nonferromagnetic cobalt-base alloy, and a 5-mm-diameter stent typically weighs about 1.4 mg per millimeter of length. The stent is flexible along its long axis, and for coronary implants, its length varies between 15 and 50 mm and its diameter between 3.0 and 6.5 mm in the fully expanded state. For any given lesion, a stent is selected so that its fully expanded diameter is somewhat larger than the estimated normal lumen of the recipient vessel; it is then stable once it is positioned and exerts a residual radial pressure on the arterial wall. For implantation (Fig. 43–1), the stent is compressed and thereby elongated on a delivery system. This is introduced via a standard 8-French guiding catheter over an exchange guide wire after completion of balloon angioplasty. The delivery system used for coronary arteries has an outer diameter of 1.57 mm and can accommodate stents of up to 6.5 mm in diameter. A doubled-over membrane or a tubular retractable sheath ("Magic Wallstent") maintains the stent constrained in an elongated state. The space between the inner and the outer layers of the doubled-over membrane is filled with contrast medium at approx-

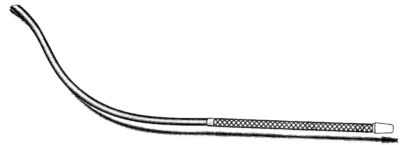

FIGURE 43–1. Stent compressed by a retaining membrane on the delivery catheter.

imately 3 bars of pressure to ensure both lubrication and x-ray visualization. Trapped air may escape through a distally located microscopic pinhole. Retraction of the membrane allows the stent to be progressively released into the vascular lumen.

Modifications of the stent design have brought the braiding angle from 130 degrees to 110 degrees. This has reduced the exerted radial force by about 30% and the amount of metal per millimeter of stented vessel by about 7%. Advances in polymer technology have allowed the simple retractable sleeve ("unistep") without the somewhat delicate and—from the operator standpoint—not always straightforward banana skin peel-away principle.

## HISTOLOGY

Experimental evidence from several different animal studies shows that a thin fibrin and platelet layer is deposited on a metallic stent within minutes of implantation.[8–11] The stent slowly becomes embedded in thickened intima, and the endoluminal surface is eventually covered by neoendothelium. The neoendothelial covering is completed within 1 to 8 weeks, depending on the type of stent and the animal model studied. Using a balloon-expandable stent in the rabbit model, Palmaz and colleagues[12] observed an immature endothelial cover with a "crazy-paving" appearance after 1 week and normal-appearing endothelium with flat, elongated cells at 8 weeks. Using the same stent deployed in a dog's peripheral artery, these investigators observed that the development of neoendothelium took 3 weeks.[13]

We have made similar observations with the self-expanding stent.[1, 8] Forty-seven stents were inserted in dogs and sheep. They were covered within the first few hours of deployment by a thin fibrin and platelet layer. Complete endothelial covering was observed at 3 weeks (Fig. 43–2). The mesh design allowed islands of endothelium to grow between the stainless steel strands and eventually coalesce. The thickness of the neointima varied between 50 and 500 μm. Pressure necrosis was not seen, but thinning and slight fibrosis of the underlying media

were observed with all stent devices. Side branches covered by these stents remained patent.

## DEPLOYMENT OF THE SELF-EXPANDING MESH STENT

During elective stenting procedures, angioplasty of the target lesion is carried out by use of standard procedures with any 8-French guiding catheter. Because until 1995 no rapid exchange system existed for the deployment of this stent, the balloon catheter was withdrawn over an 300-cm exchange guide wire. The stent is sized so that its unconstrained diameter is 10% to 20% larger than the reference diameter. This size differential not only exerts some residual radial force on the vessel wall but also ensures that the stent will be in intimate wall contact. The stent length ought to exceed the length of the diseased segment or cover the entire dissection.

The "classic" introducing system (Fig. 43–3) is prepared by aspiration preparation of the space between the outer and the inner membrane of the doubled-over constraining system. When undiluted contrast under 3 to 4 bars of pressure arrives at the

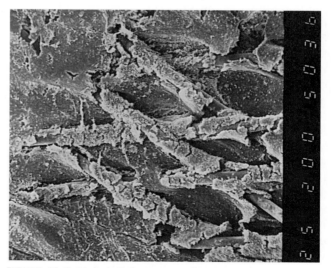

FIGURE 43–2. Endothelial coverage of stent struts 3 weeks after implantation.

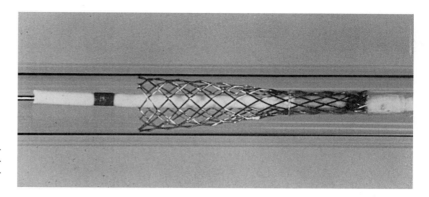

FIGURE 43–3. Original Wallstent during deployment in a glass tube. Note the constraining one-way peel-away membrane. The distal marker continuously moves leftward during deployment.

distal pinhole, the side arm stopcock may be closed and the wire lumen flushed with saline. Numerous side openings in the shaft underlying the stent allow for rinsing of the stent itself, especially if the distal wire lumen is temporarily occluded by gentle finger pressure. The new "unistep" system simply requires a saline flush through the side arm. The so-prepared stent is then advanced over the guide wire with the stent carefully positioned across the predilated area. Because the stent shortens as its diameter expands, the operator must visually estimate where the fully expanded stent will finally be positioned, and considerable experience is required for this maneuver. The constraining membrane of the classic system is inflated under a pressure of 3 bars; the new unistep sheath does not need any further preparation. Either one is then slowly withdrawn under fluoroscopic guidance. This action releases the stent into the vascular lumen. The position of the constraining membrane of the classic introducing system can be estimated by virtue of the undiluted contrast used to fill the space, but superior digital fluoroscopy is required. Three markers on the delivery catheter also help at deployment: the distal and proximal markers indicate the end of the elongated stent on the deployment instrument, and the middle marker helps to predict the extremity of the expanded stent. Because of the higher radio-opacity of the Magic Wallstent and some confusion about its appropriate position, the third marker has been eliminated on the new system. The Magic Wallstent can easily be recaptured for repositioning as long as the constraining sheath has not been retracted more than two thirds of the stent length. In order to minimize trauma, it is important not to try to correct the stent position without properly constraining the partially deployed device (Fig. 43–4). After successful deployment, the carrier catheter jumps slightly forward and can easily be moved back and forth. Finally, a balloon catheter is reintroduced over the guide wire into the stented segment, and a final inflation is performed to fully expand the stent to its desired size and embed the metal struts as thoroughly as possible into the arterial wall (sometimes

referred to as the *Swiss kiss*). Numerous angiographic and ultrasonic studies have shown that the improved appearance after stenting correlates with an abolition of the translesional gradient and with a reduction in postoperative events, such as subacute thrombosis and restenosis.

The classic rolling membrane introducing system negotiates tortuous segments more easily than the new unistep deployment catheter, which is slightly stiffer. The tapered tip design facilitates primary stenting in friable vein grafts without prior balloon dilatation. Large-diameter arteries or vein grafts can be treated with the same 1.57-mm diameter introducing catheter used for small vessels because the expansion ratio of the stent is excellent (2:4.1, corresponding to 3.0 to 6.5 mm). We have not had problems of stent migration or premature stent release, and embolization has not occurred. Apart from difficult release, in some cases, the only important problem with the classic rolling membrane has been trauma from other intravascular stents, resulting in nondeployment, and, in one case, even vessel perforation from proximal wire endings.[14]

## INDICATIONS FOR CORONARY STENTING

### Abrupt Closure

Abrupt occlusion probably arises from major intimal flaps, which reduce flow and promote thrombus formation, as well as from vessel wall recoil.[15–18] Stenting is now the standard management of this complication (Fig. 43–5). The Wallstent may well have a role to play in this indication, in particular if the dissection is long and occurs in a relatively large vessel (see Fig. 43–4). The new Magic Wallstent presents a certain advantage with respect to rapid preparation and precise placement. Newer clinical data are sparse in the literature.

### Coronary Artery Restenosis

The mechanism of restenosis is under intense investigation, but our knowledge is still limited. Patho-

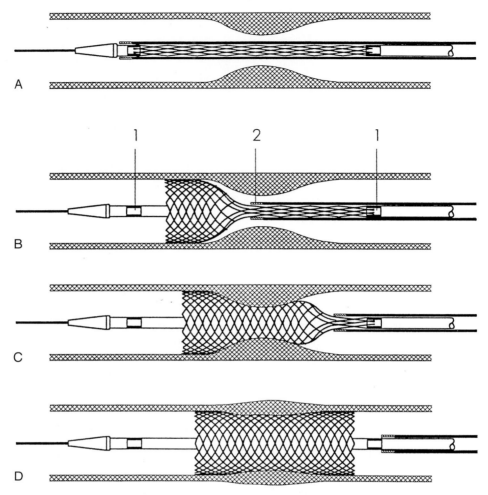

FIGURE 43–4. Deployment of the "Magic" Wallstent. *A*, The stent fully constrained on the delivery catheter. *B*, Initial deployment showing the distal and proximal radiopaque markers (1) on the delivery catheter and the distal extremity of the constraining sheath. (2) At this point, the partially deployed stent can easily be retrieved by advancing the constraining sheath. *C*, Further sheath retraction results in almost complete stent deployment. It may even be possible to reposition the stent when only a small portion is still constrained by the retractable sheath. *D*, Full, irreversible deployment of the stent within the lesion requiring further balloon dilatation. Note the relative, continuously changing position of the radiopaque markers in relation to the stent during the deployment process.

logic studies in animals and humans have shown that angioplasty involves fissuring of plaque material, sometimes not only to the level of the internal elastic membrane but also deep into the media.[16, 19] The initial plaque disruption and the rheologic consequences of a suboptimal balloon dilatation lead to the deposition of platelets and fibrin along the vessel wall. Mitogens are released both by the vessel wall and by platelets, which causes migration of smooth muscle cells to the damaged area.[20] The compromised flow and the amount of intimal and medial damage may be among the early triggers that initiate the fibromuscular proliferation that leads to restenosis.[21] Early restenosis typically occurs in the first 6 weeks after the procedure and is usually due to vascular recoil at the site of the original balloon dilatation, coronary spasm, or a major intimal flap that limits flow and is further compromised by fresh thrombus. Standard balloon dilatations with var-

ious sized balloons inflated with either low- or high-pressure inflations, for a short or prolonged duration, have not altered the incidence of restenosis.[22, 23] Apart from a trial using platelet antibodies, adjunctive medical therapy also has had little effect on rates of restenosis.[24, 25] Therefore, investigators have turned to mechanical alternatives to balloon angioplasty. There is a growing consensus that achieving the largest possible lumen diameter at the time of the procedure (acute gain) decreases the incidence of clinically significant lumen reduction, even if the unavoidable fibrointimal proliferation (late loss) is more pronounced.[26]

Depending on its design, a stent can produce a smooth surface and normal flow and prevents the elastic recoil, making it a logical device for this problem. However, any intravascular foreign body may contribute to smooth muscle cell proliferation. The stent could act as a mechanical irritant, causing

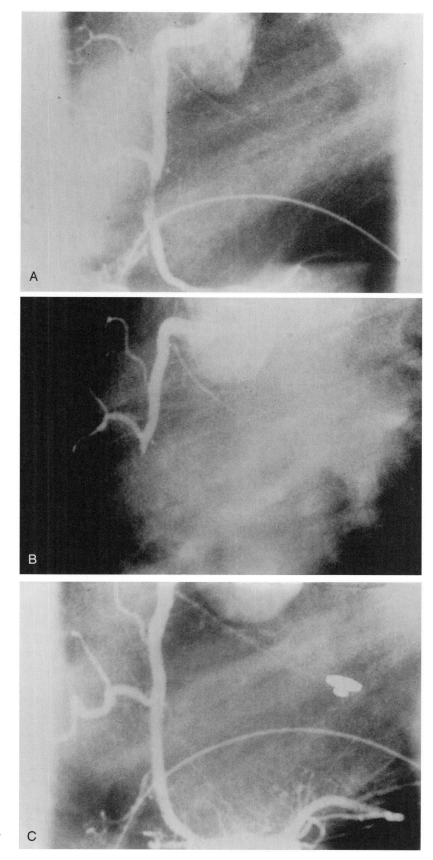

FIGURE 43–5. Abrupt closure of the right coronary artery.

the release of mediators from the adjacent endothelium, stimulating coronary spasm or intimal hyperplasia. Although initially less aggressive, self-expanding stents may exert more mechanical irritation than balloon expandable stents over time. Perhaps most worrisome, the device can become a nidus for the development of thrombus.

## Saphenous Vein Graft Stenosis

Balloon angioplasty within venous bypass grafts is well documented as having a higher restenosis rate than that in native coronary arteries. If the lesion is in the body of the graft, restenosis rates as high as 60% have been reported.[27] Stenting grafts appears to be an attractive alternative to these high restenosis rates. It is especially appealing because repeat coronary artery bypass surgery has a lower likelihood of success and an increased morbidity and mortality when compared with a first operation.[28] The Wallstent is particularly suited for this indication for several reasons: it is long and flexible, it has a high expansion rate, it has a tapered tip for primary passage without predilatation, and it has a relatively good structural support with small pores preventing tissue protrusion in friable substrates (Fig. 43–6). There is good documentation of short-term and long-term results in saphenous vein grafts.[29–31]

## CLINICAL STUDIES UTILIZING THE SELF-EXPANDING MESH STENT FOR ABRUPT OCCLUSION

We reported our early experience from Lausanne in which the intracoronary stent was used for situations of abrupt closure.[1, 2, 32–34] In the early days of

this experimental procedure, we did not have stents available at the hospital. Each situation in which a stent was indicated required us to call the company and have a device brought to the catheter laboratory. The time delay led us to the use of intracoronary urokinase in hopes of preventing the formation of thrombus along the guide wire, which remained across the occluded area. Once the procedure became more routine, a supply of stents was kept in the laboratory, decreasing the time between occlusion and stent implantation. At that time, we stopped using intracoronary urokinase.

In the early days of stenting, the median hospital stay after stent deployment for abrupt closure was 7 days. The initial angiographic follow-up of this patient subgroup suggested that the combined restenosis and late occlusion rates were lower after emergency stenting than after angioplasty alone. The angiographic rate of restenosis was 3/17 (18%) for the patients who underwent late control angiography.[1] During a mean follow-up period of 7 months, two patients had a myocardial infarction, and there were two noncardiac deaths.

Since that original report, we have deployed the self-expanding mesh stent for abrupt closure in many more patients. There was considerable variability in the rate of acute stent thrombotic complications between the operations performed in Lausanne (12%) and those done in the other sites (20%). These differences probably reflected differing anticoagulation regimens, patient selection criteria, and an important learning curve effect. The Thoraxcentre group in Rotterdam implanted 44 new, less shortening Wallstents in 35 native coronary arteries in 35 patients with acute or threatened closure after balloon angioplasty, according to a strategy of oversizing and complete coverage of the lesion

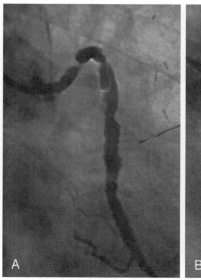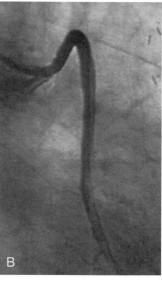

FIGURE 43–6. Wallstent implantation in a degenerate saphenous vein graft.

length. The initial and 6-month follow-up angiograms were analyzed with a quantitative coronary angiography system. Acute gain (minimal luminal diameter [MLD] after minus MLD before) and late loss (MLD after minus MLD at follow-up) were examined. Stent deployment was successful in 44 of 44 attempts (100%). The nominal stent diameter used was 1.40 mm larger than the maximal vessel diameter. One patient (3%) with a dilated but unstented lesion proximal to the stented segment sustained a subacute occlusion on day 1 that was associated with myocardial infarction. Event-free survival at 30 days after stent implantation was 97% (34 of 35 patients). Of the 34 patients eligible for 6-month angiographic follow-up, three who were asymptomatic declined repeat angiography. MLD and percent diameter stenosis changed from 0.83 ± 0.50 mm (72%) before the procedure through 3.06 ± 0.48 mm (15%) after the procedure to 2.27 ± 0.74 mm (28%) at follow-up. Acute gain was 2.23 ± 0.63 mm, and late loss was 0.78 ± 0.61 mm. Angiographic restenosis (>50 percent diameter stenosis) was observed in five of 31 patients (16%) at 6 months, all of whom underwent repeat angioplasty. Thus, the overall event-free survival at 6-month follow-up was 83%.[35]

The investigators concluded that oversized Wallstents with complete coverage of the lesion length conferred a favorable 6-month clinical and angiographic outcome. The large acute gain obtained by the Wallstent afforded greater accommodation of the subsequent late loss.

## CLINICAL RESULTS WITH THE WALLSTENT FOR DOCUMENTED RESTENOSIS

The initial 50 elective stenting procedures of native coronary arteries for restenosis in Lausanne were performed in patients with a mean of 1.6 previous angioplasties at the same site (range, 1 to 4).[3] In 46 cases, a single stent was deployed, and in four cases, two or more stents were implanted. All implants were technically successful. Temporary thrombotic occlusion occurred in two cases (4%), and permanent occlusion was observed in two additional cases (4%) during the hospital stay. Two of these patients underwent emergency surgery; one of them died after surgery from surgical complications (unrecognized tamponade). The major complication rate (Q-wave infarction, emergency surgery, or death) was 6% in hospital. After a mean follow-up period of 8 months, angiography was repeated in 34 patients from the study group. Restenosis within the stented segment occurred in four patients (12%), and stent occlusion was documented in three other patients (9%). There were three late deaths (6%). One death

occurred during elective surgery for a new left main stem coronary lesion, which occurred proximal to a stent placed near the origin of the left anterior descending artery. Two patients from this group required elective surgery for restenosis within the stent.[36]

In the multicenter experience with the self-expanding stent, the overall results were not optimal,[37] but they represent the very early learning curve of several centers, at a time when indications, technique, and postimplantation management were still not well defined.

## THE SELF-EXPANDING MESH STENT IN SAPHENOUS VEIN GRAFTS

In the initial Lausanne-London series, 56 patients received stents for stenosis within a saphenous vein bypass graft.[38] On several occasions, stenting was performed in old grafts that were diffusely diseased and would not have been considered appropriate targets for balloon angioplasty alone (see Fig. 43–6). The implantation procedure for bypass grafts sometimes varied from the one we described for native coronary arteries. To avoid the potential embolization of friable plaque material or thrombus, the stent was inserted before any dilatations were made with a standard balloon catheter. In this series, we attempted implantation of 78 self-expanding stents in bypass grafts of 56 patients during 60 separate procedures. The stent diameter ranged from 3.5 to 6 mm (mean, 4.7 mm), and the length from 15 to 30 mm (mean, 24 mm). Angiographic success was achieved in 59 procedures (98%). There was one case of subacute stent occlusion and one in-hospital death. Transfusion or surgical repair of the vascular access site was required for five procedures (8%) because of bleeding. At follow-up, restenosis was documented in four patients (7%), and myocardial infarction occurred in one patient. There were two late deaths (34%).

The Rotterdam experience with the Wallstent in saphenous vein grafts[39] comprised 69 patients with a 100% implantation success rate. There were four deaths, seven patients had a myocardial infarction, and coronary artery bypass grafting was required for six. The overall early clinical success was 87%, and the restenosis rate was 47%.

The immediate and long-term results for elective stenting of venous bypass grafts with the self-expanding device were better than the results for stenting native coronary vessels. This is probably due to the larger diameter of vein grafts, which allows larger stents to be implanted. Perhaps the lack of vasomotor tone and the generally higher compliance of venous bypass grafts also play a role. Anecdotal observations from explanted grafts with stents seem to indicate that there are many fewer degenerative changes in the stented segment than in the rest of the vessel. The combination of an acceptably low complication rate and the low rate of restenosis makes elective stenting of venous bypass grafts probably the best indication for the use of the self-expanding mesh stent at this time.

## WALLSTENTS FOR CHRONIC TOTAL OCCLUSIONS

Although the use of Wallstents after recanalization of chronic occlusions is common clinical practice, only one study has been published to date.[14] The goal of the trial was to examine whether oversized Wallstents of the new type provide a more favorable outcome and lower restenosis rate than balloon angioplasty alone.

Wallstents were implanted in 20 patients (20 lesions) and postdilated with pressures averaging 14 bars. The acute gain was significantly larger than in the balloon-only group consisting of 249 patients (266 lesions), but the late loss was equally large in the Wallstent group. The net result, however, was still in favor of stenting, and restenosis was seen in 29% of the Wallstent group and in 45% of the balloon group. This difference must be viewed with some caution because of the sample size.

## CONTRAINDICATIONS FOR CORONARY USE OF WALLSTENTS

Relative contraindications to coronary stenting with the self-expanding device should be considered whenever possible:

- Vessel size below 3 mm
- Markedly funnel-shaped segments (currently available stents are cylindrical)
- Very tight bend in the target segment (because it would promote important shear forces at both stent extremities)
- Insufficient flow anticipated through the prosthesis after implantation caused by either poor distal runoff or extensive collateralization (stasis at stent level favors thrombus formation)
- Anticipated difficulty with the antiplatelet medication regimen.

## RESTENOSIS AFTER STENT PLACEMENT

Experimental animal data, histologic data from percutaneous atherectomy,[40] and surgical material excised from stented segments all have documented that stent restenosis is due to excessive fibrointimal proliferation. One predictor for stent restenosis appears to be the timing of the deployment after the original angioplasty procedure. In a group of patients treated for restenosis in Lausanne, the recurrence rate was 6% in patients who were stented more than 3 months after their initial angioplasty, but it was 41% for those stented within 3 months. Similar observations have been made with other stents and other techniques, such as percutaneous directional atherectomy. These findings and the well-known time course for restenosis after standard balloon dilatation suggest that the process of fibrointimal proliferation may have a period of hyperactivity that would be difficult to alter with mechanical interventions alone.

Restenosis in the area covered by a self-expanding stent cannot be dealt with as successfully as in the case of balloon expandable stents. The reason for this difference lies in the fact that a firmly embedded self-expanding stent cannot easily be enlarged any further: if the stent has reached its nominal (i.e., maximal) diameter (either passively, by intrastent balloon inflation at the time of implantation, or actively, through its self-expanding property during the first weeks of follow-up), further expansion is impossible. Even if the stent has not reached its nominal diameter, further stent enlargement would produce shortening that cannot be achieved because of the lack of axial elasticity of the arterial wall. High-pressure balloon inflations, sometimes requiring 20 bars or more, may effectively enlarge the lumen by pressing the fibromuscular encroachment through the metal skeleton. Debulking with atherectomy, rotablation, or laser is feasible and may result in a reasonably good long-term outcome. Conversely, coronary stenting does not jeopardize the patient's chances of benefiting from elective surgical revascularization, should it become necessary.

## COMPLICATIONS

The process of inserting the self-expanding mesh stent is not normally a source of complications. The stent deployment adds only a few minutes to the procedure's time. Removing the classic doubled-over retaining membrane, which holds the self-expanding stent on the introducer catheter, can be difficult. In most situations, this problem responds to increasing the pressure beyond 3 bars between the membranes, but rarely, the position of the guide catheter must also be changed before the membrane can be fully withdrawn. The new coated sheath currently used should contribute to a smoother retraction.

Occasionally, partially deployed stents have been

removed without important sequelae. Investigators have not seen evidence of side branch occlusion, except in the case in which a stent was placed in an area of fresh thrombus that involved a side branch. There have been no reported cases of stent erosion or infectious complications. One complication involved deployment failure and coronary perforation.[41]

The major morbidity associated with stent implantation is the potential for a thrombotic event occurring acutely or, unpredictably, in the first 4 weeks (or even longer) after the procedure. This is in contradistinction to balloon angioplasty, in which complications are generally not seen beyond the first 24 hours after the procedure. A short-term antiplatelet regimen is mandatory. The previous use of oral anticoagulation with warfarin (Coumadin) has led to local bleeding complications at the arterial puncture site (8% of cases in Lausanne). Some of these patients required blood transfusions and surgical repair of the femoral artery. Optimal femoral compression after the procedure is important. A pneumatic compression device (Femostop, Radi Medical; Uppsala, Sweden), which allows prolonged pressure without compromising arterial flow, is now being used in all our cases. Other, newer hemostatic devices may also help overcome arterial bleeding problems and may even allow outpatient stenting.

Several risk factors for acute stent thrombosis have become apparent. Small-diameter stents carry a greater risk of thrombosis than do large ones. This observation probably explains the lower complication rate observed when vein grafts are stented. Generally, bypass grafts are at least 3.5 mm in diameter and allow placement of stents at least 4 mm in their unconstrained diameter. We do not recommend stenting of arteries that are smaller than 3 mm in diameter as measured by quantitative coronary angiography or intravascular ultrasound with self-expanding Wallstents.

Certain clinical situations promote thrombotic complications. Investigators have noted that patients with increased platelet counts are more likely to experience thrombotic complications. Systemic hypotension, poor distal runoff, untreated significant proximal lesions, uncovered dissection flaps proximal or distal to the stent, and well-developed collaterals can all decrease flow through the stented vessel and therefore potentiate thrombus formation.

With increasing experience and better patient selection, acute thrombotic events have become less frequent. During the first half of the Lausanne series, we observed thrombotic events in 14% of the procedures, versus 6% for the following 49 cases. Provided that a catheterization laboratory is immediately available, acute stent thrombosis can often be treated effectively by balloon angioplasty and thrombolytic agents. When it is reversed, it does not appear to compromise the long-term results. The procedure is fairly straightforward if thrombosis occurs during the first hours after implantation, when the femoral sheath is still in place. The situation is more complex after the sheath has been removed because a second arterial puncture becomes necessary. If a thrombotic event occurs more than 2 days after stent deployment, our experience indicates that systemic thrombolysis can be beneficial; a pneumatic compression device, however, must be placed on the puncture site.

In animal studies, a diameter mismatch (ratio >1.5) between the self-expanding stent and the recipient vessel was associated with thrombotic occlusion. Although this degree of mismatch has not been reported in clinical practice, the turbulent flow induced at the stent's extremities could contribute to thrombus formation. This makes optimal sizing an important factor, especially because good strut impaction is probably equally important for preventing thrombus formation.[42]

## ADJUNCT MEDICATION

Early experimental evidence showed that heparin significantly decreased the rate of acute thrombotic occlusions when it was given perioperatively for stenting of normal canine arteries.[1] Other workers using balloon-expandable stents in animals showed that aspirin was superior to warfarin in preventing subsequent stent thrombosis.[9] The evidence favoring the use of low molecular weight dextran during the implantation procedure is debatable. At present, no study has been performed that proves a beneficial effect of low molecular weight dextran in this context.

The drug regimen we previously employed with Wallstents required a high degree of patient compliance. Before the stent procedure, patients still received aspirin in addition to their usual medication. In the catheterization laboratory, intravenous heparin, normally 10,000 to 15,000 U, was administered, and the activated clotting time (ACT) was to be at least 300 seconds at all times. After the procedure, the arterial sheath was removed as soon as possible, normally after 4 to 5 hours, and a Femostop was placed onto the puncture site for at least 3 hours at low pressure. In the early years, heparin used to be reinstituted 12 hours after the procedure and continued until oral anticoagulation was effective (International Normalized Ratio for prothrombin time ≥ 2.3). Aspirin, 100 mg daily, and dipyridamole, 100 mg three times daily, were also prescribed for all patients. Medication was usually continued for 3 to 6 months, until control angiography was performed. All patients received calcium blocking agents to prevent the possibility of stent-induced coronary spasm. Current management, based on the relatively recent notion that antiplatelet medication is more efficient and safer than typical oral anticoagulation,[43] includes the combination of aspirin and ticlopidine or clopidogrel for just 3 weeks.

## ONGOING WALLSTENT TRIALS

The Wallstent is still being tested in a number of ongoing investigations. Some are conducted in the United States and are intended to provide material for U.S. Food and Drug Administration approval processes. The Wallstent Study, led by the Atlanta Cardiology Group, is one of these trials: It is an open-label, multicenter investigation randomly assigning patients with documented restenosis to balloon angioplasty or Wallstent implantation in target lesions less than 20 mm long in vessels of at least 3.0 mm in diameter. Four hundred fifty patients are to be enrolled to test the safety and efficacy of this stent in reducing subsequent restenosis after the first occurrence of restenosis. The results of the Magic SL Study have not yet been formally published. They indicate a linear relationship between stent length and restenosis.

The Wallstent is equally one of the devices used in the SOS (Stent or Surgery) Trial which compares, in a randomized multicenter prospective study, the outcome of two treatment strategies: coronary artery bypass surgery versus stenting in multivessel disease in 1000 patients.[44] This trial finished recruiting patients in December 1999 and reported its findings for the first time in March 2001. In comparison with bypass surgery, multivessel stent implantation resulted in a slightly lower survival rate. Complete follow-up and formal study publication has not occurred.

## CONCLUSIONS

After more than 10 years of clinical study, coronary stenting has given us good reason for optimism. The Wallstent was the first such device used in clinical medicine. Wallstents can be inserted under circumstances of abrupt closure in almost all coronary segments. These self-expanding stents are now much easier to use and constitute a reasonable alternative to other balloon-expandable stents. Although no randomized data exist, the observations with self-expanding devices suggest that restenosis may be favorably influenced by stent implantation in selected subgroups, particularly for patients with saphenous vein graft lesions. Subacute thrombosis has lost much of its menace and is no longer the dreaded

complication of coronary stenting. Despite the encouraging low rates of recurrence, late restenosis has now become the "Achilles heel" of coronary stenting.

We believe that coronary stents are the most promising development in the field of interventional cardiology. Many researchers now believe that the fight against restenosis will have to include the use of pharmacologic weapons and possibly physical energy. Whether a combination of these approaches will finally prove optimal is an unresolved issue, but it does seem likely that new devices will be forthcoming that will be less thrombogenic and less likely to stimulate intimal hyperplasia.

## REFERENCES

1. Sigwart U, Puel J, Mirkovitch V, et al: Intravascular stents to prevent occlusion and restenosis after transluminal angioplasty. N Engl J Med 316:701–770, 1987.
2. Sigwart U, Urban P, Golf S, et al: Emergency stenting for acute occlusion following coronary balloon angioplasty. Circulation 78:1121–1127, 1988.
3. Sigwart U, Kaufmann U, Goy JJ, et al: Prevention of coronary restenosis by stenting. Eur Heart J 9(suppl C):31–37, 1988.
4. Urban P, Sigwart U, Golf S, et al: Intravascular stenting for stenosis of aorto-coronary venous bypass grafts. J Am Coll Cardiol 13:1085–1091, 1989.
5. Maass D, Demierre D, Deaton D, et al: Transluminal implantation of self-adjusting expandable prostheses: Principles, techniques and results. Prog Artif Org 27:979–987, 1983.
6. Wright KC, Wallace S, Charnsangavej C, et al: Percutaneous endovascular stents: An experimental evaluation. Radiology 156:69–72, 1985.
7. Charnsangavej C, Carrasco CH, Wallace S, et al: Stenosis of the vena cava: Preliminary assessment of treatment with expandable metallic stents. Radiology 161:295–298, 1986.
8. Rousseau H, Puel J, Joffre F, et al: Self-expanding endovascular prosthesis: An experimental study. Radiology 164:709–714, 1987.
9. Roubin GS, Robinson KA, King SB, et al: Early and late results of intracoronary arterial stenting after coronary angioplasty in dogs. Circulation 76:891–897, 1987.
10. Palmaz JC, Garcia OJ, Kopp DT, et al: Balloon expandable intra-arterial stents: effect of anticoagulation on thrombus formation [Abstract]. Circulation 76(suppl IV):IV–45, 1987.
11. Schatz RA, Palmaz JC, Tio FO, et al: Balloon-expandable intracoronary stents in the adult dog. Circulation 76:450–457, 1987.
12. Palmaz JC, Sibbitt RR, Tio FO, et al: Expandable intraluminal vascular graft: A feasibility study. Surgery 99:199–205, 1986.
13. Palmaz JC: Balloon-expandable intravascular stents. Am J Radiol 150:1263–1269, 1988.
14. Ozaki Y, Violaris AG, Hamburger J, et al: Short and long term results with the new, less shortening Wallstent for vessel reconstruction in chronic total occlusion: A quantitative angiographic study J Am Coll Cardiol 28:354–360, 1996.
15. Waller BF: Coronary luminal shape and the arc of disease free wall: Morphologic observations and clinical relevance. J Am Coll Cardiol 6:1100–1108, 1985.
16. Waller BF: Crackers, breakers, stretchers, shavers, burners, welders and melters: The future treatment of atherosclerotic coronary artery disease? A clinical and morphological assessment. J Am Coll Cardiol 13:969–987, 1989.
17. Cragg A, Amplatz K: Vascular pathophysiology of transluminal angioplasty. In Jang GD (ed): Angioplasty, pp 145–155. New York: McGraw-Hill, 1986.
18. Block PC: Mechanism of transluminal angioplasty. Am J Cardiol 53:69C–78C, 1984.
19. Liu MW, Roubin GS, King SB: Restenosis after coronary angioplasty: Potential biologic determinants and role of intimal hyperplasia. Circulation 79:1374–1387, 1989.

20. Steele PM, Chesebro JH, Stanson AW, et al: Balloon angioplasty: Natural history of the pathophysiological response to injury in a pig model. Circ Res 57:105–112, 1985.
21. Carter AJ, Laird JR, Farb A, et al: Morphologic characteristics of lesion formation and time course of smooth muscle cell proliferation in a porcine proliferative restenosis model. J Am Coll Cardiol 24:1398–1405, 1994.
22. Roubin GS, Douglas TJ, King SB, et al: Influence of balloon size on initial success, acute complications, and restenosis after percutaneous transluminal coronary angioplasty: A prospective randomized study. Circulation 78:557–565, 1988.
23. Meier B, Grüntzig A, King SB, et al: Higher balloon dilatation pressure in coronary angioplasty. Am Heart J 107:619–622, 1984.
24. Kuntz RE, Safian RD, Carrozza JP, et al: The importance of acute luminal diameter in determining restenosis after coronary atherectomy or stenting. Circulation 86:1827–1835, 1992.
25. Côté G, Myler RK, Stertzer SH, et al: Percutaneous transluminal angioplasty of stenotic coronary artery grafts: 5 years' experience. J Am Coll Cardiol 9:8–17, 1987.
26. Loop FD, Cosgrove DM, Kramer JR: Late clinical and arteriographic results in 500 coronary artery reoperations. J Thorac Cardiovasc Surg 81:675–685, 1981.
27. Strauss BH, Serruys PW, Bertrand ME, et al: Quantitative angiographic follow-up of the coronary Wallstent in native vessels and bypass grafts: The evolving European experience from March 1986 to March 1990. Am J Cardiol 69:475–481, 1992.
28. Stewart JT, Williams MG, Goy JJ, et al: Self-expanding stents for diseased saphenous vein coronary artery bypass grafts [Abstract]. J Am Coll Cardiol 19:49, 1992.
29. Kelly PA, Kurbaan AS, Sigwart U: Total endovascular reconstruction of occluded saphenous vein grafts using coronary or peripheral Wallstents [Abstract]. Circulation 94:258, 1996.
30. Urban P, Sigwart U: The self-expanding mesh stent. In Sigwart U, Frank GI (eds): Coronary Stents, pp 24–44. New York: Berlin-Heidelberg, 1992.
31. Goy JJ, Sigwart U, Vogt P, et al: Long-term clinical and angiographic follow-up of patients treated with the self-expanding coronary stent for acute occlusion during balloon angioplasty of the right coronary artery. J Am Coll Cardiol 19:1593–1596, 1992.
32. Nordrehaug JE, Priestley KA, Chronos N, et al: Self-expanding stents for emergency treatment of acute vessel closure following coronary angioplasty: Immediate and long term results. J Intervent Cardiol 7:161–164, 1994.
33. Goy JJ, Sigwart U, Vogt P, et al: Long term follow-up of the first 56 patients treated with intracoronary self-expanding stents (the Lausanne experience). Am J Cardiol 67:569–572, 1991.
34. Serruys PW, Strauss BH, de Feyter P, et al: The Wallstent, a self-expanding stent. J Invasive Cardiol 3:127–134, 1991.
35. Ozaki Y, Keane D, Ruygrok P, et al: Six-month clinical and angiographic outcome of the new, less shortening Wallstent in native coronary arteries. Circulation 93:2114–2120, 1996.
36. Stewart JT, Williams MG, Goy JJ, et al: The use of self-expanding stents for coronary graft stenoses [Abstract]. Eur Heart J 12(suppl):243, 1991.
37. de Scheerder IK, Strauss BH, de Feyter PJ, et al: Stenting of venous bypass grafts: A new treatment modality for patients who are poor candidates for reintervention. Am Heart J 123:1046–1054, 1992.
38. Strauss BH, Umans VA, van Suylen RJ, et al: Directional atherectomy for treatment of restenosis within coronary stents: Clinical, angiographic, and histological results. J Am Coll Cardiol 20:1465–1473, 1992.
39. Sigwart U, Kaufmann U, Golf S, et al: L'incidence et le traitement de la résténose coronairienne malgré l'implantation d'une endoprothèse. Schweiz Med Wochenschr 118:1715–1718, 1988.
40. Selmon M, Robertson G, Hinohara T, et al: Factors associated with restenosis following successful peripheral atherectomy [Abstract]. J Am Coll Cardiol 13:13A, 1989.
41. Mendzelevski B, Sigwart U: Rupture of coronary artery and cardiac tamponade complicating Wallstent implantation. Cathet Cardiovasc Diagn 40:1–4, 1997.
42. Nath FC, Muller DWM, Ellis SG, et al: Thrombosis of a flexible coil coronary stent: Frequency, predictors and clinical outcome. J Am Coll Cardiol 21:622–627, 1993.
43. Schömig A, Neuman FJ, Kastrati A, et al: A randomised comparison of antiplatelet and anticoagulant therapy after the placement of coronary artery stents. N Engl J Med 334(17):1126–1128, 1996.
44. Stables R, and SOS Trial Investigators: Design of the "Stent or Surgery" (SOS) Trial. Semin Interv Cardiol 4:201–207, 1999.

# 44

# The AVE Microstent: Evolutions in Design and Clinical Utility

*Jeffrey Moses      Issam Moussa      Antonio Colombo*

The practice of invasive cardiology has undergone a revolution as it has moved from a purely diagnostic subspecialty to one with well-documented potential for improving the health of patients. Beginning with the innovative development of the angioplasty technique by Andreas Gruentzig in the late 1970s,[1] the field has evolved tremendously. However, despite experienced operators and improved catheter technology, acute vessel closure and late restenosis are inherently associated with percutaneous transluminal coronary angioplasty (PTCA) and continue to compromise its overall efficacy.[2–5] Acute closure, thought to be a combination of dissection, recoil, spasm, and thrombus formation, occurs in 2% to 10% of patients and is associated with significant morbidity and mortality.[6–8] Even with emergency coronary artery bypass surgery, acute coronary occlusion is associated with a 2% to 10% mortality and an occurrence of myocardial infarction in 25% to 44% of patients.[9]

A second generation of new devices has been developed to remedy problems with traditional PTCA. One of these devices is the intracoronary stent. Beginning with Dotter's work on a stainless steel endoluminal prosthesis in the late 1960s,[10] the development of stents has progressed steadily. At present, a number of different stents are available, each with its own specific design, physicochemical characteristics, and mode of implantation. Distinction can be made between self-expanding[11, 12] and balloon-expandable stents.[13] The former can be constrained to a small diameter, which then expands to a predetermined dimension when the constraint is removed. The latter relies on plastic deformation of metal beyond its elastic limits. Stents are beneficial to treat vessel closure after failed coronary intervention[14, 15] and to reduce restenosis in simple lesions.[16, 17]

## ACHIEVEMENTS AND LIMITATIONS OF CORONARY STENTING

Significant progress has been made with coronary stenting, from the use of intravascular ultrasound guidance and high balloon inflation pressure for stent optimization[18–21] to advances in pharmacologic therapy after stenting.[22–24] This progress in addition to the availability of new stent designs has expanded indications for coronary stenting to more complex disease.[25–33]

The ideal stent is expected to fulfill the promise of expanding the indications of catheter-based coronary interventions with a high degree of success and low number of complications; this stent would be of low profile and flexible enough to allow easy placement; biocompatible with the coronary artery, that is, nonthrombogenic; of sufficient radial strength and metal surface area to prevent acute recoil, plaque prolapse, and chronic vessel remodeling; and available in several lengths to accommodate various clinical settings with mild radiopacity or edge markers to enable precise placement.

The introduction of the Applied Vascular Engineering (AVE) Microstent and its evolution to the present design represent significant progress toward fulfilling the promise of an ideal stent that could be utilized in simple as well as complex coronary abnormalities. The purpose of this chapter is to review the development, design, and clinical utility of the AVE Microstent.

## STENT DESIGN, HISTORY, AND DEVELOPMENT

The initial clinical evaluation of the AVE Microstent began in August 1993 with the prototype (Microstent PL). This stent is made of 316L stainless steel with strut thickness of 0.008 inches and consists of four-crown, 4-mm units, unconnected and premounted on a semicompliant delivery system (Fig. 44–1A). The major limitations with this design are stent unit separation and the lack of appropriate lesion coverage. In August 1994, the Microstent I was released (Fig. 44–1B,C). This second-generation stent is also made of 316L stainless steel, formed of four-crown, 4-mm subunits (half-connected to form

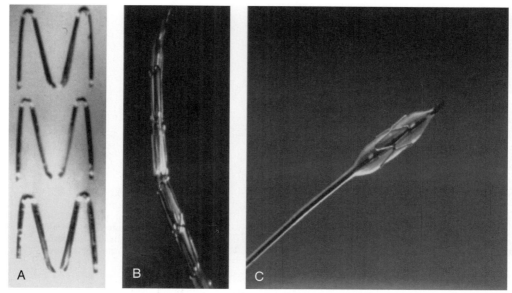

FIGURE 44–1. *A*, Microstent PL, unconnected four-crown, 4-mm segments. *B*, Microstent I, half-connected 8-mm segments consisting of four-crown, 4-mm subunits mounted on a semicompliant delivery system. *C*, Magnified image of an 8-mm Microstent I.

8-mm segments) premounted on a semicompliant delivery system. However, stent migration and large mass (strut thickness 0.008 inches) are still a limitation with this design.

Therefore, in October 1995 the Microstent II was introduced to the clinical arena. This design is characterized by having proprietary 3-mm sinusoidal subunits with continuous helical connections and thinner struts (0.006 inches), with no sharp edges or corners and smooth electropolished surface (Fig. 44–2). The delivery system has a usable length of 135 cm, compatible with 0.014-inch guide wires, has distal and proximal radiopaque balloon markers, and is available in rapid-exchange and over-the-wire systems. This design is characterized by improved flexibility and a lower profile and eliminates the risk of subunit migration. However, to expand the applicability of this design to long lesions and small vessels, two other designs were introduced in January 1996: the Microstent II XL and the Microstent 2.5. The Microstent II XL is available in 30- and 39-mm lengths mounted on a

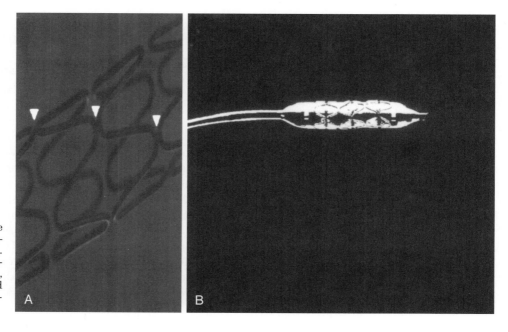

FIGURE 44–2. *A*, Microstent II; the *white arrows* point to the connections between the stent subunits. *B*, Magnified image of the Microstent II illustrating the four-crown, 3-mm subunits, fully connected and premounted on a semicompliant delivery system.

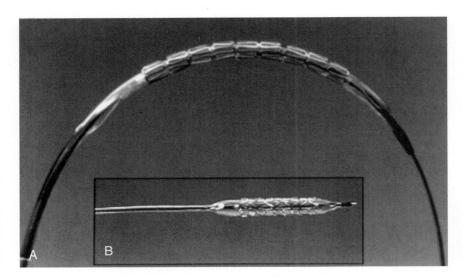

FIGURE 44–3. *A*, Microstent GFX in its elliptorectangular six-crown design and 2-mm subunits fully connected and premounted on a semicompliant delivery system in an unexpanded state. *B*, Microstent GFX in an expanded state.

delivery system with low-rated burst pressure. The Microstent 2.5 was designed to treat small vessels; this stent is compatible with 6-French guiding catheters (0.064-inch ID), has various lengths (6, 9, 12, and 18 mm), and has a lower crossing profile (0.069 inches).

The latest evolution in design was the introduction of the GFX Microstent (Fig. 44–3) in August 1996. This stent has even thinner struts (0.005 inches), which translates into a lower profile than previous designs; shorter subunits (2 mm), which leads to increased flexibility; and six crowns, which provide better plaque. Each stent length is the same design, with the deployment balloon the only variable that determines the diameter at expansion with no shortening and minimal recoil (4%). A radiopaque gold marker is located at the proximal and distal end of the stent to assist in precise placement. A comparison among all stent designs is shown in Table 44–1.

## CLINICAL STUDIES: THE COLUMBUS CLINIC AND LENOX HILL HOSPITAL EXPERIENCE

## Methods

### Patient Population

From November 1993 to September 1996, a total of 137 patients (159 lesions) underwent implantation of AVE stents (199 stents). In 87 patients (63%), the AVE stent was the only stent implanted at the culprit lesion (106 lesions, 126 stents). In 50 patients (37%), the AVE stent was used as a bailout device after implanting other stents (50 lesions, 70 stents). Therefore, two distinct scenarios are discussed: the use of the AVE Microstent for de novo lesions and its use as a bailout device after implantation of other stents.

### Stent Implantation Procedure

Intracoronary stenting was performed using techniques previously described.[18] Several designs of the Microstent were used. In our early experience, 4-mm separate unconnected units (Microstent PL) were used; then fully connected or half-connected stents (Microstent I) were utilized. The introduction of the Microstent II family (12, 16, 18, and 24-mm) was followed by Microstent II XL (30 and 39 mm) and finally the GFX Microstent (18 mm).

After stent implantation, high-pressure balloon inflations were performed to achieve an acceptable angiographic result with less than 20% residual stenosis by visual estimate. After the angiographic result was considered acceptable, intravascular ultrasonography was performed in only 47 lesions (44%), mainly because of the complex anatomic locations in which the use of intravascular ultrasonography seemed unsafe. Subsequent treatment decisions were based on the ultrasound results (if obtained) and the angiographic assessment.

### Angiographic Analysis

Coronary angiography was done in a routine manner. Patients received intracoronary nitroglycerin before initial, final, and follow-up angiograms to achieve maximal vasodilatation. Angiographic measurements were done with digital electronic calipers (Brown and Sharp) from an optically magnified image in the view that shows the most severe narrowing by an experienced angiographer blinded to the intravascular ultrasound measurements. The guiding catheter was used as the reference for magnification calibration. Previous studies have shown that digital calipers correlate closely with computer-assisted methods, with a low interobserver and intraobserver variability.[34]

Lesions were classified according to the modified

**TABLE 44–1.    A COMPARISON AMONG VARIOUS GENERATIONS OF THE AVE MICROSTENT**

|  | MICROSTENT PL | MICROSTENT I | MICROSTENT II* | GFX MICROSTENT |
|---|---|---|---|---|
| Generation | 1st | 2nd | 3rd | 4th |
| Material | 316L stainless steel | 316L stainless steel | 316L stainless steel | 316L stainless steel |
| Design | Single elements with no connections | 8-mm segments | Sinusoidal continuous elements | Elliptorectangular continuous elements |
| Strut thickness (in.) | 0.008 | 0.008 | 0.006–0.008 | 0.005 |
| Diameter (mm) | 3–4 | 3–4 | 2.5–4 | Limited release: 3–4 |
| Lengths (mm) | 8 and 12 | 4, 8, and 16 | 6, 9, 12, 18, 24, 30, and 39 | 18 |
| Number of crowns | 4 | 4 | 4 | 6 |
| Subunit length (mm) | 4 | 4 | 3 | 2 |
| Minimal guide catheter ID (in.) | 0.076 | 0.076 | 0.064–0.076 | 0.064 |
| Profile (in.) | — | 0.070 | 0.069 | 0.060 |
| Shortening | — | — | 2 | None |
| Metal surface area (%) | — | — | 8.5 | 20 |
| Recoil (%) | — | 5 | 6 | 4 |

AVE, Applied Vascular Engineering; ID, internal diameter.
*Includes Microstent II, Microstent II XL, and Microstent 2.5.

American Heart Association–American College of Cardiology (AHA-ACC) classification. Long lesions were defined as a single continuous narrowing longer than 15 mm. Bifurcational lesions were defined as lesions that are located at a bifurcation involving a branch at least 1.5 mm in size. The presence of proximal tortuosity, angiographic calcifications, and lesion location at a bend was recorded and analyzed.

### Postprocedural Pharmacologic Therapy

After a successful procedure, patients were treated only with antiplatelet agents (85 patients), either aspirin 325 mg/day alone (16 patients) or in combination with ticlopidine 250 mg orally twice daily for 1 month (67 patients). Only two patients received warfarin (Coumadin). One-month follow-up was performed in all patients by an interview or a telephone conversation with the patient or the referring physician.

## Results

### Patient and Lesion Characteristics

Baseline clinical and angiographic characteristics are shown in Table 44–2. Clearly, there was a high frequency of complex lesions in this cohort. Severe proximal tortuosity was present in 10 lesions (9%), location at a bend greater than 45 was present in 15 lesions (14%), severe calcifications requiring rotablation were present in 11 lesions (10%), and location at bifurcation was present in 42 lesions (40%).

### Indications for Stenting and Procedural Characteristics

Coronary stenting was elective in 38 lesions (35%), for restenosis in 13 lesions (12%), for chronic total

occlusions in 3 lesions (3%), for a suboptimal result after PTCA in 26 lesions (25%), and for bailout after PTCA in 26 lesions (25%). In 12 lesions, the AVE Microstent was used after failure of delivery of other stents (six Palmaz-Schatz (PS), four NIR, two BeStent). In addition, bifurcational stenting with the AVE stent was performed in 12 lesions (11%).

The mean number of stents per lesion was 1.2 ±

**TABLE 44–2.    BASELINE CLINICAL AND ANGIOGRAPHIC CHARACTERISTICS**

| PATIENTS (MEAN AGE = 61 ± 9 y) | NUMBER (%) |
|---|---|
| Clinical characteristics (patient N = 86) | |
| Male gender | 72 (84) |
| Previous myocardial infarction | 45 (52) |
| LVEF (mean %) | 57 ± 10 |
| Unstable angina* | 24 (29) |
| Multivessel disease | 57 (70) |
| Angiographic characteristics (lesion N = 106) | |
| Vessel dilated | |
| LAD | 33 (31) |
| LCX | 34 (32) |
| RCA | 35 (33) |
| Left main | 2 (2) |
| SVG | 2 (2) |
| Lesion site | |
| Ostial | 16 (15) |
| Proximal | 23 (22) |
| Midvessel | 35 (33) |
| Distal | 32 (30) |
| Modified AHA/ACC lesion type | |
| A | 3 (3) |
| B1 | 26 (25) |
| B2 | 50 (47) |
| C | 27 (25) |

AHA/ACC, American Heart Association/American College of Cardiology classification; LAD, left anterior descending; LCX, left circumflex; LVEF, left ventricular ejection fraction; RCA, right coronary artery; SVG, saphenous vein graft.
*Canadian Cardiovascular Society angina classification.

0.7 (range, one to five stents) and per vessel 2 ± 2. The final balloon size used for stent optimization was 3.28 ± 0.38 mm with a balloon/vessel ratio of 1.2 ± 0.2 and maximal balloon inflation pressure of 15 ± 4 atm.

### Angiographic and Intravascular Ultrasound Analysis

Baseline and postprocedural angiographic measurements are shown in Table 44–3. A total of 47 lesions (44%) underwent intravascular ultrasound–guided stenting. The postprocedural intrastent minimal lumen cross-sectional area was 5.97 ± 1.87 mm², that is, smaller than the average reference lumen cross-sectional area of 6.87 ± 2.37 mm² ($p = 0.02$) and similar to the distal reference lumen cross-sectional area of 6.16 ± 2.27 mm² ($p = 0.08$). The postprocedural intrastent minimal lumen diameter was 2.55 ± 0.43 mm.

### Procedural Success, Complications, and 1-Month Outcome

Initial stent implantation was angiographically successful in 103 lesions (97%). Delivery failure was encountered in three lesions, migration in five stents (all were first-generation Microstents), recoil requiring implantation of a second stent in one lesion, and significant plaque prolapse in two lesions.

Procedural complications occurred in four patients (4.5%). One patient (1.1%) underwent emergency bypass surgery, one patient (1.1%) had Q-wave myocardial infarction, one patient (1.1%) had non–Q-wave myocardial infarction, and one patient (1.1%) had a vascular complication. At 1-month follow-up after hospital discharge, only one patient (1.1%) had subacute stent thrombosis, but there were no deaths.

### Incidence and Predictors of Restenosis

A total of 41 out of 106 lesions (40%) had angiographic follow-up at 4.6 ± 1.5 months. Angio-graphic restenosis (defined by >50% diameter stenosis) occurred in 19 lesions (46%). However, angiographic follow-up was not performed in a routine manner, and only patients with symptoms returned for a repeat angiogram; therefore, the angiographic restenosis presented here is artifactually skewed toward a high restenosis rate. Patients with restenosis had smaller mean reference vessel diameters (2.48 ± 0.47 mm vs. 2.86 ± 0.58 mm, $p = 0.03$) but no difference in lesion length (6.25 ± 4.14 mm vs. 6.39 ± 2.99 mm, $p = 0.9$) and the number of stents per lesion (1.2 ± 0.5 vs. 1.2 ± 0.4, $p = 0.99$). In addition, final stent expansion in the restenosis group was done using balloons with a higher balloon/vessel ratio compared with the no-restenosis group (1.3 ± 0.2 vs. 1.2 ± 0.2, $p = 0.03$), which resulted in a similar postprocedural minimal lumen diameter (2.63 ± 0.39 mm vs. 2.81 ± 0.60 mm, $p = 0.26$) in the restenosis and no-restenosis group, respectively. Table 44–4 shows factors predictive of restenosis using simple logistic regression analysis, but when these factors were entered into a multivariate logistic regression model, none had a significant predictive value. However, it is important to keep in mind that such an analysis is of limited value because of the small number of observations.

### The Microstent as a Bailout Device After Implantation of Other Stents

The Microstent was used to treat complications that had arisen after using other stents in 50 patients (50 lesions): 17 patients treated initially with the PS stent, 16 patients treated with Gianturco-Roubin stent, 6 patients treated with Wiktor stent, 4 patients treated with BeStent, 3 patients treated with Cordis stent, 2 patients treated with the NIR stent, 1 patient treated with ACS stent, and 1 patient treated with the Wallstent.

Reasons for Microstent implantation in these cases included distal dissections (16 patients), plaque prolapse (3 patients), gap between stents (2 patients), recoil inside other stents (3 patients), and uncovered disease distal to stents (24 patients). Delivery failure of the Microstent occurred in only 2 patients (4%).

## Discussion

### A Review of Currently Available Data

Prospective randomized trials comparing the AVE stent to other stent designs are in progress. The SMART trial is a multicenter prospective randomized study that was initiated in November 1995 comparing the PS stent to the Microstent. Enrollment was closed in November 1996. AVE stents

**TABLE 44–3. QUANTITATIVE ANGIOGRAPHIC MEASUREMENTS**

| LESIONS (N = 106) | MEAN ± SD |
|---|---|
| Preprocedural | |
|   Reference diameter (mm) | 2.79 ± 0.51 |
|   Minimal lumen diameter (mm) | 1.05 ± 0.66 |
|   Diameter stenosis (%) | 63 ± 21 |
|   Lesion length (mm) | 9.08 ± 7.06 |
| Postprocedural | |
|   Minimal lumen diameter (mm) | 2.76 ± 0.56 |
|   Diameter stenosis (%) | 4.3 ± 18 |

**TABLE 44–4.    PREDICTORS OF RESTENOSIS: SIMPLE REGRESSION ANALYSIS**

| VARIABLE | PARAMETER ESTIMATE ± STANDARD ERROR | $p$ VALUE |
|---|---|---|
| Mean reference vessel diameter | 1.63 ± 0.70 | 0.02 |
| Balloon/vessel ratio | −4.3 ± 2.08 | 0.04 |
| Postprocedural MLD | 1.21 ± 0.67 | 0.07 |
| Number of stents/lesion | 0.69 ± 0.85 | 0.41 |
| Lesion length | 0.03 ± 0.09 | 0.76 |

MLD, minimal lumen diameter; $p < 0.05$ is considered significant.

have been placed in 91 patients and PS stents in 84 patients. Postprocedural angiographic data are available for 38 patients with the AVE Microstent and 32 patients with the PS stent. There was no difference in the lesion location, lesion length (9.13 ± 3.64 mm vs. 9.69 ± 4.14 mm), and lesion complexity score. The postprocedural mean quantitative coronary angiography (QCA) diameter was 3.23 ± 0.37 mm (AVE) versus 3.32 ± 0.43 mm (PS). There was no difference in stent recoil (−5.48 ± 16.82% vs. 1.37 ± 18.67%, $p$ = nonsignificant [NS]) between AVE and PS, respectively (Heuser, personal communication). Six-month angiographic and clinical follow-up data are still pending at the time of writing.

There are several observational studies reported in abstract format. The unifying feature of these studies is the high rate of bailout stenting and the anatomic complexity of patients treated.

Verheye and colleagues reported on 459 AVE Microstents implanted in 357 lesions in 344 patients.[35] Lesion types B2 and C were present in 54% of cases, and the reference vessel diameter was 3.04 mm. Stenting was elective in 28%, after suboptimal PTCA in 36%, for nonocclusive dissections in 23%, for bailout situations in 9%, for bailout after the use of other stents in 1%, and for primary PTCA in acute myocardial infarction in 3%. Immediate angiographic success was achieved in 94% of cases. Aspirin and ticlopidine were used in all but 2% of the cohort, in which warfarin was used. Subacute stent thrombosis occurred in six patients (1.7%), death in three patients, myocardial infarction in six patients, and coronary artery bypass grafting (CABG) in one patient. Angiographic follow-up was obtained in 182 patients at a mean duration of 5.5 months. Angiographic restenosis occurred in 44 patients (24%).

Hass and associates reported on 150 patients who had 186 stents implanted.[36] The stents were elective in 28%, for suboptimal PTCA in 24%, and for dissection or acute closure in 48%. Proximal vessel tortuosity (>60) was present in 22%, bend lesions were present in 14%, and the Microstent was implanted after unsuccessful delivery of the PS stent in eight cases. In eight other cases (4.4%) the

Microstent was used to seal a dissection distal to a previously implanted stent of a different type. Stents were deployed at a mean inflation pressure of 11 ± 3 atm. Visible separation in stent elements (1 ± 1 mm) was seen in 28 patients. Successful stent deployment was achieved in 182 stents (98%). Stent thrombosis occurred in 2 patients (1.4%), major bleeding complications in 8 patients (5.3%), emergency bypass surgery in 1 patient (0.7%), and in-hospital death in 1 patient (0.7%). Angiographic follow-up was performed in 124 patients (83%) at 3 months, with restenosis occurring in 43 (34.7%).

Rau and colleagues reported a comparison between 40 lesions treated with the Microstent (53 stents) and 65 lesions treated with the PS stent (97 stents).[37] All stents were deployed with high pressure, and all patients were taking only antiplatelet agents. Angiographic follow-up was performed at least 12 weeks after the procedure. Restenosis occurred in 20% of the PS cohort versus 28% in the Microstent cohort ($p$ = 0.51).

Saito and coworkers performed a retrospective comparison between 20 patients (23 lesions) treated with the Microstent and 294 patients (324 lesions) treated with the PS stent.[38] Delivery success was achieved in 96% in the Microstent group versus 91% in the PS stent group ($p$ = NS). There was no event of stent thrombosis in either group. The restenosis rate was 39% (9 lesions) for the Microstent and 20% (65 lesions) for the PS stent.

Valeix and colleagues reported on 565 patients who underwent an attempt at AVE stent implantation.[39] Stenting was elective in 45.5%, for restenosis in 12%, for nonocclusive dissection in 27%, for suboptimal PTCA in 15%, and for bailout stenting in 0.5%. A total of 756 stents were implanted (1.42 per patient) using an inflation pressure of 6 to 10 atm. Angiographic success was achieved in 522 patients (98%). At 1-month follow-up, subacute stent thrombosis occurred in 10 patients (1.8%).

Schiele and associates reported on 109 patients (120 lesions, 127 stents) undergoing AVE stent implantation.[40] Stenting was for abrupt closure in 16% and dissections in 31%. The mean reference diameter was 2.95 ± 0.65 mm; all stents were deployed using high inflation pressure, and angiographic success was achieved in 95% of the lesions. All patients were treated with antiplatelet therapy only after the procedure. Procedural complications included CABG in two patients secondary to stent migration and death in one patient. At 1-month follow-up, two patients had subacute stent thrombosis.

### Stent Delivery and Scaffolding Properties

Coronary stents have been extensively used as scaffolding devices to treat acute or threatened closure after coronary angioplasty[14, 15] and to reduce late restenosis.[16, 17] However, the inability to deliver a stent with good scaffolding properties to the culprit lesion and uncertainty about the precise placement have been reported.[41] The distinctive advantages of the Microstent in its present design are (1) ease of delivery in the most complex anatomy (because of its superior flexibility and low profile), (2) appropriate lesion coverage because of the availability of a wide range of lengths, (3) accurate placement because of its moderate radiopacity and edge markers, and (4) its superior radial strength when compared with other stent designs, as shown in Table 44–5. Figures 44–4 through 44–6 are case examples illustrating the use of the Microstent in various clinical and anatomic scenarios (chronic total occlusions, calcified lesions, and stent recoil). The implantation success rate of 97% to 98% with the Microstent in a population with complex anatomy and in bailout situations confirms the uniqueness of this design. In addition, a comparison between the AVE stent and other stents in regard to delivery success should take into account the issue of selection bias, because almost all available studies reporting experiences with the AVE stent have selected highly complex anatomy and bailout situations for implantation of this stent.

### Thrombogenicity

In the era of optimal stent implantation and only antiplatelet therapy, stent thrombosis has significantly decreased, as have bleeding complications.[22–24] The available prospective and retrospective data indicate that the incidence of stent thrombosis with the AVE stent is no different from that of other stents. This is in spite of the fact that this stent was more often used in dissections and bailout situations.[35–40] Therefore, it is reasonable to state that stent design per se does not have a significant impact on stent thrombosis if the stent was successfully deployed and appropriate antiplatelet therapy was used.

### Restenosis

Angiographic restenosis with the Microstent (I and II) has been reported to range between 24% and 40%.[35–40] However, it is critical to keep in mind that these studies included patients with small vessels and complex lesions, which are inherently associated with a high restenosis rate irrespective of the modality of catheter-based intervention. In addition, the low rate of angiographic follow-up may artifactually lead to a higher restenosis rate because more patients with symptoms tend to come back for a repeat angiogram. A meaningful comparison with other stents should await the results of prospective randomized trials.

It is clear from histologic studies that any injury to the vessel wall will be associated with neointimal hyperplasia, leading to restenosis when excessive. In regard to intrastent restenosis, experimental data suggest that metal density could lead to a higher degree of neointimal hyperplasia,[42] and preliminary intravascular ultrasound data suggest that the plaque volume before stent placement could increase the degree of late loss independent from the immediate results.[43] Other investigators have shown the relation between the final lumen obtained and restenosis.[44, 45] Data on predictors of restenosis with the AVE stent are limited. In our database, univariate predictors of restenosis included a smaller vessel diameter and a higher balloon/vessel ratio, but when these factors were entered into a multivariate

### TABLE 44–5.  MICROSTENT RADIAL STRENGTH: COMPARISON WITH OTHER STENT DESIGNS*

| | STENT DIAMETER (mm) ACCORDING TO EXTERNAL PRESSURE APPLIED (mm Hg) | | | | |
| | 50 | 100 | 200 | 300 | 400 |
|---|---|---|---|---|---|
| AVE | 3.00 | 3.00 | 2.98 | 2.97 | 2.95 |
| J & J (153) | 2.98 | 2.94 | 2.86 | n/a | n/a |
| (154) | 2.99 | 2.96 | 2.88 | 2.83 | n/a |
| ACS | 2.97 | 2.91 | 2.83 | 2.77 | n/a |
| Wiktor | 2.97 | 2.92 | 2.84 | 2.79 | n/a |
| Cordis | 2.95 | 2.85 | 2.77 | n/a | n/a |
| WallStent | 2.85 | 2.66 | n/a | n/a | n/a |

*All figures are based on an initial deployed stent internal diameter of 3 mm.
n/a, no figures available.
These figures are extrapolated from Coronary stenting, by David Kenne.

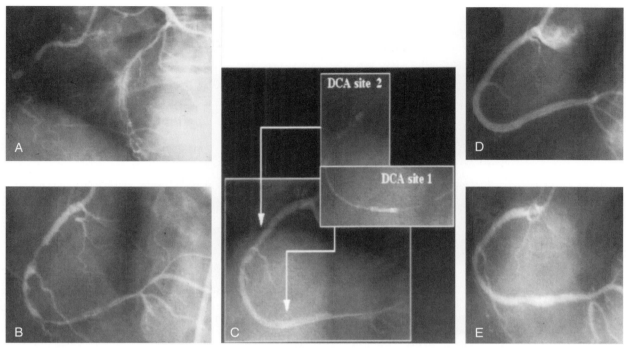

FIGURE 44–4. *A,* Coronary angiogram of the right coronary artery (RCA) with a contralateral injection of the left coronary artery showing a long total occlusion in the mid-RCA. *B,* Coronary angiogram of the RCA after lesion crossing and balloon predilatation; note the length of the lesion and the large plaque burden. *C,* Coronary angiogram of the RCA after directional coronary atherectomy. *D,* Coronary angiogram of the RCA after implantation of three (3.5-mm), 39-mm-long Microstent II's; note the large lumen obtained and the smooth vessel borders. *E,* Coronary angiogram of the RCA at 5.5-month follow-up. DCA, directional atherectomy catheter.

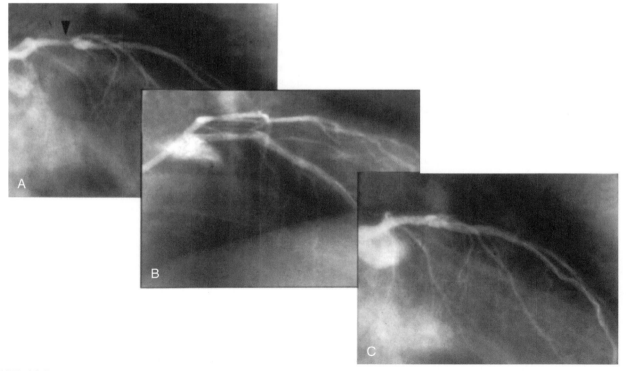

FIGURE 44–5. *A,* Coronary angiogram of the left anterior descending artery (LAD) showing a calcified long lesion *(white arrow).* *B,* Coronary angiogram of the LAD after rotablation. *C,* Coronary angiogram of the LAD after stenting.

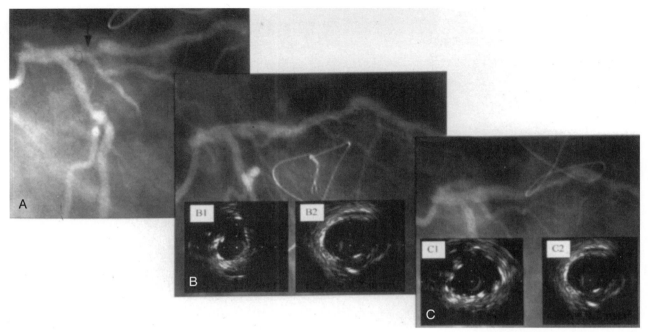

FIGURE 44–6. *A*, Coronary angiogram of the left anterior descending artery (LAD) showing a calcified proximal lesion *(arrow)*. *B*, Coronary angiogram of the LAD after stent implantation (non-AVE stent) using a 3.5 balloon at 20 atm; note the indentation at the lesion site indicating a suboptimal result. *B1*; Intravascular ultrasound (IVUS) scores of the smallest intrastent cross-sectional area (5.6 mm²) indicating suboptimal stent expansion. *B2*, IVUS image of the distal reference lumen cross-sectional area (9.2 mm²). *C*, Coronary angiogram of the LAD after implantation of a 6-mm Microstent II inside the first stent inflated with a 4 balloon at 20 atm; note the optimal angiographic result. *C1*, IVUS image of the smallest intrastent cross-sectional area (10.7 mm²). *C2*, IVUS image of the distal reference lumen cross-sectional area (9.2 mm²). Note that the deployment of the AVE stent has led to a 100% increase in lumen size.

model, none predicted restenosis. The importance of vessel size in influencing restenosis is well known. The fact that a balloon with larger balloon/vessel ratio was used to optimize stents in the restenosis group is most likely because of the smaller vessel size in this group and because the operator chose this strategy to obtain the largest lumen possible.

## CONCLUSIONS

The new-generation AVE Microstents have expanded the horizons of coronary stenting. At present, this stent provides an excellent balance among several functions: excellent radial strength, superior flexibility, adequate radiopacity, and availability in a wide range of diameters and lengths. These characteristics extend the applicability of this stent to areas that were not in the domain of coronary stenting in the past. Therefore, in addition to elective stenting, we find this stent very useful in the following situations:

1. Bailout after PTCA
2. The presence of any of the following proximal to the culprit lesion:
   - Moderate to severe tortuosity
   - Other stents
   - Moderate to severe calcifications
3. Suboptimal result after stenting due to
   - Residual lesion distal to the stent
   - Dissection distal to the stent
   - Plaque prolapse inside the stent
   - Recoil
   - Gaps in between stents
4. Bifurcational stenting. This area is still under active clinical investigation; the favorable characteristics of the Microstent GFX make it an ideal stent for this complex anatomy.

## REFERENCES

1. Grüntzig AR, Senning A, Siegenthaler WE: Nonoperative dilatation of coronary artery stenosis: Percutaneous transluminal coronary angioplasty. N Engl J Med 301:61, 1979.
2. Detre K, Holubkov R, Kelsey S, et al: Percutaneous transluminal angioplasty in 1985–1986 and 1977–1981. The National Heart, Lung, and Blood Institute Registry. N Engl J Med 318:265, 1988.
3. Leimgruber P, Roubin GS, Hollman J, et al: Restenosis after successful coronary angioplasty in patients with single-vessel disease. Circulation 73:710, 1986.
4. Dorros G, Cowley MJ, Simpson J, et al: Percutaneous transluminal coronary angioplasty: Report of complications from the National Heart, Lung and Blood Institute PTCA Registry. Circulation 67:723, 1983.
5. Popma JJ, Califf RM, Topol EJ: Clinical trials of restenosis after coronary angioplasty. Circulation 84:1426, 1991.
6. Lincoff AM, Popma JJ, Ellis SG, et al: Abrupt vessel closure complicating coronary angioplasty: Clinical angiographic and therapeutic profile. J Am Coll Cardiol 19:926, 1992.
7. Ellis SG, Roubin GS, King SB, et al: In-hospital cardiac mor-

tality after acute closure after coronary angioplasty: Analysis of risk factors from 8207 procedures. J Am Coll Cardiol 11:211, 1988.

8. Ellis SG, Roubin GS, King SB III, et al: Angiographic and clinical predictors of acute closure after native vessel coronary angioplasty. Circulation 77:372, 1988.

9. Golding LAR, Loop FD, Hollman JL, et al: Early results of emergency surgery after coronary angioplasty. Circulation 3(suppl):S26, 1986.

10. Dotter CT: Transluminally placed coil spring material tube grafts: Long-term patency in canine popliteal artery. Invest Radiol 4:329, 1969.

11. Sigwart U, Puel J, Mirkovitch V, et al: Intravascular stents to prevent occlusion and restenosis after transluminal angioplasty. N Engl J Med 316:701, 1987.

12. Serruys PW, Strauss BH, Beatt KJ, et al: Angiographic follow-up after placement of a self-expanding coronary artery stent. N Engl J Med 324:13, 1991.

13. Schatz RA, Baim DS, Leon M, et al: Clinical experience with the Palmaz-Schatz coronary stent. Initial results of a multicenter study. Circulation 83:148, 1991.

14. Lincoff AM, Topol EJ, Chapekis AT, et al: Intracoronary stenting compared with conventional therapy for abrupt vessel closure complicating coronary angioplasty: A matched case-control study. J Am Coll Cardiol 21:866, 1993.

15. Roubin GS, Cannon AD, Agrawal SK, et al: Intracoronary stenting for acute or threatened closure complicating percutaneous transluminal coronary angioplasty. Circulation 85:916, 1992.

16. Fischman DL, Leon M, Baim D, et al: A randomized comparison of coronary stent placement and balloon angioplasty in the treatment of coronary artery disease. N Engl J Med 331:496, 1994.

17. Serruys P, Jaegere P, Kiemeneij F, et al: A comparison of balloon expandable stent implantation with balloon angioplasty in patients with coronary artery disease. N Engl J Med 331:489, 1994.

18. Colombo A, Hall P, Nakamura S, et al: Intracoronary stenting without anticoagulation accomplished with intravascular ultrasound guidance. Circulation 91:1676, 1995.

19. Nakamura S, Colombo A, Gaglione S, et al: Intracoronary ultrasound observations during stent implantation. Circulation 89:2026, 1994.

20. Moussa I, Di Mario C, Di Francesco L, et al: Subacute stent thrombosis and the anticoagulation controversy: Changes in drug therapy, operator technique, and the impact of intravascular ultrasound. Am J Cardiol 3A(suppl):S13, 1996.

21. Moussa I, Di Mario C, Di Francesco L, et al: Stents don't require systemic anticoagulation . . . but the technique (and results) must be optimal. J Invasive Cardiol Suppl E:3E, 1996.

22. Barragan P, Sainsous J, Silvestri M, et al: Ticlopidine and subcutaneous heparin as an alternative regimen following coronary stenting. Catheter Cardiovasc Diagn 32:133, 1994.

23. Schomig A, Neumann FJ, Kastrati A, et al: A randomized comparison of antiplatelet and anticoagulant therapy after the placement of coronary artery stents. N Engl J Med 334:1084, 1996.

24. Karrillon GJ, Morice MC, Benveniste E, et al: Intracoronary stent implantation without ultrasound guidance and with replacement of conventional anticoagulation by antiplatelet therapy. Circulation 94:1519, 1996.

25. Goldberg SL, Colombo A, Maiello L, et al: Intracoronary stent insertion after balloon angioplasty of chronic total occlusions. J Am Coll Cardiol 26:713, 1995.

26. Moussa I, Di Mario C, Di Francesco L, et al: Coronary stenting of chronic total occlusions without anticoagulation: Immedi-

ate and long-term outcome [Abstract]. Eur Heart J 17:P2451, 1996.

27. Medina A, Melian F, Suarez de Lezo J, et al: Effectiveness of coronary stenting for the treatment of chronic total occlusion in angina pectoris. Am J Cardiol 73:1222, 1994.

28. Sirnes PA, Golf S, Myreng Y, et al for the SICCO Study Group: Stenting in chronic coronary occlusions (SICCO): A Multicenter, Randomized, Controlled study [Abstract]. J Am Coll Cardiol 27(suppl A):139A, 1996.

29. Thomas M, Hancock J, Holmberg S, et al: Coronary stenting following successful angioplasty for total occlusions: Preliminary results of a randomized trial [Abstract]. J Am Coll Cardiol 27(suppl A):153A, 1996.

30. Itoh A, Hall P, Maiello L, et al: Coronary stenting of long lesions (greater than 20 mm): A matched comparison of different stents, abstracted. Circulation 92(suppl 2):688, 1995.

31. Moussa I, Di Mariio C, Blengino S, et al: Coronary stenting after rotational atherectomy in calcified and complex lesions: Angiographic and clinical follow-up results [Abstract]. Eur Heart J 17:P2456, 1996.

32. Laham R, Cohen D, Carrozza J: Multivessel Palmaz-Schatz stenting: Acute results and one year outcome [Abstract]. Circulation 94:1506, 1996.

33. Moussa I, Di Mario C, Di Francesco L, et al: Multivessel stenting without anticoagulation: Immediate and short term outcome [Abstract]. Eur Heart J 17:P1251, 1996.

34. Scoblianco DP, Brown G, Mitten S: A new digital electronic caliper for measurement of coronary arterial stenosis: A comparison with visual and computer assisted measurements. Am J Cardiol 53:689, 1984.

35. Verheye S, Wittemberg O, Eeckhout E, et al: Early and late clinical and angiographic results of the coronary micro stent. I. A multicenter experience [Abstract]. Eur Heart J 17:P992, 1996.

36. Hasse J, Geimer M, Semmler N, et al: Micro stent implantation without anticoagulation: Initial outcomes and 3 months' follow-up [Abstract]. Eur Heart J 17:P993, 1996.

37. Rau T, Tschirner BI, Mathey DG, Schofer J: Comparison of restenosis rates after placement of Palmaz-Schatz stents and AVE micro stents [Abstract]. Eur Heart J 17:P993, 1996.

38. Saito S, Hosokawa G, Tanaka S: Comparison of initial and late angiographic results after AVE micro and Palmaz-Schatz stent implantation [Abstract]. J Am Coll Cardiol 27:110A, 1996.

39. Valeix B, Morice MC, Dumas P, et al: Early results with the AVE micro stent [Abstract]. J Am Coll Cardiol 27:53A, 1996.

40. Schiele F, Meneveau N, Vuillemenot A, et al: A single center prospective experience with two generations of coronary AVE micro-stent: Acute clinical and angiographic results [Abstract]. Circulation 94:508, 1996.

41. Baim DS, Schatz R, Cleman M, Curry C: Predictors of unsuccessful placement of the Schatz-Palmaz coronary stents. Circulation 80:174, 1989.

42. Rogers C, Edelman E: Endovascular stent design dictates experimental restenosis and thrombosis. Circulation 91:2195, 1995.

43. Moussa I, Di Mario C, Moses J, et al: The impact of preintervention plaque area as determined by intravascular ultrasound on luminal renarrowing following coronary stenting [Abstract]. Circulation 94:1528, 1996.

44. Kuntz R, Safian R, Carrozza J, et al: The importance of acute luminal diameter in determining restenosis after coronary atherectomy or stenting. Circulation 86:1827, 1992.

45. Carrozza J, Kuntz R, Schatz R, et al: Inter-series differences in the restenosis rate of Palmaz-Schatz coronary stent placement: Differences in demographics and post-procedure lumen diameter. Catheter Cardiovasc Diagn 31:173, 1994.

**VI**

# New Approaches to Restenosis and Thrombosis

# 45

# Local Drug Delivery

*Gregory S. Pavlides*

*Local drug delivery* refers to the local action of a medication, usually delivered locally or with localizing properties, which specifically affects the biologic response of the targeted organ, in this case the arterial wall. Although many physiologic properties of the arterial wall can be modified by local drug delivery, the response to interventional injury and restenosis are the main targets of this intervention.[1] Other potential cardiac applications of local drug delivery are arterial thrombus prevention, and thrombus resolution.[2]

The application of local drug delivery arose from oncology experience in developing therapeutic agents that exhibit cell or site-selective toxicity. In cardiology, several systemic therapies targeting coronary pathologic processes, such as thrombolysis for acute myocardial infarction, are extremely effective; however, they carry the price of significant systemic side effects.[3] In response to this, local drug delivery has the potential advantage to achieve high, and in some cases sustained, local concentration while avoiding systemic side effects. This benefit is especially important for highly toxic drugs. Paradigms of locally delivered drugs existed even before the invention of catheters used for local drug delivery, both for extracardiac and cardiac settings. Extracardiac cases include the intra-articular use of yttrium to treat synovitis, the intraocular slow-release pilocarpine reservoir for chronic glaucoma, polymer implants containing low doses of tetracyclines to treat periodontal disease, and others. A cardiac example of local drug delivery is the steroid-eluting pacemaker lead, which prevents the rising pacing thresholds associated with myocardial fibrosis after lead placement. The modalities used today for local drug delivery are the perivascular approach and the intraluminal approach, which is possible with catheter-based local drug delivery systems. Although there are other ways for achieving local drug effects, their description is beyond the scope of this chapter. This discussion will be limited to catheter-based local drug delivery systems, as is the case for interventional cardiology.

## FUNDAMENTAL ISSUES IN LOCAL DRUG DELIVERY

Since the invention of the first catheter by Wolinsky in 1987,[4] local drug delivery has made great strides, and it constitutes a viable treatment modality in clinical practice. There are a number of important questions, however, which have been only partially answered, and a number of questions awaiting their answer, as research in the field is progressing. The issues they address are important for both the catheters and techniques of local drug delivery used today. The early issues pertaining to local drug delivery included the establishment of a sound basis of the approach, the time period necessary for local delivery to be accomplished, the way to achieve treatment of the whole thickness of the arterial wall, the modality to be used, the definition of the time during which the drug is present in the arterial wall, and of course the way to assess the biologic effect of the delivered material on wall processes. These issues have already been addressed, and to an extent answered. The current questions of local drug delivery arose partly from the existing experience in experimental and clinical settings. They include questions about species variation (humans vs. experimental animals), pressure variations for catheters using pressure-based delivery, location variations such as adventitial or periadventitial delivery, effects of spillage of the delivered drug into the general circulation, and the pursuit of an effective modality to be delivered with the existing catheters. Most of these questions still await an answer.

## VASCULAR BIOLOGY OF THE ARTERIAL WALL RESPONSE TO INJURY

Because the main target of local drug delivery today is the arterial response to interventional injury, including restenosis, a brief review of the subject is appropriate to this discussion. The vascular response to injury includes three phases. The first or acute initiating phase occurs minutes to hours after the arterial injury. During this phase platelets adhere to the injured surface and aggregate, forming a platelet thrombus.[5–9] Thrombin is generated, and platelet and vessel wall interactions begin with the release of a number of biologically active mediators.[10–14] A number of these mediators are growth-promoting substances, including platelet-derived growth factors AA, AB, and BB, fibroblast growth factors, insulin-like growth factor-I, endothelium-derived growth factors, interleukin-1, angiotensin II, and endothelin. Growth-inhibitory substances are also released, including prostacyclin, nitric oxide, heparan sulfate, and transforming growth factor-α1. The released vasoactive substances with growth-regulatory properties are angiotensin II, endothelin, bradykinin, nitric oxide, prostacyclin, and type C natriuretic peptide. This first phase is followed by the second or intermediate phase, which lasts days to weeks. The main event in this phase is the activation and replication of medial smooth muscle cells, which later migrate to the intima.[15–17] This activation and replication of the smooth muscle cells is the response to the substances released in the first phase. The third and final phase completes the response to injury weeks to months after the initiating event. During this phase, replication of the intimal smooth muscle cells occurs,[18] with production and modulation of the extracellular matrix.[19] During this phase vascular remodeling also occurs[20] and plays an important role in determining the final vascular lumen area and the presence or not of the final restenosis.[21]

## GENERAL PROPERTIES OF CATHETERS USED FOR LOCAL DRUG DELIVERY

The first catheter devised and used intravascularly was the double balloon catheter by Wolinsky, and it was soon followed by others. The majority of these catheters deliver the desired drug intraluminally, with only a fraction of it entering the arterial wall. New devices have appeared recently with the capability to inject and deposit drugs directly into the arterial wall. The catheters used today can be classified either by generation, according to their development or by their mechanism of achieving drug entry into the arterial wall.[22] They are shown in Table 45–1 and Figure 45–1.

There are five mechanisms of wall entry of the locally delivered drugs by the existing devices:

1. Passive diffusion or movement of drug down a concentration gradient
2. Active infusion or movement of drug down a pressure gradient
3. Iontophoresis

4. Direct intramural injection
5. Local radiation

For the majority of the catheter systems, both passive diffusion and active infusion contribute to the wall entry of the delivered substances. The spectrum varies from mainly passive diffusion, as in the case of the hydrogel-coated balloon, to solely active infusion, as in the case of the infiltrator catheter.

## LOCAL DELIVERY CATHETER SYSTEMS

### Double Balloon Catheter

The double balloon catheter is a 3.5-French polyethylene shaft catheter with two urethane compliant balloons bonded at the distal tip. The balloons inflate independently, creating a chamber into which fluid is infused via a separate port. When adequate pressure within the chamber is applied the fluid penetrates through the media of the vessel wall. An early version of this catheter was the first one to be used for local drug delivery by Wolinsky[4] and Kerenyi[23] independently. These investigators were able with this catheter to deliver experimentally marked molecules into the arterial wall, or to dissolve atherosclerotic plaques by collagenase. Active compounds including heparin, r-hirudin,[24] and tissue-type plasminogen activator (tPA)[25] have also been delivered by this catheter. Also, this catheter was used to deliver the β-galactosidase gene incorporated in a retroviral vector into the arterial wall of the nonatherosclerotic porcine femoral arteries.[26] It has also been used to locally deliver transfected endothelial cells and smooth muscle cells.[27, 28]

The main advantages of this catheter are its simplicity, and the fact that it can deliver microparticles. However, it has several disadvantages, including balloon inflation in normal segments, loss of the delivered material down side branches, and the requirement of long inflations (>3 minutes) for effective drug wall penetration.

### Porous Balloon Catheter

The porous balloon catheter is a balloon catheter that has a 3.5-French polyethylene shaft, with a polyethylene terephthalate (PET) noncompliant balloon bonded at the distal tip. The balloon has 28 25-μm laser-drilled holes distributed radially around its center. When the balloon is inflated at 4 atm and at 1.2:1 balloon-to-vessel ratio, local delivery of 1 to 2 mL is achieved at 45 seconds. The administered fluid penetrates the vessel wall through the media and into the adventitia, depending on the pressure applied. This catheter has been used to deliver successfully a number of agents, including horseradish peroxidase,[29] hepa-

**TABLE 45–1.  CLASSIFICATION OF LOCAL DRUG DELIVERY CATHETERS**

| FIRST GENERATION: FEASIBILITY CATHETERS | SECOND GENERATION: LESS TRAUMATIC EFFICIENT CATHETERS | THIRD GENERATION: INCREASED EFFICIENCY CATHETERS |
|---|---|---|
| Double balloon<br>Porous balloon | Microporous balloon<br>Transport catheter<br>Channeled balloon<br>Dispatch catheter<br>Infusion sleeve<br>Hydrogel-coated balloon<br>Border infusion catheter | Annular balloon<br>Infiltrator catheter<br>Iontophoresis catheter<br>Needle device (NIC) |

rin,[30] recombinant plasminogen activator (r-PA), methotrexate,[31] doxorubicin, colchicine,[32] thiol protease inhibitor, angiopeptin,[33] antisense oligonucleotides to c-myc,[34] as well as genes, such as β-galactosidase marked gene.[35] The advantages of this catheter are also its simplicity, and that microparticles can be delivered. Serious concerns have been raised about the safety of this catheter because it has been shown that the fluid jets can cause vascular trauma, which is sometimes quite extensive.

## Microporous Infusion Catheter

The microporous infusion catheter is a porous balloon covered by outer microporous membrane in order to avoid jetting and vascular trauma during local drug delivery. Specifically, the catheter has a 3.5-French shaft, with a Duralyn balloon at its tip, which has 64 holes (8 × 8) 50 to 75 μm, covered by a polyester membrane containing pores 0.8 μm in diameter. This allows for a large pressure drop-off within the catheter, and as a result the contents of the catheter are oozed out of the membrane, decreasing arterial injury.[36] The current-generation microporous infusion catheter III is also known as the Endeavor OTW infusion catheter. Nominal in vitro flow rate for this catheter is 4.25 mL/minute at the specified operating pressure of 3 atm.[37] Horseradish peroxidase, as well as heparin, and low molecular weight heparin (LMWH) have been delivered successfully with this catheter. The catheter is currently being utilized in the IMPRESS clinical trial, to deliver low molecular weight heparin after stenting, and also in the Biostent clinical trial. Its main advantage is the limited vascular trauma with its use; disadvantages remain the long inflation time required for effective drug delivery, and the coupled balloon inflation drug delivery.

## Transport Coronary Dilation-Infusion Catheter

The transport catheter system is a 3.2-French shaft device, with dual balloons at its tip, one inside the other. The inner balloon is a semicompliant polyethylene (PE) angioplasty balloon with a nominal pressure of 6 atm. The outer balloon wall has 36 holes 250 μm in diameter each, holes large enough to avoid a local jet effect. Different ports for each balloon disconnect balloon inflation from local drug delivery. Flow rates of 1 to 6 mL/minute are achieved with infusion pressures of 1 to 3 atm, while the inner balloon is inflated at 2 atm. The catheter has been used successfully for percutaneous transluminal coronary angioplasty (PTCA) and local delivery of heparin and thrombolytics. Currently, the transport catheter is being utilized in the Investigation by the Thoraxcenter on Antisense DNA Given by Local Delivery and Assessed by Intravascular Ultrasound after Coronary Stenting (ITALICS) trial, which is looking at the effect of locally delivered antisense oligonucleotides to c-*myc* on restenosis, and in the Polish Intramural Low Molecular Weight Heparin Outpatient Stent Trial (PILOT), which is investigating the delivery of low molecular weight heparin before stent implantation. The main advantages of this catheter are its capacity to be used both as a PTCA catheter and a local delivery device, and the dissociation between balloon inflation and drug delivery. The main limitations of the catheter are its limited perfusion capability and the fairly long inflation time required for effective drug delivery.

## Channeled Balloon Drug Delivery Catheter

The channeled balloon is a 3.4-French shaft catheter, with an inner angioplasty balloon, which is surrounded by an array of 18 discrete channels. The channels are connected to an infusion port, and each contains one or more clusters of holes in the outer wall, distributed over the dilation length of the balloon. Flow rates are independent of balloon size and inner balloon pressure, when the balloon is unconstrained. Because of the configuration of the exit holes in the outer balloon wall, the flow occurs by "sweating" from the balloon surface.[38] For the coronary device, infusion pressures of 1 to 3 atm result in flow rates of 2 to 7 mL/minute.[39] Suc-

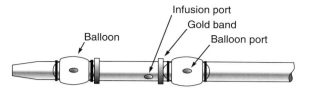

**A** Schematic of the double balloon catheter.

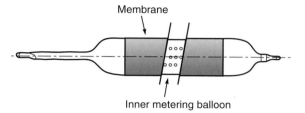

**B** Schematic of the microporous infusion catheter.

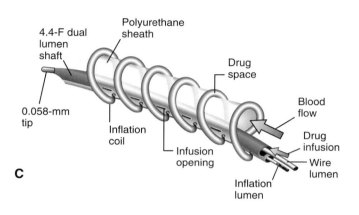

**C**

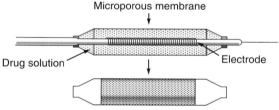

**D** The scheme illustrates the microporous membrane surrounding the electrode, which consists of a very fine wire wrapped around the inner shaft.

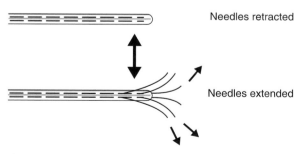

**E** Schematic of the needle injection catheter.

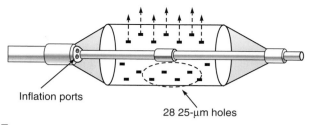

**F** Schematic of the porous balloon catheter.

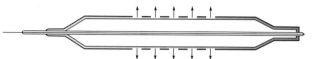

**G** Diagrammatic representation of the structure of the transport catheter. The shaded area represents the lumen between the inner PTCA balloon and the outer balloon.

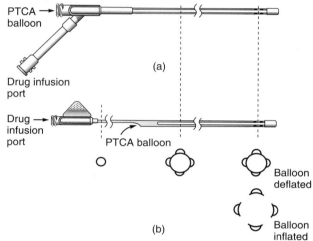

**H** Schematic drawing of the (a) first-generation and (b) second-generation infusion sleeve catheters.

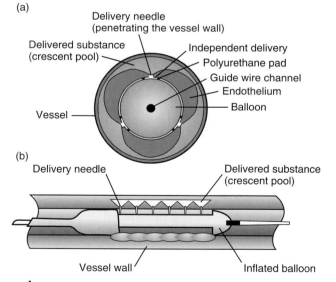

**I** Schematic (a) cross section and (b) longitudinal section of the intramural drug delivery device.

FIGURE 45–1. *A*, Double-balloon catheter. *B*, Microporous balloon catheter. *C*, Dispatch catheter. *D*, Iontophoretic catheter. *E*, Needle injection catheter. *F*, Porous balloon catheter. *G*, Transport catheter. *H*, Infusion sleeve catheter. *I*, Infiltrator balloon catheter. (The schematics for this figure are from Camenzind E, Kutryk MJ, Serruys PW: Use of locally delivered conventional drug therapies. Semin Interv Cardiol 1(1):67–76, 1996.)

cessful in vivo delivery of horseradish peroxidase,[38] heparin,[38] low molecular weight heparin,[40] urokinase,[41] and genes have been accomplished with this catheter in animal models. The advantage of this catheter is that balloon inflation is dissociated from drug delivery, which can be accomplished in fairly low pressures. Its main disadvantage is the long inflation required for effective drug delivery.

## Dispatch Coronary Perfusion and Infusion Catheter

The dispatch or coil balloon catheter is a system designed to allow infusion of drug solutions while maintaining distal blood flow. The distal end of the catheter consists of a nondilatational inflatable coil wrapped around a nonporous polyurethane sheath. When inflated, the coil balloon deploys an internal conduit, allowing blood flow through the distal coronary artery. The inflated configuration defines a series of individual chambers, produced by the sheath itself, the inflated coils, and the arterial wall. An infusion port allows for the infusion of agents through a central lumen connected to the chambers. Prolonged agent infusion can be accomplished because blood flow occurs through the central core. Distal flow through the central sheath is 55% or more of normal vessel flow. This catheter has been utilized by different centers for prolonged infusion of heparin[42] or urokinase[43] to reduce thrombus formation in patients with unstable angina or acute myocardial infarction.[44, 45] It has also been used experimentally for delivery of methylene blue, horseradish peroxidase, heparin, hirudin, urokinase, tPA, and several genes. The main advantage of this catheter is that it maintains distal coronary flow, allowing for prolonged intracoronary delivery. Its limitations include its low radial strength and potential side branch obstruction. The catheter was approved by the U.S. Food and Drug Administration (FDA) in 1993.

## Infusion Sleeve Catheter

The infusion sleeve (Local Med; Palo Alto CA) is an "over the balloon" style catheter designed for use with standard PTCA balloons for delivery of drugs to the angioplasty arterial segment. It consists of a multilumen catheter with a proximal infusion port, a main catheter shaft, and a distal infusion region with multiple side holes. The catheter has a central lumen for the PTCA catheter and guide wire access as well as four separate outer lumens for drug delivery. Side holes (nine 40-$\mu$m, in each of the four drug delivery tubes) are located within the infusion region near the catheter's distal end. The distal infusion region fit within the arterial segment is deter-

mined by the balloon support pressure, while the rate of agent delivery by the infusion pressure. With an infusion pressure of 7 atm, more than 4 mL of agent is delivered in about 30 seconds. Animal studies demonstrated successful intramural delivery of horseradish peroxidase, heparin, and urokinase. Preliminary clinical studies in Europe demonstrated the feasibility of this approach in delivering heparinized saline.[46] With this system, the Local Primary Angioplasty in Myocardial Infarction (PAMI) study, evaluating the safety of heparin delivery in the setting of acute myocardial infarction, has been completed. Ongoing studies with the infusion sleeve catheter include the Local Infusion of Heparin Prior to Stenting (LIHIPS), for the evaluation of the safety of heparin in "bail-out" stenting, and the Heparin Infusion Prior to Stenting (HIPS), for the evaluation of the efficacy of heparin delivery in reducing restenosis.

The main advantage of this system is the fact that it can be used over all conventional PTCA balloon catheters. In its current form it is limited by the occasional difficulty to advance it to the targeted segment, and its delivery efficiency. In December 1994 the device was approved by the FDA.

## Hydrogel-Coated Balloon Catheter

The hydrogel-coated balloon (SCIMED, Boston Scientific; Minneapolis MN) consists of a standard polyethylene balloon, coated with an interlacing network of polyacrylamide acid chains, which are adherent to the balloon surface (Hydroplus). When the balloon comes into contact with aqueous environment, water is absorbed by the hydrogel coating and the lattice begins to swell and form a stable matrix of polymer and water. Any agents that are dissolved in the water will also be incorporated into this matrix. Intramural drug delivery is achieved with this system during balloon inflation when the hydrogel polymer comes in contact with the arterial intimal surface. Drugs may be loaded onto the hydrogel balloon surface either by immersion of the inflated balloon into a concentrated drug solution, or by "painting" the balloon surface with known aliquots of the drug. There is experimental evidence with this balloon in delivering in vivo horseradish peroxidase,[47] heparin,[48] urokinase,[49] PPACK,[50] antisense oligonucleotides, and various genes.[51]

The major advantage of this hydrogel system is that it results in homogeneous atraumatic drug delivery at the same time that an arterial lesion is being dilated. Limitations include the rapid washout of drug from the balloon surface, the relative small amount of drug that can be loaded onto the hydrogel coating, and the need for prolonged balloon inflations for effective transmural drug delivery.

## Border Infusion Catheter

The use of the border infusion catheter is based on the boundary layer flow theory, which suggests that localized delivery of solutions along the vessel wall in the platelet-rich, low-flow boundary region results in prolonged residence time, and therefore, prolonged wall entry. The border infusion catheter is a single continuous lumen catheter that is formed into a distal three-dimensional coil. The catheter is delivered over a regular PTCA guide wire, which eliminates the coils for the delivery. When the catheter is in position, the guide wire is removed, and the distal tip of the catheter takes its preformed coil shape, coming in contact circumferentially with the vessel wall. Multiple holes (0.0085 inch) are arranged along the coil surface, pointing downstream. Delivery of the desired solution through those holes is controlled by a low-pressure infusion pump. Feasibility trials of this catheter are currently under way.

## Annular Balloon Catheter

The annular balloon catheter is a rapid exchange system designed to allow local drug delivery to the vessel wall while maintaining distal blood flow. The distal or working part of the catheter has an inflatable structure, and a membrane is fixed to it. When inflated, the structure defines a channel for blood flow, with the vessel wall being an annular leak-tight cavity containing the drug to be delivered. This catheter resembles the dispatch catheter, with larger chambers between the membrane and the vessel wall and a better fit. The catheter is currently under investigation. Its theoretical advantages are the minimal systemic leakage and the capability for prolonged inflation time, because distal flow is maintained. The presence of side branches is a disadvantage.

## Infiltrator Angioplasty Balloon Catheter

The Infiltrator angioplasty balloon catheter (IABC) is a third-generation local drug delivery catheter that delivers the drug directly into the vessel wall. It is therefore a very effective catheter. The catheter is an over-the-wire system with three lumens: one for the guide wire, one for the angioplasty balloon, and a third for drug infusion. On the surface of the balloon there are three strips of injection needles (seven in each strip for the currently available device), 120 degrees apart. Upon inflation of the balloon the needles extend 0.25 mm above the balloon surface and, in appropriately sized balloons, enter the arterial wall. They are connected to the infusion part. The balloon is advanced to the delivery site and then is inflated at 1 to 2 atm. Then a total of 0.4 mL of substance in injected through the needles by hand into the arterial wall. The injection requires less than 10 seconds, allowing for very short balloon inflation time. The safety and its superb efficacy have been demonstrated in animals.[52] The first clinical trial with this catheter (the Infiltrator Safety Trial) has been successfully completed using low molecular weight heparin delivery in the wall of coronary arteries after PTCA or stent implantation.[53] The advantages of this catheter are many. It is currently the only catheter capable of direct intramural drug delivery, balloon inflation and drug delivery are uncoupled, and it requires very short balloon inflations and delivery time. Particles and genes can be delivered by this catheter also. Its main limitation is the potential for vascular trauma, although the initial animal data have not supported this.

## Iontophoretic Drug Delivery System

*Iontophoresis* is the term used to describe the process of local delivery of ionized drugs to target tissue under the influence of electric current.[54] This method has found widespread application in transdermal drug delivery. The iontophoretic drug delivery system (CorTrak Medical, Inc.; Minneapolis MN) consists of a catheter upon which a microporous membrane balloon is mounted at the distal end. Within the balloon, an electrode wire is coiled around the inner catheter shaft. When the membrane balloon is inflated at low pressure and an electric current is applied by the power source, charged drug molecules inside the balloon flow through the balloon pores into the arterial wall in response to the voltage differential between the catheter electrode and return electrode (skin electrode). During iontophoresis, the penetration of charged drug molecules into arterial tissue is predicted by the Nernst-Planck equation. Laboratory studies have shown that the primary driving mechanism of drug delivery with this catheter is determined by the electric field.

Successful in vivo delivery of hirudin and heparin has been accomplished with the iontophoresis catheter.[55] The potential advantages of this catheter include the efficient uniform drug delivery throughout all three layers of the arterial wall and the enhanced drug retention and cellular uptake. Its main limitation is the required long inflation time.

## Needle Device

The needle injection catheter (NIC) is a device designed to deliver drugs into the perivascular space. The device is a 4.3- to 7-French flexible catheter with a central guide wire lumen and six 205-$\mu$m (31 gauge) needles, which can be extended laterally into media or perivascular area for local drug deposition. Experimental data demonstrate a large perivascular space drug deposition.[56] Its safety remains an issue for clinical use.

## PHARMACOLOGIC AGENTS USED IN EXPERIMENTAL STUDIES

A plethora of pharmacologic agents have been administered experimentally in various animal models site specifically by various catheter based systems. The majority of these agents were administered in order to control the neointimal formation in various models of restenosis after vascular injury.

## Antithrombin Agents
### Standard Heparin

Heparin is the most widely studied pharmacologic agent for the prevention of restenosis. It has been known for some time that heparin has antiproliferative actions, independent from its anticoagulant properties, the mechanism of which is not clearly understood.[57] The seminal study of Clowes and Karnovsky first demonstrated the ability of heparin to reduce neointimal formation after vascular injury, mainly through inhibition of smooth muscle cell proliferation.[58] Favorable results on inhibiting smooth muscle cell proliferation were achieved by local perivascular delivery of heparin.[59] Wolinsky and Thung first administered heparin locally by the porous balloon catheter in canine brachial arteries.[30] Atherosclerotic rabbit femoral arteries have also been used. In these studies with intra-arterial delivery, heparin failed to show any effect on restenosis. However, the issue of heparin and restenosis remains open, with several clinical studies under way. It appears that the therapeutic potential of this agent is influenced by the technique of local delivery used, the quantity of drug that can be intramurally deposited, as well as the localization and persistence of the drug in the arterial wall following delivery.

### Low Molecular Weight Heparin

LMWH has several properties that make its use for preventing restenosis attractive. It has a longer half-life than standard heparin and has potent anti–factor Xa activity. The latter may be important, because experimental inhibition of factor Xa by recombinant tick anticoagulant peptide (rTAP) in a porcine model resulted in a decrease of neointimal thickness.[60] In an animal study when administered systemically, it has been shown to reduce restenosis following balloon angioplasty.[61] LMWH has been delivered locally by the porous balloon in athero-sclerotic rabbit carotid arteries. Its use was associated with less proliferation of smooth muscle cells and subsequent intimal thickening.[62] Disappointing results were obtained when LMWH was administered by the Dispatch catheter in the rabbit iliac artery model.[40] Administration of LMWH by the porous balloon in dog coronary arteries resulted in a marked decrease of intimal and residual thrombus following PTCA.[63] LMWH is currently used in several clinical trials of local drug delivery.

### Hirudin

Hirudin, a direct thrombin inhibitor, was tested in porcine and rabbit carotid arteries, where it was administered locally by the iontophoretic catheter system. Fifty-fold higher tissue levels were achieved compared to those obtained by passive diffusion or therapeutic systemic doses. Its effects on tissue proliferation still remain to be determined. Regarding platelet deposition in injured vessels, the administration of r-hirudin in a porcine carotid artery model of vascular injury by a double balloon perfusion catheter has as an effect a significant reduction in platelet deposition.[64]

### PPACK

The specific antithrombin agent D-phenylalanyl-propyl-arginine chloromethyl ketone (PPACK) administered locally by the hydrogel balloon in Dacron graft shunts in pigs was found to inhibit platelet dependent thrombosis of those shunts.[65] Site-specific administration of PPACK via a porous balloon catheter in an ex vivo model of arterial damage has also been shown to reduce platelet deposition at the site of balloon injury.[66]

## Antiproliferative Agents
### Angiopeptin

Angiopeptin is a synthetic analogue of somatostatin, which is an endogenous growth hormone inhibitor. Angiopeptin has been shown to be able to inhibit smooth muscle cell replication experimentally, although its exact inhibitory mechanism is not known.[67] In another study, Hong and associates used the porous balloon to administer angiopeptin in a rabbit abdominal aorta balloon injury model.[33] Although they failed to show any effect on neointimal hyperplasia, they did demonstrate inhibition of intimal hyperplasia at sites downstream from the site at drug delivery. Santoian and colleagues also administered locally angiopeptin with the porous balloon with equally discouraging results, despite its favorable effects when it was administered systemically.[68] Preliminary results with angiopeptin-loaded stents, however, seem more promising.

### Colchicine

Colchicine is a drug with antimitotic, anti-inflammatory, and antifibrotic actions. It also inhibits platelet aggregation and the release of secretory products, and reduces neointimal proliferation in animals. Local delivery of colchicine by the porous balloon in rabbit femoral arteries, however, had no effect on restenosis. When polymeric microspheres with colchicine were administered in the same manner, severe muscle atrophy and chronic inflammation ensued, but there was no reduction in restenosis.[32]

## Antineoplastic Agents

### Methotrexate

Methotrexate, a potent antiproliferative, anti-inflammatory, and antifibrotic drug, was tested in the porcine carotid model of injury; a porous balloon was the delivery device. It failed to prevent neointimal thickening in this model.[31]

### Doxorubicin

The antracycline agent doxorubicin was tested in the rabbit iliac model of balloon injury, delivered locally by the porous balloon. There was no difference in vessel response of the treated vessels compared to the vessel response after balloon injury only.

## Cytochalasin B

Cytochalasins are compounds that bind to the actin molecule and inhibit its polymerization. They may suppress smooth muscle cell contraction and alter vascular remodeling, which may affect restenosis. Preliminary data from porcine femoral and coronary models support this hypothesis. Using this model, Kuntz and colleagues delivered locally cytochalasin with a microporous balloon and found larger luminal areas after treatment, without a reduction of neointimal formation.[69]

## Nitrates

Nitrates, as potent vasodilators, may affect the initial response to injury and may have an effect on restenosis. In a porcine model, Hebert and coworkers showed decreased platelet deposition and a reduced vasoconstriction with nitroglycerin administration using an infusion sheath device.[70] The inhibition of platelet deposition was confirmed in another study by Folts and associates by using nitric oxide donors delivered via a porous balloon in a canine coronary model.[71] Nitric oxide donors, administered locally by the infusion sleeve, were found recently to be associated with reduction of neointimal hyperplasia. This finding is different from the recently reported results of nitric oxide donors linsidomine and molsidomine on angiographic restenosis after coronary balloon angioplasty. In this study of systemic administration of nitric oxide donors, there was no benefit in the late luminal loss following angioplasty.[72]

## Calcium Antagonists

There is one study of local perivascular delivery of calcium antagonists in a rat carotid artery model. It was found that diltiazem was effective in suppressing intimal hyperplasia after balloon injury.[73]

## Steroids

The strong anti-inflammatory properties of the steroid compounds were tested by administering perivascularly dexamethasone in the rabbit model of vascular injury. In this model, a depot form of dexamethasone inhibited intimal hyperplasia. In contrast, in porcine carotid arteries with stents, extravascular dexamethasone was found ineffective in inhibiting intimal hyperplasia. The different animal models could be responsible for this discrepancy. Steroids have been administered also clinically (Depo-Medrol) by using the infiltrator catheter in patients undergoing stent placement. Preliminary results were negative in reducing restenosis.

## SPECIFIC CLINICAL TRIALS FOR LOCAL DRUG DELIVERY

Following the experience developed with catheter delivery systems and the initial experimental data, a number of clinical studies of local drug delivery have started, beginning in 1993. Some of these studies have been completed; others are on-going. However, the available data are scarce because very little has been published. The local drug delivery clinical trials can be classified according to (1) intention of treatment, (2) type of pharmacologic agent used, and (3) delivery modality. The currently complete and ongoing trials are shown in Table 45–2. These trials will be commented on briefly here because they will become the basis on which future clinical research in local drug delivery will be based.

*The Cohort of Rescue Angioplasty in Myocardial Infarction II (CORAMI II) trial* is a French trial by Steg and colleagues designed to compare the angiographic complications and maximum CK-MB release in patients with acute myocardial infarction undergoing primary angioplasty with or without urokinase delivery via the hydrogel-coated balloon. The study involves a total of 120 patients, with

## TABLE 45–2. LOCAL DRUG DELIVERY CLINICAL TRIALS

| COMPLETED | ONGOING |
|---|---|
| CORAMI II | EDGE |
| Local PAMI | BIOSTENT |
| Euro DISPATCH | PILOT |
| VEGF gene therapy study | IMPRESS |
| HIPS | ITALICS |
| LIHIPS | BORDER |
| Infiltrator Safety Study | |
| Hydroplus-Urokinase Study | |

CORAMI II, Cohort of Rescue Angioplasty in Myocardial Infarction II; EDGE, Evaluation of Dispatch for Vein Graft Recanalization; HIPS, Heparin Infusion Prior to Stenting; ITALICS, Investigation by the Thoraxcenter on Antisense DNA Given by Local Delivery and Assessed by Intravascular Ultrasound After Coronary Stenting; LIHIPS, Local Infusion of Heparin Prior to Stenting; PAMI, Primary Angioplasty in Myocardial Infarction; PILOT, Polish Intramural Low Molecular Weight Heparin Outpatient Stent Trial; VEGF, Vascular Endothelial Growth Factor.

encouraging preliminary results regarding the urokinase hydroplus balloon. The main benefit of the urokinase hydroplus balloon use was the lower percentage of no-reflow phenomenon following the angioplasty (3.7% vs. 24.6%, $p < 0.01$).[74]

*The local PAMI trial* was conducted by Grines and associates and its objective was to assess the safety and efficacy of intramural heparin infusion using the Infusasleeve after primary angioplasty in patients with acute myocardial infarction. The study used a total of 120 "low-risk" patients, who were randomized. The study has been completed and has confirmed the feasibility of local heparin infusion following primary angioplasty. A modest benefit was conferred in terms of recurrent ischemic events. Unfortunately, because of the need for large-bore–delivery catheters and difficulty with device tracking, widespread clinical use is unlikely.

*The Heparin Dispatch trial* was performed by Camenzind and coworkers in 22 patients after balloon angioplasty. By using the Dispatch catheter, heparin was delivered intracoronary. The study mainly confirmed the feasibility and safety of this approach.[44] A multicenter registry of local delivery of heparin by the Dispatch catheter, for the prevention of restenosis, has been established as a result (EuroDispatch). The study included a total of 105 patients and failed to demonstrate a decrease in restenosis.

*The Vascular Endothelial Growth Factor (VEGF) gene therapy study* has been conducted by Isner and colleagues. Its main objective was to assess the arterial neovascularization resulting from VEGF gene plasmid delivery to totally occluded superficial femoral arteries via the hydrogel balloon.[75] Fifteen patients have been treated, and enormous promise as well as controversy has been generated by these early gene therapy trials.

*The Heparin Infusion Prior to Stenting (HIPS) trial* is a prospective, multicenter, randomized study, conducted by Wilensky and associates.[75a] The study's purpose was to compare the late clinical and angiographic outcome of patients receiving locally delivered intramural heparin via the Infusasleeve versus intracoronary heparin prior to elective stenting. The study design was based on a previous smaller single-center trial, which had encouraging results.[76] HIPS trial has been completed, using a total of 179 patients and, in contrast to the smaller pilot, no difference in active treatment or placebo restenosis rates occurred (12.5% vs. 12.7%, $p =$ NS).

A fairly similar study is *the Local Infusion of Heparin Prior to Stenting (LIHIPS) trial* by E. M. Ohman at Duke University. In this study the objective is also to compare the acute clinical outcome of patients undergoing local delivery of intramural heparin using the Infusasleeve versus no local delivery, prior to stenting for suboptimal PTCA results, or abrupt or threatened closure. The study used a total of 57 patients, who had been randomized, and demonstrated a disturbing trend toward greater complications in the heparin-treated group.[76a]

*The Infiltrator Safety Study* is the first clinical trial with the Infiltrator, the only local drug delivery catheter with the capability for direct intramural delivery of agents. This trial was performed in patients undergoing PTCA or stent implantation.[53] The purpose of the study was to directly inject into the vessel wall low molecular weight heparin (nadroparin calcium), after conventional PTCA and before stent implantation in order to test the feasibility and safety of such an approach, as well as the short-term and long-term effects of it. The delivery was performed successfully in 20 patients (12 with stents) without complications. No adverse clinical events were recorded in short- and long-term (>2 years) follow-up. Of the 20 patients, 2 experienced renewal of symptoms within 6 months, when restenosis was confirmed. Of the remaining 18, 1 patient was found to have angiographic restenosis. The other patients remained asymptomatic, with improved exercise capacity. Our study showed the safety of the Infiltrator for clinical use and the effects of direct intramural delivery of LMWH. Further studies with this very promising catheter are under way, including the use of 15% absolute alcohol to decrease restenosis after de novo stenting or after treatment of in-stent restenosis.

*The Hydroplus-Urokinase study* is a serial case study in which a total of 95 patients with angiographically apparent intracoronary thrombus were treated with urokinase-coated hydrogel balloons. The results showed that angioplasty with urokinase-coated hydrogel balloons is an excellent treatment for thrombus-containing lesions, because the thrombus disappeared in 78, and improved in 14 patients. Thrombolysis In Myocardial Infarction (TIMI) flow grade increased from $1.4 \pm 1.2$ mm to $2.9 \pm 0.4$ mm.[77]

*The ongoing Evaluation of Dispatch for Vein Graft Recanalization (EDGE) trial* is being conducted by E. M. Ohman from Duke University. Its objectives are to assess the capability of local administration of heparin or abciximab (ReoPro or c7E3), via the Dispatch catheter, to prevent complications during saphenous vein graft intervention. A total of 58 patients were randomized. This small pilot study suggests a decrease in thrombus burden after locally administered abciximab.[77a]

*The Biostent trial*, conducted by Wilensky, is a dose-escalating double-blind, randomized, multicenter, prospective study, evaluating the agent cytochalasin B in reducing restenosis. It has as a primary objective to assess vessel recoil and remodeling after administration of cytochalasin B with the microporous infusion catheter, after elective PTCA. A trend toward improved clinical outcome and a slight decrease in angiographic restenosis was reported.[77b]

*The PILOT study* by Deutsch and coworkers has as an objective to evaluate whether intramural local delivery of enoxaparin, via the transport catheter after stent implantation, reduces restenosis. The intention is to include 200 patients.

*The IMPRESS trial* is conducted by J. P. Bassano in France, with the intention to assess the effects of LMWH, delivered locally by the microporous infusion catheter, before stent implantation. It is a randomized trial of stent implantation with and without local delivery of LMWH.

*The ITALICS trial* is conducted by P. Serruys and associates, with an intention to include 80 patients. It is a randomized trial with an objective to compare neointimal formation identified by intravascular ultrasound (IVUS) study in patients receiving locally delivered antisense DNA (LR-3280) versus placebo, after Wallstent implantation in native coronaries.

*The BORDER trial* will compare the effect of locally delivered heparin versus glycoprotein IIb/IIIa antagonist with the border infusion catheter, after PTCA and stent implantation.

The preceding studies are the most important clinical trials in local drug delivery as of this writing. It is obvious that intracoronary thrombus and restenosis after PTCA or stenting are the main targets in all. The most commonly administered drugs are heparinoids, mainly for reasons of safety. The end points are either clinical or angiographic or IVUS lately. Angiographic or IVUS end points will eventually reduce the number of patients required for clinical studies, a very important fact for their completion.

## LOCAL DRUG DELIVERY FOR MOLECULAR THERAPEUTIC APPROACHES AND GENE THERAPY

Local drug delivery is perfectly suited for the delivery of substances aiming at molecular levels, and for gene therapy of all forms of accelerated arteriopathies, including restenosis after coronary intervention. The identification of a number of genes and molecular pathways involved in the pathogenesis of these lesions allowed the development of novel therapeutic strategies to control these processes.[10, 78] These results can be achieved by means of one of three main strategies: (1) antisense technology, (2) cell targeting, or (3) gene therapy.

## Antisense Technology

The first strategy is the inhibition of expression of proteins important for lesion development, using antisense technology. Antisense technology refers to the use of synthetic oligonucleotides (relatively short DNA molecules) or RNA transcripts designed to interrupt synthesis of specific proteins by targeting specific mRNA molecules. In the process of protein synthesis, genetic information encoded in a double-stranded DNA molecule is transcribed into a single-stranded (sense) messenger RNA chain (mRNA), which is then translated into a protein. Introducing oligonucleotides can specifically bind to coding (sense) mRNA (antisense oligonucleotides) and inhibit the subsequent process. There are other approaches aiming to disrupt DNA transcription (anti-DNA strategy). For control of restenosis the replication of smooth muscle cells is targeted.[79] Although the specific mitogens for smooth muscle cell replication are not appealing targets, the final common stage of cell replication and specifically the certain cell cycle-specific genes represent good targets. Such targets are the nuclear transcription factors c-*myc* and c-*myb* proto-oncogenes, G/S and G2/S cyclins (cdc2 and cdk2 kinases), proliferating cell nuclear antigen (PCNA), and nonmuscle myosin.[80–82]

## Cell Targeting

This strategy is intended to prevent lesion and neointima formation by selective targeting of cells involved in these processes. The targets for this approach can be smooth muscle cells themselves, cell adhesion molecules, or the extracellular matrix. This goal can be achieved by targeting specific receptors by toxins or monoclonal antibodies.[83–85]

## Gene Therapy

This approach utilizes gene transfer and therapy by expressing proteins capable of inhibiting the process of smooth muscle cell proliferation, and deposition of extracellular matrix.[86] Local drug delivery catheters allow local gene transfer to the vessel wall, where the expression of the gene is most needed. The two methods by which new genetic material may be transferred into the vessel wall are (1) indirect, cell-based, ex vivo gene transfer and (2) direct, vector-based, in vivo gene transfer. The cell-based gene-transfer technique includes several steps of cell harvest, in vitro gene transfer, and cell implantation (either by local delivery catheters or stents).[27] All steps must be optimized before this becomes a practical approach. The direct, vector-based method is an efficient approach to gene transfer. Both nonviral and viral vectors have been used to perform in vivo arterial gene transfer. The nonviral vectors include naked DNA[87] and liposome-DNA complexes.[26] They are relatively simple methods, but gene transfer efficiency with these vectors is rather low. Efficient gene transfer can be achieved with viral vectors. The viral vectors are genetically modified in order to prevent their replication in the infected target cells. In the viral genome the replication genes are replaced by a gene that encodes the protein we want to express in the infected cell. The viral vectors most commonly used are retroviral and adenoviral vectors.[88–92] The retroviral vectors are small vectors. They carry the genetic information as RNA molecule and have the ability to introduce the transgene only into dividing cells. The transgene is reverse transcribed to DNA, and it is incorporated into the host cell genomic DNA, leading eventually to stable transgene expression. The main disadvantge of retroviral-based vectors is their low efficiency. Adenoviral-based vectors are larger vectors and contain the genetic information of the transgene as DNA. They are highly infective and therefore very efficient vectors. The transgene is expressed by the infected cells, but it has only limited duration of expression in the host cell because the expression of the viral proteins initiates immunogenic reaction that leads to local inflammation and termination of the transgene expression. The ideal viral vector still remains to be produced.

## LIMITATIONS AND FUTURE OF LOCAL DRUG DELIVERY

### Limitations

Despite the tremendous progress of the field of local drug delivery during the 1990s, several limitations remain. The first limitation remains the safety of the catheters used. Early studies with the porous balloon demonstrated the presence of dissection planes following local delivery. Although the currently used catheters have been greatly improved, the possibility of inducing vascular trauma, in addition to the one induced by PTCA, remains and might offset some of the benefits of the local treatment. Reducing local trauma, therefore, should remain a top priority. The second limitation is the site-specific efficiency of delivery. Pharmacokinetically, this can be divided

into peak delivery efficiency and retention time. Most of the currently used catheters have low efficiency. Efficiency has clearly been improved by the introduction of new direct injection catheters, such as the Infiltrator catheter.[93] In a comparison study by Camenzind and coworkers, the delivery efficiency of Dispatch, Channeled, and Infiltrator catheters was assessed. Both Dispatch and Channeled balloons had low efficiency (2% of the delivered agent entered the wall), but the Infiltrator had a much better efficiency rate (>50%).

## Future Directions

Local drug delivery has evolved into a very fast moving and dynamic field, and no one can predict what the future will be. However, certain trends are clear. The conceptual premises of the field are sound and have been validated. The understanding of mechanisms of local events and their manipulation will rebound to understanding of atherogenesis. Development of other technologies such as drug-coated stents has been helped by local drug delivery, and there are already clinical benefits. The delivery systems will continue to improve, although the quest will remain for the effective agents to be identified and delivered. Gene therapy and local transfer will evolve further. It is possible that an ideal viral vector will be produced that will be highly efficient, targeted to a specific cell type, and without immunogenic properties. Such a vector delivered locally might change the way patients are treated in the future.

## REFERENCES

1. Lincoff AM, Topol EJ, Ellis SG: Local drug delivery for the prevention of restenosis: Fact, fancy and future. Circulation 90:2070–2084, 1994.
2. Mckay RG: Use of local drug delivery for treating intracoronary thrombus and thrombus-containing stenoses. Semin Intervent Cardiol 1:53–59, 1996.
3. The GUSTO investigators: The effects of tissue plasminogen activator, streptikinase, or both on coronary-artery patency, ventricular function, and survival after acute myocardial infarction. N Engl J Med 329:1615–1622, 1993.
4. Goldman B, Blanke H, Wolinsky H: Influence of pressure on permeability of normal and diseased muscular arteries to horseradish peroxidase. Atherosclerosis 65:215–225, 1987.
5. Steele PM, Chesebro JH, Stanson AW, et al: Balloon angioplasty: Natural history of the pathophysiological response to injury in a pig model. Circ Pres 57:105–112, 1985.
6. Wilents JR, Sanborn TA, Sanson AW, et al: Platelet accumulation in experimental angioplasty: Time course and relation to vascular injury. Circulation 75:636–642, 1987.
7. Gasperetti CM, Gonias SL, Gimple LW, et al: Platelet activation during coronary angioplasty in humans. Circulation 88:2728–2734, 1993.
8. Schwartz RS, Edwards WD, Huber KC, et al: Coronary restenosis: Prospects for solution and new perspectives from a porcine model. Mayo Clin Proc 68:54–62, 1993.
9. Harker LA: Role of platelet and thrombus in mechanisms of acute occlusion and restenosis after angioplasty. Am J Cardiol 60(suppl B):20B–28B, 1987.

10. Okazaki H, Majesky MW, Harker LA, et al: Regulation of platelet-derived growth factor ligand and receptor gene expression by alpha-thrombin in vascular smooth muscle cells. Circ Res 71:1285, 1992.

11. Graham DJ, Alexander JJ: The effects of thrombin on bovine aortic endothelial and smooth muscle cells. J Vasc Surg 11:307, 1990.

12. Ross R: Platelet-derived growth factor. Lancet 1:1179, 1989.

13. Linder V, Majack RA, Reidy MA: Basic fibroblast growth factor stimulates endothelial regrowth and proliferation in denuded arteries. J Clin Invest 85:2004, 1990.

14. Linder V, Reidy MA: Proliferation of smooth muscle cells after vascular injury is inhibited by an antibody against fibroblast growth factor. Proc Natl Acad Sci U S A 88:3739, 1991.

15. Clowes AW, Schwartz SM: Significance of quiescent smooth muscle cell migration in the injured rat carotid artery. Circ Res 56:139, 1985.

16. Ohara T, Nanto S, Asada S, et al: Ultrastructural study of proliferating and migrating smooth muscle cells at the site of PTCA as an explanation for restenosis. Circulation 74(suppl II):II-290, 1988.

17. Casscells N: Migration of smooth muscle and endothelial cells. Critical events in restenosis. Circulation 86:723–729, 1992.

18. Gravans MB, Roubin GS: Histopathological phenomena at the site of percutaneous transluminal coronary angioplasty: The problem of restenosis. Hum Pathol 20:477, 1989.

19. Wight TN: Cell biology of arterial proteoglycans. Arteriosclerosis 9:1, 1989.

20. Mintz GS, Popma JJ, Pichard AD, et al: Arterial remodeling after coronary angioplasty: A serial intravascular ultrasound study. Circulation 94:35–43, 1996.

21. Nobuyoshi M, Kimura T, Nosaka H, et al: Restenosis after successful PTCA: Serial angiographic follow-up of 229 patients. J Am Coll Cardiol 12:616–623, 1988.

22. Hofling B, Jeuhns TY: Clinical perspective: Intravascular local drug delivery after angioplasty. Eur Heart J 16:437–440, 1995.

23. Kerenyi T, Merkel V, Szabolcs Z, et al: Local enzymatic treatment of atherosclerotic plaques. Exp Mol Pathol 49:330–338, 1988.

24. Meyer BJ, Fernandez-Ortiz A, Mailhal, et al: Local delivery of r-hirudin by a double-balloon perfusion catheter prevents mural thrombosis and minimizes platelet deposition after angioplasty. Circulation 90:2474–2480, 1994.

25. Jorgenson B, Tonnesen KH, Bulow L, et al: Femoral artery recanalization with percutaneous angioplasty and segmentally enclosed plasminogen activator. Lancet 1:1106–1108, 1989.

26. Nabel EG, Plautz G, Nabel GJ: Site-specific gene expression in vivo by direct gene transfer into the arterial wall. Science 249:1285–1288, 1990.

27. Nabel EG, Plautz G, Boyce FM, et al: Recombinant gene expression in vivo within endothelial cells of the arterial wall. Science 244:1342–1344, 1989.

28. Plautz G, Nabel EG, Nabel GJ: Introduction of vascular smooth muscle cells expressing recombinant genes in vivo. Circulation 83:578–583, 1991.

29. Wolinsky H, Lin CS: Use of the perforated balloon catheter to infuse marker substances into diseased coronary artery walls after experimental postmorten angioplasty. J Am Coll Cardiol 17(suppl B):174B–178B, 1991.

30. Wolinsky H, Thung SN: Use of a perforated balloon catheter to deliver concentrated heparin into the wall of the normal canine artery. J Am Coll Cardiol 15:475–481, 1990.

31. Muller DWM, Topol EJ, Abrams GD, et al: Intramural methotrexate therapy for prevention of neointimal thickening after balloon angioplasty. J Am Coll Cardiol 20:460–466, 1992.

32. Gradus-Pizlo I, Wilensky RL, March KL, et al: Local delivery of biodegradable microparticles contaning colchicine or a cochicine analogue. Effects on restenosis and implications for catheter-based durg delivery. J Am Coll Cardiol 26:1549–1557, 1995.

33. Hong MK, Bhatti T, Matthews BJ, et al: The effect of porous infusion balloon-delivered angiopeptin on myointimal hyperplasia after balloon injury in the rabbit. Circulation 88:638–648, 1993.

34. Shi Y, Fard A, Galeo A, et al: Transcatheter delivery of c-myc antisense aligomers reduces neointimal formation in a porcine model of coronary artery balloon injury. Circulation 90:944–951, 1994.

35. Flugelman MY, Jaklitsch MT, Newman KD, et al: Low level in vivo gene transfer into the arterial wall through a perforated balloon catheter. Circulation 85:1110–1117, 1992.

36. Lambert CR, Leone JE, Rowland SM: Local drug delivery catheters: Functional comparison of porous and microporous designs. Coron Art Dis 4:469–475, 1993.

37. Lambert CR, Taylor S, Smith T: Pressure and volume control for local drug delivery catheters: Development of a new microprocessor-controlled system. Coron Art Dis 5:163–167, 1994.

38. Hong MK, Wong SC, Farb A, et al: Feasibility and drug delivery efficiency of a new balloon angioplasty catheter capable of performing simultaneous local drug delivery. Coron Art Dis 4:1023–1027, 1993.

39. Hong MK, Wong SC, Farb A, et al: Localized drug delivery in atherosclerotic arteries via a new balloon angioplasty catheter with intramural channels for simultaneous local drug delivery. Catheter Cardiovasc Diagn 34:263–270, 1995.

40. Hong MK, Wong SC, Barry JJ, et al: Feasibility and efficacy of locally delivered enoxaparin via the channeled balloon catheter on smooth muscle cell proliferation following balloon injury in rabbits. Catheter Cardiovasc Diagn 41:241–245, 1997.

41. Mitchel JH, Barry JJ, Bow L, et al: Local urokinase delivery with the channel balloon. Catheter Cardiovasc Diagn 41:254–260, 1997.

42. Fram DB, Mitchel JF, Azrin MA, et al: Local delivery of heparin to balloon angioplasty sites with a new angiotherapy catheter. Catheter Cardiovasc Diagn 41:275–286, 1997.

43. Mitchel JF, Fram DB, Palme DF, et al: Enhanced intracoronary thrombolysis with urokinase using a novel, local drug delivery system: In vitro, in vivo and clinical studies. Circulation 91:785–793, 1995.

44. Camenzind E, Kint PP, DiMario C, et al: Local intracoronary heparin delivery in man: Acute feasibility and long-term result. Circulation 92:2463–2472, 1995.

45. Glazier JJ, Kiernan FJ, Bauer HH, et al: Treatment of thrombotic saphenous vein bypass grafts using local urokinase infusion therapy with the Dispatch catheter. Catheter Cardiovasc Diagn 41:261–267, 1997.

46. Moura A, Lam DJ, Hebert JR, et al: Intramural delivery of agent via a novel drug delivery sleeve: Histologic and functional evaluation. Circulation 92:2299–2305, 1995.

47. Fram DB, Aretz TA, Azrin MA, et al: Localized intramural drug delivery during balloon angioplasty using hydrogel-coated balloons and pressure-augmented diffusion. J Am Coll Cardiol 23:1570–1577, 1994.

48. Azrin MA, Mitchel JF, Fram DB, et al: Decreased platelet deposition and smooth muscle cell proliferation following intramural heparin delivery with hydrogel-coated balloons. Circulation 90:433–441, 1994.

49. Mitchel JF, Azrin MA, Fram DB, et al: Inhibition of platelet deposition and lysis of intracoronary thrombus during balloon angioplasty with urokinase-coated hydrogel balloons. Circulation 90:1979–1988, 1994.

50. Nunes GI, Hanson SR, King SB, et al: Local delivery of a synthetic antithrombin with a hydrogel-coated angioplasty balloon inhibits platelet-dependent thrombosis. J Am Coll Cardiol 23:1578–1583, 1994.

51. Riessen R, Rahimizadeh H, Blessing E, et al: Arterial gene transfer using pure DNA applied directly to a hydrogel-coated angioplasty balloon. Hum Gene Ther 4:749–758, 1993.

52. Barath P, Popov A, Dillehay GL, et al: Infiltrator angioplasty balloon catheter: A device for combined angioplasty and intramural site-specific treatment. Catheter Cardiovasc Diagn 41:333–341, 1997.

53. Pavlides GS, Barath P, Manginas A, et al: Intramural drug delivery by direct injection within the arterial wall. First clinical experience with a novel intracoronary delivery-infiltrator system. Catheter Cardiovasc Diagn 41:287–292, 1997.

54. Chien YW, Banga AK: Iontophoretic delivery of drugs: Overview of historical development. J Pharm Sci 78:353–354, 1989.

55. Fermandez Ortiz A, Meyer BJ, Mailhal A, et al: A new approach for local intravascular drug delivery. The iontophoretic balloon. Circulation 89:1518–1522, 1994.

56. Gonschior P, Goetz AE, Huehnst Y, et al: A new catheter for prolonged drug application. Coron Art Dis 6:329–334, 1995.

57. Guyton JR, Rosenburg RD, Clows AW, et al: Inhibition of rat arterial smooth muscle cell proliferation by heparin: In vivo studies with anticoagulant and nonanticoagulant heparin. Circ Res 46:625–634, 1980.

58. Clowes AW, Karnovsky MJ: Suppression by heparin of smooth muscle cell proliferation in injured arteries. Nature 265:625–626, 1977.

59. Edelman ER, Adams DH, Karnovsky MJ: Effect of controlled adventitial heparin delivery on smooth muscle proliferation following endothelial injury. Proc Natl Acad Sci U S A 87:3373–3377, 1990.

60. Schwartz RS, Holder DJ, Holmes DR, et al: Neointimal thickening after severe coronary artery injury is limited by short-term administration of a factor Xa inhibitor. Circulation 93:1542–1548, 1996.

61. Currier JW, Pow TK, Haudenschild C, et al: Low molecular weight heparin reduces restenosis after iliac angioplasty in the hypercholesterolemic rabbit. J Am Coll Cardiol 17(suppl B):118B–125B, 1991.

62. Oberhoff M, Herdeg C, Baumbach A, et al: Time course of smooth muscle cell proliferation after local proliferation after local drug delivery of low molecular weight heparin using a porous balloon catheter. Catheter Cardiovasc Diagn 41:268–274, 1997.

63. Baumbach A, Oberhoff M, Rubsamenk K, et al: Porous balloon delivery of low molecular weight heparin in the dog coronary artery. A safety study. Eur Heart J 17:1538–1545, 1996.

64. Meyer BJ, Fernandez Oritz A, Mailac A, et al: Local delivery of r-hirudin by a double-balloon perfusion catheter prevents mural thrombosis and minimizes platelet deposition after angioplasty. Circulation 90:2474–2480, 1994.

65. Nunes GL, Hanson SR, King SB, et al: Local delivery of a synthetic antithrombin with a hydrogel-coated angioplasty balloon catheter inhibits platelet dependent thrombosis. J Am Coll Cardiol 23:1578–1583, 1994.

66. Leung WH, Kaplan AV, Grant GW, et al: Local delivery of antithrombin agent by an infusion balloon catheter reduces platelet deposition at the site of balloon angioplasty. Coron Art Dis 2:699–706, 1991.

67. Foegh ML, Asotra S, Conte JV, et al: Early inhibition of myointimal proliferation by angiopeptin after balloon injury in the rabbit. J Vasc Surg 19:1084–1091, 1994.

68. Santoian ED, Sohnneider JE, Gravanis MB, et al: Angiopeptin inhibits intimal hyperplasia after angioplasty in porcine coronary arteries. Circulation 88:11–14, 1993.

69. Kuntz KK, Anderson PG, Schroff RW, et al: Efficacy of cytochalasin B in inhibiting coronary restenosis caused by chronic remodelling after balloon trauma in swine [Abstract]. J Am Coll Cardiol 24:302A, 1995.

70. Hebert D, Lam JYT, Moura A, et al: Local intramural nitroglycerin delivery improves vascular response to balloon arterial injury [Abstract]. J Am Coll Cardiol 25:286A, 1995.

71. Folts JD, Kaeney JF, Loscalzo J: Local delivery of nitrosated albumin to stenosed and damaged coronary arteries inhibits platelet deposition and thrombosis [Abstract]. J Am Coll Cardiol 25:377A, 1995.

72. Lablanche JM, Grollier G, Lusson JR, et al: Effect of the direct nitric oxide donors linsidomine and molsidomine on angiographic restenosis after coronary balloon angioplasty. The ACCORD study. Circulation 95:83–89, 1997.

73. Hadeishi H, Mayberg MR, Seto M: Local application of calcium antagonists inhibits intimal hyperplasia after arterial injury. Neurosurgery 34:114–121, 1994.

74. Steg GP, Spaulding C, Makowski S, et al, for the CORAMI-2 study group: A double blind randomized trial of hydrogel balloon delivery of urokinase during primary angioplasty for acute myocardial infarction [Abstract]. Circulation 92:I-543, 544, 1995.

75. Isner JM, Walsh K, Symes J, et al: Arterial gene transfer for the therapeutic angiogenesis in patients with peripheral artery disease. Hum Gene Ther 7:959–988, 1996.

75a. Wilensky RL, Tanguay JF, Ito S, et al: Heparin Infusion

Prior to Stenting (HIPS) trial: Final results of a prospective, randomized, controlled trial evaluating the effects of local vascular delivery on intimal hyperplasia. Am Heart J 139:1061–1070, 2000.

76. Bartonelli AL, Kaplan AV, De Cesare N, et al: Feasibility and safety of local heparin delivery prior to coronary stenting: Initial and six month care angiographic evaluation. J Invas Cardiol 8:60, 1996.

76a. Tanguay JF, Cantor WJ, Drucoff MW, et al: Local delivery of heparin post-PTCA: A multicenter randomized pilot study. Catheter Cardiovasc Interv 49:461–467, 2000.

77. Glazier JJ, Hirst JA, Kiernan FJ, et al: Site-specific intracoronary thrombolysis with urokinase-coated hydrogel balloons: Acute and follow-up studies in 95 patients. Catheter Cardiovasc Diagn 41:246–253, 1997.

77a. Barsness GW, Buller C, Ohman EM, et al: Reduced thrombus burden with abciximab delivered locally before percutaneous intervention in saphenous vein grafts. Am Heart J 139:824–829, 2000.

77b. Lehmann KG, Popma JJ, Werner JA, et al: Vascular remodeling and the local delivery of cytochalasin B after coronary angioplasty in humans. J Am Coll Cardiol 35:583–591, 2000.

78. Miano JM, Vlastic N, Tota RR, et al: Smooth muscle-cell immediate-early gene and growth factor activation follows vascular injury. Arterioscler Thromb 13:211–219, 1993.

79. Benneth M, Schwartz S: Antisense therapy for angioplasty restenosis. Circulation 92:1981–1993, 1995.

80. Bennett M, Anglin J, McEwan R, et al: Inhibition of vascular smooth muscle cell proliferation in vitro and in vivo by c-myc antisense oligodeoxynucleotides. J Clin Invest 93:820–828, 1994.

81. Morishita RG, Gibbons K, Ellison M, et al: Single intraluminal delivery of antisense cdc 2 kinase and proliferating-cell nuclear antigen oligonucleotides results in chronic inhibition of neointimal hyperplasia. Proc Natl Acad Sci U S A 90:8474–8478, 1993.

82. Stein C, Cheng Y: Antisense oligonucleotides as therapeutic agents—Is the bullet really magical? Science 261:1004–1012, 1993.

83. Epstein SE, Siegall CB, Biro S, et al: Cytotoxic effects of a recombinant chimeric toxin on rapidly proliferating vascular smooth muscle cells. Circulation 84:778–787, 1991.

84. Pickering JG, Bacha PA, Weir L, et al: Prevention of smooth muscle cell outgrowth from human atherosclerotic plaque by a recombinant cytoxin specific for the epidermal growth factor receptor. J Clin Invest 91:724–729, 1993.

85. Topol EJ, Califf RM, Weisman HF, et al: Randomized trial of coronary intervention with antibody against platelet IIb/IIIa integrin for reduction of clinical restenosis: Results at six months. Lancet 343:881–889, 1994.

86. Malligan RC: The basic science of gene therapy. Science 260:926–932, 1993.

87. Chapman GD, Lim CS, Gammon RS, et al: Gene transfer into coronary arteries of intact animals with a percutaneous balloon catheter. Circ Res 71:27–33, 1992.

88. Lemarchand P, Jaffe HA, Danel C, et al: Adenovirus-mediated transfer of a recombinant human alpha-1 antitrypsin cDNA to human endothelial cells. Proc Natl Acad Sci U S A 89:6482–6486, 1992.

89. Lemarchand P, Jones M, Yamada I, et al: In vivo gene transfer and expression in normal uninjured blood vessels using replication deficient recombinant adenovirous vectors. Circ Res 72:1132–1138, 1993.

90. Lee SW, Trapnell BC, Rade JJ, et al: In vivo adenoviral vector-mediated gene transfer into balloon-injured rat carotid arteries. Circ Res 73:797–807, 1993.

91. Guzman RJ, Lemarchand P, Crystal RG, et al: Efficient and selective adenovirus-mediated gene transfer into vascular neointima. Circulation 88:2838–2848, 1993.

92. Chang ME, Barr ML, Barton K, et al: Adenovirus-mediated overexpression of the cyclin/cyclin-dependent kinase inhibitor p21 inhibits vascular smooth muscle cell proliferation and neointima formation in the rat carotid artery model of balloon angioplasty. J Clin Invest 96:2260–2268, 1995.

93. Camenzind E, Bakker WH, Reijs A, et al: Site-specific intravascular administration of drugs: History of a method applicable to humans. Catheter Cardiovasc Diagn 41:342–347, 1997.

# 46

# Vascular Radiation Therapy to Reduce Restenosis

*Spencer B. King III*     *Keith A. Robinson*     *Ian R. Crocker*

Restenosis after coronary interventions remains an unsolved limitation. The multiplicity of approaches to the problem reflects the imprecise understanding of what the restenotic process is. Since Gruentzig's first coronary interventions in 1976,[1–3] restenosis has been variously viewed as related to coronary spasm, elastic recoil, endovascular thrombosis, accelerated atherosclerosis, and a wound-healing phenomenon. Clinical interventions, often based on meager experimental evidence, were applied to attack these physiologic mechanisms. Clinical trials of anticoagulants, antiplatelet agents, antispasmodics, angiotensin-converting enzyme (ACE) inhibitors, lipid-lowering agents, corticosteroids, antioxidants, somatostatin analogues, and others have not resulted in a clinical recommendation.

Because several of these therapies have been shown to have an effect in animal models in higher concentrations, a field of locally delivered compounds has emerged. Problems have been a lack of adequate tissue concentrations and rapid washout regardless of the mode of delivery. Genetic signals to interrupt the proliferating cell cycle have also been attempted.

The concept of restenosis as a wound-healing process led to an interest in using agents that have been shown to interfere with cellular proliferation and subsequent wound contracture. Two clinical examples of exuberant scar formation are keloid scars on the skin and pterygium on the sclera of the eye. After excision of both these scars, localized radiation therapy interferes with fibroblast-mediated scar formation and helps prevent rescarring. Low-dose endovascular radiation is a similar approach for inhibiting the localized "scar" that forms after coronary interventions. This chapter reviews the research evidence that this may be an effective antirestenosis strategy, the radiation physics and biology that underlie this approach, and the available clinical evidence to date.

## PRINCIPLES OF BIOLOGY AND RADIATION PHYSICS APPLIED TO ENDOVASCULAR BRACHYTHERAPY

The biologic effect of radiation is due to damage of cellular DNA.[4] Cells suffer mitotic death when they attempt to divide or undergo programmed cell death (apoptosis). No mammalian cells are entirely resistant to radiation. The sensitivity of cells depends in part on the kinetics of the cell population. Well-differentiated cells that are postmitotic have the least sensitivity to radiation, whereas dividing cells are most sensitive. Continuous or fractionated radiation doses take advantage of the fact that cells may be in different phases of the cycle and therefore will be killed more effectively as they enter the more sensitive phases of the cell cycle. The rate of delivery of a radiation dose is also important. A dose delivered over an extended time is less effective than a dose delivered in a more concentrated time frame. Hypoxic tissue may be less sensitive to radiation than well-oxygenated tissue, which may be relevant when radiation is given to tissue undergoing balloon compression or stenting.

X-rays and gamma rays are nonparticulate, and electrons, protons, neutrons, and alpha particles are particulate radiation. Electrons and protons (charged particles) produce their ionizing effect directly on nuclear DNA, and neutrons and photons (noncharged) produce their effect indirectly. X-rays and electrons are indistinguishable regarding their biologic effect. Electrons are produced by beta emitters and deposit energy with each interaction with tissue directly. Photons are produced by gamma emitters and ionize indirectly by producing fast-moving electrons. For the same energy, electrons (produced by beta emitters) have a much shorter path in tissue. This results in a more circumscribed distribution of radiation in the near field with less penetration to other parts of the body than with photons (produced by gamma emitters). The amount of energy delivered to a mass of tissue is referred to as a gray (Gy) (1 Gy = 1 joule/kg).

Certain adverse effects of radiotherapy should be mentioned. Most important is the potential for inducing cancers. Tissues that are particularly sensitive to radiation include thyroid, breast, bone marrow, and lymphoid tissues. It is anticipated that the very small total body dose received from vascular brachytherapy, especially using beta radiation, would be of no significant consequence in affecting the incidence of malignancy because the incidence of spontaneous cancers in the vascular tissues that would be radiated is very low, and very little radiation reaches other tissues. Background radiation affects everyone, and the average dose received by the U.S. population is 3.6 mrem/year. In contrast, the effective total body dose for a beta emitter used in vascular brachytherapy is approximately 1 mrem.

Radiation protection in the catheterization laboratory might depend on the type of radiation and shielding employed. Diagnostic x-rays are easily shielded by thin lead aprons and thin lead covering of the walls of the laboratory. There should be no need to increase this protection with pure beta emitters; however, the question needs to be addressed with the use of gamma emitters. Gamma-radiation therapy, as currently practiced, has been done with removal of the laboratory personnel from the room during the radiation therapy. However, the group in Geneva reported no excess radiation to the operators who remained at the patient's side while using beta radiation.

## ENDOVASCULAR BRACHYTHERAPY IN ANIMAL MODELS OF RESTENOSIS

There is a strong rationale for the idea of delivering ionizing radiation energy to the sites of coronary angioplasty and stenting for the purpose of preventing restenosis. Radiation therapy for the treatment of tumors is designed to either kill cells or prevent them from replicating; cellular hyperplasia is a major mechanism of postangioplasty restenosis and is virtually the only mechanism of in-stent restenosis. In vitro, appropriate doses of radiation inhibit serum-stimulated growth of arterial smooth muscle cells (SMCs) and fibroblasts and decrease collagen synthesis by fibroblasts.

A number of approaches for testing this hypothesis have been applied in preclinical models of vascular lesion formation. Even before the advent of angioplasty, Friedman and colleagues demonstrated that endovascular irradiation with [192]Ir suppressed the formation of hyperplastic atherosclerotic intimal lesions in cholesterol-fed rabbits.[5] More recently, a number of investigators have used both externally

delivered x-irradiation and various catheter- and stent-based endovascular approaches with diverse isotopes to determine whether such systems might affect neointima formation and cellular proliferation after angioplasty and stenting in animal models of restenosis. The design of all these studies was roughly similar: bilateral angioplasty or stenting was performed in a pair of arteries, and radiation was delivered to one of these either immediately before or afterward (in some cases radiation was given up to 5 days afterward). At a later time point, the tissue was harvested and histomorphometric and/or immunocytochemical analysis was performed to determine any differences in the healing responses to the vascular interventional procedures.

The concept of external beam irradiation is an attractive possibility: if radiation delivered to the chest using a linear accelerator were effective, the requirements for an intracoronary radiation catheter (with its small but real associated risk) and prolonged angioplasty procedures would be eliminated. Results using the external approach have been mixed, however. Schwartz and colleagues found slightly increased neointima formation in stented pig coronary arteries 4 weeks after the delivery of 8 Gy from a linear accelerator.[6] Using a nonatherosclerotic rabbit iliac artery angioplasty model, Abbas and coworkers showed a reduction in neointima formation using 12 Gy but not 6 Gy from a 6-mV linear accelerator 5 days after arterial injury.[7] Similarly, Shimotakahara and Mayberg showed a reduction in neointimal hyperplasia in rat carotid arteries after balloon deendothelialization, using a telecesium unit.[8] It is difficult to reconcile these conflicting results, but it may be that the dose, volume of tissue irradiated, and timing of the treatment are crucial. Also, the nature of the injuries (balloon vs. stent) and their consequent healing response are different.

We have performed studies of external beam irradiation in the pig coronary balloon angioplasty. Marijianowski and associates[9] and Styles and coworkers[10] reported that external beam irradiation after balloon injury was effective in decreasing the absolute size of the neointima. However, the luminal and vessel cross-sectional areas were smaller for the irradiated groups despite the arteries having an initially similar size as determined by angiograms taken immediately before angioplasty. Increased collagen content of the externally irradiated vessels was demonstrated by Picrosirius red staining. Finally, the myocardium was substantially damaged by the 14-Gy external irradiation as evidenced by increased myocyte necrosis, inflammatory infiltrates, and interstitial fibrosis. This was in contrast to the myocardium adjacent to the epicardial artery in samples that received 14 Gy by an endovascular approach. These showed no detectable differences in appearance from control arteries given balloon angioplasty alone. Thus, it would seem that although external irradiation can be effective against restenosis-like neointima formation after angioplasty, potential risks of myocardial damage may counteract the possible procedure-related advantages.

On the other hand, numerous studies have consistently demonstrated remarkable suppression of neointima formation using radiation energy from various isotopes delivered by an endoluminal approach. At least three groups have documented similar results in the pig coronary artery model of restenosis after balloon angioplasty, using the gamma emitter [192]Ir at roughly comparable doses. Wiedermann and coworkers found suppression of neointima 4 weeks after angioplasty when 20 Gy was delivered at a radial depth of 1.5 mm just before arterial injury.[11] These same researchers demonstrated a persistence of this effect in arteries harvested at 6 months.[12] Similarly, our group demonstrated profound suppression of neointima using [192]Ir with a dose-response effect in vessels treated with 3.5, 7, and 14 Gy at a radial depth of 2 mm, and continued benefit at 6 months in arteries treated with 14 Gy.[13] Using a high–dose afterloader (in contrast to the previously cited experiments, which used manual delivery of lower-activity sources), Mazur and colleagues found that 10 to 25 Gy of [192]Ir gamma energy at 1.5 mm inhibited the 4-week postinjury loss of lumen diameter and suppressed intimal thickening in the balloon-injured left circumflex (LCX) and left anterior descending (LAD) coronary arteries but had no effect on the stented right coronary artery.[14]

The findings of Mazur and colleagues regarding stented vessels are in contrast with our own results in stented arteries. We found significant inhibition of neointima and increased lumen size in stented LAD and LCX arteries using 14 Gy at 2 mm from both [192]Ir and the beta emitter [90]Sr/Y.[15] This discrepancy may be due to either differences in biologic effects of the dose rate for stented arteries, variance in the healing response of the right coronary artery to stent injury, or some combination of the two factors. An alternative approach for irradiation of stented arteries is the use of radioactive stents, which are covered in more detail later, but next the discussion of catheter-based endoluminal brachytherapy in animal models of balloon angioplasty are completed with a description of studies using the beta-emitting isotopes [90]Y and [90]Sr/Y.

Verin and coworkers reported the use of a flexible yttrium coil, activated in the neutron flux of a nuclear reactor and deployed at the end of a guide wire using a balloon catheter–centering device, after balloon injury in the carotid and iliac arteries of hypercholesterolemic rabbits.[16] Cellular prolifera-

tion at 8 days was measured by bromodeoxyuridine (BrdU) injection and immunocytochemical analysis, and neointimal formation at 8 weeks was assessed by histomorphometry. They demonstrated a reduction in BrdU-positive cells in the intima and media of arteries receiving 6, 12, or 18 Gy compared with controls; however, at 2 months, only the 18-Gy dose was effective for reduction of neointima formation. This device has been applied in a clinical feasibility study.[17]

Our group examined the delivery of stainless steel–encapsulated seeds containing [90]Sr/Y.[18] This isotope has the advantage over [90]Y of a much longer half-life (27 years as opposed to 64 hours) and has sufficient energy to deliver therapeutic doses within a few minutes. The effects of the beta emitter at doses of 7 and 14 Gy (again at a 2-mm depth) on 2-week postangioplasty coronary artery healing were similar to our previous findings using [192]Ir. The neointimal size was decreased and the luminal area was increased to approximately the same dimensions as in the previous study. Scanning electron microscopy of 14-Gy–irradiated arteries showed no morphologic differences from controls at 2 weeks; a confluent layer of endothelial or endothelial-like cells was present throughout the region of angioplasty injury. At 28 and 56 Gy, neointima formation was nearly eradicated; the overall vessel size was also increased in the 28-Gy group.

The final mode of local endovascular radiation therapy to be considered is the use of radioactive stents. There are two basic means for producing such devices: one is neutron bombardment of the stent to render all the elements of the stent metal radioactive, and the other is the implantation of radioactive particles into the surface of the metallic prosthesis. The latter can be achieved by activation of the embedded ions either before or after implantation.

Hehrlein and coworkers initially studied implantation of stents made radioactive by neutron-bombardment.[19] These devices produced mainly beta-particle radiation but also lower doses of gamma- and x-radiation from the plethora of isotopes generated from the stent metal alloy (i.e., [55]Fe, [55]Co, [56]Co, [51]Cr, [52]Mn, and [57]Ni). The stents were highly effective at inhibiting neointima formation but might conceivably be problematic for permanent implantation as some of the isotopes created have very long half-lives. Consequently, this same group of researchers investigated the effects of stents bombarded with [32]P ions by means of a mass separator.[20] In that study, stents with 4-μCi activity had less neointimal cross-sectional area than controls at 4 and 12 weeks, whereas 13-μCi stents had less only at 12 weeks. Cellularity of the neointima was markedly reduced in irradiated groups at 4 and 12 weeks, yet reendothelialization as determined by circumferential von Willebrand factor (vWF) staining was complete in all samples at 4 weeks.

A similar technique was independently developed and tested by Fischell and colleagues; [32]P ion bombardment produced a radioactive wire that inhibited SMC proliferation in vitro.[21] Subsequently, this stent was tested in pig coronary arteries at various levels of radioactivity.[22] Curiously, it was found that low-activity (0.15- to 0.5-μCi) and high-activity (3- to 23-μCi) stents inhibited neointima formation compared with control nonradioactive stents, but those of intermediate activity (1 μCi) had nearly twice as much neointima. The authors speculated that either delayed endothelialization or a stochastic effect on extracellular matrix production might be responsible for this puzzling finding.

Despite differences in isotopes and variations in doses and dose-rate strategies, the biologic effects demonstrated in all these studies are similar. Primarily, the formation of a proliferative neointima as a consequence of balloon or stent injury is greatly reduced or even eliminated (Fig. 46–1). In many cases, mural thrombi and intramural hemorrhages created by the angioplasty injury, which are normally resorbed and incorporated into the vessel wall by 2 to 4 weeks, persist and are readily identifiable at even the 4-week time point (Fig. 46–2). This has led some investigators to conclude that irradiation creates hemorrhagic injury[14]; however, it seems more likely that radiation delays the healing process, resulting in the formation of an "immature" neointima[22] because of suppression of multiple events in vascular wound healing including cell proliferation and fibrinolysis. Similar findings are observed in stented arteries examined at 4 weeks (Fig. 46–3).

Our group has investigated potential mechanisms of the effects of endovascular radiation we had previously detected, specifically suppression of neointima formation and inhibition of postangioplasty

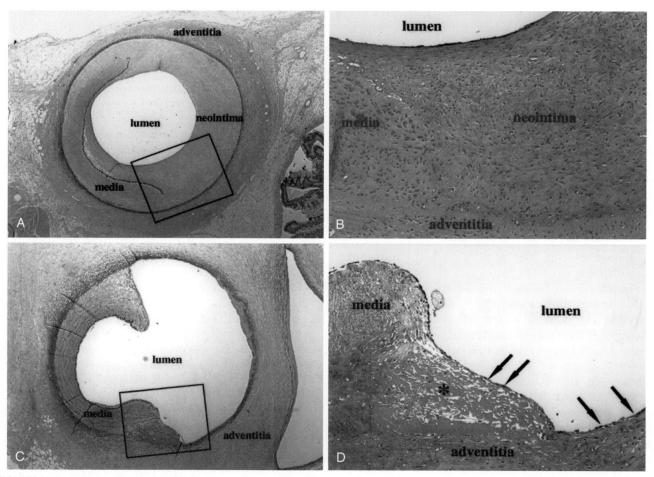

FIGURE 46–1. Light microscopy of control *(A and B)* and 14-Gy beta-irradiated *(C and D)* pig coronary arteries fixed 4 weeks after balloon overstretch angioplasty injury. *A*, Control artery. There is extensive neointima in this section, which shows severe injury with approximately 60% of the artery circumference showing a gap or fracture of the tunica media. (VVG-elastin, ×20.) *B*, Region shown in box *A*. Note abundant proliferative neointima of spindle-shaped and round cells. (H&E, ×100.) *C*, Irradiated artery. There is virtually no neointima in this section, which shows injury comparable to that of the control artery. (VVG-elastin, ×20.) *D*, Region shown in box in *C*. There is an unresolved submedial hemorrhage (*), but the neointima is limited to a single layer of endothelial or endothelial-like cells *(arrows)*. (H&E, ×100.)

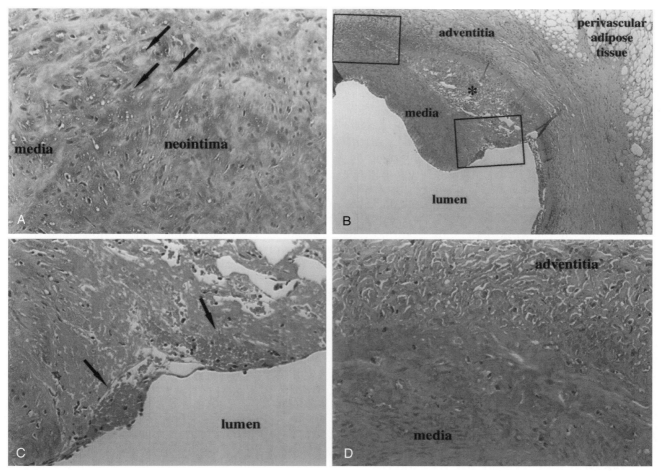

FIGURE 46–2. Light microscopy of H&E-stained control *(A)* and 14-Gy beta-irradiated *(B, C,* and *D)* pig coronary arteries fixed 4 weeks after balloon overstretch angioplasty injury. *A,* Neointima from the control at the dissected edge of the media. Only small rare erythrocyte fragments are seen in the tissue *(arrows).* (×200.) *B,* Irradiated artery. Boxes outline fields shown in *(C)* and *(D).* There is an unresolved submedial hemorrhage (*). (×40.) *C,* Dissected medial edge shows pockets of hemorrhage *(arrows),* which incorporate erythrocytes and leukocytes. (×200.) *D,* Hemorrhage in deep media and adventitia. (×200.)

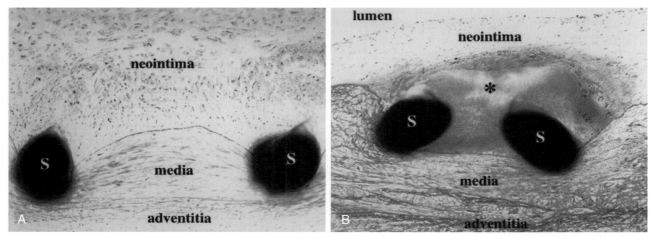

FIGURE 46–3. Light microscopy of toluidine blue-stained methacrylate sections of control *(A)* and 14-Gy beta-irradiated *(B)* pig coronary arteries fixed 4 weeks after endovascular stent (Cordis JJIS) placement. (×100.) *A,* Control shows substantial neointima composed of spindle-shaped and round cells with abundant extracellular matrix. *B,* Irradiated artery has markedly decreased neointima incorporating a pocket of unresolved mural thrombus (*). S, stent wire.

vessel chronic constriction or overall shrinkage ("negative remodeling").[23] It was found that in the pig coronary arteries treated with 14 or 28 Gy at 2 mm, whether from a [192]Ir or [90]Sr/Y source, DNA synthesis at 3 days measured by BrdU uptake was decreased throughout the vessel wall, whereas apoptosis as determined by TUNEL staining was not different from that of controls. Furthermore, SMC α-actin staining in the adventitia, a marker of the acquisition of a contractile or myofibroblastic phenotype of these cells thought to be responsible for chronic vessel constriction, was decreased in irradiated arteries particularly with 28 Gy. There also was a significantly larger vessel perimeter in the treated animals than in the controls, lending support to the idea that it is the adventitial myofibroblast that causes negative remodeling after angioplasty, and showing a potential role for brachytherapy to inhibit this phenomenon as well as the purely proliferative aspect of restenosis, neointima formation.

In summary, the animal studies of endovascular radiation therapy have consistently documented some of the most profound effects yet observed on restenosis in animal models. There is much remaining basic and applied research to be done, however. In particular, effects of brachytherapy on functional aspects of vascular biology and on the extracellular matrix have yet to be determined. These are especially important factors in the clinical and long-term outcomes of patients undergoing percutaneous transluminal coronary angioplasty (PTCA).

## EVALUATION OF ENDOVASCULAR BRACHYTHERAPY IN PATIENTS

Although the animal research has been very encouraging, it is evident that the normal rabbit iliac or pig coronary artery is not equivalent to the human atherosclerotic coronary vessel. Will the effect be the same in patients? Important questions are: What is the role of intimal hyperplasia in human restenosis? Does radiation also affect the late vessel contracture known to play a role in nonstented arteries? What is the target tissue? What is the dose and will a range of doses (unavoidable with brachytherapy) be effective? Will single-dose radiation exposure be the preferred method or will retained radioactive stents be the answer? If effective, will radiation also produce undesirable complications such as coronary aneurysms, thrombosis, or malignancies?

## CLINICAL EXPERIENCE

Although these questions should be considered before embarking on human trials, they are not com-

pletely answerable. The first attempt at vascular brachytherapy was by Liermann and associates in Frankfurt.[24] Patients undergoing angioplasty and stent placement for restenotic lesions in superficial femoral arteries had endovascular radiation applied. The Liermann group reported on 30 patients who underwent repeat angioplasty followed by the insertion of an iridium source by a high–dose-rate afterloading device. The dose was calculated to be 12 Gy at the vascular wall and required treatment times of approximately 200 seconds. The patients have now been followed from 4 to 68 months. These physicians were encouraged by the clinical improvement to an asymptomatic level in 22 of the patients. They state that reocclusion occurred in 16% during the long-term follow-up.

The first clinical coronary procedures were performed by Condado and colleagues in Venezuela.[25] Twenty-one patients were treated with 18 to 25 Gy of gamma radiation delivered with a radioactive [192]Ir wire after coronary angioplasty. Angiographic restenosis was demonstrated in four patients (19%) with angiographic late lumen loss of 0.19 mm. One of the patients developed an aneurysm that has been reexamined at 2 years and found essentially unchanged.[25a]

The proof of the principle that brachytherapy can improve late results of interventions was established by Teirstein, Jani, Massullo, and coworkers in the first randomized trial of endovascular brachytherapy.[26] Patients with prior restenosis, many with multiple restenoses, underwent radiation at the time of their repeat intervention. The procedures involved the use of a commercially available [192]Ir source embedded in a nylon ribbon (Best Medical Interventional; Springfield VA). This isotope decays by emitting photons as gamma radiation. The ribbon, consisting of five or nine seeds with 0.1-cm spacing, was chosen to match the length of the tissue to be irradiated. A hollow catheter was inserted into the coronary artery spanning the segment to be irradiated. At this point, the cardiologist and the catheter laboratory technical personnel left the room and the radiation oncologist delivered the radioactive source into the catheter, placing it into the predetermined segment within the hollow coronary catheter.

A determination of the dosing was achieved by performing intravascular ultrasonography before initiating the radiation therapy. Measurements of the artery were used to estimate the dwell time required to achieve a dose of 800 cGy at the most distant point of the media. This dose was reduced if the radiation to the closest wall of the artery would have exceeded 3000 cGy. It was assumed that the position of the radioactive source would be similar to the position of the ultrasound catheter;

however, it was not possible to utilize this computation for every interval along the dilated segment. The dwell time in the coronary artery ranged from about 20 to 40 minutes, when the oncologist removed the ribbon from the catheter and the cardiologist and catheter team returned to the room for the completion of the procedure. Radiation exposure for the radiation oncologist was measured at 32 mrem/hour, whereas the catheter team received very little radiation because they were not in the room during the procedure.

Fifty-five patients were randomized to receive radiation or a color-coded nonradioactive ribbon. Teirstein[26a, 26b] reported the results of the 53 patients who have undergone follow-up angiographic assessment. The restenosis rate, defined as 50% stenosis at follow-up, was reduced from 54% in the dummy seed group to 16% in the irradiated group. This effect was achieved by a reduction in the loss index (the initial gain minus the late loss divided by the initial gain), which was reduced from 0.6 in the nonirradiated group to 0.12 in the radiated group. This 80% reduction in new tissue within the stent correlates very well with previous evidence in animals.

Despite these encouraging results, for radiation to be a practical adjunct, it will be necessary to develop methods that allow its use as part of the routine catheter laboratory procedure. Gamma radiation as used in these trials is highly penetrating and therefore raises important concerns about exposure to laboratory personnel and increases whole-body radiation for the patient as well. Radiation sources free from these concerns have been sought and until now have been those that produce beta radiation. The absorption pattern of these electrons is highly suited for small vessels such as coronary arteries. The vast majority of radiation is absorbed in a 4- to 5-mm-diameter cylinder around the radiation source without radiating distant sensitive tissues such as bone marrow, lymph nodes, and breast tissue. The radiation leaving the patient's body is hardly greater than background radiation.

The first clinical study employing beta radiation was performed by Verrin, Urban, and associates in Geneva.[17] Their system consisted of a beta-radiation source contained inside a centering balloon. Dosing may have been inadequate due to the effect of the centering balloon placing target tissues such as media and adventitia at a greater distance from the source. The restenosis process was not significantly impacted, perhaps for this reason.

Several investigators have studied the effect of producing beta-emitting radioactive stents as described previously.[19, 26] Continuing dose-finding studies utilizing the radioactive stents are ongoing. Potential advantages are that the stent could apply the radiation directly to the arterial wall and the short distance between the stent and the affected tissue might be advantageous utilizing a beta source. A short half-life is essential because this is a permanent implant, and therefore $^{32}P$ might be ideal. On the other hand, a short half-life also creates problems for the shelf life of the stent, resulting in a lesser degree of radioactivity even over a few days on the shelf. In addition, the radiation will only be effective where the stent wires are, and there will be no effect or little effect beyond the ends of the stent, which may also participate in the restenotic process. This radioactive stent has now received Food and Drug Administration (FDA) investigational device exemption to begin some feasibility studies, which should shed additional light on proper dosing in order to find an effect in patients.

The beta-radiation catheter was developed by the Novoste Company (Atlanta GA), in collaboration with our group at Emory University. Our requirements for the system were a beta-radiation source; a catheter-based system that would allow easy introduction over the existing angioplasty guide wire; catheter features of trackability and flexibility, which would enable placement in all treated segments of the coronary tree; a system that would allow a short exposure time similar to balloon inflation times; and one that could, if possible, maintain antegrade flow during the treatment.

The system that evolved employs specially designed $^{90}Sr/Y$ cannisters fitting without gaps in a trainlike configuration. The components of the system are a catheter that contains a guide wire lumen but is otherwise closed from the circulation. The source train is delivered hydraulically within the closed catheter to the tip in order to span the treated segments. Reversal of fluid flow powers the source train back out of the catheter into the delivery device. The lucite delivery device houses the radiation source train before and after delivery and virtually completely shields the operators from radiation. Radiation 2 mm from the source in a dose of 12 to 16 Gy was delivered in about 2 to 3 minutes dwell time. In porcine coronary experiments, the beta-radiation system was found equally effective to gamma radiation, and therefore it was deemed suitable for human trials.[27]

The first FDA approval for a device using radiation for restenosis was given, and a feasibility trial was begun in January 1996. Approval was granted for use in 23 patients undergoing their first coronary angioplasty procedure. The purpose of this trial was to understand the operational specifications of the system and to identify any problems related to its use. Although underpowered to establish safety or efficacy, the results were closely scrutinized to observe any adverse events, and 6-month angiographic follow-up was scheduled to observe if the residual lesions differed from historical controls. Measurements made at follow-up were the minimal lumen diameter, the percentage stenosis, late lumen loss, the loss index, and the percentage of patients showing restenosis at the treatment site by the 50% dichotomous definition.

The preliminary results of this feasibility trial were encouraging regarding the renarrowing of the treated segments.[28, 29] The first 18 patients undergoing repeat angiography at 6 months showed a late lumen loss of only 0.1 mm and a loss index (late loss divided by initial gain) of 0.05. This means that of the initial gain in lumen diameter after angioplasty, 95% was retained at the 6-month follow-up. The final results of the feasibility study have answered two important questions.[29] The effect of radiation observed in animal studies and in patients with in-stent restenosis is also present in patients treated with balloon angioplasty alone, and beta radiation seems at least as effective as previously used gamma radiation.

## FUTURE CLINICAL TRIALS

Based on the encouraging results found with endovascular brachytherapy, clinical trials will be undertaken. The beta-catheter system used in our institution is now poised to undergo a multicenter randomized trial under an investigational device exemption (IDE) from the FDA. The trial will involve patients with both de novo and restenotic native coronary lesions undergoing angioplasty and stent placement. The basic premise is that endovascular beta radiation with both balloon angioplasty and stent placement will result in a late lumen loss that will be sufficiently low to decrease the overall restenosis rates in both populations. Patients will undergo balloon angioplasty with subsequent angiographic examination. Patients meeting certain criteria of an adequate postangioplasty lumen without significant dissection (<30% residual stenosis) will undergo angioplasty alone. Patients with significant luminal recoil or dissection will undergo coronary stenting. After the initial balloon angioplasty, both groups will receive placement of the beta-catheter system. The source train will be randomized to a radioactive source or a nonradioactive source. The randomization will be blinded from the operators and the patient and will only be known to the radiation oncologist participating in the study. The delivery of the source will be accomplished by the cardiologist for the prescribed treatment time in order to achieve a dose of approximately 14 Gy at a depth of 2 mm, giving an effective cylinder of radiation with a diameter of 4 mm. After the delivery of

the beta catheter, the catheter will be removed and final angiograms obtained. In the stent group, the stents will be placed at the completion of the procedure.

It is anticipated that the trial will consist of approximately 1000 patients, approximately 500 in the angioplasty-alone group and 500 in the stent group. Major adverse clinical events will be monitored throughout a 6-month follow-up period, and coronary arteriography will be obtained on all patients at the completion of the 6-month follow-up. Important angiographic end points will be the minimal lumen diameter of the lesion before the procedure, after the procedure, and at follow-up, and the derivatives of this measurement. Of importance is that the late lumen loss and the loss index will be computed for each patient. The lesion will also be compared with a reference segment that is most normal in appearance. The percentage diameter stenosis will be computed before the procedure, after the procedure, and at follow-up, and the dichotomous 50% definition will be applied in follow-up as well.

To complement this study, a substudy utilizing intravascular ultrasonography will be performed in approximately 100 patients. With the use of this technique, it should be possible to identify the amount of reduction in neointima formation that is achieved with radiation and the distribution of any neointima formation.

These angiographic and ultrasound studies will enable the identification of the effect of intravascular ultrasound on neointima formation and remodeling, and because the use of radiation will be completely blinded, there will be the opportunity for the first time to perform a device study that will mimic a drug study. There will be no opportunity to influence the therapy or follow-up of the patients based on knowledge of treatment assignment. Clinical follow-up will be focusing on the incidence of any major adverse clinical events and the incidence of target lesion revascularization. Any change in total revascularization will be reflected in resource utilization, and this will also be an important component of the trial.

## IMPLICATIONS FOR THE TECHNOLOGY AND CONCLUSIONS

If the clinical trials show a significant reduction in restenosis in a broad range of patients undergoing interventional procedures, there are several possible effects on the field. If restenosis in stented lesions not eligible for the Stent Restenosis Study (STRESS)[30] or the Belgium-Netherlands Stent (BENESTENT) Study,[31] such as long lesions, small vessels, bifurcations, restenotic and vein graft lesions, is 25% to 40%, then an adjunct such as endovascular radiation may be of significant benefit. If brachytherapy can prevent late lumen loss in adequately dilated segments, then stenting can be avoided in those patients treated with balloon angioplasty or atherectomy. A reduction in restenosis could markedly offset the added cost of these new technologies. The economic differences found in the multivessel angioplasty versus surgery trial, such as EAST (Emory Angioplasty versus Surgery Trial)[32] and Bypass Angioplasty Revascularization Investigation (BARI),[33] were small at 5 years despite a significant early advantage for angioplasty. This late attrition and cost benefit was entirely driven by the restenosis problem. A significant reduction in restenosis already demonstrated with stents for some lesions would make revascularization much more affordable to patients and payors alike. Only well-designed clinical trials will tell if these hopes can be realized.

## REFERENCES

1. Grüntzig AR, Senning A, Siegenthaler WE: Nonoperative dilatation of coronary artery stenosis: Percutaneous transluminal coronary angioplasty. N Engl J Med 301:61–68, 1979.
2. Gruentzig AR, King SB, Schlumpf M, et al: Long-term follow-up after percutaneous transluminal coronary angioplasty: The early Zurich experience. N Engl J Med 316:1127–1132, 1987.
3. King SB III, Schlumpf M. Ten-year completed follow-up of percutaneous transluminal coronary angioplasty: The early Zurich experience. J Am Coll Cardiol 22:353–360, 1993.
4. Johns H, Cunningham J: The Physics of Radiology, 4th ed. Springfield IL: Charles C Thomas, 1983.
5. Friedman M, Felton L, Byers S. The antiatherogenic effect of Iridium-192 upon the cholesterol-fed rabbit. J Clin Invest 43:185–192, 1964.
6. Schwartz RS, Koval TM, Edwards WD, et al: Effect of external beam irradiation on neointimal hyperplasia after experimental coronary artery injury. J Am Coll Cardiol 19:1106–1113, 1992.
7. Abbas MA, Afshari NA, Stadius ML, et al: External beam irradiation inhibits neointimal hyperplasia following balloon angioplasty. Int J Cardiol 44:191–202, 1994.
8. Shimotakahara S, Mayberg MR: Gamma irradiation inhibits neointimal hyperplasia in rats after arterial injury. Stroke 25:424–428, 1994.
9. Marijianowski MMH, Styles T, Crocker IR, et al: Epicardial artery and myocardial response to irradiation in the pig coronary artery model of balloon angioplasty: Comparison of the histopathologic consequences of endovascular vs external beam irradiation techniques [Abstract]. Proceedings from Advances in Cardiovascular Radiation Therapy 1997.
10. Styles T, Marijianowski MMH, Robinson KA, et al: Effects of external irradiation of the heart on the coronary artery response to balloon angioplasty injury in pigs. Proceedings from Advances in Cardiovascular Radiation Therapy 1997.
11. Wiedermann JG, Marboe C, Schwartz A, et al: Intracoronary irradiation reduces restenosis after balloon angioplasty in a porcine model. J Am Coll Cardiol 23:1491–1498, 1994.
12. Wiedermann JG, Marboe C, Amols H, et al: Intracoronary irradiation markedly reduces neointimal proliferation after balloon angioplasty in swine: Persistent benefit at 6-month follow-up. J Am Coll Cardiol 25:1451–1456, 1995.
13. Waksman R, Robinson KA, Crocker IR, et al: Endovascular low dose irradiation inhibits neointima formation after coronary artery balloon injury in swine: A possible role for radiation therapy in restenosis prevention. Circulation 91:1553–1539, 1995.
14. Mazur W, Ali MN, Khan MM, et al: High dose rate intracoronary radiation for inhibition of neointimal formation in the stented and balloon-injured porcine model of restenosis: Angiographic, morphometric, and histopathologic analyses. Int J Radiat Oncol Biol Phys 36:777–788, 1996.
15. Waksman R, Robinson KA, Crocker IR, et al: Intracoronary radiation prior to stent implantation inhibits neointima formation in stented porcine coronary arteries. Circulation 92:1383–1386, 1995.
16. Verin V, Popowski Y, Urban P, et al: Intra-arterial beta irradiation prevents neointimal hyperplasia in a hypercholesterolemic rabbit restenosis model. Circulation 92:2284–2290, 1995.
17. Verin V, Urban P, Popowski Y, et al: Feasibility of intracoronary β-irradiation to reduce restenosis after balloon angioplasty: A clinical pilot study. Circulation 95:1138–1144, 1997.
18. Waksman R, Robinson K, Crocker I, et al: Intracoronary low dose β-irradiation inhibits neointima formation after coronary artery balloon injury in the swine restenosis model. Circulation 92:3025–3031, 1995.
19. Hehrlein C, Gollan C, Donges K, et al: Low-dose radioactive endovascular stents prevent smooth muscle cell proliferation and neointimal hyperplasia in rabbits. Circulation 92:1570–1575, 1995.
20. Hehrlein C, Stintz M, Kinscherf R, et al: Pure β-particle–emitting stents inhibit neointima formation in rabbits. Circulation 93:641–645, 1996.
21. Fischell TA, Kharma BK, Fischell DR, et al: Low dose β-particle emission from "stent" wire results in complete, localized inhibition of smooth muscle cell proliferation. Circulation 90:2956–2963, 1994.
22. Carter AJ, Laird JR, Bailey LR, et al: Effects of endovascular radiation from a β-particle–emitting stent in a porcine coronary restenosis model: A dose-response study. Circulation 94:2364–2368, 1996.
23. Waksman R, Rodriquez JC, Robinson KA, et al: Effect of intravascular irradiation on cell proliferation, apoptosis, and vascular remodeling after balloon overstretch injury of porcine coronary arteries. Circulation 96:1944–1952, 1997.
24. Liermann D, Bottcher HD, Kollath J, et al: Prophylactic endovascular radiotherapy to prevent intimal hyperplasia after stent implantation in femoropopliteal arteries. Cardiovasc Intervent Radiol 17:12–16, 1994.
25. Condado JA, Popma JJ, Lansky AJ, et al: Effect of intracoronary 192-iridium on late quantitative angiographic outcomes after PTCA. J Am Coll Cardiol 29(suppl A):418A, 1997.
25a. Condado JA, Waksman R, Gurdiel O, et al: Long-term angiographic and clinical outcome after percutaneous transluminal coronary angioplasty and intracoronary radiation therapy in humans. Circulation 96:727–732, 1997.
26. Teirstein PS, Massullo V, Jani S, et al: Radiation therapy following coronary stenting: 6-month follow-up of a randomized clinical trial. Circulation 94(suppl I):I-210, 1996.
26a. Teirstein PS, Massullo V, Jani S, et al: Catheter-based radiotherapy to inhibit restenosis after coronary stenting. N Engl J Med 336:1697–1703, 1997.
26b. Teirstein PS, Massullo V, Jani S, et al: Three-year clinical and angiographic follow-up after intracoronary radiation: Results of a randomized clinical trial. Circulation 101:360–365, 2000.
27. Carter AJ, Laiord JR, Bailey LR, et al: Effects of endovascular radiation from a β-particle–emitting stent in a porcine coronary restenosis model: A dose-response study. Circulation 94:2364–2368, 1996.
28. King SB III, Crocker IR, Hillstead RA, et al: Coronary endovascular beta-radiation for restenosis using a novel catheter system: Initial clinical feasibility study. Circulation 94(suppl I):I-619, 1996.
29. King SB 3rd, Williams DO, Chougule P, et al: Endovascular beta-radiation to reduce restenosis after coronary balloon angioplasty: Results of the Beta Energy Restenosis Trial (BERT). Circulation 97:2025–2030, 1998.
30. Fishman DL, Leon MB, Baim DS for the Stent Restenosis Study Investigators: A randomized comparison of coronary stent placement and balloon angioplasty in the treatment of coronary artery disease. N Engl J Med 331:496–501, 1994.

31. Serruys PW, de Jaegere P, Kiemeneij F for the BENESTENT Study Group. A comparison of balloon expandable stent implantation with angioplasty in patients with coronary artery disease. N Engl J Med 331:489–495, 1994.

32. King SB III, Lembo NJ, Weintraub WS, et al: A randomized trial comparing coronary angioplasty with coronary artery bypass surgery. Emory Angioplasty versus Surgery Trial (EAST). N Engl J Med 331:1044–1050, 1994.

33. The BARI investigators. Comparison of coronary bypass surgery with angioplasty in patients with multivessel disease. N Engl J Med 335:217–225, 1996.

# 47

# Cutting Balloon Angioplasty

*Olivier F. Bertrand      Raoul Bonan*

Since its introduction in 1977, balloon angioplasty has been limited mainly by early vessel closure and late restenosis.[1, 2] Among the several devices developed during this period, none has been capable of significantly reducing these two complications.[3, 4] More recently, intracoronary stenting appeared as an invaluable procedure to reduce acute ischemic complications due to vessel dissections.[5, 6] As scaffolding wall supports, stents provide optimized lumen contour and restore adequate blood flow. At the same time, stenting also reduces the restenosis rate in selected lesions.[7, 8] Balloon dilatation leads to complex vascular wall lesions that include mechanical deformation of the vessel, a wide range of injury of the three vessel layers, and the immediate formation of thrombus. Restenosis appears as a response to injury and involves a complex interplay between thrombus formation and organization, smooth muscle cell proliferation, and vessel remodeling.[9, 10]

Despite the known proportional neointimal response to injury in animal models, the search to decrease the restenosis phenomenon initially focused on debulking devices known to produce an immediate improved residual lumen diameter after the coronary intervention ("Bigger is Better").[3, 11, 12] It was later shown that this improved acute luminal gain was followed by an exaggerated luminal loss.[12, 13] Accordingly, the beneficial effect of coronary stenting is presumably due to a better or larger vessel geometry after dilation because stenting has proved to induce more neointimal reaction when compared with balloon angioplasty.[14, 15] The concept of the cutting balloon catheter (InterVentional Technologies, San Diego, CA) developed by Peter Barath hypothesizes a reduction in the acute vessel wall injury that would allow a decrease in acute complications and late restenosis.[16] This chapter covers the proposed mechanisms of cutting balloon angioplasty, presents the current clinical experience, and discusses potential applications. Finally, a recent evolution of the cutting balloon manufacturing technology as an efficient local drug delivery system is briefly described.

## DEVICE DESCRIPTION AND MECHANISMS OF DILATION

The cutting balloon catheter has been developed from a conventional over-the-wire balloon catheter (Fig. 47–1). The cutting balloon catheter has three microblades (Fig. 47–2) on smaller balloon sizes and four microblades on balloon sizes above 3.5-mm diameter. These atherotomes (Fig. 47–3), approximately 0.25 mm in height, are three to five times sharper than conventional surgical blades. About one half of the total blade height is used in the fabrication of a microtome edge, whereas the other half is used for attachment to the balloon. In order to increase its flexibility, a specific process that creates a series of keyholes on the blade base has been developed. These keyholes remove about one third of the blade mass and provide multidimensional flexibility. To ensure definite fixation to the balloon, unique bonding processes have been developed. This results in a blade-to-balloon bond strength that exceeds the tensile strength of the atherotome itself. To prevent inadvertent exposure of the microblades, special folding techniques have been perfected (Fig. 47–4). This allows exposure of the microblades only when the balloon is inflated at the lesion site. Similarly, this system allows safe retrieval of the cutting balloon once it is deflated. During insertion and withdrawal, the microtomes have little, if any, contact with the surrounding vessel tissue or the guid-

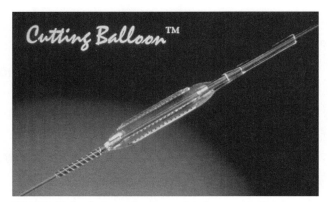

FIGURE 47–1. Photograph of an inflated cutting balloon.

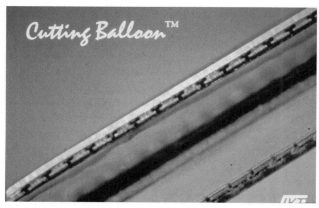

FIGURE 47–2. Magnification of the inflated cutting balloon showing the atherotome blades with its series of keyholes at the base of the blades. These keyholes reduce the blade mass and provide multidimensional flexibility.

# CUTTING BALLOON™ FOLDING ACTION

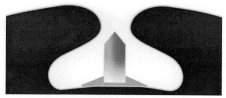

FIGURE 47–4. Atherotome blade protection during insertion/withdrawal: the balloon material has been specially engineered to cause the atherotome blades to consistently withdraw into the "folds" of the deflated balloon.

ing catheter.[17] The balloon itself is made of polyethylene terephthalate (PET) and is noncompliant. The dual shaft of the balloon catheter is made from polyethylene sulfone (PES). According to the manufacturer, the rated burst pressure is 10 atm. The cutting balloon catheter is made available with a range of inflation diameters from 2 to 4 mm in 0.25-mm increments. Nominal blades lengths of 10 and 15 mm are provided. Two platinum alloy bands are mounted symmetrically on the inner shaft tubing within the balloon and serve as radiopaque markers. These markers are nominally 10 to 15 mm apart, so their position approximates the ends of the blades. This spacing facilitates the cutting balloon positioning, as the microblades are not visible under fluoroscopy. The microsurgical dilation concept combines the features of conventional balloon angioplasty with advanced microsurgical technique.

It is intended to minimize the vessel wall trauma traditionally associated with conventional balloon angioplasty.

When the cutting balloon is inflated, the atherotomes are exposed. As inflation continues and the balloon expands, the microtomes incise (making a *cut, incision* or *score*) the plaque, relieving its hoop stress (Fig. 47–5).[18, 19] These cuts are limited to the immediate vicinity of the atherotome, developing a controlled fault line along which dilation will occur, and, unlike the situation with conventional angioplasty, random tearing of the surrounding tissue is avoided. It is expected that these incisions facilitate maximum dilation of the target lesion with the least amount of dilating force, thus minimizing trauma to the artery. The concept is therefore to *cut* first and dilate afterward.[20]

This is in contrast to conventional balloon dilation angioplasty, which typically applies 8 to 20 atm of unfocused force and propagates uncontrolled ruptures of plaque at the site or sites of least resis-

# ATHEROTOME™ DIMENSIONS

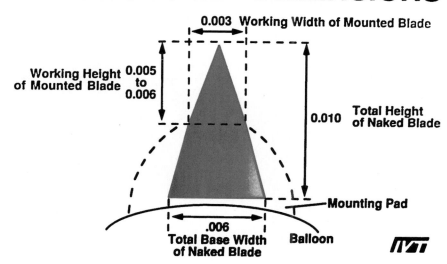

FIGURE 47–3. Size of the atherotome blades: the cutting balloon atherotome blades are approximately ten thousandths of an inch in height (approximately 0.25 mm). About one half of the total height is used for the fabrication of a microtome edge, whereas the base half is used for attachment to the balloon.

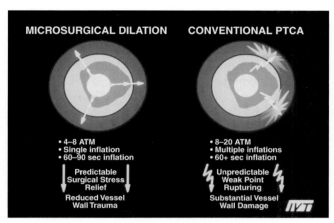

FIGURE 47–5. Schematic representations of the microsurgical dilation and conventional percutaneous transluminal coronary angioplasty (PTCA) dilation.

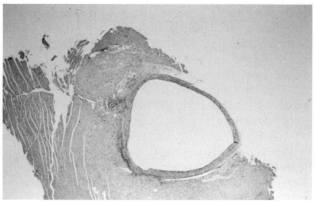

FIGURE 47–6. Effect of the cutting balloon angioplasty on normal porcine left anterior descending (LAD) artery after 14 days. Angiographic dilatation was 6.4%. Wide separation of the media is recognizable. The luminal surface area is completely endothelialized. The minimal proliferation is not sufficient even to completely fill dimpling caused by the medial separation. (H&E, × 2)

tance as evidenced by tearing, ripping, and dissecting of the lesion or the artery.[16] Conventional balloon angioplasty creates a high level of injury by tearing, splitting the inner vessel wall and stretching the vessel. It was shown in a porcine coronary model that the neointimal formation is proportional to the initial vessel injury generated by the balloon inflation.[21] It was expected that the cutting balloon would yield predictable stress relief with less pressure and that a single short inflation would ultimately translate into a reduced vessel wall trauma.

## ANIMAL STUDIES

To test the hypothesis that the microblades would score the intimal and medial layers, initial testing was performed in porcine peripheral and coronary arteries. Using angioscopy in peripheral pig arteries, Barath and associates showed that at low-pressure inflation, cutting balloon microblades initially produced sharp incisions into the vessel wall without separation of the incision's edges.[16] As the inflation pressure increased, the edges of the incisions became widely separated, exposing the media. Comparing cutting balloon angioplasty with standard balloon angioplasty, Barath and associates described endothelial denudation in 45% and 100% of the cases respectively.[16] Three days after cutting balloon angioplasty, a complete endothelialization had already occurred. Similarly, internal elastic lamina disruption and severe intimal tears that were present in more than 80% of the cases after conventional balloon angioplasty were absent after cutting balloon angioplasty. Angiographic control, 4 hours after 30% overstretch balloon angioplasty, showed the recoil to be limited at 2% after cutting balloon versus 5% after conventional balloon angioplasty.[16] These results suggested the possibility of limited

recoil after cutting balloon angioplasty compared with conventional balloon angioplasty. Histologically, vessels treated by the cutting balloon showed sharp incisions extending into one third to two thirds of the medial layer of the vessel wall (Fig. 47–6). Subsequent study, 14 days later, showed intimal proliferation to be limited to the cut area after cutting balloon angioplasty (Fig. 47–7) in contrast with a more diffuse proliferation seen after conventional balloon angioplasty.[22] Importantly, experiments conducted in porcine normal coronary arteries did not show any vessel perforation. In a series of experiments using oversized cutting balloon catheters (balloon/artery ratio of 1.3) no angiographic dissection or contrast extravasation was demon-

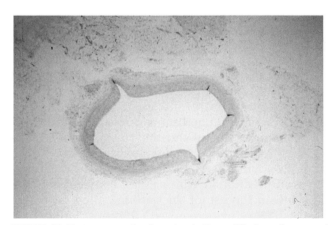

FIGURE 47–7. Acute result of cutting balloon dilation of a normal porcine left anterior descending (LAD) artery. Dilatation was 32%. Note the two incisions at 5 and 11 o'clock that penetrate into the media. (Other *black lines* are artifacts of the fixation process.) There is no intramural or perivascular bleeding present, in contrast to the artery dilated by conventional balloon angioplasty. (The incision did not remain completely open because of the fixation process, but in vivo incisions increased the luminal circumference significantly.) (H&E, × 2)

strated. In this last series of six animals, histologic examination showed dissections in two cases and no thrombus formation in any case. Therefore, in these experiments conducted in normal coronary pig arteries, the cutting balloon appeared safe as incisions were limited to the intimal and medial layers of the vessel wall. Three days after the procedures, proliferating cell nuclear antigen (PCNA) staining was markedly limited to the cut area after cutting balloon angioplasty but distributed around the entire dilated segment after balloon angioplasty. Fourteen days later, cellular proliferation was found to cover a mean value of 71% of the original vessel medial area with the conventional balloon versus only 4.6% with cutting balloon angioplasty.[23]

## CADAVERIC EXPERIMENTS

The cadaveric heart experiments were designed to show that the cutting balloon catheter could be used in diseased human coronary arteries without causing dissections, flaps, or significant damage to the vessel wall. These experiments were performed on nine different coronary arteries.[24] Overall, diameter stenoses were reduced from 68% to 12% by the cutting balloon. Postprocedural hearts were immersed in formalin for 24 hours. Then dilated segments were dissected, decalcified, embedded, and stained with hematoxylin and eosin to illustrate the cutting balloon catheter's mechanism of actions. Incisions of atherosclerotic plaque as well as incisions of the free wall were recognized. However, no incision extended beyond the media. Therefore, the cutting balloon microblades appeared well suited to incise the atherosclerotic plaque in human coronary arteries.

## EARLY CLINICAL EXPERIENCE

In 1993, Unterberg and colleagues reported the first clinical study of cutting balloon angioplasty.[25] The cutting balloon was inflated once, and inflation pressure was held constant at 4 atm for 60 seconds. In 12 patients out of 25, the cutting balloon was used as the sole device, and stenoses were reduced from 84% ± 8% to 28% ± 11%. Two patients required predilation with a small conventional balloon before the use of the cutting balloon catheter. The last 13 patients required additional balloon angioplasty because of a residual lesion greater than 50% after cutting balloon angioplasty. Then stenoses were reduced from 78% ± 8% to 29% ± 11%. At 6-month angiographic follow-up, three restenoses were noted from 14 controlled patients. All restenoses presented in lesions that were either pre- or postdilated with a conventional balloon, and

none were present in stand-alone cutting balloon procedures. Technical difficulty advancing the catheter balloon occurred in three patients, and balloon leakage was recognized. Electron microscopy revealed that damage to the balloon was caused by one distal end of a microtome. A minor balloon design modification resolved this early product failure. One patient suffered an acute vessel occlusion and required stent implantation for severe postangioplasty dissection. Overall, angiographic dissections were visible on two occasions, including the case followed by vessel closure.

Hosakawa and Suzuki reported their experience with cutting balloon angioplasty in 177 patients and 236 lesions.[26] The cutting balloon was used in any type of lesion provided the operator's judgment was that the lesion was accessible to cutting balloon. Lesion characteristics included mostly type B (80%) and type C (16%). In addition, 35% were restenotic lesions, 19% were calcified, 14% included diffuse lesions, 2% were ostial, 2% had thrombus, and 4% were chronic total occlusions. Technical data revealed large differences in operators' practice, with the number of inflations ranging from one to six (mean 1.5), maximal inflation pressure varying from 4 to 15 atm (mean 8), and mean inflation time from 50 to 1040 seconds (mean 205). Moreover, balloon/artery ratio was largely distributed from 0.8 to 1.6 (mean 1.2). The average reference vessel diameter was 2.8 ± 0.5 mm, and lesion length was 11 ± 6 mm. The minimal lumen diameter increased from 0.8 ± 0.3 mm to 1.6 ± 0.4 mm, and the percentage diameter stenosis decreased from 66% to 31%. Procedural success, defined as a residual lesion less than 50% without a major complication, was obtained in 81% of stand-alone cutting balloon angioplasty and 90% after adjunctive conventional balloon angioplasty. No lesion characteristics were significantly associated with treatment failure. The investigators reported failure in 24 cases, 38% of which were due to an inability to cross the lesion and 62% due to an inability to successfully dilate the lesion. Complications occurred in 29 cases. Major complications included one myocardial infarction, but no death or emergency bypass surgery was reported. Minor complications occurred in 12% of the cases, with complex dissections (23 of 28) most frequent. Of note, one coronary perforation occurred and was successfully treated by percutaneous pericardial drainage and prolonged inflation with an autoperfusion balloon catheter. In this preliminary experience, the restenosis rate at 3 months was 36% in 36 patients. Extending their experience to 374 patients, they reported a restenosis rate of 31% with an acute gain of 1.05 ± 0.5 mm and a late loss of 0.55 ± 0.56 mm. In this series, predictors of restenosis were found to be predilation diameter

**TABLE 47–1.    MULTICENTER EXPERIENCE—EFFICACY MEASURES**

| | I<br>N = 20*<br>n = 20* | II<br>N = 13†<br>n = 13† | III<br>N = 110†<br>n = 115† | IV<br>N = 155†<br>n = 166† | TOTAL<br>N = 298<br>n = 314 |
|---|---|---|---|---|---|
| Success/patients | 19/20 | 13/13 | 79/110 | 128/155 | 239/298 |
| (%) | (95) | (100) | (71.8) | (82.6) | (80.2) |
| Success/lesions | 19/20 | 13/13 | 83/115 | 134/166 | 249/314 |
| (%) | (95) | (100) | (72.2) | (80.7) | (79.3) |
| CB alone/lesions | 6/20 | 9/13 | 77/115 | 115/166 | 207/314 |
| (%) | (30) | (69.2) | (67) | (69.3) | (65.9) |
| Success/CB alone | 6/6 | 9/9 | 52/77 | 94/115 | 161/207 |
| (%) | (100) | (100) | (67.5) | (81.7) | (77.8) |

I, phase I, United States[25]; II, restenosed lesions; III, phase II, international[29]; IV, phase III, United States/global nonrandomized[28]; CB, cutting balloon; n, number of lesions; N, number of patients.
\*Catheter laboratory data.
†Core laboratory data.

stenosis and postprocedural minimal lumen diameter.[27, 28]

## MULTICENTER EXPERIENCE

Before the initiation of a large randomized trial comparing balloon angioplasty and cutting balloon angioplasty, four nonrandomized trials were performed. These included a total of 333 patients with type A or B lesions (Table 47–1). These patients were enrolled at 43 sites, of which 23 were located in the United States, 14 in Europe, and five in Canada. Angiographic core laboratory data are available for 294 lesions out of 314, from 298 patients treated with the cutting balloon device. Of these 314 lesions, 207 (66%) were treated by the cutting balloon catheter as sole device, whereas 107 (34%) required additional devices. As later in the randomized trial, only type A or B lesions (Fig. 47–8), 20 mm long or shorter were selected. Patients were treated with a single cutting balloon inflation using up to 8 atm and an inflation time up to 90 seconds. Physicians were encouraged not to use subsequent balloon angioplasty if the residual lesion after cutting balloon angioplasty was 40% or less. The overall lesion success after cutting balloon angioplasty was 249 of 314 (79.3%). In 207 stand-alone cutting balloon procedures, success was obtained in 161 (77.8%), and after additional balloon angioplasty in 107 cases, success was obtained in 88 (82.2%). In these multicentric experiences, no death, emergency bypass surgery or Q-wave myocardial infarction was reported during the hospitalization period. Non–Q-wave myocardial infarction occurred in 5 of 333 (1.5%) of the patients. No vessel perforations were reported, whereas abrupt vessel closure occurred in 5 of 349 (1.4%) lesions and dissections type B or greater were seen in 50 of 349 (14.3%) of the lesions (Table 47–2).

Popma and colleagues analyzed angiographic data from 150 of the Global Learning Curve Registry.[28] Overall, reference diameters were 2.80 ± 0.42 mm. The minimal lumen diameter increased from 1.02 ± 0.3 mm to 2.01 ± 0.42 mm ($p < 0.001$), and

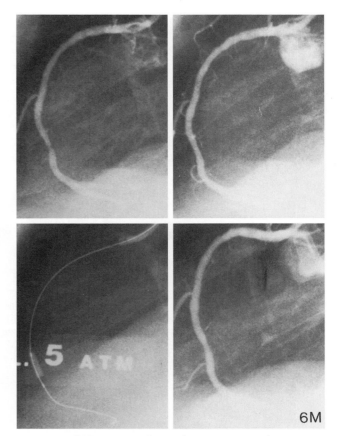

CB 2.75/10 (2.58 mm)
Ø Ref. = 2.75 mm
lesion 1.09 → 2.21mm

FIGURE 47–8. Lateral projection of a right coronary artery (RCA). Type A lesion at the midportion of the RCA. A 2.75-mm-diameter 10-mm-long cutting balloon inflated at 5 atm. Immediate result. *6M*, Result of the 6-month angiographic control.

**TABLE 47–2.    MULTICENTER EXPERIENCE—COMPLICATIONS**

| | I<br>N = 20*<br>n = 20* | II<br>N = 13*<br>n = 13† | III<br>N = 140*<br>n = 150* | IV<br>N = 160*<br>n = 166† | TOTAL<br>N = 333<br>n = 349 |
|---|---|---|---|---|---|
| No clinical events | 20/20 | 13/13 | 139/140 | 151/160 | 323/333 |
| (%) | (100) | (100) | (99.3) | (94.4) | (97.0) |
| Death | 0/20 | 0/13 | 0/140 | 0/160 | 0/333 |
| (%) | (0) | (0) | (0) | (0) | (0) |
| CABG | 0/20 | 0/13 | 0/140 | 0/160 | 0/333 |
| (%) | (0) | (0) | (0) | (0) | (0) |
| Nonfatal MI (Q-wave and non–Q-wave) | 0/20 | 0/13 | 2/140 | 3/160 | 5/333 |
| (%) | (0) | (0) | (1.4) | (1.9) | (1.5) |
| Dissections ≥ type B | 1/20 | 2/13 | 6/150 | 41/166 | 50/349 |
| (%) | (5.0) | (15.4) | (4.0) | (24.7) | (14.3) |
| Perforations | 0/20 | 0/13 | 0/150 | 0/166 | 0/349 |
| (%) | (0) | (0) | (0) | (0) | (0) |
| Abrupt closure | 0/20 | 0/13 | 4/150 | 1/166 | 5/349 |
| (%) | (0) | (0) | (2.7) | (0.6) | (1.4) |

I, phase I, United States[21]; II, restenosed lesions; III, phase II, International[28]; IV, phase III, United States/global nonrandomized[236]; CABG, coronary artery bypass graft; MI, myocardial infarction; n, number of lesions; N, number of patients.
*Catheter laboratory data.
†Core laboratory data.

diameter stenoses were reduced from 64% ± 9% to 29% ± 12% ($p < 0.001$). The minimal lumen diameter, after cutting balloon angioplasty alone (N = 106), was lower than after additional techniques (N = 44), 1.93 ± 0.37 mm versus 2.22 ± 0.46 mm, respectively. Similarly, residual stenoses after cutting balloon angioplasty alone were significantly larger than after complementary techniques, 31% ± 10% versus 24% ± 14% ($p < 0.0006$). The average cutting balloon/artery ratio was 0.88 ± 0.12 (range 0.64 to 1.34), which could be considered somewhat suboptimal given the protocol-recommended 1.1 to 1.2:1 ratio. Interestingly, no difference in the cutting balloon/artery ratio was found in lesions with dissections type B or greater and those lesions without dissections (1 ± 0.11 versus 0.97 ± 0.13). A weak inverse correlation was found between the cutting balloon/artery ratio and the final diameter stenosis ($r = 0.33$).

In the international phase II trial, the angiographic analysis of the 120 lesions (core laboratory: Cardialysis) showed a late loss in the group treated by cutting balloon alone of 0.24 mm (Fig. 47–9) compared with 0.36 mm in the group requiring addi-

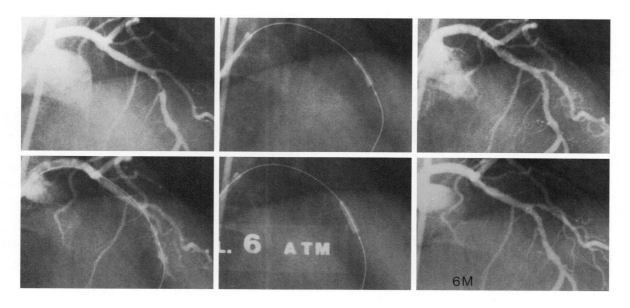

## CB 3.25/15 (3.10 mm), Ø Ref. = 2.72 mm, lesion .99 → 1.86 mm

FIGURE 47–9. Cutting balloon angioplasty of the LAD in the right anterior oblique and cranial projections. Type A lesion of the midportion of the LAD. Cutting balloon 3.25 mm in diameter and 15 mm long in position before inflation. Balloon inflated at low pressure with the waist still present and fully expanded at 6 atm. Immediate angiographic result with type B dissection. *6M*, Angiographic 6-month follow-up.

tional inflations.[29] In preliminary data comparing absolute and relative angiographic parameters from the international phase II trial with those from the Canadian Coronary Atherectomy Trial (CCAT), a lower loss index was found after cutting balloon angioplasty than after cutting balloon and additional angioplasty or directional atherectomy.[30] This in turn may suggest that cutting balloon angioplasty, by limiting the extent of vessel trauma, may reduce the neointimal formation and hence restenosis (Fig. 47–10). From these data, it appeared that the cutting balloon could be used as the sole device in about two thirds of the cases, with a primary angiographic success similar to that of balloon angioplasty. In these selected lesions, complications were kept low and initial angiographic follow-up suggested a possible advantage of cutting balloon angioplasty over conventional balloon angioplasty. To directly compare restenosis rates between cutting balloon angioplasty and conventional balloon angioplasty, the

Global Randomized Cutting Balloon Trial was designed.

## GLOBAL RANDOMIZED CUTTING BALLOON TRIAL

The Global Randomized Cutting Balloon Trial was designed to compare acute procedural results and 6-month outcomes using 1244 patients treated with cutting balloon or conventional balloon angioplasty. As illustrated (Fig. 47–11), the protocol targets short, type A, $B_1$, and $B_2$ lesions in native coronary arteries. If the patient is allocated to conventional balloon angioplasty, the operator is authorized to use multiple balloons and multiple inflations, as necessary (Fig. 47–12). Furthermore, there is no restriction in terms of inflation pressure or duration. If the patient is assigned to the cutting balloon arm, initial dilation is performed with a single inflation of maximum 8 atm for 90 seconds. The operator is

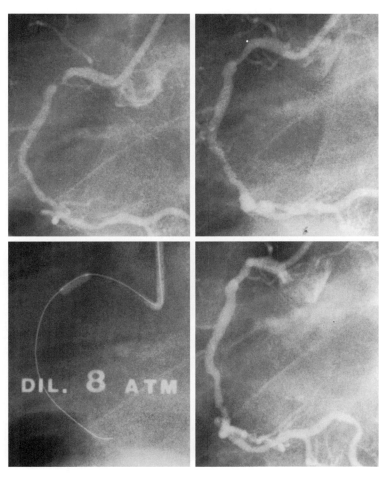

FIGURE 47–10. Treatment of a type B lesion with a 3.5-mm-diameter 10-mm-long cutting balloon. *Upper right panel,* Immediately after treatment. *Lower right panel,* Wider lumen at 6 months.

CB 3.5/10 (3.30mm), Ø Ref. = 3.78 mm, lesion 1.09 mm → 1.71 mm ↓ 2.66 mm

# Global Randomized Cutting Balloon™ Trial

**Study Design:** The Global Randomized Cutting Balloon Trial will compare acute procedural results and six-month outcomes between 1244 patients treated with Cutting Balloon or Conventional PTCA (POBA).

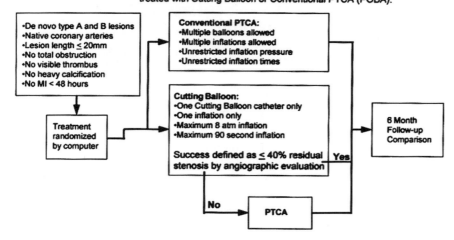

FIGURE 47–11. Global Randomized Cutting Balloon Trial protocol.

strongly encouraged not to use subsequent conventional balloon angioplasty if the residual stenosis is 40% or less (Fig. 47–13).

By November 1996, 1245 patients had been enrolled at 30 centers in North America and Europe. Designed interim analysis results of the first 299 patients were available in 1997.[31] Baseline demographic and clinical characteristics are shown in Table 47–3. Core laboratory data are available for 169 lesions in the cutting balloon group and 179 lesions in the conventional balloon group (lesion types and localization are shown in Tables 47–4 and 47–5). Overall, in the cutting balloon group, the minimal lumen diameter increased from 0.9 ± 0.3 mm to 1.9 ± 0.5 mm and diameter stenosis de-

creased from 67% ± 11% to 30% ± 16%. In the conventional group, minimal lumen diameter increased from 0.9 ± 0.3 mm to 2.1 ± 0.5 mm and diameter stenosis decreased from 66% ± 11% to 28% ± 13%. Lesions treated with the cutting balloon as the sole device numbered 113 of 169 (66.9%) with a treatment success (residual lesion ≤50% without complications) of 95 of 113 lesions (84%); as opposed to conventional angioplasty using a single percutaneous transluminal coronary angioplasty (PTCA) balloon as sole device in 93 of 148 lesions (62.8%). In the cutting balloon group, 35 patients had complementary dilation with conventional PTCA. Stenting was necessary in 13 of 149 patients (8.7%) in the cutting balloon group and 18

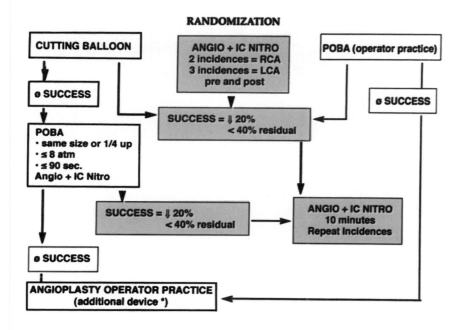

FIGURE 47–12. Decision tree in the catheter laboratory.

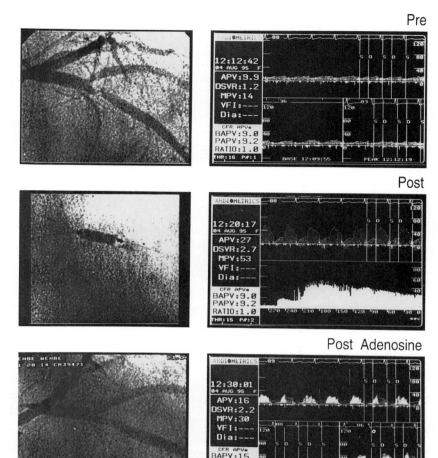

FIGURE 47–13. Cutting balloon and coronary flow. Treatment of the mid-LAD lesion with a 3.5-mm-diameter 10-mm-long cutting balloon inflated at 6 atm for 90 seconds. Moderate residual stenosis. Coronary flow reserve (CFR) was unchanged after adenosine pretreatment *(upper right panel). Mid right panel* shows the increase in the flow immediately after balloon deflation. *Lower right panel* shows normalization of the coronary flow reserve after adenosine with a CFR = 2.

of 150 (12%) in the PTCA group ($p$ = nonsignificant [ns]). No death occurred in either group, whereas bypass surgery was needed in 1.3% of both groups. Q-wave myocardial infarctions were identical in the two groups (1.3%), whereas non–Q-wave myocardial infarctions were slightly more frequent in the cutting balloon group (3.2% vs. 2.6% in the PTCA group [$p$ = ns]). Abrupt vessel closures, as recognized by the angiographic core laboratory, were reported at the same level in the two groups (4%), and one perforation occurred in the cutting balloon group. No difference was found in dissections of type B or greater (30%) in the two groups.

Interestingly, the incidence of target lesion revascularization at 6 months was reduced by 45% in the cutting balloon group with 10% (14 of 140 patients) versus 18.3% for conventional PTCA (24 of 131

**TABLE 47–3. BASELINE DEMOGRAPHIC AND CLINICAL CHARACTERISTICS**

|  | CB | PTCA | TOTAL |
|---|---|---|---|
| Patients (no.) | 149 | 150 | 299 |
| Lesions (no.) | 169 | 179 | 348 |
| Age (y) | 57 ± 10 | 59 ± 10 | 58 ± 0 |
| Male (%) | 67.1 | 72.7 | 69.9 |
| Diabetes (%) | 15.5 | 12.1 | 13.8 |
| Hyperlipidemia (%) | 47.3 | 51.7 | 49.5 |
| High blood pressure (%) | 34.4 | 38.9 | 36.7 |
| Smoking history (%) | 60.1 | 62.7 | 61.4 |
| Prior MI (%) | 35.2 | 41.4 | 38.3 |
| Prior CABG (%) | 3.4 | 4.0 | 3.7 |
| LVEF (%) | 60.4 ± 13.1 | 62.0 ± 11.0 | 61.2 ± 12.8 |

CABG, coronary artery bypass graft; CB, cutting balloon angioplasty; MI, myocardial infarction; LVEF, left ventricular ejection fraction; PTCA, percutaneous transluminal coronary angioplasty.

**TABLE 47–4. ANATOMIC CHARACTERISTICS— LOCALIZATION**

|  | CB | PTCA | TOTAL |
|---|---|---|---|
| No. of lesions | 169 | 179 | 348 |
| RCA (%) | 28.4 | 32.4 | 30.4 |
| LAD (%) | 46.2 | 44.1 | 45.1 |
| CX (%) | 25.4 | 23.5 | 24.4 |

CB, cutting balloon angioplasty; CX, circumflex artery; LAD, left anterior descending artery; PTCA, percutaneous transluminal coronary angioplasty; RCA, right coronary artery.

**TABLE 47–5. ANATOMIC CHARACTERISTICS— LESION TYPE**

|  | CB | PTCA | TOTAL |
|---|---|---|---|
| No. of lesions | 169 | 179 | 348 |
| A (%) | 23 | 22 | 22 |
| $B_1$ (%) | 44 | 39 | 42 |
| $B_2$ (%) | 29 | 37 | 33 |
| C (%) | 4 | 2 | 3 |

CB, cutting balloon angioplasty; PTCA, percutaneous transluminal coronary angioplasty.

patients). Major cardiac events were also lower at 6 months in the cutting balloon group 14.9% (17 of 114 patients) against 24.8% ($p = 0.07$) (27 of 109 patients) in the PTCA group.

Overall, these preliminary data suggest that acute results with cutting balloon angioplasty are similar to those of conventional balloon angioplasty. In particular, microblades do not induce more angiographic or clinical complications.

## OTHER STUDIES IN PROGRESS

### CUBA

The CUBA (CUtting Balloon vs. Angioplasty) study in Spain randomized 300 patients between microsurgical dilation and conventional angioplasty (Principal Investigator: J. Goicolea, Hospital San Carlos, Madrid, Spain).[32] Of interest, it also subrandomized 50 patients (25 each cohort) to intravascular ultrasonography.

The designed interim analysis presented at the European Society of Cardiology meeting in 1996 looked at the acute and follow-up results of the first 100 patients as well as the first 24 acute intravascular ultrasound (IVUS) verifications. The acute demographics and results for all patients showed no differences between the cohorts. However, although acute angiographic interpretation ascribed equal amounts of dissection to both groups, the IVUS analysis showed 70% less "true" dissection for the cutting balloon ($p < 0.05$) and also demonstrated that the cutting balloon morphology had a consistent "star-shaped" geometry of dilatation.[33] Finally, for equal angiographic postprocedural residual lumens, the cutting balloon cohort showed about 50% less vessel area increase ($p < 0.01$). Both these findings point to a validation of the acute effect concept of microsurgical dilation. The angiographic restenosis (50% definition) interim analysis of 85 patients showed the cutting balloon at 28% and conventional balloon angioplasty at 44% but did not reach significance ($p = 0.10$).

## BRIT

The BRIT (British Randomised Incisional Treatment) study randomizes 360 patients between cutting balloon and conventional balloon angioplasty exclusively in vessels 2.75 mm or less (principal Investigator: D. Cumberland, Sheffield, UK). Indeed, small vessel outcomes remain a concern with continuing unacceptable restenosis rates even with stents. This study aimed to confirm a body of observational data that cutting balloons may improve late outcomes in such small vessels. The trial was scheduled to complete patient enrollment in the latter part of 1997.

## REDUCE

The REDUCE (REstenosis reDUCtion by cutting balloon Evaluation) study will randomize 800 patients between cutting balloon and PTCA (Principal Investigator: T. Suzuki, Toyohashi, Japan). Half the sample size will receive IVUS verification. The major difference from the Global Randomized Cutting Balloon Trial is that REDUCE will allow multiple inflations of the cutting balloon in the same lesion to optimize acute residuals. Besides restenosis data, this study should yield insight into the tradeoff between less residual stenosis and potentially more damage.

### Other Trials

Several randomized protocol projects of cutting balloon angioplasty for in-stent restenosis as an alternative to radiation therapy are planned.

## OTHER POTENTIAL APPLICATIONS OF CUTTING BALLOON ANGIOPLASTY

### Resistant Coronary Lesions

Resistant coronary lesions remain a challenge for modern angioplasty. Classical approaches to dilate these lesions include high-pressure inflations, prolonged inflations, and balloon oversizing. Other alternatives include the buddy-wire dilation with one or two guide wires passed alongside a conventional balloon catheter.[34, 35] Once inflated, the guide wire exerts a focused force onto the resistant plaque. Another approach, the hugging balloon technique, involves simultaneous inflations of two balloon catheters at the critical stenosis level.[36] New technologies like rotablation, atherectomy, or laser angioplasty have also been proposed in case of failed angioplasty or for lesions that seem unsuitable for balloon angioplasty.[37–39] With a multidevice approach, Leon and coworkers reported 98% angiographic success in 85 undilatable lesions.[40, 41]

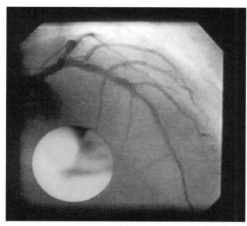

FIGURE 47–14. Angioscopic image of a cut with its angiographic equivalent of the LAD immediately after the first diagonal post–cutting balloon treatment.

Using the cutting balloon catheter (Fig. 47–14), we have reported our initial experience in six resistant lesions recruited from a total of 3090 coronary angioplasties performed over a period of 19 months.[38] Three lesions were located in saphenous vein grafts and three lesions in native coronary arteries. Reference diameters were 3.30 ± 0.68 mm. Initial attempts using conventional balloons with a maximal balloon/artery ratio of 1.14 ± 0.27, maximal inflation pressure of 20 ± 3 atm, and total inflation time of 11 ± 5 minutes failed. With the use of cutting balloon catheters and a balloon/artery ratio of 0.99 ± 0.23, a maximal inflation pressure of 8 ± 1 atm, and a duration of 3 ± 0.6 minutes, minimal lumen diameters increased from 0.85 ± 0.63 mm to 2.49 ± 0.55 mm. Additional balloon angioplasty or stenting performed in five cases led to a final minimal lumen diameter of 3.16 ± 0.97 mm. Therefore, we believe that cutting balloon angioplasty could be a special application for the treatment of resistant coronary lesions (Fig. 47–15). A multicenter registry has been initiated to further explore this new indication.

## Ostial Lesions

Balloon angioplasty of ostial lesions has been associated with an unfavorable outcome. In a multicenter trial of ostial right coronary lesions, Topol and associates reported an overall 79% procedural success, and about 10% of the patients were sent to emergency bypass surgery.[42] Technical difficulties usually were related to a lack of backup support; lesion resistance; and recoil. Moreover, multiple balloon exchanges were usually required. Clinical follow-up usually revealed a restenosis rate above 50%.[43, 44] To improve these limited results, directional, rotational, or extraction atherectomy have been put forward in limited series.[44, 45] More re-

cently, stenting appeared to significantly reduce the acute recoil and produce improved results.[46]

Ostial lesions represent one kind of resistant lesion, resistant to the balloon itself with a persistent waist or to the treatment by balloon with important recoil. After our experience with the cutting balloon in resistant lesions, an ostial stenosis of the left anterior descending artery was treated successfully with a single inflation of 3.25-mm-diameter/10-mm-long cutting balloon (Fig. 47–16).

Sigwart and his group reported similar success on aorto-ostial lesions when they used the cutting balloon before stenting in three native and five vein graft aorto-ostial lesions.[47] These lesions were resistant to conventional high-pressure balloon angioplasty and responded to cutting balloon angioplasty at a mean pressure of 7.5 ± 0.5 atm. All procedures were completed by stenting and displayed a 100% event-free survival.

## Hemodialysis Arteriovenous Fistula Lesion

Reports are coming from Europe about using the cutting balloon to treat resistant lesions in hemodialysis arteriovenous fistula.[48] Vorwerk and colleagues describe 15 patients with 19 discrete venous lesions in hemodialysis fistula (15) and grafts (4) treated by a cutting balloon 3 to 6 mm in diameter.[48] The stenosis was reduced from 65% ± 15% to 14% ± 9%, and failure to obtain residual stenosis less than 20% was experienced in two cases in which the cutting balloon was markedly undersized. Two minor complications were reported. In one patient, a fine layer of extravasation was temporarily shown along the dilated segment of the brachial cephalic vein, but shunt flow was sufficient, and the course was uneventful. Another patient presented with a rupture of the antebrachial cephalic vein at the site of dilatation resulting in a medium-sized, self-limited hematoma. Shunt flow was high, however, and further follow-up was uneventful. It was concluded that the principle of "cut then dilate" can be effectively applied in the thin-walled venous system without creating complications; moreover, after a mean follow-up of 5.4 months, 14 lesions showed no restenosis and remained widely patent.

## Creation of Atrial Septal Defects

Coe and coworkers described in 1996 a novel indication for the cutting balloon.[49] They used it for the creation of an atrial septal defect in a young piglet. Balloon atrial septotomy is a life-saving procedure that is relatively effective in infants younger than 1 month. As the atrial septum thickens beyond the neonatal period, and certainly for older children,

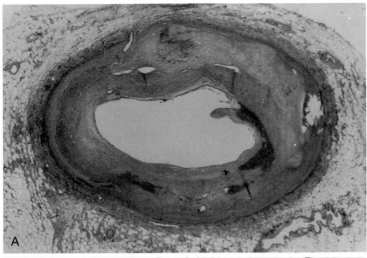

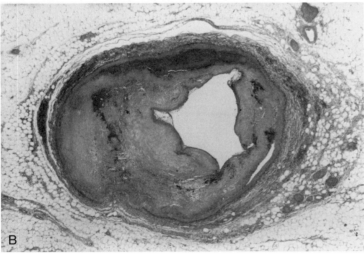

FIGURE 47–15. Histomorphology after cutting balloon angioplasty of a patient who died shortly after cutting balloon and conventional balloon angioplasty of the right coronary artery (RCA). *A*, Distal site of the RCA, which was dilated with conventional balloon angioplasty and showed classical aspects. In this concentric lesion, moderate plaque compression and a small intimal flap surrounded by some intraplaque hemorrhage are recognized. *B*, Proximal RCA (resistant lesion) dilated with two cutting balloons and one conventional balloon at high pressure. Six different small incisions into the plaque resulting from the two different cutting balloons used are easily recognized. In this non–pressure-fixed artery, the lumen enlargement resulted from widening these initial cuts through balloon expansions. The presence of the mild intraplaque hemorrhage may be the consequence of the high-pressure dilation used before the cutting balloon. (*A* and *B*, Hematoxylin-phloxine-safran, × 64)

who may need an atrial septotomy for palliation of their cardiac malformation, the atrial septum is not amenable to a simple balloon atrial septotomy. In older infants and children, an atrial septal defect may be created surgically (Blalock-Hanlon procedure) or without a thoracotomy using the Park blade septotomy catheter. Atrial septal defects were created using a cutting balloon (2.5 to 4 mm in diameter) on a 300-cm coronary angioplasty wire passed in the left atrium through the Brockenbrough needle. The atrial septal defect was then enlarged with a valvuloplasty balloon 8 mm in diameter.

## INFILTRATOR ANGIOPLASTY BALLOON CATHETER

The fabrication process developments that made cutting balloons a possibility were transitioned into the realization of a novel local drug delivery device: the Infiltrator angioplasty balloon catheter.

Local drug delivery represents an interesting challenge in interventional cardiology. Before the "magic drug" that will resolve all remaining effects of the restenosis phenomenon is discovered, the search for an adequate delivery mechanism must be completed.[50] Indeed, it has been postulated that many promising formulations have not demonstrated restenosis reduction after intervention simply because their concentration and residence time in the target tissue have been insufficient to modify the restenosis mechanism or mechanisms. To correct this deficiency, one would require a rapid and efficient delivery of low-mobility compounds directly into the lesion and/or vessel wall.

A number of studies with actual catheters have demonstrated the shortcomings of wall-oriented intraluminal designs to be slow delivery (up to 30 minutes), substantial systemic washout with potential side effects, low delivery efficiency with limited intrawall uptake (<25%), and no intrawall volume control.[51] Most of the devices developed during the last decade are intraluminal, denoting that they infuse the drug into the vessel lumen and depend on various mechanisms to migrate the infusate into the

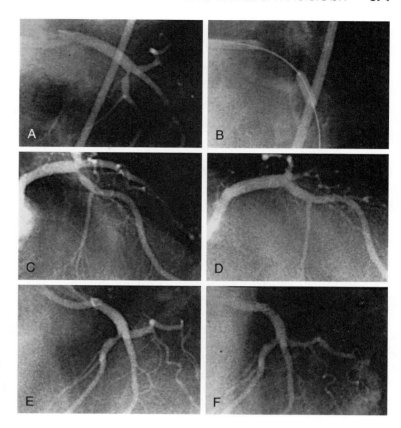

FIGURE 47–16. Ostial stenosis of the LAD treated by single inflation of a 3.25-mm-diameter 10-mm-long cutting balloon. *A,* Left anterior oblique (LAO) cranial projection of the LAD ostial stenosis. *B,* Single cutting balloon inflation. *C, D,* Pre– and post–cutting balloon in right anterior oblique (RAO) cranial projection. *E, F,* Pre– and post–cutting balloon in LAO cranial projection.

vessel wall. Most of these intraluminal designs depend on the presence of postdilation tears in the arterial wall to obtain intramural delivery. This results in variable distribution and low delivery efficiency, and it almost never produces circumferential delivery. So, although intraluminal devices are useful with thrombus treatment, they do not appear to overcome the challenge of intramural delivery as posed by the restenosis model.[52]

To date, only two devices are known as intramural devices: the Needle Injection Catheter (Bavaria Medizin Technologie GmbH; Munich, Germany) and the Infiltrator (Interventional Technologies, Inc.; San Diego CA). The Infiltrator angioplasty balloon catheter (Fig. 47–17) originates from the cutting balloon concept and was designed by Peter Barath.

This over-the-wire catheter features a conventional noncompliant balloon and several series of microminiaturized delivery ports. The balloon is 15 mm long, and the effective delivery area is identified with two radiopaque markers. Its rated burst pressure is 8 atm, and the available diameters are 2 to 4 mm in 0.5-mm increments. With a shaft diameter of 4.2-French on a 127-cm length, its crossing profile is between 0.054 and 0.059 inches, and it has to be used with a 0.014 inch or less guide wire through an 8-French guiding catheter. The delivery part consists of three U-shaped longitudinal, proximally open polyurethane troughs, mounted onto the sur-

face of the balloon with 120 degrees of separation between each. Mounted on each channel are a series of seven microports with articulated metallic plate roofs. Each microport is 0.254 mm high with an 0.102-mm micropore exit width. A separate delivery lumen feeds all three channels and carries a drug lumen priming volume of approximately 0.7 mL. Like the cutting balloon, the Infiltrator balloon is folded in such a manner that the injector ports are covered until deployment, offering a safe manipulation in the artery. When positioned, the balloon is inflated at low pressure (≤2 atm), minimizing vessel damage; the microports are uncovered, radially ex-

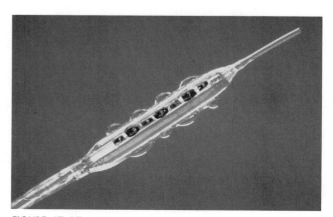

FIGURE 47–17. Infiltrator: intramural drug delivery system.

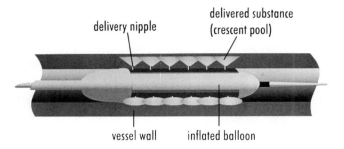

delivery nipple

delivered substance
(crescent pool)

vessel wall      inflated balloon

## DELIVERY PHASE (LONGITUDINAL SECTION)

FIGURE 47–18. Schematic representation of the Infiltrator.

tended, and penetrate the media of the artery, where the "solution" can be directly delivered by microliter precision and without a jet effect (Fig. 47–18).

The animal experimentation was conducted in pig coronary arteries (117 normal coronary arteries of 58 farm pigs). The low-profile injector port punches a well-defined hole in the intima and the elastic lamina, opening a free channel for the delivery of substance into the media at a required minimal push pressure of 0.6 atm. Delivery of 0.4 mL normal saline occurred without angiographic signs of damage. By histologic examination, a fluid edema was recognized at the injector port site without separation of layers or dissection (Fig. 47–19).

Fluorescence material delivered through the Infiltrator documented the rapid circumferential distribution of the substance (Fig. 47–20). The use of $^{99m}$Tc-labeled sulfur colloid showed no perivascular or downstream escape detected by gamma-camera analysis and recorded the high delivery efficiency. Moreover, the low injury provoked by the Infiltrator correlated with no appreciable angiographic steno-

sis at 14 days and a well-recognized injection site with interrupted internal elastic lamina and minimal intimal proliferation localized to the penetration area (Fig. 47–21). Finally, when oversized, the device is also suitable for primary dilation and performs similarly to a conventional PTCA balloon.[53]

Two feasibility and safety studies in humans have already been conducted in Europe. Pavlides and colleagues (Athens, Greece) enrolled 17 patients.[54] The Infiltrator was used after conventional angioplasty and delivered 0.4 mL (6000 IU) of low molecular weight heparin. The IABC was inflated to 1 to 2 atm for 30 to 45 seconds, and the heparin was injected by hand in 5 seconds. In 10 patients, stent placement followed IABC use. The decision to proceed to stent placement was made after the initial dilation with a conventional balloon, and it was not influenced by the IABC use. The hospital course for all patients was uneventful, with no electrocardiographic change and normal cardiac enzymes.

Colombo and colleagues (Milan, Italy) enrolled 24

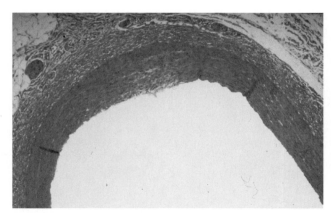

FIGURE 47–19. Cross section of a pig artery after an acute experiment with slow hand injection of 0.4 mL rhodamine with three plated normal-sized (1:1 balloon/artery ratio) Infiltrator balloons. There is some edema from the delivered fluid. The internal elastic lamina is interrupted only at the injection site. No separation or dissection of the arterial wall layer is seen. (H&E)

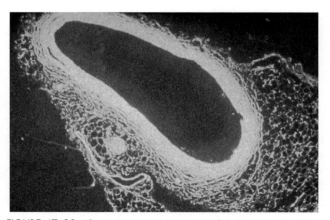

FIGURE 47–20. Fluorescence microscopy of a pig coronary artery 120 minutes after delivery of 0.4 mL of rhodamine with a three-plated balloon. By that time, the three areas of delivery became completely confluent; however, they already started to become confluent by 10 minutes after the injection. Homogeneous distribution of the dye in the media and adventitia with some perivascular escape was seen.

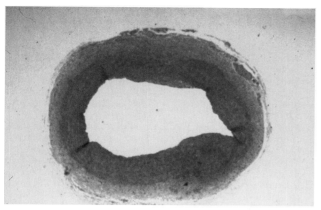

FIGURE 47–21. Cross section of a pig coronary artery after a chronic (14-day) experiment with slow hand injection of 0.4 mL of normal saline with a three-plated 30% oversized Infiltrator balloon. (H&E)

patients with 40 complex lesions (47% of type C) in a study of local intrawall drug delivery of methylprednisolone acetate before stenting implantation using the Infiltrator.[55] Delivery was realized in 36 lesions (21 patients). In the remaining 4 lesions, the Infiltrator did not cross the lesion site. After drug delivery, 46 stents were implanted at high pressure. No procedural or intrahospital complications were recorded. One subacute stent thrombosis occurred 7 weeks later, without myocardial infarction. After complete angiographic follow-up (100%), the investigators concluded that local delivery of long-acting steroid did not improve the restenosis rate (target lesion revascularization was performed in 44% of the cases) in this subset of unfavorable lesions with high risk for restenosis. Currently, two other feasibility trials employing ethyl alcohol and anti-Myc antisense administration are being conducted with the Infiltrator catheter. From these preliminary experiences, the Infiltrator catheter appears well suited and safe for local drug delivery.

## ADVANTAGES AND INCONVENIENCES

The cutting balloon angioplasty definitively offers a different mechanism of dilation. The concept of "cutting first and then dilating" permits a different approach in dilation, "controlling" the inevitable dissection and relieving the hoop stress, allowing maximal dilatation with less trauma. This has been confirmed with its favorable use in resistant and ostial lesions. The low loss index found after cutting balloon angioplasty may suggest reduced neointimal formation and hence restenosis, which needs to be confirmed by the randomized trial. Finally, the technique of a short single inflation could bring technical and economic benefits to the catheter laboratory: less procedural time per case, less fluoroscopy time

(less radiation) per case, less contrast use per case, and finally less stent use per case.

Some inconveniences are evident and directly related to the concept itself. The microblades, even small, not only increase the balloon profile but also, specifically the 15-mm-long balloon, reduce its tractability with potential failure to reach distal lesions in small tortuous vessels. The single inflation emphasizes the need to have an optimal balloon/artery ratio at once, which can often be achieved with the actual availability of the on-line quantitative coronary angiography (QCA).

## CONCLUSION

Few areas of medical specialty device application fields have undergone as rapid a transformation as the interventional cardiology discipline. Although the field is still primarily driven by angioplasty, other transluminal coronary interventions are rapidly gaining importance. Virtually all the new technologies find their origin in the persistent restenosis conumdrum and, in spite of recent advances, the perfect treatment remains elusive.

The cutting balloon represents a mechanical solution attempt to dealing simultaneously with vascular recoil/remodeling and with smooth muscle cell proliferation. In microsurgical dilation, stress fracture mechanics are employed to alter the vessel's contractility capabilities by scoring through the intima and into the media, while simultaneously reducing barotrauma by lowering inflation pressures, inflation times, and the number of inflations through localization of the dilation forces in small sections of the treatment area. Although this concept certainly represents a radical departure from present thinking, we should not forget that coronary dilation was rather unthinkable just 20 years ago.

## ACKNOWLEDGMENTS

The authors thank all the catheterization laboratories' staff of the Institut de Cardiologie de Montréal, particularly Doctor Michel Joyal, Mrs. Jacynthe Théberge, R.N., and Mrs. Suzanne Morissette, R.N., for their outstanding coordinating assistance, and Mrs. Suzanne Taillefer for her expert preparation of the manuscript.

## REFERENCES

1. Gruentzig A: Transluminal dilatation of coronary-artery stenosis. Lancet 1:263, 1978.
2. Topol EJ: Promises and pitfalls of new devices for coronary artery disease. Circulation 84:689–694, 1991.
3. Appelman YE, Piek JJ, Strikwerda S, et al: Randomised trial of excimer laser angioplasty versus balloon angioplasty for treatment of obstructive coronary artery disease. Lancet 347:79–84, 1996.
4. Adelman AG, Cohen EA, Kimball BP, et al: A comparison of directional atherectomy with balloon angioplasty for lesions of the left anterior descending coronary artery. N Engl J Med 329:228–233, 1993.
5. Schömig A, Kastrati A, Mudra H, et al: Four-year experience with Palmaz-Schatz stenting in coronary angioplasty compli-

cated by dissection with threatened or present vessel closure. Circulation 90:2716–2724, 1994.

6. Roubin GS, Cannon AD, Agrawal SK, et al: Intracoronary stenting for acute and threatened closure complicating percutaneous transluminal coronary angioplasty. Circulation 85:916–927, 1992.

7. Serruys PW, de Jaegere P, Kiemeneij F, et al: A comparison of balloon-expandable-stent implantation with balloon angioplasty in patients with coronary artery disease. N Engl J Med 331:489–495, 1994.

8. Fischman DL, Leon MB, Baim DS, et al: A randomized comparison of coronary-stent placement and balloon angioplasty in the treatment of coronary artery disease. N Engl J Med 331:496–501, 1994.

9. Forrester JS, Fishbein MM, Helfant R, Fagin J: A paradigm for restenosis based on cell biology: Clues for the development of new preventive therapies. J Am Coll Cardiol 17:758–769, 1991.

10. Mintz GS, Popma JJ, Pichard AD, et al: Arterial remodeling after coronary angioplasty: A serial intravascular ultrasound study. Circulation 94:35–43, 1996.

11. Topol EJ, Leya F, Pinkerton CA, et al: A comparison of directional atherectomy with coronary angioplasty in patients with coronary artery disease. N Engl J Med 329:221–227, 1993.

12. Kuntz RE, Baim DS: Defining coronary restenosis. New clinical and angiographic paradigms. Circulation 88:1310–1323, 1994.

13. Kuntz RE, Gibson M, Nobuyoshi M, Baim DS: Generalized model of restenosis after conventional balloon angioplasty, stenting and directional atherectomy. J Am Coll Cardiol 21:15–25, 1993.

14. Painter JA, Mintz GS, Wong SC, et al: Serial intravascular ultrasound studies fail to show evidence of chronic Palmaz-Schatz stent recoil. Am J Cardiol 75:398–400, 1995.

15. Dussaillant GR, Mintz GS, Pichard AD, et al: Small stent size and intimal hyperplasia contribute to restenosis: A volumetric intravascular ultrasound analysis. J Am Coll Cardiol 26:720–724, 1995.

16. Barath P, Fishein MC, Vari S, Forrester JM: Cutting balloon: A novel approach to percutaneous angioplasty. Am J Cardiol 62:1249–1252, 1991.

17. Michiels R: Cutting balloon system technology: The engineering perspective. J Invasive Cardiol 8(suppl A):6A–8A, 1996.

18. Blake A: Practical Fracture Mechanics in Design, pp 323–326. Marcel Dekker, 1990.

19. Blake A: A Mechanical Evaluation of the Dilatation of Atherosclerotic Disease with the Barath Surgical Dilatation Balloon System. IVT Technical Report Series, vol 2, no 2, 1992.

20. Lary BG: Coronary artery incision and dilation. Arch Surg 115:1478–1480, 1980.

21. Bonan R, Paiement P, Scortichini D, et al: Coronary restenosis: Evaluation of a restenosis injury index in a swine model. Am Heart J 126:1334–1340, 1993.

22. Barath P: Microsurgical dilatation concept: Animal data. J Invasive Cardiol 8(suppl A):2A–5A, 1996.

23. Leong HC, Schmidt D, Czer LSC: Growth factor expression, DNA synthesis and cellular proliferation after cutting balloon coronary angioplasty [Abstract]. Circulation 86(suppl 1):1331, 1996.

24. Barath P, Radish H: Personal communication, 1996.

25. Unterberg C, Buchwald A, Barath P, et al: Cutting balloon coronary angioplasty—Initial clinical experience. Clin Cardiol 16:660–664, 1993.

26. Hosakawa H, Suzuki T: Large single center experience with cutting balloon. J Invasive Cardiol 8:69, 1996.

27. Suzuki T, Hosakawa H, Yokoya K, et al: Acute and follow-up results with cutting balloon angioplasty. J Invasive Cardiol 8:72, 1996.

28. Popma J, Lansky A, Purkayastha D, et al: Angiographic and clinical outcome after cutting balloon angioplasty. J Invasive Cardiol 8(suppl A):12A–19A, 1996.

29. Bonan R: Multicentric non-randomized experience with cutting balloon. J Invasive Cardiol 8(suppl A):9A–11A, 1996.

30. Bonan R, Bertrand O, Adelman A: Different propensity of coronary restenosis: Comparison between cutting balloon, conventional balloon and atherectomy [Abstract]. J Am Coll Cardiol 27(suppl A):292, 1996.

31. Bertrand O, Roose PCH, Suttorp MJ, et al: Cutting balloon versus balloon angioplasty: Initial results from a multicenter randomized trial. Acta Cardiol LII:86–87, 1997.

32. Goicolea J, Auge J, Martinez D, et al: In-hospital results of cutting balloon versus conventional balloon angioplasty: Interim results of the CUBA study [Abstract]. Eur Heart J 17:188, 1996.

33. Martinez D, Giocolea J, Alfonzo F, et al: Intravascular ultrasound findings after cutting balloon angioplasty [Abstract]. Eur Heart J 17:180, 1996.

34. Yazdanfar S, Ledley GS, Alfieri A, et al: Parallel angioplasty dilatation catheter and guide wire: A new technique for the dilatation of calcified coronary arteries. Cathet Cardiovasc Diagn 28:72–75, 1993.

35. Bertrand O, Bonan R, Bilodeau L, et al: Management of resistant coronary lesions by the cutting balloon: Initial experience. Cathet Cardiovasc Diagn, 41:173–184, 1997.

36. Feld H, Valerio L, Shani J: Two hugging balloons at high pressures successfully dilate a lesion refractory to routine coronary angioplasty. Cathet Cardiovasc Diagn 24:105–107, 1991.

37. Heuser R, Mehta S: Holmium laser angioplasty after failed coronary balloon dilation: Use of a new solid state, infrared laser system. Cathet Cardiovasc Diagn 23:107–109, 1991.

38. Höfling B, Gonschior P, Simpson L, et al: Efficacy of directional coronary atherectomy in cases unsuitable for percutaneous transluminal coronary angioplasty and after unsuccessful PTCA. Am Heart J 124:341–348, 1992.

39. Iyer S, Hall P, King J, Dorros G: Successful rotational coronary ablation following failed balloon angioplasty. Cathet Cardiovasc Diagn 24:65–68, 1991.

40. Leon MB, Kent KM, Satler LF, et al: A multi-device lesion-specific approach for unfavorable coronary anatomy [Abstract]. J Am Coll Cardiol 19:93A, 1992.

41. Popma J, Leon M: A lesion-specific approach to new-device angioplasty. In Topol E (ed): Textbook of Interventional Cardiology, 2nd ed., vol 1, pp 973–985. Philadelphia, WB Saunders, 1994.

42. Topol E, Ellis S, Fishman J, et al: Multicenter study of percutaneous transluminal angioplasty for right coronary artery ostial stenoses. J Am Coll Cardiol 9:1214–1218, 1987.

43. Tan KH, Sulke N, Taub N, Sowton E: Percutaneous transluminal coronary angioplasty of aorta ostial, non-aorta ostial, and branch ostial stenoses: Acute and long-term outcome. Eur Heart J 16:631–639, 1995.

44. Franco I, Ellis SG, Topol E: Percutaneous revascularization of ostial saphenous vein graft stenoses. J Am Coll Cardiol 26:955–960, 1995.

45. Koller PT, Freed M, Grines CL, et al: Success, complications, and restenosis following rotational and transluminal extraction atherectomy of ostial stenoses. Cathet Cardiovasc Diagn 31:255–260, 1994.

46. Rocha-Singh K, Morris N, Wong SC: Coronary stenting for treatment of ostial stenoses of native coronary arteries or aortocoronary saphenous venous grafts. Am J Cardiol 75:26–29, 1995.

47. Kurbaan AS, Kelly PA, Sigwart U: Cutting balloon angioplasty and stenting for aorto-ostial lesions [Abstract]. J Am Coll Cardiol 30:1012–1018, 1997.

48. Vorwerk D, Adam G, Müller-Leisse C, et al: Hemodialysis fistulas and grafts: Use of cutting balloons to dilate venous stenoses. Radiology 201:864–867, 1996.

49. Coe J, Chen R, Timinsky J, et al: A novel method to create arterial septal defect using a cutting balloon in piglets. Am J Cardiol 787:47–50, 1996.

50. Scott NA: Current status and potential applications of drug delivery balloon catheters. J Intervent Cardiol 8:406–419, 1995.

51. Bonan R: Local drug delivery for the treatment of thrombus and restenosis. J Invasive Cardiol 8:399–402, 1996.

52. Serruys PW: Local drug delivery In Camenzind E (ed): Seminars in Interventional Cardiology, vol 1, issue 1. London: WB Saunders, 1996, pp 67–76.

53. Barath P, Popov A, Dillehay G, et al: Infiltrator angioplasty balloon catheter: A device for combined angioplasty and intramural site specific treatment. Cathet Cardiovasc Diagn 41:333–341, 1997.

54. Pavlides GS, Barath P, Maginas A, et al: Intramural drug delivery by direct injection within the arterial wall. First clinical experience with a novel intracoronary delivery-infiltrator system. Cathet Cardiovasc Diagn 41:287–292, 1997.

55. Reimers B, Roussa I, Akiyama T, et al: Persistent high restenosis after local intrawall delivery of long acting steroids before coronary stent implantation. J Invasive Cardiol 10: 323–331, 1998.

# VII

# Peripheral Vascular Intervention

# 48

# Management of Renal Artery Stenosis

*James J. Crowley*    *Renato M. Santos*    *Peter J. Conlon*

Obstruction of blood flow to the kidney is responsible for two major clinical syndromes: renovascular hypertension and ischemic renal failure. Patients with renovascular hypertension may have hemodynamically significant bilateral or unilateral renal artery stenoses (RASs). When the condition is unilateral, there is usually no clinically important reduction in renal function, because the contralateral kidney generally compensates unless it has parenchymal damage as a result of hypertensive or atherosclerotic disease. The demonstration of an RAS in a hypertensive patient does not necessarily establish a diagnosis of renovascular hypertension because essential hypertension may accelerate the development of atheromatous plaques. Ischemic renal disease is defined as a significant reduction in glomerular filtration rate (GFR) in patients with hemodynamically significant renovascular occlusive disease affecting the total functioning renal parenchyma (i.e., bilateral significant RAS or unilateral stenosis in a solitary kidney).

Three distinct pathologic entities commonly affect the main renal arteries and may lead to renovascular obstruction: atheromatous disease, fibromuscular dysplasia, and, much less common, Takayasu's arteritis. Atheromatous disease is the most common cause of RAS and may be part of a generalized vascular atherosclerosis. Fibromuscular dysplasia is the most common cause of RAS in children and young adults. Takayasu's arteritis is a rare disease that affects mainly young women and occurs predominantly in the Orient. It may cause discrete stenosis of the aorta and major renal arteries.[1]

RAS is frequently asymptomatic; therefore, its prevalence and natural history in the general population have not been defined. Cases of RAS probably account for between 0.2% and 5% of patients with hypertension and have been reported in 35% to 42% of patients with renovascular hypertension.[2–4] The reported incidence among patients with renal failure is 1% to 14%, but this may be an underestimation in some studies because the etiology of renal failure is not known in many patients when they begin renal replacement therapy.[5–8] As the index of suspicion for atherosclerotic renal disease has risen, this disease has been diagnosed in increasing numbers of patients.[9, 10] It has been estimated that between 3000 and 6000 of the patients currently on dialysis in the United States have ischemic nephropathy.[9]

## PATHOPHYSIOLOGY OF RENOVASCULAR HYPERTENSION AND ISCHEMIC NEPHROPATHY

Renal blood flow is threefold to fivefold greater than the perfusion to other metabolically active organs, such as the liver or heart. This level of perfusion is necessary for driving glomerular capillary filtration. Both glomerular capillary hydrostatic pressure and renal blood flow are important determinants of GFR. Renal blood flow and GFR are kept constant through wide variations in systemic arterial blood pressure by alteration in tone of the afferent and efferent glomerular resistance.

The role of the renin-angiotensin system in renovascular hypertension and ischemic renal disease is paramount and is outlined in Figure 48–1. Renin is an enzyme secreted by the juxtaglomerular cells of the kidney in response to decreased renal perfusion pressure.[11] Renin acts on circulating angiotensinogen to convert it into angiotensin I (Ang-I). Predominantly in the lungs but also in the plasma, Ang-I is converted by angiotensin-converting enzyme (ACE) into its biologically active component, angiotensin II (Ang-II). Ang-II exerts its effect on the vascular smooth muscle via Ang-II receptors. The physiologic effect of Ang-II may be inhibited pharmacologically by the inhibition of the conversion of Ang-I into Ang-II by ACE (ACE inhibitors include captopril and enalapril), and the effect of Ang-II may be inhibited by a new class of drugs, Ang-II receptor antagonists (such as losartan). In addition to having

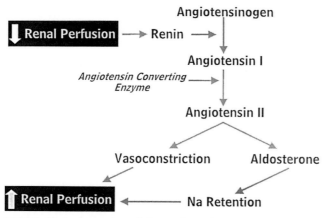

FIGURE 48–1. Activation of the renin-angiotensin system by renal ischemia.

direct vasoconstrictor effects on the vascular smooth muscle, Ang-II has potent effects on the secretion of aldosterone by the adrenal cortex. In the presence of RAS, the resistance of the efferent renal arteriole is particularly dependent on Ang-II. Inhibition of Ang-II in this setting can result in dramatic reductions in renal efferent arteriole resistance and thus in GFR. What thus ensues is the well-recognized clinical syndrome of the development of acute renal failure in the setting of either bilateral RAS or unilateral RAS of a solitary kidney with the initiation of ACE or Ang-II receptor antagonists.[8, 10]

In experimental animals, two distinct models of renovascular hypertension can be produced[12]: (1) the one-clip two-kidney model (in which a clip is placed on one kidney to induce a functional stenosis), which is analogous to unilateral RAS and in which hypertension is renin dependent and responds to ACE inhibitor therapy, and (2) the one-clip one-kidney model (in which a clip is put on one kidney and the other kidney is removed), which is analogous to either severe bilateral stenosis or RAS of a solitary kidney. In this model, hypertension is volume dependent, and ACE inhibitors have little effect on blood pressure unless the patient has undergone volume depletion.

## FIBROMUSCULAR DYSPLASIA

Fibromuscular dysplasia is the most common cause of renovascular hypertension in children and young adults. This syndrome can be classified into four types according to the histologic level of the artery that is involved[13–16]: intimal fibromuscular dysplasia, medial fibromuscular dysplasia, perimedial dysplasia, and the fourth and least common entity, which comprises the hypoplastic and dysplastic developmental lesions of the abdominal aorta and renal arteries.

Intimal fibromuscular dysplasia accounts for approximately 5% of all dysplastic RAS in children and young adults. Primary intimal fibromuscular dysplasia affects the main renal artery, usually occurring as smooth focal stenosis. This disease is characterized by a circumferential accumulation of collagen inside the internal elastic lumen. The cause of primary intimal fibromuscular dysplasia is unknown but may represent vestiges of fetal arterial musculoelastic cushions. Without intervention, progressive renal artery obstruction and ischemic atrophy of the involved kidney invariably occur.

Medial fibromuscular dysplasia accounts for nearly 85% of all dysplastic renovascular stenosis. More than 90% of affected patients are women, and the disease usually develops between the ages of 25 and 50 years. The disease is frequently bilateral and may affect other arterial systems, including the carotid, iliac, and femoral arteries. Medial fibromuscular dysplasia of the renal arteries may manifest as a solitary arterial stenosis but more commonly manifests as multiple stenoses and intervening small aneurysms, producing the classic radiographic "string of beads" sign (Fig. 48–2). Histology of involved vessels reveals that the internal elastic membrane is focally and variably thinned and, in the later stages of the disease, lost. In the thickened areas, muscle is replaced by collagen. In other areas, thinning of the media progresses to the point of complete loss, which can lead to aneurysm formation. Among patients who undergo serial angiography, medial fibromuscular dysplasia has been observed to progress in 33%, although there was no loss of renal parenchyma or function.

Perimedial fibromuscular dysplasia occurs predominantly in young women between the ages of

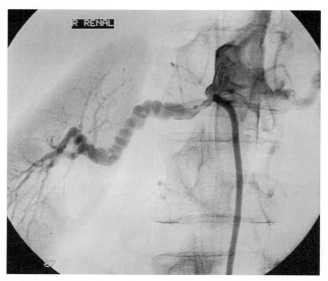

FIGURE 48–2. Renal arteriogram with medial fibromuscular dysplasia. Note the characteristic beaded appearance of the artery.

25 and 30 years and accounts for 10% of the fibrous lesions affecting the renal artery. Pathologically, the lesions consist of a ring of dense collagen encircling the renal artery, in the outer portion of the media. Arteriography demonstrates focal stenosis or multiple constrictions involving the midportion of the main renal artery without mural aneurysms. Without revascularization, progressive obstruction with ischemic atrophy occurs in the majority of patients managed medically.

## ATHEROMATOUS LESIONS

Approximately 70% of all renal arterial lesions are atherosclerotic in nature. The disease may be limited to the renal arteries; however, it is far more likely that atherosclerotic RAS is just one manifestation of a systemic disease. It is frequently an incidental finding in patients being evaluated for concomitant coronary artery, cerebrovascular, or peripheral arterial disease.[7, 17–21] Atherosclerotic stenosis usually occurs in the proximal 2 cm of the renal arteries, and in up to 80% of cases, it involves the ostia of the renal arteries.

## EPIDEMIOLOGY AND NATURAL HISTORY OF ATHEROSCLEROTIC RENAL ARTERY STENOSIS

Atherosclerotic renovascular disease, unlike fibromuscular dysplasia, is a manifestation of generalized arterial disease. The prevalence within the general population is unknown because the definitive tests for RAS are invasive. The reported prevalence of hemodynamically significant RAS at autopsy has varied from 4.3% to 73% of cases studied, with a prevalence as high as 86% of hypertensive persons over the age of 75 years at the time of death (Table 48–1).[22–25] The increasing frequency of RAS with advancing age has been observed by many authors.

Of the patients with severe hypertension who are treated at hypertension clinics, up to 36% have been reported to have angiographically significant RAS. Since 1990, a large number of studies have reported on the prevalence of RAS among patients undergoing angiography for other indications, such as peripheral arterial disease or coronary angiography (see Table 48–1).[20, 26–34] In one of the largest series reported from our institution, 1235 patients underwent abdominal aortography for the evaluation of atherosclerotic RAS, and 30% had RAS.[31] Increased age, severity of coronary artery disease, presence of congestive heart failure, presence of peripheral arterial disease, and female gender were each independently associated with the probability of having RAS. It has been estimated that there may be as many as 105 patients per million population per year with newly diagnosed, hemodynamically significant RAS.

There has been no prospective angiographic study of RAS to assess deterioration in renal function or progression of stenosis severity. A number of investigators studied the long-term follow-up documentation of selected subjects with known RAS (Table 48–2). Most of the studies were retrospective or included only patients with known disease at the outset[35] and hence do not provide an indication of the disease prevalence in the general population. However, these studies are useful because they frequently represented patients with evidence of generalized atherosclerotic disease or other risk factors who might be expected to have a higher incidence of RAS. Angiographic progression of the lesion in atherosclerotic renovascular disease was established in the early studies of Meaney and coworkers,[36]

## TABLE 48–1. STUDIES ON THE PREVALENCE OF RENAL ARTERIAL DISEASE (RAS)

| AUTHOR | YEAR | PATIENTS | STUDY/INDICATION | % WITH RAS |
|---|---|---|---|---|
| Crowley et al[41] | 1998 | 14,152 | CC | 6% |
| Uzu et al[24] | 1997 | 297 | Autopsy | 12% |
| Missouris et al[20] | 1994 | 127 | PVD | 16% |
| Jean et al[34] | 1994 | 196 | CC | 18% |
| Valentine et al[33] | 1993 | 346 | AAA/PVD | 28% |
| Harding et al[31] | 1992 | 1302 | CC | 11% |
| Swartbol et al[32] | 1992 | 450 | PVD | 3% |
| Olin et al[28] | 1990 | 395 | AAA/PVD | 33%–39% |
| Choudhri et al[83] | 1990 | 100 | PVD | 42% |
| Wilms et al[29] | 1990 | 100 | PVD | 22% |
| Salmon and Brown[30] | 1990 | 374 | PVD | 14% |
| Sawicki et al[25] | 1991 | 5194 | Autopsy | 4.3% |
| Vetrovec et al[27] | 1989 | 118 | CC | 23% |
| Brewster et al[26] | 1975 | 190 | AAA | 22% |
| Schwartz and White[22] | 1964 | 154 | Autopsy | 14% |
| Holley et al[23] | 1964 | 295 | Autopsy | 53% |

AAA, abdominal aortic aneurysm; CC, cardiac catheterization; PVD, peripheral venous disease.

**TABLE 48–2.    STUDIES ON THE PROGRESSION OF RENAL ARTERY STENOSIS**

| AUTHOR | MODALITY YEAR | | PATIENTS | FOLLOW-UP (MONTHS) | PROGRESSION | OCCLUSION |
|---|---|---|---|---|---|---|
| Crowley et al[41] | 1998 | Angiography | 1189 | 72 | 25% | 0.001% |
| Zierler et al[35] | 1994 | Doppler ultrasonography | 80 | 6–24 | 42% | 11% |
| Tollefson and Ernst[38] | 1991 | Angiography | 48 | 15–180 | 71% | 15% |
| Schreiber et al[10] | 1984 | Angiography | 85 | 12–60 | 44% | 16% |
| Dean et al[84] | 1981 | Angiography | 35 | 6–102 | 29% | 11% |
| Meaney et al[36] | 1968 | Angiography | 39 | 6–120 | 36% | 8% |
| Wollenweber et al[37] | 1968 | Angiography | 30 | 12–88 | 63% | Not reported |

Wollenweber and colleagues,[37] Schreiber and associates,[10] and others.[38, 39] These authors showed in retrospective analyses that atherosclerotic RAS progressed in 44% of patients and that progression to complete occlusion could occur in up to 16% after a mean follow-up period of 52 months.[10] Occlusion can occur without associated symptoms and with only very modest changes in serum creatinine levels (raised serum creatinine level is an indication of deterioration in renal function; however, in patients with progression of RAS, there may not be an increase of creatinine).[40]

In an effort to further define the natural history of renal arterial disease, we have studied the rate of angiographic progression of RAS in a series of 1200 patients undergoing repeat abdominal angiography (after an interval of at least 6 months) at the time of cardiac catheterization.[41] We specifically selected patients because of their need for a repeat cardiac catheterization, rather than because of any suspicion of changes in the renal arterial disease. By 12 months after the first catheterization, 12% of patients demonstrated a 25% or greater progression in severity of RAS, and by 50 months the proportion of such patients had increased to 22%. Factors that were independently associated with the probability of showing angiographic progression included advanced age, female sex, severity of coronary artery disease, and longer time between baseline screening and follow-up. Furthermore, subjects who demonstrated high degrees of angiographic progression also demonstrated significant declines in renal function.

Renal arterial disease appears to be a risk factor for premature cardiac death. In a study of patients attending the Glasgow and Newcastle hypertension clinics, the 5-year survival rate among patients with atherosclerotic RAS was found to be 83%, and the 10-year survival rate was 67%, in comparison with 90% and 79%, respectively, of subjects with essential hypertension.[42] Conlon and associates prospectively studied the 1300 patients who underwent an abdominal aortogram at the time of diagnostic cardiac catheterization and observed a 5-year survival rate of 86% among subjects without renal arterial disease, in comparison with a 5-year survival rate of 65% among those who had 50% or greater renal arterial stenosis.[43] Patients with atherosclerotic renal vascular disease are more likely to demonstrate coronary artery disease than are age- and gender-matched controls, and the presence of RAS appeared to be an independent predictor of long-term mortality. When the cause of death in this group was analyzed, we found that only 4 patients died in renal failure; the majority of deaths were due to cardiovascular disease. Thus, atherosclerotic renal arterial disease appears to be a manifestation of more severe generalized atherosclerotic disease.

## CLINICAL MANIFESTATIONS OF RENOVASCULAR DISEASE

There are few specific clinical manifestations of renovascular hypertension; however, certain features may raise clinical suspicion of the presence of RAS. Patients are more likely to have shorter duration of hypertension; accelerated hypertension; peripheral, coronary artery, or cerebrovascular disease; abdominal or flank bruits on physical examination; and retinal hemorrhages on fundoscopy. They are also more likely to require multiple medications for blood pressure control (Table 48–3).[3, 44]

**TABLE 48–3.    CLINICAL FEATURES SUGGESTIVE OF RENOVASCULAR DISEASE**

Onset of hypertension before the age of 30 years or after 50 years
Absence of family history of hypertension
Shorter duration of hypertension or recent worsening
Severe hypertension or retinopathy
Hypertension resistance to multiple medications
Symptoms or signs of vascular disease elsewhere
Elevation in plasma creatinine after initiation of ACE inhibitor
Epigastric bruit
Hypokalemia
Neurofibromatosis

ACE, angiotensin-converting enzyme.

One of the cardinal features of renovascular hypertension is severe hypertension that is refractory to most lines of medications (see Table 48–3).[45] In contrast, rapid blood pressure control after initiation of ACE inhibitor therapy may indicate RAS. An epigastric systolic bruit is audible in 50% to 60% of patients with RAS; however, up to 10% of subjects with essential hypertension may also have an abdominal bruit. Low levels of proteinuria (<1 g/dL) are more common in patients with RAS than in patients with essential hypertension. Higher levels associated with renal insufficiency are more suggestive of intrinsic renal disease. Hyperreninemia leads to associated hypokalemia through secondary hyperaldosteronism in approximately 15% of patients with RAS. In a patient with hypertension and hypokalemia (in the absence of diuretic use), both primary and secondary hyperaldosteronism must be considered. To distinguish between these two entities, it is necessary to measure circulating renin and aldosterone: Primary hyperaldosteronism results in elevated aldosterone levels and reduced plasma renin levels, whereas secondary hyperaldosteronism results in increased renin and aldosterone levels.

Renal arterial disease must be considered in any patient with either acutely or chronically impaired renal function. The development of severe renal failure shortly after the beginning of ACE inhibitor therapy is highly suggestive of bilateral RAS; lesser rises in serum creatinine levels (of ≤0.5 mg/dL) after initiation of ACE inhibition are manifestations of a reduced perfusion pressure without RAS. However, in only 6% to 38% of patients with significant renovascular disease does acute renal failure develop in response to ACE inhibition. Typically, acute renal failure in these situations is reversible, but patients should undergo evaluation for RAS after recovery of renal function. Patients with bilateral RAS may present acutely with severe, uncontrolled hypertension, recurrent pulmonary edema, and renal insufficiency.[46, 47]

## DIAGNOSTIC EVALUATION OF RENAL ARTERY STENOSIS

The definitive diagnosis of RAS can be established only by defining the anatomy of the renal arterial supply. The algorithm for the evaluation of RAS should be quite different for evaluating patients with renal vascular disease (severe hypertension with normal renal function) from that for ischemic renal disease (elevated serum creatinine levels that may be related to renal arterial disease). For ischemic renal disease, the noninvasive tests (such as captopril tests and renal scintigraphy) are much less useful because of renal insufficiency, and the bilateral nature of the disease makes the tests much less sensitive and specific.

Of the patients with proven renovascular hypertension, 75% have increased levels of plasma renin activity; however, so also do 15% of patients with essential hypertension. Therefore, the utility of plasma renin estimation in diagnosing RAS is limited.[48, 49] As discussed earlier, plasma renin levels may be depressed in the presence of bilateral arterial disease with a volume-expanded state.

Renal scintigraphy may be performed with a variety of radiopharmaceuticals, including technetium 99m–labeled mercaptoacetyltriglycine ($^{99m}$Tc MAG$_3$) and technetium-labeled diethylenetriaminepentaacetic acid (Tc-DTPA). Differences in renal perfusion between sides may be observed with these agents, and these effects may be accentuated with the administration of ACE inhibitors. Captopril renography, in which a renal scan is performed with $^{99}$Tc MAG$_3$ before and after the administration of oral captopril, has been found to have more than 90% sensitivity and specificity in the detection of RAS among high-risk patients with suspected renal vascular hypertension.[50] Captopril renography is not useful, however, in assessing ischemic renal disease, inasmuch as it depends on a comparison of perfusion between both kidneys. If both kidneys have arterial disease, it is of poor diagnostic value.

Renal ultrasonography allows assessment of renal size, and asymmetric kidneys may indicate RAS. Doppler ultrasonography has been used with variable success to detect RAS.[51] Major limitations exist with the use of Doppler ultrasonography, including lack of reproducibility of results between medical institutions. The technique is highly dependent on operator skill. Although some institutions have reported high degrees of sensitivity and specificity, others have not been able to reproduce these results. Obesity and overlying gas pattern also frequently make locating accessory renal arteries and ultrasonic interrogation of a renal artery impossible over their entire lengths.

Computed tomographic (CT) angiography, in which spiral computed tomography is used with three-dimensional reconstruction, has been reported to be highly sensitive and specific in the diagnosis of RAS. However, it requires a large volume of contrast material, which carries a risk of nephrotoxicity in patients with preexisting renal insufficiency. The amount of contrast material may be higher than the contrast load used in a carefully performed, selective renal angiographic study. In subjects with normal renal function who carry a low risk of contrast material–induced nephrotoxicity, CT angiography may be useful.

Magnetic resonance angiography has the ability to visualize the renal arteries noninvasively and with

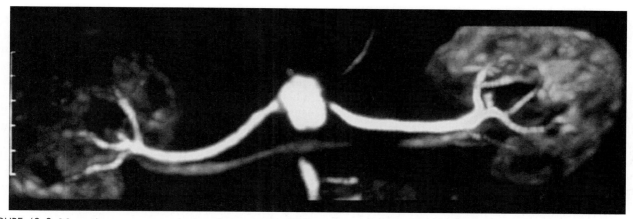

FIGURE 48–3. Magnetic resonance angiogram demonstrating high-grade ostial stenosis of the left renal artery. Note also the course of the arteries. The left renal artery arises from the posterolateral wall, whereas the right renal artery is more anterior. The ostium of the arteries lies in a more oblique plane than does the body of the arteries. This is why different angulations of the image intensifier are sometimes required to assess the ostium and the body of the artery.

a contrast agent that is not nephrotoxic (Fig. 48–3). It is highly sensitive in detecting stenosis of proximal main renal arteries; its sensitivity, however, becomes poorer for detecting stenosis in more distal branches or in accessory renal arteries.[52] Magnetic resonance angiography, although expensive, is an excellent test for screening patients with a moderate probability of having atherosclerotic renal arterial disease in which it is desirable to avoid nephrotoxicity from radiographic contrast material (see Fig. 48–3). In patients with previous stent implantation, however, imaging the area within the stent is not possible because of artifact from the stent itself.

Renal arteriography remains the best method for defining renal arterial anatomy. However, the severity of lesions may be underestimated, and multiple views may be necessary for questionable lesions. Patients with renal insufficiency should receive intravenous hydration, should discontinue diuretic therapy and other nephrotoxins before renal angiography, and should receive minimal contrast material during the study in order to avoid contrast material–induced acute renal failure.

## TECHNIQUE OF RENAL ANGIOGRAPHY, ANGIOPLASTY, AND STENT IMPLANTATION

### Patient Preparation

A complete history and examination is performed, with the focus on history of hypertension, pulmonary edema, coronary artery disease, and systemic atherosclerosis. Signs of end-organ damage from hypertension or vascular disease are noted. Routine laboratory data, including a complete blood cell count, electrolyte and creatinine measurements, and prothrombin time, are obtained. Before surgery, the patient is informed about the procedure itself but

also, of more importance, about the expected goals and possible complications. To patients with atheromatous renal disease, it is explained that blood pressure control can be expected in approximately 70% of patients and that this includes cure in a smaller proportion (depending on the nature and distribution of the renal disease). In patients with renal insufficiency, the aim is to retard or stop the process of renal deterioration and preserve remaining renal function. The patient is also informed about the small risk of losing the kidney, the possible need for emergency surgery, and other complications such as renal artery perforation and hemorrhage, distal cholesterol embolization, and allergic reactions to contrast material. The benefits of alternative therapies such as surgery or medical therapy are also discussed.

In some institutions, all antihypertensive medications are withheld before the procedure because of the risk of hypotension after the procedure; however, this is not done routinely at our laboratory. We have not seen any serious sequelae of hypotension in over 500 cases.

### Renal Arteriography

If previous studies have not been performed, renal aortography should be conducted. After arterial access is obtained, abdominal aortography is performed with a Tennis Racquet catheter or a pigtail catheter. It is important to position the catheter correctly in order to obtain adequate visualization and filling of the renal arteries. If the catheter is positioned too proximally, the superior mesenteric and celiac arteries opacify and tend to obscure the origins of the renal arteries and their distal branches. Alternatively, too distal a catheter displacement results in poor or no opacification of the renal arteries. The renal arteries usually arise in the region of the lower border of the body of the first lumbar vertebra. The tip of the catheter should be positioned just above this level so that the contrast jet is centered on the renal arteries. Accessory renal arteries are usually more distal to this position; therefore, it is unlikely that any renal branches will be missed if the injection is not more proximal. Abdominal aortography in the anteroposterior projection usually provides adequate visualization of the body of the renal arteries and their extrarenal and intrarenal branches, and it allows identification of any accessory branches and estimation of renal size. However, in order to image the ostia and proximal segments adequately, it is frequently necessary to obtain oblique views.[48–55] The left renal artery usually arises from the posterolateral wall of the aorta, and the right renal artery is somewhat more anterior; therefore, opacification of the aorta with contrast material in the anteroposterior view frequently obstructs the proximal and ostial segments of the arteries (Fig. 48–4; see Fig. 48–3). In addition, tortuosity of the aorta, which may occur particularly in atherosclerotic disease, may distort the normal anatomic relationships and course of the vessels. In patients with fibromuscular dysplasia, which usually affects the middle and distal segments of the vessel, the typical beaded appearance may be underestimated in the anteroposterior projection: As the vessel courses posteriorly and laterally, the beaded segments of the vessel may overlap each other. Ipsilateral oblique views allow imaging in a plane more perpendicular to the arteries, demonstrating the true extent of disease.[54]

For diagnostic purposes, it may not be necessary to perform selective renal angiography. Selective injection of contrast material into a diseased artery may cause dissection or occlusion of the vessel, or both, so it should be performed only when it is not possible to obtain all the information from aortography. However, in some patients it is not possible to clearly demonstrate a stenotic lesion. In these cases, selective injection allows better visualization of the artery and also allows measurement of a pressure gradient across the lesion.

The use of digital angiography has allowed the use of smaller volumes of contrast media. This is particularly important for studying patients with renal artery disease and renal insufficiency. Amounts vary from 12 to 50 mL at rates ranging from 6 to 20 mL/second.[56] A typical aortic injection with 40 mL at 20 mL/second is used in our laboratory to delineate the arteries and also to allow imaging of the aorta and proximal iliac vessels. However, smaller volumes are probably satisfactory, particularly when angiography is used only to determine the site of the ostia before intervention.

## Renal Artery Angioplasty
### General Principles
#### Arterial Access

Renal angioplasty may be performed through a femoral, brachial, or axillary approach. The choice is dependent on the operator's experience and preference. Femoral access is the route most commonly used by cardiologists and is used in most of the cases at our institution. The femoral technique avoids the need for cutdown and repair and thus decreases the infection rate. When a guide catheter is used, less manipulation is required. In a brachial

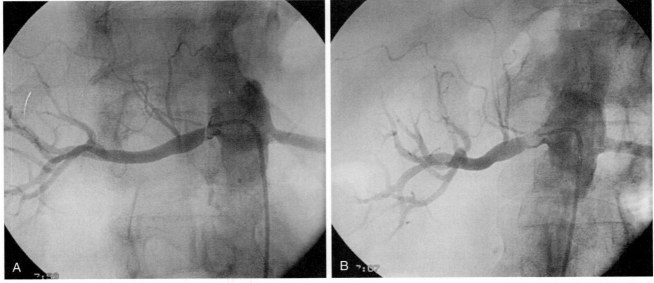

FIGURE 48–4. Effect of different angulations on ability to visualize an ostial renal artery stenosis. *A,* In the 20-degree right anterior oblique view, the lesion is seen only as a thin defect close to the ostium. *B,* In the anteroposterior view, the stenosis is clearly seen.

artery cutdown, direct arterial repair allows full anticoagulation with less periaccess bleeding. It allows early patient ambulation and discharge after the procedure. A brachial percutaneous approach may also be used; however, only 5- to 6-French sheaths should be employed, and adequate anticoagulation is required. In order to permit satisfactory hemostasis, heparin must be reversed with protamine if a cutdown is avoided.

The advantage of the axillary artery approach is that the collateral vessels from the shoulder are excellent. They are frequently sufficient to prevent limb ischemia even if large-caliber equipment is used. In cases in which there is sharp caudal angulation of the proximal renal artery, the axillary (or brachial) approach facilitates intubation of the ostium of the artery. The major risk with this approach is of damage to the brachial plexus; consequently, familiarity with this technique is important. Careful palpation of the axillary artery over the proximal humerus is made just at the lateral axillary crease. If the axillary artery can be compressed against the humerus, any hematoma that occurs is less likely to injure the brachial plexus. Local anesthesia should be administered intradermally so that diffusion to the brachial plexus does not occur. The artery should be fixed between two fingers, and a relatively shallow angle of approach taken. When arterial blood returns, a small atraumatic wire should be inserted under fluoroscopic guidance and positioned in the left subclavian or descending aorta. The axillary or brachial approach should always be taken from the left side because this is the most direct route to the abdominal aorta. When the right axillary artery is used, buckling in the brachiocephalic vessels may occur, and access to the descending aorta is extremely difficult. Because the axillary artery is smaller than vessels of the lower extremities, the lowest profile balloon should generally be employed when this form of access is used.

If bleeding occurs with the brachial or axillary percutaneous approach, it is much more difficult to control than from the femoral artery, and surgical closure may be necessary. Therefore, angioplasty of complex lesions and procedures for which prolonged access is necessary are best done via the femoral artery or with a brachial cutdown if femoral access is not available.

## Balloon Sizing

The size of the balloon is estimated according to the size of the normal vessel proximal and distal to the stenosis. It is important to recognize the presence of poststenotic dilatation so that the normal size of the vessel will not be overestimated. The ratio of the balloon to vessel diameter should be no more than 1.1:1. The aim is to achieve a residual stenosis that is less than 30% of the reference vessel diameter, because lesions more severe than this have a higher rate of restenosis.[57–59] If there is significant residual stenosis, a further dilatation is made with the same balloon. In some cases, it may be necessary to use a slightly larger diameter balloon if it is not possible to obtain a significant reduction in stenosis severity. Use of a larger balloon, however, increases the risk of dissection and requirement for stent implantation. Spasm of the main renal artery is a frequent complication and can be relieved either by intra-arterial nitroglycerin or a calcium channel blocker.

When renal artery stent implantation is planned from the outset, it is usually not necessary to obtain an ideal result with angioplasty. The primary function of the predilatation with the balloon is to dilate the lesion sufficiently so that it will be possible to advance the stent across it. Therefore, in our institution the balloon is dilated to a low pressure only until the "waist" of the balloon disappears.

### Approaches to Renal Artery Angioplasty

There are three approaches to renal angioplasty. The approach preferred in our institution is the guide catheter–supported approach. One of the specially shaped renal guide catheters is used to cannulate the renal artery. The lesion is crossed by a floppy-tipped 0.035- or 0.018-inch stiff-shaft guide wire that is positioned in the distal interlobular artery. Occasionally, for extremely severe stenoses, a coronary (0.014-inch) wire may be required initially. If a bifurcation stenosis is present, the jeopardized side branch is crossed with a 0.018-inch soft wire. The lesion is dilated to nominal pressure with a balloon that is sized appropriately to the vessel. In very severe stenoses, it may be necessary to perform an initial dilatation with an undersized balloon to create a lumen for a more appropriately sized balloon. The balloon is inflated slowly to its nominal pressure for about 30 seconds and then deflated. The balloon is then pulled back into the guide catheter, and a selective image is taken through the guide catheter. If there is significant residual stenosis, a further dilatation is made with the same or a larger balloon.

During balloon inflations, the patient may experience mild or moderate flank pain, which should resolve as soon as the balloon is deflated. Continued intense pain may indicate severe renal artery injury such as rupture or occlusion. Any degree of pain, however, should be viewed as a warning signal. The balloon should be removed from the artery and a low-pressure contrast injection into the artery performed. Vessel rupture, although unusual, may lead to catastrophic retroperitoneal hematoma. If this is detected, a balloon should be inflated at low pressure across the area where extravasation of blood was detected, and the patient should be prepared for emergency vascular surgery. In the future, covered stents may have a role in resolving the emergency.

The second approach is to use a diagnostic catheter to direct the wire across the lesion. An appropriate 5-French diagnostic catheter is advanced into the abdominal aorta. The catheter is used to select the ostium of the renal artery. The lesion is crossed by a soft, flexible 0.018- to 0.035-inch guide wire. The diagnostic catheter is then advanced across the lesion. The soft wire is exchanged for a stiff wire (such as a 0.035-inch Rosen guide wire), which will provide more support for the balloon catheter. The diagnostic catheter is then exchanged for the balloon catheter, which is inflated for about 30 seconds. The 0.035-inch wire is exchanged for a 0.018-inch wire, and a Tuohy-Bost Y-connector is attached to the balloon catheter. The balloon catheter is withdrawn across the lesion, and a pressure gradient is measured if necessary. This allows injection of contrast material through the lumen of the catheter to outline the renal artery. If further dilatation is required, the catheter is advanced again across the lesion. If a larger balloon is needed, the balloon catheter exchange is performed across a long 0.035-inch exchange wire.

The third approach is the use of a Simmons Sidewinder or cobra catheter. Access to the renal artery is accomplished through the femoral approach. These catheters have a steep primary curve to facilitate engagement of the ostium from above. This configuration takes advantage of the natural downward curve of the renal artery. Selective engagement of the artery by these catheters may be difficult, particularly when there is aorto-ostial disease. There is also potential risk of distal embolization of atherosclerotic debris, caused by scraping the catheter tip against the wall of an atherosclerotic aorta. A soft-tipped 0.035-inch wire is used to cross the lesion. The catheter is exchanged for a balloon catheter, and the procedure is performed as described earlier.

### Assessment of Different Approaches to Renal Angioplasty

We advocate the use of guide catheters. The guide catheter approach provides a stable position for traversing the lesion with a guide wire and balloon catheter. It is less difficult to lose wire position across the lesion during balloon catheter exchanges. In many cases, 0.018-inch wires can be used throughout the procedure without the necessity of wire exchanges. It allows injection of contrast through the guide catheter during the procedure so that progress can be monitored. If stent implantation is required, the guide catheter is already in place and avoids a difficult exchange at a time when it is critical not to lose wire position. The disadvantages of this technique include the requirement for an 8- or 9-French–size femoral artery puncture and the fact that the guiding catheter is stiff, so that it may traumatize the arterial wall or cause distal cholesterol or atheromatous embolization.

Traditionally, before the widespread use of stents, a direct balloon approach to renal angioplasty was used. This allows the use of a 5- to 7-French–size femoral artery puncture with reduction in the incidence of femoral artery complications. The small size of the catheters also makes this approach amenable to a brachial or axillary incision. This upper limb approach takes advantage of the caudal angulation of the renal arteries from the aorta, allowing relatively easy wiring of the vessel. However, should stent implantation be required after angioplasty, exchange to a long sheath or guide catheter must be performed over the wire, which is placed across an unstable lesion.

## Renal Artery Stent Implantation

The major reason for renal angioplasty failure has been the ostial involvement of the renal artery in the lesion. Because of the high restenosis rate of these lesions (up to 80%), other technologies have been attempted. The use of lasers and atherectomy devices has not as yet shown lasting benefit. In contrast, studies on the use of stents in renal arteries have shown promising results.

Stent implantation is usually performed through the femoral approach, although the brachial artery can also be used. In contrast to renal angioplasty, in which the balloon is usually longer than the lesion, the positioning of the stent is critical. With ostial lesions it is important that the stent extend 1 to 2 mm into the aorta so that it covers any plaque that may protrude over the proximal end of the stent. Atherosclerotic lesions of the renal artery ostium differ from those at other sites because they consist of atheroma from both the renal artery and the aorta (Fig. 48–5). Atheroma from the aorta may overhang into the renal artery.[60] It is therefore essential to use the proper view to visualize the ostium. Because of the posterior location and angulation, oblique views are almost always required. In general, contralateral views provide appropriate visualization; however, because of individual variations, ipsilateral or anteroposterior views are sometimes necessary.

### Femoral Artery Approach to Stent Implantation

Before intervention, systemic heparin is administered to achieve an activated clotting time of more

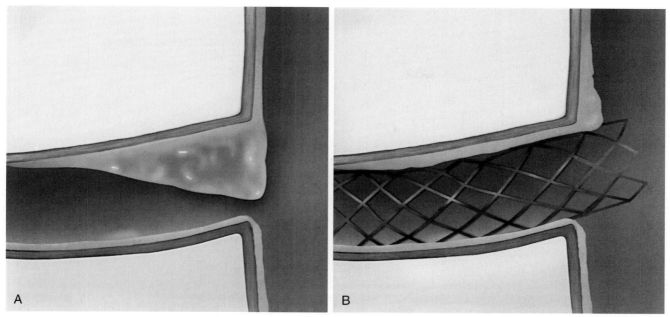

FIGURE 48–5. Artist's rendition of an ostial renal artery lesion. *A,* The lesion is really an extension of plaque in the wall of the aorta. Angioplasty may push the plaque along the wall of the aorta. The plaque may re-form rapidly within the renal artery. *B,* Stent implantation is used to buttress the walls and, by extending slightly into the aorta, prevents plaque from falling back across the arterial lumen.

than 250 seconds. An appropriately sized sheath is placed in the femoral artery, and a renal guiding catheter is positioned at the ostium of the renal artery. If stent implantation is planned as an elective procedure, the lesion is crossed with a wire as described earlier for angioplasty. The balloon is inflated to low pressure until the "waist" of the balloon is dilated (Fig. 48–6). After deflation, the balloon is withdrawn, and selective angiography is performed to document vessel patency and to determine the extent of any dissection. The wire is replaced with a 0.035-inch stiff wire through a 4-French multipurpose catheter to provide greater support for stenting. Although this wire may straighten the vessel, it also has a greater propensity to distort its natural course, leading to pseudolesions and difficulty in determining the limits of the stenosis and any dissection.

The stent-balloon combination is advanced through the guide catheter until the tip of the balloon extends out of the distal end. It is important that the stent is completely within the guide catheter so that it cannot be displaced by contact with the wall of the vessel. The guide-stent-balloon combination is advanced as a unit across the lesion until the distal end of the stent is distal to the lesion. The stent shortens by a small amount when it is deployed, and this must be taken into account during positioning. With the balloon and stent kept in place, the guide catheter is partially retracted until it covers only the proximal part of the stent. An

angiogram is performed through the guide catheter to confirm exact positioning. When the position is satisfactory, the guide catheter is fully withdrawn, and a further angiogram is obtained before balloon inflation. The stent is expanded by inflating the balloon to nominal pressure. The balloon is then deflated and withdrawn so that its distal end is within the distal end of the stent, and it is reinflated to high pressure to ensure that the stent is adequately deployed. The balloon is then deflated and withdrawn, with care taken not to move the stent during withdrawal. In this way, the guide catheter can be advanced so that it buttresses the stent during balloon catheter withdrawal. In some cases, it is difficult to remove the balloon through the stent because of the acute angle between the renal artery and the aorta. In these cases, it may be necessary to advance the guide catheter into the stent over the balloon. The balloon can usually be removed without difficulty. If the stent does not cover the entire lesion, a second stent is placed to overlap with the first. It is therefore important to ensure that the distal end of the lesion is covered by the first stent so that it is not necessary to deploy further stents through it.

Most centers use balloon-expandable stents, although the early experience with the self-expanding Wallstent was limited. In these cases, the stent is advanced across the lesion after predilatation with a balloon. When a satisfactory position is obtained, the sheath is partially removed so that about 50%

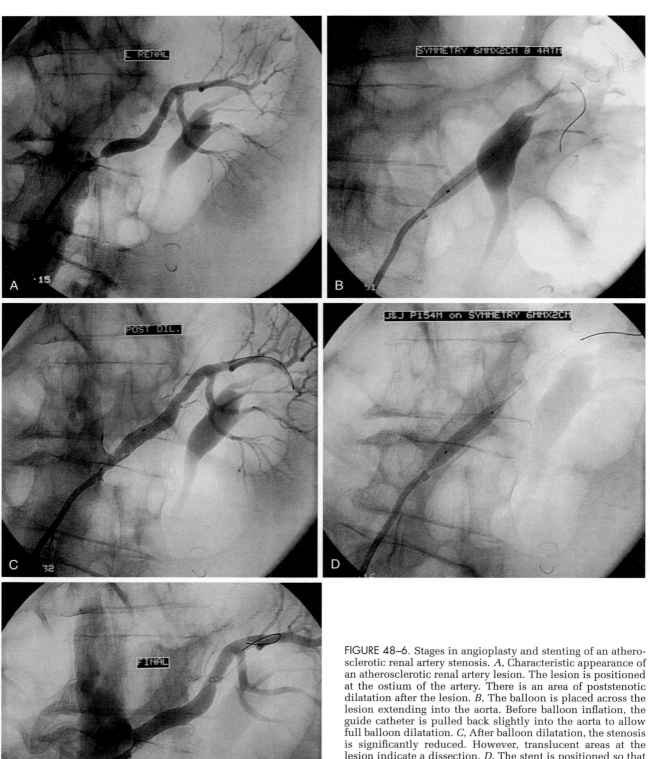

FIGURE 48–6. Stages in angioplasty and stenting of an athero-sclerotic renal artery stenosis. *A*, Characteristic appearance of an atherosclerotic renal artery lesion. The lesion is positioned at the ostium of the artery. There is an area of poststenotic dilatation after the lesion. *B*, The balloon is placed across the lesion extending into the aorta. Before balloon inflation, the guide catheter is pulled back slightly into the aorta to allow full balloon dilatation. *C*, After balloon dilatation, the stenosis is significantly reduced. However, translucent areas at the lesion indicate a dissection. *D*, The stent is positioned so that it extends 1 to 2 mm into the aorta to ensure that the lesion is fully covered. *E*, After final balloon dilatation, the vessel has a near-normal appearance.

of the stent is unsheathed. Renal angiography is performed through the guide catheter to ensure adequate positioning. Because of the marked shortening of this stent as it expands, it is particularly important to obtain further angiograms during stent deployment to allow repositioning if necessary. The sheath is then fully retracted into the guide catheter and removed. The balloon catheter is advanced into the stent, with the distal end kept proximal to the distal end of the stent and inflated to high pressure.

A modification of this technique is to use a stiff 0.018-inch wire (e.g., the Roadrunner) from the outset. No exchange is necessary after balloon dilatation, and the smaller diameter wire is less likely to cause pseudolesions. In our practice, most lesions can undergo stent implantation through this approach. Exchanging for a stiff 0.035-inch wire is reserved for highly tortuous vessels, for arteries that form acute angles with the aorta (because there may be difficulty passing the stent into the vessel), and for large vessels in which balloons require larger wires for support.

### Brachial Artery Approach

A similar technique can be used from the brachial artery, although a smaller caliber (6- to 7-French) sheath may be required. Some operators have used a long arterial sheath instead of a guide catheter.[61, 62] This method necessitates a number of exchanges. Angioplasty is performed from the brachial approach as outlined previously. Before balloon dilatation, the arterial sheath is removed from the brachial artery, leaving the stiff wire across the lesion. A 6-French long stent sheath is introduced and positioned so that its distal tip is in the aorta, proximal to the renal artery ostium. The lesion is dilated with a balloon catheter as described earlier. The balloon catheter is removed, and the stent sheath is advanced across the lesion. A balloon-expandable stent and delivered across the lesion through the sheath. The stent is then partly unsheathed, and a renal angiogram is obtained through the stent sheath side arm to determine the position. The sheath is withdrawn to uncover the stent, and the stent is deployed. The balloon is deflated and pulled back so that its distal end is within the distal end of the stent, and high-pressure dilatation of the balloon is performed. A final renal angiogram is obtained to confirm adequate deployment and positioning of the stent.

## Adjunctive Therapy

Patients are treated with daily aspirin therapy indefinitely. In addition, all patients at our institution receive clopidogrel daily for 4 weeks after the procedure. No extra heparin is administered after the procedure; however, the effect of heparin is not reversed. Blood pressure is monitored closely for 24 hours. This may fluctuate considerably immediately after the procedure.

## RESULTS OF INTERVENTIONAL PROCEDURES

### Angioplasty in Fibromuscular Dysplasia

The results of angioplasty for fibromuscular dysplasia are summarized in Table 48–4. Overall, the technical success rates are high, usually greater than 85%. Amelioration of hypertension occurs in up to 80% of patients, with cure in 25% to 58%. Patients with fibromuscular dysplasia are usually younger than those with atherosclerotic disease and have fewer associated risk factors. The rate of restenosis of fibromuscular dysplasia lesions after percutaneous transluminal coronary angioplasty is approximately 11%.[63] Recurrent lesions are usually easier to dilate than the initial lesions because the bands have been disrupted already. It is likely that in many

### TABLE 48–4. ANGIOPLASTY OF FIBROMUSCULAR DYSPLASIA (SERIES WITH 20 PATIENTS OR MORE)

| AUTHOR | YEAR | PATIENTS | TECHNICAL SUCCESS | FOLLOW-UP (MONTHS) | BLOOD PRESSURE | | |
| --- | --- | --- | --- | --- | --- | --- | --- |
| | | | | | CURE | IMPROVEMENT | BENEFIT |
| Jensen et al[85] | 1995 | 30 | 29 (97%) | 12 | 11/28 (39%) | 13/28 (46%) | 86% |
| Rodriguez-Perez et al[86] | 1994 | 27 | 25 (92%) | 96 | 6/12 (50%) | 3/12 (25%) | 75% |
| Tegtmeyer et al[87] | 1991 | 66 | 66 (100%) | 1–121 | 26/99 (39%) | 39/66 (59%) | 98% |
| Baert et al[88] | 1990 | 22 | 19 (86%) | 6–72 | 11/19 (58%) | 4/19 (21%) | 79% |
| Greminger et al[89] | 1989 | 34 | 30 (88%) | 6–48 | 14/30 (47%) | 16/30 (53%) | 100% |
| Klinge et al[90] | 1989 | 52 | 47 (90%) | — | 18/47 (38%) | 26/47 (55%) | 93% |
| Grim et al[91] | 1986 | 26 | 26 (100%) | 1 | 15/26 (58%) | 9/26 (35%) | 93% |
| Martin et al[92] | 1985 | 20 | 20 (100%) | 3–36 | 5/20 (25%) | 12/20 (60%) | |
| Kuhlmann et al[93] | 1985 | 24 | 22 (92%) | — | 11/22 (50%) | 7/22 (32%) | 82% |
| Sos et al[59] | 1983 | 31 | 27 (87%) | 4–40 | 16/27 (59%) | 9/27 (33%) | 92% |
| Geyskes et al[94] | 1983 | 21 | 21 (100%) | — | 10/21 (48%) | 10/21 (48%) | 96% |

**TABLE 48–5.   EFFECT OF ANGIOPLASTY OF ATHEROSCLEROTIC LESIONS ON HYPERTENSION**

| AUTHOR | YEAR | ARTERIES | PATIENTS | OSTIAL LESIONS (%) | TECHNICAL SUCCESS (%) | SERIOUS COMPLICATIONS (%) | DEATH | RESTENOSIS AT FOLLOW-UP | FOLLOW-UP (MONTHS) | BLOOD PRESSURE CURE | BLOOD PRESSURE IMPROVEMENT | BLOOD PRESSURE BENEFIT |
|---|---|---|---|---|---|---|---|---|---|---|---|---|
| Van de Ven et al[77] | 1999 | 51 | 42 | 100 | 63 | 4.8 | 0 | 11/31 (35%) | 6 | — | — | 49% |
| Tullis et al[95] | 1997 | 52 | 41 | 56 | — | — | 0 | 3/13 (23%) | 33 (mean) | 2/18 (11%) | 6/18 (33%) | 44% |
| von Knorring et al[96] | 1996 | 38 | 38 | 24 | 92 | 16 | 0 | — | 2–108 | 3/27 (11%) | 20/27 (74%) | 85% |
| Jensen et al[85] | 1995 | 147 | 107 | 10 | 82 | 6 | 1 | — | 12 | 11/90 (12%) | 36/90 (40%) | 62% |
| Karagiannis et al[97] | 1995 | 76 | 62 | — | 72 | — | — | — | 13–106 | 9/48 (19%) | 25/48 (52%) | 71% |
| Bonelli et al[66] | 1995 | 242 | 190 | 22 | 78 | 4.3 | 7* | 15/188† (8%) | 0–38 | 16/190 (8%) | 117/190 (62%) | 70% |
| Rodriguez-Perez et al[86] | 1994 | 50 | 37 | 48 | 78 | 8 | 0 | — | 96 | 1/28‡ (4%) | 21/28‡ (75%) | 79% |
| Losinno et al[67] | 1994 | — | 153 | 50 | 95 | 6§ | 0 | — | 1 | 18/153 (12%) | 78/153 (51%) | 63% |
| Weibull et al[74] | 1993 | 29 | 29 | — | 89 | — | 0 | 6/24 (25%) | 24 | 3/24 (13%) | 17/24 (71%) | 84% |
| Tykarski et al[98] | 1993 | 39 | 26 | 41 | 80 | 3 | 0 | 3/31‖ (10%) | 4–24 | 8/20 (40%) | 6/20 (30%) | 70% |
| Martin et al[99] | 1992 | 160 | 110 | 81 | 36 | 13 | 0 | 16/110† (15%) | 12–97 | 11/110 (10%) | 53/110 (48%) | 58% |
| Martin et al[99] | 1992 | — | 94 | 0 | — | — | — | — | — | 21/94 (22%) | 43/94 (46%) | 68% |
| Tegtmeyer et al[58] | 1984 | — | 65 | — | 94 | 1 | 0 | — | ≤60 | 15/65 (23%) | 46/65 (71%) | 94% |

Dashes indicate not reported.

*30-Day all-cause mortality rate. †Not all patients underwent repeat angiography. ‡At 12-month follow-up. §Includes 42 patients with fibromuscular dysplasia. ‖Assessed by renal Duplex ultrasonography.

cases the cause of recurrence is incomplete dilatation at the first attempt. Follow-up angiograms show that the arteries tend to smooth out and lose their beaded appearance. Patients with focal smooth lesions have a slightly less successful technical and clinical result. The lesions of perimedial or intimal fibroplasia may be more difficult to dilate, necessitating higher balloon inflation pressures. However, in a review of the literature, Archibald and associates reported an overall success rate of 81% in these patients.[64]

Angioplasty of segmental branches of the main renal artery has also been performed. Although this is a more difficult procedure, the technical success rate has been reported at 84%, with a recurrence rate of 9%.[65]

The results of angioplasty for fibromuscular dysplasia are therefore comparable with those of surgical revascularization, making it the treatment of choice for this condition.

## Angioplasty in Atherosclerotic Disease
### Technical Results

The technical and clinical success rates of angioplasty in patients with atherosclerotic renal artery stenosis are lower than in those with fibromuscular dysplasia. Technical failures may result from failure to cross the lesion; from failure to reduce the stenosis to less than 50%; or from complications such as perforation, dissection, and renal artery thrombosis. The incidence of technical failures varies considerably between studies, from 0% to 44%. This variation is probably attributable to differences in patient selection. The overall incidence is probably about 10%. The incidence has also decreased with the advent of better devices and greater experience. The results of angioplasty for atherosclerotic lesions clearly are significantly different for patients with ostial disease and those with nonostial disease. The technical success rate for ostial lesions is 25% to 60%.[59, 66, 67] Primary success rates for atherosclerotic lesions of main renal arteries have ranged from 85% to 96%, with restenosis rates of 10% to 30%. These lesions can undergo further angioplasty. However, nonostial disease occurs in only 20% of patients with atherosclerotic renal artery stenosis. Both early and more recent reports have demonstrated that angioplasty is less effective for ostial lesions; restenosis is the primary cause of failure in these patients as a result of intimal hyperplasia, elastic recoil of the dilated artery, or recurrent atherosclerosis.[59, 66, 67] Other factors that contribute to a lower technical success rate include occluded vessels, longer lesions, and advanced age.[59, 68]

### Effect on Blood Pressure

The clinical effect of angioplasty on chronic hypertension in patients with atherosclerotic renal artery stenosis is variable. In comparison to fibromuscular dysplasia, the results are less favorable. There are a number of reasons why clinical improvement may not occur: Patients with atheromatous disease may have underlying essential hypertension; contralateral hypertensive renal disease may be present, contributing to residual hypertension; cholesterol embolization may occur in the affected or contralateral kidney; and in patients with contralateral renal artery occlusion, there may be continued production of renin by the kidney. Table 48–5 shows the results of the most recent studies. To date, only one small randomized trial has been conducted.[68a] Van Jaarsveld and associates found no effect on patients treated with balloon angioplasty. This study must be replicated with stent therapy. In patients in whom the procedure was a technical success, cure of hypertension occurred in 4% to 23%, and up to 70% overall experienced benefit. The mortality in patients with renal artery stenosis is caused primarily by coronary artery disease and stroke. Because even modest reductions in blood pressure are asso-

**TABLE 48–6.  EFFECT OF ANGIOPLASTY OR STENT IMPLANTATION IN ATHEROSCLEROTIC LESIONS ON CHRONIC RENAL FAILURE**

| AUTHOR | YEAR | PATIENTS | DEATH | RENAL FAILURE | | |
| | | | | IMPROVED | STABLE | WORSE |
| --- | --- | --- | --- | --- | --- | --- |
| Dorros et al[100]* | 1998 | 54 | — | 23 (45%) | — | 28 (55%)† |
| Harden et al[73]* | 1997 | 32 | 0 | 11 (34%) | 11 (34%) | 9 (32%) |
| Tullis et al[95] | 1997 | 10 | — | 5 (50%) | 4 (40%) | 1 (10%) |
| Tykarski et al[98] | 1993 | 16 | 0 | 11 | 3 | 0 |
| O'Donovan et al[101] | 1992 | 17 | 5 | 9 (53%) | 2 (12%) | 6 (35%) |
| Canzanello et al[102] | 1989 | 69 | 2 | 36 (52%) | — | 33 (48%) |
| Martin et al[103] | 1988 | 79 | 1 | 34 (43%) | — | 45 (57%)† |
| Bell et al[104] | 1987 | 20 | 0 | 7 (35%) | 10 (50%) | 3 (15%) |
| Pickering et al[105] | 1986 | 55 | — | 26 (47%) | 19 (35%) | 10 (18%) |
| Luft et al[106] | 1983 | 12 | 0 | 3 (25%) | 5 (42%) | 4 (33%) |

Dashes indicate not reported.
*All patients received a Palmaz stent. †Includes patients who were stable or worse.

**TABLE 48–7. EFFECT OF RENAL ARTERY STENTING ON HYPERTENSION**

| AUTHOR | YEAR | ARTERIES | PATIENTS | INDICATIONS | OSTIAL LESIONS | STENT | TECHNICAL SUCCESS (%) | MAJOR COMPLICATIONS | IN-HOSPITAL DEATH | RESTENOSIS AT FOLLOW-UP | FOLLOW-UP (MONTHS) | BLOOD PRESSURE CURE | BLOOD PRESSURE IMPROVEMENT | BLOOD PRESSURE BENEFIT |
|---|---|---|---|---|---|---|---|---|---|---|---|---|---|---|
| Lederman et al[78] | 1999 | 358 | 300 | — | 278 (76%) | Palmaz | 100 | 3 (1.0%) | 1 | 23/102 (22.5%) | 10 | 2 (0.06%) | 210 (70%) | 70% |
| Van de Ven et al[77] | 1999 | 52 | 42 | — | 42 (100%) | Palmaz | 90 | 3 (5.8%) | 0 | 11/50 (22%) | 6 | — | — | 58% |
| Dorros et al[100] | 1998 | — | 163 | — | — | Palmaz | 99 | 3 (2%) | 3 | — | 36* | 1 (1%) | 41 (56%) | 57% |
| Blum et al[107] | 1997 | 74 | 68 | Unsuccessful PTRA (63) Restenosis (10) Dissection (1) | 74 (100%) | Palmaz | 100 | 0 (0%) | 0 | 8/74 (10.8%) | 60 | 11 (16%) | 15 (22%) | 38% |
| White et al[62] | 1997 | 133 | 100 | Ostial lesion (107) Unsuccessful PTRA (16) Restenosis (10) | 107 (80%) | Palmaz | 99 | 2 (2%) | 1† | 15/67 (22.4%) | 9 ± 5 | — | — | — |
| Harden et al[73] | 1997 | 33 | 33 | Ostial lesion (24) Unsuccessful PTRA (6) Dissection (1) Restenosis (1) | 24 (73%) | Palmaz | 100 | 4 (12%) | 1 | 3/24 (12.5%) | 6 | — | — | — |
| Boisclair et al[108] | 1997 | 35 | 33 | Unsuccessful PTRA (29) Restenosis (6) | — | Palmaz | 100 | 7 (21%) | 0 | — | 1–34 | 2 (6%) | 20 (61%) | 67% |
| Van de Ven et al[109] | 1995 | 28 | 24 | — | 28 (100%) | Palmaz | 100 | 2 (8.3%) | 0 | 3/19 (16%) | 6 | 0 | 16 (67%) | 67% |
| Iannone et al[110] | 1996 | 83 | 63 | — | 51 (61%) | Palmaz | 99 | 21 (33%) | 0‡ | 10/83 (14%) | 11 | 2 (3%) | 22 (35%) | 38% |
| Henry et al[111] | 1996 | 64 | 59 | Unsuccessful PTRA (42) Restenosis (20) Dissection (2) | 34 (53%) | Palmaz | 100 | 1 (2%) | 0 | 1/64 (1.6%) | 6 | 10 (17%) | 31 (53%) | 70% |

| Study | Year | Col3 | Col4 | Indication | Col6 | Stent | Col8 | Col9 | Col10 | Col11 | Col12 | Col13 | Col14 | Col15 |
|---|---|---|---|---|---|---|---|---|---|---|---|---|---|---|
| Rundback and Jacobs[112] | 1996 | 24 | 20 | Unsuccessful PTRA (24) | 22 (92%) | Palmaz | 96 | 1 (4%) | 0 | 3/16 (18.8%) | 6 | 0 | 9 (40%) | 40% |
| MacLeod et al[113] | 1995 | 28 | 28 | Unsuccessful PTRA (28) | 22 (79%) | Palmaz | 100 | 0% | 0 | 4/24 (16.7%) | 7 | 0 | 7 (25%) | 25% |
| Raynaud et al[114] | 1994 | 18 | 18 | Unsuccessful PTRA (12) Dissection (2) Restenosis (4) | 4 (22%) | Wallstent | 100 | 3 (17%) | 0 | 2/18 (11.1%) | 11 | — | — | — |
| Strecker et al[115] | 1994 | 27 | 27 | — | — | Strecker | 74 | 1 (4%) | 0 | 3/20 (15%) | 6–12 | — | — | — |
| Hennequin et al[116] | 1994 | 21 | 21 | Unsuccessful PTRA (8) Restenosis (13) | 7 (33%) | Wallstent | 100 | — | 0 | 4/21 (19%) | 12–66 | 3 (14%) | 18 (86%) | 100% |
| Dorros et al[61] | 1993 | 21 | 21 | — | — | Palmaz | 100 | 2 (1%) | 0 | — | — | — | — | — |
| Joffre et al[79] | 1992 | 17 | 16 | Unsuccessful PTRA (6) Restenosis (11) | — | Wallstent | 100 | 1 (6%) | 0 | 1/15 (6.7%) | 1–36 | 3 (19%) | 8 (50%) | 69% |
| Wilms et al[80] | 1991 | 11 | 10 | Unsuccessful PTRA§ Restenosis§ | — | Wallstent | 100 | 3 (27%) | 0 | — | 6 | 3 (30%) | 4 (40%) | 70% |
| Rees et al[117] | 1991 | 28 | 28 | Unsuccessful PTRA (8) Ostial lesion (20) | 20 (71%) | Palmaz | 96 | 5 (18%) | 0 | 7/18 (39%) | 2–18 | 3 (11%) | 15 (54%) | 65% |
| Kuhn et al[118] | 1991 | 10 | 10 | Unsuccessful PTRA (8) Dissection (1) Restenosis (1) | 1 (10%) | Strecker | 80 | 0 | 0 | — | 6–12 | 2 (20%) | 3 (30%) | 50% |

Dashes indicate not reported.
PTRA, percutaneous transluminal renal angioplasty.
*Follow-up was at 1, 2, 3, and 4 years; results at 3 years are shown here. †Sudden ischemic cardiac death 2 days after hospital discharge. ‡Ten patient deaths at follow-up. §Exact numbers not available.

ciated with greater reductions in the incidence of stroke and coronary events, the efficacy of renal angioplasty should be assessed with regard to the incidence and amount of improvement in blood pressure rather than the incidence of cure.[69–71] It is likely that these results can be improved with careful patient selection.

A distinct subgroup of patients are those with acute or recurrent pulmonary edema in the setting of poorly controlled hypertension and renal insufficiency. These findings appear to be a marker of severe bilateral atherosclerotic renal artery stenosis. Management with medical therapy may cause exacerbation of renal dysfunction without improvement in hypertension control. Revascularization provides effective resolution of pulmonary edema and control of hypertension and frequently also provides improvement in renal function.[46, 47, 72]

### Effect on Renal Failure

The effects of angioplasty on renal function have been reported in a series of retrospective studies, each involving small numbers of patients. The renal outcomes are summarized in Table 48–6. Overall, these studies have reported an improvement in renal function in about 25% to 53% of patients, with deterioration occurring in approximately 0% to 30%. However, even in patients without significant change in serum creatinine levels, there may be a reduction in the rate of deterioration of renal function. In a study of 23 patients who underwent stent implantation, Harden and coauthors reported a reduction in the rate of progression of renal failure in 18 (78%).[73] There has been only one prospective randomized trial comparing angioplasty and surgery. In this study of 58 patients, there was no significant difference between surgery and angioplasty with regard to improvement in hypertension or renal function.[74]

## Renal Transplantation and Bypass Graft Angioplasty

Angioplasty of renal transplant arteries has been performed, and in a review of 90 patients, Lohr and associates reported a success rate of 84%.[75] These results are similar to those of surgical vascular repair. There have been anecdotal reports of angioplasty of renal artery saphenous vein grafts without complications.[58, 76]

## The Role of Renal Artery Stents

A number of studies have reported the preliminary success with stents for treatment of atherosclerotic renal artery stenosis. In these studies, the most common indications for stent use have been an inadequate angioplasty result, the presence of dissection, and an ostial lesion or restenosis after previous angioplasty (Table 48–7). Therefore, these patients represent a group in which conventional angioplasty has failed or is known to have had a poor outcome. The technical success rates of these studies were usually greater than 90%. In most cases it was possible to deploy the stent satisfactorily without leaving residual stenosis or dissection. Stent implantation usually abolishes the translesional gradient in the majority of patients and produces a larger lumen diameter than does angioplasty alone.[61] Unlike angioplasty, the primary result is not influenced by the site of the lesion. Stent implantation for ostial lesions appears to be as successful as stent implantation in the main vessel. The incidence of complications in preliminary studies is low. Although only one small randomized trial of 85 patients has compared stent implantation for ostial lesions with angioplasty alone, results were clearly better with stents.[77] The rate of technical success was 57% for angioplasty in comparison with 88% after stent implantation. Restenosis after successful primary stent implantation occurred in 14% of patients, in comparison with 48% after angioplasty alone.

The overall effects on blood pressure and renal function after stent implantation are similar to those of *successful* balloon angioplasty: 60% of patients have clinical improvement in blood pressure, and 15% to 40% have improved renal function. The incidence of restenosis has been lowered with greater experience with this technique. Early studies reported an incidence of 20% to 35%; however, the incidence in more recent studies is 8% to 15%. Lederman and colleagues reviewed the incidence of restenosis in 102 of 300 patients who underwent repeat angiography for suspected restenosis or as part of another angiographic study.[78] Restenosis after stent implantation was related to the size of the reference vessel before stenting. The restenosis rate was 36% for a reference diameter less than 4.5 mm, in comparison with 15.8% for vessels 4.5 to 6.0 mm ($p = 0.068$) and 6.5% in vessels greater than 6.0 mm ($p = 0.007$). These data are reassuring because most vessels are greater than 5 mm in diameter. As with coronary stent implantation, the use of antiplatelet regimens without the use of warfarin (Coumadin) and the use of high-pressure deployment may have reduced the long-term restenosis rates. In most centers, a balloon-expandable stent is used because it can be placed more precisely than the Wallstent, which shortens considerably as it expands.[79, 80]

Stent implantation provides a significant advantage over angioplasty alone in most patients with atherosclerotic renal artery stenosis. When lesions involve the ostium, stent implantation has a significantly lower incidence of restenosis. It is therefore likely that it will be the treatment of choice for all atherosclerotic renal artery lesions. Stent implantation is probably not indicated in most patients with fibromuscular dysplasia because the results of angioplasty alone are excellent. Currently, a number of multicenter trials are assessing the role of primary stent implantation for atherosclerotic renal artery disease.

## CURRENT INDICATIONS FOR ANGIOPLASTY AND STENT IMPLANTATION

The management of patients with renal artery stenosis, particularly in the setting of chronic renal failure, is evolving. With the advent of newer percutaneous techniques that are less invasive than surgery, there is a potential for providing benefit to a wider spectrum of patients. There is a need for considerable research to increase our understanding of the pathophysiologic mechanisms involved in ischemic renal disease. Methods are needed for determining the contribution of an RAS to renal failure in patients with multifactorial causes of renal parenchymal disease. Nevertheless, certain groups of patients who are likely to benefit from this procedure can be identified.

In patients with bilateral high-grade RAS or in those with RAS of a solitary kidney, there is a significant risk of developing renal failure, and they should be referred for angioplasty and/or stent implantation or revascularization. Data from studies of surgical revascularization indicate that improvement in renal function can be expected in 50% to 85% of these patients.[81, 82] There is controversy over the management of patients with unilateral disease. In the presence of renal failure, which indicates bilateral renal disease and therefore probable parenchymal involvement of the contralateral kidney, it is possible that renal function may be improved by restoration of normal renal blood flow to the affected side. However, the data currently available are insufficient for guiding management of patients with this problem.

Patients with a significant RAS in the presence of severe hypertension that is unresponsive or only partly responsive to multiple medications should be considered for intervention. As discussed earlier, it is difficult with currently available tests to predict improvement in blood pressure control in these patients before the procedure. Most studies show some benefit in more than 70% of patients who undergo revascularization. In this regard, angioplasty and stent implantation may confer some advantages over surgery because they allow revascularization in patients who may be considered unsuitable for surgical intervention.

Finally, patients who have unilateral renal artery stenosis without renal failure or hypertension probably do not require intervention. However, the incidence of progression of these lesions to occlusion is high. Atherosclerotic renal artery disease is progressive in nature and may progress rapidly in arteries without evidence of disease at initial catheterization.[41] Therefore, it is particularly important to assess the lesions in the context of the patient. Young patients with evidence of atherosclerosis elsewhere may be at risk of developing further restenosis of the contralateral artery; therefore, preservation of renal function may be important in this age group. In older patients with fewer risk factors or who have other comorbidities, the risk of development of renal failure may be less and intervention may not be indicated. Trials are needed to further refine the management of this diverse group of patients.[119]

## REFERENCES

1. Toma H: Takayasu's arteritis. *In* Novick A, Scoble J, Hamilton G (eds): Renal Vascular Disease, pp 47–62. London: WB Saunders, 1996.
2. Horvath JS, Waugh RC, Tiller DJ, et al: The detection of renovascular hypertension: A study of 490 patients by renal angiography. Q J Med 51:139–146, 1982.
3. Maxwell MH, Bleifer KH, Franklin SS, et al: Cooperative study of renovascular hypertension. Demographic analysis of the study. JAMA 220:1195–1204, 1972.
4. Carmichael DJS, Mathias CJ, Snell ME, et al: Detection and investigation of renal artery stenosis. Lancet 1:667–670, 1986.
5. Mailloux LU, Bellucci AG, Mossey RT, et al: Predictors of survival in patients undergoing dialysis. Am J Med 84:855–862, 1988.
6. Meyrier A, Buchet P, Simon P, et al: Atheromatous renal disease. Am J Med 85:139–146, 1988.
7. O'Neill EA, Hansen KJ, Canzanello VJ, et al: Prevalence of ischemic nephropathy in patients with renal insufficiency. Am Surg 58:485–490, 1992.
8. Kalra PA, Mamtora H, Holmes AM, et al: Renovascular disease and renal complications of angiotensin-converting enzyme inhibitor therapy. Q J Med 77:1013–1018, 1990.
9. Jacobson HR: Ischemic renal disease: An overlooked clinical entity. Kidney Int 34:729–743, 1988.
10. Schreiber MJ, Pohl MA, Novick AC: The natural history of atherosclerotic and fibrous renal artery disease. Urol Clin North Am 11:383–392, 1984.
11. Pickering TG, Blumenfield JD, Laragh JH: Renovascular hypertension and ischemic nephropathy. *In* Brenner BM (ed): The Kidney, pp 2106–2126. Philadelphia: WB Saunders, 1996.
12. Textor SC: Pathophysiology of renal failure in renovascular disease. Am J Kidney Dis 24:642–651, 1994.
13. Stanley JC: Pathologic basis of macrovascular renal artery disease. *In* Stanley JC, Ernst CB, Fry WJ (eds): Renovascular Hypertension, pp 46–74. London: WB Saunders, 1984.
14. Stanley JC, Gewertz BL, Bove EL, et al: Arterial fibrodysplasia. Histopathologic character and current etiologic concepts. Arch Surg 110:561–566, 1975.
15. Stanley JC, Wakefield TW: Arterial fibrodysplasia. *In* Rutherford RB (ed): Vascular Surgery, pp 264–285. Philadelphia: WB Saunders, 1995.
16. Stanley JC: Renal artery fibroplasia. *In* Novick A, Scoble J, Hamilton G (eds): Renal Vascular Disease, pp 21–33. London: WB Saunders, 1996.
17. Connolly JO, Higgins RM, Walters HL, et al: Presentation, clinical features and outcome in different patterns of atherosclerotic renovascular disease. Q J Med 87:413–421, 1994.

18. Louie J, Isaacson JA, Zierler RE, et al: Prevalence of carotid and lower extremity arterial disease in patients with renal artery stenosis. Am J Hypertens 7:436–439, 1994.

19. Mailloux LU, Napolitano B, Bellucci AG, et al: Renal vascular disease causing end-stage renal disease, incidence, clinical correlates, and outcomes: A 20-year clinical experience. Am J Kidney Dis 24:622–629, 1994.

20. Missouris CG, Buckenham T, Cappuccio FP, et al: Renal artery stenosis: A common and important problem in patients with peripheral vascular disease. Am J Med 96:10–14, 1994.

21. Rimmer JM, Gennari FJ: Atherosclerotic renovascular disease and progressive renal failure. Ann Intern Med 118:712–719, 1993.

22. Schwartz CJ, White TA: Stenosis of the renal artery: An unselected necropsy study. BMJ 2:1415–1421, 1964.

23. Holley KE, Hunt JC, Brown AL, et al: Renal artery stenosis: A clinical-pathological study in normotensive and hypertensive patients. Am J Med 37:14–22, 1964.

24. Uzu T, Inoue T, Fujii T, et al: Prevalence and predictors of renal artery stenosis in patients with myocardial infarction. Am J Kidney Dis 29:733–738, 1997.

25. Sawicki PT, Kaiser S, Heinemann L, et al: Prevalence of renal artery stenosis in diabetes mellitus—An autopsy study. J Intern Med 229:489–492, 1991.

26. Brewster DC, Retana A, Waltman AC, et al: Angiography in the management of aneurysms of the abdominal aorta: Its value and safety. N Engl J Med 292:822–825, 1975.

27. Vetrovec GW, Landwehr DM, Edwards VL: Incidence of renal artery stenosis in hypertensive patients undergoing coronary angiography. J Intervent Cardiol 2:69–76, 1989.

28. Olin JW, Melia M, Young JR, et al: Prevalence of atherosclerotic renal artery stenosis in patients with atherosclerosis elsewhere. Am J Med 88:46N–51N, 1990.

29. Wilms G, Marchal G, Peene P, et al: The angiographic incidence of renal artery stenosis in the arteriosclerotic population. Eur J Radiol 10:195–197, 1990.

30. Salmon P, Brown MA: Renal artery stenosis and peripheral vascular disease: Implications for ACE inhibitor therapy [Letter]. Lancet 336:321, 1990.

31. Harding MB, Smith LR, Himmelstein SI, et al: Renal artery stenosis: Prevalence and associated risk factors in patients undergoing routine cardiac catheterization. J Am Soc Nephrol 2:1608–1616, 1992.

32. Swartbol P, Thorvinger BO, Parsson H, et al: Renal artery stenosis in patients with peripheral vascular disease and its correlation to hypertension. A retrospective study. Int Angiol 11:195–199, 1992.

33. Valentine RJ, Myers SI, Miller GL, et al: Detection of unsuspected renal artery stenoses in patients with abdominal aortic aneurysms: Refined indications for preoperative aortography. Ann Vasc Surg 7:220–224, 1993.

34. Jean WJ, al-Bitar I, Zwicke DL, et al: High incidence of renal artery stenosis in patients with coronary artery disease. Cathet Cardiovasc Diagn 32:8–10, 1994.

35. Zierler RE, Bergelin RO, Isaacson JA, et al: Natural history of atherosclerotic renal artery stenosis: A prospective study with duplex ultrasonography. J Vasc Surg 19:250–257, 1994.

36. Meaney TF, Dustan HP, McCormack LJ: Natural history of renal arterial disease. Radiology 91:881–887, 1968.

37. Wollenweber J, Sheps SG, Davis GD: Clinical course of atherosclerotic renovascular disease. Am J Cardiol 21:60–71, 1968.

38. Tollefson DF, Ernst CB: Natural history of atherosclerotic renal artery stenosis associated with aortic disease. J Vasc Surg 14:327–331, 1991.

39. Cohen LS, Friedman EA: Losartan-induced azotemia in a diabetic recipient of a kidney transplant [Letter]. N Engl J Med 334:1271–1272, 1996.

40. Weibull H, Bergqvist D, Andersson I, et al: Symptoms and signs of thrombotic occlusion of atherosclerotic renal artery stenosis. Eur J Vasc Surg 4:159–165, 1990.

41. Crowley JJ, Santos RM, Peter RH, et al: Progression of renal artery stenosis in patients undergoing cardiac catheterization. Am Heart J 136:913–918, 1998.

42. Isles C, Main J, O'Connell J, et al: Survival associated with renovascular disease in Glasgow and Newcastle: A collaborative study. Scott Med J 35:70–73, 1990.

43. Conlon PJ, Athirakul K, Kovalik R, et al: Survival in renal vascular disease. J Am Soc Nephrol 9:252–256, 1998.

44. Simon N, Franklin SS, Bleifer KH, et al: Clinical characteristics of renovascular hypertension. JAMA 220:1209–1218, 1972.

45. Albers FJ: Clinical characteristics of atherosclerotic renovascular disease. Am J Kidney Dis 24:636–641, 1994.

46. Pickering TG, Herman L, Devereux RB, et al: Recurrent pulmonary oedema in hypertension due to bilateral renal artery stenosis: Treatment by angioplasty or surgical revascularisation. Lancet 2:551–552, 1988.

47. Messina LM, Zelenock GB, Yao KA, et al: Renal revascularization for recurrent pulmonary edema in patients with poorly controlled hypertension and renal insufficiency: A distinct subgroup of patients with arteriosclerotic renal artery occlusive disease. J Vasc Surg 15:73–80, 1992.

48. Harward TR, Poindexter B, Huber TS, et al: Selection of patients for renal artery repair using captopril testing. Am J Surg 170:183–187, 1995.

49. Mann SJ, Pickering TG: Detection of renovascular hypertension. State of the art: 1992. Ann Intern Med 117:845–853, 1992.

50. Nally JV Jr, Olin JW, Lammert GK: Advances in noninvasive screening for renovascular disease. Cleve Clin J Med 61:328–336, 1994.

51. Olin JW, Piedmonte MR, Young JR, et al: The utility of duplex ultrasound scanning of the renal arteries for diagnosing significant renal artery stenosis. Ann Intern Med 122:833–838, 1995.

52. Gedroyc W: Magnetic resonance angiography of the renal arteries. In Novick A, Scoble J, Hamilton G (eds): Renal Vascular Disease, pp 91–106. London: WB Saunders, 1996.

53. Gerlock AJ Jr, Goncharenko V, Sloan OM: Right posterior oblique: The projection of choice in aortography of hypertensive patients. Radiology 127:45–48, 1978.

54. Dean RH, Burko H, Wilson JP, et al: Deceptive patterns of renal artery stenosis. Surgery 76:872–881, 1974.

55. Harrington DP, Levin DC, Garnic JD, et al: Compound angulation for the angiographic evaluation of renal artery stenosis. Radiology 146:829–831, 1983.

56. Reidy J: Contrast arteriography. In Novick A, Scoble J, Hamilton G (eds): Renal Vascular Disease, pp 77–90. London: WB Saunders, 1990.

57. Tegtmeyer CJ, Teates CD, Crigler N, et al: Percutaneous transluminal angioplasty in patients with renal artery stenosis: Follow-up studies. Radiology 140:323–330, 1981.

58. Tegtmeyer CJ, Kellum CD, Ayers C: Percutaneous transluminal angioplasty of the renal artery. Results and long-term follow-up. Radiology 153:77–84, 1984.

59. Sos TA, Pickering TG, Sniderman K, et al: Percutaneous transluminal renal angioplasty in renovascular hypertension due to atheroma or fibromuscular dysplasia. N Engl J Med 309:274–279, 1983.

60. Cicuto KP, McLean GK, Oleaga JA, et al: Renal artery stenosis: Anatomic classification for percutaneous transluminal angioplasty. AJR Am J Roentgenol 137:599–601, 1981.

61. Dorros G, Prince C, Mathiak L: Stenting of a renal artery stenosis achieves better relief of the obstructive lesion than balloon angioplasty. Cathet Cardiovasc Diagn 29:191–198, 1993.

62. White CJ, Ramee SR, Collins TJ, et al: Renal artery stent placement: Utility in lesions difficult to treat with balloon angioplasty. J Am Coll Cardiol 30:1445–1450, 1997.

63. Martin LG, Rees CR, O'Bryant T: Percutaneous angioplasty of the renal arteries. In Strandness DE, van Breda A (eds): Vascular Disease: Surgical and Interventional Therapy, pp 721–741. New York: Churchill Livingstone, 1994.

64. Archibald GR, Beckmann CF, Libertino JA: Focal renal artery stenosis caused by fibromuscular dysplasia: Treatment by percutaneous transluminal angioplasty. AJR Am J Roentgenol 151:593–596, 1988.

65. Cluzel P, Raynaud A, Beyssen B, et al: Stenoses of renal branch arteries in fibromuscular dysplasia: Results of percu-

taneous transluminal angioplasty. Radiology 193:227–232, 1994.

66. Bonelli FS, McKusick MA, Textor SC, et al: Renal artery angioplasty: Technical results and clinical outcome in 320 patients. Mayo Clin Proc 70:1041–1052, 1995.

67. Losinno F, Zuccala A, Busato F, et al: Renal artery angioplasty for renovascular hypertension and preservation of renal function: Long-term angiographic and clinical follow-up. AJR Am J Roentgenol 162:853–857, 1994.

68. Julien J, Jeunemaitre X, Raynaud A, et al: Influence of age on the outcome of percutaneous angioplasty in atheromatous renovascular disease. J Hypertens Suppl 7:S188–S189, 1989.

68a. van Jaarsveld BC, Krijnen P, Pieterman H, et al: The effect of balloon angioplasty on hypertension in atherosclerotic renal-artery stenosis. N Engl J Med 342:1007–1014, 2000.

69. 1993 guidelines for the management of mild hypertension. Memorandum from a World Health Organization/International Society of Hypertension meeting. Guidelines Subcommittee of the WHO/ISH Mild Hypertension Liaison Committee. Hypertension 22:392–403, 1993.

70. MacMahon S, Peto R, Cutler J, et al: Blood pressure, stroke, and coronary heart disease: Part 1. Prolonged differences in blood pressure: Prospective observational studies corrected for the regression dilution bias. Lancet 335:765–774, 1990.

71. Collins R, Peto R, MacMahon S, et al: Blood pressure, stroke, and coronary heart disease: Part 2. Short-term reductions in blood pressure: Overview of randomised drug trials in their epidemiological context. Lancet 335:827–838, 1990.

72. Ying CY, Tifft CP, Gavras H, et al: Renal revascularization in the azotemic hypertensive patient resistant to therapy. N Engl J Med 311:1070–1075, 1984.

73. Harden PN, MacLeod MJ, Rodger RS, et al: Effect of renal-artery stenting on progression of renovascular renal failure. Lancet 349:1133–1136, 1997.

74. Weibull H, Bergqvist D, Bergentz SE, et al: Percutaneous transluminal renal angioplasty versus surgical reconstruction of atherosclerotic renal artery stenosis: A prospective randomized study. J Vasc Surg 18:841–850, 1993.

75. Lohr JW, MacDougall ML, Chonko AM, et al: Percutaneous transluminal angioplasty in transplant renal artery stenosis: Experience and review of the literature. Am J Kidney Dis 7:363–367, 1986.

76. Hayes JM, Risius B, Novick AC, et al: Experience with percutaneous transluminal angioplasty for renal artery stenosis at the Cleveland Clinic. J Urol 139:488–492, 1988.

77. van de Ven PJG, Kaatee R, Beutler JJ, et al: Arterial stenting and balloon angioplasty in ostial atherosclerotic renovascular disease: A randomised trial. Lancet 353:282–286, 1999.

78. Lederman RJ, Mendelsohn FO, Greenbaum AB, et al: Renal artery stents: Characteristics and outcomes after 369 procedures. J Am Coll Cardiol 33(suppl A):22A, 1999.

79. Joffre F, Rousseau H, Bernadet P, et al: Midterm results of renal artery stenting. Cardiovasc Intervent Radiol 15:313–318, 1992.

80. Wilms GE, Peene PT, Baert AL, et al: Renal artery stent placement with use of the Wallstent endoprosthesis. Radiology 179:457–462, 1991.

81. Novick AC, Ziegelbaum M, Vidt DG, et al: Trends in surgical revascularization for renal artery disease. Ten years' experience. JAMA 257:498–501, 1987.

82. Dean RH, Kieffer RW, Smith BM, et al: Evolution of renal insufficiency in ischemic nephropathy. Ann Surg 213:446–456, 1991.

83. Choudhri AH, Cleland JG, Rowlands PC, et al: Unsuspected renal artery stenosis in peripheral vascular disease. BMJ 301:1197–1198, 1990.

84. Dean RH, Kieffer RW, Smith BM, et al: Renovascular hypertension: Anatomic and renal function changes during drug therapy. Arch Surg 116:1408–1415, 1981.

85. Jensen G, Zachrisson BF, Delin K, et al: Treatment of renovascular hypertension: One year results of renal angioplasty. Kidney Int 48:1936–1945, 1995.

86. Rodriguez-Perez JC, Plaza C, Reyes R, et al: Treatment of renovascular hypertension with percutaneous transluminal angioplasty: Experience in Spain. J Vasc Intervent Radiol 5:101–109, 1994.

87. Tegtmeyer CJ, Selby JB, Hartwell GD, et al: Results and complications of angioplasty in fibromuscular disease. Circulation 83:I-155–I-161, 1991.

88. Baert AL, Wilms G, Amery A, et al: Percutaneous transluminal renal angioplasty: Initial results and long-term follow-up in 202 patients. Cardiovasc Intervent Radiol 13:22–28, 1990.

89. Greminger P, Steiner A, Schneider E, et al: Cure and improvement of renovascular hypertension after percutaneous transluminal angioplasty of renal artery stenosis. Nephron 51:362–366, 1989.

90. Klinge J, Mali WP, Puylaert CB, et al: Percutaneous transluminal renal angioplasty: Initial and long-term results. Radiology 171:501–506, 1989.

91. Grim CE, Yune HY, Donohue JP, et al: Renal vascular hypertension. Surgery vs. dilation. Nephron 44:96–100, 1986.

92. Martin LG, Price RB, Casarella WJ, et al: Percutaneous angioplasty in clinical management of renovascular hypertension: Initial and long-term results. Radiology 155:629–633, 1985.

93. Kuhlmann U, Greminger P, Gruentzig A, et al: Long-term experience in percutaneous transluminal dilatation of renal artery stenosis. Am J Med 79:692–698, 1985.

94. Geyskes GG, Puylaert CB, Oei HY, et al: Follow up study of 70 patients with renal artery stenosis treated by percutaneous transluminal dilatation. BMJ 287:333–336, 1983.

95. Tullis MJ, Zierler RE, Glickerman DJ, et al: Results of percutaneous transluminal angioplasty for atherosclerotic renal artery stenosis: A follow-up study with duplex ultrasonography. J Vasc Surg 25:46–54, 1997.

96. von Knorring J, Edgren J, Lepantalo M: Long-term results of percutaneous transluminal angioplasty in renovascular hypertension. Acta Radiol 37:36–40, 1996.

97. Karagiannis A, Douma S, Voyiatzis K, et al: Percutaneous transluminal renal angioplasty in patients with renovascular hypertension: Long-term results. Hypertens Res 18:27–31, 1995.

98. Tykarski A, Edwards R, Dominiczak AF, et al: Percutaneous transluminal renal angioplasty in the management of hypertension and renal failure in patients with renal artery stenosis. J Hum Hypertens 7:491–496, 1993.

99. Martin LG, Cork RD, Kaufman SL: Long-term results of angioplasty in 110 patients with renal artery stenosis. J Vasc Intervent Radiol 3:619–626, 1992.

100. Dorros G, Jaff M, Mathiak L, et al: Four-year follow-up of Palmaz-Schatz stent revascularization as treatment for atherosclerotic renal artery stenosis. Circulation 98:642–647, 1998.

101. O'Donovan RM, Gutierrez OH, Izzo JLJ: Preservation of renal function by percutaneous renal angioplasty in high-risk elderly patients: Short-term outcome. Nephron 60:187–192, 1992.

102. Canzanello VJ, Millan VG, Spiegel JE, et al: Percutaneous transluminal renal angioplasty in management of atherosclerotic renovascular hypertension: Results in 100 patients. Hypertension 13:163–172, 1989.

103. Martin LG, Casarella WJ, Gaylord GM: Azotemia caused by renal artery stenosis: Treatment by percutaneous angioplasty. AJR Am J Roentgenol 150:839–844, 1988.

104. Bell GM, Reid J, Buist TA: Percutaneous transluminal angioplasty improves blood pressure and renal function in renovascular hypertension. Q J Med 63:393–403, 1987.

105. Pickering TG, Sos TA, Saddekni S, et al: Renal angioplasty in patients with azotemia and renovascular hypertension. J Hypertens 4(suppl 6):S667–S669, 1986.

106. Luft FC, Grim CE, Weinberger MH: Intervention in patients with renovascular hypertension and renal insufficiency. J Urol 130:654–656, 1983.

107. Blum U, Krumme B, Flugel P, et al: Treatment of ostial renal artery stenoses with vascular endoprostheses after unsuccessful balloon angioplasty. N Engl J Med 336:459–465, 1997.

108. Boisclair C, Therasse E, Oliva VL, et al: Treatment of renal angioplasty failure by percutaneous renal artery stenting

with Palmaz stents: Midterm technical and clinical results. AJR Am J Roentgenol 168:245–251, 1997.

109. Van de Ven PJ, Beutler JJ, Kaatee R, et al: Transluminal vascular stent for ostial atherosclerotic renal artery stenosis. Lancet 346:672–674, 1995.

110. Iannone LA, Underwood PL, Nath A, et al: Effect of primary balloon expandable renal artery stents on long-term patency, renal function, and blood pressure in hypertensive and renal insufficient patients with renal artery stenosis. Cathet Cardiovasc Diagn 37:243–250, 1996.

111. Henry M, Amor M, Henry I, et al: Stent placement in the renal artery: Three-year experience with the Palmaz stent. J Vasc Intervent Radiol 7:343–350, 1996.

112. Rundback JH, Jacobs JM: Percutaneous renal artery stent placement for hypertension and azotemia: Pilot study. Am J Kidney Dis 28:214–219, 1996.

113. MacLeod M, Taylor AD, Baxter G, et al: Renal artery stenosis managed by Palmaz stent insertion: Technical and clinical outcome. J Hypertens 13:1791–1795, 1995.

114. Raynaud AC, Beyssen BM, Turmel-Rodrigues LE, et al: Renal artery stent placement: Immediate and midterm technical and clinical results. J Vasc Intervent Radiol 5:849–858, 1994.

115. Strecker EP, Hagen B, Liermann D, et al: Current status of the Strecker stent. Cardiol Clin 12:673–687, 1994.

116. Hennequin LM, Joffre FG, Rousseau HP, et al: Renal artery stent placement: Long-term results with the Wallstent endoprosthesis. Radiology 191:713–719, 1994.

117. Rees CR, Palmaz JC, Becker GJ, et al: Palmaz stent in atherosclerotic stenoses involving the ostia of the renal arteries: Preliminary report of a multicenter study. Radiology 181:507–514, 1991.

118. Kuhn FP, Kutkuhn B, Torsello G, et al: Renal artery stenosis: Preliminary results of treatment with the Strecker stent. Radiology 180:367–372, 1991.

119. Safian RD, Textor SC: Medical progress: Renal-artery stenosis. N Engl J Med 344:431–442, 2001.

# 49

# Carotid Artery Intervention

*Gary S. Roubin    Jiri J. Vitek    Sriram S. Iyer    Gishel New*

## HISTORY AND BACKGROUND

Carotid artery stenting (CAS) (Fig. 49–1) represents one of the final frontiers for percutaneous endoluminal intervention. Although the idea of balloon angioplasty of the major aortic arch vessels was frequently entertained in the earliest days of intervention, it was only occasionally performed (A. Gruentzig and F. Mahler, personal communication, 1984). With the subsequent improvement in equipment and experience, many radiologists and neuroradiologists have been able to treat stenotic lesions in the subclavian and innominate arteries, and less frequently at the origin of the common carotid arteries (CCAs).[1-3] However, the most common site for carotid atherosclerotic disease, the carotid bifurcation, was thought to be unsuitable for percutaneous intervention. Two reasons were proposed for this. First, the potentially friable nature of the atherosclerotic plaque at this site and the risk of brain embolization were well recognized. Second, the carotid bifurcation was reasonably accessible by surgical operation. In comparison with the location of the coronary arteries, aortic arch vessels, renal arteries, and even iliac arteries, the superficial location of the carotid bifurcation was considered ideal for operative intervention. As a result, during the 1960s and 1970s, carotid endarterectomy (CEA) was one of the most commonly performed and successful procedures undertaken by vascular surgeons, neuro-

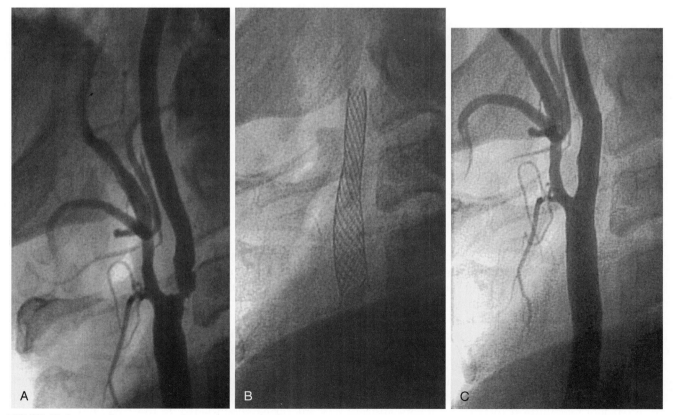

FIGURE 49–1. Carotid artery stenting. *A,* This significant stenosis at the origin of the internal carotid artery (ICA) is not tortuous nor a "kinked" vessel. The common carotid artery (CCA) is also a straight artery and free of atherosclerosis. *B,* A 10 × 20 Wallstent. *C,* Angiography after stenting. Complete obliteration of the lesion is seen.

surgeons, and general surgeons.[4] The initial results of the first prospective randomized controlled trial comparing the results of CEA with standard medical therapy in symptomatic patients with bifurcation disease were reported in 1991.[5] Despite the acknowledged limitations of this study, the strong positive results made the study a landmark in the evolution of treatment of carotid artery disease.

Throughout the 1980s, the field of interventional neuroradiology was cultivated.[6, 7] By the early 1990s, pioneering work on the carotid bifurcation was begun in Europe by two groups led by Théron[8] and Mathias,[9] and in 1992, Ferguson began exploring the possibility of a national registry to document the increasing experience with angioplasty of the extracranial and intracranial carotid arteries.[10] The early 1990s were also an era of increased interest in the mechanical and pharmacologic management of acute ischemic stroke. Many neurologists, neuroradiologists, and neurosurgeons were frustrated with the lack of treatment for this devastating event. Thrombolysis and primary angioplasty had already become standard therapies for acute myocardial infarction, and there was growing interest in applying these techniques to the carotid artery and its branches. Despite the important differences between the cerebral and coronary circulations, the following years proved that there would be more similarity in the therapeutic approaches than many physicians had believed.

The final determining factors that precipitated the "coming out" of carotid intervention were (1) the development of arterial stent technology and the understanding of optimal stenting techniques and (2) the increasing role of cardiologists in the treatment of peripheral vascular disease.[2]

Elective stenting of carotid bifurcation lesions was begun at the University of Alabama at Birmingham in March, 1994, by a multidisciplinary group comprising Jiri J. Vitek (neuroradiology), Gary S. Roubin (cardiology and radiology), and Sriram S. Iyer (cardiology), in collaboration with Jay Yadav, a board-certified neurologist with an interest in stroke intervention. The first series of stented patients was reported in 1995.[11] Live demonstration courses by the authors at the University of Alabama Hospital, individual proctoring, and participation in a large number of international meetings have been pivotal in the increasing widespread application of this percutaneous approach for treating extracranial carotid stenoses.

The success of CAS is intimately related to the training and experience of the operator. A "learning curve" is associated with the clinical, cognitive, and technical factors required to perform a safe and effective procedure. In this chapter, we present the current indications, patient selection factors, and technical and procedural details required for performing safe CAS.

## General Indications for Carotid Intervention

The goal of CAS is the same as that of CEA: that is, the prevention of stroke. Because the risk of stroke is related to the nature of the lesion to be treated, it requires establishing the risk/benefit ratio for any individual patient. Because the late outcomes from both CEA and CAS seem to be favorable and similar (see later section) the critical issues are (1) the periprocedural risk (stroke or death rate) associated with the procedure, and (2) the natural history of the lesion if the patient continues to be managed with conservative medical therapy.

A carotid stenosis may cause a stroke by the generation of emboli or the propagation of thrombus originating from plaque in the internal carotid artery (ICA). This may subsequently lead to occlusion of an intracerebral vessel and cerebral infarction. The presence of adequate collateral filling and/or associated contralateral disease also determines the extent of infarction and clinical deficit that prevail. It is also known that the risk of stroke is increased in patients with more severe stenoses, ulcerated lesions, and thrombotic lesions and when there are unstable neurologic symptoms, such as those caused by recent stroke or transient ischemic attacks.

The NASCET (North American Symptomatic Carotid Endarterectomy Trial),[12, 13] ACAS (Asymptomatic Carotid Atherosclerosis Study),[14] and ECST (European Carotid Surgery Trial)[15, 16] provide the guidelines on which we base recommendations for revascularization therapy. In symptomatic patients, revascularization is indicated for 60% of lesions in women and 50% of lesions in men (using NASCET angiographic criteria) if the revascularization can be done with a periprocedural stroke or death rate of 6% or less. Interestingly, the ECST study did not demonstrate as great a benefit from CEA in women compared with men because of the increased perioperative complications that occurred in women and the lower incidence of late strokes in women in the control arm. In asymptomatic patients, revascularization can be recommended in 70% of lesions in women and 60% of lesions in men only if the revascularization can be done with a 3% or lower complication rate.[13] For these data to be applied to CAS, there must be an assumption that the late results from both CEA and stenting are equivalent. Intermediate-term outcomes to date from multiple stent series suggest this is the case, but additional follow-up studies and randomized controlled trials are required to confirm these observations.

# Complications of Carotid Endarterectomy

On the basis of these three landmark randomized trials comparing CEA with the best (at that time) medical therapy,[12–16] CEA is currently considered the standard revascularization therapy for the treatment of both symptomatic and asymptomatic extracranial carotid stenosis. To appreciate the proper indications for CEA, one must review the populations enrolled in these trials and the results obtained. First, the NASCET was conducted over a 10-year period by a preselected group of vascular surgeons who could only qualify as operators if they could demonstrate a complication (death and stroke) rate of 5% or less in their last 100 patients. In addition, the patient population studied represented a relatively low risk cohort, with many patients excluded for a variety of clinical and anatomic reasons (Table 49–1).[17]

These exclusions are important, because it can be argued that the NASCET results cannot be extrapolated to the overall general population.[18] Wennberg and associates have suggested that the risks of CEA are likely to be significantly higher in a general Medicare population, and as such, the actual benefit of CEA in this population may not be the same as that seen in the randomized population.[18]

Interestingly, in the NASCET study, the benefit of CEA was directly related to the severity of stenosis.[13, 19] That is, the benefit was greatest for patients with 90% lesions as opposed to a less significant benefit in those with 50% or 60% lesions. Also, the method that was used to measure stenosis severity

**TABLE 49–1.** **CONDITIONS CAUSING PATIENTS TO BE EXCLUDED FROM NORTH AMERICAN SYMPTOMATIC CAROTID ENDARTERECTOMY TRIAL**

No clear and adequate selective angiographic visualization of the carotid arteries or intracranial branches
Carotid stenosis intracranially that was more severe than the surgically accessible lesion
Older than 79 years
Renal, liver, heart, or lung failure
Prior disabling stroke
Cardiac valve disease, atrial fibrillation, or other cardiac disease likely to cause cardioembolic symptoms
Prior ipsilateral carotid endarterectomy
Recent uncontrolled diabetes or hypertension*
Unstable angina or myocardial infarction within prior 6 months*
Progressive neurologic symptoms*
Contralateral endarterectomy within 4 months*
Any major surgical procedure within last 30 days*
Symptoms attributable to nonatherosclerotic disease, e.g., tumor

*Temporarily ineligible.
From North American Symptomatic Carotid Endarterectomy Trial. Methods, patient characteristics, and progress. Stroke 22:711–720, 1991.

**TABLE 49–2.** **PERIOPERATIVE MORBIDITY AND MORTALITY FROM CAROTID ENDARTERECTOMY (NORTH AMERICAN SYMPTOMATIC CAROTID ENDARTERECTOMY TRIAL)**

| COMPLICATION | RATE (%) |
|---|---|
| Death or stroke* | 5.8 |
| Carotid nerve palsy | 7.6 |
| Neck wound hematoma | 5.5 |
| Wound infection | 3.4 |
| Nonfatal myocardial infarction | 0.9 |
| Congestive heart failure | 0.6 |
| "Arrhythmias" | 1.2 |
| Other significant cardiac problems | 1.2 |
| **Total** | **26.2** |

From Beneficial effect of carotid endarterectomy in symptomatic patients with high-grade carotid stenosis. North American Symptomatic Carotid Endarterectomy Trial Collaborators. N Engl J Med 325:445–453, 1991.

is important. The precise angiographic definition was based on the percentage diameter narrowing at the lesion site compared with a nontapering segment of the more distal ICA. It is of note that no correlative carotid duplex data were collected in the NASCET study.[13] Given the widely disparate results between routine community-based carotid duplex studies and angiographic measurements,[20] the current trend toward operating on carotid stenoses based on duplex studies alone is probably inappropriate. It can be strongly argued that this current strategy of operating based on ultrasound reports has no proven basis, and it may lead to unnecessary surgery in low-risk (by NASCET definition) carotid disease. The ACAS investigators demonstrated that even in accredited laboratories, the duplex finding of a 50% to 75% lesion will be incorrect and overestimates the angiographic severity of disease in a large number of patients (G. Howard, personal communication).

The NASCET study provides us with a somewhat unique insight into the outcome of CEA when performed in centers of excellence.[12] It represents the largest and most rigorous prospectively collected data with neurologic oversight. In this relatively low risk subset that excluded very elderly (older than 79 years) persons, those with significant cardiac or pulmonary comorbidities, and those who had any of a large number of other common conditions, the 30-day mortality and morbidity from stroke was 5.8%. In addition, there was a 7% rate of cranial nerve palsies and a 13% incidence of local wound or medical complications (Table 49–2).

This trial also demonstrated a significantly higher incidence of death and stroke (14%) in those who underwent CEA in the presence of an occluded contralateral carotid artery. Regardless, the 2-year outcome for CEA with respect to freedom from any ipsilateral stroke or death (92%) was significantly better than the outcome from medical management (72% free from any ipsilateral stroke or death).

The second landmark study that examined the benefit of CEA in symptomatic patients was the ECST.[15] This large prospective randomized study demonstrated a clear benefit of surgery over medical management. At 3 years, the risk of stroke and death in the control group was 26.5% compared with 14.9% in the CEA group. The overall complication rates in the ECST were similar to those seen in NASCET (Table 49–3). The periprocedural neurologic and nonneurologic complication rates in the NASCET and ECST studies underscores the need to pursue alternative potentially safer methods for treating bifurcation disease. The complications listed in Table 49–2 rarely occur in those patients undergoing CAS. Hence, this procedure may have specific application in those subsets of patients found to be "high risk" for CEA.

Although CEA can be performed under regional anesthesia, 90% of surgeries are still performed under general anesthesia. Many patients with carotid disease also have coronary artery disease (CAD); hence, general anesthesia in these patients may be associated with an increased risk of myocardial infarction and cardiac death. Patients with heart failure, pulmonary disease, and poorly controlled diabetes are also at risk. Stenting requires no general anesthesia or sedation of the patient. CAS is performed in a nonsedated but relaxed patient. Only local anesthesia around the femoral artery is required for sheath insertion. This enables close monitoring for neurologic sequelae. Because the patient is awake and in the angiographic suite, if a neurologic event occurs, it can be investigated immediately by intracranial angiography, and appropriate

treatment can be implemented. On the other hand, when patients undergo CEA, angiography is not immediately available and neurologic complications may only be apparent after the patient recovers from the anesthesia.

The ACAS trial examined the role of CEA in those patients with asymptomatic disease.[14, 21] In this trial, the 30-day perioperative risk of stroke or death was 2.5%. In this study, surgical revascularization also produced a significant reduction in the incidence of ipsilateral stroke at 5 years (4.7% vs. 9.4%) with the benefit less significant in women and in those with less severe (50% to 70%) stenoses. In this trial, there was a carotid duplex correlative study with accredited noninvasive laboratories. Despite this, correlation with angiography was poor for lesions of 50% to 70%, modest for stenoses of 70% to 80%, and only good in stenoses greater than 80% (G. Howard, personal communication).

The actual incidence of stroke and death from CEA in the community is not surprisingly higher than that recorded in multicenter randomized trials. Brott and coworkers reviewed the hospital records of all patients having CEA in a major North American metropolitan area.[22] The combined stroke and death rate was 8.6%. The stroke rate was 5.6% for asymptomatic patients and 11.6% for symptomatic patients. Importantly, 57% of the operative strokes occurred after a neurologically intact postoperative period. There have been other contemporary reports supporting the observation that in the community, CEA is performed with a higher perioperative risk than that reported in the NASCET and ACAS studies. Approximately 80% of CEAs are performed in low-volume hospitals where the overall risk of stroke or death for asymptomatic and symptomatic patients is 7% (higher in symptomatic patients) and surgeons who perform fewer than 20 operations per year perform 90% of endarterectomies.[23]

Rothwell and associates reviewed several published series on CEA to determine if there was a reporting bias.[24] In their study, they acknowledged that their analysis probably provides a favorable picture of CEA because reporting bias would favor better results.[24] The average risk of death and stroke was 6.8%: that is, very similar to the NASCET study results. They identified a difference between results reported by single surgeons (2.2%) and those reported when neurologists were involved in the authorship of the study (7.7%; Table 49–4). In addition, they noted that there was a consistent finding of a ratio of strokes to deaths between 5:1 and 3:1 depending on the rigor of postprocedural neurologic assessment.[24]

Accordingly, with the use of reliable Medicare mortality statistics, an assessment of the risk of death and stroke can be made. Medicare data on in-

**TABLE 49–3.** **PERIOPERATIVE MORBIDITY AND MORTALITY FROM CAROTID ENDARTERECTOMY (EUROPEAN CAROTID SURGERY TRIAL)**

| COMPLICATION | RATE (%) |
|---|---|
| Death and major stroke* | 7.1 |
| Minor stroke | 2.0 |
| Cranial nerve palsy | 6.4 |
| Wound hematoma | 3.1 |
| Nonfatal myocardial infarction | 0.2 |
| Other (pulmonary complications, etc.) | 0.3 |
| **Total** | **19.3** |

*Disabling stroke lasting more than 7 days.
From MRC European Carotid Surgery Trial: Interim results for symptomatic patients with severe (70–99%) or with mild (0–29%) carotid stenosis. European Carotid Surgery Trialists Collaborative Group. Lancet 337:1235–1243, 1991.

**TABLE 49-4.    OVERALL REPORTED STROKE AND DEATH FOR CAROTID ENDARTERECTOMY**

| DEATH AND STROKE | RATE (%) |
|---|---|
| Average | 6.8 |
| Surgeon as author | 2.2 |
| Neurologist as author | 7.7 |

From Rothwell PM, Slattery J, Warlow CP: A systematic review of the risks of stroke and death due to endarterectomy for symptomatic carotid stenosis. Stroke 27:260–265, 1996.

**TABLE 49-5.    ACTUAL MORTALITY AND STROKE RISK ESTIMATES FROM CAROTID ENDARTERECTOMY IN THE UNITED STATES—1998**

| | DEATH (%) | DEATH* AND STROKE (%) | DEATH† AND STROKE (%) |
|---|---|---|---|
| NASCET/ACAS centers | 1.4 | 5.6 | 8.4 |
| High–CEA-volume centers | 1.9 | 7.8 | 11.4 |
| Low–CEA-volume centers | 2.5 | 10 | 14 |

ACAS, Asymptomatic Carotid Atherosclerosis Study; CEA, carotid endarterectomy; NASCET, North American Symptomatic Carotid Endarterectomy Trial.
*Assuming a 3:1 stroke/death ratio.
†Assuming a 5:1 stroke/death ratio (extrapolated from data of Rothwell and colleagues[24]).

hospital mortality (not the more rigorous 30-day mortality) show the following results[18]: NASCET hospitals, 1.4%; high-volume centers, 1.9%; low-volume centers, 2.5%. Thus, the risk of in-hospital procedural stroke and death is in the range of 5% to 14% depending on the volume of surgery performed (Table 49–5). These represent average results over a range of high- and low-risk CEA patients. The periprocedural risks of CEA are intimately dependent on the risk profiles of the population treated. This was first described in the seminal work of Thor Sundt. His work is particularly renowned for the characterization of risk profiles and complications from the procedure.[4] Sundt identified three groups of factors that increased the risks of CEA: medical, neurologic, and angiographic (Table 49–6).

Sundt categorized patients according to the presence or absence of these risk factors as follows:

Grade I: Neurologically stable—no risk factors
Grade II: Neurologically stable—angiographic risk factors
Grade III: Neurologically stable—medical risk factors
Grade IV: Neurologically unstable
Grade V: Acute carotid occlusion—evolving stroke
Grade VI: Restenosis after CEA

The risk of stroke and death increases significantly as the risk factor grade increases. Patient se-

lection, operator experience, and methods of auditing results complicate the literature on risk factors associated with CEA. Rothwell and colleagues published in 1997 the first systematic review of the clinical and angiographic factors associated with an increased perioperative risk from CEA.[25] Thirteen potential risk factors were examined, eight of which were identified as being significantly associated with increased perioperative risk (Table 49–7).

Rothwell and colleagues found no relationship between a history of stroke, diabetes, angina pectoris, or myocardial infarction and increased risk from CEA. These findings most likely relate to the exclusion of patients with recent or evolving stroke, severe diabetes, and severe CAD from major randomized trials. Of particular interest is that women had an increased operative stroke and mortality rate. The overall risk of death or stroke was increased by 44% in women. In 1729 patients in the ECST study, a multivariate analysis was performed to determine factors that increase the operative risks of CEA.[26] Independent risk factors were (1) cerebral instead of ocular symptoms, (2) female gender, (3) systolic hypertension greater than 180 mm Hg, and (4) pe-

**TABLE 49-6.    RISK FACTORS FOR CAROTID ENDARTERECTOMY**

| MEDICAL | NEUROLOGIC | ANGIOGRAPHIC |
|---|---|---|
| Angina pectoris | Progressive neurologic deficit | Contralateral occlusion |
| Age >70 y | Recent cerebral infarction (≥7 d) | Stenosis in region of siphon |
| Congestive heart failure | Generalized cerebral ischemia | Plaque extending 3 cm distally or 5 cm proximally into CCA |
| Severe hypertension (SBP >180 mm Hg) | Recently resolved neurologic deficit (≥24 h) | High bifurcation at level of second cervical vertebra |
| Chronic obstructive lung disease | Frequent TIAs not controlled by medications | Thrombus extending from ulcerated lesion |
| Recent MI (≥6 mon) | | Diffuse narrowing of entire distal ICA 2 degrees to subtotally occluded ICA |
| Uncontrolled diabetes | | |
| Severe obesity | | |
| Advanced PVD | | |

CCA, common carotid artery; ICA, internal carotid artery; MI, myocardial infarction; PVD, peripheral vascular disease; SBP, systolic blood pressure; TIA, transient ischemic attack.

**TABLE 49–7.    PERIOPERATIVE RISK FACTORS**

| RISK FACTOR | NO. OF STUDIES | ODDS RATIO DEATH AND STROKE | 95% CONFIDENCE INTERVAL | $p$ VALUE |
|---|---|---|---|---|
| Cerebral vs. ocular ischemia | 7 | 0.49 | 0.37–0.66 | <0.00001 |
| Women vs. men | 7 | 1.44 | 1.14–1.83 | <0.005 |
| Age > 75 y | 10 | 1.36 | 1.09–1.71 | <0.01 |
| Systolic BP >180 mm Hg | 4 | 1.82 | 1.37–2.41 | <0.0001 |
| Peripheral vascular disease | 1 | 2.19 | 1.40–3.60 | <0.0005 |
| Contralateral occlusion | 14 | 1.91 | 1.35–2.69 | <0.0001 |
| Ipsilateral ICA siphon stenosis | 1 | 1.56 | 1.03–2.36 | <0.02 |
| Ipsilateral ECA stenosis | 1 | 1.61 | 1.05–2.47 | <0.03 |

BP, blood pressure; ECA, external carotid artery; ICA, internal carotid artery.

ripheral vascular disease. The baseline risk profile of patients undergoing CEA is also relevant. Only a small percentage were at low risk, about half could be considered at acceptable risk by AHA guidelines for symptomatic patients, and a large percentage were at moderate to high risk from the procedure (Table 49–8 and P. M. Rothwell, personal communication).

The overall risk of stroke/death for women in the ECST was 10.6%; for systolic blood pressure (BP) greater than 180 mm Hg, it was 12.3%; and for the presence of peripheral vascular disease, it was 12.3%. In a study at major academic centers, McCrory and associates reported an increased risk of a major complication (24%) when CEA was combined with coronary bypass surgery, when patients had had a prior CEA (11%), and when they had a contralateral occlusion (9%).[27] In the relatively low risk ACAS population, the risk of perioperative stroke was associated with the presence of diabetes mellitus, ipsilateral siphon stenosis, and the length of the external carotid artery (ECA) plaque. A history of prior stroke and the presence of a 60% contralateral stenosis was also associated with an increased risk of complications.[19]

In addition to strokes, the other major risk associated with CEA is myocardial infarction and/or cardiovascular death. The coexistence of carotid artery disease and CAD is well recognized, and the general risks in CEA, particularly under general anesthesia, are well known.[4] Although CEA can be performed

under regional anesthesia, the procedure with the anesthesia is not well tolerated by most patients.[28]

Technical limitations of CEA such as when carotid revascularization requires a more difficult and extensive exposure of the artery are also factors that increase risks (Table 49–9). In those patients with high bifurcation or stenoses that extend more than 3 cm distally, extensive dissection frequently includes subluxation and mobilization of the mandible. It is also more difficult for the surgeon to tack down the distal extremity of the plaque and expose the artery for shunt placement. This definitely requires general anesthesia, may increase the risk of cranial nerve damage, and prolongs wound healing.

Similarly, lesions in the CCA, particularly near the origin, require an extensive surgical procedure that may include bypassing the stenosis and entering the chest cavity. Patients with radiation-induced scarring of the neck with or without prior radical neck dissections for head and neck carcinomas are also technically challenging. Similarly, patients with restenosis after CEA are at higher risk too.[4, 19] The scarring external to the artery increases the duration of the dissection and generally requires greater manipulation of the bifurcation, which is associated with an increased risk of plaque embolization. Cranial nerve palsies from the extensive dissection are also common. In some patients, an endarterectomy cannot be performed, the diseased segment must be excised, and an interposition graft is required. Finally, surgery may be more difficult

**TABLE 49–8.    EUROPEAN CAROTID SURGERY TRIAL POPULATION RISK PROFILE FOR CAROTID ENDARTERECTOMY***

| NO. OF RISK FACTORS | NO. OF PATIENTS | PERCENTAGE OF POPULATION | INCIDENCE OF DEATH OR STROKE (LASTING >7 d) (%) |
|---|---|---|---|
| 0 | 149 | 8.31 | 2.0 (0.4–5.8)† |
| 1 | 911 | 50.7 | 4.5 (3.3–6.1) |
| 2 | 577 | 32.1 | 8.3 (6.2–11) |
| 3 or more | 162 | 9.5 | 18.5 (13–25) |

*Presence of risk factors: female gender; cerebral event; age >75 y; systolic blood pressure >180 mm Hg; or contralateral occlusion.
†95% confidence intervals.

## TABLE 49–9. HIGH ANATOMIC RISK CANDIDATES FOR CAROTID ENDARTERECTOMY

| | |
|---|---|
| Contralateral occlusion | Short obese necks |
| High lesion/bifurcations | Spinal immobility |
| Low or ostial CCA lesions | Stenosis involving the ipsilateral siphon |
| Neck radiation | Severe stenosis of the ipsilateral ECA |
| Prior radial neck dissection | Prior CEA |

CCA, common carotid artery; CEA, carotid endarterectomy; ECA, external carotid artery.

in some obese patients or those with short necks. In general, none of these conditions are problems with the endovascular approach, and accordingly, CAS may be clearly preferable.

In a meta-analysis of over 8000 patients, Rothwell and colleagues calculated an overall 10.7% incidence of stroke or death in patients with contralateral occlusion compared with a 3% incidence if this risk factor was not present.[26] In the NASCET trial, the incidence of stroke (at 30-day adjudication) and death in patients with contralateral occlusion was 14%,[29] and in the ECST study the incidence was 12.5%.[15] Repeat CEA is also associated with an increased risk of complications ranging from 9% to 11%.[4, 27, 30] A number of studies have documented a higher perioperative risk of stroke and death for patients with restenosis (Table 49–10).

## TABLE 49–10. RISK FACTOR FOR CAROTID ENDARTERECTOMY

| STUDY | RISK FACTOR FOR CEA | INCIDENCE OF DEATH/STROKE (%) |
|---|---|---|
| Gasecki et al, 1995[29] | Contralateral occlusion | 14 |
| Rothwell et al, 1997[25, 26] | Contralateral occlusion | 12.3 |
| Rothwell et al, 1996[24] | Contralateral occlusion | 10.7 |
| McCrory et al, 1993[27] | Contralateral occlusion | 9.0 |
| McCrory et al, 1993[27] | Prior ipsilateral CEA | 11 |
| Meyer et al, 1994* | Prior ipsilateral CEA | 10.6 |
| Das et al, 1995[30] | Prior ipsilateral CEA | 7.6 |
| McCrory et al, 1993[27] | Severe CAD | 10 |
| Hertzer et al, 1997† | High comorbidity | 7.4 |

CAD, coronary artery disease; CEA, carotid endarterectomy.
*Meyer FB, Peipgras DG, Fode NC: Surgical treatment of recurrent carotid artery stenosis. J Neurosurg 80:781–787, 1994.
†Hertzer NR, O'Hara PJ, Mascha EJ, et al: Early outcome assessment for 2228 consecutive carotid endarterectomy procedures. The Cleveland Clinic from 1989 to 1995. J Vasc Surg 26:1–10, 1997.

## CAROTID STENTING: EVOLVING INDICATIONS

The application of CAS is evolving as the technique, stent, and catheter technology improve. Ultimately, prospective randomized trials will be necessary to determine the role of both CAS and CEA in comparable subsets of patients. Currently, the experience and results of the operator predominantly determine the eligibility for stenting. In patients deemed to be low-risk candidates for CEA, there should be no contraindication to proceed with stenting providing the procedure can be performed with complication rates as low as that recommended for CEA: that is, less than a 5% complication rate in symptomatic patients and less than a 3% complication rate in asymptomatic patients.[31] Similarly, based on current knowledge of the natural outcome of carotid bifurcation disease, stenting in general should only be applied to high-grade asymptomatic lesions (60% in men and 70% in women),[14] and based on NASCET results, 50% or greater lesions in symptomatic patients.[13] The indications for stenting may also be determined by the availability of skilled vascular surgeons. Because results of CEA (and stenting) correlate with operator experience and patient volume, claims of low perioperative complication rates by any surgeon or interventionalist should be carefully scrutinized.[24]

There are also factors that may increase the risk of a complication (usually an embolic event during CAS). During the initial learning curve phase of the operator, cases associated with higher periprocedural risk should be avoided. Many of the factors that increase the risks of CEA also increase the risks of endovascular intervention. These include advanced age, a history of stroke (particularly large deficits), and recent unstable neurologic symptoms (Table 49–11).

The stent type used in our early experience has influenced the incidence of restenosis. In general, restenosis has been extremely uncommon, particularly since changing from the Palmaz stent to the self-expanding Wallstent.[1] The ability of stents to prevent embolic stroke originating from the bifurcation should not be surprising. Fifteen years of experience with metallic stents in arterial sites has taught us that, particularly in high-flow systems, the healing response is densely fibrotic and remarkably stable after the first 3 to 6 months. Accordingly, the ability of stents to exclude the necrotic, thrombotic plaque from the circulation should not be surprising. We now have follow-up for 5 years, and as expected, there has been no indication that the stented site is unstable in the long term.

Several of the risk factors listed later were determined based on our learning curve experience. As

**TABLE 49–11. PATIENTS AT HIGH RISK FOR STENTING**

Clinical
  Advanced age (≥80 years)
  Prior stroke (large neurologic deficit)
  Cerebral atrophy/dementia
  Unstable neurologic symptoms (transient ischemic attacks /
    recent stroke)
  Diffuse, severe PVD (involving aortic arch vessels)
Anatomic
  Severely tortuous, calcified, and atherosclerotic arch vessels
  Coexistent proximal CCA lesions
  High-grade and sub–total occlusion lesions
  Severe concentric calcification
  Angiographic evidence of large amounts of thrombus
  Long, severe, complex lesions extending into the distal ICA,
    "string sign" (see Fig. 49–6)
  Severe tortuosity just distal to the bifurcation

CCA, common carotid artery; ICA, internal carotid artery; PVD, peripheral vascular disease.

experience and technology improve (including the availability of cerebral protection devices) these factors may alter.

The current contraindications to stenting include

- Severely tortuous, calcified, and atheromatous aortic arch vessels that make access to the carotid bifurcation difficult (Fig. 49–2).
- Pedunculated thrombus at the lesion site. This type of thrombus is best seen using 15-frame/ second coronary angiography.
- Severe renal impairment precluding safe use of contrast agents.
- Recent (3 weeks) stroke. These patients are best placed on antiplatelet agents and possibly anticoagulants in order to stabilize.
- Patients unable to tolerate appropriate doses of antiplatelet agents.

Low-risk patients (Figs. 49–3 and 49–4) should be selected at the beginning of the operators' experience. In our experience, low-risk patients can be stented with a 3% or less minor complication rate. The higher-risk subsets require much greater experience and expertise to achieve these types of results (Fig. 49–5). Although there is a temptation to accept patients deemed to be at high risk for complications of CEA, this should be avoided if the patient has one or more features to suggest that he or she is at high risk for CAS (see Table 49–10). Increasing the periprocedural complication rate because of high-risk subgroups may cause a program to be discontinued before the operator has had the chance to develop the necessary expertise and skill to perform this procedure on these patients.

A number of patients with a high risk of complications from CEA may in fact have a low risk of complications from CAS. These patients are ideal for CAS.[32, 33] These include post-CEA restenosis

(Figs. 49–6 to 49–8), discrete stenoses in those with prior neck radiation or radical neck dissections, cervical spine disease (Fig. 49–9), discrete proximal or ostial CCA lesions, and discrete lesions in the distal ICA or involving high bifurcations (Table 49–12 and Fig. 49–10).

In general, mainly systemic factors and comorbidities increase the risk of CEA, whereas local anatomic and lesion factors may increase the risk of stenting. However, these risk factors may only become apparent after detailed initial angiography or during the procedure when attempting to gain access into the carotid artery. The operator should be prepared to abandon the procedure at this point and consider elective CEA or continuing medical therapy. Such operator judgment is critical in maintaining low complication rates. Because there are usually reasonable alternative therapies, it must also be emphasized that failure to complete the procedure is acceptable, but an avoidable complication is not.

## CAROTID STENTING: CLINICAL APPROACH

Patients usually present with carotid duplex and/ or magnetic resonance angiography (MRA) studies suggesting evidence of either unilateral or bilateral carotid bifurcation disease. Less frequently, patients are directly referred for assessment with four-vessel cerebral angiograms.

As in all cardiovascular practice, patients are assessed for the presence of arteriovascular disease with a thorough history and physical examination. The history of prior stroke, transient ischemic attacks, amaurosis fugax, or CEA should prompt a detailed assessment for carotid disease. Clinical examination should document the presence or absence of carotid bruits and evidence of peripheral vascular disease. The large association between coronary disease, peripheral vascular disease, and cerebrovascular disease should raise suspicion and prompt carotid duplex ultrasound studies.

Patients with a history of stroke or transient ischemic attacks and those with an abnormal neurologic examination should have a computed tomographic (CT) scan or magnetic resonance imaging (MRI) study of the brain to document baseline cerebral abnormalities. All patients are referred for formal assessment by a neurologist to document the preprocedural clinical neurologic status. In our practice, all patients have a National Institutes of Health (NIH) Stroke Scale completed by a board-certified neurologist. Because all patients must undergo a complete four-vessel carotid angiogram, MRA is not obligatory.

The risks and benefits of carotid stenting, and

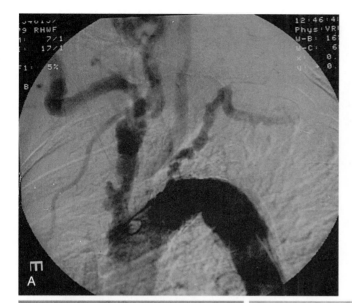

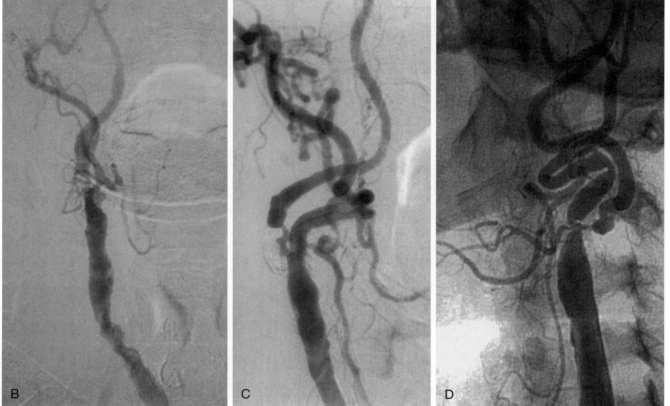

FIGURE 49–2. *A,* Contraindication to carotid stenting: a severely tortuous, calcified, ulcerated, and atheromatous aortic arch. *B,* Contraindication to carotid stenting: a diffusely ulcerated and atheromatous CCA. *C,* Contraindication to carotid stenting: a critical, heavily calcified lesion in an 85-year-old man. This is a difficult lesion to treat safely because of the crossing profile of current devices and the tendency for such a lesion to recoil after balloon dilatation. *D,* Type C lesion for experienced operators. This lesion has five adverse morphologic features; 90-degree angulation of the ICA from the CCA, heavy calcification, severe distal tortuosity, complex plaque morphology, and a severe stenosis below the bifurcation.

the availability of alternative surgical therapy, are discussed in detail with all patients. In particular, we explain to our patients that major complications are rare and occur in less than 0.5% to 1% of the patients. We discuss the risk of minor stroke (in the 3% to 4% range), by which they may expect minor weakness of a limb, mild confusion, or dysphasia, and should this occur, complete recovery is usually the rule. It is important to inform family members of this unlikely but possible outcome. We carefully

point out that although our medium-term (5-year) outcomes appear favorable,[34] long-term data are not yet available.

The details of the procedure are carefully explained. We inform the patients that they will receive no sedation or general anesthesia, but that the only discomfort is related to local anesthesia at the femoral access site. Patients can expect to spend one night in the hospital and leave early the next day. If necessary, they can return to work and full

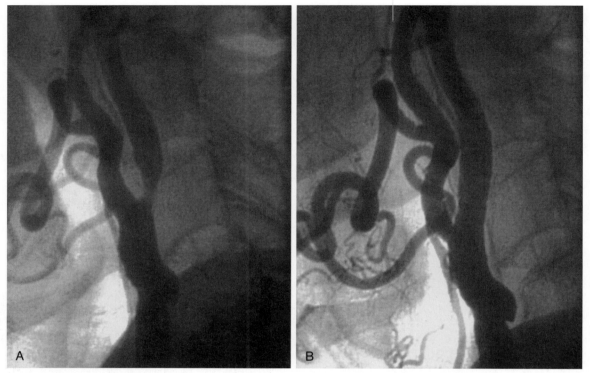

FIGURE 49–3. *A,* Ideal (type A) lesion for carotid stenting. The lesion is discrete with minimal calcification and no evidence of thrombus. The CCA is a straight vessel, and its body is free of disease. The lesion is in a nonangulated segment, and the distal ICA is not tortuous or kinked. *B,* Angiography after stenting with a 10 × 20 mm Wallstent.

activities after 72 hours. We are now performing CAS as day case procedures in selected low-risk patients.

Patients are started on antiplatelet therapy, soluble aspirin, 325 mg bid (with meals), and clopidogrel (Plavix), 75 mg qd preferably for 4 days, before the procedure. In all cases, patients should have received a *total* dose of 300 mg of clopidogrel before the intervention.

We usually arrange for patients to undergo a four-vessel cerebral angiogram and, providing the anatomy is favorable, stenting in the same procedure. Carotid duplex studies often overestimate the angiographic severity of the lesion, which may only be realized at the time of angiography.[20] Occasionally, anatomic features dictate that surgical therapy is the preferred option.

Patients are usually admitted the morning of the procedure. Standard hematologic and chemical profiles are performed as well as an electrocardiogram. All medications including antiplatelet therapy are administered the morning of the procedure.

In preparation for the procedure, patients are brought into the interventional laboratory with intravenous access. Their head is cradled in a commercially available foam head constraint. They are asked to remain as still as possible and focus on the ceiling. A six-lead electrocardiogram monitors the heart rate (HR), BP is monitored via the access

sheath, and pulse oximetry is also utilized. Dentures and eyeglasses are removed. Heparin is available for anticoagulation, as well as an activated clotting time (ACT)-monitoring system. We do not routinely administer the IIb/IIIa platelet inhibitors for carotid stenting.

Other intravenous drugs such as atropine are available for bradycardia, metaraminol bitartrate (Aramine) and dopamine for hypotension, and nitroglycerin for control of hypertension and arterial spasm. Temporary transvenous pacemakers and other standard resuscitation equipment should also be available. Patients are well hydrated before the procedure to prevent contrast-induced nephrotoxicity.

We utilize single-plane angiographic equipment with 9-, 7-, and 5-inch image magnification. Ideally, the equipment should have road mapping and digital subtraction capability to allow detailed examination of intracranial vessels and minimize the contrast load. A variety of subtracted and coronary mode (7.5 frames/second) modalities are utilized. In a routine procedure, initial four-vessel cerebral angiography takes approximately 15 to 20 minutes and the stenting procedure is completed within another 20 minutes.

After the procedure, the patient is monitored in the holding area with hemodynamic (HR and BP), groin, and neurologic observations every 15 minutes

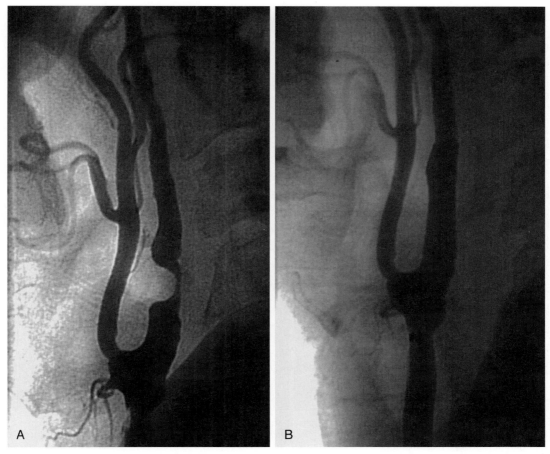

FIGURE 49–4. *A*, Lesion suitable for stenting. The ICA has a severe eccentric stenosis with minimal calcification. The CCA and distal ICA are not atheromatous and do not have bends or kinks. *B*, Angiography after stenting with a 10 × 20 mm Wallstent.

for the first hour, and hourly for the next 6 hours. Sheaths are removed the same day as the procedure after ACT measurements document the appropriate time for sheath removal. In our most recent experience, femoral puncture sites have been closed on the table with a 6- or 8-French percutaneous arteriotomy suture system (Perclose, Inc.; Menlo Park CA). This allows patients to sit up and move their limbs immediately after the procedure and is helpful in counteracting the hypotensive effect of stenting on the carotid baroreceptor. Closure devices have also enabled us to send patients home on the same day of the procedure.

## CAROTID STENTING: TECHNIQUE

### Four-Vessel Cerebral Angiography

In the vast majority of elderly patients, only one 5-French VTK catheter is required to catheterize all brachiocephalic arteries. The distal end of this catheter is shaped into a double curve with the tip, when located in the aortic arch, pointing upward. The proximal curve of this catheter is opened; this facilitates advancement of the 0.038-inch Glide Wire

into brachiocephalic arteries, even in arteries with significant tortuosity. The distal end of this catheter is at the same level as the proximal curve when reshaped in the aortic arch. This helps locate the origin of the left CCA in an elongated arch, when the origin of the left CCA migrates posteriorly or when it originates from the innominate artery. The sequence of catheterization of brachiocephalic vessels is from left to right; first the left subclavian artery, then the left CCA, and finally the innominate artery is cannulated. Straight anteroposterior (AP) fluoroscopic projection is used. Once the catheter is placed with the left subclavian artery, only slight, slow advancing movements are required to enter the left CCA and to slip the catheter into the innominate artery. After the origin of the vessel is found, the 0.038-inch Glide Wire is advanced into the left CCA or the innominate artery. Slight rotation of the catheter within the innominate artery often helps to distinguish between the right CCA and right subclavian artery. Medial rotation of the wire tip directs it into the right CCA. Road mapping can be used. The catheter should never be advanced into the artery alone, only by advancing it over the wire. The catheter is advanced into the artery over the wire slowly,

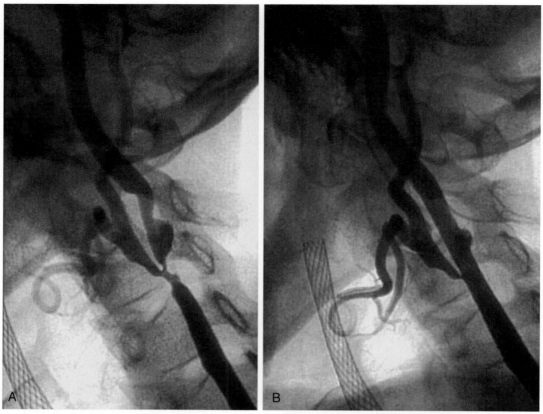

FIGURE 49–5. *A*, A more complex lesion with some calcification and ulceration involving the ICA, CCA, and external carotid artery (ECA). Note that the contralateral side has previously been stented. *B*, Angiography after stenting with a 10 × 20 mm Wallstent. Note that the ECA is "jailed" but there is Thrombosis In Myocardial Infarction (TIMI)-3 flow, and therefore the ECA required no further treatment.

sometimes using the formation of a "good" curve in the aortic arch and left upper wall of the thoracic aorta as support. A slow, "push-pull" technique over 0.5 to 1 minute may be necessary with difficult and angulated origins of vessels. A deep inspiration by the patient is sometimes helpful. Occasionally, in extremely dilated aortic arches, a sidewinder-curved catheter is needed (Simmons 3 curve). For routine cases, other operators prefer less shaped 5F $H_1$, HINK, or Berenstein diagnostic catheters. The $HN_5$ curve is occasionally useful in the left CCA or left subclavian artery.

### Cerebrovascular Anatomy

In children and young adults, the aortic arch is a symmetrically curved vascular structure tilted from the right anterior to the left posterior upper mediastinal compartment. Origins of the brachiocephalic arteries are nicely aligned in straight lines and course superiorly. The aging process and especially the atherosclerotic degenerative process elongate the aortic arch, displace the aortic knob more superiorly and posteriorly, and shift the ostia of brachiocephalic arteries. The most common congenital anomaly of the aortic arch is the joint origin of the

left CCA and innominate artery. The second most common is the left CCA originating from the innominate artery itself. In this instance, it can originate close to the aortic arch but also deeply, resembling truncus bicaroticus. In young adults, the left CCA courses superiorly, but with the aging process, it can become elongated and then courses to the left with a sharp superior turn. This anatomic variation can make selective catheterization of the left CCA very difficult. Other anomalies of the aortic arch and origins of the brachiocephalic arteries are rare, the most common being anomalous origin of the right subclavian artery. In this instance, there is a separate origin of the right CCA from the aortic arch, and the right subclavian artery is the last brachiocephalic artery with its origin distal to the left subclavian artery. There are racial and gender differences in the origins of the vessels of the aortic arch and tortuosities of the brachiocephalic arteries. In the United States, these differences are most common in black females.

As already mentioned, aging and the atherosclerotic process elongate and distend the aortic arch and shift the ostia of the brachiocephalic arteries. Because the aortic knob becomes more superior and

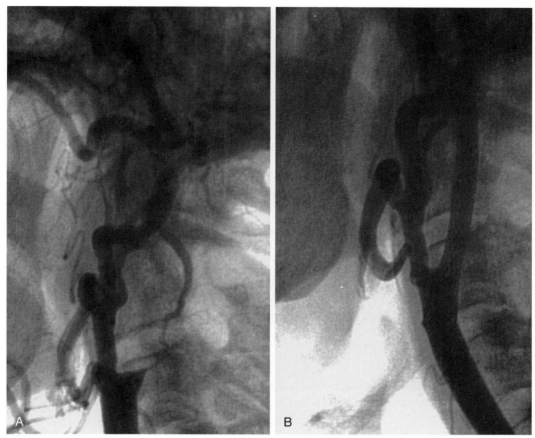

FIGURE 49–6. *A,* "String sign," a long complex restenosis after carotid endarterectomy involving the ICA, CCA, and ECA. Note that the contralateral side has previously been stented. *B,* Angiography after stenting with a 10 × 20 mm Wallstent. Note that the ECA is "jailed," but there is TIMI-3 flow.

posterior to the ostia of the brachiocephalic arteries, it is more difficult to selectively catheterize these vessels and advance the catheter deeper into these arteries. With aging, the brachiocephalic arteries tend to tilt from right to left, which also increases the disadvantageous angulation for selective catheterization. If the origin of the innominate artery is well below the level of aortic knob, the innominate artery is tilted to the left and the proximal right CCA is tortuous, making it almost impossible to selectively advance the catheter deep into the right CCA. With aging and atherosclerotic elongation of the aortic arch, the ostium of the left CCA is displaced posteriorly and the origins of brachiocephalic arteries form a triangle when looking down onto the aortic arch. It is more common to fail to selectively catheterize the right CCA compared with the left CCA.

The bifurcation of the CCAs is usually located at the level of the C3 and C4 vertebral bodies; however, higher or lower bifurcations can occur. Rarely, bifurcations within the upper thoracic or lower cervical levels have been described. In both instances, bifurcation presents a technical problem for CEA. Within the common carotid bifurcation, the origin of the

ICA usually points medially and posteriorly. The origin of the ECA points anteriorly and laterally. For these anatomic reasons, the best projections to separate the origins of the internal and external carotid arteries are lateral oblique and pure lateral projections. Occasionally, the bifurcation is congenitally overrotated: that is, if lateral-projection internal and external carotid arteries are superimposed. In this arrangement, the best projection to separate internal and external carotid arteries is straight AP or the contralateral oblique projections.

The ECA supplies the facial and meningeal structures. It can also become an important source of collateral blood supply to the brain if the ICA is occluded (by the ophthalmic artery or s.c. rete mirabile). ECA–to–vertebral artery steal is not uncommon in the stenosis or occlusion of the proximal subclavian artery.

The ICA can have kinks, coils, and tortuosities. Coils and tortuosities are congenital; kinks are related to the aging process. However, all three are exaggerated by the aging process, atherosclerosis, and shortening of the cervical spine. Kinks can turn into significant stenotic lesions with hyaline wall degeneration. All these conditions are prone to pro-

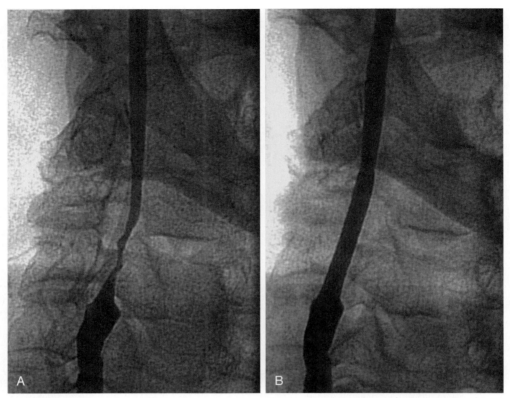

FIGURE 49–7. *A*, Postcarotid endarterectomy. The ICA has a critical restenosis. The ECA is occluded. *B*, Angiography after stenting with a 10 × 20 mm Wallstent.

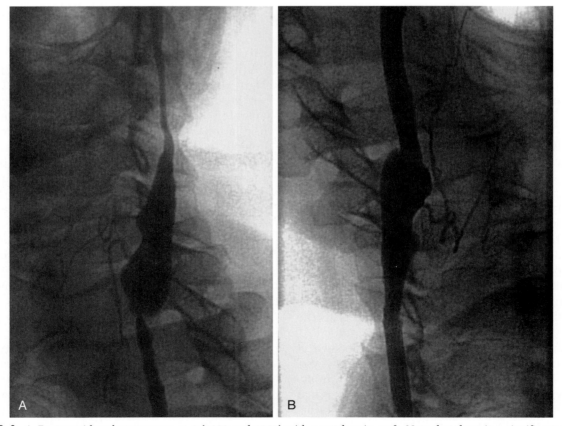

FIGURE 49–8. *A*, Postcarotid endarterectomy × 2 (1993 and 1997) with a patch vein graft. Note that there is a significant stenosis in the distal CCA as well as a long tight stenosis in the ICA. *B*, Postcarotid stenting angiogram reveals that the lesions are obliterated.

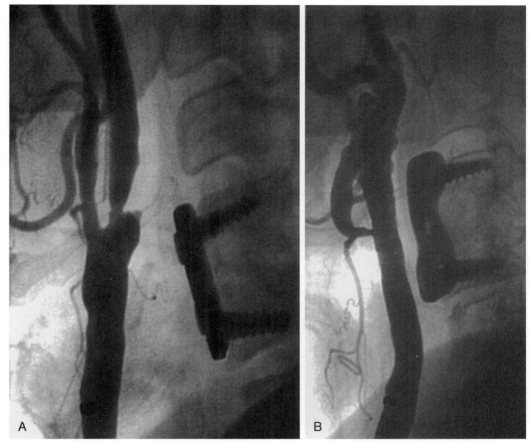

FIGURE 49–9. *A*, Prior cervical spine surgery. Note the vertebral body prosthesis. There is a short discrete stenosis in the proximal portion of the ICA. *B*, Postcarotid stenting angiogram. Note the vertebral body prosthesis. The patient is at high risk for needing intubation during general anesthesia.

duce spasm from guide wire or catheter manipulation. The cervical segment of the ICA does not have any branches. With rare exceptions, the occipital or ascending pharyngeal artery can originate from this artery (and extremely rarely the hypoglossal and proatlantal arteries). The cervical segment of the ICA may develop fibromuscular dysplasia. This is a rare condition seen more in females and is ex-

tremely prone to vascular spasm. The cavernous segment of the ICA can be straight or very tortuous. Rarely, the primitive trigeminal artery originates at this level, supplying the upper third of the basilar artery.

The intracranial segment of the ICA is divided into the clinoid and supraclinoid segments. The ophthalmic artery is the first intracranial branch of the ICA from within the clinoid segment. The posterior communicating and anterior choroidal arteries originate more distally. The posterior communicating artery can be absent or developed to a degree that it may exclusively supply the posterior cerebral artery. The supraclinoid segment terminates in the bifurcation, where the ICA divides into smaller anterior and larger middle cerebral arteries. The horizontal segments of the anterior cerebral arteries (A1 segments) can communicate across the midline through the anterior communicating artery. The horizontal segment of the middle cerebral artery (M1 segment) terminates within the trifurcation in the proximal sylvian fissure. Distal branches of the middle cerebral artery are the ascending frontoparietal artery, parietal artery, and anterior temporal ar-

### TABLE 49–12. PATIENTS AT LOW RISK FOR CAROTID STENTING

Clinical
    Younger (<80 years)
    No recent prior stroke
    Neurologically intact
    Asymptomatic
    No severe peripheral vascular disease
Anatomic
    Straight, noncalcified, "smooth arch vessels"
    No common carotid disease
    Less severe stenosis
    No thrombus
    Short lesions
    No severe kinks or bends at lesion site
    Nontortuous bifurcation
    Prior ipsilateral carotid endarterectomy

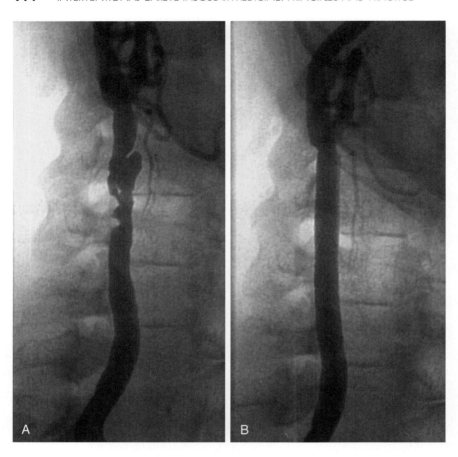

FIGURE 49–10. *A,* Long, severe, and ulcerated mid-CCA stenosis. Note that the carotid bifurcation is normal. *B,* Postcarotid stenting angiogram showing complete elimination of the lesion.

tery. The lenticulostriate arteries whose terminal branches supply anterior basal ganglions originate from the M1 segment of the middle cerebral artery.

The most important collateral pathways are through the anterior and posterior communicating arteries. These with anterior, middle, posterior cerebral, and basilar arteries form the circle of Willis. This collateral channel can readily compensate for occluded internal carotid or vertebral arteries. The circle of Willis is not always developed in all people. Both anterior and posterior communicating arteries can be hypoplastic or absent. The hemispheric blood supply can be completely isolated and can depend only on the ipsilateral ICA in this situation. Even a short, temporary occlusion of this ICA can result in significant consequences. Another, but somewhat less important, brain collateral supply is through the leptomeninges. The small branches of the anterior, middle, and posterior cerebral arteries are connected within pia mater and can supply peripheral branches of these vessels through retrograde flow. This collateral system unfortunately functions much better in early life than in advanced age. The collateral brain supply through the external carotid artery has been previously mentioned.

### Techniques

The most important aspect in determining the success of catheterization of brachiocephalic arteries is the shape of the catheter.[6, 7] The shape of the VTK catheter we use was described in the section "Four-Vessel Cerebral Angiography." The catheter is placed in the junction of the aortic arch and upper thoracic aorta with its tip pointing to the left. By the advancement of the catheter into the aortic arch, the catheter reshapes and attains its double curve with the tip pointing cephalad. In most instances, the tip of the catheter first enters the left subclavian artery. If the catheter does not reshape, folds, or twists to the right, the guide wire is used to reposition the catheter. The guide wire can be also used to "stiffen" the catheter. The guide wire should not be advanced beyond the distal tip of the catheter as this may prevent the tip of the catheter from entering into the vessel ostium and disturb and distend the preshaped catheter curve. After the catheter is placed within the proximal subclavian artery, this vessel is studied angiographically. It is essential to carefully aspirate the catheter every time the Glide Wire is removed in order to withdraw blood from the catheter to prevent air embolism. A hand injection is performed using a 6-mL control syringe with the speed of injection adjusted so that the catheter is not ejected from the subclavian artery. This angiogram shows the origin of the left vertebral artery. The 0.038-inch Glide Wire with an angled tip is then used to enter the left vertebral artery. The wire should always enter the artery first, followed by the catheter. To change the direction in which the guide wire is advanced, the catheter can be rotated, pushed forward, or slightly retracted. These movements with rotation of the angled guide wire give innumerable possibilities to change the direction and angulation in advancing the Glide Wire (road mapping is useful). Once the guide wire enters the vertebral artery, the catheter is slipped cephalad over the Glide Wire. Holding the wire while advancing the catheter performs this. When the wire starts to slip proximally, it is advanced cephalad. Advancement of the catheter (pushing the catheter over the guide wire) is done slowly while taking advantage of pulsating blood flow. This maneuver is performed several times until the moment when the catheter is securely placed in the vertebral artery. If there is tortuosity of the proximal vertebral artery, it often straightens with the guide wire. The same technique of placing the wire in the desired vessel: that is, slowly advancing the catheter over the wire, advancing the wire deeper into the vessel if it slips proximally, is used to catheterize both the CCA and the right vertebral artery. After the catheter enters the desired artery, slow hand injection is done to confirm the position of the catheter, to make sure that good blood flow is maintained and that there is no subintimal entry of the contrast agent. Then the intracranial vasculature is studied angiographically. Injections of contrast agent into all brachiocephalic arteries should be done by hand and with small amounts of contrast material (no more then 6 mL/injection). (Larger volumes create a mixture of arterial, intermediate, and venous faces, thus obscuring arteries with early-filling veins and other abnormalities.)

After completion of the vertebral artery angiogram, the catheter is withdrawn into the proximal subclavian artery, but not into the aortic arch. Keeping the catheter in the subclavian artery reforms the shape of the catheter. At this point, the catheter is gently advanced forward up to the moment when it slips into the ostium of the left CCA. Slow injections of contrast agent can be used to confirm the catheter position. The same technique is used to find an anomalous origin of the left vertebral artery from the aortic arch (8% to 10%). In distended and elongated aortic arches, the origin of the left CCA migrates posteriorly. In this case, the catheter can be rotated so that the tip of the catheter is located more posteriorly. All these maneuvers are performed using a straight AP projection. Once the origin of the left CCA is found, the same technique as described for catheterizing the left vertebral artery is employed. The trick is to advance the catheter slowly over the Glide Wire while maintaining the wire deep inside the carotid artery. The left wall of the upper thoracic

aorta can be used to support advancement of the catheter into the carotid artery. Learning to recognize "good" and "bad" curves of the catheter that form within the aortic arch while the catheter is being advanced into the CCA is important. If the wire is deep in the carotid artery, the catheter can also be rotated while being advanced to straighten out a "bad" curve. Whether clockwise or counterclockwise rotation is used depends on the curve formation in the aortic arch.

After angiography of the left CCA has been completed, the catheter is withdrawn proximally, so the tip is still in the left CCA and the curve of the catheter has reformed. Then the catheter is advanced up to the point where it enters into the innominate artery. Again, a small injection of contrast agent confirms the position. The same technique as described in catheterizing the left vertebral artery and left CCA is used to selectively catheterize the right CCA, right subclavian artery, and right vertebral artery. All four brachiocephalic arteries are usually catheterized with the one catheter. It is the exception to have to change the VTK catheter for one with a different distal curve.

## Carotid Sheath Placement

Once the diagnostic study is completed and the stenotic internal carotid artery is identified, the 5-French catheter is advanced, using the 0.038-inch Glide Wire, into the ipsilateral ECA. The Glide Wire is then withdrawn and replaced with an extra-stiff 0.038-inch exchange-length Amplatz wire. The 7-French 90-cm Shuttle sheath is then advanced into the CCA over the Amplatz wire (Fig. 49–11). The sheath is thin walled and kink and pressure resistant with good flexibility. The radiopaque band is incorporated into the distal end for accurate positioning. The proximal end of the sheath has an open-ended Tuohy-Borst manual-adjusting valve seal that permits unimpeded catheter or guide wire introduction. The side arm attachment allows intermittent or continuous flushing and contrast injection as well as continuous intra-arterial BP monitoring. The sheath (sheath OD, 3 mm [9-French]) can also be used as a reference diameter for measuring the diameter of the ICA and CCA (quantitative carotid angiography [QCA]). The sheath accepts 7-French OD devices.

If the four-vessel diagnostic cerebral angiography has previously been performed and the target lesion identified before the procedure, the 7-French 90-cm sheath is advanced over a guide wire into the upper thoracic aorta immediately after femoral puncture. After withdrawing the inner dilator from the sheath and carefully flushing the sheath and administering heparin, the operator introduces the 125-cm 5-

*Text continued on page 920*

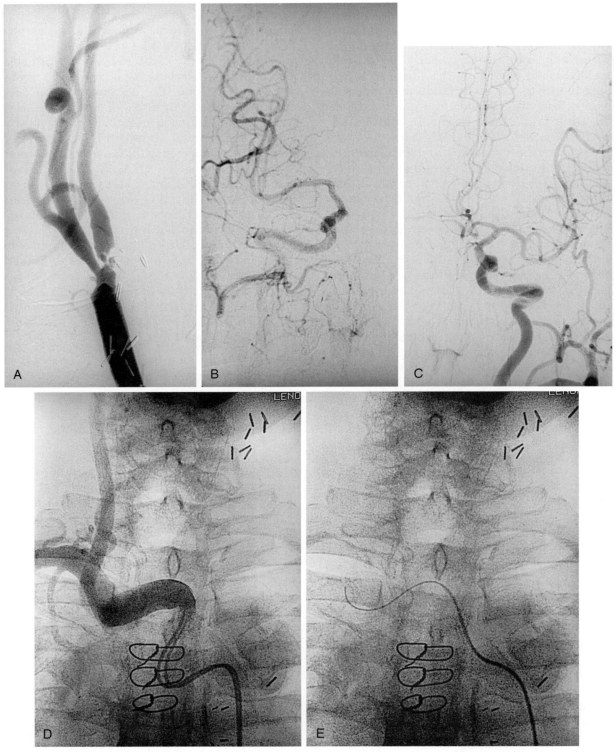

FIGURE 49–11. *A*, Critical ulcerated lesion involving the origin of the right ICA and carotid bifurcation. *B*, Digital subtracted intracranial angiogram demonstrates poor filling of the distal ICA and middle cerebral artery (MCA) and absent flow into the anterior cerebral artery (ACA). *C*, Injection into the left CCA shows filling of the right ICA (ACA and MCA). This confirms the critical nature of the left ICA stenosis and provides important information about collateral supply via the circle of Willis. *D*, Injection into the origin of the tortuous innominate artery and proximal right CCA. Note the correct positioning of the VTK 5-French diagnostic catheter (anteroposterior projection). *E*, A 0.038-inch angle-tipped Glide Wire is advanced into the right CCA.

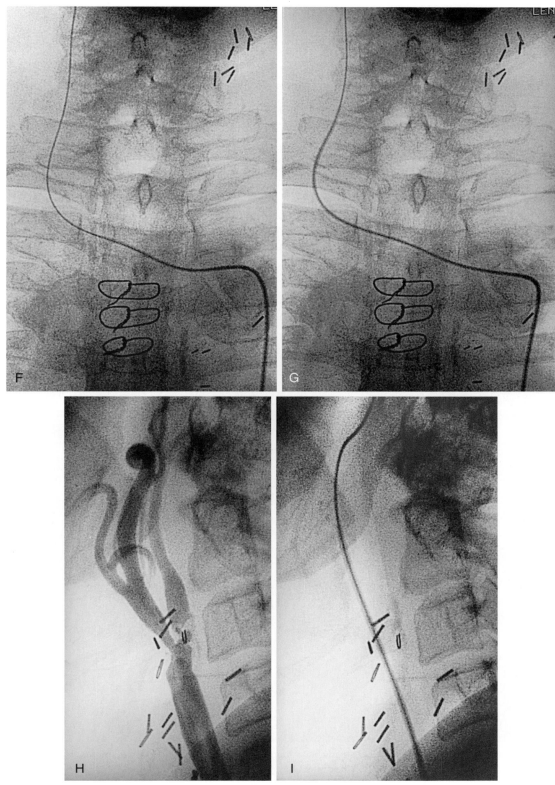

FIGURE 49–11 *Continued.* *F,* The wire is advanced to just below the carotid bifurcation, and a slow, gentle, push-pull maneuver is used to move the 5-French diagnostic catheter into the CCA. *G,* The 5-French diagnostic catheter "slips" up into the CCA with the use of a push-pull technique (anteroposterior projection). A deep breath from the patient and time allow the catheter to slowly "slide" up the artery with each arterial pulsation. *H,* A "road map" or "freeze frame" angiogram is taken to show the origin of the ECA (lateral projection). *I,* The 0.038-inch angle-tipped Glide Wire is advanced into the ECA, and the 5-French diagnostic catheter follows (lateral projection). The Glide Wire is then removed for placement of a 0.038-inch Amplatz wire.

*Illustration continued on following page*

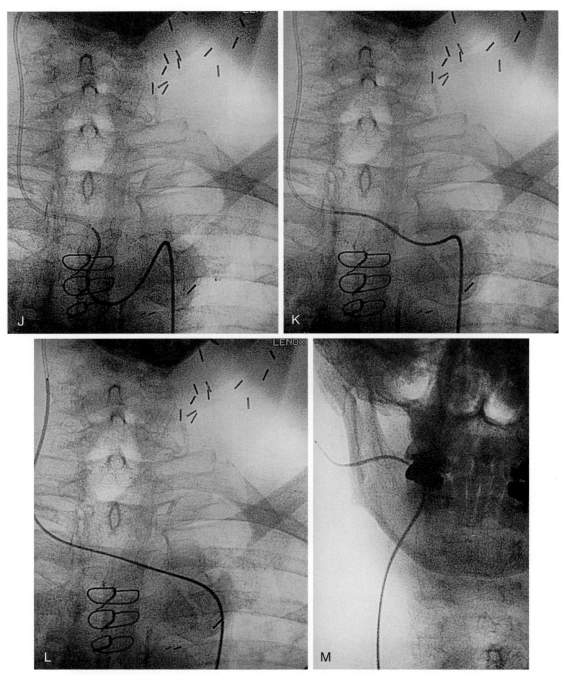

FIGURE 49–11 *Continued. J,* As the Amplatz wire is advanced, a loop has formed in the aortic arch (anteroposterior projection). *K,* To prevent the Amplatz wire from prolapsing the 5-French catheter out of the ECA, gentle "pulling" of the diagnostic catheter straightens out the loop. *L,* The Amplatz wire now easily advances through the VTK 5-French catheter up into the ECA (anteroposterior projection). *M,* The tip of the Amplatz wire is in the distal ECA, and the 5-French VTK catheter has been removed (anteroposterior projection).

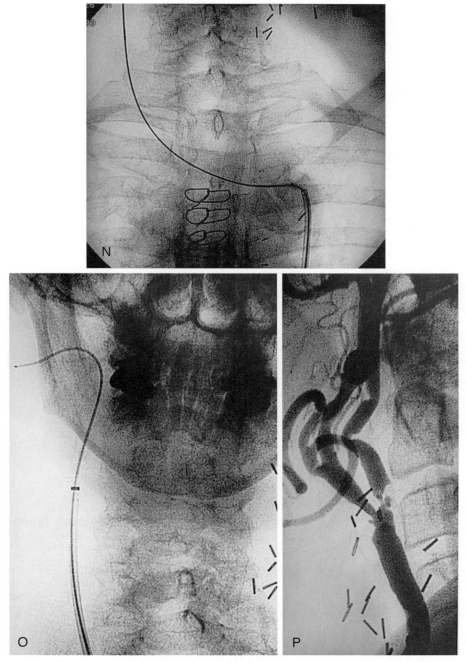

FIGURE 49–11 *Continued. N,* The 7-French Cook 90-cm Shuttle sheath with introducer is advanced slowly over the Amplatz wire to the CCA. Note how the Amplatz wire straightens the innominate artery and provides support for the sheath. *O,* The sheath is advanced to a position just below the bifurcation. It is important not to allow the sheath to "snowplow" into the diseased bifurcation. Once in position, the Amplatz wire and sheath introducer are removed. The operator should hold back on the sheath at this time to prevent the tendency for it to move cephalad into the bifurcation. The operator should allow the sheath to back bleed, flush carefully, and administer heparin to the patient. *P,* A careful guiding angiogram is now obtained to define the lesion anatomy. Note that the straightening effect of the sheath in the CCA has accentuated the distal kinks in the ICA (lateral projection).

*Illustration continued on following page*

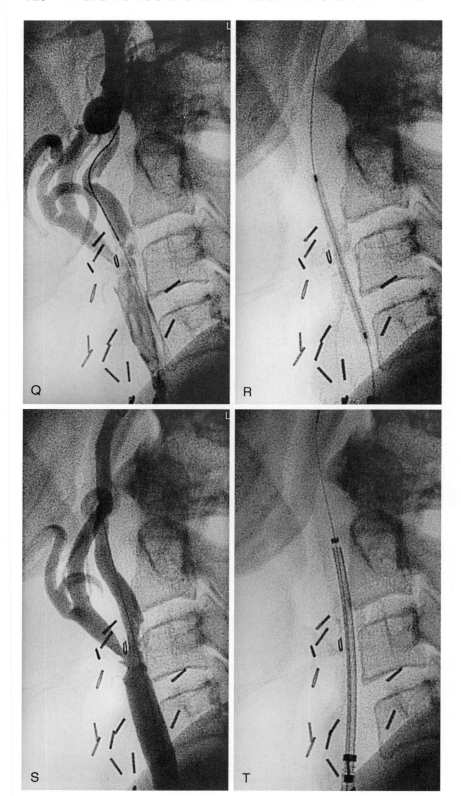

FIGURE 49–11 *Continued. Q,* A soft 0.014-inch coronary guide wire is carefully advanced through the lesion. *R,* The lesion is first dilated with a 2-mm balloon followed by a 4 × 40 mm, 0.018-in wire–compatible coronary balloon. *S,* The 0.014-inch wire is replaced with a more supportive 0.018-inch Roadrunner wire through the wire lumen of the coronary balloon. The 0.018-inch wire is shown in the dilated lesion. *T,* A 10 × 20 mm non-reconstrainable Wallstent is advanced over the 0.018-inch wire (lateral projection). The distal end of the stent is positioned 5 to 10 mm distal to the lesion using bony landmarks and lesion calcification as a guide.

French VTK catheter into the 7-French sheath. Care must be taken not to advance the 7-French sheath too close to the aortic arch as this may decrease the maneuverability of the 5-French catheter. Then the appropriate CCA is catheterized. The tip of the catheter is advanced over the appropriate guide wire (either 0.038-inch Glide Wire or extra stiff 0.038-inch Amplatz wire, depending on the arch extension and tortuosity of the carotid artery), into the ECA. Road mapping can be very useful in identi-

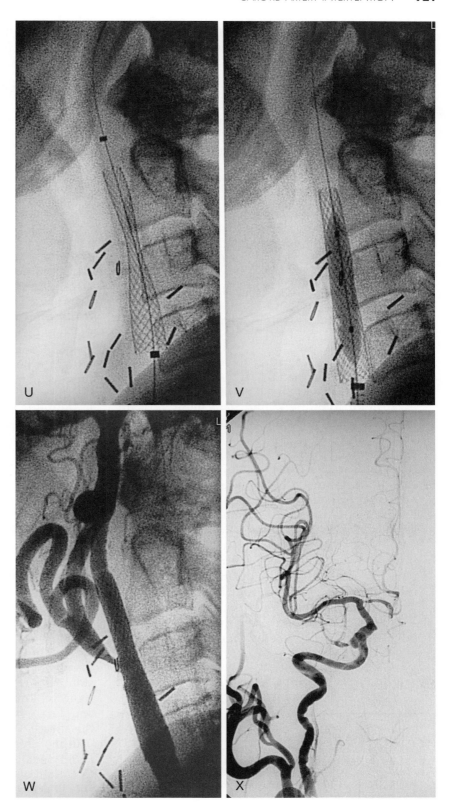

FIGURE 49–11 *Continued. U,* Note that the Wallstent is constrained in the 5-mm ICA, leaving a small stent pore size that excludes plaque from the bloodstream. The stent expands fully across the bifurcation reaching 8 to 10 mm in the CCA. The effective stent length is approximately 30 mm. *V,* The stent is carefully postdilated using a low-profile 5 × 20 mm balloon. *W,* Final angiography shows some mild distal spasm of the ICA and some compromise of the ECA. The ECA has good flow and requires no further intervention. *X,* Poststent intracranial angiograms show good filling of the right MCA and ACA.

fying the ECA. The 7-French sheath is slipped over the VTK catheter into the CCA and positioned just below the stenosis. If the pelvic arteries and pelvic abdominal aorta are tortuous, first the appropriate 5-French catheter is placed in the upper thoracic aorta, and using the 0.038-inch stiff Amplatz exchange wire, the 7-French sheath is advanced into the upper thoracic aorta. There are slight modifications of this technique, especially if the stenosis is located in mid or distal segments of the CCA. Of note, when placing the 7-French sheath in the CCA, particularly if it is tortuous, the vessel may be displaced upward, and kinks can be created in the ICA. These usually disappear once the sheath is withdrawn.

### Troubleshooting for Difficult Carotid Access

With experience, 95% of bifurcations can be accessed using the VTK catheter–0.038-inch Glide Wire system. However, severely tortuous and calcified arteries may be difficult to access using our standard approach. We have developed alternative strategies in those arteries in which the Glide Wire will not advance without prolapsing the VTK out of the artery (Table 49–13). If the CCA is diffusely atherosclerotic along its course, it may be prudent to refer the patient for surgery because the excessive manipulation may produce embolic complications. If not, we have found the following techniques successful:

1. Use a Simmons-3 catheter to advance the Glide Wire distally into the ECA. If the 0.038-inch wire will not advance, try a 0.035-inch wire. In either case, rapid torquing of the wire helps forward movement. A 0.035-inch movable core wire is also often useful.
2. Remove the Simmons catheter. This may pull the wire out if it is not very distal in the ECA.
3. Advance a 4-French multipurpose Slip Catheter or similar catheter distally into the ECA.
4. Exchange the Glide Wire or movable core wire for a 0.035-inch Amplatz wire (a 0.038-inch wire will "pull" the 4-French catheter out). Sometimes it is prudent to use a less stiff 0.035-inch wire, for example, Supra Core. The 4-French catheter is then exchanged for a 5-French catheter, for example, multipurpose, vertebral, or H$_1$. The 0.035-inch wire can now be replaced with a 0.038-inch Amplatz wire that is finally posi-

### TABLE 49–13.   WIRES AND CATHETERS FOR DIFFICULT ACCESS

Wires
    0.035-in. Glide Wire (Boston Scientific Corp.; Watertown MA)
    0.035-in. Movable core guide wire (Medtronic; Danvers MA)
    0.035-in. Supra Core (Guidant; Temecula CA)
    0.038-in. Glide Wire (Boston Scientific Corp.; Watertown MA)
    0.038-in. Amplatz (Cook Inc.; Bloomington IN)
    0.035-in. Amplatz (Cook Inc.; Bloomington IN)
    0.018-in. Roadrunner (Cook Inc.; Bloomington IN)
Catheters
    5-Fr VTK Torocon Advantage (Cook Inc.; Bloomington IN)
    5-Fr Simmons-3 (Cook Inc.; Bloomington IN)
    4-Fr SlipCath (Cook Inc.; Bloomington IN)
    5-Fr Glide Cath (Terumo Inc., Scimed Inc.; Maple Grove MN)
    5-Fr Berenstein (Angiodynamics Inc.; Queensbury NY)
    5-Fr 125-cm MP (Cook Inc.; Bloomington IN)

tioned in the distal ECA ready for access sheath insertion. In these cases, put the introducer back into the access sheath to transition the curves over the 0.038-inch Amplatz wire. If necessary, before removing the introducer, replace the Amplatz wire with a 0.018-inch Roadrunner wire to give extra support to the sheath. Note that deep breaths may help to straighten out the great vessels during each maneuver. Another tip is to gently ease back on the catheter curve in the arch as you attempt to advance successive wires. This reduces the curve in the arch and prevents the successively stiffer wires from prolapsing the catheter back into the ascending aorta.

### Carotid Access in the Presence of an Occluded External Carotid Artery; Common Carotid Artery Lesions Below the Bifurcation; Ostial Common Carotid Artery Lesions; Ostial Innominate Artery Lesions

Placing the access sheath into the CCA may present special challenges when the ECA is occluded, a critical lesion is situated below the bifurcation, or there is a critical ostial CCA lesion.

In these situations, we try to avoid crossing the lesion with a stiff 0.038-inch wire as this may disrupt the necrotic plaque material and cause distal embolization.

If possible, we advance the VTK catheter over the 0.038-inch Glide Wire in the usual fashion. The tip of the Glide Wire is carefully kept proximal so as not to cross the lesion. The Glide Wire is then exchanged for a 0.038-inch extra-stiff Amplatz wire. If necessary, we shape a pigtail curve to the tip of the wire. The sheath is then advanced without having to cross the lesion. If the proximal CCA is very tortuous or angulated and more support is required, the Amplatz wire may have to be placed more distally. In this situation, the Glide Wire and 5-French catheter are first advanced through the lesion. This maneuver should be performed only in patients considered to be at high risk from carotid surgery, and for whom the risk/benefit ratio remains in favor of stenting. Alternately, a 6- or 7-French diagnostic right Judkins catheter can be advanced over the Amplatz wire to give more transitional support to the sheath.

In the presence of a common carotid ostial lesion or an ostial innominate artery lesion (Fig. 49–12), the origin of the CCA should be first dilated to allow sheath access. The ICA bifurcation lesion should be stented first, and then the ostium of the CCA stented, usually with a balloon expandable stent on the way out.

### Predilatation of the Lesion

Heparin, usually 5000 to 6000 U, is given through the sheath to raise the ACT to approximately 200

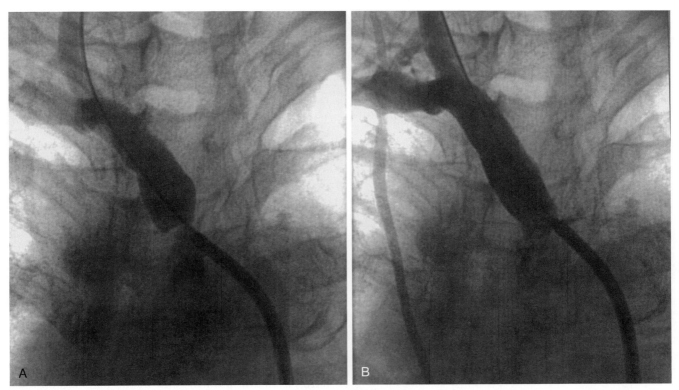

FIGURE 49–12. *A,* Short discrete stenosis at the origin of the innominate artery. *B,* Angiography after stenting with a P154 Palmaz stent.

to 250 seconds (Hemotec method). Arteriography through the sheath, in the appropriate angulation, is performed to maximize the angulation of the bifurcation and severity of the stenosis. QCA is performed in this projection to measure the diameter of the CCAs and the percentage diameter stenosis. Then the optimal angulation in which to perform the intervention is identified. This projection is not necessarily the one that demonstrates the maximal stenosis severity but one that ideally separates the internal and external carotid arteries and identifies bony landmarks. The stenotic lesion is crossed with a steerable 0.014-inch coronary guide wire. Selection of the wire depends on the severity, location, length, angulation, and eccentricity of the stenosis and on the anatomy of the bifurcation. The tip of the 0.014-inch wire is shaped appropriately to match the angle of the origin of the ICA. After crossing the stenosis, the tip of the wire is placed close to the base of the skull. If the ICA has kinks, coils, or tortuosities, the wire is passed distal to the stenosis, again to the level of the base of the skull. For predilation of the stenosis, we routinely use a Cobra-18 4 × 40 mm coronary balloon. The long length of this balloon has the advantage of preventing the balloon from slipping during the inflation. If the stenosis is preocclusive or the artery is occluded, we first predilate with a 2 × 40 mm coronary balloon. After this first predilation, a second dilation using a 4-mm balloon is performed. Usually, 4-mm

balloon predilation is sufficient to pass the stent smoothly, without encountering major resistance through the stenosis. After predilation, the Cobra-18 balloon catheter is advanced distally into the ICA and the 0.014-inch wire is changed for a 0.018-inch stiffer exchange-length wire such as a Roadrunner. Again, the position of the tip of the 0.018-inch wire is very important. It should be placed close to the base of the skull and certainly must be advanced through all kinks and tortuosities in the ICA while not allowing it to pass intracranially. It is easier to advance the stent over the stiffer and larger-diameter wire, which straightens the ICA, facilitating the delivery and deployment of the stent. Maintaining the position of this wire will enable deployment of another stent if a distal dissection develops. The nitinol tip of the Roadrunner wire is ideal: radiopaque, soft, flexible, and nontraumatic to the carotid siphon. In nontortuous ICAs when the newer low-profile delivery systems are used, extra-support 0.014-inch coronary wires (Platinum-Plus, Iron Man) can also be used as an alternative to a 0.018-inch wire. Very rarely, usually in heavily calcified lesions, the stent will not pass through the stenosis after predilation with the 4-mm balloon. In this situation, a 5-mm balloon should be used for predilation; a stent should never be forced across a stenosis. In our experience, predilation with a coronary balloon is rarely, if ever, associated with significant embolus release. It is necessary, however, to use a balloon that rewraps efficiently without residual wings and to allow full deflation before carefully withdrawing the balloon. Primary stenting without predilation is not recommended because it is our impression that later postdilation of the constricted stent is associated with more "scissoring" of the stent wires on plaque and subsequent distal embolization.

## Stent Deployment

In our early experience, we worked with balloon-expandable stents. This practice has now been abandoned with three exceptions: (1) the ostium of the common carotid artery is treated and the proximal end of the stent has to be placed with precision, (2) the lesion is in the distal segment of the ICA (present delivery systems for self-expanding stents cause dissections in the petrous portion of the ICA), and (3) the self-expanding stent delivery system will not pass through a calcified, "recoiling" lesion. Forcing the current high-profile delivery systems may break off plaque and cause distal embolization. In this situation, a short Palmaz (P104) stent or AVE-Medtronic (5-mm) stent is placed to hold the lesion open before passing a definitive self-expanding stent.

The balloon-expandable stent has several disadvantages when deployed within the carotid bifurcation. First, more then one stent is often required. Second, the stent has to be differentially expanded to accommodate to the different sizes of the ICA, bifurcation, and CCA; thus, more than one balloon is required for appropriate stent expansion. Third, the balloon can rupture while deploying the stent. Fourth, there may be difficulties in advancing the balloon-stent assembly (especially a 20-mm stent) through the guiding sheath if the aortic arch is distended or the proximal CCA is tortuous. Finally, balloon-expandable stents tend to occlude the ECA. It is our impression that more soft plaque may extrude through the stent struts of balloon-expandable stents.

In the last 500 patients, we have almost exclusively used self-expanding stents (Wallstent). These stents have several advantages. First, only one stent is usually required. Second, they are easily deployed using vertebral bodies as landmarks (the distal end of the stent can be deployed from within the healthy part of the ICA distal to the stenosis while the proximal end of the stent will end up across the bifurcation and in the CCA). The unconstrained diameter of the self-expanding stent to be deployed should be at least 1 to 2 mm larger than the largest vessel segment to be covered by the stent. Usually, we use 10 × 20 mm stents based on the fact that the surface area of artery covered by the stent is greater than in a smaller-diameter stent, which may

reduce the size of emboli that may be "sliced off" during the postdilation. Although the ICA is commonly 2 to 3 mm smaller then the CCA, angiographic follow-up studies have shown that oversizing the stent in the ICA does increase restenosis rates.[35] Most recently, we have gained experience with the nonshortening nitinol self-expanding stents (Memotherm, Smart Stent). These devices are ideal for lesions that do not involve the carotid bifurcation. They can be precisely placed using the distal and proximal markers. An important technical point is to release 3 to 5 mm of stent distally and wait for the stent to expand fully and stabilize against the wall before slight proximal retraction and release of the remainder of the stent. Longer nitinol stents can be deployed completely in the ICA with suitable 6- and 8-mm diameters. If the stent is to be deployed across the bifurcation, 8- to 10-mm stents should be utilized.

## Postdilatation

The self-expandable stent is postdilated with either 5 or 5.5 × 20 mm balloons (over the 0.018-inch wire), depending on the size of the ICA. We believe that it is safer to underdilate than overdilate. Overdilation may squeeze the atherosclerotic material through the stent mesh and cause emboli. A 10% to 15% residual stenosis has not been shown to cause any problems. Importantly, it is not necessary to overexpand the stent to produce a 0% residual diameter narrowing. Furthermore, it is not necessary to dilate the stent to obliterate segments of contrast-filled ulcerated areas external to the stent. This angiographic appearance after stenting is of no prognostic significance, and follow-up angiography has documented complete healing of these "pockets" over time. Covering the ECA with a stent may cause some "jailing" of the ECA. However, on follow-up arteriograms, the ECA is usually seen to remain patent with only rare exceptions. If the ECA becomes preocclusive and there is less than Thrombosis In Myocardial Infarction (TIMI)-3 flow or it is completely occluded after postdilation of the stent, this vessel can be accessed through the stent mesh with a 0.014-inch wire and reopened with a 2- to 4-mm coronary balloon. The equipment used and the 10 steps to CAS are outlined in Tables 49–14 and 49–15.

## Procedural Monitoring

All carotid angiograms and interventions are performed under only local anesthesia so that the neurologic status of the patient can be continuously monitored. A "squeeze toy" is placed in the contralateral hand to monitor upper extremity motor functions after each step in the procedure. In addition,

## TABLE 49–14. EQUIPMENT REQUIRED FOR CAROTID STENTING

| EQUIPMENT | DIAMETER | LENGTH | COMPANY, LOCATION |
|---|---|---|---|
| VTK Torocon Advantage (catheter) | 5-Fr | 100, 125 cm | Cook, Inc.; Bloomington IN |
| Glide Wire, angled tip (wire) | 0.038 in. | 190, 260 cm | Meditech; Boston MA |
| Amplatz wire, extra stiff (wire) | 0.038 in. | 180, 260 cm | Cook, Inc.; Bloomington IN |
| Balance (wire) | 0.014 in. | 190, 260 cm | Guidant, Inc.; Temecula CA |
| Platinum-Plus (wire) | 0.014 in. | 190, 260 cm | Scimed, Inc.; Maple Grove MN |
| Iron Man (wire) | 0.014 in. | 190, 260 cm | Guidant, Inc.; Temecula CA |
| Roadrunner (wire) | 0.018 in. | 190, 260 cm | Cook, Inc.; Bloomington IN |
| Shuttle Sheath (catheter) | 6-Fr, 7-Fr | 90 cm | Cook, Inc.; Bloomington IN |
| Ranger (balloon) | 2 mm | 4 cm | Scimed, Inc.; Maple Grove MN |
| Cobra-18 (balloon) | 4 mm | 4 cm | Scimed, Inc.; Maple Grove MN |
| Wallstent* (stent) | 10 mm | 20 mm | Boston Scientific Corp.; Watertown MA |
| Smart Stent (stent) | 10 mm | 20–40 mm | Cordis Endovascular; Warren NJ |
| Memotherm (stent) | 8–10 mm | 20–40 mm | CR Bard, Inc.; Murray Hill NJ |
| Endotex (stent) | 10 mm | 20 mm | Endotex Interventional Systems, Inc.; Cupertino CA |
| Savvy (balloon) | 5–5.5 mm | 20 mm | Cordis Endovascular; Warren NJ |
| Symmetry (balloon) | 5–5.5 mm | 20 mm | Meditech; Natick MA |
| Jupiter (balloon) | 5–5.5 mm | 20 mm | Cordis Endovascular; Warren NJ |
| Mega-Titan (balloon) | 5–5.5 mm | 20 mm | Cordis Endovascular; Warren NJ |

*Avoid reconstrainable sheath system with 7-French sheath—not compatible.

the patients are asked to speak and move the contralateral foot to confirm that they are neurologically intact. Continuous monitoring of the HR and BP throughout the intervention is mandatory. Bradycardia and even asystole are not uncommon, especially when the bulb of the ICA is stretched. When self-expanding stents are used, they always respond to deflation of the balloon. Atropine (0.6 to 1 mg) prophylactically can help. For the rare occurrence, internal heart pacing should be available. If bradycardia persists, atropine is the treatment of choice. Hypotension is managed aggressively with fluid boluses, metaraminol boluses (100 to 200 μg by push

injection), and, if necessary, a dopamine infusion.[36] Loss of consciousness rarely occurs with balloon inflation when the ipsilateral hemispheric blood supply is isolated or if the contralateral carotid artery is occluded. Consciousness is regained spontaneously after immediate deflation of the balloon. Occasionally, spasm can develop, especially after placement of the 0.018-inch wire, with stretching of the artery, or after stent placement. This usually resolves with removal of the wire, intra-arterial administration of nitroglycerin (100 to 200 μg), and retraction of the sheath into the arch (Fig. 49–13).

## CAROTID STENTING: EARLY EXPERIENCE

Our clinical experience with carotid intervention continues to be a work in progress. The neurology, neuroradiology, and interventional cardiology collaboration has resulted in the development of a rigorous protocol with prospective collection of data on our patient population, technical details, and outcomes. Prospective, independent, neurologic evaluation is an important aspect of the protocol, as was institutional ethics review board approval. After reviewing the early radiology experience and discussing options with Robert Ferguson, principal investigator of the North American Carotid Percutaneous Transluminal Angioplasty Registry (NACPTAR), we began our series using 9-French multipurpose guiding catheters and peripheral transluminal angioplasty (PTA) balloons. Elective stenting was not employed in our first five patients. Our experience with the fifth patient changed our subsequent approach. The details of this case are instructive.

The patient was a 55-year-old woman who had

## TABLE 49–15. TEN STEPS TO CAROTID STENTING

| | |
|---|---|
| Step 1 | Place sheath in thoracic aorta. Treat patient with heparin. |
| Step 2 | Cannulate CCA with VTK catheter over Glide Wire. |
| Step 3 | "Road map" to display origin of ECA. |
| Step 4 | Advance Glide Wire into ECA and follow with VTK catheter. |
| Step 5 | Replace Glide Wire with Amplatz wire and advance sheath into CCA to just below bifurcation. |
| Step 6 | Remove Amplatz wire and VTK catheter, "back bleed" and flush carefully, and take "guiding" images of lesion by injecting contrast medium through sheath side arm. |
| Step 7 | Advance Cobra balloon over coronary wire across lesion and dilate slowly and carefully. |
| Step 8 | Replace coronary wire for Roadrunner wire—remove balloon and take a further angiogram to relocate vertebral body landmarks. |
| Step 9 | Advance stent across lesion and deploy by precisely placing distal stent margin. |
| Step 10 | Postdilate conservatively (size and pressure) depending on ICA diameter. |

CCA, common carotid artery; ECA, external carotid artery; ICA, internal carotid artery.

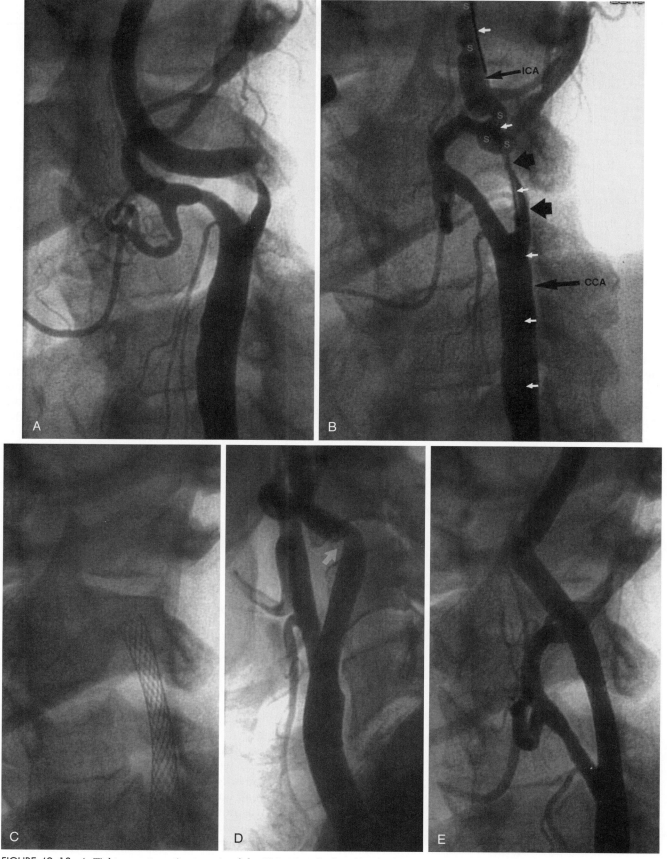

FIGURE 49–13. *A*, Tight symptomatic stenosis of the ICA. Note the bend at the lesion site. *B*, Note the distal spasm and pseudospasm after straightening the ICA with an extra support wire. S, spasm. *C*, A 10 × 20 mm Wallstent. *D*, Angiography after stenting. Note that most of the spasm has resolved after the administration of nitroglycerin. *E*, After retraction of the sheath, the spasm has completely resolved. A distal bend remains.

suffered a previous disabling stroke and had an occluded right ICA. She had recovered a significant degree of function but began having transient ischemic attacks (TIAs) from a long and complex left internal carotid lesion. The length and distal extension of the lesion and associated coronary disease placed her at increased risk from endarterectomy. Long discussion with the patient and her family preceded the written informed consent, and the patient underwent balloon angioplasty of the lesion with good initial angiographic and clinical results. One hour after the procedure, the patient lost consciousness and was urgently returned to the interventional suite. The artery had undergone acute closure. It was recrossed and stented, producing a good angiographic result. The patient, however, had an intracranial hemorrhage after reopening of the artery, did not regain consciousness, and died some days later. The study was suspended for a number of weeks while the investigators considered the options. After consultation with our hospital's institutional review board, it was determined that we should proceed cautiously with the protocol and elective stenting of all lesions. Now with over 600 vessels electively stented, we have observed only one (0.1%) periprocedural stent thrombosis and none in the last 500 procedures.

## Overall Results

### Patient Population

Our series of CAS encompasses a wide variety of patients who may not have been included in randomized trials of CEA.[37–39] In fact, a large percentage of the patients were referred to us because they had a variety of baseline features that put them at higher risk from CEA. In general, they include elderly persons (12.5% ≥80 years) and those with CAD (71%). Their mean age ± SD was 69 ± 10 years. Their ages ranged from 35 years (patients with diffuse fibromuscular dysplasia) to 89 years. Over 70% had hypertension, 67% had a history of smoking, and 32% had diabetes. One third of the patients were female. Fifty-two percent of the population were symptomatic with recent stroke, TIAs, or amaurosis fugax. Forty-eight percent were asymptomatic.

Patients are also referred to us because they have specific anatomic features that place them at increased risk from endarterectomy. The risk factors include contralateral occlusion in 10% (43 patients); prior ipsilateral endarterectomy in 77 vessels (17%); a variety of distal lesions; high bifurcations; common carotid disease; previous radical neck dissection; and radiation treatment.

Over the last 4 years, we challenged this new technique by accepting almost all referrals for carotid stenting. During our first 3 years, only two patients with angiographically evident mobile thrombus at the lesion site were refused an attempt at stenting. All lesion subsets were treated including severely ulcerated or calcified lesions and totally occluded vessels. Similarly, all types of severely diseased aortic arch vessels including tortuous, calcified, atherosclerotic, and stenotic CCAs were accessed in order to complete the procedure.

Indications for carotid stenting were discussed in a previous section. Over our 5-year experience, we have modified our eligibility criteria and now reject approximately 5% of our referrals because we consider that they may be at lower risk from an endarterectomy procedure (see previous list of contraindications to stenting). We now believe strongly that given current technology and taking into account the experience of the operator, careful patient selection is critical in maintaining complication-free results.

### Technical Success

From the outset, we have been able to achieve a technical success rate of greater than 98%. We define this as our ability to access the carotid bifurcation and place a stent producing a less than 30% residual diameter narrowing (NASCET criteria). In our long-term follow up of 528 patients (604 vessels) (September 1994 to September 1999), we have failed in 12 (2%) cases (nine failures to access or deliver a stent; two air embolizations, causing abandonment of the procedure in that session; and one inability to cross a lesion with wire). All these procedures occurred in our early experience. Air embolization occurred when we attempted to use long sheaths with "fixed" hemostasis valves. In our current experience, technical success is 99%.

### Immediate (30-Day) Outcomes and Complications

The total elective stenting experience is shown in Table 49–16. As of September 1999, we had per-

**TABLE 49–16.    IMMEDIATE OUTCOMES AND COMPLICATIONS**

| EVENT | HEMISPHERES (N = 604) NO. (%) | PATIENTS (N = 528) NO. (%) |
|---|---|---|
| Minor nonfatal strokes | 29* (4.8) | 29* (5.5) |
| Major nonfatal strokes | 6 (1.0) | 6 (1.0) |
| Fatal strokes | | 3 (0.6) |
| Nonneurological deaths | | 5 (1.0) |
| Major nonfatal strokes and all deaths | 14 (2.6) | 14 (2.6) |
| All nonfatal strokes and all deaths | 43 (7.4) | 43 (8.1) |

*One retinal artery embolus 2 weeks after the procedure.

formed carotid stenting on 528 patients and 604 vessels in a total of 576 procedures. Seventy-six patients (14%) had bilateral stenting. Of these, 30 were done in the same procedure.

### Deaths

We had a total of four procedural deaths (three neurologic). Of the three neurologic deaths, two were associated with stenting of total occlusions. In the first patient, a cerebral hemorrhage occurred after aggressive balloon dilation and administration of urokinase in attempts to recanalize a residual intracranial stenosis distal to the occlusion. In the other occluded vessel, a posterior communicating artery aneurysm not evident on the suboptimal referral films ruptured after opening the short ICA occlusion and exposing the aneurysm to systemic pressure. The third neurologic death was caused by carotid rupture with a 7-mm balloon in an early misguided attempt to obtain a perfect angiographic result. The perforation was sealed with prolonged balloon inflation and reversal of anticoagulation. The patient subsequently had a nondisabling embolic stroke but died from aspiration pneumonia. The fourth procedure-related death was caused by a retroperitoneal bleed in a patient with severe peripheral vascular disease in whom aggressive cannulation of the iliac vessel was required to gain access to the complex ostial common carotid and critical bifurcation disease.

Four nonneurologic deaths occurred, not immediately after the procedure but within 30 days. Three were cardiac related; the remaining patient died after a peripheral vascular surgical procedure, a week after successful carotid stenting. Given the risk profile and associated comorbidity of the patient cohort, the total 30-day mortality (1.6%) appears very low. No deaths occurred among the next 230 patients treated.

### Major (Disabling) Strokes (30 Days)

There have been only six (1%) disabling strokes in our entire stenting experience associated with procedural distal embolization. The first was in the single case of stent thrombosis. This patient lost consciousness just after leaving the procedure room. Emergent repeat angiography and recanalization of the stent restored patency, but the patient had a residual disabling neurologic deficit due to distal embolic debris. The next patient had an embolic stroke with an increase in the NIH stroke scale greater than 3 at 30 days despite attempts at neurovascular rescue during the procedure. Both these events occurred during our early experience.

The third stroke was secondary to a cardiac arrest and prolonged resuscitation in an elderly woman who went into cardiac arrest during a Rotablator coronary procedure 5 days after carotid stenting. The fourth stroke was due to an embolus in a woman with severe lung disease with failure to deliver a stent due to severe tortuosity. The fifth stroke was embolic during postdilation. There was one major contralateral stroke due to an embolus from a prosthetic mitral valve in a patient with atrial fibrillation; it was not procedure related.

### Minor (Nondisabling) Strokes (30 Days)

There have been a total of 29 (4.8%) nondisabling strokes. A nondisabling stroke was defined as any neurologic deficit (detected after a protocol physical examination by a board-certified neurologist) that persisted for more than 24 hours but resolved by 30 days. These events included neurologic abnormalities such as left upper extremity drift lasting 72 hours; mild aphasia; partial hemianopia; mild left hand weakness; left hand numbness, and receptive dysphasia. They also include nonhemispheric emboli such as a retinal artery occlusion. It is important to note that few CEA patient cohorts have been subjected to this level of early postprocedural scrutiny. Certainly, these events would not have been recorded as stroke events in the NASCET or ACAS studies, in which detailed independent neurologic examination was delayed until 30 days.

### Learning Curve and Current Experience

As in coronary stenting, there is a learning curve of the technique of CAS. Table 49–17 shows the results of our series annualized over the last 5 years of experience. The overall incidence of procedure-related major neurologic complications has been low throughout the experience. The majority of these complications were isolated events directly related to practical technical decision making based on the nondedicated equipment availability and our naiveté concerning patient selection factors. We have learned that these problems can be avoided using the meticulous technique described in this chapter. This has contributed to a progressive fall in minor neurologic events (Table 49–17) as the team's experience has increased. The most recent results of our team are shown in Table 49–18. This represents 407 consecutive patients (443 vessels) with an overall total stroke and death rate of 4.4%.

### Analysis of High- and Low-Risk Subsets

Over the last 4 years, we have repeatedly analyzed our outcomes to examine the risk of complications in a variety of patient subsets (Table 49–19). The results have provided guidance to patient selection, but these results may be confounded by improved

**TABLE 49–17.    PROGRESSION OF EXPERIENCE**

| | NO. | | | | |
|---|---|---|---|---|---|
| | 9/94–9/95 | 9/95–9/96 | 9/96–9/97 | 9/97–9/98 | 9/98–9/99 |
| Patients | 86 | 96 | 118 | 83 | 145 |
| Vessels/hemispheres | 99 | 120 | 131 | 93 | 161 |
| Minor nonfatal strokes | 7 (7.1%) | 7 (5.8%) | 7 (5.3%) | 3* (3.2%) | 5 (3.1%) |
| Major nonfatal strokes | 1 (1%) | 2 (1.7%) | 1 (0.8%) | 0 | 2 (1.2%) |
| Fatal strokes | 0 | 0 | 3 (2.5%) | 0 | 0 |
| Nonneurologic deaths | 1 (1.2%) | 0 | 4 (3.9%) | 0 | 0 |
| All nonfatal strokes/ deaths | 9 (9.3%) | 9 (7.5%) | 15 (12.5%) | 3 (3.2%) | 7 (4.3%) |

*One retinal artery embolus 2 weeks after the procedure.

operator experience, modification of techniques and equipment, and the use of new antiplatelet agents.

The first subsets of patients who may benefit from this procedure are those with restenosis after CEA.[40] In our initial group of 25 vessels, we had one minor stroke for a complication rate of 4%. We have now treated 102 such vessels with one major stroke complication (1%) and a nondisabling stroke rate of 4 of 102 (3.9%). Most importantly, we have had no cranial neuropalsies and no anesthetic complications. These results compare favorably with those of reported series of CEA for postendarterectomy restenosis.[40]

The second group comprises those patients with contralateral occlusions of the ICA. In our initial series of 26 patients, we had no major complications and one minor stroke (3.8%).[37] In our total series including our recent experience until April 2000, we have had one (1.6%) death and two minor strokes (3.1%).

Similarly, in the minority of patients in our series who would have been eligible for inclusion in the NASCET study, we have had excellent results (including our learning curve experience).[39] In this subset of symptomatic NASCET-eligible younger (<80 years) patients with no severe cardiac or pulmonary comorbidity, we have observed a 30-day risk of stroke or death of 3.6%.[39]

During our early experience, we noted a number of factors that were associated with embolic stroke.

These were increased lesion severity, long or multiple stenosis, and advanced age (Tables 49–20, 49–21, and 49–22). There was also a notable trend toward more embolic events in more calcified lesions, eccentric lesions, ulcerated lesions, and lesions with markedly irregular borders. Using multivariable analysis, only age and long or multiple lesions proved to be significant variables. In particular, patients older than 80 years showed the greatest risk, and the long and multiply diseased segments reflected complications in severe vasculopathic patients with aortic arch, common carotid, and internal carotid disease.

### Late Outcomes

#### General Comments

The primary indication for carotid stenting is the prevention of embolic stroke. Rigorous follow-up of our patients has been of great importance. Important end points are the incidence of embolic events during the vessels' healing phase after stent placement (i.e., in the first 3 to 4 weeks); the incidence of stent thrombosis; the restenosis rates; and, importantly, the incidence of ipsilateral stroke 2 to 5 years after the procedure.

Periprocedural embolic events are invariably evident immediately or within 1 to 2 hours after the procedure. Embolic events within the first 4 weeks after the procedure have been very rare. This is in

**TABLE 49–18.    CURRENT EXPERIENCE (PERIPROCEDURAL OUTCOMES), NOV. 1997–SEPT. 2000**

| | NO. OF PATIENTS (%) (N = 407) | NO. OF VESSELS (%) (N = 443) |
|---|---|---|
| Death | 1 (0.3) | 1 (0.3) |
| Minor stroke | 12 (3.0) | 12 (2.7) |
| Major stroke | 5 (1.2) | 5 (1.1) |
| Total strokes/deaths | 18 (4.4) | 18 (4.1) |

**TABLE 49–19.    RESULTS IN LOW-RISK SUBSETS**

| | MINOR STROKE (%) |
|---|---|
| NASCET eligible | 2.7 |
| CEA restenosis | 3.9 |
| Age <70 y | 4.2 |
| Lesion severity <70% | 3.5 |

CEA, carotid endarterectomy; NASCET, North American Symptomatic Carotid Endarterectomy Trial.

**TABLE 49–20. CORRELATION OF DEMOGRAPHICS AND CLINICAL CHARACTERISTICS WITH POSTPROCEDURAL EVENTS**

| | NO. OF PATIENTS (%) | NO. OF MINOR STROKES (%) | | NO. OF MAJOR STROKES (%) | NO. OF TOTAL EVENTS (%) | p VALUE |
|---|---|---|---|---|---|---|
| | | CATEGORY 1 | CATEGORY 2 | | | |
| Total | 231 | 8 (3.5) | 8 (3.5) | 1 (0.4) | 17 (7.4) | |
| Age (y) | | | | | | |
| <70 | 119 (51.5) | 3 (2.6) | 2 (1.7) | 0 | 5 (4.2) | |
| 70–79 | 86 (37.2) | 3 (3.5) | 4 (4.7) | 0 | 7 (8.1) | 0.001* |
| ≥80 | 26 (11.3) | 2 (7.7) | 2 (7.7) | 1 (3.8) | 5 (19.2) | |
| Sex | | | | | | |
| Male | 165 (71.4) | 7 (4.2) | 6 (3.6) | 0 | 13 (7.9) | 0.842 |
| Female | 66 (28.6) | 1 (1.5) | 2 (3.0) | 1 (1.5) | 4 (6.1) | |
| Symptomatic | | | | | | |
| Yes | 139 (60.2) | 5 (3.6) | 4 (2.9) | 1 (0.7) | 10 (7.2) | 0.883 |
| No | 92 (39.8) | 5 (5.4) | 2 (2.2) | 0 | 7 (7.6) | |
| Coronary disease | | | | | | |
| Yes | 164 (71.0) | 6 (3.7) | 7 (4.3) | 0 | 13 (7.9) | 0.811 |
| No | 67 (29.0) | 2 (2.9) | 1 (1.5) | 1 (1.5) | 4 (5.9) | |
| Hypertension | | | | | | |
| Yes | 179 (77.5) | 8 (4.5) | 6 (3.4) | 0 | 14 (7.8) | 0.423 |
| No | 52 (22.5) | 0 | 2 (3.9) | 1 (1.9) | 3 (5.8) | |
| Smoking | | | | | | |
| Yes | 145 (62.8) | 6 (4.1) | 7 (4.8) | 0 | 13 (8.9) | 0.340 |
| No | 86 (37.2) | 2 (2.3) | 1 (1.2) | 1 (1.2) | 4 (4.7) | |
| Bilateral disease | | | | | | |
| Yes | 91 (39.4) | 5 (5.5) | 1 (1.1) | 0 | 6 (6.6) | 0.352 |
| No | 140 (60.6) | 3 (2.1) | 7 (5.0) | 1 (0.7) | 11 (7.9) | |
| Contralateral occlusion | | | | | | |
| Yes | 28 (12.1) | 1 (3.6) | 0 | 0 | 1 (3.6) | 0.860 |
| No | 203 (87.9) | 7 (3.5) | 8 (3.9) | 1 (0.5) | 16 (7.9) | |

*χ² test for linear trend.

**TABLE 49–21. CORRELATION OF MORPHOLOGIC FEATURES WITH POSTPROCEDURAL EVENTS**

| | NO. OF PATIENTS (%) | NO. OF MINOR STROKES (%) | | NO. OF MAJOR STROKES (%) | NO. OF TOTAL EVENTS (%) | p VALUE |
|---|---|---|---|---|---|---|
| | | CATEGORY 1 | CATEGORY 2 | | | |
| Total | 271 | 8 (2.9) | 8 (2.9) | 1 (0.4) | 17 (6.3) | |
| Post-CEA | | | | | | |
| Yes | 59 (21.8) | 2 (3.4) | 1 (1.7) | 0 | 3 (5.1) | 0.890 |
| No | 212 (78.2) | 6 (2.8) | 7 (3.3) | 1 (0.5) | 14 (6.6) | |
| Lesion severity | | | | | | |
| <70% | 85 (31.4) | 1 (1.2) | 2 (2.4) | 0 | 3 (3.5) | |
| 70%–89% | 137 (50.6) | 4 (2.9) | 2 (1.5) | 1 (0.7) | 7 (5.1) | 0.007* |
| ≥90% | 47 (17.3) | 3 (6.4) | 4 (8.5) | 0 | 7 (14.9) | |
| Long/multiple stenoses | | | | | | |
| Yes | 88 (32.5) | 4 (4.6) | 5 (5.7) | 1 (1.1) | 10 (11.4) | 0.012 |
| No | 183 (67.5) | 4 (2.2) | 3 (1.6) | 0 | 7 (3.8) | |
| Eccentric | | | | | | |
| Yes | 209 (77.1) | 7 (3.3) | 8 (3.8) | 1 (0.5) | 16 (7.7) | 0.168 |
| No | 62 (22.9) | 1 (1.6) | 0 | 0 | 1 (1.6) | |
| Ulcerated | | | | | | |
| Yes | 66 (24.4) | 2 (3.0) | 3 (4.6) | 1 (1.5) | 6 (9.1) | 0.212 |
| No | 205 (75.6) | 6 (2.9) | 5 (2.4) | 0 | 11 (5.4) | |
| Calcified | | | | | | |
| Yes | 87 (32.1) | 6 (6.9) | 2 (2.3) | 0 | 8 (9.2) | 0.108 |
| No | 184 (67.9) | 2 (1.1) | 6 (3.3) | 1 (0.5) | 9 (4.9) | |
| Residual irregularity | | | | | | |
| Yes | 87 (32.1) | 3 (3.5) | 5 (5.8) | 0 | 8 (9.2) | 0.108 |
| No | 184 (67.9) | 5 (2.7) | 3 (1.6) | 1 (0.5) | 9 (4.9) | |
| NASCET eligible | | | | | | |
| Yes | 37 (13.7) | 1 (2.7) | 0 | 0 | 1 (2.7) | 0.582 |
| No | 234 (86.3) | 7 (2.9) | 8 (3.4) | 1 (0.4) | 16 (6.8) | |

CEA, carotid endarterectomy; NASCET, North American Symptomatic Carotid Endarterectomy Trial.
*χ² test for linear trend.

**TABLE 49–22. CORRELATION OF PROCEDURAL VARIABLES WITH NEUROLOGIC EVENTS**

| | NO. OF PATIENTS (%) | NO. OF MINOR STROKES, (%) | | NO. OF MAJOR STROKES (%) | NO. OF TOTAL EVENTS (%) | p VALUE |
| | | CATEGORY 1 | CATEGORY 2 | | | |
|---|---|---|---|---|---|---|
| Total | 231 | 8 (3.5) | 8 (3.5) | 1 (0.4) | 17 (7.4) | |
| Combined procedure | | | | | | |
| Yes | 32 (13.9) | 3 (9.4) | 0 | 0 | 3 (9.4) | 0.404 |
| No | 199 (86.1) | 5 (2.5) | 8 (4.0) | 1 (0.5) | 14 (7.0) | |
| Bilateral procedure | | | | | | |
| Yes | 19 (8.2) | 1 (5.3) | 0 | 0 | 1 (5.3) | 0.926 |
| No | 212 (91.8) | 7 (3.3) | 8 (3.8) | 1 (0.5) | 16 (7.6) | |

contrast to CEA, in which 50% of embolic events are seen up to 7 days after the procedure.[19] Similarly, stent thrombosis after carotid stenting has been remarkably rare. After placement of more than 600 stents, we have seen one perioperative thrombosis. We have also observed a fatal stent thrombosis in a female patient who had a long (4-cm) segment of CCA stented for postradiation stenosis. This event occurred 6 weeks after the procedure without preceding symptoms.

Early experience with the balloon-expandable Palmaz stent is worthy of comment. In our first 120 Palmaz stent placements, we observed stent deformation in 10 stents.[41] Usually, this involved the distal end of the stent and was not associated with symptoms. Severe stent compression has, however, been observed. Even placement of the stent behind the angle of the jaw was not protective. We now avoid the use of Palmaz or any balloon-expandable stents, except when we are treating lesions at the ostium of the CCA. Stent compression can be treated by repeat balloon dilation, and with the placement of a self-expanding stent within the previous balloon-expandable device. The incidence of stent restenosis in our series is confounded by the effect of stent compression or angiographic restenosis in our initial series. We have not yet seen stent deformation with the use of self-expanding stents.

### In-Stent Restenosis

Of our first 225 successfully stented patients, we were able to perform carotid follow-up angiography in 121 and follow-up duplex studies in an additional 29. Of these 150 patients, restenosis (using a 50% diameter-narrowing definition) was present in 8 (5.3%). Only 4 of these patients (2.7%) had binary restenosis (>50%) that warranted repeat intervention. Restenosis in carotid stents should be treated with repeat balloon dilation. This can be done through a long 6-French sheath or guiding catheter and can be accomplished as an outpatient procedure.

### Late Clinical Outcome

We had 99.6% follow-up on our first 528 patients with 604 successfully stented arteries. At a mean follow-up of 17 ± 12 months, we have observed 75 nonneurologic deaths mainly attributed to cardiac disease. Regarding neurologic events, there were two fatal ipsilateral strokes, one nonfatal ipsilateral major stroke, one nonfatal minor ipsilateral stroke, two fatal contralateral or vertebrobasilar strokes, four nonfatal major contralateral or vertebrobasilar strokes, four nonfatal minor contralateral or vertebrobasilar strokes, one stroke of unknown hemisphere or severity, and two deaths of indeterminate cause. The results compare very favorably with outcomes seen in the NASCET.[12]

## Complications

The success of carotid stenting depends on the ability of the operator to minimize periprocedural complications. Performing carotid stenting through percutaneous access and without the need for general anesthesia minimizes the wound and anesthetic complications associated with CEA. Our evolving techniques over the last 4 years have been associated with a variety of complications that were encountered, analyzed, and subsequently avoided with modifications in our technique (Table 49–23). The meticulous step-by-step technique that we have

**TABLE 49–23. CAROTID STENTING COMPLICATIONS**

| MINOR | MAJOR |
|---|---|
| Puncture site complications | Carotid dissection |
| Carotid artery spasm | Carotid perforation |
| Transient bradycardia | Acute thrombosis |
| Poststenting hypotension | Cerebral hemorrhage |
| Transient cerebral ischemia (intraprocedural) | Major embolic stroke |
| Transient seizure or loss of consciousness | Fatal stroke |
| Minor embolic stroke | |
| Stenosis of the external carotid | |

developed has allowed us to avoid complications and perform carotid stenting as safely as the best practice of CEA. An important factor in avoiding complications is related to patient selection as discussed in conjunction with complications.

Major complications are rare when carotid stenting is performed using meticulous technique. In this section, we detail a variety of complications we have encountered mainly during the early phase of our experience with this procedure. We describe the modifications of our technique that we have implemented in order to avoid these complications and how to troubleshoot if they occur.

### Puncture Site Complications

Carotid stenting should only be undertaken within an interventional (endovascular) program in which personnel are familiar with discomfort-free, efficient, and safe arterial sheath removal. Puncture site complications can be minimized by careful anterior wall cannulation of the femoral artery, with the use of the 6- or 7-French long sheath that is exchanged for a short sheath at the end of the procedure, and with conservative use of periprocedural anticoagulation.

Sheaths are routinely removed by experienced personnel under additional local anesthesia 3 to 4 hours after the procedure, when the ACT falls to less than 150 seconds. Manual compression is used to initially control the site, after which a compression device can be used. A good intravenous line, adequate hydration, and pretreatment with atropine are used to prevent and treat hypotension commonly observed with the vasovagal response to sheath removal. Patients require bed rest for at least 2 to 4 hours after sheath removal, depending on the size of the sheath.

### Carotid Artery Spasm and Pseudospasm

The occurrence of spasm (Figs. 49–14 and 49–15) in the distal ICA is a common angiographic anomaly that usually resolves spontaneously after the guide wire and/or sheath have been retracted. Severe spasm may be a potential hazard in the presence of contralateral carotid artery occlusion. To date, we have not encountered this problem. Use of 0.018- or 0.014-inch soft-tipped wires minimized the occurrence of spasm. Injections of 100 to 200 μg of nitroglycerin through the carotid access sheath may help resolve the spasm. Spasm that is sometimes discovered in the ECA after removal of the Amplatz wire is benign and should be ignored.

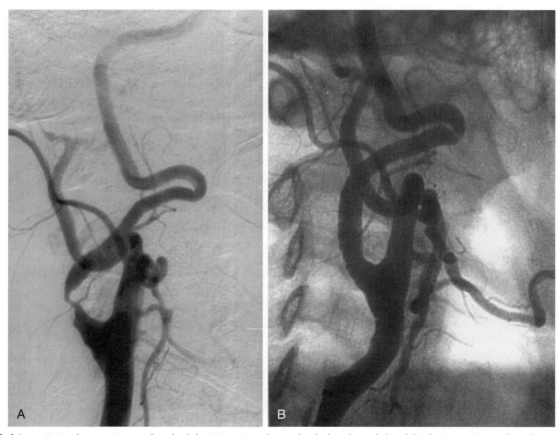

FIGURE 49–14. *A,* Critical stenosis on a bend of the ICA. Note the multiple bends and distal kinks *B,* Angiography after stenting with a 10 × 20 mm Wallstent. Note the spasm in the ICA and CCA. This is of no clinical consequence.

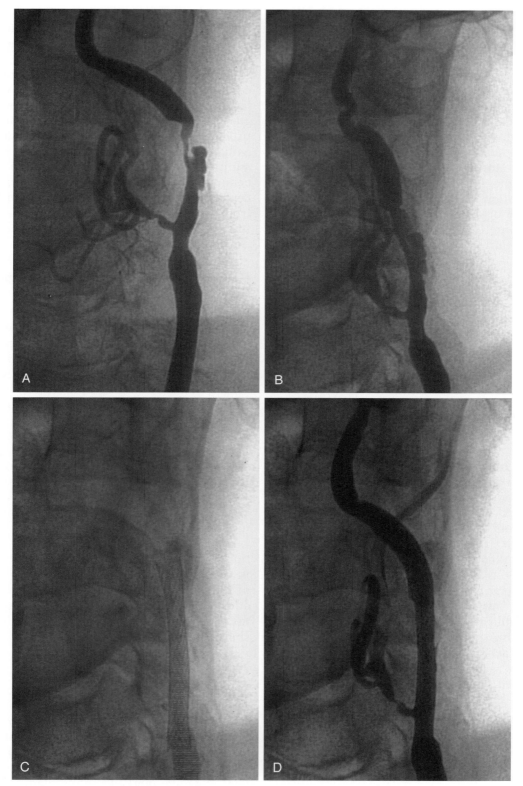

FIGURE 49–15. *A*, Critical ulcerated complex stenosis involving the ICA, CCA, and ECA. *B*, Note the distal spasm after predilation. *C*, The 10 × 20 mm Wallstent. *D*, Angiography after stenting. There is minimal residual spasm.

Spasm must be differentiated from kinking of the carotid artery. In many patients, normal carotid anatomies include redundant tortuous segments and even complete loops that can be seen in the proximal CCA near the bifurcation or in the distal ICA below the siphon. The placement of stiff wire guides and the cephalad pressure placed on the CCA by the access sheath accentuate those "loops and kinks" and temporarily shift them more cephalad. These kinks should be ignored, as they will resolve completely when the wire and sheath are removed. The operator must not be tempted to dilate or stent distal kinks. However, a special situation arises when a tortuous loop occurs just distal (cephalad) to the bifurcation. A "bend point" at this site can be the source of distal dissection, and techniques to avoid this are discussed in the section "Carotid Dissection." Current stent designs, however, may unavoidably "straighten out" a tortuous area that is adjacent to a lesion and leave a "new" kink just distal to the stent. Occasionally, in one angiographic view the kink may look like a stenosis. These angiographic findings should be ignored. Follow-up angiographic studies in our patients have confirmed that these anomalies are benign and are not associated with an adverse outcome. Distal ICA kinks often resolve when the guiding sheath is retracted.

### Transient Bradyarrhythmias and Hypotension

Bradycardia and episodes of transient asystole are common during dilation at the carotid bifurcation. They are due to pressure from the balloon and stent on the carotid baroreceptors. More prolonged hypotension and bradycardia are seen with balloon-expandable stents that place more sustained pressure on the receptors or in cases in which bilateral stenting is undertaken during the same procedure. Interestingly, this phenomenon is not seen when treating post-CEA lesions in which the receptors have been denervated during previous dissection.

Initially in our experience, when we used balloon-expandable stents, we routinely used temporary transvenous pacemakers. We have since abandoned this practice and only rarely acquire femoral venous access as a routine precaution. Patients who exhibit marked bradycardia are administered atropine, 0.5 to 1 mg. Large doses of atropine are avoided in elderly patients, as this can result in confusion and make accurate neurologic assessment more difficult. Asystole that is seen during balloon inflation in a minority of patients is always transient and responds to balloon deflation.

### Poststenting Hypotension

Hypotension is common after carotid stenting and may last hours to days, depending on the sensitivity of the baroreceptors, the type of stent used, and the presence of bilateral stents. The degree of hypotension appears to be more pronounced in heavily calcified lesions. Usually, there are no clinical sequelae and the modest fall in BP requires no specific intervention.

In patients with additional intracranial stenosis, contralateral occlusion, or significant vertebrobasilar disease, hypotension should be treated more aggressively. Similarly, when patients develop periprocedural cerebral ischemia secondary to an embolic event, hypotension should be corrected in addition to ensuring good hydration. In the postprocedural period, hypotension due to carotid baroreceptor pressure should be carefully differentiated from relatively masked retroperitoneal bleeding from the femoral puncture site or other less benign causes of hypotension.

### Poststenting Hypertension—Hyperperfusion Syndrome

In many patients, carotid stenting has no effect on BP. In hypertensive patients with critical lesions greater than 90%, we have observed a transient postprocedural confusional state, occasionally associated with transient localizing symptoms, that is observed with no angiographic, CT, or MRI/MRA abnormalities. The syndrome resolves over 24 hours with good control of BP. The syndrome is seen most often when bilateral high-grade lesions are treated in the same session. Accordingly, in particularly elderly patients with bilateral high-grade disease, we now perform stenting in a staged approach, separating the procedures by days or weeks. The most critical, symptomatic, or angiographically threatening vessel is usually treated first.

Hypertension and anticoagulation, in combination with good antiplatelet therapy, can rarely result in cerebral hemorrhage after stenting. The presence of intracranial aneurysms may place the patient at additional risk. In elderly patients, hypertension must be carefully controlled and anticoagulation should be used conservatively.

### Contrast Encephalopathy

Contrast encephalopathy is a rare syndrome observed in a few of our patients. The Washington Hospital Center has experienced a similar case (M. Leon, personal communication). Patients developed a profound neurologic deficit associated with the hemisphere at risk but with no CT scan abnormalities, except for marked contrast staining in the basal ganglion and in the cortex. There were no angiographic abnormalities on subtracted intracranial angiograms. We saw this event after a complicated prolonged procedure in which a large volume of contrast material was used. Because contrast material should not leak through the blood-brain barrier, it has been suggested that this phenomenon is caused by the combination of fine particulate embolization and excessive local contrast injection. Leaky capillaries due to hyperperfusion have also been suggested as the cause. Importantly, patients recover fully within 24 hours with no permanent neurologic sequelae.

### Carotid Dissection

Carotid dissection is a rare but important complication of the carotid stenting procedure. We have seen this associated with two situations. The first and most important is distal dissection, which may occur when attempting to stent a lesion that is adjacent to a severe distal kink or bend point.

Dissection associated with very tortuous internal carotid arteries (Figs. 49–16 and 49–17) can be avoided by careful technique. When we have experienced dissection, it has been caused by trying to force stiff peripheral balloons or stiff-ended stent delivery systems through the bends in the ICA while trying to position the balloon or stent across the lesion. Attempting to deliver a stent over too-flexible nonsupportive guide wire has precipitated the problem in every case.

To avoid this complication, we recommend the following procedural maneuvers:

1. Cross the lesion with a soft 0.014-inch coronary guide wire and advance the tip close to the siphon.
2. Advance a 0.018-inch wire–compatible low-profile coronary balloon over this wire to just below the siphon.
3. Exchange the 0.014-inch wire for an extra-support 0.018-inch wire. Dilate the lesion as usual, but have the tip of the Roadrunner wire 0.018 inch in the siphon to keep the vessel straight. (Note: spasm, pseudospasm, and distally displaced kinks should be ignored.)
4. Advance the stent so that it just covers the lesion. Do not attempt to straighten the bend with the stent as this will compress the kinks toward the base of the skull.
5. Postdilate before allowing the wire to come back to let the artery relax. (Note: Distal kinks are enhanced by upward thrust of the access sheath or guide. Kinks will improve after the sheath is withdrawn to the proximal part of the CCA.)

The second, less common site for dissection is in the CCA, caused by the tip of the guiding sheath. This complication can be treated, if necessary, by

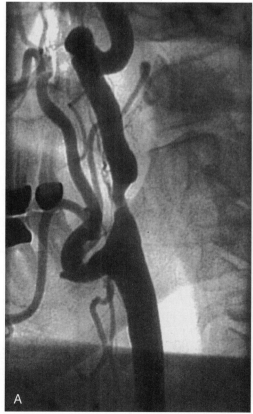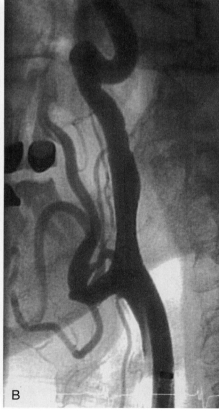

FIGURE 49–16. *A,* Severe kink well distal to a critical stenosis of the ICA. In this case, there is sufficient distance to allow passage of the delivery system without risking dissection. *B,* Angiography after stenting. The kink remains distal to the site of stent deployment.

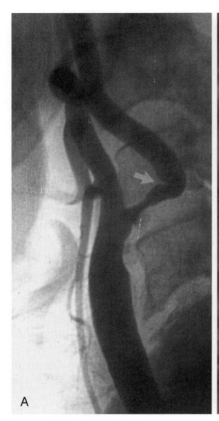
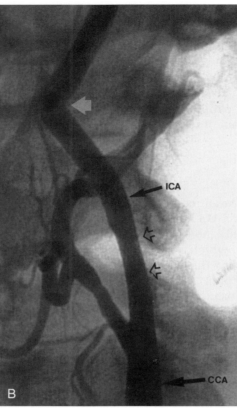

FIGURE 49–17. *A*, Severe kink *(arrow)* just distal to the lesion. The 0.018-inch guide wire should be placed well distal to the lesion and kink in the ICA to straighten out this segment of the ICA. *B*, Angiography after stenting with a 10 × 20 mm Wallstent. Note that the segment has been straightened by the Wallstent and the kink *(solid arrow)* has now shifted distally. This is of no clinical significance.

deploying another Wallstent across the dissection in the CCA before removing the guide sheath.

### Treating Dissections

If you suspect a dissection has occurred distal to the stent, maintain the position of the wire and stent across the area. Distal dissections are best treated using flexible coronary stents, for example, Magic Wallstent (6-mm diameter). Start distally and stent in a retrograde manner into the stent at the bifurcation.

### External Carotid Occlusion

The ECA is frequently involved with disease in the bifurcation (Fig. 49–18). During CEA, surgeons attempt to maintain patency of this vessel, but many follow-up angiograms show that the vessel has occluded. Acute occlusion of the ECA is usually tolerated well; however, in the absence of good collaterals from the contralateral external artery or vertebral system, some patients experience jaw muscle angina. This usually resolves over time as collaterals develop. More importantly, the ECA can, in some patients, supply important collaterals to the brain via the ophthalmic artery and pial collateral branches. Accordingly, its patency should be maintained if possible but not at the expense of excess

manipulation that causes embolic complications or compromise of the ICA. The procedure for avoiding jailing and dilating of the ECA is described in the Postdilatation Technique section. Note that it is not necessary to produce a wide opening, but just sufficient to establish TIMI-3 flow. Even moderately compromised ECAs will be patent on angiographic follow-up.

### Carotid Perforation

Carotid perforation is a rare event. We have had one case in over 600 vessels stented. This perforation occurred because of aggressive balloon sizing in a misguided attempt to optimize the luminal appearance of the stented segment. We now appreciate that luminal irregularities or "pockets" of contrast material in residual ulceration external to the stent are of no prognostic significance and disappear over time (Fig. 49–19). Our approach is to conservatively size all balloons and expect that vessel perforation can be completely avoided. We now rarely postdilate with a balloon larger than 5 mm.

### Acute Stent Thrombosis

Stent thrombosis is also a rare event in the carotid bifurcation. The low rate of stent thrombosis and periprocedural embolic events is predicated on the

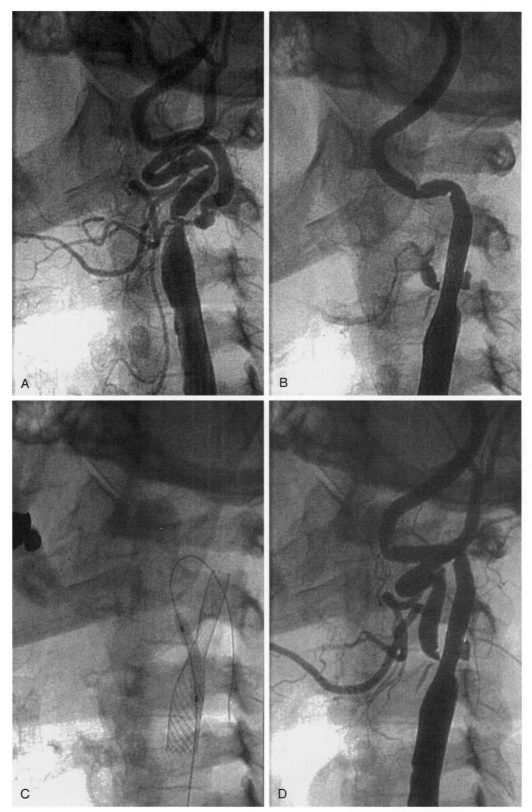

FIGURE 49–18. *A,* High-grade complex (type C) stenosis involving the ICA, CCA, and ECA. Note that the lesion is on a bend, and note the distal kinking of the ICA. *B,* The ECA is occluded after stent deployment. *C,* Balloon dilation of the ECA with a 2 × 20 mm Ranger (Scimed) followed by a 3.5 × 20 mm Ranger at the origin of the ECA. *D,* Angiography after stenting. The stenosis remains but there is TIMI-3 flow.

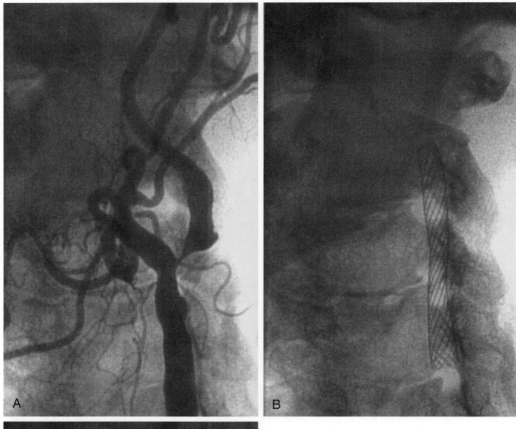

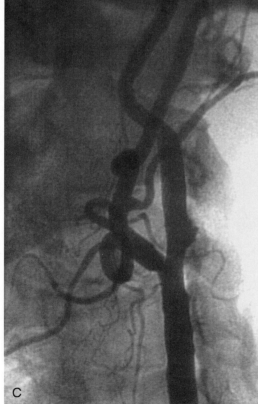

FIGURE 49–19. *A,* High-grade stenosis with ulceration involving the ICA and the CCA. *B,* The 10 × 20 mm Wallstent. *C,* Angiography after stenting. Note the small filling defect external to the stent and the residual stenosis. This is of no prognostic significance, and attempts should not be made to obliterate the ulceration or residual stenosis by overdilating. Minor jailing of the ECA is also noted but not treated.

correct and strict use of appropriate doses of adjunctive antiplatelet therapy. Basic stenting techniques must be adhered to. These include (1) only stenting in the presence of brisk flow without significant inflow or outflow obstruction, (2) stenting from "normal" segment to "normal" segment if possible, and (3) ensuring proper stent sizing (oversizing in the case of self-expanding stents) and careful apposition to the wall. Our practice is not to dilate segments of the stent deployed in "normal" segments of artery as long as the stent is at least 1 to 2 mm larger than the reference vessel diameter. When edges of the stent are dilated, this is done carefully at low pressures to avoid edge dissection. The high-flow, low-resistance carotid circulation is the interventionist's friend, but good basic stenting techniques are essential for complication-free results.

### Cerebral Hemorrhage

Cerebral hemorrhage is a devastating, usually fatal but fortunately rare, complication of carotid stenting. In our experience cerebral hemorrhage has been associated with at least one, but usually a combination, of the following factors:

■ Excessive anticoagulation
■ Poorly controlled hypertension
■ Overaggressive attempts at intracranial rescue
■ The presence of a vulnerable Berry aneurysm
■ Stenting in the presence of a recent (<3 weeks) ischemic stroke

The first two issues are the most important. Anticoagulation should be monitored carefully with the use of ACT measurements. We currently use weight-adjusted doses of heparin between 5000 and 6000 U to achieve an ACT of around 200 to 250 seconds. Glycoprotein IIb/IIIa inhibitors are not used routinely. We have employed these agents selectively when ticlopidine or clopidogrel have been omitted or when we have had residual distal dissections that could not be controlled by stenting in the presence of visible thrombus or distal embolization seen after the procedure. In these cases, we control hypertension with intravenous nitroglycerin and ensure that the ACT is below 200 seconds. During intracranial rescue, we are extremely cautious with guide wire manipulation and the use of thrombolytics in the presence of elevated ACT levels and/or the use of IIb/IIIa inhibitors.

If a cerebral hemorrhage is suspected, the procedure should be terminated. Anticoagulation should be reversed with protamine and an emergency CT scan performed. Operators should be familiar with the angiographic features of an intracranial mass effect. Sudden loss of consciousness preceded by a severe headache in the absence of intracranial vessel occlusion should alert the operator to this devastating event. Fortunately, with careful patient selection and strict attention to these technical and anticoagulation issues, cerebral hemorrhage should be a very rare occurrence.

## DISTAL EMBOLIZATION

Distal embolization that manifests clinical symptoms is an important complication of carotid stenting. It is caused by the release of thrombotic, necrotic, or other atherosclerotic material from the lesion. Careful patient selection and meticulous technique can minimize this complication. The future availability of distal neuroprotection devices will, we hope, make this complication a very rare event. Transient rapidly resolving (minutes to 1 hour) neurologic events may occur in no more than 3% of patients. Major or fatal strokes can be almost completely avoided with appropriate and careful technique. The potential causes of distal embolization are listed in Table 49–24.

It is essential to monitor the neurologic status at every step of the procedure. Very transient changes in neurologic status should prompt the operator to optimize the BP and hydration and clarify the status of the intracranial vasculature. This is best done after completion of the procedure. If the change in neurologic status is associated with slow flow from lesion recoil, guide wire spasm, or, rarely, dissection, it is important to rapidly place the stent, remove the guide wire, and complete the procedure. Clearly, optimal treatment requires the operator to be proficient with the technique so this can be accomplished quickly. A significant change in neurologic status that does not resolve immediately should initiate the steps described in the following sections.

## Managing Distal Embolization

General resuscitative care of the patient should be instituted. This includes maintaining normal BP,

**TABLE 49–24.  CAUSES OF DISTAL EMBOLIZATION**

| MOST IMPORTANT | LESS IMPORTANT |
|---|---|
| Predilation with oversized balloon | Initial angiographic access |
| Forcing high-profile stent across heavily calcified lesion | Guide wire crossing |
| Postdilating "aggressively" with oversized balloon | |
| Persistent and aggressive attempts to access tortuous, highly atherosclerotic CCA | |

CCA, common carotid artery.

normal HR, and a patent airway and administering oxygen. The stenting procedure should be quickly and efficiently completed including poststent dilation as additional maneuvers may involve passing neurovascular rescue equipment through the stented segment to access the distal vasculature.

If the patient becomes uncooperative or agitated or if the airway is compromised, conscious sedation may be required.

Intracranial angiography is performed in AP and lateral projections. If possible, angiography of the contralateral carotid artery and at least one vertebral artery should be performed to determine the status of anterior and posterior communicating arteries and leptomeningeal anastomoses. The arteriograms are carefully examined to determine the site and extent of intracranial vessel embolism. Because of anatomic arrangements and flow patterns, the most likely site of intracranial embolism is the distal ICA, the middle cerebral artery, and its branches. Large vessel occlusion is usually obvious (especially in lateral projection), but embolism in the smaller branches requires careful scrutiny. Acute occlusion of a small branch vessel may be noted only in comparison with preprocedural angiography. The availability of a good preprocedural intracranial angiogram is therefore essential in all patients undergoing carotid stenting. A change of neurologic status can ensue not only from occlusive phenomena such as embolus, but also from intracerebral hemorrhage or hyperperfusion syndrome (especially if a very tight stenosis or totally occluded artery has been opened). Appropriate steps are taken to recanalize the occluded vessel as soon as possible. Time is brain. If there is a residual neurologic deficit and small branch occlusions, remember the three H's— hydrate, heparinize, and higher BP. If on the diagnostic arteriogram there are no signs of embolism, the heparin should be reversed with protamine and a CT scan should be performed immediately. An intracerebral hemorrhage may rarely occur. Angiography can indicate this diagnosis if the middle cerebral artery is displaced, there is leakage of contrast material into the brain parenchyma, or the sylvian triangle is displaced inferiorly on the lateral view.

## Technique

The 7-French sheath within the CCA is the pivotal catheter for guiding of the variable-stiffness microcatheter into the intracranial circulation. Through this sheath, the 6-French 120-cm multipurpose guide catheter (Table 49–25) is advanced into the ICA over the 0.038-inch Glide Wire. This catheter should not be advanced deep into the ICA if there are tortuosities or coils in this vessel. This may produce spasm or even dissections. The variable-

**TABLE 49–25.   EQUIPMENT AND ADJUNCTIVE MEDICATIONS FOR NEUROVASCULAR RESCUE**

6-Fr 120-cm multipurpose guiding catheter
0.018-in. variable-stiffness microcatheter, Tracker-18 (Target Therapeutics; Fremont CA)
Guide wires, 0.016 in. Taper wire (Target Therapeutics; Fremont CA)
0.014-in. Balance wire (Guidant Inc.; Temecula CA)
0.014-in. Dasher wire (Target Therapeutics; Fremont CA)
PTA balloon catheters, 1.5–4 mm Predator (Cordis Endovascular; Warren NJ)
Tuohy-Borst adaptors
Pressurized bags with heparinized normal saline
Air filters
1 and 3-mL Luer-Lok syringes
Intra-arterial spasmolytics (papaverin, adenosine, nicardepine)
Urokinase 250,000–1 million U
Glycoprotein IIb/IIIa inhibitors

PTA, percutaneous transluminal angioplasty.

stiffness microcatheter is advanced through the 6-French catheter. All catheters should be continuously perfused with heparinized saline, which should be passed through an air filter. The variable-stiffness microcatheter (0.018-inch) is advanced over the wire (0.016-inch) into the intracranial segment of the ICA. There are a variety of guide wires that can be used. The most commonly used wire is one with good ability to be torqued and a soft malleable distal tip. If the position of the embolus is obvious (in the ICA or horizontal M1 segment of the middle cerebral artery), no additional arteriography is needed. If the occlusive lesion is within the trifurcation of the middle cerebral artery or distally, an arteriogram with injection through the variable-stiffness microcatheter is obtained (using a 1- to 3-mL syringe). Both AP and lateral projections are used so the occluded branch of the middle cerebral artery can be clearly identified and cannulated. Road mapping is useful. Before the recanalization is attempted, the length of the occluded segment should be determined. This can be done by careful analysis of the diagnostic arteriogram by looking for retrograde flow into the occluded artery. If there is no retrograde flow, the variable-stiffness microcatheter is passed through the embolus over the wire distally. Continuous rotating movement of the distal curved end of the wire usually allows penetration through the embolus. The wire is withdrawn, and slow injection of contrast material through the microcatheter is undertaken while the catheter is simultaneously and slowly pulled back. This determines the distal end of the embolus. Embolic debris produced during carotid angioplasty with stenting can be both soft and hard. Soft emboli consist of blood coagula and are prone to lysis. Hard emboli consist of stenotic debris (plaque with cholesterol and calcium) and cannot be lysed but may be mechanically disrupted.

There are three techniques to reopen an acutely occluded intracranial artery:

- Thrombolysis
- Mechanical disruption
- Removal of the embolus

### Thrombolysis

Thrombolysis involves injecting a thrombolytic agent into the embolus, with the hope of dissolving it. Thrombolysis should start at the proximal end of the embolus. The distal end of the microcatheter is positioned within or close to the proximal end of the embolus, and injection of the thrombolytic agent begins. It can be injected by continuous infusion or in pulses though the syringe. The latter is our practice. Most currently used thrombolytic agents are urokinase and recombinant tissue-type plasminogen activator (r-tPA). Both agents are appropriately diluted. To follow the progress of the thrombolysis, control angiograms are obtained through the microcatheter. The position of the microcatheter is adjusted depending on the progress of the thrombolysis, always inserting the distal tip into the thrombus. The usual dose of urokinase is between 250,000 and 500,000 U and should not exceed 1 million U.

### Mechanical Disruption

Mechanical disruption of the embolus improves the success rate of thrombolysis; however, this may also increase the risk of further distal embolization and/or vessel perforation. The embolus can be fragmented with several passages of the guide wire and catheter through its length; by twisting the curved end of the guide wire within the embolus while the wire is pulled back; and by saline injections into the embolus through the microcatheter. A more specialized form of mechanical disruption of the embolus and vessel recanalization is to perform balloon angioplasty. After placing a variable-stiffness microcatheter such as the Tracker-18 intracranially, an angioplasty balloon catheter can be simply advanced over the guide wire (0.014- or 0.016-inch). The tip of the 0.014-inch exchange wire should be distal to the embolus in the secondary branches of the middle cerebral artery. The diameter of the balloon should not exceed 1.5 mm for middle cerebral artery branches, 2.5 mm for the horizontal segment of the middle cerebral artery, and 4 mm for the distal ICA. Only gentle low-pressure inflations should be used. The most rewarding method to reopen an intracranially occluded artery by embolus is the combination of thrombolysis and mechanical disruption with a microcatheter/wire combination and angio-plasty. It usually achieves success faster than thrombolysis alone and decreases the need for large amounts of thrombolytic agent, thus reducing the risk of postrecanalization intracerebral hemorrhage.

We have found the local injection of nicardipine, 200 to 400 μg, to be very useful in treating distal spasm and improving distal flow. Occasionally, we have used low doses of IIb/IIIa, but great caution must be exercised in combining potent antiplatelet and thrombolytic agents. When good flow has been rapidly reestablished, we have occasionally reversed the anticoagulation with protamine to reduce the risk of hemorrhagic conversion.

### Removal of the Embolus

The embolus may also be removed with a snare or by funnel attached to the end of specially designed nitinol wire.

A potential risk of neurovascular rescue is brain hemorrhage. This is directly related to the length of time the vessel is occluded. Reperfused ischemic brain parenchyma is very prone to hemorrhage. Ischemically damaged terminal branches, especially lenticulostriate basal ganglionic arteries, are also very prone to rupture. The risk is increased in these arteries, as they are terminal with no availability of a collateral circulation. If the horizontal M1 segment of the middle cerebral artery is recanalized, causing reperfusion of ischemic brain parenchyma, and this, in combination with ischemic damage to small vessels, increases the risk of postrecanalization hemorrhage into the basal ganglia.

## FUTURE DEVELOPMENTS

CAS even using nondedicated equipment can be performed with remarkably low complication rates. Multiple centers have demonstrated excellent results,[42] whereas there have been only anecdotal reports of poor outcomes and at least one notable very small series with negative results published in the surgical literature.[43] Clearly, there is an urgent need to train operators who would like to do this work. The next 5 years should be focused on education and technical training through symposia, workshops, and live demonstration courses. It is our view that the most successful results can be attained through collegial collaboration between cardiology, radiology, and neuroradiology personnel.

## Technical Developments

There is an ongoing and urgent need to improve the equipment available for carotid stenting. Invariably, when we encounter a technical problem, it is related to the inadequacy of the devices currently available.

There is a need for lower-profile stent delivery systems, better access sheaths, and specially designed guide wires and balloons. It is likely that a variety of different stent designs will be required for optimal treatment of the variable carotid bifurcation anatomy.

The major challenge from a technical perspective is the development of devices that will reliably prevent any mobile particulate matter that is produced during the intervention from reaching the brain. Clinical experience and work from the Ohki ex vivo model has taught us that embolic particles can be released from aggressive guide wire manipulation, large-diameter guide wire, balloon dilatation, stent deployment, and poststent dilatation.[44]

It is also well known that emboli are released during surgical exposure of the carotid bifurcation, during shunt placement, immediately after clamp release, and for up to 1 week after endarterectomy.[45] In the ACAS study, more than half the periprocedural strokes and TIAs occurred between postsurgical days 2 and 7.

## Neuroprotection

Data from intraprocedural transcranial Doppler monitoring studies have shown that high-intensity transients (HITS) representing emboli are seen during the carotid stent implantation as well as during carotid endarterectomy.[46, 47] Although embolization is universal, clinically evident strokes do not always occur. The rationale for the use of neuroprotection devices is to reduce the number of embolic HITS and consequently reduce the risk of a clinically relevant event. Neuroprotection devices are similar to the devices used during percutaneous treatment of saphenous vein graft disease. Three forms of devices have been developed. The first, pioneered by Jacques Théron, involves the use of a distal occlusion balloon that interrupts flow during critical maneuvers likely to release particles.[48] The column of blood containing embolic material is aspirated using a variety of techniques before deflating the balloon. This approach occludes flow and excludes the use of contrast injections to guide balloon and stent placement. In addition, occlusion of the ICA may produce significant cerebral ischemia in approximately 5% of patients, in particular those with contralateral occlusion, critical contralateral disease, or an incomplete circle of Willis. Preliminary studies suggest that embolic events are fewer with this device.[49]

The second approach involves the deployment of a low-profile embolic filter that is placed distally at the beginning of the procedure and removed after completion of stent positioning and postdilation. The filter provides constant cerebral perfusion allowing more time for careful and precise interven-

tion of the lesion. Currently available devices are the Mednova, Angioguard, and Epi Filter, deployed and retrieved on a 0.014- or 0.018-inch wire that serves as the guide wire for delivery of balloons and stents. Studies in ex vivo models have shown 90% capture of particles of 200 μm and 100% capture of particles greater than 500 μm.[44] The third neuroprotection system, Parodi, involves a common carotid artery–guiding sheath with an external circumferential balloon that occludes antegrade flow and facilitates reversal of flow, which is subsequently filtered and channeled in a retrograde manner into the femoral vein. A supplementary occlusion balloon is placed into the external carotid artery to augment this reversal of flow.[50] Clinical trials are currently in progress. These protection devices are user-friendly and do not add significant time to the current procedure. Carotid filter devices have the potential to greatly enhance the safety of carotid stenting.

## Clinical Trials

If carotid stenting is to attain superiority by providing a less traumatic, safe, and effective alternative to endarterectomy, it must be validated in rigorous, randomized controlled trials.

One such trial, Carotid and Vertebral Artery Transluminal Angioplasty Study (CAVATAS), has been completed, a second industry-sponsored trial is in progress, and a third, larger National Institutes of Health (NIH)-sponsored study, Carotid Revascularization Endarterectomy Versus Stent Trial (CREST), is planned. The CAVATAS trial was a prospective randomized controlled trial conducted in Great Britain through a collaborative effort between neurologists, radiologists, and vascular surgeons.[51] In general, the trial included a high-risk symptomatic population of patients with high-grade carotid stenosis. Inclusion criteria were much broader than those of the NASCET trial, and accordingly this study represents the first prospective evaluation of CEA in higher-risk patients by independent neurologic assessment. The study was undertaken at large regional centers in Britain by experienced vascular surgeons. In contrast, the radiologists involved in the trial were operating within their learning curves for carotid intervention. Only 20% of the patients received a stent as a bailout for inadequate angioplasty results. The stents that were used were suboptimal, and the technical approach with 0.035-inch wires, no carotid sheath, and peripheral balloons is now considered an outdated suboptimal approach. Despite these differences in operator experience and the relative maturity of the techniques, both early and late outcomes were similar. The 30-day incidences of major stroke and death were approximately 5% for both procedures. The incidences of all strokes (disabling and nondisabling) were approximately 11% for both procedures, and follow-up events were also similar.

The CREST trial is an NIH-sponsored multicenter randomized study that plans to recruit 2500 patients with symptomatic stenosis of 50% or greater diameter narrowing (NASCET angiographic criteria).[52] Initial entry into the study and randomization will be on the basis of carotid angiography if available or carotid duplex assessment if this study shows a 70% to 99% lesion. Patients randomized to CEA may undergo an angiographic evaluation, but this will not be required.

Independent neurologic assessment will be undertaken at 24 hours for both stent and CEA patients. This will be the first time such rigorous evaluation of CEA patients has been undertaken.

Primary endpoints will be

1. Incidence of death, any stroke, or myocardial infarction at 30 days
2. Incidence of ipsilateral stroke at 4 years

Recruitment of patients was scheduled to begin in the first quarter of 2001. Credentialing of both surgeons and stent operators will be required before recruitment commences.

Credentialing of stent operators will require the close collaboration with stent manufacturers. Because stent technology is evolving rapidly and operator experience with the new generations of carotid stents is very limited, operators will need to be credentialed on each new device before it can be used in the randomized trial. The final results of CREST, assuming optimal recruitment rates, will not be available for 5 to 6 years. In the interim, there are sufficient multicenter data to support the use of stenting by experienced operators, particularly in those subsets of patients known to be at higher risk from CEA.[42] Many observers have stated the compelling public health need for the availability of a safe alternative to CEA in these high-risk subsets. It needs to be emphasized that a large proportion of the patients currently undergoing CEA have never been shown to benefit from CEA on the basis of randomized controlled trials. The CREST investigators in collaboration with industry sponsors are planning a coordinated, rigorous prospective evaluation of stenting in these patients (Table 49–26) under Food and Drug Administration–Investigational Device Exemption (IDE) regulations and CREST-NIH oversight. It is hoped that satisfactory outcomes in this registry will facilitate the availability of devices and the technique and appropriate Health Care Financing Administration (HCFA) reimbursement for the treatment of patients at higher risk from CEA.

Carotid stenting represents the natural progression toward a less invasive approach to treating a critical carotid stenosis. The potential benefit for a large number of patients at risk of stroke is great. The availability of the method will depend on the dedication of operators in gaining the necessary expertise and experience and the dedication of all physicians involved to rigorous scientific evaluation.

**TABLE 49–26. PROPOSED PATIENT POPULATION IN HIGH CAROTID ENDARTERECTOMY RISK CREST REGISTRY**

Anatomic surgical access problems
  ICA lesions higher than cervical vertebrae $C_2$ or $C_3$
  Lesions at ostium or origin of CCA
  Patients with cervical spine disease or fixation preventing extension beyond neutral
  Prior radical neck dissection
  Prior cervical radiation with tissue injury
  Prior CEA surgery
Comorbid conditions increasing risk of CEA
  Unstable angina pectoris (defined as rest angina in association with ECG changes)
  Myocardial infarction within prior 1 mon
  Critical CAD (left main; left main equivalent, proximal three-vessel disease) requiring revascularization
  Congestive heart failure (classes III and IV)
  Severe pulmonary disease ($FEV_1 \leq 1$)
  Uncontrolled or poorly controlled diabetes (blood glucose $\geq 400$ mg/dL)
  Bleeding diathesis increasing the risk of wound hematoma or hemorrhage

CAD, coronary artery disease; CCA, common carotid artery; CEA, carotid endarterectomy; CREST, Carotid Revascularization Endarterectomy Stent Trial; ECG, electrocardiogram; $FEV_1$, forced expiratory volume in 1 second; ICA, internal carotid artery.

## REFERENCES

1. Vitek JJ. Angioplasty of arteries in the carotid territory [Letter; Comment]. AJNR Am J Neuroradiol 12:1024, 1991.
2. Vitek JJ, Raymon BC, Oh SJ: Innominate artery angioplasty. Am J Neuroradiol 5:113–114, 1984.
3. McNamara TO, Greaser LE, Fischer JR, et al: Initial and long-term results of treatment of brachiocephalic arterial stenoses and occlusions with balloon angioplasty, thrombolysis, stents. J Invasive Cardiol 9:372–383, 1997.
4. Sundt TMJ, Meyer FB, Piepgras DG, et al: Risk factors and operative results. In Meyer FB (ed): Sundt's Occlusive Cerebrovascular Disease, vol 1, pp 241–247. Philadelphia: WB Saunders, 1994.
5. Clinical alert: Benefit of carotid endarterectomy for patients with high-grade stenosis of the internal carotid artery. National Institute of Neurological Disorders and Stroke and Trauma Division. North American Symptomatic Carotid Endarterectomy Trial (NASCET) investigators. Stroke 22:816–817, 1991.
6. Vitek JJ, Powel DF, Anderson RD: Damage of the brachiocephalic vessels due to catheterization. Neurology 9:63–67, 1975.
7. Vitek JJ: Femoro-cerebral angiography: Analysis of 2,000 consecutive examinations: Special emphasis on carotid arteries catheterization in older patients. Am J Roentgenol Radium Ther Nucl Med 118:633–647, 1973.
8. Théron J, Raymond J, Casasco A, et al: Percutaneous angioplasty of atherosclerotic and postsurgical stenosis of carotid arteries. AJNR Am J Neuroradiol 8:495–500, 1987.
9. Mathias K: Catheter treatment of arterial occlusive disease of supraaortic vessels [in German]. Radiologe 27:547–554, 1987.

10. Ferguson RD, Ferguson JG: Carotid angioplasty. In search of a worthy alternative to endarterectomy. Arch Neurol 53:696–698, 1996.

11. Yadav SS, Roubin GS, Iyer SS, et al: Application of lessons learned from cardiac interventional techniques to carotid angioplasty. J Am Coll Cardiol 25:380A, 1995.

12. Beneficial effect of carotid endarterectomy in symptomatic patients with high-grade carotid stenosis. North American Symptomatic Carotid Endarterectomy Trial Collaborators. N Engl J Med 325:445–453, 1991.

13. Barnett HJ, Taylor DW, Eliasziw M, et al: Benefit of carotid endarterectomy in patients with symptomatic moderate or severe stenosis. North American Symptomatic Carotid Endarterectomy Trial Collaborators. N Engl J Med 339:1415–1425, 1998.

14. Endarterectomy for asymptomatic carotid artery stenosis. Executive Committee for the Asymptomatic Carotid Atherosclerosis Study. JAMA 273:1421–1428, 1995.

15. MRC European Carotid Surgery Trial: Interim results for symptomatic patients with severe (70–99%) or with mild (0–29%) carotid stenosis. European Carotid Surgery Trialists' Collaborative Group. Lancet 337:1235–1243, 1991.

16. Randomised trial of endarterectomy for recently symptomatic carotid stenosis: Final results of the MRC European Carotid Surgery Trial (ECST). Lancet 351:1379–1387, 1998.

17. North American Symptomatic Carotid Endarterectomy Trial. Methods, patient characteristics, and progress. Stroke 22:711–720, 1991.

18. Wennberg DE, Lucas FL, Birkmeyer JD, et al: Variation in carotid endarterectomy mortality in the Medicare population: Trial hospitals, volume, and patient characteristics [see Comments]. JAMA 279:1278–1281, 1998.

19. Young B, Moore WS, Robertson JT, et al: An analysis of perioperative surgical mortality and morbidity in the asymptomatic carotid atherosclerosis study. ACAS Investigators. Asymptomatic Carotid Atherosclerosis Study [see Comments]. Stroke 27:2216–2224, 1996.

20. New G, Roubin GS, Oetgen ME, et al: Validity of duplex ultrasound as a diagnostic modality for internal carotid artery disease. Catheter Cardiovasc Interven 52(1):9–15, 2001.

21. Results of a randomized controlled trial of carotid endarterectomy for asymptomatic carotid stenosis. Mayo Asymptomatic Carotid Endarterectomy Study Group. Mayo Clin Proc 67:513–518, 1992.

22. Brott T, Thalinger K: The practice of carotid endarterectomy in a large metropolitan area. Stroke 15:950–955, 1984.

23. Cebul RD, Snow RJ, Pine R, et al: Indications, outcomes, and provider volumes for carotid endarterectomy [see Comments]. JAMA 279:1282–1287, 1998.

24. Rothwell PM, Slattery J, Warlow CP: A systematic review of the risks of stroke and death due to endarterectomy for symptomatic carotid stenosis. Stroke 27:260–265, 1996.

25. Rothwell PM, Slattery J, Warlow CP: Clinical and angiographic predictors of stroke and death from carotid endarterectomy: Systematic review. BMJ 315:1571–1577, 1997.

26. Rothwell PM, Robertson G: Meta-analyses of randomised controlled trials [Letter; Comment]. Lancet 350:1181–11822, 1997.

27. McCrory DC, Goldstein LB, Samsa GP, et al: Predicting complications of carotid endarterectomy. Stroke 24:1285–1291, 1993.

28. Michenfelder JD: Anaesthetic and pharmacological management. In Meyer FB (ed): Sundt's Occlusive Cerebrovascular Disease, vol 1, pp 171–180. Philadelphia: WB Saunders, 1994.

29. Gasecki AP, Eliasziw M, Ferguson GG, et al: Long-term prognosis and effect of endarterectomy in patients with symptomatic severe carotid stenosis and contralateral carotid stenosis or occlusion: Results from NASCET. North American Symptomatic Carotid Endarterectomy Trial (NASCET) Group. J Neurosurg 83:778–782, 1995.

30. Das MB, Hertzer NR, Ratliff NB, et al: Recurrent carotid stenosis. A five-year series of 65 reoperations. Ann Surg 202:28–35, 1985.

31. Bettmann MA, Katzen BT, Whisnant J, et al: Carotid stenting and angioplasty: A statement for healthcare professionals from the Councils on Cardiovascular Radiology, Stroke, Cardio-Thoracic and Vascular Surgery, Epidemiology, and Prevention, and Clinical Cardiology, American Heart Association. Circulation 97:121–123, 1998.

32. Al-Mubarak N, Roubin GS, Gomez CR, et al: Carotid stenting for severe radiation-induced extracranial carotid artery occlusive disease. J Endovasc Surg 7:36–40, 2001.

33. Al-Mubarak N, Roubin GS, Liu MW, et al: Early results of percutaneous intervention for severe coexisting carotid and coronary artery disease. Am J Cardiol, in press.

34. New G, Iyer SS, Roubin GS, et al: Long-term outcomes following carotid artery stenting. Circulation 100(suppl I):674, 1999.

35. Piamsomboon C, Roubin GS, Liu MW, et al: Relationship between oversizing of self-expanding stents and late loss index in carotid stenting. Cathet Cardiovasc Diagn 45:139–143, 1998.

36. Al-Mubarak N, Liu MW, Dean LS, et al: Incidence and outcomes of prolonged hypotension following carotid artery stenting [Abstract]. J Am Coll Cardiol 33:65A, 1999.

37. Mathur A, Roubin GS, Gomez CR, et al: Elective carotid artery stenting in the presence of contralateral occlusion. Am J Cardiol 81:1315–1317, 1998.

38. Mathur A, Roubin GS, Yadav JS, et al: Combined coronary and bilateral carotid stenting: A case report. Cathet Cardiovasc Diagn 40:202–206, 1997.

39. Mathur A, Roubin GS, Iyer SS, et al: Predictors of stroke complicating carotid artery stenting. Circulation 97:1239–1245, 1998.

40. Yadav JS, Roubin GS, Iyer S, et al: Elective stenting of the extracranial carotid arteries. Circulation 95:376–381, 1997.

41. Mathur A, Dorros G, Iyer SS, et al: Palmaz stent compression in patients following carotid artery stenting. Cathet Cardiovasc Diagn 41:137–140, 1997.

42. Wholey MH, Wholey M, Bergeron P, et al: Current global status of carotid artery stent placement. Cathet Cardiovasc Diagn 44:1–6, 1998.

43. Naylor AR, Bolia A, Abbott RJ, et al: Randomized study of carotid angioplasty and stenting versus carotid endarterectomy: A stopped trial. J Vasc Surg 28:326–334, 1998.

44. Ohki T, Marin ML, Lyon RT, et al: Ex vivo human carotid artery bifurcation stenting: Correlation of lesion characteristics with embolic potential. J Vasc Surg 27:463–471, 1998.

45. Muller M, Reiche W, Langenscheidt P, et al: Ischemia after carotid endarterectomy: Comparison between transcranial Doppler sonography and diffusion-weighted MR imaging [see Comments]. AJNR Am J Neuroradiol 21:47–54, 2000.

46. Jordan WD Jr, Voellinger DC, Doblar DD, et al: Microemboli detected by transcranial Doppler monitoring in patients during carotid angioplasty versus carotid endarterectomy. Regarding "A comparison of carotid angioplasty with stenting versus endarterectomy with regional anesthesia." Cardiovasc Surg 7:33–38, 1999.

47. Crawley F, Stygall J, Lunn S, et al: Comparison of microembolism detected by transcranial Doppler and neuropsychological sequelae of carotid surgery and percutaneous transluminal angioplasty. Stroke 31:1329–1334, 2000.

48. Théron JG, Payelle GG, Coskun O, et al: Carotid artery stenosis: Treatment with protected balloon angioplasty and stent placement. Radiology 201:627–636, 1996.

49. Théron JG: Protected angioplasty and stenting of atherosclerotic stenosis at the carotid artery bifurcation. In Connors JJI, Wojak JC (eds): Interventional Neuroradiology. Philadelphia, WB Saunders Co., 1998:466–473.

50. Ohki T, Parodi J, Veith FJ, et al: Efficacy of a proximal occlusion catheter with reversal of flow in the prevention of embolic events during carotid artery stenting: An experimental analysis. J Vasc Surg 33:504–509, 2001.

51. Brown M: Results of the Carotid and Vertebral Artery Transluminal Angioplasty Study (CAVATAS). Cerebrovasc Dis 8(suppl 4):21, 1998.

52. Hobson RW 2nd, Brott T, Ferguson R, et al: CREST: Carotid revascularization endarterectomy versus stent trial. Cardiovasc Surg 5:457–458, 1997.

# 50

# Endovascular Therapies for Diseases of the Aorta

*William B. Hillegass*      *William D. Jordan, Jr.*

The aorta is subject to diseases that produce aneurysms, occlusion, emboli, and dissection. Until the late 1990s, therapeutic options consisted of medicines and conventional surgery. The limited efficacy of medicines and the risks of conventional surgery have spurred the development of new endovascular therapies.

## ABDOMINAL AORTIC ANEURYSMS

An aneurysm is a circumscribed dilatation of an artery in contact with the lumen that has, in general, enlarged to at least twice the transverse diameter of an adjacent, uninvolved vessel. Enlargement to a lesser degree is usually referred to as ectasia. A true aneurysm involves all three layers of the arterial wall, whereas a false aneurysm (pseudoaneurysm) is at least partially contained by tissue other than arterial wall. Beyond these basic definitions, aneurysms are classified by their pathogenesis and location. The pathogenetic types are atherosclerotic (degenerative), mycotic (infected), traumatic, congenital, inflammatory, arteritic, and dissecting. Aortic aneurysms are classified further by location: ascending, arch, descending thoracic, and abdominal. Aneurysms of the aorta are the most common arterial aneurysms that come to medical attention. In one contemporary series, 78% of all aneurysms undergoing surgical therapy were aortic (68% infrarenal aortoiliac and 10% suprarenal and thoracoabdominal).[1]

The incidence of abdominal aortic aneurysm (AAA) has been estimated at 21 per 100,000 person-years or an annual incidence of 55,000 cases in the United States.[2] The prevalence of AAAs is unknown with observed ranges from 1% to 16%, depending on the population examined. Men are twice as likely to have an AAA as women. Infrarenal AAAs frequently involve the aortic bifurcation and common iliac arteries. They usually manifest as an asymptomatic pulsatile mass found by the patient or incidentally by the physician during an evaluation for another medical problem. In rare cases, they present with abdominal, lumbar, or flank pain. Once a patient is symptomatic, the risk of rupture is high. Acutely symptomatic ruptured AAA usually manifests with acute back or abdominal pain and hemodynamic collapse. Rupture is associated with a 50% to 70% mortality rate.[3] Infrequently, a ruptured AAA manifests with high-output congestive heart failure and venous hypertension due to rupture into the inferior vena cava. Occasionally, AAA manifests with distal embolization.

Once the asymptomatic AAA is diagnosed, its diameter, which can be accurately measured with ultrasound scanning or computed tomography, is the critical determinant of the risk for rupture. The annual risk of rupture appears to be quite low at a diameter of 4 cm or less but is extraordinarily high at 6 cm or more.[4] In a recent prospective, population based study in England, the maximum potential rupture rate (actual rupture plus elective surgery rate) was 2.1% per year for 3.0 to 4.0 cm aneurysms and 10.2% per year for aneurysms of 4.5 to 5.9 cm diameter.[4a] This has led to the general rule of thumb to seek repair at a diameter of 5 cm.[5] Abdominal aortic aneurysms have been estimated to increase in diameter at a mean rate of 0.39 cm/year.[6]

## Surgical Therapy

The mainstay of treatment has been surgical repair with a Dacron or polytetrafluoroethylene (PTFE) synthetic graft through a midline, traverse, low left thoracoabdominal, or left flank incision. Effort is made to preserve the autonomic plexus crossing the left iliac artery and hypogastric perfusion in sexually active male patients. The inferior mesenteric artery is reimplanted if colonic circulation is compromised. The major predictors of patient outcome include the elective versus nonelective nature of the operation and the patient's comorbidities, particularly concomitant coronary, pulmonary, and renal disease. Emergency operation for symptomatic or ruptured AAA carries a 19% to 50% mortality rate.

Elective operation had a reported early mortality rate of 5.6% in 1990.[7] Between January 1989 and February 1995, the Cleveland Clinic reported a 1.8% early postoperative mortality rate in asymptomatic aneurysms, compared to 15% for symptomatic aneurysms. Six-year survival rate is reported at 60% in asymptomatic patients with most deaths being cardiac in origin. Similarly, the Cleveland Clinic reported an early postoperative mortality rate of 8% in octogenarians undergoing elective repair between 1989 and 1993.[8] In Finland, the 30-day mortality for patients undergoing elective AAA repair between 1993 and 1997 was 5.1%.[8a] Similarly, in Maryland, the in-hospital mortality rate for elective AAA repair between 1990 and 1995 was 3.5%.[8b]

## Endovascular Therapy

In the late 1980s, the concept of an endovascular graft for AAA repair was pioneered and developed, culminating in the first human implantation by Parodi and colleagues in 1989.[9, 10] On the basis of the initial concept, several devices and techniques are being developed and refined. Approximately 12 different devices have been implanted in over 1000 patients. Several devices are in phase III studies in the United States, and the U.S. Food and Drug Administration (FDA) approved two devices (Guidant Ancure and Medtronic AneuRx) in 1999 for general use.

There are several designs for AAA exclusion devices, which can be classified as straight tube endografts, aorto-uni-iliac endografts with a contralateral iliac occluder (requiring femorofemoral bypass), and bifurcated endografts (Fig. 50–1). Bifurcated or tube endografts are the only approved devices available at this time and can be subdivided into two other categories: unibody and modular (Fig. 50–2A [Guidant Ancure] and B [Medtronic AneuRx]). A stent graft has two basic components: a metallic stent skeleton and a graft fabric. The stent skeleton is usually self-expanding, with good radial strength. The fabric needs to be thin and strong, and must have low water permeability. Some of the devices available or being developed are listed in Table 50–1.

## Patient Evaluation and Selection

Preprocedural evaluation requires precise definition of the extent of disease, involvement of the renal and visceral vessels, and the dimensions of the aneurysm and attachment zones. Vascular access sites are evaluated with particular attention to the calcification, tortuosity, caliber, and occlusive disease in the iliac vessels. Several techniques have been used to gather this information including computed tomography (CT), spiral CT, angiography, and intravascular ultrasound.

These preprocedural imaging studies determine patient suitability, approach, and device selection. The preprocedural evaluation at most centers includes spiral CT and angiography. Spiral CT is performed with 3-mm slices and a pitch between 1.0

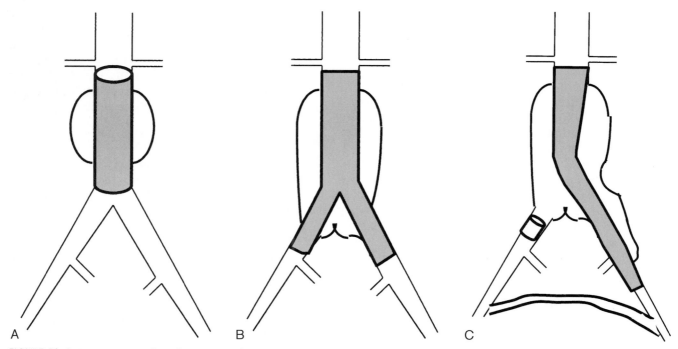

FIGURE 50–1. Basic aortic endografting approaches. *A,* Straight or tube graft. *B,* Bifurcated graft. *C,* Uni-iliac tube graft with contralateral occluder and femorofemoral bypass graft.

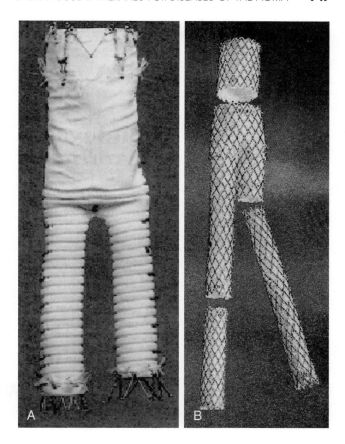

FIGURE 50–2. U.S. Food and Drug Administration–approved aortic devices. *A*, Ancure, by Guidant, is a unibody bifurcated device as well as availability of a straight graft. *B*, AneuRx, by Medtronic, is a modular device.

and 1.8. After a test injection of iodinated contrast material to estimate peak opacification, 120 mL of iodinated contrast medium are injected intravenously at 3 to 4 mL/second. The first slice is performed 1 cm above the celiac artery with imaging distal to the femoral vessels. Important dimensional characteristics include the diameter and length of the proximal neck, the length of the aneurysm, the angulation between the proximal neck and aneurysm, the diameter and length of the distal landing zones whether they be distal aortic or iliac, and the angulation between the aneurysm and the iliac

## TABLE 50–1.　TYPES OF STENT GRAFTS

| MANUFACTURER/PRODUCT | COMPOSITION | SIZE | FIXATION | BODY | "TWIST" |
|---|---|---|---|---|---|
| ***Approved Devices*** | | | | | |
| Guidant Ancure | Unibody | 24.5 Fr | Hooks | Unsupported | Most tested |
| Medtronic AneuRx | Modular | 21.5 Fr | Radial Force | Supported | Smaller size |
| ***Investigational Devices*** | | | | | |
| World Medical TALENT straight stent graft TALENT bifurcated graft | | | | | Uni-iliac graft |
| W.L. Gore & Assoc Excluder endoprosthesis | Modular | 18 Fr | Radial Force | Supported | PTFE graft |
| Cook Zenith graft | | | | | |
| Sulzer Vascutek Anaconda graft | Modular | 18 Fr | Radial Force | Supported | Recoverable deployment |
| Bard–Impra Endologix | Unibody | | Radial Force | Supported | Retrograde deployment |
| Edwards Life Sciences Lifepath | Modular | | | | |
| Boston Scientific Vanguard III | Modular | | | | |

PTFE, polytetrafluoroethylene.

arteries. Figure 50–3 shows the preprocedural anatomic worksheet. Additional morphologic features such as the presence of thrombus, iliac stenosis, eccentric plaque of the proximal neck, heavy calcification, and iliac tortuosity may affect successful implantation.

Abdominal angiography should be performed in anteroposterior (AP) and lateral projections. The renal arteries need to be assessed for device selection and positioning. The celiac and superior mesenteric arteries need to be visualized to determine the effect of inferior mesenteric occlusion on collateral intestinal circulation. The iliac and common femoral arteries should be imaged in AP and oblique projections. A calibrated pigtail or tennis racket catheter helps confirm the length and diameter measurements from the spiral CT.

Although the anatomy suitable for each device varies slightly and will change with further miniaturization and advances, the following anatomic inclusion parameters generally apply:

1. Aneurysm greater than 4.5 cm in diameter
2. Proximal neck diameter between 14 and 25 mm
3. Proximal neck length 10 mm or more
4. Less than 60-degree angle between the proximal neck and the aneurysm
5. At least one external iliac artery 7 mm or more in diameter
6. Iliac diameter 14 mm or less

Anatomic findings that generally make the patient unsuitable include:

1. Proximal neck less than 10 mm length
2. Excessive tapering of the proximal neck (over 4 mm dilatation from the proximal to distal end of the neck)
3. Small and severely diseased iliac arteries

Ancure™ ENDOGRAFT® System

**SIZING WORKSHEET**

Hospital: ______

Physician: ______

Patient ID: ______

Date of Birth: ______

Case Date: ______

**Imaging Information**

Diameter measurements were taken from
☐ Spiral CT ☐ Angiogram

Length measurements were taken from
☐ Spiral CT ☐ Angiogram

**Anatomical Specifications**

- Accessory renal artery ☐ Yes ☐ No
  If yes, treatment ☐ Cover ☐ Coil ☐ Deploy Endograft below
- Stenotic SMA ☐ Yes ☐ No
- Large patent IMA ☐ Yes ☐ No
  If large IMA is present and SMA is stenotic do not use ENDOGRAFT® Vascular Graft
- Internal iliac arteries patent
  Right ☐ Yes ☐ No
  Left ☐ Yes ☐ No
- Angled superior neck
  ☐ <30° ☐ 30-60° ☐ >60°
- Tortuous/stenotic iliacs
  Right ☐ Yes ☐ No
  Left ☐ Yes ☐ No

**Measurements 1–10**

**Tube and Bifurcated Endograft** mm

1. Diameter, superior neck ______
2. Length, superior neck ______
3. Diameter, inferior neck ______
4. Length, inferior neck ______
5. Length, infrarenal aorta ______
   - From planned superior attachment site to aortic bifurcation
   - Please allow for vascular angulation

**Bifurcated Endograft**
Measure at planned attachment site

6. Diameter, R common iliac ______
7. Diameter, L common iliac ______
8. Distance from aortic bifurcation to Iliac attachment site
   Right ______
   Left ______
9. Length, R common Iliac* ______
10. Length, L common Iliac* ______

*Length from aortic bifurcation to iliac bifurcation

**Treatment Plan**

- Graft type ☐ Tube ☐ Bifurcated
- Graft size ______
- Planned access site ☐ Right ☐ Left
- Indicate the placement of attachment systems on the drawing below with arrows
  - Tube, superior/inferior attachment system
  - Bifurcated, superior/right iliac and left iliac attachment system

**Comments:** ______

The information contained on this form is confidential patient information. Do not disclose this information to any third party or use it for any purpose other than its intended purpose.

FIGURE 50–3. Ancure worksheet for patient evaluation. The worksheet details the anatomic measurements required from the spiral computed tomography and angiography that are essential for determining the patient's anatomic suitability and sizing for the Ancure device. IMA, inferior mesenteric artery; SMA, superior mesenteric artery.

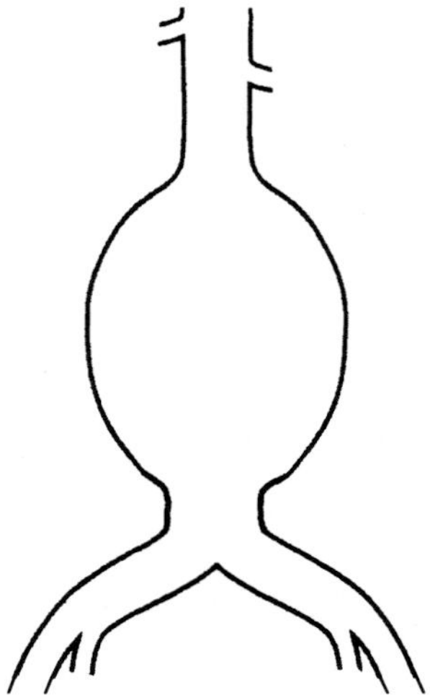

In addition to deployment failures, these features can lead to iliac artery dissection and endoleaks from stent malalignment or malposition. Nonetheless, some centers have reported success with adjunctive maneuvers in the presence of these unfavorable characteristics. In 33 high-risk cases with anatomic challenges such as short proximal necks, excessive neck angulation, and severe iliac tortuosity, Chuter and coworkers achieved success with no conversions to open surgery by adjunctive maneuvers including percutaneous transluminal angioplasty (PTA), additional stent placement, and additional stent graft placement.[11] Clinical factors that are generally felt to exclude the patient are systemic infection, congenital connective tissue disease, and intolerance of anticoagulation. Ruptured aneurysms can also sometimes be treated with stent grafts.[12]

Intravascular ultrasound may also prove to be a valuable preprocedural evaluation modality. Van Essen and colleagues examined 15 normal, atherosclerotic, and aneurysmal abdominal aortic specimens with intravascular ultrasound followed by three-dimensional reconstruction.[13] Diameter and length measurements determined from this technique were highly accurate, with r values of 0.93 to 0.99. Intravascular ultrasound (IVUS) information may help guide device selection and sizing while limiting contrast requirements. Similarly, a study comparing dimension determinations in 61 patients with spiral CT, digital subtraction angiography, and gadolinium-enhanced magnetic resonance angiography showed no significant difference in the measurements.[14]

## Description of the Graft Procedure

The placement of a bifurcated abdominal aortic endograft is described to give a general understanding of the procedure. The precise details and approach vary between devices and operators. After appropriate access sites are secured (usually femoral), the vessel is then punctured with an access needle, a 0.035-inch J wire is advanced, and an angiogram is performed to confirm the anatomic characteristics and critical vessel location (Fig. 50–4A). Then the wire is exchanged through a catheter for a stiff wire. Heparin is administered. Access is then obtained in the contralateral groin. A wire is passed for control of the contrallateral limb, whether by cannulation of a "gate" or manipulation of the contralateral limb. An arteriotomy is performed followed by introduction of an 18- to 27-French delivery sheath, depending on the appropriate device diameter. The delivery system is advanced until the endoluminal graft is in an appropriate position for deployment below the renal arteries. The initial proximal deployment is a critical step that usually requires angiographic confirmation of the renal artery location prior to "release" of the endograft. If balloon fixation is used, then inflation is typically undertaken at this time to secure the proximal attachment. Attention is then directed to the contralateral limb for deployment or cannulation to insert an additional modular component. The rest of the stent graft is deployed sometimes during or after a balloon inflation is performed to unfold the material, secure the distal attachments, and model the stents into the vessel.

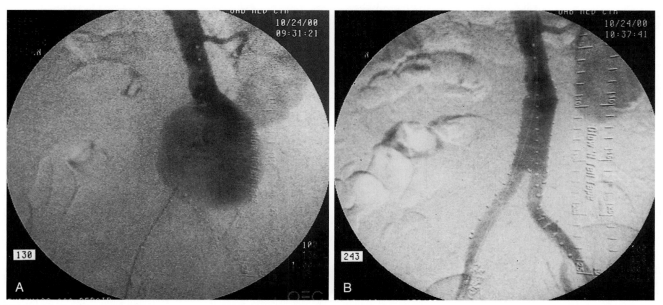

FIGURE 50–4. *A*, Intraoperative angiogram of a 10.0-cm fusiform abdominal aortic aneurysm involving the aortoiliac bifurcation and proximal common iliac arteries. *B*, Completion intraoperative angiogram after deployment of the Ancure device, demonstrating aneurysm exclusion without apparent endoleak.

Angiograms are performed above and in the graft to check for leaks (Fig. 50–4*B*). The delivery sheaths are removed with closure of the arteriotomies.

## Procedural and Clinical Results

The results of reported series examining endovascular exclusion for AAA are shown in Table 50–2. Important considerations are the deployment success rates, early complications, primary and secondary conversion rates to open repair, and endoleaks. A small incidence of aneurysm rupture after stent graft has been reported, suggesting a rate of less than 1% per year.[15]

Some of the technical limitations, such as inadequate proximal neck for fixation, and access limitations are being studied and addressed. The limitation of an inadequate proximal neck below the renal arteries for secure attachment of the stent graft led to the development of stent grafts with an uncovered proximal portion that can be placed across one or more renal arteries, a placement labeled *transrenal fixation*. Duda and coworkers compared the outcome of seven patients with a proximal neck less than 15 mm (range, 3 to 14 mm) with seven patients with a proximal neck over 15 mm.[19] The patients with a short proximal neck of the infrarenal aorta received juxtarenal implantation of a polyester-nitinol co-knit stent graft with a 12-mm proximal length of uncovered stent. These were placed across one or more renal artery orifices. The other seven patients received standard infrarenal stent graft placement. The patients were followed for a mean of 10.1 months. Measurement of creatinines, captopril renography, and follow-up CT showed no evidence of impaired renal function or perfusion. In 18 patients with 25 renal arteries "jailed" by uncovered Z-stents to secure the device in patients with short proximal necks, Malina and associates reported no change in creatinine or blood pressure control.[20]

In addition to lowering the profile of the delivery systems for covered stents, an alternative approach has been to deliver lower profile uncovered self-expanding stents with or without injection of coils into the excluded aneurysm sac to promote thrombosis. Smalling and associates reported their initial experience with treating six patients with infrarenal AAA employing uncovered 12-French Wallstents.[21] The mean patient age was 75.3 years, and mean AAA diameter was 4.3 cm. Four patients required reconstruction of the aortic bifurcation with kissing stents. Four patients received coil embolization through the stent into the aneurysm sac. The coiled patients had minimal flow outside the stent by Doppler scanning at 2 months.

## Pathophysiologic Considerations and Mechanism of Action

An underlying assumption in endovascular aneurysm exclusion is that the device will prevent fur-

**TABLE 50–2.** **RESULTS OF SERIES INVESTIGATING ENDOVASCULAR EXCLUSIONS FOR ABDOMINAL AORTIC ANEURYSMS**

| CENTER | ATTEMPTED PROCEDURES | DEPLOYMENT SUCCESS | FOLLOW-UP | OPEN CONVERSIONS |
|---|---|---|---|---|
| MGH, 1998[16] | N = 30<br>8 tube grafts<br>8 bifurcated<br>12 aortouni-iliac with femorofemoral bypass | 28/30 (93%) | 11 months | Primary, 2/30 (access difficulties)<br>Secondary, 5/28 (endoleak, 3; aneurysm expansion, 1; rupture, 1) |
| U. of Sydney, 1998 | N = 156 | Overall, 142/156 (91%)<br>Last 2.5 years: 95/97 (98%) | 2 years | Primary conversions 14/156 (access difficulties, 2; balloon problems, 2; migration, 4; thrombosis, 1; failed deployment in bifurcated artery, 5)<br>Secondary conversions, 9/142 (6.3%) (renal obstruction, 2; aneurysm expansion, 1; endoleak, 6) |
| EVT Phase I Trial[17] 1996 | N = 46<br>46 tube grafts | 39/46 (85%)<br>EGS-I 10/15 (67%)<br>EGS-II 29/31 (94%) | 14 months | Primary conversions, 7/46 (15%) (iliac stenosis, 4; subintimal deployment, 1; proximal deployment, 1; short distal neck, 1) |
| AneuRx Phase I and II[18], 1999 | N = 190<br>190 bifurcated grafts | 185/190 (97%) | 12 months | Primary conversion, 0/190 (0%) (5 patients: the procedure was abandoned because of inadequate iliac access [4] and myocardial infarction during anesthesia [1]) |

ther enlargement and subsequent rupture of the aneurysm. The putative mechanism for this is a reduction in the transmission of systemic blood pressure to the aneurysm wall. Malina and colleagues examined this question by comparing ultrasound pulsatile wall motion of the aneurysm pre-procedure with that seen postprocedure and at 1, 3, 6, 12, 18, and 24 months follow-up.[22] Median follow-up was 12 months with an interquartile range of 5 to 24 months. They treated 47 patients with endovascular stent grafts for AAA. The preoperative pulsatile wall motion (PWM) was 1.0 mm (range, 0.8 to 1.3 mm). This motion was reduced 25% after stent graft placement in patients without endoleaks. Similarly, the aneurysm diameter decreased 8 mm over 18 months in patients with complete exclusion of the aneurysm. No further reduction was seen in aneurysm diameter after 18 months. Among the 15 patients with endoleaks, there was no reduction in aneurysm diameter and less reduction in PWM. In five patients with transient endoleaks, the PWM was reduced after the leak ceased. A disturbing finding was that three patients without endoleaks had enlargement of their aneurysm. This enlargement was associated with a lesser reduction in PWM after the procedure. These data suggest that a successful clinical result may be predicted by a reduction in postprocedure PWM, implying successful reduction of the pressure transmitted to the aortic wall. Failure to observe a reduction in PWM and aneurysm diameter is associated with endoleaks. However, some patients fail to have a reduction in PWM despite the absence of an endoleak. Not only do these patients appear to be at higher risk for further aneurysm enlargement, but it implies that *the absence of an endoleak is a necessary but not sufficient condition to predict success in reducing the transmission of pressure to the aneurysm wall.* Therefore, patients need to be monitored serially with some type of imaging study after their endoluminal graft is placed.

## Other Reported Uses for Aortic Endografts

1. Aortocaval fistula between an aneurysm of the distal aorta and the inferior vena cava causing high-output cardiac failure.[23]
2. Aneurysmal aortitis in Behçet's disease[24]
3. Traumatic pseudoaneurysm of the abdominal aorta

White and associates reported a patient who developed a pseudoaneurysm of the abdominal aorta between the superior mesenteric artery and the renal arteries secondary to a gunshot wound. The pseudoaneurysm could not be detected by aortography but was seen by spiral CT and IVUS, which allowed construction of a customized stent graft, which in turn was subsequently deployed with successful exclusion of the pseudoaneurysm.[25]

## Procedural Outcomes and Complications

### Conversion to Open Operation

Conversions to an open operation can be divided into two categories. *Primary conversion* refers to the necessity of open repair at the initial procedure, and *secondary conversion* refers to an open repair in follow-up that is needed because of a late complication or failure to achieve the desired therapeutic end. The reasons for and frequency of conversion to an open repair after attempted endovascular stent grafting of AAA are changing over time. Among 156 patients undergoing endoluminal repair of AAA in 5 years at the University of Sydney, 14 patients underwent primary conversion (during the initial procedure) to open repair while 9 required open repair at a subsequent procedure.[26] The reasons for primary conversion were access problems (2), balloon problems (2), endograft migration (4), endograft thrombosis (1), and failed deployment of a bifurcated endograft (5). Twelve of the 14 primary conversions occurred in the first 59 patients treated. The reduced frequency of primary conversion can be attributed to increased experience and improved devices and techniques for overcoming obstacles. Only 2 of 97 patients required primary conversion in the last 2.5 years. Secondary conversion was required for covering the renal arteries (2), increasing aneurysm diameter despite no endoleak (1), and persistent endoleak (6).

### Endograft Attachment Site Dilatation

Enlargement of the aorta at the proximal and distal attachment zones could effect device stability and efficacy, yet this concern remains a theoretical one and long-term data are not yet available to determine its clinical significance. Longitudinal studies after surgical infrarenal AAA repair have demonstrated continued enlargement and aneurysm formation in the aortic segment proximal to the surgical repair. Lipski and Ernst reviewed 800 translumbar aortograms in 272 patients before and after conventional AAA repair to measure the change in the diameter and length of the infrarenal aortic segment. The mean follow-up time was 42 months.[27] The length of the native infrarenal aorta cephalad to the proximal anastomosis increased from 23 to 26 mm ($p = 0.001$). In 115 patients (43%), the aortic segment elongated by over 5 mm, and in 63 patients (24%) it elongated by more than 10 mm. The diameter of the segment proximal to the anastomosis increased from 23 to 24 mm ($p = 0.001$) but increased over 5 mm in 21 (8%) patients. The diameters of the proximal anastomosis and graft did not change. The knowledge that a significant number of patients have enlargement of both the diameter and length of the infrarenal aortic segment proximal to the conventional anastomosis raises concern about the long-term integrity of the anastomoses of endovascular devices. Examining 59 patients treated successfully with straight endografts and followed for 24 months, Matsumura and Chaikof reported the annual expansion rate of both proximal and distal neck sizes.[28] The proximal necks enlarged by 0.7 ± 2.1 mm and 0.9 ± 1.9 mm in the first and second years after implantation, respectively. Distal neck expansion was 1.7 ± 2.9 mm and 1.5 ± 2.5 mm in the first and second years. The expansion rates did not have a statistically significant correlation with initial neck size, aneurysm size change, the presence of an endoleak, endograft dimensions, or attachment system fracture. Migration of the distal attachment was observed in three of the five patients in whom the minor diameter of the distal neck expanded by at least 6 mm. Because of this potential for dimensional changes of the aorto-iliac segment, most clinicians have preferred to use bifurcated systems to increase the security of the distal attachment site.

### Endoleaks

Endoleaks result from incomplete endovascular graft exclusion of the aneurysm or side branch flow. Some studies have shown an association between endoleaks and continued aneurysm growth and rupture.[29] Endoleaks remain one of the greatest limitations of endovascular exclusion devices in the aorta. Anatomic, chronologic, and physiologic classification of endoleaks has been advocated to help understand and treat them.[30]

Endoleak classification:

Anatomic: proximal or distal
Chronologic: immediate, late, transient, persistent
Physiologic: sidebranch, aortic inflow, aortic outflow

The classification system shown in Figure 50–5 has gained wide acceptance. In the abdominal aorta, several characteristics have been associated with endoleaks, including a proximal neck length between the renal arteries and the proximal end of the AAA of 2 cm or less, severe neck calcification, patent side branches, and the absence of iliac occlusive disease.

## Endoleak Frequency and Management

The presence of an endoleak at the conclusion of the graft implantation procedure is an important

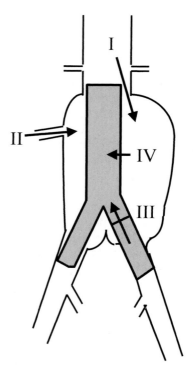

FIGURE 50–5. Endoleak classification. Type I involves the proximal and distal attachments. Type II results from backbleeding of a branch vessel into the aneurysm sac. Type III is at the junction of modular components of the device. Type IV is a transgraft leak secondary to porosity of the graft material.

part of the postimplantation evaluation. Most type I endoleaks, particularly proximal type I, are treated at the time of their discovery. Type II endoleaks are typically followed and treated if the aneurysm grows in size or becomes suspicious for an unstable state. Type III endoleaks are treated at time of discovery if found at the initial implantation. Early type IV leaks are typically followed unless there is known failure of the graft material. Some thin graft material may have a transgraft "seepage" that appears as an endoleak at implantation. If there is known graft material disruption, further intervention is typically required.

The frequency of endoleaks has been estimated in several studies. In the North American EndoVascular Technology phase I trial, 17 of 39 tube grafts (44%) had an immediate endoleak on CT scan. Nine of the 17 closed spontaneously during approximately 6-month follow-up. Eight patients had persistent endoleaks, of which one was fixed with subsequent PTA and another required later surgical conversion. The remaining six patients had no further enlargement of the aneurysm sac and are being carefully followed. Within this series, 15 of 17 endoleaks were type I, with the majority (10) being at the distal attachment site. This finding has led most operators to prefer a bifurcated device instead of a straight tube graft. The remaining 2 of 17 endoleaks were felt to be type II (backbleeding from side-branch vessels). In the phase II trial of the same graft, 40 of 149 bifurcated grafts (32%) had endoleaks at the 12 months postoperative CT scan, but only 2 of 34 patients with type II endoleaks had an increase in the aneurysm diameter. In the bifurcated series implanted since December 1995, only 3 of 383 patients have required conversion for expansion of the aneurysm or endograft failure. There were no ruptures in this entire series. In the AneuRx trial, 39 of 185 bifurcated grafts (21%) had immediate endoleaks. Seventeen patients had a type I endoleak at the proximal or distal anastamosis. Seven of the 17 had proximal leaks. Three were sealed with extender cuffs, and four sealed spontaneously. Ten had distal attachment leaks, of which seven sealed spontaneously within 6 months and three were sealed with iliac extender cuffs before discharge. Twelve were type II leaks, of which six spontaneously closed at 1 month and one was closed with coiling of a lumbar artery. Five of these 12 have persistent endoleaks and are being closely followed. Ten of the 12 with type IV transgraft "seepage" leaks were spontaneously sealed at 1 month. By 6 months, the endoleak rate was 9%. Of these 15 patients, nine had no change in their aneurysm size, five have had decrease in aneurysm size, and one has been too ill for further evaluation.

## Patient Follow-up after Aortic Stent Grafting

Appropriate follow-up of patients after endovascular repair of aortic aneurysms is critical given the small but important rate of residual endoleaks as well as the lack of assurance that a technically successful stent graft will prevent aneurysm enlargement. Several techniques have been reported as useful for follow-up (Fig. 50–6). Schurink and coworkers created an ex vivo aneurysm model with a catheter of known diameter simulating a lumbar artery. The aneurysms were excluded with a stent graft followed by systemic and aneurysm sac pressure measurements. With 0.41-mm, 1.00-mm, or 2.33-mm "lumbar arteries," pressure in the aneurysm sac exceeded systemic diastolic pressure, although the waveform was damped. Imaging with digital subtraction angiography, CT angiography, and delayed CT angiography were also performed. The small endoleaks (0.41 mm) were not detected with digital subtraction angiography or CT angiography, but were detected with delayed CT angiography.[31] Thompson and colleagues were able to define the renal arteries, prosthetic lumen, attachment sites, and aneurysm wall in 17 patients with ultrasound. Color Doppler allowed detection of an endoleak in one patient at a distal attachment site. Another study compared the results of 20 patients followed with both CT and duplex sonography at 6-month intervals after procedure.[32] CT and duplex sonography both detected four patients with endoleaks. The site of endoleak was better localized with duplex scanning than CT. In three of four patients with endoleaks, the aneurysm continued to enlarge. Among the 16 that had no endoleak detected, the aneurysm shrank at 0.40 cm/year (range, 0.13 to 0.8 cm/year) with duplex measurements and by 0.43 cm/year (range, 0 to 1.0 cm/year) by CT measurement. In another series of

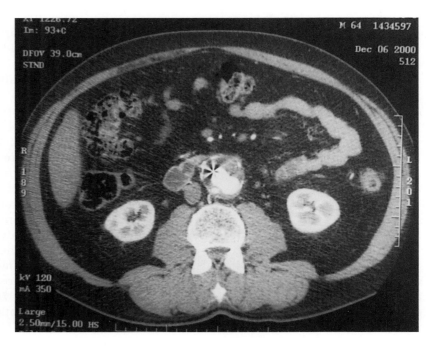

FIGURE 50–6. Spiral CT with intravenous contrast material 30 days after endograft implantation for an abdominal aortic aneurysm. There is enhancement in the aneurysm sac at the 7 o'clock position, as well as a side-branch artery, consistent with a type II persistent endoleak.

26 patients in which 7 had persistent endoleaks, serial CT measurements showed a median shrinkage of 0.41 mm/month in patients with no endoleak as opposed to aneurysm expansion at 0.30 mm/month in the patients with persistent endoleaks.[33]

Aneurysm rupture has been reported after endoluminal grafting.[34, 35] These reports highlight the need for continued surveillance of the aneurysm after endograft implantation and the correlation of expanding aneurysm with the risk of rupture. The EUROpean collaborators registry on Stent-graft Techniques for abdominal aortic Aneurysm Repair (EUROSTAR) group followed 2464 patients over 4 years and found the risk of aneurysm rupture to be 1% per year. Factors associated with a risk of rupture included proximal type I or type III endoleaks, graft migration, and postoperative kinking. The risk factors for late conversions (2.1% per year) included type I, II, or III endoleaks, graft migration, and graft kinking.[36]

## Economic and Quality-of-Life Outcomes from Endovascular Aortic Stenting

Endovascular treatment of aortic disease offers the promise of lower medical costs due to less morbidity and faster patient recovery than conventional open repairs. Holzenbein and associates retrospectively compared procedure length, length of stay, and hospital cost between 44 patients receiving either stent graft or open repair.[37] Endovascular treatment took 207.6 minutes, versus 229.1 minutes for open repair. Intensive care unit stay and hospital days were 22.7 hours versus 55.0 hours and 5.6 days versus 13.3 days, respectively, for endovascular versus open repair. Overall, open surgery was more expensive (25,374 European Currency Units [ECU] vs. 22,269 ECU) despite the more expensive evaluation and endovascular procedure (10,699 ECU vs. 4,032 ECU). The greater cost of the procedure was more than offset by the lower cost of patient recovery. In the United States, the Massachusetts General Hospital group showed that the length of stay was 3.9 days for endovascular repair, versus 10.3 days for open repair. On average, complete patient recovery took 11 days with endovascular therapy, versus 47 days with open repair.

## ABDOMINAL AORTIC OCCLUSIVE DISEASE

Stenosis and chronic occlusion of the aorta have usually been treated surgically. The distal aorta and aortic bifurcation are frequently an area of severe stenosis or occlusion leading to limiting bilateral intermittent claudication. Endovascular techniques including thrombolysis, balloon angioplasty, covered stents, and uncovered stents have been developed with approximately 90% immediate technical success rates in occlusions and 95% for stenoses. Five-year primary patency rates are estimated at 70% to 80% for percutaneous distal aortic and aortoiliac bifurcation interventions. Kissing angioplasty and stenting of the distal aorta and bilateral ostial/proximal common iliac arteries are often required (Fig. 50–7). In patients who are poor surgical candidates with severe distal aortic stenosis coupled with bilateral iliac artery stenoses, the distal aorta and both iliac arteries can frequently be percutaneously revascularized. With occlusions, the success rate is lower. Not infrequently, only one iliac artery can be percutaneously revascularized because of long, chronic total flush occlusion of the contralateral iliac. In these cases, percutaneous treatment of the distal aorta and one iliac artery with minimal residual pressure gradient to the femoral artery can be coupled with femoral-to-femoral artery bypass surgery at relatively low risk. The following series demonstrate the technical success rates, patency rates, and complications of these approaches.

Henry and colleagues reported their experience treating 28 patients with claudication or distal embolic lesions.[38] Ten of the patients had isolated infrarenal aortic stenosis (9) or occlusion (1). Eighteen had aortoiliac disease with 38 stenoses (aorta, 13; iliac 25) and 16 occlusions (aorta, 5; iliac, 11). Using a combination of thrombolysis (7), kissing PTA, and stent implantation for residual stenosis or dissection, complete technical success was achieved in 26 of 28 patients without immediate complications. Ankle-brachial indices (ABIs) increased from 0.62 ± 0.12 to 0.94 ± 0.11. Mean follow-up was 2 years with 100% patency for isolated aortic lesions and 83% primary patency overall. In a broader population with aortic bifurcation disease, Henry and colleagues also reported their experience in 72 symptomatic patients with 162 arteries treated.[39] The population included 54 patients (108 arteries) with bilateral proximal common iliac obstruction and 18 patients (54 lesions) with associated abdominal aortic lesions; 162 lesions (34 occlusions: 30 iliac, 4 aortic) were treated in 128 arteries (114 iliac, 14 aortic) with fibrinolysis in 8 patients, PTA alone in 25 lesions, and stents in 137 lesions. Complete technical success was achieved in 70 of 72 patients with two requiring femoral-femoral artery bypass because only one iliac artery was successfully recanalized. There were no immediate complications. Mean follow-up was 30 months. Twelve patients had restenosis in 21 arteries, requiring PTA in 7, stenting in 7, and surgery in 7. At 6-year follow-up primary patency was 74% and secondary patency was 90% for all lesions. Primary and secondary

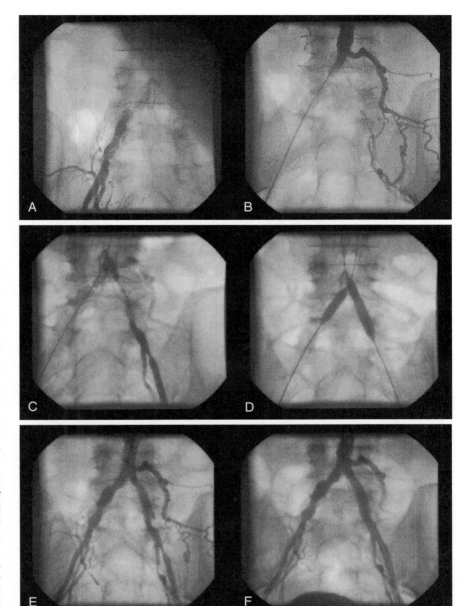

FIGURE 50–7. *A* and *B*, A patient with distal aortic disease and chronic total occlusion of the left common iliac artery extending into the distal aorta, as well as subtotal occlusion of the right common iliac artery. *C*, After obtaining access in the reconstituted left femoral artery, a glide wire is used to cross the left iliac occlusion with a retrograde approach. Given the patient's increased left lower extremity symptoms in the past 3 months, a multi–side hole local infusion catheter is placed across the lesion, and pulse-spray urokinase is administered with restoration of patency and better definition of the underlying atherosclerotic disease. *D*, Kissing percutaneous transluminal angioplasty is performed at the aortoiliac bifurcation. *E*, The post–percutaneous transluminal angioplasty image shows patent vessels with residual stenosis and dissection of the left common iliac artery. *F*, Kissing self-expanding nitinol stents are deployed to reconstruct the distal aortoiliac bifurcation. The final angiogram shows a widely patent aortoiliac bifurcation and iliac arteries with minimal residual stenosis. Less than 5 mm Hg residual mean pressure gradient was demonstrated between the abdominal aorta and the bilateral femoral sheaths.

patency for patients with isolated common iliac disease was 76% and 96%, respectively. In patients with associated distal aortic disease, the patency rates were 93% and 98%, respectively. There was no association between occlusion versus stenosis or stenting versus unstented lesions and patency rates. Similarly, Sievert and associates have reported their experience in 76 consecutive patients with 83 chronically occluded iliac arteries or distal aortas.[40] Technical success was achieved in 76 of 83 lesions (91%) employing local thrombolytic therapy in 26, PTA, stenting in 2, and stent grafts in 5 patients. Complications included distal embolization in four treated with local fibrinolysis or catheter aspiration and iliac perforation in three treated with prolonged balloon inflation in one, stent graft in one, and sur-

gery in the third. There is a case report of early pseudoaneurysm formation at the proximal end of an aortic stent requiring aortobifemoral bypass grafting and exclusion of the aneurysm.[41]

## THORACIC AORTIC DISEASE

A variety of thoracic aortic diseases have now been approached with endovascular therapies. These diseases include relatively common conditions such as descending aortic aneurysms, aortic arch aneurysms, and acute aortic dissection. Less common conditions treated include mycotic descending thoracic aneurysms, aorto-caval fistula, post-traumatic false aneurysms, and congenital aortic coarctation.

## Descending Thoracic Aortic Aneurysms

Experience to date in treating descending thoracic aortic aneurysms with endovascular stent grafts has yielded 90% to 100% deployment success rates, complete exclusion without endoleak in 80% to 90%, and 6% to 10% 30-day mortality rates (Fig. 50–8). Although no randomized comparisons with conventional surgery have been performed, the results compare favorably with conventional surgery, even in high-risk groups. The early Stanford experience in 44 high-risk patients who were poor candidates for conventional surgery has been favorable.[42] They deployed Z-stents covered with polyester fabric by way of a 22- to 24-French delivery catheter through a femoral arteriotomy or a left retroperito-

neal flank incision under fluoroscopic guidance. Technical success was 100% with aneurysm thrombosis in 88%. There were no intraprocedural deaths, stent migration, or open surgical conversions. Two patients who underwent simultaneous open repair of infrarenal AAAs developed paraplegia. The 30-day perioperative mortality rate was 6.8%, with an 82% 35-month actuarial survival rate.

Ehrlich and coworkers reported their experience with conventional versus stent graft treatment of aneurysms of the descending thoracic aorta.[43] They compared 58 patients receiving conventional surgery who would have been suitable candidates for stent grafting with 10 patients treated with stent grafts. The mean aneurysm diameter was 7 cm. The 30-day mortality rate was 31% in the conventional group versus 10% in the stent group. Five of the 10

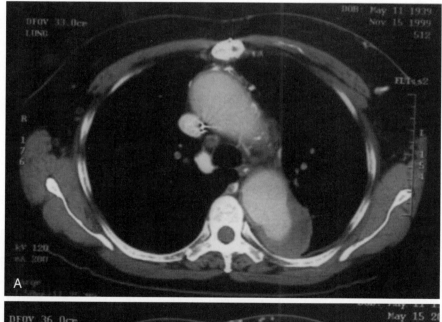

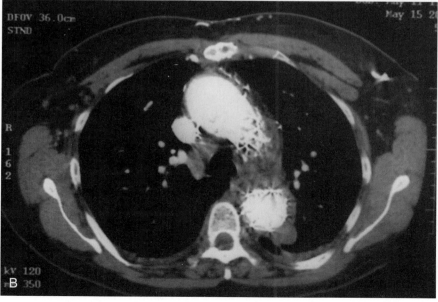

FIGURE 50–8. *A*, The patient has a 7.5-cm saccular aneurysm of the descending thoracic aorta, demonstrated by contrast-enhanced CT. *B*, Thirty-day postoperative CT demonstrates shrinkage of the aneurysm with no evidence of endoleak after treatment with a stent graft. Left carotid to left subclavian artery bypass was performed before the stent graft procedure.

patients required transposition of the left subclavian artery to achieve an adequate proximal neck for stent placement. Five of the 58 patients undergoing surgery experienced spinal cord injury. None of the 10 stented patients experienced neurologic complications. Two of the stented patients required additional stent implantation procedures because of an endoleak.

A subsequent report concerned the experience with the first 108 patients treated with stent grafts for thoracic aneurysms. Complete aneurysm thrombosis was achieved primarily in 103 of 108 patients (95%). Mortality rate at 30 days was 9.25% (10 of 108), and four of the deaths were directly attributable to the procedure. Four patients had periprocedural strokes, and four developed paraplegia. With a mean follow-up of 21.8 months, there have been two late stent graft failures. In summary, the endovascular approach to thoracic aortic aneurysms appears promising given the extensive comorbidities encountered in this patient population as well as the mortality and morbidity rates associated with open repair via left thoracotomy.

Additional unusual situations with thoracic aneurysms include mycotic and post-traumatic false aneurysms. Although standard therapy for mycotic aneurysms of the descending aorta includes thoracotomy with in situ graft placement or extra-anatomic bypass, stent grafts have been used as an alternative treatment. Stanford has reported three such patients they treated with polyester fabric–covered Z-stents. Median follow-up period was 24 months. There were no complications of persistent bacteremia, reinfection, paraplegia, delayed rupture, surgical conversion, or distal emboli.[44]

Patients with thoracic false aneurysms secondary to trauma have been successfully treated with endoluminal stent grafts, including bifurcated grafts to major visceral vessels such as the celiac artery.[45, 46] Stanford has reported ten cases of traumatic thoracic aortic aneurysm they have treated.[47] Three patients experienced complications, including perigraft leak treated with subsequent coil embolization, left arm ischemia requiring transposition of the left subclavian artery, and left mainstem bronchus compression requiring bronchial stenting. All ten patients were alive without complication after a mean follow-up period of 15 months.

## Acute Aortic Dissection

Shimono and associates reported successful treatment of acute type A aortic dissection with an endovascular stent graft.[48] A case-control study comparing surgical versus transluminal placement of a self-expanding endovascular stent graft in distal arch and thoracic aortic dissections compared 24 patients with similar pathoanatomic features receiving surgery (12) versus stent grafts (12).[49] Surgery was associated with three deaths (25%) and five (42%) serious adverse events at 6 months follow-up. There were no deaths or serious adverse events in the stent graft group. Follow-up magnetic resonance angiography (MRA) at 6 months showed no endoleaks and thrombosis of the false lumen. Full physical recovery was seen in all patients with a stent graft compared to 8 of 12 patients (67%) with conventional surgery ($p < 0.05$).

## Technical Issues and Complications

Thoracic aortic surgery and stent grafts, particularly in the middle and descending segment of the thoracic aorta, can cause spinal cord ischemia and injury due to interruption of spinal cord blood flow. This complication has been reported in approximately 10% of patients undergoing descending thoracic aorta aneurysm surgery and 4% of endovascular stent grafts. A novel approach is the initial deployment of a retrievable device with measurement of evoked spinal cord potentials. Ishimaru and colleagues placed the Retriever device in 17 thoracic aneurysms in 16 patients, followed by permanent stent graft placement with continuous spinal evoked response monitoring throughout the procedure as well as 24 hours after the procedure. The Retriever was placed to exclude the aneurysms for 20 minutes. No change in spinal cord potentials were seen. Permanent stent grafts were then deployed with no neurologic sequelae or change in the spinal potentials.

## SUMMARY

The common aortic diseases are aneurysm, occlusion, and dissection. Patients with these conditions are usually older with multiple comorbidities including diffuse atherosclerotic vascular disease involving the coronary, cerebral, visceral, and peripheral circulations. Chronic renal insufficiency and pulmonary disease are also frequently present in these patients. Medical therapies generally have limited efficacy for aortic diseases. Conventional surgical therapies have been lifesaving and technically successful but sometimes limited by patients' advanced comorbidities. In the last decade, endovascular therapies for aortic diseases have rapidly developed, becoming an increasingly feasible and important mode of treatment. Further refinements in techniques, devices, and patient selection need to be coupled with the collection of long-term outcome data as the role of endovascular therapy for aortic diseases evolves.

# REFERENCES

1. O'Hara PJ: Arterial aneurysms. *In* Young JR, Olin JW, Bartholomew JR (eds): Peripheral Vascular Diseases, pp 343–357. St. Louis: Mosby, 1996.
2. Bickerstaff LK, Hollier LH, Van Peenen HJ, et al: Abdominal aortic aneurysms, the changing natural history. J Vasc Surg 1:6, 1984.
3. Cronenwett JL, Murphy TF, Zelenock GB, et al: Actuarial analysis of variables associated with rupture of small abdominal aortic aneurysms. Surgery 98:472, 1985.
4. Crane C: Arteriosclerotic aneurysm of the abdominal aorta. N Engl J Med 253:954, 1955.
4a. Scott RA, Tisi PV, Ashton HA, et al: Abdominal aortic aneurysm rupture rates: A 7-year follow-up of the entire abdominal aortic aneurysm population detected by screening. J Vasc Surg 28(1):124–128, 1998.
5. Hollier LH, Taylor LM, Ochsner J: Recommended indications for operative treatment of abdominal aortic aneurysms. Report of a subcommittee of the Joint Council of the Society for Vascular Surgery and the North American Chapter of the International Society for Cardiovascular Surgery. J Vasc Surg 15:1046, 1992.
6. Wolf YG, Bernstein EF: A current perspective on the natural history of abdominal aortic aneurysms. Cardiovasc Surg 2:16, 1994.
7. Katz DJ, Stanley JC, Zelenock GB: Operative mortality rates for intact and ruptured abdominal aortic aneurysm in Michigan: An eleven-year statewide experience. J Vasc Surg 19:804, 1994.
8. O'Hara PJ, Hertzer NR, Krajewski LP, et al: Ten-year experience with abdominal aortic aneurysm repair in octogenarians: early results and late follow-up. J Vasc Surg 21:830, 1995.
8a. Kantonen I, Lepantalo M, Salenius JP, et al: Mortality in abdominal aortic aneurysm surgery—the effect of hospital volume, patient mix and surgeon's case load. Eur J Vasc Endovasc Surg 14(5):375–379, 1997.
8b. Dardik A, Lin JW, Gordon TA, Williams GM, Perler BA: Results of elective abdominal aortic aneurysm repair in the 1990s: A population-based analysis of 2335 cases. J Vasc Surg 30(6):985–995, 1999.
9. Parodi JC: Endovascular repair of abdominal aortic aneurysms and other arterial lesions. J Vasc Surg 21:549, 1995.
10. Lazarus HM: Endovascular grafting for the treatment of abdominal aortic aneurysms. Surg Clin North Am 72:959, 1992.
11. Chuter TA, Reilly LM, Kerlan RK, et al: Endovascular repair of abdominal aortic aneurysm: getting out of trouble. Cardiovasc Surg 6(3):232, 1998.
12. Seelig MH, Berchtold C, Jakob P, et al: Contained rupture of an infrarenal abdominal aortic aneurysm treated by endoluminal repair [published erratum appears in Eur J Vasc Endovasc Surg 19(5):560, 2000.
13. Van Essen JA, van der Lugt A, Gussenhoven EJ, et al: Intravascular ultrasonography allows accurate assessment of abdominal aortic aneurysm: An in vitro validation study. J Vasc Surg 27(2):347–353, 1998.
14. Thurnher SA, Dorffner R, Thurnher MM, et al: Evaluation of abdominal aortic aneurysm for stent-graft placement: Comparison of gadolinium-enhanced MR angiography versus helical CT angiography and digital subtraction angiography. Radiology 205(2):341–352, 1997.
15. Harris PL, Vallabhaneni SR, Desgranges P, et al: Incidence and risk factors of late rupture, conversion, and death after endovascular repair of infrarenal aortic aneurysms: The EUROSTAR experience. J Vasc Surg 32(4) 739–749, 2000.
16. Brewster DC, Geller SC, Kaufman JA, et al: Initial experience with endovascular aneurysm repair: Comparison of early results with outcome of conventional open repair. J Vasc Surg 27(6):992–1003, 1998.
17. Moore WS, Rutherford RB, EVT Investigators: Transfemoral endovascular repair of abdominal aortic aneurysm: Results of the North American EVT phase I trial. J Vasc Surg 23:543–553, 1996.
18. Zarins CK, White RA, Schwarten D, et al: AneuRx stent graft versus open surgical repair of abdominal aortic aneurysms: Multicenter prospective clinical trial. J Vasc Surg 29:292–308, 1999.
19. Duda SH, Raygrotzki S, Wiskirchen J, et al: Abdominal aortic aneurysms: Treatment with juxtarenal placement of covered stent-grafts. Radiology 206(1):195–198, 1998.
20. Malina M, Brunkwall J, Ivancev K, et al: Renal arteries covered by aortic stents: Clinical experience from endovascular grafting of aortic aneurysms. Eur J Vasc Endovasc Surg 14(2):109–113, 1997.
21. Smalling RW, Denktas AE, Cafri CJ, et al: Abdominal aortic aneurysm repair by percutaneous implantation of uncovered wire mesh stents and coil embolization of the aneurysm. J Am Coll Cardiol 33(2):22A, 1999.
22. Malina M, Lanne T, Ivancev K, et al: Reduced pulsatile wall motion of abdominal aortic aneurysms after endovascular repair. J Vasc Surg 27(4):624–631, 1998.
23. Beveridge CJ, Pleass HC, Chamberlain J, et al: Aortoiliac aneurysm with arteriocaval fistula treated by a bifurcated endovascular stent-graft. Cardiovasc Intervent Radiol 21(3):244–246, 1998.
24. Vasseur MA, Haulon S, Beregi JP, et al: Endovascular treatment of abdominal aneurysmal aortitis in Behçet's disease. J Vasc Surg 27(5):974–976, 1998.
25. White R, Donayre C, Walot I, et al: Endograft repair of an aortic pseudoaneurysm following gunshot wound injury: Impact of imaging on diagnosis and planning of intervention. J Endovasc Surgery 4(4):352–353, 1997.
26. May J, White GH, Yu W, et al: Endovascular grafting for abdominal aortic aneurysms: Changing incidence and indication for conversion to open operation. Cardiovasc Surg 6(2):194–197, 1998.
27. Lipski DA, Ernst CB: Natural history of the residual infrarenal aorta after infrarenal abdominal aortic aneurysm repair. J Vasc Surg 27(5):805–811, 1998.
28. Matsumura JS, Chaikof EL: Continued expansion of aortic necks after endovascular repair of abdominal aortic aneurysms. EVT Investigators. J Vasc Surg 28(3):422–430, 1998.
29. Harris PL, Vallabhaneni SR, Desgranges P, et al: Incidence and risk factors of late rupture, conversion, and death after endovascular repair of infrarenal aortic aneurysms: The EUROSTAR experience. J Vasc Surg 32(4):739–749, 2000.
30. Wain RA, Marin ML, Ohki T, et al: Endoleaks after endovascular graft treatment of aortic aneurysms: Classification, risk factors, and outcome. J Vasc Surg 27(1):69–78, 1998.
31. Schurink GW, Aarts NJ, Wilde J, et al: Endoleakage after stent-graft treatment of abdominal aneurysms: Implications on pressure and imaging—An in vitro study. J Vasc Surg 28(2):234–241, 1998.
32. Thompson MM, Boyle JR, Hartshorn T, et al: Comparison of computed tomography and duplex imaging in assessing acute morphology following endovascular aneurysm repair. Br J Surg 85(3):346–350, 1998.
33. Broeders IA, Blankensteijn JD, Gvakharia A, et al: The efficacy of transfemoral endovascular aneurysm management: A study on size changes of the abdominal aorta during midterm follow-up. Eur J Vasc Endovasc Surg 14(2):84–90, 1997.
34. Harris PL, Vallabhaneni SR, Desgranges P, et al, for the EUROSTAR Collaborators: Incidence and risk factors of late rupture, conversion, and death after endovascular repair of infrarenal aortic aneurysms: The EUROSTAR experience. J Vasc Surg 32:739–749, 2000.
35. Zarins CK, White RA, TJ Fogarty: Aneurysm rupture after endovascular repair using the AneuRx stent graft. J Vasc Surg 31:960–973, 2000.
36. Harris PL, Vallabhaneni SR, Desgranges P, et al, for the EUROSTAR Collaborators: Incidence and risk factors of late rupture, conversion, and death after endovascular repair of infrarenal aortic aneurysms: The EUROSTAR experience. J Vasc Surg 32:739–749, 2000.
37. Holzenbein J, Kretschmer G, Glanzl R, et al: Endovascular AAA treatment: Expensive prestige or economic alternative. Eur J Vasc Endovasc Surg 14(4):265–272, 1997.
38. Henry M, Amor M, Henry I, et al: Percutaneous endovascular treatment of abdominal aortic occlusive diseases. J Am Coll Cardiol 33(2):65A, 1999.
39. Henry M, Amor M, Henry I, et al: Percutaneous endovascular

treatment of aortic bifurcation occlusive diseases. J Am Coll Cardiol 33(2):23A, 1999.

40. Sievert H, Schultze HJ, Peters J, et al: Recanalization of chronic total occlusions of the abdominal aorta and the iliac arteries. J Am Coll Cardiol 33(2):65A, 1999.

41. Cutry AF, Whitley D, Patterson RB: Midaortic pseudoaneurysm complicating extensive endovascular stenting of aortic disease. J Vasc Surg 26(6):58–62, 1997.

42. Semba CP, Mitchell RS, Miller DC, et al: Thoracic aortic aneurysm repair with endovascular stent-grafts. Vasc Med 2(2):98–103, 1997.

43. Ehrlich M, Grabenwoegner M, Cartes-Zumelzu F, et al: Endovascular stent graft repair for aneurysms on the descending thoracic aorta. Ann Thorac Surg 66(1):19–24, 1998.

44. Semba CP, Sakai T, Slonim SM, et al: Mycotic aneurysms of the thoracic aorta: Repair with use of endovascular stent-grafts. J Vasc Interv Radiol 9(1):33–40, 1998.

45. Deshpande A, Mossop P, Gurry J, et al: Treatment of traumatic false aneurysm of the thoracic aorta with endoluminal grafts. J Endovasc Surg 5(2):120–125, 1998.

46. Inoue K, Iwase T, Sato M, et al: Transluminal endovascular branched graft placement for a pseudoaneurysm: Reconstruction of the descending thoracic aorta including the celiac axis. J Thorac Cardiovasc Surg 114(5):859–861, 1997.

47. Kato N, Dake MD, Miller DC, et al: Traumatic thoracic aortic aneurysm: Treatment with endovascular stent grafts. Radiology 205(3):657–662, 1997.

48. Shimono T, Kato N, Tokui T, et al: Endovascular stent-graft repair for acute type A aortic dissection with an intimal tear in the descending aorta. J Thorac Cardiovasc Surg 116(1):171–173, 1998.

49. Nienaber CA, Fattori R, Lund G, et al: Nonsurgical reconstruction of thoracic aortic dissection. J Am Coll Cardiol 33(2):311A, 1999.

# INDEX

Note: Page numbers followed by f refer to figures; those followed by t refer to tables.

ISBN 0-443-07979-X